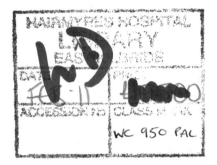

Oxford Textbook of
Zoonoses

Oxford Textbook of
Zoonoses
Biology, Clinical Practice, and Public Health Control

SECOND EDITION

Edited by

S. R. Palmer

Lord Soulsby

P. R. Torgerson
and
David W. G. Brown

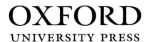

OXFORD
UNIVERSITY PRESS

OXFORD

UNIVERSITY PRESS

Great Clarendon Street, Oxford OX2 6DP

Oxford University Press is a department of the University of Oxford.
It furthers the University's objective of excellence in research, scholarship,
and education by publishing worldwide in

Oxford New York

Auckland Cape Town Dar es Salaam Hong Kong Karachi
Kuala Lumpur Madrid Melbourne Mexico City Nairobi
New Delhi Shanghai Taipei Toronto

With offices in

Argentina Austria Brazil Chile Czech Republic France Greece
Guatemala Hungary Italy Japan Poland Portugal Singapore
South Korea Switzerland Thailand Turkey Ukraine Vietnam

Oxford is a registered trademark of Oxford University Press
in the UK and in certain other countries

Published in the United States
by Oxford University Press, Inc., New York

© Oxford University Press 2011

Chapter 41 © Elsevier

British Library Cataloguing in Publication Data
Data available

Library of Congress Cataloging in Publication Data
Data available

Typeset by Glyph International, Bangalore, India

Printed in Slovakia
by Neografia

ISBN: 978-0-19-857002-8

1 3 5 7 9 10 8 6 4 2

Contents

Preface

Definitions

Zoonoses are defined by the World Health Organization as 'Diseases and infections which are naturally transmitted between vertebrate animals and man' (WHO 1959), but there has been debate on this definition. Some believe there is not sufficient evidence in all accepted zoonoses for natural transmission, even though epidemiological evidence would appear to be strong. Others point out the desirability of including 'unnatural' opportunistic infections of severely immunosuppressed patients by organisms of invertebrate origin. Some would include intoxications, such as snake and spider venoms or botulism. The definition excludes the deliberate transmission of human infectious agents to animals, usually for experimental purposes.

Zoonoses cover a broad range of diseases with very different clinical and epidemiological features and control measures. The fundamental reason for grouping these diseases together is that successful control requires joint veterinary and medical efforts. While the concept of 'zoonoses' is anthropocentric (Nelson 1960), the epidemiological study and their control is not. However, too frequently the medical and veterinary aspects of a zoonotic disease are studied separately, and funding for work often is derived from separate sources. In many cases, the infection in animals is unapparent or mild, causing little or no animal health or economic concern, so that winning resources to study the veterinary sources is often difficult. This book is aimed at developing the co-ordinated medico-veterinary approach to investigation and control.

Classification of zoonoses

Various classifications of the zoonoses have been proposed largely based on epidemiological features and whether the reservoir hosts are man or lower vertebrate animals. Hence the term anthropozoonoses refers to infections transmitted to man from lower animals and zooanthroponoses to infections transmitted from man to lower vertebrates. Where infections can be maintained in both man and animals and transmitted in either direction, the term amphixenoses has been applied. However, such terms have led to confusion and sometimes have been used indiscriminately. They will not be used in this volume.

For teaching purposes Schwabe (1964) has suggested that a classification based on the type of life cycle of the infecting agent may be useful and proposes four categories:

(1) Direct zoonoses: transmission is by direct contact, by contact with a fomite or mechanical vector, the agent undergoing little or no propagative changes or development during transmission (e.g. rabies, brucellosis).

(2) Cyclo-zoonoses: requiring more than one species or vertebrate host, but not invertebrate host, to complete the developmental cycle of the agent (e.g. echinococcosis).

(3) Meta-zoonoses: transmission is by invertebrate vector in which the agent develops and/or multiples and there is an extrinsic incubation period before an infective stage is produced (e.g. arbovirus infection, plague, schistosomosis).

(4) Sapro-zoonoses: both a vertebrate host and a non-animal developmental site or reservoir is required. Organic matter, including food, soil, and plants, is considered non-animal (e.g. larva migrans, mycoses).

Nomenclature of diseases

There have been several attempts to standardize the nomenclature of diseases caused by parasitic infections (reviewed by Kassai *et al.* 1988). The disease entity is usually designated by adding the suffixes *-iasis* or *-osis* after the proper name, but this has varied to include *-asis* and *-iosis*. Whitlock (1955) had previously proposed that the suffix *-iasis* be applied to parasitic infections where clinical manifestations were not apparent and *-osis* where they were. One difficulty in accepting such a proposal is that as pathophysiological measurements of parasitic disease become more capable of measuring clinical effects, the point where *-iasis* becomes *-osis* is increasingly difficult to decide. However, Whitlock's proposal has not met with general favour. The most recent proposal, increasingly accepted by scientific organizations, journals and international bodies is the 'Standardized Nomenclature of Animal Parasitic Diseases (SNOAPAD)' (Kassai *et al.* 1988) which consists of adding the suffix *-osis* to the name of the parasite (e.g. echinococcosis, fasciolosis, sarcocystosis, trypanosomosis). The SNOAPAD recommendations, which are considered as a logical approach to nomenclatures of disease, are adopted in this volume. Nevertheless, there are some workers who feel very strongly that this change is unacceptable and, with the agreement of the editors, have continued to use the -iasis suffix (e.g. Chapter 43).

There are several diseases where -osis has not been added to the taxon and their names are either specifically descriptive of the diseases or are named after the discoverer or in honour of a person (e.g. plague, yellow fever, Chagas disease, Rocky mountain spotted fever, hydatid disease, malaria, visceral larva migrans, cat-scratch disease). These names are well established but even so they do not necessarily specifically indicate the disease-producing agent and it is likely that more specific designations will be applied in the future.

Trends in zoonoses

The close association of people with their animals in large areas of the world and often in unsatisfactory sanitary conditions continues to promote the opportunity for zoonotic infections. Animals continue to provide a substantial contribution to the energy requirements of agriculture in terms of converting poor-quality cellulose to first-class protein, in the provision of draught power by cultivation of crops and transport, and the provision of fuel. The need to care for these valuable animals, which represent a major capital investment to the peasant farmer, exposes millions of rural people to contact with zoonotic disease. The tropical parts of the world are high-risk areas, especially where the zoonotic infection is arthropod-borne.

The situation may become acutely worse when political or social instability occurs and normal sanitary arrangements are disrupted, disease control programmes discontinued, and medical and veterinary services cease to function.

Certain occupational groups may be at greater risk such as the rural agriculturist or pastoralist and including forest workers, hunters, and wildlife workers. Such groups may accentuate the problem through the expansion of rural and even urban settlement into undeveloped woodland, marginal land, or waste land.

While it might be thought that zoonoses are essentially a rural problem, the urban dimension must also be considered important in several respects. Wildlife can become established in suburban and recreation areas, in some cases encouraged by householders, which may enhance these as a source of zoonotic infection (e.g. foxes and *Echinococcus multilocularis*). However, the companion animal in the urban scene is an important source of zoonotic diseases, especially of parasitic infections. The population of dogs and cats as companion animals continues to grow, and it has been estimated in the United Kingdom that of the 22.56 million households at least 50 per cent own a companion dog or cat. In 1994 the companion animal populations in the United Kingdom were 6.65 million dogs and 7.18 million cats. Increasingly, the dangers of zoonotic diseases associated with these companion animals are recognized and national and local laws and regulations are enacted to control where animals can be taken and the fouling of the environment.

A new dimension of zoonotic diseases has been manifest by the growing numbers of immunosuppressed people, either through the use of immunosuppression in therapy as in transplantation, or through immunosuppressive diseases, particularly in the acquired immunodeficiency syndrome (AIDS). Infections which in the normal individual are inapparent, or at most, minor, self-limiting conditions, may become life threatening during immunosuppression or in AIDS patients (e.g. toxoplasmosis, cryptosporidiosis). There are increasing reports of unusual opportunistic zoonotic infections in immunosuppressed patients, such as *Microspondium* spp and *Pleistophora*, a fish parasite (Eckert 1989).

With the possible advent of xenotransplantation, fears have been expressed that unknown infectious agents (viruses, prions, etc.) of a donor animal (pig) could be transmitted to the human recipient to cause clinical disease or even an epidemic.

These latter instances of infections being transmitted to human patients may not be regarded strictly as zoonoses since they would not meet the criterion of being 'naturally transmitted'. Should such infections become more commonplace then the definition of a zoonoses may require reconsideration.

Finally we should point out that many of the newly emerging or re-emerging infections which are causing concern, and for which global surveillance systems are being developed, are zoonoses. Important recent examples include Ebola virus in Africa, and Hantavirus in the United States of America, *Escherichia coli* O157 in Japan, the new equine morbillivirus in Australia, and brucellosis in the Middle East.

Zoonotic infections reviewed

This volume deals with the major zoonoses; however, it does not attempt to be all-inclusive in its coverage. Minor or occasional infections in man with animal infectious agents have been excluded.

References

Eckert, J. (1989). New aspects of parasitic zoonoses. *Vet. Parasitol.*, **32**: 37–55.

Kassai, T., Cordero Del Campillo, M., *et al.* (1988). Standardised Nomenclature of Animal parasitic diseases (SNOAPAD). *Vet. Parasitol.*, **29**: 299–326.

Nelson, G. S. (1960). Schistosome infections as Zoonoses in Africa. *Trans. R. Soc. Trop. Med. Hyg.*, **54**: 301–24.

Schwabe, C. N. (1964). *Veterinary medicine and human health.* Baltimore: William and Wilkins.

Whitlock, J. H. (1955). Trichostrongylosis in sheep and cattle. *Proceedings 92nd Annual meeting American Veterinary Medical Associations*, pp. 123–31.

World Health Organization (1959). *Zoonoses:* Second report of the Joint WHO/FAO Expert Committee.

Contributors

Abo-Shehada, Mahmoud N., Department of Basic Medical Veterinary Sciences, Faculty of Veterinary Medicine, Jordan University of Science and Technology, P.O. Box 3030, Irbid 22110, Jordan

Alexander, D. J., Veterinary Laboratory Agency, Addlestone, Surrey, UK

Angelakis, Emmanouil, Unité des Rickettsies, CNRS UMR 6020, IFR 48, Faculté de Médecine, Université de la Méditerranée, France

Baillie, Les, Welsh School of Pharmacy, Cardiff University, UK

Banyard, Ashley C., Rabies Wildlife and Zoonoses Group, Veterinary Laboratories Agency, Weybridge, Surrey, UK

Bell, Diana J., Senior Lecturer, School of Biological Sciences, University of East Anglia, Norwich, UK

Bellini, William J., Measles, Mumps Rubella, and Herpesvirus Laboratory Branch, Division of Viral Diseases, National Center Immunizations and Respiratory Diseases, Centers for Disease Control and Prevention, Atlanta, GA, USA

Birtles, Richard, School of Environment and Life Sciences, University of Salford, M5 4WT, UK

Blasco, José M., Gobierno de Aragón, Unidad de Sanidad Animal, Edificio Torre, Alfonso, Zaragoza, Spain

Bowman, Dwight D., Professor of Parasitology, Cornell University College of Veterinary Medicine, USA

Brown, David W. G., Virus Reference Department, London, UK

Brown, I. H., Veterinary Laboratory Agency, Addlestone, Surrey, UK

Budke, Christine M., Department of Veterinary Integrative Biosciences, College of Veterinary Medicine & Biomedical Sciences, Texas A&M University, College Station, TX, USA

Carabin, Hélène, Department of Biostatistics and Epidemiology, College of Public Health, University of Oklahoma Health Sciences Center, Oklahoma, USA

Chai, Jong-Yil, Department of Parasitology and Tropical Medicine, Seoul National University College of Medicine, Seoul 110-799, Korea

Chalmers, Rachel M., Head, UK Cryptosporidium Reference Unit, NPHS Microbiology Swansea, Singleton Hospital, Swansea, UK

Chitkara, Rajinder K., MB, MD, Staff Physician, United States Department of Veterans Affairs Palo Alto Health Care System, Associate Professor of Medicine, Division of Pulmonary and Critical Care Medicine, Stanford University School of Medicine, USA

Cox, F. E. G., Department of Infectious and Tropical Diseases, London School of Hygiene and Tropical Medicine, London, UK

Craig, Philip S., Cestode Zoonoses Research Group, School of Environmental and Life Sciences, University of Salford, M5 4WT, UK

Cross, John H., Uniformed Services University of the Health Sciences, Bethesda, MD 20814, USA

Dagleish, Mark P., Head of Pathology, Moredun Research Institute, Edinburgh

Dalton, John P., Institute for the Biotechnology of Infectious Diseases (IBID), University of Technology, Sydney, Australia

Dance, David A. B., Health Protection Agency, Regional Microbiologist's Office, Plymouth, Devon

Dawson, Susan, University of Liverpool, UK

De Zoysa, Aruni, Respiratory and Systemic Infection Laboratory, HPA Centre for Infections, London, UK

Deplazes, P., Institute for Parasitology, University of Zurich, Switzerland

Drancourt, Michel, Unité de Recherche sur les Maladies Infectieuses et Tropicales Emergentes CNRS 6236 IRD 198, IFR 48, Faculté de Médecine, Université de la Méditerranée, Marseille, France

Dubey, J. P., United States Department of Agriculture, Agricultural Research Service, Animal Natural Resources Institute, Animal Parasitic Diseases Laboratory, Beltsville, USA

Eckert, J., Institute for Parasitology, University of Zurich, Switzerland

Evans, Merion, Senior Lecturer in Epidemiology and Public Health, Cardiff University, UK

Flisser, Ana, Departamento de Microbiologia y Parasitologia, Facultad de Medicina, Universidad Nacional Autonoma de Mexico, Mexico

Fooks, Anthony R., Rabies Wildlife and Zoonoses Group, Veterinary Laboratories Agency, Weybridge, Surrey, UK

Friedman, Jennifer F., Center for International Health Research, Rhode Island Hospital, Providence, RI 02906, USA

Gasser, Robin B., Department of Veterinary Science, The University of Melbourne, Werribee, Victoria, Australia

Gibson, W., School of Biological Sciences, University of Bristol, Bristol BS8 1UG, UK

Gould, E. A., Unité des Virus Emergents, Faculté de Médecine Timone, France and Centre for Ecology and Hydrology, Oxford, UK

Gramiccia, Marina, Section of Vector-borne Diseases and International Health, MIPI Department, Istituto Superiore di Sanità, Rome, Italy

Guptill, Lynn, Department of Veterinary Clinical Sciences, School of Veterinary Medicine, Purdue University, West Lafayette, IN, USA

Hjelle, Brian, Department of Pathology, University of New Mexico HSC, Albuquerque, New Mexico, USA

Hope, James, Veterinary Laboratories Agency Lasswade, Midlothian, UK

Howard, Colin R., DSc, FRCPath, School of Immunity and Infection, College of Medicine and Dentistry, University of Birmingham, UK

Huwar, Theresa, Battelle, Columbus, Ohio, USA

Ito, Akira, Department of Parasitology, Asahikawa Medical University, Midorigaoka Higashi 2-1, Asahikawa, 078-8510 Hokkaido, Japan

Jex, Aaron R., Department of Veterinary Science, The University of Melbourne, Werribee, Victoria, Australia

Johansen, Maria V., Centre for Health Research and Development, Department of Disease Biology, Faculty of Life Sciences, University of Copenhagen, Thorvaldsensvej 57, DK-1870 Frederiksberg C, Denmark

Karmali, Mohamed A., Laboratory for Foodborne Zoonoses, Public Health Agency of Canada, and the Department of Pathology and Molecular Medicine, McMaster University, Canada

Kern, P., Division of Infectious Diseases and Clinical Immunology, Comprehensive Infectious Diseases Center, University Hospitals, Ulm, Germany

Kirkbride, Hilary, Consultant Epidemiologist, Health Protection Agency, Colindale, UK

Kurkela, Satu, Virus Reference Department, HPA Centre for Infection, London, UK

Lane, C., Health Protection Agency, Gastrointestinal, Emerging and Zoonotic Infections, Centre for Infections, London, UK

Lawson, A. J., Laboratory of Gastrointestinal Pathogens, Health Protection Agency, London UK

Lloyd, Graham, Special Pathogens Reference Unit, Porton Down

Lloyd, Sheelagh, Department of Clinical Veterinary Medicine, Cambridge University, UK

Longbottom, David, Moredun Research Institute, Pentlands Science Park, Edinburgh, UK

Lord Soulsby of Swaffham Prior, House of Lords, London

Lun, Zhao-Rong, Center for Parasitic Organisms, School of Life Sciences, Sun Yat-Sen University, Guangzhou, P.R. China

Lysons, Ruth, Deputy Director, Veterinary Science Team, Defra, Nobel House, 17 Smith Square, London SW1P 3JR, UK

Macpherson, C. N. L., St George's University, Grenada, West Indies

Madsen, Henry, DBL - Centre for Health Research and Development, Faculty of Life Sciences, University of Copenhagen, Thorvaldsensvej 57, DK1871 Frederiksberg C, Denmark

Marrie, Thomas J., Faculty of Medicine, Dalhousie University, Halifax, Nova Scotia, Canada

McDonald, Vincent, Barts and the London School of Medicine and Dentistry, Blizard Institute of Cell and Molecular Science, Centre for Digestive Diseases, Queen Mary, University of London, London, UK

McGarvey, Stephen T., International Health Institute, Brown University School of Medicine, Providence, RI 02912, USA

McLauchlin, J., Food Water and Environmental Microbiology Laboratory, Health Protection Agency, London, UK

Mehlhorn, Heinz, Parasitology, Heinrich- Heine- Universität, D- 40225- Düsseldorf, Germany

Meng, X. J., Center for Molecular Medicine and Infectious Diseases, Department of Biomedical Sciences and Pathobiology, College of Veterinary Medicine, Virginia Polytechnic Institute and State University, Blacksburg VA, USA

Mignon, Bernard, DVM, PhD, Dip ECVD, Department of Infectious and Parasitic Diseases, Faculty of Veterinary Medicine, University of Liège, Belgium

Mills, James N., Viral Special Pathogens Branch, Division of High-Consequence Pathogens and Pathology, National Center for Emerging and Zoonotic Infectious Diseases, Centers for Disease Control and Prevention, Atlanta, GA, USA

Monath, Thomas P., Partner, Kleiner Perkins Caufield & Byers, Harvard, USA

Monod, M., Service de Dermatologie et Vénéréologie, Laboratoire de Mycologie, BT422, Centre Hospitalier Universitaire Vaudois, 1011 Lausanne, Switzerland

Morgan, Dilys, Head, Gastrointestinal, Emerging and Zoonotic Infections, Health Protection Agency, Colindale, London, UK

Morgan, Eric R., School of Biological Sciences, University of Bristol, UK

Morgan, Marina, Royal Devon & Exeter hospital, Exeter, Devon, UK

Moriyón, Ignacio, Professor, Depto. Microbiología–Edificio de Investigación, Universidad de Navarra, Pamplona, Spain

Mounsey, K. E., University of Queensland, Queensland Institute of Medical Research, Division of Infectious Diseases, Brisbane, Queensland, Australia

Müller, Borna, DST/NRF Centre of Excellence for Biomedical Tuberculosis Research/MRC Centre of Molecular and Cellular Biology, Division of Molecular Biology and Human Genetics, Faculty of Health Sciences, Stellenbosch University, Cape Town, South Africa

Nithikathkul, Choosak, Faculty of Medicine, Mahasarakham University, Thailand

Nolan, T. J., Laboratory of Parasitology, School of Veterinary Medicine, University of Pennsylvania, Philadelphia, USA

Nutman, T. B., Laboratory of Parasitic Diseases, National Institute of Allergy and Infectious Diseases, National Institutes of Health, Bethesda, USA

Nuttall, Patricia A., Centre for Ecology and Hydrology, Oxfordshire, UK

O'Connell, Sue, Consultant Medical Microbiologist, Head, Health Protection Agency Lyme Borreliosis Unit, Southampton University Hospitals Trust, Southampton, UK

O'Neill, Sandra M., School of Nursing, Dublin City University, Glasnevin, Ireland

Paintal, Harman S., Staff Physician, United States Department of Veterans Affairs Palo Alto Health Care System, Clinical Assistant Professor of Medicine, Division of Pulmonary and Critical Care Medicine, Stanford University School of Medicine, USA

Palmer, Stephen, Cochrane Professor of Epidemiology and Public Health, Cardiff University, Cardiff, UK

Parkinson, Michael, School of Biotechnology, Dublin City University, Glasnevin, Ireland

Pavlik, Ivo, Veterinary Research Institute, Department of Food and Feed Safety, Mycobacteriology Unit, OIE Reference Laboratories for Paratuberculosis and Avian Tuberculosis, Brno, The Czech Republic

Paweska, J. T., National Institute for Communicable Diseases, Sandringham 2131, South Africa

Peacock, Sharon J., Department of Medicine, University of Cambridge, Cambridge Microbiology and Public Health Laboratory, Addenbrooke's Hospital, Cambridge, UK

Pearson, Andrew, Department of Advanced Computational Biology, University of Maryland, USA

Phin, N., Consultant Epidemiologist, Centre for Infections, London, UK

Pozio, Edoardo, Istituto Superiore di Sanità, Rome, Italy

Prentice, Michael B., Department of Microbiology, University College Cork, Cork, Ireland

Puthia, Manoj K., Laboratory of Molecular and Cellular Parasitology, Department of Microbiology, Yong Loo Lin School of Medicine, National University of Singapore, and Defence Medical and Environmental Research Institute, DSO National Laboratories, Singapore

Raoult, Didier, Unité des Rickettsies, CNRS UMR 6020, IFR 48, Faculté de Médecine, Université de la Méditerranée, France

Reid, Hugh W., Moredun Research Institute, Edinburgh, UK

Riley, Steven, Department of Community Medicine and School of Public Health, Li Ka Shing Faculty of Medicine, The University of Hong Kong, Hong Kong Special Administrative Region, China

Rota, Paul A., Measles, Mumps Rubella, and Herpesvirus Laboratory Branch, Division of Viral Diseases, National Center Immunizations and Respiratory Diseases, Centers for Disease Control and Prevention, Atlanta, GA, USA

Royal, Louis, Huachiew Chalermprakiet University, Thailand

Saichua, Prasert, Thammasat University, Thailand

Salmon, Roland L., Communicable Disease Surveillance Centre, Public Health Wales, The Temple of Peace and Health, Cathays Park, Cardiff, UK

Sargeant, Jan M., Laboratory for Foodborne Zoonoses, Public Health Agency of Canada and Department of Clinical Epidemiology and Biostatistics, McMaster University, Canada

Schad, G. A. (now deceased), Laboratory of Parasitology, School of Veterinary Medicine, University of Pennsylvania, Philadelphia, USA

Schelling, Esther, DVM, PhD, Department of Epidemiology and Public Health, Swiss Tropical and Public Health Institute, Basel, Switzerland

Schofield, C. J., ECLAT Coordinator, Department of Infectious and Tropical Diseases, London School of Hygiene & Tropical Medicine, London, UK

Sillis, Margaret, Norfolk and Norwich University Hospital, Norwich, UK

Smith, Huw V., Scottish Parasite Diagnostic Laboratory, Stobhill Hospital, Glasgow, UK

Smith, Robert M., Communicable Disease Surveillance Centre, Public Health Wales, The Temple of Peace and Health, Cathays Park, Cardiff, UK

Sohn, Woon-Mok, Department of Parasitology and Institute of Health Sciences, Gyeongsang National University School of Medicine, Jinju 660-751, Korea

Solera, Javier, Servicio de Medicina Interna y Unidad de Investigación, Hospital General Universitario, Albacete, Spain

Spiropoulou, Christina F., Viral Special Pathogens Branch, Division of High-Consequence Pathogens and Pathology, National Center for Emerging and Zoonotic Infectious Diseases, Centers for Disease Control and Prevention, Atlanta, GA, USA

Staples, J. Erin, Medical Epidemiologist, Arboviral Disease Branch, Division of Vectorborne Infectious Diseases, Centers for Disease Control and Prevention, Fort Collins, USA

Swanepoel, R., National Institute for Communicable Diseases, Sandringham 2131, South Africa

Tan, Kevin S. W., Laboratory of Molecular and Cellular Parasitology, Department of Microbiology, Yong Loo Lin School of Medicine, National University of Singapore, and Infectious Disease Programme, Life Science Institute, National University of Singapore

Thomas, Daniel Rh., Communicable Disease Surveillance Centre, Public Health Wales, The Temple of Peace and Health, Cathays Park, Cardiff, UK

Thompson, R. C. Andrew, WHO Collaborating Centre for the Molecular Epidemiology of Parasitic Infections, School of Veterinary and Biomedical Sciences, Murdoch University, Australia

Threlfall, E. J., Health Protection Agency, Gastrointestinal, Emerging and Zoonotic Infections, Centre for Infections, London, UK

Torgerson, Paul R., Professor of Epidemiology, Vetsuisse Faculty, Zurich University, Switzerland

Vaheri, Antti, Department of Virology, Haartman Institute, University of Helsinki, Finland

Vuitton, D. A., WHO Collaborating Centre on Prevention and Treatment of Echinococcosis, Université de Franche-Comté et CHU de Besançon, France

Wain, J., Health Protection Agency, Gastrointestinal, Emerging and Zoonotic Infections, Centre for Infections, London, UK

Walton, S. F., University of the Sunshine Coast, School of Health and Sports Science, Maroochydore, Queensland, Australia

Wang, Qiao-Ping, Center for Parasitic Organisms, School of Life Sciences, Sun Yat-Sen University, Guangzhou, P.R. China

Weiss, Louis M., MD, MPH, Albert Einstein College of Medicine, New York, USA

Wheat, L. Joseph, MiraVista Diagnostics & MiraBella Technologies, 4444 Decatur Blvd; Suite 300 Indianapolis, IN 46241, USA

Widmer, Giovanni, Tufts Cummings School of Veterinary Medicine, Division of Infectious Diseases, North Grafton, Massachusetts, USA

Xiao-Nong, Zhou, National Institute of Parasitic Diseases, Chinese Center for Disease Control and Prevention, P.R. China

Zinsstag, Jakob, DVM, PhD, Department of Epidemiology and Public Health, Swiss Tropical and Public Health Institute, Basel, Switzerland

Zochowski, Wendy J., Leptospira Reference Unit, Department of Microbiology and Immunology, County Hospital, Hereford, UK

Zuckerman, M., Consultant Virologist, Kings College Hospital NHS Foundation Trust, London, UK

Abbreviations

ABC	ATP-binding cassette		BHK	Baby hamster kidney cells
ABLV	Australian bat lyssavirus		BLS	Big liver spleen disease
ABZ	Albendazole		BPSU	British Paediatric Surveillance Unit
AC	Adenyl cyclase		BRDC	Bovine Respiratory Disease Complex
ACAF	Advisory Committee on Animal Feeding		BSE	Bovine Spongiform Encephalopathy
ACIP	Advisory Committee on Immunization Practices		BSL	Biosafety level
ACMSF	Advisory Committee on the Microbiological Safety of Food		BTB	Bovine Tuberculosis
			CAM	Choriollantoic membrane
AD	Anchoring disk		CAT	Computer-aided tomography
Ado	Adenosine		CATT	Card agglutination test for Trypanosomosis
ADPG	Animal Disease Policy Group		CBPP	Contagious Bovine Pleuropneumonia
AE	Alveolar echinococcosis		CCHF	Crimean-Congo haemorrhagic fever
AE	Attached and Effacing		CDC	Centers for Disease Control and Prevention
AFLP	Amplified Fragment Length Polymorphism		CE	Cystic echinococcosis
AHT	Animal Health Trust		CEP	Counter electrophoresis
AI	Avian influenza		CF	Complement fixation
AIDS	Acquired Immune Deficiency Syndrome		CFA	Case fatality rate
ALP	Alkaline phosphatase		CFT	Complement Fixation Test
ALT	Alanine transaminase		CFU	Colony Forming Units
AMCHA	Amazonian Chagas Initiative		CHCA	Cholangio carcinoma
AMP	Adenosine monophosphate		CHOCV	Choclo virus
AMP	Antimicrobial peptides		CIC	Circulating immune complexes
AMR	Antimicrobial resistance		CJD	Creutzfeldt-Jakob Disease
ANDV	Andes virus		CK	Creatine kinase
ANON	Anonymous		CL	Cystic lesion
AOX	Alternative oxidase		CL	Cutaneous leishmania
APTT	Activated partial thromboplastin		CLSI	Clinical Laboratory Standards Institute
APUA	Alliance for the Prudent use of Antibiotics		CMI	Cell mediated immune
ARAV	Aravan virus		CNS	Central Nervous System
ARC	Alliance for Rabies Control		Cpn60	Chaperone 60
ART	Anti-retrovirus therapy		CRP	C-reactive protein
ASF	African Swine Fever		CSF	Cerebrospinal fluid
AST	Aspartate transaminase		CSF	Classical Swine Fever
ATCC	American type culture collection		CT	Computerized tomography
BAL	Broncho-alveolar lavage		CVED	Common Veterinary Entry Documents
BAYV	Bayo virus		Cyd	Cytidine
BCCV	Black Creek Canal virus		DALY	Disability Adjusted Life Year
BEFV	Bovine ephemeral fever virus		DARD NI	Department of Agriculture and Rural Affairs Northern Ireland
BEVA	British Empire Veterinary Association			
BF	Bursa of Fabricus		DAT	Direct agglutination test
BFV	Barmah Forest virus		DAT	Diphtheria Antitoxin

DCL	Diffuse cutaneous leishmania
DEC	Diethycarbamazine
Defra	Department for Environment, Food and Rural Affairs
DENV	Dengue virus
DFA	Direct immunofluorescent antibody
DHF	Dihydrofolate
DI	Defective interfering
DIC	Differential interface
DNA	Deoxyribonucleic Acid
DRC	Democratic Republic of Congo
dThd	Deoxythymidine
DTM	Dermatophyte test medium
DUVV	Duvenhage virus
DWSP	Drinking water safety plans
E. coli	Escherichia coli
EAE	Enzootic abortion of ewes
EB	Elementary Body
EBLV	European bat lyssaviruses
ECDC	European Centre for Disease Prevention and Control
ECMO	Extra corporeal membrane oxygenation
EFIG	Epidemiology of Food-Borne Infections Group
EFSA	European Food Safety Agency
EGD	Endo-gastroduodenoscopy
EHEC	Enterohaemorrhagic E. coli
EHF	Ebola haemorrhagic fever
EIA	Enzyme immunoassay
ELISA	Enzyme-linked Immunosorbent Assay
EMJH	Ellinghausen and McCullough Medium
En	Endospore
EPEC	Entropathogenic E. coli
Epg	Eggs/gm
ER	Endoplasmic reticulum
ERCP	Endoscopic Retrograde Cholangiopancreatography
ERIC	Enterobacterial Repetitive Intergenic Consensus
ESBL	Extended Spectrum β-lactamase Producing Bacteria
ESR	Erythrocyte sedimentation rate
ET	Edema Toxin
ETIB	Immuno-electrotransfer blot
EU	European Union
EUCALB	EU Concerted action on Lyme Borreliosis
Ex	Exosphere
FAD	Flea Allergy Dermatitis
FAO	Food and Agriculture Organization of the UN
FAT	Fluorescent antibody test
FAUN	Fluorescent antibody virus neutralization
FBSF	Flea-borne Spotted Fever
FDA	US Food and Drugs Administration
FMD	Foot-and-mouth disease
FMDV	Foot-and-mouth disease virus
FMS	Fast Sedimentation Method
FPA	Fluorescence Polarization Assay
FPSR	False positive serological reaction
FSA	Food Standards Agency
FSME	Frut-Sommer-meningo-encephalitis
GAE	Granulomatous amoebic encephalitis

GBD	Global Burden of Disease
GLEWS	Global Early Warning and Response System
GMP	Guanosine monophosphate
GOT	Glutamic oxaloacetic transaminase
GPI	General paralysis of the insane
GPI	Glycophosphatidylinositol
GPT	Glutamic pyruvic transaminase
GS	Gravity sedimentation technique
GTM	Genetic transformation methods
HA	Haemagglutinin
HACCP	Hazard Analysis and Critical Control Point
HAIRS	Human Animal Infections and Risks Surveillance Group
HALY	Health Adjusted Life Year
HCPS	Hantavirus cardiopulmonary syndrome
HCT-8	Human colonic tumour cells
HDCV	Human diploid cell vaccine
HEE	Human Ewingii Ehrlichiosis
HEL	Human Embryonic Lung
HeV	Hendra virus
HEV	Hepatitis E virus
HFL	Halofuginone lactate
HFL	Human fetal lung
HFMD	Hand, foot, and mouth disease
HFRS	Haemorrhagic fever with renal syndrome
HGA	Human Granulocytic Anaplasmosis
HIV	Human Immunodeficiency virus
HME	Human Monocytic Ehrlichiosis
HN	Haemagglutinin
HOOF	Hypervariable octameric oligonucleotide fingerprints
HPA	Health Protection Agency
HPS	Hantavirus Pulmonary Syndrome
HRT	Human rectal tumour
HSE	Health and Safety Executive
Hsp70	Heat-shock protein 70
HSV	Human Herpes Simplex viruses
HTC	Haematocrit
HTNV	Hantaan virus
HUS	Haemolytic Uraemic Syndrome
IAAT	Immunoabsorbent agglutination assay test
IBS	Irritable Bowel Syndrome
ICTV	International Committee for the Taxonomy of Viruses
ICVP	International certificate of vaccination or prophylaxis
IFA	Immunufluorescence assay
IFAA	Indirect fluorescent antibody assay
IFAT	Indirect fluorescent antibody test
IgG	Immunoglobulin G
IHT	Indirect haemagglutination test
IHA	Indirect haemagglutination assay
IHR	International Health Regulations
IID	Infectious Intestinal Disease
IM	Immediate hypersensitivity
IMS	Immunomagnetic Separation
INCOSUR	Southern Cone Initiative against Chagas disease
INKV	Inkoo virus
InsP3	Inositol phosphate

IPCA	Initiative of the Central American countries to interrupt transmission of Chagas Disease
IRIS	Immune reconstitution inflammatory syndrome
IRKV	Irkut virus
IS	Insertion sequence
ISRE	IFN stimulated response element
IST	Intestinal scraping technique
JEV	Japanese encephalitis virus
JICA	Japanese international cooperation
KFDV	Kyasanur forest disease virus
KHUJV	Khujand virus
L1	First stage larva
L2	Second stage larva
L3	Third stage larva
L4	Fourth stage larva
LACV	La Crosse virus
LAMP	Loop mediated isothermal amplification
LANV	Laguna Negra virus
LBV	Lagos bat virus
LDH	Lactate dehydrogenase
LEE	Locus of Enterocyle Effacement
LGTV	Langat virus
LIPS	Luciferase immunoprecipitation assays
LIV	Louping ill virus
LOS	Lipooligosaccharide
LP	Low pathogenicity
lpg	Larvae per g
LPS	Lipopolysaccharide
LRN	Laboratory Response Network
LT	Lethal Toxin
LT	Liver transplant
M	manubrium
MAC	*M. avium* Complex
MAPK	Mitogen-Activated Protein Kinases
MAT	Microscopic agglutination test
MBG	Marbug virus
MBZ	Mebendazole
mCCDA	Modified Charcoal Cefoperazone Desoxycholate Agar
MCL	Mucocutaneous leishmaniosis
MDBK	Madin-Darby bovine kidney
MDCK	Madin-Darby canine kidney
MDR	Multi-drug Resistance
MDRP	Multiple-drug-resistance protein
MenV	Menagle virus
MIF	Micro-immunofluorescence
MIT	Mouse inoculation test
MLEE	Multilocus enzyme electrophoresis
MLST	Multilocus Sequence Typing
MLVA	Multiple Locus Variable
MMWR	Morbidity and Mortality Weekly Report
MOKV	Mokola virus
MOMP	Major outer membrane protein
MOTT	Mycobacteria other than Tubercile bacilli
MR	Magnetic resonance
MRC	Medical Research Council
MRI	Magnetic resonance imaging
MRSA	Methicillin Resistance *Staphylococcus aureus*
MTC	*M. tuberculosis* Complex
MYA	Million years ago
NA	Neuraminidase
NADH DH	NADH dehydrogenase
NAHD	Nicolinamide adenine dinucleotide
NAHMS	National animal health monitoring system
Narf-like	Nuclear prelamin A recognition factor-like protein
NASPHV	National Association State Public Health Veterinarians
NCAM	Neural cell adhesion molecule
NCBI	National Center for Biotechnology Informatics
NCCR	National Center for Competence – North-South
NCP	National Control programme
ND	Newcastle Disease
NDV	Newcastle Disease Virus
NE	Nephropathia Epidemica
NEPNEI	National Expert Panel on New and Emerging Infections
NHS	National Health Service
NI	Neuramindase inhibitors
NIAID	National Institute of Allergy and Infectious Disease
NiV	Nipah virus
NK	Natural killer cells
NKV	No known vector
NL	Newborn larvae
NLS	Nuclear localizational signal
NMR	Nuclear magnetic resonance
NS	Non-structural
NTB	Nerve tissue based
NTS	Non-typhoidal Salmonella
Nu	Nucleus
NWS	New world screwworm
NxCpl	Ciprofloxacin
NYV	New York virus
OEA	Ovine enzootic abortion
OECD	Organization for Economic Cooperation and Development
OHFV	Omsk haemorrhagic fever virus
OIE	World Organization for Animal Health
OLM	Ocular larva migrans
OM	Outer Membrane
OMI	Office of the Medical Investigator
ONNV	O'Nyong Nyong virus
ORF	Open-reading frames
OSF	Oriental Spotted Fever
OVS	Official Veterinary Surgeon
OWS	Old world screwworm
p.i.	post-infection
P1	Lamellar polaroplast
PAHO	Pan-American Health Organization
PAI	Pathogenicity Island
PAM	Primary amoebic meningo enchaphalitis
PAS	Periodic Acid Schiff
PCECV	Purified chick embryo cell vaccine
PCK	Primary chicken kidney
PCP	*Pneumocystis* pneumonia
PCR	Polymerase Chain Reaction
PEP	Phosphoenolpyruvate phosphatase
PFGE	Pulsed Field Gel Electrophoresis

PHLSSG	Public Health Laboratory Service Study Group	SARS-CoV	Severe acute respiratory syndrome – Coronavirus
PI(3)K	Phosphatidylinositol 3-kinase	SC	Suspension concentrates
PKC	proteinkinase C	SCF	Soluble complement fixing
PKDL	Post Kala-azar dermal leishmania	SCID	Severe combined immunodifficiency syndrome
PLC	Phospholipase C	SCT	Sedimentation counting techniques
Plos	Public Library of Sciences	SEOV	Seoul virus
Pm	Plasma membrane	SESV	Southern elephant seal virus
PMP	Polymorphic membrane protein	SFG	Spotted Fever Group
PMQR	Plasmid Mediated Quinolone Resistance	SGDIA	Surveillance Group on Diseases and Infections in Animals
PNM	Liver neighbouring organs and metastasis	SICCT	Single Intra-dermal Comparative Cervical Tuberculin
PNO–CPR	Pyruvate:NADPþ oxidoreductase fused to cytochrome P450reductase domain	SIT	Sterile insect technique
POWV	Powassan virus	SLT	Shiga-like Toxin
PP	Pathogenic polycystic	SNP	Single Nucleotide Polymorphism
PPE	Personal protective equipment	SNT	Serum neutralization tests
PPM	Potentially Pathogenic Mycobacteria	SNV	Sin Nombre virus
PPR	Peste des Petits Ruminants	Sp	Sporoplasm
PRP	Partnership for Rabies Prevention	SPDV	Salmon pancreatic disease virus
PRR	Pattern recognition receptors	SPS	Sanitary and phytosanitary measures
PT	Phage Type	SSHV	Snowshoe hare virus
PUUV	Puumala virus	SSR	Simple sequence repeats
PV	Posterior vacuole	SSU	Small subunit
PVI	Post mortem interval	STARI	Southern tick-associated illness
PVL	Panton-Valentine Leukocidin	STEC	Shiga Toxin Producing *E. coli*
PVM	Parasitophorous vascular membrane	SWDV	Swine vesicular disease virus
PVRV	Purified vero rabies vaccine	T4SS	Type 4 secretion systems
QALY	Quality Adjusted Life Year	TAHV	Tahyna virus
QBC	Quantitative buffy coal	TBEV	Tick-borne encephalitis virus
RADAR	Rapid Analysis and Detection of Animal-related Risks	TES	Toxocara larval excretions/secretions
RANTES	Regulated upon Activation, Normal T-cell Expressed and Secreted	THF	Tetrahydrofolate
		TIM17	Translocase of the inner mitochondrial membrane 17
RAPD	Randomly amplified polymorphic DNA	TiV	Tioman virus
RB	Reticular Body	TLR	Toll-like receptors
RBT	Rose Bengal Test	TLR4	Toll-like receptor 4
RDEC	Rabbit diarrheagenic *E. coli*	TM	Teleman centrifugation technique
ReA	Reactive Arthritis	TOM40	Translocase of the outer mitochondrial membrane 40
REP	Repetitive Extragenic Palindramic		
RFFIT	Rapid Fluorescent focus inhibitor test	TPMV	Thottapalayam virus
RFLP	Restriction fragment length polymorphism	TRACES	Trade Control and Expert Systems
RIDDOR	Reporting of Injuries, Diseases and Dangerous Occurrences Regulations	TSE	Transmisible Spongiform Encephalopathies
		TTSS	Type III Secretion System
RIVM	Netherlands Environmental Assessment Agency	TULV	Tula virus
RMSF	Rocky Mountain Spotted Fever	UE	Unicystic echinococcosis
RMT	Milk Ring Test	UK	United Kingdom
RNA	Ribonucleic acid	UKZADI	UK Zoonoses, Animal Diseases and Infections Group
RNP	Ribonucleoprotein complex		
ROAR	Reservoirs of Antibiotic Resistance Network	ULN	Upper limit of normal
RREID	Rapid rabies enzyme immunodiagnosis	ULV	Ultra low volume
RRV	Ross River virus	UN	United Nations
RSSE	Russian spring-summer encephalitis	UQ	Ubiquinone
RTCIT	Rabies tissue culture inoculation test	Urd	Uridine
RT-PCR	Reverse transcription-polymerase chain reaction	US	Ultrasound
RVF	Rift Valley Fever	USA	United States of America
SA8	Simian agent	US-EPA	US Environment Protection Agency
SAC	Scottish Agricultural Colleges	USSR	Union of the Soviet Socialist Republics
SACAR	Scientific Advisory Committee on Antibiotics Resistance	USUV	Usulu virus
SARS	Severe acute respiratory syndrome	UTS	Untranslated regions

vCJD	Variant Creutzfeldt-Jakob Disease		WEEV	Western equine encephalitis virus
VELI	Rabbit chondrocyte cell line		WHO	World Health Organization
VIDA	Veterinary Investigation Diagnosis Analysis		WHO-IWGE	WHO Informal Working Group
VLA	Veterinary Laboratory Agency		WNV	West Nile virus
VLM	Visceral larva migrans		WP	Wettable powders
VNC	Viable non-culturable		WTO	World Trade Organization
VNTR	Variable Number Tandem Repeats		YEL-AND	Yellow fever vaccine-associated neurotropic disease
Vpl	Vesiculotubular polaroplast			
VS	Vesicular stomatitis		YEL-AVD	Yellow fever vaccine-associated viscerotropic disease
VSV	Vesicular stomatitis virus			
VT	Verocytotoxin		YFV	Yellow fever virus
VTEC	Verocytotoxin-producing *Escherichia coli* O157		YLD	Years lived with a certain level of disability
WAHID	World Animal Health Information Database		YLL	Years of Life Lost
WCBV	West Caucasian bat virus		ZO	Zonula-occludens

PART 1

Introduction

CHAPTER 1

The global challenge of zoonoses control

Stephen Palmer

Summary

Zoonotic diseases are now recognized as a major global threat to human health and sustainable development and a major concern for national and international agencies (Marano *et al.* 2006). There was a period in the 1960s and 70s when it was widely expected that the antibiotic and vaccine era would relegate infectious diseases to footnotes of history, and in many countries communicable control systems were neglected (Keusch *et al.* 2009) but the frequent and often dramatic appearance of new infectious agents or the re-appearance of well recognized zoonoses has changed perceptions (Table 1.1). 'A wide variety of animal species, domesticated, peri-domesticated and wild, can act as reservoirs for these pathogens, which may be viruses, bacteria, parasites or prions. Considering the wide variety of animal species involved and the often complex natural history of the pathogens concerned, effective surveillance, prevention and control of zoonotic diseases pose a real challenge to public health' (WHO 2004). No country has been able to anticipate the sudden and sometimes devastating impact of novel agents, and international trade and transport of people, animals and goods have ensured that wherever zoonoses emerge they have to be considered as global issues. The cost of zoonoses can be enormous. The H1N1v pandemic which began in pig herds on the Mexico-US border resulted in major losses to the pork industry amounting to US$25 million per week; fear that transmission could occur from meat led to the banning of importation of pigs and pork products by at least 15 countries (Keusch *et al.* 2009). And in addition to these 'natural' threats, several zoonoses are prime agents for deliberate release by disaffected groups. A more esoteric threat, though nonetheless a real cause of concern, is the possibility of zoonotic emergence from xenotransplantation (Mattiuzzo *et al.* 2008).

Emerging zoonoses

In a recently published landmark study, Jones *et al.* (2008) identified 335 emergent events between 1940 and 2004 and sought to identify where the emergence first occurred. The definition of events included pathogens that crossed species for the first time (e.g. HIV-1, SARS) and established pathogens which have recently increased in incidence (e.g. Lyme disease). A degree of subjectivity in listing such events is perhaps inevitable but nevertheless this

work represents the most complete attempt to date to map emerging diseases. 54% of events were due to bacteria or rickettsiae, 25% to viruses and prions, 11% to protozoa, 6% to fungi and 3% to helminths. 60% were zoonotic. Despite improving diagnosis and reporting the authors conclude that there has been a real increase in events (Fig. 1.1), particularly in the 1980s, which may be related to the emergence of new diseases associated with the HIV/AIDS pandemic. Of the zoonotic events, Jones *et al.* (2008) report that 72% were pathogens of wildlife origin (such as Nipah virus in Malaysia and SARS in China) and that the rate of the new wildlife events is increasing. They also report a significant rise in vector-borne events related possibly to 'climate anomalies occurring during the 1990s'. Not surprisingly human population density and growth was a powerful predictor of all events and of non-wildlife zoonotic events. The world map of the location of first emergence shows that the most likely places are the least well served by resources for surveillance, investigation and control (Fig. 1.2).

A major initiative to address emerging zoonotic diseases was made by the Government of the Netherlands during their presidency of the European Union in 2004. A joint consultation by WHO, FAO and OIE (WHO 2004) in collaboration with the Health Council of the Netherlands concluded that emerging zoonotic diseases are global threats and that an upward trend is likely to continue. Consequently, 'coordinated international responses are therefore essential across veterinary and human health sectors, regions and countries to control and prevent emerging zoonoses'. They acknowledged that prediction is extremely difficult but that anthropogenic factors are major drivers. Surveillance and field investigation are important in understanding causes but 'shortfalls in public health infrastructure and policy and in scientific studies to answer public health questions and to build expertise were identified as contributing risk factors for emergence, along with a lack of integration between human and animal health surveillance'. New technology should be applied to surveillance, investigation and response and new international networks created. A sister Report on Zoonoses in Europe from the Netherlands RIVM (van der Giessen *et al.* 2004), thoroughly reviewed threats of individual zoonoses and then sought to prioritize these using criteria including likelihood of spread, case fatality rates, availability of prevention or treatment, economic impact and risk perception.

Table 1.1 Zoonotic Outbreaks of Global Significance Reported by WHO Global Alert and Response Network (as of 11.3.11) (www.who.int/csr/don/archive/year/en/index.html)

Year	Outbreak	Region
2011	Avian Influenza	Egypt, Indonesia, Cambodia
2010	Avian Influenza	Egypt, Indonesia, China, Cambodia, Vietnam
	Crimean Congo Hemorrhagic fever	Pakistan
	Plague	Peru
	Pandemic (H1N1) Influenza	Global
	Rift Valley fever	South Africa
2009	Pandemic (H1N1) Influenza	Global
	Avian Influenza	Cambodia, Vietnam, Egypt, China
	Plague	China
	Ebola Reston virus	Philippines
	Ebola Hemorrhagic fever	Democratic Republic of Congo
2008	Ebola Hemorrhagic fever	Democratic Republic of Congo
	Avian Influenza	Cambodia, Indonesia, Vietnam, China, Bangladesh, Egypt, Pakistan
	New Arenavirus	South Africa, Zambia
	Marburg Hemorrhagic fever	Netherlands, Uganda
	Rift Valley fever	Madagascar, Sudan
	Ebola Hemorrhagic fever	Uganda
2007	Avian Influenza	Egypt, Vietnam, Pakistan, Indonesia, Myanmar, China, UK, Cambodia, Lao, Nigeria
	Rift Valley fever	Sudan, Kenya, Somalia, Tanzania
	Ebola Hemorrhagic fever	Uganda, Democratic Republic of Congo
2006	Avian Influenza	Egypt, Indonesia, Turkey, Thailand, Iraq, China, Azerbaijan, Cambodia, Germany, Nigeria, Niger, India
	Rift Valley fever	Kenya
	Plague	Democratic Republic of Congo
	Chikungunya	India, Mauritius, Seychelles, Mangyotte, La Reunion Island
	Crimean Congo Hemorrhagic fever	Turkey
	Lassa fever	Germany

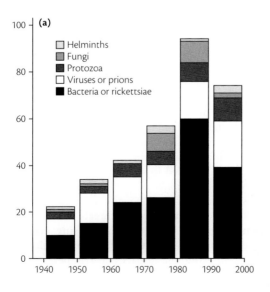

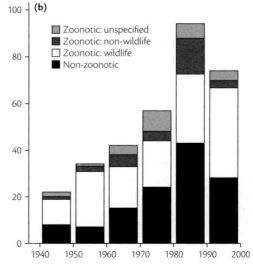

Fig. 1.1 Number of EID events per decade. EID events (defined as the temporal origin of an EID, represented by the original case or cluster of cases that represents a disease emerging in the human population) are plotted with respect to **a**, pathogen type, and **b**, transmission type (keys for details).
Reproduced from Jones *et al.* (2008), by permission from Macmillan Publishers Ltd

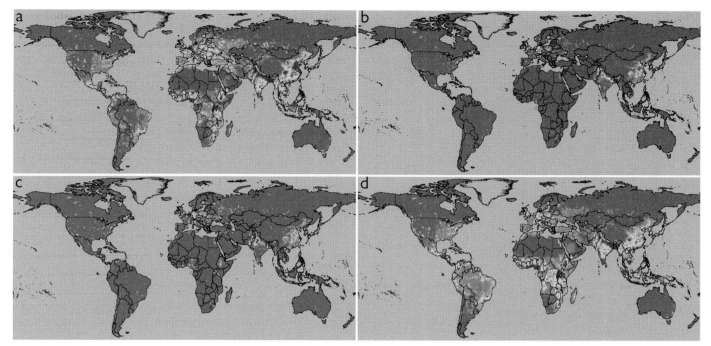

Fig. 1.2 Maps are derived for EID events caused by **a**, zoonotic pathogens from wildlife, **b**, zoonotic pathogens from non-wildlife, **c**, drug-resistant pathogens and **d**, vector-borne pathogens. The relative risk is calculated from regression coefficients and variable values in Table 1 in Jones *et al.* (2008) (omitting the variable measuring reporting effort), categorized by standard deviations from the mean and mapped on a linear scale from green (lower values) to red (higher values). This figure is reproduced in colour in the colour plate section. Reproduced from Jones *et al.* (2008), by permission from Macmillan Publishers Ltd.

The RIVM Report summarizes the EUs zoonoses directives which have focussed attention on monitoring disease incidence within each member country (Defra 2010), as well as seeking to ensure that effective measures are taken to control them.

International concern about the impact of emerging zoonoses has led to proposals to establish new global surveillance and response systems. In 2008, the World Health Organization (WHO), the Food and Agriculture Organization of the United Nations (FAO) and the World Organization for Animal Health (OIE) set up a Global Early Warning System for Major Animal Diseases, including Zoonoses (GLEWS) to improve early warning and response (www.GLEWS.net). There are 25 diseases on its priority list, 19 of which are zoonoses (Table 1.2).

In the USA the Committee on Achieving Sustainable Gobal Capacity for Surveillance and Response to Emerging Diseases of Zoonotic Origin was convened by the Institute of Medicine and the National Research Council at the request of the US Agency for International Development. The Report published in 2009 by the National Academy of Sciences (Keusch *et al.*) is a major assessment of zoonoses worldwide, and the factors for emergence. In making the case for surveillance the report sets out the rapidly increasing trends in global trade in livestock and animal products (Fig. 1.3) and wildlife and products. It documents the economic impact in detail. For example, during the course of the 1994 outbreak of plague in India, trade and travel restrictions were imposed and this led to losses on the stock markets of nearly US$2 billion. The EUs total ban on beef and cattle exports from the UK in the 1996, Bovine Spongiform Encephalophathy (BSE) epidemic led to losses of trade of £700 million per year. The Report identifies

the need for international leadership to strengthen capacity and win international finance for surveillance, investigation and governance in those countries most likely to see emergent events. One barrier to better surveillance is the reluctance of countries to admit to infections that may result in significant loss of trade or restriction of movement of people imposed by other countries. Clearly such protection is short sighted but understandable. A local farmer facing culling of his animals may be reluctant to report without the reassurance of compensation. At national level a government may fear the economic cost of trade embargoes and therefore wish to cover an emerging problem. 'A global zoonotic disease surveillance and response strategy that does not address the fundamental incentives and disincentives of reporting is likely to be unproductive'.

Increasing knowledge and rumours about emerging infections will challenge the ability of health agencies and governments to accurately assess risks to public health in the short time frame of an emergent event. Better surveillance will take public health agencies from not knowing enough to knowing too much and having to separate rumour from fact by rapid verification processes. For such surveillance to be useful for prevention it will need to be set within a risk assessment framework which can trigger early action when necessary but also allow countries to avoid committing resources inefficiently on theoretical or unlikely threats (Palmer *et al.* 2005).

Drivers for emergence

The drivers for emergence are complex (Wolfe *et al.* 2007) and need to be better understood if events are to be anticipated and

Table 1.2 Global Early Warning and Response System (GLEWS) Disease Priority List (www.GLEWS.net)

Non zoonotic
· African Swine Fever (ASF)
· Classical Swine Fever (CSF)
· Contagious Bovine Pleuropneumonia (CBPP)*
· Foot and Mouth Disease (FMD)*
· Peste des Petits Ruminants (PPR)
· Rinderpest–Stomatitis/Enteritis
Zoonotic
· Anthrax
· Bovine Spongiform Encephalopathy (BSE)
· Brucellosis (B. melitensis)
· Crimean-Congo Hemorrhagic Fever (CCHF)
· Ebola Virus
· Food borne diseases
· Highly Pathogenic Avian Influenza (HPAI)
· Japanese Encephalitis
· Marburg Hemorrhagic Fever
· New World Screwworm
· Nipah Virus
· Old World Screwworm
· Q fever
· Rabies
· Rift Valley Fever (RVF)
· Sheep Pox/Goat Pox
· Tularemia
· Venezuelan Equine Encephalomyelitis
· West Nile Virus

Reproduced from GLEWS (Global Early Warning and response System for major animal diseases, including zoonoses) website http://www.glews.net/index.php?option=com_content&view=article&id=64&Itemid=68, with permission

their impacts mitigated. Cutter *et al.* (2010) have recently summarized causal factors, which, in addition to mutation and recombinant events in the organisms themselves, range from climate change that affects vector abundance and distribution to cultural and socio-economic factors such as movement of infected animals and people, tourism, changes in land use, changes in livestock management practices and a developing taste for exotic pets and meats. As is clear from the examples set out by the WHO (Table 1.3), such drivers usually interact in complex pathways. Common themes at a population level are the growth in world population and the increasing demand for animal protein leading to intensive rearing, congested live animal markets, and encroachment into new ecosystems by farming, logging and mining. Set alongside this there is a growing population of immuno-compromised people who are susceptible to opportunistic zoonotic infections.

The interplay of causal factors in a complex pathway is not a new phenomenon. For example, the Black Death in Europe can be traced back to 1347 when the Mongols of the Golden Horde swept westwards from Central Asia and besieged a Genoese trading post, Kaffa in the Crimea. Plague broke out among the Mongols, probably from marmots killed for their pelts. Contemporary accounts report that the corpses of plague victims were thrown over the city walls, deliberately spreading plague. Plague subsequently spread along the trade routes to Europe and killed 20–25% of Western Europe's 80 million population in four years. The causal pathway from marmot to pandemic involved culture, the migration of peoples, warfare and international trade.

The following are a few more recent illustrations:

BSE: Variant CJD infection in humans was the result of exposure to BSE in cattle. The BSE epidemic itself appears to have been the result of feeding cattle protein derived from meat and bone of previously slaughtered animals and thereby recycling the prion agent throughout the cattle industry in the UK. The origins of the BSE agent appear to have been the introduction of scrapie from sheep into this food chain. Possibly changes in rendering practices contributed (see Chapter 3).

E. coli 0157: This infection was first recognized as a major threat in the early 1980s after several outbreaks from contaminated fast food hamburgers. The organism was shown to be a widespread commensal of cattle with contamination of carcasses and meat a common problem. Control measures to cook hamburgers thoroughly have greatly reduced fast food outbreaks but outbreaks from a wide range of other foods have been identified (Rangel *et al.* 2005). A recently recognized problem has been associated with the growth of petting farms as a result of farmers diversifying under economic pressures, and where children have been exposed to contaminated animals and environments. In one outbreak cases in children were associated with sticky hands from eating ice-cream and candy floss (Payne *et al.* 2003).

HIV/AIDS: HIV-1 (from chimpanzees) and HIV-2 (from sooty mangabeys) appear to have hopped from animal species to humans on a handful of occasions decades ago as a result of hunting for bush meat (Morens *et al.* 2004). Transmission from person to person did not become epidemic until the social disruption caused by regional political upheavals and military action, the movement of soldiers, new routes of transport, the movement of rural people to unprepared cities with poverty, prostitution and the loss of social controls (Haln *et al.* 2000). Rapid global spread resulted from global travel and sexual promiscuity. Other zoonotic diseases as a result of the immuno-suppression of HIV then came to the fore including cryptosporidium and toxoplasmosis.

Q fever: The recent unprecedented epidemic of Q fever in the Netherlands (van der Hoek *et al.* 2010) appears to be the result of diversification of the farming industry over the last 10 years. European Union policies on restriction of cows' milk production led farmers there to move into goats' milk production with unusually high intensity methods. The result has been outbreaks of Q fever in goats and massive contamination of the environment. Cases in humans have occurred well outside of farmers and their families suggesting widespread dissemination by wind or fomites.

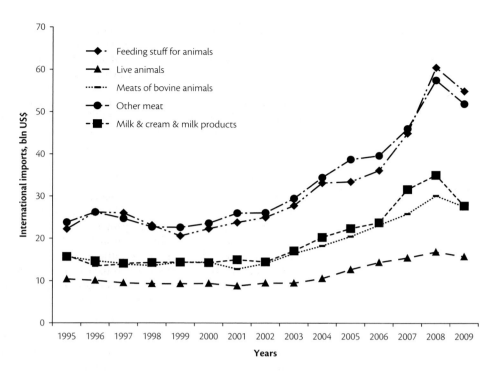

Fig. 1.3 International trade in live animals and meats and dairy products valued as imports in billions of US$. (Source: United Nations International Merchandise Trade Statistics. http://comtrade.un.og/pb/CommodityPagesNew.aspx?y=2009.)

Table 1.3 Risk factors for the emergence and spread of selected zoonoses (WHO, 2004)

Risk factors				
Disease, disease category or causation agent	**Social**	**Technological**	**Ecological**	**Microbial**
Leishmaniasis (*Leishmania* spp.)	Peri-urban settlements in slum areas (e.g. Afghanistan, Central America) Intravenous drug use (e.g. Spain)	—	Deforestation (e.g. South America) Global Warming (Italy)	—
Arthropod-borne disease (pathogen carried by flies, mosquitoes, ticks and midges)	Human encroachment on natural environments (e.g. forests) Tourism and air travel Live animal trade and traffic	Ruminant husbandry	Climate change (e.g. increase in temperature)	—
Lyme disease	People being outdoors Introduction of deer into parks (the Netherlands)	—	Movements of ticks	Possible adaptation of bacterial agent to other arthropod vectors
Monkeypox virus	Increased trade of wild animals Increased air travel Waning human immunity as a result of vaccinations being stopped	—	Introduction of non-native animals to a country	—
Foodborne diseases	Consumption of new or wild animal species (e.g. civets) Population growth and increased demand for meat Lack of quality controls Changes in consumer demand Risk-seeking behaviour	Globalization Food-chain control mostly focused on bacteria, not viruses Current risk assessment cannot incorporate changes rapidly	Experiments in food production (e.g. co-cropping of rice and ducklings) Immune-deficient populations	Recombination of viruses possible following faecal contamination of food with multiple pathogens

(Continued)

Table 1.3 (Cont'd) Risk factors for the emergence and spread of selected zoonoses (WHO, 2004)

Risk factors				
Disease, disease category or causation agent	**Social**	**Technological**	**Ecological**	**Microbial**
Alveolar echinococcosis (Echinococcus multilocularis)	Increased movement of pets in the European Union resulting in increased contact between humans and animals Control measures not implemented uniformly for dogs Increased trade in fresh mushrooms and berries	Difficult to detect emergence as long lag time between infection and onset of symptoms and diagnosis Humans hard to treat (require liver transplants)	Increase in fox population	—
Severe acute respiratory syndrome	Consumption of wildlife Mobility Air travel Population density Social economic status Increased wealth and protein consumption Lack of infrastructure (relative)	Medical interventions (e.g. intubation) Food production	Increased close contact of humans with wild animals through wildlife farming and at markets Close contact between animal species in markets and farms	Virulence Host range
Avian influenza	Mobility of people, animals, animal products and faeces Increased wealth and protein consumption Lack of infrastructure in public health and animal health and lack of integration Expanded markets for poultry exports	Food production (e.g. large poultry plants) Agricultural practices (e.g.*open* production, multiple species)	Contact between wild and domestic species Climate change Migration routes of possible reservoir hosts	Virus changes and reassortment
Human immunodeficiency virus	Promiscuity Lack of compliance with recommended precautions Social economic status Bush-meat consumption (factor emergence)	Blood transfusion	—	—
Ebola virus	Bush-meat consumption Specific practices leading to human-to-human transmission	Nosocomial transmission	Reservoir unknown	—
Mycobacterium	Changes in food preferences (e.g. consumption of raw milk)	—	Increased contact between deer and badgers (carriers of the pathogen) Human contact with zoo animals	—
West Nile virus	Air travel Illegal marketing in wild animals Lack of adequate quarantine for exotic birds Insufficient infrastructure and expertise for vector control	—	Climate change Adaptation of vector species to new areas continents	Different degrees of virulence between strains (e.g. highly virulent strain that invaded North America)

Reproduced from World Health Organization (2004) Report of the WHO/FAO/OIE joint consultation on emerging zoonotic disease, 3–5 May 2004, Geneva, Switzerland, with permission

Salmonella enteritidis pt 4: The narrow base of the international trade in poultry breeding stock has meant that infection in the elite flocks led to the whole industry being affected (ACMSF 2001). Intensive control involving slaughter of infected flocks and quality assurance schemes that prevent reintroduction with a strain of salmonella that may have special features that allow transovanarium transmission has brought infection under control in many countries. Nevertheless egg-borne outbreaks still occur from international trade in eggs from countries that have not vigorously implemented such control schemes.

Neglected zoonoses

Emerging zoonoses are clearly a topic of increased public health and government interest, but the ongoing burden from established zoonoses has been identified as a neglected area. Paradoxically, giving priority to some high profile zoonoses may lead to increased morbidity from prominent endemic zoonoses (Etter *et al.* 2006). Even zoonoses that have been successfully controlled may re-emerge as the result of loss of focus or disinvestment in control measures. In the European region, WHO has been involved in outbreaks of Crimean Congo Haemorrhagic Fever in south-eastern

Europe, Tularaemia in Albania and Kosovo, Anthrax in Romania and Leishmaniasis in Mediterranean countries. Some of these problems are a consequence of civil strife and disruption to traditional economies and life styles. Even in the UK *Echinococcous granulous* persists. A successful supervised dog dosing control programme in Wales was prematurely ended because of the difficulty of funding dog dosing when the disease was a human not animal problem (Buishi *et al.* 2005). A replacement health education programme clearly failed since prevalence of the tapeworm in dogs in the control area quickly returned to pre-control levels justifying a reintroduction of supervised dosing.

In order to keep the importance of zoonoses at the forefront of international attention, the WHO has identified 'neglected zoonoses' that have a major impact on households in developing countries that are dependent upon animals for feed, transport and farm work. Of particular concern are sleeping sickness, cystic echnococcosis, rabies, bovine tuberculosis, chagas disease, leishmaniasis, anthrax and cystercercosis (Maudlin *et al.* 2009). Poor people in developing economies are much more likely to live in close proximity to animals that harbour zoonoses. Those who keep livestock, estimated by WHO to be in excess of 500 million people, are likely to be exposed to bovine tuberculosis, anthrax and brucellosis. The poor are more likely to consume meat that is unfit because of the presence of cysts, or meat that has been taken from dying or fallen animals. Zoonotic infections in these households can be devastating, especially since several such as sleeping sickness, tuberculosis and brucellosis affect active adults. Zoonoses such as cystercercosis also exacerbate poverty because of the losses of income, or as in the case of anthrax, high mortality in livestock. Endemic zoonoses 'are amongst the most seriously underdiagnosed of all human diseases'. Symptoms are shared with many other common diseases, and diagnosis is complex and expensive. The peoples affected have poor knowledge of the diseases and their prevention and little or no access to medical care for themselves or their animals.

Endemic zoonoses can therefore be seen as a major impediment to achieving the Millennium goals to reduce world poverty. WHO (2006) has identified four elements for successful control:

- A legal framework,
- A policy framework,
- Institutional structures,
- A programme implementation plan.

But in many countries zoonoses do not have sufficient priority to command political support and often fall through the gap between veterinary and medical responsibilities. Yet the economic benefits of preventing zoonoses are easily demonstrated. The cost per DALY averted by vaccination against rabies in Tanzania was estimated at just US$10, and the cost per DALY averted by mass vaccination of livestock against brucellosis in Mongolia was US$19.

One Health approach to control

Given the complex causal pathways of zoonoses it is clear that prevention and control need to be exerted at multiple points. Successful zoonoses control requires coordinated action across the traditional professional lines of veterinary and human medicine and science

(Bell and Palmer 1983). WHO has identified the One Health approach as the key to tackling endemic zoonoses in poor communities. Improving animal health will reduce exposure of humans to infection as well as increase relative prosperity by reducing livestock losses and condemnation of meat. The veterinary contribution to the prevention of human infection for tuberculosis, brucellosis and other major infections has been enormous. However, in many countries responsibility for animal and human health are vested in different government ministries so that effective control has to overcome the difficulties of intersectoral working. In the UK eventual control of BSE and SE4 required new cross government approaches. Difficulties can arise when animal health budgets are required to control disease only of major significance to human health (e.g. hydatid disease, Campylobacter). Slowness in identification of a threat to human health from bovine BSE was severely criticized by a Government Enquiry in the UK.

Achieving international leadership in the age of globalization is a challenge addressed by the UK's House of Lords Committee on Intergovernmental Organizations. The growth of agencies and organizations means that 'the landscape of international health' has become 'crowded and poorly coordinated' (House of Lords 2008). The Committee concluded that leadership must come from WHO. They saw that 'there is little coordination between the intergovernmental systems for conducting surveillance of human and animal diseases'. The 'one medicine' or 'one health' approach must be underpinned by coordinated national and international planning and response. Good examples of such coordination do exist. At international level there is good cooperation between WHO, FAO and OIE but such cooperation needs to be translated at national and local levels. One such initiative is the Mediterranean Zoonoses Control Programme which was established in 1978 and has programmes for brucellosis, salmonellosis, Echinococcosis and rabies. At the European level excellent scientific cooperation across professional boundaries has been undertaken through the Med-Vet-Net collaboration (Belcher and Newell 2005).

New approaches to prediction and control

The growth of human population and the demand for animal protein is rising relentlessly. Zoonoses are therefore going to continue to be major threats to sustainable development. Recent developments in prediction of emerging events may play a significant part in the future for mitigating the consequences of emergence and re-emergence of zoonoses (Rogers and Randolph 2003). Techniques in Health Impact Assessment of policies are now well developed. An example of its application is the assessment of the Three Gorges Dam across the Yangtze River which predicted significant ecological impact on the future transmission and control of schistosomiasis (Li *et al.* 2007). New approaches to mathematical modelling of zoonotic dynamics will play an increasingly prominent role (Lloyd-Smith *et al.* 2009). A particularly exciting development is the use of satellite data to better understand the ecology of zoonotic disease and also predict the changes in epidemiology as a result of climate change. For example, understanding the link between El Nino/ Southern Oscillation climate anomalies and Rift Valley fever in East Africa consequent upon elevated rainfall led to successful prediction of an outbreak in 2006/7. The predictions provided a 2 to 6 week period of warning for the Horn of Africa during which time resources could be mobilized to contain the epidemic (Anyamba *et al.* 2008). Another example is the use of satellite data to understand the local conditions that allow tick borne encephalitis transmission and the use of climate change predictions to anticipate the moving pattern of TBE (Randolph 2010).

But even better surveillance and prediction will not in themselves lead to control of zoonoses. Hard choices will need to be faced since control will involve the restriction on trade and movement of animals and products and sometimes of people. Controls need to be exerted on the legal and illegal trade in wildlife and products such as bush meat and the exotic pet trade. In one study in the USA of mammals imported from 2000–2005, 246,772 mammals in 190 genera were recorded with clear potential to import numerous zoonoses (Parlin *et al.* 2009). The growth of global markets needs to take into account the encroachment into ecosystems that harbour zoonotic agents consequent upon the economic pressure to expand agriculture for international consumption. Even in developed economies the risks of endemic zoonoses cannot be ignored. For example, recent outbreaks of E. coli 0157 and cryptosporidium in children visiting petting farms and agricultural shows has focussed attention on the difficult balance to be struck between the clear benefits of increasing exposure of children to animals and the risk of zoonotic infections (NASPHV 2009).

References

Advisory Committee on the Microbiological Safety of Food (2001). Second Report on Salmonella in Eggs. London: The Stationery Office.

Anyamba, A., Chretien, J. P., Small, J., Tucker, C. J., Formenty, P. B., *et al.* (2009). Prediction of Rift Valley Fever Outbreak. *Proceedings of the National Academy of Sciences USA,* **106**(3): 955–59.

Belcher, T., and Newell, D.G. (2005). Crossing the Boundaries. *Vet. Rec.,* **157**(22): 682–84.

Bell, J. C., and Palmer, S. R. (1983). Control of Zoonoses in Britain: past, present and future. *BMJ,* **287**: 591–93.

Buishi, I., Walters, T., Guildea, Z., Craig, P., and Palmer, S. (2005). Reemergence of canine Echinococcus granulosus infection, Wales. *Emerg. Infect. Dis.,* **11**(4): 568–71.

Cleri, D. J., Ricketti, A. J., and Vernaleo, J. R. (2010). Severe acute respiratory syndrome (SARS). *Infect. Dis. Clin. North Am.,* **24**(1): 175–202.

Cutler, S. J., Fooks, A. R., and van der Poel, W. H. M. (2010). Public Health Threat of New, Reemerging, and Neglected Zoonoses in the Industrialized World. *Emerg. Infect. Dis.,* **16**(1): 1–7.

Dalton, H. R., Bendall, R., Ijaz, S., and Banks, M. (2008). Hepatitis E: an emerging infection in developed countries. *Lancet Infect. Dis.,* **8**(11): 698–709.

Department for Environment Food and Rural Affairs (2008). Zoonoses Report. www.defra.gov.uk.

Etter, E., Donado, P., Jori, F., Caron, A., Goutard, F., *et al.* (2006). Risk Analysis and Bovine Tuberculosis, a Re-emerging Zoonosis. *Ann. NY Acad. Sci.,* **1081**: 61–73.

Guernier, V., Hochberg, M. E., and Guegan, J. F. (2004). Ecology drives the worldwide distribution of human diseases. *PLoS Biol.,* **2**: 740–46.

Hahn, B. H., Shaw, G. M., De Cock, K. M., and Sharp, P. M. (2000). AIDS as a Zoonosis: Scientific and Public Health Implications. *Science,* **287**: 607–614.

House of Lords, Select Committee on Intergovernmental Organizations (2008). Diseases know no frontiers: How effective are intergovernmental organizations in controlling their spread? First Report of the Session 2007–2008. London, UK: The Stationery Office.

Jones, K. E., Patel, N. G., Levy, M. A., Storeygard, A., Balk, D., *et al.* (2008). Global Trends in Emerging Infectious Diseases. *Nature,* **451**: 990–93.

Krause, R. M. (1981). The Restless Tide: The Persistent Challenge of the Microbial World Washington DC: *National Foundation for Infectious Diseases.*

Keusch, G., Pappaioanou, M., Gonzalez, M. C., Scott, K. A., and Tsai, P. (2009). Sustaining Global Surveillance and Response to Emerging Zoonotic Disease. Washington DC: The National Academies Press. www.nap.edu/catalog/12625.htlm.

Lederberg, J., Shope, R. E., Oaks, S. C. (eds.) (1992). Emerging Infections, Microbial Threats to the Health in the United States. Committee on Emerging Microbial Threats to Health. Washington DC: National Academy Press.

Li, Y. S., Raso, G., Zhao, Z., He, Y., Ellis, M., *et al.* (2007). Large Water Management Projects and Schistosomiasis Control, Dongting Lake Region, China. *Emerg. Infect. Dis.,* **13**(7): 973–78.

Lloyd Smith, J. O., George, D., Pepin, K. M., Pitzer, V. E., Pulliam, J. R. C., *et al.* (2009). Epidemic Dynamics at the Human–Animal Interface. *Science,* **326**: 1362–67.

Marano, N., Arguin, P., Pappaioanou, M., Chomel, B., Schelling, E., *et al.* (2006). International Attention for Zoonotic Infections. *Emerg. Infect. Dis.* **12**(12): 1813–15.

Mattiuzzo, G., Scobie, L., and Takeuchi, Y. (2008). Strategies to enhance the safety profile of xenotransplantation: minimising the risk of viral zoonoses. *Curr. Opin. Organ Transplant.* **13**(2): 184–88.

Maudlin, I., Eisler, M. C., and Welburn, S. C. (2009). Neglected and endemic zoonoses. *Phil. Trans. R. Soc. Biol.* **364**: 2777–87.

Med-Vet-Net (2009). Building a European Community to Combat Zoonoses. www.medvetnet.org.

Meng, X. J. (2010). Hepatitis E virus: animal reservoirs and zoonotic risk. *Vet. Microbiol.* **140**(3–4): 256–65.

Morens, D. M., Folkers, G. K., and Fauci, A. S. (2004). The Challenge of Emerging and Re-emerging Infectious Diseases. *Nature* **430**: 242–49.

National Association of State Public Health Veterinarians (2009). Compendium of Measures to Prevent Disease Associated with Animals in Public Settings. *Morbid. Mortal. Wkly. Rep.* **58**: RR–5.

Palmer, S. R., Brown, D., and Morgan, D. (2005). Early qualitative risk assessment of the emerging zoonotic potential of animal diseases. *BMJ,* **331**(7527): 1256–60.

Pavlin, B. I., Schloegel, L. M., and Daszak, P. (2009). Risk of Importing Zoonotic Diseases through Wildlife Trade, United States. *Emerg. Infect. Dis.* **15**(11): 1721–26.

Payne, C. J. I., Petrovic, M., Roberts, R., Paul, A., Linnane, E., *et al.* (2003). Vero Cytotoxin-Producing *Escherichia coli* 0157 Gastroenteritis in Farm Visitors. *Emerg. Infect. Dis.,* **9**(5): 526–30.

Randoph, S. E. (2010). To what extent has climate change contributed to the recent epidemiology of tick borne diseases? *Vet. Parasitol.* **167**: 92–94.

Rangel, J. M., Sparling, P. H., Crowe, C., Griffin, P. M., and Swerdlow, D. L. (2005). Epidemiology of *Escherichia coli* 0157: H7 Outbreaks, United States, 1982–2002. *Emerg. Infect. Dis.* **11**(4): 603–609.

Rogers, D. J., and Randolph, S. E. (2003). Studying the global distribution of infectious diseases using GIS and RS. *Nature Rev. Microbiol.* **1**: 231–37.

Taylor, L. H., Latham, S. M., and Woolhouse, M. E. J. (2001). Risk factors for human disease emergence. *Phil. Trans. R. Soc. Lond. B. Biol. Sci.,* **356**: 983–89.

Van der Giessen, J. W. B., Isken, L. D., *et al.* (2004). Zoonoses in Europe: a risk to public health *RIVM, Microbiological Laboratory for Health*

Protection, Center for Infectious Disease Epidemiology. Netherlands Environmental Assessment Agency (RIVM) report number: 330200002/2004.

Van der Hoek, W., Dijkstra, F., Schimmer, B. *et al.* (2010). Q Fever in the Netherlands: An Update on the Epidemiology Measures. *Eurosurveillance* **15:** 12.

Wolfe, N. D., Dunavan, C. P., Diamond, J. (2007). Origins of Major Human Infectious Diseases. *Nature,* **447:** 279–83.

World Health Organization (2006). The control of neglected zoonotic disease: A route to poverty alleviation. www.who.int/zoonoses. ISBN: 92 4 159430 6.

World Health Organization (2004). Report of the WHO/FAO/OIE joint consultation on emerging zoonotic disease, 3–5 May 2004, Geneva, Switzerland: WHO.

CHAPTER 2

Deliberate release of zoonotic agents

Stephen Palmer

Summary

Since 9/11 2001, international attention has once again focused on the risks to human and animal health from the deliberate release of infectious or toxic chemical agents. In theory any agent could be used by terrorists and disaffected people, but the most serious risk for infectious agents are mainly zoonotic (Franz *et al.* 1997). Three modes of exposure may be anticipated, inhalation of powder or spray or dust from explosives, direct contact or inoculation from an explosion, and ingestion. Centers for Disease Control (CDC) list 19 bioterrorism agents or groups of agents of which 14 are zoonotic (http://emergency.cdc.gov/bioterrorism). In Category A are 6 agents which can be easily disseminated or transmitted from person to person, that result in high mortality rates and have the potential for major public health impact, which might cause public panic and social disruption and which require special action from public health preparedness. Of these 6, four are zoonoses—Anthrax, Plague, Tularaemia and Viral Haemorrhagic Fevers. In Category B, are 12 groups of agents, which are moderately easy to disseminate and cause moderate morbidity. Of these 12 groups, 8 contain zoonoses:

- Brucellosis,
- Food Safety threats (e.g. Salmonella, E.coli 0157, Campylobacter),
- Meliodiosis,
- Psittacoccosis,
- Q fever,
- Typhus,
- Viral encephalitis,
- Water safety threats (e.g. Cryptosporidium).

Biological warfare

In the twentieth century the main concern was biological warfare perpetrated by states. In the twenty-first century the concern is non-state deliberate release by disaffected groups. Leintenberg (2001) has published a comprehensive review of biological weapons in the twentieth century. In World War I, Germany targeted draft animals (horses and mules) with anthrax and glanders, but apparently without much effect. Following World War I several countries developed biological weapons, including France, USSR, UK, USA, Japan, Germany, Italy, Hungary and Canada. It is reported that only Japan actually used biological weapons, in China in the 1930s, and these included plague, typhoid, cholera and anthrax. The Japanese allegedly experimented with biological agents on at least 3,000 prisoners of war. The USA-UK-Canadian BW programme in which anthrax featured heavily was cancelled before the end of the war. However the USA did manage to develop small particle size aerosol dissemination of wet or dry precipitations of pathogens. Effective delivery of an aerosol requires particle sizes of 1–10 micros in order to reach alveoli.

Following the Second World War, the USSR/Russia, USA, Iraq, UK and South Africa appear to have continued biological weapons programmes. The USA programme up to 1969 produced weaponized Anthrax, Tularaemia, Borreliosis, Q fever, Yellow fever, and Venezuelan Equine Encephalitis. The USSR programme was the most extensive and included weaponization of Tularaemia, Anthrax, Brucellosis, Marburg, Smallpox, Plague, Anthrax and Venezuelan Equine Encephalitis and included research on Ebola, Bolivian and Argentinian Haemorrhagic Fever, Lassa Fever, Japanese and Russian Spring-Summer Encephalitis. In 1979 an epidemic of anthrax affected people and animals in a narrow 4 km zone downwind of a USSR military bio-weapons facility at Sverdlovsk. 77 cases were identified with certainty and 66 died. The weight of spores released as an aerosol appear to have been less than a gram (Henderson 1998).

In 1992 the United Nations (UN) set up the Biological and Toxic Weapons Convention but several countries mainly in the Middle East and South East Asia are believed to have still sought to acquire biological weapons. Stockpiles of agents will exist in many laboratories throughout the world and more recent concern has focused on the role of states that might sponsor terrorism.

Non-state groups

Databases have been compiled of non-state groups using or threatening to use biological weapons, and Leitenberg summarizes these as containing nearly 1,000 events, although real events were extremely rare.

The potential destructive power of infectious agents is clear. The World Health Organization (WHO) has estimated that a release of 50 kg of anthrax in a population of 5 million people could produce

100,000 deaths, of plague 36,000 deaths, and of tularaemia 19,000 deaths. Preparedness for such eventualities is challenging. Two scenarios are usually considered—an overt release which will initially be difficult to distinguish from hoaxes and false alarms, and covert release which will only become manifest once health care staff make the diagnosis. The delay in recognition is a major impediment to effective control, and therefore attention has focussed on developing surveillance systems that collect data on syndromes rather than just confirmed diagnosis. The WHO Global Outbreak Alert and Response Network links more than 70 separate information and diagnostic networks around the world. An important aspect of this system is the use of informal sources to both alert and verify information. Rumours of outbreaks and scanned and early warning of for example Ebola in Uganda in 2009, and yellow fever in West Africa in 2010 were picked up early. The GLEWS for animal disease and zoonoses is a complementary surveillance and early warning network. Ryan (2008) has argued for the use of animal disease as an early warning of bioterrorism attack and integration of veterinary and human health surveillance, a constant theme of this book.

Complacency is discouraged by the fact that there have been notable episodes of malicious release of zoonotic agents. The Aum Shinrikyo Group in Japan who released Sarin in Tokoyo in 1995 also attempted but failed to produce Botulism toxin and anthrax. However, a more successful venture was perpetrated in October 2001 in the USA when letters carrying anthrax spores and mailed through the USA postal system caused 18 cases of anthrax over 8 weeks. The public health response monitored by the USA was unprecedented. Chemoprophylaxis was given to 32,000 potentially exposed people, and those considered at higher risk were on 60 day courses. 120,000 environmental and chemical samples were processed during the acute phase.

International contamination of food was perpetuated by members of a religious cult in the USA in September 1984. *Salmonella typhimurium* was sprinkled on salad bars and 751 people developed illness (Tovok *et al.* 1997). Sobel, Khan and Sverdlow (2002) identify episodes of deliberate contamination of food by *Shigella dysentiae* and *Ascaris Suis* which caused severe pulmonary disease. Clearly all food supplies are vulnerable, as is proven by the frequent accidental contamination incidents of 'normal' food-borne diseases. Detection of a covert attack would be challenging since outbreaks are common. In the Dallas, Oregon, Salmonella Outbreak it was the size and nature of the outbreak that led to an crucial investigation in which a vial of the outbreak strain of salmonella was discovered in the cult's laboratory. The restaurants affected by the same strain of salmonella did not have common food suppliers and epidemiologic analyses of food consumption revealed multiple food vehicles.

Dembek *et al.* (2006) suggest eleven clues to detecting an unnatural outbreak:

i. A highly unusual event with large numbers of casualties, especially when there is no plausible natural explanation.

ii. Higher morbidity or mortality than is expected. This may suggest altered pathogenicity or a higher inoculum than is normal.

iii. Uncommon disease. The most serious agents are mainly extremely rare diseases in developed economies.

Table 2.1 Potential agents of bioterrorism: US Centres for Disease Control (Agents highlighted in bold are zoonoses)

Category A
Anthrax (*Bacillus anthracis*)
Botulism (*Clostridium botulinum* toxin)
Plague (*Yersinia pestis*)
Smallpox (Virola Major)
Tularemia (*Francisella tularensis*)
Viral hemorrhagic fevers (filoviruses [e.g. Ebola, Marburg] and arenaviruses [e.g. Lassa, Machupo])
Category B
Brucellosis (*Brucella* species)
Epsilon toxin of *Clostiridum perfringens*
Food safety threats (e.g. *Salmonella* species, *Escherichia coli* O157:H7, *Shigella*)
Glanders (*Burkholderia mallei*)
Melioidosis (*Burkholderia pseudomallei*)
Psittacosis (*Chlamydia psittaci*)
Q fever (*Coxiella burnetii*)
Ricin toxin from *Ricinus communis* (castor beans)
Staphylococcal enterotoxin B
Typhus fever (*Rickettsia prowazekii*)
Viral encephalitis (alphaviruses [e.g. Venezuelan equine encephalitis, eastern equine encephalitis, western equine encephalitis])
Water safety threats (e.g. *Vibrio cholerae*, *Cryptosporidium parvum*)
Category C
Emerging Infectious Diseases such as Nipah virus and hantavirus.
HPA list
Biological agents
The organisms which are most likely to be used as biological threat agents can be grouped as Category A or B.
Category A Diseases/Agents
◆ Are easily disseminated or transmitted from person-to-person
◆ Have high mortality rates and potential for major public health impact
◆ Might cause public panic and social disruption
◆ Require special action for public health preparedness
Diseases in this category include:
◆ Anthrax
◆ Smallpox
◆ Botulism
◆ Plague
◆ Tularemia
◆ Viral Haemorrhagic Fevers
Category B Diseases/Agents
◆ Are moderately easy to disseminate
◆ Have moderate morbidity rates and low mortality rates
◆ Require enhancement of both diagnostic capacity and disease surveillance

(Continued)

Table 2.1 (Cont'd) Potential agents of bioterrorism: US Centres for Disease Control (Highlighted agents are zoonoses)

Diseases in this category include:
◆ Glanders
◆ Melioidosis
◆ Brucellosis
◆ Q fever
◆ Psittacosis

Links to further information for some of these agents can be found on the disease specific guidance pages.

See also: biological releases page and Cardinal Signs and Tips (PDF, 140 KB). Unusual Illness, including Deliberate or Accidental Releases: Cardinal Signs and Tips for key Biological Agents v1.0 Oct 2007.

iv.   Point-source outbreak. A single release will be manifest as a cluster of cases with onset within one incubation period of the release.

v.   Multiple epidemics. This would be the result of multiple discrete releases or multiple organisms of different incubation period released at the same time.

vi.   Lower attack rates in protected individuals. This applies to military populations where some are wearing protective equipment or are in protected buildings.

vii. Dead animals. Animals dying in local areas, as occurred in the West Nile Virus encephalitis outbreak in 1999 in New York, may be a sentinel for deliberate release.

viii. Reverse spread. Human disease that precedes animal disease or occurs simultaneously with animal disease may suggest unnatural spread.

ix.   Unusual disease manifestation. Inhalation anthrax, for example, is very unusual and suggested an unusual source.

x.   Downwind plume pattern. Malicious release to create maximum impact may utilize the airborne route.

xi.   Direct evidence. This would include unusual vectors such as letters or spray devices.

In addition to these clues, Dembek *et al.* (2007) draw attention to Grunow and Finke's (2002) procedure for differentiating between the unnatural release of agents and natural outbreaks.

Effective to deliberate release will require effective response routine diagnostic and surveillance systems, capacity for rapid and expert field epidemiological investigation and good public health communication systems. It is generally recognized that the best way to deal with deliberate release is to use well tried and tested public health systems that are applied to naturally occurring infectious diseases. For some infections, stockpiles of antibiotics/antitoxins and vaccines are appropriate. However, it is clear that most public health systems, especially in conflict areas, are under resourced and could not reasonably be expected to cope with early detection of deliberate release. The field epidemiological skills required to investigate and interpret findings with the precision required in applying Grunow and Finke's (2002) procedure would challenge even the best public health units. Continued investment in 'One Health' surveillance and field investigation should be a priority for all countries.

References

Dembek, Z. F., Kortepeter, M. G., and Pavlin, J. A. (2007). Discernment between deliberate and natural infectious disease outbreaks. *Epidemiol. Infect.*, 135: 353–71.

Grunow, R., and Finke, E. J. (2002). A procedure for differentiating between the international release of biological warfare agents and natural outbreaks of disease: its use in analysing the tularaemia outbreak in Kosovo in 1999 and 2000. *Clin. Microbiol. Infect.*, 8: 510–21.

Franz, D. R., Jahrling, P. B., Friedlander, A. M., McClain, D. J., Hoover, D. L., *et al.* (1997). Clinical recognition and management of patients exposed to biological warfare agents. *JAMA*, 278: 399–411.

Henderson, D. A. (1998). Bioterrorism as a Public Health Threat. *Emerg. Infect. Dis.*, 4: 488–92.

Leitenberg, M. (2001). Biological Weapons in the Twentieth Century: A Review and Analysis. *Crit. Rev. Microbiol.*, 27(4): 267–320.

Ryan, C. P. (2008). Zoonoses Likely to be used in Bioterrorism. *Pub. Heal. Rep.*, 123: 276–81.

Sobel, J., Khan, A. S., and Swerdlow, D. L. (2002). Threat of a biological terrorist attack on the US food supply: the CDC perspective. *Lancet*, 359: 874–80.

Torok, T., Tauxe, R. V., Wise, R. P., *et al.* (1997). A large community outbreak of Salmonellosis caused by international contamination of restaurant salad bars. *JAMA*, 278: 389–95.

CHAPTER 3

Veterinary and human health surveillance and risk analysis of zoonoses in the UK and Europe

Dilys Morgan, Ruth Lysons and Hilary Kirkbride

Summary

Surveillance (derived from the French word *surveiller,* meaning *to watch over*) is the 'ongoing scrutiny, generally using methods distinguished by their practicability, uniformity, and frequently their rapidity, rather than by complete accuracy. Its main purpose is to detect changes in trend or distribution in order to initiate investigative, (preventive) or control measures' (Last 1988). Understanding the burden and detecting changes in the incidence of human and animal infections utilizes a number of surveillance mechanisms, which rely on voluntary and/or statutory reporting systems. These include international as well as national surveillance schemes for outbreaks of infectious disease and laboratory-confirmed infections, enhanced surveillance schemes for specific zoonoses and notification of specified infectious diseases.

Purpose of disease surveillance

Surveillance comprises a number of steps including data collection, analysis, interpretation and dissemination of information in order to inform appropriate action. It involves the assessment of disease occurrence in the context of the 'at risk' human or animal population. It is not an end in itself, but a tool to guide decision-making.

Measuring the burden of endemic diseases

One of the principle uses of surveillance data is to monitor trends in incidence. For example surveillance in humans shows a gradual increase in laboratory confirmed cases of Lyme borreliosis in the UK since the mid 1990s, thought to be due to a combination of increased awareness, changes in leisure pursuits, expansion of deer habitat and environmental conditions. Surveillance data may also demonstrate geographical and seasonal variations in diseases such as the peak in laboratory confirmed reports of verocytotoxin-producing *Escherichia coli* 0157 (VTEC) in humans during late summer and early autumn (Department for the Environment, Food and Rural Affairs, a).

Monitoring of trends may lead to a better understanding of the burden of zoonoses. Even non-statutory endemic diseases of animals (i.e. those that are not required to be notified by law) can have implications for the cost and environmental impact of livestock production, for occupational health of farm workers and others, or may pose food safety concerns. Therefore an understanding of the endemic disease burden is an important factor for farmers in achieving safe and efficient farm businesses. Most of these diseases are asymptomatic in animals but are monitored for public health purposes. For example, a UK baseline survey of Q fever seroprevalence was carried out in sheep and goats in 2010 to inform the assessment of the likely benefit from possible interventions in animals, in the light of a large outbreak of human disease associated with goats in the Netherlands in 2009.

Detection of outbreaks and incidents

Surveillance may allow early detection and characterization of outbreaks and incidents, especially those with cases occurring over a wider geographical area. Local outbreaks are usually detected by alert veterinarians or health care professions recognizing an unusual pattern or links between individual cases. Exceedance scores can be used to calculate whether excess reporting is above the expected baseline level and are flagged as a possible outbreak (Farrington *et al.* 1996). An example of this is shown in Fig. 3.1 which demonstrates the detection of a national outbreak of Salmonella Agona associated with meat products from the Republic of Ireland in June 2008 (O'Flanagan *et al.* 2008).

The detection of zoonotic disease incidents in farm animals tends to be at the flock or herd level, since there are likely to be far stronger epidemiological links between animals in the same flock or herd, than with other animals in the locality. This is due to the constraints on individual animal movements which result from conventional farming practices where biosecurity and prevention of introduction of infectious disease into a farm is very important in assuring animal health and welfare. That said, for organisms such as Campylobacter or VTEC, animals may be carriers, but rarely, if ever, display signs of illness. In this situation, the animal infection would most often be detected through targeted surveillance in animals for the organism concerned, or, through identification of an epidemiological association with animals during the investigation of an outbreak of human illness. Scanning surveillance can more readily identify patterns of zoonotic disease where there are signs of illness. For example, in sheep, which are seasonal breeders, *Chlamydophila abortus* and *Toxoplasma gondii* are most commonly diagnosed during the winter and early spring, and are the first and

SALMONELLA AGONA
Week no. 2008 24

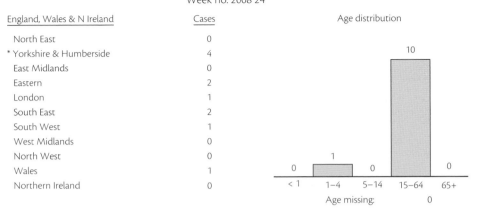

England, Wales & N Ireland	Cases
North East	0
* Yorkshire & Humberside	4
East Midlands	0
Eastern	2
London	1
South East	2
South West	1
West Midlands	0
North West	0
Wales	1
Northern Ireland	0

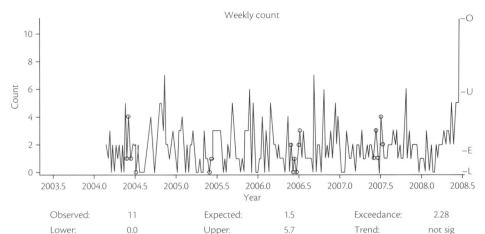

Fig. 3.1 Exceedance score for *Salmonella Agona*

Observed:	11	Expected:	1.5	Exceedance:	2.28
Lower:	0.0	Upper:	5.7	Trend:	not sig

second most commonly diagnosed cause of ovine abortion in Great Britain (Veterinary Laboratories Agency (VLA)).

Characterization of isolates identifies outbreak strains and allows the recognition of linked cases and often the source of infection. This was demonstrated when, in August 2009, a marked upsurge in the number of non-travel human isolates of *Salmonella Enteritidis* phage type (PT) 14b was noted in England and Wales. The increase was dominated by one antibiotic resistance profile that showed resistance to naladixic acid and low-level resistance to ciprofloxacin (NxCpl). Between 1 September and 31 December 2009, 489 cases of *S. Enteritidis* 14b NxCpl were identified in England and Wales, including 16 discrete outbreaks of infection. Investigations found that infection was associated with the consumption of eggs sourced from an establishment in Spain (Health Protection Agency (HPA 2009 & 2010)).

Detection of newly emerging disease, infection or toxicity

In the early 1970s, many scientists considered that the major threat from infectious diseases had been overcome, through technical advances such as vaccines and antimicrobial medicines. This was exemplified by the opinion 'The most likely forecast about the future of infectious disease is that it will be very dull. There may be some wholly unexpected emergence of a new and dangerous infectious disease, but nothing of the sort has marked the past fifty years' (Burnet and White 1972). Unfortunately, this prediction has proved incorrect and new diseases have continued to emerge. Since 1980 new pathogen species have been discovered at an average of over 3 per year (Woolhouse and Gaunt 2007). Furthermore, 73% of emerging pathogens are known to be zoonotic (Taylor *et al.* 2001).

In Great Britain, the VLA's Scanning Surveillance system raised 160 alerts of possible new animal disease between 2005 and 2008, which on further investigation led to the identification of 26 emerging (or re-emerging) animal diseases or syndromes over this period (Table 3.1).

In humans, most established surveillance systems are designed to detect known diseases and therefore these are unlikely to detect newly emerging infections. Syndromic surveillance systems including the Royal College of General Practitioners Weekly Returns Service (http://www.rcgp.org.uk/clinical_and_research/rsc.aspx) and NHS Direct (Baker *et al.* 2003) are used in primary care to detect increases in common presentations such as influenza like illness and other respiratory conditions. Surveillance of emerging infections is undertaken through horizon scanning or event-based surveillance, a system designed to detect incidents of potential public health significance including emerging infections via systematic review of informal and formal reports. Events are then verified, assessed and investigated as necessary (Kaiser *et al.* 2006).

Table 3.1 New and re-emerging diseases/syndromes identified through scanning surveillance and referred to HAIRS, 2006–2009

Cattle	Sheep & Goats	Pigs	Poultry	Other Species
	Infectious venereal disease (? Herpes virus) 2006	CNF *E. coli* 2006	Hepatitis E in poultry 2007	Respiratory disease in rooks 2007
Neurological illness in cattle and sheep 2006		Congenital tremor 'Dancing pigs' 2007	Avian Influenza H7N2 2007	Tuberculosis in a dog (M. Avium) 2007
Fasciolosis in calves 2007	'Kangaroo gait' in sheep 2008	Cryptosporidiosis 2007	Intestinal spirochaetosis in layers 2008	Brucella in marine mammals 2008
Bovine Influenza A 2007	Bovine TB in goats 2008	Neurological disease (porcine enterovirus-8) 2008		Ljungan virus (equivocal diagnosis in fox) 2008
Toxocara vitulorum in cattle and bison 2007		Streptococcus suis (unusual serotypes) pigs & cattle 2009		Trichomonosis in garden birds 2008
Paramphistomum (Rumen fluke) in cattle and reindeer 2008				Mycobacterial infection in cats 2008
Virulent Psoroptic mange in cattle 2008				Polioencephalomyelitis (foxes) 2008
Bleeding calf syndrome 2009				Vibrio cholera (swans) 2009

Source: A Review of the Implementation of the Veterinary Surveillance Strategy, March 2010, Defra. www.defra.gov.uk/foodfarm/farmanimal/diseases/vetsurveillance/strategy/index.htm

Early detection of an inherently new disease offers particular challenges, as diagnostic tests will often not be available at the time of first suspicion of disease. In most cases, a new disease event is a self-limiting, sporadic event, confined to a single species, but occasionally such conditions can have far wider adverse implications, spanning human and animal health and well-being, food safety, food supply, the rural economy, and triggering international movement or trade restrictions. An example is the emergence of Bovine Spongiform Encephalopathy (BSE) in England in 1986, as a serious neurological disorder of cattle, which led to a major statutory control programme and caused the imposition of substantial livestock trade restrictions. In 1996 BSE was implicated as the cause of a severe new variant Creutzfeldt-Jakob Disease (vCJD) in people. Although subsequently the disease occurrence was relatively rare, at the time the impact was unknown and considerable numbers of cases were predicted (Ghani *et al.* 2000).

Surveillance to enable early identification and characterization of potential new disease threats is therefore vital to facilitate timely risk assessment and appropriate interventions.

Monitoring prevention and control measures

Endemic diseases may be subject to statutory controls. For example within the European Union (EU), legislation has been put in place to ensure the harmonised monitoring and control of salmonella (Directive 2003/99/EC and Regulation (EC) No 2160/2003). This legislation sets out a framework for the reduction and control of salmonella in specific farming sectors through various defined measures. These include the implementation of species-specific National Control Programmes (NCPs) in all EU member states, to manage the risk principally at the level of primary production (the farm) and monitor the progress towards achieving an agreed flock prevalence reduction target. The overall aim of this EU legislation is to reduce the level of salmonella infection of public health significance at the farm level in the EU and in turn reduce the level of human infection caused by salmonella across the EU. This requirement applies in all member states and in the specified livestock sectors in third countries that export to the EU. To date, NCPs are now in place for breeding, laying and meat-producing flocks of domestic fowl (Defra b, c) The programmes include ongoing surveillance which is an essential component to measure the effectiveness of the control measures. The impact of controls in livestock can also be monitored through surveillance of salmonellosis in humans, although this is dependent on sufficient attribution of source of infection to human cases, and there may be a notable time lag before a reduction in human disease is observed.

Informing policy

Surveillance of vCJD has identified four cases associated with blood transfusion, three of whom developed symptoms of vCJD (Turner and Ludlam 2009). All four cases had received transfusions of non-leucodepleted red blood cells between 1996 and 1999 and the donors subsequently developed vCJD 17 months to 3.5 years after donation. The first case of vCJD associated with blood transfusion was identified in December 2003 and the second case was identified a few months later in a recipient of red cells. The same donor donated the vCJD-implicated blood transfused to the third and fourth cases. In March 2004 the Department of Health announced that people who had received a blood transfusion in the UK since 1980 would no longer be able to give blood. This change was implemented on 5 April 2004 (HPA a).

The *S. Enteritidis* epidemic in England and Wales began in the early 1980s, and in the mid 1980s *S. Enteritidis* PT4 emerged and rapidly became the most prevalent salmonella strain in humans. Subsequent epidemiological studies confirmed an association with the consumption of hens eggs. Early control measures such as health education and compulsory slaughter of infected flocks had little impact on the numbers of cases of infection, which reached a peak in 1997. It was only after the introduction of vaccination for broiler breeder flocks and commercial laying flocks in the mid 1990s (Advisory Committee on the Microbiological Safety of Food 2001), improved bio-security in layer grandparent birds (Ward *et al.* 2000) and the adoption of industry-led health schemes such as the Lion Brand that the incidence of human disease dropped dramatically (HPA b).

Providing assurance of freedom from specified diseases in animals

The international movement of animals and animal products is beneficial to global economic development and assurance of food supplies. However, it carries the risk of unwanted spread of disease. To strike a balance between these issues many countries, including all EU member states, are signatories to an international framework drawn-up by the World Trade Organization (WTO) on the Application of Sanitary and Phytosanitary (SPS) Measures. Details of the SPS agreement can be found at www.wto.org. The agreement seeks to liberalise trade in animals and their products by requiring its signatories to define their import policies based on risk posed to human or animal health by livestock or their products from the exporting country, and to avoid protectionist measures. For such risk assessments to be meaningful, they require robust evidence from disease surveillance.

Ongoing disease surveillance in livestock provides the evidence to confirm national or regional freedom from specified animal diseases. This has important consequences in relation to official certification of health status of animals (or animal products), prior to export, and in negotiating the animal health requirements for international trade. Such surveillance also enables the disease reporting obligations of EU and World Organization for Animal Health (OIE) member countries to be met.

Detection of incursion of a disease which is not usually present

Surveillance is also crucial for early identification of known diseases that are not normally present in a country or region. For some designated animal diseases there is a defined policy to contain and eradicate them, should an incursion occur. An example is highly pathogenic Avian Influenza which causes severe disease and high mortality in susceptible birds. Although this strain does not readily transmit to people, it has infrequently been associated with severe human illness in people in close contact with live infected poultry. The virus was first detected in Asia in 1997 and spread globally, reaching Europe in 2006, probably through the migration of infected wild waterfowl. In 2007, it was confirmed in wild birds in four member states (Germany, Czech Republic, France and Poland) and in domestic poultry in six member states (Hungary, UK, Czech Republic, Germany, Romania and Poland) and Turkey (OIE 2008). In 2008 H5N1 activity in Europe was very low. A series of positive wild birds were associated with a single cluster of infection in Dorset. The UK has maintained a high vigilance for avian influenza in recent years with targeted and scanning surveillance of wild birds and poultry, as well as mandatory reporting of suspicion of the disease in birds. All incursions of this disease have been promptly detected in the UK and speedily 'stamped out' through a robust policy of movement controls, tracing epidemiological links, killing of infected flocks, cleansing of depopulated sites and structured surveillance to ensure no residual pockets of disease remained (Defra a).

Mechanisms for surveillance

There are a variety of mechanisms by which surveillance can be carried out, the choice of which depends on the objective of the surveillance, the urgency of the requirement, the degree of precision and accuracy needed, the available sources of information, and the extent of the resources available. Surveillance may be active in which special efforts are made to collect data and confirm the diagnosis, or passive i.e. reliant on routine sources of information.

In humans the main data sources used to estimate the burden of zoonotic infection in the population and monitor trends in incidence are:

- Statutory notifications systems for specified diseases (i.e. notification required by law).
- Statutory reporting of specified laboratory confirmed infections. This was introduced in Scotland, England and Wales (but not Northern Ireland) in 2010, to replace national voluntary reporting for laboratory-confirmed infections.
- National surveillance for general outbreaks of zoonotic illness, mainly gastrointestinal infections.
- Enhanced surveillance for specific zoonoses (e.g. Lyme disease, leptospirosis, vCJD), often coordinated through relevant national reference laboratories.
- Additional routine data sources may be used such as primary care physician records, hospital episode statistics and mortality records.

In addition local and regional surveillance systems may exist that provide more detailed local information.

For animals the main sources include:

- Statutory notifications systems.
- Statutory reporting of Salmonella and Brucella isolates.
- Surveillance of post-mortem conditions found in slaughterhouses by the Meat Hygiene Service.
- Voluntary reporting schemes for disease in different animal species.
- Scanning surveillance through VLA Regional Laboratories.

None of these gives a complete picture, and the data generated will have biases that need to be taken into account in analysis and interpretation.

Statutory notification and reporting of zoonotic diseases

A number of zoonotic infections are statutorily notifiable under national veterinary and/or human legislation and a summary of these is shown in Table 3.2. However, not all zoonotic diseases in animals and humans are notifiable, and some diseases are notifiable in humans but not animals, and vice versa. Statutory notification systems are well suited for syndromes with easily recognized clinical signs, particularly if there are high levels of awareness of the requirement. They enable rapid investigations and intervention, and allied legal powers underpin public health action. The statutory requirement can include age, sex, location, and, for animals, species which may enable population-based prevalence to be calculated, as well as temporal and spatial trends. They may provide useful comparison with other data sources and the legal obligation on clinicians should ensure completeness. However, under-reporting may occur if the reporting procedure is unclear or unduly time-consuming, if there is lack of awareness amongst clinicians, or if the consequences of making a report are a disincentive (for example, imposition of animal movement restrictions).

Animals

In the United Kingdom, there is an obligation for any animal keeper who suspects that their animal may have a notifiable disease (as listed in the Specified Diseases (Notification and Slaughter) Order 1992 and the Specified Diseases (Notification) Order 1996) to immediately notify the Animal Health Agency. Procedures for notification and control of specified diseases are outlined in the Animal Health Act 1981 (Amendment) regulations 2005, the Zoonoses

Order 1989 and the Specified Animal Pathogens (Amendment) (England) Order 2006, and the equivalent legislation for Wales, Scotland and Northern Ireland. Under the Zoonoses Order 1989 laboratories have a statutory requirement to report the isolation of Salmonella and Brucella from animals (referred to as reportable diseases). In addition, laboratory work with a number of designated animal pathogens (as specified in the Specified Animal Pathogens Order 2008) must be notified to the Health and Safety Executive. A single regulatory framework has recently been proposed to cover work with human and animal pathogens that currently fall under different regulations. This is expected to come into force in 2011. An important aspect of surveillance with respect to food-borne disease is carried out by the Meat Hygiene Service who collect and communicate post-mortem conditions found in slaughterhouses

Table 3.2 Notifiable[a,b] and reportable[c] zoonotic diseases and organisms in humans and animals in UK

Disease	Requirements for Humans			Requirements for Animals		
	Notifiable Diseases in England, Wales, Scotland and NI[a]	Notifiable causative agents in England, Wales and Scotland[b]	Reportable to HSE under RIDDOR	Notifiable[a] (to Animal Health)	Reportable[c]	Notifiable under SAPO[g]
Anthrax	√	√	√	√		√
Avian Influenza		√		√		√
Bovine spongiform encephalopathy				√		
Brucellosis	√ (Not NI)	√	√			
Brucella abortus, B. melitensis				√		√
Brucella ovis (contagious epididymitis, sheep)				√		√
Brucella suis (pigs) and all other *Brucella* species					√	√
Chlamydiosis • *Chlamydophila abortus* • *C. psittaci*	(√) [d]	√	√ √	e		
Clinical syndrome due E coli 0157/infectious bloody diarrhoea	√ (Not NI)	√				
Diphtheria (includes toxigenic *C. ulcerans*)	√	√				
Encephalitis (acute)	√ (not Scotland)					
Equine viral encephalomyelitis				√		√
Echinococcus multilocularis and *granulosus*		√ (Scotland only)				√
Equine morbillivirus (Hendra)						√
"Food poisoning" (all causes)	√ (not Scotland)	√				
Foot And Mouth Disease				√		√
Glanders and Farcy (*Burkholderia mallei*)		√ (not Scotland)		√		√
Hanta virus		√				
Leptospirosis	√ (NI only)	√	√			
Lyme disease			√			
Meningitis (acute)	√ (not Scotland)					
Newcastle disease and paramyxovirus infection				√		√

(Continued)

Table 3.2 (Cont'd) Notifiable[a,b] and reportable[c] zoonotic diseases and organisms in humans and animals in UK

Disease						
Plague (*Yersinia pestis*)	√	√				
Q fever (*Coxiella burnetii*)		√	√			
Rabies • Classical rabies virus (genotype 1) • Other rabies virus genotypes (e.g. European Bat Lyssavirus)	√	√	√	√		√
Rift valley Fever		√		√		√
Salmonella spp		√			√	
Streptococcus suis			√			
Trichinella spiralis		√ (Scotland only)				√
Toxoplasmosis		√ (Scotland only)				
Tuberculosis	√	√	√	√[f]		
Tularemia (*Francisella tularensis*)	√ (Scotland only)	√				
Vesicular Stomatitis				√		√
Viral haemorrhagic fevers (all)	√	√				
Viral hepatitis (acute)	√ (not Scotland)	√	√			
West Nile Fever	√ (Scotland only)	√		√		

a Notifiable diseases are those where there is a statutory requirement to report clinical cases of disease (both human and animal).

b Notifiable causative agents are those where there is a statutory requirement to report laboratory confirmed isolates of organisms. Humans only and does not apply in NI.

c Reportable diseases (in animals) are those where there is a statutory requirement to report laboratory confirmed isolation of organisms of the genera *Salmonella* and *Brucella* under the Zoonoses Order 1989. The report is to be made by the laboratory which isolated the organism from an animal derived sample.

d A local anomaly exists in Cambridgeshire where psittacosis is reportable to the local CCDC under a local bylaw.

e Legislative veterinary powers under The Psittacosis or Ornithosis Order 1953 (S.I. 1953 No. 38) give discretionary powers to serve notices to impose movement restrictions and require cleansing and disinfection of affected premises, and so Animal Health may be involved in the control of Psittacosis, even though it is not actually a notifiable disease in animals or birds.

f Under the Tuberculosis (England) Order 2007, the Tuberculosis (Wales) Order 2006, and the Tuberculosis (Scotland) Order 2007, there is a statutory requirement to notify the suspected presence of TB in the carcase of any bovine, deer, farmed or companion (pet) mammal to nearest Animal Health Divisional Veterinary Manager (DVM). Furthermore, identification of *M. bovis* in samples taken from any mammal (other than man) is also notifiable to Animal Health unless the organism was present in the sample as a result of an agreed research procedure. Notifying the suspicion of TB in a living domestic animal in the course of clinical examination, surgery, by radiography or in biopsy material is not mandatory (except for cattle or deer), but submission of clinical samples from such cases to VLA is encouraged.

g Under the Specified Animal Pathogens Order 1998 anyone with reasonable grounds for suspecting the presence of these specific zoonoses should notify a veterinary inspector forthwith, unless they are held under licence made under this legislation. This requirement only relates to avian influenza viruses and Newcastle Disease viruses which are either uncharacterised or have been found to be of higher pathogenicity (set out in the legislation), or for avian influenza type A viruses H5 or H7 subtypes with specified nucleotide sequences. *Echinococcus* and *Trichinella* are only notifiable under this Order.

to primary producers under the Meat Hygiene Regulations (EC) 852/2004, (EC) 853/2004, and (EC) 854/2004, which are implemented in the UK by The Food Hygiene (England) Regulations (2006) and equivalent legislation in Wales, Scotland and Northern Ireland. The Meat Hygiene Service also notifies suspect cases of notifiable disease found at abattoirs to Animal Health.

In EU member states, statutory surveillance is closely interrelated with regulation of animal movements into the EU and between member states. From 1 January 2005 it became compulsory for all member states to use the internet-based Trade Control and Expert System (TRACES), introduced by EU Decision 2004/292/EC, for export health certification for intra-community trade in live animals, germplasm (semen and embryos), poultry, hatching eggs and some animal products. When these commodities are exported from one member state to another, the veterinary authorities of that member state are required to enter the details of the movement into TRACES so that the member state of receipt is made aware of the movement. TRACES is also used for monitoring and conducting checks on such consignments, and to generate individually numbered Common Veterinary Entry Documents (CVED) which are used for imports from third countries into the EU. CVED is a

certificate required to be signed by Official Veterinary Surgeon (OVS) confirming that veterinary checks have been carried out on animal(s) and/or products of animal origin.

In addition, there is EU legislation in relation to surveillance for various named animal diseases. This includes important zoonoses such as Transmissible Spongiform Encephalopathies (TSE), Bovine tuberculosis (bTB), and Salmonellosis. EU member states are required to undertake active surveillance for TSEs in cattle, sheep and goats, as laid down in Commission Regulation 999/2001 (as amended), as well as completing a time-limited active surveillance programme for TSEs in wild and farmed red deer in accordance with Commission Decision 2007/182/EC. The requirements for routine testing of cattle for TB are set out in EU Directive 64/432/EEC, a trade directive covering health requirements for cattle and pigs.

EU Directive 2003/99/EC and Regulation (EC) 2160/2003 sets out a framework for the reduction and control of *Salmonella* in specific farm industry sectors, through various defined measures including the implementation of National Control Programmes in all EU member states, and in third countries which export to the EU. The objective is to reduce the level of human Salmonella infections across the EU, through achieving a reduction in prevalence at the farm level.

Human

In the UK, statutory reports of specified infections in humans are collated as Notifications of Infectious Disease. The primary purpose of the notification system is to identify possible cases and outbreaks and initiate appropriate action as soon as possible. Accuracy of diagnosis is secondary, and generally *clinical suspicion* is all that is required. If the diagnosis later proves incorrect, there is no requirement to denotify. Under the Public Health (Control of Disease) Act 1984 and Public Health (Infectious Diseases) Regulations 1988, clinically diagnosed cases of notifiable disease in humans should be reported by the responsible clinician to the proper officer of the local authority (this is usually the Consultant for Communicable Disease Control). In Northern Ireland the equivalent legislation is the Public Health Notifiable Disease Order (Northern Ireland (1989) and in Scotland the Public Health (Notification of infectious diseases) Scotland) Regulations 1988.

Amendments to the 1984 (Control of Disease) Act were made in 2010 in England, Wales and Scotland with improved powers available to both local authorities and justices of the peace, for the control of disease and the protection of public health. The Notification Regulations introduced significant amendments to the notification system with a revised list of notifiable diseases and, for the first time, diagnostic laboratories have a duty to notify specified causative agents. In addition the new legislation adopts an all hazards approach, and includes a requirement to notify cases of other infections or contamination which could present a significant risk to human health. The list of notifiable organisms contains many of the indigenous and exotic zoonoses, and includes time limits within which laboratory diagnoses and notifications must be made. However, the specified notifiable organism list varies slightly between Scotland, England and Wales. For more details of the lists of specified notifiable diseases and causative organisms see: Scotland http://www.legislation.gov.uk/asp/2008/5/contents; Wales http://www.legislation.gov.uk/wsi/2010/1546/contents/made; England http://www.legislation.gov.uk/uksi/2010/659/contents/made.

Under the Reporting of Injuries, Diseases and Dangerous Occurrences Regulations 1995 (RIDDOR) employers, the self-employed and those in control of premises must report specified workplace incidents, work-related deaths, major injuries or over-three-day injuries, work related diseases, and dangerous occurrences (near miss accidents) which arise 'out of or in connection with work'. The Regulations apply to Great Britain but not to Northern Ireland, where separate Regulations have been made, and are administered by the Health and Safety Executive (HSE). Reportable Diseases under Schedule 3 include infections listed in Table 3.3 plus 'Any infection reliably attributable to.... work with microorganisms; work with live or dead human beings in the course of providing any treatment or service or in conducting any investigation involving exposure to blood or body fluids; work with animals or any potentially infected material derived from any of the above' (http://www.hse.gov.uk/riddor/).

European statutory reporting

Directive 2003/99/EC of the European Parliament and of the Council (the Zoonoses Monitoring Directive 2003/99/EC) requires member states of the European Union (EU) to collect, evaluate and report data on zoonoses, zoonotic agents, antimicrobial resistance and food-borne outbreaks to the European Commission each year (Directive 2003/99/EC) (European Commission 2003). The data required covers both zoonoses that are important for public health in the whole European Community as well as zoonoses that are relevant on the basis of the national epidemiological situation (see Table 3.3). The member states have to send their national report on zoonoses to the Commission each year (European Food Standards Agency 2009). These reports are collated by the European Food Safety Authority (EFSA) and published in collaboration with the European Centre for Disease Prevention and Control (European Commission 2004) in the *Community Summary Report on Trends and Sources of Zoonoses and Zoonotic Agents and Food-borne Outbreaks in the European Union* (European Food Safety Authority).

The Directive also covers the mandatory epidemiological investigation and reporting of food-borne outbreaks in the member states. Thorough investigation of food-borne outbreaks aims to identify the pathogen, the food vehicle involved, and the factors in the food preparation and handling contributing to the outbreak. The Zoonoses Directive makes provisions for such investigations and for close co-operation between various authorities. The competent authority of each member state must provide the Commission with a minimum dataset and summary report of the results of the investigations of food-borne outbreaks, which is sent to the EFSA on an annual basis.

National surveillance centres receive preliminary reports of outbreaks of infectious disease from laboratories, health protection staff and local authority environmental health (Public Protection) departments. These are frequently of intestinal infections but can include other zoonotic agents. For the food-borne outbreaks, a minimum dataset on each outbreak is then collected from the appropriate health authority/board as required under the Zoonoses Directive 2003/99/EC. Surveillance of this kind provides information on specific risk factors associated with different pathogens and also trends in the importance of these factors.

In addition member states are required to report certain zoonotic diseases in humans to the European Centre for Disease Prevention and Control (ECDC). A list of these can be found in Table 3.4. These are published in the *ECDC Annual Epidemiological Report on Communicable Diseases in the European Union* (European Centre for Disease Prevention and Control).

Voluntary notification

Voluntary notification involves the co-ordinated capture and systematic reporting of disease events. This collaborative approach is particularly effective if the data providers are strongly motivated, and can be a highly cost-effective mechanism for data capture. However it is likely to suffer from lack of specificity of case details and from under-reporting, since the submission of information will be influenced by the motivation of the reporting clinician.

Animals

The UK Veterinary Surveillance Strategy (Defra 2003) set out five principles for effective surveillance, which would enable earlier warning and detection of animal-related threats, and faster better targeted control measures. Progress with implementation of the

Table 3.3 Mandatory reporting and reporting based on epidemiological situation in animals and humans (reportable to the European Food Safety Authority)

In accordance with the Zoonoses Directive 2003/99/EC, all Member States (MSs) have to report on the following zoonoses, zoonotic agents (Annex 1) and other subjects

- Brucellosis and agents thereof;
- Campylobacteriosis and agents thereof;
- Echinococcosis and agents thereof;
- Listeriosis and agents thereof;
- Salmonellosis and agents thereof;
- Trichinellosis and agents thereof;
- Tuberculosis due to *Mycobacterium bovis*;
- Verotoxigenic *Escherichia coli*;
- Antimicrobial resistance in *Salmonella* and *Campylobacter* isolates from poultry, pigs and cattle and foodstuffs derived from these species;
- Food-borne outbreaks;
- Susceptible animal populations.

Other zoonoses are to be included in the monitoring and reporting according to the epidemiological situation in each MS. This means that if a certain zoonoses is of public health importance in a MS, this MS should report on that zoonoses, but the other MSs do not have the same obligation to report on it, if it is of minor importance in their MSs.

The zoonoses to be reported based on the epidemiological situation are listed in Annex I to Directive 2003/99/EC:

Viral zoonoses:

- Calicivirus;
- Hepatitis A virus;
- Influenza virus;
- Rabies;
- Viruses transmitted by arthropods.

Bacterial zoonoses:

- Borreliosis and agents thereof;
- Botulism and agents thereof;
- Leptospirosis and agents thereof;
- Psittacosis and agents thereof;
- Tuberculosis other than in point A;
- Vibriosis and agents thereof;
- Yersiniosis and agents thereof.

Parasitic zoonoses:

- Anisakiasis and agents thereof;
- Cryptosporidiosis and agents thereof;
- Cysticercosis and agents thereof;
- Toxoplasmosis and agents thereof.

Other zoonoses and zoonotic agents

---

strategy was reviewed in 2007 (Lysons *et al.* 2007) and the strategy was revised in 2010. Under the first principle, collaboration, two examples of collaborative voluntary surveillance have been established, to enhance veterinary surveillance coverage of equine and small companion animal diseases.

The Equine Quarterly Surveillance report is co-ordinated by a charity, the Animal Health Trust (AHT) (http://www.aht.org.uk/), in conjunction with Defra, the British Equine Veterinary Association (BEVA) and a network of different laboratories and specialist equine practices. Each participant provides anonymized disease information that, since 2004, has been collated by the AHT into quarterly reports, available on the Defra, AHT and BEVA websites.

The newly created Small Animal Veterinary Surveillance Network, co-ordinated by the Liverpool University Veterinary School (http://www.liv.ac.uk/savsnet/The_Project/index.htm) aims to describe the disease status of the small companion animal population of the United Kingdom through collection of data from diagnostic laboratories and from veterinary practices with production of quarterly reports.

The National Animal Disease Information Service is a sentinel network of 60 veterinary practices and 6 veterinary colleges monitoring endemic diseases in cattle, sheep and pigs in the UK and reporting observations of interest to farmers and veterinarians, on a regional basis and via their website: http://www.nadis.org.uk.

Humans

Laboratory reports are an important source of data for those zoonoses that rely on laboratory confirmation for their diagnosis, and species, subspecies and subtypes of microbial pathogens are reported if appropriate. All laboratories are asked to report electronically any clinically significant infections and isolates as soon as these are identified. From 2010 all laboratories in England, Scotland and Wales are required to report the identification of specified causative agents as listed in their respective revised notification regulations. However, since not all zoonoses of public health significance are included, voluntary laboratory reporting will remain an important aspect of surveillance.

As with most infections, laboratory confirmed cases of zoonotic infections may only represent the 'tip of the disease iceberg' and account for only a small proportion of the true number of cases of infection that are occurring. This is because a series of steps must be undertaken for data to be recorded in a national surveillance database. An infected individual must be sufficiently concerned about their symptoms to consult a clinician, who then arranges for a specimen to be taken and referred to a microbiology laboratory, which must isolate or positively identify a pathogen, and either the laboratory or clinician then report the finding to the national surveillance centre. These factors lead to under-reporting, and sampling tends to be biased towards more clinically severe cases in high-risk groups. However, it does give a precise diagnosis and is useful for monitoring trends in the incidence of the infection and identifying outbreaks and incidents.

Structured surveys targeted at specific conditions

Targeted surveys can be useful for determining baseline prevalence of a condition. Provided comparable methodologies are used in subsequent surveys, this can be useful for measuring effectiveness of disease control policies. The disadvantages with this approach are that denominator data is needed, if the survey is to be made representative of the population being studied, and that it can be very costly to design and implement.

Animal

In farm animals, structured surveys are usually carried out either to provide evidence of freedom from a disease, to establish prevalence and/or to inform government policy. The annual UK survey of sheep and goats for Brucella melitensis is an example of the former. European Commission Decision 93/52 recognized the United Kingdom as free from Brucella melitensis, but required that to retain this status, testing must be carried out each year to demonstrate with 95% confidence that fewer than 0.2% of holdings are infected, or to test each year at least 5% of sheep and goats in the country over the age of six months. In contrast, the salmonella NCPs were founded on baseline prevalence surveys conducted by all EU member states, and against which target levels for each country were determined by the European Commission, advised by EFSA.

Human

The Infectious Intestinal Disease (IID) study was established following recommendations by the Committee on the Microbiological Safety of Food in 1989, with the aim of establishing the 'true incidence' of infectious intestinal disease in the community (Food Standards Agency 2000). The study took place between 1993 and 1996 and was the largest microbiological epidemiological and economic study of IID undertaken to date. Two methods were used to estimate the factor by which national surveillance data should be multiplied to describe the incidence of IID in the population and the number of cases presenting to GPs, the so-called reporting pyramid. In the first, a direct method, names of those cases for whom positive stools were obtained were reconciled with the national database and the degree of under-reporting calculated. In the second, an indirect method, the rates of IID estimated to occur in the whole population of England were compared with the rates appearing in national surveillance figures and the degree of under-reporting was calculated.

The former method estimated that for every 136 cases of IID in the community 23 presented to a GP, 6.2 had a stool sent routinely for microbiological examination, 1.4 had a positive result, and one was reported to the National Surveillance Centre. The indirect method estimated that there was a ratio of 88 cases in the community for every one reported to the national centre.

The proportion of different target organisms causing IID identified in the population and presenting to GPs varied, and these proportions were different again from those that were routinely identified in laboratories and reported to the national surveillance scheme. This reporting pyramid and 'multiplier' to estimate the true number of cases of specific intestinal infections from number of laboratory reports was calculated, and has been used for policy development and prioritizing interventions since then. The second Infectious Intestinal Disease (IID2) study is currently underway and will report in 2011.

The British Paediatric Surveillance Unit (BPSU) undertakes epidemiological surveillance and research into uncommon childhood infections and disorders. Previous studies include Haemolytic Uraemic Syndrome (HUS) (Lynn *et al.* 2005) and congenital toxoplasmosis (Ryan *et al.* 1995).

Surveillance systems specific to animals
Scanning surveillance through outbreak investigation in animals

Scanning surveillance involves surveillance of a sample of the population of interest, for the presence of diseases of concern. This is the primary approach used for detecting new and emerging infections in animals in the United Kingdom. Animal populations are monitored by the VLA and the Animal Health Agency for the appearance of notifiable or novel diseases or changing trends in existing diseases, including actual and potential zoonoses. The VLA undertakes scanning surveillance through the collection, collation and analysis of disease data, based on submissions to VLA Regional Laboratories, which are included in the Veterinary Investigation Diagnosis Analysis (VIDA) database. The reporting of Salmonella isolations from defined animal species, their environment and animal feeding stuffs is mandatory under the Zoonoses Order 1989. VLA is responsible for the laboratory testing, reporting, data management, analysis and investigation of Salmonella incidents in animals and receives reports of isolations from other veterinary laboratories.

Surveillance systems specific to humans
Enhanced surveillance systems

Enhanced surveillance, whereby patients with a specific infection are followed up, can be established either short-term or longer-term, nationally or locally, to provide information on aspects of a zoonoses such as risk factors and how these might change between different groups and over time.

For selected diseases including Leptospirosis and Lyme disease in England and Wales routinely collected data is supplemented with additional information as part of enhanced surveillance. Additional information collected for these includes travel and other potential risk factors. In Scotland, cases of HUS are reported to the National Surveillance Centre, who follow up for risk factors and outcome, irrespective of whether a verocytotoxin-producing *Escherichia coli* (VTEC) has been isolated (Health Protection Scotland).

Reporting and surveillance outputs for zoonoses

Surveillance information is only useful if it is reported promptly and effectively to those who can benefit from it. There are various approaches for reporting surveillance information, and the most appropriate will depend on the target audience, and the type of action or intervention they might take as a result.

Official data on human cases of zoonotic infections
National

Details and number of notifications of infectious disease, laboratory-confirmed infections, outbreak surveillance and other enhanced surveillance systems are reported by each of each of the national surveillance centres in England (HPA Centre for Infections www.hpa.org.uk), Wales (Public Health Wales http://www.publichealthwales.wales.nhs.uk, Scotland (Health Protection Scotland http://www.hps.scot.nhs.uk) and Northern Ireland (Public Health Agency Northern Ireland http://www.publichealth.hscni.net/).

International

As described above, ECDC collates reports on a wide range of infections, including food-borne and other zoonoses (Table 3.4) and these are published in their *Annual Epidemiological Report on Communicable Diseases in Europe*. Although ECDC has undertaken work on standardization of case definitions there are still variations in reporting practices reflecting different surveillance systems in member states (European Centre for Disease Prevention and Control).

Table 3.4 List of Zoonotic diseases in humans for European Union surveillance (reportable to the European Centre for Disease Prevention and Control)

Annex I of Commission Decision 2000/96/EC of 22 December 1999 on the communicable diseases to be progressively covered by the Community network under Decision No 2119/98/EC of the European Parliament and of the Council, as amended by Decisions 2003/534/EC, 2003/542/EC, 2007/875/EC and 2009/312/EC.
1. Communicable diseases and special health issues to be progressively covered by the community network as referred to in Article 1 [of Decision 2000/96/EC]
1.1 For the communicable diseases and special health issues listed in the Annex, epidemiological surveillance within the Community network is to be performed by the standardised collection and analysis of data in a way that is to be determined for each communicable disease and special health issue when specific surveillance networks are put in place.
Diseases
Food- and waterborne diseases and diseases of environmental origin
Anthrax
Botulism
Campylobacteriosis
Cryptosporidiosis
Giardiasis
Infection with Enterohaemorrhagic *E.coli*
Leptospirosis
Listeriosis
Salmonellosis
Shigellosis
Toxoplasmosis
Trichinosis
Yersinosis
Diseases transmitted by non-conventional agents
Transmissible spongiform encephalopathies, variant Creutzfeldt-Jakob's disease
Zoonoses (other than those listed in 2.4)
Brucellosis
Echinococcosis
Rabies
Q Fever
Tularaemia
Avian influenza in humans
West Nile virus infection

Official data on zoonoses and other diseases in animals

The RADAR veterinary surveillance information management system

Surveillance information is held by many individual databases. The Rapid Analysis and Detection of Animal-related Risks (RADAR) data warehouse, an initiative of the UK Government's Veterinary Surveillance Strategy, enables data to be extracted from different sources and transformed into a format that enables collation, analysis and report production. Figures 3.2 and 3.3 depict the RADAR technical architecture and a sample output.

The system currently receives regular 'downloads' of data from 15 different databases, which enables rapid production of many different kinds of reports, with the latest available source data, in a variety of formats (such as maps, charts and tables), and accompanied by a quality statement describing the completeness, age and biases which pertain to the underlying data. RADAR reports are primarily intended to assist UK Government policy makers by presenting evidence about animal-related disease and risk factors, in an accessible way, to enable effective decisions on disease control measures. Extracts of data are also available to the research community for purposes of veterinary surveillance and disease control in the UK. Due to the sensitive nature of some of the source data, the need for data security, and the need to regulate access in accordance with all relevant legislation, data users are required to comply with data confidentiality agreements and an overarching data sharing protocol. However, in many cases, data can usefully be reported in an anonymized way, and many of these RADAR reports are published at:

http://www.defra.gov.uk/foodfarm/farmanimal/diseases/vetsurveillance/reports/index.htm.

Veterinary Laboratories Agency and Scottish Agricultural College monthly and quarterly summaries

Information on trends in animal diseases (including zoonoses and new or emerging conditions) is published regularly. A monthly summary report for England and Wales is compiled from data gathered by the VLA, published by Defra (Defra d) at http://www.defra.gov.uk/vla/reports and an equivalent report is produced for Scotland by the Scottish Agricultural Colleges (SAC) Veterinary Services Division at http://www.sac.ac.uk/consulting/services/s-z/veterinary/publications/monthlyreports/. In Northern Ireland the Department of Agriculture and Rural Development, Northern Ireland (DARD NI) is the official source of information on zoonoses in animals.

Quarterly reports describing trends in the major endemic diseases are published by the VLA for poultry, cattle, miscellaneous captive exotic species (such as alpacas and llamas), pigs, sheep, goats and wildlife. There is also a quarterly report for non-statutory zoonoses, covering the main food-borne zoonoses (other than salmonella) and the miscellaneous environmental zoonoses.

Veterinary Investigation Diagnosis Analysis (VIDA)

The *VIDA Report* is published annually by the VLA. This is produced from data within the VIDA database (launched in 1975) which contains a record of every submission made for diagnostic purposes to the regional laboratory network of the VLA (in England and Wales) and of the SAC in Scotland. Diagnoses throughout this network are made using standardized 'case definitions' and recorded on VIDA. The VIDA report details the total number of

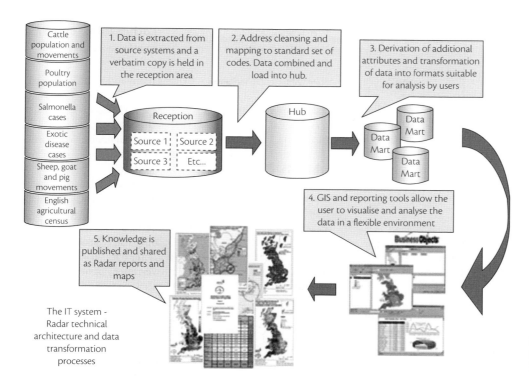

Fig. 3.2 Schematic illustration of the RADAR Surveillance Information Management System

diagnoses reached, and records those submissions where no diagnosis was reached.

There are inherent biases in VIDA data, which should be considered when interpreting individual figures or apparent disease trends. Total numbers of submissions recorded by VIDA represent only the material submitted for investigation to VLA Regional Laboratories and SAC Disease Surveillance Centres. This bias is influenced by many factors including, for example, the particular clinical presentation of a suspected disease, the level of awareness of a disease and its perceived importance, the value of the animal or animals affected, and the general economic climate. Particular diagnoses may be affected by improved scientific methods, and knowledge of this may also affect rates of submission; these factors will usually vary differentially with time. This bias should be considered when interpreting both individual figures, and apparent trends, from VIDA data.

Annual report on salmonella in livestock

The annual report on *Salmonella in Livestock Production in Great Britain* presents data on *Salmonella* reports from livestock species in Great Britain (England, Wales and Scotland) collected and collated by the Department for Environment, Food and Rural Affairs (Defra c) and available at http://www.defra.gov.uk/vla/reports/rep_salm_rep07.htm. It also provides data from previous years for comparative purposes. The report includes information on the reason and place of sampling, with separate sections on Salmonella isolates from each livestock species, from wildlife, livestock products and animal feeding stuffs. It also describes patterns of antimicrobial sensitivity of salmonella (England and Wales only).

International disease surveillance reports

International disease surveillance reports, preliminary assessments of animal disease outbreaks outside the UK, and qualitative risk assessments based on information from the veterinary administrations of UK trading partners, the EC, OIE, veterinary reference laboratories and overseas embassies, are published by Defra (Defra d) and available at: http://www.defra.gov.uk/food-farm/farmanimal/diseases/monitoring/index.htm.

The monthly surveillance reports and the Quarterly International Disease Surveillance reports are also published in the Veterinary Record (http://veterinaryrecord.bvapublications.com/).

Official reports and publications on zoonoses in animals and humans

The UK Zoonoses Report

The *Zoonoses Report: United Kingdom* is published by Defra annually and includes a summary of all zoonoses surveillance data, utilizing information from all agencies that are involved in monitoring zoonoses (Defra a). This comprehensive report is intended for professionals who deal with zoonotic disease but also seeks to give an insight into the burden and importance of zoonoses for the non-specialist. It provides an overview of both food-borne and non-food-borne zoonoses covering the more important ones in greater detail.

Trends and sources of specified zoonotic agents in animals, feeding stuffs, food and man in the UK

The annual report *Trends and sources of specified zoonotic agents in animals, feeding stuffs, food and man in the UK* is published by Defra (Defra d) and contains information which covers both zoonoses that are important for the public health in the whole EU, as well as zoonoses which are relevant on the basis of the national epidemiological situation as required by the Zoonoses Monitoring Directive 2003/99/EC. The reports contain information covering the occurrence of these diseases and agents in humans, animals, foodstuffs and in some cases also in feeding stuffs. In addition the report includes data on antimicrobial resistance in some zoonotic

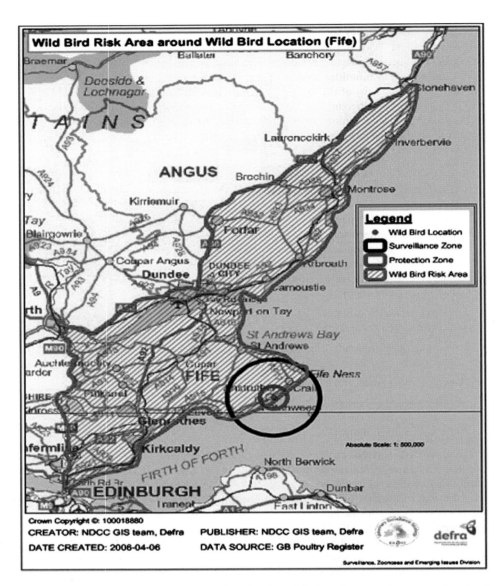

Fig. 3.3 Use of RADAR system: Control zones which were imposed following detection of Avian Influenza in a wild bird

agents and commensal bacteria as well as information on epidemiological investigations of food-borne outbreaks.

Community summary report on trends and sources of zoonoses and zoonotic agents in the European Union

Surveillance data from member states contributes to the annual *Community Summary Report on Trends and Sources of Zoonoses and Zoonotic Agents* in the European Union. In addition to the zoonoses of public health importance (Table 3.3), this includes data on a varying number of zoonoses and comprehensive datasets from most MS are included as annexes. This report is produced in collaboration with the ECDC, who are responsible for collation of data on human infections as outlined before (Table 3.4).

Risk analysis and communication for zoonoses

United Kingdom

The following groups collectively are responsible for the identification, assessment, management and communication of zoonotic risks.

They are the foci for formal liaison between human and animal health professionals, and consider other issues relating to zoonoses across the UK.

The UK Zoonoses, Animal Diseases and Infections (UKZADI) Group

The UK Zoonoses, Animal Diseases and Infections (UKZADI) Group is an independent committee made up of experts from across the agricultural and public health departments. The Group was formed by the amalgamation of the UK Zoonoses Group (UKZG) and the Surveillance Group on Diseases and Infections in Animals (SGDIA) in late 2008. The Group's role is to provide a strategic overview and means of ensuring overall co-ordination of public health action at the UK, national and local level with regard to existing and emerging zoonotic infections. The Group also advises as appropriate the Chief Medical Officers and Chief Veterinary Officers, government departments and key agencies for England, Wales, Scotland and Northern Ireland on important trends and observations which impact on animal and public health including where necessary preventative and remedial action may be required.

The Animal Disease Policy Group (ADPG)

The role of the ADPG is to provide disease control policy advice based on scientific evidence to UK Government Ministers and the Civil Contingencies Committee, and to ensure that policies across the four administrations of the United Kingdom are consistent, although they may be different. For zoonotic diseases, membership of the group comprises senior representatives from the four UK government administrations, Defra, Animal Health Agency, Cabinet Office, HPA and Department of Health (Defra e).

National expert panel on new and emerging infections

The Chief Medical Officer for England's Infectious Disease Strategy—'Getting Ahead of the Curve' (2002) proposed the establishment of a National Expert Panel to assess the threat from new and emerging infectious diseases. It was envisaged that this would be an over-arching horizon scanning panel, reporting to the Chief Medical Officer and advising the Department of Health. The Panel's terms of reference include identifying key areas for action and advising on priorities by:

- Identifying emerging and potential infectious threats to public health both nationally and internationally.

- Placing emerging infections in the wider clinical and public health contexts.

- Advising on prevention and control measures.

Since the majority of emerging infections are zoonoses, the Panel provides an overview of the threats posed by emerging zoonoses or new infections with zoonotic potential.

Human Animal Infections and Risk Surveillance Group

The Human Animal Infections and Risk Surveillance (HAIRS) Group was established in 2004, and is an HPA, Defra, VLA and Department of Health horizon scanning group chaired by the HPA. The Chair of the National Expert Panel on New and Emerging Infections (NEPNEI) and representatives from the Public Health Wales, Food Standards Agency, Animal Health Agency, Health Protection Scotland, the Scottish Government and Public Health Agency Northern Ireland are also members.

The HAIRS group meets monthly and acts as a forum to discuss and assess potential threats to UK public health. The group carries out horizon scanning for emerging and potentially zoonotic infections by systematic examination of formal and informal reports on infectious incidents in animal and human populations nationally and internationally. Potential hazards, such as new or unusual syndromes or infections in animals, or increases in endemic disease are brought to the group for discussion and assessment. The multidisciplinary nature of the HAIRS group enables objective and scientific assessment of potential threats, and the group to assess these reports in an objective and scientific manner.

The HAIRS group uses three different risk assessment procedures, depending on the nature of the incident under discussion and the extent of the information available. These are: Defra's triage profiles which are produced as part of their prioritization programme; assessment of the zoonotic potential of emerging animal diseases (Palmer *et al.* 2005) or the level of threat from emerging infections (Morgan *et al.* 2009). The group reports to the NEPNEI and UKZADI and in addition, members of the group communicate any finding back through their respective organizations (HPA c).

Regional zoonoses liaison groups

These are networks which operate in each of the countries of the UK variously comprising members of Health Protection Teams/ Local Health Boards, VLA, Animal Health Agency, Defra, Local Authorities and other partners. They meet to discuss local zoonotic issues, and to strengthen links, share expertise and contribute to the effective prevention and control of zoonotic infections through joined up working across their regions.

Cross departmental groups co-ordinated by the Food Standards Agency (FSA)

The FSA is an independent Government department set up by an Act of Parliament in 2000 to protect the public's health and consumer interests in relation to food. Most food-borne pathogens are zoonotic, and reducing the risks means close liaison with those responsible for animal and human health. The FSA co-ordinates three cross departmental groups on food-borne zoonoses. These are: the *Epidemiology of Foodborne Infections Group* (EFIG) which brings together UK surveillance data in humans and animals; the *Advisory Committee on the Microbiological Safety of Food* (ACMSF) and the *Advisory Committee on Animal Feeding stuffs* (ACAF) which assess the risk to humans of microorganisms which are used, or occur, in or on food or animal feeds, respectively, and advise the FSA on any matters relating to the microbiological safety of food.

International

The European Food Safety Authority (EFSA)

The EFSA was formally set up in January 2002, as an independent source of scientific advice and communication on risks associated with the food chain (http://www.efsa.europa.eu/). EFSA's main work is to assess and communicate on all risks associated with the food chain. Examples of this include an EU-wide baseline study on the prevalence of Salmonella in laying hen flocks, and the European summary report on zoonoses.

European Centre of Disease Prevention and Control (ECDC)

The ECDC is an EU agency established in 2005 to strengthen Europe's defences against infectious diseases (http://www.ecdc. europa.eu/). According to Regulation EC 851/2004 founding the European Centre for Disease Prevention and Control 'the Centre's mission should be to identify, assess, and communicate regarding current and emerging threats to human health from communicable diseases'. ECDC works in partnership with national health protection bodies across Europe to strengthen and develop continent-wide disease surveillance and early warning systems. By working with experts throughout Europe, ECDC pools Europe's health knowledge to develop authoritative scientific opinions about the risks posed by current and emerging infectious diseases (European Commission 2004).

World Organization for Animal Health (OIE)

The Office International des Epizooties was established in 1924 in order to fight animal diseases at global level and was renamed the World Organization for Animal Health in 2003 (http://www.oie. int/). The OIE is the intergovernmental organization responsible for improving animal health worldwide and has a number of objectives including collection, analysis and dissemination of veterinary scientific information, encouraging international solidarity in the control of animal diseases, sanitary safety, promotion of veterinary services and food safety and animal welfare.

World Health Organization (WHO)

WHO (http://www.who.int/en/) is the directing and coordinating authority for health within the United Nations (UN) system. It is responsible for providing leadership on global health matters, shaping the health research agenda, setting norms and standards, articulating evidence-based policy options, providing technical support to countries and monitoring and assessing health trends.

WHO and OIE are key stakeholders in the Global Early Warning System for Major Animal Diseases (**GLEWS**) (http://www.glews.net/). This is a joint system that builds on the added value of combining and coordinating alert mechanisms of WHO, OIE and the Food and Agriculture Organization of the United Nations (FAO), while linking networks from the international community and stakeholders, to assist in prediction, prevention and control of zoonotic disease threats through sharing of information, epidemiological and risk analysis.

Conclusion

National and international surveillance systems are essential for public health control of both emerging and endemic zoonoses but giving priority to and identifying scarce resources to support this activity requires strong leadership at Government and inter-Government levels. Medical and veterinary scientists must cooperate to work across traditional boundaries to share information and undertake joint risk assessments if surveillance is to be for public health action. In this chapter we have described how such systems have been established and report in the UK and in Europe.

References

Advisory Committee on the Microbiological Safety of Food (ACMSF) (2001). Second report on *Salmonella* in eggs. London: The Stationery Office.

Baker, M., Smith, G.E., and Cooper, D. *et al.* (2003). Early warning and NHS Direct: a role in community surveillance? *J. Pub. Health. Med.* **25**: 362–68.

Burnet, F.M. and White, D. (1972). *Natural History of Infectious Disease.* Cambridge University Press, Cambridge.

Defra a: Zoonoses Report: United Kingdom 2008 available at: http://www.defra.gov.uk/foodfarm/farmanimal/diseases/atoz/zoonoses/index.htm (Accessed 9 February 2011.)

Defra b: UK National Control Programme for *Salmonella* in chickens (*Gallus gallus*) reared for meat (Broilers). Available at: http://www.defra.gov.uk/foodfarm/farmanimal/diseases/atoz/zoonoses/ncp.htm (Accessed 9 February 2011.)

Defra c: UK National Control Programme for *Salmonella* in layers (*Gallus gallus*) reared for meat (Layers). Available at: http://www.defra.gov.uk/foodfarm/farmanimal/diseases/atoz/zoonoses/ncp.htm (Accessed 9 February 2011.)

Defra d: Trends and sources of specified zoonotic agents in animals, feeding stuffs, food and man in the UK. Available at: http://www.defra.gov.uk/foodfarm/farmanimal/diseases/atoz/zoonoses/trends-sources.htm (Accessed December 2009.)

Defra e: Framework Response Plan for Exotic Diseases of Animals, December 2009, Defra, London. Available at www.defra.gov.uk/foodfarm/farmanimal/diseases/control/ (Accessed 9 February 2011.)

Defra f: Partnership, Priorities and Professionalism: a Strategy for Enhancing Veterinary Surveillance in the UK (2003). Available at: http://www.defra.gov.uk/foodfarm/farmanimal/diseases/vetsurveillance/strategy/index.htm (Accessed 9 February 2011.)

European Centre for Disease Prevention and Control. Annual epidemiological report on communicable diseases in Europe. Available at: http://www.ecdc.europa.eu/en/publications/surveillance_reports/annual_epidemiological_report/Pages/index.aspx (3 January 2011.)

European Commission (2003). Directive 2003/99/EC of the European Parliament and of the Council of 17th November 2003 on the monitoring of zoonoses and zoonotic agents, amending Council Decision 90/424/EEC and repealing Council Directive 92/117/EEC. *Official Journal of the European Union* December.Available at http://eur-lex.europa.eu/LexUriServ/LexUriServ.do?uri=OJ:L:2003:325:0031:0040:EN:PDF (Accessed 3 January 2011.)

European Commission 2004 Regulation (EC) no 851/2004 of the European Parliament and of the Council of 21 April 2004 establishing a European centre for disease prevention and control *Official Journal of the European Union* http://ecdc.europa.eu/en/aboutus/Key%20Documents/0404_KD_Regulation_establishing_ECDC.pdf. (Accessed 4 January 2011)

European Food Safety Authority (2008). Community Summary Report on Trends and Sources of Zoonoses and Zoonotic Agents and Food-borne Outbreaks in the European Union in 2008. EFSA Journal. 8:1496–1906 Available at: http://www.efsa.europa.eu/en/efsajournal/pub/1496.htm (Accessed 3 January 2011.)

European Food Safety Authority (2009). Manual on Reporting on Zoonoses, 2008 *EFSA Journal* 255: 1–90. Available at: http://www.efsa.europa.eu/en/scdocs/doc/zoon_report_ej255_manual2008_en.pdf (Accessed 3 January 2011.)

Farrington, C.P., Andrews, N.J., Beale, A.D. and Catchpole, M.A. (1996). A statistical algorithm for the early detection of outbreaks of infectious disease. *J. R. Stat. Soc.* 159: 547–63.

Foods Standards Agency (2000). *A report of the study of infectious intestinal disease in England.* London: The Stationery Office.

Ghani, A.C., Ferguson, N.M., Donnelly, C.A. and Anderson, R.M. (2000). Predicted vCJD mortality in Great Britain. *Nature,* **406:** 583–84.

Health Protection Agency (2010). Health Protection Report 2010 Volume 4 No 6, 12 February. Available at: http://www.hpa.org.uk/hpr/archives/2010/news0610.htm#pt14b (Accessed 4 January 2011.)

Health Protection Agency (2009). Health Protection Report Volume 3 No 47, 27 November. Available at: http://www.hpa.org.uk/hpr/archives/2009/news4709.htm (Accessed 4 January 2011.)

Health Protection Agency a: Variant CJD and blood. Available at: http://www.hpa.org.uk/Topics/InfectiousDiseases/InfectionsAZ/CreutzfeldtJakobDisease/VariantCJDAndBlood (Accessed 4 January 2011.)

Heath Protection Agency b: Salmonella Epidemiological data 1990–2009. Available at: http://www.hpa.org.uk/Topics/InfectiousDiseases/InfectionsAZ/Salmonella/EpidemiologicalData/ (Accessed 4 January 2011.)

Heath Protection Agency c: Human Animal Infection and Risk Surveillance group http://www.hpa.org.uk/Topics/InfectiousDiseases/InfectionsAZ/EmergingInfections/HAIRS/ (Accessed 10 January 2011.)

Health Protection Scotland. Enhanced surveillance of thrombotic microangiopathies in Scotland, 2003–2008. Available at: http://www.hps.scot.nhs.uk/giz/wrdetail.aspx?id=40709&wrtype=9. (Accessed 10 January 2011.)

Kaiser, R., Coulombier, D., Baldari, M., Morgan, D. and Paquet, C. (2006). What is epidemic intelligence, and how is it being improved in Europe? *Eurosurv.* **11**(5) Available at: http://www.eurosurveillance.org/ViewArticle.aspx?ArticleId=2892 (Accessed 10 January 2011.)

Last, J.M. (1988). *A Dictionary of Epidemiology.* New York: Oxford University Press.

Lynn, R.M., O'Brien, S.J., Taylor, C.M., *et al.* (2005). Childhood hemolytic uremic syndrome, United Kingdom and Ireland. *Emer. Infect. Dis.,* **411:** 590–96.

Lysons, R., Gibbens, J. and Smith, L. (2007). Progress with enhancing veterinary surveillance in the United Kingdom. *Vet. Rec.,* **160:** 105–12.

Morgan, D., Kirkbride, H., Hewitt, K., Said, B. and Walsh, A. (2009). Assessing the Risk from Emerging Infections. *Epidemiol. and Infect.,* **137:** 1521–30.

O'Flanagan, D., Cormican, M., McKeown, P. *et al.* (2008). A multi-country outbreak of Salmonella Agona, February–August 2008. *Eurosurveillance*; 13, 33. Available at: http://www.eurosurveillance.org/ViewArticle.aspx?ArticleId=18956 (Accessed 8 February 2011.)

Palmer, S., Brown, D., and Morgan, D. (2005) Early Qualitative Risk Assessment of the Emerging Zoonotic Potential of Animal Diseases. *BMJ,* **331:** 1256–60.

Ryan, M., Hall, S.M., Barrett, N.J., Balfour, A.H., Holliman, R.E. and Joynson, D.H. (1995). Toxoplasmosis in England and Wales 1981–1992. *Communic. Dis. Rev.,* **3**(5): R13–21.

Taylor, L.H., Latham S.M., and Woolhouse M.E.J. (2001). Risk factors for human disease emergence. *Phil. Trans. R. Soc. Lond.,* **356:** 983–89.

Turner, M.L., and Ludlam, C.A. (2009) An update on the assessment and management of the risk of transmission of variant Creutzfeldt-Jakob disease by blood and plasma products. *Brit. J. Haematol.,* **144:** 14–23.

Veterinary Laboratories Agency. Non Statutory Zoonoses (Project FZ2100) Annual Report 2008. Available at: http://www.defra.gov.uk/vla/reports/docs/rep_zoo0408.pdf (Accessed 1 March 2010.)

Ward, L.R., Threlfall, J., Smith, H.R., and O'Brien, S.J. (2000). *Salmonella enteritidis* epidemic. *Science,* **287:** 1753–54.

Woolhouse, M.E.J. and Gaunt, E. (2007). Ecological origins of novel pathogens. *Crit. Rev. Microbiol.,* **33:** 231–42.

CHAPTER 4

Health impact assessment and burden of zoonotic diseases

Christine M. Budke, Hélène Carabin and Paul R. Torgerson

Summary

Numerous zoonotic diseases cause morbidity, mortality and productivity losses in both humans and animal populations. Recent studies suggest that these diseases can produce large societal impacts in endemic areas. Estimates of monetary impact and disease burden provide essential, evidence-based data for conducting cost-benefit and cost-utility analyses that can contribute to securing political will and financial and technical resources. To evaluate burden, monetary and non-monetary impacts of zoonoses on human health, agriculture and society should be comprehensively considered. This chapter reviews the framework used to assess the health impact and burden of zoonoses and the data needed to estimate the extent of the problem for societies. Case studies are presented to illustrate the use of burden of disease assessment for the zoonotic diseases cystic echinococcosis, *Taenia solium* cysticercosis, brucellosis and rabies.

Introduction

Numerous zoonotic infections result in ill health and economic losses in humans and animals. The challenge in assessing the burden of a zoonotic infection is that most approaches will estimate the impact of the infection in one species at a time. In addition, some approaches are only applicable to measuring human health impact, and are not applicable to animal health impact. To overcome this challenge, a number of large-scale initiatives and individual researchers have endeavoured to assess the burden of these infections in both non-monetary and monetary terms. Non-monetary assessment can include measures of mortality, morbidity (which often includes reduction in productivity in animals), and health adjusted life year (HALY) measures which include the quality adjusted life year (QALY) and the disability adjusted life year (DALY). Monetary assessment of these conditions should include both direct and indirect costs associated with disease in both human and animal hosts.

Measuring burden

Mortality as a measure of burden

Mortality has traditionally been used to measure and compare the health status of populations (Hyder and Morrow 2001). For humans, vital statistics data have been shown to be available from only 115 out of 192 member states of the World Health Organization (WHO) (Mathers *et al.* 2005). Of those 115 member states, death registration was considered complete in only 64 (33%). In addition, among 106 countries with recent data at least 50% complete, the quality of the data on classification of the causes of death was considered as high, medium and poor in 23, 55 and 28 countries, respectively. These data underline the difficulty of measuring burden across states even using what is usually considered an objective and reliable measure, death.

There is no systematic data collection on causes of animal deaths, except in the case of the occurrence of an outbreak. In livestock, slaughterhouse data, when available, may be used to estimate the prevalence of infections (see later), but do not reflect causes of death nor natural (non-slaughter) death rates. There is no vital statistics system for pet animals. Therefore, while there is a way to compare human death rates across countries, even if they are not completely accurate, such measures are not available for animal populations.

Morbidity as a measure of burden

Causes of death data may accurately measure the impact of deadly diseases, but ignore those diseases that may be chronic and disabling, but not or rarely fatal. In humans, such data can be estimated from clinical records systems, health insurance claims databases or notifiable disease or cancer registries. Medical records systems will only reflect the incidence rates of diseases among people seeking medical care, even in countries with universal health coverage. Notifiable disease surveillance data are known to underestimate the true frequency of infectious diseases, but are helpful to detect outbreaks and analyse temporal and spatial trends (Trottier *et al.* 2006; Giesecke 2002; Chorba 2001; Nelson and Sifakis 2007). In addition, models have been developed for some diseases, such as measles, to adjust for under-reporting (Fine and Clarkson 1982). The reliability of the classification of diseases from medical records is often poor (De Coster *et al.* 2006). Finally, availability of medical record data is limited to only a few developed countries.

In animals, data from slaughterhouses or official carcass inspections in markets can be used, where available, to estimate frequency of diseases in animals. Such data are only useful in countries where home slaughter is uncommon and where the majority of carcasses will be inspected. The advantage of these data is that most animals will be eventually slaughtered thus providing reliable estimates of the frequency of lesions associated with infections under surveillance. For example, slaughterhouse data were used in a recent publication aimed at estimating the monetary burden of cystic echinococcosis in Spain (Benner *et al.* 2010). Unfortunately, reliable abattoir data are only available from developed countries and are very limited elsewhere.

Companion animals can be the source of a number of zoonoses. Unfortunately, accurate data on diseases in such animals are rarely available except with certain notifiable diseases (e.g. rabies). However, an initiative to address this problem, the National Companion Animal Surveillance Program, is being undertaken in the USA using the electronic records of over 500 small animal hospitals and the electronic reports from diagnostic laboratories serving over 18,000 private veterinary practices (Glickman *et al.* 2006). This initiative aims to provide better information about zoonotic and emerging diseases in companion animals. These data will, however, still present the same limitations in that they only represent those animals under care that were accurately diagnosed, but this is a considerable improvement on the current lack of information.

Surveillance data may also be used in animals. The World Organization for Animal Health (OIE) recently launched the World Animal Health Information Database (WAHID), which aims at collecting data on notifiable animal diseases, including zoonoses. Even though an improvement from what has been traditionally available, this source of data has the same limitation as human notifiable disease data, in that it is highly dependent on the willingness of people to report cases of disease. Also, for several of these notifiable infections, only outbreaks are being reported and information on endemic infections is not available. Another common limitation in estimating the frequency of infection in animals is the lack of accurate estimates of animal populations, leading to the absence of valid denominators to estimate frequency measures such as incidence rates or prevalence proportions.

In the absence of reliable data from surveillance or medical records in humans and slaughterhouse or surveillance data in animals, estimates of prevalence can be obtained through surveys conducted by independent researchers. However, these types of surveys are problematic because they are often conducted in areas known to be endemic for the infection of interest, which leads to an overestimation of the true frequency of the infection. In addition, estimates of disease prevalence are often obtained via serological testing (e.g. to diagnose cystic echinococcosis or *T. solium* infection in humans and livestock). These tests are developed to detect exposure to the infectious agent (tests designed to measure antibodies) or to detect the presence of the infectious agent (tests designed to measure the agent itself or its antigens). Exposure to the agent may have occurred in the past and its association with the development of symptoms, which cause disability, may be very weak. Similarly, the presence of the agent in an infected individual will not always result in the development of symptoms. For example, not all larvae of *T. solium* will migrate and cause lesions in the brain and not all brain lesions will be associated with symptoms. In a cross-sectional survey of people with epilepsy in South Africa, an ELISA test for the detection of the antigens to the larval stages of *T. solium* was estimated to have a sensitivity of only 17.4% to detect lesions of neurocysticercosis identified by CT-scan (Foyaca-Sibat *et al.* 2009). In a cross-sectional survey conducted among healthy

volunteers in Mexico, 9.1% demonstrated asymptomatic lesions of neurocysticercosis on a brain CT-scan (Fleury *et al.* 2003).

The poor performance of serological tests to detect symptomatic cases is due to the fact that several zoonotic infections remain asymptomatic and have variable incubation periods. More expensive and intrusive methods may be available, but are often not accessible or not usable in the field. For example, both echinococcosis and neurocysticercosis rely heavily on advanced imaging to make a definitive diagnosis in humans. These techniques can incur more than minimal risk to the subjects, which limit their use in large scale surveys. Regardless of the diagnostic test(s) used, error will occur and must be accounted for in the analysis of frequency data. Latent class analysis methods, including Bayesian methods, have been applied to obtain disease frequency estimates based on imperfect tests (Dorny *et al.* 2004; McGarvey *et al.* 2006; Carabin *et al.* 2005). However, such approaches can only be used if some prior knowledge is available on the accuracy of the test specific to the region where it is being used. Indeed, due to cross-reactions with other agents, the specificity of some tests can vary extensively from region to region. To better estimate the risk (or cumulative incidence) of infection over time or the incidence rates of infection per person-time at risk, a cohort study is needed. In this design, a group of individuals initially free of infection are followed-up for a set period and new infections are identified. Unfortunately, these types of studies are very expensive and may be cost-prohibitive in the communities where they are most needed. The additional need to follow both animals and humans further reduces their use in the context of zoonotic infections.

Productivity measures

In order to assess losses associated with health impact assessment of zoonotic conditions, productivity losses must be measured in addition to estimates of disease frequency (e.g. mortality and morbidity). An example of productivity losses, in humans, is the inability of an individual to work due to the symptoms associated with the sequelae of an infection such as cystic echinococcosis or neurocysticercosis. For individuals currently in the work force, actual estimates of salary losses can be used. However, for individuals, and especially women, who are not formally employed, losses in productivity due to illness are much more difficult to estimate. Nevertheless, it is important to account for productivity losses for all affected members of society. For example, Majorowski *et al.* (2005) estimated that women not formally economically active and retired individuals were considered 30% and 10% as productive as a formally employed individual, respectively. In a study estimating the monetary burden of cysticercosis in the Eastern Cape Province of South Africa, a sensitivity analysis was conducted to estimate the effect of three alternative methods to value time of unemployed or unofficially employed individuals (Carabin *et al.* 2006). In animals, productivity losses can be measured in terms of reductions in milk or wool production, reproduction indices and growth (Majorowski *et al.* 2005; Benner *et al.* 2010).

HALYS—QALYs and DALYs

Non-financial methods have been developed to estimate human disease burden and are often referred to under the umbrella term of Health Adjusted Life Years (HALYs) (Gold *et al.* 2002). HALYs are summary measures of population health that combine the impact of morbidity and death. HALYs aim at comprehensively measuring the impacts associated with all aspects (domains) of an ill-health condition. Hence, in contrast to measures of morbidity or mortality, they are designed to capture the impact of all aspects of an infection, including more subtle manifestations which may not be diagnosed with usual methods. However, the use of HALYs does have a number of disadvantages and may not always be appropriate when estimating the societal burden of zoonoses. For one, no HALYs are applicable to animal disease.

Disability Adjusted Life Years (DALYs) are the WHO's preferred measure of disease burden and were utilized in the Global Burden of Disease (GBD) Study (Murray 1994; Murray and Lopez 1996). The goal of the original and subsequent versions of the GBD Study was to consistently assess burden across diseases, risk factors and regions. In other words, the goal of DALYs was to assess the burden of human diseases, assuming that these diseases caused the same level of 'disability' across cultures. While the assumption that the same level of condition-specific disability exists regardless of culture or socioeconomic status is a key feature of the DALY, it is also one of the largest points of contention. It has been argued that an individual's ability to adapt to a disability can vary greatly based on the socioeconomic status of the region. For example, Allotey *et al.* (2003) discussed the differences in the ability to adapt and cope with a condition such as paraplegia for an individual living in Australia as compared to an individual living in Cameroon. Their conclusion was that the DALY undervalues the burden of disease in less developed countries. However, even with this and other shortcomings, the DALY continues to be an important and widely used burden of disease metric.

The DALY is estimated as the sum of the number of years of life lost due to mortality (YLL) and the number of years lived with a certain level of disability (YLD) associated with a specific disease or infection. To quantify DALYs, the frequency of symptoms and sequelae associated with each infection must be known. Those symptoms and sequelae are assigned specific disability weights for as long as they persist, and, therefore, their duration must also be known. Disability weights were developed to capture relative 'disabilities' of health states on a 0 to 1 scale. For example, a healthy individual has a disability weight of 0 and no loss of DALYs, whereas a fatal condition has a disability weight of 1 (Table 4.1).

While the DALY is the most well known and most employed burden of disease metric, other HALYs do exist. These methods

arose due to a concern that measuring morbidity or mortality alone did not capture all aspects of a health condition. Another important rationale for the development of quality of life measures was the possible side effects of treatment for diseases which may outweigh their benefits, but could not be measured through morbidity alone. Health outcome measures first appeared in the late 1960s and early 1970s (Klarman *et al.* 1968; Fanshel and Bush 1970; Bush *et al.* 1972; Torrance *et al.* 1976), with the term quality adjusted life year (QALY) coined by Weinstein and Stason in 1977. QALYs are often considered the precursors to DALYs and are conceptually similar to DALYs, but use different scales. In general, index scores are calculated with QALY standard questionnaires and these are linked to a 'utility' value, which aims at evaluating the 'value' of a health status and were originally designed to be the equivalent of the concept of utility of goods in economics. Thus, interventions would aim to minimize DALYs but maximize QALYs.

The effectiveness of intervention strategies can be calculated as the number of DALYs estimated to occur due to a given condition in the absence of intervention minus the number of DALYs expected if control measures were implemented. However, this disregards any additional benefits of disease control to agriculture (i.e. anthelmintic treatment of dogs reduces cystic echinococcosis incidence in both humans and sheep). Nevertheless, if a total societal financial analysis is undertaken, the true cost-effectiveness of control, in terms of DALYs saved, can be estimated by implementation of cost sharing between sectors proportional to each sector's overall benefit (Roth *et al.* 2003).

Official burden of disease estimates, in terms of DALYs, for zoonotic diseases are limited. For example, until recently, human cysticercosis, cystic echinococcosis, and rabies were not officially evaluated as part of the GBD Study or other international project to evaluate non-monetary disease burden. Research is, however, underway to overcome this deficit and include all three conditions in the upcoming re-evaluation of the GBD Study. In addition, cystic echinococcosis and *T. solium* cysticercosis are both being evaluated as part of the WHO's assessment of the global burden of food-borne diseases (WHO 2010).

Monetary losses

Monetary losses associated with zoonoses can be calculated by the following expression (Majorowski *et al.* 2005).

Table 4.1 Examples of disability weights used to calculate DALYs

Description	Disability weight
Healthy	0
Limited ability to perform at least one activity in one of the following areas: recreation, education, procreation or occupation.	0.096
Limited ability to perform most activities in one of the following areas: recreation, education, procreation or occupation.	0.220
Limited ability to perform most activities in two or more of the following areas: recreation, education, procreation or occupation.	0.400
Limited ability to perform most activities in all of the following areas: recreation, education, procreation or occupation.	0.600
Needs assistance with instrumental activities of daily living such as meal preparation, shopping or housework.	0.810
Needs assistance with activities of daily living such as eating, personal hygiene or toilet use.	0.920
Dead	1

Adapted from Murray , C. J. L. (1994) Quantifying the burden of disease: the technical basis for disability-adjusted life years. Bulletin of the World Health Organization, 72, 429–445, with permission

Equation 1.

$$\sum_{s=1}^{S} \sum_{a=1}^{A} \left[N_{a,s} \beta_{a,s} \left(\sum_{x=1}^{X} \pi_{x,a,s} C_{x,a,s} \right) \right]$$

This equation corresponds to the additive societal costs for all affected species (S) across all age groups (A). For the age-species-specific population of size ($N_{a,s}$), with the age-species-specific annual incidence ($\beta_{a,s}$), there is an age-species proportion ($\pi_{x,a,s}$) of infected individuals with symptoms X. The treatment and consequences of each of these symptoms have a cost of $C_{x,a,s}$. Ideally, the whole spectrum of symptoms and losses in humans and animals is included.

Human losses

Both direct and indirect costs should be included in monetary estimates of human disease burden. Direct costs include costs associated with resources expended for health care (e.g. diagnostics, medications, surgical treatment, etc.). Indirect costs include costs of the resources forgone either to participate in an intervention or as the result of a health condition (e.g. earnings lost because of loss of time from work, costs of transportation to and from treatment, earning losses for a family member while taking care of the sick individual). As discussed earlier, indirect losses associated with productivity losses can be difficult to assess for those not formally employed.

Animal losses

Animal-associated monetary losses can also be divided into direct and indirect costs. Direct costs can stem from monetary losses due to condemnation of an infected carcass or parts thereof. For example, the condemnation of a pig carcass heavily infected with

T. solium cysticerci or the condemnation of a sheep liver infected with cystic echinococcosis are direct costs. Indirect costs would encompass other disease-related production losses. For example, decreased carcass weight linked to a reduction in growth, decreased hide value, decreased milk production, and decreased fecundity due to cystic echinococcosis infection in a sheep. Even though estimates of these losses are sometimes uncertain and have very little available data, studies incorporating estimates of indirect costs for livestock-associated losses have shown that these losses are likely to be significant. For example, monetary losses associated with cystic echinococcosis in Spanish livestock contributed to an estimated 10.4% of cystic echinococcosis total costs, with indirect costs contributing to 10.3% and direct costs contributing to only 0.12% of losses (Benner *et al.* 2010).

Including uncertainty

As mentioned above, several parameters that need to be used to estimate the monetary losses of zoonotic infections are poorly described. This leads to a large level of uncertainty as to what the true value of several of the components of the monetary value in Equation 1 actually are. One approach which has been used to reflect this uncertainty is that of stochastic models where the range of possible values for each uncertain parameter is repetitively sampled using a Latin Hypercube or Monte Carlo sampling technique (Majorowski *et al.* 2005; Knobel *et al.* 2005; Carabin *et al.* 2006; Benner *et al.* 2010).

The various measures of disease burden discussed above all have their positive and negative aspects. Table 4.2 provides comparisons between mortality, morbidity, QALYs, DALYs and monetary losses in terms of what is being assessed and the current availability of quality data.

Table 4.2 Comparisons of the main measures of disease burden

Measure of burden	Items	Availability/quality of data	
		Humans	**Animals**
Mortality	Cause-specific death rates	Quality highly variable between countries	Rarely available except for notifiable diseases
Morbidity	Disease-specific incidence rates	Notifiable/registry disease data Quality/completeness highly variable	Research studies only Acute, non-recurrent and notifiable diseases (i.e. rabies) if denominator known
	Disease-specific prevalence	National/special survey data Special survey data often overestimate the truth	Abattoir data where home slaughtering is rare Special survey data often overestimate the truth
QALYs	Cause-specific death rates	Quality highly variable between countries	Not applicable
	Life expectancy	Largely available	
	Disease-specific incidence rates	Notifiable/registry disease data Quality/completeness highly variable	
	Time evolution of disease states	Knowledge of natural history of disease needed	
	Quality of life measure at various disease states	Special studies Place/time specific	

(Continued)

Table 4.2 (Cont'd) Comparisons of the main measures of disease burden

Measure of burden	Items	Availability/quality of data	
		Humans	**Animals**
DALYs	Cause-specific death rates	Quality highly variable between countries	Not applicable
	Disease-specific incidence rates	Notifiable/registry disease data Quality/completeness highly variable	
	Distribution of sequela associated with disease in treatment free individuals	Knowledge of natural history of disease needed	
	Duration of each sequela in treatment free individuals	Knowledge of natural history of each sequela needed	
	Distribution of sequela associated with disease among people under treatment	Special studies required	
	Duration of each sequela in people under treatment	Special studies required	
	Disability weights for each sequela (treated/ non treated)	Available from GBD initiative Not all sequelae have been attributed disability weights	
Monetary burden	Cause-specific death rates	Quality highly variable between countries	Rarely available except for notifiable diseases
	Disease-specific prevalence	National/special survey data Special survey data often overestimate the truth	Abattoir data where home slaughtering is rare Special survey data often overestimate the truth
	Distribution of sequelae associated with disease	Knowledge of natural history of disease needed	Knowledge of natural history of disease needed
	Frequency of care/treatments/diagnoses and productivity losses for each sequela	Special studies Expert opinion	Special studies Expert opinion
	Costs associated with care/treatments/ productivity losses of each sequela	Country-level health/labour statistics Special surveys	Agricultural statistics Special surveys

Use of decision trees and mathematical models

Decision trees are a useful aid to help estimate frequency of infection or other outcomes when data are not readily available (Haddix *et al.* 2003). A decision tree is a decision support tool that uses a tree-like graph of decisions and their possible consequences, including chance event outcomes, resource costs, and utility. Figure 4.1 is an example of a decision tree for estimating the monetary burden of cystic echinococcosis in Tunisia (Majorwoski *et al.* 2005). A decision tree commonly consists of 3 different types of nodes:

1. 'decision' nodes which are usually represented by squares,

2. 'chance' notes which are usually represented by circles,

3. 'end' nodes which are usually represented by triangles.

The value at the end of each 'branch' is an estimation of the prevalence of that particular end-point.

Once frequency data from official sources and data obtained using tools such as decision trees have been collected, an uncertainty analysis can be conducted as described above. Sensitivity analyses can also be conducted to determine which parameters have the largest impact on the overall estimates.

Cost utility and cost benefit analyses

An important aspect of undertaking disease burden studies is to compare the ability of alternative control strategies to reduce such burden. Public health and monetary resources are often scarce and hence intervention strategies should be designed to maximize cost benefit or cost utility of a control programme. In purely human health terms, cost utility (e.g. the cost per DALY averted or QALY saved) can be undertaken. For example, the WHO defines interventions with the best incremental cost utility ratios as those interventions costing less than US$25 per DALY averted. Incremental cost utility ratios of less than US$125 per DALY averted (WHO 1996) are considered as second tier. The impact of zoonotic diseases can be underestimated when solely human health metrics, such as DALYs or QALYs, are used since these measures ignore the often considerable economic impact of these diseases in animals. Such economic impact may be a considerable additional societal burden and can be very important in assessing the cost effectiveness of disease intervention.

Animals usually have an economic value and hence monetary losses can be calculated for animal diseases. A cost benefit analysis can then be performed in terms of money saved per money invested. The challenge occurs when attempting to obtain the overall societal benefit in terms of improvement of both human and animal health. The methods to assess the monetary burden of a zoonotic disease discussed above can be used to obtain an overall societal burden, including animal health losses. From this information, a cost benefit analysis can be conducted for comparing alternative intervention strategies. Cost sharing ideas can also be used

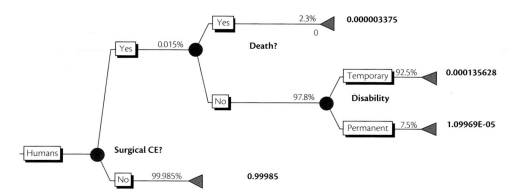

Fig. 4.1 Example of a decision tree for assessing the outcome of cystic echinococcosis in humans in Tunisia. Reproduced from Majorwoski *et al.* (2005), with permission from Elsevier.

to assess the cost utility of control where the costs are shared between public health and agricultural sectors in terms of relative benefits. If cost sharing of the control of echinococcosis in western China were to be undertaken, the cost effectiveness to the public health sector would be in the most cost effective band at less than US$25 per DALY averted. In addition, the programme would also have a positive cost benefit in terms of reduction in agricultural losses (Budke *et al.* 2005). Brucellosis control in Mongolia was also predicted to be highly cost effective (in terms of DALYs averted per cost invested) for the public health sector if cost sharing was undertaken with the agricultural sector (Roth *et al.* 2003).

Cost analyses can also be used to examine ongoing disease control programmes. For example, as purely a public health intervention strategy, the present bovine tuberculosis control programme in the UK and the *Trichinella* surveillance programme in the European Union (EU) are not considered as having good cost utility ratios in terms of cost per DALY averted (Torgerson and Torgerson 2010; Speybroek *et al.* 2010). In contrast, diseases such as toxoplasmosis result in a considerable human disease burden, but potential food safety interventions are not implemented (Kijlstra and Jongert 2009). Cost utility, in terms of DALYs averted, is one tool to drive public health policies to maximize health with the resources available.

Burden of zoonotic disease case studies

Cysticercosis

Cysticerocis and neurocysticercosis (NCC) are caused by the taeniid-type zoonotic tapeworm *Taenia solium*. The parasite has a human definitive host and a pig intermediate host. Pigs contain cysticerci in different parts of the body (cysticercosis). Humans become infected with the tapeworm form (taeniasis) by ingesting undercooked pork containing *T. solium* cysticerci. Eggs and/or mature proglottids of the tapeworm are regularly excreted by human tapeworm carriers. Humans can also act as accidental hosts by ingesting food or water contaminated with the eggs of *T. solium* leading to cysticercosis and/or NCC, when cysts are located in the central nervous system. Common clinical manifestations associated with NCC include epilepsy, severe headaches, dementia, and stroke. A more complete overview of *T. solium* cysticercosis can be found in Chapter 51 of this volume.

Regional study: Cameroon

The first estimates of both the monetary and non-monetary burden of disease, due to *T. solium* cysticercosis, were carried out in the African country of Cameroon (Praet *et al.* 2009). Parameters for costs associated with cysticercosis were estimated for both humans and pigs. Decision tree analysis was used to identify the proportion of the population with epilepsy due to NCC, with or without injury and with or without treatment by a medical doctor or traditional healer. Costs for visiting a physician or traditional healer, drugs, and salary losses were estimated from available data. In addition, losses due to porcine cysticercosis were estimated based on tongue inspection, with the average value on an adult pig and price reduction of pigs diagnosed with cysticercosis estimated based on available local data. Parameters for the estimation of DALYs lost were based on GBD Study estimates for disability weights associated with epilepsy and average duration of disability by age and gender. Monte Carlo methods were then used to estimate the annual socioeconomic costs and numbers of DALYs lost due to *T. solium* cysticercosis in Cameroon.

Based on a 3.6% prevalence of epilepsy, 50,326 (credibility interval (95% CR) 37,299–65,929) people were estimated to be suffering from NCC-associated epilepsy, which equals approximately 1% of the population. The total estimated cost associated with *T. solium* cysticercosis, was estimated at €19,255,202 (6,889, 048–14,754,044), with 4.7% of this value due to pig-associated losses and the remaining due to direct and indirect human losses. The average number of DALYs lost was 9.0 per thousand persons per year (95% CR 2.8–20.4).

Cystic echinococcosis

Cystic echinococcosis is caused by the taeniid-type zoonotic tapeworm *Echinococcus granulosus*. It has a cosmopolitan distribution, but is most prevalent in resource-constrained livestock rearing areas. The parasite has a dog definitive host and a variety of livestock (e.g. sheep, goats, cattle) intermediate hosts. Parasitic cysts develop in infected intermediate hosts, especially in the liver and lungs, which can result in substantial livestock production losses. Humans become infected upon ingestion of parasite eggs shed in the faeces of infected dogs, with humans also developing slow-growing cystic lesions, most commonly in the liver or lungs, which can be fatal if not treated with the appropriate chemotherapeutic and/or surgical therapy. A more complete overview of cystic echinococcosis can be found in Chapter 53 of this volume.

Regional study: China

A monetary and non-monetary burden of disease assessment was performed for Shiqu County, which is located in western Sichuan

Province, China. Shiqu County has a population of approximately 63,000 with the vast majoring of inhabitants being ethnically Tibetan (Budke *et al.* 2005). DALYs were applied to human cystic echinococcosis cases in Shiqu County in a stochastic manner utilizing disability weights for conditions with similar symptomology (e.g. hepatic carcinoma). Based on human ultrasound prevalence, an estimated 17,995 (95% CI 14,268–22,128) DALYs were lost due to cystic echinococcosis (Budke *et al.* 2004). Since this region is also endemic for the zoonotic parasite *Echinococcus multilocularis*, the causative agent of alveolar echinococcosis, the number of DALYs lost was also estimated for this condition. Based on human ultrasound prevalence, an additional 32,978 (95% CI 25,019–42,422) DALYs were lost due to alveolar echinococcosis. This equates to approximately 0.81 DALYs lost (or 0.81 healthy year of life lost) per resident of Shiqu County due to echinococcosis, illustrating the substantial health impact of echinococcosis on this community.

In addition to non-monetary estimates of disease burden, an estimate of monetary losses, due to echinococcosis, was also performed for Shiqu County (Budke *et al.* 2005). Assuming that humans were treated for echinococcosis primarily via chemotherapeutic treatment, US$218,676 (95% CI 189,850–247,871) was estimated to be lost annually if only direct livestock-associated losses (i.e. only liver-related losses) were taken into account. This value could, however, reach as high as approximately US$1,000,000 if livestock CE-associated production losses (e.g. decreased hide value, decrease carcass weight, decreased fecundity) were assumed.

Brucellosis

Brucellosis is a bacterial zoonoses with humans becoming infected via contact with an infected animal or animal product. There are a number of *Brucella* species that can infect humans including *B. melitensis*, which is commonly found in small ruminants, *B. abortus*, which is common in cattle, *B. suis*, which is found in pigs, and *B. canis* which is found in dogs. Brucellosis is considered endemic in livestock and humans in parts of the Mediterranean, Asia, Africa, and Latin America (Pappas *et al.* 2006). A more complete overview of brucellosis can be found in Chapter 7 of this volume.

Regional study: Mongolia

The cost-utility and economic benefit of a brucellosis vaccination campaign was modelled for the country of Mongolia (Roth *et al.* 2003). The number of DALYs lost due to human brucellosis was estimated. In addition, monetary losses associated with human and livestock brucellosis were estimated as were the costs of a planned 10-year livestock mass vaccination campaign. The authors determined that a vaccination campaign that could reduce brucellosis transmission between livestock by 52% would result in 49,027 DALYs being averted. It was also estimated that the proposed vaccination programme would cost US$3.3 million, but would have an overall benefit of US$26.6 million, resulting in a net present value of US$18.3 million and an average benefit-cost ratio of 3.2 (95% CI 2.3–4.4). This study went on to propose how a brucellosis prevention programme could be even more attractive to the various public health and agricultural agencies if the intervention costs were shared proportionally by the sectors which the condition impacts.

Rabies

Rabies is a neuro-invasive viral disease most commonly transmitted via the bite of an infected warm-blooded animal. A more complete overview of rabies can be found in Chapter 35 of this volume.

Regional study: Africa and Asia

The burden of canine-associated rabies has been evaluated for Africa and Asia in terms of monetary losses and DALYs lost (Knobel *et al.* 2005). First, the number of human rabies deaths was estimated using a dog-bite probability model. Costs associated with rabies were then estimated as were direct and indirect costs associated with post-exposure treatment, dog vaccination and population control, livestock losses, and surveillance. DALY estimates were conducted that not only included mortality due to rabies, but also mortality and morbidity due to the use of post-exposure treatments using crude nerve-tissue vaccines. Regional monetary and non-monetary burden estimates were estimated for both Africa and Asia using Monte Carlo sampling methods to model uncertainty.

Endemic rabies was estimated to cause 55,000 deaths per year in Africa and Asia (95% CI 24,000–93,000). The annual costs of rabies was estimated at US$20,500,000 (95% CI 19,300,000–21,800,000) for Africa and US$563,000,000 (95% CI 520,000,000–605,800,000) for Asia. This study also estimated 747,558 (95% CI 217,690–1,448,514) DALYs lost in Africa and 994,607 (95% CI 257,275–1,393,125) DALYs lost in Asia due to canine-associated rabies.

Conclusions

Zoonotic diseases such as cystic echinococcosis, *Taenia solium* cysticercosis, brucellosis and rabies contribute to high levels of human morbidity, human mortality, and livestock losses in endemic regions. While control of these conditions should be prioritized, in many areas of the developing world, a lack of accurate estimates of disease burden hampers these efforts. In industrialised countries, such estimates can more easily be made and used to compare cost effectiveness of current and proposed disease control programmes.

Glossary

Cystic echinococcosis: an infection or disease of humans or animals caused by the larvae of *Echinococcus granulosus*.

Cysticercosis: an infection or disease of humans or animals caused by the larvae of *Taenia* spp. In this chapter, the term refers to infection of humans or pigs with *Taenia solium* cysticercosis.

Decision tree analysis: a method of organizing epidemiological data into infections and the frequency of their consequences.

Disability adjusted life year: in simplest terms, this can be considered a lost healthy year of life and is a non-monetary measure of disease burden. It takes into account the severity of the syndrome and its duration, thus levelling the playing field when comparing acute and chronic conditions. A DALY also has the same value in poor and rich countries.

Disability weight: a score between 0 and 1 that is assigned to a condition depending on the degree of debilitation.

Direct costs: costs such as carcass condemnation or medical costs arising directly from the treatment of infection.

Health adjusted life year: an umbrella term for a family of measures of population health that includes, for example, DALYs and QALYs.

Indirect costs: costs such as production deficits or wage losses arising indirectly from infection.

Monte Carlo sampling technique: a method that can be employed in cost analysis when exact estimates are unknown. Repeated samples are taken over a probability distribution based on the known information.

Nerve tissue vaccines: nerve tissue vaccines are an older type of rabies vaccine made from inactive virus cultivated in a sheep's or goat's brain. These vaccines are no longer available in most countries in the developed world since they can cause severe immune reactions against the neural tissue.

Neurocysticercosis: a neurological disease caused by invasion of the CNS by larvae of *T. solium*.

Quality adjusted life year: a population measure of health. A year of full health is equivalent to 1 QALY, whereas death corresponds to 0 QALYs. Disease conditions are graded on a continuous scale between these two extremes.

References

Allotey, P. *et al.* (2003). The DALY, context and the determinants of the severity of disease: an exploratory comparison of paraplegia in Australia and Cameroon. *Soc. Sci. & Med.*, **57:** 949–58.

Benner, C. *et al.* (2010). Analysis of the economic impact of cystic echinococcosis in Spain. *Bull. World Heal. Org.* **88:** 49–57.

Budke, C. M. *et al.* (2004). Utilization of DALYs in the estimation of the disease burden of echinococcosis for a high endemic region of the Tibetan plateau. *Am. J. Trop. Med. and Hyg.*, **71:** 56–64.

Budke, C. M. *et al.* (2005). Economic effects of echinococcosis on a highly endemic region of the Tibetan plateau. *Am. J. Trop. Med. and Hyg.*, **73:** 2–10.

Bush *et al.* (1972). Analysis of a tuberculin testing program using a health status index. *Socio-Econ. Plan. Sci.*, **6:** 49–68.

Carabin, H. *et al.* (2005). Estimating sensitivity and specificity of a faecal examination method for Schistosoma japonicum infection in cats, dogs, water buffaloes, pigs, and rats in Western Samar and Sorsogon Provinces, The Philippines. *Int. J. Parasitol.*, **35:** 1517–24.

Carabin, H. *et al.* (2006). Estimation of the monetary burden of Taenia solium cysticercosis in the Eastern Cape, South Africa. *Trop. Med. Int. Health*, **11:** 906–916.

Chorba, T. L. (2001). Disease Surveillance. In: J. C. Thomas and D. J. Weber (ed.). *Epidemiologic methods for the study of infectious diseases*, pp. 138–62, Oxford: Oxford University Press.

De Coster, C. *et al.* (2006). Identifying priorities in methodological research using ICD-9-CM and ICD-10 administrative data: report from an international consortium. *BMC Health Ser. Res.*, **6:** 77.

Dorney, P. *et al.* (2004). A Bayesian approach for estimating values for prevalence and diagnostic test characteristics of porcine cysticercosis. *Int. J. Parasitol.*, **34:** 569–76.

Fanshel, S. and Bush, M. D. (1970). A health status index and its application to health services outcomes. *Oper. Res.*, **18:** 1021–66.

Fine, P. E. and Clarkson, J. A. (1982). Measles in England and Wales - II: The impact of the measles vaccination programme on the distribution of immunity in the population. *Int. J. Epidemiol.*, **11:** 15–25.

Fleury, A. *et al.* (2003). High prevalence of calcified silent neurocysticercosis in a rural village of Mexico. *Neuroepidemiol.*, **22:** 139–45.

Foyaca-Sibet, H. *et al.* (2009). Accuracy of serological testing for the diagnosis of prevalent neurocysticercosis in outpatients with epilepsy,

Eastern Cape Province, South Africa. *PLoS Negl. Trop. Dis.*, **8:** e562 Doi: 10.11371/journal.pntd.0000562.

Giesecke, J. (2002). Routine surveillance of infectious disease. In: J. Giesecke (ed.). *Modern infectious disease epidemiology*, (2nd edn.), pp. 148–59. New York: Arnold.

Glickman, L. T. *et al.* (2006). Purdue University-Banfield National Companion Animal Surveillance Program for emerging and zoonotic diseases. *Vect. Borne Zoonot. Dis.*, **6:** 14–23.

Gold, M. R. *et al.* (2002). HALYs and QALYs and DALYS, Oh my: similarities and differences in summary measures of population health. *Ann. Rev. Publ. Heal.*, **23:** 115–34.

Haddix, A. C. *et al.* (2003). *Prevention Effectiveness. A Guide to Decision Analysis and Economic Evaluation.* Oxford: Oxford University Press.

Hyder, A. A. and Morrow, R. H. (2001). Disease burden measurements and trends. In: M. H. Merson, R. E. Black and A. J. Mills (ed.). *International Public Health. Diseases, programs, systems, and policies*, pp. 1–52, Gaithersburg: An Aspen Publication.

Kijlstra, A. and Jongert, E. (2009). Toxoplasma-safe meat: close to reality. *Trends in Parasitol.*, **25:** 18–22.

Klarman *et al.* (1968). Cost-effectiveness analysis applied to the treatment of chronic renal disease. *Med. Care*, **6:** 48–54.

Knobel, D. L. *et al.* (2005). Re-evaluating the burden of rabies in Africa and Asia. *Bull. World Heal. Orga.*, **83:** 360–68.

McGarvey, S. T. *et al.* (2006). Cross-sectional associations between intensity of animal and human infection with Schistosoma japonicum in Western Samar province, Philippines. *Bull. World Heal. Orga.*, **84:** 446–52.

Majorwoski, M. M. *et al.* (2005). Echinococcosis in Tunisia: a cost analysis. *Trans. R. Soc. Trop. Med. Hyg.*, **99:** 268–78.

Mathers, C. D. *et al.* (2005). Counting the dead and what they died from: an assessment of the global status of cause of death data. *Bull. World Heal. Orga.*, **83:** 171–77.

Murray, C. J. L. (1994). Quantifying the burden of disease: the technical basis for disability-adjusted life years. *Bull. World Heal. Orga.*, **72:** 429–45.

Murray, C. J. L. and Lopez, A. D. (1996). The Global Burden of Disease: A Comprehensive Assessment of Mortality and Disability from Disease, Injuries, and Risk Factors in 1990 and Projected to 2020. Boston: Harvard University Press.

Nelson, K. E. and Sifakis, F. (2007). Surveillance. In: K.E. Nelson and C. Masters Williams (ed.). *Infectious disease epidemiology, theory and practice.* (2nd edn.), pp. 119–46 Sudbury: Jones and Bartlett Publishers.

Pappas, G. *et al.* (2006). The new global map of human brucellosis. *Lancet Infect. Dis.*, **6:** 91–99.

Praet, N. *et al.* (2009). The disease burden of Taenia solium cysticercosis in Cameroon. *PLoS Negl. Trop. Dis.*, **3**(3): e406. Doi:10.1371/journal. pntd.000406.

Roth, F. *et al.* (2003). Human health benefits from livestock vaccination for brucellosis: case study. *Bull. World Heal. Orga.*, **81:** 867–76.

Speybroeck, N. *et al.* (2010). *The impact of neglected tropical zoonoses: a viewpoint from an interactive workshop.* (manuscript submitted)

Torrance, G. W. (1976). Health status index models: A unified mathematical view. *Manage. Sci.*, **22:** 990–1001.

Torgerson, P. R. and Torgerson, D. J. (2010). Public health and bovine tuberculosis: what's all the fuss about? *Trends in Microbiol.*, **18:** 67–72.

Trottier, H. *et al.* (2006). Measles, pertussis, rubella and mumps completeness of reporting. Literature review of estimates for industrialized countries. *Revue Epidemiol. Sante. Publiq.*, **54:** 27–39.

Weinstein, M. and Stason, W. (1977). Foundations of cost-effectiveness analysis for health and medical practices. *N. Engl. J. Med.*, **296:** 716–21.

WHO (1996). Report of the Ad Hoc Committee on Health Research Relating to Future Intervention Options, 1996. *Investing in Health Research and Development.* Geneva: World Health Organization TDR/Gen, 96.1.

WHO (http://www.who.int/foodsafety/foodborne_disease/ferg/en/index. html). (Accessed 12 March 2010.)

CHAPTER 5

Antimicrobial resistance: animal use of antibiotics

Lord Soulsby

Summary

International concerns

The evolution of resistance to microbes is one of the most significant problems in modern medicine, posing serious threats to human and animal health. The early work on the use of antibiotics to bacterial infections gave much hope that infectious diseases were no longer a problem, especially in the human field. However, as their use, indeed overuse, progressed, resistance (both mono-resistance and multi-resistance), which was often transferable between different strains and species of bacteria, emerged. In addition, the situation is increasingly complex, as various mechanisms of resistance, including a wide range of β-lactamases, are now complicating the issue. The use of antibiotics in animals, especially those used for growth promotion, has come in for serious criticism, especially those where their use should be reserved for difficult human infections. To lend control, certain antibiotic growth promoters have been banned from use in the EU and the UK.

It is now a decade since the UK House of Lords Science and Technology Committee (1998) highlighted concerns about antimicrobial resistance and the dangers to human health of resistant organisms derived from animals fed antibiotics for growth promotion or the treatment of infectious diseases. The concern expressed in the House of Lords report was similar to that in other major reports on the subject, for example from the World Health Organization, the Wellcome Foundation, the Advisory Committee on the Microbiological Safety of Food and the Swann Report (1969) in which it was recommended that antibiotics used in human medicine should not be used as growth promoters in animals. At the press conference to launch the Lord's Report it was emphasized that unless serious attention was given to dealing with resistance 'we may find ourselves returning to a pre-antibiotic era'. The evolution of resistance is one of the significant problems in modern medicine, a much changed situation when the early work on antibiotics gave hope that infectious diseases were no longer a problem, especially in the human field. Optimism was so strong that the Surgeon General of the USA, William H. Stewart, in 1969 advised the US Congress that 'it is time to close the book on infectious diseases and to declare that work against the pestilence is over'. This comment was not only mistaken but it was also damaging to human health undertakings and also reduced funding for research on infectious diseases.

Despite the widespread support for and dependence on antibiotics, resistance was increasingly reported worldwide and to recognize the global problem a group of medical workers established in 1981, at Tufts University, the Alliance for the Prudent Use of Antibiotics (APUA). This now has affiliated chapters in over 60 countries, many in the developing world. APUA claims to be the 'world's leading organization conducting antimicrobial resistance research, education, capacity building and advocacy at the global and grass roots levels'.

Antibiotic use in growth promotion

The House of Lords Report (1998) was well received by the UK Government. Advice to medical practitioners to show prudence in prescribing antibiotics was provided via information documents and cartoons for clients. The comments in the Report on animal use of antibiotics, especially their use as growth promoters, were less well received, especially by the pharmaceutical industry. Growth promotion in young animals, such as chickens, piglets and calves, consisted of adding small qualities of antibiotics, well below the normal therapeutic dose, to enhance growth, a fact discovered in the USA in 1940 when chickens were fed a fermented ration containing the microorganism *Streptomyces aureofaciens* used in the production of chlortetracycline. Since then antibiotic growth promoters have been used extensively in livestock production, it being claimed by some that not only do they enhance growth but they may also be a substitute in part for poor husbandry practices.

The use of antibiotics for growth promotion which were also used in human medicine (e.g. virginiamycin) and the potential for multi-resistance derived from growth promoters has occasioned much debate. Indeed concern was expressed in the UK several years ago in the Swann Report (1969) which recommended the setting up of a specialist advisory committee on antimicrobial use in man, animals and horticulture. Such a committee was not established until after the House of Lords Report, some 20 years later (1998), this being the Scientific Advisory Committee on Antibiotic Resistance (SACAR) (Wise 2007). Much debate has ensued regarding the health importance and economic impact of growth promoters. In 1998 an EU-wide ban on the use of four growth promoting antibiotics came into effect. These were spiramycin, tylosin, bacitracin zinc and virginiamycin. This ban was later ratified by the UK. There was a dramatic fall in the sales of antimicrobial growth promoters: in 1998, 141 tonnes of active growth promoting ingredient were sold, but by 2005 this had reduced to 14. Remaining antibiotic growth promoters (monensin, avilamycin, salinomycin and flavomycin) came under the EU-wide ban in 2006. Whereas the concern about antibiotic use in growth promotion has been attended to, the overall sales of antimicrobials for therapeutic use in food animals has remained much the same over the last 10 year period. SACAR has now been replaced by the Advisory Committee on Antimicrobial Resistance and Healthcare Associated Infections.

Antibiotic use in animals has shown the same dramatic increase as in humans, many serious infections of farm livestock are now amenable to treatment and cure. Examples are mastitis due to Staphylococci and Streptococci, pneumonia due to Pasteurella spp and the various enteritides due to Salmonella spp and other Gramnegator organisms. There is also widespread use of antibiotics in companion animals, including fish, and also in horticulture.

β-lactamases

The changing face of antimicrobial resistance is illustrated by the appearance of b-lactamases of which multiple types of extended spectrum β-lactamase producing bacteria (ESBLs) have now been recognized; a classification based on hydrolytic profiles has been published by Livermore (2008, a,b) and Livermore et al. (2007). The β-lactam antibiotics are the most flexible compounds being versatile and diverse in terms of chemical properties, antibacterial spectra and administrative requirements. Hence they remain the most commonly used antibacterial agents in the present chemotherapeutic armamentarium. The β-lactamases, the enzymes that hydrolyse the β-lactam antibiotics, are the major cause of resistance to these compounds. A major threat is the ever growing diversification and proliferation of β-lactamases, there being more than 350 identified and one third are able to hydrolyse broad spectrum cephalosporins. Ambler (1980) classifies the β-lactamases into four classes. Class A generally prefer penicillins as substrates, whereas Class C β-lactamases attack cephalosporins more effectively. Class B hydrolyse a broad range, including carbapenims which are generally resistant to most other enzymes. Class D are efficient oxicillin type β-lactamases. Since the recognition of ESBLs the new additional concern is the CTX-M enzymes, including CTX-M type β-lactamase, which is particularly widespread in the UK and other countries. CTX-M, a new family of ESBLs, was detected in humans in Germany and Argentina (Canton and Coque 2006) and the CTX-M enzymes have shown a dramatic increase, being the most prevalent ESBLs worldwide.

The CTX-M family can be subdivided into several clusters and mutational events lead to emergence of variants within each cluster. These encoding genes are highly mobile, mobility and expression being further promoted by the association, for example, of many of the CRX-M genes with insertion sequences. A further issue is that of co-resistance whereby the genes encoding ESBLs are often physically linked in integrons, transposons and/or plasmids with genes encoding resistance to other structurally unrelated resistance genes.

ESBLs initially were of particular concern in nosocomial situations and little attention was paid to the spread of these antibiotic resistant bacteria in the food chain (but see Andreoletti et al. 2008) and other routes such as water and effluent. Drug resistant bacteria and their genes including those encoding CTX-M and CMY beta lactamases are widespread and have spread rapidly in the Enterobacteriaceae in many parts of the world. Third generation cephalosporins such as ceftiofur are widely used in many different food animals and there are often minimal restrictions placed on their use. Recently a fourth generation cephalosporin (cefquinone) was approved in the EU and it is likely to be approved shortly by the US Food and Drug Administration without label restriction.

Poultry production in the USA relies extensively on lactams such as ceftiofur which may be given by direct injection of eggs before chickens hatch or by dipping eggs in beta lactams. In Canada probably the majority of hatcheries use the injecting of hatching eggs with ceftiofur. This may be why there has been a marked increase in ESBL *E.coli* (Pitout et al. 2009) isolates causing infections in people with a community onset around the world. The role of poultry in the spread of resistant organisms, especially *E.coli*, is probably unappreciated in view of the extensive movement of chicken meat under the World Trade Agreements. Chicken meat as a potential source of quinolone-resistant *E.coli* producing ESBLs in the UK has been reported. With respect to red meat, monitoring of ESBLs in the UK showed that all ESBLs detected in *E.coli* from clinical diagnostic samples have originated from cattle (Liebana et al. 2002). The Veterinary Laboratory Agency (VLA) has identified ESBL producing *E.coli* in horses and sheep on a farm visited following the detection of *E.coli* producing CTX-M-15 from cattle. The isolates of recently recovered *E.coli* carrying ESBLs have come from different counties of the UK so that these enzymes are widespread. Most of the isolates in the UK were from calves under two weeks of age, of which 15 were positive for the CTX-M-15 enzyme and 8 for the CTX-M-14 enzyme. The former is the most common ESBL *E.coli* in the UK, while CTX-M-14 is the next most common. Other types also found in cattle are CTX-M-1, -3-20- and 32. The *E.coli* strains in cattle and humans are generally different but analysis of the plasmids carrying the resistant genes suggests they have been transferring between human and bovine *E.coli*. The authors point out that that if human *E.coli* can transfer ESBL resistant plasmids to bovine *E.coli*, transfer may also be occurring in the opposite direction and thus the spread of resistant plasmids among bovine *E.coli* may therefore pose a serious threat to human health.

Use of antibiotics in animals

As the use of antibiotics in human patients expanded so did the use in animals for infections difficult to treat such as mastitis and pneumonia in farm livestock but also other injections in companion animals. But a particular aspect of use in animals referred to in the introduction was the use of antibiotics as growth promoters in growing livestock such as pigs, calves and chickens. A major concern was the possibility of the use of antibiotics as growth promoters leading, via the food chain, to resistance to antibiotics used for the treatment of human infections. The Swann Committee in 1969 set up to report on antimicrobial use in man and animals, concluded there was a significant problem, particularly in antibiotics use in animal feed as a growth promoter. Swann recommended that a Committee be set up with authority to review and recommend antibiotic use in man, animals and horticulture. Such a committee was not established until the UK House of Lords Scientific and Technology Committee on Resistance to Antibiotics and other Antimicrobial Agents in 1998 reminded the UK Government of the situation and pressed for the long awaited 'Swann Committee'. The Scientific Advisory Committee on Antibiotic Resistance (SACAR) was the result (see previous comments).

Resistance derived from growth promoters

The concern over the transfer of multi-resistance derived from growth promoters via the food chain to human patients has occasioned much debate and though clear evidence of antibiotic resistance in man deriving from growth promoter use has been sparse, nevertheless all authorities believe the prudent use of antibiotics in food producing animals should have high priority. The EU-wide ban on the use of four growth promoting antibiotics, namely spiramycin, tylosin, bacitracin zinc and virginiamycin, was later ratified by the UK. The remaining antibiotic growth promoters (monensin, avilamycin, salinomycin and flavomycin) came under EU-wide ban in January 2006.

The important concern of antibiotic use in growth promotion, and the possibility of resistance developing to human pathogens, has been dealt with by banning the use of certain antibiotics for growth promotion. Nevertheless, antibiotics are much in use for the treatment of infections in production animals and the overall sales of therapeutic antimicrobials for food animals has remained much the same over the last eight year period.

MRSA in animals

An important bacterial infection is that caused by Staphylococcus Aureus and its associated resistance to methicillin—hence methicillin resistance (MRSA). Hitherto MRSA was a human pathogen almost exclusively but it has now been reported in livestock and companion animals by the European Food and Safety Authority (EFSA). It is reported that food producing animals such as pigs, calves and broiler chickens often carry without clinical signs a specific strain of MRSA named CC398, but there is no evidence to date that eating or handling food contaminated with MRSA is a health risk for humans. However, people in contact with live animals that carry 398 are at risk of infection.

Some strains of community acquired MRSA (CA-MRSA) are thought to have originated in hospitals and then been taken into the community but most workers consider the strain to have developed independently (Coombs *et al.* 2004). Now CA-MRSA strains have become firmly established, especially in the USA, and a report by Penn (2005) showed that 70% of all MRSA strains have been reported globally. Patients with CA-MRSA infections are significantly younger than those with hospital acquired infections, those with CA-MRSA with a medium age of 30 compared with 70 with hospital acquired MRSA, in a Minnesota study (Naimi *et al.* 2003).

Of particular concern is that CA-MRSA is often more virulent and can spread more easily than hospital acquired MRSA. But in addition MRSA which produces the Panton-Valentine leukocidin (PVL) toxin is much more common in CA-MRSA strains, although in 2006 PVL-MRSA was reported in hospitals in the UK (Labandeira-Rey *et al.* 2007). PVL-MRSA is associated with necrotizing pneumonia as well as necrotizing fasciitis. In addition to CA-MRSA a further MRSA has been recognized, namely

farm-animal MRSA. CA-MRSA and farm animal MRSA differ from hospital acquired MRSA in that they differ in the antibiotic resistance. (For a detailed account of the genetics of these strains see Nunan and Young (2007).)

As with MRSA in man, CA-MRSA and farm animal MRSA are increasingly found in pigs, due to increasing use of antibiotics in animal husbandry. However, the extent of the threat to human health of animal derived MRSAs is uncertain. People living on pig farms (in the Netherlands) have carriage rates of about 50% and some patients have infections due to these MRSAs. But an important question is whether the strain will spread from those living on pig farms to others in the community. If so, animal derived MRSA may pose an important source of MRSA as a zoonoses (Kluytmans 2007).

Recently, companion animals such as cats, dogs and horses have been reported to carry both human-type MRSA as well as animal associated strains of MRSA (Hawkey 2008). Hawkey (2008) also mentions that MRSA strains have been identified in food animals and he mentions that there has been spread to humans in the Netherlands (de Neeling *et al.* 2007). Also Hawkey (2008) refers to the clonal strain 398 that has been associated with dog, pig and horse (see also Witte *et al.* 2007).

In a recent study of MRSA in slaughter pigs in Germany 49 to 70% of various batches of pigs from various regions in Germany were positive for MRSA showing a wide range of resistances to terythromycin, clindamycin, oxacillin, tetracycline, and other antimicrobials. Most isolates from pigs belong to the multilocus sequence type (MLST) ST 398 which the authors state is increasing and is more prevalent in rural than urban locations (Tenhagen *et al.* 2009).

Responding to the threat

International concern over the threat from antibiotic resistance has led to a number of initiatives to mobilize action.

Responsible Use of Medicines in Agriculture (RUMA): The livestock sector of agriculture has responded to criticism by the formation of RUMA, a consortium of veterinarians, agriculturists and pharmaceutical organizations. As well as the collection and analysis of data referring to antimicrobial sales and usage, it produces guidelines and advice on antimicrobial use. This is a welcome illustration of private sector concern and action, addressing the nexus between animal and humans use of antibiotics.

Committee for Medicinal Products for Veterinary Use (CVMP): This Committee of the European Medicines Agency (2009) has produced a reflective paper on the use of third- and fourth-generation cephalosporins in food-producing animals in the EU with reference to the development of resistance and impact on human and animal health. This paper discusses cephalosporins with a focus on substances of the third- and fourth-generation and food-producing animals but excludes these compounds in aquaculture. The paper gives a good account of the mechanism in action, classification and spectrum of activity. It gives a useful list of the various generative cephalosporins (first through fourth) and the resistance of various organisms to cephalosporins.

Reservoirs of Antibiotic Resistance Network (ROAR): This network originated from the Alliance for the Prudent Use of Antibiotics (AUPA) recognizing the misuse of antibiotics in medicine, veterinary medicine and agriculture, and also their use in non-medical areas such as horticulture for the control of fungal infestation on fruit, etc. ROAR (2002) made the case that commensal bacteria are reservoirs of resistance and the microbes are everywhere, in water and soil and in the bodies, mainly the digestive tract, of humans and animals. The vast majority do not cause disease but they may not be completely innocuous. Disease causing bacteria have frequent contact with these commensals from a multitude of sources and they then can serve as reservoirs for resistance genes exchanging resistance information and holding that information for future transmission to disease causing bacteria. ROAR states that bacteria in every environment where antibiotics are used are constantly exchanging genes that confer resistance to antibiotics. When a human or animal patient is treated with an antibiotic the pathogenic organism causing the disease may well be controlled by this antibiotic but commensal bacteria in the gut of the patient are also exposed to the antibiotic and these then exchange resistant genes with other commensals and subsequently with pathogens. ROAR maintains that even if a bacterium occupies a person's intestine for only a short period, gene exchange between two bacteria may take less than one hour. Evidence is said to be growing that extensive horizontal transfer of antibiotic resistance genes is occurring between clinical and non-clinical bacteria, between animal and human intestinal bacteria and intestinal and soil bacteria. Indeed Salyers, Shoemaker and Schlesinger (2008) comment that the movement of antibiotic resistant genes, as opposed to movement of resistant bacterial strains, has become an issue in connection with clinical and agricultural antibiotic use. They state that evidence suggests that extensive DNA transfer in occurring in natural settings includes cross genes lines and is probably mediated mainly by conjugative transfer of plasmids and transposons. Hence reservoir bacteria may be important in the spread and maintenance of resistant genes.

Conclusion

Hawkey (2008) has well summarized the present antibiotic resistance issue. He states that we live in a microbiologically interlinked world in which resistance genes derived from animals can colonize human bowel flora which are then excreted and via sewage systems find their way back into land and water and then to animals. Cycling of resistance genes in hospitals and then via the faecal oral route in the community and then via sewage systems to water and soil, is another example of inter-linkage. An additional concern is that some compounds such as quaternary ammonium compounds used in fabric conditioning, and which are not thought of as having antimicrobial activity can select for antibiotic resistance genes (Gaze *et al.* 2005). Hawkey (2008) comments that we live in a world where there is greater mobility of people and food and other goods that can lead to the greater probability of the spread of resistant clones that may emerge in distant locations. He quotes the carriage of CTX-M beta lactamase genes in the faecal flora of persons in China and India, where estimates are as high as 10% in a combined population of 2.5 billion and which must represent the largest reservoir of antimicrobial resistance genes capable of conferring resistance to important antibiotics used to treat Gram-negative infection, 'It is only through the prudent use of antimicrobial drugs and the introduction of new and effective agents, particularly against multi-drug-resistant strains as a

worldwide effort, that the march of antibiotic resistance will be slowed down'.

Finch (2007) in looking to the future voices the concerns that antibiotic resistance holds for the future health of mankind. He notes that 'the speed with which resistance is currently escalating among community as well as hospital microorganisms is extremely worrisome'. A strategy to contain resistance and prolong the useful life of existing therapies is not unrealistic. He concludes that 'to do nothing is not an option'.

References

Ambler, R.P. (1980). The structure of beta-lactamases. *Philos. Trans. R. Soc. Lond. Bio. Sci.* **289**: 321–31.

Andreoletti, O., Budka, H., Buncic, S., *et al.* (2008). Food-borne antimicrobial resistance as a biological hazard. Draft Scientific Opinion of the Panel on Biological Hazards, European Food Safety Authority, pp. 1–91.

Canton, R., and Coque, T.M. (2006). The CTX-M beta-lactamase pandemic. *Curr. Opin. Microbiol.* **9**: 466–75.

Coombs, G.W., Nimmo, G.R., Bell J.M., Huygens, E., O'Brien, E.G., *et al.* and the Australian group for Antimicrobial Resistance (2004). Genetic Diversity among community methicillin-resistant Staphylococcus aureus strains causing outpatient infections in Australia. *J. Clin. Microbiol.* **42**: 4735–44.

de Neeling, A.J., van den Broek, M.J., Spalburg, E.C., Santen-Verheuvel, M.G., Dam-Deisz, W.D., *et al.* (2007). High prevalence of methicillin resistant Staphylococcus aureus in pigs. *Vet. Microbiol.* **12**: 366–72.

Finch, R. (2007). Innovation - drugs and diagnostics. *J. Antimicrob. Chemother.* **60** (Suppl 1.): 79–82.

Gaze, W.H., Abdouslam, N., Hawkey, P.M., and Wellington, E.M. (2005). Incidence of Class 1 integrons in a quaternary ammonium compound-polluted environment. *Antimicrob. Agents Chemother.*, **49**: 182–7.

Hawkey, P.M. (2008). Review. molecular epidemiology of clinically significant antibiotic resistant genes. *Brit. J. Pharmacol.*, **153**: S406–13.

House of Lords Select Committee on Science and Technology Session 1997–8, 7th Report. Resistance to antibiotics and other antimicrobial agents. Chairman Lord Soulsby, London, The Stationary Office.

Kluytmans, J. (2007). Quoted by Nunan, C. and Young, R., (2007). MRSA in Farm Animals and Meat.

Labandeira-Rey, M., Couzon, F., Boisset, S., Brown, E.L., Bes, M., Benito, Y., Barbu, E.M., *et al.* (2007). Staphylococcus aureus Panton-Valentine leukocidin causes necrotic pneumonia. *Science*, **315**: 1130–33.

Liebana, E., Batchelor, M., Hopkins, K.L., Clifton-Hadley F.A., Teale C.J., *et al.* (2006). Longitudinal farm study of extended spectrum B-Lactamase-mediated resistance. *J. Clin. Microbiol.*, **44**(5): 1630–34.

Livermore, D.M. (2008a). Defining an extended -spectrum beta lactamase. *Clin. Microbiol. Infect.*, **14**(Suppl 1): 3–10.

Livermore, D.M. (2008b). The Zeitgeist of Resistance. *J. Antimicrob. Chemother.* **60**(Suppl.): 59–61.

Livermore, D.M., Canton, R., Gniadkowski, M., *et al.* (2007). CTX-M: Changing face of ESBLs in Europe. *J. Antimicrob. Chemother.*, **59**: 165–75.

Naimi, T.S., LeDell, K.H., Como-Sabetti, K., Borchardt, S.M., Boxrud, D.J., *et al.* (2003). Comparison of community and healthcare-associated methicillin-resistant Staphylococcus aureus infection. *JAMA*, **290**: 2976–84.

Nunan, C., and Young, R. (2007). MRSA in farm animals and meat. A new threat to human health. Rept 5: The use and misuse of antibiotics in UK agriculture. Soil Association.

Penn, C. (2005). Pandemic bug returns as community MRSA strain. New Scientist News Service, 1 April.

Pitout, J.D., Gregson, D.B., Campbell, L, and Laupland, K.B. (2009). Molecular characterisitics of extended-spectrum-beta-lactamase-producing Escherichia coli isolates causing bacteremia in the Calgary

Health Region from 2000 to 2007: emergence of clone ST131 as a cause of community acquired infections. *Antimicrob. Agents Chemother.*, **53**(7): 2846–51.

ROAR (2002). Reservoirs of Antibiotic Resistance. 22 March 1998 Meeting. Building a Scientific Network to Monitor Antibiotic Resistance Genes in Non Clinical Bacteria http://www.tufts.edu./med/apua/ROAR/Meeting.htm

Salyers, A.A., Shoemaker, N., and Schlesinger, D. (2008). Ecology of Antibiotic Resistant Genes. In: R.G. Wax, K. Lewis, A. Salyers, and H. Taber,: Bacteria Resistance to Antimicrobials (2nd ed.) (eds.) pp. 11–21. Baca Raton, London, New York: CRC Press.

Soulsby, L. (2008). The 2008 Garrod Lecture: Antimicrobial resistance—animals and the environment. *J. Antimicrob. Chemother.*, **62**(2): 229–33.

Swann, M.M., Baxter, K.C., Field, H.L. *et al.* (1969). Report of the Joint Committee on the Use of Antibiotics in Animal Husbandry and Veterinary Medicine. London, HMSO.

Tenhagen, B.A., Fetsch, A., Stuherenberg, B., Schleuter, G., Guerra, B., *et al.* (2009). Prevalence of MRSA types in slaughter pigs in different German abattoirs. *Vet. Rec.*, **165**: 589–93.

Wise, R. (2007). An Overview of the Specialist Advisory Committee on Antimicrobial Resistance (SACAR). *J. Antimicrob. Chemother.*, **60**:(Suppl 1): 5–7.

Witte, W., Strommenger, R., Stanek, G. and Cuny, C. (2007). Methicillin resistant Staphylococcus aureus ST398 in humans and animals, Central Europe. *Emerg. Infect. Dis.*, **13**: 255–58.

PART 2

Bacterial, chlamydial, and rickettsial zoonoses

CHAPTER 6

Anthrax

Les Baillie and Theresa Huwar

Summary

Anthrax is caused by the bacterium *Bacillus anthracis*, a Gram-positive aerobic spore-forming bacillus, primarily infecting herbivores. Although rare in the developed world, the organism remains a threat to livestock in African and Asian countries where control depends on appropriate animal husbandry approaches such as vaccination and disposal/decontamination of carcasses. Animals are thought to contract anthrax by ingesting spores from contaminated soil while humans become infected via contact with diseased animals, their products or as a consequence of acts of bioterrorism such as occurred in 2001. This unprecedented act has stimulated a burst of research, shedding new light on the biology of the organism and its ability to cause disease. It is to be hoped that through this renewed interest anthrax will once again regain the status of an exotic disease of antiquity.

History and background

Anthrax has been a scourge of man and animals since the first written history of disease. It may have been one of the plagues of Egypt in the time of Moses (*c.* 1250 BC) and accounts of its symptoms can be found in the writings of ancient scholars such as Homer (*c.* 1000 BC) and Galen (*c.* AD 200) demonstrating the disease was well known to the Greeks and Romans. The earliest scientific (as opposed to historical) reports are the descriptions of malignant pustules by Maret in 1752 and of the disease in animals by Chabert in 1780 (Wilson and Miles 1946). The nineteenth century work on anthrax has more than usual significance, underpinning a major turning point in the history of medicine. It was the first disease of man (Woolsorter's disease) and animals shown to be caused by a microorganism, enabling Koch to established his postulates in 1877 by proving *Bacillus anthracis* (named by Cohn in 1875) was the cause of anthrax. Subsequent researchers such as Greenfield and Pasteur in the early 1880s demonstrated the feasibility of using attenuated live vaccines to protect livestock, establishing histories second bacterial vaccine. At the turn of twentieth century Metchnikoff employed *B. anthracis* to characterize the ability of macrophages to kill microbes and helped establish the field of immunology.

During the twentieth century the scientific fruits of these endeavours, particularly the development and extensive use of animal vaccines, saw the status of the organism reduced to an exotic disease responsible for occasional outbreaks in animals and rare secondary infections in humans. It is ironic that while science developed the tools to manage the threat posed by anthrax, it also facilitated its development as a biological weapon.

While there are reports of the use of anthrax against cavalry horses during the First World War, serious efforts to develop anthrax weapons did not begin until the outbreak of World War II. In 1942 trials off the coast of Scotland demonstrated the feasibility of using *B. anthracis* spores as a biological weapon, and while the Allies sought to develop anthrax bombs they were never used in anger. The UK offensive program was terminated in the 1950s, with the USA program following suite in 1969. The Japanese and Soviets also had offensive biological weapons programs during the war and though the Japanese program terminated, the Soviet effort continued (Zilinskas 2006).

B. anthracis has been weaponized by various nations, most recently Iraq in 1991. The simplicity of the production technology and the availability of the organism in nature have made anthrax an attractive terror option for extremist groups such as the Aum Shinrikyo cult (Keim *et al.* 2001). The ability of a small scale attack to disrupt the infrastructure of a whole country was amply demonstrated by the 2001 postal attacks in the USA.

The agent

Taxonomy

Bacillus anthracis is the only obligate pathogen within the genus *Bacillus*, comprising the Gram-positive aerobic or facultative anaerobic spore-forming, rod-shaped bacteria. It is a member of the genetically closely related '*Bacillus cereus* group' comprised of *B. cereus*, *B. anthracis*, *B. thuringiensis*, *B. mycoides*, *B. pseudomycoides*, and *B. weinhenstephanensis*. However, it can be clearly identified by phenotypic traits such as virulence (which can be lost), lack of motility, absence of haemolysis on sheep and horse blood agar, susceptibility to penicillin, and sensitivity to the diagnostic gamma bacteriophage.

At the genetic level *B. anthracis* can be clearly distinguished by a range of DNA-based approaches, such as multilocus sequence typing (MLST), which targets chromosomal sequences (Priest *et al.* 2004). While snap shot techniques such as MLST enable the relationship of large numbers of isolates to be rapidly assessed, it is now feasible economically to determine the entire genetic sequence of the bacterium. Analysis of the genome of the Ames strain of *B. anthracis* revealed a 5.23 megabase chromosome essentially identical to *B.cereus* and *B.thuringiensis*, suggesting a common insect pathogen ancestor that acquired additional plasmid borne virulence factors (Read *et al.* 2003). The diversity of phenotypes within this group is often mediated by plasmid encoded factors. In the case of *B. anthracis* these comprise two plasmids, pXO1 (182 kb) and pXO2 (96 kb), both encoding major virulence factors (Fig. 6.1).The ability of these virulence plasmids to be transferred to other members of the *B.cereus* group has been reported. An example of this is *B.cereus* G9241, which was isolated from individuals presenting with an infection clinically indistinguishable from inhalational anthrax (Hoffmaster *et al.* 2004). Genetic analysis revealed the presence of a homolog to pXO1 and a second plasmid, which although genetically distinct from pXO2, encoded a phenotypically similar anti-phagocytic capsule.

Given the central role of virulence plasmids in pathogenicity and their ability to move between closely related strains we should take care in dismissing all clinical isolates of *B.cereus* as environmental contaminants.

Life cycle

Under conditions that favour growth, *B. anthracis* forms large, non-motile Gram-positive square ended rods which produce opaque, white, non-haemolytic colonies when grown on sheep blood agar. The colony has a rough surface with an irregular edge appearing filamentous when viewed using a hand lens. In contrast, if cultured in the presence of 5% CO_2 the organism forms a capsule (Uchida *et al.* 1993) and the resulting colonies are smooth and mucoid.

Unfavourable growth conditions, such as nutrient limitation, result in the formation of highly resistant, oval spores clearly visible in the centre of the bacilli in stained smears (Fig. 6.2). Spore formation is a survival strategy which enables the organism to persist for decades and survive exposure to physical and chemical insults. The spore is constructed as an internal double membrane-bound compartment, called the forespore, over the course of several hours. Dormancy and resistance depend in part on the partial dehydration of the inner compartment of the spore, known as the core, which houses the chromosome. This core is surrounded by a thick layer of peptidoglycan, known as the cortex, which is further enveloped by the spore coat. The outer most layer of the spore, which is separated by a gap, is called the exosporium.

The various proteinaceous layers which comprise the spore protect the cortex from damage by mechanisms which still remain unclear. It is possible that the exosporium and spore coat act as a permeability barrier to some chemicals or that toxic agents react with the various layers reducing the amount of agent available to attack essential molecules such as enzymes and DNA located in the spore core.

In addition to contributing to physical protection, the exosporium also contains biologically active enzymes thought to play a role in the intracellular survival of the vegetative bacterium within the phagolysosome of the macrophage (Kang *et al.* 2005). These include enzymes which subvert the production of antibacterial radicals, such as superoxide and nitric oxide, in addition to enzymes that regulate *in vivo* germination (Baillie *et al.* 2005; Raines *et al.* 2006; Weaver *et al.* 2007).

The ability to regulate germination is due to presence of enzymes such as alanine racemase and an inosine preferring nucleoside hydrolase. Alanine racemase, an inhibitor of germination, converts L-alanine to D-alanine, a form not recognized by the alanine specific germination receptor of *B. anthracis*. It has been proposed that spores employ this mechanism to prevent germination under

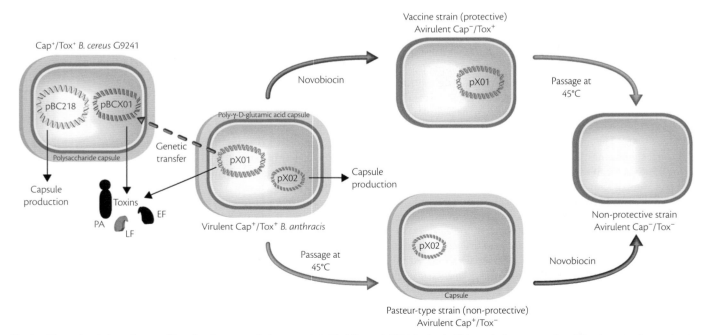

Fig. 6.1 The major virulence factors of *B.anthracis* are encoded on two plasmid, pXO1 and pXO2, both of which can be lost or transferred to other organisms, as is thought to be the case with *B.cereus* G9241

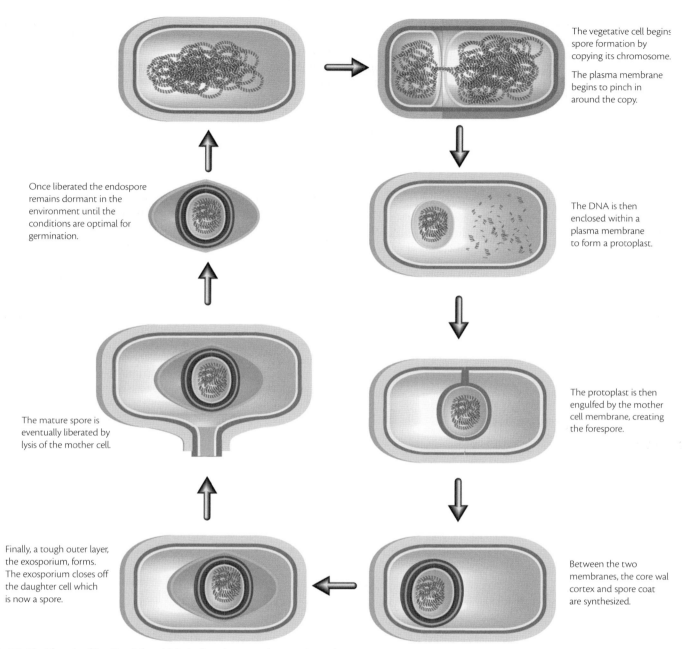

The vegetative cell begins spore formation by copying its chromosome.

The plasma membrane begins to pinch in around the copy.

Once liberated the endospore remains dormant in the environment until the conditions are optimal for germination.

The DNA is then enclosed within a plasma membrane to form a protoplast.

The mature spore is eventually liberated by lysis of the mother cell.

The protoplast is then engulfed by the mother cell membrane, creating the forespore.

Finally, a tough outer layer, the exosporium, forms. The exosporium closes off the daughter cell which is now a spore.

Between the two membranes, the core wall cortex and spore coat are synthesized.

Fig. 6.2 The life cycle of *B.anthracis* from biologically active vegetative organism to inert spore

sub-optimal conditions such as high spore numbers in soil or non-permissive environments encountered during infection (Hu *et al.* 2006; Titball and Manchee 1987).

Environmental growth and survival

There is debate concerning the ability of *B. anthracis* to replicate outside an infected host. As a consequence, it has been regarded as an obligate pathogen whose environmental presence reflects contamination from an animal source rather than self-maintenance in the environment. The ability of the organism to germinate and replicate greatly depend on the local conditions such as availability of germinants and nutrients, pH, temperature, moisture, and the presence of microbial competitors and predators such as bacteriophages. However, while replication is uncommon, germination, gene transfer, and spore formation can occur under certain environmental conditions such as those found in the immediate vicinity of plant roots and in organically rich soils (Saile and Koehler 2006; Baillie Labs, unpublished data). However, once spores have been formed, it is well established that they can survive for long periods, and the time interval between host infection can be decades.

Detection

While culture based methods have been developed to identify the presence of *B. anthracis* in environmental samples, they are time consuming and can lack sensitivity due to the need to eliminate other closely related members of the *B. cereus* group. For this reason rapid antibody and DNA based assays have been developed which target unique signatures associated with the major virulence factors (toxins and capsule), the chromosome and the spore surface. While these assays are considerably faster than culture, giving results in hours versus days, there are concerns over sensitivity and specificity—particularly against environmental samples.

An additional complication is that the organism is normally present as a spore in nature. This means that the majority of rapid DNA based assays include an additional step to crack open the spore and access the DNA target. The methodologies adopted to achieve this focus primarily on physical and chemical disruption and while effective, they can detect <10 spores in a sample, the multi-step processes required are labour intensive and time consuming.

Alternative approaches target spore surface located factors such as *BclA*, a major glycoprotein of the exosporium, and cellular debris derived from the mother cell which includes both protein and DNA encoding virulence factors. By employing the polymerase chain reaction (PCR) to detect surface located DNA one can identify as few as 10^2 spores within 2 hrs. Indeed it is now feasible to detect DNA on the surface of a spores in as little as 30 seconds (Kadir *et al.* 2007).

Molecular and genetic aspects of pathogenesis

The organism has two major virulence factors, a tripartite toxin and an antiphagocytic capsule encoded by genes carried on two plasmids pXO1 and pXO2. The loss of either plasmid results in a marked reduction in virulence (Little and Ivins 1999). Plasmid pXO1 encodes a tripartite toxin comprising Lethal Factor (LF-776 amino acids) a metaloprotease, Oedema Factor (EF-767 amino acids) a cyclic AMP modulator, and Protective Antigen (PA-735 amino acids) the non-toxic, cell binding component responsible for transporting LF and EF into the cell. This toxin accounts for the majority of the pathology, while pXO2 encodes an antiphagocytic capsule composed of poly-D-glutamic acid, thought to inhibit uptake by immune effector cells such as macrophages (Makino *et al.* 2002).

The tripartite toxin follows the AB model where the A moiety is comprised of catalytic subunits LF and EF, and the B moiety, PA, translocates EF or LF into the cytosol. The B moiety is named due to its role as the key protective immunogen in the current human vaccine. It binds to ubiquitous cell surface receptors, two of which have been identified; anthrax toxin receptor/tumour endothelial marker 8 and capillary morphogenesis protein 2. Upon binding, PA is cleaved by the cell-surface protease furin to expose the A moiety binding site (Bradley *et al.* 2001; Rainey and Young 2004). Following proteolytic activation, PA forms a membrane-inserting heptamer that translates LF and EF into the cytosol (Petosa *et al.* 1997). The current working model (Leppla 1991) of *in vivo* toxin uptake is shown in Fig. 6.3.

Experimental evidence indicates that this is not the only model of toxin interaction and uptake (Panchal *et al.* 2005). PA and LF can form biologically active complexes in serum capable of killing susceptible macrophages.

Irrespective of how the toxin complex enters the cell, Lethal Toxin (LT), the combination of LF and PA, is the central effector of shock and death (Smith and Keppie 1954). The toxin contains a thermolysin-like active site and zinc-binding consensus motif HExxH, which acts as a Zn^{2+} metalloprotease on a range of substrates, including peptide hormones and Mitogen-Activated Protein Kinases (MAPK) (Duesbery *et al.* 1998; Pellizzari *et al.* 1999). The MAPK cascade is essential for full induction of the oxidative burst and pro-inflammatory cytokine expression, and its disruption neutralizes macrophage activation favouring bacterial escape from lymph nodes during the initial phase of infection (Baldari *et al.* 2006).

The combination of EF and PA results in oedema toxin (ET) causing oedema through the elevation of cellular cyclic AMP (cAMP) concentrations in affected tissues. Once in contact with the

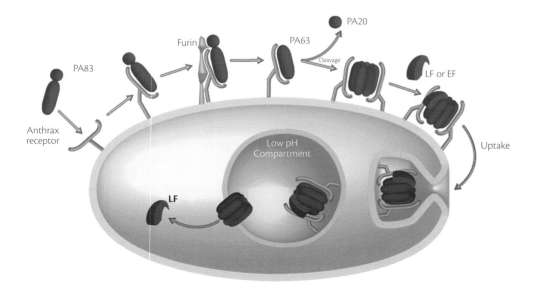

Fig. 6.3 The current working model of *in vivo* toxin uptake (Leppla 1991)

cytoplasm, EF binds calmodulin (a eukaryotic calcium-binding protein) becoming enzymatically active, converting ATP to cAMP. The effects are the same as those caused by cholera toxin, with intoxicated cells secreting large amounts of fluid (Leppla 1991).

The overall contribution of ET to the infective process is ill defined. It is generally considered that the pathological changes seen in infected animals are due to the LT and that these acute effects mask any cAMP-mediated responses. However, purified ET has been shown to inhibit chemotactic response of polymorpho-nuclear leukocytes and subsequent phagocytosis (O'Brien *et al.* 1985; Wright and Mandell 1986).

Both LT and ET are expressed soon after germination and suppress superoxide and nitric oxide production, which are key antibacterial killing mechanisms of the macrophage (O'Brien *et al.* 1985; Pellizzari *et al.* 1999). Following escape from the macrophage the two toxins target all the cells of the innate and adaptive immune system, subverting cell signalling so as to suppress their ability to mount a protective immune response against the bacteria, resulting in massive bacteremia and toxemia (Baldari *et al.* 2006).

As infection progresses the accumulation of toxin induces the development of cytokine independent shock. This is thought to be related to the direct injurious effects of LT on the endothelial cell function which ultimately contributes to death (Moayeri and Leppla 2004; Sherer *et al.* 2007).

While the toxins play an important role in virulence, to be fully pathogenic an infecting strain of *B. anthracis* must also produce a capsule. This structure is composed of a polypeptide, poly-D-glutamic acid which is thought to inhibit phagocytosis and opsonisa-tion of the bacilli by virtue of its negative charge. The genes controlling capsule synthesis, *capB*, *capC* and *capA*, are present as an operon on the pXO2 plasmid. Their expression is in part regulated by serum, CO_2 and temperature via an unclear mechanism involving the product of the *atxA* and *acpA* genes, which also regulate toxin expression.

In addition to the major factors already described, the bacterium expresses other plasmid and chromosome encoded genes which contribute to the overall pathogenesis of the organism (Baillie and Read 2001). Differential expression of any or all of these genes may explain why wild type strains differ in virulence. Candidate virulence factors include chromosomally encoded extracellular proteases, phospholipases such as cereolysin and S layer proteins. Interestingly PlcR, a global transcription regulator of a virulence regulon thought to play a major role in insect virulence is defective in *B. anthracis*, possibly due to the acquisition of pXO1 (Mignot *et al.* 2001).

Disease mechanisms

Infection commences subsequent to entry of the spore into the body by one of a number of routes and is followed by germination and multiplication locally or after transport to the regional lymph nodes. Germination *in vivo* plays a key role in pathogenicity; while spores germinate poorly in serum, the process is considerably more efficient within professional phagocytic cells such as alveolar mac-rophages. Recent data suggests that exposure to antibacterial free radicals generated within the phagolysosome triggers germination by inactivating negative regulators of germination such as alanine racemase located on the surface of the spore (Baillie *et al.* 2005).

In cutaneous infections, germination, multiplication and production of the toxin result in the characteristic eschar invariably accompanied by extensive oedema. Neutrophils, rather than mac-rophages, are the first white blood cells recruited to the site of a cutaneous infection (Mayer-Scholl *et al.* 2005). These cells are particularly adept at combating *B. anthracis* and their effectiveness is thought to account for why the majority of cutaneous infections spontaneously resolve.

Inhalational anthrax differs from cutaneous infection because inhaled spores are taken up by alveolar macrophages and pulmonary dendritic cells rather than neutrophils and are then carried to mediastinal lymph nodes. Following germination bacteria are released and lymphadenitis develops with minor, often unreported symptoms including malaise, mild fever and a mild cough. Bacteria frequently overcome the lymph-node filter, and enter lymphatic and blood circulation, causing massive bacteremia and toxemia. This blood borne phase is accompanied by major symptoms including fever, enlarged lymph nodes, pulmonary oedema with acute dyspnea (laboured respiration) and cynosis (bluish discoloration of the skin caused by poor blood oxygenation). As infection progresses accumulation of toxin and other bacterial derived factors inactivate the innate and adaptive immune systems, damage endothelial cell function and induce cytokine independent shock which ultimately results in death.

The primary role of toxin in causing death has been demonstrated experimentally in laboratory animals. There is an inverse relationship between susceptibility to infection and susceptibility to toxin. Guinea-pigs are highly susceptible to infection, yet quite resistant to toxin, while the opposite is true for rats. Toxin sensitivity could be linked to polymorphisms in a gene called *Nalp1b* which has been identified in toxin sensitive laboratory mice. The gene encodes a protein involved in the recognition of microbial components and danger-associated host molecules (Boyden and Dietrich 2006). In contrast to mice and rats, human and primate cells have been reported to be relative resistant to lethal toxin possibly due to variations in the coding sequence of the primate version of *Nalp1*.

Hosts

Anthrax is primarily a disease of warm blooded animals such as herbivores, particularly human food animals, and has a world-wide distribution. Prior to the advent of effective animal vaccines it caused heavy losses in cattle, sheep, goats, horses and donkeys. In 1923 in South Africa it was estimated that 30,000–60,000 animals died of anthrax (Sterne 1967). Species vary in their susceptibility to different aspects of the infectious agent, for example, while dogs are relatively resistant to spore challenge they are extremely sensitive to anthrax toxin (Lincoln *et al.* 1967).

The pathogenic process in humans is, understandably, ill defined. The extrapolation of disease responses in experimental animals to man is complex, although the limited data available indicate that the infective process in humans is similar to that seen in animals (Phipps *et al.* 2004).

Healthy individuals can tolerate low level exposure to anthrax spores. A study of mill workers found that individuals could inhale 600–1,300 spores during the working day with no ill effect, although no indication was given as to the size of the particles inhaled (Dahlgren *et al.* 1960). This is an important factor—animals studies have demonstrated that to gain access to the body via the lungs, aerosol particles should be <5 μm. Attempts to use primate data to determine an infectious dose for humans has proved challenging, not least because of the outbred, diverse nature of the general population with regards to age, size, and health status. As a general guide, a dose of spores lethal for 50% of the individuals challenged via the aerosol route has been estimated at between 250–5,500 spores (Inglesby *et al.* 2002). It should be noted that this is an average dose, it is estimated that Ottilie Lundgren, aged 94, the last fatal victim of the anthrax postal attacks, was exposed to a single spore.

Clinical manifestations and diagnosis in animals

Sudden death in a herbivore without prior symptoms or following a brief period of fever and disorientation should lead to suspicion of anthrax, and bloody fluid exuding from the nose, mouth, or anus of the dead animal is particularly suggestive. In pigs and carnivores, local oedemas, particularly in the neck region, are pathognomonic signs. At death, in most susceptible species, the blood contains 10^7–10^9 bacilli mL^{-1}, provided the animal has not been treated (numbers may also be lower in immunized animals which succumb to the disease). Pigs are noted for being an exception and the bacterium may be undetectable in their blood at death.

The blood of an anthrax victim clots poorly and usually the small volume of blood necessary for a diagnostic smear and culture can be drawn with a syringe from a vein in reasonably fresh carcass. Where that is not possible, a small piece of tissue, traditionally (but not necessarily) an ear clipping because of its high capillary content, preferably with signs of blood on it, can be excised and used to make a smear and for culture.

Smears should be stained with polychrome methylene blue (M'Fadyean's stain); large numbers of blue-black-staining bacilli, often square ended and in short chains, surrounded by a clearly demarcated pink capsule is fully diagnostic. Specimens for culture should be submitted to the appropriate diagnostic laboratory (Defra 2007).

If anthrax is suspected, the carcass should not be opened thus avoiding environmental contamination. In pigs, where confirmation may depend on obtaining the relevant lymph nodes (submandibular, suprapharyngeal, or mesenteric) for culture, appropriate precautions should be taken before dissection to avoid environmental contamination. For differential diagnosis, blackleg, botulism, toxicosis (e.g. toxic plants, heavy metals, snake bite), lightning strike, and peracute babesiosis may cause symptoms similar to those of anthrax (Turnbull 1998).

Clinical manifestations and diagnosis in humans

Three forms of the disease are recognized in humans: cutaneous, inhalational and gastrointestinal. The latter two forms are regarded as being most frequently fatal due to being unrecognized until it is too late to instigate effective treatment (Dixon *et al.* 1999). An occasional complication is meningitis. Subsequent infections in the same individual are rare (Heyworth *et al.* 1975).

Human anthrax is frequently differentiated into non-industrial or industrial anthrax depending on whether the disease is acquired directly from animals or indirectly during the handling and processing of contaminated animal products. Non-industrial anthrax usually affects people who work with animals or animal carcasses, such as farmers, abattoir workers, knackers, butchers, and veterinary personnel, and is almost always cutaneous, although occasionally intestinal if, as occurs in developing countries, the owners' skin, butcher, and eat the meat (Baillie 1999).

Industrial anthrax, occurring as a result of contact with contaminated animal products is usually cutaneous but has a higher chance of being inhalational through exposure to spore-laden dust.

Analysis of the aerosolized spore content of a goat hair processing mill in the USA, where cases of inhalational anthrax had previously occurred, found that the spore load varied from day to day with workers being exposed to significant numbers of spores without ill effects suggesting that other factors contribute to susceptibility (Dahlgren *et al.* 1960). Indeed the unfortunate bongo drum maker in Scotland who contracted a fatal case of inhalational anthrax from untanned animals hides in 2006 suffered from an underlying health problem which is likely to have increased his susceptibility to infection (Anaraki *et al.* 2008).

Cutaneous anthrax

Entry of infecting spores occurs via a lesion in the skin with a small pimple occurring 3–5 days later. Over the next 2–3 days, the centre of the pimple ulcerates to become a dry, black, firmly adherent scab, surrounded by a ring of vesicles, the typical anthrax eschar. Despite its angry appearance, there is little pain; pain and pus only develop if there is secondary infection. Lesions vary greatly in size from about 2 cm to several centimetres across and are accompanied by pronounced oedema, which can become life threatening if located on the face or neck. In uncomplicated cases, the eschar begins to resolve about 10 days after the appearance of the initial papule; resolution takes 2–6 weeks, regardless of treatment leaving little trace. Complications arise when the organism spreads to the bloodstream resulting in an overwhelming infection in ~20% of untreated cutaneous cases. Diagnosis is made by M'Fadyean-stained smears and/or culture of pretreatment specimens of vesicular fluid obtained from under the edge of the eschar. For differential diagnosis, boil, orf, primary syphilitic chancre, erysipelas, plague, glanders, and tropical ulcer should be considered (Turnbull 1998).

Inhalational and intestinal anthrax

In pulmonary (due to inhalation of spores) and intestinal (due to ingestion of contaminated meat) forms of anthrax, the illness has an incubation period of 1–6 days, during which nonspecific symptoms of fever, sweats, fatigue, dyspenea, non-productive cough, and nausea can occur (Abramova *et al.* 1993; Jernigan *et al.* 2002). These symptoms persist for 2 or 3 days, and in some cases there is a short period of clinical improvement. This is followed by the sudden onset of increasing respiratory distress with dyspenea, stridor, cyanosis, increased chest pain, and sweating. Respiratory distress is typically followed by rapid onset of shock and death within 24–36 hours. Mortality rates of 45 to 100% have been reported (Jernigan *et al.* 2002; Phipps *et al.* 2004). The recent 'outbreak' of human anthrax in the USA in 2001 saw 22 cases of laboratory confirmed anthrax, half of which were inhalational in nature with five cases proving fatal (45% case fatality ratio).

Early recognition of individuals with inhalational anthrax is difficult as its prodrome is similar to many common acute respiratory illnesses. While there are significant chest radiograph differences between inhalational anthrax and community—acquired pneumonia such as mediastinitis, none of the changes taken alone are highly predictive of infection with *B. anthracis* in the absence of evidence of previous contact with the organism (Kyriacou *et al.* 2007).

In recent years a number of laboratory based assays have been developed to supplement the diagnostic potential of M'Fadyean-stained smears and microbiological culture. These approaches include PCR based detection of genes encoding virulence factors, immunohistochemical and ELISA based detection of toxin proteins, and detection of enzymically active lethal factor protein in biological samples by mass spectroscopy (Walsh *et al.* 2007).

Pathology

The characteristics of human infection, as seen by gross and microscopic observation, are largely similar to those seen in multiple animal models (for a review see Phipps *et al.* 2004). Studies of the pathology of human inhalation anthrax have focused primarily on mediastinal, hemi-lymphatic, and pulmonary changes. Events in the lung are unspectacular, being limited to haemorrhage, oedema, and atelectasis. This is due to it not being a primary site of infection but rather a portal of entry into the body, although secondary infection can occur once septicaemia has been established. Spores are taken up from the alveoli by macrophages and transported to a regional lymph node. Once there, they multiple and lyse their host cells, and escape in to the bloodstream to establish a systemic infection (Barnes 1947; Ross 1957). In contrast, mediastinal changes in humans are more pronounced, consisting primarily of oedema and haemorrhage with similar changes within the parenchyma of mediastinal lymph nodes which exhibit haemorrhage, necrosis, and the presence of Gram-positive bacteria as a consequence of lymphocytolysis. Vasculitis within the mediastinal lymph nodes is characterized by fibrinoid necrosis and infiltration by neutrophils and histiocytes.

The basic disease mechanism is vascular injury with oedema, haemorrhage, and thrombosis. Vascular injury is probably the result of toxin acting directly on the endothelial cell membrane, making them highly permeable to plasma, and causing adhesion of the leucocytes and platelets with widespread intravascular thrombosis (Dalldorf *et al.* 1971). Lesions in other organs beside lymphoid tissue, lungs, and brain have been described, but many appear to be secondary to shock and agonal changes.

Treatment
Antibiotics

Most strains are sensitive to penicillin, erythromycin, chloramphenicol, gentamicin, ciprofloxacin and tetracycline. It is important that chemotherapy is administered early regardless of the antibiotic chosen, due to the accumulation of toxin. Cutaneous anthrax responds well to treatment, however eschar formation may still occur due to the presence of toxin in the primary lesion.

In contrast, the treatment of inhalation anthrax is usually ineffective as the disease is rarely recognized prior to the onset of bacteremia. Once treatment has commenced it must continue for prolonged periods. Spores can persist in the lungs of infected primates for 60 days and reinitiate infection if treatment is prematurely terminated. Thus exposed individuals should be vaccinated on commencement of antibiotic treatment to enable antibiotic cover to be halted once protective immunity has be established (Friedlander *et al.* 1993).

Following the postal attacks in the USA ~32,000 individuals were given ciprofloxacin and then, when antimicrobial sensitivities became available, where encouraged to change to doxycycline (Jernigan *et al.* 2002). Amoxicillin was provided for pregnant women, breast feeding mothers, and children, due to concerns over the potential toxicity of the first two agents. While adverse events associated with antimicrobial prophylaxis were common (57%), serious events requiring hospitalization were rare (7%). Only 44% of over 10,000 individuals recommended to complete a 60 day course of treatment did so, suggesting that relapse may be an issues in the event of future attacks (Shepard *et al.* 2002).

Antitoxins

Numerous animal studies have demonstrated that inhibiting toxin activity prevents morbidity. The development of antitoxins to treat anthrax has been recently reviewed by Rainey and Young (2004). Approaches currently being pursued include antibodies (the approach closest to a product), receptor decoys, dominant-negative inhibitors of translocation, small molecule inhibitors and substrate analogues.

Prognosis

Until recently sub-clinical cases of anthrax in animals could not be diagnosed and as a consequence, infection was regarded as inevitably fatal. The development and application of antibody based assays have shown that sub-clinical infections do occur in animals that appear healthy. Humans are thought to be relatively resistant to anthrax when compared to herbivores, and data from cutaneously or orally exposed but untreated individuals suggest that sub-clinical infection is not uncommon (Heyworth *et al.* 1975).

Due to the scarcity of human infection there is little data concerning the long term health consequences of infection. Follow up of a significant proportion of the 22 infected individuals who survived the USA Postal attacks revealed that 53% had not returned to work a year after the event and that all were receiving psychiatric supports. Many of the survivors reported significant health problems, psychological distress, poor life adjustment, and loss of functional capacity (Reissman *et al.* 2004).

Epidemiology
Occurrence

While few countries are truly enzootic for anthrax, most have some cases of the disease in their livestock in any one year. Countries experiencing relatively high incidence are those in sub-Saharan Africa, the Indian subcontinent and Indonesia, certain provinces of China, parts of Turkey, and various countries of the former USSR. The incidence of the disease declined dramatically in Britain due to the adoption of control measures such as vaccination and an increase in the use of man-made alternatives to animal products. Nevertheless, specialized leather and woollen industries continue to depend on hides and wool from particular species or breeds raised in countries where anthrax is still endemic (Turnbull 1998).

Transmission in animals

Epidemics are of the point source type with animals acquiring infection as a consequence of grazing on spore contaminated land. Animal to animal transmission appears to be a rare event and when it does occur it is believed to be mediated by biting flies. Outbreaks have been linked to environmental changes, particularly flooding, which may result in the redistribution and concentration of anthrax spores in particular areas. Little is known as to how animals become infected or indeed the factors that determine why some animals in the same herd survive while others succumb to infection. It is likely that underlying host specific factors are important. Experimental infection studies have shown that spore levels far higher than those encountered in nature are required to initiate infection events in susceptible, healthy animals.

Transmission in humans

Human-to-human transmission is exceedingly rare but exceptions have been recorded (Heyworth *et al.* 1975). As indicated earlier, man normally contracts anthrax directly or indirectly from animals. The most common, cutaneous form of the disease occurs as a result of spores gaining access to the body via a lesion. Workers who carry hides or carcasses on their shoulders are susceptible to infection on the back of the neck; handlers of other animal materials or products tend to be infected on the hands, arms, or wrists. Gastrointestinal infection can also occur as a result of the consumption of contaminated meat when the nutritional value of meat outweighs the perceived risks of serious illness from eating.

Prevention and control

Control of anthrax for both livestock and humans lies in the well supervised disposal of infected animals carcasses, the application of biocides which reduce spore numbers to an undetectable level, and the immediate vaccination/and or prophylactic treatment of other members of the affected herd or at risk individuals. Although official recommendations in most countries are that anthrax carcasses be buried or burnt, the legacy of contaminated land from past burials (often decades ago) shows that incineration is the only truly satisfactory option. Mobile blowtorch incinerators are available but complete destruction of a bovine carcass can take more than 24 hours. Some countries prefer rendering, although the problem of preventing contamination of environment and equipment during transport and loading into the rendering plant has to be addressed.

Decontamination strategies for anthrax spores have centred on the use of toxic biocides (formaldehyde, chlorine releasing agents such chlorine dioxide and hydrogen peroxide) or gamma radiation. While effective these approaches suffer from the dual handicap of toxicity to man and the environment and/or are extremely expensive.

Control in wildlife

The application of control criteria designed for domestic animals to wildlife is impractical particularly with regards to the disposal of infected carcasses, many of which die unobserved. As to vaccination of wildlife in enzootic areas there are number of hurdles, not least of which is the argument that vaccination would interfere with the natural balance of the ecosystem. At present, immunization depends on the use of the livestock vaccines which requires either direct dart gun administration or immobilization of the animals followed by administration using a syringe. Either approach is expensive, traumatic for the animals, and can only give cover to a small core of susceptible animals. Also, it must be remembered that the duration of effectiveness of the vaccine is thought to be only about a year. Considerations are being given to the development of suitable oral vaccines for this purpose, although numerous obstacles must be overcome before oral vaccines satisfy concerns over safety, environmental contamination, and efficacy.

Vaccines

Vaccination is the most cost-effective form of prophylactic treatment. For this reason a considerable amount of time and effort has been expended on developing safe and effective animal and human vaccines.

The Sterne attenuated live spore vaccine which comprises a toxin expressing (pXO1+) but capsule deficient (pXO2−) isolate derived from a case of bovine anthrax has been employed extensively to control the disease in livestock (Turnbull 2000). Immunization of humans with live spores similar to the Sterne vaccine has been limited to the former USSR and China. The UK and the USA use non-living subunit vaccines based primarily on PA due to concerns over the possibility of residual virulence. The UK vaccine, which is similar in principle to its US counterpart, is produced from an alum precipitate of the cell-free culture filtrate of the Sterne strain of *B. anthracis*. In addition to containing large amounts of PA, the UK vaccine also comprises trace amounts of LF and other bacterially derived, immunogenic antigens, which have been shown to stimulate antibody responses in recipients and may contribute to protection and the transient side effects reported by some individuals (Baillie 2006).

Given the shortfalls of the current vaccine, research is in progress to develop a next generation replacement which will be fully defined and thus free from any adverse effects. In addition, vaccine formulations capable of self administration via the oral, nasal, or dermal routes, which induce immunity following a single dose and are stable at room temperature, would be extremely attractive to authorities seeking to build stockpiles to respond to a large scale future threat (Baillie 2006).

References

Abramova, F. A., Grinberg, L. M., Yampolskaya, O. V. and Walker, D. H. (1993). Pathology of Inhalational Anthrax in 42 Cases from the Sverdlovsk Outbreak of 1979. *Proc. Nat. Acad. Sci.,* **90:** 2291–94.

Anarki, S., Addiman, S., Nixon, G., Krahe, D., Ghosh, R., *et al.* (2008). Investigations and control measures following a case of inhalation anthrax in East London in a drum maker and drummer, October. *Eurosurveillance,* **13**(51): 1–3.

Baillie, L., Hibbs, S., Tsai, P., Cao, G. L. and Rosen, G. M. (2005). Role of Superoxide in the Germination of *Bacillus anthracis* Endospores. *FEMS Microbiol. Lett.,* **245:** 33–38.

Baillie, L., and Read, T. D. (2001). *Bacillus anthracis,* a Bug with Attitude! *Curr. Opin. Microbiol.,* **4:** 78–81.

Baillie, L. W. J. (1999). *Bacillus anthracis*. In: C. A. Batt, R. K. Robinson and P. D. Patel (eds.) *Encyclopedia of Food Microbiology,* pp. 129–35. Oxford: Academic Press.

Baillie, L. W. J. (2006). Past, Imminent and Future Human Medical Countermeasures for Anthrax. *J. Appl. Microbiol.,* **101:** 594–606.

Baldari, C. T., Tonello, F., Paccani, S. R., and Montecucco, C. (2006). Anthrax Toxins: A Paradigm of Bacterial Immune Suppression. *Trends in Immunol.,* **27:** 434–40.

Barnes, J. M. (1947). The Development of Anthrax Following the Adminstration of Spores by Inhalation. *Brit. J. Experi. Pathol.,* **28:** 385–94.

Boyden, E. D. and Dietrich, W. F. (2006). Nalp1b Controls Mouse Macrophage Susceptibility to Anthrax Lethal Toxin. *Nature Genet.,* **38:** 240–4.

Bradley, K. A., Mogridge, J., Mourez, M., Collier, R. J. and Young, J. A. T. (2001). Identification of the Cellular Receptor for Anthrax Toxin. *Nature,* **414:** 225–29.

Dahlgren, C. M., Buchanan, L. M., Decker, H. M., Freed, S. W., Phillips, C. R., *et al.* (1960). *Bacillus anthracis* Aerosols in Goat Hair Processing Mills. *Am. J. Hyg.,* **72:** 24–31.

Dalldorf, F. G., Kaufmann, A. F. and Brachman, P. S. (1971). Woolsorters' Disease. An Experimental Model. *Arch. Pathol.,* **92:** 418–26.

Defra (2007). *Anthrax: Culture and Identification of Bacillus anthracis from Field Cases in Animals: UK National Reference Method.* NRM 007. The

Veterinary and Public Health Test Standardisation Group: UK Surveillance Group for Diseases and Infections of Animals, London.

Dixon, T. C., Meselson, M., Guillemin, J., and Hanna, P. C. (1999). Anthrax. *N. Engl. J. Med.,* **341:** 815–26.

Duesbery, N. S., Webb, C. P., Leppla, S. H., *et al.* (1998). Proteolytic Inactivation of Map-Kinase-Kinase by Anthrax Lethal Factor. *Science,* **280:** 734–37.

Friedlander, A. M., Welkos, S. L., Pitt, M. L., *et al.* (1993). Postexposure Prophylaxis against Experimental Inhalation Anthrax. *J. Infect. Dis.,* **167:** 1239–43.

Heyworth, B., Ropp, M. E., Voos, U. G., Meinel, H. I., and Darlow, H. M. (1975). Anthrax in the Gambia: An Epidemiological Study. *BMJ,* **4:** 79–82.

Hoffmaster, A. R., Ravel, J., Rasko, D. A., *et al.* (2004). Identification of Anthrax Toxin Genes in a *Bacillus cereus* Associated with an Illness Resembling Inhalation Anthrax. *Proc. Nat. Acad. Sci.,* **101:** 8449–54.

Hu, H., Sa, Q., Koehler, T. M., Aronson, A. I., and Zhou, D. (2006). Inactivation of *Bacillus anthracis* Spores in Murine Primary Macrophages. *Cell. Microbiol.,* **8:** 1634–42.

Inglesby, T. V., O'Toole, T., Henderson, D. A., *et al.* (2002). Anthrax as a Biological Weapon, 2002: Updated Recommendations for Management. *J. Am. Med. Assoc.,* **287:** 2236–52.

Jernigan, D. B., Raghunathan, P. L., Bell, B. P., *et al.* (2002). Investigation of Bioterrorism-Related Anthrax, United States, 2001: Epidemiologic Findings. *Emerg. Infect. Dis.,* **8:** 1019–28.

Kang, T. J., Fenton, M. J., Weiner, M. A., *et al.* (2005). Murine Macrophages Kill the Vegetative Form of *Bacillus anthracis. Infect. and Immun.,* **73:** 7495–7501.

Keim, P., Smith, K. L., Keys, C., Takahashi, H., Kurata, T., *et al.* (2001). Molecular Investigation of the Aum Shinrikyo Anthrax Release in Kameido, Japan. *J. Clin. Microbiol.,* **39:** 4566–67.

Kyriacou, D. N., Yarnold, P. R., Stein, A. C., *et al.* (2007). Discriminating Inhalational Anthrax from Community-Acquired Pneumonia Using Chest Radiograph Findings and a Clinical Algorithm. *Chest,* **131:** 489–96.

Leppla, S. H. (1991). *The Anthrax Toxin Complex.* In J. E. Alouf and J. H. Freer (eds.) *Sourcebook of Bacterial Protein Toxins,* pp. 277–302. New York: Academic Press.

Lincoln, R., Walker, J., and Klein, F. (1967). Value of Field Data for Extrapolation in Anthrax. *Fed. Proc.,* **26:** 1558–62.

Little, S. F., and Ivins, B. E. (1999). Molecular Pathogenesis of *Bacillus anthracis* Infection. *Microbes and Infect.,* **1:** 131–39.

Makino, S.-I., Watarai, M., Cheun, H.-I., Shirahata, T., and Uchida, I. (2002). Effect of the Lower Molecular Capsule Released from the Cell Surface of *Bacillus anthracis* on the Pathogenesis of Anthrax. *J. Infect. Dis.,* **186:** 227–33.

Mayer-Scholl, A., Hurwitz, R., Brinkmann, V., *et al.* (2005). Human Neutrophils Kill *Bacillus anthracis. PLoS Path.,* **1:** e23.

Mignot, T., Mock, M., Robichon, D., Landier, A., Lereclus, D., *et al.* (2001). The Incompatibility between the PlcR- and Atxa-Controlled Regulons May Have Selected a Nonsense Mutation in *Bacillus anthracis. Molec. Microbiol.,* **42:** 1189–98.

Moayeri, M. and Leppla, S. H. (2004). The Roles of Anthrax Toxin in Pathogenesis. *Curr. Opin. Microbiol.,* **7:** 19–24.

O'Brien, J., Friedlander, A., Dreier, T., Ezzell, J., and Leppla, S. (1985). Effects of Anthrax Toxin Components on Human Neutrophils. *Infect. Immun.,* **47:** 306–10.

Panchal, R. G., Halverson, K. M., Ribot, W., *et al.* (2005). Purified *Bacillus anthracis* Lethal Toxin Complex Formed in Vitro and During Infection Exhibits Functional and Biological Activity. *J. Biolog. Chem.,* **280:** 10834–39.

Pellizzari, R., Guidi-Rontani, C., Vitale, G., Mock, M., and Montecucco, C. (1999). Anthrax Lethal Factor Cleaves Mkk3 in Macrophages and Inhibits the Lps/Ifn-γ-Induced Release of No and Tnfα. *FEBS Lett.,* **462:** 199–204.

Petosa, C., Collier, R. J., Klimpel, K. R., Leppla, S. H., and Liddington, R. C. (1997). Crystal Structure of the Anthrax Toxin Protective Antigen. *Nature,* **385:** 833–8.

Phipps, A. J., Premanandan, C., Barnewall, R. E., and Lairmore, M. D. (2004). Rabbit and Nonhuman Primate Models of Toxin-Targeting Human Anthrax Vaccines. *Microbiol. Molec. Biol. Rev.,* **68:** 617–29.

Priest, F. G., Barker, M., Baillie, L. W. J., *et al.* (2004). Population Structure and Evolution of the *Bacillus cereus* Group. *J. Bacter.,* **186:** 7959–70.

Raines, K. W., Kang, T. J., Hibbs, S., *et al.* (2006). Importance of Nitric Oxide Synthase in the Control of Infection by *Bacillus anthracis. Infect. Immun.,* **74:** 2268–76.

Rainey, G. J. A., and Young, J. A. T. (2004). Antitoxins: Novel Strategies to Target Agents of Bioterrorism. *Nature Rev. Microbiol.,* **2:** 721–26.

Read, T. D., Peterson, S. N., Tourasse, N., *et al.* (2003). The Genome Sequence of *Bacillus anthracis* Ames and Comparison to Closely Related Bacteria. *Nature,* **423:** 81–86.

Reissman, D. B., Whitney, E. A. S., Taylor Jr., T. H., *et al.* (2004). One-year Health Assessment of Adult Survivors of *Bacillus anthracis* Infection. *JAMA,* **291:** 1994–98.

Ross, J. M. (1957). The Pathogenesis of Anthrax Following the Administration of Spores by the Respiratory Route. *J. Pathol. Bacteriol.,* **73:** 485–94.

Saile, E., and Koehler, T. M. (2006). *Bacillus anthracis* Multiplication, Persistence, and Genetic Exchange in the Rhizosphere of Grass Plants. *Appl. Environ. Microbiol.,* **72:** 3168–74.

Shepard, C. W., Soriano-Gabarro, M., Zell, E. R., *et al.* (2002). Antimicrobial Postexposure Prophylaxis for Anthrax: Adverse Events and Adherence. *Emerg. Infect. Dis.,* **8:** 1124–32.

Sherer, K., Li, Y., Cui, X., and Eichacker, P. Q. (2007). Lethal and Edema Toxins in the Pathogenesis of *Bacillus anthracis* Septic Shock: Implications for Therapy. *Am. J. Respirat. Critic. Care Med.,* **175:** 211–21.

Smith, H., and Keppie, J. (1954). Observations on Experimental Anthrax; Demonstration of a Specific Lethal Factor Produced in vivo by Bacillus anthracis. *Nature,* **173:** 869–70.

Sterne, M. (1967). Distribution and Economic Importance of Anthrax. *Fed. Proc.,* **26:** 1493–5.

Titball, R. W., and Manchee, R. J. (1987). Factors Affecting the Germination of Spores of *Bacillus anthracis. J. Appl. Bacteriol.,* **62:** 269–73.

Turnbull, P. C. (2000). Current Status of Immunization against Anthrax: Old Vaccines May Be Here to Stay for a While. *Curr. Opin. Infect. Dis.,* **13:** 113–20.

Turnbull, P. C. B. (1998). *Anthrax.* In: S. R. Palmer, Lord Soulsby and D. I. H. Simpson (eds.) *Zoonoses: Biology, Clinical Practice, and Public Health Control,* pp. 3–16. Oxford: Oxford University Press.

Uchida, I., Hornung, J. M., Thorne, C. B., *et al.* (1993). Cloning and Characterization of a Gene Whose Product Is a Trans-Activator of Anthrax Toxin Synthesis. *J. Bacteriol.,* **175:** 5329–38.

Walsh, J. J., Pesik, N., Quinn, C. P., *et al.* (2007). A Case of Naturally Acquired Inhalation Anthrax: Clinical Care and Analyses of Anti-Protective Antigen Immunoglobulin G and Lethal Factor. *Clinic. Infect. Dis.,* **44:** 968–71.

Weaver, J., Kang, T. J., Raines, K. W., *et al.* (2007). Protective Role of *Bacillus anthracis* Exosporium in Macrophage-Mediated Killing by Nitric Oxide. *Infect. Immun.,* **75:** 3894–3901.

Wilson, G. S., and Miles, A. A. (1946). *Topley and Wilsons Principles of Bacteriology, Virology and Immunity.* London: Edward Arnold.

Wright, G. G., and Mandell, G. L. (1986). Anthrax Toxin Blocks Priming of Neutrophils by Lipopolysaccharide and by Muramyl Dipeptide. *J. Experim. Med.,* **164:** 1700–1709.

Zilinskas, R. A. (2006). The Anti-Plague System and the Soviet Biological Warfare Program. *Critic. Rev. Microbiol.,* **32:** 47–64.

CHAPTER 7

Brucellosis

J. Zinsstag, E. Schelling, J. Solera,
J. M. Blasco and I. Moriyón

Summary

Animal brucellosis is the source of *Brucella* infection in humans. The disease can be eliminated from animals through costly and technically cumbersome test and slaughter strategies. Accordingly, only well developed economies able to cover the costs of compensation for culled animals have been successful with Brucellosis elimination. Today, brucellosis is affecting mainly low income and transition countries. There has been significant progress in knowledge of the molecular biology of Brucella. Significantly more efficacious and safe animal vaccines in terms of reduction of transmission are still lacking. Control strategies that have been successful in western countries are not directly applicable to low income and transition countries because their national governments do not have the finance to compensate farmers and lack the technical capacity for effective control campaigns. However, new staged control approaches in developing economies are proving effective.

Current status

Brucellosis is one of the world's major zoonoses, alongside bovine tuberculosis and rabies (Boschiroli *et al.* 2001). Human brucellosis can result from direct contact with infected animals and can be transmitted to consumers through contaminated raw milk and milk products. Human-to-human transmission of the infection does not occur significantly. The most important causative bacteria in decreasing order are: *Brucella melitensis* (small ruminants), *B. abortus* (cattle), *B. suis* (pigs), and *B. canis* (dogs). Brucellosis has been successfully controlled or eliminated by effective and well managed vaccination and test-slaughter strategies in Australia, the USA, and European countries. The cost of control was essentially borne by national governments including the cost of acceptable compensation for culled animals. Brucellosis is, however, endemic in humans and livestock in the Mediterranean region, Africa, the Near East, and South and Central America and Mexico and is re-emerging as a major epidemic in countries of the former Soviet Union and Mongolia (Roth *et al.* 2003). In most countries the importance of brucellosis in terms of burden of disease and societal cost is not known but brucellosis can have a considerable impact on both human and animal health, as well as wide socioeconomic impact in countries in which rural income relies largely on livestock breeding and dairy products. Human brucellosis can, ultimately, only be eliminated by its control in animals. This chapter summarizes the current best practices for human brucellosis prevention and treatment and emphasizes socio-economic and ecological conditions and practical aspects of the control of brucellosis in livestock.

History

In 1887, Bruce reported the isolation of *Micrococcus melitensis* from a human case in Malta. The connection between goats and milk consumption was established by Zammit and Horrock seventeen years later (Vassallo 1996). In 1897, Bang described *Bacterium abortus* which he isolated from the uterus of a cow that had aborted. Evans showed the close relationship of these two bacteria in 1918 (Evans 1918) and, following her suggestions, Meyer and Shaw proposed the genus *Brucella* two years later for *B. melitensis* and *B. abortus* (Meyer and Shaw 1920). The swine isolates were considered atypical *B. abortus* strains until Huddleson noted the differences and proposed the species *B. suis* (Huddleson 1929). This better understanding of the genus paved the way for the description of *B. neotomae*, that was isolated from the desert wood rat (*Neotoma lepida*) (Stoenner and Lackman 1957). However, the surface differences (see below) of *B. ovis* (Buddle 1956) and *B. canis* (Carmichael and Bruner 1968) made these two species controversial until several analyses proved their placement in the genus (Díaz *et al.* 1967; Díaz *et al.* 1968; Hoyer and McCullough 1968a, 1968b). The *Brucella* Taxonomy Subcommittee approved the return to the classical species in 2006 (Osterman and Moriyón 2006). New species for marine mammals and common vole isolates have been proposed recently. All *Brucella* species are classified as group 3 pathogens and their handling requires biosafety Level 3 precautions.

The agent

Structural and antigenic characteristics

The bacterium *Brucella* follows a Gram-negative architecture: a cytoplasm encased in a cell envelope made of an inner membrane, a periplasm and an outer membrane (OM). The OM contains peculiar free lipids, proteins (Omp) and a lipopolysaccharide (LPS). The LPS is the dominant OM molecule and is critical in *Brucella's* virulence and as an antigen. Whereas *B. ovis* and *B. canis* have a rough type LPS (R-LPS) made of a lipid A linked to an oligosaccharide, other *Brucella* spp. have a smooth (S) type LPS with an O-polysaccharide (or O-chain) linked to the oligosaccharide. This is manifested in the surface of the colonies: R in *B. ovis* and *B. canis* and S in other brucellae. The S brucellae can dissociate to yield mixtures of S and R colonies and cells as a result of mutations affecting the O-polysaccharide. Dissociation hampers species identification and its control is essential in vaccine and antigen production (Alton *et al.* 1988).

Brucella O-polysaccharides create three basic epitopes: A (Abortus; ≥5 contiguous sugars in α 1–2 linkages); C (or A=M; common to all S-brucellae); and M (Melitensis) (Douglas and Palmer 1988; Perry and Bundle 1990). They are distributed in various proportions among S species and biovars so that neither A nor M is characteristic of *B. abortus* or *B. melitensis*, respectively. In addition to the S-LPS, S brucellae produce a free polysaccharide (native hapten [NH]) with a structure similar to that of the O-polysaccharide (Aragón *et al.* 1996). Bacteria cross-reacting with S brucellae include *Stenotrophomonas maltophilia*, group N (O:30) *Salmonella* spp., *Vibrio cholerae*, *E. coli* O:157, some *Escherichia hermanii* strains and *Yersinia enterocolitica* O:9. The soluble fraction contains proteins common to all brucellae but not to the S-LPS cross-reacting bacteria, which make them useful for discriminating *Brucella* spp. infections from false positive serological reactions (FPSR) caused by the latter.

Genetic characteristics

All brucellae except *B. suis* biovar 3, have two circular chromosomes of about 1.85–2.1 and 1.15 Mb. They carry neither plasmids nor lysogenic phages (Moreno 1992). Significant polymorphism affect several Omps and LPS genes (Ferrao-Beck *et al.* 2006; Vizcaíno and Cloeckaert 2004; Zygmunt *et al.* 2009). Variations in the position and number of the *Brucella* characteristic insertion sequence IS*711* (IS*6501*) and of two extragenic elements (repetitive extragenic palindromic [REP] sequences and the enterobacterial repetitive intergenic consensus (ERIC) also generate interspecies differences. Moreover, taxonomically and epidemiologically valuable polymorphism has been found by the analysis of restriction fragments (Al Dahouk *et al.* 2005; Vizcaíno and Cloeckaert 2004; Whatmore *et al.* 2005), hypervariable octameric oligonucleotide fingerprints (HOOF prints) (Bricker and Ewalt 2006), multiplex single nucleotide polymorphism (SNP) (Gopaul *et al.* 2008; Scott *et al.* 2007) and multiple locus variable number tandem repeats (MLVA, VNTR) (Huynh *et al.* 2008; Le Fléche *et al.* 2006; Whatmore *et al.* 2006).

Culture and selective media

Farrell's selective medium, originally developed to test milk for *B. abortus* is widely used (Alton *et al.* 1988) but inhibits *B. ovis* and many *B. melitensis* strains. The modified Thayer-Martin's medium, although less selective, gives better results with the latter species. The optimal strategy is to use both media simultaneously (Marin *et al.* 1996). These media have been recommended for the isolation of *B. abortus*, *B. melitensis* and *B. ovis* and, although unquestionably useful, inhibit some strains. This combination is also probably satisfactory for other *Brucella* species.

Identification and typing

The brucellae are gram-negative coccobacilli or short rods of 0.5–0.7 by 0.6–1.5 μm (some strains produce larger cells) commonly arranged most often as individual, non-motiles without capsules. They stain positive in Stamp's modification of the Ziehl-Neelsen method. Colonies have an entire edge and are transparent, convex and small (0.5–1.0 mm after 2–3 days of incubation). All species are catalase positive, all but *B. ovis* and *B. neotomae*, are oxidase postive, and all but *B. ovis* reduce nitrate to nitrite and show urease activity (Alton *et al.* 1988). Since bacteria that cause FPSR are easily differentiated using bacteriological tests, slide agglutination with anti-S sera readily identifies S brucellae and distinguishes it from the R forms. Species identification requires experience, specific anti-A and anti-M sera and phage and dye sensitivity assays. Biovar level typing is similarly difficult to perform and to reproduce.

Molecular tests advantageously substitute for the classical methods for species and vaccine typing. Most can be applied to colonies on isolation plates, thus avoiding dangerous manipulations. This is a rapidly evolving field (Al Dahouk *et al.* 2005; Bricker 2002), and some tests are presented in Table 7.1. Methods like Bruce-ladder for species identification or MLVA for finer analyses (Table 7.1) will probably be used extensively in the future.

Ecology and epidemiology

Brucellosis due to *B. abortus* and *B. melitensis* circulates predominantly in ruminant livestock (mostly in cattle, sheep and goats, but also in camels). Wildlife reservoirs of brucellosis exist in wild

Table 7.1 Selected molecular tests for *Brucella* identification and typing

Level of Identification	Test	Description (references)
Species	AMOS-PCR	A multiplex PCR assay based on IS711-related polymorphism that differentiates *B. abortus* (biovars 1, 2, and 4), *B. melitensis* (biovars 1, 2, and 3), *B. ovis*, *B. suis* (biovar 1), plus vaccines *B. abortus* S19 and RBT51 (Bricker *et al.* 2003b)
	Bruce-ladder-PCR	A single-step multiplex PCR assay that identifies *B. abortus* biovars 3, 5, 6, 7, 9, *B. melitensis*, *B. ovis*, *B. suis* biovars 2, 3, 4, *B. canis*, *B. neotomae*, *B. pinnipedialis* and *B. ceti* as well as the vaccine strains *B. abortus* S19, *B. abortus* RBT51 and *B. melitensis* Rev.1. (Lopez-Goñi *et al.* 2008)
	MLSA-SNP	MLSA-SNP identifies the six classical *Brucella* species plus the marine strains as a group (Scott *et al.* 2007)
Species and strain	MLVA-16	It uses a set of 8 minisatellite markers to discriminate *Brucella* species, including *B. microti*, plus a second set of 8 microsatellite markers for fine discrimination (Al Dahouk *et al.* 2007; Scholz *et al.* 2008).
Strain	HOOF prints	Method based on multilocus hypervariable octameric oligonucleotide fingerprints (HOOF) analysis (Bricker *et al.* 2003a)

ruminants like bison or red deer (Arenas-Gamboa *et al.* 2009) and can act as a reservoir for transmission to livestock (Forbes and Tessaro 1996). Transmission to humans occurs almost exclusively from domestic ruminants through occupational exposure (livestock and abattoir workers, veterinarians) and the consumption of raw milk and milk products. A model of livestock to human brucellosis transmission has been developed for Mongolia to assess the effect of different intervention strategies (Zinsstag *et al.* 2005).

Hosts

Animal brucellosis

Animal brucellosis is characterized by epidemic late stage abortions. Brucella may be shed for prolonged periods in the milk upon the cessation of clinical signs, representing a major risk for public health. Little is known about how brucellosis affects animal production quantitatively. The main clinical feature of brucellosis is late abortion in cattle, sheep and goats. In one study, among the sero-positive animals, it is estimated that 10–50% have aborted, of which 20% of cattle remained sterile (Bernues *et al.* 1997). The same authors estimate a loss of 10–25% of total milk yield among the sero-positive. Having aborted, animals are often not milked and the entire lactation is lost. Besides abortions, perinatal mortality is estimated at 5–20%, and 1% of cows with abortions may die.

Diagnosis

Brucellosis is a stealthy disease lacking pathognomonic clinical symptoms. Abortion, infertility and other manifestations are not specific and laboratory tests are necessary in diagnosis. Although Stamp's staining of smears of vaginal swabs, placentas or aborted foetuses is useful to reveal the presence of bacteria compatible with *Brucella*, isolation is the only unequivocal diagnostic method. Culture should always be attempted to both confirm the disease and to determine the *Brucella* species and biovar involved. Culture is however slow, expensive and cumbersome, and sensitivity depends on the type and number of samples, their adequate conservation and the amount of bacteria shed in the collected sample. Sampled abortions taken from the field are usually heavily contaminated and yield poor diagnostic results. Milk and vaginal swabs taken in the weeks that follow abortion are appropriate and often yield isolates of *B. melitensis* and *B. abortus.* Upon necropsy, the spleen and the iliac, mammary, cranial and prefemoral lymph nodes are the most adequate diagnostic samples. Selective media are necessary. Several direct PCR protocols have been proposed for diagnostic purposes. These protocols have been optimized in laboratory experiments for analytical sensitivity and specificity. However, there are only fragmentary studies to assess their diagnostic sensitivity and specificity and these protocols as such require further validation.

Brucella triggers both humoral and cell-mediated responses. However, these responses may not be detected at early stages of infection, in old animals and some animals born to infected mothers[1] do not develop antibodies until pregnancy (Plommet 1977). Moreover, an immune-response proves exposure to *Brucella* (or to cross-reacting bacteria) but not necessarily infection. Setting up adequate standardization protocols to avoid conflicting situations

is important because of the implications for livestock trade. In a proficiently managed programme, when used judiciously and with awareness of their properties, the existing tests are good enough to monitor the disease and to assist efficiently in elimination.

Classical tests

The Rose Bengal Test (RBT) and the Complement Fixation test (CFT) have been standardized for the diagnosis of cattle brucellosis (Alton *et al.* 1988). The former is a rapid and low cost plate agglutination test with a stained *B. abortus* suspension at pH 3.6–3.7. Depending on the route of administration and age at vaccination RBT is positive in vaccinated animals for a period of time and it is used for screening in this context. Combined with RBT, CFT has been the most widely used serological test but has several drawbacks. These classical tests are not optimal for the serodiagnosis in small ruminants. RBT shows lower sensitivity than in cattle and, although the problem is greatly reduced by increasing the proportion of serum:antigen to 3:1, standardization needs reassessment (Blasco *et al.* 1994a; Blasco *et al.* 1994b; Díaz-Aparicio *et al.* 1994; Ferreira *et al.* 2003). In dairy cattle, milk and whey are suitable samples for individual diagnosis or for monitoring pooled milk. The milk ring test (MRT) was designed for these purposes. It is moderately sensitive and easy to perform but it is useful only in cattle.

Elisa

Several indirect (i-ELISA) and competitive (c-ELISA) protocols have been developed for the diagnosis of brucellosis in cattle, goats and sheep (Alonso-Urmeneta *et al.* 1998; Muñoz *et al.* 2005; Nielsen 2002). The i-ELISAs show sensitivity equal or higher than that of RBT, higher than that of the CFT, can be automated and are suitable for goat, sheep and cattle blood serum and milk (Chand *et al.* 2005). Nevertheless, their specificity is curtailed by vaccination with S19 or Rev1, or by cross-reacting bacteria. To improve the specificity of S-LPS tests, c-ELISA was developed in the context of vaccination with S19 or Rev 1. Whereas the specificity in the vaccination contexts is improved with regard to i-ELISA, c-ELISA does not eliminate the problem created by cross-reacting bacteria and there are conflicting results on the sensitivity in cattle and sheep. In sheep, it does not outperform CFT and has lower sensitivity than the i-ELISA or the RBT (Marin *et al.* 1999; Minas *et al.* 2008).

Fluorescence polarization assay (FPA)

FPA uses *B. abortus* polysaccharide obtained from S-LPS labelled with fluorescein and measurements can be performed in a few minutes (Nielsen and Gall 2001). Its performance in the absence of vaccination is very similar to that of i-ELISA, RBT or RBT-like tests and, depending upon the study, of c-ELISA (McGiven *et al.* 2003; Nielsen and Gall 2001). The same conclusions probably apply to sheep and goats (Minas *et al.* 2007; Ramirez-Pfeiffer *et al.* 2007). Some studies have indicated that FPA has specificity greater than that of other S-LPS in vaccinated cattle (Aguirre *et al.* 2002). Further studies are required in sheep (Stournara *et al.* 2007).

Human brucellosis

Clinical manifestations

Clinical manifestations of human brucellosis vary with the population studied and the *Brucella* species. In general terms, *B. melitensis* causes more severe disease, followed by *B. suis* and then *B. abortus.* It is also important to keep in mind that not all *Brucella* contacts

---

1 In brucellosis, there is congenital transmission.

are followed by disease. In endemic areas over 50% of slaughter-house workers and up to 33% of veterinarians may have anti-*Brucella* antibodies in the absence of recognized clinical infection. Those who develop acute, symptomatic brucellosis may manifest a wide spectrum of symptoms including fever (undulant or not), sweats, malaise, anorexia, headache, arthralgias, myalgias, backache and weight loss. Lymphadenopathy, splenomegaly, and hepatomegaly are found in some cases. Complications can occur anywhere in the body (Table 7.2). Apart from abscesses, they include spondylitis, sacroiliitis, osteomyelitis, meningitis and orchitis. Endocarditis is the primary cause of mortality. The most important factor leading to a poor prognosis is probably the delay in effective antimicrobial therapy. Increased rates of spontaneous abortion, premature delivery and intrauterine infection with foetal death have been described in women with clinical evidence of brucellosis, but it is unclear whether these occur at rates higher than in other bacterial diseases.

Diagnosis

Because the clinical manifestations are variable and unspecific, a keen awareness of possible infection and a thorough occupational and travel history are necessary to reach a suspicion of brucellosis. Clinical suspicion has to be confirmed using laboratory tests.

Cultures should be performed whenever possible in the pyretic phase. Isolation can be attempted from articular, cerebrospinal and other fluids or some tissues in focal forms, but broth blood culture under 10% CO_2 is the routine culture method. Modern bacterial growth detecting systems or Ruiz-Castañeda's biphasic system are recommended. In either case, prolonged incubation (up to 21 and 45 days, respectively) is necessary before discarding a suspicious culture. Large (5–10 ml) samples in duplicate flasks and two or three independent blood samplings at adequate intervals are advisable. The leukocyte lysis-concentration procedure or the use of bone marrow may improve detection.

Seroconversion in any test is rarely observed and is a poor criterion because patients are diagnosed once the infection becomes established, and incubation times can be long. Whereas in acute (short evolution) brucellosis the agglutinating activity dominates, it is superseded by the non-agglutinating activity as the disease progresses. Lateral flow immuno-chromatography requires little skill and is perhaps the most appropriate and simple method to directly assess IgM and IgG (Irmak *et al.* 2004). Non-agglutinating

Table 7.2 Important clinical complications of human brucellosis[1]

Syndrome or focal complication	Comments
Osteoarticular (arthritis, spondylitis, sacroiliitis, osteomyelitis, bursitis, tenosynovitis).	In 20–85% of cases. In children, arthritis of the hip and knee joints are the most common diagnosis. Unilateral sacroiliitis is common in young adults. Spondylitis is not infrequent in older patients, and is the most serious osteoarticular complication; paraspinal and epidural abscesses not infrequent.
Neurological and psychiatric (meningitis, meningoencephalitis, cerebral abscess, myelitis, neuritis, depression and psychosis, cerebral venous thrombosis).	Meningitis is the most common here (<2% of cases). Cerebrospinal fluid shows lymphocytic pleocytosis with elevated protein but normal or low glucose levels. Gram stains and culture show low sensitivity. PCR is more sensitive than culture or serology. Computerized tomography may demonstrate basal ganglia calcification and abscesses.
Genitourinary (epididymo-orchitis, prostatitis, cystitis, interstitial nephritis, glomerulonephritis).	Unilateral epididymo-orchitis is frequent in young men. Renal involvement is uncommon but interstitial nephritis, pyelonephritis, and membranous glomerulonephritis, massive proteinuria, and caseating granulomas have all been reported. Increased rates of abortion, premature delivery, and intrauterine infection with foetal death has been described in pregnant women with clinical evidence of brucellosis.
Cardiovascular (endocarditis, myocarditis, pericarditis, endarteritis, thrombophlebitis).	Endocarditis (the most common cause of death) in <2% of cases. Aortic valve involvement is the most frequent endocarditis subtype. Embolic phenomena is common. Valve replacement is warranted in most cases. Mycotic aneurysms of the aorta and large vessels is rare.
Hepatobiliary (non-granulomatous and granulomatous hepatitis, hepatic abscesses, cirrhosis, acute cholecystitis).	Abnormal liver function tests in 30%–90% of cases. Percutaneous drainage and prolonged course of antibiotics.
Spleen (splenomegaly, abscesses, calcifications).	Surgical drainage of localized suppurative lesions and splenectomy may be of value if antimicrobial treatment is ineffective.
Pulmonary (bronchitis, bronchopneumonia, biliar adenopathy, perihiliar infiltrates, nodular lesions, lung abscesses, interstitial pattern, empyema, pleural effusions).	Cough and other pulmonary symptoms documented in about 15–25% of patients. Less than 40% of cases with a cough have normal chest X-ray pictures.
Haematological (anaemia, leukopenia, thrombocytopenia and pancytopenia, haemophagocytosis, disseminated intravascular coagulation).	More common in patients with *Brucella melitensis*. Erythrocyte sedimentation reaction (ESR) is normal frequently.
Cutaneous (rashes, papules, petechiae, purpura, cutaneous granulomatous vasculitis, erythema nodosum).	Occurs in <5% of patients. Many are transient and often non-specific skin lesions are described.
Other (ocular infection, thyroiditis, mastitis, colitis).	Ophthalmologic complications of *Brucella* infection include uveitis, keratitis, endophthalmitis, dacryo-cystitis and optic neuritis.

[1] Brucellosis can involve any organ or organ system and rare complications have been described.

and blocking antibodies, common in brucellosis, become agglutinating at pH ≤ 5, and can be detected by Brucellacapt and RBT. RBT (pH 3.6–3.7) detects IgM, IgG and IgA. RBT is often considered a qualitative test (positive or negative) not effectively discriminating exposure from active infection in endemic areas. This problem is overcome when RBT is used to test serum dilutions that allows for a diagnostic titre to be established. Brucellacapt and RBT titres increase with the time of evolution (Casanova *et al.* 2009). RBT is the test of choice in rural settings and in small or understaffed hospitals. However, antibodies to this antigen persist in recovered patients for a long time.

PCR-based methods have been developed in the past two decades to detect *Brucella* DNA in human samples. Presently, the variety of protocols, reproducibility problems, and quick advances in this area preclude specific recommendations. It is expected that kits for diagnosis will be available in the near future (Navarro *et al.* 2004).

Treatment and relapses

Treatment recommendations are summarized in Table 7.3 (Ariza *et al.* 2007). Adults with acute brucellosis and no complications or focal disease (Table 7.2) should be treated as outpatients with doxycycline-streptomycin or doxycycline-gentamicin combinations. Alternative regimes, necessary when tetracyclines are contraindicated, are less satisfactory. In focal forms, the preferred regimen is the same as for uncomplicated brucellosis but duration of therapy must be individualized. Surgery should be considered for patients with endocarditis, cerebral, epidural, spleen, hepatic or other abscesses not resolving with antibiotic therapy. Pregnancy poses a special problem as tetracyclines and streptomycin must be avoided and a rifampin monotherapy is considered the regimen of choice. Trimethoprim-sulfamethoxazole (cotrimoxazole) plus rifampin is an alternative regimen but it can be teratogenic if used before pregnancy week 13, and may induce kernicterus after week 36. Children often have fewer or milder symptoms. Since tetracyclines are generally contraindicated for children less than 8 years old, rifampin-cotrimoxazole is recommended. Alternatively, rifampin or cotrimoxazole plus gentamicin can be used. Some studies reported good results with long (>6 months) cotrimoxazole treatment. Depending upon the therapy, relapses occur in 5 to 30% of patients, usually 1 to 6 months after treatment and tend to be more mild than the original attack. The bacteria isolate from a relapsed patient maintain the same antibiotic-susceptibility. Consequently, nearly all relapses respond to a repeated course of antimicrobial therapy.

Burden of disease estimation

Even in the latest global comparative assessments that qualifies brucellosis as a neglected disease, an estimate of the burden of disease for brucellosis is not readily available. Estimating DALYs (disability adjusted live years) for brucellosis requires specifications of several parameters (Murray and Lopez 1994). Roth *et al.* (2003) considered that brucellosis is associated with a class II (0.2) disability weight, as the disease is perceived as very painful affecting occupational ability even during periods of remission and a median duration of untreated brucellosis of 3.1 years. They point out the need for consensus on these parameters.

Brucellosis vaccines

Small ruminant vaccines

B. melitensis Rev 1 is the best sheep and goat vaccine available and one that induces strong immunity. Under controlled conditions,

Table 7.3 Treatment of human brucellosis[1]

Clinical syndromes	Recommended	Alternative
Acute brucellosis (adults and children above 8 years of age).	Doxycycline 100 mg orally twice a day for 45 days plus either streptomycin 15 mg/kg intramuscularly daily for14–21 days, or gentamicin 3–5 mg/kg intravenously daily for 7–14 days. Or Doxycycline 100 mg orally twice a day for 45 days plus rifampin 600–900 mg orally daily for 45 days.	Rifampin 600 mg orally daily for 42 days plus quinolone (ofloxacin 400 mg orally twice a day or ciprofloxacin 750 mg orally twice a day) for 42 days. Or Doxycycline 100 mg orally twice a day plus trimethoprim-sulfamethoxazole, one double strength tablet twice a day for 2 months.
Children less than 8 years old.	trimethoprim-sulfamethoxazole 5 mg/kg (of trimethoprim component) orally twice a day for 45 days plus gentamicin 5–6 mg/kg intravenously daily for 7 days. Rifampin 15 mg/kg orally daily 45 days plus gentamicin 5–6 mg/kg intravenously daily for 7 days.	Monotherapy with doxycycline or rifampin 15mg/kg orally daily for 3–6 weeks.
Brucellosis during pregnancy.	Rifampin 600 mg orally daily for 45 days plus trimethoprim-sulfamethoxazole one double strength tablet twice a day for 45 days.	Rifampin 600–900 mg orally daily for 45 days.
Focal infections (endocarditis, spondylitis, meningitis, paraspinous abscesses).[2]	Doxycycline 100 mg orally twice a day and rifampin 600 mg orally daily for 6–52 weeks plus either streptomycin 1 g intramuscular daily or gentamicin 3–5 mg/kg intravenously daily for 14–21 days.	Consider trimethoprim-sulfamethoxazole, ciprofloxacin 750 mg orally twice a day or ofloxacin 400 mg orally twice a day as substitute for doxycycline or rifampin. Surgery should be considered for patients with endocarditis, cerebral or epidural abscess, spleen or hepatic abscess, or other abscesses that are antibiotic resistant.

[1] The choice of regimen/duration should be based on the presence of focal disease and underlying conditions that may contraindicate certain antibiotic therapy.

[2] Patients with focal disease (such as spondylitis or endocarditis) may require long courses of therapy depending on the clinical evolution. Aminoglycoside and quinolone dosage should be adjusted in patients with poor renal function.

rates of protection by the standard dose ($1–2 \times 10^9$ viable bacteria-colony forming units [CFU])/animal) can be as high as 80–100% against challenges (1.5×10^9 virulent bacteria) while infecting 100% of unvaccinated controls (Barrio *et al.* 2009; Jacques *et al.* 2007). Indeed, it has been successfully used in several countries and regions. Nevertheless, Rev 1 has some drawbacks. Rev 1 shows some instability and is virulent in humans, requires quality control and precaution when handling. If Rev 1 infection is suspected, treatment should not include streptomycin (Table 7.3).

The standard dose administered subcutaneously induces a protracted serological response that interferes in serological tests. This effect is more marked when applied to animals more than 4 months old (or adults of any age). The same dose administered by conjunctival instillation confers similar immunity and markedly reduces the serological response, particularly in young animals. Indeed, this is the only procedure fully compatible with combined elimination programmes (see below) (Blasco 1997; Fensterbank *et al.* 1985). Although Rev 1 has no undesirable effects in young rams, billy goats and lactating animals, vaccination of pregnant females can produce high numbers of abortions and vaccine excretion in milk (Blasco 1997; Zundel *et al.* 1992). This is a problem when mass vaccination is applied (see below). *B. suis* S2 was proposed as an alternative to Rev 1 but controlled experiments showed that is not protective (Garin-Bastuji *et al.* 1998). *B. abortus* RB51 (see Cattle vaccines) does not protect sheep and similarly negative results have been obtained with *B. melitensis* VTMR1 (like RB51, a *wboA* mutant) in goats (Moriyón *et al.* 2004). Other *B. melitensis* R vaccines are also inferior to Rev 1 (Barrio *et al.* 2009).

Cattle vaccines

With a few exceptions, all successful control and elimination programmes in cattle have been carried out with 19, an attenuated S strain. In heifers (vaccination of males is counter indicated) vaccinated subcutaneously with the standard dose (10×10^{10} CFU/animal), it induces an infection that is usually cleared in a few months. In adult females vaccinated similarly, however, about 2% of the animals develop udder infections and shed the vaccine in the milk for several years (Nicoletti 1990). Although more stable than Rev 1, S19 occasionally dissociates so that quality control is necessary (Grilló *et al.* 2000). S19 is not as dangerous as Rev 1, but it can also infect humans and therefore minimal biosafety precautions are necessary when handling this vaccine (Meyer 1985). The rate of abortion caused in adults by the reduced doses (see below) of S19 applied subcutaneously is generally low (up to 5%; less than 1% in a large study involving over 10 000 cows which were 7 to 8 months pregnant (Nicoletti 1990)). This procedure can induce udder infections and vaccine shedding in milk in a very low proportion of animals (Nicoletti 1990). However, both problems are significantly minimized when the same reduced doses are applied conjunctivally.

Cattle may become infected by *B. melitensis* upon contact with sheep and goats. This has prompted some research on the use of Rev 1 in cattle, but taking into account that *B. melitensis* infections in cattle can be controlled with the help of S19 (Jiménez de Bagüés *et al.* 1991), the use of the latter vaccine should be recommended for the prophylaxis of both *B. abortus* and *B. melitensis* infection in cattle. *B. abortus* RB51 is an R mutant obtained by repeated passage on media with rifampin and penicillin to develop a vaccine that would not interfere in the S-LPS serological tests. The properties of

RB51 have been the subject of recent reviews (Moriyón *et al.* 2004; Schurig *et al.* 2002). RB51 has been used in several countries (Martins *et al.* 2009; Schurig *et al.* 2002) but its efficacy under field conditions is controversial and it is less protective than S19 in controlled experiments (Moriyón *et al.* 2004; Schurig *et al.* 2002).

Control and elimination

There are four points that need to be considered before implementing any brucellosis control and elimination programme. These are:

1 Identification of all flocks and herds and the proficiency of veterinary services to vaccinate the whole population in a short time frame.

2 Sufficient public resources to cover intervention costs and for the compensation of culled animals at market value if elimination is the goal.

3 Active involvement and cooperation of the farming community through awareness campaigns.

4 Well known disease status from randomized cross-sectional cluster surveys proportional to size and stratified by geographical regions, possibly involving cross-border assessments and the occurrence in humans (Schelling *et al.* 2003; Zinsstag *et al.* 2009). Knowledge of the circulating *Brucella* species and biovars in the different livestock species involved is also important.

If greater than 10% of flocks and/or herds are infected, mass vaccination is the method of choice. At this stage interference with serological tests is not a major concern because the goal is to control the disease and to reduce the economical losses, human contagion and the prevalence of the disease. If between 5–10% of flocks and/or herds are infected, a combined strategy of vaccination of young replacements and test and slaughter of adults can eliminate the disease at medium to long term. If less than 1–2% of flocks and/or herds are infected, a test-slaughter program (serological testing and culling of seropositive animals) along with the ban of vaccines can eliminate the disease in the near future.

Control strategies

In countries with elementary veterinary services and limited economic resources, or where prevalence is high, immunization of the whole population is the strategy of choice. Bulls should not be vaccinated (side effects have been reported), but mass vaccination of the whole female population (over 4 months of age) with a single reduced dose (5×10^9 UFC/animal) of S19 administered conjunctivally, and repeated yearly or at two year intervals (see below) is the method of choice for controlling *B. melitensis* and *B. abortus* in cattle. In the case of small ruminants, mass vaccination with Rev 1 may cause abortions. Safer alternatives include vaccination of only the 3–4 month old replacements (both male and female) every year, assuming that the total population would be immunized in an acceptable period of time (4–10 years) (Blasco 1997). Since implementation of this programme often fails, as an alternative the conjunctival vaccination could be repeated in the whole ruminant population (except bulls) every two years with Rev 1 (sheep and goats) or S19 (cattle) vaccines at a time period when the risk of vaccine-induced abortions is minimal.

Elimination

Once prevalence decreases, and provided the basic requirements are met, elimination could be attempted by conjunctival vaccination of 3–4 months old replacements (Rev 1 in both male and female lambs and kids, and S19 in heifers alone) plus the test of adults and slaughter of seropositive animals. To avoid the entry of infected animals into healthy flocks or herds, compulsory individual identification and movement control are essential collateral measures. As a final step, vaccination is banned and test and slaughter (with partial of full depopulation of infected flocks and herds) can lead to complete elimination.

Surveillance

Once elimination is achieved, a surveillance system has to be implemented to detect outbreaks or reintroduction. Passive surveillance systems based, for example, on the compulsory declaration by farmers of abortions are both inefficient and ineffective for early detection. Therefore, active surveillance is necessary. In ruminants, it should be based on the regular (at least once a year) serological screening (RBT or i-ELISA are optimal for this purpose) of a representative cluster sample proportional to size (Bennett *et al.* 1991). Systematic sampling of large numbers of animals should be avoided.

Economics

In industrialized countries, an important part of successful brucellosis control has been compensating farmers for culled livestock. However, many resource-limited countries would not be able to conduct such programs. To attempt control, and possibly the elimination of brucellosis, benefits to public health and society need to be demonstrated, particularly in countries with scarce resources. Documented economic analyses of brucellosis control are rare. Roth *et al.* (2003) estimated a benefit-to-cost ratio of 3.2 for a livestock mass vaccination campaign in Mongolia. If the costs of the intervention were shared amongst the public health and livestock sectors in proportion to the benefit to each, the public health sector would contribute 12%, with a cost-effectiveness ratio of US$19 per DALY averted. If costs of vaccinating livestock are allocated proportionally to all benefits, the intervention is cost-saving and cost-effective for the agricultural and the public health sectors. With such an allocation of costs to benefits per sector, brucellosis control becomes a very cost-effective intervention (<US$25 per DALY gained) in the public health sector, compared to cost-effectiveness of vaccinating women and children or treating tuberculosis.

Acknowledgement

This work has been supported by the EU-FP 7 funded project Integrated Control of Zoonoses (ICONZ).

References

Aguirre, N. P., Vanzini, V. R., Torioni-de-Echaide, S., Valentini, B. S., De-Lucca, G., *et al.* (2002). Antibody dynamics in holstein friesian heifers vaccinated with *Brucella abortus* strain 19, using seven serological tests. *J. Immunoassay Immunochem.*, **23**: 471–78.

Al Dahouk, S., Tomaso, H., *et al.* (2005). Identification of Brucella species and biotypes using polymerase chain reaction-restriction fragment length polymorphism (PCR-RFLP). *Crit. Rev. Microbiol.*, **31**: 191–96.

Al Dahouk, S., Fleche, P. L., Nockler, K., Jacques, I., Grayon, M., *et al.* (2007). Evaluation of *Brucella* MLVA typing for human brucellosis. *J. Microbiol. Methods*, **69**: 137–45.

Alonso-Urmeneta, B., Marín, C. M., *et al.* (1998). Evaluation of lipopolysaccharides and polysaccharides of different epitopic structures in the indirect enzyme-linked immunosorbent assay for diagnosis of brucellosis in small ruminants and cattle. *Clin, Diagn. Lab. Immunol.*, **5**: 749–54.

Alton, G. G., Jones, L. M., Angus, R. D., and Verger, J. M. (1988). 'Techniques for the brucellosis laboratory.' Paris, France: INRA.

Aragón, V., Díaz, R., Moreno, E., and Moriyón, I. (1996). Characterization of *Brucella abortus* and *Brucella melitensis* native haptens as outer membrane O-type polysaccharides independent from the smooth lipopolysaccharide. *J. Bacteriol.*, **178**: 1070–79.

Arenas-Gamboa, A. M., Ficht, T. A., *et al.* (2009). Enhanced immune response of red deer (*Cervus elaphus*) to live rb51 vaccine strain using composite microspheres. *J. Wildlife Dis.*, **45**: 165–73.

Ariza, J., Bosilkovski, M., Cascio, A., Colmenero, J. D., *et al.* (2007). Perspectives for the treatment of brucellosis in the 21st century: the Ioannina recommendations. *PloS Med.*, **4**: e317.

Barrio, M. B., Grillo, M. J., Munoz, P. M., Jacques, I., Gonzalez, D., *et al.* (2009). Rough mutants defective in core and O-polysaccharide synthesis and export induce antibodies reacting in an indirect ELISA with smooth lipopolysaccharide and are less effective than Rev 1 vaccine against *Brucella melitensis* infection of sheep. *Vaccine*, **27**: 1741–49.

Bennett, S., Woods, T., Liyanage, W. M., and Smith, D. L. (1991). A simplified general method for cluster-sample surveys of health in developing countries. *Rapp. Timest. Stat. Sanit. Mond.*, **44**: 98–106.

Bernues, A., Manrique, E., and Maza, M. T. (1997). Economic evaluation of bovine brucellosis and tuberculosis eradication programmes in a mountain area of Spain. *Prev. Vet. Med.*, **30**: 137–49.

Blasco, J. M. (1997). A review of the use of *B. melitensis* Rev 1 vaccine in adult sheep and goats. *Prev. Vet. Med.*, **31**: 275–83.

Blasco, J. M., Garin-Bastuji, B., Marín, C. M., Gerbier, G., Fanlo, J., *et al.* (1994a). Efficacy of different rose bengal and complement fixation antigens for the diagnosis of *Brucella melitensis* infection in sheep and goats. *Vet. Rec.*, **134**: 415–20.

Blasco, J. M., Marín, C. M., Jiménez de Bagüés, A., *et al.* (1994b). Evaluation of allergic and serological tests for diagnosing *Brucella melitensis* infection in sheep. *J. Clin. Microbiol.*, **32**: 1835–40.

Boschiroli, M. L., Foulongne, V., and O'Callaghan, D. (2001). Brucellosis: a worldwide zoonosis. *Curr. Opin. Microbiol.*, **4**: 58–64.

Bricker, B. J. (2002). PCR as a diagnostic tool for brucellosis. *Vet. Microbiol.*, **90**: 435–46.

Bricker, B. J. and Ewalt, D. R. (2006). HOOF prints: *Brucella* strain typing by PCR amplification of multilocus tandem-repeat polymorphisms. *Methods Mol. Biol.*, **345**: 141–73.

Bricker, B. J., Ewalt, D. R., and Halling, S. M. (2003a). *Brucella* 'Hoof-Prints': strain typing by multi-locus analysis of variable number tandem repeats (VNTRs). *BMC Microbiol.*, **3**: 15.

Bricker, B. J., Ewalt, D. R., Olsen, S. C., and Jensen, A. E. (2003b). Evaluation of the *Brucella abortus* species-specific polymerase chain reaction assay, an improved version of the *Brucella* AMOS polymerase chain reaction assay for cattle. *J. Vet. Diagn. Invest.*, **15**: 374–78.

Buddle, M. B. (1956). Studies on *Brucella ovis* (n.sp.), a cause of genital disease of sheep in New Zealand and Australia. *J. Hyg. (Lond)*, **54**: 351–64.

Carmichael, L. E. and Bruner, D. W. (1968). Characteristics of a newly-recognized species of *Brucella* responsible for infectious canine abortions. *Cornell Vet.*, **48**: 579–92.

Casanova, A., Ariza, J., Rubio, M., Masuet, C., and Díaz, R. (2009). Brucellacapt vs. classical tests in the serological diagnosis and management of human brucellosis. *Clin. Vaccine Immuno.*, **6**(6): 844–51.

Chand, P., Rajpurohit, B. S., Malhotra, A. K., and Poonia, J. S. (2005). Comparison of milk-ELISA and serum-ELISA for the diagnosis of *Brucella melitensis* infection in sheep. *Vet. Microbiol.*, **108:** 305–311.

Díaz, R., Jones, L. M., and Wilson, J. B. (1967). Antigenic relationship of *Brucella ovis* and *Brucella melitensis*. *J. of Bacteriol.*, **93:** 1262–68.

Díaz, R., Jones, L. M., and Wilson, J. B. (1968). Antigenic relationship of the gram-negative organism causing canine abortion to smooth and rough brucellae. *J. Bacteriol.*, **95:** 618–24.

Díaz-Aparicio, E., Marín, C. M., Alonso-Urmeneta, B., *et al.* (1994). Evaluation of serological tests for diagnosis of *Brucella melitensis* infection of goats. *J. Clin. Microbiol.*, **32:** 1159–65.

Douglas, J. T. and Palmer, D. A. (1988). Use of monoclonal antibodies to identify the distribution of A and M epitopes on smooth *Brucella* species. *J. Clin. Microbiol.*, **26:** 1353–56.

Evans, A. C. (1918). Further Studies on Bacterium Abortus and Related Bacteria: I. The Pathogenicity of Bacterium Lipolyticus for Guinea-Pigs. *J. Infect. Dis.*, **22:** 576–79.

Fensterbank, R., Pardon, P., and Marly, J. (1985). Vaccination of ewes by a single conjunctival administration of *Brucella melitensis* Rev. 1 vaccine. *Ann. Rech. Vet.*, **16:** 351–56.

Ferrao-Beck, L., Cardoso, R., Muñoz, P. M., de Miguel, M. J., Albert, D., *et al.* (2006). Development of a multiplex PCR assay for polymorphism analysis of *Brucella suis* biovars causing brucellosis in swine. *Vet. Microbiol.*, **115:** 269–77.

Ferreira, A. C., Cardoso, R., Dias, I. T., Mariano, I., Belo, A., *et al.* (2003). Evaluation of a modified Rose Bengal test and an indirect Enzyme-Linked Immunosorbent Assay for the diagnosis of *Brucella melitensis* infection in sheep. *Vet. Res.*, **34:** 297–305.

Forbes, L. B. and Tessaro, S. V. (1996). Infection of cattle with *Brucella abortus* biovar 1 isolated from a bison in Wood Buffalo National Park. *Can. Vet. J.*, **37:** 415–491.

Garin-Bastuji, B., Blasco, J. M., Grayon, M., and Verger, J. M. (1998). *Brucella melitensis* infection in sheep: present and future. *Vet. Res.*, **29:** 255–74.

Gopaul, K. K., Koylass, M. S., Smith, C. J., and Whatmore, A. M. (2008). Rapid identification of *Brucella* isolates to the species level by real time PCR based single nucleotide polymorphism (SNP) analysis. *BMC Microbiol.*, **8:** 86.

Grilló, M. J., Bosseray, N., and Blasco, J. M. (2000). In vitro markers and biological activity in mice of seed lot strains and commercial *Brucella melitensis* Rev 1 and *Brucella abortus* B19 vaccines. *Biologicals*, **28:** 119–27.

Hoyer, B. H. and McCullough, N. B. (1968a). Homologies of deoxyribonucleic acids from *Brucella ovis*, canine abortion organisms, and other *Brucella* species. *J. Bacteriol.*, **96:** 1783–90.

Hoyer, B. H. and McCullough, N. B. (1968b). Polynucleotide homologies of *Brucella* deoxyribonucleic acids. *J. Bacteriol.*, **95:** 444–48.

Huddleson, I. F. (1929). 'The differentiation of the species in the genus *Brucella*.' East Lansing, Michigan, Agricultural Experimental Station, Michigan University.

Huynh, L. Y., Van Ert, M. N., Hadfield, T., Probert, W. S., Bellaire, B. H., *et al.* (2008). Multiple Locus Variable Number Tandem Repeat (VNTR) Analysis (MLVA) of *Brucella* spp. Identifies Species-Specific Markers and Insights into Phylogenetic Relationships. pp. 47–54.

Irmak, H., Buzgan, T., Evirgen, O., Akdeniz, H., Demiroz, A. P., *et al.* (2004). Use of the *Brucella* IgM and IgG flow assays in the serodiagnosis of human brucellosis in an area endemic for brucellosis. *Am. J. Trop. Med. Hyg.*, **70:** 688–94.

Jacques, I., Verger, J. M., Laroucau, K., Grayon, M., Vizcaino, N., *et al.* (2007). Immunological responses and protective efficacy against *Brucella melitensis* induced by bp26 and omp31 B. melitensis Rev. 1 deletion mutants in sheep. *Vaccine*, **25:** 794–805.

Jiménez de Bagüés, M. P., Marín, C. M., and Blasco, J. M. (1991). Effect of antibiotic therapy and strain-19 vaccination on the spread of *Brucella melitensis* within an infected dairy herd. *Prev. Vet. Med.*, **11:** 17–24.

Le Flèche, P., Jacques, I., Grayon, M., Al Dahouk, S., Bouchon, P., *et al.* (2006). Evaluation and selection of tandem repeat loci for a *Brucella* MLVA typing assay. *BMC Microbiol.*, **6:** 9.

Lopez-Goni, I., Garcia-Yoldi, D., Marin, C. M., de Miguel, M. J., Munoz, P. M., *et al.* (2008). Evaluation of a multiplex PCR assay (Bruce-ladder) for molecular typing of all *Brucella* species, including the vaccine strains. *J. Clin. Microbiol.*, **46:** 3484–87.

Marin, C. M., Jiménez de Bagüés, M. P., Barberán, M., and Blasco, J. M. (1996). Comparison of two selective media for the isolation of *Brucella melitensis* from naturally infected sheep and goats. *Vet. Rec.*, **138:** 409–11.

Marin, C. M., Moreno, E., Moriyón, I., Díaz, R., and Blasco, J. M. (1999). Performance of competitive and indirect enzyme-linked immunosorbent assays, gel immunoprecipitation with native hapten polysaccharide, and standard serological tests in diagnosis of sheep brucellosis. *Clin. Diagn. Lab. Immunol.*, **6:** 269–72.

Martins, H., Garin-Bastuji, B., Lima, F., Flor, L., Pina, F. A., *et al.* (2009). Eradication of bovine brucellosis in the Azores, Portugal-Outcome of a 5-year programme (2002–2007) based on test-and-slaughter and RB51 vaccination. *Prev. Vet. Med.*, **90:** 80–89.

McGiven, J. A., Tucker, J. D., Perrett, L. L., Stack, J. A., Brew, S. D., *et al.* (2003). Validation of FPA and cELISA for the detection of antibodies to *Brucella abortus* in cattle sera and comparison to SAT, CFT, and iELISA. *J. Immunol. Methods*, **278:** 171–78.

Meyer, K. F. and Shaw, E. B. (1920). A comparison of the morphologic, cultural and biochemical characteristics of *B. abortus* and *B. melitensis*: Studies on the genus Brucella Nov. Gen. I. *The J. Infect. Dis.*, **27:** 173–84.

Meyer, M. E. (1985). Characterization of *Brucella abortus* strain 19 isolated from human and bovine tissues and fluids. *Am. J.Vet. Res.*, **46:** 902–904.

Minas, A., Stournara, A., Christodoulopoulos, G., and Katsoulos, P. D. (2008). Validation of a competitive ELISA for diagnosis of *Brucella melitensis* infection in sheep and goats. *Vet. J.*, **177:** 411–17.

Minas, A., Stournara, A., Minas, M., Stack, J., Petridou, E., *et al.* (2007). Validation of a fluorescence polarization assay (FPA) performed in microplates and comparison with other tests used for diagnosing *B. melitensis* infection in sheep and goats. *J. Immunol. Methods*, **320:** 94–103.

Moreno, E. (1992). Evolution of Brucella. In: M. Plommet (ed.) *Prevention of brucellosis in the Mediterranean countries*, pp. 198–218. Wageningen: Pudoc Scientific Publishers.

Moriyón, I., Grilló, M. J., Monreal, D., Gonzalez, D., Marín, C., *et al.* (2004). Rough vaccines in animal brucellosis: structural and genetic basis and present status. *Vet. Res.* **35:** 1–38.

Muñoz, P. M., Marín, C. M., Monreal, D., González, D., Garin-Bastuji, B., *et al.* (2005). Efficacy of several serological tests and antigens for diagnosis of bovine brucellosis in the presence of false-positive serological results due to *Yersinia enterocolitica* O:9. *Clin. Diagn. Lab. Immunol.*, **12:** 141–51.

Murray, C. J. L. and Lopez, A. D. (1994). Global comparative assessments in the health sector: disease burden, expenditures and interventions packages. *Bull. World Heal. Organ.*, **1:** 1–196.

Navarro, E., Casao, M. A., and Solera, J. (2004). Diagnosis of human brucellosis using PCR. *Expert. Rev. Mol. Diagn.*, **4:** 115–23.

Nicoletti, P. L. (1990). Vaccination. In: K. H. Neilsen and J. R. Duncan (eds.) *Animal Brucellosis*, pp. 283–99. Boca Raton: CRC Press.

Nielsen, K. (2002). Diagnosis of brucellosis by serology. *Vet. Microbiol*, **90:** 447–59.

Nielsen, K. and Gall, D. (2001). Fluorescence polarization assay for the diagnosis of brucellosis: a review. *J. Immunoassay Immunochem.*, **22:** 183–201.

Osterman, B. and Moriyón, I. (2006). International Committee on Systematics of Prokaryotes; Subcommittee on the taxonomy of *Brucella*: Minutes of the meeting, 17 September 2003, Pamplona, Spain. *Int. J. Syst. Evol. Microbiol.*, **56:** 1173–75.

Perry, M. B. and Bundle, D. R. (1990). Lipopolysaccharide antigens and carbohydrates of *Brucella*. In: L. G. Adams (ed.) *Advances in brucellosis research*, pp. 76–88. College Station: Texas A&M University Press.

Plommet, M. (1977). Studies on experimental brucellosis in cows in France. In: R. P. Crawford and R. J. Hidalgo (eds.) *Bovine brucellosis. An International Symposium*, pp. 116–34. College Station and London: Texas A&M University Press.

Ramirez-Pfeiffer, C., Nielsen, K., Smith, P., Marin-Ricalde, F., Rodriguez-Padilla, C., *et al.* (2007). Application of the fluorescence polarization assay for detection of caprine antibodies to *Brucella melitensis* in high vaccination areas. *Clin. Vaccine Immunol.*, **14**(3): 299–303.

Roth, F., Zinsstag, J., Orkhon, D., Chimed-Ochir, G., Hutton, G., *et al.* (2003). Human health benefits from livestock vaccination for brucellosis: case study. *Bull. World Heal. Organ.*, **81**: 867–76.

Schelling, E., Diguimbaye, C., Daoud, S., Nicolet, J., Boerlin, P., *et al.* (2003). Brucellosis and Q-fever seroprevalences of nomadic pastoralists and their livestock in Chad. *Prev. Vet. Med.*, **61**: 279–93.

Scholz, H. C., Hubalek, Z., Sedlacek, I., Vergnaud, G., Tomaso, H., *et al.* (2008). *Brucella microti* sp. nov., isolated from the common vole *Microtus arvalis. Int. J. Syst. Evol. Microbiol.*, **58**: 375–82.

Schurig, G. G., Sriranganathan, N., and Corbel, M. J. (2002). Brucellosis vaccines: past, present and future. *Vet. Microbiol.*, **90**: 479–96.

Scott, J. C., Koylass, M. S., Stubberfield, M. R., and Whatmore, A. M. (2007). A multiplex single nucleotide polymorphism (SNP) based assay to rapidly speciate *Brucella* isolates. *Appl. Environ. Microbiol.*, doi:10.1128/AEM.00976-07.

Stoenner, H. G. and Lackman, D. B. (1957). A new species of *Brucella* isolated from the desert wood rat, *Neotoma lepida* Thomas. *Am. J. Vet. Res.*, **18**: 947–51.

Stournara, A., Minas, A., Bourtzi-Chatzopoulou, E., Stack, J., Koptopoulos, G., *et al.* (2007). Assessment of serological response of young and adult sheep to conjunctival vaccination with Rev-1 vaccine by fluorescence polarization assay (FPA) and other serological tests for *B. melitensis. Vet. Microbiol.*, **119**: 53–64.

Vassallo, D. J. (1996). The saga of brucellosis: controversy over credit for linking Malta fever with goats' milk. *The Lancet,* **348**: 804–808.

Vizcaíno, N. and Cloeckaert, A. (2004). DNA polymorphism and taxonomy of *Brucella* species. In: I. López-Goñi, and I. Moriyón (eds.) *Brucella: Molecular and Cellular Biology*, pp. 1–24. Wymondham, Norfolk: Horizon Bioscience.

Whatmore, A. M., Murphy, T. J., Shankster, S., Young, E., Cutler, S. J., *et al.* (2005). Use of amplified fragment length polymorphism to identify and type *Brucella* isolates of medical and veterinary interest. *J. Clin. Microbiol.*, **43**: 761–69.

Whatmore, A. M., Shankster, S. J., Perrett, L. L., Murphy, T. J., Brew, S. D., *et al.* (2006). Identification and Characterization of Variable-Number Tandem-Repeat Markers for Typing of *Brucella* spp. *J. Clin. Microbiol,* **44**: 1982–93.

Zinsstag, J., Roth, F., Orkhon, D., Chimed-Ochir, G., Nansalmaa, M., *et al.* (2005). A model of animal-human brucellosis transmission in Mongolia. *Prev. Vet. Med.*, **69**: 77–95.

Zinsstag, J., Schelling, E., Bonfoh, B., Fooks, A. R., Kasymbekov, J., *et al.* (2009). Towards a 'one health' research and application tool box. *Vet., Ital.* **45**: 121–33.

Zundel, E., Verger, J. M., Grayon, M., and Michel, R. (1992). Conjunctival vaccination of pregnant ewes and goats with *Brucella melitensis* Rev 1 vaccine: safety and serological responses. *Ann. Rech. Vet.* **23**: 177–88.

Zygmunt, M. S., Blasco, J. M., Letesson, J. J., Cloeckaert, A., and Moriyón, I. (2009). DNA polymorphism analysis of *Brucella* lipopolysaccharide genes reveals marked differences in O-polysaccharide biosynthetic genes between smooth and rough Brucella species and novel species-specific markers. *BMC Microbiol.*, **9**: 92–105.

CHAPTER 8

Verocytotoxin-producing *Escherichia coli* (VTEC) infections

Mohamed A. Karmali and Jan M. Sargeant

Summary

Verocytotoxin (VT)-producing *Escherichia coli* (VTEC), also known as Shiga toxin producing *E. coli* (STEC), are zoonotic agents, which cause a potentially fatal illness whose clinical spectrum includes diarrhoea, haemorrhagic colitis, and the haemolytic uraemic syndrome (HUS). VTEC are of serious public health concern because of their association with large outbreaks and with HUS, which is the leading cause of acute renal failure in children. Although over 200 different OH serotypes of VTEC have been associated with human illness, the vast majority of reported outbreaks and sporadic cases of VTEC-infection in humans have been associated with serotype O157:H7.

VTs constitute a family of related protein subunit exotoxins, the major ones implicated in human disease being VT1, VT2, and VT2c. Following their translocation into the circulation, VTs bind to endothelial cells of the renal glomeruli, and of other organs and tissues via a specific receptor globotriosylceramide (Gb_3), are internalized by a process of receptor-mediated endocytosis, and cause subcellular damage that results in the characteristic microangiopathic disease observed in HUS.

The incubation period of VTEC-associated illness is about 3–5 days. After ingestion VTEC (especially of serotype O157:H7) multiply in the bowel and colonize the mucosa of probably the large bowel with a characteristic attaching and effacing (AE) cytopathology. Colonization is followed by the translocation of VTs into the circulation and the subsequent manifestation of disease.

The majority of patients with uncomplicated VTEC infection recover fully with general supportive measures. Historically, the case-fatality rate was high for HUS. However, improvement in the treatment of renal failure and the attendant biochemical disturbances has substantially improved the outlook, although long-term sequelae may develop.

Ruminants, especially cattle, are the main reservoirs of VTEC. Human infection is acquired through the ingestion of contaminated food, especially under-cooked hamburger, through direct contact with animals, via contaminated water or environments, or via person-to-person transmission.

The occurrence of large outbreaks of food-borne VTEC-associated illness has promoted close scrutiny of this zoonoses at all levels in the chain of transmission, including the farm, abattoir, food processing, packaging and distribution plants, the wholesaler, the retailer and the consumer. While eradication of VTEC O157 at the farm may not be an option, interventions to increase animal resistance or to decrease animal exposure are being developed and validated. Hazard Analysis and Critical Control Programmes are being implemented in the processing sector and appear to be associated with temporal decreases in VTEC serotype O157 illness in humans. Education programmes targeting food handling procedures and hygiene practices are being advocated at the retail and consumer level. Continued efforts at all stages from the farm to the consumer will be necessary to reduce the risk of VTEC-associated illness in humans.

History

Konowalchuk and colleagues in Canada conducted the pioneering work in the late 1970s that led to the discovery of Verocytotoxins (VTs) (Konowalchuk *et al.* 1977; Konowalchuk *et al.* 1978). During an investigation of the usefulness of Vero (African green monkey kidney) cells for detecting the heat-labile enterotoxin (labile toxin (LT)) of *E. coli* they observed that culture filtrates from some *E. coli* strains produced a profound irreversible cytopathic effect in Vero cells, in contrast to the reversible cytotonic effect of LT. VT was detected in culture filtrates from 10 strains (belonging to 9 different serotypes) of 136 test strains from various sources; 7 of the VT+ strains were from infants with diarrhoea, one was from a weanling pig, and two strains were from cheese which provides the earliest suggestion of food as a source for these bacteria. Konowalchuk and colleagues speculated that VTs had a role in the genesis of diarrhoea.

O'Brien and LaVeck (1983) purified and characterized the VT from Konowalchuk's prototype VT-producing *Escherichia coli* (VTEC) strain, H.30, showed that it was a polypeptide subunit toxin that was structurally and antigenically similar to Shiga toxin produced by *Shigella dysenteriae* type 1, and referred to it as Shiga-like toxin (SLT). There has been some controversy about the nomenclature of these toxins, which are referred to as Shiga toxins (Calderwood *et al.* 1996), Verotoxins (Karmali *et al.* 1985) and Verocytotoxins (Karmali 1989; Konowalchuk *et al.* 1977).

The clinical significance of VTEC in human disease remained uncertain until the early 1980s when Riley *et al.* (1983), and Karmali *et al.* (1983, 1985) linked these bacteria with two diseases of hitherto unknown etiology, hemorrhagic colitis and HUS, respectively. In a report of two outbreaks of a poorly understood condition referred to as 'haemorrhagic colitis' in 1983, Riley and colleagues from the Centers for Disease Control (CDC), Atlanta, found a close link between disease, consumption of undercooked hamburger patties from a commercial fast-food outlet, and infection by a hitherto 'rare' *E. coli* serotype, O157:H7 which was later shown to produce VT. The outbreak strain was subsequently recovered from a preserved quality-control sample of hamburger meat from the batch implicated in the outbreaks.

Also in 1983, Karmali *et al.* (1983) in Toronto, established a link between infection by VTEC belonging to several serotypes, including O157:H7, and HUS, a condition of unknown aetiology that was first described in 1955 (Gasser *et al.* 1955). Karmali *et al.* (1983) suggested that VT was of direct significance in the genesis of HUS because VT was present *in vivo* (in faecal filtrates of HUS patients), it was a common denominator in strains belonging to several different *E. coli* serotypes that were associated with HUS, and significant antibody responses to VT were observed in the sera of several patients. They postulated that VT was responsible for the damage to capillaries in the glomeruli and other organs, probably through a direct cytotoxic action on endothelial cells, to produce the characteristic microangiopathic features of HUS.

These initial observations by Riley *et al.* and Karmali *et al.* were subsequently confirmed in several centres throughout the world (Griffin 1995; Griffin and Tauxe 1991; Karch *et al.* 1999; Karmali 1989; Nataro and Kaper 1998).

Significant advances were subsequently made in understanding the epidemiology and pathogenesis of infection by VTEC, which have become widely recognized as major zoonotic pathogens of humans (Griffin 1995; Griffin and Tauxe 1991; Karch *et al.* 1999; Karmali 1989; Nataro and Kaper 1998).

The hosts

Human

Incubation period
The majority of reported outbreaks of VTEC infection have been associated with VTEC serotype O157:H7. Estimates of the incubation period in these outbreaks have ranged from about 1 to 9 days, with an average of about 3–5 days (Griffin and Tauxe 1991).

Clinical features
VTEC infection is associated with a wide spectrum of clinical manifestations that include non-specific diarrhoea, haemorrhagic colitis, and HUS (Griffin 1995; Griffin and Tauxe 1991; Karch *et al.* 1999; Karmali 1989; Nataro and Kaper 1998).

Haemorrhagic colitis
This illness is characterized by the sudden onset of severe abdominal cramping, followed within hours by watery diarrhoea (Riley *et al.* 1983; Riley 1987). Patients may experience nausea, but vomiting is not a distinctive feature. Watery diarrhoea progresses rapidly to a phase characterized by profuse bloody discharge resembling lower gastrointestinal haemorrhage. Fever is typically absent or low-grade. The white blood cell count may be elevated with a slight left shift. Barium enema examination, if performed early, shows a 'pseudotumour' or 'thumbprinting' pattern, suggesting submucosal oedema or haemorrhage, usually in the ascending or transverse colon. Colonoscopy may show erythema, haemorrhage, and oedema in the ascending and proximal transverse colon. An inflammatory exudate may also be seen. Most patients recover fully. Severe illness may be complicated by HUS, and rarely, by bowel stricture.

Haemolytic uraemic syndrome (HUS)
The triad of features that define HUS are: acute renal failure, thrombocytopenia, and microangiopathic haemolytic anaemia. Although there are different varieties of HUS, the most common form, by far, is 'classical,' or D+ (diarrhoea associated) HUS, which has its highest incidence in children. It presents, typically, a few days after the onset of an acute diarrhoeal 'prodromal' illness, which is often bloody with features indistinguishable from those of haemorrhagic colitis. The other, very uncommon, forms of HUS, also referred to as D-HUS, include the 'atypical' HUS of childhood (in which the prodrome is typically a respiratory illness), childhood forms that are inherited, and adult forms that occur in association with pregnancy, oral contraceptive usage, malignant hypertension, and various chronic illnesses.

Classical, VTEC-associated, HUS is a leading cause of acute renal failure in childhood (Fong *et al.* 1982; Karmali 1989; Taylor and Monnens 1998). The incidence of HUS in outbreaks of VTEC serotype O157:H7 infection has been typically about 7–10% (Griffin and Tauxe 1991) although it was as high as 25% (Carter *et al.* 1987) in an outbreak in a nursing home. HUS may also occur as a complication of VTEC-associated urinary tract infection (Tarr *et al.* 2005). The severity of HUS varies from an incomplete and/or clinically mild condition (McLaine *et al.* 1992; Tarr *et al.* 2005) to a severe and fulminating illness with multiple organ involvement including the gastrointestinal tract, heart, lungs, pancreas, and central nervous system (CNS) (Richardson *et al.* 1988; Upadhyaya *et al.* 1980).

HUS is also a major complication of Shiga dysentery associated with *Shigella dysenteriae* type 1 (Butler *et al.* 1987; Raghupathy *et al.* 1978). The central factor responsible for the genesis of HUS following both VTEC infection and Shiga dysentery is likely the identical protein exotoxin, referred to as VT1 or Shiga toxin, that is elaborated by VTEC and *Sh. dysenteriae* type 1, respectively (Karmali 1992).

Treatment and prognosis
Most patients with uncomplicated VTEC infection recover fully with general supportive measures (Griffin *et al.* 1988; Karmali 1989). In the USA the number of cases of VTEC infection annually was estimated to be 110,220 (73,480 associated with VTEC serotype O157:H7 and 36,740 cases associated with non-O157 serotypes) (Mead *et al.* 1999), with a hospitalization rate of about 30% and a case fatality rate of about 1%, the fatal cases being associated with complications such as HUS.

HUS used to have a very high case-fatality rate of about 50% (Gianantonio *et al.* 1964, 1973). But improvement in the treatment of renal failure and the attendant biochemical disturbances, largely through the use of peritoneal dialysis, has substantially improved the outlook; the case-fatality rate is now greatly reduced to 5% or less. However, up to 40% of survivors may develop long-term residual disability in the form of end-stage renal disease (ESRD), hypertension, diabetes (Garg *et al.* 2003, 2005; Suri *et al.* 2005), or a neurological deficit (Garg *et al.* 2003; Trompeter *et al.* 1983). The severity of acute illness, especially CNS symptoms, and the need for initial dialysis is strongly associated with a worse long-term prognosis (Garg *et al.* 2003). Lynn and colleagues (Lynn *et al.* 2005) observed that the case-fatality rate of diarrhoea-associated HUS during the acute illness in the UK and Ireland was 1.8% (of 389 patients) during the period 1997 to 2001 compared to 5.6% (of 252 patients) during the period 1985 to 1988.

Tarr and colleagues (Tarr *et al.* 2005) recommend that patients with confirmed VTEC infection and bloody diarrhoea should be initially admitted to hospital to observe for any signs of progression to HUS and also to limit spread of the infection to the community. There are no specific therapies for HUS and patients should, as far as possible, be managed by specialists with experience in the management of renal failure, and of any other complications such as CNS symptoms, with strategies, including dialysis, to ensure optimal renal perfusion, blood pressure control, and fluid and electrolyte balance.

Although the role of antimicrobial agents in ameliorating the symptoms of VTEC infection, or preventing complications such as HUS, remains controversial (Ikeda *et al.* 1999; Safdar *et al.* 2002; Wong *et al.* 2000), Tarr and colleagues recommend avoidance of antimicrobial use (Tarr *et al.* 2005) based on a number of considerations including enhancement of toxin production by these agents (Grif *et al.* 1998a; Karch *et al.* 1986). Anti-motility drugs, opiates, and non-steroidal anti-inflammatory agents also should be avoided (Cimolai *et al.* 1992, 1994; Tarr *et al.* 2005). The possibility that immunotherapy using humanized monoclonal antibody against VTs might be useful clinically if administered soon after exposure, or after onset of symptoms, is under investigation (Tzipori *et al.* 2004). Non-antibody ligands, such VT receptor analogues offer the theoretical possibility for absorbing VT in the bowel and thus reducing toxin translocation and the development of systemic toxaemic complications such as HUS (Armstrong *et al.* 1995; Karmali 2004; Paton *et al.* 2001; Watanabe *et al.* 2004). In a phase-II clinical trial, one receptor analogue, Synsorb (Pk trisaccharide) was shown to be very safe, but evidence for its efficacy in preventing HUS was inconclusive (Trachtman *et al.* 2003).

Pathology

Post-mortem findings in fatal cases of HUS with haemorrhagic colitis typically include pale swollen kidneys with petechial capsular haemorrhages (Richardson *et al.* 1988). Oedematous thickening and haemorrhage is seen affecting parts or all of the colon and the small intestine, and also may be evident in other organs, such as the central nervous system, lungs, heart, and pancreas. In severe cases the entire bowel may appear necrotic and gangrenous (Richardson *et al.* 1988).

The renal histopathology is characterized by glomerular thrombotic microangiopathy with endothelial cell swelling and subendothelial deposits (Habib *et al.* 1982; Richardson *et al.* 1988). Afferent arterioles and small- and medium-sized arteries also may be involved (Habib *et al.* 1982; Richardson *et al.* 1988). Similar thrombotic microangiopathy may be seen in the capillaries of the brain, gastrointestinal tract, and other organs (Richardson *et al.* 1988; Upadhyaya *et al.* 1980).

Histopathological appearances in the bowel include mucosal and submucosal oedema and haemorrhage, patchy ulceration, thrombotic occlusion of vessels, and, occasionally, pseudomembrane formation (Morrison *et al.* 1985; Richardson *et al.* 1988). Inflammatory changes vary from mild and non-specific (Richardson *et al.* 1988) to acute inflammation resembling ischaemic colitis or infectious colitis (Griffin *et al.* 1990; Kelly *et al.* 1987). Severe cases may exhibit marked ileal mucosal ulceration or full-thickness necrosis of the bowel wall (Richardson *et al.* 1988).

Colonoscopy or sigmoidoscopy in patients with haemorrhagic colitis may show a friable oedematous mucosa with evidence of inflammation, haemorrhage, ulceration, or pseudomembrane formation (Morrison *et al.* 1985). Histological examination of biopsies is often inconclusive, showing non-specific changes or variable features of both infectious colitis and ischaemic colitis.

Diagnosis

The optimal strategy for the laboratory diagnosis of VTEC infection involves the detection and isolation of VTEC, especially of serotype O157:H7, from the faeces of patients with a compatible clinical illness. A variety of methods are now available for rapid detection including genetic methods using the polymerase chain reaction (PCR) (Bellin *et al.* 2001; Karch and Meyer 1989; Paton and Paton 1998a, 1998b; Pollard *et al.* 1990; Pulz *et al.* 2003) and various immunospecific methods to detect VT antigen in faeces, either directly or after broth-culture enrichment, or in bacterial culture filtrates (Karmali *et al.* 1994; Kehl *et al.* 1997; Mackenzie *et al.* 1998). Rapid isolation of VTEC in pure culture provides an opportunity to investigate the role of the isolated strain in outbreaks, especially of serotype O157:H7, by pulsed-field gel electrophoresis (Bohm and Karch 1992; Swaminathan *et al.* 2001). Suitably-adapted culture methods as well as genetic and immunospecific assays are used for detecting VTEC in animal, food and environmental samples (Karch *et al.* 1999; Paton and Paton 1998b).

We recommended that clinical laboratories use both the sorbitol-MacConkey agar to isolate VTEC serotype O157:H7, from faeces, as well as a rapid screening method, either PCR or an immunospecific assay, to detect non-O157 VTEC in faeces.

Isolation of VTEC O157:H7 in culture

Sorbitol MacConkey agar: VTEC serotype, O157:H7 (and also O157:H–) is typically isolated from faeces on sorbitol-containing MacConkey (SMAC) agar (March and Ratnam 1986). The selectivity of the SMAC medium is based on the fact that most *E. coli* O157:H7 strains, unlike 95% of other *E. coli*, do not ferment sorbitol within 24 hours of incubation and thus appear colourless on this medium (March and Ratnam 1986). Non-sorbitol-fermenting colonies need to be confirmed as *E. coli* by biochemical tests, and serotyped by anti-serum to the O157 and H7 antigens using commercial reagents that are widely available. Isolates should be tested for VT production by genetic or immunospecific methods (Mackenzie *et al.* 1998; Pulz *et al.* 2003). While easily incorporated in most diagnostic laboratories, the SMAC medium is limited because it:

1 Is insensitive for detecting low inocula,

2 Cannot diagnose infection due to non-O157 VTEC.

The emergence of a clone of sorbitol-fermenting VTEC O157 in Central Europe further compromises the utility of the SMAC medium in diagnosing VTEC infections (Gunzer *et al.* 1992; Karch *et al.* 1999). The technique of immunomagnetic separation has been found to be useful in selectively isolating *E. coli* O157 from foods and animals (Chapman and Siddons 1996).

Detection and isolation of non-O157 VTEC serotypes

Over 200 serotypes of VTEC other than O157 have been associated with human disease. Non-O157 VTEC serotypes are probably best detected using one of a variety of very sensitive and specific immunoassays (Karmali *et al.* 1994; Kehl *et al.* 1997; Mackenzie *et al.* 1998) or PCR protocols, including real-time PCR (Bellin *et al.* 2001; Karch and Meyer 1989; Paton and Paton 1998a, 1998b; Pollard *et al.* 1990; Pulz *et al.* 2003), that are available to detect VTs or

VT genes either directly in faeces or faecal filtrates, after broth culture enrichment, or in colony sweeps. Growing evidence indicates that not all non-O157 VTEC serotypes are human pathogens. The more virulent serotypes (seropathotypes) can be distinguished from the non-virulent and less virulent forms on the basis of the presence of specific genomic islands (Karmali *et al.* 2003b; Coombes *et al.* 2008).

Typing methods

Typing and subtyping of strains is essential for investigating and identifying outbreaks and for establishing the sources, reservoirs, and routes of transmission of pathogens. The main methods currently used for typing and subtyping *E. coli* O157:H7 strains (Karmali *et al.* 2010) include pulsed-field gel electrophoresis (PFGE) (Swaminathan *et al.* 2006), phage-typing (Ahmed *et al.* 1987) and MLVA (Hyytia-Trees *et al.* 2006). Following its development in the United States, the PulseNet network has been implemented in Canada, Europe, the Asia Pacific region, and Latin America to facilitate sharing of molecular epidemiological information internationally (Swaminathan *et al.* 2006).

Serological methods

Serological diagnosis of VTEC infection using antibodies against VTs is not useful because such antibodies are found in both cases as well as control samples (Karmali *et al.* 2003a). However, serological responses to the O157 lipopolysaccharide correlate well with recent infection by *E. coli* O157:H7, and are thus useful in diagnosing VTEC infection associated with this particular serotype (Barrett *et al.* 1991; Chart *et al.* 1991; Reymond *et al.* 1996). VTEC serotype O157 infections also may be diagnosed by assaying saliva for serological response to O157 (Ludwig *et al.* 2002a).It should be noted, however, that the O157 lipopolysaccharide (LPS) cross-reacts with the LPS of other bacteria, such as *Brucella abortus* (Corbel *et al.* 1983; Notenboom *et al.* 1987). Serological responses to LPS of serotypes other than O157 may be helpful in establishing the pathogenetic significance of these strains (Ludwig *et al.* 1994).

Animal

Animals may be asymptomatic carriers of VTEC or may develop specific syndromes, depending on the host species and the characteristics of the infecting VTEC. A highly fatal syndrome affecting weanling pigs, oedema disease, is associated with specific VTEC serotypes O138, O139 and O141 and is characterized by anorexia, oedema of the eyelids, and neurological involvement (Dobrescu 1983; MacLeod *et al.* 1991; Shanks 1938). However, the majority of VTECs of public health significance are shed in the faeces of asymptomatic cattle which constitute the main reservoir of strains implicated in human disease (Beutin *et al.* 1993, 1995; Mohammed *et al.* 1985; Montenegro *et al.* 1990; Shanks 1938; Suthienkul *et al.* 1990; Wells *et al.* 1991). A growing number of non-O157 VTEC serotypes have been isolated from animals, and many of these serotypes have been associated with human disease (Beutin *et al.* 1998; Wilson *et al.* 1996; World Health Organization (WHO) 1999).

Cattle

Escherichia coli O157 (*E.coli* O157) has been the most widely studied VTEC serotype in cattle. Cattle shed these bacteria transiently in their faeces without clinical symptoms (Besser *et al.* 1997; Mechie *et al.* 1997; Rahn *et al.* 1997; Shere *et al.* 1998; Zhao *et al.* 1995). VTEC serotype O157 strains also have been isolated from raw milk (Sandhu *et al.* 1996; Wells *et al.* 1991). Because *E. coli* O157 are not associated with clinical illness in cattle, and there are no established

strategies to eliminate faecal shedding, diagnostic testing is generally conducted for research purposes. The concentration of faecal shedding is often low, requiring the use of selective enrichment and immunomagnetic separation (IMS) to detect the pathogen (Moxley 2003). Most testing in cattle faeces involves identifying the presence or absence of *E. coli* O157. Culture methods typically involve the use of enrichment, immunomagnetic separation, and selective media such as SMAC containing cefixime and tellurite, with latex agglutination used to detect the presence of the O157 antigen (Meyer-Broseta *et al.* 2001; Moxley 2003).

Estimates of the prevalence of *E. coli* O157 in cattle vary among studies, between countries, and among cattle production types. Nonetheless, *E. coli* O157 is common in cattle (Gannon *et al.* 2002; Gansheroff and O'Brien 2000). Prevalence estimates in peri-parturient cows and their calves in one herd in Alberta, Canada, ranged from 16 to 26% (Gannon *et al.* 2002) and serological evidence from cattle in the USA suggests that most range-fed beef calves have been exposed to *E. coli* O157 by the time of weaning (Laegreid *et al.* 1999). Point prevalence estimates of *E. coli* O157 in North American feeder cattle range from 10 to 28% and most, if not all, farms have positive animals at some time (Elder *et al.* 2000; National Animal Health Monitoring System (NAHMS) 2001; Sargeant *et al.* 2003; Smith *et al.* 2001). Within pen prevalence in feedlot cattle shows temporal peaks with 80% or more of the cattle shedding *E. coli* O157 at some points in time (Khaitsa *et al.* 2003; Smith *et al.* 2001). Previous exposure to *E. coli* O157 does not appear to confer protection against reinfection, even with the same genetic strain (Cray and Moon 1995; Johnson *et al.* 1996; Sanderson *et al.* 1999; Wray *et al.* 2000). It has been proposed that faecal shedding may be either transient, wherein cattle shed the pathogen briefly following exposure, or more long term, resulting from colonization of the gastrointestinal tract (Rice *et al.* 2003). Mathematical disease models (Matthews *et al.* 2006) and studies quantifying the concentration of *E. coli* O157 in cattle at slaughter (Low *et al.* 2005; Omisakin *et al.* 2003) suggest that a proportion of positive animals may shed *E. coli* O157 at much higher concentrations than others—the so-called super-shedders (Naylor *et al.* 2003). High concentration of *E. coli* O157 in faeces or prolonged shedding may result from colonization in the terminal rectum (Low *et al.* 2005; Naylor *et al.* 2003; Rice *et al.* 2003). These animals may be important in the maintenance of infection and the occurrence of temporal peaks in cattle herds. Animals shedding *E. coli* O157 at a high concentration also may be important from a public health standpoint; process risk modelling has identified the concentration of *E. coli* O157:H7 in cattle faeces as a highly important risk for human illness, whereas prevalence in cattle was not nearly as highly correlated with risk (Cassin *et al.* 1998).

Sorbitol-fermenting *E. coli* O157:H- associated with human disease in Central Europe have been isolated from cattle (Bielaszewska *et al.* 2000; Karch *et al.* 1999).

Non-bovine species

E. coli O157 also have been isolated from the faeces of numerous non-bovine species. These include, but likely are not limited to, sheep (Chapman *et al.* 1997; Kudva *et al.* 1996), deer (Fischer *et al.* 2001; Renter *et al.* 2001; Sargeant *et al.* 1999), rats (Cizek *et al.* 1999), birds, horses, and dogs (Hancock *et al.* 1998), raccoons (Shere *et al.* 1998), and possums (Renter *et al.* 2003). As with cattle, clinical illness does not appear to be associated with *E. coli* O157 in any of these species. The significance of faecal shedding of *E. coli* O157 in non-bovine species is not known. However, it is plausible that non-bovine species may be involved in the transmission of the pathogen to cattle within shared environments. *Escherichia coli* O157 also have been isolated from flies (Alam and Zurek 2004; Hancock *et al.* 1998; Iwasa *et al.* 1999; Rahn *et al.* 1997), which may serve as a mechanical vector. The public health significance of *E. coli* O157 in non-bovine species is not clear, although disease in humans associated with flies and with deer has been reported (Keene *et al.* 1997b; Moriya *et al.* 1999) and identical genetic strains have been identified in wildlife and cattle within the same agricultural environment (Renter *et al.* 2003).

Non-O157 VTEC in animals

Less research has been conducted to determine the prevalence and epidemiology of non-O157 VTEC in ruminants. However, non-O157 VTEC strains with the potential to cause disease in humans, such as O26, O103, O111, and O145, have been isolated from healthy cattle (Cobbold *et al.* 2004; Hussein and Sakuma 2005; Jenkins *et al.* 2003; Renter *et al.* 2005). VTEC also have been isolated from water sources available to cattle (Renter *et al.* 2005) and identical VTEC strains have been identified in wildlife and cattle in close proximity (Nielsen *et al.* 2004; Renter *et al.* 2005). The full extent of the prevalence of non-O157 VTEC, of human clinical significance, in domestic animals and wildlife is not known.

The agent (VTEC)

Taxonomy and classification

Taxonomically the genus *Escherichia*, in the family Enterobacteriaceae, is very closely related to, if not identical with, the genus *Shigella* (Donnenberg and Whittam 2001). VT1, in VTEC is virtually identical to Shiga toxin produced by *Sh. dysenteriae* type 1. Both toxins are phage-mediated (Schmidt 2001).

The property of VT-production distinguishes VTEC from other pathogenic enteric *E. coli*, enterotoxigenic *E. coli*, enteroinvasive *E. coli*, enteropathogenic *E. coli* (EPEC) serotypes, and enteroaggregative *E. coli* (Nataro and Kaper 1998).

Over 200 different VTEC OH serotypes have now been associated with human disease and many others have been recovered exclusively from animals (WHO 1999). The term enterohaemorrhagic *E. coli* (EHEC) has been applied to those VTEC serotypes that have the same clinical, epidemiological, and pathogenetic features associated with the prototype strain *E. coli* O157:H7 (Levine *et al.* 1987).

Population genetics of VTEC

Whittam and colleagues investigated the clonal origin of VTEC serotype O157:H7 strains by assaying allelic variation at up to 20 different enzyme loci by multilocus enzyme electrophoresis. Strains of *E. coli* O157:H7 from a diversity of sources were found to constitute a genetically distinct clonal group that is only distantly related to VTEC of other serotypes (Whittam *et al.* 1988). The O157:H7 clone was shown to be most closely related to a clone of EPEC serotype O55:H7 that has long been associated with worldwide outbreaks of infantile diarrhoea (Whittam *et al.* 1993). A model has been developed (Feng *et al.* 1998; Wick *et al.* 2005) for the stepwise evolution of *E. coli* O157:H7 from a non-toxigenic EPEC serotype O55:H7 progenitor strain with the sequential acquisition of a VT2-encoding bacteriophage, the O157 antigen, and the large pO157 plasmid. Further lineages then developed with, in one, the classical *E. coli* O157:H7 clone, the loss of the properties of sorbitol

fermentation (Sor) and beta-glucuronidase (GUD) activities and gain of a VT1 phage, and in another, the retention of Sor and GUD activites, but the loss of motility. The latter clone represents the Sor+ O157:H-clone which is becoming increasingly prevalent in Central Europe (Karch *et al.* 1999). There is growing evidence that O157 genomes are rapidly diverging and radiating into new niches as the pathogen disseminates (Kim *et al.* 2001; Wick *et al.* 2005). Using Octamer-Based Genome Scanning, Kim *et al.* (Kim *et al.* 1999; Kim *et al.* 2001a) showed that GUD- and Sor-*E. coli* O157:H7 strains have diverged into two distinct lineages, I and II, with distinct ecological characteristics and that lineage I strains are more commonly associated with human disease than lineage II strains. Comparative genomic studies (Zhang *et al.* 2007) have identified significant differences in the genomic content of the two lineages thus supporting the notion that the two lineages have differences in virulence characteristics, including transmissibility. An analysis of strains associated with a very severe, spinach-associated outbreak, resulted in the identification of a unique clade, clade 8 that was associated with severe disease (Manning *et al.* 2008). This clade corresponds to a lineage that is intermediate between lineages I and II and is referred to as lineage I/II (Ziebell *et al.* 2008).

Disease mechanisms

Current knowledge of VTEC's disease mechanisms is based primarily on studies with VTEC serotype O157:H7 (Nataro and Kaper 1998). The low infectious dose (~ 100–500 organisms) (Griffin 1998) of *E. coli* O157:H7 is a major determinant of its ability to cause severe and epidemic disease, although the underlying mechanisms for this are not fully understood. However resistance of the organism to gastric acid (Lin *et al.* 1996) probably contributes to this.

Following passage through the stomach the two key virulence strategies of VTEC are VT-production and colonization of the bowel. While bowel colonization is likely a complex process requiring several mechanisms, the only established process involves colonization of the mucosal epithelial cells of, probably, the large bowel (Nataro and Kaper 1998) with a characteristic 'attaching and effacing' (AE) cytopathology, which is encoded for by genes on the LEE (Locus of Enterocyte Effacement) pathogenicity island (PAI) (Jerse *et al.* 1990; McDaniel *et al.* 1995; McDaniel and Kaper 1997; Nataro and Kaper 1998). Many other factors are postulated to be virulence factors and the list has expanded greatly with the publication of the genome sequences of two epidemic strains of *E. coli* O157:H7 by scientists from the USA (Perna *et al.* 2001) and Japan (Hayashi *et al.* 2001) respectively, and also from the sequence of the plasmid pO157 of *E. coli* O157:H7 (Brunder *et al.* 1999; Burland *et al.* 1998; Karch *et al.* 1998; Makino *et al.* 1998).

Verocytotoxins and the pathogenesis of HUS

Human VTEC strains elaborate at least four potent bacteriophage-mediated VTs: VT1, VT2, VT2c, and VT2d (Melton-Celsa and O'Brien 1998; Nataro and Kaper 1998). Each may be present alone, or in a combination of two or three different VTs. VT1 is virtually identical to Shiga toxin, but is serologically distinct from VT2s (Karmali 1989; O'Brien *et al.* 1992). The toxins share a common polypeptide subunit structure consisting of an enzymatically-active A subunit (~ 32 kDa) linked to a pentamer of B subunits (~ 7.5 kDa). VT's are produced in the bowel and are translocated intact into the circulation although the mechanism of translocation is not fully understood (Hurley *et al.* 1999; Philpott *et al.* 1997). The toxins are thought to be transported by leukocytes (te Loo *et al.* 2001) to capillary endothelial cells (Obrig *et al.* 1988) in the renal glomeruli, gastrointestinal tract, pancreas, and other organs and tissues (Monnens *et al.* 1998; Richardson *et al.* 1992). After binding to the glycolipid receptor, globotriaosylceramide (Gb3) (Lingwood *et al.* 1987, 1998) on the target endothelial cell, the toxins are internalized by receptor-mediated endocytosis (Sandvig and van Deurs 1996). They then target the endoplasmic reticulum via the Golgi by a process termed 'retrograde transport' (Sandvig and van Deurs 1996). Inside the host cell, the A subunit is proteolytically nicked to give an enzymatically active A_1 fragment (O'Brien *et al.* 1992), which cleaves the N-glycosidic bond at position A^{4324} of the 28S rRNA of the 60S ribosomal subunit (Endo *et al.* 1988). This blocks EF 1-dependent aminoacyl tRNA binding, resulting in the inhibition of protein synthesis (O'Brien *et al.* 1992). VTs may also damage eukaryotic cells by apoptosis (Monnens *et al.* 1998). Cytokines, especially TNF- α and IL 1- β, potentiate toxin action through upregulation of the cellular receptor; Gb3 (Monnens *et al.* 1998). It is thought that increased cytokine production might be the result of VT action on monocytes (Monnens *et al.* 1998).

While the injurious action of VTs on endothelial cells appears to be crucial to the development of HUS, the precise cellular events that result in the associated pathophysiological changes, including thrombotic microangiopathy, hemolytic anemia and thrombocytopenia, remain to be fully elucidated (Proulx *et al.* 2001; Tarr *et al.* 2005).

The attaching and effacing (AE) lesion and the locus of enterocyte effacement

First coined by Moon and colleagues in the early 1980s (Moon *et al.* 1983) the AE lesion is a characteristic phenotype of enteropathogenic *E. coli* (EPEC), enterohemorrhagic *E. coli* (EHEC), a small subset of enteropathogenic *Hafnia alvei*, rabbit diarrheagenic *E. coli* (RDEC) and strains of *Citrobacter rodentium* that cause murine colonic hyperplasia (Nataro and Kaper 1998). The AE lesion of *E. coli* O157:H7 and other EHEC serotypes resembles that associated with enteropathogenic *E. coli* (EPEC) and consists of the destruction of microvilli, an intimate effacing adherence of the organism to the enterocyte membrane, and changes in the cytoskeletal structure of the enterocyte associated with the accumulation of polymerized actin and other cytoskeletal proteins beneath the site of bacterial attachment (Knutton *et al.* 1987; Moon *et al.* 1983; Nataro and Kaper 1998; Sherman *et al.* 1988). All of the virulence factors necessary for the formation of the AE lesion, in EHEC and EPEC, are encoded by the LEE PAI (Jerse *et al.* 1990; McDaniel *et al.* 1995; McDaniel and Kaper 1997; Nataro and Kaper 1998) which encodes the structural, accessory, and effector molecules of a type III secretion system (TTSS) (Foubister *et al.* 1994; Goosney *et al.* 2001; Jarvis *et al.* 1995; Jarvis and Kaper 1996; Knutton *et al.* 1994), a macromolecular complex spanning both bacterial membranes that is used by many Gram-negative bacterial pathogens to inject virulence factors directly into host cells to subvert host cellular function for the benefit of the pathogen (Hueck 1998).

The LEE of VTEC serotype O157:H7 reference strain EDL 933, which is ~ 43.4 kb in size, contains 41 open-reading frames (ORFs) which are organized in five polycistronic operons (LEE 1, LEE 2, LEE 3, LEE 5, and LEE 4) (Nataro and Kaper 1998). LEE 1, LEE 2, and LEE 3 encode structural and regulatory components of the TTSS (Nataro and Kaper 1998). LEE 5 contains the *eae* gene, which encodes the outer membrane adhesin, intimin (Nataro and Kaper 1998), and genes that encode the translocated intimin receptor known as Tir (Kenny *et al.* 1997) or EspE (Deibel *et al.* 1998) and

the Tir chaperone, CesT (Abe *et al.* 1999; Elliott *et al.* 1999). The LEE 4 operon encodes the structural needle protein, EscF (Wilson *et al.* 2001), the translocator proteins EspA, EspB, and EspD (Garmendia *et al.* 2005; Nataro and Kaper 1998), and the effector protein EspF (McNamara and Donnenberg 1998).

About 40 different effector molecules, encoded for within LEE as well as on PAIs outside LEE have been recognized which are secreted by the LEE-encoded TTSS and progress is being made in understanding how they disrupt the host cellular machinery to cause pathology (Tobe *et al.* 2006; Dean and Kenny 2009). The first gene (Ler), in the LEE 1 operon, activates transcription of the LEE 2, 3, and 4 operons (Elliott *et al.* 2000; Mellies *et al.* 1999; Sperandio *et al.* 2000), which, in *E. coli* O157:H7, are also activated by a complex network of regulatory molecules (Dean and Kenny 2009; Garmendia *et al.* 2005) and processes such as quorum sensing through activation of autoinducer-2 (Sperandio *et al.* 1999).

Plasmid-mediated putative virulence factors

Escherichia coli O157:H7 and other EHEC contain a large 92-kb F-like plasmid, pO157, which contains 100 ORFs of which 20 encode putative virulence factors (Brunder *et al.* 1999; Burland *et al.* 1998; Karch *et al.* 1998; Makino *et al.* 1998). These include: the EHEC hemolysin (hlyCABD operon); catalase-peroxidase (katP); a serine protease (espP) which is secreted by a type IV secretion system; a 13 gene cluster (etpC-etpO) related to the type II secretion pathway; and an ORF encoding a 3169 aa predicted product that shares homology with large clostridial toxins. None of these genes has been shown to have a role in pathogenesis. The large plasmid is present in several other EHEC serotypes, but its composition is very heterogeneous (Brunder *et al.* 1999). Plasmids from strains causing HUS have lacked one or more of hly, katP, and espP, suggesting that the latter are not, by themselves, critical for the development of severe disease (Bielaszewska *et al.* 2000).

The genome of *E. coli* O157:H7

The publication of the genome sequences of two epidemic strains of *E. coli* O157:H7, EDL 933 and the Sakai strain in 2001, by investigators from the United States (Perna *et al.* 2001) and Japan (Hayashi *et al.* 2001), respectively led to a rapid growth of knowledge about new potential virulence factors of VTEC and EHEC. The sequences of at least four *E. coli* O157:H7 genomes and selected non-O157 VTEC genomes are available from PubMed (http://www.ncbi.nlm.nih.gov/genomes/lproks.cgi).

The EDL 933 and Sakai genomes have a size of 5.5 Mb, compared to the 4.6-Mb genome size of *E. coli* K-12 strain MG1655. The O157 and K-12 genomes share a common backbone of 4.1 Mb, which is co-linear except for one 422-kb inversion spanning the replication terminus in EDL 933, but not in the Sakai genome.

Differences between the EDL 933 and MG 1655 genomes are reflected by K-islands (KI), which are DNA segments present in MG 1655, but not in EDL933, and O-islands (OI), which are unique segments in EDL933 (Perna *et al.* 2001). In the Sakai genome, the *E. coli* K-12 specific segments are referred to as K-loops and those specific to the Sakai genome are referred to as S-loops (Hayashi *et al.* 2001).

In the EDL 933 genome, OIs total 1.34 Mb of DNA and KIs total 0.53 Mb. There are 177 OIs and 234 KIs greater than 50 bp. Overall, EDL933 contains 1,387 new genes, encoded in strain-specific clusters of diverse sizes. Several of the 177 OIs encode putative virulence factors (Perna *et al.* 2001) and thus may be pathogenicity islands (PAIs) (Hacker and Kaper 2001). Eighteen multigenic regions are related to known bacteriophages, including the *VT-2* converting phage BP-933W and the *VT-1* converting phage CP-933V (Perna *et al.* 2001).

The major OI, other than the VT-1 and VT-2-converting phages, of known pathogenetic significance is LEE which, as discussed in the previous section, encodes the structural, accessory, and effector molecules of a type III secretion system (TTSS) whose actions result in the characteristic AE lesion. Investigation of the biology of the AE lesion in a mouse model of infection by the LEE-positive *Citrobacter rodentium* revealed that the LEE-encoded TTSS is employed for the secretion of several effector molecules encoded outside LEE on other OIs (Deng *et al.* 2004). These effector molecules include NleC and NleD (OI-36), NleF, NleG, and NleA (OI-71), and OI-122 (effectors NleB and NleE). A systematic analysis of the Sakai genome by experimental and biochemical approaches has further expanded the number of TTSS effector molecules encoded outside the LEE-locus to 39 proteins encoded on >20 exchangeable effector loci (EEL) scattered throughout the chromosome (Tobe *et al.* 2006).

At least three newly-identified O-Islands, including OI-122, OI-57, and OI-71 are associated with VTEC serotypes/seropathotypes that are associated with severe and/or epidemic disease (Karmali *et al.* 2003b; Coombes *et al.* 2008). OI-122, OI-57, and OI-71 are thus key markers, together with LEE (Nataro and Kaper 1998), of non-O157 VTEC serotypes of clinical and public health significance.

Immunity and vaccines

The nature of protective immunity to VTEC infection is not well understood (Karmali 1998). The two main virulence strategies of VTEC are their ability to colonize the bowel and to produce VTs. Antibodies that are most likely to be protective are those that inhibit bowel colonization by VTEC and/or those that neutralize the toxins before they reach their target sites.

The peak age-related incidence of HUS is in childhood (Karmali 1989; Rowe *et al.* 1991). The incidence then declines with age, but appears to rise again during old age (Griffin *et al.* 1988). Seroepidemiological studies show that the age-related frequencies of immunoglobulin G antibodies to VT1 and VT2 are inversely related to the age-specific incidence of HUS (Karmali *et al.* 2003a), suggesting strongly that the presence of such antibodies is associated with anti-toxin immunity. Support for the concept that such antibodies are protective against the development of systemic illness such as HUS come from experimental and clinical findings. Rabbits immunized with VT1 or VT2 toxoid develop anti-toxin antibodies, and are protected from disease when challenged intravenously by toxin (Bielaszewska *et al.* 1997; Ludwig *et al.* 2002b; Richardson *et al.* 1992). A sero-epidemiological study of two outbreaks of VTEC infection found that individuals who were seropositive for antibodies to VT did not develop disease whereas those that were seronegative became symptomatic (Karmali *et al.* 1994). A Canadian study (Karmali *et al.* 2003a) found that the frequency of anti-VT1 antibodies and anti-VT2 antibodies was substantially higher in rural dairy farm residents compared to urban residents, an observation consistent with the higher expected exposure to VTEC in the dairy farm environment compared to the urban setting.

Antibodies to LEE-encoded type III secretion proteins have been detected in human sera (Jarvis and Kaper 1996; Jenkins *et al.* 2000;

Karpman *et al.* 2002) but their duration and possible role in protective immunity is not known.

Patients with *E. coli* O157:H7 infection develop strong IgG and IgM responses to the O157 lipopolysaccharide antigen but the antibody levels decline to background levels within several weeks after infection suggesting that they do not have a role in immunity (Bitzan *et al.* 1993; Morooka *et al.* 1995).

Despite *in vitro* (Bielaszewska *et al.* 1997; Ludwig *et al.* 2002b; Richardson *et al.* 1992) and *in vivo* (Karmali *et al.* 2003a) evidence that antibody responses to the VTs are associated with protective immunity, little progress has been made in developing VT toxoid immunization for human populations. However, an *E. coli* O157 O-specific polysaccharide conjugate vaccine, in which the O-specific polysaccharide is conjugated to *Pseudomonas aeruginosa* exotoxin A, was found to be safe and immunogenic in young children (Ahmed *et al.* 2006). A phase-III trial of the latter is planned.

Growth and survival requirements

VTEC grow well under aerobic or facultatively anaerobic conditions. They normally inhabit the intestinal tract, where they can multiply to large numbers when host factors facilitate growth. As with other enteric pathogens, such as *Salmonella*, the normal host flora probably plays an important role in inhibiting growth of VTEC in the intestinal environment. Most information on growth and survival is currently based on studies with VTEC serotype O157:H7. Information on environmental survival is limited (USDA:APHIS:VS 1994), but it has been demonstrated that *E. coli* O157 can survive for long periods (>40 days) in water (Wang and Doyle 1998). Laboratory models suggest that *E. coli* O157 may survive and persist in soil (Gagliardi and Karns 2000; Maule 1999; Ogden *et al.* 2001). VTECs may survive for extended periods in manure (Fukushima *et al.* 1999; Kudva *et al.* 1998; Wang *et al.* 1996), and it is likely that environments contaminated with faecal material will be sources of the organisms for prolonged periods (USDA:APHIS:VS 1994). Prolonged persistence of VTEC in the environment has been linked to survival in soil protozoa (Brown *et al.* 2002). There also is evidence that these organisms may persist for prolonged periods on various farm surfaces such as wood and steel (Williams *et al.* 2005).

In food, *E. coli* O157 strains are killed by routine pasteurization of milk and cooking temperatures (Line *et al.* 1991; USDA:APHIS:VS 1994), similar to many other bacterial pathogens. Recovery of *E. coli* O157 strains from frozen, ground beef after many months suggests that these organisms may persist in the environment under winter conditions for prolonged periods. The ability of some strains to survive low pH (4.5) conditions, coupled with outbreaks associated with apple cider and mayonnaise, has prompted investigation of survival of these organisms under various food-processing methods. The organisms appear to survive dessication and may persist in dry foods such as chocolate for prolonged periods (Hiramatsu *et al.* 2005). Further investigations of the ecology and survival of this complex group of pathogens will be essential for effective public health control methods.

Epidemiology

Outbreaks

There have been numerous outbreaks of *E. coli* O157 throughout the world, in some cases involving hundreds or thousands of cases

(Ahmed and Donaghy 1998; CDC 1993; Effler *et al.* 2001; Michino *et al.* 1999). In the USA between 1982 and 2002, there were 350 outbreaks (more than 2 cases with a common epidemiological exposure) of *E. coli* O157, representing over 8,500 cases with 17% of cases resulting in hospitalization, and 0.5% in death (Rangel *et al.* 2005; Wallace *et al.* 2000). The median number of cases per outbreak in this study was 8, although this number appeared to decline over the 20-year period. Attack rates in outbreaks of *E. coli* O157:H7 have ranged from 0.1 to 71% (Griffin and Tauxe 1991).

Current food production practices may increase the risk of widespread outbreaks (Altekruse *et al.* 1997; Armstrong *et al.* 1996). The mixing of ground hamburger from multiple animals to produce large lots of product, and the widespread distribution of foods from large suppliers means that a single incident of contamination could lead to human illness over a large geographic area. In the USA, consumption of contaminated hamburgers led to a four state outbreak of *E. coli* O157:H7 in 1992–1993 (Davis *et al.* 1993) and alfalfa sprouts from a common lot contaminated with *E. coli* O157:H7 resulted in illness in multiple states (Breuer *et al.* 2001). The increased globalization of food production and dissemination may result in the inadvertent importation of contaminated foods (Kaferstein *et al.* 1997). In the United Kingdom large food-borne outbreaks have occurred from cooked meats cross contaminated from raw meat in commercial kitchens (Cowden *et al.* 2001; Salmon *et al.* 2005). A notable feature has been high secondary household transmission rates in children (Werber *et al.* 2008). Outbreaks associated with petting farms have become a cause of growing concern (NASPHV 2009).

Sporadic cases

Sporadic cases of VTEC, usually *E. coli* O157:H7 from cases of bloody diarrhoea or HUS, have been reported from several countries and occur more frequently than outbreak cases (Griffin and Tauxe 1991; Willshaw *et al.* 2001).

The annual average incidence of sporadic VTEC in Ontario, Canada, between 1997 and 2001 was 3.7 per 100,000 persons. In a major 2-year prospective study of over 5,000 cases of diarrhoea presenting to hospitals in Calgary, Alberta, (Pai *et al.* 1988) found VTEC (mostly serotype O157:H7) in 3.7% of patients, compared to *Salmonella* spp. in 2.7% and *Campylobacter* spp. in 2.0%. In other studies, VTEC serotype O157:H7 has been isolated from 0.6 to 2.5% of submitted stools, usually representing the second or third most frequent bacterial pathogen isolated. The isolation rate in bloody stools has ranged from 15 to 37% (Griffin and Tauxe 1991).

Seasonal occurrence

The number of outbreak and sporadic cases of VTEC O157 and non-O157 VTEC typically peak in the summer months (Brooks *et al.* 2005; Lee and Middleton 2003; Rangel *et al.* 2005; Wallace *et al.* 2000; Willshaw *et al.* 2001). This may be related to factors such as increased consumption of barbequed hamburgers, increased shedding of VTEC by cattle, higher bacterial loads in ground beef, or increased environmental contamination or survival.

Age-related incidence

The peak age-related frequency of VTEC-associated diarrhoea and HUS is in young children (Brooks *et al.* 2005; Eklund *et al.* 2005; Willshaw *et al.* 2001), although the elderly also are at increased risk (Griffin and Tauxe 1991). In a nationwide survey of HUS in children in Australia, HUS was significantly higher in children under 5 years of age compared to those between 5 and 15 years of age (Elliott *et al.* 2001a).

Occurrence of complications

The main complication of VTEC infection is HUS, which has been reported to occur with a frequency of about 8% in several outbreaks of *E. coli* O157:H7 (Karmali 1989) although in one outbreak affecting elderly residents in a nursing home it was as high as 22% (Carter *et al.* 1987). The frequency of sporadic cases of HUS in North America is about 2–3 cases per 100,000 children below 5 years of age (Tarr and Hickman 1987) and 1.5 cases per 100,000 children below 5 years of age in the UK (Lynn *et al.* 2005). However, within the UK, the incidence of childhood HUS is considerably higher in Scotland (3.4 cases per 100,000 children under 5 years of age) (Lynn *et al.* 2005). The incidence in young children in Argentina is roughly tenfold higher than North American rates (Lopez *et al.* 1989).

Sources

Cattle are the main animal reservoirs of VTEC strains implicated in human disease, and foods of bovine origin, especially undercooked ground beef patties and unpasteurized milk, constitute the major sources of human infection (Griffin and Tauxe 1991; Rangel *et al.* 2005). In 2 US studies conducted in the summer months, 53.9 to 64.9% of beef carcasses were positive for non-O157 VTEC strains prior to evisceration, with prevalence reduced to 4–8.3% following safety interventions (Arthur *et al.* 2002; Barkocy-Gallagher *et al.* 2003). In studies of retail ground beef in North America and Thailand, the prevalence of VTEC ranged from 9 to 36.4%, with *E. coli* O157 isolated from 0–3.7% of the samples tested (Doyle and Schoeni 1987; Read *et al.* 1990; Sekla *et al.* 1990; Suthienkul *et al.* 1990). In the same studies, VTEC were detected in retail pork (1–10.6%), poultry (0–1.5%), and lamb (2%), with *E. coli* O157:H7 prevalence in these products of 0–1.5, 0–1.5, and 2%, respectively. Whether the presence of VTEC in foods of non-bovine origin represents carriage in these species or cross-contamination from beef sources during processing is not clear. VTEC also have been detected in about 1% of milk filters in dairy farms (Clarke *et al.* 1989), and unpasteurized milk has been the source of outbreaks (Allerberger *et al.* 2003; Duncan *et al.* 1987; Karmali *et al.* 1994).

Other foods have served as vehicles of VTEC infection, either as primary sources or through cross-contamination with a primary source (Griffin and Tauxe 1991; Morgan *et al.* 1993). These include lettuce (Ackers *et al.* 1998; Hilborn *et al.* 1999), alfalfa sprouts (Breuer *et al.* 2001), radish sprouts (Michino *et al.* 1999), unpasteurized milk (Keene *et al.* 1997a), and apple cider (Besser *et al.* 1993; Cody *et al.* 1999). Transmission of *E. coli* O157 to lettuce plants from manure and irrigation water has been documented (Solomon *et al.* 2002).

Outbreaks of *E. coli* O157 also have been linked to consumption or recreational use of water (Anon 2000; Effler *et al.* 2001; Jackson *et al.* 1998; Keene *et al.* 1994; Swerdlow *et al.* 1992), direct contact with cattle (Crump *et al.* 2002; Wilson *et al.* 1996) or animal excreta (Locking *et al.* 2001), attendance at agricultural fairs (Crump *et al.* 2003; Durso *et al.* 2005), and recreational use of pastures (Ogden *et al.* 2002). Case-controls studies have identified hamburger consumption, lack of hand washing by food preparers, and exposure to a farm environment as major risk factors for sporadic infection with *E. coli* O157 (Mead *et al.* 1997; O'Brien *et al.* 2001). A case of *E. coli* O157:H7 infection in a lacto-vegetarian was thought to be due to the consumption of vegetables from a garden fertilized with cattle faeces (Cieslak *et al.* 1993).

Persons infected with *E. coli* O157 may serve as a source of infection to others and secondary transmission following outbreaks is common (Rowe *et al.* 1993). Numerous outbreaks in day-care centres (Belongia *et al.* 1993; Galanis *et al.* 2003; Spika *et al.* 1986) and within families (Eklund *et al.* 2005) have been documented. A case of laboratory-acquired infection in a technician has been reported (Booth and Rowe 1993) and a severe case of HUS in a nurse was acquired from a patient she was tending (Karmali *et al.* 1988).

Transmission and communicability

Due to the variety of potential sources, there are a large number of potential pathways by which VTEC can be transmitted to individuals and between individuals. Detecting and investigating outbreaks is an important means of determining which sources are most problematic (Tauxe 2006). Molecular subtyping is a valuable aid to increase the ability of surveillance to identify outbreaks and detect them at an earlier stage, increase the specificity of case definition, develop and test hypothesis related to cause, and compare strains across public health jurisdictions (Tauxe 2006). A variety of methods are available for subtyping *E. coli* O157 strains, including biotyping, phage typing, plasmid profiling, chromosomal restriction fragment length polymorphism, and pulsed-field gel electrophoresis (PFGE) (Grif *et al.* 1998b). PulseNet USA is a network of federal and state public health agencies that use a standardized PFGE protocol to subtype *E. coli* O157 (Gerner-Smidt *et al.* 2006; Swaminathan *et al.* 2001, 2006). The network was established in 1996 and achieved full national participation in 2001. The PulseNet network has been implemented in Canada, Europe, the Asia Pacific region, and Latin America who, along with the USA, work together to share molecular epidemiological information (Gerner-Smidt *et al.* 2006; Swaminathan *et al.* 2001, 2006).

Prevention and control

Prevention and control strategies

Optimum control of food-borne pathogens such at VTEC involves efforts at all stages of food production, from farm to fork. Quantitative risk assessments and simulation models are available which describe stages in the farm-to-fork continuum that contribute to an increased risk of food-borne illness and allow potential control measures to be assessed (Cassin *et al.* 1998; Ebel *et al.* 2004; Jordan *et al.* 1999).

Controlling VTEC at the farm level is important not only to reduce the risk of contamination at slaughter, but also to reduce human illness due to direct animal contact, environmental contamination, or contamination of crops following manure fertilization or contamination via water irrigation or run-off. There is a special concern about prevention of transmission on farms that are open to the general public (NASPHV 2009). The complex on-farm ecology, as evidenced by the presence of *E. coli* O157 in non-bovine species within the farm environment (Sargeant and Smith 2003), and in cattle water (Hancock *et al.* 1998; LeJeune *et al.* 2001; Van Donkersgoed *et al.* 2001), and feed (Dodd *et al.* 2003), will need to be considered in designing control efforts.

Contamination of carcasses during the slaughter process is unavoidable, which poses a significant challenge to food safety (Edwards and Fung 2006). Contamination can occur when gut contents or faecal matter come into contact with meat surfaces.

There is a significant correlation between the prevalence of *E. coli* O157 in faeces and hides and carcass contamination (Elder *et al.* 2000). Cross-contamination between carcasses may occur and the extent of contamination can be magnified during processing (Brabban *et al.* 2004; Edwards and Fung 2006). The current trend for concentration and rapid distribution systems in the food-processing sector has resulted in plants that produce vast quantities of product on a daily basis with distribution to large geographic areas (Altekruse *et al.* 1997). This can result in large outbreaks when coupled with improper cooking and handling procedures at the retail or consumer level. However, such concentration of volume can facilitate the implementation of control strategies, resulting in the production of large volumes of high-quality, safe food.

In the home, high-risk food-handling, preparation, and consumption practices are common, revealing the need for food safety education of consumers (Redmond and Griffith 2003). Person-to-person transmission of VTEC infection necessitates effective infection control procedures in hospitals, day-care centres, and other institutions and in families where a family member is experiencing illness.

Methods/Programmes/Evaluation
On-farm

Conceptually, there are a number of means by which pathogens can be controlled in live cattle: eradication by identifying and removing positive animals, pre-harvest testing of cattle prior to marketing, herd level management interventions aimed at reducing animal exposure, and interventions aimed at increasing resistance to infection in animals (Besser *et al.* 2003; Gyles 1998; Hancock *et al.* 2001). While these principles can apply to any pathogen, the majority of research into on-farm control strategies for VTEC has been conducted for *E. coli* O157. The transient nature of faecal shedding of *E. coli* O157 in cattle, the ubiquitous occurrence in cattle and their environments, and the carriage in non-bovine species mean that eradication of this pathogen in cattle is unlikely to be a viable control option. Testing cattle before shipping to market for the purpose of screening-out positive cattle or pens is also an impractical solution due to the transient nature of shedding, the current lack of real-time diagnostic tests, and the high on-farm and pen-level prevalence.

Management practices

Identifying management strategies that enhance or allow faecal shedding, and modifying these practices to reduce the prevalence or concentration of faecal shedding, would reduce animal exposure and transmission. An advantage of this approach is that it tends to target management practices related to faecal-oral transmission, and thus could conceivably have the potential to impact enteric pathogens in general, rather than specifically *E. coli* O157. Numerous studies in dairy and beef cattle have investigated associations between management practices and *E. coli* O157 (Dewell *et al.* 2005; Garber *et al.* 1999; Herriott *et al.* 1998; Sargeant *et al.* 2004a, 2004b; Smith *et al.* 2001). However, management factors that could be manipulated to reduce *E. coli* O157 have not been consistently identified.

Increasing animal resistance

Another option for controlling *E. coli* O157 in cattle is to target intervention efforts at increasing animal resistance to infection.

Examples of interventions using this approach include probiotics, vaccination, antimicrobials, sodium chlorate, and bacteriophages (reviewed in Callaway *et al.* 2004; Lonergan and Brashears 2005).

Probiotics are commensal bacteria fed to reduce pathogenic bacteria in the gastro-intestinal tract through competitive inhibition (Fuller 1989). Randomized controlled trials using these products have produced variable results (Brashears *et al.* 2003; Folmer *et al.* 2003; Peterson *et al.* 2005; Ransom 2004; Younts-Dahl *et al.* 2004, 2005). Randomized controlled trials in small groups of feedlot cattle using a combination of *L. acidophilus* NP51 and *P. freudenreichii* found a significant reduction in the prevalence of *E. coli* O157 (Younts-Dahl *et al.* 2004, 2005), although the same combination was not significantly associated with faecal prevalence in a commercial feedlot (Ransom 2004). This probiotic combination is currently licensed in the USA as Bovamine Culture Complex Probiotic (Nutrition Physiology Corp).

Progress is occurring in understanding the biology of VTEC colonization in cattle, and this has the potential to open up avenues for immunizing cattle against VTEC colonization (Dziva *et al.* 2004; Jordan *et al.* 2004; Naylor *et al.* 2005a; Stevens *et al.* 2002). The LEE PAI is responsible for the colonization of the bovine recto-sigmoid junction by VTEC serotype O157:H7, which is associated with high levels of excretion of this organism by cattle (Low *et al.* 2005; Naylor *et al.* 2005b). Vaccinations utilizing LEE-encoded type III secreted proteins (Tir, EspA, and EspB) have been developed and are being evaluated for use in cattle. In a randomized controlled trial, Potter and colleagues reported a significant reduction in the faecal prevalence of *E. coli* O157:H7 when the vaccine was administered 3 times (Potter *et al.* 2004). However, using a different adjuvant and 2 doses of the vaccine, which may be more practical in commercial feedlot operations, Van Donkersgoed and colleagues did not find a significant reduction in prevalence (Van Donkersgoed *et al.* 2005). The faecal prevalence of *E. coli* O157:H7 was much lower in the latter study, which would have impacted the power to detect small treatment differences. Recent studies have shown reduction in fecal shedding of *E. coli* O157 with 3 doses of a type II vaccine (Moxley *et al.* 2009; Rich *et al.* 2010; Peterson *et al.* 2007). Results with 2 doses of vaccine are more variable, with some trials reporting a significant reduction in *E. coli* O157 (Peterson *et al.* 2007; Smith *et al.* 2008; Smith *et al.* 2009a; Smith *et al.* 2009b) and others reporting no significant effect (Moxley *et al.* 2009). Siderophore Receptor and Porin Protein (SRP) vaccines also have been evaluated in field trials. Thompson *et al.* (2009) reported a significant reduction in fecal shedding of *E. coli* O157 with both 2 and 3 doses of vaccine. Fox *et al.* (2009) reported a significant reduction in fecal shedding with 2 doses of 3 ml of vaccine and a numeric, but not statistically significant, reduction with 2 doses containing 2 ml of vaccine. Vaccines are beginning to be licensed for use in commercial cattle in some countries.

Antimicrobial products may directly affect bacterial populations in the gastro-intestinal tract. The antibiotic neomycin sulfate has been shown to significantly decrease faecal shedding of *E. coli* O157:H7 in cattle (Elder *et al.* 2002; Ransom 2004). However, the use of antibiotics in food animals is controversial due to concerns about the potential for development of antibiotic resistance and neomycin has not been approved in cattle for use as an intervention for *E. coli* O157. Inoculation studies and a randomized control trial in cattle and sheep found a significant reduction in *E. coli* O157 when sodium chlorate was used in the feed or water (Anderson *et al.* 2005; Callaway *et al.* 2002, 2003; Edrington *et al.*

2003). Bacteriophages active against *E. coli* O157:H7 have been identified in ruminants (Kudva *et al.* 1999). However, the effectiveness of bacteriophages in natural conditions has been extremely variable and more research is needed to determine whether this is a viable intervention strategy in ruminants (Callaway *et al.* 2004).

The potential to use interventions that reduce *E. coli* O157 in ruminants by increasing animal resistance is an active area of research. More research is needed to determine efficacy under commercial conditions. Additionally, the use of combinations of intervention strategies needs to be evaluated.

Abattoir

Meat inspection programmes worldwide are undergoing a change from a sensory-based approach to the implementation of strategies with an emphasis on total quality management. Food safety in the processing sector is based on a Hazard Analysis and Critical Control Point (HACCP) approach (Hulebak and Schlosser 2002; Ropkins and Beck 2000). This approach is not specific to the control of VTEC, but broadly addresses biological, chemical, and physical hazards. The specific methods used in the processing sector to meet HACCP requirements vary, but fall into the categories of hide interventions, carcass interventions, or trim interventions (Koohmaraie *et al.* 2005). Interventions include the use of chemicals or antimicrobial products, knife trimming, vacuuming, washing, stream pasteurization, multiple hurdle interventions, low-dose low-penetrating radiation, and good manufacturing practices in the processing line (Edwards and Fung 2006; Koohmaraie *et al.* 2005). In the past, the largest problem with irradiation as an intervention has been consumer acceptance. Recent marketing of irradiated chicken in the USA has shown that consumer attitudes are changing and that irradiation may be a viable approach to reduce VTEC contamination of retail foods (Basaran *et al.* 2004; Oteiza *et al.* 2005).

Retail and consumer

In many countries public health regulations dictate minimal cooking temperatures that must be achieved and good food hygiene practices to ensure that 'ready to eat' food sold at the retail level is safe. Basic elements of food hygiene in the home and institutional setting need to be advocated aggressively in public education campaigns, especially through the popular media. Programmes aimed at consumer food-safety education, such as FightBac™ (www.fightbac.org), have been developed. These programmes tend to emphasize the need for frequent washing of hands and surface areas in contact with food, separation of foods during storage and preparation to avoid cross-contamination, proper cooking temperatures to kill pathogens that may be present, and prompt refrigeration of purchased and leftover foods.

Evaluation

Evaluating the public health impact of interventions at various stages of the farm to fork continuum is complicated by difficulties in traceability of product from farm to consumers, under-reporting of disease, and difficulties in confirming source identification due to the potential time lag between contamination and recognition of a case or outbreak. At the farm level, control programmes generally do not include testing for VTEC due to the transient nature of faecal shedding and a current lack of effective intervention strategies. Evaluation of the effectiveness of control programmes is hampered by the difficulties of quantifying the concentration of pathogen in cattle faeces. When the outcome is measured as the presence or absence of VTEC, the intervention must eliminate the pathogen, or at least reduce it to below detection levels, to appear efficacious. Thus, interventions that reduce pathogen concentration, but do not eliminate shedding, may not appear to be effective. At present, existing on-farm control programmes are voluntary and tend to consist of general good production practices that are not targeted specifically at VTEC control (Haines 2004).

HACCP programmes in the processing sector include microbial testing of product for indicator bacteria and/or specifically for *E. coli* O157. There is some evidence from temporal analyses that intervention strategies may be having an impact. Changes over time should be interpreted with caution due to coinciding advances in diagnostic tests and disease reporting. Nonetheless, although outbreaks remain common, the median number of cases per outbreak and HUS and case-fatality rates declined in the USA between 1982 and 2002 (Rangel *et al.* 2005). The incidence of *E. coli* O157 in the USA decreased 42% between 1996 and 2004 (CDC 2005) and the annual number of domestically acquired VTEC infections declined in Finland between 1998 and 2002 (Eklund *et al.* 2005).

A systematic review of retail and consumer food safety programmes found evidence that food handler training, food premise inspections, and community-based education programmes promoting proper food handling and preparation techniques are effective components in reducing public exposure to food-borne pathogens (Campbell *et al.* 1998).

Legislation

Currently VTEC infection in animals is not a reportable or 'named' disease in agricultural regulations worldwide. Investigations are usually the result of trace-backs from food-borne outbreaks. This may change in some countries as farm-level control programmes for VTEC, especially serotype O157:H7, are implemented. In many countries, the sale of unpasteurized milk is illegal, thereby providing an effective regulatory measure to reduce VTEC-related milkborne outbreaks. Most of the regulatory focus on the prevention of VTEC has been in the processing sector (Brabban *et al.* 2004). *Escherichia coli* O157:H7 is considered a legal adulterant of meat in the USA. HACCP is mandatory in some countries and other countries are moving towards mandatory implementation. Internationally, food inspection systems are under increasing trade pressure to comply with international standards such as the ISO 9000 series. Many nations and municipalities have guidelines and regulations setting standards for internal cooking temperatures and sanitary measures at the retail level, that, when properly enforced, also serve as critically important barriers to human infection.

Public health surveillance of VTEC infection can play a major role in devising and implementing control measures. Whereas reporting of human cases of VTEC infection (or only O157:H7 infection) to public health authorities is mandatory in some countries, it is not so in others. Consistent reporting by all countries can make a vital contribution to surveillance at the international level and allow more global strategies of control to be developed.

References

Abe, A., de Grado, M., Pfuetzner, R. A., Sanchez-Sanmartin, C., DeVinney, R., *et al.* (1999). Enteropathogenic *Escherichia coli* translocated intimin receptor, Tir, requires a specific chaperone for stable secretion. *Mol. Microbiol.*, **33**: 1162–75.

Ackers, M. L., Mahon, B. E., Leahy, E., Goode, B., Damrow, T., *et al.* (1998). An outbreak of *Escherichia coli* O157:H7 infections associated with leaf lettuce consumption. *J. Infect. Dis.*, **177**: 1588–93.

Ahmed, A., Li, J., Shiloach, Y., Robbins, J. B., and Szu, S. C. (2006). Safety and immunogenicity of *Escherichia coli* O157 O-specific polysaccharide conjugate vaccine in 2–5-year-old children. *J. Infect. Dis.*, **193**: 515–21.

Ahmed, R., Bopp, C., Borczyk, A., and Kasatiya, S. (1987). Phage-typing scheme for Escherichia coli O157:H7. *J. Infect. Dis.*, **155**: 806–9.

Ahmed, S., and Donaghy, M. (1998). An outbreak of *Escherichia coli* O157:H7 in Central Scotland. In: J. B. Kaper and A. D. O'Brien (eds.). *Escherichia coli O157:H7 and other Shiga toxin-producing E. coli strains*, pp. 59–65. Washington, D.C.: ASM Press.

Alam, M. J., and Zurek, L. (2004). Association of Escherichia coli O157:H7 with houseflies on a cattle farm. *Appl. Environ. Microbiol.*, **70**: 7578–80.

Allerberger, F., Friedrich, A. W., Grif, K., Dierich, M. P., Dornbusch, H. J., *et al.* (2003). Hemolytic-uremic syndrome associated with enterohemorrhagic Escherichia coli O26:H infection and consumption of unpasteurized cow's milk. *Int. J. Infect. Dis.*, **7**: 42–45.

Altekruse, S. F., Cohen, M. L., and Swerdlow, D. L. (1997). Emerging foodborne diseases. *Emerg. Infect. Dis.*, **3**: 285–93.

Anderson, R. C., Carr, M. A., Miller, R. K., King, D. A., Carstens, G. E., *et al.* (2005). Effects of experimental chlorate preparations as feed and water supplements on Escherichia coli colonization and contamination of beef cattle and carcasses. *Food Microbiol.*, **22**: 439–47.

Anon. (2000). Waterborne outbreak of gastroenteritis associated with a contaminated municipal water supply, Walkerton, Ontario, May–June 2000. *Can. Commun. Dis. Rep.*, **26**(20): 170–73; 10–15.

Armstrong, G. D., Rowe, P. C., Goodyear, P., Orrbine, E., Klassen, T. P., *et al.* (1995). A phase-1 study of chemically-synthesized verotoxin (Shiga-like toxin) Pk-trisaccharide receptors attached to chromosorb for preventing hemolytic uremic syndrome. *J. Infect. Dis.*, **171**: 1042–45.

Armstrong, G. L., Hollingsworth, J., and Morris Jr., J. G., (1996). Emerging foodborne pathogens: Escherichia coli O157:H7 as a model of entry of a new pathogen into the food supply of the developed world. *Epidemiol. Rev.*, **18**: 29–51.

Arthur, T. M., Barkocy-Gallagher, G. A., Rivera-Betancourt, M., and Koohmaraie, M. (2002). Prevalence and characterization of non-O157 Shiga toxin-producing Escherichia coli on carcasses in commercial beef cattle processing plants. *Appl. Environ. Microbiol.*, **68**: 4847–52.

Barkocy-Gallagher, G. A., Arthur, T. M., Rivera-Betancourt, M., Nou, X., Shackelford, S. D., *et al.* (2003). Seasonal prevalence of Shiga toxin-producing Escherichia coli, including O157:H7 and non-O157 serotypes, and Salmonella in commercial beef processing plants. *J. Food Prot.*, **66**: 1978–86.

Barrett, T. J., Green, J. H., Griffin, P. M., Pavia, A. T., Ostroff, S. M., *et al.* (1991). Enzyme-linked immunosorbent assays for detecting antibodies to Shiga-like toxin I, Shiga-like toxin II, and Escherichia coli O157:H7 lipopolysaccharide in human serum. *Curr. Microbiol.*, **23**: 189–95.

Basaran, N., Quintero-Ramos, A., Moake, M. M., Churey, J. J., and Worobo, R. W. (2004). Influence of apple cultivars on inactivation of different strains of Escherichia coli O157:H7 in apple cider by UV irradiation. *Appl. Environ. Microbiol.*, **70**: 6061–65.

Bellin, T., Pulz, M., Matussek, A., Hempen, H. G., and Gunzer, F. (2001). Rapid detection of enterohemorrhagic Escherichia coli by real-time PCR with fluorescent hybridization probes. *J. Clin. Microbiol.*, **39**: 370–74.

Belongia, E. A., Osterholm, M. T., Soler, J. T., Ammend, D. A., Braun, J. E., *et al.* (1993). Transmission of Escherichia coli O157:H7 infection in Minnesota child day-care facilities. *JAMA*, **269**: 883–88.

Besser, R. E., Lett, S. M., Weber, J. T., Doyle, M. P., Barrett, T. J., *et al.* (1993). An outbreak of diarrhea and hemolytic uremic syndrome from Escherichia coli O157:H7 in fresh-pressed apple cider. *JAMA*, **269**: 2217–20.

Besser, T. E., Hancock, D. D., Pritchett, L. C., McRae, E. M., Rice, D. H., *et al.* (1997). Duration of detection of fecal excretion of Escherichia coli O157:H7 in cattle. *J. Infect. Dis.*, **175**: 726–29.

Besser,T. E., LeJeune, J. T., Rice, D., and Hancock, D. D. (2003). Prevention and control of Escherichia coli O157:H7. In: M. E. Torrance and R. E. Isaacson (eds.). *Microbial Food Safety in Animal Agriculture: Current topics*, pp. 167–74. Ames, Iowa: Iowa State Press.

Beutin, L., Geier, D., Steinrück, H., Zimmerman, S., and Scheutz, F. (1993). Prevalence and some properties of verotoxin (shiga-like toxin)-producing Escherichia coli in seven different species of healthy domestic animals. *J. Clin. Microbiol.,* **31**: 2483–88.

Beutin, L., Geier, D., Zimmerman, S., and Karch, H. (1995). Virulence markers of shiga-like toxin-producing Escherichia coli strains originating from healthy domestic animals of different species. *J. Clin. Microbiol.,* **33**: 631–635.

Beutin, L., Zimmermann, S., and Gleier, K. (1998). Human infections with Shiga toxin-producing Escherichia coli other than serogroup O157 in Germany. *Emerg. Infect. Dis.,* **4**: 635–39.

Bielaszewska, M., Clarke, I., Karmali, M. A., and Petric, M. (1997). Localization of intravenously administered verocytotoxins (shiga-like toxins) 1 and 2 in rabbits immunized with homologous and heterologous toxoids and toxin subunits. *Infect. Immun.,* **65**: 2509–2516.

Bielaszewska, M., Schmidt, H., Liesegang, A., Prager, R., Rabsch, W., et al. (2000). Cattle can be a reservoir of sorbitol-fermenting shiga toxin-producing escherichia coli O157:H(-) strains and a source of human diseases. *J. Clin. Microbiol.,* **38**: 3470–73.

Bitzan, M., Ludwig, K., Klemt, M., König, H., Büren, J., et al. (1993). The role of Escherichia coli infections in the classical (enteropathic) haemolytic uraemic syndrome: Results of a Central European, multicentre study. *Epidemiol. Infect.,* **110**: 183–96.

Bohm, H., and Karch, H. (1992). DNA fingerprinting of Escherichia coli O157: H7 strains by pulsed-field gel electrophoresis. *J. Clin. Microbiol.,* **30**: 2169–72.

Booth, L., and Rowe, B. (1993). Possible occupational acquisition of Escherichia coli O157 infection. *Lancet,* **342**: 1298–99.

Brabban, A. D., Nelsen, D. A., Kutter, E., Edrington, T. S., and Callaway, T. R. (2004). Approaches to controlling *Escherichia coli* O157:H7, a foodborne pathogen and an emerging environmental hazard. *Environ. Pract.,* **6**: 208–29.

Brashears, M. M., Galyean, M. L., et al. (2003). Prevalence of *Escherichia coli* O157:H7 and performance by beef feedlot cattle given *Lactobacillus* direct-fed microbials. *J. Food Prot.,* **66**: 748–54.

Breuer, T., Benkel, D. H., Shapiro, R. L., Hall, W. N., Winnett, M. M., et al. (2001). A multistate outbreak of Escherichia coli O157:H7 infections linked to alfalfa sprouts grown from contaminated seeds. *Emerg. Infect. Dis.,* **7**: 977–82.

Brooks, J. T., Sowers, E. G., Wells, J. G., Greene, K. D., Griffin, P. M., et al. (2005). Non-O157 Shiga toxin-producing Escherichia coli infections in the United States, 1983–2002. *J. Infect. Dis.,* **192**: 1422–29.

Brown, M. R., Smith, A. W., Barker, J., Humphrey, T. J., and Dixon, B. (2002). E. coli O157 persistence in the environment. *Microbiology,* **148**: 1–2.

Brunder, W., Schmidt, H., Frosch, M., and Karch, H. (1999). The large plasmids of Shiga-toxin-producing Escherichia coli (STEC) are highly variable genetic elements. *Microbiology,* **145**(Pt 5): 1005–1014.

Burland, V., Shao, Y., Perna, N. T., Plunkett, G., Sofia, H. J., et al. (1998). The complete DNA sequence and analysis of the large virulence plasmid of Escherichia coli O157:H7. *Nucleic Acids Res.,* **26**: 4196–4204.

Butler, T., Islam, M. R., Azad, M. A. K., and Jones, P. K. (1987). Risk factors for development of hemolytic uremic syndrome during shigellosis. *J. Pediatr.,* **110**: 894–97.

Calderwood, S., Acheson, D. W. K., Keusch, G. T., Barrett, T. J., Griffin, P. M., et al. (1996). Proposed New Nomenclature for SLT (VT) Family. *Am. Soc. Microbiol. News,* **62**: 118–119.

Callaway, T. R., Anderson, R. C., Edrington, T. S., et al. (2004). What are we doing about Escherichia coli O157:H7 in cattle? *J. Anim. Sci.,* **82** E-Suppl: E93–99.

Callaway, T. R., Anderson, R. C., Genovese, K. J., et al. (2002). Sodium chlorate supplementation reduces E. coli O157:H7 populations in cattle. *J. Anim. Sci.,* **80**: 1683–89.

Callaway, T. R., Edrington, T. S., Anderson, R. C., et al. (2003). Escherichia coli O157:H7 populations in sheep can be reduced by chlorate supplementation. *J. Food Prot.,* **66**: 194–99.

Campbell, M. E., Gardner, C. E., Dwyer, J. J., et al. (1998). Effectiveness of public health interventions in food safety: a systematic review. *Can. J. Public Health,* **89**: 197–202.

Carter, A. O., Borczyk, A. A., Carlson, J. A. K., Harvey, B., Hockin, J. C., et al. (1987). A severe outbreak of Escherichia coli O157:H7-associated hemorrhagic colitis in a nursing home. *N. Engl. J. Med.,* **317**: 1496–1500.

Cassin, M. H., Lammerding, A. M., Todd, E. C., Ross, W., and McColl, R. S. (1998). Quantitative risk assessment for Escherichia coli O157:H7 in ground beef hamburgers. *Int. J. Food Microbiol.,* **41**: 21–44.

Centers for Disease Control (1993). Update: Multistate Outbreak of Escherichia coli O157:H7 infections from Hamburgers - Western United States, 1992–1993. *J. Amer. Med. Assoc.,* **269**: 2194–96.

Centers for Disease Control (2005). Preliminary FoodNet data on the incidence of infection with pathogens transmitted commonly through food - 10 sites, Unites States, 2004. *Morb. Mort. Wkly. Rep.,* **54**: 352–56.

Chapman, P. A., and Siddons, C. A. (1996). A comparison of immunomagnetic separation and direct culture for the isolation of verocytotoxin-producing Escherichia coli O157 from cases of bloody diarrhoea, non-bloody diarrhoea and asymptomatic contacts. *J. Med. Microbiol.,* **44**: 267–71.

Chapman, P. A., Siddons, C. A., Gerdan Malo, A. T., and Harkin, M. A. (1997). A 1-year study of Escherichia coli O157 in cattle, sheep, pigs and poultry. *Epidemiol. Infect.,* **119**: 245–50.

Chart, H., Smith, H. R., Scotland, S. M., Rowe, B., Milford, D. V., et al. (1991). Serological identification of Escherichia coli O157 infection in haemolytic uraemic syndrome. *Lancet,* **337**: 138–40.

Cieslak, P. R., Barrett, T. J., Griffin, P. M., et al. (1993). Escherichia coli O157:H7 infection from a manured garden. *Lancet,* **342**: 367.

Cimolai, N., Basalyga, S., Mah, D. G., Morrison, B. J., and Carter, J. E. (1994). A continuing assessment of risk factors for the development of Escherichia coli O157:H7-associated hemolytic uremic syndrome. *Clin. Nephrol.,* **42**: 85–89.

Cimolai, N., Morrison, B. J., and Carter, J. E. (1992). Risk factors for the central nervous system manifestations of gastroenteritis-associated hemolytic-uremic syndrome. *Pediatrics,* **90**: 616–21.

Cizek, A., Alexa, P., Literak, I., Hamrik, J., Novak, P., et al. (1999). Shiga toxin-producing Escherichia coli O157 in feedlot cattle and Norwegian rats from a large-scale farm. *Lett. Appl. Microbiol.,* **28**: 435–39.

Clarke, R. C., McEwen, S. A., Gannon, V. P., Lior, H., and Gyles, C. L. (1989). Isolation of verocytotoxin-producing Escherichia coli from milk filters in south-western Ontario. *Epidem. Inf.,* **102**: 253–60.

Cobbold, R. N., Rice, D. H., Szymanski, M., Call, D. R., and Hancock, D. D. (2004). Comparison of shiga-toxigenic Escherichia coli prevalences among dairy, feedlot, and cow-calf herds in Washington State. *Appl. Environ. Microbiol.,* **70**: 4375–78.

Cody, S. H., Glynn, M. K., Farrar, J. A., Cairns, K. L., Griffin, P. M., et al. (1999). An outbreak of Escherichia coli O157:H7 infection from unpasteurized commercial apple juice. *Ann. Intern. Med.,* **130**: 202–209.

Coombes, B. K., Wickham, M. E., Mascarenhas, M., Gruenheid, S., Finlay, B. B., and Karmali, M. A. (2008). Molecular analysis as an aid to assess the public health risk of non-O157 Shiga toxin-producing Escherichia coli strains. *Appl. Environ. Microbiol.,* **74**: 2153–60.

Corbel, M. J., Stuart, F. A., and Brewer, R. A. (1983). Observations on serological cross-reactions between smooth Brucella species and organisms of other genera. *Devel. Biol. Stand.,* **56**: 341–48.

Cowden, J. M., Ahmed, S., Donaghy, M., and Riley, A. (2001). Epidemiological investigation of the central Scotland outbreak of Echerichia coli 0157 infection, November to December 1996. *Epidemiol. Infect.,* **126**: 335–41.

Cray, W. C., and Moon, H. W. (1995). Experimental infection of calves and adult cattle with Escherichia coli O157:H7. *Appl. Environ. Microbiol.,* **61**: 1586–90.

Crump, J. A., Braden, C. R., Dey, M. E., Hoekstra, R. M., Rickelman-Apisa, J. M., et al. (2003). Outbreaks of Escherichia coli O157 infections at multiple county agricultural fairs: a hazard of mixing cattle, concession stands and children. *Epidemiol. Infect.,* **131**: 1055–62.

Crump, J. A., Sulka, A. C., Langer, A. J., *et al.* (2002). An outbreak of Escherichia coli O157:H7 infections among visitors to a dairy farm. *N. Engl. J. Med.,* **347**: 555–60.

Davis, M., Osaki, C., Gordon, D., Mottram, E. K., Winegar, C., *et al.* (1993). Multistate outbreak of Escherichia coli O157:H7 infection from hamburgers — Western United States, 1992–1993. *Morb. Mort. Wkly. Rep.,* **42**: 258–63.

Dean, P., and Kenny, B. (2009). The effector repertoire of enteropathogenic E. coli: ganging up on the host cell. *Current Opin. Microbiol.,* **12**: 101–9.

Deibel, C., Kramer, S., Chakraborty, T., and Ebel, F. (1998). EspE, a novel secreted protein of attaching and effacing bacteria, is directly translocated into infected host cells, where it appears as a tyrosine-phosphorylated 90 kDa protein. *Molec. Microbiol.,* **28**: 463–74.

Deng, W., Puente, J. L., Gruenheid, S., Li, Y., Vallance, B. A., *et al.* (2004). Dissecting virulence: systematic and functional analyses of a pathogenicity island. *Proc. Nat. Acad. Sci. USA,* **101**: 3597–3602.

Dewell, G. A., Ransom, J. R., Dewell, R. D., McCurdy, K., Gardner, I. A., *et al.* (2005). Prevalence of and risk factors for Escherichia coli O157 in market-ready beef cattle from 12 U.S. feedlots. *Foodborne Pathog. Dis.,* **2**: 70–76.

Dobrescu, L. (1983). New biological effect of edema disease principle (Escherichia coli neurotoxin) and its use as an in-vitro assay for this toxin. *Am. J. Vet. Res.,* **44**: 31–34.

Dodd, C. C., Sanderson, M. W., Sargeant, J. M., Nagaraja, T. G., Oberst, R. D., *et al.* (2003). Prevalence of Escherichia coli O157 in cattle feeds in Midwestern feedlots. *Appl. Environ. Microbiol.,* **69**: 5243–47.

Donnenberg, M. S. and Whittam, T. S. (2001). Pathogenesis and evolution of virulence in enteropathogenic and enterohemorrhagic Escherichia coli. *J. Clin. Invest.,* **107**: 539–48.

Doyle, M. P. and Schoeni, J. L. (1987). Isolation of Escherichia coli O157:H7 from retail fresh meats and poultry. *Appl. Environ. Microbiol.,* **53**: 2394–96.

Duncan, L., Mai, V., Carter, A., Carlson, J. A. K., Borczyk, A., *et al.* (1987). Outbreak of gastrointestinal disease - Ontario. *Can. Comm. Dis., Report,* **13**: 5–8.

Durso, L. M., Reynolds, K., Bauer, N., Jr., and Keen, J. E. (2005). Shiga-toxigenic Escherichia coli O157:H7 infections among livestock exhibitors and visitors at a Texas County Fair. *Vector Borne Zoonot. Dis.,* **5**: 193–201.

Dziva, F., van Diemen, P. M., Stevens, M. P., Smith, A. J., and Wallis, T. S. (2004). Identification of Escherichia coli O157: H7 genes influencing colonization of the bovine gastrointestinal tract using signature-tagged mutagenesis. *Microbiology,* **150**: 3631–45.

Ebel, E., Schlosser, W., Kause, J., Orloski, K., Roberts, T., *et al.* (2004). Draft risk assessment of the public health impact of Escherichia coli O157:H7 in ground beef. *J. Food Prot.,* **67**: 1991–99.

Edrington, T. S., Callaway, T. R., Anderson, R. C., Genovese, K. J., Jung, Y. S., *et al.* (2003). Reduction of E. coli O157:H7 populations in sheep by supplementation of an experimental sodium chlorate product. *Small Ruminant Res.,* **49**: 173–81.

Edwards, J. R. and Fung, D. Y. C. (2006). Prevention and decontamination of *Escherichia coli* O157:H7 on raw beef carcasses in commercial beef abattoirs. *J. Rapid Meth. and Automat. Microbiol.,* **14**: 1–95.

Effler, E., Isaacson, M., Arntzen, L., Heenan, R., Canter, P., *et al.* (2001). Factors contributing to the emergence of Escherichia coli O157 in Africa. *Emerg. Infect. Dis.,* **7**: 812–19.

Eklund, M., Nuorti, J.P., Ruutu, P., and Siitonen, A. (2005). Shigatoxigenic Escherichia coli (STEC) infections in Finland during 1998–2002: a population-based surveillance study. *Epidemiol. Infect.,* **133**: 845–52.

Elder, R. O., Keen, J. E., Siragusa, G. R., Barkocy-Gallagher, G. A., Koohmaraie, M., *et al.* (2000). Correlation of enterohemorrhagic Escherichia coli O157 prevalence in feces, hides, and carcasses of beef cattle during processing. *Proc. Nat. Acad. Sci. USA,* **97**: 2999–3003.

Elder, R. O., Keen, J. E., Wittum, T. E., Callaway, T. R., Edrington, T. S., *et al.* (2002). Intervention to reduce fecal shedding of enterohemorrhagic Escherichia coli O157:H7 in naturally infected cattle using neomycin sulfate. *J. Anim. Sci.,* **80**: 15.

Elliott, E. J., Robins-Browne, R. M., O'Loughlin, E. V., Bennett-Wood, V., Bourke, J., *et al.* (2001a). Nationwide study of haemolytic uraemic syndrome: clinical, microbiological, and epidemiological features. *Arch. Dis. Child.,* **85**: 125–31.

Elliott, S. J., Hutcheson, S. W., Dubois, M. S., Mellies, J. L., Wainwright, L. A., *et al.* (1999). Identification of CesT, a chaperone for the type III secretion of Tir in enteropathogenic Escherichia coli. *Mol. Microbiol.,* **33**: 1176–89.

Elliott, S. J., Sperandio, V., Giron, J. A., Shin, S., Mellies, J. L., *et al.* (2000). The locus of enterocyte effacement (LEE)-encoded regulator controls expression of both LEE- and non-LEE-encoded virulence factors in enteropathogenic and enterohemorrhagic escherichia coli. *Infect. Immun.,* **68**: 6115–26.

Endo, Y., Tsurugi, K., Yutsudo, T., Takeda, Y., Ogasawara, T., *et al.* (1988). Site of action of a Vero toxin (VT2) from Escherichia coli O157:H7 and of shiga toxin on eukaryotic ribosomes; RNA N-glycosidase activity of the toxins. *Eur. J. Biochem.* **171**: 45–50.

Feng, P., Lampel, K. A., Karch, H., and Whittam, T. S. (1998). Genotypic and phenotypic changes in the emergence of Escherichia coli O157:H7. *J. Infect. Dis.,* **177**: 1750–53.

Fischer, J. R., Zhao, T., Doyle, M. P., Goldberg, M. R., Brown, C. A., *et al.* (2001). Experimental and field studies of Escherichia coli O157:H7 in white-tailed deer. *Appl. Environ. Microbiol.,* **67**: 1218–24.

Folmer, J., Macken, C., Moxley, R., Smith, D., Brashears, M. M., *et al.* (2003). Intervention strategiesfor reduction of Escherichia coli O157:H7 in feedlot steers, pp. 22–23. University of Nebraska. Nebraska Beef Report.

Fong, J. S. C., de Chadarevian, J. P., and Kaplan, B. (1982). Hemolytic Uremic Syndrome. Current Concepts and Management. *Pediatr. Clin. North Amer.,* **29**: 835–56.

Foubister, V., Rosenshine, I., Donnenberg, M. S., and Finlay, B. B. (1994). The eaeB gene of enteropathogenic Escherichia coli is necessary for signal transduction in epithelial cells. *Infect. Immun.,* **62**: 3038–40.

Fox, J. T., Thomson, D. U., Drouillard, J. S., Thornton, A. B., Burkhardt, D.T., Emery, D. A., and Nagaraja, T. G. (2009). Efficacy of *Escherichia coli* O157:H7 Siderophore Receptor/Porin Proteins-Based vaccine in feedlot cattle naturally shedding *E. coli* O157. *Foodborne Pathog. and Dis.,* **6**: 893–9.

Fukushima, H., Hoshina, K., and Gomyoda, M. (1999). Long-term survival of shiga toxin-producing Escherichia coli O26, O111, and O157 in bovine feces. *Appl. Environ. Microbiol.,* **65**: 5177–81.

Fuller, R. (1989). Probiotics in man and animals. *J. Appl. Bacteriol.,* **66**: 365–78.

Gagliardi, J. V. and Karns, J. S. (2000). Leaching of Escherichia coli O157:H7 in diverse soils under various agricultural management practices. *Appl. Environ. Microbiol.,* **66**: 877–83.

Galanis, E., Longmore, K., Hassleback, P., Swann, D., Ellis, A., *et al.* (2003). Investigation of an *Escherichia coli* O157:H7 outbreak in Brooks, Alberta, June-July, 2002: The role of occult cases in the spread of infection within a daycare setting. *Can. Commun. Dis. Report,* **29**: 21–28.

Gannon, V. P., Graham, T. A., King, R., Michel, P., Read, S., *et al.* (2002). Escherichia coli O157:H7 infection in cows and calves in a beef cattle herd in Alberta, Canada. *Epidemiol. Infect.,* **129**: 163–72.

Gansheroff, L. J. and O'Brien, A. D. (2000). Escherichia coli O157:H7 in beef cattle presented for slaughter in the U.S.: higher prevalence rates than previously estimated. *Proc. Nat. Acad. Sci. USA, A* **97**: 2959–61.

Garber, L., Wells, S., Schroeder-Tucker, L., and Ferris, K. (1999). Factors associated with fecal shedding of verotoxin-producing Escherichia coli O157 on dairy farms. *J. Food Prot.,* **62**: 307–312.

Garg, A. X., Moist, L., Matsell, D., Thiessen-Philbrook, H. R., Haynes, R. B., *et al.* (2005). Risk of hypertension and reduced kidney function after acute gastroenteritis from bacteria-contaminated drinking water. *Can. Med. Assoc. J.,* **173**: 261–68.

Garg, A. X., Suri, R. S., Barrowman, N., Rehman, F., Matsell, D., et al. (2003). Long-term renal prognosis of diarrhea-associated hemolytic uremic syndrome: a systematic review, meta-analysis, and meta-regression. *JAMA,* **290:** 1360–70.

Garmendia, J., Frankel, G., and Crepin, V. F. (2005). Enteropathogenic and enterohemorrhagic Escherichia coli infections: translocation, translocation, translocation. *Infect. Immun.,* **73:** 2573–85.

Gasser, C., Gautier, E., Steck, A., Siebenmann, R. E., and Oechslin, R. (1955). Hämolytisch-ürämische syndrome: bilaterale nierenindennekrosen bei akuten erworbenen hämolytischen Anämien. *Schweiz. Med. Wochenschr.,* **85:** 905–909.

Gerner-Smidt, P., Hise, K., Kincaid, J., Hunter, S., Rolando, S., et al. (2006). PulseNet USA: a five-year update. *Foodborne Pathog. Dis.,* **3:** 9–19.

Gianantonio, C., Vitacco, M., Mendilaharzu, F., Gallo, G. E., and Sojo, E. T. (1973). The hemolytic uremic syndrome. *Nephron,* **11:** 174–92.

Gianantonio, C., Vitacco, M., Mendilaharzu, F., Rutty, A., and Mendilaharzu, J. (1964). The hemolytic-uremic syndrome. *J. Pediatr.,* **64:** 478–91.

Goosney, D. L., DeVinney, R., and Finlay, B. B. (2001). Recruitment of cytoskeletal and signaling proteins to enteropathogenic and enterohemorrhagic Escherichia coli pedestals. *Infect. Immun.,* **69:** 3315–22.

Grif, K., Dierich, M. P., Karch, H., and Allerberger, F. (1998a). Strain-specific differences in the amount of Shiga toxin released from enterohemorrhagic Escherichia coli O157 following exposure to subinhibitory concentrations of antimicrobial agents. *Eur. J. Clin. Microbiol. Infect. Dis.,* **17:** 761–66.

Grif, K., Karch, H., Schneider, C., Daschner, F. D., Beutin, L., et al. (1998b). Comparative study of five different techniques for epidemiological typing of Escherichia coli O157. *Diagn. Microbiol. Infect. Dis.,* **32:** 165–76.

Griffin, P. M. (1995). Escherichia coli O157:H7 and other enterohemorrhagic Escherichia coli. In: M. J. Blaser, P. D. Smith, J. L. Ravdin, H. B. Greenberg and R. L. Guerrant (eds.) *Infections of the Gastrointestinal Tract,* pp. 739–61. New York: Raven Press, Ltd.

Griffin, P. M. (1998). Epidemiology of shiga toxin-producing Escherichia coli infections in humans in the United States. In: J. B. Kaper and A. D. O'Brien (eds.). *Escherichia coli O157:H7 and other Shiga toxin-producing E. coli strains,* pp. 15–22. Washington, D.C.: ASM Press.

Griffin, P. M., Olmstead, L. C., and Petras, R. E. (1990). Escherichia coli O157:H7-associated colitis. A clinical and histological study of 11 cases. *Gastroenterology,* **99:** 142–49.

Griffin, P. M., Ostroff, S. M., Tauxe, R. V., Greene, K. D., Wells, J. G., et al. (1988). Illnesses Associated with Escherichia coli 0157:H7 Infections: A Broad Clinical Spectrum. *Ann. Int. Med.,* **109:** 705–12.

Griffin, P. M. and Tauxe, R. V. (1991). The epidemiology of infections caused by Escherichia coli O157:H7, other enterohemorrhagic E. coli, and the associated hemolytic uremic syndrome. *Epidemiol. Rev.,* **13:** 60–98.

Gunzer, F., Bohm, H., Russman, H., Bitzan, M., Aleksik, S., et al. (1992). Molecular detection of sorbitol-fermenting Escherichia coli O157 in patients with the hemolytic uremic syndrome. *J. Clin. Microbiol.,* **30:** 1807–10.

Gyles, C. L. (1998). Vaccines and Shiga toxin-producing *Escherichia coli* in animals. In: J. B. Kaper and A. D. O'Brien (eds.). *Escherichia coli O157:H7 and other Shiga toxin-producing E. coli strains,* pp. 434–44. Washington, D.C.: ASM Press.

Habib, R., Levy, M., Gagnadoux, M. F., and Broyer, M. (1982). Prognosis of the hemolytic uremic syndrome in children. *Adv. Nephrol.,* **11:** 99–128.

Hacker, J. and Kaper, J. (2001). The Concept of Pathogenicity Islands. In: J. B. Kaper and J. Hacker (eds.). *Pathogenicity Islands and Other Mobile Virulence Elements,* pp. 1–11. Washington, D.C.: ASM Press.

Haines, R. J. (2004). *Farm to fork: A strategy for meat safety in Ontario.* Report of the Meat Regulatory and Inspection Review. Ministry of the Attorney General, Ontario Publications, Toronto, Canada.

Hancock, D. D., Besser, T., LeJeune, J., Davis, M., and Rice, D. (2001). Control of VTEC in the animal reservoir. *Int. J. Food Microbiol.,* **66:** 71–78.

Hancock, D. D., Besser, T. E., Rice, D. H., Ebel, E. D., Herriott, D. E., et al. (1998). Multiple sources of Escherichia coli O157 in feedlots and dairy farms in the northwestern USA. *Prev. Vet. Med.,* **35:** 11–19.

Hayashi, T., Makino, K., Ohnishi, M., Kurokawa, K., Ishii, K., et al. (2001). Complete genome sequence of enterohemorrhagic Escherichia coli O157:H7 and genomic comparison with a laboratory strain K-12. *DNA Res.,* **8:** 11–22.

Herriott, D. E., Hancock, D. D., Ebel, E. D., Carpenter, L. V., Rice, D. H., and Besser, T. E. (1998). Association of herd management factors with colonization of dairy cattle by Shiga toxin-positive Escherichia coli O157. *J. Food Prot.,* **61:** 802–807.

Hilborn, E. D., Mermin, J. H., Mshar, P. A., Hadler, J. L., Voetsch, A., et al. (1999). A multistate outbreak of Escherichia coli O157:H7 infections associated with consumption of mesclun lettuce. *Arch. Intern. Med.,* **159:** 1758–64.

Hiramatsu, R., Matsumoto, M., Sakae, K., and Miyazaki, Y. (2005). Ability of Shiga toxin-producing Escherichia coli and Salmonella spp. to survive in a desiccation model system and in dry foods. *Appl. Environ. Microbiol.,* **71:** 6657–63.

Hueck, C. J. (1998). Type III protein secretion systems in bacterial pathogens of animals and plants. *Microbiol. Mol. Biol. Rev.,* **62:** 379–433.

Hulebak, K. L. and Schlosser, W. (2002). Hazard analysis and critical control point (HACCP) history and conceptual overview. *Risk Anal.,* **22:** 547–52.

Hurley, B. P., Jacewicz, M., Thorpe, C. M., Lincicome, L. L., King, A. J., et al. (1999). Shiga toxins 1 and 2 translocate differently across polarized intestinal epithelial cells. *Infect. Immun.,* **67:** 6670–77.

Hussein, H. S. and Sakuma, T. (2005). Prevalence of shiga toxin-producing Escherichia coli in dairy cattle and their products. *J. Dairy Sci.,* **88:** 450–65.

Ikeda, K., Ida,O., Kimoto, K., Takatorige, T., Nakanishi, N., et al. (1999). Effect of early fosfomycin treatment on prevention of hemolytic uremic syndrome accompanying Escherichia coli O157:H7 infection. *Clin. Nephrol.,* **52:** 357–62.

Iwasa, M., Makino, S., Asakura, H., Kobori, H., and Morimoto, Y. (1999). Detection of Escherichia coli O157:H7 from Musca domestica (Diptera: Muscidae) at a cattle farm in Japan. *J. Med. Entomol.,* **36:** 108–112.

Jackson, S. G., Goodbrand, R. B., Johnson, R. P., Odorico, V. G., Alves, D., et al. (1998). Escherichia coli O157:H7 diarrhoea associated with well water and infected cattle on an Ontario farm. *Epidemiol. Infect.,* **120:** 17–20.

Jarvis, K. G., Giron, J. A., Jerse, A. E., McDaniel, T. K., Donnenberg, M. S., et al. (1995). Enteropathogenic Escherichia coli contains a putative type III secretion system necessary for the export of proteins involved in attaching and effacing lesion formation. *Proc. Nat. Acad. Sci. USA,* **92:** 7996–8000.

Jarvis, K. G. and Kaper, J. B. (1996). Secretion of extracellular proteins by enterohemorrhagic Escherichia coli via a putative type III secretion system. *Infect. Immun.,* **64:** 4826–29.

Jenkins, C., Chart, H., Smith, H. R., Hartland, E. L., Batchelor, M., et al. (2000). Antibody response of patients infected with verocytotoxin-producing Escherichia coli to protein antigens encoded on the LEE locus. *J. Med. Microbiol.,* **49:** 97–101.

Jenkins, C., Pearce, M. C., Smith, A. W., Knight, H. I., Shaw, D. J., et al. (2003). Detection of Escherichia coli serogroups O26, O103, O111 and O145 from bovine faeces using immunomagnetic separation and PCR/DNA probe techniques. *Lett. Appl. Microbiol.,* **37:** 207–12.

Jerse, A. E., Yu, J., Tall, B. D., and Kaper, J. B. (1990). A genetic locus of enteropathogenic Escherichia coli necessary for the production of attaching and effacing lesions on tissue culture cells. *Proc. Nat. Acad. Sci.,* **87:** 7839–43.

Johnson, R. P., Cray, W. C., and Johnson, S. T. (1996). Serum antibody responses of cattle following experimental infection with Escherichia coli O157: H7. *Infect. Immun.,* **64:** 1879–83.

Jordan, D., McEwen, S. A., Lammerding, A. M., McNab, W. B., and Wilson, J. B. (1999). A simulation model for studying the role of pre-slaughter factors on the exposure of beef carcasses to human microbial hazards. *Prev. Vet. Med.,* **41**: 37–54.

Jordan, D. M., Cornick, N., Torres, A. G., Dean-Nystrom, E. A., Kaper, J. B., *et al.* (2004). Long polar fimbriae contribute to colonization by *Escherichia coli* O157:H7 in vivo. *Infect. Immun.,* **72**: 6168–71.

Kaferstein, F. K., Motarjemi, Y., and Bettcher, D. W. (1997). Foodborne disease control: a transnational challenge. *Emerg. Infect. Dis.,* **3**: 503–510.

Karch, H., Bielaszewska, M., Bitzan, M., and Schmidt, H. (1999). Epidemiology and diagnosis of Shiga toxin-producing *Escherichia coli* infections. *Diagn. Microbiol. Infect. Dis.,* **34**: 229–43.

Karch, H. and Meyer, T. (1989). Single Primer Pair for Amplifying Segments of Distinct Shiga-Like-Toxin genes by Polymerase Chain Reaction. *J. Clin. Microbiol.,* **27**: 2751–57.

Karch, H., Schmidt, H., and Brunder, W. (1998). Plasmid-encoded determinants of *Escherichia coli* O157:H7. In: J. B. Kaper and A. D. O'Brien (eds.). *Escherichia coli O157:H7 and other Shiga toxin-producing E. coli strains,* pp. 183–94. Washington, D.C.: ASM Press.

Karch, H., Strockbine, N. A., and O'Brien, A. D. (1986). Growth of *Escherichia coli* in the presence of trimethoprim-sulfamethoxazole facilitates detection of Shiga-like toxin producing strains by colony blot assay. *FEMS Microbiol. Lett.,* **35**: 141–45.

Karmali, M. A. (1989). Infection by Verocytotoxin-producing Escherichia coli. *Clin. Microbiol. Rev.,* **2**: 15–38.

Karmali, M. A. (1992). The association of verocytotoxins and the classical hemolytic uremic syndrome. In: B. S. Kaplan (ed.). *Hemolytic Uremic Syndrome and Thrombotic Thrombocytopenic Purpura,* pp. 199–212. New York: Marcel Dekker, Inc.

Karmali, M. A. (1998). Human immune response and immunity to Shiga toxin (verocytotoxin)-producing *Escherichia coli* infection. In: J. B. Kaper and A. D. O'Brien (eds.). *Escherichia coli O157:H7 and other Shiga toxin-producing E. coli strains,* pp. 236–48. Washington, D.C.: ASM Press.

Karmali, M. A. (2004). Prospects for preventing serious systemic toxemic complications of Shiga toxin-producing Escherichia coli infections using Shiga toxin receptor analogues. *J. Infect. Dis.,* **189**: 355–59.

Karmali, M. A., Arbus, G. S., Petric, M., Patrick, M. L., Roscoe, M., *et al.* (1988). Hospital-acquired Escherichia coli O157:H7-associated hemolytic uremic syndrome in a nurse. *Lancet,* i: 526.

Karmali, M. A., Gannon, V., and Sargeant, J. M. (2010). Verocytotoxin-producing *Escherichia coli* (VTEC). *Vet Microbiol.,* **140**: 360–70.

Karmali, M. A., Mascarenhas, M., Petric, M., Dutil, L., Rahn, K., *et al.* (2003a). Age-Specific Frequencies of Antibodies to Escherichia coli Verocytotoxins (Shiga Toxins) 1 and 2 among Urban and Rural Populations in Southern Ontario. *J. Infect. Dis.,* **188**: 1724–29.

Karmali, M. A., Mascarenhas, M., Shen, S., Ziebell, K., Johnson, S., *et al.* (2003b). Association of genomic O island 122 of Escherichia coli EDL 933 with verocytotoxin-producing Escherichia coli seropathotypes that are linked to epidemic and/or serious disease. *J. Clin. Microbiol.,* **41**: 4930–40.

Karmali, M. A., Petric, M., Lim, C., Fleming, P. C., Arbus, G. S., *et al.* (1985). The association between hemolytic uremic syndrome and infection by Verotoxin-producing Escherichia coli. *J. Infect. Dis.,* **151**: 775–82.

Karmali, M. A., Petric, M., Steele, B. T., and Lim, C. (1983). Sporadic cases of hemolytic uremic syndrome associated with fecal cytotoxin and cytotoxin-producing Escherichia coli. *Lancet,* i: 619–20.

Karmali, M. A., Petric, M., Winkler, M., Bielasczewska, M., Brunton, J., *et al.* (1994). Enzyme-linked immunosorbent assay (ELISA) for detection of IgG antibodies to *Escherichia coli* Verocytotoxin 1. *J. Clin. Microbiol.,* **32**: 1457–63.

Karpman, D., Bekassy, Z. D., Sjogren, A. C., Dubois, M. S., Karmali, M. A., *et al.* (2002). Antibodies to intimin and Escherichia coli secreted proteins A and B in patients with enterohemorrhagic Escherichia coli infections. *Pediatr. Nephrol.,* **17**: 201–211.

Keene, W. E., Hedberg, K., Herriot, D. E., Hancock, D. D., McKay, R. W., *et al.* (1997a). A prolonged outbreak of Escherichia coli O157:H7 infections caused by commercially distributed raw milk. *J. Infect. Dis.,* **176**: 815–818.

Keene, W. E., McAnulty, J. M., Hoesly, F. C., Williams, L. P., Jr., Hedberg, K., *et al.* (1994). A swimming-associated outbreak of hemorrhagic colitis caused by Escherichia coli O157:H7 and Shigella sonnei. *N. Engl. J. Med.,* **331**: 579–84.

Keene, W. E., Sazie, E., Kok, J., Rice, D. H., Hancock, D. D., *et al.* (1997b). An outbreak of Escherichia coli O157:H7 infections traced to jerky made from deer meat. *JAMA.,* **277**: 1229–31.

Kehl, K. S., Havens, P., Behnke, C. E., and Acheson, D. W. (1997). Evaluation of the premier EHEC assay for detection of Shiga-toxin producing Escherichia coli. *J. Clin. Microbiol.,* **35**: 2051–54.

Kelly, J. K., Pai, C. H., Jadusingh, I. H., Macinnis, M. L., Shaffer, E. A., *et al.* (1987). The histopathology of rectosigmoid biopsies from adults with bloody diarrhea due to verotoxin-producing Escherichia coli. *Am. J. Clin. Pathol.,* **88**: 78–82.

Kenny, B., DeVinney, R., Stein, M., Reinscheid, D. J., Frey, E. A., *et al.* (1997). Enteropathogenic E. coli (EPEC) transfers its receptor for intimate adherence into mammalian cells. *Cell,* **91**: 511–20.

Kenny, B., Ellis, S., Leard, A. D., Warawa, J., Mellor, H., *et al.* (2002). Co-ordinate regulation of distinct host cell signalling pathways by multifunctional enteropathogenic Escherichia coli effector molecules. *Mol. Microbiol.,* **44**: 1095–1107.

Khaitsa, M. L., Smith, D. R., Stoner, J. A., Parkhurst, A. M., Hinkley, S., *et al.* (2003). Incidence, duration, and prevalence of Escherichia coli O157:H7 fecal shedding by feedlot cattle during the finishing period. *J. Food Prot.,* **66**: 1972–77.

Kim, J., Nietfeldt, J., and Benson, A. K. (1999). Octamer-based genome scanning distinguishes a unique subpopulation of Escherichia coli O157:H7 strains in cattle. *Proc. Nat. Acad. Sci. USA,* **96**: 13288–93.

Kim, J., Nietfeldt, J., Ju, J., Wise, J., Fegan, N., *et al.* (2001). Ancestral divergence, genome diversification, and phylogeographic variation in subpopulations of sorbitol-negative, beta-glucuronidase-negative enterohemorrhagic Escherichia coli O157. *J. Bacteriol.,* **183**: 6885–97.

Knutton, S., Baldwin, T. J., Haigh, R. D., Williams, P. H., Manjarrez, A., *et al.* (1994). Intracellular changes in 'attaching and effacing' adhesion. In: M. A. Karmali and A. Goglio (eds.). *Recent Advances in Verocytotoxin-producing Escherichia coli infections.* pp. 215–22. Amsterdam: ELSEVIER Science.

Knutton, S., Lloyd, D. R., and McNeish, A. S. (1987). Adhesion of enteropathogenic Escherichia coli to human intestinal enterocytes and cultured human intestinal mucosa. *Infect. Immun.,* **55**: 69–77.

Konowalchuk, J., Dickie, N., Stavric, S., and Speirs, J. I. (1978). Properties of an Escherichia coli cytotoxin. *Infect. Immun.,* **20**: 575–77.

Konowalchuk, J., Speirs, J. I., and Stavric, S. (1977). Vero response to a cytotoxin of Escherichia coli. *Infect. Immun.,* **18**: 775–79.

Koohmaraie, M., Arthur, T. M., Bosilevac, J. M., Guerini, M., Shackelford, S. D., *et al.* (2005). Post-harvest interventions to reduce/eliminate pathogens in beef. *Meat Sci.,* **71**: 79–91.

Kudva, I. T., Blanch, K., and Hovde, C. J. (1998). Analysis of Escherichia coli O157:H7 survival in ovine or bovine manure and manure slurry. *Appl. Environ. Microbiol.,* **64**: 3166–74.

Kudva, I. T., Hatfield, P. G., and Hovde, C. J. (1996). Escherichia coli O157:H7 in microbial flora of sheep. *J. Clin. Microbiol.,* **34**: 431–33.

Kudva, I. T., Jelacic, S., Tarr, P. I., Youderian, P., and Hovde, C. J. (1999). Biocontrol of *Escherichia coli* O157 with O157-specific bacteriophages. *Appl. Environ. Microbiol.,* **65**: 3767–73.

Laegreid, W. W., Elder, R. O., and Keen, J. E. (1999). Prevalence of Escherichia coli O157:H7 in range beef calves at weaning. *Epidemiol. Infect.,* **123**: 291–98.

Lee, M. B. and Middleton, D. (2003). Enteric illness in Ontario, Canada, from 1997 to 2001. *J. Food Prot.,* **66**: 953–61.

Lee, M. S., Kaspar, C. W., Brosch, R., Shere, J., and Luchansky, J. B. (1996). Genomic analysis using pulsed-field gel electrophoresis of Escherichia coli O157: H7 isolated from dairy calves during the United State National Dairy Heifer Evaluation Project (1992–1992). *Vet. Microbiol.,* **48**: 223–30.

LeJeune, J. T., Abedon, S. T., Takemura, K., Christie, N. P., and Sreevatsan, S. (2004). Human Escherichia coli O157:H7 genetic marker in isolates of bovine origin. *Emerg. Infect. Dis.*, **10**: 1482–84.

LeJeune, J. T., Besser, T. E., and Hancock, D. D. (2001). Cattle water troughs as reservoirs of Escherichia coli O157. *Appl. Environ. Microbiol.*, **67**: 3053–57.

Levine, M. M., Xu, J-G., Kaper, J. B., Prado, V., Tall, B., *et al.* (1987). A DNA probe to identify enterohemorrhagic Escherichia coli of O157:H7 and other serotypes that cause hemorrhagic colitis and hemolytic uremic syndrome. *J. Infect. Dis.* **156**: 175–82.

Lin, J., Smith, M. P., Chapin, K. C., Baik, H. S., Bennet, G. N., *et al.* (1996). Mechanisms of acid resistance in enterohemorrhagic Escherichia coli. *Appl. Environ. Microbiol.*, **62**: 3094–3100.

Line, J. E., Fain, A. R. Jr., and Moran, A. B. (1991). Lethality of heat to Escherichia coli O157:H7: D-value and Z-value determinations in ground beef. *J. Food Prot.*, **54**: 762–66.

Lingwood, C. A., Law, H., Richardson, S. E., Petric, M., Brunton, J. L., *et al.* (1987). Glycolipid binding of natural and recombinant Escherichia coli produced Verotoxin in-vitro. *J. Biolog. Chem.*, **262**: 8834–39.

Lingwood, C. A., Mylvaganam, M., Arab, S., Khine, A. A., Magnusson, C., *et al.* (1998). Shiga toxin (Verotoxin) binding to its receptor glycolipid. In: J. B. Kaper and A. D. O'Brien (eds.). *Escherichia coli O157:H7 and other Shiga toxin-producing E. coli strains,* pp. 129–39. Washington, D.C.: ASM Press.

Locking, M. E., O'Brien, S. J., Reilly, W. J., Wright, E. M., Campbell, D. M., *et al.* (2001). Risk factors for sporadic cases of Escherichia coli O157 infection: the importance of contact with animal excreta. *Epidemiol. Infect.*, **127**: 215–20.

Lonergan, G. H. and Brashears, M. M. (2005). Preharvest interventions to reduce carriage of Escherichia coli O157:H7 by harvest-ready feedlot cattle. *Meat Sci.*, **71**: 72–78.

Lopez, E. L., Diaz, M., Grinstein, S., Devoto, S., Mendilaharzu, F., *et al.* (1989). Hemolytic uremic syndrome and diarrhea in Argentine children: the role of Shiga-like toxins. *J. Infect. Dis.*, **160**: 469–75.

Low, J. C., McKendrick, I. J., McKechnie, C., Fenlon, D., Naylor, S. W., *et al.* (2005). Rectal carriage of enterohemorrhagic Escherichia coli O157 in slaughtered cattle. *Appl. Environ. Microbiol.*, **71**: 93–97.

Ludwig, K., Bitzan, M., Zimmerman, S., Kloth, M., Mueller-Wiefel, D. E., *et al.* (1994). Antibody response to non-O157 verotoxin-producing Escherichia coli lipopolysaccharide in children with classical hemolytic uremic syndrome. In: M. A. Karmali and A. Goglio (eds.). *Recent Advances in Verocytotoxin-producing Escherichia coli infections,* pp. 89–91. Amsterdam: ELSEVIER Science.

Ludwig, K., Grabhorn, E., Bitzan, M., Bobrowski, C., Kemper, M. J., *et al.* (2002a). Saliva IgM and IgA are a sensitive indicator of the humoral immune response to Escherichia coli O157 lipopolysaccharide in children with enteropathic hemolytic uremic syndrome. *Pediatr. Res.*, **52**: 307–313.

Ludwig, K., Karmali, M. A., Smith, C. R., and Petric, M. (2002b). Cross-protection against challenge by intravenous Escherichia coli verocytotoxin 1 (VT1) in rabbits immunized with VT2 toxoid. *Can. J. Microbiol.*, **48**: 99–103.

Lynn, R. M., O'Brien, S. J., Taylor, C. M., Adak, G. K., Chart, H., *et al.* (2005). Childhood hemolytic uremic syndrome, United Kingdom and Ireland. *Emerg. Infect. Dis.*, **11**: 590–90.

Mackenzie, A. M., Lebel, P., Orrbine, E., Rowe, P. C., Hyde, L., *et al.* (1998). Sensitivities and specificities of premier E. coli O157 and premier EHEC enzyme immunoassays for diagnosis of infection with verotoxin (Shiga-like toxin)-producing Escherichia coli. The SYNSORB Pk Study investigators. *J. Clin. Microbiol.*, **36**: 1608–1611.

MacLeod, D. L., Gyles, C. L., and Wilcox, B. P. (1991). Reproduction of Edema Disease of Swine with purified Shiga-like toxin-II variant. *Vet. Pathol.*, **28**: 66–73.

Makino, K., Ishii, K., Yasunaga, T., Hattori, M., Yokoyama, K., *et al.* (1998). Complete nucleotide sequences of 93-kb and 3.3-kb plasmids of an enterohemorrhagic Escherichia coli O157:H7 derived from Sakai outbreak. *DNA Res.*, **5**: 1–9.

Manning, S. D., Motiwala, A. S., Springman, A. C., Qi, W., Lacher, D. W., Ouellette, L. M., Mladonicky, J. M., Somsel, P., Rudrik, J. T., Dietrich, S. E., Zhang, W., Swaminathan, B., Alland, D., and Whittam, T. S. (2008). Variation in virulence among clades of Escherichia coli O157:H7 associated with disease outbreaks. *Proc. Natl. Acad. Sci. USA,* **105**: 4868–73.

March, S. B. and Ratnam, S. (1986). Sorbitol MacConkey medium for detection of Escherichia coli O157:H7 associated with hemorrhagic colitis. *J. Clin. Microbiol.*, **23**: 869–72.

Matthews, L., McKendrick, I. J., Ternent, H., Gunn, G. J., Synge, B., *et al.* (2006). Super-shedding cattle and the transmission dynamics of Escherichia coli O157. *Epidemiol. Infect.*, **134**: 131–142.

Maule, A. (1999). Environmental aspects of *Escherichia coli* O157:H7. *Int. Food Hyg.*, **9**: 21–23.

McDaniel, T. K., Jarvis, K. G., Donnenberg, M. S., and Kaper, J. B. (1995). A genetic locus of enterocyte effacement conserved among diverse enterobacterial pathogens. *Proc. Nat. Acad. Sci. USA,* **92**: 1664–68.

McDaniel, T. K. and Kaper, J. B. (1997). A cloned pathogenicity island from enteropathogenic Escherichia coli confers the attaching and effacing phenotype on *E. coli* K-12. *Mol. Microbiol.*, **23**: 399–407.

McLaine, P. N., Orrbine, E., and Rowe, P. C. (1992). Childhood Hemolytic Uremic Syndrome in Canada: A multicenter study. In: B. S. Kaplan (ed.). *Hemolytic Uremic Syndrome and Thrombotic Thrombocytopenic Purpura,* pp. 61–69. New York: Marcel Dekker, Inc.

McNamara, B. P. and Donnenberg, M. S. (1998). A novel proline-rich protein, EspF, is secreted from enteropathogenic Escherichia coli via the type III export pathway. *FEMS Microbiol. Lett.,* **166**: 71–78.

Mead, P. S., Finelli, L., Lambert-Fair, M. A., Champ, D., Townes, J., *et al.* (1997). Risk factors for sporadic infection with Escherichia coli O157:H7. *Arch. Intern. Med.,* **157**: 204–208.

Mead, P. S., Slutsker, L., Dietz, V., McCaig, L. F., Bresee, J. S., *et al.* (1999). Food-related illness and death in the United States. *Emerg. Infect. Dis.,* **5**: 607–25.

Mechie, S. C., Chapman, P. A., and Siddons, C. A. (1997). A fifteen month study of Escherichia coli O157:H7 in a dairy herd. *Epidemiol. Infect.,* **118**: 17–25.

Mellies, J. L., Elliott, S. J., Sperandio, V., Donnenberg, M. S., and Kaper, J. B. (1999). The Per regulon of enteropathogenic Escherichia coli: identification of a regulatory cascade and a novel transcriptional activator, the locus of enterocyte effacement (LEE)-encoded regulator (Ler). *Mol. Microbiol.,* **33**: 296–306.

Melton-Celsa, A. R. and O'Brien, A. D. (1998). Structure, biology, and relative toxicity of Shiga toxin family members for cells and animals. In: J. B. Kaper and A. D. O'Brien (eds.). *Escherichia coli O157:H7 and other Shiga toxin-producing E. coli strains,* pp. 121–28. Washington, D.C.: ASM Press.

Meyer-Broseta, S., Bastian, S. N., Arne, P. D., Cerf, O., and Sanaa, M. (2001). Review of epidemiological surveys on the prevalence of contamination of healthy cattle with Escherichia coli serogroup O157:H7. *Int. J. Hyg. Environ. Health,* **203**: 347–61.

Michino, H., Araki, K., Minami, S., Takaya, S., Sakai, N., *et al.* (1999). Massive outbreak of Escherichia coli O157:H7 infection in schoolchildren in Sakai City, Japan, associated with consumption of white radish sprouts. *Am. J. Epidemiol.,* **150**: 787–96.

Mohammed, A., Peiris, J. S. M., Wijewanta, E. A., Mahalingam, S., and Gunasekara, G. (1985). Role of verocytotoxigenic Escherichia coli in cattle and buffalo calf diarrhea. *FEMS Microbiol. Lett.,* **26**: 281–83.

Monnens, L., Savage, C. O., and Taylor, C. M. (1998). Pathophysiology of hemolytic-uremic syndrome. In: J. B. Kaper and A. D. O'Brien (eds.). *Escherichia coli O157:H7 and other Shiga toxin-producing E. coli strains,* pp. 287–92. Washington, D.C.: ASM Press.

Montenegro, M., Bülte, M., Trumpf, T., Aleksic, S., Reuter, G., *et al.* (1990). Detection and characterization of fecal verotoxin-producing Escherichia coli from healthy cattle. *J. Clin. Microbiol.,* **28**: 1417–21.

Moon, H. W., Whipp, S. C., Arzenio, R. A., Levine, M. M., *et al.* (1983). Attaching and effacing activities of rabbit and human enteropathogenic Escherichia coli in pig and rabbit intestines. *Infect. Immun.,* **41**: 1340–51.

Morgan, D., Newman, C. P., Hutchinson, D. N., Walker, A. M., Rowe, B., et al. (1993). Verotoxin-producing Escherichia coli O157 infections associated with consumption of yoghurt. Epidemiol. Infect., 111: 181–87.

Moriya, K., Fujibayashi, T., Yoshihara, T., Matsuda, A., Sumi, N., et al. (1999). Verotoxin-producing Escherichia coli O157:H7 carried by the housefly in Japan. Med. Vet. Entomol., 13: 214–216.

Morooka, T. H., Matano, A., Umeda, T., Amako, K., and Karmali, M. A. (1995). Indirect hemagglutination assay for antibodies to Escherichia coli lipopolysaccharides O157, O111, and O26 in patients with hemolytic uremic syndrome. Acta Paediatr. Japonica, 37: 469–73.

Morrison, D. M., Tyrell, D. L. J., and Jewell, L. D. (1985). Colonic biopsy in Verotoxin-induced hemorrhagic colitis and thrombotic thrombocytopenic purpura (TTP). Am. J. Clin. Pathol., 86: 108–112.

Moxley, R. A. (2003). Detection and diagnosis of Escherichia coli O157:H7 in Food-producing animals. In: M. E. Torrance and R.E. Isaacson (eds.). Microbial Food Safety in Animal Agriculture: Current Topics, pp. 143–54. Ames, Iowa: Iowa State Press.

Moxley, R. A., Smith, D. R., Luebbe, M., Erickson, G. E., Klopfenstein, T. J., and Rogan, D. (2009). Escherichia coli O157:H7 vaccine dose-effect in feedlot cattle. Foodborne Pathog. Dis., 6: 879–84.

NASPHV, Centers for Disease Control and Prevention (2009). Commercial of State and Territorial Epidemiologists, American Veterinary Medical Association. Compendium of measures to prevent disease associated with animals in public settings, 2009. National Association of State Public Health Veterinarians, Inc (NASPHV). MMWR Recomm. Report, 58 (RR-5):1–21.

Nataro, J. P. and Kaper, J. B. (1998). Diarrheageneic Escherichia coli. Clin. Microbiol. Rev., 11: 142–201.

Nataro, J. P., Seriwatana, J., Fasano, A., Maneval, D. R., Guers, L. D., et al. (1995). Identification and cloning of a novel plasmid-encoded enterotoxin of enteroinvasive Escherichia coli and Shigella strains. Infect. Immun., 63: 4721–28.

National Animal Health Monitoring System (NAHMS)(2001). Escherichia coli O157 in United States feedlots. United States Department of Agriculture.

Naylor, S. W., Gally, D. L., and Low, J. C. (2005a). Enterohaemorrhagic E. coli in veterinary medicine. Int. J. Med. Microbiol., 295: 419–41.

Naylor, S. W., Low, J. C., Besser, T. E., Mahajan, A., Gunn, G. J., et al. (2003). Lymphoid follicle-dense mucosa at the terminal rectum is the principal site of colonization of enterohemorrhagic Escherichia coli O157:H7 in the bovine host. Infect. Immun., 71: 1505–1512.

Naylor, S. W., Roe, A. J., Nart, P., Spears, K., Smith, D. G., et al. (2005b). Escherichia coli O157: H7 forms attaching and effacing lesions at the terminal rectum of cattle and colonization requires the LEE4 operon. Microbiology, 151: 2773–81.

Nielsen, E. M., Skov, M. N., Madsen, J. J., Lodal, J., Jespersen, J. B., et al. (2004). Verocytotoxin-producing Escherichia coli in wild birds and rodents in close proximity to farms. Appl. Environ. Microbiol., 70: 6944–47.

Notenboom, R. H., Borczyk, A., Karmali, M. A., and Duncan, L. M. C. (1987). Clinical relevance of a serological cross-reaction between Escherichia coli O157 and Brucella abortus. Lancet, ii: 745.

O'Brien, A. D. and LaVeck, G. D. (1983). Purification and characterization of a Shigella-dysenteriae 1-like toxin produced by Escherichia coli. Infect. Immun., 40: 675–83.

O'Brien, A. D., Tesh, V. L., Donohue-Rolfe, A., Jackson, M. P., Olsnes, S., et al. (1992). Shiga toxin: Biochemistry, Genetics, Mode of Action. and Role in Pathogenesis. Curr. Topics Microbiol. Immunol., 180: 65–94.

O'Brien, S. J., Adak, G. K., and Gilham, C. (2001). Contact with farming environment as a major risk factor for Shiga toxin (Vero cytotoxin)-producing Escherichia coli O157 infection in humans. Emerg. Infect. Dis., 7: 1049–51.

Obrig, T. G., Vecchio, P. J. D., Brown, J. E., Moran, T. P., Rowland, B. M., et al. (1988). Direct Cytotoxic Action of Shiga Toxin on Human Vascular Endothelial Cells. Infect. Immun., 56: 2373–78.

Ogden, I. D., Hepburn, N. F., MacRae, M., Strachan, N. J., Fenlon, D. R., et al. (2002). Long-term survival of Escherichia coli O157 on pasture following an outbreak associated with sheep at a scout camp. Lett. Appl. Microbiol., 34: 100–104.

Ogden, L. D., Fenlon, D. R., Vinten, A. J., and Lewis, D. (2001). The fate of Escherichia coli O157 in soil and its potential to contaminate drinking water. Int. J. Food Microbiol., 66: 111–17.

Omisakin, F., MacRae, M., Ogden, I. D., and Strachan, N. J. (2003). Concentration and prevalence of Escherichia coli O157 in cattle feces at slaughter. Appl. Environ. Microbiol., 69: 2444–47.

Oteiza, J. M., Peltzer, M., Gannuzzi, L., and Zaritzky, N. (2005). Antimicrobial efficacy of UV radiation on Escherichia coli O157:H7 (EDL 933) in fruit juices of different absorptivities. J. Food Prot., 68: 49–58.

Pai, C. H., Ahmed, N., Lior, H., Johnson, W. M., Sims, H. V., et al. (1988). Epidemiology of sporadic diarrhea due to verocytotoxin-producing Escherichia coli: a two-year prospective study. J. Infect. Dis., 157: 1054–57.

Paton, A. W. and Paton, J. C. (1998a). Detection and characterization of shiga toxigenic Escherichia coli by using multiplex PCR assays for stx1, stx2, eaeA, enterohemorrhagic E. coli hlyA, rfbO111, and rfbO157. J. Clin. Microbiol., 36: 598–602.

Paton, J. C. and Paton, A. W. (1998b). Pathogenesis and diagnosis of Shiga toxin-producing Escherichia coli infections. Clin. Microbiol. Rev., 11: 450–79.

Paton, J. C., Rogers, T., Morona, R., and Paton, A. W. (2001). Oral administration of formaldehyde-killed recombinant bacteria expressing a mimic of the Shiga toxin receptor protects mice from fatal challenge with Shiga-toxigenic Escherichia coli. Infect. Immun., 69: 1389–93.

Perna, N. T., Plunkett III, G., Burland, V., Mau, B., Glasner, J. D., et al. (2001). Genome sequence of enterohaemorrhagic Escherichia coli O157:H7. Nature, 409: 529–33.

Peterson, R. E., Klopfenstein, T. J., Moxley, R. A., Erickson, G. E., Hinkley, S., Bretschneider, G., Berberov, E. M., Rogan, D., Smith, D. R. (2007a). Effect of a vaccine product containing type III secreted proteins on the probability of Escherichia coli O157:H7 fecal shedding and mucosal colonization in feedlot cattle, J. Food Prot.,70: 2568–77

Peterson, R. E., Klopfenstein, T., Smith, D. R., Folmer, J. D., et al. (2005). Direct-fed microbial products for Escherichia coli O157:H7 in market-ready feedlot cattle, pp. 64–65. Lincoln, University of Nebraska. Nebraska Beef Report.

Philpott, D. J., Ackerley, C. A., Kiliaan, A. J., Karmali, M. A., Perdue, M. H., et al. (1997). Translocation of verotoxin-1 across T84 monolayers: mechanism of bacterial toxin penetration of epithelium. Am. J. Physiol., 273: G1349–58.

Pollard, D. R., Johnson, W. M., Lior, H., Tyler, S. D., and Rozee, K. R. (1990). Rapid and specific detection of Verotoxin genes in Escherichia coli by the polymerase chain reaction. J. Clin. Microbiol., 28: 540–45.

Potter, A. A., Klashinsky, S., Li, Y., Frey, E., Townsend, H., et al. (2004). Decreased shedding of Escherichia coli O157:H7 by cattle following vaccination with type III secreted proteins. Vaccine, 22: 362–69.

Proulx, F., Seidman, E. G., and Karpman, D. (2001). Pathogenesis of Shiga toxin-associated hemolytic uremic syndrome. Pediatr. Res., 50: 163–71.

Pulz, M., Matussek, A., Monazahian, M., Tittel, A., Nikolic, E., et al. (2003). Comparison of a shiga toxin enzyme-linked immunosorbent assay and two types of PCR for detection of shiga toxin-producing Escherichia coli in human stool specimens. J. Clin. Microbiol., 41: 4671–75.

Raghupathy, P., Date, A., Shastry, J. C. M., Sudarsanam, A., and Jadhav, M. (1978). Haemolytic-ureaemic syndrome complicating shigella dysentery in south Indian children. BMJ, 1: 1518–21.

Rahn, K., Renwick, S. A., Johnson, R. P., Wilson, J. B., Clarke, R. C., et al. (1997). Persistence of Escherichia coli O157:H7 in dairy cattle and the dairy farm environment. Epidemiol. Infect., 119: 251–59.

Rangel, J. M., Sparling, P. H., Crowe, C., Griffin, P. M., and Swerdlow, D. L. (2005). Epidemiology of Escherichia coli O157:H7 outbreaks, United States, 1982–2002. Emerg. Infect. Dis., 11: 603–609.

Ransom, J. R. (2004). Cattle feedlot management practices to reduce Escherichia coli O157:H7 contamination. In: Pre-harvest and post-harvest intervention strategies to reduce prevalence of pathogens in beef and beef products, pp. 33–49. Fort Collins, CO: Department of Animal Science, Colorado State University.

Read, S. C., Gyles, C. L., Clarke, R. C., Lior, H., and McEwen, S. (1990). Prevalence of verocytotoxigenic Escherichia coli in ground beef, pork, and chicken in southwestern Ontario. *Epidemiol. Infect.*, **105**: 11–20.

Redmond, E. C. and Griffith, C. J. (2003). Consumer food handling in the home: a review of food safety studies. *J. Food Prot.*, **66**: 130–61.

Renter, D. G., Morris, J. G.Jr., Sargeant, J. M., Hungerford, L. L., Berezowski, J., *et al.* (2005). Prevalence, risk factors, O-serogroups, and virulence profiles of shiga-toxin producing bacteria from cattle production environments. *J. Food Prot.*, **68**: 1556–65.

Renter, D. G., Sargeant, J. M., Hygnstorm, S. E., Hoffman, J. D., and Gillespie, J. R. (2001). Escherichia coli O157:H7 in free-ranging deer in Nebraska. *J. Wildl. Dis.*, **37**: 755–60.

Renter, D. G., Sargeant, J. M., Oberst, R. D., and Samadpour, M. (2003). Diversity, frequency, and persistence of Escherichia coli O157 strains from range cattle environments. *Appl. Environ. Microbiol.*, **69**: 542–47.

Reymond, D., Johnson, R. P., Karmali, M. A., Petric, M., Winkler, M., Johnson, S., *et al.* (1996). Neutralizing antibodies to Escherichia coli Vero cytotoxin 1 and antibodies to O157 lipopolysaccharide in healthy farm family members and urban residents. *J. Clin. Microbiol.*, **34**: 2053–57.

Rice, D. H., McMenamin, K. M., Pritchett, L. C., Hancock, D. D., and Besser, T. E. (1999). Genetic subtyping of Escherichia coli O157 isolates from 41 Pacific Northwest USA cattle farms. *Epidemiol. Infect.*, **122**: 479–84.

Rice, D. H., Sheng, H. Q., Wynia, S. A., and Hovde, C. J. (2003). Rectoanal mucosal swab culture is more sensitive than fecal culture and distinguishes Escherichia coli O157:H7-colonized cattle and those transiently shedding the same organism. *J. Clin. Microbiol.*, **41**: 4924–29.

Rich, A. R., Jepson, A. N., Luebbe, M., Erickson, G., Klopfenstein, T., Smith, D. R., and Moxley, R. A. (2010). Vaccination to reduce the prevalence of *Escherichia Coli* O157:H7 in feedlot cattle fed wet distillers grains plus solubles. *Nebraska Beef Cattle Report*, 94–5.

Richardson, S. E., Karmali, M. A., Becker, L. E., and Smith, C. R. (1988). The Histopathology of the Hemolytic Uremic Syndrome Associated With Verocytotoxin-Producing Escherichia coli Infections. *Hum. Pathol.*, **19**: 1102–1108.

Richardson, S. E., Rotman, T. A., Jay, V., Smith, C. R., Becker, L. E., *et al.* (1992). Experimental verocytotoxemia in rabbits. *Infect. Immun.*, **60**: 4154–67.

Riley, L. W. (1987). The epidemiologic, clinical, and microbiologic features of hemorrhagic colitis. *Ann. Rev. Microbiol.*, **41**: 383–407.

Riley, L. W., Remis, R. S., Helgerson, S. D., McGee, H. B., Wells, J. G., *et al.* (1983). Hemorrhagic colitis associated with a rare Escherichia coli serotype. *New Engl. J. Med.*, **308**: 681–85.

Ropkins, K. and Beck, A. J. (2000). Evaluation of worldwide approaches to the use of HACCP to control food safety. *Trends in Food Sci. Techn.*, **11**: 10–21.

Rowe, P. C., Orrbine, E., Lior, H., Wells, G. A., and McLaine, P. N. (1993). Diarrhoea in close contacts as a risk factor for childhood haemolytic uraemic syndrome. *Epidemiol. Infect.*, **110**: 16.

Rowe, P. C., Orrbine, E., Wells, G. A., and McLaine, P. N. (1991). Epidemiology of hemolytic-uremic syndrome in Canadian children from 1986 to 1988. The Canadian Pediatric Kidney Disease Reference Centre. *J. Pediatr.*, **119**: 218–24.

Safdar, N., Said, A., Gangnon, R. E., and Maki, D. G. (2002). Risk of hemolytic uremic syndrome after antibiotic treatment of Escherichia coli O157:H7 enteritis: a meta-analysis. *JAMA*, **288**: 996–1001.

Salmon, R., Outbreak Control Team (2005). Outbreaks of verotoxin producing E. coli 0157 infections involving over forty schools in South Wales, September 2005. *Euro. Surv.*, **10**: 40.

Sanderson, M. W., Besser, T. E., Gay, J. M., Gay, C. C., and Hancock, D. D. (1999). Fecal Escherichia coli O157:H7 shedding patterns of orally inoculated calves. *Vet. Microbiol.*, **69**: 199–205.

Sandhu, K. S., Clarke, R. C., McFadden, K., Brouwer, A., Louie, M., *et al.* (1996). Prevalence of the eaeA gene in verotoxigenic Escherichia coli strains from dairy cattle in Southwest Ontario. *Epidemiol. Infect.*, **116**: 1–7.

Sandvig, K. and van Deurs, B. (1996). Endocytosis, intracellular transport, and cytotoxic action of Shiga toxin and ricin. *Physiol. Rev.*, **76**: 949–66.

Sargeant, J. M., Hafer, D. J., Gillespie, J. R., Oberst, R. D., and Flood, S. J. (1999). Prevalence of Escherichia coli O157:H7 in white-tailed deer sharing rangeland with cattle. *J. Am. Vet. Med. Assoc.*, **215**: 792–94.

Sargeant, J. M., Sanderson, M. W., Griffin, D. D., and Smith, R. A. (2004a). Factors associated with the presence of Escherichia coli O157 in feedlot-cattle water and feed in the Midwestern USA. *Prev. Vet. Med.*, **66**: 207–37.

Sargeant, J. M., Sanderson, M. W., Smith, R. A., and Griffin, D. D. (2003). Escherichia coli O157 in feedlot cattle feces and water in four major feeder-cattle states in the USA. *Prev. Vet. Med.*, **61**: 127–35.

Sargeant, J. M., Sanderson, M. W., Smith, R. A., and Griffin, D. D. (2004b). Associations between management, climate, and Escherichia coli O157 in the faeces of feedlot cattle in the Midwestern USA. *Prev. Vet. Med.*, **66**: 175–206.

Sargeant, J. M. and Smith, D. R. (2003). The epidemiology of Escherichia coli O157:H7. In: M. E. Torrance and R. E. Isaacson (ed.). *Microbial Food Safety in Animal Agriculture: Current topics*, pp. 131–141. Ames, Iowa: Iowa State Press.

Schmidt, H. (2001). Shiga-toxin-converting bacteriophages. *Res. Microbiol.*, **152**: 687–95.

Sekla, L., Milley, D., Stackiw, W., Sisler, J., Drew, J., *et al.* (1990). Verotoxin-producing Escherichia coli in ground beef,Manitoba. *Can. Commun. Dis. Rep.*, **16**: 103–105.

Shanks, P. L. (1938). An unusual condition affecting the digestive organs of the pig. *Vet. Rec.*, **50**: 356–58.

Shere, J. A., Bartlett, K. J., and Kaspar, C. W. (1998). Longitudinal study of Escherichia coli O157:H7 dissemination on four dairy farms in Wisconsin. *Appl. Environ. Microbiol.*, **64**: 1390–99.

Sherman, P., Soni, R., and Karmali, M. (1988). Attaching and effacing adherence of Verocytotoxin producing Escherichia coli to rabbit intestinal epithelium in vivo. *Infect. Immun.*, **56**: 756–61.

Smith, D., Blackford, M., Younts, S., Moxley, R., Gray, J., *et al.* (2001). Ecological relationships between the prevalence of cattle shedding Escherichia coli O157:H7 and characteristics of the cattle or conditions of the feedlot pen. *J. Food Prot.*, **64**: 1899–1903.

Smith, D. R., Moxley, R. A., Klopfenstein, T. J., and Erickson, G. E. (2009a). A randomized longitudinal trial to test the effect of regional vaccination within a cattle feedyard on *Escherichia coli* O157:H7 rectal colonization, fecal shedding, and hide contamination. *Foodborne Pathog. Dis.*, **6**: 885–92.

Smith, D. R., Moxley, R. A., Peterson, R. E., Klopfenstein, T. J., Erickson, G .E., Bretschneider, G., Berberov, E. M., and Clowser, S. (2009b). A two-dose regimen of a vaccine against Type III Secreted Proteins reduced *Escherichia coli* O157:H7 colonization of the terminal rectum in beef cattle in commercial feedlots. *Foodborne Pathog. Dis.*, **6**: 155–61.

Smith, D. R., Moxley, R. A., Peterson, R. E., Klopfenstein, T. J., Erickson, G .E., and Clowser, S. L. (2008). A two-dose regimen of a vaccine against *Escherichia coli* O157:H7 Type III Secreted Proteins reduced environmental transmission of the agent in a large-scale commercial beef feedlot clinical trial. *Foodborne Pathog. Dis.*, **5**: 589–98.

Solomon, E. B., Yaron, S., and Matthews, K. R. (2002). Transmission of Escherichia coli O157:H7 from contaminated manure and irrigation water to lettuce plant tissue and its subsequent internalization. *Appl. Environ. Microbiol.*, **68**: 397–400.

Sperandio, V., Mellies, J. L., Delahay, R. M., Frankel, G., Crawford, J. A., (2000). Activation of enteropathogenic Escherichia coli (EPEC) LEE2 and LEE3 operons by Ler. *Molec. Microbiol.*, **38**: 781–93.

Sperandio, V., Mellies, J. L., Nguyen, W., Shin, S., and Kaper, J. B. (1999). Quorum sensing controls expression of the type III secretion gene transcription and protein secretion in enterohemorrhagic and enteropathogenic Escherichia coli. *Proc. Nat. Acad. Sci. USA*, **96**: 15196–201.

Spika, J. S., Parsons, J. E., Nordenberg, D., and Gunn, R. A. (1986). Hemolytic uremic syndrome and diarrhea associated with Escherichia coli O157:H7 in a day-care center. *J. Pediatr.*, **109**: 287–91.

Stevens, M. P., van Diemen, P. M., Dziva, F., Jones, P. W., and Wallis, T. S. (2002). Options for the control of enterohaemorrhagic Escherichia coli in ruminants. *Microbiology*, **148**: 3767–78.

Suri, R. S., Clark, W. F., Barrowman, N., Mahon, J. L., Thiessen-Philbrook, H. R., *et al.* (2005). Diabetes during diarrhea-associated hemolytic uremic syndrome: a systematic review and meta-analysis. *Diabetes Care,* **28**: 2556–62.

Suthienkul, O., Brown, J. E., Seriwatana, J., Tienthongdee, S., Sastravaha, S., *et al.* (1990). Shiga-like-toxin-producing Escherichia coli in retail meats and cattle in Thailand. *Appl. Environ. Microbiol.,* **56**: 1135–39.

Swaminathan, B., Barrett, T. J., Hunter, S. B., and Tauxe, R. V. (2001). Pulsenet: the molecular subtyping network for foodborne bacterial disease surveillance, US. *Emerg. Infect. Dis., 7*: 382–89.

Swaminathan, B., Gerner-Smidt, P., Ng, L. K., Lukinmaa, S., Kam, K. M., *et al.* (2006). Building PulseNet International: an interconnected system of laboratory networks to facilitate timely public health recognition and response to foodborne disease outbreaks and emerging foodborne diseases. *Foodborne Pathog. Dis.,* **3**: 36–50.

Swerdlow, D. L., Woodruff, B. A., Brady, R. C., Griffin, P. M., Tippen, S., *et al.* (1992). A waterborne outbreak in Missouri of Escherichia coli O157:H7 associated with bloody diarrhea and death. *Annals Int. Med., 117*: 812–19.

Tarr, P. I., Gordon, C. A., and Chandler, W. L. (2005). Shiga-toxin-producing Escherichia coli and haemolytic uraemic syndrome. *Lancet,* **365**: 1073–86.

Tarr, P. I. and Hickman, R. O. (1987). Hemolytic uremic syndrome epidemiology: a population-based study in King County, Washington, 1971–1980. *Pediatrics,* **80**: 41–45.

Tauxe, R. V. (2006). Molecular subtyping and the transformation of public health. *Foodborne Pathog. Dis.,* **3**: 4–8.

Taylor, C. M. and Monnens, L. A. (1998). Advances in haemolytic uraemic syndrome. *Arch. Dis. Child.,* **78**: 190–93.

te Loo, D. M., Hinsbergh, V. W., Heuvel, L. P., and Monnens, L. A. (2001). Detection of verocytotoxin bound to circulating polymorphonuclear leukocytes of patients with hemolytic uremic syndrome. *J. Am. Soc. Nephrol., 12*: 800–806.

Thomson, D. U., Loneragan, G. H., Thornton, A. B., Lechtenberg, K. F., Emery, D. A., Burkhardt, D. T., and Nagaraja, T. G. (2009). Use of a Siderophore Receptor and Porin Proteins-Based vaccine to control the burden of *Escherichia coli* O157:H7 in feedlot cattle. *Foodborne Pathog. Dis., 6*: 871–7.

Trachtman, H., Cnaan, A., Christen, E., Gibbs, K., Zhao, S., *et al.* (2003). Effect of an oral shiga toxin-binding agent on diarrhea-associated hemolytic uremic syndrome in children. *JAMA, 290*: 1337–44.

Trompeter, R. S., Schwartz, R., Chantler, C., Dillon, M. J., Haycock, G. B., (1983). Haemolytic uraemic syndrome: an analysis of prognostic features. *Arch. Dis. Child.,* **58**: 101–105.

Tzipori, S., Sheoran, A., Akiyoshi, D., Donohue-Rolfe, A., and Trachtman, H. (2004). Antibody therapy in the management of shiga toxin-induced hemolytic uremic syndrome. *Clin. Microbiol. Rev.,* **17**: 92641.

Upadhyaya, K., Barwick, K., Fishaut, M., Kashgarian, M., and Segal, N. J. (1980). The importance of nonrenal involvement in hemolytic uremic syndrome. *Pediatr.,* **65**: 115–20.

USDA:APHIS:VS. (1994). Escherichia coli O157:H7 issues and ramifications Fort Collins, Colorado, USA, 80521: Centers for Epidemiology and Animal Health.

van de Kar, N. C. and Monnens, L. A. (1998). The haemolytic-uraemic syndrome in childhood. *Baillieres Clin. Haematol.,* **11**: 497–507.

Van Donkersgoed, J., Berg, J., Potter, A., Hancock, D., Besser, T., *et al.* (2001). Environmental sources and transmission of Escherichia coli O157 in feedlot cattle. *Can. Vet. J.,* **42**: 714–20.

Van Donkersgoed, J., Hancock, D., Rogan, D., and Potter, A. A. (2005). Escherichia coli O157:H7 vaccine field trial in 9 feedlots in Alberta and Saskatchewan. *Can. Vet. J.,* **46**: 724–28.

Wallace, D. J., Van Gilder, T., Shallow, S., Fiorentino, T., Segler, S. D., *et al.* (2000). Incidence of foodborne illnesses reported by the foodborne diseases active surveillance network (FoodNet)-1997. FoodNet Working Group. *J. Food Prot.,* **63**: 807–9.

Wang, G. and Doyle, M. P. (1998). Survival of enterohemorrhagic Escherichia coli O157:H7 in water. *J. Food Prot.,* **61**: 662–67.

Wang, G., Zhao, T., and Doyle, M. P. (1996). Fate of enterohemorrhagic Escherichia coli O157:H7 in bovine feces. *Appl. Environ. Microbiol.,* **62**: 2567–70.

Watanabe, M., Matsuoka, K., Kita, E., Igai, K., Higashi, N., *et al.* (2004). Oral therapeutic agents with highly clustered globotriose for treatment of Shiga toxigenic Escherichia coli infections. *J. Infect. Dis.,* **189**: 360–68.

Wells, J. G., Shipman, L. D., Green, K. D., Sowers, E. G., Green, J. H., *et al.* (1991). Isolation of Escherichia coli serotype O157:H7 and other Shiga-like-toxin-producing Escherichia coli from dairy cattle. *J. Clin. Microbiol.,* **29**: 985–89.

Werber, D., Mason, B. W., Evans, M. R., and Salmon, R. L. (2008). Preventing household transmission of Shiga toxin-producing Escherichia coli 0157 infection: promptly separating siblings might be the key. *Clin. Infect. Dis., 46*, 1189–96.

Whittam, T. S., Wachsmuth, I. K., and Wilson, R. A. (1988). Genetic evidence of clonal descent of Escherichia coli O157:H7 associated with hemorrhagic colitis and hemolytic uremic syndrome. *J. Infect. Dis.,* **157**: 1124–33.

Whittam, T. S., Wolfe, M. L., Wachsmuth, I. K., Orskov, F., Orskov, I., *et al.* (1993). Clonal relationships among Escherichia coli strains that cause hemorrhagic colitis and infantile diarrhea. *Infect. Immun.,* **61**: 1619–29.

Wick, L. M., Qi, W., Lacher, D. W., and Whittam, T. S. (2005). Evolution of genomic content in the stepwise emergence of Escherichia coli O157:H7. *J. Bacteriol.,* **187**: 1783–91.

Williams, A. P., Avery, L. M., Kilham, K., and Jones, D. L. (2005). Persistence of Escherichia coli O157 on farm surfaces under different environmental conditions. *J. Appl. Microbiol.,* **98**: 1075–83.

Willshaw, G. A., Cheasty, T., Smith, H. R., O'Brien, S. J., and Adak, G. K. (2001). Verocytotoxin-producing Escherichia coli (VTEC) O157 and other VTEC from human infections in England and Wales: 1995–1998. *J. Med. Microbiol.,* **50**: 135–42.

Wilson, J. B., Clarke, R. C., Renwick, S., Rahn, K., Johnson, R. P., *et al.* (1996). Verocytotoxigenic Escherichia coli infection in dairy farm families. *J. Infect. Dis.,* **174**: 1021–27.

Wilson, R. K., Shaw, R. K., Daniell, S., Knutton, S., and Frankel, G. (2001). Role of EscF, a putative needle complex protein, in the type III protein translocation system of enteropathogenic Escherichia coli. *Cell Microbio., 3*: 753–62.

Wong, C. S., Jelacic, S., Habeeb, R. L., Watkins, S. L., and Tarr, P. I. (2000). The risk of the hemolytic-uremic syndrome after antibiotic treatment of Escherichia coli O157:H7 infections. *N. Engl. J. Med., 342*: 1930–36.

World Health Organization (1998). Zoonotic non-O157 Shiga toxin-producing Escherichia coli (STEC). Report of a WHO Scientific Working Group Meeting, Berlin, Germany, 22–23 June. *WHO/CSR/APH/98.8,* pp. 1–30. Geneva: WHO.

Wray, C., McLaren, I. M., Randall, L. P., and Pearson, G. R. (2000). Natural and experimental infection of normal cattle with Escherichia coli O157. *Vet. Rec., 147*: 65–68.

Younts-Dahl, S. M., Galyean, M. L., Lonergan, G. H., Elam, N. A., and Brashears, M. M. (2004). Dietary supplementation with Lactobacillus and Propionibacterium based direct-fed microbials and prevalence of *Escherichia coli* O157 in beef feedlot cattle and on hides at harvest. *J. Food Prot.,* **67**: 889–93.

Younts-Dahl, S. M., Osborn, G. D., Galyean, M. L., Rivera, J. D., Lonergan, G. H., *et al.* (2005). Reduction of *Escherichia coli* O157 in finishing beef cattle by various doses of Lactobacillus acidophilus in direct-fed microbials. *J. Food Prot.,* **68**: 6–10.

Zhang, Y., Laing, C., Steele, M., Ziebell, K., Johnson, R., Benson, A. K., *et al.* (2007). Genome evolution in major *Escherichia coli* O157:H7 lineages. *BMC Genomics, 8*: 121.

Zhao, T., Doyle, M. P., Shere, J., and Garber, L. (1995). Prevalence of enterohemorrhagic Escherichia coli O157:H7 in a survey of dairy herds. *Appl. Environ. Microbiol., 61*: 1290–93.

Ziebell, K., Steele, M., Zhang, Y., Benson, A., Taboada, E. N., Laing, C., McEwen, S., Ciebin, B., Johnson, R., and Gannon, V. (2008). Genotypic characterization and prevalence of virulence factors among Canadian Escherichia coli O157:H7 strains. *Appl. Environ. Microbiol.,* **74**: 4314–23.

CHAPTER 9

Lyme borreliosis

Sue O'Connell

Summary

Lyme borreliosis is the most common vectorborne bacterial infection in the temperate northern hemisphere. In the USA over 35,000 confirmed or probable cases were reported by state health departments to the Centers for Disease Control and Prevention (CDC) in 2008. It is likely that well over 100,000 cases occur in Europe each year. Lyme borreliosis is caused by several genospecies of *Borrelia burgdorferi* sensu lato, which are transmitted by ticks of the *Ixodes ricinus* complex. The infection occurs most commonly in forested, woodland and heathland habitats that support the lifecycles of *Ixodes* ticks and the small mammals and birds that are reservoir-competent hosts for *B burgorferi*. The most common presenting feature of Lyme borreliosis is erythema migrans, a slowly spreading rash. The spirochaetes can disseminate through the bloodstream and lymphatics to other organs and tissues and cause later manifestations, most commonly affecting the nervous and musculoskeletal systems. The infection responds to appropriate antibiotic treatment at any stage of disease, with excellent outcomes in most cases, but patients with severe tissue damage from previously untreated late stage disease may recover incompletely. A small proportion of patients can have persistent nonspecific symptoms following treatment, without evidence of continuing active infection. This has been termed 'post-Lyme syndrome' and appears to be similar to other post-infection syndromes. Prevention relies mainly on personal protection measures against tick bites.

History

The term Lyme arthritis was first used in the mid-1970s following recognition of a cluster of cases in children living in Old Lyme and neighbouring areas of Connecticut. Two mothers reported their concerns about the apparent high incidence of 'juvenile rheumatoid arthritis' to the local public health authorities (Edlow 2003). This prompted a series of investigations by the Connecticut State Public Health Department and researchers from Yale University (Steere *et al.* 1977a). They showed that the arthritis was not typical of juvenile rheumatoid arthritis but predominantly affected large joints, mainly the knee, and presented with recurrent attacks of swelling and pain, with onset mostly in the summer and fall. Some patients reported a history of erythematous skin lesions associated with insect bites prior to the onset of arthritis, leading investigators to suspect an arthropod-borne infection, which was initially thought to be viral in origin. It also became apparent that other systems and tissues could be involved, including the nervous system and the heart. The term 'Lyme disease' was used to denote this expanded clinical spectrum (Steere *et al.* 1977b).

Epidemiological and ecological investigations indicated that deer ticks (*Ixodes scapularis*) were the most likely vectors of the disease. Some patients recalled tick bites preceding their illness, and findings from tick population surveys correlated with areas of markedly higher focal geographic incidence of disease. The incidence of disease was 13 times higher in communities living near the eastern bank of the Connecticut River compared to those residing near the western side. The causative agent, a previously unidentified spirochaete, was isolated, initially from ticks and subsequently from blood and skin biopsy samples from patients (Burgdorfer *et al.* 1982; Benach *et al.* 1983) and the organism was named *Borrelia burgdorferi* in 1984 (Johnson *et al.* 1984).

Investigators related the clinical appearance of the rash to that of a condition termed erythema migrans or erythema chronicum migrans, which had been described in the European medical literature from the early years of the twentieth century and had been related to *Ixodes ricinus* tick bites (Afzelius 1921). Tick bites and erythema migrans had also been linked to other clinical presentations in Europe, including lymphocytic meningitis, facial palsy and radiculopathy, from 1922 onwards (Garin and Bujadoux 1922; Bannwarth 1941). Throughout the twentieth century cases had been reported from many parts of Europe that are now known to be highly endemic for Lyme borreliosis. The spirochaetal aetiology of European erythema migrans and other skin manifestations including acrodermatitis chronica atrophicans, a presentation of longstanding infection, was confirmed by the isolation of the organisms from skin biopsies of Swedish patients (Asbrink *et al.* 1984). The terms Lyme borreliosis or Lyme disease are now used to encompass all manifestations of the infection in Europe and North America. Lyme borreliosis also occurs throughout forested temperate regions of Asia, including Japan.

Agent

Lyme borreliosis is caused by several genospecies of the *Borrelia burgdorferi* sensu lato complex. At least fifteen genospecies have been identified, but most appear to be non-pathogenic; disease has been attributed to only four or five at the present time (EUCALB 2011). In North America Lyme borreliosis is caused exclusively by *B burgdorferi* sensu stricto. In Europe several other pathogenic genospecies also occur, predominantly *B afzelii* and *B garinii,* but *B burgdorferi* sensu stricto is found in some areas. Another genospecies, *B bavariensis,* previously thought to be a part of the *B garinii* group has recently been recognized as a separate entity, and another genospecies, *B spielmanii,* has also been shown to cause occasional cases of erythema migrans. Rare case reports have linked *B valaisiana* and *B lusitaniae* with clinical illness, but pathogenicity of these two genospecies has not been confirmed.

All pathogenic strains can cause erythema migrans, the early skin lesion. There is evidence for some genospecies-dependent variations in later disease manifestations and also for within-genospecies variations in pathogenicity. *B burgdorferi* sensu stricto is strongly linked with arthritic and neurological complications, *B garinii* and *B bavariensis* with neuroborreliosis and *B afzelii* with acrodermatitis chronica atrophicans (ACA), a late skin manifestation which was first described by Buchwald, a German dermatologist, in 1883. These variations in clinical presentations are linked to the genospecies' differences in tissue tropisms. Genospecies differences also have implications for vaccine development.

There is evidence for associations between specific borrelial genospecies and reservoir hosts. For example, *B afzelii* is associated with rodents, *B garinii* and *B valaisiana* with birds, and *B burgdorferi* sensu stricto with both rodents and birds (EUCALB 2011). These findings appear to be linked to differing susceptibilities of the borrelial genospecies to serum complement of the host animals.

Variations in the geographic distribution of European borrelial genospecies affect the incidence and types of clinical presentations of later disease seen in different locations. For example, ACA is more frequently seen in Scandinavia and central Europe, where *B afzelii* is commonly found. The condition occurs infrequently in the UK and Ireland, where *B afzelii* is uncommon. The most frequently identified pathogenic genospecies in the UK is *B garinii,* and acute neuroborreliosis is the main complication seen there. A high proportion of infected ticks in the UK and Ireland carry *B valaisiana,* which is essentially non-pathogenic. This has some bearing on the lower overall incidence of clinically significant disease in these countries compared to some other parts of Europe where a higher proportion of infected ticks carry more pathogenic genospecies (EUCALB 2011).

Microbiology

Borrelia burgdorferi sensu lato is a helically shaped bacterium measuring about 10 to 30 um long and about 0.2 to 0.5 um wide, with about three to ten loose coils and 7 to 11 periplasmic flagella extending along the length of the organism. Its ultrastructure comprises an outer surface layer, a trilaminar outer membrane which surrounds the periplasmic space containing the flagella and an inner compartment, the protoplasmic cylinder, consisting of a peptidoglycan layer and a cytoplasmic inner membrane enclosing the cytoplasmic contents. The flagella and the organism's loose coiled shape enable it to be highly motile in viscous fluids, aiding dissemination through host tissues. Its optimal mobility is seen in collagen-like viscosity (Bergstrom *et al.* 2001). The hidden nature of the flagella, beneath the outer membrane, helps to protect their highly conserved and immunogenic proteins from the host's immune system. The outer membrane has a

very large number of lipoproteins, including the plasmid-encoded outer-surface proteins (Osps) A–F.

The organism has an unusual genetic structure consisting of a linear chromosome and multiple linear and circular plasmids. The complete genome of the B31 reference strain has been sequenced and it has been shown that the organism lacks genes encoding enzymes for functions such as synthesis of amino acids, fatty acids, enzyme co-factors and nucleotides and energy pathways. It is an obligate parasite, relying on its host for many nutrients. It does not possess virulence factors such as the toxins, lipopolysaccharides and enzymes found in many other bacterial pathogens (Tilly *et al.* 2008). Its major virulence factors appear to be those of motility and the ability of surface-exposed lipoproteins to attach to mammalian cells.

Because of their complex life-cycles borreliae must adapt to life in very different environments: the midgut of the tick vector at ambient temperature and the mammalian or avian natural reservoir host from about 35º to 39°C. They vary gene expression, leading to production of different protein components. Some of these variations help the organisms to evade the initial defences of the host's innate immune system and others contribute to evasion of the subsequent acquired immune response. For example, borreliae express an outer surface protein (Osp), OspA, within the tick, but another outer surface protein, OspC, is expressed preferentially during the early stages of mammalian infection. There is variability in OspC proteins amongst different strains of *B burgdorferi,* and only some strains are associated with disseminated disease (Tilly *et al.* 2008; Bergstrom *et al.* 2002).

Expression of another protein, VlsE, which has an elaborate system for extensive variation over time, is required to maintain persistent infection. Synthesis of VlsE starts at about the time that OspC production ceases and helps the organism to evade the host's humoral immune response, at least for some time. The specific IgG antibody response to an increasing array of borrelial antigens gradually develops over months, as shown by immunoblot (western blot) findings on sera from patients at various stages of clinical infection (Aguero-Rosenfeld *et al.* 2005).

Pathogenesis

Many clinical manifestations of Lyme borreliosis occur largely as a consequence of the human immunopathologic response to infection. Some borrelial lipoproteins can activate a variety of cells, including macrophages, B cells, dendritic cells and endothelial cells, triggering inflammatory responses that contribute to pathogenesis. There is also some *in vitro* evidence that antibodies produced in response to *B burgdorferi* infection may also bind to human neural and other antigens (Tilly *et al.* 2008; Rupprecht *et al.* 2008; Kannian *et al.* 2007).

Ecology

Hard-bodied ticks of the *Ixodes ricinus* complex are the only vectors for Lyme borreliosis. Although borrelial DNA has been detected in other arthropods, including other tick genera such as *Dermacentor* or *Amblyomma* species, there has been no experimental or epidemiological evidence to suggest that they are vector-competent. In North America the infection is transmitted mainly by the black-legged or deer tick, *I scapularis,* and by *I pacificus,* the western black-legged tick, in the Pacific coastal states (CDC 2011).

The main European vector is *Ixodes ricinus* (commonly called the deer, sheep or castor bean tick) (Anon. 2004). In Russia and the Baltic republics the range of *I ricinus* overlaps with that of another vector, *I persulcatus* (the taiga tick), which is also widespread throughout temperate Asia to the Far East including Sakhalin Island, Japan, Korea and China.

Ixodid ticks are very susceptible to desiccation and require a high relative humidity (Gray *et al.* 2009). The most favourable tick habitats are forested areas and heath land where leaf litter and undergrowth provide protection against drying. These habitats also support animals and birds that are the natural feeding hosts for ticks. Ticks have a three-stage lifecycle (larva, nymph and adult), usually over two to three years (see Fig. 9.1). At each stage they take a single blood meal lasting from about three to seven days. In Europe the common feeding hosts for larvae and nymphs are small and medium sized mammals such as field mice, voles, squirrels and hares, and ground-feeding birds including blackbirds, robins and pheasants (EUCALB 2011). The most common feeding hosts for larval and nymphal *I scapularis* ticks in North America are white-footed mice, *Peromyscus leucopus*. These creatures are reservoir-competent hosts for *B burgdorferi*. The main feeding hosts for *I pacificus* ticks are lizards, which are not competent reservoir hosts

for borreliae, so borrelial infection rates in *I pacificus* ticks are very much lower than those found *in I scapularis* (CDC 2011). Ticks can become infected during the course of a blood meal taken from a spirochaetemic animal and in turn can transmit infection to hosts during feeds at later stages in their lifecycle, thus maintaining the spirochaetal reservoir in nature. Spring and early summer is the peak period for tick feeding and there can be a secondary peak during autumn in some regions.

Deer are strongly associated with the presence of ticks. They are the preferred feeding hosts for adult female ticks, who mate after feeding, drop back into the undergrowth and lay between 1,000 and 2,000 eggs before dying. Deer are important in the maintenance and expansion of tick populations because of their feeding role at the tick's reproductive stage but they are not competent reservoir hosts for *B burgdorferi*. Increased numbers and geographic ranges of deer in some regions of Europe and North America have been linked to significant increases in tick populations and to rising incidence of Lyme borreliosis. In some regions changes in land use, particularly agricultural and forestry practice, have had profound effects on deer populations and in creating the ecological conditions that favour ticks and their small mammal and avian feeding hosts which are also reservoir-competent for borreliae. The most

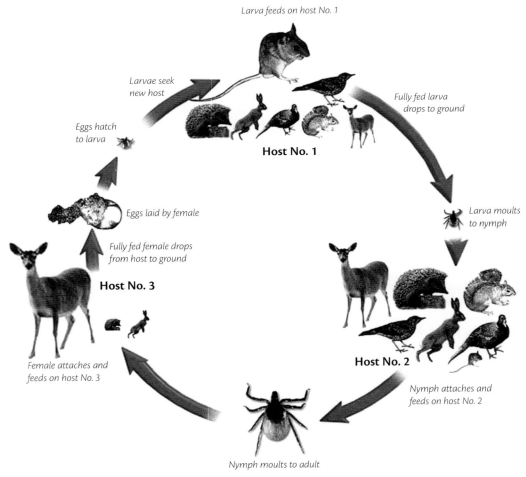

Fig. 9.1 Lyme borreliosis transmission dynamics
Courtesy of Dr Jeremy Gray and Bernard Kaye

dramatic example is the loss of farming and the return of forested areas in parts of the New England states in the mid-twentieth century, coupled with residential developments in these areas, leading to the explosive appearance of Lyme borreliosis in this region.

Human beings can be incidental feeding hosts for ticks. Larval ticks pose minimal risk for borrelial transmission, as it is rare for them to have been infected transovarially. Nymphal ticks are most likely to transmit infection to people, as they are very small (about the size of a poppyseed), and may not be noticed, even after feeding. Their major feeding period is during late spring and early summer, when human outdoor recreational activity is also likely to be at its peak. The larger adult ticks are more likely to be spotted and removed before completing their feeds.

In most areas only a minority of ticks carry borreliae. Infected *I ricinus* ticks are unlikely to transmit infection in the first 18–24 hours of feeding and *I scapularis* ticks within the first 36 hours, but transmission risk rises steadily as feeding continues. Early removal of attached ticks greatly reduces human infection risk (CDC 2011; EUCALB 2011). There is some evidence that transmission may take place at an earlier stage during *I persulcatus* blood meals.

Epidemiology

To a large extent the epidemiology of Lyme borreliosis can be predicted through assessment of ecological, environmental and human behavioural factors, which include residential, recreational and occupational risks, and readiness (or otherwise) of acceptance of risk reduction measures. Ecological and epidemiological studies have shown no evidence for disease presence in tropical or equatorial regions and it is not endemic in Australia or New Zealand. Limited studies in South America have not given robust evidence for endemicity in that region.

The epidemiology of Lyme borreliosis is now well documented in both North America and Europe and in some parts of Asia. Case definitions for surveillance purposes in the USA were revised in 2008 (CDC 2011). Case definitions for clinical and epidemiological use in Europe have also recently been updated (Stanek *et al.* 2011).

Lyme borreliosis is a notifiable disease in the USA. In 2008 over 35,000 confirmed or probable cases were reported, but it is recognized that there is a significant degree of under-reporting, and the actual annual number of cases may be as high as 100,000 (CDC 2011). The disease is highly focal, with over 90% of cases reported from the north-eastern and north-central states. The ten highest incidence states are Connecticut, Delaware, Massachusetts, Maryland, Minnesota, New Jersey, New York, Pennsylvania, Rhode Island and Wisconsin. These ten states had an average annual incidence rate of 29.3/100,000 between 2003 and 2005, but within each state there were considerable variations between different counties, reflecting ecological and residential factors contributing to focal high-endemicity. Active surveillance in coastal northern California suggested an incidence rate of 5.5/100,000, reflecting the very much lower borrelial carriage rates in *I pacificus* ticks.

A USA surveillance report covering the years 1992 to 2006 showed a bimodal distribution in age at acquisition, with peaks occurring in children aged five to nine and adults between 55–59 years, at rates of 8.6 and 7.8/100,000 respectively (CDC 2011). The lowest rate was reported in the 20–24 year old age group (3/100,000). In most age groups there is a slight preponderance of males, with an average annual rate/100 000 of 6.3 for males and 5.4 for females.

There is marked seasonality to case reporting, with the majority occurring in the three months June to August, reflecting the peak times that ticks quest for feeds and when human outdoor activity is likely to be at its peak. Erythema migrans was reported in about 70% of cases, arthralgia or arthritis in 32%, and neurological presentations in about 12%. Cardiac manifestations were present in 1% of patients. More than one clinical manifestation was reported in 12.8% of cases.

Fewer cases are reported in Canada but the demographic data, clinical presentations and seasonality of cases reported in Canada are similar to those of the USA. The main endemic area is in southern Ontario, where *I scapularis* is present. Very few cases are reported from British Columbia, where borrelial infection rates of *I pacificus* are very low. However, there is some evidence of focal expansions of tick populations, possibly due to changing climatic conditions Ecological risk assessment studies are ongoing (Ogden *et al.* 2008).

About 85,000 cases are reported annually in Europe but this is a considerable underestimate, both because of inconsistent case reporting mechanisms and under-recognition of disease manifestations, particularly erythema migrans (Lindgren and Jaenson 2006). There is no standardized or centralized method of collecting epidemiological data on Lyme borreliosis in Europe and there are currently no plans to add Lyme borreliosis to the listed diseases covered by European Community-coordinated disease surveillance (Smith and Takkinen 2006). Epidemiological evidence is obtained piecemeal from numerous sources, including national or regional mandatory notification schemes in a few countries, surveillance schemes in some endemic regions, regional prospective incidence studies, primary care surveys, seroprevalence studies and reporting systems based on laboratory-confirmed cases. In 2002 it was estimated that at least 60,000 cases occur annually in Germany alone, giving an approximate incidence rate of 75/100,000 in that country. Prospective studies in endemic regions of France and Germany have shown annual incidences 180–232/100,000 and 111/100,000 respectively. About 90% of the cases in both studies consisted of erythema migrans only (Anon 2008; Huppertz *et al.* 1999).

Disease incidence increases from the west to the east of the continent of Europe, and decreases from south to north in Scandinavia and from north to south in Italy, Spain, Portugal and Greece. The highest prevalence regions are included in the area extending eastwards from a longitude of about 5° East and southwards between latitudes 62° and 42° North, particularly in Central Europe, southern Scandinavia and the Baltic Republics, but there focal areas of high prevalence elsewhere (EUCALB 2011; Lindgren and Jaenson 2006). It is interesting that the early descriptions of various clinical presentations of Lyme borreliosis originated from physicians working in the areas of Europe where more recent ecological, epidemiological and clinical studies have indicated high infection prevalence.

It is possible to assess trends from year to year in countries or regions that have stable reporting systems, whether they are based on mandatory notification, regional clinical reporting or laboratory surveillance. Epidemiological data from a variety of sources indicate that in most European countries there is a bimodal age effect for disease acquisition, with peaks occurring in the 5–15 and 40–60 age groups. Peak periods for the diagnosis of erythema migrans are late spring and summer, following the peak tick feeding periods. Acute neuroborreliosis cases peak 1–2 months later, but may be diagnosed at any time through the year.

The age at which a person acquires infection can have some bearing on the clinical features of disseminated disease. The most common complication of Lyme borreliosis reported in children is facial palsy. Painful radiculopathy is more commonly diagnosed in older adults, and is rare in children. Acrodermatitis chronica atrophicans is principally seen in older people, and is reported more frequently in women than in men (Stanek and Strle 2003).

Data on neuroborreliosis incidence is particularly valuable as a sentinel for monitoring trends and for informing public health activities. Neurological manifestations are the most common and potentially most serious complications of European-acquired Lyme disease, and are likely to have a high degree of diagnostic specificity. Neuroborreliosis is notifiable in Norway and Denmark and is also well represented in data based on laboratory reporting because of high laboratory diagnostic sensitivity in these circumstances.

Reported incidence has increased very significantly throughout Europe in recent years for several reasons. Public health efforts and media attention have led to far greater awareness of the disease, leading to diagnoses of cases that might otherwise have been unrecognized. There has also been a significant genuine increase in incidence, related to expansion in density and range of tick populations and increased recreational and residential human activities in tick habitats.

Asymptomatic or minimally symptomatic infections are common in many endemic areas. Seroprevalence in high risk occupational groups is significant in many parts of Europe, and increases with age and years of exposure risk, but incidence of occupationally acquired clinical disease seems to be low.

Hosts

Communicability

Lyme borreliosis is transmitted only by *Ixodes spp* ticks. Other arthropods are not vector-competent, although they may contain borrelial DNA as a result of ingesting blood from infected hosts. The infection is not transmitted person-to-person, sexually or through contact with blood or other body fluids. There is a small theoretical risk of transmission through blood transfusion but no cases associated with transfusion have been well documented. It is not transmitted through ingestion of meat from deer or other mammalian or avian species, nor from contact with blood from these species. It is unfortunate that some internet sites promulgate misinformation about the communicability of Lyme borreliosis.

Lyme borreliosis in pregnancy

A few early case reports of pregnant women with untreated Lyme borreliosis described adverse outcomes, with babies stillborn or dying within 48 hours of birth, but no set pattern of abnormality was found. Subsequent large population studies showed no increased risks of adverse outcomes of pregnancies in women with Lyme borreliosis who received appropriate treatment, and large population studies of pregnancy outcomes in Lyme high-endemic areas and non-endemic areas showed no excess of adverse outcomes in high-endemic areas. A review concluded that adverse outcomes of Lyme borreliosis were rare events (Elliott *et al.* 2001). Most treatment guidelines for treatment of Lyme borreliosis recommend that infections in pregnancy are treated similarly to

those in non-pregnant women, with the exception that doxycycline is contraindicated.

Clinical manifestations of Lyme borreliosis

Infection can be asymptomatic or minimally symptomatic, as shown by prospective studies in highly endemic areas. Symptomatic infections can be localized to the site of infection or can affect various organs and tissues, most commonly the nervous and musculoskeletal systems following dissemination via the bloodstream and lymphatics. It has been customary to divide manifestations of disseminated infection into early and late disease, however these are not clear-cut stages but form a continuum which occurs only in some untreated patients. Late stage complications have become rare in recent years because of recognition and appropriate treatments of earlier manifestations.

Early localized Lyme borreliosis

The most common presenting feature of Lyme borreliosis is erythema migrans, estimated to occur in about 90% of cases (Dandache and Nadelman 2008; Huppertz *et al.* 1999). It usually presents about 3–10 days (range 2–30 days) after a tick bite, which may have gone unnoticed. The rash is a slowly enlarging erythematous skin lesion, usually round or oval, which expands from the site of tick attachment and is not usually significantly pruritic or painful Spirochaetes gradually migrate outwards from the inoculation site, and the size of the rash is dependent on the duration of the infection. With increasing duration the skin at the centre can return to a more normal appearance, giving an annular or target-like appearance. This 'bull's-eye' appearance was a characteristic feature of many early descriptions of erythema migrans in the USA, but it is less frequently seen now because greater familiarity of the condition in endemic areas has led to earlier diagnosis and treatment in many cases. Some patients also have malaise, headaches, fever, myalgias, and arthralgias.

Erythema migrans caused by *B burgdorferi* sensu stricto is more rapidly progressive that that caused by *B afzelii*, which can cause more indolently developing lesions that are less inflamed in appearance. They can become quite large in diameter (greater than 50 centimetres) if untreated, and develop central clearing (Strle *et al.* 1999). Rashes caused by *B afzelii* are also less likely to be accompanied by systemic symptoms than infections caused by *B burgdorferi* sensu stricto or *B garinii*, reflecting the lower virulence of *B afzelii*. Erythema migrans lesions eventually clear even if left untreated, but appropriate antibiotic treatment results in rapid resolution of rash and excellent long-term outcomes.

The differential diagnosis of erythema migrans includes hypersensitivity reactions to arthropod bites, which usually present within 24 hours of the bite, expand rapidly and are itchy. Other conditions that have been mistaken for erythema migrans include staphylococcal and streptococcal cellulitis, tinea infections, urticaria, erythema annulare, and in the USA, brown recluse spider bites and southern tick-associated illness (STARI), also called Masters' disease (Dandache and Nadelman 2008; Tibbles and Edlow 2007). The cause of STARI is currently unknown but is associated with bites of *Amblomma americanum* ticks, and it does not appear to lead to significant systemic complications.

Borrelial lymphocytoma is an uncommon presentation of early localized infection that is almost exclusively seen in Europe and is strongly associated with *B afzelii* infection (Stanek and Strle 2003). It is a localized lesion with an intense bluish red appearance and most commonly occurs on the earlobe, nipple and scrotum. It responds well to antibiotics but if untreated it can last for several months, and histologically can be mistaken for a cutaneous lymphoma, as it has a dense lymphocytic infiltrate.

Disseminated Lyme borreliosis

Infection with *B burgdorferi* sensu stricto can cause multiple erythema migrans, resulting from spirochaetaemic spread to other areas of skin. The affected patches are usually smaller than a primary lesion and the patients often have significant systemic symptoms and other complications of disseminated infection such as carditis, meningitis, facial palsy, or arthritis (Dandache and Nadelman 2008). Multiple erythema migrans occur less commonly in Europe than in North America.

Lyme carditis is an uncommon complication which usually presents within a few weeks to several months of infection in previously untreated patients, and other symptoms of disseminated disease are frequently present. The most common manifestation of cardiac involvement is a self-limited conduction defect, usually varying degrees of atrioventricular conduction delay (Fish *et al.* 2008; Stanek and Strle 2003).

Nervous system involvement causes a well described spectrum of presentations, most commonly one or more elements of a triad termed Garin-Bujadoux-Bannwarth syndrome, initially described in Europe and comprising lymphocytic 'viral-like' meningitis, cranial neuritis, and radiculoneuritis (Garin and Bujadoux 1922; Bannwarth 1941; Halperin 2008; Rupprecht *et al.* 2008). These presentations usually occur within a few weeks to several months of infection. Facial palsy is the most common neurological presentation, and can be bilateral in a minority of cases. Neuroborreliosis is one of the most common causes of bilateral facial palsies. Other cranial nerves, mainly the oculomotor (III) and abducens (VI) are occasionally affected. Radiculoneuritis usually affects the trunk or a limb and presents with altered sensation or severe pain that can be similar to shingles or nerve entrapments such as sciatica. Antibiotic treatment usually results in rapid reduction of analgesia requirements, and this can be a helpful adjunctive diagnostic sign. In Europe a more indolent form of radiculopathy has also been reported, with symptoms gradually developing over many months. It may be caused by direct spread of organisms, principally *B garinii*, along the affected nerves to the nerve roots (Rupprecht *et al.* 2008). Encephalomyelitis is a rare complication and can cause a multiple sclerosis-like presentation, which will respond to antibiotics. The outcomes of treated neuroborreliosis are good, but complete resolution of symptoms, particularly in older patients, can be slow and incomplete, especially if treatment had been delayed.

Lyme arthritis is particularly associated with *B burgdorferi* sensu stricto infection, although other pathogenic genospecies have also been occasionally implicated in Europe. It presents initially with migratory arthralgias early in infection, developing later into mono- or oligo-arthritis of large joints, predominantly affecting the knee (Steere *et al.* 1987; Stanek and Strle 2003, Steere and Angelis 2006). Small joints are rarely affected. The arthritis is relapsing/remitting in nature, with marked synovial effusion causing swelling out of proportion to the degree of pain. The condition responds to antibiotic treatment but a proportion of patients have slower resolution of symptoms and signs. This so-called 'antibiotic-refractory' arthritis is thought to have an autoimmune component and there is evidence for failure of down-regulation of the inflammatory response following eradication of the organism. There appear to be significant host genetic susceptibility factors in the development of this complication, as it is seen predominantly in patients who have HLA-DR4 and/or HLA-DR2 haplotypes (Steere and Angelis 2006). As with other complications of Lyme borreliosis it is less frequently seen now because of greater recognition and treatment of early-stage infection.

Acrodermatitis chronica atrophicans is a skin manifestation of longstanding, previously untreated infection, almost exclusively seen in Europe and caused by *B afzelii* (Stanek and Strle 2003). It usually occurs on extensor surfaces of the extremities, with bluish red discolouration and doughy swelling of the affected skin, which can gradually progress to hyperpigmented atrophic lesions giving a cigarette paper-like appearance. The underlying vasculitis can cause an accompanying peripheral neuropathy. Appropriate antibiotic treatment will eradicate infection but severely damaged skin may not return to a completely normal appearance.

Persisting symptoms following treated Lyme borreliosis (post-infection symptoms; post-Lyme syndrome)

There have been only rare cases of patients who have objective evidence of persistent infection (microbiological treatment failure) following treatment with currently recommended regimens. Erythema migrans resolves rapidly with appropriate treatment. Later clinical manifestations may not have resolved completely by the end of antibiotic therapy, but will continue to improve in the following weeks to months. Patients with severe tissue damage prior to treatment may have incomplete clinical recovery despite resolution of the infective process.

Following appropriate treatment a small proportion of patients (estimated 5–10%) continue to experience non-specific symptoms such as fatigue, musculoskeletal pain and cognitive difficulties, without objective evidence of treatment failure. A case definition for post-Lyme disease syndrome has been proposed to aid further research and understanding of this condition (Wormser *et al.* 2006). The occurrence of post-Lyme disease symptoms appears to correlate with disseminated disease, greater illness severity at presentation and delayed antibiotic treatment (Marques 2008). The condition appears to be similar in incidence and clinical pattern to post-infection syndromes triggered by other infections (Hickie *et al.* 2006). The mechanisms contributing to the development of these syndromes are unknown. Four randomized placebo-controlled double-blinded studies have found no evidence for persistent infection and showed that prolonged antibiotic therapy does not provide sustained benefit but has potential serious adverse effects.

'Chronic Lyme disease'

This term has been used to encompass widely different patient groups, including those with objective manifestations of late Lyme borreliosis, patients with post-Lyme symptoms, those who have a previous history of Lyme borreliosis and an unrelated current illness, and patients with no credible evidence of current or past *B burgdorferi* infection (Feder *et al.* 2007; Marques 2008). This lack of specificity has contributed greatly to public and professional confusion. Studies at referral centres have shown that about 50–60% of patients who had been given a diagnosis of chronic Lyme disease had no credible evidence of *B burgodorferi* infection, and many of them fulfilled diagnostic criteria for chronic fatigue syndrome or fibromyalgia (Marques 2008). Some had a variety of other conditions, which included multiple sclerosis, rheumatoid arthritis and systemic lupus erythematosus. Many of these patients had been diagnosed as a result of false-positive serology or the use of non-validated laboratory tests. A cause for concern is the use of inappropriate and potentially dangerous treatments for 'chronic Lyme disease', which have resulted in deaths and serious adverse events (Whelan 2007). This has become a widespread problem in North America and Europe, even in regions where Lyme disease is not endemic, and is a serious concern for public health and regulatory authorities.

Diagnosis

Case definitions for Lyme disease were published for epidemiological purposes in the USA by the Centers for Disease Control and have recently been updated (CDC 2011). The Infectious Diseases Society of America has produced guidelines for the assessment and management of Lyme disease (Wormser *et al.* 2006). The European Union Concerted Action on Lyme Borreliosis (EUCALB) study group developed clinical case definitions for use in Europe and the European Society of Clinical Microbiology and Infectious Diseases developed guidelines for laboratory diagnosis (Stanek *et al.* 2011; Brouqui *et al.* 2004). Guidelines for diagnosis and treatment of neuroborreliosis have also been developed by the American Academy of Neurology and the European Federation of Neurological Societies (Halperin *et al.* 2007; Mygland *et al.* 2010). Laboratory tests are not required by any guidelines to confirm a diagnosis of erythema migrans, but laboratory support is necessary for a diagnosis of later stage infection, since none of the presentations of disseminated or late Lyme borreliosis is unique to the infection.

Direct diagnostic methods

Ideally, direct methods of organism detection (bacterial culture or DNA detection) and diagnostic tests for the laboratory confirmation of Lyme borreliosis would be the preferred, However, they have serious limitations for routine use. Borrelial culture requires complex media that can be difficult to standardize, and it is also slow, because of the organism's prolonged generation time (7 to 20 hours in log-phase growth) (Aguero-Rosenfeld *et al.* 2005). The method is generally available only in research-orientated facilities. It has the advantage of providing unequivocal proof of active infection and also enabling researchers to obtain strains of proven pathogenicity. It is very insensitive as a routine diagnostic tool for specimens other than skin biopsies of erythema migrans and acrodermatitis chronica atrophicans. Culture of skin biopsies from previously untreated patients with erythema migrans is likely to have about a 70% success rate. This rate is probably lower in patients with more longstanding erythema migrans caused by *B afzelii*, but culture of biopsies from untreated ACA can be successful in over 90% of cases, reflecting the high organism load found in these lesions. Culture of CSF is successful in less than 20% of cases of acute neuroborreliosis and there have been only isolated reports of successful culture from synovial fluid or membrane.

Detection of borrelial DNA through nucleic acid amplification test (NAAT) methods has some advantages over culture, as results can be provided very much more rapidly. Primers detecting a variety of gene targets are available (Aguero-Rosenfeld *et al.* 2005). Overall sensitivities of NAAT tests on skin biopsy samples

appear to be similar to that of culture, but they have only limited diagnostic value, as erythema migrans is primarily a clinical diagnosis. They are more sensitive than culture on CSF samples from patients with acute neuroborreliosis, but detection rates remain disappointing, at less than 40%. This reflects a low level of free DNA target in CSF rather than an inherent lack of methodological sensitivity. DNA detection is potentially very valuable in the assessment of synovial fluid from patients with Lyme arthritis. Detection rates of borrelial DNA in synovial samples from previously untreated patients are greater than 95%, and the method can be helpful in assessing the need for re-treatment of patients with persistent arthritis (Steere and Angelis 2006). As with any DNA detection test, care must be taken to avoid laboratory contamination, as NAAT methods are extremely sensitive and are vulnerable to false-positive results from extraneous target DNA (Molloy *et al.* 2001).

Indirect diagnostic methods

Antibody tests remain the mainstay of laboratory support for the diagnosis of Lyme borreliosis. The antibody response to *B burgdorferi* infection is slow to develop compared to many other acute bacterial or viral infections, reflecting the organism's slow replication cycle, and early treatment can abrogate an antibody response. Antibody positivity rates in erythema migrans range from 30–80% depending on duration of infection and, to a certain extent, on infecting genospecies. Infection with *B burgdorferi* sensu stricto appears to generate a brisker antibody response than infection caused by the other pathogenic genospecies. Between 70% and 90% of patients with early disseminated infection are seropositive at clinical presentation, and the remainder usually seroconvert within several weeks. Patients with late stage Lyme borreliosis are very rarely seronegative; seropositivity is in excess of 99% (Aguero-Rosenfeld *et al.* 2005; Wilske *et al.* 2007; Stanek *et al.* 2011). The great majority of patients with late stage infections, including ACA, Lyme arthritis and late neuroborreliosis are very strongly seropositive, and have developed antibodies to a wide range of borrelial antigens as a result of the organisms' expanding range of surface protein expression over time.

Most current antibody screening tests are based on enzyme-linked immunosorbent assay (ELISA) methods. There are significant issues with specificities of these tests, related to the complex antigenic structure of *B burgdorferi* sensu lato. Some antigens are shared with other spirochaetes and also with other flagellated organisms. False-positive reactions can occur in tests on sera from patients with syphilis, leptospirosis and enteric bacterial infections, presumably caused by high levels of antibodies produced to common antigens, particularly those associated with flagella. Non-specific reactions, especially in IgM tests, have been well documented to occur in the presence of other acute infections including Epstein-Barr virus and parvovirus B19 and also with some autoimmune conditions such as rheumatoid arthritis and lupus, which can cause diagnostic confusion, especially when tests are applied in situations of low pre-test probability.

Accordingly, authorities in North America and Europe have recommended using a two-stage testing process to minimize risk of false-positive results. Serum samples are screened in a first stage test, using a sensitive ELISA method. Specimens giving reactive or indeterminate results are then tested with a second method, usually immunoblot (western blot), which allows a visual evaluation of the sample's reactions to a broad range of *B burgdorferi* antigens, only some of which are specific to the organism. This assessment minimizes the risk of false-positive results overall. There are some differences in assay preparation and immunoblot interpretive criteria between North America and Europe, reflecting the differences in distributions of pathogenic genospecies, but the overall principles of antibody testing are similar (Aguero-Rosenfeld 2005; Wilske *et al.* 2007).

Adherence to the two-stage recommendation is important, as some commonly used screening ELISAs have specificities of less than 90% and the predictive value of positive results can be very low when tests are applied in a situation where there is a low prior probability of *B burgdorferi* infection, leading to misdiagnosis. Unfortunately, inappropriate testing frequently occurs. Numerous studies have shown that misdiagnosis is a major cause of non-response to treatment for presumed Lyme borreliosis, usually resulting from false-positive tests or from the application of poorly-specific clinical diagnostic criteria (Reid *et al.* 1998, Feder *et al.* 2007; Hassett *et al.* 2009). An additional factor to be considered when evaluating serological results is the high background seroprevalence in populations living in highly endemic areas, so it is important that true-positive antibody results are carefully assessed for clinical relevance (Wilske *et al.* 2007). Antibody tests are also useful in CSF assessment. Most patients with acute neuroborreliosis have detectable antibodies to *B burgdorferi* in CSF at time of presentation, and intrathecal antibody synthesis can be assessed. This is particularly useful in the evaluation of suspected late neuroborreliosis (Wilske *et al.* 2007; Mygland *et al.* 2010).

There have been steady improvements in antibody tests since the first generation assays became available in the late 1980s. The development of recombinant and peptide antigens may reduce the need for immunoblotting in the future, as EIAs based on these antigens are more specific than whole-cell lysate-based EIAs. There is also some evidence that recently developed assays, particularly the C6 peptide and VlsE recombinant assays, may be helpful in assessing response to treatment but further work is required to validate this approach (Aguero-Rosenfeld *et al.* 2005).

Diagnostic tests that are not recommended

A number of poorly standardized and unvalidated methods are marketed, mainly from commercial specialty laboratories. They include live blood microscopy, antigen detection tests in body fluids, PCR of urine, lymphocyte transformation tests, CD-57 lymphocyte measurements and immunoblots interpreted using non-standard criteria. These tests have contributed to many misdiagnoses in North America and Europe (Anon. 2005; Wormser *et al.* 2006).

Treatment

Evidence-based treatment guidelines have been prepared by specialist societies and expert groups in North America and Europe (Wormser *et al.* 2006; Halperin *et al.* 2007; Societe Pathologie Infectieuse de Langue Francaise 2007; Mygland *et al.* 2010). There is broad consensus on antibiotic agents of choice, with only minor differences in dosages and durations of treatment (O'Connell, 2010). Doxycycline or amoxicillin are the most commonly recommended oral agents, and ceftriaxone is the parenteral agent of choice, because of its convenient once-daily dosing.

Doxycycline is contraindicated for children under the age of nine years (less than 12 years in the UK) and for pregnant and breast-feeding women. Cefuroxime axetil is an effective second-line choice in cases where doxycycline or amoxicillin are contra-indicated. Azithromycin can be used as a third-line oral antibiotic but patients require careful follow-up, as treatment failures occur more frequently than with first- and second-line choices. Erythromycin is not recommended for treating any stage of Lyme borreliosis as it has a high failure rate.

Prognosis

Lyme borreliosis is rarely if ever fatal, and the overall prognosis for appropriately treated patients is excellent. The very few fatalities reported in the medical literature have been associated with cardiac dysrythmia or co-infections with babesiosis, a tick-transmitted parasitic infection. Several large studies have shown excellent long-term outcomes for adult and paediatric patients treated for erythema migrans (Nadelman *et al.* 1996; Gerber *et al.* 1996; Lipsker *et al.* 2002; Cerar *et al.* 2010). Patients with disseminated infections also have good overall outcomes, but full recovery may take some weeks to months after completing treatment. Patients with severe or longstanding infection prior to treatment may have incomplete clinical recovery, despite microbiological cure, because of the degree of tissue damage sustained (Kruger *et al.* 1989; Hansen and Lebech 1992; Thorstrand *et al.* 2002; Ljostad *et al.* 2008).

Prevention and control

Personal protection measures

No vaccine is currently available against Lyme borreliosis, although research efforts are continuing in both Europe and North America. Personal protection against tick bites is the main measure for protection against borrelial infection and other ixodid tick-transmitted infections (Hayes and Piesman 2003). The avoidance of tick habitats is undoubtedly the most robust way of avoiding infection but this is not practical or desirable for many people for residential, occupational or recreational reasons. Raising awareness of ticks, the risks associated with tick bites and the personal protection measures that can reduce risks are important goals for public health practitioners.

Protective clothing such as long trousers tucked into socks, and long-sleeved shirts with buttoned cuffs are recommended for people venturing into tick-infested habitats, and these measures can be enhanced by the use of DEET-containing insect repellents on skin (Hayes and Piesman 2003; CDC 2011; EUCALB 2011). Permethrin can be applied to clothing as an additional protection, and this can be very useful for people who are at heavy occupational risk, such as forestry workers, gamekeepers or military personnel. Permethrin kills ticks on contact, through its effects on their nerve tissue. It is not approved for use directly on human skin.

Additional important risk reduction measures are regular checks for attached ticks on exposed skin during the day and a thorough full-body inspection of the skin for attached ticks at the end of each day of possible exposure, bearing in mind that ticks with as shower or bath are very small and are easily be overlooked unless a careful search is carried out. Because their saliva contains substances that act as local anaesthetic and anti-inflammatory agents tick bites are not usually particularly itchy or painful. Infected ticks are very unlikely to transmit borreliae during the early stages of their feed, so prompt removal is an effective protection strategy. Areas that deserve special attention include skin folds, which can have a degree of humidity attractive to ticks. These include the groins, armpits, waistband area, backs of knees, and under the breasts. It is particularly important to check the head and neck regions, including scalps, of young children, as they are significantly more likely than adults to sustain tick bites on the upper body.

Ticks can be removed using fine-pointed tweezers or forceps, grasping the tick as close to the skin as possible and gently pulling straight up until the tick detaches (CDC 2011). Ideally, a skin disinfectant should be applied to the site after removal to minimize risk of pyogenic infection. Retained tick mouth-parts do not increase the risk of borrelial transmission, and are likely to be spontaneously discharged from the skin over the following few days. Proprietary tick removal devices are also commercially available but are not more effective than tweezers.

Post-exposure antibiotic prophylaxis

Single-dose prophylaxis with doxycycline is recommended only under certain restricted circumstances in the USA (Wormser *et al.* 2006; Shapiro 2001). The conditions for prescribing are:

◆ A nymphal or adult tick bite, with duration of attachment greater than 36 hours;

◆ Ecologic information suggesting that the tick bite occurred in an area where at least 20% of ticks are likely to be infected;

◆ Prophylaxis can be given within 72 hours of tick removal and doxycycline is not contraindicated.

If all of these conditions are fulfilled the recommended dose of doxycycline for adults is 200mg and 4 mg/kg (maximum 200mg) for children older than eight years. Antibiotic prophylaxis is currently not recommended in European guidelines (Kahl and Stanek 1999; SPILF 2006; EUCALB 2011).

Environmental measures

Various methods to reduce tick populations have been developed, mainly in North America, but have had only limited success (Hayes and Piesman 2003). These include area-wide application of acaricides to kill nymphal ticks at the start of their feeding season, but this approach is not generally acceptable to the public. Other methods include application of acaricides to tick-feeding hosts including deer and small mammals, but are of limited value. Vegetation management around residences in Lyme-endemic areas is probably the most practical and cost-effective environmental measure to reduce risk of tick exposure in the peri-domestic situation. Measures include regular mowing of grass, clearance of leaf litter and removing bushes and other vegetation around the perimeter of gardens that back on to woodland or other tick habitats and replacing with a wide band of bark chippings or similar material (Stafford 2004). These measures can help to reduce ticks' protection against desiccation and lower the risk of tick bites within the residential environment.

References

Afzelius, A. (1921). Erythema chronicum migrans. *Acta Derm. Venereol.*, **2**: 120–5.

Aguero-Rosenfeld, M. E., Wang, G., Schwarz, I., and Wormser, G. P. (2005). Diagnosis of Lyme borreliosis. *Clin. Microbiol. Rev.*, **18**: 484–509.

Anon, (2004). The vectorborne human diseases of Europe: their distribution and burden on public health. Geneva: *World Health Organization Regional Office for Europe.*

Anon, (2005). Centers for Disease Control and Prevention. Notice to readers: caution regarding testing for Lyme disease. *Morb. Mortal. Wkly. Rep.*, **54**: 125.

Anon, (2008). La maladie de Lyme: Donnees de reseau du surveillance de la maladie en Alsace Mars 2001-Fev 2003. *Institut Veille Sanitaire.* Accessed 3 June 2009, at http://www.invs.sante.fr/publications/2005/lyme_alsace/index.html.

Asbrink, E., Hovmark, A., and Hederstedt, B. (1984). The spirochetal etiology of acrodermatitis chronica atrophicans Herxheimer. *Acta Derm. Venereol.*, **64**: 506–12.

Bacon, R. M., Kugeler, K. J., and Mead, P. S. (2008). Surveillance for Lyme disease – USA 1992–2006. *Morbid. Mortal. Wkly. Rep.*, **57**(SS10): 1–9.

Bannwarth, A. (1941). Chronische lymphocytare Meningitis, entzunliche Polyneuritis und "Rheumatismus". *Arch. Psychiatr. Nervenkr.*, **113**: 284–376.

Benach, J. L., Bosler, E. M., and Hanrahan, J. P. *et al.* (1983). Spirochetes isolated from the blood of two patients with Lyme disease. *N. Engl. J. Med.*, **308**: 740–42.

Bergstrom, S., Noppa, L., Gylfe, A., and Ostberg, Y. (2002). Molecular and cellular biology of *Borrelia burgdorferi* sensu lato. In: J. S. Gray, O. Kahl, R. S. Lane and G. Stanek, (eds.) *Lyme Borreliosis, Biology, Epidemiology and Control*, pp. 47–90. Wallingford, Oxon: CABI Publishing.

Brouqui, P., Bacellar, F., Baranton, G. *et al.* (2004). Guidelines for the diagnosis of tick-borne bacterial diseases in Europe. *Clin. Microbiol. Infect.*, **10**: 1108–32.

Burgdorfer, W., Barbour, A. G., Hayes, S. F. *et al.* (1982). Lyme disease–a tick-borne spirochaetosis? *Science*, **216**: 1317–9.

Centers for Disease Control and Prevention http://www.cdc.gov/ncidod/dvbid/lyme/index.htm. Accessed, 5th February 2011.

Cerar, D., Cerar, T, Ruzic-Slabjic, E. *et al.* (2010). Subjective symptoms after treatment of Lyme disease. *Am. J. Med.*, **123**: 79–86.

Dandache, P., and Nadelman, R. (2008). Erythema migrans. *Infect. Dis. Clin. N. Am.*, **22**: 235–60.

Edlow, J. A. (2003). *Bull's Eye: unraveling the medical mystery of Lyme disease.* (2nd ed.). New Haven: Yale University Press.

Elliott, D. J., Eppes, S. C., and Klein, J. L. (2001). Teratogen update: Lyme disease. *Teratology*, **64**: 276–81.

European Union Concerted Action on Lyme Borreliosis: http://meduni09.edis.at/eucalb/cms/index.php?lang=en. Accessed 5th February 2011.

Feder, H. M., Johnson, B. J. B., O'Connell, S. *et al.* (2007). A critical appraisal of 'chronic Lyme disease'. *N. Engl. J. Med.*, **357**: 1422–30.

Fish, A. E., Pride, Y., and Pinto, D. S. (2008). Lyme carditis. *Infect. Dis. Clin. N. Am.*, **22**: 275–88.

Garin, C., and Bujadoux, C. (1922). Paralysie par les tiques. *J. Med. Lyon*, **71**: 765–67.

Gerber, M. A., Shapiro, E. D., Burke, G. S. *et al.* (1996). Lyme disease in children in southeastern Connecticut. *N. Engl. J. Med.*, **335**: 1270–74.

Gray, J. S., Dautel, H., Estrada-Pena, A. *et al.* (2009). Effects of climate change on ticks and tick-borne diseases in Europe. *Interdiscipl. Perspect. Infect. Dis.*, doi :10.1155/2009/593232.

Halperin, J. J. (2008). Nervous system Lyme disease. *Infect. Dis. Clin. N. Am.*, **22**: 261–74.

Halperin, J. J., Shapiro, E. D., Logigian, E. *et al.* (2007). Practice Parameter: Treatment of nervous system Lyme disease (an evidence-based review) Report of the Quality Standards Subcommittee of the American Academy of Neurology. *Neurol.*, **69**: 91–102.

Hansen, K., and Lebech, A. M. (1992). The clinical and epidemiological profile of Lyme neuroborreliosis in Denmark 1985–1990. A prospective study of 187 patients with Borrelia burgdorferi-specific intrathecal antibody production. *Brain*, **115**: 399–423.

Hassett, A. L., Radvanski, D. C., Buyske, S. *et al.* (2009). Psychiatric co-morbidity and other psychological factors in patients with 'chronic Lyme disease'. *Am. J. Med.*, **122**: 843–50.

Hayes, E. B., and Piesman, J. (2003). How can we prevent Lyme disease? *N. Engl. J. Med.*, **348**: 2424–30.

Hickie, I., Davenport, T., Wakefield, D. *et al.* (2006). Post-infective and chronic fatigue syndromes precipitated by viral and non-viral pathogens: prospective cohort study. *BMJ*, **333**: 575.

Huppertz, H. I., Bohme, M., Standaert, S. M., Karch, H., and Plotkin, S. A. (1999). Incidence of Lyme borreliosis in the Wurzburg region of Germany. *Eur. J. Clin. Microbiol. Infect. Dis.*, **18**: 697–703.

Johnson, R. C., Hyde, F. W., Steigerwalt, A. G., and Brenner, D. J. (1984). Borrelia burgdorferi sp. nov.: Etiologic agent of Lyme disease. *Internat. J. System. Bacteriol.*, **34**: 496–97.

Kahl, O., and Stanek, G. (1999). Chemoprophylaxis for Lyme borreliosis? *Zentralbl. Bakteriol.*, **289**: 655–65.

Kannian, P., McHugh, G., Johnson, B. J. B. *et al.* (2007). Antibody responses to Borrelia burgdorferi in patients with antibiotic-refractory, antibiotic-responsive or non-antibiotic-treated Lyme arthritis. *Arth. Rheum.*, **56**: 4216–25.

Krüger, H., Reuss, K., Pulz, M., Pflughaupt, K. W. *et al.* (1989). Meningoradiculitis and encephalomyelitis due to Borrelia burgdorferi: a follow-up study of 72 patients over 27 years. *J. Neurol.*, **236**: 322–28.

Lindgren, E., and Jaenson, T. G. T. (2006). Lyme borreliosis in Europe: influences of climate and climate change, epidemiology, ecology and adaptation measures. Geneva: World Health Organization Regional Office for Europe.

Lipsker, D., Antoni-Bach, N., Hansmann, Y., and Jaulhac, B. (2002). Long term prognosis of patients treated for erythema migrans in France. *Brit. J. Dermatol.*, **146**: 872–76.

Ljostad, U., Skogvoll, E., Eikelund, R. *et al.* (2008). Oral doxycycline versus intravenous ceftriaxone for European Lyme borreliosis: a multicentre, noninferiority, double-blind, randomised trial. *Lancet Neurol.*, **7**: 690–95.

Marques, A. (2008). Chronic Lyme disease: a review. *Infect. Dis. Clin. N. Am.*, **22**: 341–60.

Molloy, P. J., Persing, D. H. and Berardi, V. P. (2001). False-positive results of PCR testing for Lyme disease. *Clin. Infect. Dis.*, **33**: 412–413.

Mygland, A., Ljostad, U., Fingerle, V. *et al.* (2010). EFNS guidelines on the diagnosis and management of European Lyme neuroborreliosis. *Eur. J. Neurol.*, **17**: 8–16.

Nadelman, R. B., Nowakowski, J., Forseter, G. *et al.* (1996). The clinical spectrum of early Lyme borreliosis in patients with culture-confirmed erythema migrans. *Am. J. Med.*, **100**: 502–8.

O'Connell, S. Recommendations for diagnosis and treatment of Lyme borreliosis: guidelines and consensus papers from specialist societies and expert groups in Europe and North America. http://www.hpa.org.uk/Topics/InfectiousDiseases/InfectionsAZ/LymeDisease/Guidelines/

Ogden, N. H., Lindsay, L. R., Morshed, M., Sockett, P. N., and Artsob, H. (2008). The rising challenge of Lyme borreliosis in Canada. *Can. Commun. Dis. Rep.*, **34**: 1–19.

Puius, Y. A., and Kalish, R. A. (2008). Lyme arthritis: pathogenesis, clinical presentation and management. *Infect. Dis. Clin. N. Am.*, **22**: 289–300.

Reid, M. C., Schoen, R. T., Evans, J., Rosenberg, J. C., and Horwitz, R. I. (1998). The consequences of overdiagnosis and overtreatment of Lyme disease: an observational study. *Ann. Intern. Med.*, **128**: 354–62.

Rupprecht, T. A., Koedel, U., Fingerle, V., and Pfister, H-W. (2008). The pathogenesis of Lyme neuroborreliosis–from infection to inflammation. *Mol. Med.*, **14**: 205–12.

Seltzer, E. G., and Shapiro, E. D. (1996). Misdiagnosis of Lyme disease: when not to order serologic tests. *Pediatr. Infect. Dis. J.*, **15**: 762–63.

Shapiro, E. D. (2001). Doxycline for tick bites?–Not for everyone. *N. Engl. J. Med.*, **345**: 133–34.

Smith, R., and Takkinen, J. (2006). Lyme borreliosis: Europe-wide coordinated surveillance and action needed? *Euro. Surveill.*, **11**: E060622 1.

Societe de Pathologie Infectieuse de Langue Francaise (2007). Lyme borreliosis: diagnostic, therapeutic and preventive approaches. *Med. Mal. Infect.*, **37**(S3): 8153–74. http://www.infectiologie.com/site/medias/_documents/consensus/2006-lyme-long.pdf.

Stafford, K. C., (2007). Tick Management Handbook. (3rd ed.) In: T.C.A.E. Station, (ed.) *The Connecticut Agricultural Experiment Station New Haven: The Connecticut Agricultural Experiment Station*, pp. 1–80. Available in PDF format from the CDC website: http://www.cdc.gov/ncidod/dvbid/lyme/index.htmCDC.

Stanek, G., and Strle, F. (2003). Lyme borreliosis. *Lancet*, **362**: 163947.

Stanek, G., Fingerle, V., Hunfeld, K-P. *et al.* (2011). Lyme borreliosis: clinical case definitions for diagnosis and management in Europe. *Clin. Microbiol. Infect.*, **17**: 69–79.

Steere, A. C., Malawista, S. E., Snydman, D. R. *et al.* (1977a). Lyme arthritis: an epidemic of oligoarticular arthritis in children and adults in three Connecticut communities. *Arthritis Rheum.*, **20**: 7–17.

Steere, A. C., Malawista, S. E., Hardin, J. A. *et al.* (1977b). Erythema chronicum migrans and Lyme arthritis: the enlarging clinical spectrum. *Ann. Intern. Med.*, **86**: 685–98.

Steere, A. C., Schoen, R. T., and Taylor, E. (1987). The clinical evolution of Lyme arthritis. *Ann. Intern. Med.*, **107**: 725–31.

Steere, A. C., and Angelis, S. (2006). Therapy for Lyme arthritis. Strategies for the treatment of antibiotic-refractory arthritis. *Arthr. Rheum.*, **54**: 3079–86.

Strle, F., Nadelman, R., Cimperman, J. *et al.* (1999). Comparison of culture-confirmed erythema migrans caused by Borrelia burgdorferi sensu stricto in New York and by Borrelia afzelii in Slovenia. *Ann. Intern. Med.*, **130**: 32–36.

Thorstrand, C., Belfrage, E., Bennet, R. *et al.* (2002). Successful treatment of neuroborreliosis with ten day regimens. *Pediatr. Infect. J.*, **21**: 1142–45.

Tibbles, C. D., and Edlow, J. A. (2007). Does this patient have erythema migrans? *JAMA*, **297**: 2617–27.

Tilly, K., Rosa, P. A., and Stewart, P. E. (2008). Biology of Infection with Borrelia burgdorferi. *Infect. Dis. Clin. N. Am.*, **22**: 217–34.

Wilske, B., Fingerle, V., and Schulte-Spechtel, U. (2007). Microbiological and serological diagnosis of Lyme borreliosis. *FEMS Immunol. Med. Microbiol.*, **49**: 13–21.

Whelan, D. (2007). Lyme Inc. *Forbes Magazine*; 12 March 2007, pp. 96–97.

Wormser, G. P., Dattwyler, D. J., Shapiro, E. D. *et al.* (2006). The clinical assessment, treatment and prevention of Lyme disease, human granulocytic anaplasmosis and babesiosis. Clinical Practice Guidelines by the Infectious Diseases Society of America. *Clin. Infect. Dis.*, **43**: 1089–134.

CHAPTER 10

Tick-borne rickettsial diseases

Emmanouil Angelakis and Didier Raoult

Summary

Bacteria of the genus *Rickettsia* belong to the family *Rickettsiaceae* in the order *Rickettsiales* and have for long been described simply as short, Gram-negative, strict intracellular rods that retain basic fuchsin when stained by the method of Gimenez (Raoult and Roux 1997). These bacteria are associated with ticks, lice, fleas, or mites. To date the *Rickettsia* genus contains 24 recognized species classified into three groups based on their antigenic, morphological, and ecologic patterns:

1   The typhus group,

2   The spotted fever group,

3   *Rickettsia bellii* (Fournier and Raoult 2007).

   Most spotted fever group (SFG) rickettsiae are closely associated with ticks belonging to the family *Ixodidae* (also called 'hard' ticks) (Parola *et al.* 2005). Ticks can act as vectors, reservoirs, and/or amplifiers of SFG rickettsiae and require optimal environmental conditions which determine the geographic distribution of the vectors and consequently the risk areas for rickettsioses. Many *Rickettsia* species are strictly associated with one genus of ticks and the transmission to people is made through the tick bite, which generally implies that the *Rickettsia* can localize to their salivary glands. Therefore, since larvae, nymphs, and adults may all be infective for susceptible vertebrate hosts, the ticks must be regarded as the main reservoir host of rickettsiae. Humans are not considered as good reservoirs for *Rickettsiae*, as they are seldom infested with ticks for long periods and rickettsiaemia has normally short duration, especially with antibiotic intervention.

Introduction

During most of the twentieth century, the epidemiology of tick-borne Rickettsioses was understood as the occurrence of a single pathogenic *Rickettsia* on each continent, *R. rickettsii* for the America, *R. conorii* for Europe, Asia and Africa with the addition of *R. sibirica* (in the former USSR and China), and *R. australis* (in Australia) (Parola and Raoult 2006). In recent years with the introduction of cell culture and molecular biological testing methods new species or subspecies within the spotted fever group of the genus *Rickettsia* have been described. As a result, around the Mediterranean area seven more species or subspecies have been identified including *R. conorii israelensis, R. conorii caspia, R. aeschlimannii, R. slovaca, R. sibirica mongolitimonae, R. massiliae,* and *R. helvetica* (Brouqui *et al.* 2007). *R. heilongjiangensis* has been reported in Asia, *R. parkeri* in the USA, when *R. japonica* and *R. honei* have been reported in islands where spotted fever was previously unknown (Parola *et al.* 2005) (Table 10.1).

Rocky Mountain spotted fever

R. rickettsii, is the agent of Rocky Mountain spotted fever (RMSF), one of the oldest known tick-borne rickettsioses that was first described by Maxey as a specific clinical entity in 1899 (Ricketts 1909). The disease is transmitted in rural areas by ticks of the genus *Amblyomma, Rhipicephalus, Dermacentor,* and *Ixodes* (Jensenius *et al.* 2004). Several other tick species have been found to be naturally infected with rickettsiae but they rarely attack humans (Table 10.1) (Raoult and Roux 1997). In its acarine host *R. rickettsii* infects and replicates in several cell types, including ovaries, salivary gland, midgut epithelium and haemocytes (Sonenshine 1993). The disease has been reported from Canada to Argentina and is endemic to regions of North, Central and South America, with the greatest number of RMSF fatalities reported from the USA and Brazil (Parola *et al.* 2005). Approximately 90% of cases of RMSF occur during the months of April to September in the temperate USA (Childs and Paddock 2007).

   RMSF has been considered as the most severe SFG rickettsiosis which can involve endothelial cells of capillaries and small-to-medium-sized vessels of small tissues and organs (Childs and Paddock 2007). After a mean incubation period of about 7 days, (range, 2 to 14 days) (Masters *et al.* 2003) following the tick bite RMSF, begins with abrupt onset of fever (39–41°C) usually accompanied by malaise, chills, headache, myalgia, anorexia, generalized or focal abdominal pain, and diarrhoea (Walker 1995). *R. rickettsii* does not elicit an eschar at the tick bite site and about 40% of the patients do not mention the bite of a tick (Parola *et al.* 2005). The characteristic spotted rash is generally observed in 90% of the patients after the fourth day of illness and heralds progression of the infection to more severe disease (Childs and Paddock 2007). The rash usually begins on the wrists, ankles and forearms but in 24 hours it spreads centrally to involve the legs, buttocks, arms, axillae, truck, neck, and face (Childs and Paddock 2007). In approximately 10% of patients the rash may be absent,

Table 10.1 Current classification of tick borne rickettsioses reported to date: epidemiological data

Spotted fever group	*Rickettsia*	Principal vectors	Distribution
Rocky Mountain spotted fever	*R. rickettsii*	Ticks which rarely attack humans:	North America, Brazil
		Hemaphysalis leporispalustris, Dermacentor parumapertus, Ixodes dentatus, I. brunneus, I. texanus.	
		Ticks which attack humans:	
		Amblyomma americanum, A. maculatum, A. cajennense, A. aureolatum, Dermacentor occidentalis, D. andersoni, D. variabilis, Ixodes scapularis, I. pacificus, I. cookie, Rhipicephalus sanguineus,	
Tick-borne rickettsioses around the Mediterranean area			
Mediterranean spotted fever	*R. conorii conorii*	*Rhipicephalus sanguineus*	Mediterranean area
African tick bite fever	*R. africae*	*Amblyomma hebraeum, A. variegatum*	Sub-Saharan Africa, Caribbean, India
Israeli spotted fever	*R. conorii israelensis*	*Rhipicephalus sanguineus*	Israel, Portugal, Sicily
Astrakhan fever	*R. conorii caspia*	*Rhipicephalus pumilio, Rh. Sanguineus*	Astrakhan, Kosovo
Siberian tick typhus	*R. sibirica*	*Dermacentor nuttalli, D. marginatus, D. silvarum, Haemaphysalis concinna*	Northern Asia
TIBOLA- DEBONEL	*R. slovaca*	*Dermacentor marginatus, D. reticulates*	From western Europe to central Asia
Unspotted rickettsial fever	*R. helvetica*	*Ixodes ricinus*	Europe, Asia
Marseilles' fever	*R. massiliae*	*Rhipicephalus turanicus, Rh. Sanguineus*	France, Greece, Spain, Italy, Portugal
Unnamed	*R. aeschlimannii*	*Hyalomma marginatum, Hy. M. rufipes, R. appendiculatus, Ha. Punctata*	Africa, Europe
Lymphangitis-associated rickettsiosis (LAR)	*R. sibirica mongolotimonae*	*Hyalomma asiaticum, H. truncatum, H. anatolicum Excavatum*	Southern France, northern Africa, China
Tick-borne rickettsioses around the world			
Queensland tick typhus	*R. australis*	*Ixodes holocyclus, I. tasmani*	Eastern Australia
Flinders Island spotted fever	*R. honei*	*Ixodes granulatus, I. tasmanii, Aponomma cajennense, A. hydrosauri*	Australia, Southeast Asia, northwestern North America
Japanese spotted fever	*R. japonica*	*Ixodes ovatus, Dermacentor taiwanensis, Haemaphysaliss longicornis, H. flava*	Japan
Far Eastern spotted fever	*R. heilongjiangensis*	*Haemaphysalis concinna, Dermacentor silvarum*	Russia and Kazakhstan
Unexpected American spotted fever	*R. parkeri*	*Amblyomma maculatum, A. americanum, A. triste*	USA

and this may delay diagnosis and therapy (Parola *et al.* 2005). RMSF may result in various neurological manifestations, including deafness, convulsions, and hemiplegia. Severe clinical manifestation of RMSF may include pulmonary oedema and haemorrhage, cerebral oedema, myocarditis, renal failure, disseminated intravascular coagulopathy, and gangrene (Doyle *et al.* 2006; Zavala-Castro *et al.* 2006; Parola *et al.* 2005). RMSFs fatality rate has been reported as 2.4% during 1993–1996 (Treadwell *et al.* 2000) and 1.4% during 1997–2002 (Chapman *et al.* 2006) compared with 65–90% at the beginning of the century, in the USA. Geographical variation in severity of RMSF has also been reported. In active surveillance in the USA during 1997–2002 the overall case-fatality rate was 1.4% (Chapman *et al.* 2006), although in Brazil, the average case-fatality during 1995–2004 was 29% (Dantas-Torres 2007).

Tick-borne rickettsioses around the Mediterranean area

Mediterranean spotted fever

Mediterranean spotted fever (MSF) due to *R. conorii conorii* was described at the beginning of the twentieth century and was thought to be the only tick-borne rickettsial disease prevalent in the Mediterranean area (Raoult and Roux 1997). The disease is endemic in the Mediterranean area, including northern Africa and southern Europe and is transmitted by the brown dog tick *Rhipicephalus sanguineus* with most cases encountered in the summer when the tick vectors are highly active (Rovery and Raoult 2007). *Rh. sanguineus* can also survive in colder places of Europe and cases of MSF have been reported in northern and central Europe, including Switzerland, Belgium, northern France and the

Alpine region (Rehacek 1993; Rovery and Raoult 2007). Sporadic cases of MSF in non-endemic countries are also observed (Jensenius *et al.* 2004). Males are more frequently ill than females possibly as a result of occupation, tick contact or specific susceptibility.

The onset of MSF is abrupt usually after an asymptomatic incubation of 6 days. Typical cases present with high fever (39°C), flu-like symptoms, a black eschar (tache noire) at the tick bite site (Fig. 10.1). The Eschar is indolent and is usually localized on the trunk, the legs and the arms. Patients must be carefully examined as eschars can occasionally be localized on the scrotum or in an inguinal or axillar area (Rovery and Raoult 2007). One to 7 days (median, 4 days) following the onset of fever, a generalized maculopapular rash develops that often involves the palms and soles but spares the face (Raoult *et al.* 1986a). Regional adenopathy is more frequent in children, 33–74% of cases in one case series (Rovery and Raoult 2007). Headache, myalgia, and arthralgia are characteristic symptoms of boutonneuse fever. MSF was thought to be a benign illness with a case fatality less than 1% before the antibiotics era. However in active surveillance of MSF in Marseilles and the surrounding area in 1983–1984, 7 of 142 (5%) patients had a severe form of MSF (Raoult *et al.* 1986a). At the same time, severe cases of MSF were described in Spain (Ruiz Beltran *et al.* 1985). Elderly patients, and patients presenting with cirrhosis, chronic alcoholism, and glucose-6-phosphate dehydrogenase (G6PD) deficiency were more likely to have severe complications (Raoult *et al.* 1986b). Severe cases of MSF developed purpuric rash associated, neurological manifestations and multi-organ dysfunction syndrome with thrombosis of the deep venous vessels and acute pericarditis (Drancourt *et al.* 1991). At the time, *R. conorii conorii* was the sole agent isolated from clinical samples such as eschar biopsy of severe spotted fever in endemic countries. However, it is possible that some of these severe cases could have been due to other spotted rickettsial species.

African tick bite fever

R. africae is the etiological agent of African tick bite fever, a disease that has been discovered twice. The first time was during the 1930s, when Pijper described a mild tick bite disease with or without rash caused by an isolate than was not *R. conorii*. Unfortunately, all the

data were lost (Gear 1938). In 1990, Kelly, for a second time, isolated a new rickettsial strain, in Zimbabwe which was named *R. africae* (Jensenius *et al.* 2007). *R. africae* is transmitted by ixodid ticks of the genus *Amblyomma* with *A. hebraeum* as the main vector and reservoir (Jensenius *et al.* 2007). *R. africae* has been also isolated in *A. variegatum, A. lepidum,* and *Rhipicephalus* (*Boophilus*) *decoloratus* ticks (Parola *et al.* 2005; Portillo *et al.* 2007). Cattle, wild game and other ungulates constitute the principal hosts, although tick larvae and nymphs may also parasitize birds and rodents. The disease is endemic in large parts of rural sub-Saharan Africa, eastern Caribbean and Reunion island (Indian Ocean) (Parola *et al.* 2005; Parola and Barre 2004) (Fig. 10. 2). Sporadic cases of infection by *R. africae* have been described around the world among travellers, military personnel, game hunters, sports participants, and school students who had visited endemic areas (Jensenius *et al.* 2006).

Between 1983 and 2003, 171 published cases have been microbiologically confirmed as African tick bite fever, and another 78 cases could be classified retrospectively as probable African tick bite fever (Parola *et al.* 2005). *R. africae* infections are symptomatic in less than 50% of cases (Jensenius *et al.* 2007). The time lag from tick bite to symptom onset is usually 5–7 days but may be as long as 10 days. Most patients present with abrupt flu-like symptoms such as fever, nausea, fatigue, headache, and myalgia. An inoculation eschar, a black crust surrounded by a red halo at the site of the tick bite, is present in most cases but may easily be overlooked, particularly on dark skin, in the hair, or in the anogenital region. Up to 54% of patients with African tick bite fever have multiple eschars, a pathognomonic clinical sign which indicates the aggressive behaviour of the implicated tick vectors (Jensenius *et al.* 2003). Enlargement of lymph nodes draining area of the eschar (s) is common (43%) but it may be seen also in the absence of a frank eschar (Parola *et al.* 2005). A generalized cutaneous rash, sometimes vesicular and usually best seen close to the eschar, is present in 15–46% of the patients (Jensenius *et al.* 2003). The disease is usually self-limited and complications such as long lasting fever, reactive arthritis, myocarditis, and neuropsychiatric symptoms are rarely seen (Jensenius *et al.* 2007). To date no deaths or severe manifestations have been reported in patients with African tick bite fever (Jensenius *et al.* 2007).

Israeli spotted fever

R. conorii israelensis is the agent of Israeli spotted fever, a disease that was first described in Haifa Bay area in 1946 (Valero 1949). In 1999 *R. conorii israelensis* was also isolated in three patients living in semi-rural areas of Portugal (Bacellar *et al.* 1999). In Sicily, *R. conorii israelensis* was isolated in *Rh. sanquineus* ticks, and in a retrospective review of patients presenting from 1987 to 2001, 5 patients were identified with Israeli spotted fever (Giammanco *et al.* 2005). The disease may be acquired even without direct contact with animals, through exposure to ticks in places with dogs (Rovery *et al.* 2003). Israeli spotted fever appears as a typical spotted fever, but the eschar at the inoculation site was absent in more than 90% of cases and resembles a small pinkish papule rather than a real eschar (Gross and Yagupsky 1987). Splenomegaly and hepatomegaly are seen in 30 to 35% of patients. The disease may be severe and fatal cases have been reported especially in children and in people with glucose-6-phosphate dehydrogenase deficiency (Parola *et al.* 2005). However, clinical characteristics of 10 fatal

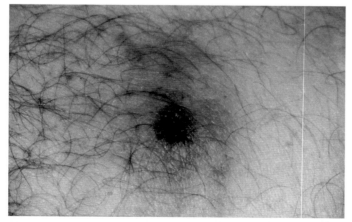

Fig. 10.1 Eschar at the tick bite site from a patient with Mediterranean spotted fever

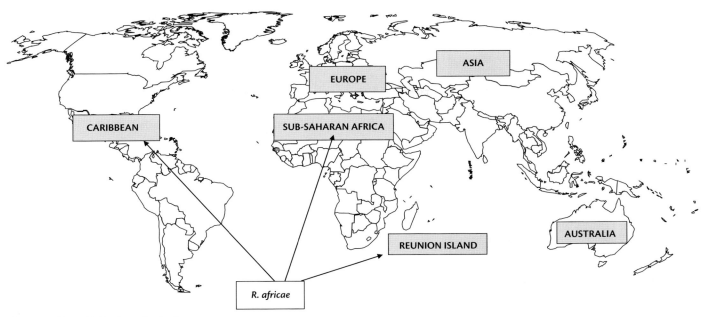

Fig. 10.2 African tick bite fever distribution

cases of Israeli spotted fever in Portugal were similar to those of 44 patients infected with *R. conorii israelensis* in the same period (De-Sousa *et al.* 2005).

Astrakhan fever

Astrakhan fever is a summer spotted fever endemic in Astrakhan and caused by *R. conorii caspia*. Astrakhan fever has been known since 1983 and was thought to have emerged as a result of environmental changes (Raoult and Roux 1997). Prospective surveillance from 1983 to 988 identified 321 cases, mostly during summer months (85%, including 43% in August) with most patients being adults (94%), males (61%), and owners of dogs (Tarasevich *et al.* 1991). The disease is mild and characterized by high fever, headaches, a papular rash with spontaneous remission of signs in 2 to 3 weeks (Parola *et al.* 2005) (Fig. 10.3). About 20% of the patients present 'tache noire' and about 32% have conjunctivitis. No fatal cases have been reported (Rovery and Raoult 2007).

Infection due to *Rickettsia slovaca* (TIBOLA)

R. slovaca was first isolated in 1968 from *Dermacentor marginatus* ticks in Czechoslovakia (Rehacek 1984). *R. slovaca* has been detected or isolated from ticks in all European countries where *D. marginatus* and *D. reticulatus* have been studied for rickettsiae (Parola *et al.* 2005). *R. slovaca* had been considered for more than 20 years as 'non-pathogenic' but in 1997 a woman with a single eschar at the site of the tick bite surrounded by an erythema and painful regional lymphadenopathy was found to be infected by *R. slovaca* (Raoult *et al.* 1997a) (Fig. 10.4). Clinically similar cases had been previously described in France, Slovakia, and Hungary, where this clinical syndrome had been named 'TIBOLA' (for tick-borne lymphadenopathy) by Lakos (Mediannikov *et al.* 2007). In Spain, a similar clinical syndrome was called 'DEBONEL' (for *Dermacentor*-borne necrosis-erythema-lymphadenopathy) (Parola

et al. 2005). The disease is mild and appears most likely in children and in patients who were bitten during the colder months of the year. Fever and rash were uncommon, and sequelae included localized alopecia at the tick bite site and chronic fatigue (Mediannikov *et al.* 2007).

Spotted fever due to Rickettsia sibirica mongolitimonae

R. sibirica mongolitimonae was first isolated in 1991 from *Hyalomma* ticks in Inner Mongolia (China) and the first case of human infection by *R. sibirica mongolitimonae* was reported in 1996 in a woman with a febrile rash and a single inoculation eschar in the groin (Raoult *et al.* 1996). Nine more cases of spotted fever due to *R. sibirica mongolitimonae* have been reported in active surveillance from January 2000 to June 2004 in France (Fournier *et al.* 2005).

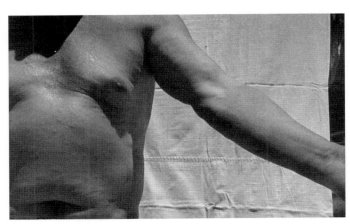

Fig. 10.3 Papular rash to a patient with Astrakhan fever

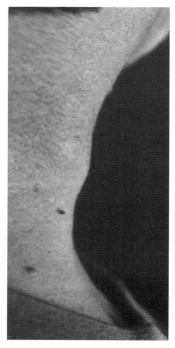

Fig. 10.4 Lymphadenopathy by *Rickettsia slovaca*

Eschars were observed in 22% of the patients, draining lymph node in 55% of the patients, and lymphangitis expanding from the inoculation eschar to the draining node in 44% of the patients. Fournier *et al.* (2005) proposed the nickname, 'lymphangitis-associated rickettsiosis' for the clinical features of this new rickettsiosis.

Other tick-transmitted rickettsioses around the Mediterranean area

R. aeschlimannii was first isolated from *Hyalomma marginatum* ticks collected in Morocco in 1997 (Beati *et al.* 1997). Since then *R. aeschlimannii* has been isolated from various ticks (Table 10.1) but *Hyalomma* spp. ticks are more actively questing and more likely to bite humans in Europe (Mediannikov *et al.* 2007). The first human infection caused by *R. aeschlimannii* was reported in 2002 in a patient returning from Morocco to France. The symptoms are similar to those of MSF with high fever, inoculation eschar at the side of the bite and a generalized maculopapular rash (Mediannikov *et al.* 2007).

R. massiliae was first isolated in 1992 from *Rh. sanguineus* ticks collected near Marseille. From then *R. massiliae* has been detected in various ticks around the Mediterranean, central Africa, and recently in Arizona (Mediannikov *et al.* 2007) (Table 10.1). The first human infection by *R. massiliae* was reported in 2005, 20 years after the isolation of rickettsia from the patient (Vitale *et al.* 2006).

R. helvetica has been isolated from *I. ricinus* in Switzerland in 1979 (Gilot 1985) and has since been isolated in many European countries. Recently it was found that the distribution of the bacterium extends to Asia (Mediannikov *et al.* 2007). *R. helvetica* was considered a 'non-pathogenic rickettsia' during approximately 20 years after its. Recently, *R. helvetica* has been incriminated with cases of a mild form of rickettsiosis (without skin rash and characterized by fever, headache, and myalgia) as three patients in 2004 were serologically attributed to *R. helvetica* (Fournier *et al.* 2004).

Tick-transmitted rickettsioses around the world

Japanese or Oriental spotted fever

R. japonica is the causative agent of Japanese or Oriental spotted fever (OSF) and was first isolated from patients in Shikoku in 1985 (Uchida 1993). OSF was first identified in three patients with high fever and rash during the summer of 1984 by the Japanese physician Fumihiko Mahara (Mahara 1984). The disease was thought to be endemic in Japan but a recent report from South Korea shows that closely related rickettsia may cause diseases in humans (Mediannikov *et al.* 2007). *R. japonica* has been detected from 6 species of ticks in Japan but only *H. flava*, *H. longicornis*, *D. taiwanensis* and *I. ovatus* commonly feed on humans and are considered to be the most likely vectors of the disease (Parola *et al.* 2005). OSF occurs from April to October and approximately 30 to 40 cases have been reported annually (Mahara 1997). OSF has an abrupt onset with high fever (39 to 40°C), headache, chills and an inoculation eschar in 90% of cases. Severe cases of encephalitis, disseminated intravascular coagulopathy, multi-organ failure, and acute respiratory distress syndrome have been reported (Mediannikov *et al.* 2007).

Queensland tick typhus

Queensland tick typhus (QTT) was clinically recognized in 1946 with the first cases observed among Australian troops; *R. australis* was named in 1950. *R. australis* has been identified in *I. holocyclus*, a common human-biting tick in Queensland, and from *I. tasmani*, a species that rarely bites humans but may play a role in the enzootic maintenance of *R. australis* in small animals (Parola *et al.* 2005). QTT is characterized by a sudden onset characterized by fever, eschar (65% of patients), headache, lymphadenopathy (71% of cases) and myalgia, followed within 10 days by maculopapular or vesicular rash (Baird *et al.* 1996). The disease ranges from mild to severe and two fatal cases have been described (Mediannikov *et al.* 2007).

Flinders Island spotted fever

Flinders Island spotted fever was described in 1991 by R. S. Stewart as a febrile eruptive disease with 26 patients observed over 12 years. An eschar was noted in 25% of cases and enlarged local lymph nodes were present in 55%. All cases occurred in spring and summer, predominantly during December and January, which corresponds with tick activity (Parola *et al.* 2005). The isolation of *R. honei* as the agent of Flinders Island spotted fever was identified in 1992 from two patients (Stewart 1991). *R. honei* was first identified in *Aponomma hydrosauri* a tick that usually bites reptiles. *A. hydrosauri* is widespread in south Australia, New South Wales, and Tasmania and it is therefore possible that *R. honei* also exists in these places (Mediannikov *et al.* 2007). The usual features of Flinders Island spotted fever are a sudden onset of fever, headache, arthromyalgias with joint swelling, and slight cough. However, the rash which appeared a few days later, as maculopapular with no vesiculation, in contrast to QTT caused by *R. australis* (Mediannikov *et al.* 2007).

Siberian tick typhus or North Asian tick typhus

R. sibirica is the agent of Siberian tick typhus (STT), a spotted fever group rickettsiosis that was first described in Primorye in 1934 by Shmatikov (Parola *et al.* 2005). *R. sibirica* has been found in several species of ticks, and some of them are thought to be principal vectors (Table 10.1). Siberian tick typhus is well documented in the former USSR but infection due to *R. sibirica* is also prevalent in northern China where it is known as North Asian tick typhus (Yu *et al.* 1993). The disease is strongly associated with the distribution of its natural reservoirs, with the most cases occurring in the spring-summer season (Parola *et al.* 2005). Few descriptions are available in the English medical literature but from officially published data available from the Ministry of Health of the Russian Federation the annual morbidity rates from 1995–2004 varied from 1.5 to 2.4 per 100,000 and in endemic areas rates were as high as 40 or even 120 per 100,000 (Mediannikov *et al.* 2007). The onset of STT is acute, after an incubation period of usually 4 to 7 days following a tick bite. High fever (40°C), severe headache, myalgia, and digestive disturbances are concomitant symptoms. The eschar typically appears in 62–77% of cases, often accompanied by regional lymphadenopathy and rash 2 to 4 days after the onset of the symptoms. Without antibiotics STT usually lasts for 7–9 days but in some cases the duration may be more than 20 days (Mediannikov *et al.* 2007).

American spotted fever caused by *R. parkeri*

R. parkeri was first isolated by Parker in 1939 from Gulf Coast ticks (*Amblyomma maculatum*) collected from cows in south Texas (Parker *et al.* 1939) and was generally considered as a non-pathogenic species. It received relatively little attention for the rest of the twentieth century. However, in 2004 the first recognized case of infection with *R. parkeri* was reported in a 40 year-old from Virginia (Paddock *et al.* 2004). The patient did not have a travel history and presented with fever, headache, diffuse myalgias and arthralgias, and multiple eschars on his lower extremities (Parola *et al.* 2005). A second case of infection with *R. parkeri* was reported for a man with a febrile illness and an eschar that developed at the site of a tick bite (Whitman *et al.* 2007). Recent cases considered to be RMSF were retested for as *R. parkeri* infection (Raoult and Paddock 2005). *R. parkeri* has also been detected on a few occasions in the lone star tick (*A. americanum*), and one study suggests that this rickettsia may be transovarially and transstadially transmitted in this widely distributed tick (Parola *et al.* 2005). Preliminary studies also suggest that *A. cajennense* will support the growth and survival of *R. parkeri* (Mediannikov *et al.* 2007). *R. parkeri* has been also been isolated in *A. triste* (formerly *A. maculatum*) ticks in Uruguay and more recently *R. parkeri* was isolated in Brazil (Labruna *et al.* 2007).

Far-Eastern tick-borne rickettsiosis

R. heilongjanghensis is the agent of Far-Eastern tick-borne rickettsiosis and was isolated in 1982 from *Dermacentor silvarum* ticks collected in Suifenhe in the Heilongjiang Province of China (Fan *et al.* 1999). Genomic analysis allowed a definitive characterization of this rickettsia which is closely related to *R. japonica*. Until recently, infections caused by *R. heilongjanghensis* were attributed to *R. sibirica* (Parola *et al.* 2005). In 2002, *R. heilongjiangensis* was diagnosed in 13 patients from the Russian Far East. In 2006,

R. heilongjanghensis was found in the skin biopsy of an acutely ill patient, and the tick was removed prior to the disease development (Mediannikov *et al.* 2006, 2007). The clinical symptoms are similar to other SFG rickettsioses and all patients with Far-Eastern tick-borne rickettsiosis have had a history of tick bite, tick exposure, or have been in an epidemiologically suspected area. In most cases a macular or maculopapular rash appeared but was faint in most cases. Most patients had eschars, and conjunctival papulae were noticed in some patients (Mediannikov *et al.* 2007). Two patients were shown to have lymphangitis and regional lymphadenopathy (Parola *et al.* 2005).

Diagnosis

Diagnosis is a challenge for the physicians because most clinicians are not familiar with Rickettsial diseases and symptoms during the early stages of illness are non-specific (O'Reilly *et al.* 2003). Although the advent of novel diagnostic tools such as cell culture and molecular amplification, has dramatically improved the efficiency of diagnosing rickettsioses, its important to mention that SFG rickettsioses have been initially described solely on the basis of clinical evidence. Careful clinical examination and epidemiologic investigation of patients with potential rickettsioses is critical. Clinically, the presence of a characteristic rash, associated with high fever and headache should lead to the suspicion of SFG rickettsioses. The presence of eschar is crucial for some SFG rickettsioses and Table 10.2 presents an up to date summary of the clinical characteristics of the most common SFG rickettsioses. Common non-specific laboratory abnormalities in rickettsioses include mild leukopenia, anemia, and thrombocytopenia. Hyponatremia, hypoalbuminemia, and hepatic and renal abnormalities may also occur (Parola *et al.* 2005).

Direct diagnosis

Culture and isolation of *Rickettsia* sp. must only be carried out in Biosafety level 3 laboratories and can be done in cell cultures (Vero, L929, HEL, XTC-2, or MRC5 cells) (Parola *et al.* 2005). The immunofluorescence technique allows the detection of *rickettsiae* in blood or other tissues before seroconversion (Woodward *et al.* 1976). Techniques have improved and in several cases the specificity approaches 100% for the diagnosis of both RMSF and MSF, though the sensitivity remains low, between 53 and 75% (La Scola and Raoult 1997). Polymerase chain reaction (PCR) is also used for the diagnosis of spotted fever with primers to amplify sequences of several genes, including 16S rDNA, outer membrane proteins *ompA*, *ompB*, *gltA*, and gene D (Parola *et al.* 2005). Recently, a nested PCR assay using single-use primers targeting single-use gene fragments present in the genomes of *R. conorii* was proposed by our laboratory and named 'suicide' PCR. 'Suicide' PCR is 2.2 times more sensitive than culture and 1.5 times more sensitive than regular PCR (Fournier and Raoult 2004).

Indirect diagnosis

Serology is a useful method for the diagnosis of *Rickettsia* infections and serological tests are the most frequently used and widely available methods for diagnosis. Micro-immunofluorescence (MIF) is the most used technique for the diagnosis of *Rickettsia* infections (Raoult and Roux 1997). Usually IgM and IgG antibodies

Table 10.2 Symptoms of Tickborne rickettsioses reported to date

Spotted fever group	Fever (%)	Rash (%)	Eschar (%)	Enlarged local nodes (%)	Fatality rate without treatment (%)
Rocky Mountain spotted fever	Yes	90%	rarely	No	20–25%
Mediterranean spotted fever	100%	Maculopapular, 87%	53%	Rare	1–2.5%
African tick bite fever	80%	Yes, but less common	53–98% multiple	49–57%	No
Israeli spotted fever	Yes	Maculopapular, 100%	90%	No	0–3.5%
Astrakhan fever	Yes	Papular rash 94%	20%	?	No
Siberian tick typhus	Yes	Yes	62–77%	regional	?
TIBOLA- DEBONEL	24%	Uncommon	Yes, scalp	Yes, cervical, painful	No
Marseille's fever	Yes	Yes	Yes	?	No
Unspotted rickettsial fever	Yes	Yes	Yes	?	No
R. aeshlimani's fever	Yes	Maculopapular	Yes	?	?
Lymphangitis-associated rickettsiosis	Yes	Maculopapular	75%	25%	?
Queensland tick typhus	Yes	Maculopapular or vesicular rash	65%	71%	2 fatal cases
Flinders Island spotted fever	Yes	Maculopapular	25%	55%	No
Japanese spotted fever	Yes	No	91%	No	No
Far Eastern spotted fever	Yes	macular or maculopapular	Yes	Yes	No
Unexpected American Spotted fever	Yes	Yes	Yes	?	?

are detected between 7 and 15 days after the onset of the disease except the infection with African tick-bite fever in which the seroconversion in patients is 28 and 25 days after the onset of the disease (Brouqui *et al.* 2007). That is the reason for patients with African tick-bite fever the definitive serological diagnosis should be made using sera collected 4 weeks after the onset of the illness; because sensitivity is low during the early stages of the disease (Brouqui *et al.* 2007). Serology does not allow differentiation of infection among the spotted fever group rickettsiae (Hechemy *et al.* 1989) and one of the major limitations is the cross-reacting antibodies that often exists among antigens of pathogens within the same genus and, occasionally, between different genera (La Scola and Raoult 1997). When differences in titers between several antigens are lower than 2 dilutions, Western blot assays and, if needed, cross-absorption studies are performed (Parola *et al.* 2005). Western blot detects two types of antigens, two high-molecular-weight proteins (rOmpA and rOmpB) which are species specific (Raoult *et al.* 1997b) and provide the basis for rickettsial serotyping and lipopolysaccharide (Philip *et al.* 1978). Western blotting and MIF have the same sensitivity for the detection of antibodies directed against the rOmpA and rOmpB proteins but Western blotting is more useful in detecting antibodies early in the course of MSF, and these tend to be reactive to lipopolysaccharide (Brouqui *et al.* 2007).

Ticks

Ticks are mostly used for epidemiological purposes, but the amplification or the culture of *Rickettsia* spp. from the engorged ticks removed from patients can be useful for xenodiagnosis, which can be performed several days before development of the disease.

Ticks should be disinfected with iodinated alcohol and then rinsed with sterile water and crushed before being inoculated onto a shell vial (Parola *et al.* 1999). Ticks can be kept alive in a box which retains moisture prior to testing (Garcia and Bruckner 1993) or may be frozen (Kelly *et al.* 1991).

Treatment

Antimicrobial susceptibility

SFG rickettsia are susceptible to tetracycline, doxycycline, chloramphenicol, and the new ketolides in cell culture models but resistant to erythromycin and spiramycin (Rolain 2007; Raoult and Drancourt 1991). Rifampin is effective against the most SFG rickettsia with the exception of *R. montanensis*, *R. massiliae*, *R. rhipicephali*, and *R. aeschlimannii* which are resistant (Rolain 2007).

Antibiotic therapy

Early antibiotic therapy should be prescribed in any suspected spotted fever patient before confirmation of the diagnosis. Doxycycline is the gold standard antibiotic for treatment of tick-transmitted rickettsioses, and a single dose of oral doxycycline 200 mg have been proven effective in most cases of MSF (Raoult and Roux 1997). However, the duration of the treatment depends on the clinical manifestations, and is usually contracted for at least 3 days after the offset of clinical manifestations (Parola *et al.* 2005). Chloramphenicol can be used as an alternative in patients who are tetracycline allergic, but it is generally reserved for situations in which doxycycline is contraindicated (Raoult and Drancourt 1991). Children treated with azithromycin and clarithromycin required shorter duration of

Table 10.3 Guidelines and recommendations for the treatment of SFG rickettsioses

Clinical feature	Patient cohort	Treatment	Duration	References
Rocky Mountain Fever	adults	doxycycline 200mg/day (100mg/12hours)	5–10 days	(Raoult and Roux 1997)
	children	doxycycline 2,2mg/kg/12 hours	5–10 days	(Sexton and Kaye 2002a)
	alternative for children or adults	chloramphenicol 12.5 to 25 mg/kg/6 hours	5–10 days	(Sexton and Kaye 2002b)
	pregnant women	doxycycline 200mg/day (100mg/12hours)	5–10 days	(Parola *et al.* 2005d)
Mediterranean spotted fever	adults	doxycycline 200 mg/day	1–15 days	(Raoult and Roux 1997)
		ciprofloxacin 1.5 g/day	5 days	(Parola *et al.* 2005c)
		chloramphenicol 2 g/day.	7–10 days	(Raoult and Drancourt 1991)
	pregnant women	josamycin 3g/day		(Raoult and Roux 1997)
	children	doxycycline 5mg/kg	single dose	(Purvis and Edwards 2000)
		josamycin 100 mg/kg/day	5 days	(Bella *et al.* 1990)
		azithromycin 10 mg/kg/day	3 days	(Parola *et al.* 2005b)
		clarithromycin 15/mg/kg/day	7 days	(Parola *et al.* 2005a)
		chloramphenicol 2mg/day	7–15 days	(Raoult and Roux 1997)

therapy and fever disappeared in less than seven days (Cascio *et al.* 2002). Rifampin, has not been successful in children with MSF (Bella *et al.* 1991) and Fluoroquinolones not compared well with tetracyclines and chloramphenicol (Raoult and Drancourt 1991). Josamycin has been used for the treatment of pregnant women and children (Raoult and Roux 1997). Table 10.3 presents the guidelines and recommendations for the treatment of SFG rickettsioses.

Prevention and control

The prevention or control of any tick-borne disease is most effectively achieved by personal protection measures to reduce the probability of a tick attaching and feeding on a human host. For that reason people should avoid contact with rodents, dogs, and domestic livestock in tick-infested areas. People living or travelling to endemic areas should wear protective clothing, preferably impregnated with permethrin or another pyrethroid when walking in high grass. The prompt inspection for removal of crawling or attached ticks on skin or clothing plays a crucial role for the prevention of tick-borne infectious diseases. No licensed vaccine exists for SFG rickettsioses.

References

Bacellar, F., Beati, L., Franca, A., Pocas, J., Regnery, R., *et al.* (1999). Israeli spotted fever rickettsia (Rickettsia conorii complex) associated with human disease in Portugal. *Emerg. Infect. Dis.*, **5**: 835–36.

Baird, R. W., Stenos, J., Stewart, R., Hudson, B., Lloyd, M., *et al.* (1996). Genetic variation in Australian spotted fever group rickettsiae. *J. Clin. Microbiol.*, **34**: 1526–30.

Beati, L., Meskini, M., Thiers, B., and Raoult, D. (1997). *Rickettsia aeschlimannii* sp. nov., a new spotted fever group rickettsia associated with *Hyalomma marginatum* ticks. *Int. J. Syst. Bact.*, 548–54.

Bella, F., Espejo-Arenas, E., Uriz, S., Serrano, J. A., Alegre, M. D., *et al.* (1991). Randomized trial of five-day rifampin versus one-day doxycycline therapy for Mediterranean spotted fever. *J. Infect. Dis.*, **164**: 433–34.

Bella, F., Font, B., Uriz, S., *et al.* (1990). Randomized trial of doxycycline versus josamycin for Mediterranean spotted fever. *Antimicrob. Agents Chemother.*, **34**: 937–38.

Brouqui, P., Parola, P., Fournier, P. E., and Raoult, D. (2007). Spotted fever rickettsioses in southern and eastern Europe. *FEMS Immunol. Med. Microbiol.*, **49**: 2–12.

Cascio, A., Colomba, C., Antinori, S., Paterson, D. L., and Titone, L. (2002). Clarithromycin versus azithromycin in the treatment of Mediterranean spotted fever in children: a randomized controlled trial. *Clin. Infect. Dis.*, **34**: 154–58.

Chapman, A. S., Murphy, S. M., Demma, L.J., *et al.* (2006). Rocky mountain spotted fever in the United States, 1997–2002. *Ann. N. Y. Acad. Sci.*, **1078**: 154–55.

Childs, J. and Paddock, C. (2007). Rocky Mountain Spotted Fever. In: D. Raoult and P. Parala (eds.) *Rickettsial Diseases*, pp. 97–116. New York: Informa Health Care.

Conor, A. and Bruch, A. (1910). Une fièvre éruptive observée en Tunisie. *Bull. Soc. Pathol. Exot. Filial.*, **8**: 492–96.

Dantas-Torres, F. (2007). Rocky Mountain spotted fever. *Lancet Infect. Dis.*, **7**: 724–32.

De-Sousa, R., Ismail, N., Doria-Nobrega, S., *et al.* (2005). The presence of eschars, but not greater severity, in Portuguese patients infected with Israeli spotted fever. *Ann. N. Y. Acad. Sci.*, **1063**: 197–202.

Doyle, A., Bhalla, K. S., Jones III, J. M., and Ennis, D. M. (2006). Myocardial involvement in Rocky mountain spotted fever: a case report and review. *Am. J. Med. Sci.*, **332**: 208–210.

Drancourt, M., Brouqui, P., Chiche, G., Raoult, D. (1991). Acute pericarditis in Mediterranean Spotted Fever. *Trans. R. Soc. Trop. Med. Hyg.*, **85**: 799.

Fan, M. Y., Zhang, J. Z., Chen, M., and Yu, X. J. (1999). Spotted fever group rickettsioses in China. In: D. Raoult and P. Brouqui (eds.) *Rickettsiae and rickettsial diseases at the turn of the third millenium*, pp. 247–57. Paris: Elsevier.

Fournier, P. E., Allombert, C., Supputamongkol, Y., Caruso, G., Brouqui, P., *et al.* (2004). Aneruptive fever associated with antibodies to *Rickettsia helvetica* in Europe and Thailand. *J. Clin. Microbiol.*, **42**: 816–18.

Fournier, P. E., Gouriet, F., Brouqui, P., Lucht, F., and Raoult, D. (2005). Lymphangitis-associated rickettsiosis, a new rickettsiosis caused by

Rickettsia sibirica mongolotimonae: seven new cases and review of the literature. *Clin. Infect. Dis.*, **40**: 1435–44.

Fournier, P. E. and Raoult, D. (2007). *Bacteriology, Taxonomy, and Phylogeny of Rickettsia.* In: D. Raoult and P. Parala (eds.) *Rickettsial Diseases*, pp. 1–13. New York: Informa Health Care.

Fournier, P. E. and Raoult, D. (2004). Suicide PCR on skin biopsy specimens for diagnosis of rickettsioses. *J. Clin. Microbiol.*, **42**: 3428–34.

Garcia, L. S. and Bruckner, D. A. (1993). *Diagnostic medical parasitology*. Washington, D.C.: American Society for Microbiology.

Gear, J. H. S. (1938). South African typhus. *South Afri. J. Med. Sci.*, **3**: 134–60.

Giammanco, G. M., Vitale, G., Mansueto, S., Capra, G., Caleca, M. P., *et al.* (2005). Presence of *Rickettsia conorii* subsp. *israelensis*, the causative agent of Israeli spotted fever, in Sicily, Italy, ascertained in a retrospective study. *J. Clin. Microbiol.*, **43**: 6027–31.

Gilot, B. (1985). *Bases biologiques, écologiques et cartographiques pour l'étude des maladies transmises par les tiques (Ixodidae et Argasidae) dans les Alpes françaises et leur avant pays*. 1–535. Université de Grenoble/ France. Ref Type: Thesis/Dissertation.

Gross, E. M., and Yagupsky, P. (1987). Israeli rickettsial spotted fever in children. A review of 54 cases. *Acta Trop.*, **44**: 91–96.

Hechemy, K. E., Raoult, D., Fox, J., Han, Y., Elliott, L. B., *et al.* (1989). Cross-reaction of immune sera from patients with rickettsial diseases. *J. Med. Microbiol.*, **29**: 199–202.

Jensenius, M., Fournier, P. E., Kelly, P., Myrvang, B., and Raoult, D. (2003). African tick bite fever. *Lancet Infect. Dis.*, **3**: 557–64.

Jensenius, M., Fournier, P. E., and Raoult, D. (2004). Tick-borne rickettsioses in international travellers. *Int. J. Infect. Dis.*, **8**: 139–46.

Jensenius, M., Ndip, L. M., and Myrvang, B. (2007). African Tick-Bite Fever. In: D. Raoult and P. Parala (eds.) *Rickettsial Diseases*, pp. 117–23. New York: Informa Health Care.

Jensenius, M., Parola, P., and Raoult, D. (2006). Threats to international travellers posed by tick-borne diseases. *Travel. Med. Infect. Dis.*, **4**: 4–13.

Kelly, P. J., Raoult, D., and Mason, P. R. (1991). Isolation of spotted fever group rickettsias from triturated ticks using a modification of the centrifugation-shell vial technique. *Trans. R. Soc. Trop. Med. Hyg.*, **85**: 397–98.

La Scola, B. and Raoult, D. (1997). Laboratory diagnosis of rickettsioses: current approaches to the diagnosis of old and new rickettsial diseases. *J. Clin. Microbiol.*, **35**: 2715–27.

Labruna, M. B., Horta, M. C., Aguiar, D. M., *et al.* (2007). Prevalence of *Rickettsia* infection in dogs from the urban and rural areas of Monte Negro municipality, western Amazon, Brazil. *Vector. Borne. Zoonotic. Dis.*, **7**: 249–55.

Mahara, F. (1984). Three Weil-Felix reaction OX2 positive cases with skin eruptions and high fever. *J. Anan Med. Assoc.*, **68**: 4–7.

Mahara, F. (1997). Japanese spotted fever: Report of 31 cases and review of the literature. *Emerg. Infect. Dis.*, **3**: 105–111.

Masters, E. J., Olson, G. S., Weiner, S. J., and Paddock, C. D. (2003). Rocky mountain spotted fever: a clinician's dilemma. *Arch. Intern. Med.*, **163**: 769–74.

Mediannikov, O., Parola, P., and Raoult, D. (2007). Other Tick-Borne Rickettsioses. In: D. Raoult and P. Parala (eds.) *Rickettsial Diseases*, pp. 139–62. New York: Informa Health Care.

Mediannikov, O., Sidelnikov, Y., Ivanov, L., Fournier, P. E., Tarasevich, I., *et al.* (2006). Far eastern tick-borne rickettsiosis: identification of two new cases and tick vector. *Ann. N. Y. Acad. Sci.*, **1078**: 80–88.

O'Reilly, M., Paddock, C., Elchos, B., Goddard, J., Childs, J., *et al.* (2003). Physician knowledge of the diagnosis and management of Rocky mountain spotted fever: Mississippi, 2002. *Ann. N. Y. Acad. Sci.*, **990**: 295–301.

Paddock, C. D., Sumner, J. W., Comer, J. A., *et al.* (2004). *Rickettsia parkeri*: a newly recognized cause of spotted fever rickettsiosis in the United States. *Clin. Infect. Dis.*, **38**: 805–11.

Parker, R. R., Kohls, G. M., Cox, G. W., and Davis, G. E. (1939). Observations on an infectious agent from *Amblyomma maculatum*. *Public Health Rep.*, **54**: 1482–84.

Parola, P. and Barre, N. (2004). *Rickettsia africae*, the agent of African tick-bite fever: an emerging pathogen in the West Indies and Reunion Island (Indian Ocean). *Bull. Soc. Pathol. Exot.*, **97**: 193–98.

Parola, P., Davoust, B., and Raoult, D. (2005). Tick- and flea-borne rickettsial emerging zoonoses. *Vet. Res.*, **36**: 469–92.

Parola, P., Paddock, C. D., and Raoult, D. (2005). Tick-Borne Rickettsioses around the World: Emerging Diseases Challenging Old Concepts. *Clin. Microbiol. Rev.*, **18**: 719–56.

Parola, P. and Raoult, D. (2006). Tropical rickettsioses. *Clin. Dermatol.*, **24**: 191–200.

Parola, P., Vestris, G., Martinez, D., Brochier, B., Roux, V., *et al.* (1999). Tick-borne rickettsiosis in Guadeloupe, the French West Indies: isolation of *Rickettsia africae* from *Amblyomma variegatum* ticks and serosurvey in humans, cattle and goats. *Am. J. Trop. Med. Hyg.*, **60**: 888–93.

Philip, R. N., Casper, E. A, Burgdorfer, W., Gerloff, R. K., Hugues, L. E., Bell, E. J. (1978). Serologic typing of rickettsiae of the spotted fever group by micro immunofluoresence. *J. Immunol.*, **121**: 1961–68.

Portillo, A., Perez-Martinez, L., Santibanez, S., Blanco, J. R., Ibarra, V., *et al.* (2007). Detection of *Rickettsia africae* in *Rhipicephalus* (*Boophilus*) *decoloratus* ticks from the Republic of Botswana, South Africa. *Am. J. Trop. Med. Hyg.*, **77**: 376–77.

Purvis, J. J. and Edwards, M. S. (2000). Doxycycline use for rickettsial disease in pediatric patients. *Pediatr. Infect. Dis. J.*, **19**: 871–74.

Raoult, D., Berbis, P., Roux, V., Xu, W., and Maurin, M. (1997a). A new tick-transmitted disease due to *Rickettsia slovaca*. *Lancet*, **350**: 112–13.

Raoult, D., Brouqui, P., and Roux, V. (1996). A new spotted-fever-group rickettsiosis. *Lancet*, **348**: 412.

Raoult, D. and Drancourt, M. (1991). Antimicrobial therapy of Rickettsial diseases. *Antimicrob. Agents Chemother.*, **35**: 2457–62.

Raoult, D. and Paddock, C. D. (2005). *Rickettsia parkeri* infection and other spotted fevers in the United States. *N. Engl. J. Med.*, **353**: 626–27.

Raoult, D. and Roux, V. (1997). Rickettsioses as paradigms of new or emerging infectious diseases. *Clin. Microbiol. Rev.*, **10**: 694–719.

Raoult, D., Roux, V., Ndihokubwaho, J. B., *et al.* (1997b). Jail fever (epidemic typhus) outbreak in Burundi. *Emerg. Infect. Dis.*, **3**: 357–60.

Raoult, D., Weiller, P. J., Chagnon, A., Chaudet, H., Gallais, H., *et al.* (1986a). Mediterranean spotted fever: clinical, laboratory and epidemiological features of 199 cases. *Am. J. Trop. Med. Hyg.*, **35**: 845–50.

Raoult, D., Zuchelli, P., Weiller, P. J., *et al.* (1986b). Incidence, clinical observations and risk factors in the severe form of Mediterranean spotted fever among patients admitted to hospital in Marseilles 1983–1984. *J. Infection*, **12**: 111–16.

Rehacek, J. (1984). *Rickettsia slovaca*, the organism and its ecology. *Acta SC. Nat. Brno.*, **18**: 1–50.

Rehacek, J. (1993). Rickettsiae and their ecology in the Alpine region. *Acta Virol.*, **37**: 290–301.

Ricketts, H. T. (1909). Some aspects of Rocky mountain spotted fever as shown by recent investigations. *Med. Rec.*, 843–55.

Rolain, J. M. (2007). Antimicrobial Susceptibility of Rickettsial Agents. In: D. Raoult and P. Parala (eds.) *Rickettsial Diseases*, pp. 361–69. New York: Informa Health Care.

Rovery, C. and Raoult, D. (2007). *Rickettsia conorii* Infection (Mediterranean Spotted Fever, Israeli Spotted Fever, Indian Tick Typhus, Astrakhan Fever). In: D. Raoult and P. Parala (eds.) *Rickettsial Diseases*, pp. 125–37. New York: Informa Health Care.

Rovery, C., Rolain, J. M., Raoult, D., and Brouqui, P. (2003). Shell vial culture as a tool for isolation of *Brucella melitensis* in chronic hepatic abscess. *J. Clin. Microbiol.*, **41**: 4460–61.

Ruiz Beltran, R., Herrerro-Herrero, J. I., Martin-Sanchez, A. M., *et al.* (1985). Formas graves de fiebre exantematica mediterranea. Analisis prospectivo de 71 enfermos. *Ann. Med. Interna. (Madrid)*, **2**: 365–68.

Sexton, D. J. and Kaye, K. S. (2002). Rocky mountain spotted fever. *Med. Clin. North Am.*, **86:** 351–60.

Sonenshine, D. E. (1993). *Biology of ticks.* New York: Oxford University Press.

Stewart, R. S. (1991). Flinders Island spotted fever: a newly recognised endemic focus of tick typhus in Bass Strait. Part 1. Clinical and epidemiologiocal features. *Med. J. Australia*, **154:** 94–99.

Tarasevich, I. V., Makarova, V., Fetisova, N. F., *et al.* (1991). Astrakhan fever: new spotted fever group rickettsiosis. *Lancet*, **337:** 172–73.

Treadwell, T. A., Holman, R. C., Clarke, M. J., Krebs, J. W., Paddock, C. D., *et al.* (2000). Rocky Mountain spotted fever in the United States, 1993–1996. *Am. J. Trop. Med. Hyg.*, **63:** 21–26.

Uchida, T. (1993). *Rickettsia japonica*, the etiologic agent of oriental spotted fever. *Microbiol. Immunol.*, **37:** 91–102.

Valero, A. (1949). Rocky Mountain spotted fever in Palestine. *Harefuah*, **36:** 99.

Vitale, G., Mansuelo, S., Rolain, J. M., and Raoult, D. (2006). *Rickettsia massiliae* human isolation. *Emerg. Infect. Dis.*, **12:** 174–75.

Walker, D. H. (1995). Rocky mountain spotted fever: a seasonal alert. *Clin. Infect. Dis.*, **20:** 1111–17.

Whitman, T. J., Richards, A. L., Paddock, C. D. *et al.* (2007). *Rickettsia parkeri* infection after tick bite, Virginia. *Emerg. Infect. Dis.*, **13:** 334–36.

Woodward, T. E., Pedersen Jr., C. E., Oster, C. N., Bagley, L. R., Romberger, J., *et al.* (1976). Prompt confirmation of Rocky mountain spotted fever: identification of rickettsiae in skin tissues. *J. Infect. Dis.*, **134:** 297–301.

Yu, X., Fan, M., Xu, G., Liu, Q., and Raoult, D. (1993). Genotypic and antigenic identification of two new strains of spotted fever group rickettsiae isolated from China. *J. Clin. Microbiol.*, **31:** 83–88.

Zavala-Castro, J. E., Zavala-Velazquez, J. E., Walker, D. H., *et al.* (2006). Fatal human infection with *Rickettsia rickettsii*, Yucatan, Mexico. *Emerg. Infect. Dis.*, **12:** 672–74.

CHAPTER 11

Flea-borne rickettsial diseases

Emmanouil Angelakis and Didier Raoult

Summary

R. felis has been identified in cats and cat fleas and is now considered to be the cause of flea-borne spotted fever (cat flea typhus). Cases of fever, rash and lymphadeopathy have been reported from Europe and the Americas. Diagnosis is based on serology and treatment with doxycycline.

History

Bacteria of the order Rickettsiales are Gram-negative microorganisms that grow in association with eukaryotic cells. 'Rickettsia' has long been used as a generic term for many small bacteria that could not be cultivated and were not otherwise identified. However, the progress in taxonomy that was made over the last 35 years with the introduction of molecular techniques resulted in the term 'rickettsia' applying only to arthropod-borne bacteria belonging to the genus Rickettsia within the family Rickettsiaceae, in the order Rickettsiales (Brenner *et al.* 1993). The *Rickettsia* genus is currently made of 24 recognized species, and also contains several dozens of as yet uncharacterized strains or tick amplicons (Fournier and Raoult 2007). At present the family *Rickettsia* is divided into three groups, namely the spotted fever group (SFG), the Typhus group, and *Rickettsia bellii*.

Flea-borne bacterial diseases include cat-scratch disease, plague, murine typhus and flea-borne spotted fever (FBSF) due to *R. felis*. The first description of a *Rickettsia* in a cat flea *Ctenocephalides felis* was in 1918 and it was named *R. ctenocephali*. It was rediscovered in 1990, when *C. felis* ticks were examined in California as potential vectors of *R. typhi*, the agent of murine typhus (Adams *et al.* 1990). A new rickettsia was observed to these ticks by electronic microscopy and named the ELB agent after the EL laboratory in Soquel, California (Adams *et al.* 1990). Later in 1994, the bacterium was detected by polymerase chain reaction (PCR) and genomic sequence comparison based on the 17-kDa protein gene sequencing, and was considered to be a new SFG *Rickettsia* named *R. felis* (Higgins *et al.* 1996). These first attempts to define the classification of *R. felis* have proved problematic and not confirmed since the first isolations were contaminated by *R. typhi* (Znazen and Raoult 2007). *R. felis* was definitely characterized and validated as a unique SFG *Rickettsia* in 2001 when culture conditions using *Xenopis laevis* tissue cells and mosquito cells at 28°C were established (La Scola *et al.* 2002).

The agent

R. felis is a small (0.8–2µm in length and 0.3–0.5µm in diameter) rod-shaped, Gram-negative bacillus that retains basic fuchsin when stained by the Gimenez method (Znazen and Raoult 2007). *R. felis* presents pili, probably involved in the attachment of the bacteria to other cells and in conjugation (Ogata *et al.* 2005). The genome of *R. felis* has been recently sequenced and a number of rickettsial genetic specificities were found. The genome of *R. felis* (1485 Mb) is circular and larger than other previously sequenced rickettsiae (i.e. *R. prowazekii*, *R. conorii*, *R. sibirica*, *R. rickettsii*, *R. akari*, and *R. typhi*). In *R. felis* were surprisingly found 2 plasmids (63 kb pRF and 39 kb pRFδ), with one of them to contain the equipment to allow conjugative plasmid transfer (Ogata *et al.* 2005). When *R. felis* was compared to other published genomes (*R. prowazekii*, *R. typhi*, *R. conorii*, and *R. sibirica*) 530 specific open-reading frames (ORFs) were found (Ogata *et al.* 2005). In addition, *R. felis* have 22 ankyrin (*ank*) repeats which are more than any prokaryotes sequenced so far (Ogata *et al.* 2005).

A high number of transposase (*tnp*) genes on *pRF* are also presented and this high occurrence of transposases suggests that *pRF* genes have been frequently rearranged through recombination mediated by *tnp* elements (Gillespie *et al.* 2007). Moreover, *R. felis* carries 14 *spoT* genes for its adaptation to the environment (Ogata *et al.* 2005). Also, 11 tetratricopeptide repeat-containing protein genes, *tpr*, and 5 families of toxin-antitoxin (TAT) system genes (16 toxins and 14 antitoxin genes) were found (Ogata *et al.* 2005). The TAT system was considered exceptional in intracellular organisms before its identification in *R. felis* and is associated with the increase of cell survival during nutritional stress (Ogata *et al.* 2005). *R. felis rel* BE has been demonstrated to stabilize plasmid efficiently even when it is chromosomal which may indicate its role in *R. felis* plasmid maintenance (Ogata *et al.* 2005).

Epidemiology

R. felis is the only known species of SFG that is transmitted by fleas. Today several species of fleas have been associated with *R. felis* and Table 11.1 illustrates these species and the continent of their isolation. From all these species, the cat flea *C. felis* (Fig. 11.1) is one of the most frequent external parasites of companion animals worldwide. *C. felis* is generally regarded as the predominant species to

Table 11.1 Species of flea that have been associated with *R. felis* and the continent of their isolation

Species of flea	Continents of isolation	References
C. felis	Europe, USA, South America, Asia, Africa, Australia	(Rolain *et al.* 2003; Venzal *et al.* 2006; Jiang *et al.* 2006; Marquez *et al.* 2006; Marie *et al.* 2006; Bitam *et al.* 2006; Schloderer *et al.* 2006; Horta *et al.* 2006a; Hawley *et al.* 2007)
C. canis	South America, Africa	(Venzal *et al.* 2006; Horta *et al.* 2006a)
Xenopsylla cheopis	Asia	(Jiang *et al.* 2006)
Pulex irritans	Europe	(Brouqui *et al.* 2007)
Archaeopsylla erinacei	Africa, Europe	(De *et al.* 2006; Bitam *et al.* 2006)
Ctenophtalmus sp	Europe	(De *et al.* 2006)
Anomiopsyllus nudata	USA	(Stevenson *et al.* 2005)

find on dogs, cats and opossums. *R. felis* DNA have been determined in *C. felis* in the USA with an infection rate of 3.8% and 7.6% in Israel and up to 12% in the UK (Bauer *et al.* 2006; Znazen and Raoult 2007). Antibodies to *R. felis* have been detected in cats but current infection by PCR assay or culture have not been described (Case *et al.* 2006; Hawley *et al.* 2007). Although, data suggest that *R. felis* infection may be prevalent worldwide and

humans can be infected after flea bites, the role of mammals, including rodents, hedgehogs, cats, and dogs, in the life cycle and circulation of *R. felis* is still unclear (Parola *et al.* 2005a).

Hosts

Human pathogenicity and clinical manifestations

R. felis is now known as the agent of FBSF (also called cat flea typhus) a disease with similar clinical manifestations with murine typhus (Schriefer *et al.* 1994). Cases of FBSF have been reported in Europe including Spain, Canary Islands, Germany, France and the UK, in Asia including Thailand and New Zealand, in Africa including Tunisia and Ethiopia, in America including Brazil and Mexico (Parola *et al.* 2005b). Debate over the pathogenicity of *R. felis* for humans was fuelled in 2000 in Mexico when three patients with fever, exanthema, headache, and central nervous system involvement were diagnosed with *R. felis* infection (Zavala-Velazquez *et al.* 2000). In 2002, FBSF was found in an adult couple in Germany with high fever (39°C), associated with marked fatigue and headache generalized maculopapular rash of 4 and 2 days. The man had enlarged, painful lymph nodes in the inguinal region and 5 days before the onset of the symptoms patients mentioned a single black, crusted, cutaneous lesion surrounded by a livid halo (on the woman's right thigh and the man's abdomen) (Richter *et al.* 2002). Recently in Spain, an adult couple, having visited a forest area two days before, presented with itching skin lesions, mainly located on flexion areas of the lower extremities, malaise, arthralgia, and pruritic papular rash over the lower extremities, abdomen, and chest. Both patients showed the same clinical picture, although fever was absent in the male. *R. felis* was identified by PCR (Oteo *et al.* 2006). *R. felis* can cause severe debilitating disease in some people—a 34 year old woman from rural eastern Yucatán developed central nervous system involvement with Brudzinski and Kernig signs (Zavala-Velazquez *et al.* 2000) and a 18 year old man presented severe case of pneumonia following *R. felis* infection (Zavala-Velazquez *et al.* 2006). To date no fatal cases have been reported (Znazen and Raoult 2007). However, more studies are needed to determine the real clinical spectrum of symptoms present in FBSF as well as the epidemiology including the role of vectors, reservoirs, hosts, and the case:fatality ratio of this disease.

Diagnosis

The mildness of the disease, together with the non specific clinical manifestations, that may be the same in all rickettsioses, leads to the fact that the illness is difficult to recognize. Mild leucopenia, anemia, and thrombocytopenia are usually presented and hyponatremia, hypoalbuminemia, and hepatic and renal abnormalities may also occur (Znazen and Raoult 2007).

Direct diagnosis

R. felis is an obligate intracellular bacterium and its culture and isolation must only be carried out in Biosafety level 3 laboratories. *R. felis* isolation and establishment can be obtained in XTC-2 cells at low temperature (27°C), on mosquito cell lines (C6/36 cell line) and on Ixodes scapularis-derived tick cell line (ISE6) (Pornwiroon *et al.* 2006; Horta *et al.* 2006b; Znazen and Raoult 2007). *R. felis* can be detected and identified by PCR and sequencing methods

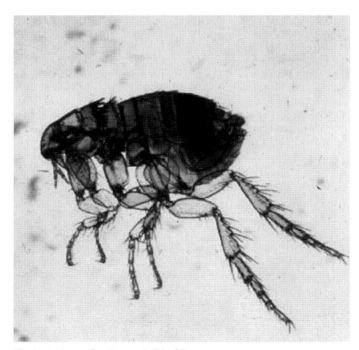

Fig. 11.1 The cat flea *Ctenocephalides felis*

targeting the citrate synthase (*gltA*), the 16S rRNA, the rickettsia genus-specific 17-kDa antigen, and SFG-specific outer membrane protein A (*ompA*) or protein B (*ompB*) genes (Pornwiroon *et al.* 2006; Znazen and Raoult 2007). Recently a quantitative real-time polymerase chain reaction (qPCR) assay, detecting outer membrane protein B genes (*ompB*) was proposed for the detection of the *R. felis* (Henry *et al.* 2007).

Indirect diagnosis

Serological tests are the most frequently used and widely available methods for the diagnosis. The Weil-Felix test was developed 90 years ago but continues to be used by many laboratories around the world. Microimmunofluorescence (MIF) is widely accepted as the reference method and is reliable but does not allow differentiation of infection among the SFG rickettsiae (Hechemy *et al.* 1989). One limitation of serology is the cross-reactivity that might occur between the antigens of organisms within the same genus and occasionally in different genera. *R. felis* harbors the antigenic profile of an SFG rickettsia and, by a neighbour-joining analysis based on MIF *R. felis*, was found to be related to SFG rickettsiae antigenically, clustering with *R. australis*, *R. akari*, and *R. montanensis* (Fang and Raoult 2003). Moreover, antisera to *R. felis* have low cross-reactivities with *R. rickettsii*, *R. conorii*, and *R. typhi*, which are the only commercially available antigens (Fang and Raoult 2003).

Western blot assays and, if needed, cross absorption studies can be used when differences in titers between several antigens are lower than two dilutions and in cases of cross-reactivity. However these techniques are time and antigen consuming (Znazen and Raoult 2007).

Fleas

Fleas can also be used as epidemiological tools in order to detect the presence of a pathogen in a specific area. The fleas should be disinfected with iodinated alcohol and then rinsed with sterile water and be crushed before being inoculated onto a shell vial for culture or being processed using molecular methods (Parola *et al.* 1999). Arthropods which are sent to a reference centre for PCR analysis should be stored dry or frozen at −80°C before transport in dry ice (Gouriet *et al.* 2005).

Treatment

Antimicrobial susceptibility

The evaluation of antibiotic susceptibility for *R. felis* showed that doxycycline, fluoroquinolones, telithromycin, and rifampin are effective against the organism but trimethoprim-sulfamethoxazole, β-lactams, and erythromycin are not (Rolain *et al.* 2002). In fact, genome of *R. felis* was found to carry a gene coding to β-lactamases of class C and D, streptomycin-resistant protein, and multidrug transport-system protein (Znazen and Raoult 2007).

Antibiotic therapy

The conventional antibiotic regimen for SFG rickettsioses is a 7–14 day oral course of doxycycline (200 mg/day) and all reported cases of FBSF rickettsioses have been treated with doxycycline (Znazen and Raoult 2007).

Prevention and control

Prevention efforts are aimed at reducing conditions associated with contact with the fleas of cats, dogs, rodents, and hedgehogs. To date no vaccine is available.

References

Adams, J. R., Schmidtmann, E. T., and Azad, A. F. (1990). Infection of colonized cat fleas, *Ctenocephalides felis* (Bouché), with a rickettsia-like microorganism. *Am. J. Trop. Med. Hyg.*, **43**: 400–409.

Bauer, O., Baneth, G., Eshkol, T., Shaw, S. E., and Harrus, S. (2006). Polygenic detection of *Rickettsia felis* in cat fleas (*Ctenocephalides felis*) from Israel. *Am. J. Trop. Med. Hyg.*, **74**: 444–48.

Bitam, I., Parola, P., De La Cruz, K. D. *et al.* (2006). First molecular detection of *Rickettsia felis* in fleas from Algeria. *Am. J. Trop. Med. Hyg.*, **74**: 532–35.

Brenner, D. J., O'Connor, S., Winkler, H. H., and Steigerwalt, A. G. (1993). Proposals to unify the genera *Bartonella* and *Rochalimaea*, with descriptions of *Bartonella quintana* comb. nov., *Bartonella vinsonii* comb. nov., *Bartonella henselae* comb. nov., and *Bartonella elizabethae* comb.nov., and to remove the family *Bartonellaceae* from the order *Rickettsiales*. *Inter. J. System. Bacteriol.*, **43**: 777–86.

Brouqui, P., Parola, P., Fournier, P. E., and Raoult, D. (2007). Spotted fever rickettsioses in southern and eastern Europe. *FEMS Immunol. Med. Microbiol.*, **49**: 2–12.

Case, J. B., Chomel, B., Nicholson, W., and Foley, J. E. (2006). Serological survey of vector-borne zoonotic pathogens in pet cats and cats from animal shelters and feral colonies. *J. Feline. Med. Surg.*, **8**: 111–17.

De Sousa, R., Edouard-Fournier, P., Santos-Silva, M., Amaro, F., Bacellar, F., *et al.* (2006). Molecular detection of *Rickettsia felis*, *Rickettsia typhi* and two genotypes closely related to *Bartonella elizabethae*. *Am. J. Trop. Med. Hyg.*, **75**: 727–31.

Fang, R. and Raoult, D. (2003). Antigenic classification of *Rickettsia felis* by using monoclonal and polyclonal antibodies. *Clin. Diagn. Lab Immunol.*, **10**: 221–28.

Fournier, P. E. and Raoult, D. (2007). Bacteriology, Taxonomy, and Phylogeny of *Rickettsia*. In: D. Raoult and P. Parala (eds.) *Rickettsial Diseases*, pp. 1–13. New York: Informa Health Care.

Gillespie, J. J., Beier, M. S., Rahman, M. S. *et al.* (2007). Plasmids and rickettsial evolution: insight from *Rickettsia felis*. *PLoS. ONE*, **2**: e266.

Gouriet, F., Fenollar, F., Patrice, J. Y., Drancourt, M., and Raoult, D. (2005). Use of shell-vial cell culture assay for isolation of bacteria from clinical specimens: 13 years of experience. *J. Clin. Microbiol.*, **43**: 4993–5002.

Hawley, J. R., Shaw, S. E., and Lappin, M. R. (2007). Prevalence of *Rickettsia felis* DNA in the blood of cats and their fleas in the United States. *J. Feline. Med. Surg.*, **9**: 258–62.

Hechemy, K. E., Raoult, D., Fox, J., Han, Y., Elliott, L. B., *et al.* (1989). Cross-reaction of immune sera from patients with rickettsial diseases *J. Med. Microbiol.*, **29**: 199–202.

Henry, K. M., Jiang, J., Rozmajzl, P. J., Azad, A. F., Macaluso, K. R., *et al.* (2007). Development of quantitative real-time PCR assays to detect *Rickettsia typhi* and *Rickettsia felis*, the causative agents of murine typhus and fleaborne spotted fever. *Mol. Cell. Probes.*, **21**: 17–23.

Higgins, J. A., Radulovic, S., Schriefer, M. E., and Azad, A. F. (1996). *Rickettsia felis*: a new species of pathogenic rickettsia isolated from cat fleas. *J. Clin. Microbiol.*, **34**: 671–74.

Horta, M. C., Chiebao, D. P., De Souza, D. B., *et al.* (2006a). Prevalence of *Rickettsia felis* in the fleas *Ctenocephalides felis* and *Ctenocephalides canis* from two Indian villages in Sao Paulo Municipality, Brazil. *Ann. NY Acad. Sci.*, **1078**: 361–63.

Horta, M. C., Labruna, M. B., Durigon, E. L., and Schumaker, T. T. (2006b). Isolation of *Rickettsia felis* in the mosquito cell line C6/36. *Appl. Environ. Microbiol.*, **72**: 1705–7.

Jiang, J., Soeatmadji, D. W., Henry, K. M., Ratiwayanto, S., Bangs, M. J., *et al.* (2006). *Rickettsia felis* in *Xenopsylla cheopis*, Java, Indonesia. *Emerg. Infect. Dis.*, **12**: 1281–83.

La Scola, B., Meconi, S., Fenollar, F., Rolain, J. M., Roux, V., *et al.* (2002). Emended description of *Rickettsia felis* (Bouyer *et al.* 2001) a temperature-dependent cultured bacterium. *Int. J. Syst. Evol. Microbiol.*, **52**: 2035–41.

Marie, J. L., Fournier, P. E., Rolain, J. M., Briolant, S., Davoust, B., *et al.* (2006). Molecular detection of *Bartonella quintana*, *B. Elizabethae*, *B. Koehlerae*, *B. Doshiae*, *B. Taylorii*, and *Rickettsia felis* in rodent fleas collected in Kabul, Afghanistan. *Am. J. Trop. Med. Hyg.*, **74**: 436–39.

Marquez, F. J., Muniain, M. A., Rodriguez-Liebana, J. J., Bernabeu-Wittel, M., and Pachon, A. J. (2006). Incidence and distribution pattern of *Rickettsia felis* in peridomestic fleas from Andalusia, Southeast Spain. *Ann. NY Acad. Sci.*, **1078**: 344–46.

Ogata, H., Renesto, P., Audic, S., *et al.* (2005). The genome sequence of *Rickettsia felis* identifies the first putative conjugative plasmid in an obligate intracellular parasite. *Ann. NY Acad. Sci.*, **1063**: 26–34.

Oteo, J. A., Portillo, A., Santibanez, S., Blanco, J. R., Perez-Martinez, L., *et al.* (2006). Cluster of cases of human *Rickettsia felis* infection from Southern Europe (Spain) diagnosed by PCR. *J. Clin. Microbiol.*, **44**: 2669–71.

Parola, P., Davoust, B., and Raoult, D. (2005a). Tick- and flea-borne rickettsial emerging zoonoses. *Vet. Res.*, **36**: 469–92.

Parola, P., Paddock, C. D., and Raoult, D. (2005b). Tick-Borne Rickettsioses around the World: Emerging Diseases Challenging Old Concepts. *Clin. Microbiol. Rev.*, **18**: 719–56.

Parola, P., Vestris, G., Martinez, D., Brochier, B., Roux, V., *et al.* (1999). Tick-borne rickettsiosis in Guadeloupe, the French West Indies: isolation of *Rickettsia africae* from *Amblyomma variegatum* ticks and serosurvey in humans, cattle and goats. *Am. J. Trop. Med. Hyg.*, **60**: 888–93.

Pornwiroon, W., Pourciau, S. S., Foil, L. D., and Macaluso, K. R. (2006). *Rickettsia felis* from cat fleas: isolation and culture in a tick-derived cell line. *Appl. Environ. Microbiol.*, **72**: 5589–95.

Richter, J., Fournier, P. E., Petridou, J., Haussinger, D., and Raoult, D. (2002). *Rickettsia felis* Infection Acquired in Europe and Documented by Polymerase Chain Reaction. *Emerg. Infect. Dis.*, **8**: 207–208.

Rolain, J. M., Franc, M., Davoust, B., and Raoult, D. (2003). Molecular detection of *Bartonella quintana*, *B. koehlerae*, *B. henselae*, *B. clarridgeiae*, *Rickettsia felis* and *Wolbachia pipientis* in cat fleas, France. *Emerg. Infect. Dis.*, **9**: 338–42.

Rolain, J. M., Stuhl, L., Maurin, M., and Raoult, D. (2002). Evaluation of antibiotic susceptibilities of three rickettsial species including *Rickettsia felis* by a quantitative PCR DNA assay. *Antimicrob. Agents Chemother.*, **46**: 2747–51.

Schloderer, D., Owen, H., Clark, P., Stenos, J., and Fenwick, S. G. (2006). *Rickettsia felis* in fleas, Western Australia. *Emerg. Infect. Dis.*, **12**: 841–43.

Schriefer, M. E., Sacci, J. B. Jr., Dumler, J. S., Bullen, M. G., and Azad, A. F. (1994). Identification of a novel rickettsial infection in a patient diagnosed with murine typhus. *J. Clin. Microbiol.*, **32**: 949–54.

Stevenson, H. L., Labruna, M. B., Montenieri, J. A., Kosoy, M. Y., Gage, K. L., *et al.* (2005). Detection of Rickettsia felis in a New World flea species, Anomiopsyllus nudata (Siphonaptera: Ctenophthalmidae). *J. Med. Entomol.*, **42**: 163–67.

Venzal, J. M., Perez-Martinez, L., Felix, M. L., Portillo, A., Blanco, J. R., *et al.* (2006). Prevalence of *Rickettsia felis* in *Ctenocephalides felis* and *Ctenocephalides canis* from Uruguay. *Ann. NY Acad. Sci.*, **1078**: 305–308.

Zavala-Velazquez, J., Laviada-Molina, H., Zavala-Castro, J., *et al.* (2006). *Rickettsia felis*, the agent of an emerging infectious disease: Report of a new case in Mexico. *Arch. Med. Res.*, **37**: 419–22.

Zavala-Velazquez, J. E., Ruiz-Sosa, J. A., *et al.* (2000). *Rickettsia felis* rickettsiosis in Yucatan. *Lancet*, **356**: 1079–80.

Znazen, A. and Raoult, D. (2007). Flea-Borne Spotted Fever. In: D. Raoult and P. Parala (eds.) *Rickettsial Diseases*, pp. 87–96. New York: Informa Health Care.

CHAPTER 12

Epidemic and murine typhus

Emmanouil Angelakis and Didier Raoult

Summary

Epidemic typhus is now a rare disease, but previously it was worldwide in distribution. Typically epidemic typhus occurred during instances in which humans were forced to live in crowded, cold, and unhygienic conditions (e.g. aboard ships, in jails, and during military operations). Until recently man was considered to be the only reservoir for *R.prowazekii*, but in 1975, a new sylvatic cycle involving the flying squirrel and its ectoparasites was discovered in the eastern USA.

Murine typhus occurs throughout the world. Its epidemiology is primarily linked to the distribution of rats and the rat flea, *Xenopsylla cheopis*. However, recently both a new reservoir (opossums in southern California) and a new potential vector (the cat flea) have been discovered.

Control or avoidance of the vectors are the cornerstones of strategies to prevent morbidity and mortality.

Introduction

Bacteria of the order *Rickettsiales* were first described as short Gram-negative bacillary microorganisms that retained basic fuchsin when stained by the method of Gimenez and grew in association with eukaryotic cells (Raoult and Roux 1997). In 1993, *Rickettsiales* was divided into three families, namely, *Rickettsiaceae*, *Bartonellaceae*, and *Anaplasmataceae* (Raoult and Roux 1997). To date the *Rickettsia* genus is currently made of 24 recognized species, and also contains several dozens of as yet uncharacterized strains or tick amplicons (Fournier and Raoult 2007). These 24 species are classified into three groups:

- Includes *Rickettsia bellii*.
- The typhus group, which includes the agent of the louse-borne epidemic typhus, *Rickettsia prowazekii*, and the agent of the flea-borne murine typhus, *R. typhi*.
- The spotted fever group (SFG), whose members are associated mainly with ticks, but also with fleas and mites (Fournier and Raoult 2007).

Epidemic typhus

History

The life-threatening louse-borne epidemic typhus, also named 'jail fever', is caused by a *Rickettsia* of the typhus group, *R. prowazekii*, with the human body louse as vector. The first description of epidemic typhus was in the sixteenth century in the Mediterranean area and the name typhus was first used in 1760 (Andersson and Andersson 2000). From the sixteenth century until the Second World War, the disease is mentioned to afflict each army moving up through Europe caused by the low hygienic conditions which normally exist during wars. It is estimated that 30 million cases occurred in the Soviet Union and Eastern Europe between 1918 and 1922, with an estimated 3 million deaths (Saah 1995). After the Second World War, foci of the disease remained restricted to the cooler mountainous countries of Africa and epidemic typhus was considered a disease of the past (Parola and Raoult 2006). However, cases of epidemic typhus are still reported in situations of poverty, lack of hygiene (Mokrani *et al.* 2004; Zanetti *et al.* 1998), and among homeless people who are particularly exposed to ectoparasites—they often present with the hallmarks of epidemic typhus and relapsing fever (Badiaga *et al.* 2005).

Agent

R. prowazekii belongs to the alpha subgroup of *Proteobacteria* and is short (0.8–2 μm long and 0.3–0.5 μm diameter), Gram-negative bacillary organism, classified as a category B bioterrorism agent. The genome of *R. prowazekii* (1.1 Mb) consists of a single circular chromosome (Andersson *et al.* 1998), contains a high proportion of non-coding DNA (24%) (Andersson *et al.*1998). *R. prowazekii* is related antigenically to *R. typhi* (Baxter 1996).

Epidemiology

The disease is transmitted by the body louse (*Pediculus humanus corporis*) which lives in clothes (Gross 1996) (Fig. 12.1) but *R. prowazekii* has been also found in African-*Hyalomma* ticks (Reiss-Gutfreund 1966), *Amblyomma* ticks from Mexico (Medina-Sanchez *et al.* 2005) and in flying squirrels (Bozeman *et al.* 1975). Lice live in clothing and their prevalence is determined by the weather, humidity, poverty, and lack of hygiene. As a result, *R. prowazekii* is transmitted to people when the infected faeces of lice contaminate their feeding sites or when conjunctivae or mucous membranes are exposed to the crushed bodies or faeces of infected lice. Infected lice usually die within 1 to 3 weeks due to obstruction of the alimentary tract and do not transmit the organism to their offspring. Transmission might also result from the inhalation of infected faeces and this is thought to be the main route of infection for health workers attending patients (Parola and Raoult 2006).

Infection through aerosols of faeces-infected dust has been reported and provides the main risk of contraction of typhus for the physicians who are in contact with the patients infected with the infected lice (Houhamdi and Raoult 2007).

Hosts

Human pathogenesis-genetics

After inoculation, *R. prowazekii* spreads throughout the body via the bloodstream and enters the endothelial cells of capillaries and small blood vessels producing vasculitis usually in the skin, heart, central nervous system, skeletal muscle, and kidneys (Baxter 1996). In severe cases, endothelial damage results in permeability changes and the passage of plasma and plasma proteins from the intravascular compartments to the interstitium. As a result, tissue biopsy reveals perivascular infiltration with lymphocytes, plasma cells, polymorphonuclear leukocytes, and histiocytes, with or without necrosis of the vessel (Houhamdi and Raoult 2007).

Clinical manifestations

Epidemic typhus occurs in two clinical forms: the primary febrile illness and recrudescent infection (Brill-Zinsser disease). The primary febrile illness has an incubation period from 10 to 14 days. Most patients develop malaise and vague symptoms before the abrupt onset of nonspecific symptoms of high fever (100%), headaches (100%), and severe myalgias (70–100%) (Parola and Raoult 2006). In a recent investigation in Burundi, a crouching attitude due to myalgia, named 'sutama', was reported (Houhamdi and Raoult 2007). A petechial rash may appear in 20% to 60% of cases (Parola and Raoult 2006). In Africa the rash is observed more rarely (20 to 40%) (Perine *et al.* 1992). Typically, the rash begins in the axillary folds and upper trunk on about the fifth day of illness and spreads to the extremities. The rash initially appears as non-confluent erythematous macules that blanch on pressure, but after several days becomes maculopapular and petechial, affecting the trunk and extremities and sparing the face, palms, and soles (Baxter 1996). Other manifestations include nausea or vomiting (42%–56%) and coughing-pneumonia (38%–70%) (Parola and Raoult 2006). Many patients manifest various abnormalities of the central nervous system (CNS), ranging from confusion to stupor (18%–80%), drowsiness, hearing loss, and coma (4%) (Parola and Raoult 2006).

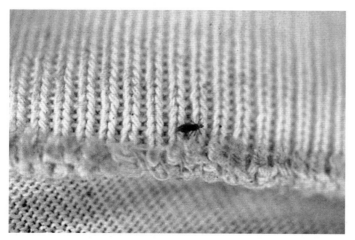

Fig. 12.1 Body louse in clothes

Myocarditis, pulmonary involvement, mild thrombocytopenia, jaundice, and abnormal liver function test may occur in severe cases. In uncomplicated epidemic typhus, fever usually resolves after 2 weeks of illness if untreated, but recovery usually takes 2 to 3 months (Baxter 1996). Without treatment, the disease is fatal in 13 to 30% of the cases (Raoult and Roux 1997).

People who survive epidemic typhus remain infected with *R. prowazekii* for life and under conditions of stress or of a waning immune system may experience a recrudescence, known as Brill-Zinsser disease. Brill-Zinsser disease is generally milder but the patients may become the source of a new epidemic if they become infected with body lice (Weissmann 2005). Patients with Brill-Zinsser has a fatality rate of 1.5% (Houhamdi and Raoult 2007).

Diagnosis

Careful clinical examination and epidemiologic investigation of patients with potential rickettsioses is critical. Typical findings of epidemic typhus such as fever, headaches and skin rash in patients infected with body louse or in persons who are living in poverty and lack of hygiene, can suggest the diagnosis. Thrombocytopenia and an increase of the hepatic enzymes may be observed particularly in severe cases.

Direct diagnosis

As with other rickettsial diseases the diagnosis of epidemic typhus can be confirmed by culture on to shell vials containing human embryonic lung (HEL) fibroblasts grown on coverslips, in a biosafety level 3 containment laboratory (Birg *et al.* 1999). Immuno-detection, in blood or other tissues, allows the confirmation of infection in patients before their seroconversion and thus permits early prescription of specific treatment. *R. prowazekii* can be detected by PCR amplification from an array of samples that include eschars, paraffin-embedded tissues, slide-fixed specimens, peripheral blood mononuclear cells, and arthropod tissues (Parola and Raoult 2006). If PCR-based diagnosis is delayed for more than 24 hours, the samples should be stored at –20°C or lower. Blood should be collected before antimicrobial therapy either in a citrate-containing vial for culture or in EDTA. Recently a nested PCR assay, 2.2 times more sensitive than culture and 1.5 times more sensitive than regular PCR using single-use primers targeting single-use gene fragments present in the genomes of *R. prowazekii*, was proposed by our laboratory and named 'suicide' PCR (Fournier and Raoult 2004).

Indirect diagnosis

The Weil-Felix test is the oldest serological assay for rickettsioses test but it has poor sensitivity and specificity (Ormsbee *et al.* 1977). Patients with Brill-Zinsser disease usually have no agglutinating antibodies detectable by the Weil-Felix test (La Scola and Raoult 1997). The rickettsial IFA adapted to a micromethod format is the test of choice for the serodiagnosis of rickettsial diseases. The diagnosis of recent epidemic typhus can be established by demonstrating a fourfold or greater rise in titer of antibody in acute and convalescent serum samples (Houhamdi and Raoult 2007). However, *R. prowazekii*'s antibodies cross-react with those of *R. typhi* and their differentiation is difficult by serology (Raoult and Roux 1997). As a result epidemic and murine typhus cannot be differentiated by serology. Cross-adsorption followed by IFA and Western blotting can increase the identification of the etiological agent but the high costs of such studies limit their use (La Scola *et al.* 2000).

Enzyme-linked immunosorbent assay (ELISA) has been introduced for detection of *R. prowazekii* antibodies. The use of this technique is highly sensitive and reproducible, allowing the differentiation of IgG and IgM antibodies (La Scola and Raoult 1997).

Lice

Lice may be tested by molecular biology and used as an epidemiologic tool. Lice are easy to collect and to transport to reference laboratories where suitable molecular biological approaches can be used. For example, *R. prowazekii* detected in lice collected from refugees in Burundi was sent to our laboratory in Marseille to confirm the presence of epidemic typhus (Roux and Raoult 1999).

Treatment

Antimicrobial susceptibility

Cells models presented the efficacy of chloramphenicol, tetracycline, doxycycline, minocycline, and rifampin against *R. prowazekii* (Raoult and Drancourt 1991). Erythromycin, rifampin and the new ketolide, telithromycin were also effective (Rolain 2007). However, new quinolones were found only to be moderately active and beta-lactams and aminoglycosides were not effective (Raoult and Drancourt 1991).

Antibiotic therapy

Because antibiotic therapy does not eradicate rickettsia in lice-infested patients, delousing is essential in the management of a typhus outbreak. If appropriate treatment is begun promptly, complications, including mortality, can be avoided in most cases. Doxycycline remains the treatment of choice for epidemic typhus. A single dose of oral doxycycline 200 mg usually leads to defervescence within 48 to 72 hours in most cases. Chloramphenicol is widely used as an empirical treatment in places where diagnostic facilities are unavailable but it can be also administered in cases of allergy to tetracyclines. Fluoroquinolones should be avoided for the treatment of epidemic typhus as a patient who, misdiagnosed as having typhoid, died from typhus after treatment with ciprofloxacin (Houhamdi and Raoult 2007). Finally, co-trimoxazole is reported to be ineffective for the treatment of epidemic typhus (Huys *et al.* 1973). Table 12.1 presents the guidelines for the treatment of epidemic typhus.

Prevention

Prevention efforts aimed at reducing conditions associated with contact with the human body louse and at minimizing the risk of arthropod bites should be taken. These measures include regular bathing and washing of clothes and the use of long-acting insecticides. Dusting of all clothing with 10% DDT, 1% malathion, or 1% permethrin is a rapid and effective method of killing body lice and reduces the risk of reinfestation (Raoult and Roux 1999). Doxycycline as chemoprophylaxis to visitors at high risk areas can also provide protection. Vaccines using crude antigen and/or inactivated rickettsia are partially protective against epidemic typhus but have been accompanied with undesirable toxic reactions and difficulties in standardization (Coker *et al.* 2003).

Murine typhus

History

Murine typhus (also called endemic typhus) is caused by *R. typhi* (formely *R. mooseri*). It is classified as a typhus-group rickettsia,

transmitted by fleas and has rodents as its main reservoirs. The disease was probably reported in Mexico in 1570 by Bravo (Parola and Raoult 2006). Paullin made the first clinical description of a 'milder form of typhus' without mortality in 1913 in Atlanta (Tselentis and Gikas 2007). In 1917, Neil noted that male guinea pigs inoculated with the blood of typhus patients in south Texas often developed a scrotal swelling and inflammation, along with haemorrhage beneath the tunica, similar to the lesions elicited by *R. rickettsii* (Tselentis and Gikas 2007). His results confirmed in 1928 by Mooser, showed that the American and European variety could be clearly differentiated by their reactions in the guinea pigs (Tselentis and Gikas 2007). These studies contributed in distinguishing the endemic from the classic typhus. In 1923, in the Annual Reports of the Department of Health of Palestine, there was a reference to a mild course of typhus fever, similar to Brill's disease and different from the classic form of typhus (Tselentis and Gikas 2007). In 1925, an outbreak of 200 cases of endemic typhus occurred in Australia. Plazy, Marcandier, and Pirot observed the first Mediterranean cases of murine typhus on sailors on the warships of Toulon (Tselentis and Gikas 2007). In the period 1931–1946 in the USA, 42,000 cases were reported. Late reports established the worldwide distribution of endemic typhus. In 1940, Lewthwaite and Savoor reiterated the important distinction between the *Xenopsylla cheopsis* borne murine typhus ('shop typhus') and the chigger-borne scrub typhus ('tsutsugmushi' or 'rural typhus') (Lewthwaite 1952).

Agent

R. typhi is a small (0.4 × 1.3 μm), Gram-negative, obligate intracellular bacterium which belongs to the alpha subgroup of *Proteobacteria*. The genome of *R. typhi* (1,111,496 bp) is nearly identical to its close relative *R. prowazekii* and highly similar to *R. conorii* and other spotted fever group *Rickettsia*. A 12-kb insertion in the genome of *R. prowazekii*, a large inversion close to the origin of replication with no loss of genes in the region, several pseudogenes for which functional homologs are found in *R. prowazekii* and the fact that *R. typhi* has lost the complete cytochrome *c* oxi-

Table 12.1 Guidelines for the treatment of Epidemic and Murine typhus

Clinical feature	Patient cohort	Treatment	Duration
Epidemic typhus	Adults	doxycycline, 200 mg/day	7–15 days
		chloramphenicol, 2 g/day	7–15 days
	Children	chloramphenicol, 150 mg/kg/day	5 days
Murine typhus	Adults	doxycycline, 200 mg/day	7–15 days
		chloramphenicol, 2 g/day	7–15 days
	Children	chloramphenicol, 150 mg/kg/day	5 days

dase system are some of the few differences between the two rickettsiae (McLeod *et al.* 2004).

Epidemiology

Murine typhus is one of the most prevalent rickettsial diseases. *R. typhi* strains have a worldwide distribution, but the number of reported cases does not reflect the current prevalence. The disease occurs on every continent except Antarctica, in a variety of environments, ranging from hot and humid to cold and montane or semi-arid (Traub and Wisseman 1978). Cases are regularly documented in the USA, Mexico, and Europe. Murine typhus have also been reported in tourists returning from countries including China, Indonesia, India, Morocco, Canaries Isles, Africa, Malaysia, Southeast Asia, and Thailand (Parola and Raoult 2006). Recently, murine typhus, which had never been reported in Japan since the 1950s, re-emerged in that country (Parola and Raoult 2006). Although murine typhus is most prevalent in warmer countries, the fact that the disease is mild and non-specific suggests that its incidence is probably largely unrecognized or misdiagnosed in these.

The rat flea *X. cheopis* and the rat louse (*Polyplax spinulosa*) are the principal vectors of murine typhus (Azad *et al.* 1997). Occasionally, other flea species or arthropods vectors have been reported to transmit *R. typhi*, including the cat flea *Ctenocephalides felis*, the mouse flea *Leptopsyllia segnis,* and lice, mites, and ticks (Boostrom *et al.* 2002). The fleas remain infected for life, but neither their lifespan nor their reproductive activity are affected (Tselentis and Gikas 2007). Rats belonging to the subgenus *Rattus*, mainly *R. norvegicus* and *R. rattus* are the primary reservoirs (Azad 1990) and the widespread distribution of murine typhus in many coastal areas is attributed to the introduction of infected rats and their fleas from ships. However, various rodents and other wild and domestic animals, such as house mice, cats, opossums, shrews, and skunks can also act occasionally as hosts (Azad 1990). The classical cycle of infection is rat-to-rat flea after a rickettsemic blood meal from an infected rat. Beside the classical cycle of infection, *R. typhi* is rarely transmitted transovarially from flea to uninfected flea (Azad 1990). Rickettsiae can persist into the flea faeces for several years and they infect humans by feeding or more rarely via inhalation or contamination of the conjuctiva (Azad 1990).

Hosts

Human pathogenesis

Infection of endothelial cells lining vessel walls, and the resultant vascular inflammation and haemostatic alterations are salient pathogenetic features of *R. typhi* (Walker *et al.* 1989). In fatal cases, organ damage secondary to vasculitis has been described in the lungs, kidneys, myocardium, brain, and liver parenchyma. Interstitial myocarditis is believed to be a major risk factor for death in these patients (Baxter 1996). Obliterative thrombovasculitis and perivascular nodules of the skin at autopsy resemble lesions of murine typhus. Widespread infection of the hepatic sinusoidal lining cells and the endothelium of vessels in portal regions results in injury to adjacent hepatocytes and may cause localized symptoms or liver function abnormalities (Baxter 1996).

Clinical manifestations

The disease is usually mild with a group of symptoms that is shared with an array of other infectious diseases, including several bacterial and viral infections. As a result, many cases of murine typhus can be overlooked without a laboratory-confirmed diagnosis (WHO Working Group on Rickettsial Diseases 1982). Usually, after an incubation period of 6 to 14 days, patients with scrub typhus usually present an abrupt onset of symptoms like fever, rash, cough, headaches, maculopapular exanthema on the trunk to the half patients, chills, as well as with myalgias and hepatomegaly (Raoult and Roux 1997). Less common manifestations of murine typhus are lymphadenopathy (4%) (Gikas *et al.* 2002), splenomegaly (5%) (Silpapojakul *et al.* 1993). The rash is non-specific and its reported prevalence varies from 20% of patients from Thailand, 38% of patients from Laos, 49% of patients from Texas and 80% of patients from Greece (Silpapojakul *et al.* 1993; Phongmany *et al.* 2006; Gikas *et al.* 2002; Whiteford *et al.* 2001). Most cases of murine typhus are mild, and signs in untreated patients last for 7 to 14 days, when there is usually a rapid return to health, but aseptic meningitis, deafness, deep venous thrombosis, and even death have been reported with a fatality rate which may be as high as 4% (Dumler *et al.* 1991).

Diagnosis

Murine typhus should be considered for patients from places with high rat populations such as tropical countries, but also from northern countries late in summer or early in autumn. As a result murine typhus should be considered in patients with prolonged fever and rash with or without lymphadenopathy during the summer or early autumn months (Koliou *et al.* 2007; Nogueras *et al.* 2006).

Direct diagnosis

During recent years, the development of cell culture systems for viral isolation has led to an increase in the number of laboratories suitably equipped to isolate rickettsiae. Murine typhus can be confirmed by culture onto shell vials containing Vero or L929 cells (La Scola and Raoult 1997). Detection of rickettsiae by using immunofluorescence allows the confirmation of infection in patients prior to their seroconversion. *R. typhi* has successfully been detected in the organs of a patient with a fatal case of murine typhus. Biopsy specimens of the skin with a rash around the lesion and preferably petechial lesions are the most common samples used for digital immunodetection (La Scola and Raoult 1997). PCR and sequencing methods are useful, sensitive, and rapid tools to detect and identify rickettsiae in blood and skin biopsies. Four genes have been proposed for use in the identification of rickettsia, namely, those encoding 16S rDNA, a protein of 17 kDa, citrate synthase, and OmpB (La Scola and Raoult 1997).

Indirect diagnosis

Because specific antibodies are frequently absent during the acute illness, serologic diagnosis can be made by obtaining acute and convalescent serum during the acute illness, serologic diagnosis can be made by obtaining acute and convalescent serum for specific rickettsial antibodies. The rickettsial IFA adapted to a micromethod format is the reference method for serodiagnosis of *R. typhi* in most laboratories. The micro-IFA has the advantage that it can simultaneously detect antibodies to a number of rickettsial antigens (up to nine antigens) with the same drop of serum in a single well containing multiple rickettsial antigen dots. An immunoperoxidase assay has been developed as an alternative to IFA *R. typhi*. The procedure is the same as IFA, but fluorescein is replaced by peroxidase (La

Scola and Raoult 1997). The advantage of the immunoperoxidase assay is that the results can be read with an ordinary light microscope. In addition, the immunoperoxidase assay provides a permanent slide record. Cross-absorption studies are useful, especially if complemented by Western blotting. This is the case for typhus because in 50% of patients, the sera had the same level of antibodies to both *R. prowazekii* and *R. typhi* (Schriefer *et al.* 1994).

Enzyme-linked immunosorbent assay (ELISA) has also been introduced for the detection of antibodies against *R. typhi*. The use of this technique is highly sensitive and reproducible, allowing the differentiation of IgG and IgM antibodies (La Scola and Raoult 1997).

Treatment

Antimicrobial susceptibility

Fibroblasts and Vero cells have been used for the determination of the antibiotic susceptibility *R. typhi in vitro* testing. Chloramphenicol, tetracycline, doxycycline, minocycline, and rifampin were effective against *R. typhi* (Raoult and Drancourt 1991). *R. typhi* was also found to be susceptible to erythromycin, rifampin and the new ketolide, telithromycin (Rolain 2007). New quinolones were found to be moderately active when beta-lactams and aminoglycosides were not effective (Raoult and Drancourt 1991).

Antibiotic therapy

Complete clinical recovery is observed over a period of 15 days from initiation of symptoms, even in untreated murine typhus. Infection confers long-lasting immunity to reinfection (Tselentis and Gikas 2007). Doxycycline 200 mg/day is the recommended treatment for murine typhus and a single dose of oral doxycycline 200 mg usually leads to defervescence within 48 to 72 hours in most cases. However, of 7–15 day course is recommended. In patients with severe hypersensitivity to the tetracyclines, 2 gm per day of chloramphenicol has been considered an alternate therapy, but its use is limited by side effects. Chloramphenicol is the drug of choice for pregnant patients, except for the parturient, due to the danger of gray syndrome to the infant (Tselentis and Gikas 2007). Chloramphenicol relapses have been reported in patients with murine typhus (Shaked *et al.* 1989).

Prevention

The control of the flea vector and mammalian reservoirs of infection is the main step for the prevention of murine typhus. As a result, the reduction of rat populations and the insecticide dusting campaigns has decreased the incidence of murine typhus. No effective vaccine is available for murine typhus but recovery from natural infection confers long-lasting immunity to reinfection (Baxter 1996).

References

Andersson, J. O. and Andersson, S. G. E. (2000). A century of typhus, lice and *Rickettsia. Res. Microbiol.*, **151:** 143–50.

Andersson, S. G. E., Zomorodipour, A., Andersson, J. O. *et al.* (1998). The genome sequence of *Rickettsia prowazekii* and the origin of mitochondria. *Nature*, **396:** 133–40.

Azad, A. F. (1990). Epidemiology of murine typhus. *Ann. Rev. Entomol.*, **35:** 553–69.

Azad, A. F., Radulovic, S., Higgins, J. A., Noden, B. H., and Troyer, J. M. (1997). Flea-borne rickettsioses: ecologic considerations. *Emerg. Infect. Dis.*, **3:** 319–27.

Badiaga, S., Brouqui, P., and Raoult, D. (2005). Autochthonous epidemic typhus associated with Bartonella quintana bacteremia in a homeless person. *Am. J. Trop. Med. Hyg.*, **72:** 638–39.

Baxter, J. D. (1996). The typhus group. *Clinics in Dermatology*, **14:** 271–78.

Birg, M. L., La Scola, B., Roux, V., Brouqui, P., and Raoult, D. (1999). Isolation of *Rickettsia prowazekii* from blood by shell vial cell culture. *J. Clin. Microbiol.*, **37:** 3722–24.

Boostrom, A., Beier, M. S., Macaluso, J. A. *et al.* (2002). Geographic association of Rickettsia felis-infected opossums with human murine typhus, Texas. *Emerg. Infect. Dis.*, **8:** 549–54.

Bozeman, F. M., Masiello, S. A., Williams, M. S., and Elisberg, B. L. (1975). Epidemic typhus rickettsiae isolated from flying squirrels. *Nature*, **255:** 545–47.

Coker, C., Majid, M., and Radulovic, S. (2003). Development of *Rickettsia prowazekii* DNA vaccine: cloning strategies. *Ann. NY Acad. Sci.*, **990:** 757–64.

Dumler, J. S., Taylor, J. P., and Walker, D. H. (1991). Clinical and laboratory features of Murine Typhus in South Texas, 1980 through 1987. *JAMA*, **266:** 1365–70.

Fournier, P. E. and Raoult, D. (2007). Bacteriology, Taxonomy, and Phylogeny of *Rickettsia*. In: D. Raoult and P. Parala (eds.) *Rickettsial Diseases*, pp. 1–13. New York: Informa Health Care.

Fournier, P. E. and Raoult, D. (2004). Suicide PCR on skin biopsy specimens for diagnosis of rickettsioses. *J. Clin. Microbiol.*, **42:** 3428–34.

Gikas, A., Doukakis, S., Pediaditis, J., Kastanakis, S., Psaroulaki, A., *et al.* (2002). Murine typhus in Greece: epidemiological, clinical, and therapeutic data from 83 cases. *Trans. R. Soc. Trop. Med. Hyg.*, **96:** 250–53.

Gross, L. (1996). How Charles Nicolle of the Pasteur Institute discovered that epidemic typhus is transmitted by lice: Reminiscences from my years at the Pasteur Institute in Paris. *Proc. Nat. Acad. Sci. USA*, **93:** 10539–40.

Houhamdi, L. and Raoult, D. (2007). Louse-Borne Epidemic Typhus. In: D. Raoult and P. Parala (eds.) *Rickettsial Diseases*, pp. 51–61. New York: Informa Health Care.

Huys, J., Freyens, P., Kayihigi, J., and Van den Berghe, G. (1973). Treatment of epidemic typhus. A comparative study of chloramphenicol, trimethoprim-sulphamethoxazole and doxycycline. *Trans. R. Soc. Trop. Med. Hyg.*, **67:** 718–21.

Koliou, M., Psaroulaki, A., Georgiou, C., Ioannou, I., Tselentis, Y., *et al.* (2007). Murine typhus in Cyprus: 21 paediatric cases. *Eur. J. Clin. Microbiol. Infect. Dis.*, **26:** 491–93.

La Scola, B. and Raoult, D. (1997). Laboratory diagnosis of rickettsioses: current approaches to the diagnosis of old and new rickettsial diseases. *J. Clin. Microbiol.*, **35:** 2715–27.

La Scola, B., Rydkina, L., Ndihokubwayo, J. B., Vene, S., and Raoult, D. (2000). Serological differentiation of murine typhus and epidemic typhus using cross-adsorption and western blotting. *Clin. Diag. Lab. Immunol.*, **7:** 612–16.

Lewthwaite, R. (1952). The typhus group of fevers. *BMJ*, **2:** 826–28.

McLeod, M. P., Qin, X., Karpathy, S. E., *et al.* (2004). Complete genome sequence of *Rickettsia typhi* and comparison with sequences of other rickettsiae. *J. Bacteriol.*, **186:** 5842–55.

Medina-Sanchez, A., Bouyer, D. H., Cantara-Rodriguez, V., *et al.* (2005). Detection of a typhus group *Rickettsia* in *Amblyomma* ticks in the state of Nuevo Leon, Mexico. *Ann. NY Acad. Sci.*, **1063:** 327–32.

Mokrani, K., Fournier, P. E., Dalichaouche, M., Tebbal, S., Aouati, A., *et al.* (2004). Reemerging threat of epidemic typhus in Algeria, *J. Clin. Microbiol.*, **42:** 3898–3900.

Nogueras, M. M., Cardenosa, N., Sanfeliu, I., Munoz, T., Font, B., *et al.* (2006). Evidence of infection in humans with *Rickettsia typhi* and *Rickettsia felis* in Catalonia in the Northeast of Spain. *Ann. NY Acad. Sci.*, **1078:** 159–61.

Ormsbee, R., Peacock, M., Philip, R., *et al.* (1977). Serologic diagnosis of epidemic typhus fever. *Am. J. Epidemiol.*, **105:** 261–71.

Parola, P. and Raoult, D. (2006). Tropical rickettsioses. *Clinics in Dermatol.*, **24:** 191–200.

Perine, P. L., Chandler, B. P., Krause, D. K., *et al.* (1992). A clinico-epidemiological study of epidemic typhus in Africa. *Clin. Infect. Dis.*, **14:** 1149–58.

Phongmany, S., Rolain, J.M., Phetsouvanh, R., *et al.* (2006). Rickettsial infections and fever, Vientiane, Laos. *Emerg. Infect. Dis.*, **12:** 256–62.

Raoult, D. and Drancourt, M. (1991). Antimicrobial therapy of Rickettsial diseases. *Antimicrob. Agents Chemother.*, **35:** 2457–62.

Raoult, D. and Roux, V. (1997). Rickettsioses as paradigms of new or emerging infectious diseases, *Clin. Microbiol. Rev.*, **10:** 694–719.

Raoult, D. and Roux, V. (1999). The body louse as a vector of reemerging human diseases. *Clin. Infect. Dis.*, **29:** 888–911.

Reiss-Gutfreund, R. J. (1966). The isolation of *Rickettsia prowazeki* and *mooseri* from unusual sources. *Am. J. Trop. Med. Hyg.*, **15:** 943–49.

Rolain, J. M. (2007). Antimicrobial Susceptibility of Rickettsial Agents. In: D. Raoult and P. Parala (eds.) *Rickettsial Diseases*, pp. 361–69. New York: Informa Health Care.

Roux, V. and Raoult, D. (1999). Body lice as tools for the diagnosis and surveillance of reemerging diseases. *J. Clin. Microbiol.*, **37:** 596–99.

Saah, A. J. (1995). *Rickettsia prowasekii* (Epidemic or Louse-Borne Typhus). In: G. L. Mandell, J. E. Bennett, and R. Dolin (eds.) *Principles and Practice of Infectious Diseases*, pp. 1735–1736. New York: Churchill Livingstone.

Schriefer, M. E., Sacci Jr., J. B., Dumler, J. S., Bullen, M. G., and Azad, A. F. (1994). Identification of a novel rickettsial infection in a patient diagnosed with murine typhus. *J. Clin. Microbiol.*, **32:** 949–54.

Shaked, Y., Samra, Y., Maier, M. K., and Rubinstein, E. (1989). Relapse of rickettsial Mediterranean spotted fever and murine typhus after treatment with chloramphenicol. *J. Infect.*, **18:** 35–37.

Silpapojakul, K., Chayakul, P., and Krisanapan, S. (1993). Murine typhus in thailand:clinical features, diagnosis and treatment. *Quart. J. Med.*, **86:** 43–47.

Traub, R. and Wisseman, C. L. (1978). The ecology of murine typhus-a critical review. *Trop. Dis. Bull.*, **75:** 237–317.

Tselentis, Y. and Gikas, A. (2007). Murine Typhus. In: D. Raoult and P. Parala (eds.) *Rickettsial Diseases*, pp. 37–49. New York: Informa Health Care.

Walker, D. H., Parks, F. M., Betz, T. G., Taylor, J. P., and Muehlberger, J. W. (1989). Histopathology and immunohistologic demonstration of the distribution of *Rickettsia typhi* in fatal murine typhus. *Am. J. Clin. Path.*, **91:** 720–24.

Weissmann, G. (2005). Rats, lice, and Zinsser. *Emerg. Infect. Dis.*, **11:** 492–96.

Whiteford, S. F., Taylor, J. P., and Dumler, J. S. (2001). Clinical, laboratory, and epidemiologic features of murine typhus in 97 Texas children. *Arch. Pediatr. Adolesc. Med.*, **155:** 396–400.

WHO Working Group on Rickettsial Diseases (1982). Rickettsioses: a continuing disease problem. *Bull. Wor. Heal. Organ.*, **60:** 157–64.

Zanetti, G., Francioli, P., Tagan, D., Paddock, C. D., and Zaki, S. R. (1998). Imported epidemic typhus. *Lancet*, **352:** 1709.

CHAPTER 13

Scrub typhus

Emmanouil Angelakis and Didier Raoult

Summary

Bacteria of the genus *Rickettsia* are obligate intracellular rods that retain basic fuchsin when stained by the method of Gimenez. This genus has long been used as a generic term of small intracellular bacteria. However, taxonomic progress made over the last years has deeply modified the definition of 'rickettsia'. As a result, in 1995 the position of *R. tsutsugamushi* has been reclassified from the genus *Rickettsia* into a separate new genus, *Orientia* (Tamura *et al.* 1995).

Scrub typhus, also known as 'tsutsugamushi fever', occurs only in Asia and is a chigger-borne zoonoses. The disease is acute, febrile, potentially fatal and has been known for centuries in China where it was probably described as early as the fourth century BC (Parola and Raoult 2006). In recent years this infection has been re-emerging because of descriptions of strains of *O. tsutsugamushi* with reduced susceptibility to antibiotics and of the surprising interactions between scrub typhus and the human immunodeficiency virus (HIV). It is estimated that more than a million cases of scrub typhus are transmitted annually in Asia and more than a billion people are at risk (Rosenberg 1997).

History

The presence of tsutsugamushi disease and its association with chigger bites has been recognized by some of the native populations of Japan and China for centuries. The term 'akamushi', the origin of the Japanese name for this rickettsiosis, means 'red chigger'. Rural residents of these countries often knew that the best way to avoid being infected was to avoid areas infested by these arthropods (Weiss 1981; Walker 1991). Early Chinese and Japanese investigators suspected that the illness was related to small mites. In 1920 Hayashi isolated an agent from mites that he called 'Theileria tsutsugamushi'. In retrospect, this agent was not the cause of scrub typhus, but the term 'tsutsugamushi' (for 'noxious mite') has persisted. In retrospect, the first identification of the causative agent of scrub typhus was by Nagayo and co-workers in 1930 (Nagayo *et al.* 1930). They called this organism *Rickettsia orientalis* but the name was changed to *R. tsutsugamushi* in 1948 (Bengston 1948) and then to *Orientia tsutsugamushi* in 1996. Prior to Nagyo's isolation of *O. tsutsugamushi,* investigators working with what is now Malaysia used epidemiological data to classify locally occurring disease into urban (or 'shop') typhus or rural typhus. Rural typhus,

which occurred predominately in grass or shrub land, later came to be called scrub typhus by the British and Amercians during the Second World War. The term scrub typhus is now used throughout the world except Japan where the name 'tsutsugamushi disease' is preferred. However, other symptoms have also been used, including chigger-borne rickettsioses, Kedani (hairy mite) fever, akamushi (red mite) fever, flood fever, Japanese river fever, and tropical typhus.

The interest of physicians and scientists in this disease increased during the Second World War, when more than 15,000 cases of infection were diagnosed among the allied forces, with a mortality rate varying from 1 to 35% (Weiss 1981). However, the disease cannot be associated with war conditions or natural disasters as is the case with epidemic typhus. The high incidence of scrub typhus during the Second World War and, to a lesser extent during the Vietnam War, can be ascribed to the fact that, during military field operations, larger numbers of non-immune individuals were introduced into ecological niches inhabited by trombidulid mites. Therefore, scrub typhus should not be directly associated to the lack of hygiene and health care, which are characteristic features of war conditions. The term 'scrub' typhus was adopted because it was thought that the vectors were mainly found on scrub vegetation.

Although the high incidence of scrub typhus among the allied troops may be partly due to false-positive serologiclal results, its occurrence led to a better description of the epidemiology and clinical features of the disease, and to the introduction of appropriate treatments. The disease shares common features with epidemic typhus, for example fever, headache, and rash, but the presence of an eschar and generalized lymphadenopathies is distinctive of scrub typhus.

In 1982, the WHO pointed out that, based on specific serological tests, a high proportion of fevers of unknown origin in endemic areas were probably undiagnosed scrub typhus cases even though the characteristic clinical signs, fever, eschar and adenopathies, are often lacking (Groupe de travail OMS 1982). In 1993, a WHO meeting on global surveillance of rickettsial disease reported that, if the amount of epidemiological data collected on rickettsioses was considered rather inadequate in developing countries, then the information on scrub typhus was downright non-existent (WHO 1993). Emergence of scrub typhus has recently been observed in Australia and Japan, proving that endemic foci of the disease persist and that the disease should not be underestimated (Yamshita *et al.* 1988, 1994; Currie *et al.* 1993).

Agent

O. tsutsugamushi is an obligate intracellular Gram-negative bacterium that has a different cell wall structure and genetic make-up from those of rickettsiae. Compared to other species belonging to the genus *Rickettsia*, *O. tsutsugamushi* presents a lack of peptidoglycan and lipopolysaccharide (Ohashi *et al.* 1990) that make a thicker outer leaflet of the cell wall (Silverman *et al.* 1978). This difference makes the bacteria very soft, fragile and more resistant to growth in penicillin (Miyamura *et al.* 1989). *Orientia* has also a unique profile of antigenic variation and this heterogeneity among strains is greater than that encountered in other Rickettsiales. *O. tsutsugamushi* has a variable 56-kDa protein as a major surface protein antigen, which accounts for 10 to 15% of its total protein. As a result there are three classical antigenically distinct prototype strains of *O. tsutsugamushi*, (Karp, Kato and Gilliam) isolated from New Guinea, Japan, and Burma respectively (Chattopadhyay and Richards 2007). However, other strain types have been found in Thailand and it has also reported that Shimokoshi, Kawasaki, and Kuroki strains, which were isolated from patients in Japan, were antigenically distinguishable from the prototype strains of Gilliam, Karp, and Kato (Tamura *et al.* 1999). This antigenic variation depends largely on the diversities of the immunodominant 56-kDa type-specific antigen located on the surface of this microorganism.

Recently, the complete genome of *O.tsutsugamushi* strain Boryong was sequenced by Cho *et al.* (2007) which is a single circular chromosome consisting of 2,127,051 bp with an average G+C content of 30.5%. The genome size and estimated number of genes are the largest among the currently sequenced genomes in the order *Rickettsiales*. The repeat density of the scrub typhus pathogen is 200-fold higher than that of its close relative *R. prowazekii*, the agent of epidemic typhus. A total of 359 *tra* genes for components of conjugative type IV secretion systems were identified at 79 sites in the genome. A unique feature is the presence of 4,197 identical repeats >200 bp, which represents 37.1% of the *O. tsutsugamushi* genome. Additionally, the *O. tsutsugamushi* genome contains >400 transposases, 60 phage integrases, and 70 reverse transcriptases.

Epidemiology

Scrub typhus and is one of the most common infectious diseases of rural south, south-eastern Asia and the western Pacific. The endemic region of scrub typhus is often referred as the 'tsutsugamushi triangle' bounded to the north by Siberia and the Kamchatka Peninsula, to the south by Australia, to the east by Japan and to the west by Afghanistan and India (Fig. 13.1). Endemic areas range from typical tropical secondary growth (scrub) vegetation to temperate zones and even the Himalayas (Jensenius *et al.* 2004).

The disease is transmitted by the bites of larval trombiculid mites (chiggers) of the genus *Leptotrombidium* which live in forests and areas with tall grass. These mites only feed on mammalian tissue fluid once in their lifetime and constitute the reservoir of infection through transovarial transmission. Chiggers usually feed on rats but may readily bite humans on any part of the body and feed for 2 to 10 days. Several species can act as vectors, which are also known as reservoirs of the disease with *Leptotrombidium* deliense to be the

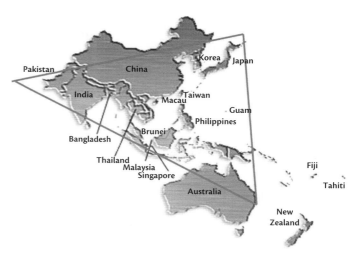

Fig. 13.1 The tsutsugamushi triangle

most important vector species in Southeast Asia and southern China, whereas *L. akamushi*, *L. scutellare* and *L. pallidum* are main vectors in Korea and Japan and *L. chiangraiensis* was found in cultivated rice fields in Thailand (Watt and Kantipong 2007).

Humans usually become infected when they accidentally encroach on a zone in which there are infected chiggers. That is the reason that disease transmission has been reported in suburban area during clearing of land, logging, and road building, when residents of city centers are not at risk. The transmission depends on the seasonal activities of both chiggers and humans with most scrub typhus cases occurring during the rice-planting and rice-harvesting seasons, although infected chiggers and rodents can be found in rice fields all through the year (Watt and Kantipong 2007). Co-infection by leptospirosis and scrub typhus is also possible and rice farmers in north-eastern Thailand are commonly infected with both diseases (Watt and Parola 2003). Military personnel are also at risk and it is estimated that during the Second World War, there were 18,000 cases of scrub typhus and during the Vietnam war, the ratio was one case of scrub typhus to 50 to 100 cases of malaria (Baxter 1996; Bavaro *et al.* 2005). Travellers visiting rural areas in order to engage in activities like camping, trekking, or rafting may be also in danger. Since 1986 about 20 cases of travel-associated scrub typhus have been reported to people returning from scrub typhus endemic areas and mainly from Thailand (Jensenius *et al.* 2004).

The disease

Pathogenesis—clinical manifestations

Much remains to be learned about the pathogenesis of scrub typhus. Several recent investigations have focused on the survival of *O. tsutsugamushi* in the intracellular milieu and on the host response to infection. *O. tsutsugamushi* invades host cells by induced phagocytosis and escapes from the phagosome to the cytosol (Watt and Kantipong 2007). The bacteria can induce apoptosis in a variety of host cells, including lymphocytes and endothelial cells by retarding the release of intracellular calcium (Watt and Parola 2003). Moreover in murine macrophages, *O. tsutsugamushi* produces inflammatory cytokines tumour necrosis factor (TNF)-alpha and interleukin-6. TNF-α production appears to be inhibited by the production of interleukin-10 (Watt and Kantipong 2007).

O. tsutsugamushi disseminates from the skin to target organs, and the bacteria can be demonstrated in peripheral white blood cells taken from patients presenting to hospital with acute scrub typhus (Watt and Parola 2003). *O. tsutsugamushi* produces vasculitis and perivasculitis of the small blood vessels of the skin, lungs, heart and brain. Endovasculitis and focal haemorrhage may be present but less prominent than in Rocky Mountain spotted fever and epidemic typhus (Watt and Kantipong 2007). The basic histopathological lesions, disseminated perivasculitis, and focal interstitial mononuclear infiltrations associated with oedema suggest that macrophages are a more important target cell than the endothelium (Watt and Kantipong 2007).

The onset of symptoms occurs usually 7 to 10 days after the chiggers bite and is usually abrupt, with fever, a drainage lymphadenopathy, chills, myalgia, a macular or maculopapular eruption, and headache. Rash, gastrointestinal manifestations, cough, and other respiratory symptoms are also frequent (Parola and Raoult 2006). In a recent study from Laos scrub typhus was the most common rickettsiosis identified and the patients presented with fever, headache, nausea, myalgia, lymphadenopathy, and a palpable liver (Phongmany *et al.* 2006). Moreover, in a review of 87 American soldiers who were infected with scrub typhus in South Vietnam, all were reported to have fever, headache, and anorexia (Berman and Kundin 1973). Other symptoms were chills (80%), cough (45%), myalgia (32%), and nausea (28%). The most common physical finding was generalized lymphadenopathy (85%), and an eschar was found in 46% of these. The eschar is primarily detected in males but it may be absent or innocuous (Kim *et al.* 2007a). The prevalence of eschars varies and patients from Laos with serologically confirmed scrub typhus had a prevalence of about 50% (Phongmany *et al.* 2006) but in patients from Japan the prevalence was 87% (Phongmany *et al.* 2006), in Korea, 92% (Kim *et al.* 2007a) and South Vietnam, 48% (Berman and Kundin 1973). The eschar is often hidden in skin folds, beneath the beltline, under the axilla, or around the buttock region. Most cases of scrub typhus are mild, but without treatment it may progress to severe organ dysfunction, meningismus, dyspnea, pneumonitis, acute respiratory distress syndrome (ARDS), Guillain-Barré, meningoencephalitis, disseminated intravascular coagulation, or renal failure (Pandey *et al.* 2006; Wang *et al.* 2007; Lee *et al.* 2007; Chen *et al.* 2006; Phongmany *et al.* 2006). The fatality rate of scrub typhus ranges from 1 to 35%, depending on the virulence of the infecting strain, host factors, and treatment (Silpapojakul 1997).

Scrub typhus and HIV-1 infection

Although co-infection with the HIV-1 virus does not affect the clinical severity of scrub typhus, the discovery that acute *O. tsutsugamushi* infection was shown to suppress HIV-1 viral replication both *in vivo* and *in vitro* has spurred the development of new lines of research in HIV treatment (Parola and Raoult 2006).

Diagnosis

The clinical and laboratory features of scrub typhus are notoriously non-specific. The eschar is the single most useful diagnostic clue but it may only appear with a minority of patients and can be overlooked by physicians. Infection with *O. tsutsugamushi* should always be suspected in patients who have visited or live in endemic areas and present with fever, acute hearing loss, lymphadenopathy with or without eschars. Unfortunately, scrub typhus is an often overlooked cause of both acute undifferentiated fever and of pneumonitis of undetermined etiology (Watt and Kantipong 2007). Rice farmers in north-eastern Thailand are commonly infected with both leptospirosis and scrub typhus and dual infections should be considered in patients at risk for both who have atypical clinical features of either disease alone, and in patients responding poorly to treatment.

Direct diagnosis

O. tsutsugamushi can be grown in the yolk sac of 5–7 day old embryonated chicken eggs, in primary cultured cells of chicken embryos and established cell lines such as HeLa, Vero, BHK, McCoy and L929, and mice (Seong *et al.* 2001). PCR to peripheral blood and skin biopsy from patients with acute scrub typhus can be also used for the detection of *O. tsutsugamushi*. PCR must be performed before initiation of antibiotic treatment and before antibody becomes detectable. Recently, a real-time PCR assay has been introduced for the diagnosis of scrub typhus detecting major outer membrane antigen genes (Singhsilarak *et al.* 2005; Jiang *et al.* 2004).

Indirect diagnosis

A variety of serologic assays have been used in the diagnosis of scrub typhus such as the indirect immunoperoxidase and Weil-Felix assays. The Weil-Felix slide agglutination test lacks sensitivity but is easy to perform in less developed areas of the world (Isaac *et al.* 2004; Mahara 1984). IFA is the gold standard assay for the serologic detection of scrub typhus antibodies (La Scola and Raoult 1997) which has subsequently been modified to allow the use of smaller volumes of serum and antigens (Gan *et al.* 1972). Maximum titres of patients treated after 7 days of symptoms averaged between 1:640 and 1:1,280, compared to patients treated promptly who had maximum antibody titres between 1:40 and 1:160 (Berman and Kundin 1973). The immunoperoxidase assay has been developed as an alternative to IFA for the diagnosis of scrub typhus (La Scola and Raoult 1997). The advantage of the immunoperoxidase assay is that it provides a permanent slide record, and the results can be read with an ordinary light microscope. In cases of sera cross-reactions, Western blotting assay of the outer membrane proteins can be used for the detection of scrub typhus (Jiang *et al.* 2003). Rapid serological tests have also been developed and are positive in more than 90% of patients with scrub typhus infection during the first week of fever (Watt and Kantipong 2007).

Treatment

In tissue cell cultures, *O. tsutsugamushi* are susceptible to tetracycline, demethylchlortetracycline, doxycycline, minocycline, chloramphenicol, and rifampin (Raoult and Drancourt 1991). Quinolones such as norfloxacin, ciprofloxacin and ofloxacin were only moderately active and beta-lactams and nalidixic acid were inactive (Urakami *et al.* 1989).

Therapy with anti-rickettsial drugs is recommended whenever a case of scrub typhus is suspected. Scrub typhus is said to respond even more promptly to antibiotics than do other rickettsial diseases, with patients generally becoming afebrile within 24 to 36 hours after beginning antibiotic therapy. Prompt antibiotic therapy generally prevents death, but good supportive care and early detection of complications are important in severe cases. To date, chloramphenicol (2 g/day) has been the first effective antibiotic for the treatment of scrub typhus. Currently, however, doxycycline (200 mg daily) for not less than 7 days is regarded the drug of choice. Shorter treatment courses are often curative, but may result in relapse (Sheehy *et al.* 1973). Physicians should be aware that scrub typhus cases from Chiangrai, in Thailand have been resistant to chloramphenicol and doxycycline (Watt *et al.* 1996). Roxithromycin was as effective as doxycycline and chloramphenicol in a trial of 39 Korean children (Watt and Kantipong 2007). Recently telithromycin was also found to be effective in 92 Korean patients (800 mg/day for 5 days) (Kim *et al.* 2007b). Quinolones have been used experimentally although fever usually subsides later when ciprofloxacin is used and its efficacy remains questionable (Mathai *et al.* 2003).

In cases of co-infection with leptospirosis, doxycycline was found to be highly effective (Phimda *et al.* 2007). However, azithromycin can be used as an appropriate alternative antimicrobial treatment in areas where doxycycline-resistant scrub typhus is prevalent (Phimda *et al.* 2007). Recently, a patient infected by leptospirosis and scrub typhus, was treated by early plasma exchange and a 7 day course of moxifloxacin therapy (Chen *et al.* 2007).

Prevention and control

Chemoprophylaxis for persons with anticipated intense but transient exposure to *O. tsutsugamushi* with weekly doses of 200 mg of doxycycline has been proposed (Twartz *et al.* 1982). Soldiers and road construction crews are typically examples but chemoprophylaxis should also be considered in travellers at high risk areas. Contact with chiggers can be reduced by not sitting or lying directly on the ground and by applying repellent to the tops of boots and socks and to the hem of trousers, but this may be impractical in those exposed occupationally. The meal of mites lasts several days, but it seems that infectious organisms are not transmitted during the first 6–8 hours after attached. Thus rapid removal of attached chiggers may be helpful in avoiding infection. Because of the antigenic diversity of the various serotypes, an effective vaccine for prevention of scrub typhus has not been developed (Chattopadhyay and Richards 2007).

References

Bavaro, M. F., Kelly, D. J., Dasch, G. A., Hale, B. R., and Olson, P. (2005). History of U.S. military contributions to the study of rickettsial diseases. *Mil. Med.*, **170**: 49–60.

Baxter, J. D. (1996). The typhus group. *Clin. Dermatol.*, **14**: 271–78.

Bengston, I. A. (1948). Rickettsiales Gieszcyzkiewicz (6th edn). In: R. S. Breed, E. G. P. Murray and A. P. Hitchens (eds.) *Bergey's manual of definitive bacteriology*. Baltimore, Maryland: Williams and Wilkins.

Berman, S. J. and Kundin, W. D. (1973). Scrub typhus in South Vietnam. A study of 87 cases. *Ann. Med. Inter.*, **79**: 26–30.

Chattopadhyay, S. and Richards, A. L. (2007). Scrub typhus vaccines: past history and recent developments. *Hum. Vaccin.*, **3**: 73–80.

Chen, P. H., Hung, K. H., Cheng, S. J., and Hsu, K. N. (2006). Scrub typhus-associated acute disseminated encephalomyelitis. *Acta Neurol. Taiwan.*, **15**: 251–54.

Chen, Y. S., Cheng, S. L., Wang, H. C., and Yang, P. C. (2007). Successful treatment of pulmonary hemorrhage associated with leptospirosis and scrub typhus coinfection by early plasma exchange. *J. Formos. Med. Assoc.*, **106**: S1–S6.

Cho, N. H., Kim, H. R., Lee, J. H. *et al.* (2007). The *Orientia tsutsugamushi* genome reveals massive proliferation of conjugative type IV secretion system and host-cell interaction genes. *Proc. Natl. Acad. Sci. U. S. A.*, **104**: 7981–86.

Currie, B., O'Connor, L., and Dwyer, B. (1993). A new focus of scrub typhus in tropical Australia. *Am. J. Trop. Med. Hyg.*, **49**: 425–29.

Gan, E., Cadigan Jr., F. C., and Walker, J. S. (1972). Filter paper collection of blood for use in a screening and diagnostic test for scrub typhus using the IFAT. *Trans. R. Soc. Trop. Med. Hyg.*, **66**: 588–93.

Groupe de travail OMS (1982). Rickettsioses: un probleme de morbidite persistant. *Bull. Wor. Heal. Organ*, **60**: 693–71.

Isaac, R., Varghese, G. M., Mathai, E. J. M., and Joseph, I. (2004). Scrub typhus: prevalence and diagnostic issues in rural Southern India. *Clin. Infect. Dis.*, **39**: 1395–96.

Jensenius, M., Fournier, P. E., and Raoult, D. (2004). Tick-borne rickettsioses in international travellers. *Int. J. Infect. Dis.*, **8**: 139–46.

Jiang, J., Chan, T. C., Temenak, J. J., Dasch, G. A., Ching, W. M., *et al.* (2004). Development of a quantitative real-time polymerase chain reaction assay specific for *Orientia tsutsugamushi*. *Am. J. Trop. Med. Hyg.*, **70**: 351–56.

Jiang, J., Marienau, K. J., May, L. A. *et al.* (2003). Laboratory diagnosis of two scrub typhus outbreaks at Camp Fuji, Japan in 2000 and 2001 by enzyme-linked immunosorbent assay, rapid flow assay, and Western blot assay using outer membrane 56-kD recombinant proteins. *Am. J. Trop. Med. Hyg.*, **69**: 60–66.

Kim, D. M., Won, K. J., Park, C. Y. *et al.* (2007a). Distribution of eschars on the body of scrub typhus patients: a prospective study. *Am. J. Trop. Med. Hyg.*, **76**: 806–9.

Kim, D. M., Yu, K. D., Lee, J. H., Kim, H. K., and Lee, S. H. (2007b). Controlled trial of a 5-day course of telithromycin versus doxycycline for treatment of mild to moderate scrub typhus. *Antimicrob. Agents Chemother.*, **51**: 2011–15.

La Scola, B. and Raoult, D. (1997). Laboratory diagnosis of rickettsioses: current approaches to the diagnosis of old and new rickettsial diseases. *J. Clin. Microbiol.*, **35**: 2715–27.

Lee, S. H., Jung, S. I., Park, K. H. *et al.* (2007). Guillain-Barre syndrome associated with scrub typhus. *Scand. J. Infect. Dis.*, **39**: 826–28.

Mahara, F. (1984). Three Weil-Felix reaction OX2 positive cases with skin eruptions and high fever. *J. Anan Med. Assoc.*, **68**: 4–7.

Mathai, E., Rolain, J. M., Verghese, G. M. *et al.* (2003). Outbreak of scrub typhus in southern India during the cooler months. *Ann. N. Y. Acad. Sci.*, **990**: 359–64.

Miyamura, S., Ohta, T., and Tamura, A. (1989). Comparison of in vitro susceptibilities of *Rickettsia prowazekii*, *R. rickettsii*, *R. sibirica* and *R. tsutsugamushi* to antimicrobial agents. *Nippon. Saikingaku. Zasshi.*, **44**: 717–21.

Nagayo, M., Tamiya, T., Mitamura, T. *et al.* (1930). On the virus of tsutsugmushi disease and its demonstration by a new method. *Jap. J. Experim. Med.*, **8**: 309–18.

Ohashi, N., Tamura, A., Sakurai, H., Yamamoto, S. (1990). Characterization of a new antigenic type, Kuroki, of *Rickettsia tsutsugamushi* isolated from a patient in Japan. *J. Clin. Microbiol.*, **28**: 2111–13.

Pandey, D., Sharma, B., Chauhan, V., Mokta, J., Verma, B. S., *et al.* (2006). ARDS complicating scrub typhus in Sub-Himalayan region. *J. Assoc. Phys. India*, **54**: 812–13.

Parola, P. and Raoult, D. (2006). Tropical rickettsioses. *Clin. Dermatol.*, **24**: 191–200.

Phimda, K., Hoontrakul, S., Suttinont, C. *et al.* (2007). Doxycycline versus azithromycin for treatment of leptospirosis and scrub typhus. *Antimicrob. Agents Chemother.*, **51**: 3259–63.

Phongmany, S., Rolain, J. M., Phetsouvanh, R. *et al.* (2006). Rickettsial infections and fever, Vientiane, Laos. *Emerg. Infect. Dis.*, **12**: 256–62.

Raoult, D. and Drancourt, M. (1991). Antimicrobial therapy of Rickettsial diseases. *Antimicrob. Agents Chemother.*, **35**: 2457–62.

Rosenberg, R. (1997). Drug-resistant scrub typhus: Paradigm and paradox. *Parasitol. Today*, **13**: 131–32.

Seong, S. Y., Choi, M. S., and Kim, I. S. (2001). *Orientia tsutsugamushi* infection: overview and immune responses. *Microbes. Infect.*, **3**: 11–21.

Sheehy, T. W., Hazlett, D., and Turk, R. E. (1973). Scrub typhus. A comparison of chloramphenicol and tetracycline in its treatment. *Arch. Intern. Med.*, **132**: 77–80.

Silpapojakul, K. (1997). Scrub typhus in the Western Pacific region. *Ann. Acad. Med. Singapore*, **26**: 794–800.

Silverman, D. J., Wisseman Jr., C. L. Waddell, A. D., and Jones, M. (1978). Comparative ultrastructural study on the cell envelopes of *Rickettsia prowazekii, Rickettsia rickettsii,* and *Rickettsia tsutsugamushi. Infect. Immun.*, **21**: 1020–23.

Singhsilarak, T., Leowattana, W., Looareesuwan, S. *et al.* (2005). Short report: detection of *Orientia tsutsugamushi* in clinical samples by quantitative real-time polymerase chain reaction. *Am. J. Trop. Med. Hyg.*, **72**: 640–41.

Tamura, A., Makisaka, Y., Enatsu, T. *et al.* (1999). Isolation of Orientia tsutsugamushi from patients in Shikoku and finding of a strain which grows preferentially at low temperatures. *Mi Isolation crobiol. Immunol.*, **43**: 979–81.

Tamura, A., Ohashi, N., Urakami, H., Miyamura, S. (1995). Classification of *Rickettsia tsutsugamushi* in a new genus, *Orientia* gen nov, as *Orientia tsutsugamushi* comb. *nov. Int. J. Syst. Bact.*, **45**: 589–91.

Twartz, J. C., Shirai, A., Selvaraju, G., Saunders, J. P., Huxsoll, D. L., *et al.* (1982). Doxycycline propylaxis for human scrub typhus. *J. Infect. Dis.*, **146**: 811–18.

Urakami, H., Yamamoto, S., Tsuruhara, T., Ohashi, N., and Tamura, A. (1989). Serodiagnosis of scrub typhus with antigens immobilized on nitrocellulose sheet. *J. Clin. Microbiol.*, **27**: 1841–46.

Walker, D. H. (1991). *Biology of rickettsial diseases.* Vol I. Boca Raton, Florida: CRC Press.

Wang, C. C., Liu, S. F., Liu, J. W., Chung, Y. H., Su, M. C., *et al.* (2007). Acute respiratory distress syndrome in scrub typhus. *Am. J. Trop. Med. Hyg.*, **76**: 1148–52.

Watt, G. and Kantipong, P. (2007). *Orientia tsutsugamushi* and Scrub Typhus. In: D. Raoult and P. Parala (eds.) *Rickettsial Diseases*, pp. 237–56. New York: Informa Health Care.

Watt, G., Chouriyagune, C., Ruangweerayud, R. *et al.* (1996). Scrub typhus infections poorly responsive to antibiotics in northern Thailand. *Lancet*, **348**: 86–89.

Watt, G. and Parola, P. (2003). Scrub typhus and tropical rickettsioses. *Curr. Opin. Infect. Dis.*, **16**: 429–36.

Weiss, E. (1981). The family Rickettsiaceae: human pathogens. In: M. P. Starr, H. Stolp, H. G. Truper, A. Balows, H. G. Schlegel (eds.) *The prokaryotes. A handbook on habitats, isolation, and identification of bacteria)*, pp. 2138–60. Berlin-Heidelberg: Springer-Verlag.

WHO (1993). Global surveillance of rickettisal diseases: memorandum from a WHO meeting. *Bull. Worl. Heal. Organ.*, **71**: 293–6.

Yamshita, T., Kasuya, S., Noda, S., Nagano, I., Ohtsuka, S. *et al.* (1988). Newly isolated strains of *Rickettsia tsutsugamushi* in Japan identified by using monoclonal antibodies to Karp, Gilliam and Kato strains. *J. Clin. Microbiol.*, **26**: 1859–60.

Yamashita, T., Kasuya, S., Noda, N., Nagano, I. and Kang, J. S. (1994). Transmission of *Rickettia tsutsugamushi* strains among humans, wild rodents, and trombidulid mites in an areas of Japan in which tsutsugamushi disease is newly endemic. *J. Clin. Microbiol.*, **32**: 2780–85.

CHAPTER 14

Listeriosis

J. McLauchlin

Summary

Listeriosis occurs in a variety of animals including humans, and most often affects the pregnant uterus, the central nervous system (CNS) or the bloodstream. During pregnancy, infection spreads to the foetus, which will either be born severely ill or die in-utero. In non-pregnant animals, listeriosis usually presents as meningitis, encephalitis or septicaemia. In humans, infection most often occurs in the immunocompromised and elderly, and to a lesser extent the pregnant woman, the unborn, or the newly delivered infant. Infection can be treated successfully with antibiotics, however 20–40% of human cases are fatal.

In domestic animals (especially in sheep and goats) listeriosis usually presents as encephalitis, abortion, or septicaemia.

The genus *Listeria* comprises seven species of Gram-positive bacteria. Almost all cases of listeriosis are due to *Listeria monocytogenes* although up to 10% of cases in sheep are due to *Listeria ivanovii*.

Listeriae are ubiquitous in the environment worldwide, especially in sites with decaying organic vegetable material. Many animals carry the organism in the faeces without serious infection. The consumption of contaminated food or feed is the principal route of transmission for both humans and animals, however other means of transmission occur.

Human listeriosis is rare (<1 to >10 cases per million people in North America and Western Europe), but because of the high mortality rate, it is amongst the most important causes of death from food-borne infections in industrialized countries. In the UK, human listeriosis is the biggest single cause of death from a preventable food-borne disease. Listeriosis in domestic animals is a cause of considerable economic loss. Control measures should be directed towards both to exclude *Listeria* from food or feed as well as inhibiting its multiplication and survival. Silage which is spoiled or mouldy should not be used, and care should be taken to maintain anaerobic conditions for as long as possible.

Dietary advice is available for disease prevention, particularly targeted at 'at risk' individuals to modify their diet to avoid eating specific foods such as soft cheese and pâté.

History

The bacterium *Listeria monocytogenes* and the disease listeriosis were first recognized in 1924 as a spontaneous outbreak of infection amongst laboratory rabbits and guinea-pigs in Cambridge (England) by Murray and colleagues. The species name 'monocytogenes' was derived from the marked mononuclear leucocytosis shown by these animals. The same bacterium was isolated from infected gerbils in South Africa by Pirie in 1926, and was named *Listerella* after the surgeon and pioneer of antisepsis Lord Lister. The generic name was changed to *Listeria* in 1940 for taxonomic reasons. Gill in New Zealand is credited with the first isolation of *L.monocytogenes* from an infected domestic animal and described a type of ovine encephalitis 'circling disease'.

L.monocytogenes was isolated from the blood of humans with a mononucleosis-like infection (a rare manifestation of the disease) in Denmark in 1929. In the USA listeriosis was established as a cause of infection during the perinatal period and also as meningitis in adults. Prior to 1926 there are descriptions of disease likely to have been listeriosis, indeed a 'diphtheroid' isolated from the cerebrospinal fluid of a soldier in Paris in 1919 was later identified as *L.monocytogenes*.

During the 1980s the rise in the numbers of both human and animal listeriosis in several countries (including the UK) together with the a series of human food-borne outbreaks in North America and Europe lead to much professional interest in this disease as well as public alarm. The number of cases reduced during the 1990s but have increased again after 2000 in European countries and in North America.

The genus *Listeria*

The agent

Listeria are coccobacilli or rod-shaped, non-sporing, Gram-positive bacteria with a DNA G+C content of 36–42 mol%. The cell wall is typical for a Gram-positive organism, and contains alanine and glutamic acid cross-linked by meso-diaminopimelic acid: teichoic acids are present. The fatty acids anteiso $C_{17:0}$ and anteiso $C_{15:0}$ predominate. The metabolism is aerobic and microaerophilic, and both cytochromes and menaquinones are present. Almost all cultures are catalase positive, oxidase negative and motile below 35°C by means of peritrichate flagella. Cultures growing on carbohydrates are weakly fermentative, and lactate but no gas is produced from glucose.

DNA/DNA homology studies indicate that this genus comprises 6 species:

- *L. monocytogenes*,

- *L. grayi*,

- *L.innocua,*
- *L.ivanovii,*
- *L.seeligeri,*
- *L.welshimeri.*

Two further species, *L.marthii,* and *L.rocourtiae* were described in 2009. The different species of *Listeria* can be readily identified by means of a small number of phenotypic or genotypic characters (Table 14.1).

Genotypic data confirms the close relationship between the different species of *Listeria*, and shows the closet relationship between organisms of the genus *Brochothrix* which are included in a single family, the listeriaceae, which has a more distant relationship to members of other low G+C Gram-positive genera (i.e. *Bacillus, Enterococcus, Lactobacillus, Lactococcus,* and *Streptococcus*).

Almost all cases of human listeriosis are due to *L.monocytogenes,* although rarely *L.seeligeri* and *L.ivanovii* have been implicated. A similar pattern is seen in animals, except up to 10% of cases are due to *L.ivanovii.* Under experimental conditions using both mice or mammalian tissue culture growing *in vitro,* only *L.monocytogenes* and *L.ivanovii* are pathogenic, and these species share many factors identified with virulence.

Biology

The chromosome of *L.monocytogenes* has been estimated to be about 3,000 Kb in size and a physical and genetic map were established prior to sequencing of the genomes of several different isolates. Complete genomes are available for multiple *L.monocytogenes* strains together with *L.innocua, L.welshimeri, L.grayi* and *Listeria* phages.

Transposons Tn1545, Tn916 and Tn917 (and their derivatives) have been introduced and expressed in *L.monocytogenes* and have proved extremely useful tools in the understanding of the virulence of this bacterium. A transposon very similar to Tn917 (designated Tn5422) has been recognized in plasmids recovered from *L. monocytogenes* which also encode resistance to cadmium as well as some antimicrobial agents. Transfer of native listerial plasmids has

been demonstrated between stains of *L.monocytogenes,* between *Listeria* species, and to other species of bacteria including *Bacillus subtilis, Enterococcus faecalis, Streptococcus agalactiae,* and *Staphylococcus aureus.*

Lysogenic phage are commonly carried by *Listeria* and are generally morphologically similar with isometric heads, long noncontractile tails and correspond to the *Myoviridae* or *Styloviridae* families. The phage genomes are linear double stranded DNA of 35–42 Kb in size. Lytic properties of sets of phages have been used for subtyping *L.monocytogenes.*

As well as the use of transposon mutagenesis, plasmid complementation experiments together with the behaviour of *L.monocytogenes* either in mammalian tissue culture or in experimentally infected mouse models has lead to a great increase in the understanding of the genes involved with the virulence of this organism. Techniques to generate in-frame point mutations by allelic exchange, introduce genetic material by electroporation, and express *L.monocytogenes* genes in *L.innocua* and *Bacillus subtilis* have now also been applied with much success to the analysis of this bacterium (see later sections).

Growth survival and distribution

L.monocytogenes is widely distributed in the environment, and has been isolated from numerous sites including soil, sewage, water and decaying plant material (especially poorly fermented silage): its viability is remarkable with survival in soil or silage for >2 years. It is found in excreta from apparently healthy animals (including humans) although carriage in the gut is likely to be transitory.

Many types of raw, processed, cooked and ready to eat foods contain *L.monocytogenes,* albeit usually at low levels (<10 organisms/g). The properties of the organism favour food as an agent in transmission of listeriosis. *L.monocytogenes* grows in a wide range of foods having relatively high water activities (A_w >0.95) and over a wide range of temperatures (<0°C to 45°C). Growth occurs at refrigeration temperatures, although this is relatively slow with a maximum doubling time of about 1–2 days

Table 14.1 Phenotypic differentiation of *Listeria* species

Phenotypic test	Listeria species							
	L.monocytogenes	*L.ivanovii*	*L.innocua*	*L.welshimeri*	*L.marthii*	*L.rocourtiae*	*L.seeligeri*	*L.grayi*
β-haemolysis on blood agar	+	+	−	−	−	−	(+)	−
Lipase production	+	+	−	−	−	−	+	−
Acid production from:								
D-mannitol	−	−	−	−	−	+	−	+
L-rhamnose	+	−	+	v	−	+	−	V
D-xylose	−	+	−	+	−	+	+	−
CAMP (enhancement of haemolysis) against:								
Staphylococcus aureus	+	−	−	−	NK	−	(+)	−
Rhodococcus equi	−	+	−	−	NK	−	−	−
Amino acid peptidase	−	+	+	+	+	+	+	+

+, positive reaction; −, negative reaction; (+), weak reaction; v, variable reaction; NK, not known.

at 4°C. Multiplication in food is somewhat restricted to the pH range 5 to 9, and *L.monocytogenes* are not sufficiently heat resistant to survive mild heating including pasteurization. The tolerance of the bacterium to sodium chloride and sodium nitrite, and the ability to multiply (albeit slowly) in foods at refrigeration temperatures makes *L.monocytogenes* of particular concern as a post processing contaminant in refrigerated foods. Even when present at high levels in foods, spoilage or taints are not generally produced. The widespread distribution of *L.monocytogenes* and the ability to survive on dry and moist surfaces favours post-processing contamination of foods from both raw product and factory sites.

Primary selective isolation and detection

Prior to the mid 1980s, 'cold enrichment' utilizing the ability of *Listeria* to outgrow competing organisms at refrigeration temperatures in non-selective broths was principally used for selective isolation. However, because of the lack of specificity of this method and its slowness (some workers incubated broths for up to 6 months), procedures have been much improved.

Media have been developed which rely on a number of selective agents, including: acriflavin, lithium chloride, colistin, ceftazidime, cefotetan, fosfomycin, moxolactam, nalidixic acid, cycloheximide, and polymyxin. Furthermore, chromogenic agar based on phospholipase and glucosidase activity are now available which allows differentiate of *L.monocytogenes* colonies from other *Listeria* species on solid selective agar. Methods for identification of Listeria species are also now widely available including PCR based techniques for detection in liquid enrichment broths. These techniques have resulted in the widespread ability of microbiology laboratories (especially those involved with the examination of foods) to detect, selectively isolate and enumerate *L.monocytogenes* as well as other *Listeria* species.

The hosts

Human listeriosis

Risk factors

Listeriosis is an opportunistic infection which most often affects those with severe underlying illness, the elderly, pregnant women and both unborn and newly delivered infants. However, patients without these risk factors can also become infected. Individuals at greatest risk of contracting listeriosis include those with malignant neoplasms, or who are undergoing immunosuppressive therapy. Other predisposing conditions include those with: agents to reduce stomach acid, AIDS, alcoholism, alcoholic liver disease, diabetes, and recipients of prosthetic heart valves or articulation joints. Patients >60 years of age with concurrent pathologies are now the most common group affected in England and Wales (Fig. 14.1).

Disease presentation

Listeriosis most often affects the pregnant uterus, the central nervous system or the blood stream. The recent increase in human listeriosis in England and Wales has been almost exclusive to those >60 years of age with bacteraemia which now comprises the most common presentation (Fig. 14.1). The rate of listeriosis in the >60 age group has more than tripled between 1990 and 2009 in England and Wales. In non-pregnant individuals, listeriosis most frequently presents septicaemia without involvement of the central nervous system, or, to a lesser extent, as meningitis (with or without septicaemia). The former is generally confined to immunocompromised individuals and rarely has identifiable foci of infection. Listeric meningoencephalitis and encephalitis occur less commonly.

In the pregnant woman, listeriosis is most often recognized with one or more self-limiting influenza-like episodes during or after the latter half of the second trimester, although infection can occur

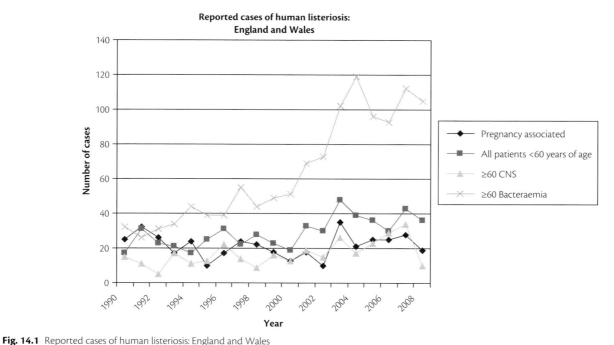

Fig. 14.1 Reported cases of human listeriosis: England and Wales
◆, all pregnancy associated cases; ■, all cases < 60 years of age; ▲, cases ≥60 years of age with involvement of the central nervous system (CNS); ✕, cases ≥60 years of age with bacteraemia and without involvement of the central nervous system.

throughout gestation. Maternal listeriosis usually presents with pyrexia and other non-specific symptoms, although some individuals may be asymptomatic. Maternal listeric meningitis during pregnancy is very rare. During pregnancy, infection spreads from the maternal circulatory system to the foetus, probably via the placenta, although this is not inevitable. Foetal infection developing before the third trimester usually results in *intra-uterine* death. The foetus has severe and overwhelming multisystem infection involving internal organs, with the widespread formation of granulomatous lesions, especially in the liver and placenta, and is named *granulomatosis infantiseptica*. Infection of the infant during the third trimester results in either intra-uterine death, or the delivery of a severely ill neonate (early onset infection).

Early-onset sepsis is characterized by non-specific signs of infection and prematurity. Cutaneous lesions may be present (sometimes with granulomas) and the neonate may have convulsions. Most early-onset cases are septicaemic, some with meningitis, however some infants appear infected only at superficial sites. The degree of severity may be partially dependant on the gestational age at infection. Surviving infants can exhibit long term sequelae, especially those delivered prematurely or with involvement of the central nervous system.

Late-onset neonatal sepsis typically occurs after uncomplicated full term pregnancies, and usually presents as meningitis about 10 days after delivery. *L.monocytogenes* is acquired either from maternal sites during or shortly after delivery (possibly during passage through the birth canal) or from the post-natal environment, including from direct or indirect contact with an early onset case of neonatal listeriosis.

Focal infections caused by *L.monocytogenes* are relatively rare, and are primarily confined to immunocompromised individuals. Deep seated infections with or without abscess formation occurs in a wide variety of sites. Listeric endocarditis also occurs, and is usually confined to patients with underlying cardiac lesions or with prosthetic heart valves. Diarrhoeal disease has also been described, although this does not appear in all cases and may be specific to some *L.monocytogenes* strains.

Non-systemic cutaneous and ocular listeriosis resulting from contact with infected animals or animal material has been described, the most common being lesions on the hand and arm after attending a bovine abortion. These superficial lesions may develop to serious systemic infection.

Since *L.monocytogenes* is common in the environment individuals must be exposed to the organism through food alone on a frequent basis: it is possible that the majority of incidents of listeriosis are subclinical. This is also supported by the relatively mild forms of the disease presenting as cutaneous infections or as bacteraemia in the pregnant woman.

During infection of the foetus, the pregnant woman often exhibits a series of pyrexial influenza-like episodes resulting from the same strain of *L.monocytogenes* invading the maternal blood stream. However in both humans and animals it is very rare for the pregnant individual with an infected foetus to develop serious infection (such as meningitis or encephalitis) despite invasion of the blood stream.

Diagnosis

Since the clinical symptoms of human listeriosis are not sufficiently characteristic to establish a diagnosis, it is necessary to isolate and identify *L.monocytogenes* from the patient's body sites. Special culture media and procedures are not usually required when examining samples from normally sterile sites.

Diagnosis of septicaemia or meningitis is made by culturing blood or cerebrospinal fluid. *L.monocytogenes* is sometimes seen in stained cerebrospinal fluid smears collected from patients with meningitis together with a moderate leucocyte reaction (usually lymphocytic), elevated protein levels and depressed sugar concentrations. Despite the species name '*monocytogenes*', monocytosis during septicaemia or meningitis is rarely observed.

During pregnancy, *L.monocytogenes* can be cultured from maternal blood, especially when collected during febrile episodes. Before delivery, an abnormal visual appearance of the amniotic fluid may give an early suggestion of listeriosis, especially when discoloured by meconium. At birth *L.monocytogenes* is present in high numbers both on multiple sites of the infected infant and in the maternal genital tract, and can be seen in stained smears. This bacterium can be readily cultured from: the placenta and lochia, the infant's blood, cerebrospinal fluid, respiratory and gastric tract, skin and other surface sites, and the maternal high vagina. Amniotic fluid and meconium should be cultured when available.

Following *intra-uterine* death and expulsion of the foetus, necropsy should be carried out. Material taken from the infant's liver, spleen, brain and other internal organs should be examined for *L.monocytogenes*. Culturing maternal high vaginal swabs may also be useful in retrospective diagnosis of *intra-uterine* infection within several weeks after delivery.

Methods to detect specific nucleic acid sequences by PCR have been described. Procedures to detect specific antibody have also been described, however interpretation is problematic and these have not led to useful diagnostic tests.

Pathology

Histological changes in human listeriosis are similar to that observed in animals. Infection causes necrosis followed by proliferative activity of cells in the reticuloendothelial system resulting in miliary granuloma formation and focal necrosis with supporation of the affected tissues. The bacterium is often present in the necrotic foci: the numbers and extent of the lesions varies with the sites infected as well as between patients.

Meningitis is characterized by supporative inflammation of the meninges with granuloma and necrosis of cerebral tissue. A thick purulent exudate may be found in the subarachnoid space. During encephalitis, gross lesions may be absent, or present in the pons and medulla oblongata. In cases of encephalomyelitis, submiliary to miliary nodules are often found in the leptomeninges.

In the newborn, the disease is characterized by a massive involvement of the liver with disseminated lesions in numerous other organs including the spleen, adrenal glands, lungs, oesophagus, posterior pharyngeal wall, and the tonsils. Cutaneous foci are often seen, especially on the back and lumbar region.

In the placenta, multiple white or grey necrotic areas occur within the villous parenchyma and decidua, the largest usually in the basal villi and decidua basalis. This gross appearance may allow a presumptive diagnosis of listeriosis. The necrotic foci are identical to those in the foetal organs. Gram-positive rods are usually seen within the necrotic centres of the villous and decidual abscesses, as well as within the membranes, umbilical cord, and surface of the foetus. The necrotic foci typically contain collections of polymorphonuclear leucocytes and are found between the trophoblast and stroma. Inflamed or necrotic chorionic villi are enmeshed in intervillous inflammatory material and fibrin.

Antimicrobial treatment

In vitro studies on the activities of various antimicrobial agents show that *L.monocytogenes* is almost always uniformly sensitive to ampicillin, penicillin, and erythromycin, although up to 10% may be resistant to tetracycline. *L.monocytogenes* is uniformly highly resistant to cephalosporins, and fluoroquinolones have insufficient activity to be recommended for the treatment of listeriosis.

There is general agreement that a combination of ampicillin or penicillin plus an aminoglycoside is superior to using either drug alone. For central nervous system listeriosis in adults, treatment with intravenous ampicillin plus an aminoglycoside for 3 to 4 weeks is recommended. During pregnancy, 2 weeks treatment with ampicillin plus an aminoglycoside should be given intravenously if amnionitis is present, or amoxicillin if not present. In cases of serious allergy to ampicillin, trimethoprime plus sulfamethoxazole may be given intravenously.

Neonatal listeriosis should be treated with intravenous ampicillin plus an aminoglycoside. Two weeks of treatment is recommended, but a longer course should be considered if a diagnosis of meningitis has been made. With late onset neonatal listeriosis, meningitis is commonly present and ampicillin plus gentamicin is recommended. The length of treatment is variable; if prompt clinical improvement occurs and the bacterium is absent from the CSF, 2 weeks treatment may be adequate. However 4 to 6 weeks should generally be considered.

Prognosis

Foetal infection and death during early gestation is a recognized complication of maternal infection, but this is not inevitable. Once infection of the pregnant uterus has occurred, successful pre-partum treatment of the mother with antimicrobial agents has resulted in the birth of apparently healthy infants. In late gestation, death of the foetus may occur, although it is more common to result in the birth of a severely ill infant. Early-onset neonatal listeriosis has a high fatality (>35%), and in those that survive, sequelae such as neurodevelopmental handicaps, hydrocephalus, ptosis, and strabismus may occur. Late-onset neonatal listeriosis also has a high mortality rate, although generally not as high as early-onset infection. The long-term prognosis for infants after late onset sepsis or meningitis has not been well studied.

Mortality rates for adult and juvenile listeriosis varies from 10 to >50%, with poor prognostic indicators including: age (>50 years), pre-existing disease, early convulsions (in cases of meningitis), and the needs for cardiovascular renal or ventilatory support. Residual disabilities may occur. Relapses of infection, some greater than two years after the original episodes, have been described.

Animal listeriosis
Disease presentation

Amongst domestic animals, sheep and goats are most susceptible, although infection also takes place in cattle (Low and Donachie 1997). Infection has been recognized in >40 other species of feral and domesticated animals, although this account will principally deal with sheep and cattle.

Listeriosis presents as a wide range of disorders which parallel much of what has already been outlined for humans, although there are some differences. *L.monocytogenes* is the major pathogen,

however some of the cases of abortion or septicaemia in sheep (but less commonly in cattle) are accounted for by *L.ivanovii*.

There are six main manifestations of the disease: abortion, septicaemia, encephalitis, diarrhoea, mastitis, and ocular infections. However the disease varies depending on the species involved. Listeriosis in primates manifests similarly to that in humans.

In sheep, goats and cattle, abortion is recognized late in pregnancy and is rarely accompanied by severe systemic disease in the dam. Aborting animals may excrete the organism in the milk without evidence of mastitis. Septicaemia in young animals occurs in the first few weeks of life: some with diarrhoea, but there is no specific symptomology. Diarrhoea and septicaemia also occur in older animals (principally ewes).

Unlike human listeriosis, the most common form of listeriosis in animals is as an encephalitis. In ruminants, this takes the form of a unilateral (or less commonly bilateral) cranial nerve paralysis effecting the eye, eyelid, ear, and lips (with consequent dropping of cud), which is often followed by ataxia, and moving in circles: hence the name circling disease. The affected animals are dull with the head standing to one side sometimes with food or cud hanging from the mouth and, because of the partial paralysis of the pharynx, saliva is often drooled. Animals sometimes stand still pressing against a fixed object, or appear recumbent. The course of the disease in bovines is quite prolonged (4–14 days), but is much more acute in sheep where death can occur within 4 to 48 hours. In sheep, the disease can resemble pregnancy toxaemia (ketosis). Encephalitis occurs in older animals (in sheep most often during late pregnancy or soon after lambing) as well as in the young.

Abortion, septicaemia and encephalitis are usually sporadic in cattle, but can occur as outbreaks amongst flocks of sheep where losses may be heavy. During outbreaks, septicaemia and abortion may occur together with cases of encephalitis, but is unusual. Experimental infection indicates the septicaemia can develop in a few days after consumption of contaminated feed, but the incubation period for encephalitis is likely to be much longer (20–30 days).

L.monocytogenes causes mastitis in cows and sheep, where large numbers of the bacterium can be shed into milk. All four quarters or only one may be affected, and the disease severity can vary markedly, sometimes appearing subclinical. Excretion of the organism into milk can persist for >3 years.

Keratoconjunctivits together with iritis occurs in both sheep and cattle. These conditions are usually unilateral. In cases of conjunctivitis, other bacterial or viral pathogens may also be present on the conjunctiva.

Listeric abortion, septicaemia and encephalitis has been recognized in pigs, horses, dogs and cats, but this is rare.

Listeriosis occurs in rodents and >20 species of birds, although is probably rare. Infection is most often recognized in those birds more commonly farmed, i.e. chickens, turkeys and ducks. Septicaemia and myocardial necrosis are the most common manifestation, and these have been suggested to be often secondary to other infections.

Risk factors

Although less commonly associated with predisposing factors (as described for humans) listeriosis in animals shows characteristics of an opportunistic pathogen. The unborn and newly delivered are more susceptible to infection, and encephalitis occurs most often in the adult pregnant animal during the later stages of gestation or shortly after delivery. Outbreaks have been associated with climatic stress (sudden drops in temperature, snow falls, drought, and shortage of food), and cases most often occur in the spring when animals may be in a poor condition. Increases in susceptibility of animals to experimental infection have been demonstrated by malnutrition, immunosuppression, viral infection, and other uncharacterized stress factors.

As with humans, the majority of animal listeriosis cases are assumed to be acquired via contaminated feed (a particular risk factor is the consumption of poor quality silage).

Diagnosis and pathology

Diagnosis of abortion is usually achieved by culturing foetal organs (liver or spleen) or stomach contents. The culturing of the organism from placenta may be difficult to interpret in the absence of histological analysis where necrosis and abscess formation will be observed. The placental lesions are pin-point, yellowish necrotic foci involving the tips of the cotyledonary villi, with a focal to diffuse intercotyledonary placentitis covered in a red/brown exudate. The foetus is usually autolytic with miliary necrotic foci scattered throughout the liver and spleen, although these are not always present. Septicaemia is often accompanied by focal hepatic necrosis (sawdust liver).

Anti-mortem diagnosis of listeric encephalitis is problematic since there are no satisfactory diagnostic tests, and listeric encephalitis may mimic other diseases. Prior to death, *L.monocytogenes* may be cultured from the brain, but in some cases is absent: the organism is invariably only isolated from the brain and not from other organs. Necropsy samples show a diagnostic pattern of histological changes and this has proved to be the only definitive means of diagnosis. It is essential that histological examination is performed to exclude the possibility of other diseases causing the condition. The typical listeric parenchimal lesions are confined to the brain stem and medulla and are composed of microabscesses which begin with the collection of neutrophils or microglial cells. Gross pathological lesions are rarely observed. The glial nodules often persist and become infiltrated by macrophages. Adjacent to the lesions is heavy perivascular cuffing composed mainly of lymphocytes and histocytes in addition to occasional neutrophils and eosinophils. Bacteria, either singly or in small clumps are sometimes seen near the periphery of the lesions, but not in the perivascular cuffs. Meningitis (affecting the cerebellum and anterior cervical cord) probably developing secondarily to the parenchimal lesions and neuritis of the trigeminal nerve may also be present. A correlation between the degree of cell mediated immunity and brain lesion suggests that immunopathological reactions are important components of this condition. *L.monocytogenes* has been isolated from brains of apparently healthy sheep, but it is not clear how commonly this occurs.

L.monocytogenes is probably rare as a cause of mastitis, but should be considered during cultural procedures as part of the investigation of this condition. The condition presents with abnormal milk secretion and swelling of the affected quarter(s).

A marked monocytosis is commonly observed in infected rodents, together with focal hepatic necrosis from which the organism can be readily cultured. A diffuse myocardial necrosis is often observed in guinea pigs.

Listeriosis in birds is characterized by conspicuous lesions of myocardial degeneration and necrosis, with necrotic foci found in the liver, spleen, and lungs from which the organism can be readily cultured. Involvement of the central nervous system also sometimes occurs.

Treatment and prognosis

Because of the disease severity and rapid onset of clinical symptoms, treatment of infected sheep or cattle is rarely attempted: infected animal may be destroyed on humanitarian grounds. During outbreaks, mortality rates are often 100%, and those surviving can exhibit permanent central nervous system disorders.

As is found with humans, the pregnant dam with an intra-uterine infection is rarely accompanied by severe systemic disease so it is not necessary to attempt treatment. A listeric abortion does not seem to effect the possibility of subsequent conceptions.

The response to antibiotic treatment in cows with listeric mastitis has been poor and the organism can be excreted for extended periods of time. Hence it is recommended that such animals should not be used for milk production and culling should be considered.

Disease mechanisms

The production of an experimental keratoconjunctivitis (Anton's eye test) performed in either guinea-pigs or rabbits by instilling a live bacterial suspension into the conjunctiva has been used to demonstrate the virulence of *L.monocytogenes* for the past 60 years. Mice and rabbits are now more frequently used and they suffer an acute fatal infection one to seven days after a sufficient dose of a virulent strain (usually $>10^4$ bacteria) is given either intravenously or intraperitoneally. Virulence can be measured by LD_{50}, by the kinetics of growth of the bacterium in tissues, or by the extent of survival in the liver and spleen. Intraperitoneal carrageenin or mineral oil may be given prior to inoculation to increase susceptibility to infection.

Ovine encephalitis accompanied by the characteristic histological features has been experimentally achieved by inoculating the organism into the dental pulp. Histological encephalitis was evident after 6 days, but the onset of clinical neurological disease varied between 20 to 40 days.

Oral inoculation of mice, rats and guinea pigs have been reported. Infection showed most consistency in gnotobiotic animals and interference of colonization by the microflora of the gastrointestinal tract has been suggested. Differences have been reported between both strains of *L.monocytogenes*, and growth condition used for the bacteria prior to inoculation which were not apparent when using the intravenous or intraperitoneal route. Oesophageal inoculation of 10^6 *L.monocytogenes* to juvenile rats showed about a 50% infection rate in the liver or spleen. A reduction in the acidity of the stomach by cimetidine treatment reduced the infective dose.

Feeding trials in cynomologous monkeys have been reported, and only those animals receiving 10^9 cells showed fever, septicaemia, loss of appetite, irritability, and occasional diarrhoea. Those animals fed $\geq 10^7$ bacteria (some of which were completely asymptomatic) shed the organism in the faeces for up to 21 days.

In chick embryos injected by the intra-allantoic route, the LD_{50} is around 10^2 organisms. Lesions occur in the chorio-allantoic membrane, liver, and heart, and the bacterium can be readily cultured from these sites.

Chronic mastitis can be induced experimentally in cows by intramammary injection. Bacteraemia could not be detected in these animals and typically 10^3 to 10^4 L.monocytogenes/ml was shed into milk for 9 to 12 months of the remaining lactation period.

L.monocytogenes is able to infect a range of mammalian cell types growing in vitro, including enterocytes, macrophages, and fibroblasts. The use of such models has contributed much to an understanding of the factors involved in intracellular invasion and growth (see later description).

It is a characteristic of the natural disease in both humans and animals in that there is usually a low attack rate. The susceptibility to infection may be increased by external factors, some of which have already been mentioned. However other factors (such as other infectious agents or products of the metabolism of other microorganisms) may yet prove to be of importance. L.monocytogenes is a somewhat marginal pathogen. Hence experimental models reflecting the natural infection may work poorly, and relatively large numbers of animals may be needed for a small proportion of these to produce clinical symptoms of disease.

There is evidence supporting the role of antacid therapy in increasing susceptibility of some patients, and in experimental animal infection. The buffering capacity of some food types may also be of importance in facilitating the survival of the organism, which may then invade at sites further along the gastrointestinal tract, although other routes of infection may occur. Experimental septicaemia in animals can be achieved via the respiratory route, and further evidence supporting this possibility comes from one of the cases (septicaemia and aspiration pneumonia) which developed after eating contaminated coleslaw salad in the 1981 Canadian outbreak.

Histopathological analysis suggests that the intestinal tract can act as the site of invasion and the M cells overlying the Peyer's patches may act as the site of penetration. Although the observation that L.monocytogenes (as well as L.ivanovii) can readily invade various epithelial and fibroblast cell types growing in vitro suggests that there may be multiple routes by which this bacterium initially invades the hosts' cells. In the caecum and colon of animals following oral inoculation, the bacteria can be observed together with an inflammatory reaction in phagocytic cells present in the underlying lamina propria. Following this phase, invasion of the uterine contents or central nervous system (for patients with shorter incubation periods), may occur probably via the circulatory system.

In the liver, the organism is cleared from the blood by the phagocytic Kupffer cells. In their non-activated state, some bacteria will survive, escape to the cell cytoplasm, and subsequently spread to hepatocytes using the process described in the following section. Formation of localized lesions occur in the liver and also in the spleen.

Intrauterine infection of the foetus results from haematogenous spread from the mother. Abscess formation takes place in the placenta, and this may spread via the umbilical vein or the amniotic fluid to the foetal internal organs. The series of pyrexial episodes observed in the mother may result from re-invasion of maternal blood stream from placental sites. L.monocytogenes is unusual in that it is able to survive and grow in amniotic fluid, and aspiration of this leads to the pathological changes in the foetal respiratory tracts. The presence of high numbers of the organism in amniotic fluid results in widespread contamination of neonatal and maternal surface sites at delivery as well as the postnatal environment and may result in cases of neonatal cross-infection.

Experimental and field studies suggest that encephalitis in sheep and cattle results from L.monocytogenes reaching the base of the brain along cranial nerves, particularly the trigeminal nerve. It is assumed that animals eat contaminated feed, particularly silage, and the organism enters the nerves after penetrating the oral mucus membrane or through pre-existing areas of trauma such as tooth root scars (which are prominent in sheep during the spring). The mechanism for travel along nerves is not well understood

Listeria genes involved with invasion and intracellular movement in mammalian cells are shown in Fig. 14.2. The cell surface listerial protein named internalin is involved with initial stages of invasion and binds to mammalian cell surface proteins including E-cadherin. Subsequently L.monocytogenes becomes encapsulated in a membrane bound compartment which dissolves by the action of a thiol activated haemolysin (hly gene). L.monocytogenes enters the host cell cytoplasm where it multiplies and becomes surrounded by polymerized host cell actin, which becomes preferentially polymerized at the older pole of the bacterium by the ActA cell surface protein. The actin polymerization confers intracellular motility to the bacterium which allows invasion of an adjacent mammalian cell. The bacterium is then encapsulated in a double membrane bound compartment which is dissolved by the action of a lecithinase which is activated by a metalloprotease (the haemolysin and a phospholipase may also contribute in this process) and the whole process is repeated. The genes are all regulated by the positive regulation factor (prfA gene) and are located in two operons located quite closely together on the bacterial chromosome.

It is of note that all the above mentioned genes (or a very similar set) are present in L.ivanovii, which follows the same general pattern of cellular invasion and movement. Unlike L.monocytogenes, L.ivanovii does not cause plaque formation in fibroblasts growing in vitro, and it has been suggested that the lower virulence of the latter species may be related to lack of as yet uncharacterized other factors. There is evidence supporting the presence of these genes in L.seeligeri, although it is only weakly invasive to mammalian cells. It is not clear if L.seeligeri too lacks additional virulence factors or if these genes are poorly functional. An alternative explanation may be that L.seeligeri is adapted to survive in quite different eukaryotic environments.

Regulation of the genes involved with the virulence of L.monocytogenes is under the control of the positive regulation factor (prfA) gene product, and other promoters have been identified which interact with this protein (Fig. 14.3), including a promoter for its own production. Listeriolysin is one of the major extracellular proteins produced by L.monocytogenes under conditions of heat shock, and there is evidence to suggest that some of the above mentioned genes are also regulated by the stage of the cell cycle and temperature. The disaccharide cellobiose represses the expression of the listeriolysin and phospholipase genes by an as yet uncharacterized mechanism. It is tempting to speculate that the absence of this environmentally ubiquitous plant-derived molecule allows the induction of genes as a pathogenic response to the environment of eukaryotic cells.

L.monocytogenes is an intracellular parasite, and it is in this environment that the pathogen gains protection and evades some of the hosts defences. However the host has a number of strategies to deal with such parasites and is beyond the scope of this chapter.

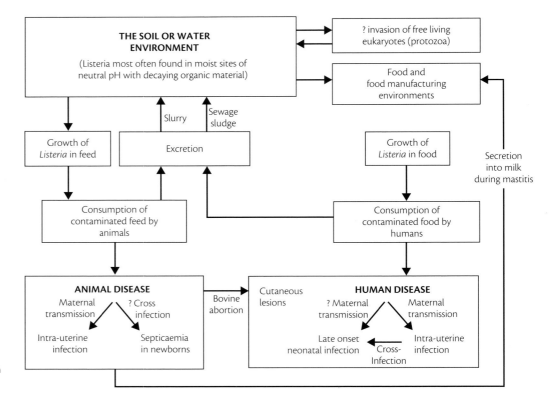

Fig. 14.2 Interactions of *Listeria* with the environment

Epidemiology

The widespread distribution of *L.monocytogenes* provides numerous potential ways in which the disease may be transmitted to both animals and humans. Although there has been much current interest in infection via the oral route, this is not the only mode of transmission (Fig. 14.2). The peak in the incidence of human listeriosis most often occurs in the end of the summer and early in the autumn. The reasons for this are not understood. Animal listeriosis principally occurs in the Spring. This is probably not only because of the physiology and condition of the animals, but also because of the provision of poorly prepared feed stuffs (see later notes).

The reported incidence of human listeriosis varies between countries from <1 to >10 cases per million of the total population. Although these in part may reflect differences in surveillance systems, they probably represent true differences in incidence. There are similar differences in the incidence of animal listeriosis in different regions: for example in the UK, listeriosis in sheep is a particular problem in Scotland and the North of England. These differences may in part be due to the ability to produce good quality feed.

Transmission of listeriosis in humans

Direct contact with infected animals

Listeriosis may be transmitted by direct contact with infected animals or animal material. In such cases the disease occurs as papular or pustular cutaneous lesions usually on the upper arms or wrists of farmers or veterinarians 1–4 days after attending bovine abortions. Since listeric infection is more common in sheep than cows, it is remarkable that such infections do not occur in association with sheep. However the duration of manipulation and extent of skin exposure is greater when dealing with bovines abortions (McLauchlin and Low 1994).

L.monocytogenes is widespread in the environment and superficial infections in humans from other sources are rare. This observation together with the likelihood that extremely high levels of the *L.monocytogenes* (10^8cfu/ml) occurring in infected bovine amniotic fluid as are found during *intra-uterine* infection in humans, suggests that the infective dose for human cutaneous listeriosis is high.

Although cutaneous listeriosis in adults are invariably a mild infection with a successful resolution (even without antimicrobial therapy), systemic involvement is suggested in some cases by fever and tenderness of the axillary lymph nodes. Indeed brucellosis has been considered as a differential cause in some cases. Furthermore, cases have also been described of acute meningitis in farmers after assisting at bovine abortions, although in these instances the route of infection is unclear.

Conjunctivitis in poultry workers has also been reported.

Cross-infection during the neonatal period

Hospital cross-infection between newborn infants occurs and these show a common pattern of an infant born with congenital listeriosis (onset within 1 day of birth). In the same hospital, and within a short period of time, an apparently healthy (or more rarely more than one) neonate is born who typically develops late onset listeriosis between the 5th and 12th day after delivery. The same strain of *L.monocytogenes* is isolated from both infants and the mother of the early onset case, but not from mother of the late onset case. In most of the episodes, the cases are either delivered or nursed in the same or adjacent rooms, and consequently staff and equipment are common to both. Two larger series have been described occurring in Sweden and Costa Rica, where 4 and 7 cases respectively resulted

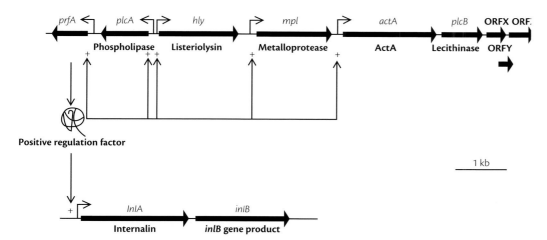

Fig. 14.3 Regulation of genes involved with the virulence of *L.monocytogenes*. The cell cycle, temperature and cellobiose are also involved in gene regulation

from single early onset cases. The likely routes of transmission here involved a contaminated rectal thermometer and a mineral oil bath. In one episode, true person to person transmission occurred where, 3 days after delivery, the mother of an early onset case was nursed in an open ward and handled a neonate from an adjacent bed who subsequently developed late onset listeriosis.

As previously outlined, *L.monocytogenes* is able to infect the pregnant uterus where extremely high levels of the organism occur (10^8/ml in amniotic fluid). At delivery, very large numbers of the organism are present on the newborn, in the maternal birth canal, and on sites, personnel and instruments contaminated during delivery in the postnatal environment. The very large numbers of organisms present during early onset neonatal infection clearly cause infection to further late onset neonatal cases.

There is little or no evidence for cross-infection or person to person transmission outside the neonatal period.

Food-borne transmission

The consumption of contaminated foods is the principal route of transmission for this disease and microbiological and epidemiological evidence supports an association with many food types (dairy, meat, vegetable, fish and shellfish) in both sporadic and epidemic listeriosis (Table 14.2). Although diverse in their constituents and manufacturing processes, foods associated with transmission often show the common features of:

- The capability of supporting the multiplication of *L.monocytogenes* (relatively high water activity and near-neutral pH);

- Relatively heavy (>10^3/g) contamination with the implicated strain;

- Processed with an extended (refrigerated) shelf life;

- Consumed without further cooking.

One food (alfalfa tablets), was quite different in that it was a dry product in which *L.monocytogenes* would not be able to grow. The most common food type associated with cases of listeriosis in the UK has been pre-prepared sandwiches served in hospitals.

The incubation period varies widely between individuals from 1 up to 90 days, with an average for intra-uterine infection of around 30 days. It is not known if these differences after oral ingestion are dose or strain dependent, or perhaps reflect unknown differences

in host susceptibility. Based on data from a very small number of cases, high levels of *L.monocytogenes* (10^3 to >10^7/g) have been found in foods consumed by patients prior to infection, suggesting that the infective dose is high. However much caution is needed here since there is likely to be much variation in susceptibility between individuals. In addition, suspect foods are generally only available for examination for relatively short periods and hence will be more likely to be collected from patients showing short incubation periods. These observations, together with the ability of *L.monocytogenes* to multiply in foods (even under ideal storage conditions) means that there are considerable difficulties in ascribing a 'safe' level of *L.monocytogenes* in food.

As has already been stated, *L.monocytogenes* is widespread in the environment, including food, although it is generally present in relatively low numbers. This feature together with the properties and types of foods associated with transmission of infection (Table 14.2), also support a dose response with very much greater

Table 14.2 Examples of ready-to-eat food types associated with human listeriosis

DAIRY PRODUCTS	VEGETABLE PRODUCTS
Soft cheese	Coleslaw salad
Milk	Vegetable rennet
Ice cream/soft cream	Salted mushrooms
Butter	Alfalfa tables
	Raw vegetables
	Pickled olives
	Rice salad
	Cut fruit

MEAT PRODUCTS	FISHERY PRODUCTS
Cooked chicken	Fish
Turkey frankfurters	Shellfish
Sausages	Shrimps
Pâté and rillettes	Smoked fish and shellfish
Pork tongue in aspic	Cod roe
Sliced meats	

COMPLEX FOODS
Pre-prepared sandwiches

risk following exposure to high numbers of the bacterium through food.

Outbreaks of human listeriosis involving >100 individuals have been recognized, however most cases are probably sporadic. Outbreaks have occurred over durations of 6 months to 5 years, and this is likely to represent a long term colonization of specific sites in the food manufacturing environment as well as the long incubation periods shown by some patients. *L.monocytogenes* has been shown to survive well in a variety of environments where food is manufactured, particularly those that are moist with organic material, and it is from such sites that contamination of food occurs during processing. Given the properties and distribution of *L.monocytogenes*, cases related by a common source may be very widely distributed both temporally and geographically.

Transmission of listeriosis in animals

Abortion and septicaemia in newborn animals results from intra-uterine infection acquired from the dam, and parallels abortion and early onset neonatal infection in humans. Septicaemia (also with meningitis in some animals) in lambs in the first few weeks of life has been attributed to umbilical infection acquired in lambing pens, possibly from contaminated soil or feed: this corresponds to late-onset neonatal infection in humans.

Iritis and keratoconjunctivitis usually occur during the winter in silage fed sheep and cattle. These may occur by direct introduction of contaminated feed into the eye, and have been particularly associated where feed is provided in holders or racks at eye level.

As in human infection, the majority of cases of animal listeriosis are assumed to be acquired via the oral route. There is a strong association between the feeding of silage and all manifestations of listeriosis in sheep and cattle, although cases do occur where this has not been used. However, the exact mechanism in which silage feeding leads or predisposes to listeriosis is not clear. Under normal conditions it is impossible to produce silage free of *Listeria*: the organism has been isolated from silage with a pH of <4, albeit in very low numbers. However, where poor quality silage has been produced and a low pH and anaerobic conditions are not achieved, proliferation of *Listeria* takes place and very high numbers can be found. Poor quality is often also due to insufficient herbage quality, or to contamination by soil or faeces. The change to production of silage in polythene bales ('big bale' silage) corresponded to increases in ovine listeriosis in the UK. Although the big bale method is more economical than the traditional use of clamps, these are more prone to spoilage and growth of *Listeria*: high numbers of the organism are often associated with sites where the damage to the bags has occurred or at the tied end. The peak in the numbers of animal listeriosis in the spring may reflect a decrease in the quality of silage used for feed. The observation that listeriosis is often associated with poor quality silage where high numbers of *L.monocytogenes* occur suggests that there is a similar dose response to humans.

Relationship between animal and human listeriosis and interactions of *Listeria* with the environment

The possible routes of infection in both human and animal disease are represented in Fig. 14.2. For both humans and animals the majority of infection probably results from ingestion of food or feed where excessive proliferation of *L.monocytogenes* has occurred.

It is not clear if there are differences in virulence between strains of *L.monocytogenes* and *L.ivanovii* in the environment, and why *L.ivanovii* is such a very rare pathogen for humans. Although some non-pathogenic cultures of *L.monocytogenes* have been identified, experimental infection of animals (albeit with rather 'unnatural' models) have indicated limited variation in virulence. However, the distribution of 'types' of *L.monocytogenes* usually varies between cultures isolated from the environment and to those causing disease. The proportion of *L.monocytogenes* types is significantly different between syndromes in both humans and animals. In addition, the majority of the strains responsible for the apparently unrelated large food-borne outbreaks of human listeriosis have been unexpectedly similar. The significance of these three observations is not clear, however they may be reflecting adaptions by strains (or species) to different environmental niches which effects virulence. For public health purposes, all strains of *L.monocytogenes* should be regarded as potentially pathogenic and capable of causing disease.

Apart from human infection acquired as a direct result of attending infected animals or from food directly contaminated from an infected animal (as may be the case with milk from an animal with listerial mastitis), it is unclear what, if any, are the connections between human and animal listeriosis. Analysis of strains causing 'sporadic' human and animal listeriosis indicates a wide range of 'types' in both groups which do not generally appear related. The seasonal peaks in human and animal listeriosis do not coincide, also suggesting that these two groups are not causally related. This perhaps should not be unexpected of a group of marginal pathogens which are probably not host adapted and occur widely in the environment as many different types.

L.monocytogenes and *L.ivanovii* are members of a group of bacteria which are adapted to saprophytic environments in soil or water and have additionally adapted to survive in eukaryotic intracellular environments. Quite how these additional factors have evolved is not clear. It may be that these factors evolved for survival in mammals, or for a free living multicellular eukaryotes living in the soil.

Prevention and control

Manufacturers of food, and food processing equipment should be aware of the properties of *Listeria*. The design of the factory and equipment should facilitate cleaning and sanitizing to reduce the possibility of contamination and colonization with *L.monocytogenes*. Producers, shippers and retailers of perishable foods must utilize good refrigeration and shelf life control, together with adequate packaging and consumer advice including 'sell by' and 'consume by' date and proper storage conditions. Application of a HACCP (hazard analysis critical control point) programme or a similar comprehensive assessment and control scheme is advised for both the safety and quality of the final product. Over the past decade, the food industry in Europe and North America has been active in investigating *Listeria* in foods and the factory environment, in implementing hazard analysis, and establishing codes of practice, and there is evidence to suggest that some foods have improved in microbiological quality with respect to contamination by *L.monocytogenes*.

L.monocytogenes can multiply (albeit slowly) at refrigeration temperatures, hence it is not only important to exclude the organism from foods, but also to inhibit its multiplication and survival. Because *L.monocytogenes* is a potential pathogen, and the detection of other species of *Listeria* can indicate environmental contamination (especially in those foods which have undergone a listericidal process), the ideal should be to exclude all *Listeria* from food, and this should be actively pursued. The achievement of this objective is probably impractical for all foods, and is clearly unattainable for raw foods or those which have not undergone a listericidal process. EU legislation (EC No. 2073/2005, Microbiological criteria for foodstuffs) defines different criteria for three categories of foods (25g samples) by:

♦ An absence of *L.monocytogenes* in foods intended for infants and for special medical purposes placed on the market during their shelf life.

♦ A limit of 100 *L.monocytogenes*/g for foods able to support the growth of *L.monocytogenes* and placed on the market during their shelf life and an absence of *L.monocytogenes* in these foods before they have left the immediate control of the food business operator.

♦ A limit of 100 *L.monocytogenes*/g foods unable to support the growth of *L.monocytogenes* and placed on the market during their shelf life.

Foods were defined as unable to support the growth of *L.monocytogenes* in this legislation by:

pH $\leq$4.4; $a_w \leq$ 0.92; pH $\leq$5.0 and $a_w \leq$ 0.94; shelf life less than 5 days

To avoid listeriosis and other food-borne infections, the general public should be educated about the use of good food and personal hygiene practices from the time the food is purchased to consumption. This includes avoiding cross-contamination between raw and cooked foods, properly maintaining refrigerators, and not over-extending the normal shelf life of foods. Since *Listeria* are widely distributed in the environment, total avoidance and complete elimination of *L.monocytogenes* from all food is not possible, and it is likely that all individuals will be exposed to *Listeria* at some time. However, pregnant women and immunocompromised individuals are at increased risk of contracting listeriosis. In a number of countries (including the UK, USA, France, New Zealand and parts of Australia) 'at risk' individuals are advised to take special precautions. Processed and ready-to-eat foods such as soft and surface-ripened cheese and pâté have been identified as being particularly hazardous, and general advice has been issued in England and Wales for vulnerable individuals not to consume these. Further general advice was issued in the USA to avoid other types of soft cheese (feta and Mexican-style), to avoid delicatessen type foods and to reheat 'cold cut' type meats. In the light of the recent outbreaks in Australasia, it might also be prudent to include similar advice to avoid types of cooked and ready to eat fish and seafood.

Susceptible individuals should also avoid consuming raw or inadequately cooked meat and seafood, wash fruits and vegetables to be consumed raw, and thoroughly reheat all pre-cooked and 'leftover' foods before consumption, especially highly processed ready-to-eat meals.

Unexplained influenza-like illness in pregnant women and the immunocompromised should be medically investigated by the culturing of blood to establish a diagnosis of listeriosis. In addition, those individuals attending infected animals should be aware of the possibility of cutaneous or ocular listeriosis, and should also seek medical attention if suspect lesions develop. It may also be prudent to advise the pregnant and immunosuppressed not to help with lambing, milking ewes that have recently given birth, touch the afterbirth, or come into contact with newborn lambs. This clearly represents a potential route of infection, although with the exception of the cutaneous and ocular lesions, significant associations have not been observed between listeriosis cases and rural backgrounds.

To prevent cross-infection during the neonatal period, strict infection control measures must be instigated at the time of delivery. Such measures include adherence to barrier nursing, use of heat sterilized or single use equipment, single use barriers and alcohol wipes for surfaces, and the wearing of gloves and aprons which are changed prior to hand-washing and attending other patients.

Because human listeriosis is a rare disease, surveillance schemes and epidemiological investigations of cases are essential to identify clusters of patients related by common source and vehicles of infection. The use of analytical studies to investigate outbreaks of listeriosis has had mixed success, and common source outbreaks may only be recognized by collection of isolates from infected patients and identification of common strains. Since *L.monocytogenes* is widespread in the environment (including foods), it is important that comparisons of isolates are made using discriminatory typing schemes.

To prevent listeriosis in animals attention should be paid to feeds, especially to silage, and this has already been discussed. Live attenuated vaccines have been developed for use in animals and it is claimed that this offers some protection although results of field trials are equivocal.

References

Barlow, R.M., and McGorum, B. (1985). Ovine Listerial encephalitis: Analysis, hypothesis and synthesis. *Vet. Rec.,* **116:** 233–36.

Cossart, P., and Toledo-Arana, A. (2008). *Listeria monocytogenes,* a unique model in infection biology: an overview. *Microbes Infect.,* **10:** 1041–50.

Denny, J., and McLauchlin, J. (2008). Human *Listeria monocytogenes* infections in Europe: An opportunity for improved pan-European Surveillance. Eurosurveillance available from http://www. eurosurveillance.org/edition/v13n13/080327_5.asp.

European Food Safety Authority (2007). *Listeria monocytogenes* risk related to ready-to-eat foods and scientific advice on different levels of *Listeria monocytogenes* in ready-to-eat foods and the related risk for human illness - Scientific Opinion of the Panel on Biological Hazards (member) published 5th December 2007. http://www.efsa.europa.eu/ EFSA/efsa_locale-1178620753812_1178680093176.htm.

Farber, J.M., and Peterkin, P.I. (1991). *Listeria monocytogenes,* a food-borne pathogen. *Microbiol. Rev.,* **55:** 476–511.

Freitag, N.R., Port, G.C., and Miner, M.D. (2009). Listeria monocytogenes—from saprophyte to intracellular pathogen. *Nat. Rev. Microbiol.,* **7:** 623–28.

Hamon, M., Bierne, H., and Cossart, P. (2006). Listeria monocytogenes: a multifaceted model. *Nat. Rev. Microbiol.,* **4:** 423–34.

Lui, D. (ed.) (2008). Handbook of *Listeria monocytogenes.* CRC Press, Boca Raton: Taylor Francis Group.

McLauchlin, J., and Low, J.C. (1994). Primary cutaneous listeriosis in adults: An occupational disease of veterinarians and farmers. *Vet. Rec.,* **24:** 615–17.

McLauchlin, J., and Rees, C.E.D. (2009). Genus *Listeria.* In: P. De Vos, G. Garrity, D. Jones, N.R. Krieg, W. Ludwig, *et al.* (eds.) Bergey's Manual of Systematic Bacteriology. Volume 3, The low G + C Gram-positive Bacteria. (2nd edn.), pp. 244–57. NY: Springer.

Ryser, E.T., and Marth, E.H. (eds.) (2007). *Listeria,* Listeriosis, and Food Safety, (3rd Edn.), Boca Raton: CRC Press Taylor Francis Group.

CHAPTER 15

Mycobacterioses

Jakob Zinsstag, Borna Müller and Ivo Pavlik

Summary

The *Mycobacterium tuberculosis* complex (MTC) is composed of several species of mycobacteria which are *M. tuberculosis*, the main cause of human tuberculosis, *M. canetti*, *M. africanum*, *M. microti*, *M. pinnipedii*, *M. caprae*, *M. bovis BCG* and *M. bovis*. Cattle are the principal host of *M. bovis*, but a large number of other ruminants and other mammals, particularly wildlife are infected. Human tuberculosis is a global problem of huge proportions. More than 95% of human tuberculosis cases occur in developing and transition countries, of which one third are in Africa but the proportion of cases caused by *M. bovis* is still not known. Today, bovine tuberculosis (BTB) is re-emerging and threatens the livestock industry in industrialized countries with wildlife reservoirs like the white-tailed deer (*Odocoileus virginianus*) in the USA or the badger (*Meles meles*) in the UK. Most developing countries lack the means and capacity for effective control of BTB. A better understanding of its epidemiology is required to identify novel, locally adapted options for control in a given context. BTB in Africa is emphasized here because of the special importance of multiple transmission interfaces between wildlife, livestock and humans.

In addition to obligatory pathogenic mycobacteria (esp. members of the MTC), potentially pathogenic mycobacteria (PPM) previously designated as 'mycobacteria other than tubercle bacilli' (MOTT) are increasingly important causes of mycobacterioses in humans and animals. Most of them are opportunistic in humans and occur mostly in immunocompromised patients. The mycobacteria that cause human disease are both the *M. avium* complex (MAC) members and other mycobacterial species MAC members have been detected in more than 95% of cases; this chapter will mainly focus on *M. avium* subsp. *avium*, *M. a. hominissuis*, and *M. intracellulare*.

History

Tuberculosis is an ancient disease with evidence of this affliction, in the form of classical spinal lesions, being seen in Eqyptian mummies dating back to 2000–3000 BC, since which time it has become a scourge of most civilizations. A variety of views were originally held as to the causation of tuberculosis. Thoughts that it was a contagious disease appear to have developed with the early Greek observers, Socrates, Aristotle, and Galen, but little progress was made until Francisus Silvus defined the pathology of tuberculosis in 1671.

In 1882 Robert Koch discovered a bacillus, coined as Koch's bacillus or *M. tuberculosis*. He established the bacterial aetiology of tuberculosis by demonstrating its presence in the sputum of all clinical phthisis patients and in all excretions from tuberculous humans and animals. In 1898 Theobald Smith distinguished *M. bovis* from *M. tuberculosis* by its culture properties and studies on their virulence. A Royal Commission set up in Britain to assess the public health significance of bovine tuberculosis found that 5% of all deaths from this disease were due to infection with bovine strains and the proportion of such infections was much higher in very young children.

In 1921, Albert Calmette and Camille Guérin attenuated the virulence of *M. bovis*, producing the first tuberculosis vaccine called BCG (Bacille Calmette Guérin), which is still largely used in humans and is currently being reconsidered for the vaccination of cattle and wildlife in modified versions.

The *M. tuberculosis* complex (MTC) is composed of several species of mycobacteria which are *M. tuberculosis*, the main cause of human tuberculosis, *M. canetti*, *M. africanum*, *M. microti*, *M. pinnipedii*, *M. caprae*, *M. bovis BCG* and *M. bovis*. Cattle are the principal host of *M. bovis*, but a large number of other ruminants and other mammals, particularly wildlife, are infected (Ayele *et al.* 2004). In the middle of the twentieth century, effective government funded control programs were carried out in most industrialized countries. Today, bovine tuberculosis (BTB) is re-emerging and threatens the livestock industry in industrialized countries with wildlife reservoirs like the white-tailed deer (*Odocoileus virginianus*) in the USA or the European badger (*Meles meles*) in the UK. However, in most developing countries, particularly in Africa, they lack the means and capacity for effective control. BTB in Africa is emphasized here because of the disproportionately high burden, the particular difficulties to control it and the distinctive importance of multiple transmission interfaces between wildlife, livestock and humans (Marcotty *et al.* 2009; Michel *et al.* 2009).

The causative agent of avian tuberculosis, *M. avium* was identified in 1891, new insights into the pathogen and taxonomical studies contributed to clarify its occurrence and significance. Several phenotypically related mycobacterial species causing disease in humans and animals have been classified in the *M. avium* complex

(MAC) since 1974 (Meissner *et al.* 1974). New molecular biological methods have established currently accepted classifications (Bartos *et al.* 2006; Mijs *et al.* 2002; Thorel *et al.* 1990):

1 *M. a. avium* (fully virulent for birds),

2 *M. a. hominissuis* (partly virulent for birds),

3 *M. intracellulare* (non-virulent for birds),

4 *M. chimaera* (virulence for birds unknown (Tortoli *et al.* 2004)),

5 *M. colombiense* (virulence for birds unknown (Murcia *et al.* 2006)).

The agent

Mycobacterium bovis

M. bovis is a slow growing, facultative intracellular, aerobic and Gram-positive bacterium with a dysgonic colony shape when cultured on Löwenstein-Jensen medium (Kubica *et al.* 2006). As all mycobacteria, *M. bovis* has an unusual cell wall surface structure characterized by the dominant presence of mycolic acids and a wide array of lipids (Glickman and Jacobs Jr. 2001). This waxy lipid envelope confers an extreme hydrophobicity, which renders the bacteria acid- and alcohol-fast, a feature that can be exploited to identify mycobacteria via the Ziehl-Neelsen staining technique. The mycobacterial surface lipids also have a potent biologic activity and are thought to play a crucial role in pathogenesis (Steingart *et al.* 2006). *M. bovis* can be identified on the basis of specific biochemical and metabolic properties e.g. *M. bovis* requires pyruvate as a growth supplement, is negative for niacin accumulation and nitrate reduction, shows microaerophilic growth on Lebek medium, and is generally resistant to pyrazinamide but sensitive to the isoniazid analogue thiophen-2-carboxylic acid (Cole 2002; Grange *et al.* 1996; Steingart *et al.* 2006). However, the unequivocal validity of these characteristics has been challenged by several studies (Kubica *et al.* 2006; Niemann *et al.* 2000).

Molecular epidemiological methods

Molecular markers allow the unambiguous identification and differentiation of mycobacteria and the members of the MTC (Boddinghaus *et al.* 1990; Durr *et al.* 2000; Huard *et al.* 2006; Pinsky and Banaei 2008) and genotyping techniques can differentiate distinct strains of MTC (Brudey *et al.* 2006; Haddad *et al.* 2004; Harris 2006; Kanduma *et al.* 2003; Mostrom *et al.* 2002). Molecular typing of isolates offer insights into the population structure and evolution of infections and pathogens (van Soolingen 2001) have helped to identify disease transmission chains, risk factors for tuberculosis infections and laboratory cross-contaminations (Haddad *et al.* 2004; Harris 2006). *Spacer oligotyping* (*Spoligotyping*) makes use of the variability of the MTC chromosomal direct repeat (DR) locus for strain differentiation (Kamerbeek *et al.* 1997). Extensive databases (www. Mbovis.org and SpolDB4) have facilitated the comparison of strains isolated in different countries. Several genomic loci within the MTC with tandemly repeated mini-satellite sequences have been identified and are used for *Variable number of tandem repeat* (VNTR) typing (Harris 2006). Large genomic deletions (also called regions of difference, RD) have been used for the phylogenetic reconstruction of MTC strains (Brosch *et al.* 2002; Gagneux and Small 2007; Muller *et al.* 2009; Smith *et al.* 2006a). *Restriction fragment length polymorphism (RFLP)* typing uses most frequently a probe for the MTC specific transposable element IS*6110* (Mostrom *et al.* 2002; van Soolingen 2001).

Evolution

The population structure of the MTC can be considered as highly clonal if *M. canetti* is excluded (Hershberg *et al.* 2008). Because of the smaller genome size of *M. bovis* compared to *M. tuberculosis* and because no significant chromosomal regions are present in *M. bovis* but absent in all strains of *M. tuberculosis*, it can be inferred that *M. bovis* emerged from an *M. tuberculosis*-like ancestor (Brosch *et al.* 2002; Hershberg *et al.* 2008; Smith *et al.* 2006a). Recently it has been suggested, that the MTC should be considered as a group of different 'ecotypes', adapted to distinct environments or hosts (Smith *et al.* 2006b).

Epidemiology

BTB was detected in Africa at the beginning of the twentieth century with reports of 1–2% intradermal test positive animals in rural areas, and 10–40% in regions of intensive farming around larger cities in South Africa (von Ostertag and Kulenkampff 1941). Whether BTB had been introduced solely during the colonial period or if there existed autochthonous reservoirs is still debated (Cousins *et al.* 2004; Muller *et al.* 2008; Njanpop-Lafourcade *et al.* 2001). Today BTB is reported in most African countries (Ayele *et al.* 2004).

Livestock

Gidel *et al.* (1969) were one of the first to isolate animal derived mycobacteria in Africa during their work in Burkina Faso. Trials on the use of BCG as a vaccine for cattle were undertaken in Malawi without success (Ellwood and Waddington 1972), but new trials are currently ongoing in Ethiopia (Hewinson pers. comm.). The isolation and molecular characterization of strains of *M. bovis* from cattle has been reported in several African countries (Diguimbaye-Djaibe *et al.* 2006; Jiwa *et al.* 1997; Muller *et al.* 2008; Rigouts *et al.* 1996; Sahraoui *et al.* 2009; Wekhe and Berepubo 1989). Mycobacteria have been isolated from the raw milk of pastoral cattle in Southern Tanzania (Kazwala *et al.* 1998). Low intradermal test prevalence <1% but a herd prevalence of 11% was found in rural Tanzania. Age and herd sizes >50 animals were risk factors for infection (Cleaveland *et al.* 2007). High prevalence in peri-urban dairy operations was confirmed again recently in Ethiopia (Ameni *et al.* 2007). The type of livestock production and husbandry affects the disease pathology and gamma interferon response of *M. bovis* (Ameni *et al.* 2006). *M. bovis* has been detected in dromedaries in Mauritania and Chad (Chartier *et al.* 1991). *M. bovis* infection patterns have been surveyed extensively in countries that have applied a test-slaughter protocol to cattle with low prevalence (Hewinson *et al.* 2006). Trans-national strain comparisons have shown the usefulness of MIRU-VNTR typing when addressing issues of cross-border transmission between Mexico and the USA (Milian-Suazo *et al.* 2008). *M. bovis* transmission chains in Belgian cattle were demonstrated by a combination of Spoligotyping, MIRU-VNTR and tracing of cattle trader and farmer contact (Allix *et al.* 2006). In the same way cattle to human transmission could be demonstrated in Mexico (Perez-Guerrero *et al.* 2008). Muller *et al.* showed that a newly identified clonal complex, called Af1 dominates the population structure of *M. bovis* in the Central West African sub-region (Muller *et al.* 2009).

Humans

Mycobacteria different from *M. tuberculosis* have been reported in Kinshasa (Congo) (Pattyn *et al.* 1967). In a study in Lagos (Nigeria) 4% of MTC strains were *M. bovis* (Idigbe *et al.* 1986). *M. bovis* infections in humans has been reported from Guinea-Bissau, Burundi, Tanzania, Madagascar, Uganda, and Ghana (Addo *et al.* 2007; Hoffner *et al.* 1993; Kazwala *et al.* 2001; Oloya *et al.* 2007; Rasolofo-Razanamparany *et al.* 1999; Rigouts *et al.* 1996). However, most of the countries in Africa lack technical capacity to differentiate *M. bovis* from the other members of MTC (Daborn *et al.* 1996). Higher proportions of *M. bovis* infections in humans are detected in rural settings compared to urban areas (Table 15.1), but little is known about tuberculosis in pastoralist communities in Africa, since they are often excluded from public health services (Zinsstag *et al.* 2006a).

Wildlife

Whilst cattle are the main host *M. bovis* has been isolated from a large number of wildlife species like wild boar (*Sus scrofa*), the common brushtail possum (*Trichosurus vulpecula*), the fallow deer (*Dama dama*) in New Zealand, and European badgers (*Meles meles*) in the UK. Bison (*Bison bison*), red deer (*Cervus elaphus*), and white-tailed deer (*Odocoileus virginianus*) were identified to be affected by *M. bovis* in the USA (Cousins *et al.* 2004). In Africa, *M. bovis* has been found in the Lechwe antelope (*Kobus leche*) (Clancey 1977), in warthog (*Phacocerus aethiopicus*) (Woodford 1982), and in olive baboon (*Papio anubis*) (Tarara *et al.* 1985). *M. bovis* has been isolated from African buffalo (*Syncerus caffer*) in the Krüger National Park in South Africa (Bengis *et al.* 1996), and from cheetah (*Acinonyx jubatus*), lion (*Panthera leo*) and Chacma baboon (*Papio ursinus*) (Keet *et al.* 1996). Most likely, infected cattle grazing close to Krüger National Park transmitted BTB to buffalo, which then spread to large carnivores. The establishment of BTB in the South African wildlife is a serious problem, as the disease can be transmitted to many different species by direct transmission along the food chain, and to other countries (Kriek 2006). A study in Zambia indicates the risk of transmission from wildlife to cattle (Munyeme 2008) and BTB has been described in blue wildebeest (*Connochaetes taurinus*), and Topi antelopes (*Damaliscus lunatus*) in Tanzania (Cleaveland *et al.* 2005).

Interfaces of wildlife, livestock and humans

Wildlife and cattle frequently use the same pasture around nature reserves and national parks in Africa. Currently there is evidence of transmission from cattle to African buffalo and Lechwe antelope in Southern Africa. Humans may be infected from cattle by the aerial and/or alimentary routes, and there can be subsequent human-to-human transmission. From a general point of view, BTB control should aim first at cattle and at the same time limit the spread in wildlife (Cousins *et al.* 2004; Renwick *et al.* 2007). Further studies should also include livestock and humans within a systemic 'one health' approach to understand the ecology of BTB (Zinsstag *et al.* 2005).

Hosts

Cattle

BTB caused by *M. bovis* is mainly a chronic respiratory disease (Fig. 15.1) with emaciation, loss of appetite, chronic cough, and other signs of pneumonia, but it can affect many other organs, notably the mammary lymph nodes; consequently, *M. bovis* is commonly excreted in milk. BTB is transmitted by aerosol and by milk consumption to other animals and humans. BTB is clinically difficult to diagnose especially in developing countries, where many other chronic, emaciating diseases, like African trypanosomiasis, chronic contagious bovine pleuro-pneumonia (CBPP), or chronic multi-parasitism are present. BTB pathology is characterized by the formation of granulomatous lesions, which can within the course of the disease regress or exhibit extensive necrosis, calcify or liquefy,

Table 15.1 A selection of reports on zoonotic tuberculosis infections in Africa

Country	Study setting	Total MTBC	M. bovis	% M. bovis	Reference
Cameroon	15 district hospitals in Ouest province	455	1	0.2%	Niobe-Eyangoh *et al.* 2003
Djibouti	Unknown	85	1	1.2%	Koeck *et al.* 2002
Egypt	Six fever hospitals in different cities	67	1	1.5%	Cooksey *et al.* 2002
Ghana	Korle-Bu Teaching Hospital	64	2	3.1%	Addo *et al.* 2007
Guinea-Bissau	Unknown	229	4	1.7%	Källenius *et al.* 1999
Madagascar	Antananarivo, Antsirabe, Fianarantsoa, Mahajanga	400	5	1.3%	Rosolofo-Razanamparany *et al.* 1999
Nigeria	2 hospitals in Ibadan	60	3	5.0%	Cadmus *et al.* 2006
Nigeria	Lagos	91	4	4.4%	Idigbe *et al.* 1986
Nigeria	3 hospitals in Jos	50	10	20.0%	Mawak *et al.* 2006
Tanzania	4 districts of Manyara (Arusha) Region	34	7	20.6%	Cleaveland *et al.* 2007
Tanzania	Pastoralist communities in the North and South	38	7	18.4%	Kazwala *et al.* 2001
Tanzania	Rural and semi-rural districts of Arusha	34	7	20.6%	Mfinanga *et al.* 2004
Uganda	Kampala	344	1	0.3%	Asiimwe *et al.* 2008
Uganda	Kampala	234	1	0.4%	Niemann *et al.* 2002
Uganda	Pastoralists of transhumant areas in Karamoya	10	3	30.0%	Oloya *et al.* 2007

and subsequently lead to cavity formation. During meat inspection tuberculous lesions are primarily found in the upper and lower respiratory tract and associated lymph nodes.

However, the bacteria can also develop a systemic infection. The main productivity losses in cattle are reduced milk and meat production and fertility (Bernues *et al.* 1997). Milk productivity is estimated to be $10 \pm 2.5\%$ less than non-infected cows. In one study, BTB was found to decrease meat production by 6–12% (Meisinger 1970).

The two most widely used tests for the diagnosis of BTB are the single intra-dermal comparative cervical tuberculin (SICCT) test and the Bovigam® test (Prionics) (de la Rua-Domenech *et al.* 2006). Both are based on the detection of the early cell mediated immune response (CMI response) in tuberculosis infection, which is also known as the Th1-type immune response (Thoen and Barletta 2006). Internationally recognized standard procedures for the diagnosis of BTB (International Office of Epizootics (OIE) 2006) exist. However, two recent studies suggest a modification in some sub-Saharan African settings (Ameni *et al.* 2008; Ngandolo *et al.* 2009).

In late stage diseased animals, the CMI response may wane, which potentially causes false negative SICCT results. Such animals are thought to be more accurately diagnosed by the detection of antibodies for *M. bovis* specific antigens (Plackett *et al.* 1989). Importantly, there is evidence that such skin test anergic animals are heavily diseased, shed higher amounts of causal agents and may be one cause of persistent and severe herd breakdowns (de la Rua-Domenech *et al.* 2006; Palmer and Waters 2006; Pollock *et al.* 2005). Some ELISA or FPA based serological tests for the diagnosis of BTB have been developed but are unlikely to replace the above tests (Amadori *et al.* 2002; de la Rua-Domenech *et al.* 2006; Jolley *et al.* 2007; Ngandolo *et al.* 2009).

Humans

Clinical *M. bovis* in humans is most often indistinguishable from human tuberculosis and cannot be diagnosed unless mycobacterial culture and molecular diagnosis is available (Ayele *et al.* 2004; Cosivi *et al.* 1998). Extra pulmonary BTB is the result of ingestion of contaminated milk and milk products. Extra pulmonary tuberculosis involves predominantly cervical lymph nodes (Kazwala *et al.* 2001) but can also involve the gastro-intestinal tract, liver, spleen, kidneys, pleura, and peritoneum together with their associated lymph nodes. *M. bovis* is resistant to pyranzinamide. For diagnosis and treatment in humans we refer here, for space reasons, to the relevant literature on human tuberculosis and the Stop-TB strategy of the World Health Organization (http://www.who.int/topics/tuberculosis/en/).

Prevention and control

Effective control and in some countries elimination of BTB has been achieved through well managed test and slaughter programmes, movement control and compensation of farmers for culled stock. Today, livestock producing countries of the developing world bear most of the global burden of BTB. The disease is virtually uncontrolled in the whole of Africa. There, surveillance is generally based on slaughterhouse meat inspection. Conventional test and slaughter schemes may not be affordable or may be ill suited for Africa. Therefore, new approaches for BTB control are being considered. From a public health perspective, the first priority with regards to BTB control is the prevention of zoonotic transmission of *M. bovis* from animals to humans. Losses from meat confiscations are most often not refunded by the government, promoting fraud and (illegal) private slaughter of animals. Milk pasteurization is used increasingly in urban African centres and has a wider benefit including prevention of other zoonoses like brucellosis or Q-fever (Bonfoh *et al.* 2003, 2004). However, in rural areas and pastoralist communities, close contact between humans and animals may pose another important risk factor for zoonotic transmission of *M. bovis*.

Economic analyses of the cost to society of *M. bovis* are required to create the necessary political awareness for its effective control (Zinsstag *et al.* 2006b). From a global perspective, the shortfalls of current control efforts in developing countries should be of interest for all countries. In a globalized world, with falling trade barriers, endemic diseases in one part of the world will always threaten the spread of disease to disease-free zones. Many developing countries, however, will not be able, by their own means, to invest in control and elimination programs for decades. A global fund, analogous to the Global Fund against *AIDS*, tuberculosis and malaria is required for worldwide control of BTB and zoonoses in general (Zinsstag *et al.* 2007).

Mycobacterium avium complex

Epidemiology and ecology

New insights into the ecology of all three MAC members and a majority of mycobacteria discovered before 2008 have recently been provided by Kazda (2002; Kazda *et al.* 2009). The main sources of *M. a. avium* are domestic and free living birds (Anz and Meissner 1969a; Meissner and Anz 1977; Thoen *et al.* 1977). Birds may spread *M. a. avium* through their faeces or infected bodies to the environment. There is little evidence of *M. a. avium* multiplication outside of the host. However, it has been shown that *M. a. avium* has the ability to survive in the environment for months or even for years compensated for this disadvantage (Kazda *et al.* 2009). People may become infected through direct contact with infected live or dead birds, or by eating raw eggs, meat and vegetables. Among 2,311 isolates obtained from patients in Australia, the USA, Canada,

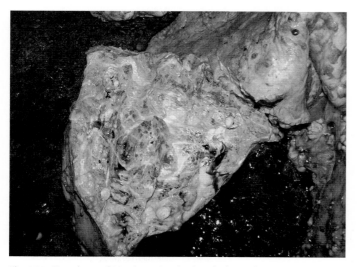

Fig. 15.1 Granuloma of *Mycobacterium bovis* in the lung of a cow in Sarh (Chad) Photo with permission by: Bongo Nare Ngandolo

Germany, and Japan, zoonotic *M. a. avium*, *M. a. hominissuis* and *M. intracellulare* were detected in 17.7%, 56.7% and 25.6% of patients, respectively (Anz and Meissner 1969; Blacklock and Dawson 1979; Meissner and Anz 1977; Miyachi *et al.* 1988; Reznikov *et al.* 1971).

The primary source of *M. a. hominissuis* and *M. intracellulare* is a contaminated environment where they multiply: sediments and biofilms in surface water, soil, peat-bogs, compost heaps etc. (Kazda *et al.* 2009). Direct transmission from animals to humans can occur through, e.g. contact of people with infected slurry, or contact of owners with infected domestic pets such as parrots (Shitaye *et al.* 2009). It follows that *M. a. hominissuis* can be considered as an agent with considerably limited zoonotic potential. Most frequent hosts are pigs and humans (Kazda *et al.* 2009; Mijs *et al.* 2002). *M. intracellulare* cannot be considered as pathogen with zoonotic potential.

Hosts
Humans

All three principal MAC members cause human mycobacteriosis, with both pulmonary and extra-pulmonary localizations. A weakened immune system is a significant precondition for mycobacterial colonization. Receiving immunosuppressive treatment is the most common cause for development of infection in non-*HIV/AIDS* patients. Furthermore, social factors like alcoholism or drug addiction can also play a role (Korvick and Benson 1996). The infection can manifest itself in several different forms:

1 Lymphadenitis,

2 Bituminosis,

3 Disseminated infection,

4 Occasional skin infection.

In the last decade, a hypersensitivity pneumonitis-like disease, also designated as 'Hot tub lung', has been described (Embil and Warren 1997; Korvick and Benson 1996).

Before the discovery of *HIV* virus and clinical manifestation of *AIDS*, four forms of pulmonary tissue lesions had been described (Teirstein *et al.* 1990):

1 Occasional nodules,

2 Chronic bronchitis or bronchiectasis,

3 Tuberculosis-like infiltrates,

4 Diffused infiltration, in immunocompromised patients (haematological malignancies, combined immunosuppression after transplantations, caused by treatment with corticoids or cytotoxic drugs etc.).

Mycobacteria have become major opportunist pathogens in HIV infected people and in such complex cases, reliability of diagnosis in identifying mycobacteria in different organs with atypical localization of infection is very low (Horsburgh Jr. *et al.* 2001).

Animals

M. a. avium causes avian tuberculosis in animals, primarily in birds, by affecting all parenchymatous organs. Hepatic lesions are present in almost 100% of cases. In cattle and pigs, intestinal lymph nodes are usually infected, but lesions in parenchymatous organs or miliary forms have been diagnosed occasionally. Clinical signs of the disease are rarely observed, and infection is usually recognized at meat inspection after slaughter. *M. a. avium* is shed in faeces, urine, eggs, ejaculate etc. which then become the most significant sources of this causative agent transmission (Dvorska *et al.* 2004; Shitaye *et al.* 2006; Thorel *et al.* 1997).

Birds exhibit considerable resistance to *M. a. hominissuis* infection. Their infection can be only elicited in the inoculated muscle. In other animals, this disease is designated as avian mycobacteriosis due to low frequency of lesions (Dvorska *et al.* 1999, 2004; Matlova *et al.* 2005; Shitaye *et al.* 2006, 2009).

M. intracellulare is uncommonly found in animals. Nevertheless, it can produce tuberculous lesions in head and intestinal lymph nodes, primarily in pigs (Kleeberg and Nel 1973; Piening *et al.* 1972). The last-mentioned two species, *M. chimaera* and *M. colombiense*, have so far only been isolated from humans, and their virulence for birds is unknown (Murcia *et al.* 2006; Tortoli *et al.* 2004).

Prevention and control

Human-to-human transmission of the three MAC members does not appear to take place and therefore it is assumed that the main sources of *M. a. avium* for humans are contaminated food and water. Prevention should focus on heat treatment of foods and thorough washing of raw fruits and vegetables.

Acknowledgement

This work has been supported by the Wellcome Trust Livestock for live initiative, the National Centre for Competence North-South (NCCR North-South) and the Swiss National Science Foundation. This work was supported by grant No. MZE0002716202 from the Ministry of Agriculture of the Czech Republic and by Grant CZ 1.05/2.1.00/01.0006-ED0006/01/01 AdmireVet from the Ministry of Education, Youth and Sports, Czech Republic.

References

Addo, K., Owusu-Darko, K., Yeboah-Manu, D., Caulley, P., Minamikawa, M., *et al.* (2007). Mycobacterial species causing pulmonary tuberculosis at the korle bu teaching hospital, Accra, Ghana. *Ghana. Med. J.*, **41**: 52–57.

Allix, C., Walravens, K., Saegerman, C., Godfroid, J., Supply, P., *et al.* (2006). Evaluation of the epidemiological relevance of variable-number tandem-repeat genotyping of *Mycobacterium bovis* and comparison of the method with IS6110 restriction fragment length polymorphism analysis and spoligotyping. *J. Clin. Microbiol.*, **44**: 1951–62.

Amadori, M., Lyaschenko, K. P., Gennaro, M. L., Pollock, J. M., and Zerbini, I. (2002). Use of recombinant proteins in antibody tests for bovine tuberculosis. *Vet. Microbiol.*, **85**: 379–89.

Ameni, G., Aseffa, A., Engers, H., Young, D., Hewinson, G., *et al.* (2006). Cattle husbandry in ethiopia is a predominant factor affecting the pathology of bovine tuberculosis and gamma interferon responses to mycobacterial antigens. *Clin. Vaccine Immunol.*, **13**: 1030–36.

Ameni, G., Aseffa, A., Engers, H., Young, D., Gordon, S., *et al.* (2007). High prevalence and increased severity of pathology of bovine tuberculosis in Holsteins compared to zebu breeds under field cattle husbandry in central Ethiopia. *Clin. Vaccine Immunol.*, **14**: 1356–61.

Anz, W. and Meissner, G. (1969). Serotypes of strains of avian mycobacteria isolated from humans and animals. *Prax. Pneumol.*, **23**: 221–30.

Ayele, W. Y., Neill, S. D., Zinsstag, J., Weiss, M. G., and Pavlik, I. (2004). Bovine tuberculosis: an old disease but a new threat to Africa. *Int. J. Tuberc. Lung Dis.*, **8**: 924–37.

Bartos, M., Hlozek, P., Svastova, P., Dvorska, L., Bull, T., *et al.* (2006). Identification of members of *Mycobacterium avium* species by Accu-Probes, serotyping, and single IS900, IS901, IS1245 and IS901-flanking region PCR with internal standards. *J. Microbiol. Meth.,* **64:** 333–45.

Bengis, R. G., Kriek, N. P., Keet, D. F., Raath, J. P., *et al.* (1996). An outbreak of bovine tuberculosis in a free-living African buffalo (*Syncerus caffer*—Sparrman) population in the Kruger National Park: a preliminary report. *The Onderstep. J. Vet. Res.,* **63:** 15–18.

Bernues, A., Manrique, E., and Maza, M. T. (1997). Economic evaluation of bovine brucellosis and tuberculosis eradication programmes in a mountain area of Spain. *Prev. Vet. Med.,* **30:** 137–49.

Blacklock, Z. M. and Dawson, D. J. (1979). Atypical mycobacteria causing non-pulmonary disease in Queensland. *Pathology,* **11:** 283–87.

Boddinghaus, B., Rogall, T., Flohr, T., Blocker, H., and Bottger, E. C. (1990). Detection and identification of mycobacteria by amplification of rRNA. *J. Clin. Microbiol.,* **28:** 1751–59.

Bonfoh, B., Roth, C., Traoré, A. N., Fané, A., Simbé, C. F., *et al.*(2004). Effect of washing and disinfecting containers on the microbiological quality of fresh milk sold in Bamako (Mali). *Food Cont.,* **17:** 153–61.

Bonfoh, B., Wasem, A., Traore, A. N., Fane, A., Spillmann, H., *et al.* (2003). Microbiological quality of cows' milk taken at different intervals from the udder to the selling point in Bamako (Mali). *Food Cont.,* **14:** 495–500.

Brosch, R., Gordon, S. V., Marmiesse, M., Brodin, P., Buchrieser, C., *et al.* (2002). A new evolutionary scenario for the *Mycobacterium tuberculosis* complex. *Proc. Natl. Acad. Sci. USA,* **99:** 3684–89.

Brudey, K., Driscoll, J., Rigouts, L., Prodinger, W., Gori, A., Al-Hajoj, S., *et al.* (2006). *Mycobacterium tuberculosis* complex genetic diversity: mining the fourth international spoligotyping database (SpolDB4) for classification, population genetics and epidemiology. *BMC Microbiol.,* **6:** 23.

Chartier, F., Chartier, C., Thorel, M. F., and Crespeau, F. (1991). Un nouveau cas de tuberculose pulmonaire à *Mycobacterium bovis* chez le dromadaire (*Camelus dromedarius*) en Mauritanie. *Revue Elev. Méd. vét. Pays Trop.,* **1:** 43–47.

Clancey, J. K. (1977). The incidence of tuberculosis in Lechwe (marsh antelope). *Tubercle.* **58:** 151–56.

Cleaveland, S., Mlengeya, T., Kazwala, R. R., Michel, A., Kaare, M. T., *et al.* (2005). Tuberculosis in Tanzanian wildlife. *J. Wildl. Dis.,* **41:** 446–53.

Cleaveland, S., Shaw, D. J., Mfinanga, S. G., Shirima, G., Kazwala, R. R., *et al.* (2007). *Mycobacterium bovis* in rural Tanzania: risk factors for infection in human and cattle populations. *Tuberculosis. (Edinb.),* **87:** 30–43.

Cole, S. T. (2002). Comparative and functional genomics of the *Mycobacterium tuberculosis* complex. *Microbiol.,* **148:** 2919–28.

Cosivi, O., Grange, J. M., Daborn, C. J., Raviglione, M. C., Fujikura, T., *et al.* (1998). Zoonotic tuberculosis due to *Mycobacterium bovis* in developing countries. *Emerg. Infect Dis.,* **4:** 59–70.

Cousins, D., Huchzermeyer, H., Griffin, J. F. T., Brückner, G., van Rensburg, I. B. J., *et al.* (2004). Tuberculosis. In: J. A. W. Coetzer and R. C. Tustin (eds.) Infectious Diseases of Livestock, pp. 1973–93. Oxford: Oxford University Press.

Daborn, C. J., Grange, J. M., and Kazwala, R. R. (1996). The bovine tuberculosis cycle—an African perspective. *Soc. Appl. Bacteriol. Symp. Ser.,* **25:** 27S–32S.

de la Rua-Domenech, R., Goodchild, A. T., Vordermeier, H. M., Hewinson, R. G., Christiansen, K. H., *et al.* (2006). *Ante mortem* diagnosis of tuberculosis in cattle: a review of the tuberculin tests, gamma-interferon assay and other ancillary diagnostic techniques. *Res. Vet. Sci.,* **81:** 190–210.

Diguimbaye-Djaibe, C., Hilty, M., Ngandolo, R., Mahamat, H. H., Pfyffer, G. E., *et al.* (2006). *Mycobacterium bovis* isolates from tuberculous lesions in Chadian zebu carcasses. *Emerg. Infect Dis.,* **12:** 769–71.

Durr, P. A., Hewinson, R. G., and Clifton-Hadley, R. S. (2000). Molecular epidemiology of bovine tuberculosis - I. *Mycobacterium bovis* genotyping. *Revue Scientift. Techni. Off. Internat. Epizoot.,* **19:,** 675–88.

Dvorska, L., Matlova, L., Bartos, M., Parmova, I., Bartl, J., *et al.* (2004). Study of *Mycobacterium avium* complex strains isolated from cattle in the Czech Republic between 1996 and 2000. *Vet. Microbiol.,* **99:** 239–50.

Dvorska, L., Parmova, I., Lavickova, M., Bartl, J., Vrbas, V., *et al.* (1999). Isolation of *Rhodococcus equi* and atypical mycobacteria from lymph nodes of pigs and cattle in herds with the occurrence of tuberculoid gross changes in the Czech Republic over the period of 1996–1998. *Vet. Med.,* **44:** 321–30.

Ellwood, D. C. and Waddington, F. G. (1972). A second experiment to challenge the resistance to tuberculosis in B.C.G. vaccinated cattle in Malawi. *Br. Vet. J.,* **128:** 619–26.

Embil, J. M. and Warren, C. P. W. (1997). Pneumonitis due to *Mycobacterium avium* complex in hot tub water - Infection or hypersensitivity? *Chest,* **112:** 1713–14.

Gagneux, S. and Small, P. M. (2007). Global phylogeography of *Mycobacterium tuberculosis* and implications for tuberculosis product development. *Lancet Infect. Dis.,* **7:** 328–37.

Gidel, R., Albert, J. P., Lefevre, M., Menard, M., and Retif, M. (1969). [Mycobacteria of animal origin isolated by the Muraz Center from 1965 to 1968: technics of isolation and identification; results]. *Rev. Elev. Med. Vet. Pays. Trop.,* **22:** 495–508.

Glickman, M. S. and Jacobs Jr., W. R. (2001). Microbial pathogenesis of *Mycobacterium tuberculosis:* dawn of a discipline. *Cell,* **104:** 477–85.

Grange, J. M., Yates, M., and de Kantor, I. N. (1996). Guidelines for speciation within the *Mycobacterium tuberculosis* complex. WHO/EMC/ZOO/96.4, pp. 1–18. Geneva: World Health Organization.

Haddad, N., Masselot, M., and Durand, B. (2004). Molecular differentiation of *Mycobacterium bovis* isolates. Review of main techniques and applications. *Res. Vet. Sci.,* **76:** 1–18.

Harris, N. B. (2006). Molecular Techniques: Applications in Epidemiologic Studies. In: C. O. Thoen, J. H. Steele and M. J. Gilsdorf (eds.) *Myctobacterium bovis* infection in animals and humans, pp. 54–62. Ames, Iowa, USA: Blackwell Publishing.

Hershberg, R., Lipatov, M., Small, P. M., Sheffer, H., Niemann, S., *et al.* (2008). High functional diversity in *Mycobacterium tuberculosis* driven by genetic drift and human demography. *PLoS. Biol.,* **6:** e311.

Hewinson, R. G., Vordermeier, H. M., Smith, N. H., and Gordon, S. V. (2006). Recent advances in our knowledge of *Mycobacterium bovis:* a feeling for the organism. *Vet. Microbiol.,* **112:** 127–39.

Hoffner, S. E., Svenson, S. B., Norberg, R., Dias, F., Ghebremichael, S., *et al.* (1993). Biochemical Heterogeneity of *Mycobacterium tuberculosis* Complex Isolates in Guinea-Bissau. *J. Clin. Microbiol.,* **31:** 2215–17.

Horsburgh Jr., C. R., Gettings, J., Alexander, L. N., and Lennox, J. L. (2001). Disseminated *Mycobacterium avium* complex disease among patients infected with human immunodeficiency virus, 1985–2000. *Clin. Infect. Dis.,* **33:** 1938–43.

Huard, R. C., Fabre, M., de Haas, P., Lazzarini, L. C., van Soolingen, D., *et al.* (2006). Novel genetic polymorphisms that further delineate the phylogeny of the *Mycobacterium tuberculosis* complex. *J. Bacteriol.,* **188:** 4271–87.

Idigbe, E. O., Anyiwo, C. E., and Onwujekwe, D. I. (1986). Human pulmonary infections with bovine and atypical mycobacteria in Lagos, Nigeria. *J. Trop. Med. Hyg.,* **89**(3): 143–48.

International Office of Epizootics (OIE) (2006). Manual of diagnostic tests and vaccines for terrestrial animals 2004. Paris: OIE.

Jiwa, S. F., Kazwala, R. R., Aboud, A. A., and Kalaye, W. J. (1997). Bovine tuberculosis in the Lake Victoria zone of Tanzania and its possible consequences for human health in the HIV/AIDS era. *Vet. Res. Commun.,* **21:** 533–39.

Jolley, M. E., Nasir, M. S., Surujballi, O. P., Romanowska, A., Renteria, T. B., *et al.* (2007). Fluorescence polarization assay for the detection of antibodies to *Mycobacterium bovis* in bovine sera. *Vet. Microbiol.,* **120:** 113–21.

Kamerbeek, J., Schouls, L., Kolk, A., van Agterveld, M., van Soolingen, D., *et al.* (1997). Simultaneous detection and strain differentiation of *Mycobacterium tuberculosis* for diagnosis and epidemiology. *J. Clin. Microbiol.,* **35:** 907–914.

Kanduma, E., McHugh, T. D., and Gillespie, S. H. (2003). Molecular methods for *Mycobacterium tuberculosis* strain typing: a users guide. *J. Appl. Microbiol.*, **94**: 781–91.

Kazda, J. (2002). The ecology of mycobacteria, pp. 211–212. Dordrecht, Boston. London: Kluwer Academic Publishers.

Kazda, J., Pavlik, I., Falkinham III, J. O., and Hruska, K. (2009).The ecology of mycobacteria: impact on animal's and human's health, pp. 1–522. NY: Springer.

Kazwala, R. R., Daborn, C. J., Kusiluka, L. J., Jiwa, S. F., Sharp, J. M., *et al.* (1998). Isolation of *Mycobacterium* species from raw milk of pastoral cattle of the Southern Highlands of Tanzania. *Trop. Anim. Health Prod.*, **30**: 233–39.

Kazwala, R. R., Daborn, C. J., Sharp, J. M., Kambarage, D. M., Jiwa, S. F., *et al.* (2001). Isolation of *Mycobacterium bovis* from human cases of cervical adenitis in Tanzania: a cause for concern? *Int. J. Tuberc. Lung Dis.*, **5**: 87–91.

Keet, D. F., Kriek, N. P., Penrith, M. L., Michel, A., and Huchzermeyer, H. (1996). Tuberculosis in buffaloes (*Syncerus caffer*) in the Kruger National Park: spread of the disease to other species. *Onderstepoort J. Vet. Res.*, **63**: 239–44.

Kleeberg, H. H. and Nel, E. E. (1973). Occurrence of environmental atypical mycobacteria in South Africa. *Ann. Soc. Belg. Med. Trop.*, **53**: 405–418.

Korvick, J. A. and Benson, C. A. (1996). *Mycobacterium avium* complex infection: Progress in research and treatment, pp. 1–316. NY: Marcel Dekker.

Kriek, N. P. (2006). Bovine tuberculosis program in South Africa: The impact of *M. bovis*-infected wild species. In: C. O. Thoen, J. H. Steele and M. J. Gilsdorf (eds.) *Mycobacterium bovis* infection in animals and humans, pp. 54–62. Ames, Iowa, USA: Blackwell Publishing.

Kubica, T., Agzamova, R., Wright, A., Rakishev, G., Rusch-Gerdes, S., *et al.* (2006). *Mycobacterium bovis* isolates with *M. tuberculosis* specific characteristics. *Emerg. Infect. Dis.*, **12**: 763–65.

Marcotty, T., Matthys, F., Godfroid, J., Rigouts, L., Ameni, G., *et al.* (2009). Zoonotic tuberculosis and brucellosis in Africa: neglected zoonoses or minor public-health issues? The outcomes of a multi-disciplinary workshop. *Ann. Trop. Med. Parasitol.*, **103**: 401–11.

Matlova, L., Dvorska, L., Ayele, W. Y., Bartos, M., Amemori, T., *et al.* (2005). Distribution of *Mycobacterium avium* complex isolates in tissue samples of pigs fed peat naturally contaminated with mycobacteria as a supplement. *J. Clin. Microbiol.*, **43**: 1261–68.

Meisinger, G. (1970). Economic effects of the elimination of bovine tuberculosis on the productivity of cattle herds. 2. Effect on meat production. *Monatsh.Veterinarmed.*, **25**: 7–13.

Meissner, G., Schroder, K. H., Amadio, G. E., Anz, W., Chaparas, S., *et al.* (1974). A co-operative numerical analysis of nonscoto- and nonphotochromogenic slowly growing mycobacteria. *J. Gen. Microbiol.*, **83**: 207–35.

Meissner, G. and Anz, W. (1977). Sources of *Mycobacterium avium* complex infection resulting in human diseases. *Am. Rev. Respir. Dis.*, **116**: 1057–64.

Michel, A. L., Muller, B., and Van Helden, P. D. (2010). *Mycobacterium bovis* at the animal-human interface: A problem, or not? *Vet. Microbiol.*, **140**(3–4): 371–81.

Mijs, W., De Vreese, K., Devos, A., Pottel, H., Valgaeren, A., *et al.* (2002). Evaluation of a commercial line probe assay for identification of Mycobacterium species from liquid and solid culture. *Eur. J. Clin. Microbiol. Infect. Dis.*, **21**: 794–802.

Milian-Suazo, F., Harris, B., Arriaga, D. C., Romero, T. C., Stuber, T., *et al.* (2008). Molecular epidemiology of *Mycobacterium bovis*: usefulness in international trade. *Prev. Vet. Med.*, **87**: 261–71.

Miyachi, T., Shimokata, K., Dawson, D. J., and Tsukumura, M. (1988). Changes of the biotype of *Mycobacterium avium-Mycobacterium intracellulare* complex causing lung disease in Japan. *Tubercle.*, **69**: 133–37.

Mostrom, P., Gordon, M., Sola, C., Ridell, M., and Rastogi, N. (2002). Methods used in the molecular epidemiology of tuberculosis. *Clin. Microbiol. Infect.*, **8**: 694–704.

Muller, B., Hilty, M., Berg, S., Garcia-Pelayo, M. C., Dale, J., *et al.* (2009). African 1; An Epidemiologically important clonal complex of *Mycobacterium bovis* dominant in Mali, Nigeria, Cameroon and Chad. *J. of Bacteriol.*, **191**(6): 1951–60.

Muller, B., Steiner, B., Bonfoh, B., Fane, A., Smith, N. H., *et al.* (2008). Molecular characterisation of *Mycobacterium bovis* isolated from cattle slaughtered at the Bamako abattoir in Mali. *BMC. Vet. Res.*, **4**: 26.

Munyeme, M., Muma, J. B., Skjerve, E., Nambota, A. M., Phiri, I. G., Samui, K. L., Dorny, P., Tryland, M., (2008). Risk factors associated with bovine tuberculosis in traditional cattle of the livestock/wildlife interface areas in the Kafue basin of Zambia. *Prev Vet Med.*, **85**: (3–4) 317–28.

Murcia, M. I., Tortoli, E., Menendez, M. C., Palenque, E., and Garcia, M. J. (2006). *Mycobacterium colombiense* sp. nov., a novel member of the *Mycobacterium avium* complex and description of MAC-X as a new ITS genetic variant. *Int. J. Syst. Evol. Microbiol.*, **56**: 2049–54.

Ngandolo, B. N. R., Müller, B., Diguimbaye-Djaïbe, C., Schiller, I., Marg-Haufe, B., *et al.* (2009). Comparative assessment of fluorescence polarization and tuberculin skin testing for the diagnosis of bovine tuberculosis in Chadian cattle. *Prev. Vet. Med.*, **89**: 81–89.

Niemann, S., Richter, E., and Rusch-Gerdes, S. (2000). Differentiation among members of the *Mycobacterium tuberculosis* complex by molecular and biochemical features: evidence for two pyrazinamide-susceptible subtypes of M. bovis. *J. Clin. Microbiol.*, **38**: 152–57.

Njanpop-Lafourcade, B. M., Inwald, J., Ostyn, A., Durand, B., Hughes, S., *et al.* (2001). Molecular typing of *Mycobacterium bovis* isolates from Cameroon. *J. Clin. Microbiol.*, **39**: 222–27.

Oloya, J., Opuda-Asibo, J., Kazwala, R., Demelash, A. B., Skjerve, E., *et al.* (2007). Mycobacteria causing human cervical lymphadenitis in pastoral communities in the Karamoja region of Uganda. *Epidemiol. Infect.*, **136**(5):636–43.

Palmer, M. V. and Waters, W. R. (2006). Advances in bovine tuberculosis diagnosis and pathogenesis: what policy makers need to know. *Vet. Microbiol.*, **112**: 181–90.

Pattyn, S. R., Van Ermengem, J., and Gatti, F. (1967). Mycobacteria other than *M. tuberculosis* isolated from clinical material in Kinshasa (Congo). *Ann. Soc. Belg. Med. Trop*, **47**: 435–41.

Perez-Guerrero, L., Milian-Suazo, F., Arriaga-Diaz, C., Romero-Torres, C., and Escartin-Chavez, M. (2008). Molecular epidemiology of cattle and human tuberculosis in Mexico. *Salud Publica. Mex.*, **50**: 286–91.

Piening, C., Anz, W., and Meissner, G. (1972). Serotyping and its significance for epidemilogical studies of porcine tuberculosis in Schleswig Holstein. *Dtsch. Tierarztl. Wochenschr.*, **79**: 316–21.

Pinsky, B. A. and Banaei, N. (2008). Multiplex real-time PCR assay for rapid identification of *Mycobacterium tuberculosis* complex members to the species level. *J. Clin. Microbiol.*, **46**: 2241–46.

Plackett, P., Ripper, J., Corner, L. A., Small, K., de Witte, K., *et al.* (1989). An ELISA for the detection of anergic tuberculous cattle. *Aust. Vet. J*, **66**: 15–19.

Pollock, J. M., Welsh, M. D., and McNair, J. (2005). Immune responses in bovine tuberculosis: Towards new strategies for the diagnosis and control of disease. *Vet. Immunol. Immunopathol.*, **108**:, 37–43.

Rasolofo-Razanamparany, V., Ménard, D., Rasolonavalona, T., Ramarokoto, H., Rakotomanana, F., Aurégan, G., Vincent, V., Chanteau, S., (1999). Prevalence of *Mycobacterium bovis* in human pulmonary and extra-pulmonary tuberculosis in Madagascar. *Int J Tuberc Lung Dis.*, **3**(7): 632–34.

Renwick, A. R., White, P. C., and Bengis, R. G. (2007). Bovine tuberculosis in southern African wildlife: a multi-species host-pathogen system. *Epidemiol. Infect.*, **135**: 529–40.

Reznikov, M., Leggo, J. H., and Dawson, D. J. (1971). Investigation by seroagglutination of strains of the *Mycobacterium intracellulare-*

M. scrofulaceum group from house dusts and sputum in Southeastern Queensland. *Am. Rev. Respir. Dis.,* **104:** 951–53.

Rigouts, L., Maregeya, B., Traore, H., Collart, J. P., Fissette, K., *et al.* (1996). Use of DNA restriction fragment typing in the differentiation of *Mycobacterium tuberculosis* complex isolates from animals and humans in Burundi. *Tuber. Lung Dis.,* **77:** 264–68.

Sahraoui, N., Muller, B., Guetarni, D., Boulahbal, F., Yala, D., *et al.* (2009). Molecular characterization of *Mycobacterium bovis* strains isolated from cattle slaughtered at two abattoirs in Algeria. *BMC. Vet. Res.,* **5:** 4.

Shitaye, E. J., Grymova, V., Grym, M., Halouzka, R., Horvathova, *et al.* (2009). *Mycobacterium avium* subsp *hominissuis* Infection in a Pet Parrot. *Emerg. Infect. Dis.,* **15:** 617–19.

Shitaye, J. E., Parmova, I., Matlova, L., Dvorska, L., Horvathova, A., *et al.* (2006). Mycobacterial and *Rhodococcus equi* infections in pigs in the Czech Republic between the years 1996 and 2004: the causal factors and distribution of infections in the tissues. *Vet. Med.,* **51:** 497–511.

Smith, N. H., Gordon, S. V., de la Rua-Domenech, R., Clifton-Hadley, R. S., and Hewinson, R. G. (2006a). Bottlenecks and broomsticks: the molecular evolution of *Mycobacterium bovis*. *Nat. Rev. Microbiol.,* **4:** 670–81.

Smith, N. H., Kremer, K., Inwald, J., Dale, J., Driscoll, J. R., *et al.* (2006b). Ecotypes of the *Mycobacterium tuberculosis* complex. *J. Theor. Biol.,* **239**(2): 220–25.

Steingart, K. R., Ng, V., Henry, M., Hopewell, P. C., Ramsay, A., *et al.* (2006). Sputum processing methods to improve the sensitivity of smear microscopy for tuberculosis: a systematic review. *Lancet Infect. Dis.,* **6:** 664–74.

Tarara, R., Suleman, M. A., Sapolsky, R., Wabomba, M. J., and Else, J. G. (1985). Tuberculosis in wild olive baboons, *Papio cynocephalus anubis* (Lesson), in Kenya. *J. Wildl. Dis.,* **21:** 137–40.

Teirstein, A. S., Damsker, B., Kirschner, P. A., Krellenstein, D. J., Robinson, B., *et al.* (1990). Pulmonary Infection with *Mycobacterium avium-intracellulare* - diagnosis, clinical-patterns, treatment. *Mount Sinai J. Med.,* **57:** 209–215.

Thoen, C. O. and Barletta, R. G. (2006). Pathogenesis of *Mycobacterium bovis*. In: C. O. Thoen, J. H. Steele, and M. J. Gilsdorf (eds.) *Mycobacterium bovis* infection in animals and humans, pp. 18–33. Ames, Iowa, USA: Blackwell Publishing.

Thoen, C. O., Richards, W. D., and Jarnagin, J. L. (1977). Mycobacteria isolated from exotic animals. *J. Am. Vet. Med. Assoc.,* **170:** 987–90.

Thorel, M. F., Huchzermeyer, H., Weiss, R., and Fontaine, J. J. (1997). *Mycobacterium avium* infections in animals. Literature review. *Vet.Res,* **28:** 439–47.

Thorel, M. F., Krichevsky, M., and Levy-Frebault, V. V. (1990). Numerical taxonomy of mycobactin-dependent mycobacteria, emended description of *Mycobacterium avium*, and description of *Mycobacterium avium* subsp. avium subsp. nov., *Mycobacterium avium* subsp. *paratuberculosis* subsp. nov., and *Mycobacterium avium* subsp. *silvaticum* subsp. nov. *Int. J. Syst. Bacteriol.,* **40:** 254–60.

Tortoli, E., Rindi, L., Garcia, M. J., Chiaradonna, P., Dei, R., *et al.* (2004). Proposal to elevate the genetic variant MAC-A, included in the *Mycobacterium avium* complex, to species rank as *Mycobacterium chimaera* sp. nov. *Int. J. Syst. Evol. Microbiol.,* **54:** 1277–85.

van Soolingen, D. (2001). Molecular epidemiology of tuberculosis and other mycobacterial infections: main methodologies and achievements. *J. Inter. Med.,* **249:** 1–26.

von Ostertag, R. and Kulenkampff, G. (1941). Tierseuchen und Herdenkrankheiten in Afrika, pp. 1–522. Berlin: Walter de Gruyter.

Wekhe, S. N. and Berepubo, N. A. (1989). Prevalence of bovine tuberculosis among trade cattle in southern Nigeria. *Trop. Anim. Heal. Prod.,* **21:**151–52.

Woodford, M. H. (1982). Tuberculosis in wildlife in the Ruwenzori National Park, Uganda (Part II). *Trop. Anim. Heal. Prod.,* **14:** 155–60.

Zinsstag, J., Ould, T. M., and Craig, P. S. (2006a). Editorial: Health of nomadic pastoralists: new approaches towards equity effectiveness. *Trop. Med. Internat. Heal.,* **11:** 565–68.

Zinsstag, J., Schelling E., Roth, F., and Kazwala, R. R. (2006b). Economics of bovine tuberculosis. In: C. O. Thoen, J. H. Steele, and M. J. Gilsdorf (eds.) Mycobacterium bovis infection in animals and humans, pp. 68–84. Ames, Iowa, USA: Blackwell Publishing.

Zinsstag, J., Schelling, E., Roth, F., Bonfoh, B., de Savigny, D., *et al.* (2007). Human benefits of animal interventions for zoonosis control. *Emerg. Infect. Dis.,* **13:** 527–31.

Zinsstag, J., Schelling, E., Wyss, K., and Mahamat, M. B. (2005). Potential of cooperation between human and animal health to strengthen health systems. *Lancet,* **366:** 2142–45.

CHAPTER 16

Campylobacteriosis

A. J. Lawson

Summary

Campylobacter jejuni and *C. coli* are frequent causes of bacterial enteritis in industrialized countries and are a major cause of childhood illness in the developing world. Although deaths due to campylobacteriosis are rare, the morbidity and public health and economic burden is high because of its very high incidence. Campylobacters normally inhabit the intestinal tract of wild birds and domestic animals. Poultry is a major source of campylobacter infection and a large proportion of retail chicken meat is contaminated. Other meats are contaminated to a lesser degree. Human infection is mostly sporadic and outbreaks are uncommon. Infections arise from the consumption of raw or inadequately cooked meat or from other foods contaminated during production or preparation. Contaminated water and raw milk can also act as vehicles of campylobacter infection and have given rise to significant outbreaks. The most effective means of controlling human campylobacteriosis would be the implementation of measures to reduce the contamination of food producing animals during slaughter and processing. Public health education regarding the principles of hygiene and safe food handling are also important.

History

Cases of campylobacteriosis were probably first observed as early as 1886 by Theodore Escherich who reported non-cultivable spiral bacteria in diarrhoeic stool specimens from kittens and human infants. However, it was not until 1906 that McFadyean and Stockman isolated 'microaerobic vibrio-like bacteria', which were later named 'Vibrio fetus', from an aborted sheep foetus. Subsequently 'Vibrio jejuni' was isolated from calves with 'winter dysentery' and 'Vibrio coli' from pigs suffering from swine dysentery, although it is now known they are part of the normal microbial flora in these animals. These 'vibrio-like' bacteria were eventually assigned to a new genus *Campylobacter* that originally consisted of *Campylobacter fetus* (the type species), *C. coli*, *C. jejuni* and *C. sputorum*.

Campylobacter were first implicated as agents of human enteritis by Levy in 1938 during an outbreak of milk-borne diarrhoea in two adjacent USA prisons. At this time campylobacters could not be grown from human faeces, but several cases developed bacteraemia which led to the culture of a 'vibrio' that was most likely *C. jejuni*. In the 1950s King made the connection between 'microaerobic vibrios' isolated from cases of bacteraemia in humans and isolates of 'V. jejuni' from poultry. She also observed that the human isolates from blood culture were all from patients with symptoms of acute diarrhoea. This work was followed up by Butzler who used filtration-based isolation techniques borrowed from veterinary microbiology to demonstrate that campylobacters were frequently present in the faeces of children with diarrhoea in the Congo (Butzler *et al.*1973). Butzler's work was expanded upon by Skirrow working in the UK, who developed an antibiotic-containing selective culture medium for *C. jejuni* and *C. coli* (Skirrow 1977). The paper describing Skirrow's work was a major turning point: it described the clinical entity, suggested appropriate antibiotic therapy and reported an easy culture method which resulted in a high isolation rate from diarrhoeal cases. It further demonstrated that there was a serological response to the infection, and confirmed the previously suspected link between disease in humans and the presence of campylobacter in poultry. Subsequently, throughout the late 1970s and 1980s, laboratories began to culture for campylobacter and the isolation rate increased dramatically as cultivation techniques were refined. In the UK the number of campylobacter isolates exceeded those of salmonella in 1981 and continued to rise reaching a peak of 58, 236 cases in 2000. In the UK and elsewhere the number of isolates reached a plateau in the late 1990s and since the mid 2000s isolate numbers have begun to decline. Nevertheless, campylobacteriosis remains the major cause of bacterial enteritis and a major public health burden worldwide.

The agent

Taxonomy

The genus *Campylobacter* together with the genera *Arcobacter* and *Sulfurospirillum* constitute the family *Campylobacteraceae* within the epsilon subdivision of the proteobacteria. This subdivision also contains the closely related genus *Helicobacter*, which includes *H. pylori* a major human pathogen associated with gastritis and stomach ulcers that was originally assigned to the genus *Campylobacter*. At present the *Campylobacter* genus comprises 21 species and 8 subspecies, most of which are inhabitants of the gastrointestinal tracts of man and animals.

Disease associations

Campylobacter are the major cause of acute bacterial enteritis in humans worldwide. The vast majority of infections are caused by *C. jejuni* and *C. coli*, which typically account for 90% and 10%, respectively, of cases. *C. jejuni* comprises two subspecies: *doylei* and *jejuni*. Subspecies *doylei* was originally isolated from the stomach of a patient with gastritis and subsequently from diarrhoeal stools from children living in poor social conditions. It is distinct from subspecies *jejuni* phenotypically and its clinical significance is uncertain. Subspecies *jejuni* accounts for nearly all the isolates of the species and is referred to as *C. jejuni* throughout this chapter.

Other *Campylobacter* species have the potential to be zoonotic pathogens but occur comparatively rarely and account for less than 0.5% of cases of campylobacter enteritis in humans in industrialized countries (Lawson *et al.* 1999): *C. upsaliensis* is associated with gastroenteritis in cats and dogs and is occasionally reported in cases of gastroenteritis from humans, particularly in children. *C. lari* was first isolated from gulls and subsequently from other animals and has been occasionally isolated from humans with gastroenteritis; *C. hyointestinalis*, originally isolated from pigs is also occasionally isolated from cases of diarrhoea in humans. *C. fetus* is usually found in the intestinal and genital tracts of cattle and sheep and accounts for less than 0.05% of campylobacter isolates from human faeces. Nevertheless, after *C. jejuni*, it is the second most common campylobacter associated with bacteraemia accounting for ~25% of isolates from blood culture. Most human infection is caused by *C. fetus* subspecies *fetus* and cases are typically elderly patients who often have an underlying condition or immunosuppression. The remainder of this chapter will focus on *C. jejuni* and *C. coli*.

Description

Campylobacter are small, non-spore forming, Gram-negative bacilli typically 0.5 to 5.0µm long and 0.2 to 0.9µm wide, with a spiral curve and tapering ends. Cells usually possess a polar flagellum at one or both ends and are highly motile. On Gram stain campylobacter cells can appear curved, S-shaped or spiral and may become coccoid in old cultures or on prolonged exposure to air. Campylobacter are microaerobic and are unable to tolerate oxygen at atmospheric levels. For optimum growth they require an atmosphere with an oxygen concentration of between 3 to 5% and a carbon dioxide concentration of 5 to 15%. The addition of hydrogen at 3 to 5% may improve growth of some strains and is a requirement for some species. Campylobacter grow well at 37°C, but certain species, such as *C. jejuni* and *C. coli*, have an optimum growth temperature of 42°C and are often termed 'thermophilic campylobacter'. Campylobacter are susceptible to pasteurization, chlorination, and other forms of disinfection. Although they are generally regarded as fastidious bacteria they are more resistant to stress and adverse conditions than previously thought. They exhibit a heat shock response and are able to survive and respire at temperatures as low as 4°C though viability is rapidly lost. The coccoid form of the bacteria has been associated with the so called 'viable non-culturable' (VNC) state, which may represent a dormant form of campylobacter capable of survival in hostile environments. However, the VNC concept remains controversial and difficult to evaluate.

Molecular biology

The genome of *C. jejuni* NCTC 11168 was sequenced in 2000 (Parkhill *et al.* 2000): it is 1.64 million nucleotide bases long and encodes 1,643 genes with an average G+C ratio of 30.6%. The genome is relatively small compared with other bacteria (for example *Salmonella enterica* has a genome of 4.68 million bases) and unlike most other sequenced bacterial genomes there is an almost complete absence of repetitive DNA such as insertion sequences and transposons. It had been estimated that approximately 94.3% of the genome encodes for proteins, a much higher proportion than that found in other bacteria. A significant proportion of this small, compact genome is given over to encoding carbohydrate surface structures (8% in NCTC 11168). These include the lipooligosaccharide (LOS) locus; the capsule locus; and the O-linked and N-linked glycosylation systems (Gundogdu *et al.* 2007) and presumably these play a major role in interactions between the cell and its host/environment. An interesting feature of the *C. jejuni* genome is the presence of intragenic homopolymeric tracts, which take the form of variable mononucleotide runs of 8 or more bases. These are thought to provide a slipped strand miss-pairing mechanism for phase variation of key genes such as the capsule, LOS and flagella glycosylation loci leading to a potentially high degree of diversity in these immunogenic structures.

Many campylobacter strains are capable of natural transformation: that is they are naturally able to incorporate homologous DNA from other strains without any specific genetic exchange mechanism. This leads to a high level of genetic exchange and campylobacter exhibit a remarkable degree of genomic plasticity. This has major consequences for the epidemiological study of these bacteria as they exhibit a 'weakly clonal' population structure. Here the normal clonal expansion of a strain, where genetic information is passed vertically from one generation to the next, is confused by the horizontal exchange of genetic material with other, often distantly related strains.

C. jejuni possesses a polysaccharide capsule, the exact function of which is unclear. It may contribute to pathogenicity, serum resistance, and survival in the environment. The capsular polysaccharide is the principal component of the Penner serotyping scheme (although epitopes from the LOS and flagella are also involved to some extent), which had long been assumed to be based on membrane-associated lipopolysaccharide (LPS) (Karlyshev *et al.* 2000). The genes encoding the capsule consist of a highly variable central region flanked by relatively conserved regions. Between different strains there appears to be a great deal of variation by means of insertion and deletion of genes in the central region (Karlyshev *et al.* 2005). The outer surface of the *campylobacter* cell membrane lipid bilayer is composed of LOS rather than the LPS found in other bacteria. Campylobacter LOS consists of two covalently linked domains: lipid A, a hydrophobic anchor, and a non-repeating core oligosaccharide, consisting of an inner and outer core region. The repeating O-chain of polysaccharide that characterizes LPS is absent. The genes encoding the biosynthesis of the outer core region vary in number and content between different strains. Campylobacter are capable of producing glycoproteins. Until recently it was presumed that only eukaryotic organisms were able to do this. *C. jejuni* possesses two distinct glycosylation pathways: an O-linked glycosylation pathway responsible of modification of the flagella and an N-linked general glycosylation system. The O-linked system is highly variable with multiple copies of some genes present in the locus suggesting that it has potential for generating structural diversity in the flagellin protein. In contrast the N-linked glycosylation is highly conserved and in *C. jejuni* it has been shown to modify upwards of thirty proteins. The role that these *N*-linked glycoproteins play in the pathogenesis of *campylobacter* infection is unclear, but disruption of the locus results in cells with a reduced capacity to invade and colonize.

Diagnosis

Detection and identification

The diarrhoeal illness caused by campylobacter is clinically indistinguishable from other forms of gastroenteritis and laboratory diagnosis is required to determine the nature of infection. Campylobacter can be readily cultured from faecal samples, which should be promptly delivered to the laboratory and examined within three days. Campylobacter are cultured on a selective media, such as modified Charcoal Cefoperazone Desoxycholate Agar (mCCDA) and incubated in micro-aerobic conditions at 42°C or 37°C for 48 hours. Campylobacter are identified by their colonial morphology, a positive oxidase test, and their appearance on Gram stain. For many laboratories this level of identification is deemed sufficient and isolates are reported as '*Campylobacter* species' with no attempt made to distinguish between species. *C. jejuni* can be readily identified by a positive hippurate hydrolysis test. Definitive identification of *C. coli* is more problematic, but most hippurate-negative, catalase-positive; indoxyl acetate-positive cultures isolated on selective media will be *C. coli*. Unfortunately, no single phenotypic test is completely infallible: hippurate-negative *C. jejuni* are known and many uncommon campylobacter and campylobacter-like species are phenotypically similar to *C. coli*.

Techniques for the detection and enumeration of campylobacter from food have been defined by the International Organization for Standardization and are described in the documents ISO 10272: Horizontal method for detection and enumeration of *Campylobacter* species Parts 1 and 2. Briefly, these describe techniques for isolation and identification of *Campylobacter* species; recovery of low numbers using an enrichment broth; and enumeration by dilution and plate count. These standardized techniques have been used to establish baseline levels of campylobacter contamination of chicken carcases in the European Union.

Accurate and timely identification of *Campylobacter* species can be achieved using PCR assays. Many assays have been developed, but there has been no systematic review of their accuracy and reliability. Although generally reliable PCR assays can be susceptible to the genomic plasticity of campylobacter and the exchange of genes between closely related species such as *C. jejuni* and *C. coli* is not uncommon. Genes that are under evolutionary or selective pressure, such as those involved in antimicrobial resistance, should be avoided as targets for PCR assays. PCR assays may also be applied to the direct detection of campylobacter from faecal samples and achieves a similar level of sensitivity to routine culture with the advantages of speed, amenability for automation, and definitive identification (Lawson *et al.* 1999). PCR is not widely used in the routine clinical laboratories, where these advantages are outweighed by cost. However, in the food industry, where rapid results are at a premium, the latest generation of real-time PCR identification assays are becoming more widely used.

Typing for epidemiological investigation

The typing of *C. jejuni* and *C. coli* for epidemiological purposes has proven problematic. The genetic diversity and weakly clonal population structure of campylobacter does not lend itself to conven-tional typing approaches. Initial attempts at typing schemes were phenotypically-based and included serotyping, phage typing, and biotyping. Of these the original serotyping schemes developed by Lior and Penner were probably the most widely used, primarily in reference laboratories. However, the performance of these schemes was poor as common serotypes were widely distributed and an unacceptably large proportion of isolates were untypable.

Theoretically DNA-based molecular typing techniques provide 100% typability and many methodologies have been developed for campylobacter including: ribotyping, Restriction Fragment Length Polymorphism (RFLP), Amplified Fragment Length Polymorphism (AFLP) and Random Amplification of Polymorphic DNA (RAPD) analysis. However, these techniques are not widely used, though they may be of use in local outbreak investigations. The most widely used molecular techniques are Pulsed Field Gel Electrophoresis (PFGE) and Multi Locus Sequence Typing (MLST).

PFGE involves the digestion of chromosomal DNA using bacterial endonucleases, which produces characteristic restriction fragment patterns when run out on an agarose gel. Many variations of PFGE exist for campylobacter, using different restriction enzymes and electrophoresis conditions and despite attempts at standardization by CampyNet in Europe and PulseNet in the USA comparisons between results from different centres are difficult. PFGE is vulnerable to genetic rearrangement which occurs relatively frequently in campylobacter and may result in major changes in PFGE profile between closely related strains.

An MLST-based typing scheme was first developed for *C. jejuni* in 2001 (Dingle *et al.* 2001) and subsequently schemes have been published for other *Campylobacter* species. The technique involves sequencing seven house-keeping genes (loci) and assigning numbers for each new sequence for each allele. The seven allelic numbers from each locus combined together for a sequence type (ST) and related STs that differ by a few base pairs grouped together in clonal complexes (CC). For *C. jejuni* basic MLST provides a comparable degree of resolution to PFGE. Greater resolution can be provided if additional, more variable loci are sequenced (Dingle *et al.* 2008). MLST sequence data are unambiguous and easily comparable with an internet-based database. MLST data provides a measure of the degree of relatedness between two strains rather than simply determining if they are the same or different and can thus be adapted to population genetics studies. As the cost of DNA sequencing has decreased over the last decade, so MLST-based typing schemes have become more widely used. For the first time truly global comparisons of campylobacter isolates from different temporal, geographic and ecological niches can be made. However, the high degree of genetic variability and weakly clonal population structure of *C. jejuni* and *C. coli* limit the usefulness of any typing scheme and MLST is no exception. MLST-based studies of *C. jejuni* typically show half as many genotypes as there are strains in the study with relatively few common types accounting for a significant proportion of the isolates (6 ST account for 63% of the isolates) with a 'long tail' of uncommon STs (Dingle *et al.* 2001).

The capacity for natural transformation that confounds conventional typing approaches can be used to provide a degree of source attribution. Campylobacter of chicken origin are likely to have acquired genes that are current among chicken campylobacter strains and it has been estimated that in an average *C. jejuni* isolate 86 of its 1643 genes will have been acquired from the gene pool of the host *campylobacter* population (McCarthy *et al.* 2007).

This effect is apparent in the loci used for MLST and it has been found that certain alleles have a host species signature. Although this approach doesn't work on some common widely distributed STs, it is able to distinguish between strains of chicken, ruminant, pig origins, and wild bird origin.

The hosts

Animal hosts

Campylobacter enteritis is primarily a human disease and *C. jejuni* and *C. coli* are considered to be part of the commensal microbial flora of food producing animals such as chickens, cattle, sheep, and pigs. Nevertheless, campylobacter do elicit an immune response in the animals that they colonize and have been associated with gastroenteritis in ruminants and pigs and 'vibrionic hepatitis' in poultry. The impact of these conditions is difficult to assess as campylobacter are so widespread in food producing animals that they are readily found in both sick and health animals. Wild birds have high carriage rates of campylobacter but are usually colonized with strains not commonly found in humans. Companion animals may act as reservoirs of campylobacter infection and there is evidence of enteric illness particularly in young animals.

Human hosts

Humans are not natural hosts of *C. jejuni* and *C. coli* and infection is usually transitory. Infections may be asymptomatic, and there is considerable variation in the severity of illness. Humans are not a significant reservoir of infection and person-to-person spread is uncommon. Not all members of the genus *Campylobacter* are pathogenic to humans and some such as *C. hominis* (Lawson *et al.* 2001) seem to be part of the normal human intestinal microbial flora.

Infection and pathology

The infectious dose of *C. jejuni* has been estimated at as few as 500 cells and the typical incubation period is between 3 to 5 days but may range from 1 to 10 days. Upon ingestion campylobacters pass through the acid environment of the stomach where their survival will be influenced by the buffering capacity of the food with which they are consumed. Initially colonization occurs in the jejunum and upper ileum and then spreads to rest of ileum and colon. Campylobacters cross the intestinal mucosa, adhere to epithelial surface and enter epithelial cells. Infected mucosa show acute inflammatory infiltration accompanied by fluid secretion which varies in extent dependent on the degree of host response and the extent of epithelial damage. Cell adherence and invasiveness are essential in campylobacter induced diarrhoea. The mechanisms involved are poorly understood, but are dependent on flagella-mediated motility and may involve other factors such as the capsule. Several host cell adhesion factors have been identified in *C. jejuni* and though their exact roles remain unclear, attachment to the host cells is required for subsequent invasion. Once internalized, *C. jejuni* cells are primarily confined to membrane bound vacuoles, termed *C. jejuni* containing vacuoles, in which they are able to survive intercellularly. The role of toxins in campylobacter pathogenesis is not fully understood, but it is now clear that, contrary to some early reports, *C. jejuni* does not produce a cholera-like endotoxin. Most strains of *C. jejuni* produce a cytolethal distending toxin, which has been shown to cause cell cycle arrest and apoptotic cell death.

Infected individuals typically show a rapid immune response with circulating antibodies detectable 6 to 7 days after the onset of illness. Specific IgA antibodies are secreted in the intestines and these give protection against the infecting strain and to some degree against other strains that share or have similar epitopes in immunogenic structures such as the capsule, flagella, and LOS.

Symptoms and signs

The symptoms of the diarrhoeal illness caused by *C. jejuni* and *C. coli* vary from asymptomatic to severe. The first signs are abdominal pain and diarrhoea or in some cases a prodomal fever with headache, flu-like illness, and myalgia. Cases with this prodome usually have a more severe illness. The abdominal pain can be severe so that it may be mistaken for appendicitis. In England 82% of patients admitted to hospital with 'food poisoning' have a campylobacter infection (Adak *et al.* 2002). Nausea is a commonly reported symptom but vomiting is rare. The diarrhoea is profuse and may be watery or bloody (Gillespie *et al.* 2006). After three to four days the diarrhoea will ease and most patients recover spontaneous within a week. Recovery is usually complete but relapse is possible. In some cases excretion of campylobacter may continue for several weeks after symptoms abate, but person to person spread is uncommon, and long-term carriage does not occur except in immunosuppressed individuals. In children the illness is usually less severe than that in adults, but bloody diarrhoea, especially in children under one year of age, and vomiting, are more commonly reported. Complications are rare but include bacteraemia, intestinal haemorrhage, toxic mega colon and haemolytic uraemic syndrome. Bacteraemia occurs more frequently in the elderly and reported rates vary from between 1 to 8 cases per 1,000. Deaths due to campylobacter are uncommon and usually associated with underlying illness.

Post infection sequalae

Campylobacter infection has been associated with the development of Irritable Bowel Syndrome (IBS), although a causal link between the two is still contentious. It is thought that a combination of the damage to the mucosa and disruption of the normal flora lead to prolonged bowel dysfunction. It has been estimated that as much as 25% of post infectious IBS could be attributable to campylobacter infection (Neal *et al.* 1997).

Campylobacter has been associated with a range of post infection rheumatological conditions, (Townes 2010) the most commonly reported being reactive arthritis (ReA). Symptoms usually occur two weeks post infection and manifest as pain and swelling in more than one joint, most typically the knees, ankles, wrists, and lower back. Symptoms may last for up to two months. The estimated incidence of ReA varies from between 1 to 15% and has been particularly associated with individuals with the HLA-B27 genotype.

Guillain-Barré Syndrome (GBS) may occur 1 to 3 weeks after infection with campylobacter and is an acute inflammatory demyelinating polyneuropathy characterized by progressive symmetrical motor weakness ranging from weakness of the extremities to complete paralysis and respiratory problems. GBS is now the major cause of flaccid paralysis worldwide since the near eradication of poliomyelitis. GBS occurs due to molecular mimicry between certain campylobacter LOS epitopes and nerve gangliosides. This causes an autoimmune response resulting in demylation of the nerve and degeneration of the axons and this is initially experienced as a tingling sensation, then as apparent weakness and ultimately flaccid paralysis. Mortality in severe cases of GBS ranges from 2 to 10% reflecting the varying quality of care available in different counties. Full recovery may take between 6 to 12 months but often there is some residual deficit (Nachamkin 2002; Wierzba *et al.* 2008). Other agents such as *Mycoplasma pneumoniae* and cytomegalovirus are associated with GBS and the proportion of cases with campylobacter as an antecedent is unclear. Estimates range from 15% in culture-based studies (Tam *et al.* 2003) to 80% where serology has been used (Van Koningsveld *et al.* 2000). The occurrence of GBS has been estimated at 1 in every 1,000 cases of campylobacter. Penner serotypes HS:19 and HS:41 are especially associated with GBS (Nachamkin 2002) and though it is now known that the serotype is derived primarily from capsular polysaccharide, the LOS of these strains possess epitopes analogous with human nerve gangliosides. Many campylobacter strains are capable of expressing LOS epitopes that are sufficiently similar to human nerve gangliosides to be able to induce GBS. Antibodies analogous to over 20 different gangliosides have been identified in the sera of cases of GBS.

Milder forms of ReA and GBS may be under reported. In a survey of patients recovering from campylobacteriosis, 37% reported musculoskeletal problem, 11% sensory problems, and 9% general weakness (Zia *et al.* 2003).

Treatment

In most cases campylobacteriosis is best treated with rest and regular dehydration to replace lost fluid and electrolytes. The use of antibiotics is rarely indicated but may be effective if given early enough and has been shown to reduce the period of faecal shedding. The most commonly used antibiotics are erythromycin and ciprofloxacin. Resistance rates vary widely between countries but generally erythromycin resistance rates for *C. jejuni* are fairly low, but higher in *C. coli*. Ciprofloxacin resistance rates have increased alarmingly especially from travellers returning from countries where fluoroquinolones are licensed for use in animal husbandry. There is some evidence to suggest that infection with resistant campylobacter strains leads to a more severe infection.

Epidemiology

Occurrence

Incidence

Campylobacter is the major cause of bacterial enteritis worldwide and the World Health Organization estimate that 1% of the population of Western Europe are infected with campylobacter each year. The reported incidence varies widely from country to country primarily due to differences in approach to laboratory culture and reporting practices. Incidence is estimated from the number of laboratory confirmed cases and the models used in different countries may vary greatly. Generally, worldwide, the picture has been one of a rise in incidence rates during the 1980s as isolation techniques were refined. There then seems to have been a more gradual increase in incidence throughout the 1990s, which seems to have peaked in most countries in the early 2000s and in some countries a subsequent decline. In the European Community the overall incidence of campylobacteriosis is 51.6 cases per 1 00,000 persons per year (Janssen *et al.* 2008).

However, the incidence in individual member states varies from 0 to over 300 per 1 00,000. In the UK laboratory confirmed cases reached a peak at 57,674 cases in 2000, declined to 44,294 cases in 2004 and have since begun to rise once more (Fig. 16.1). The estimated incidence in the UK, based on 2005 data, is 88.5 per 1 00,000 (EFSA 2006) at the same time the USA incidence was estimated at 12.7 per 1 00,000 (CDC 2005), whilst the highest incidence occurred in New Zealand with 400 per 1 00,000 persons (Baker *et al.* 2007).

In industrialized countries cases of campylobacter typically show a bimodal age distribution with the highest peak in 1 to 4 year olds and a less pronounced second peak in young adults (15 to 24 year olds). The reasons for these peaks remain unclear. Perhaps small children are over represented in samples as they are more likely to have stool samples taken. There is a slight bias amongst cases towards males (1.1 to 1.5 times higher) and this is most evident in young adults.

Recent analysis of longitudinal data in the UK suggests that underlying the gradual rise in reported campylobacter cases is a more complex story of changing incidence amongst different age groups that may reflect changes in society. Over the last twenty years the number of reported cases in the over 50's has risen by a factor of 3.8, whilst during the same period cases in the under 20's have decreased by 5% (Fig. 16.1) (Gillespie *et al.* 2009). There are probably many factors behind these changes not least the fact the UK has an increasing aging population, but also changes in access to health care, and eating habits. The wider use of immunosuppressive therapies may also be an important factor as individuals with an impaired immune system are more prone to campylobacter infection. Interestingly, the rise in campylobacter infection amongst the over 50's since the 1980s coincides with discovery of *Helicobacter pylori* as the cause of gastric ulcers and its treatment with a combination of antibiotics and a proton pump inhibitor. Gastric ulcers are seen most frequently amongst the over 50's and it has been suggested that the use of proton pump inhibitors to reduce stomach acidity during treatment of *H. pylori* infections effectively removes or reduces a significant barrier to campylobacter infection by effectively lowering the infectious dose in this group (Gillespie *et al.* 2009).

Sporadic infection

The majority of reported campylobacter cases are sporadic infections involving individuals or small family groups. Case-control studies have identified several risk factors associated with sporadic campylobacter infection these include the consumption of chicken in various forms; the consumption of barbecued or undercooked meat; the consumption of salad vegetables; drinking unpasteurized milk; drinking untreated water; swimming in natural surface water; and foreign travel (Adak *et al.* 1995; Frost *et al.* 2002; Gillespie *et al.* 2002, 2003, 2006). Interestingly, case-control studies report that handling and cooking of chicken at home have a 'protective' effect: i.e. those people who regularly eat and prepare chicken at home have a lower rate of infection presumably from acquired immunity (Adak *et al.* 1995).

Outbreaks

Campylobacter outbreaks (i.e. those affecting more than one household) are rarely recognized. There are a number of reasons why this is so: the bacterium generally survives poorly outside the host and is unable to multiply on food or to grow below 30°C; person to person transmissibility is low; campylobacter have a

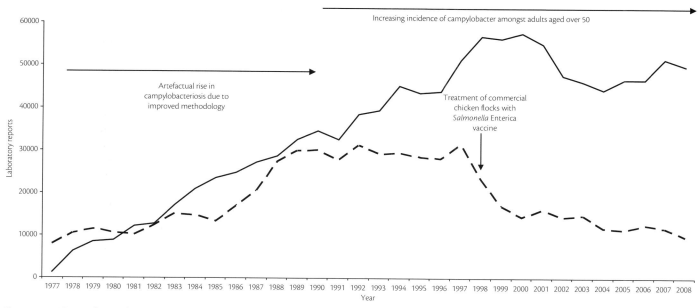

Fig. 16.1 Incidence of Campylobacter and Salmonella in the UK. – – – Salmonella isolates,——Campylobacter isolates: Data from HPA website:

relatively long incubation period and with a further 48 hours required for culture, often several days will have elapsed between infection and diagnosis, and this reduces the chances of recognition and reporting of outbreaks. Of the 2,374 general outbreaks of infectious intestinal disease reported to the Public Health Laboratory Service between 1995 and 1999 for which an aetiological agent was identified, campylobacter accounted for only 50 (2%), of which food-borne transmission was identified in 35 (Frost *et al.* 2002). Nevertheless, point source outbreaks of campylobacter may be more common than previously thought. An extended MLST-based longitudinal study has shown evidence of temporal and spatial clustering of specific types within a locale (Dingle *et al.* 2008). Detailed epidemiological questionnaires distributed to cases of campylobacter infection often reveal knowledge of people with similar symptoms (Gillespie *et al.* 2003).

When campylobacter outbreaks are successfully investigated they are commonly associated with the consumption of chicken (especially when under cooked); consumption of unpasteurized milk and drinking untreated or contaminated water. However, the investigation of outbreaks can be complicated by the fact that several campylobacter strains may be isolated from epidemiologically linked cases. This may occur when faecal material from several sources contaminates a watercourse or when material from several different animals is combined in a foodstuff: for example the livers from a number of birds combined in chicken liver paté (Forbes *et al.* 2009).

Seasonality

The incidence of campylobacter infections in humans exhibits a pronounced and consistent seasonal pattern (Nylen *et al.* 2002). In temperate countries such as the UK, incidence peaks in late spring and early summer then falls away during late summer and autumn. Elsewhere in the world seasonality is variable but the effect seems to be more pronounced with increasing latitude and is more

evident in rural than urban areas. The factors behind seasonality are not fully understood, but seem to be associated with climate factors such as temperature, sunlight, rain fall, and humidity. Of these higher temperature seems to be the best correlate (Kovats *et al.* 2005). Seasonality is also evident in animals. In the UK the prevalence of campylobacter in chickens rises sharply during late spring and early summer to reach a peak in July/August. Interestingly, in a study from Wales the seasonal peak in chickens seemed to occur a few weeks after the peak in human infections (Meldrum *et al.* 2005). The role of other animals such as flies (Nichols 2005) and migratory birds (Colles *et al.* 2008) either as sources or vectors of campylobacter has been suggested but the relative importance of these, if any, has yet to be determined.

Developing countries

A combination of the lack of chlorinated drinking water, poor sanitation, and frequent contact with animals leads to hyperendemic infection in many developing countries. The repeated exposure to campylobacter that children experience during the first few years of life results in immunity and older children and adults are generally unaffected by the disease. Nevertheless, campylobacter may contribute significantly to infant diarrhoea and mortality in some circumstances. The often unapparent high prevalence of campylobacter in developing countries may pose a high risk of infection to tourists and other visitors. Campylobacter enteritis is a common form of travellers' diarrhoea.

Economic costs

The estimate of the economic cost of campylobacteriosis varies enormously between countries. In the UK it has been estimated from data gathered between 1996 and 2000 when laboratory confirmed cases ranged from 43,978 to 57,674 (Fig. 16.1) that the average number of actual cases of campylobacter infection was 337,655. From this figure it has been extrapolated that this would have resulted in 160,788 GP consultations, 15,918 hospital admissions, 58,897 bed days spent in hospital, and 80 deaths (Adak *et al.* 2005). The impact of campylobacter infections should not be underestimated: of causes of food-borne illness in the UK campylobacter is the greatest single cause accounting for 20% of all cases, but in terms of hospital bed days needed it accounts for 58% of the total (Adak *et al.* 2005). The greater requirement for hospitalization arises from the severity of abdominal pain and sequalae. In terms of financial cost in England in 1995 the average cost of an uncomplicated case of campylobacter enteritis was estimated at £1,315. That would have given a conservative estimate of a total cost £65 million per year. However, if one considers the additional cost of hospitalization the estimate might be as much as £500 million per year (Humphrey *et al.* 2007).

Sources and transmission

Campylobacter are adapted to grow in the ruminant and avian gut and at some point the strains that cause campylobacteriosis in humans must have originated in an animal host. Recent MLST-based attribution studies suggest ~97% of *C. jejuni* isolates from humans originated from animals farmed for meat and poultry (Sheppard *et al.* 2009; Wilson *et al.* 2008). This approach suggests that for *C. jejuni* isolated from humans between 57 to 78% originated from chicken, 18 to 39% from ruminants (sheep and cattle), ~1% from pigs and between 3 to 4% from environmental sources such as wild birds and water. For isolates of *C. coli* from humans 40 to 56% originated from chicken, 42 to 54% from ruminants, and 1 to 6% from pigs (Sheppard *et al.* 2009). Detailed questionnaire-based follow up studies of cases of campylobacteriosis suggest that a food-borne vehicle was responsible for the infection in about half of the cases, the route of infection in the remainder of cases remains unknown. Table 16.1 illustrates the levels of campylobacter commonly found in food animals and the corresponding (uncooked/unpasteurized) foods that they produce.

Table 16.1 Isolation of *Campylobacter* from food animals and corresponding foodstuff

Animal	Mean % Positive Samples	% Range	Food	Mean % Positive Samples	% Range
Dairy Cows	30.0	6 – 64	Raw Milk	3.2	0–9.2
Beef Cattle	62.1	42 – 83	Beef at retail	2.7	0–9.8
Sheep	31.1	18 –44	Lamb at retail	6.0	0–12.2
Pigs	61.0	50 – 69	Pork at retail	2.0	0–5.1
Chicken Flocks	58.7	2.9 – 100	Chicken at retail	57.4	23–100
Turkey Flocks	78.0	20 – 100	Turkey at retail	47.8	14–94
Duck Flocks	38.0	0 – 88	Duck at retail	30.2	19–46

Reproduced from Humphrey *et al.* (2007) with permission from Elsevier.
Data compiled by Prof. T. Humphrey based on publications from 21 different countries

Direct transmission

The transmissibility of camplylobacter is low and survival of the cells outside the body is short. In the absence of a protective food matrix cells are unlikely to pass through the stomach's acid barrier unless consumed in large numbers. Simple hygiene measures should be sufficient to protect against direct campylobacter infection. In outbreaks and sporadic cases person to person spread does not seem to occur and secondary cases are uncommon. In the food industry there is a risk of acquiring campylobacter infection associated with the handling colonized animals or carcasses. Newly recruited poultry and abattoir workers often report illness in the first few months of employment, but thereafter do not seem to be troubled, presumably having acquired immunity though repeated exposure.

Poultry

Over the last two decades the consumption of poultry, primarily chicken, has increased dramatically. In the UK poultry production increased between 1985 and 2005 from 120 to 174 million birds, the increase being primarily due to a near doubling in the number of 'table birds' produced (Defra). Likewise in the USA over the same period yearly chicken consumption per capita increased from 53.1 to 87.4 pounds (USDA). This dramatic increase in production and consumption coincides with the increase in confirmed campylobacter cases and poultry consumption has been demonstrated to be a major risk factor in several studies. As can be seen in Table 16.1 poultry are frequently heavily contaminated with campylobacter before and after production. Various types of poultry have been implicated as a vehicle of human campylobacterosis: any type of chicken; poultry and poultry liver; raw or rare chicken; cooked chicken; processed chicken; and chicken prepared by or eaten in a commercial food establishment (ACMSF 2005). In the UK it is thought that contaminated chicken is the single most important cause of foodborne illness being responsible for an estimated 398,420 cases each year. This is equivalent to 111 cases per million servings (Adak *et al.* 2005). Further evidence of the role of poultry in human campylobacteriosis came from Belgium in 1999 when poultry meat was withdrawn from sale due to fears that chicken feed had become contaminated with dioxins. During the period of withdrawal there was a concomitant decline of ~40% of in the number of cases of human campylobacteriosis (Vellinga and Van Loock 2002). It is important to distinguish between chicken as a source of campylobacter and chicken as a vehicle for campylobacter infection. Undoubtedly chicken is a major source of campylobacter as has been shown in MLST-based attribution studies. However, epidemiological evidence suggests that actual consumption of chicken is responsible for only between 20 to 40% of cases (ACMSF 2005). A significant proportion of the campylobacter that originated in chicken must reach humans via other vehicles. Such routes might include: other foodstuffs cross-contaminated during production or in the household; companion animals; contaminated water; or other as yet to be identified routes of infection. Alternatively, the comparatively long incubation period and laboratory isolation required to detect campylobacter might confound epidemiological analysis making it difficult to attribute a vehicle in some cases.

Red meat

Campylobacter are part of the normal flora of cattle, sheep, and pigs and can readily be isolated from these animals. However, within any given herd carriage rates may vary considerably between animals with some individuals being heavily contaminated and others below the level of detection. In contrast to poultry, the process of converting cattle, sheep, and pigs to beef, mutton, and pork results in a significant reduction in the degree of campylobacter contamination (see Table 16.1). This is primarily because the slaughter process for larger animals is less automated than that for poultry and the practice of roding and bunging, whereby the gastrointestinal tract of the animal is sealed during slaughter and initial processing reduces the chance of faecal contamination of the carcass. Once prepared the carcasses are hung in chillers where a combination of cold and desiccation is effective in reducing campylobacter numbers (Humphrey et al. 1995). Despite the lower levels of contamination, red meats still pose a risk of campylobacter infection. MLST-based source attribution studies suggest that campylobacter originating in cattle and sheep are responsible for a significant proportion of human infections. In contrast, by this approach, campylobacter originating from pigs seem to be a relatively unimportant source of human campylobacteriosis with even *C. coli* of porcine origin contributing a maximum of 6% of human isolates in the UK. This may be because a significant proportion of pork often undergoes additional curing processes prior to consumption, which might further reduce campylobacter numbers. Epidemiological studies identify undercooked and barbecued red meats as a vehicle for campylobacter infection (Adak et al. 1995).

Milk

A significant proportion of dairy cattle carry campylobacter and inevitably milk may become contaminated (see Table 16.1). Faecal contamination at the time of milking is thought to be the primary means by which the bacteria get into milk, but they may also be excreted directly from infected udders in cases of campylobacter mastitis. Historically many major outbreaks of campylobacteriosis have been milk-related. These have been due to the consumption of raw or inadequately pasteurized milk and have sometimes involved thousands of people. Milk-related outbreaks are now less common due to legislation and better awareness of the risks associated with the consumption of unpasteurized milk. Also with the decline of smaller farms, milk is more likely to be pasteurized in larger centralized facilities that are well maintained. Small outbreaks have occurred due to the consumption of milk delivered to doorsteps that has been pecked by birds (usually of the crow family) (Southern et al. 1990). Typically this occurred in early summer when birds have young to feed. It is thought that the birds become contaminated whilst gathering insects from cow faeces. This route of infection has diminished with the decline in use of foil topped bottles and door step deliveries.

Water

Campylobacters are capable of survival in unchlorinated water, in planktonic suspension, in biofilms, and in the vacuoles of certain amoeba species. However, it is unlikely that they are able to multiply in water to any great extent and water must therefore be seen as a vehicle for rather than a source of campylobacteriosis. Open water is frequently contaminated with faeces from wild bird and farm animals. In some circumstances it may become more heavily contaminated with slurry run off or untreated human sewage. Sporadic infection due to recreational use of water, either inadvert-

ently through water sports activities or in cases of trekkers drinking streams or lake water has been reported. Often these types of infection are associated with uncommon campylobacter types associated with wild birds. A more significant threat to human health is the risk posed by the contamination of potable water supplies. This might be an important and underappreciated route of infection particularly in rural areas where local unchlorinated sources of potable water might be utilized and where chlorinated mains water is available the greater length of pipe required to connect properties to the mains might make them vulnerable to breakage and contamination. In Sweden an association was found between the incidence of campylobacter in different regions and the average water pipe length per person (Nygard et al. 2004). Epidemiological studies have identified consumption of bottled mineral water as a risk factor for campylobacteriosis (Gillespie et al. 2002). Although campylobacters have been shown experimentally to be capable of long term survival in refrigerated bottled water they have yet to be isolated or detected by PCR-based techniques from commercially available bottled waters. Presumably the positive association between campylobacteriosis and bottled water is due to some other as yet undetermined risk factor to which regular consumers of bottled water are more exposed than the general populace.

Other vehicles of campylobacteriosis

Ready-to-eatfoods such as vegetables, salad and fruit have occasionally been implicated as vehicles of campylobacteriosis. These food stuffs may become contaminated either during production (i.e. if irrigated or washed with water contaminated with faeces) or in the home due to cross-contamination from contaminated meat via surfaces, kitchen implements, or unwashed hands. The extent to which this route of infection contributes to overall human illness is difficult to assess.

Companion animals and animals in petting zoos and farms may also act as vehicles for campylobacteriosis. Cats and dogs have their own campylobacter species: *C. helveticus* and *C. upsaliensis* and the latter has been implicated as an uncommon cause of illness in humans. MLST analysis of *C. jejuni* isolates from dogs shows that they originated in chicken and ruminants. Studies suggest that cats and dogs are capable of acting as vehicles for *C. jejuni* and *C. coli* and sick animals, particularly puppies and kittens, may pose a risk of infection to humans especially young children.

Prevention and control

Intervention during food production

The widespread distribution of campylobacter amongst food producing animals is the most significant reservoir of infection for humans. Of all of the elements affecting the food chain, control of level of campylobacter contamination in poultry production would be likely to have the biggest impact. Even if complete eradication were not possible it has been estimated a 2 log reduction of *campylobacter* on poultry carcasses would reduce the risk of human infection 30-fold (Rosenquist et al. 2003). Broiler chickens are probably the most numerically significant poultry product and are reared on an industrial scale in high density sheds and slaughtered and prepared for retail in high throughput processing plants. Interventions could be made during production in the form of better animal husbandry, increased biosecurity and greater efforts to avoid cross contamination between flocks. During slaughter, priority possessing of campylobacter-negative or low-level contaminated flocks might be effective. During processing, carcasses identified as highly contaminated could be earmarked for freezing or decontamination with disinfectant spays or washes. The development of a campylobacter vaccine for poultry capable of achieving similar results to the *Salmonella* Enteritidis vaccine (Fig. 16.1) would have a major impact on the number of cases of human campylobacteriosis. However, at present the prospects for such a vaccine seem quite distant. For a more detailed view of intervention during food production see the review article by (Humphrey *et al.* 2007).

Protecting public health

In industrialized countries the provision of safe drinking water and adequate sanitation are vital preventative measures that are largely taken for granted. They only become apparent when the system fails. Continued public education should be undertaken regarding basic hygiene in particular the importance of hand washing after handling animals and before eating or handling food. Clear instructions on best practice in the kitchen, particularly with regard to the handling, storage and preparation of raw meat should also be available.

National clinical laboratories and epidemiology networks continue to play a major role in identifying and monitoring trends in campylobacter infection in humans. Whilst the usefulness of typing methods for campylobacter is debated, it is generally accepted that typing remains epidemiologically useful in the investigation of outbreaks.

References

ACMSF (2005). Advisory Committee on the Microbiological Safety of Food: Second Report on *Campylobacter*.

Adak, G. K., Cowden, J. M., Nicholas, S. and Evans, H. S. (1995). The Public Health Laboratory Service national case-control study of primary indigenous sporadic cases of campylobacter infection. *Epidemiol. Infect.*, **115**: 15–22.

Adak, G. K., Long, S. M. and O'Brien, S. J. (2002). Trends in indigenous foodborne disease and deaths, England and Wales: 1992 to 2000. *Gut*, **51**: 832–41.

Adak, G. K., Meakins, S. M., Yip, H., Lopman, B. A. and O'Brien, S. J. (2005). Disease risks from foods, England and Wales, 1996–2000. *Emerg. Infect. Dis.*, **11**: 365–72.

Baker, M. G., Sneyd, E. and Wilson, N. A. (2007). Is the major increase in notified campylobacteriosis in New Zealand real? *Epidemiol. Infect.*, **135**: 163–70.

Butzler, J. P., Dekeyser, P. *et al.* (1973). Related vibio in stools. *J. Paediat.*, **82**: 493–95.

CDC (2005). Centers for Disease Control and Prevention: Preliminary FoodNet data on the incidence of infection with pathogens transmitted commonly through food. *Morbid. Mortal. Wkly. Rep.*, **54**: 352–56.

Colles, F. M., Dingle, K. E., Cody, A. J. and Maiden, M. C. (2008). Comparison of Campylobacter populations in wild geese with those in starlings and free-range poultry on the same farm. *Appl. Environm. Microbiol*, **74**: 3583–90.

Department for Environment, Food and Rural Affairs: www.defra.gov.

Dingle, K. E., Colles, F. M., Wareing, D. R. *et al.* (2001). Multilocus sequence typing system for Campylobacter jejuni. *J. Clin. Microbiol.*, **39**: 14–23.

Dingle, K. E., McCarthy, N. D., Cody, A. J., Peto, T. E. and Maiden, M. C. (2008). Extended sequence typing of Campylobacter spp., United Kingdom. *Emerg. Infect. Dis.*, **14**: 1620–22.

Forbes, K. J., Gormley, F. J., Dallas, J. F. *et al.* (2009). Campylobacter immunity and coinfection following a large outbreak in a farming community. *J. Clin. Microbiol.*, **47**: 111–16.

Frost, J. A., Gillespie, I. A. and O'Brien, S. J. (2002). Public health implications of campylobacter outbreaks in England and Wales, 1995–9: epidemiological and microbiological investigations. *Epidemiol. Infect.*, **128**: 111–18.

Gillespie, I. A., O'Brien, S. J., Frost, J. A. *et al.* (2002). A case-case comparison of Campylobacter coli and Campylobacter jejuni infection: a tool for generating hypotheses. *Emerg. Infect. Dis.*, **8**: 937–42.

Gillespie, I. A., O'Brien, S. J., Adak, G. K. *et al.* (2003). Point source outbreaks of Campylobacter jejuni infection—are they more common than we think and what might cause them? *Epidemiol. Infect.*, **130**: 367–75.

Gillespie, I. A., O'Brien S, J., Frost, J. A. *et al.* (2006). Investigating vomiting and/or bloody diarrhoea in Campylobacter jejuni infection. *J. Med. Microbiol.*, **55**: 741–46.

Gillespie, I. A., O'Brien, S. J., and Bolton, F. J. (2009). Age patterns of persons with campylobacteriosis, England and Wales, 1990–2007. *Emerg. Infect. Dis.*, **15**: 2046–48.

Gundogdu, O., Bentley, S. D., Holden, M. T., Parkhill, J., Dorrell, N. *et al.* (2007). Re-annotation and re-analysis of the Campylobacter jejuni NCTC11168 genome sequence. *BMC Genom.*, **8**: 162.

Health Protection Agency: www.hpa.org.uk.

Humphrey, T., Mason, M. and Martin, K. (1995). The isolation of Campylobacter jejuni from contaminated surfaces and its survival in diluents. *Internat. J. Food Micro.*, **26**: 295–303.

Humphrey, T., O'Brien, S. and Madsen, M. (2007). Campylobacters as zoonotic pathogens: a food production perspective. *Internat. J. Food Microbiol.*, **117**: 237–57.

Janssen, R., Krogfelt, K. A., Cawthraw, S. A., van Pelt, W., Wagenaar, J. A. *et al.* (2008). Host-pathogen interactions in Campylobacter infections: the host perspective. *Clin. Microbiol. Rev.*, **21**: 505–18.

Karlyshev, A. V., Linton, D., Gregson, N. A., Lastovica, A. J. and Wren, B. W. (2000). Genetic and biochemical evidence of a Campylobacter jejuni capsular polysaccharide that accounts for Penner serotype specificity. *Molecul. Microbiol.*, **35**: 529–41.

Karlyshev, A. V., Ketley, J. M. and Wren, B. W. (2005). The Campylobacter jejuni glycome. *FEMS Microbiol. Rev.*, **29**: 377–90.

Kovats, R. S., Edwards, S. J., Charron, D., Cowden, J. *et al.* (2005). Climate variability and campylobacter infection: an international study. *Internat. J. Biomet.*, **49**: 207–14.

Lawson, A. J., Logan, J. M., O'Neill, G. L., Desai, M. and Stanley, J. (1999). Large-scale survey of Campylobacter species in human gastroenteritis by PCR and PCR-enzyme-linked immunosorbent assay. *J. Clin. Microbiol.*, **37**: 3860–64.

Lawson, A. J., On, S. L., Logan, J. M. and Stanley, J. (2001). Campylobacter hominis sp. nov., from the human gastrointestinal tract. *Internat. J. System. Evolut. Microbiol.*, **51**: 651–60.

McCarthy, N. D., Colles, F. M. and Dingle, K. E. *et al.* (2007). Host-associated genetic import in Campylobacter jejuni. *Emerg. Infect. Dis.*, **13**: 267–72.

Meldrum, R. J., Griffiths, J. K., Smith, R. M. and Evans, M. R. (2005). The seasonality of human campylobacter infection and Campylobacter isolates from fresh, retail chicken in Wales. *Epidemiol. Infect.*, **133**: 49–52.

Nachamkin, I. (2002). Chronic effects of Campylobacter infection. *Microbes Infect.*, **4**: 399–403.

Neal, K. R., Hebden, J. and Spiller, R. (1997). Prevalence of gastrointestinal symptoms six months after bacterial gastroenteritis and risk factors for development of the irritable bowel syndrome: postal survey of patients. *BMJ Clinic. Res. Edn.*, **314**: 779–82.

Nichols, G. L. (2005). Fly transmission of Campylobacter. *Emerg. Infect. Dis.*, **11**: 361–64.

Nygard, K., Andersson, Y. and Rottingen, J. A. *et al.* (2004). Association between environmental risk factors and campylobacter infections in Sweden. *Epidemiol. Infect.*, **132**: 317–25.

Nylen, G., Dunstan, F., Palmer, S. R., Andersson, Y., Bager, F., *et al.* (2002). The seasonal distribution of campylobacter infection in nine European countries and New Zealand. *Epidemiol. Infect.*, **128**: 383–90.

Parkhill, J., Wren, B. W., Mungall, K. *et al.* (2000). The genome sequence of the food-borne pathogen Campylobacter jejuni reveals hypervariable sequences. *Nature,* **403:** 665–68.

Rosenquist, H., Nielsen, N. L., Sommer, H. M., Norrung, B. and Christensen, B. B. (2003). Quantitative risk assessment of human campylobacteriosis associated with thermophilic Campylobacter species in chickens. *Internat. J. of Food Microbiol.,* **83:** 87–103.

Sheppard, S. K., Dallas, J. F., Strachan, N. J. *et al.* (2009). Campylobacter genotyping to determine the source of human infection. *Clin. Infect. Dis.,* **48:** 1072–78.

Skirrow, M. B. (1977). Campylobacter enteritis: a 'new' disease. *BMJ,* **2:** 9–11.

Southern, J. P., Smith, R. M. M., and Palmer, S. R. (1990). Bird attack on milk bottles: possible mode of transmission of Campylobacter jejuni to man. *Lancet,* **336:** 1425–27.

Tam, C. C., Rodrigues, L. C. and O'Brien, S. J. (2003). Guillain-Barre syndrome associated with Campylobacter jejuni infection in England, 2000–2001. *Clin. Infect. Dis.,* **37:** 307–10.

Townes, J. M. (2010). Reactive arthritis after enteric infections in the United States: the problem of definition. *Clin. Infect. Dis.,* **50:** 247–54.

Van Koningsveld, R., Van Doorn, P. A., Schmitz, P. I., Ang, C. W. and Van der Meche, F. G. (2000). Mild forms of Guillain-Barre syndrome in an epidemiologic survey in The Netherlands. *Neurology,* **54:** 620–25.

Vellinga, A. and Van Loock, F. (2002). The dioxin crisis as experiment to determine poultry-related campylobacter enteritis. *Emerg. Infect. Dis.,* **8:** 19–22.

Wierzba, T. F., Abdel-Messih, I. A., Gharib, B. *et al.* (2008). Campylobacter infection as a trigger for Guillain-Barre syndrome in Egypt. *PloS One,* **3:** e3674.

Wilson, D. J., Gabriel, E., Leatherbarrow, A. J. *et al.* (2008). Tracing the source of campylobacteriosis. *PLoS Genetics,* **4:** e1000203.

Zia, S., Wareing, D., Sutton, C., Bolton, E., Mitchell, D. *et al.* (2003). Health problems following Campylobacter jejuni enteritis in a Lancashire population. *Rheumat.,* **42:** 1083–88.

CHAPTER 17

Chlamydiosis

Margaret Sillis and David Longbottom

Summary

Chlamydial pathogens cause a wide-range of infections and disease, known as chlamydioses, in humans, other mammals and birds. The causative organisms are Gram-negative obligate intracellular bacteria that undergo a unique biphasic developmental cycle involving the infectious elementary body and the metabolically-active, non-infectious reticulate body. At least two species, *Chlamydophila psittaci* and *Chlamydophila abortus*, are recognized as causes of zoonotic infections in humans worldwide, mainly affecting persons exposed to infected psittacine and other birds, especially ducks, turkeys, and pigeons, and less commonly to animals, particularly sheep. Outbreaks occur amongst aviary workers, poultry processing workers, and veterinarians. Infection is transmitted through inhalation of infected aerosols contaminated by avian droppings, nasal discharges, or products of ovine gestation or abortion. Person to person transmission is rare. Control strategies have met with variable success depending on the degree of compliance or enforcement of legislation. In the UK control is secondary, resulting from protection of national poultry flocks by preventing the importation of Newcastle disease virus using quarantine measures. Improved standards of husbandry, transport conditions, and chemoprophylaxis are useful for controlling reactivation of latent avian chlamydial infection. Vaccination has had limited effect in controlling ovine infection. Improved education of persons in occupational risk groups and the requirement for notification may encourage a more energetic approach to its control.

History

The disease

The disease, psittacosis, was first recognized by Ritter in 1879 (Harris and Williams 1985) who described several cases of unusual pneumonia or 'pneumotyphus' associated with exposure to tropical pet birds in Switzerland. Morange named the disease after the Greek word for parrot, *psittakos*, having established parrots to be the source of infection in a similar outbreak in Paris in 1894. The term 'ornithosis' was suggested for infection in non-psittacine birds. Currently the term 'chlamydiosis' is used to describe chlamydial infection in all avians and mammals.

The agent

The original description of chlamydial elementary bodies is attributed to Halberstaedter and von Prowazek in 1907 who observed intracytoplasmic inclusions containing large numbers of minute particles in conjunctival epithelial cells from humans and apes with trachoma. They classified these 'Chlamydozoa' (Greek, meaning 'a mantle') between bacteria and protozoa incorrectly, but they rightly inferred that these inclusions were the aetiological agents of trachoma.

The causative organism of psittacosis was described initially in 1930 independently by three researchers (Coles 1930; Levinthal 1930; Lillie 1930). Each reported minute spherical bodies within reticuloendothelial cells in infected parrots. In 1930, Bedson and co-workers described the agent as 'an obligate intracellular parasite with bacterial affinities' (Bedson *et al.* 1930)—a concept not generally accepted for another 30 years. Thereafter, the generic name Bedsoniae was used to describe the agent. In due course the agent was cultivated in fertile hens' eggs.

In 1932, Bedson and Bland demonstrated the complex replication cycle from initial infection to the release of progeny of *Chlamydia psittaci* (Bedson and Bland 1932) (now *Chlamydophila psittaci*) (Fig. 17.1). They found two cell-type populations: the small, infectious elementary body (EB) and the larger, metabolically-active, non-infectious reticulate body (RB), subsequently recognized to be unique to all members of the family Chlamydiaceae (Fig. 17.2). It is now clear that chlamydiae are small prokaryotes that have evolved to a highly parasitic existence and do not constitute the missing link between bacteria and viruses as once thought.

Pathogenesis

The causal relationship between elementary bodies and psittacosis was demonstrated in 1932 by Bedson and co-workers. They demonstrated pathogenicity for experimental budgerigars, viable chick embryos, and mouse tissue cultures. Burnet (1935), investigating the ecology of psittacosis, showed that fledglings acquired infection from asymptomatic parent birds. Human infections were most commonly acquired via the aerosol route from inhalation of infected avian excreta or fomites. Infection in domestic mammals was first reported in 1936, following abortions in sheep (Greig 1936), although this was not confirmed as being an organism of the psittacosis group (ovine *C. psittaci* strains; now known as *C. abortus*)

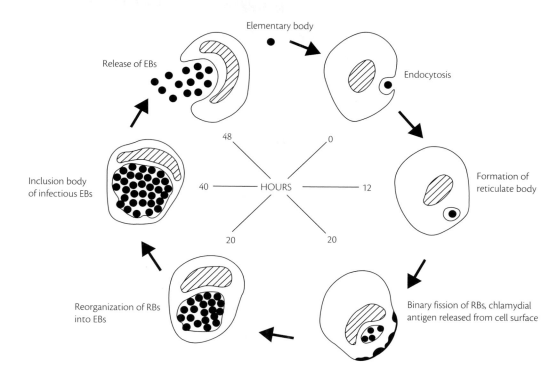

Fig. 17.1 Developmental cycle of chlamydiae.

until 1950 (Stamp *et al.* 1950). The disease was named enzootic abortion of ewes (EAE), or ovine enzootic abortion (OEA).

Chlamydia psittaci has considerable pneumopathogenic potential and is known to cause human disease ranging from asymptomatic infection to severe pneumonia and death. Haematogenous spread of the organism from the respiratory tract results in a systemic illness affecting multiple organ systems. The detailed clinical and pathological observations of 18 patients in a chlamydial outbreak in Louisiana (Treuting and Olson 1944) are noteworthy.

Human infection in pregnancy (Giroud *et al.* 1956) with EAE agent was recognized in 1967 as a zoonoses. Although human infection with the ovine strains is relatively rare in comparison to the avian strains, the risk for pregnant women and the developing fetus is considerable (Longbottom and Coulter 2003). Infection can result in spontaneous abortion and stillbirths.

Cases of conjunctivitis and atypical pneumonia in humans in close contact with infected cats have also been reported, suggesting a probable zoonotic role for the agent responsible (now known as *Chlamydophila felis*) (Longbottom and Coulter 2003).

Epidemiology

The disease, psittacosis, arises from human contact with psittacines, from which many of the early outbreaks were derived. As ownership of psittacines became fashionable, large-scale importation of South American birds into the USA and Europe occurred. This resulted in the 1929–30 pandemic with its associated high mortality and serious recognition of the disease. In 1935 chlamydiosis was also found to be prevalent in wild psittacines in Australia. Further sporadic cases of chlamydiosis occurred in the USA and Germany, incriminating domestically bred budgerigars. Nonpsittacine birds have also been implicated in the transmission of this infection. Pneumonitis infections, due to chlamydiosis, in

women in the Faroe Islands (Bedson 1940) in 1938, were probably contracted while preparing fulmar petrels for consumption. In the 1950s outbreaks occurred in turkey-processing plant employees in the USA (Irons *et al.* 1951) and later domestic ducks were implicated in outbreaks in Czechoslovakia (Strauss 1967). Poultry-associated cases were first reported in Western Europe in 1975 (in Denmark). More recently outbreaks have occurred in a veterinary teaching hospital (Heddema *et al.* 2006) and in poultry processing plants in the UK, especially among workers on eviscerating lines or who plucked birds (Newman *et al.* 1992; Gaede *et al.* 2008; Williams *et al.* 2008). Serological surveys showed that asymptomatic infections were common in persons at risk. An association between sheep contact and human abortion was noted by Giroud and coworkers, many years after the agent causing EAE was first described. Since that time a number of human *C. psittaci* infections (now known to be due to *C. abortus*) have been ascribed to contact with lambing or aborting ewes and to respiratory illness in laboratory staff, as well as workers in vaccine plants and abattoirs (Palmer and Salmon 1990; Longbottom and Coulter 2003).

Control

Recognition of the zoonotic potential of *C. psittaci* resulted in adoption of various strategies in an attempt to control the spread of chlamydial infection to humans and to protect the domestic poultry industries from the velogenic, viscerotropic Newcastle disease. National embargoes on psittacine importation were first recorded in the 1930s in the USA, UK, and Federal Republic of Germany after the pandemic in 1929–30. This resulted in an increase in bird smuggling and import bans were revoked and replaced in the 1960s with import permits, health certification, quarantine measures, and prophylactic antibiotics.

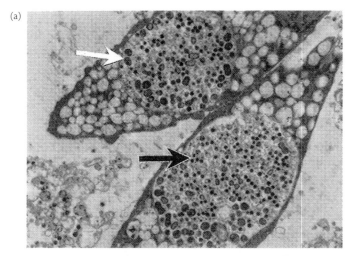

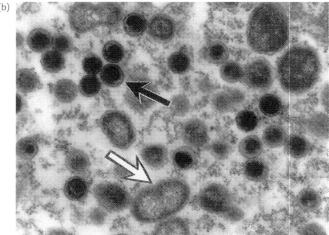

Fig. 17.2 (a) Electron micrograph of Chlamydia infected cell culture. Arrows indicate large cytoplasmic vacuole containing various stages in Chlamydia replication (× 2000). (b) Chlamydia elementary bodies (black arrow) and reticulate bodies (white arrow) within cytoplasmic vacuoles (× 17,000)

In the UK, the Psittacosis or Ornithosis Order MAFF 1953 provided statutory powers to detain and isolate affected birds and to disinfect premises. In 1976, import restrictions were re-imposed through the MAFF Importation of Captive Birds Order, because of an increase in human cases. These strategies met with limited success in some countries and have encouraged psittacines to be bred domestically. However, chlamydiosis still occurs globally and is more frequently associated with poultry industries. Commercial importation of psittacines ceased in the US in 1993 with the implementation of the Wild Bird Conservation Act. However, legal importation of pet birds, interstate quarantine of psittacines and prophylaxis with chlorotetracycline remains under USDA supervision; but there is no federal control after quarantined birds are released. Some countries made chlamydiosis a statutory notifiable disease to encourage more energetic control measures.

The disease was made notifiable in 1972 in Australia and in 1978 in Norway. Avian chlamydiosis in humans is not notifiable in the UK, except in Cambridgeshire, but in 1989 it was added to the list of prescribed industrial diseases under the Social Security Act (1975) (Industrial Injuries Advisory Council 1989). More recently

the International Animal Health Code and an EC Council Directive have stipulated animal health requirements covering international trade and importation.

Despite vaccines being available to control ovine chlamydiosis, EAE remains the most common infectious cause of abortion in sheep in the UK and many countries worldwide, responsible for over 40% of all diagnosed cases of abortion in the UK. Although there is no specific legislation relating to infection control, many farms participate in voluntary accredited health schemes, specifically the Sheep and Goat Health Scheme in England and Wales, and the Premium Health Scheme for Sheep in Scotland, as a way of controlling infection (Longbottom and Coulter 2003). However, these schemes are reliant on serological testing using the complement fixation test (CFT) which cross reacts with other chlamydial species infecting these animals and so is not 100% effective.

The agent

Taxonomy

Chlamydiae are small, coccoid, obligate, intracellular Gram-negative bacteria. Their developmental cycle is unique, involving alternation between elementary bodies (EBs) and reticulate bodies (RBs). The small (0.3 μm) spore-like infectious EB (Fig. 17.2) binds and enters the eukaryotic host cell, where it differentiates into a metabolically active RB (0.5–1.6 μm) within a cytoplasmic membrane-bound vacuole. The RB undergoes division by binary fission, followed by re-differentiation back into EBs and release from the cell to complete the cycle (Fig. 17.2) (Treharne 1991). Their metabolic repertoire is distinct from that of free-living bacteria, being partially reliant on host-derived intermediates, which is consistent with an intracellular lifestyle, a small genome size (1.0–1.3 megabase pairs) and the probability that they are undergoing a process of reductive evolution (Thomson *et al.* 2005). Structurally, the cell wall is comprised of protein and lipopolysaccharide (LPS) but lacks peptidoglycan, although genomic sequencing of chlamydiae has shown they have the full set of genes necessary for peptidoglycan biosynthesis.

In 1999 the order of Chlamydiales was reclassified based on sequence analysis of the 16S and 23S ribosomal RNA genes (Everett *et al.* 1999). Analysis identified three new distinct families (Parachlamydiaceae, Simkaniaceae and Waddliaceae), in addition to the original single family member, the Chlamydiaceae. The Chlamydiaceae, which previously comprised the single genus *Chlamydia*, was divided into two genera, *Chlamydia* and *Chlamydophila*. The emended genus *Chlamydia* included the original species *C. trachomatis* as well as two new species, *C. muridarum* and *C. suis*, whereas the new genus *Chlamydophila* comprised the original species *C. psittaci*, *C. pecorum* and *C. pneumoniae*, and three new species, *C. abortus*, *C. felis* and *C. caviae*. More recent changes have been proposed reflecting the increase in diversity of chlamydial species found in the environment, including the new families Rhabdochlamydiaceae and Criblamydiaceae, and new genera of the Parachlamydiaceae (Protochlamydia), Simkaniaceae (Fritschea) and Chlamydiaceae (Clavochlamydia) (Table 17.1). Although there is little evidence on the epidemiology, prevalence or zoonotic potential of these agents, there have been reports supporting a role for *Waddlia* and *Parachlamydia* in bovine abortion, human miscarriage, and pneumonia (Borel *et al.* 2007; Baud *et al.* 2007, 2009). *Rhabdochlamydia* has also been associated with community-acquired pneumonia in humans (Casson *et al.* 2008).

Table 17.1 Chlamydial taxonomy (as of October 2009)

Family	Genus	Species	Typical Host
Chlamydiaceae	Chlamydia	C. trachomatis	Humans
		C. muridarum	Mice, hamsters
		C. suis	Swine
	Chlamydophila	C. pneumoniae	Humans
		C. psittaci	Birds, poultry
		C. abortus	Ruminants, swine
		C. caviae	Guinea pigs
		C. felis	Cats
		C. pecorum	Ruminants, swine
	Clavochlamydia	Candidatus C. Salmonicola	Salmonid fish
Simkaniaceae	Simkania	S. negevensis	
	Fritschea	Candidatus F. eriococci	Insects
		Candidatus F. bemisiae	
	Unclassified	Chlamydial symbionts of Xenoturbella	
Waddliaceae	Waddlia	W. chondrophila	Cattle
		W. malaysiensis	Fruit bat
Parachlamydiaceae	Parachlamydia	P. acanthamoebae	Acanthamoeba
	Neochlamydia	N. hartmannellae	Hartmanella veriformis
	Protochlamydia	Candidatus P. ameobophila	Acanthamoeba
		Candidatus P. naegleriophila	Naegleria amoeba
	Unclassified	UWE1, TUME1, UWC22	
Rhabdochlamydiaceae	Rhabdochlamydia	Candidatus R. crassificans	Arthropods (Cockroach)
		Candidatus R. porcellionis	Crustacean isopod (Woodlouse)
Criblamydiaceae	Criblamydia	Criblamydia sequanensis	[River water]
		Estrella lausannensis	
Unclassified		Candidatus Piscichlamydia salmonis	Farmed atlantic salmon

Molecular biology

Molecular research of chlamydial structure has been largely focused on the outer membrane of the elementary body (EB) because of its central role in the infection process. The main constituents of the outer membrane are proteins of molecular mass 40, 57, and 12 kDa together with lipopolysaccharide (LPS). The major outer membrane protein (MOMP), composed of the 40 kDa protein, is the dominant surface-exposed protein, comprising 60% of the total membrane protein content. MOMPs from different chlamydial species exhibit high sequence homology but still contain species- (biovar-) and serovar-specific epitopes located in surface-accessible variable domains. The protein functions as a porin and structurally is composed of three protein monomers in its native form, with each protein molecule forming a separate channel through which nutrients may pass from the host cell (Wyllie *et al.* 1998).

Other major protein components are the 60 kDa and 12 kDa cysteine-rich proteins. These EB-associated proteins, unlike MOMP which is also present in the RB, are developmentally regulated and probably involved in the condensation of the RB to EB late in the developmental cycle. The 60 kDa protein is thought to be located in the periplasm, where it forms disulphide bond cross-links with itself, as well as with the 12 kDa lipoprotein anchored on the periplasmic surface of the outer membrane and with MOMP forming a supramolecular structure responsible for structural rigidity of the EB outer membrane. The final major component of the membrane complex is the deeply truncated genus-specific LPS, which forms the basis of laboratory diagnosis. LPS is overproduced during replication and can be incorporated into the host cell surface.

There are many other proteins of interest present in the chlamydial outer membrane complex, including components of the type III secretion system, the 27 kDa macrophage infectivity potentiator-like protein, which is similar to an important virulence factor of *Legionella pneumophila* and the 57 kDa heat-shock protein which may also have an important pathogenic role. This genus-specific antigen, closely related to the groEL protein of *E. coli*, can elicit delayed conjunctival hypersensitivity in guinea pigs (Watkins *et al.* 1986) and monkeys (Schachter 1978) sensitized by prior chlamydial infection. This would explain the exacerbation of disease observed in animals immunized with whole organism based vaccines following reinfection, and is an important consideration for vaccine development strategies (Longbottom and Livingstone 2006). In addition, a group of antigens and corresponding genes have been identified as minor but immunodominant components of the protective chlamydial outer membrane complex (Longbottom *et al.* 1998).

Subsequently, genome sequencing of multiple chlamydial strains has revealed a large family of these polymorphic membrane proteins or pmps, while bioinformatic analysis has suggested them to be autotransporter proteins of the type V secretion system, an important virulence system of Gram-negative bacteria (Henderson and Lam 2001). These proteins may play a role in adhesion and immune evasion. Another important group of proteins that directly interact with the host are those secreted through the type III secretion system. These include the large number of candidate inclusion membrane proteins (Inc proteins), the chlamydial protease-like activity factor (CPAF antigen), CopN and the actin-recruiting phosphoprotein Tarp.

Disease mechanisms

Chlamydiae cause a broad spectrum of clinically distinct diseases. It is unclear whether these diverse features are mediated by differences in pathogenetic characteristics or are due to variation of the host's immune response. Disease mechanisms may, in part, involve direct activity on the host cell as shown by the dose-related immediate toxic response when injected into experimental animals. This toxicity, originally thought to be associated with the endotoxic LPS, now appears to be due to the genus-specific heat-shock protein (57 kDa). Circulating chlamydial LPS immune complexes have been incriminated in the pathogenesis of some chronic disease.

Chlamydophila psittaci does not exhibit host cell-type specificity and can cause productive infection in various cell types, including mononuclear phagocytes which contribute to systemic spread. It is possible that monocytes may degrade internalized immune complexes prior to acquisition by dendritic cells, which in turn are uniquely capable of eliciting primary T-cell responses (Stagg *et al.* 1992). *In vivo*, the pivotal role of dendritic cells shapes the immunological outcome, either by T-cell stimulation or by generation of nonspecific killing mechanisms. This is observed in post-chlamydial reactive arthritis where dendritic cells drive inflammatory processes.

Protective immunity to chlamydial reinfection is associated with mucosal antibody, is serovar specific and short lived. Surface-exposed outer membrane constituents of the chlamydial EBs (MOMP, Pmps and LPS), are immunoaccessible and are likely targets of the immune response. However, LPS neutralizing antibody is not stimulated. MOMP is antigenically complex and exhibits unique and common moieties conferring species serovariation. While Pmps have been shown to be minor but immunodominant components of the chlamydial outer membrane complex of chlamydiae that has been shown to protect from infection (Longbottom *et al.* 1998).

Chlamydiae primarily infect the mucosal epithelium and resolution of infection occurs without adverse sequelae (Schachter 1992), although severe chronic inflammation may occur. Repeated exposure to chlamydial antigens may contribute to the immuno-pathology. Evidence from experimental animal work implies that multiple episodes of infection provoke hypersensitivity responses, causing irreversible tissue damage. Application of non-infectious detergent-extracted chlamydial antigens to the conjunctivae of immune guinea-pigs results in delayed hypersensitivity (Watkins *et al.* 1986). The offending protein was the genus-specific heat-shock 57 kDa antigen. Clarification of the role of the host response to this protein and its invocation of autoimmunity is required.

In humans, *C. psittaci* infects via the respiratory tract and is transported to, and replicates in, the reticuloendothelial cells of the liver and spleen. Spread via the haematogenous route to the lungs produces EB-rich fibrinous exudates. This process accounts for the long incubation period (7–20 days). Man is an incidental, dead-end host.

Maternal infection with ovine *C. psittaci* results in a predilection for, and replication in, placental trophoblasts. EBs are released into intervillous spaces and infect other chorionic villi, inducing intense inflammation. Placental insufficiency and fetal anoxic death follow. Trophoblast destruction releases large amounts of thromboplastin, and possibly chlamydial toxins, into the circulation resulting in disseminated intravascular coagulation and shock.

Avian chlamydiosis is a generalized infection affecting all major organs (Meyer 1965). Oedema, haemorrhage, and extensive lymphocytic infiltration are common. Inapparent infection is more common than overt disease, which is precipitated by stress following capture, transport, re-housing or food shortage. EBs are shed during overt and inapparent infection. Subclinical intestinal infections are common both in abortion-affected and healthy ruminants, although their pathogeneticity remains unclear (Storz 1988).

Chlamydial adhesion consists of two factors acting in unison where specific binding to cell receptors and/or non-specific physical interactions occur. Adhesion is trypsin resistant, heat- and periodate oxidation-sensitive and inhibited by heparin and heparan sulphate. Non-specific attachment of chlamydial MOMP by electrostatic and hydrophobic interactions is also likely to be important.

Endocytosis is essential for chlamydial development, although conceivably more than one route is used. This may depend on the mode of presentation, the chlamydial strain or the host cell. Endocytosis is 'parasite determined', blocked at low temperatures (4–8°C) involving local segmental responses of the host cell membrane similar to clathrin-dependent receptor-mediated endocytosis. Intracellular lysosomal fusion with the chlamydia-containing endocytic vesicle is probably inhibited, by undefined surface properties of the EBs, and occurs prior to replication. Reduction of the disulphide bonds, which cross-link the MOMP, causes loss of EB envelope rigidity and initiates the conversion of EBs to RBs. Increase in porin activity facilitates nutrient exchanges between the developing RB and host cell. Complete differentiation into metabolically active RBs occurs within 9 or 10 hours. Macromolecular synthesis of proteins and nucleic acids utilizes host cell ATP and nucleotides. RBs divide by binary fission and by 30 hours reorganize into a new generation of EBs, stimulated probably by reduction of ATP within the endocytic vesicle. Extensive cross-linking of MOMP increases the rigidity of the outer membrane. The endocytic vacuole enlarges due to EB accumulation, followed by release into the extracelluar environment.

Non-productive and persistent infections are common in chlamydial disease but the mechanism is unknown. Chlamydiae may survive in cells for long periods in a non-replicative form or, alternatively, multiply at a low level. Tissue culture studies indicate that tryptophan concentrations are critical for persistent infection, although interferon and depletion of other cell nutrients may be involved.

Drugs inhibiting *C. psittaci* replication interfere with protein synthesis or cell wall synthesis (Collier and Ridgway 1984). Rifampicin has the highest antichlamydial activity, followed by tetracyclines and macrolides, e.g. erythromycin and clarithromycin. The newer quinolones, e.g. ofloxacin, also show high antichlamydial activity. Penicillins and some cephalosporins possess moderate antichlamydial activity by their action on RBs. Inhibition of binary fission and development of abnormal forms occurs and can be reversed by removal of antibiotics. Such drugs are not recommended for therapy.

EB suspensions are thermolabile, lose infectivity within hours at 35–37°C and within days at 4°C. Survival can be improved by buffering at pH 7.2 containing 0.4 M sucrose and can be maintained for months/years at −70°C or in liquid nitrogen. Freeze-drying is variably successful.

Infectivity is destroyed or greatly reduced, within 1 min at room temperature, by chemical agents at concentrations routinely used for disinfection, e.g. alcohols, iodine, and hypochlorite, although 1% phenol was less rapid. *Chlamydophila psittaci* is stable in dust, feathers, faeces, and products of abortion at ambient temperatures, an ecologically important factor in transmission. Infectivity has been documented in canary feed for 2 months, in poultry litter for up to 8 months, straw and hard surfaces for 2–3 weeks, and in diseased turkey carcasses for more than 1 year.

The hosts

Globally, chlamydioses occur throughout the animal kingdom affecting ectothermic vertebrates, avians, mammals, and man. Common reservoirs of zoonotic avian chlamydiae include psittacine birds, pigeons, pheasants, and seabirds. Bird species of the economically important poultry industries, for example turkeys, geese, and ducks, are also natural hosts. *Chlamydophila abortus* infections are also of economic importance in farm animals, e.g. sheep, goats, cattle, and pigs. Close domestic association between symptomatic cats and humans provides ample opportunity for zoonotic *C. felis* spread.

Incubation period

Humans: usually 4–15 days, may be as long as 1 month. Avians: unknown in natural infection but experimental infection in turkeys produced symptoms in 5–10 days. Mammals: varies but in non-pregnant ruminants *C. abortus* rapidly enters a latent phase, upon becoming pregnant the organism recrudesces resulting in infection of the placenta.

Symptoms and signs

Humans

The onset of disease may be insidious or rapid, with fever, headache and generalized malaise. After a few days an irritating non-productive cough develops followed by sputum production. Chest signs are often limited to râles with little evidence of consolidation, which is at variance with the radiological findings. Epistaxis and mucocutaneous manifestations frequently occur. Complications include hepato-splenomegaly, meningitis or meningoencephalitis, myocarditis, or pericarditis (Crosse 1990). During acute illness the white cell count is often normal with leucopenia developing in about 25% of cases.

Infection with *C. abortus* is particularly significant in pregnancy as several cases of abortion, critical puerperal sepsis, and shock, including renal failure, hepatic dysfunction, disseminated intravascular coagulation, with significant mortality, have occurred in women in contact with sheep (Bloodworth *et al.* 1987). Uncommonly, neural involvement, flu-like illness, respiratory symptoms, and conjunctivitis have been reported in children and adults following sheep exposure.

Avians

Chlamydiosis is often asymptomatic but a generalized infection affecting all major organs may occur. Loss of condition with yellow-green gelatinous diarrhoea, anorexia, respiratory distress and nasal discharge occurs. Conjunctivitis may be the only symptom. Ducks typically have serous or purulent nasal and ocular discharges, whereby feathers around the eyes and nostrils become encrusted.

Mammals

Feline pneumonitis manifests febrile, depressive, and anorexic illness with mucopurulent discharge from eyes and nostrils (Storz 1988). Recovery after 2–4 weeks frequently results in a subclinical carrier state which may relapse. In very young or elderly cats pneumonitis may be fatal.

In ruminants chlamydiae can cause respiratory, intestinal, placental, and arthropathogenic manifestations. Intestinal infections cause diarrhoea in young animals, initiate pathology in other parts of the body, thus representing important transmission mechanisms. Many ruminants harbour chlamydiae in the alimentary tract without clinical symptoms. Observations in dogs and pigs are similar, and intestinal chlamydial infection in mammals is comparable to acute/persistent avian infection.

Placental and fetal infections of ruminants, with ensuing abortion, are economically important causes of reproductive failure. In experimentally infected animals, clinical observations show a clear sequence of events. Fever and marked leucopenia can occur 1–2 days after inoculation and continue for 3–5 days. The placental junction is breached and thereafter events *in utero* proceed independently of those in the dam. Abortion occurs late in gestation, usually in the last trimester at around 2–3 weeks preterm, but may be as early as day 100 of gestation. Ovine enzootic abortion spreads by contact at lambing, and infection acquired at this time remains latent until subsequent pregnancy when recrudescence results in abortion. In affected flocks, loss can be up to 30% during an abortion storm, thereafter the annual incidence falls to 5–10% (Aitken and Longbottom 2007). Infertility problems may occur after chlamydial abortion.

Bovine mastitis (Storz 1988), caused by naturally occurring infection in milking herds, causes severe reduction, or transitory cessation, of milk production. Chlamydiae can be recovered from the milk but its epidemiological significance is unknown.

Polyarthritis of lambs (stiff lamb disease) occurs in epizootic proportions in the USA and is economically important. The age of affected lambs ranges from 4 days to several weeks. Varying degrees of mobility, anorexia, and conjunctivitis are observed and, with disease progression, lambs are reluctant to bear weight on their limbs. In Germany, chlamydiae have been isolated from synovial specimens of pigs with chronic, non-purulent synovitis.

Pathology

Humans

Infection may be generalized but major changes occur in the lungs which appear congested. Typically, areas of normal alveoli containing air, interspersed with areas of affected alveoli with an EB-rich cellular fibrinous or serous exudate are seen. Interstitial infiltration and mucosal oedema is rare. Necrotic areas and Kupffer cell vacuolation occur in the liver, and the spleen is typically congested. Cardiac muscle may be oedematous with interstitial infiltration and vegetations may occur on heart valves. Occasionally, adrenals may be haemorrhagic. When the central nervous system is affected, congestion and oedema of the brain and cord is observed, sometimes with chromatolysis of nerve cells or intracytoplasmic inclusions in meningeal cells.

Pathological features of placentitis caused by chlamydiae from ovine infection reveal a focal acute microinfarction due to patchy infiltration of inflammatory cells and fibrin deposits in the intervillous spaces (Wong *et al.* 1985). Destruction and desquamation of trophoblasts in the absence of chorio-amnionitis occurs with an associated deciduitis.

Avians

Lung and air sac congestion results from focal inflammatory cell infiltration, oedema, and haemorrhage. Histiocytic and lymphatic cells accumulate in interalveolar septa and propria of the large bronchioli. Other mucous membranes are infiltrated diffusely or focally with lymphocytes, mononuclear cells, and heterophils. Similar changes occur in other major organs. Eosinophilic necrosis occurs in the liver.

Mammals

Intestinal infection can be cytocidal, resulting in atrophied, irregularly shaped, vesiculated microvilli, and ultimately cell degeneration. Oedema and cellular infiltration of the lamina propria occurs. Diarrhoea results from loss of enterocyte function.

Placental and fetal infections are complex pathological phenomena. The major pathology is localized placentitis with necrotic cotyledons and thickened, opaque periplacentomes. Margins of placental lesions consist of zones of hyperaemia and haemorrhage. Cytoplasmic inclusions are present in chorionic cells of the intercotyledonary region and endometrial cells. Exudate is present in the inter- and peri-placentome and the chorio-allantois is oedematous.

Fetal infection occurs through haematogenous spread from the placenta to the fetal circulation. Oral, conjunctival, and respiratory lesions are reported, but fetal death is associated with terminal anoxia due to placental insufficiency.

Treatment

Humans

Diagnosis is often delayed or mixed and many patients recover without specific therapy. Severely ill patients require supportive therapy, fluid level maintenance, oxygen therapy, and measures to combat shock. Tetracyclines and macrolides, particularly erthyromycin and clarithromycin, are the drugs of choice, although some quinolones, ofloxacin and ciprofloxacin, are effective. Tetracyclines have better bioavailability in the central nervous system. They are administered either orally or parenterally, dependent on clinical severity. Early therapeutic intervention results in excellent response and is particularly important in pregnancy, but inadequate regimens may lead to relapse.

Avians

Chemotherapy is identical for treatment and prophylaxis (Grimes 1985). Treatment can be affected by feed-administered chlorotetracycline or by parenteral administration. Antibiotic concentration in feed varies according to species, e.g. 2,500–5,000 p.p.m. for parrots and 500 p.p.m. for budgerigars. The prescribed time for treatment is 45 days for oral administration in parrots and 30 days for budgerigars. For injection, 75 mg/kg body weight every 5 days is recommended; however, repeated injections may result in muscle damage. Blood concentrations greater than 1 μg/ml are considered adequate. Vibramycin-calcium syrup is effective and is the treatment of choice in Europe. The efficacy of some quinolones for treating avian psittacosis is being evaluated.

Mammals

Injection of a long-acting oxytetracycline preparation will maintain ovine pregnancy until nearer the expected parturition date (Aitken *et al.* 1990). It is recommended as a 'one-off' procedure to minimize the development of resistance. Tetracyclines do not eliminate placental infectivity, and it is advisable to institute treatment of the whole flock. Ewes not close to lambing may require a further dose of tetracycline after 2 weeks. Despite treatment, some ewes still abort and remain potential sources of infection for other naïve ewes.

Prognosis

Humans

Mortality rates from avian sources were as high as 40% in the pre-antibiotic era. In the Louisiana outbreak, 8 of 19 cases died and during the 1929 pandemic 20–30% of infected cases died. Nowadays fatalities are rare, accounting for less than 5% of affected cases, but significant morbidity is common. Ovine chlamydial infection in pregnant women may result in an 80% fatality rate. Fetal or neonatal death is common.

Avians

Infection is usually inapparent with overt disease being precipitated by stress, e.g. overcrowding, inadequate nutrition, or transportation. Epizootics accompanied by high mortality rates occur among flocks of birds. Sporadic deaths occur in older birds that escaped infection as nestlings. Unchecked, mortality in domestic poultry flocks may reach 30%.

Mammals

Ovine and bovine adult infection is usually asymptomatic and rarely results in death. Infection during pregnancy can result in up to 30% of aborting ewes in flocks.

Diagnosis

There are two main approaches to diagnosing chlamydial infections in mammals and birds. One involves direct detection of the organism in swab and tissue samples by cytochemical staining of smears, histochemical detection in tissue sections, immunofluorescent detection of antigen, by the detection of nucleic acid by PCR or DNA microarray, or following isolation in tissue culture. The other involves serological methods to identify anti-chlamydial antibodies in blood samples (Sachse *et al.* 2009). With minor modification, many of the laboratory tests used for chlamydial diagnosis are applicable in all hosts. The merits of the commonly used tests are outlined in Tables 17.2 and 17.3.

Humans

The mainstay of diagnosis is the complement fixation (CF) test, but immunofluorescence tests are also used. Antigen and genome detection have been evaluated and appear to be both reliable and rapid, although not widely used (Sillis *et al.* 1992). Culture is not routinely attempted. Recently a new MOMP based nested PCR/enzyme immunoassay (EIA) has been developed that detects positive cases of human psittacosis (Vanrompay *et al.* 2007).

Avians

Available diagnostic tests are not reliable enough to allow screening or culling programmes to be 100% effective. The CF test and microimmunofluorescence test are currently used for routine diagnosis, as well as a latex agglutination test for detecting IgM (Andersen 2008). Veterinarians only accept a positive culture result

Table 17.2 Laboratory tests in routine chlamydial diagnosis: detection of the organism

Test	Specimen type	Limitations of use	Limitations of interpretation
Histology/cytology: stain with Gimenez, Geimsa, modified Ziehl-Neelsen or FITC-labelled antibody	Impression smears from tissue or post-mortem tissue from avians and mammals	Easy to perform Suitable for one-off test or can be automated Does not allow for therapeutic intervention	Depends on typical morphological appearance
Immunoassays			
1. ELISAs (enzyme-linked immunosorbent assay): plate-based (indirect enzyme immunoassays or IDEIAs) and solid-phase	Post-mortem tissue, oropharyngeal, cloacal and faecal specimens from avians Vaginal swabs, placental and fetal tissue from mammals Respiratory material from humans	Vary in sensitivity and specificity depending on the type of samples tested Faecal material may cause false positive or false negative results. Commercial solid-phase tests are subjective. May get cross-reactivity with other bacterial species.	Positive results should be confirmed by visualization of EBs by direct IF Intermittent shedding of chlamydiae, particularly in the carrier state, may necessitate repeat testing to exclude the infective state
2. Direct fluorescent antibody (DFA) tests: direct immunofluorescence (IF)	As for ELISA	Subjective and requires expertise in reading the tests. Only commercial tests are suitable for large numbers of specimens. Vary in sensitivity and specificity depending on types of samples tested. May get cross-reactivity with other bacterial species.	Absence of representative cellular material in the specimen invalidates a negative result Differentiation of species depends on the antibody used, i.e. LPS, genus-specific; MOMP, species-specific
Nucleic acid detection			
1. Polymerase chain reaction (PCR) and real-time PCR	As for ELISA	Complex method requiring rigorous technical skill and specialist equipment. Subject to extrinsic nucleic acid contamination. Useful epidemiological tool. A positive result does not necessarily indicate a current infection. Tests vary in their sensitivity and specificity.	Possibility of contamination must be excluded. A positive result may not indicate clinical relevance. Inhibitors of PCR may be present, thus invalidating a negative result. Species-specific assays are available. Real-time PCR can be used to quantify the amount of agent present in a sample.
2. DNA microarray (including genotyping)	As for ELISA	Requires specialist equipment. Sensitivity equivalent to that of real-time PCR. Expensive for large numbers of samples.	A positive result does not necessarily indicate a current infection.
Culture	As for ELISA	Contamination problems with faecal and post-mortem material. Technique is slow, difficult and special transport conditions are required to maintain chlamydial viability. Culture of avian strains presents a hazard to personnel and strict containment measures are required. Optimal sensitivity of cultures is necessary.	The predictive value of a negative result is low unless optimal conditions for transport and culture are maintained.

as a basis for complying with notification regulations and there is a great need for a test which is accurate, rapid and economical (Spencer 1989). Immunological and genomic techniques on ante-mortem specimens are becoming popular, whereas conventional histopathology is declining. Most recently, a *C. psittaci* genotyping method based on DNA microarray technology has been developed (Sachse *et al.* 2008).

Mammals

Laboratory diagnosis is generally performed by CF test on paired blood samples collected at the time of abortion and then at least three weeks later. Diagnosis can also be made by detection of chlamydiae in placentae, aborted fetal tissue or on vaginal swabs using histochemical stains such as Giemsa, Gimenez or modified Ziehl-Nielsen, or using immunological methods (Longbottom 2008). Other more sensitive and specific molecular methods of detection can be carried out in specialist laboratories.

Epidemiology

Occurrence

Confirmation of human infection may only be sought in moderate to severe cases, resulting in many unrecognized mild and asymptomatic infections. In many countries, human disease is not notifiable whereas in Norway and Sweden notification has occurred for nearly 40 years. In the USA, CDC report fewer than 50 confirmed cases a year. In Britain fewer than 40 cases were reported annually before 1966 but this has now increased to more than 400 cases per year, with periodic peaks. Bird exposure was reported in only 20% of cases. In Japan, where pet bird keeping is very popular, the annual incidence is estimated at 250–300 cases. Most countries detected an infection peak in 1981 linked to spread by migratory geese. However, the epidemiology of chlamydial respiratory infection needs re-evaluation following the recognition of C. *pneumoniae*. The CF test remains the most routinely used laboratory

Table 17.3 Laboratory tests in routine chlamydial diagnosis: detection of a serological response

Test	Limitations of use	Limitations of interpretation
Complement fixation (CF) test	Not suitable for 'one-off' testing. Technique requires optimizing for different animal species sera under test.	Cannot differentiate between species, detects genus-specific antibody only. CF antibody may be absent in some birds actively excreting chlamydiae. Presence of antibody does not necessarily indicate a current infection – testing paired samples may show current infection through rising titre.
WIF test (whole cell inclusion IF)	Detects genus- and species-specific antibody and requires expertise in interpretation. Useful in diagnosis of human infection as the genus-specific response is detected early in the infection and allows timely therapeutic intervention. IgM is applicable in primary infection.	Species-specific antibody peaks at approx. 4 weeks after onset of illness and detection is therefore of limited clinical value.
Micro-IF or MIF (micro-immunofluorescence)	Highly dependent on selection of a correct pool of chlamydial antigens.	Requires considerable interpretative skill and intuitive selection of antigens for reliable result. Cross-reactivity between chlamydial species has been reported
Latex agglutination	As sensitive as CF test in avian diagnosis but detects mainly IgM antibody	Better indicator of current or recent infection in avians. Cockatiels and budgerigars do not produce IgM in chronic infection, therefore a negative result may be unreliable in these avian species
ELISA (indirect and competitive)	A number of commercial ELISAs are available that are based on the genus specific LPS, whole EBs and Pmps, which vary in sensitivity and specificity. Other sensitive and specific tests based on Pmps and anti-MOMP monoclonal antibody have been developed but have yet to be commercialized.	Tests do not necessarily identify a current infection, just persisting antibodies. A rising titre in multiple samples a few weeks apart may indicate current infection. It is difficult to differentiate between animals infected with multiple chlamydial strains. Cannot differentiate between vaccinated and naturally infected animals.

investigation for human chlamydiosis, although it cannot differentiate between the chlamydial species. Epidemics of *C. pneumoniae* occur and the contribution of this species to the reported human cases requires definition.

The incidence data of avian and ovine infections are subject to similar distortions of underdiagnosis and under-reporting. Differences in ecology, surveillance, reporting procedures and market value of animals over time affect this data. In the UK 84–89% of reported ovine cases occur during January to March each year, hence the increased risk to pregnant women at this time.

Ovine *C. psittaci* is enzootic and large numbers of EBs are shed in fetal fluids and placentae. Ewes do not abort twice as a result of chlamydial infection, but chlamydial excretion can occur in the faeces and in fetal and placental products in subsequent pregnancies. Hence healthy sheep are a source of infection. Human infection with ovine *C. psittaci* is sporadic and no outbreaks have occurred. Bovine abortion is epizootic and poses minimal risk for humans as infection is relatively chronic with low-level excretion in aborted material. Serological evidence that stockmen and veterinarians face significant exposure to ruminant chlamydiae is available, although this may require further evaluation using more specific serology.

Seasonality has not been observed in most countries, but peaks are usual in July and August in Czechoslovakia and early in the year in Japan. This may provide information on the source of some infections. In the duck industry human infection relates to ducklings hatching in the spring and reaching a summer peak when birds are processed. Japanese observations may relate to continuous contact with pet birds indoors during the winter.

The first European chlamydiosis outbreak was related to a sick bird in a Swiss household, resulting in 50% mortality. Similar outbreaks were observed worldwide until the 1930 pandemic involving at least 1,000 cases with 20% mortality. The pandemic was due to large-scale importation of infected Amazon parrots to satisfy fashionable demand. Since then, over 70 types of psittacine birds have been found to harbour chlamydiae. In Britain infection among domestically bred budgerigars is uncommon, although a recent Slovenian outbreak did implicate budgerigars (Dov *et al.* 2007).

Infection is not confined to psittacines, as exemplified by the Louisiana outbreak where egrets were implicated (Treuting and Olson 1944). Eight of 19 affected cases died, including nurses involved in caring for primary cases. Many wild game and garden birds are also known to be infected and remain an important source of infection to humans and other birds. Periodically, epizootics of infection occur in aviaries, resulting in a high avian mortality.

Feral pigeons in towns and cities worldwide are commonly infected. However, zoonotic spread of infection from asymptomatic pigeons appears to be low. Handling sick pigeons and killing or dressing wild pigeons is a major risk. Sporadic infections acquired from racing pigeons are frequent. Stress of flying long distances, housing in insanitary lofts, competing for food, and transportation are all factors which may trigger avian disease.

Since the introduction of intensive poultry rearing, several major outbreaks of chlamydiosis affecting man have been reported, mainly associated with ducks and turkeys. These were evident in Czechoslovakia when the formation of large poultry plants and increased production was associated with an increase in pneumonia. Between 1949 and 1960, 1,072 cases were diagnosed, with a further 500 during the next 5 years. The mortality rate in humans was 0.7%.

An outbreak of psittacosis occurred in the Minnesota turkey industry in 1986 (Hedberg *et al.* 1989). The risk of acquiring infection varied by work area, with employees in the evisceration area and those in the live hang area many more times more likely to acquire infection than employees in other areas.

Ducks have been associated with a number of outbreaks of human chlamydiosis (Table 17.4). The first outbreak in the British

Table 17.4 Attack rates for human psittacosis in various outbreaks

Outbreak	Source of infection	Number exposed	Number infected	Attack rate % (range[a])	Reference
Israeli families	Psittacine and non-psittacine birds	37	30	83	Huminer, D. et al. (1988). Lancet, **8611**, 615–18.
Denmark abattoir	Ducks	142	15	11	Mordhorst, C. (1978). Ugerskrift for Laeger, **140**, 2875–80.
Minnesota turkey plant	Turkeys	1233	186	15 (5–46)	Hedberg, K. et al. (1989). American Journal of Epidemiology, **130**, 569–77.
Texas/Missouri/Nebraska Outbreak	Turkeys	645	80	12 (2–44)	Durfee, P. et al. (1975). Journal of the American Veterinary Association, **167**, 804–8.
UK Veterinarians	Ducks	34	15	44	Palmer, S. et al. (1981). Lancet, **ii**, 798–9.
UK duck plant	Ducks	190	14	8 (3–18)	Andrews, B. et al. (1981). Lancet, **i**, 632–4.
UK duck processors	Ducks	80	13	16	Newman, P. et al. (1992). Epidemiology and Infection, **108**, 203–10.
UK duck processors	Ducks	63	9	14	Williams, C.J. et al. (2008). Abstracts of International Meeting on Emerging Diseases and Surveillance, Vienna, p. 94.

[a] range, attack rate variation related to job assignment.

duck industry occurred in 1980 when a cluster of cases led to an epidemiological survey (Andrews *et al.* 1981). Seventy-two per cent of plant workers were seropositive compared with 37% of the duck farm workers. Attack rates were highest in workers on the eviscerating line. In another British duck outbreak in 1985 (Newman *et al.* 1992) new employees were three times more likely to become infected cases than established employees. An explosive outbreak of duck-associated *C. psittaci* infection among British veterinarians in 1980 (Palmer *et al.* 1981) was associated with a visit to one of the duck plants involved in the previous outbreak. The highest attack rates were associated with contact with feathers. No illness was observed in workers at the plant. The exposure of a susceptible group to a heavily contaminated environment may account for these findings. Similar findings were reported in the UK (Williams *et al.* 2008).

Transmission

Transmission to man occurs by the respiratory route from healthy and sick birds through faecal droppings and conjunctival/nasal secretions. Organisms survive well on feathers or in dust and cases have occurred in workers processing duck feathers for pillows. Ruminants and cats transmit *C. psittaci* to man via aerosols of infected body fluids. Outbreaks in poultry plant workers have implicated parenteral transmission via cuts and abrasions (Hedberg *et al.* 1989), although this is contentious.

In birds, exposure of nestlings to infection is the major mode of transmission. Vertical transmission through the egg or from parent to young through feeding by regurgitation occurs in some species. Contamination of the nesting site with infected exudates may be important in gulls and shore birds. Wild birds are important in transmission to commercial poultry. In ruminants (Stamp *et al.* 1950), infection is spread by contact at lambing and infection remains latent until the following pregnancy when recrudescence results in abortion which contaminates pastures. The theory that birds feeding on this material may act as a vector to other flocks remains to be proved.

Lice and mites have been shown to carry chlamydiae but their role in the epidemiology of psittacosis is unknown. Survival of the agent of epizootic bovine abortion on the surface of ectoparasites has been demonstrated.

Prevention and control

Regulations aimed at preventing importation of Newcastle disease virus into countries to protect the domestic poultry flocks, also prevent the importation of avian chlamydiae. Currently there are no effective vaccines available.

After the 1930 pandemic, numerous countries instituted a complete import ban of psittacine birds. However, due to inadequately controlled prohibitions, illegal smuggling became rife, resulting in the introduction in many countries of import permits with quarantine. The USA no longer imposes import restrictions as chlamydiosis is not felt to be a serious public health threat (Grimes 1985). The restriction on import permits to only a few birds per permit or to a small number of licensed premises may be more effective.

The International Animal Health Code (Office International des Epizootics) and the European Union Council Directive EC318/2007 lays down specific trade and import conditions. Psittacines must have appropriate health certification and birds must originate from one of the approved registered breeding establishments complying with appropriate transit legislation. In the US, state regulatory agencies may impose quarantine on interstate movement of diseased poultry. The US National Association of State Public Health Veterinarians published a compendium of measures to control chlamydioses in humans and pet birds in 2009.

Recrudescence frequently occurs in carrier birds due to transit stress, and overt symptoms or death may occur early in quarantine, thus eliminating infective birds. Not all carriers will be identified in the quarantine period, but healthy carriers constitute less of a human or avian health hazard. Quarantine periods vary in different countries, e.g. 35 days in the UK and Europe. In the US uninterrupted treatment of psittacines with chlortetracycline for 45 days, but only 30 days for budgerigars, is recommended by the National Association of State Public Health Veterinarians (2009); a measure designed mainly to protect the quarantine station employees. Ideally, following treatment, quarantined birds should be tested for chlamydiosis. More stringent measures apply in Germany (Gerbermann 1989).

Preventative strategies in poultry plants include the use of masks, hermetic domes over plucking machines, and installation of good ventilation to reduce spread by inhalation. Defeathering carcasses previously immersed in scalding water and heat processing of feathers/down have been used. The most effective measures focus on identifying and treating infected flocks before processing, while remembering that apparently healthy birds are infectious.

Education of exposed occupational groups is important to raise awareness and to improve husbandry. Pregnant women should avoid sheep exposure and laboratory personnel should apply good laboratory practice with strict containment measures.

Preventing domestic birds acquiring infection is difficult because of the high carriage rate in wild birds. However, poultry or pet birds kept indoors can be given prolonged antibiotic therapy. In sheep, transmission to other ewes can be reduced by isolating aborted ewes, destroying placentae, and disinfecting the area. Prophylactic tetracycline treatment of other ewes should be considered. Protective vaccines are available but they tend to give only short-lived, modest protection against disease. Formalized vaccines are of value, but the live, attenuated, vaccines have better efficacy against disease, although they do not prevent infection or shedding.

References

Aitken, D., Clarkson, M. J. and Linklater, K. (1990). Enzootic abortion of ewes. *Vet. Rec.*, **126**: 136–38.

Aitken, I. D. and Longbottom, D. (2007). Chlamydial abortion, In: I. D. Aitken (ed.) *Diseases of Sheep*, (4th ed,), pp. 105–12. Oxford: Blackwell Publishing.

Andersen, A. A. (2008). Avian chlamydiosis. In: OIE Biological Standards Commission (ed.) *Manual of Diagnostic Tests and Vaccines for Terrestrial Animals (Mammals, Birds and Bees)*, pp. 431–42. Paris: Office International des Epizooties.

Andrews, B. E., Major, R. and Palmer, S. R. (1981). Ornithosis in poultry workers. *Lancet*, **i**, 632–34.

Baud, D., Thomas, V., Arafa, A., Regan, L. and Greub, G. (2007). *Waddlia chondrophila*, a potential agent of human fetal death. *Emerg. Infect. Dis.*, **13**: 1239–43.

Baud, D., Goy, G., Gerber, S., Vial, Y., Hohlfeld, S. *et al.* (2009). Evidence of maternal-fetal transmission of *Parachlamydia acanthamoebae*. *Emerg. Infect. Dis.*, **15**: 120–21.

Bedson, S. P. (1940). Virus diseases acquired from animals. *Lancet*, **ii**: 577–79.

Bedson, S. P. and Bland, J. O. W. (1932). A morphological study of psittacosis virus, with the description of a developmental cycle. *Brit. J. Experim. Pathol.*, **13**: 461–66.

Bedson, S. P., Western, G. T. and Simpson, S. L. (1930). Observations on the aetiology of Psittacosis. *Lancet*, **1**: 235–36.

Bloodworth, D. L., Howard, A. J., Davies, A. and Mutton, K. J. (1987). Infection in pregnancy caused by *Chlamydia psittaci* of ovine origin. *Communic. Dis. Rep.*, **10**: 3–4.

Borel, N., Ruhl, S., Casson, N., Kaiser, C., Pospischil, A. *et al.* (2007). Evidence of *Parachlamydia* and related *Chlamydia*-like organisms in bovine abortion: a potential emerging zoonotic risk? *Emerg. Infect. Dis.*, **13**: 1904–7.

Burnet, F. M. (1935). Enzootic psittacosis amongst wild Australian parrots. *J. Hyg. (London)*, **35**: 412–20.

Casson, N., Entenza, J. M., Borel, N., Pospischil, A. and Greub, G. (2008). Murine model of pneumonia caused by *Parachlamydia acanthamoebae*. *Microb. Pathogen.*, **45**: 92–97.

Coles, A. C. (1930). Microorganisms in psittacosis. *Lancet*, **i**: 1011–12.

Collier, L. H. (1984). Chlamydia. In: M. T. Parker (ed.) *Topley and Wilson's Principles of bacteriology, virology and immunity*, (7th edn.), Vol. 2, pp. 510–25. London: Edward Arnold.

Collier, L. H. and Ridgway, G. L. (1984). Chlamydial diseases. In: G. R. Smith (ed.) *Topley and Wilson's principles of bacteriology, virology and immunity*, (7th edn.) Vol. 3, pp. 558–73. London: Edward Arnold.

Crosse, B. A. (1990). Psittacosis: a clinical review. *J. Infect.*, **21**: 251–9.

Dovč, A., Slavec, B., Lindtner-Knific, R., *et al.* (2007). Study of *Chlamydophila psittaci* outbreak in budgerigars. *Bull. Vet. Instit. Pulawy*, **51**: 343–6.

Everett, K. D. E., Bush, R. M. and Andersen, A. A. (1999). Emended description of the order Chlamydiales, proposal of *Parachlamydiaceae* fam. nov. and *Simkaniaceae* fam. nov., each containing one monotypic genus, revised taxonomy of the family *Chlamydiaceae*, including a new genus and five new species, and standards for the identification of organisms. *Internat. J. System. Bacteriol.*, **49**: 415–40.

Gaede, W., Reckling, K. F., Dresenkamp, B., *et al.* (2008). *Chlamydophila psittaci* infections in humans during an outbreak of psittacosis from poultry in Germany. *Zoon. Pub. Heal.*, **55**: 184–88.

Gerbermann, H. (1989). Current situation and alternatives for diagnosis and control of chlamydiosis in the Federal Republic of Germany. *J. Am. Vet. Med. Assoc.*, **195**: 1542–47.

Giroud, P., Roger, F. and Dumes, N. (1956). Certaines avortements chez la femme peuvent être dus a des agents situés a côté du groupe de la psittacose. *Compt. Rend. des Sean. de L'Acad. Sci.*, **242**: 697–99.

Grieg, J. R. (1936). Enzootic abortion in ewes: a preliminary note. *Vet. Rec.*, **48**: 1225–27.

Grimes, J. E. (1985). Enigmatic psittacine chlamydiosis: Results of serotesting and isolation attempts, 1978 through 1983, and considerations for the future. *J. Am. Vet. Med. Assoc.*, **186**: 1075–79.

Halberstaedter, L. and von Prowazek, S. (1907). Zur Ätiologie des Trachoms. *Deut. Medizinis. Wochens.*, **33**: 1285–87.

Harris, R. L. and Williams, T. W. (1985). Contributions to the origin of pneumotyphus. A discussion of the original article by J. Ritter in 1880. *Rev. Infect. Dis.*, **7**: 119–22.

Hedberg, K., White, K. E., Forfang, J. C., *et al.* (1989). An outbreak of psittacosis in Minnesota turkey industry workers: Implications for modes of transmission and control. *Am. J. Epidemiol.*, **130**: 569–77.

Heddema, E. R., van Hannen, E. J., Duim, B., *et al.* (2006). An outbreak of psittacosis due to Chlamydophila psittaci genotype A in a veterinary teaching hospital. *J. Med. Microbiol.*, **55**: 1571–75.

Henderson, I. R. and Lam, A. C. (2001). Polymorphic proteins of Chlamydia spp.—autotransporters beyond the Proteobacteria. *Trends in Microbiol.*, **9**: 573–78.

Irons, J. V., Mason, D. and White, R. F. (1951). Outbreaks of Psittacosis (ornithosis) from working with turkeys or chickens. *Am. J. Pub. Heal.*, **41**: 931–37.

Levinthal, W. (1930). Die Ätiologie der Psittacosis. *Klinis. Wochensch.*, **9**: 654.

Lillie, R. D. (1930). Psittacosis: rickettsia-like inclusions in man and in experimental animals. *Pub. Heal. Rep.*, **45**: 77–78.

Longbottom, D. (2008). Enzootic abortion of ewes (ovine chlamydiosis), In: OIE Biological Standards Commission (ed.) *Manual of Diagnostic Tests and Vaccines for Terrestrial Animals (Mammals, Birds and Bees)*, pp. 1013–20. Paris: Office International des Epizooties.

Longbottom, D. and Coulter, L. J. (2003). Animal chlamydioses and zoonotic implications. *J. Comp. Path.*, **128**: 217–44.

Longbottom, D. and Livingstone, M. (2006). Vaccination against chlamydial infections of man and animals. *Vet. J.*, **171**: 263–75.

Longbottom, D., Russell, M., Dunbar, S. M., Jones, G. E. and Herring, A. J. (1998). Molecular cloning and characterization of the genes coding for the highly immunogenic cluster of 90-kilodalton envelope proteins from the *Chlamydia psittaci* subtype that causes abortion in sheep. *Infect. Immun.*, **66:** 1317–24.

Meyer, K. F. (1965). Ornithosis. In: H. E. Biester and L. H. Schwarte (eds.), *Ornithosis diseases of poultry*, (5th edn.), pp. 675–70. Iowa: Iowa State University Press.

National Association of State Public Health Veterinarians. (2009). *Compendium of Measures to Control Chlamydophila psittaci Infection Among Humans (psittacosis) and Pet Birds (Avian Chlamydiosis)*, 2009. Available at: http://www.nasphv.org/Documents/Psittacosis.pdf (accessed 30 October 2009).

Newman, C. P., Palmer, S. R., Kirby, F. D. and Caul, E. O. (1992). A prolonged outbreak of ornithosis in duck processors. *Epidemiol. Infect.*, **108:** 203–10.

Palmer, S. R., Andrews, B. E. and Major, R. (1981). A common source outbreak of ornithosis in veterinary surgeons. *Lancet*, **ii:** 798–99.

Palmer, S. R. and Salmon, R. L. (1990). Enzootic abortion in ewes: risks to humans. *Heal. Hyg.*, **11:** 205–7.

Sachse, K., Vretou, E., Livingstone, M., Borel, N., Pospischil, A. *et al.* (2009). Recent developments in the laboratory diagnosis of chlamydial infections. *Vet. Microbiol.*, **135:** 2–21.

Schachter, J. (1978). Chlamydial infections. *N. Engl. J. Med.*, **298:** 540–9.

Schachter, J. (1992). The pathogenesis of chlamydial infection. In P. A. Mårdh, M. La Placa, and M. Ward (eds.) *Proceedings Second Meeting of the European Society for Chlamydia Research*, pp. 677–82. Uppsala, Sweden: Uppsala University.

Strauss, J. (1967). Microbiologic and epidemiologic aspects of duck ornithosis in Czechoslovakia. *Am. J. Ophthalmol.*, **63:** 1246–59.

Sillis, M., White, P., Caul, E. O., Paul, I. D. and Treharne, J. D. (1992). The differentiation of Chlamydia species by antigen detection in sputum specimens from patients with community-acquired acute respiratory infections. *J. Infect.*, **25** (Suppl. 1): 77–86.

Spencer, L. M. (1989). Chlamydiosis research and control runs regulatory obstacle course. *J. Am. Vet. Med. Assoc.*, **195:** 853–62.

Stagg, A. J., *et al.* (1992). Dendritic cells in the initiation of immune responses to Chlamydia. In: P. A. Mårdh, M. La Placa, and M. Ward (eds.) *Proceedings Second Meeting of the European Society for Chlamydia Research*, pp. 77–80. Uppsala, Sweden: Uppsala University.

Stamp, J. T., McEwen, A. D., Watt, J. A. A. and Nisbet, D. I. (1950). Enzootic abortion in ewes. Transmission of the disease. *Vet. Rec.*, **62:** 251–54.

Storz, J. (1988). Overview of animal diseases induced by chlamydial infections. In A. L. Barron (ed.) *Microbiology of Chlamydia*, pp. 168–91. Boca Raton: CRC Press.

Thomson, N. R., Yeats, C., Bell, K., *et al.* (2005). The *Chlamydophila abortus* genome sequence reveals an array of variable proteins that contribute to interspecies variation. *Genome Res.*, **15:** 629–40.

Treharne, J. D. (1991). Recent developments in the biology of the chlamydiae. *Rev. Med. Microbiol.*, **2:** 45–49.

Treuting, W. L. and Olson, B. J. (1944). An epidemic of severe pneumonitis in the Bayou region of Louisiana. *Pub. Heal. Rep., Washington*, **59:** 1299–311, 1331–50.

Vanrompay, D., Harkinezhad, T., van de Walle, M., *et al.* (2007). *Chlamydophila psittaci* transmission from pet birds to humans. *Emerg. Infect. Dis.*, **13:** 1108–10.

Watkins, N. G., Hadlow, W. J., Moos, A. B. and Caldwell, H. D. (1986). Ocular delayed hypersensitivity: a pathogenetic mechanism of chlamydial conjunctivitis in guinea pigs. *Proc. Nat. Acad. Sci. USA*, **83:** 7480–84.

Williams, C. J., Sillis, M. and Nair, P. (2008). Psittacosis outbreak in poultry processing workers in the East of England. Abstracts of International Meeting on Emerging Diseases and Surveillance, p. 94, *Vienna*.

Wong, S. Y., Gray, E. S., Buxton, D., Finlayson, J. and Johnson, F. W. (1985). Acute placentitis and spontaneous abortion caused by *Chlamydia psittaci* of sheep origin: a histological and ultrastructural study. *J. Clin. Pathol.*, **38:** 707–11.

Wyllie, S., Ashley, R. H., Longbottom, D. and Herring, A. J. (1998). The major outer membrane protein of *Chlamydia psittaci* functions as a porin-like ion channel. *Infect. Immun.*, **66:** 5202–7.

Further reading

Barron, A. L. (ed.) (1987). *Microbiology of Chlamydia*. Boca Raton: CRC Press.

Stephens, R. S. (ed.) (1999). *Chlamydia: Intracellular biology, pathogenesis and immunity*. Washington D.C.: ASM Press.

Storz, J. (1971). *Chlamydia and chlamydia-induced diseases*. Springfield, Illinois: C. Thomas.

The comprehensive reference and education site to Chlamydia and the chlamydiae. Available at http://www.chlamydiae.com/ (accessed 30 October 2009).

CHAPTER 18

Q fever

Thomas J. Marrie

Summary

Q fever is a wide spread illness affecting wild and domestic animals and man. The etiological agent *Coxiella burnetii*, has both a wildlife and domestic animal cycle. In mammals, infection localizes to the endometrium and the mammary glands. The organism is reactivated during pregnancy reaching high concentrations in the placenta. At the time of parturition the organism is aerosolized. Inhalation of *Coxiella burnetii* by a susceptible animal results in Q fever. In man, Q fever may be acute (self-limited febrile illness, pneumonia, hepatitis) or chronic (mostly endocarditis, but also osteomyelitis, endovascular infection, hepatitis [can be both acute and chronic] and Q fever in pregnancy). Abortion and stillbirth are manifestations of Q fever in domestic animals and in animal models of disease (such as a mouse model of Q fever in pregnancy). A vaccine is available for abattoir workers, veterinarians and others at high risk for acquiring Q fever.

History

In August 1935, E. H. Derrick, Director of the Laboratory of Microbiology and Pathology at the Queensland Health Department in Brisbane, Australia was asked to investigate an outbreak of undiagnosed febrile illness among abattoir workers in Brisbane (Derrick 1937). This illness he named Q for 'query fever'. Derrick sent samples of blood and urine from his patients to McFarlane-Burnet in an attempt to identify the agent responsible for this illness. Burnet and Freeman inoculated guinea-pigs, mice, monkeys, and embyronated eggs with materials that they received from Derrick. In a haematoxylin–eosin-stained section from a mouse spleen they found areas filled with lightly stained material of faint, uniformly granular texture. Smears stained by Castaneda's method and with Gimesa stain revealed bodies which appeared to be of rickettsial nature (Burnet and Freeman 1937). The organisms they saw were in the forms of tiny rods less than 1 μm in length and about 0.3 μm across—the shape varied from well-formed rods to coccoid forms. At about the same time, Cox and Davis at the Rocky Mountain Laboratory in Montana, United States, working on possible vectors of Rocky Mountain spotted fever and tularaemia, identified rickettsiae (the Nine Mile agent—because the ticks had been collected from the nearby Nine Mile Creek) from ticks. In April 1938, Burnet sent Dyer spleen specimens from mice infected with the Q fever

agent. Dyer showed that the Q fever agent was identical to the Nine Mile agent (McDade 1990). Derrick (1939) proposed the name *Rickettsia burnetii* for the Q fever agent; however, in 1948 Philip proposed that *Rickettsia burnetii* be considered as a single species of a distinct genus, *Coxiella* since it was now apparent that this organism was unique among the rickettsia. The Q fever agent is now known as *Coxiella burnetii*.

Early in the course of work with *C. burnetii* it was evident that it was highly infectious and, indeed, there were several reports of laboratory-acquired outbreaks of Q fever among employees at the National Institutes of Health from 1940 to 1946 (Hornibrook 1940; Huebner 1947; Spicknall *et al.* 1947).

In 1944, outbreaks of Q fever occurred among British troops stationed in Italy, Greece, and Corsica during the Second World War. Outbreaks were also reported among American troops returning to the USA from duty in the Mediterranean area (Robbins and Regan 1946; Robbins *et al.* 1946).

Outbreaks of Q fever were observed at meat-packing houses in Amarillo, Texas (Topping *et al.* 1947) and Chicago, Illinois (Shepard 1947). As part of these studies, Shepard implicated aerosols as the route of transmission of Q fever in Chicago.

In a series of studies from southern California, Lennette and co-workers found that Q fever was associated with exposure to sheep and goats and that *Coxiella burnetii* could be isolated from the air of premises housing infected animals (Lennette *et al.* 1949; Lennette and Welsh 1951). In 1948, Huebner and colleagues (Huebner *et al.* 1948) isolated *Rickettsia burnetii* from raw milk obtained from cows in southern California. In 1950, Luoto and Huebner were able to isolate *C. burnetii* from placentas of naturally infected parturient dairy cows.

In 1956, Stoker and Fiset described phase variation in *Rickettsia burnetii*. This observation has proven to be a sentinel one in the history of *Coxiella burnetii*. As will be discussed later, phase variation is important in the pathogenesis of Q fever. By 1959 Q fever had been found in man and animals from 16 countries in Africa, 9 in America, 23 in Europe, Asia, Australia, and Oceania (Babudieri 1959) and *C. burnetii* had been isolated from a wide variety of arthropods, wild, and domestic animals. To date New Zealand and Antarctica remain free from *C. burnetii*.

The discovery of phase variation was instrumental in vaccine studies of *C. burnetii*. In 1957, Abinanti and Marmion found that antibody against phase I antigen had a protective effect against infection in mice and guinea-pigs. Work during the 1960s examined the antibody response to inactivated whole-cell phase I vaccine in human volunteers (Bell *et al.* 1964). In 1984, Marmion and co-workers reported the results of a clinical trial of a low-dose (30 µg), formalin-inactivated *C. burnetii* phase I vaccine, Henzerling strain, that they had used in Australian abattoir workers. Knowledge of phase variation is central to the diagnosis of chronic infection where phase 1 antibody titres are higher than (usually) or equal to phase II titres.

The agent

Coxiella burnetii is a highly pleomorphic coccobacillus with a Gram-negative cell wall (Figs. 18.1 and 18.2). It measures 0.2×0.7 µm. It has a developmental cycle—this term applies to parasites that in addition to pleomorphism have developed forms with different functions to withstand physiological and biochemical variations in their habitats and immunological challenges (McCaul 1991). There are two cell types, distinguished on the basis of size, sensitivity to osmotic lysis, ability to metabolize exogenously supplied substrates, and peptidoglycan content. The development cycle of *C. burnetii* begins with attachment and ingestion of the small cell variant (SCV) by a host cell. Fusion of the primary lysosome with the phagosome containing the small cell variant occurs (Figs. 18.1 and 18.2). Following this, there is metabolic activation of the SCV starting vegetative growth, leading to differences in morphological appearance. The acid pH of the phagolysosome activates the metabolic enzymes of *C. burnetii*. During the early stage of bacterial growth the intermediate cell maintains the small cell variant morphology but loses its resistance property. Further bacterial growth leads to the development of a large cell variant in which *C. burnetii* begins to undergo sporogenesis. Upon release from the mother cell the endogenous cell undergoes further development to achieve the full resistant capability of the small resting cell.

Following lysis from the cell *C. burnetii* is released into the external environment. Spores are then also released. Both the small and large cell variants have Gram-negative cell walls. The formation of spores explains the ability of *C. burnetii* to withstand harsh environmental conditions. It survives for 7–10 months on surfaces at 15–20°C for more than 1 month on fresh meat in cold storage, and for more than 40 months in skimmed milk at room temperature (Christie 1974). *Coxiella burnetii* can be destroyed by 2% formaldehyde but the organism has been isolated from infected tissues stored in formaldehyde for up to 4–5 months. It has also been isolated from fixed paraffinized tissues. Lysol 1% and 5% hydrogen peroxide will kill *C. burnetii*.

Coxiella burnetii undergoes phase variation (Stoker and Fiset 1956). In nature and laboratory animals it exists in the phase I state in which organisms react with late (45 day) convalescent guinea-pig sera and only slightly with early (21 day) sera. Repeated passage of phase I organisms in embryonated chicken eggs leads to gradual conversion to phase II avirulent forms. There are no morphological differences between the two phases although they differ in the sugar composition of their lipopolysaccharides (Schramek and Mayer 1982), and their buoyant density in caesium chloride and in their affinity for basic fuchsin dyes. *Coxiella burnetii* lipopolysac-charide (LPS) is non-toxic to chicken embryos at doses of over 80 µg per embryo, in contrast to *Salmonella typhimurium*

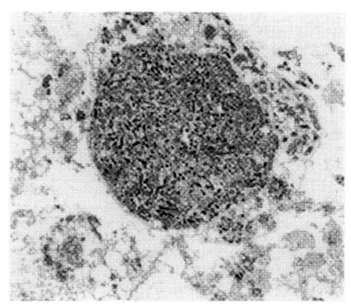

Fig. 18.1 Transmission electron micrograph of a vegetation from a patient with Q fever endocarditis. Note the many *C. burnetii* cells in a phagolysosome. (Magnification × 3865.)

smooth and rough-type LPS, which is toxic in nanogram amounts (Hacksteadt *et al.* 1985).

Plasmids have been found in both phase I and phase II cells (Samuel *et al.* 1985). Three different plasmids varying from 36 to 45 kb have been described (Sawyer *et al.* 1987). The first plasmid, named Q_pH_1 was found in a Nine Mile phase I isolate. It is 36 kb and is present at about three copies per cell. The second plasmid, designated

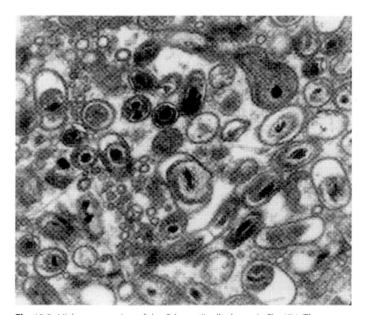

Fig. 18.2 Higher power view of the *C. burnetii* cells shown in Fig. 17.1. The electron-dense material is condensed DNA. Note the characteristic Gram-negative cell wall. (Magnification × 21 632.)

Q$_p$RS was obtained from an isolate named Priscilla which was recovered from the placenta of a goat that had aborted. This plasmid has been found in four isolates obtained from patients with Q fever endocarditis (Michael *et al.* 1990; Mallavia *et al.* 1991). Q$_p$RS has considerable homology with Q$_p$H$_1$ and is 39 kb in size. The third, a 51 kb plasmid, was obtained from feral rodent isolates near Dugway, Utah and has been designated Dugway (Stoennes and Lachman 1960). Isolates with no plasmids have plasmid DNA integrated into the genome. Stein and Raoult (1992a) examined eight new *C. burnetii* isolates from patients with chronic Q fever and found that seven of the eight had plasmids which were about 40 kb in size.

There is no correlation between plasmid type and disease caused by *C. burnetii*. The QpHj plasmid has been found in isolates from cases of acute Q fever while the QpRS plasmid and chromosomally integrated sequences with homology to this plasmid are found in isolates of patients with Q fever endocarditis (Minnick *et al.* 1991).

It has been suggested by some workers that there are at least six strains of *C. burnetii*. These are Hamilton, Bacca, Rasche, Biotzere, Corazon, and Dod. The first three strains contain the Q$_p$H$_1$ plasmid and have been associated with acute Q fever. Biotzere has plasmid QpRS and Corazon has no plasmid but plasmid-related sequences are present in the genome. These two strains are associated with chronic Q fever. The Dod strain, which contains the QpDG plasmid, is avirulent.

More recently Thiele *et al.* (1993) have used pulsed field gel electrophoresis to examine isolates of *C. burnetii* and have shown that there is considerable heterogeneity among isolates. It is very likely that there are more strains of *C. burnetii* than have been recognized to date.

Genotyping of *C. burnetii* isolates (Glazunova *et al.* (2005) was carried out by multispacer sequence typing. Ten spacers that exhibited the most variation were selected and used to examine 159 isolates from various specimens from different countries. Thirty different allelic combinations were found. Phylogenic analysis showed three major clusters.

The ability of *C. burnetii* to survive in the phagolysosome has been linked to its ability to produce superoxide dismutase which protects it from host cell generated superoxide anion and hydrogen peroxide (Akporiaye and Baca 1983). *Coxiella burnetii* inhibits the respiratory burst of phagocytosing human neutrophils, a property similar to that possessed by *Legionella* and *Leishmania* (Baca *et al.* 1993). Acid phosphatase is a possible virulence factor for *C. burnetii*.

Only a few of the *C. burnetii* genes are known; two of these comprise the heat-shock inducible *htp*AB operon (*hip*A and *htp*B genes) which encode the heat-shock protein that is homologous to similar proteins in mycobacteria and *E. coli* (Vodkin and Williams 1988). The *C. burnetii* genes for the two heat-shock proteins and for citrate synthase have been cloned and expressed in *Escherichia coli*. Hendrix *et al.*(1993) have cloned and sequenced the gene *com*1 which codes for an outer membrane protein.

The 1,995,275 base pair genome of *Coxiella burnetii* phase I, Nine Mile strain, was recently sequenced (Seshardi *et al.* 2003). It possesses 29 insertion sequence elements and 83 pseudogenes. Because *C. burnetii* can persist in the external environment the absence of pathways for synthesis of storage compounds such as glycogen, trehalose or polyhydroxybutyrate was unexpected (Seshardi *et al.* 2003).

A recent advance has been the ability to grow *C. burnetii* in cell free media (Omsland *et al.* 2009).

Taxonomy

Coxiella burnetii is the sole species of its genus (Weiss *et al.* 1991). On the basis of 16S RNA sequence similarities, it has been placed in the gamma subdivision of proteobacteria with a specific but rather distant relationship to *Legionella*. Only *Wolbachia persica* belongs in the gamma subdivision with minor relatedness to the *Coxiella-Legionella* cluster.

Pathogenicity

When guinea-pigs are inoculated intraperitoneally with *C. burnetii* granulomas develop in the liver, bone marrow, and spleen. Guinea-pigs exposed to aerosols containing *C. burnetii* develop pneumonia within the first 5 days. The pneumonia begins to resolve by day 15 following exposure and is complete by day 29. Hepatic and splenic granulomas develop. Mice inoculated with *C. burnetii* either intranasally or intraperitoneally also develop pneumonia, hepatic, and splenic granulomas, bone marrow, and liver involvement (Baca 1991).

In studies with persistently infected L929 mouse fibroblasts or macrophage cell lines such as J774 and P3881, different isolates of *C. burnetii* produce different effects. Cells infected with Q$_p$RS isolates exhibit multivacuolation and do not proliferate in suspension cultures or infect J774 cells. Proteins of *C. burnetii* are inserted into the cell membrane of these cells and this leads to the antibody-dependent cell cytotoxicity found in Q fever (Marecki *et al.*1978). Isolates implicated in short-term acute disease caused the insertion of more antigen into the host cell membrane than did isolates associated with chronic disease (Baca 1991). These observations may be a partial explanation as to why some patients develop acute Q fever and others develop chronic Q fever.

A considerable amount has been learned about the pathogenesis of *C. burnetii* infection over the past few years. The attachment of virulent forms of *C. burnetii* to monocytes is mediated by one integrin whereas the interaction of the avirulent form with monocytes requires the same integrin as the virulent forms plus complement receptor 3 (CR3) integrins (Capo *et al.* 1999). The virulent variant inhibits the internalization mediated by CR3 through the impairment of cross talk between these two integrins (Capo *et al.* 1999). Interferon γ mediates intracellular killing of *C. burnetii* by promoting apoptosis of infected monocytes through activation of caspase-3 while interleukin-4 enables monocytes to support *C. burnetii* replication (Dellacasagrande *et al.* 2002). The T-cell dependent immune response does not eliminate *C. burnetii*, and subsequent immunosuppression can lead to relapse (Sidwell *et al.* 1964a, b). Indeed, *Coxiella burnetii* DNA persists in monocytes and bone marrow years after acute Q fever and the microorganism survives in monocytes from patients with chronic infection but not in monocytes from patients with acute Q fever or from seronegative control subjects (Harris *et al.* 2000; Dellacasagrande *et al.* 2000). This defect, which appears to be due to the secretion of soluble TNF receptor 75 disappears when the patients are cured (Ghigo *et al.* 2000). In the setting of chronic Q fever IL-10 overproduction occurs and anti-IL-10 antibodies restore the microbial activity of the monocytes *in vitro* (Ghigo *et al.* 2001). In the *C. burnetii*–infected human monocytic leukemia cell line THP-1 335 genes were up-or-down-regulated at least twofold (Ren *et al.* 2003).

The hosts

Animals

Coxiella burnetii can infect a large number of animal species including livestock, but infection is usually asymptomatic. In his 1959 review Babudieri describes bronchopneumonia in goats due to Q fever and continuous fever lasting several days in infected cattle. Catarrhal mastitis in cows and bronchopneumonia in a dog have been reported. Studies from the United States suggested that there was no morbidity in cattle and sheep naturally infected with *C. burnetii* and no reports of effects on milk yields. Endocarditis, the major form of chronic Q fever in man, does not seem to occur in other animals.

Coxiella burnetii localizes to the uterus and mammary glands of infected animals. Cattle have been resistant to experimental infection by intranasal, intravenous, intravaginal inoculation, and by the feeding of contaminated bran. Intranasal infection of a pregnant cow by means by an atomizer did lead to infection. *Coxiella burnetii* has been isolated from the placentas of naturally infected cows and naturally infected and experimentally infected sheep (Lang 1990). It has been transmitted transplacentally in a guinea-pig model of infection.

Once infected, cows can shed *C. burnetii* in milk for up to 32 months. Grist (1959) in his 4-year longitudinal study of a dairy herd found that no more than 15% of the milk cows showed evidence of infection at any one time. He suggested that infection is maintained within a herd largely by infection of younger non-immune animals. Sheep have shed the organism in faeces for 11–18 postpartum (Welsh *et al.* 1958). The use of polymerase chain reaction to amply *C. burnetii* DNA has led to an increase in our understanding of shedding patterns of this organism in cattle, sheep and goats (Rodolakis *et al.* 2007). Rodolakis *et al.* (2007) studied 95 cows, 120 goats and 90 ewes using PCR. They found that cows were asymptomatic and shed almost exclusively in milk, as did goats although one of the goat herds had abortions. The ewes which came from flocks with abortions shed the bacteria mostly in the faeces and in vaginal mucus. The authors felt that their findings explained why Q fever was more common in humans following exposure to infected ovines than bovines. In a recent review, Rodolakis (2009) indicates that in asymptomatic herds cows shed *C. burnetii* almost exclusively in milk and this may persist for months and it can be intermittent or continuous. Experimentally infected ewes shed 100 to 1,000 times less bacterial cells in milk than in vaginal mucus (Rodolakis 2009).

McCaughey *et al.* (2009) tested 5,182 cows in Northern Ireland using an ELISA test and found that 6.2% of the animals and 48.4% of the herds were positive.

Outbreaks of abortion due to *C. burnetii* have been reported in goats, cattle, and sheep. Inflammation of the placenta has been demonstrated in sheep and goats in instances where *C. burnetii* has caused abortion (Palmer *et al.* 1983). Stresses such as overcrowding and pregnancy are associated with multiplication of *C. burnetii* in the placenta. The placentas of infected sheep can contain 10^9 guinea-pig infective doses per gram of tissue.

In addition to cattle, sheep, and goats, which are the traditional reservoirs of *C. burnetii*, the following domestic animal species have been found to be infected with this organism in some areas: pigs, horses, dogs, cats, camels, buffaloes, pigeons, geese, and fowl (Babudieri 1959; Marrie *et al.* 1985, 1993). Rats are implicated in

the spread of Q fever in the United Kingdom by some investigators (Webster *et al.* 1995).

Coxiella burnetii has been found in many species of ticks and in lice and flies. Sanders *et al.* (2008) examined 1,597 nymphs, 14 females and 13 male *Amblyomma* ticks collected in South Texas. Nine nymphal pools, 2 females and 3 males were positive for *Coxiella burnetii*. Five of 363 flies were positive for *C. burnetii* DNA (Nelder 2008). Positive flies were obtained from carrion, a garbage bin of animal faeces and a barn at a ranch. *Stomoxys calcitrans* in which adults feed on animal and human blood and the blow flies *Lucilia coeruleiviridis* and *L. sericata* were the species of flies that were positive. Under experimental conditions it has been possible to infect fleas and cockroaches. Infection with *C. burnetii* is widespread throughout the wild animal population and the rate of this infection varies from country to country. Where Q fever is endemic there may very well be a differential infection rate among the wildlife; hares and rabbits are more commonly infected than other animals (Marrie *et al.* 1993).

Table 18.1 summarizes studies of a variety of animals in Nova Scotia, carried out using a micro-immunofluorescence test. Experience in Nova Scotia illustrates that the data regarding infected animals has to be correlated carefully with the epidemiology of this infection in man. Several outbreaks of Q fever have followed exposure to infected parturient cats (Marrie *et al.* 1988a, b) and cases of Q fever have also followed exposure to wild rabbits and to deer (Laughlin *et al.* 1991). Only three cases (out of >300) of Q fever was associated with exposure to infected cattle despite a considerable percentage of the cattle infected. These data are in keeping with the conclusions of Rodolakis *et al.* (2007) that because cows shed the organism almost exclusively in milk the spread to man is less than following exposure to infected ovines. In a seroepidemiological survey of a random sample of the Nova Scotia population it was found that there was a statistically significant association between residence in four counties and seropositivity for *C. burnetii*. These four counties account for 75% of the cattle, sheep, and goats in our province. However, exposure to cattle, sheep, and goats as reported by questionnaire data was not a risk factor for seropositivity. It is likely that indirect exposure resulted in subclinical Q fever in this population.

Sheep and goats in the US have a higher seroprevalence for *C. burnetii* than cattle. While only one study has been published for each of these animals—the seropositivity rate among tested dogs was 53%, cats 8%, and horses 25.6% (McQuiston *et al.* 2002). McQuiston also noted an extensive wildlife reservoir for this organism in the USA. Various studies have shown varying degrees of seropositivity for coyotes, grey foxes, skunks, raccoons, rabbits, deer, mice, bears, birds and opossums (McQuiston *et al.* 2002).

One always has to consider all the facts in determining the animal source responsible for an outbreak of Q fever. Nowhere is this more applicable than an outbreak of Q fever associated with a horse-boarding ranch in Colorado (Bamberg *et al.* 2007). In fact this was due to spread of infection from two herds of goats that had been acquired by the owners. Twenty (53%) of 38 persons tested had serological evidence of infection with *C. burnetii*. Testing of the soil and goats using a PCR assay confirmed the presence of *C. burnetii* in the soil and among the goats. One hundred and thirty-eight persons who lived within 1 mile of the ranch were also tested. Eleven (8%) had evidence of *C. burnetii* infection, 8 of whom had no direct contact with the ranch.

Table 18.1 Rate of *Coxiella burnetii* infection of various animals in Nova Scotia as measured by antibodies to *C. burnetii* phase I and phase II antigens. Data are from (George and Marrie 1987; Marrie *et al.* 1985)

Animal	Number Tested	Phase I	Phase II
Domestic			
Sheep	329	0	6.7
Cattle	214	24.2	23.8
Goats	29	3.5	7.0
Cats	216	6.0	24.1
Dogs	447	0	0
Wild			
Snowshoe hare (*Lepus americanus*)	730	49	12
Moose (*Alms alces americana Clinton*)	243	16.5	11.5
White-tailed deer (*Odocoileus virginianus*)	68	1.5	4.4
Raccoon (*Procyon lotor*)	42	7.1	9.5

(Columns 2–4 grouped under: **Percent positive IFA[a] test**)

[a] IFA, indirect fluorescence antibody.

The human host

Clinical features

Humans are the only animals known to develop illness regularly as a result of *C. burnetii* infection. There are several distinct syndromes of *C. burnetii* infection in man.

Table 18.2 shows the symptoms of acute Q fever in patients from six different countries from 1948 to 1989. Fever and fatigue are the predominant manifestations in almost all of the patients in all series. Headache is also a prominent symptom, although its frequency ranges from a low of 65% in the California series to a high of 98% in the patients reported from Uruguay. Cough was reported in only 24% of the patients in the Northern California series but in

Table 18.2 Symptoms of acute Q fever in patients from six different countries

	Northern California 1948–49; 180 patients (Clark *et al.* 1951)	Australia 1962–81; 111 patients (Spelman 1981)	Switzerland 1983; 191 patients (Dupuis *et al.* 1985)	Uruguay 1975–1985; 1358 patients[a] (Somma–Moreira *et al.* 1987)	Nova Scotia 1983–1986; 51 patients (Marrie *et al.* 1988a)	West Midlands UK March–April 1989; 102 patients (Smith *et al.* 1993)	
Fever	100	100		88	98	94	99
Fatigue	100	NS[b]		97	98	98	NS
Chills	74	68		NS	NS	88	NS
Headache	65	86		77	98	73	68
Myalgia	47	60		64	NS	69	54
Sweats	31	NS		NS	98	84	NS
Cough	24	32		70	90	28	51
Nausea	22	25		25	NS	49	NS
Vomiting	13	42		25	NS	25	
Chest pain	10	NS		34	NS	28	45
Diarrhoea	5	7		NS	NS	22	NS
Sore throat	5	NS		27	NS	14	NS
Rash	4	8		5	NS	18	NS
Neurological	NS	NS		NS	NS	NS	23

(Columns grouped under: **Percentage with indicated symptom**)

[a] All cases occurred in workers at meat-processing plants.

[b] NS, not stated.

90% of the patients from Uruguay. Rash is infrequently reported. Neurological manifestations are generally uncommon but in the series from the West Midlands, UK, 23% of the patients had neurological symptoms.

Self-limited febrile illness

Where Q fever is endemic a significant percentage of the general population, often of the order of 11–12%, has been found to have antibodies to *C. burnetii*. Most of these individuals do not recall pneumonia or any other illness that could readily be attributable to this infection. The extent to which Q fever contributes to undifferentiated febrile illnesses in the population may be very high, as suggested by a study from the south of Spain wherein 21% of 505 adults who had fever of more than 1 week and less than 3 weeks' duration had Q fever (Viciana *et al.* 1992). All of these individuals had normal chest radiographs.

Pneumonia

Pneumonia is one of the predominant manifestations of acute Q fever in man, but there is tremendous variation in its reported frequency. It is the predominant manifestation of acute Q fever in Nova Scotia, but in France where hepatitis is the major manifestation of acute Q fever, pneumonia is rarely seen (Dupont *et al.* 1992). However, in the Canary Islands region of Spain both pneumonia and hepatitis are manifestations of Q fever (Velasco *et al.* 1996).

Cough may not be present even though pneumonia is evident radiographically. In most instances the pneumonia is of mild to moderate severity, but it can be rapidly progressive, resulting in respiratory failure.

Physical examination of the chest is often normal. About 5% of patients with pneumonia due to *C. burnetii* have splenomegaly. The rapidly progressive form of Q fever pneumonia mimics Legionnaires' disease, the pneumonic form of tularaemia, severe *Chlamydophila pneumoniae*, and in some cases pyogenic bacterial pneumonia.

The radiographic picture of Q fever pneumonia is variable (Figs. 18.3–18.5). Segmental and subsegmental pleural based opacities are common (Gordan *et al.* 1984) Multiple rounded opacities are seen, and in Nova Scotia this is very suggestive of Q fever that follows exposure to infected parturient cats. Pleural effusions (usually small) are found in up to one-third of cases.

The rare fatalities from *C. burnetii* pneumonia usually occur in patients with severe co-morbid illnesses. Information regarding the histology of Q fever in pneumonia in man is extremely limited. In one of our patients with severe pneumonia, the bronchial epithelial lining was denuded in part due to necrosis. The interstitium showed oedema and infiltration by lymphocytes and macrophages. Alveolar spaces were filled with macrophages and other cells resembling detached epithelium (Figs. 18.6 and 18.7). In another patient, there was a lung mass (pseudotumor) composed of mixtures of macrophages, giant cells, plasma cells, and lymphocytes (Janigan and Marrie 1983).

White blood cell count is usually normal but one-third of patients have an increased count. A slight elevation in the hepatic transaminase levels occurs in almost all patients. Rarely, the syndrome of inappropriate secretion of antidiuretic hormone complicates the pneumonia (Biggs *et al.*1984).

Diagnosis

Since most laboratories do not have the facilities required to isolate this micro-organism, the diagnosis of *C. burnetii* pneumonia is

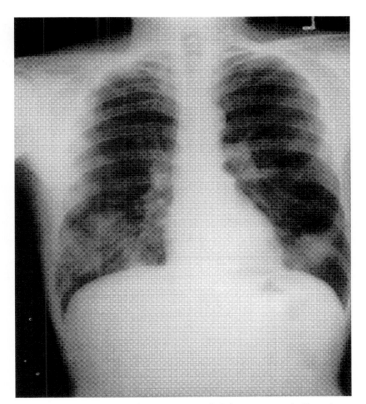

Fig. 18.3 Chest radiograph of a young man with Q fever pneumonia. Note the multiple rounded opacities

usually confirmed by demonstration of a fourfold rise in antibody titre between acute and convalescent sera. Recently, Stein and Raoult (1992b) were able to detect *C. burnetii* DNA by amplification using a polymerase chain reaction. They developed primers derived from the *C. burnetii* superoxide dismutase gene. This

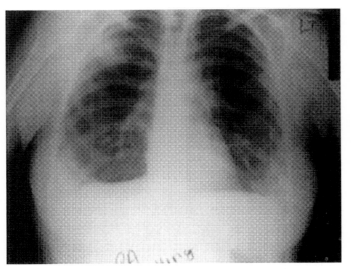

Fig. 18.4 Chest radiograph of a 20 year old female with right upper lobe pneumonia due to *C. burnetii*

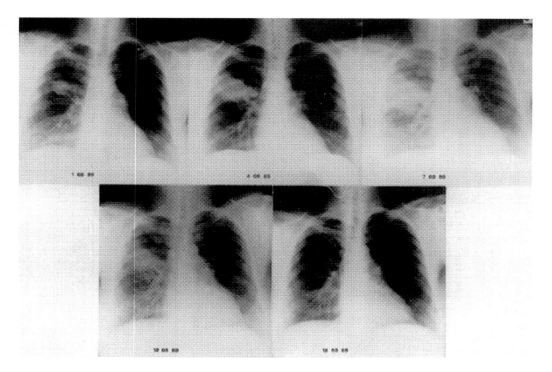

Fig. 18.5 Serial chest radiographs of a patient with Q fever pneumonia. Note the rapidity with which the opacity increases in size and the speed with which it resolves

should allow the detection of *C. burnetii* in a variety of clinical specimens although the sensitivity of this test in *C. burnetii* pneumonia is still unknown. Since *C. burnetii* is an intracellular pathogen, there may be very little in the way of *C. burnetii* DNA in respiratory secretions.

A variety of laboratory tests have been used to detect antibodies to *C. burnetii*, including microagglutination, complement fixation, microimmunofluorescence, and enzyme-linked immunoabsorbent assay. The complement fixation and microimmunofluorescence tests are most commonly used. Antibodies should be

determined to both phase I and phase II antigens. In acute Q fever, antibodies to phase II predominate while in chronic Q fever antibodies to phase I predominate.

Some authors have advocated using the indirect immunofluorescence test to detect antibodies to IgM so that a single serum sample may be used in the diagnosis of acute Q fever (Hunt *et al.* 1983). However, IgM antibodies may persist for up to 678 days following acute infection and in one study 3% of 162 patients still had significant IgM antibody levels 1 year after infection (Dupius *et al.* 1985).

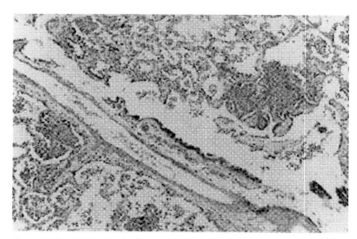

Fig. 18.6 Photomicrograph of an open lung biopsy from a patient with *C. burnetii* pneumonia. Note the extensive inflammatory response which is both alveolar and interstitial. (Magnification × 175.)

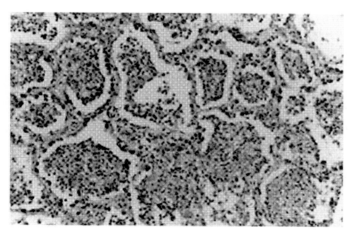

Fig. 18.7 Photomicrograph of an open lung biopsy from a patient with *C. burnetii* pneumonia. The alveoli are filled with an inflammatory exudate. There is hyperplasia of the pneumocytes lining the alveoli. (Magnification × 175.)

Treatment

The treatment of choice for *C. burnetii* pneumonia is tetracycline or doxycycline. Tetracycline is given in a dose of 500 mg every 6 hours for 7–10 days. Doxycycline is given in a dosage of 100 mg twice daily for 7–10 days. *In vitro* studies performed by Yeaman *et al.* (1987) suggest that several quinolones, including difloxacin, ciprofloxacin, levofloxacin, moxifloxacin should also be effective in the treatment of Q fever. Rifampin is the most active antibiotic *in vitro* against *C. burnetii*.

Chronic Q fever

Clinical features

The major manifestation of chronic Q fever is endocarditis, but infection of vascular prostheses, aneurysms, osteomyelitis, hepatitis, prolonged fever and purpuric eruptions are reported (Brouqui *et al.* 1993).

As with other forms of endocarditis, *C. burnetii* infection usually develops on abnormal or prosthetic cardiac valves (Raoult *et al.* 1987). The incidence of Q fever endocarditis seems to be increasing, although this may reflect increased recognition of this entity. Turck *et al.* (1976) drew attention to this form of Q fever when they reported 16 cases of chronic Q fever that they diagnosed between 1968 and 1973. Their review of the literature yielded only 55 other cases of chronic Q fever. This contrasts with 79 cases of chronic Q fever reported from the Public Health Laboratory Service's Communicable Disease Surveillance Centre in England from 1975 to 1980 (Palmer and Young 1982). From 1975 to 1981, *C. burnetii* accounted for 3% of all cases for endocarditis reported in England and Wales. In the small province of Nova Scotia, Canada with a population of 900,000, 11 cases of Q fever endocarditis were diagnosed between 1979 and 1993.

The clinical presentation is that of culture-negative endocarditis. Prolonged fever and negative blood cultures in a patient with an abnormal native valve or a prosthetic valve should suggest this diagnosis. If these findings are combined with marked clubbing of the fingers and hyperglobulinaemia one should be even more suspicious of this diagnosis. Splenomegaly and hepatomegaly are found in about half the patients, and a purpuric rash due to leucocytoclastic vasculitis occurs in about 20% of patients. The sedimentation rate is usually quite high (often >100 mm/h); anaemia and microscopic haematuria are also present. Arterial emboli complicate the course of one-third of patients.

The vegetations in chronic Q fever are different for those found in pyogenic bacterial endocarditis. In chronic Q fever the vegetation is usually smooth and may form nodules on the valve (Fig. 18.8). Microscopically there is a subacute and chronic inflammatory infiltrate and many large, foamy macrophages (Fig. 18.9) full of the characteristic micro-organisms are readily seen with electron microscopy (Figs. 18.1 and 18.2).

Diagnosis

Confirmation of the diagnosis of Q fever endocarditis is usually made serologically. A complement fixation titre of ≥1:200 to phase I antigen is said to be diagnostic of chronic Q fever, although not all patients in the series reported by Turck *et al.* (1976) had this titre. The best serological test is the indirect immunofluorescence test. Using this test phase I antibodies are invariably higher than phase II antibodies in chronic Q fever, while the reverse is true in acute Q fever. It is not unusual to see phase I antibody titres of 1:56,000 in chronic Q fever. An anti-phase I IgG titre of 1:800 or

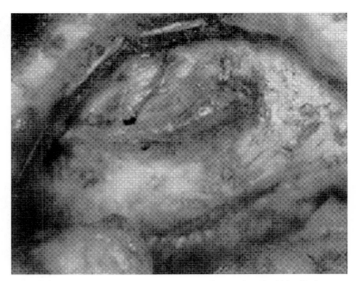

Fig. 18.8 *Coxiella burnetii* vegetation on a prosthetic valve. The 'ridge' is the vegetation (reproduced with permission from Raoult, D., Raza, A., and Marrie, T.J. (1991). Q fever endocarditis and other forms of chronic Q fever. In *Q fever. Volume 1: The disease*, (ed. T.J. Marrie pp. 179–99. CRC Press, Boca Raton, FLA).

greater has been shown to raised the post-test probability to 98% (Tissot-Dupont *et al.* 1994).

Coxiella burnetii can be isolated from the blood of patients with Q fever endocarditis by using a shell vial technique. Organisms can be detected in the valve lesions using an immunofluorescence technique (Raoult *et al.* 1994). PCR has successfully been used to detect DNA in cell cultures and clinical samples (94). Several genes have been used to generate specific primers including 16S rRNA, 23S rDNA, superoxide dismutase, plasmid based sequences, and the IS1111 multicopy insertion sequence (Fournier *et al.* 1998). LightCycler Nested PCR (LCN-PCR) using the IS111 multicopy gene, is very sensitive and can be used to amplify *C. burnetii* DNA from vegetations.

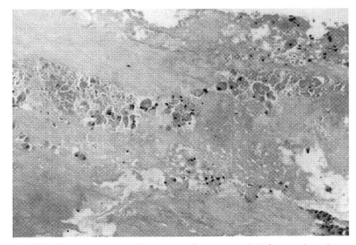

Fig. 18.9 Photomicrograph of vegetation of a patient with Q fever endocarditis. The large round cells are foamy macrophages. (Magnification × 114.)

Isolation of C. *burnetii* must be done only in a biosafety level 3 containment facility due to its extreme infectivity. This microorganism can be isolated by inoculation of specimens into conventional cell cultures (e.g. Vero cells) (Raoult *et al.* 1990), embryonated egg yolk sacs (Ormsbee 1952), or laboratory animals, such as mice or guinea pigs (Huebner *et al.* 1948). The shell vial technique, wherein material to be cultured is centrifuged onto a cell culture line which has been grown on a coverslip, has been a major advance in isolation of C.*burnetii* from clinical specimens (Raoult *et al.* 1991).

The microagglutination test (Fiset *et al.* 1969), the complement fixation test, the indirect immunofluorescent antibody (IFA) test (Field *et al.* 1983), and ELISA (Waag *et al.* 1995) have been used for the serological diagnosis of C. *burnetii* infection. Based on our experience the best serological test for the diagnosis of Q fever is the IFA.

In acute Q fever, seroconversion usually is detected 7 to 15 days after the onset of clinical symptoms. Approximately 90% of patients have detectable antibodies by the third week. IFA antibody titres reach their maximum levels 4 to 8 weeks after the onset of disease and then decrease gradually during the ensuing 12 months (Brouqui *et al.* 2007). IgM titres declined to undetectable levels after 10 to 17 weeks (Brouqui *et al.* 2007). In blood culture-negative endocarditis the sensitivity and the post-test probability of having Q fever in a single-step serological assay with a cut-off at 1/800 and greater was 100% and 99.5% respectively (Brouqui *et al.* 2007). Thus in chronic Q fever a single serum sample is diagnostic.

The persistence of high levels of anti-phase I antibodies despite appropriate treatment or the reappearance of such antibodies, should raise the suspicion of possible chronic Q fever. Patients with valvular or vascular abnormalities, those who are immunocompromised and pregnant women should have repeated C. *burnetii* serology tests if they have medical history of acute Q fever or prolonged and unexplained febrile episode. In uncertain cases, a PCR performed in blood may help to determine if the patient is convalescent (negative) or infected (positive).

The follow-up of patients treated for chronic Q fever also should be done serologically. During therapy, serologic testing should be performed once monthly for 6 months and every 3 months thereafter. The levels of antibodies decrease very slowly but this decrease correlates with the serum doxycycline level and a two-dilution decrease for anti-phase I IgG and IgA is associated with cure (Brouqui *et al.* 2007). When present, IgM antibodies disappear first, then IgA antibodies, but IgG titres remain positive for years. Antimicrobial treatment can be stopped after 18 months to 3 years if the IgG titer anti-phase I by immunofluorescence assay is below 1:400 and IgA anti-phase I is undetectable (Brouqui *et al.* 2007).

Treatment

There have been no controlled clinical trials of the treatment of Q fever endocarditis. A variety of antibiotics have been used and some authorities recommend that treatment be continued indefinitely. However, a consensus is emerging that combination antibiotic therapy is necessary to treat this severe illness successfully (Levy *et al.* 1991). The finding that the bactericidal effect of doxycycline is enhanced when alkalinization of the phagolysosome is accomplished with chloroquine or amantadine had major implications for the future treatment of endocarditis (Maurin *et al.* 1992).

The growing evidence suggests that hydroxychoroquine plus doxycycline should be first line treatment for Q fever endocarditis.

Raoult *et al.* (1999) compared the results of treatment with doxycycline 100 mg bid and hydroxychloroquine 200 mg tid (plasma levels were measured and the dose adjusted to maintain a concentration between 0.8 and 1.2 mcg/mL) for 18 months with those of their usual regimen of doxycycline and ofloxacin. The latter patients were treated from January 1987 to May 1991 and the former group from May1991 until December 1997. Twenty-one patients received doxycycline and hydroxychloroquine—1 died of a surgical complication, 2 were still receiving treatment at the time of the report and 1 was being evaluated and 17 were cured. The mean duration of treatment was 31 months. In the historical comparison group (ofloxacin and doxycycline) there were 14 patients—1 died, 1 was still on treatment at the time of the report, 7 relapsed and 5 were cured. The doxycycline-hydroxychloroquine regimen had a significantly lower relapse rate. Doxycycline levels should also be measured as the MICs of doxycycline for C. *burnetii* of 1 to 4 µg/mL are very close to serum levels. A ratio of serum level to doxycycline MIC of ≥ 1 is associated with a rapid decline in antibodies to phase 1 (Rolain *et al.* 2005). Patients who take this regimen must be advised about the photosensitivity and retinal toxicity risks. Regular follow-up by an ophthalmologist is mandatory. The ability to monitor hydroxychloroquine and doxycycline blood levels is also necessary.

An alternative regimen is ciprofloxacin (750 mg twice daily, orally) plus rifampin (300 mg daily, orally). We have now treated 12 patients with this regimen, with only one failure. We recommend at least 2 years of treatment, while others recommend 3 years (Marrie 2002). The best approach is to monitor response to treatment by determining antibody titres to phase I and phase II antigens with a microimmunofluorescence test. These antibody titres should be determined for the IgG and IgA every 3 months during treatment. Declining antibody titres reflect adequate response to treatment. When the antiphase I IgA is 1:200 or less, therapy can be stopped.

There are several reports of isolation of C. *burnetii* from heart valves following months to years of treatment, especially with single antimicrobial agents (Levy *et al.* 1991). Other antibiotic combinations that have been used successfully to treat Q fever endocarditis are: (1) doxycycline and cotrimoxazole and (2) doxycycline and quinolones (Levy *et al.* 1991).

Hepatitis

There are three main manifestations of Q fever hepatitis (Hofmann and Heaton 1982):

1   Infectious hepatitis-like picture.

2   Hepatitis as an incidental finding in a patient with acute Q fever.

3   Fever of unknown origin with characteristic granulomas on liver biopsy.

The hepatic granuloma in Q fever hepatitis, the so-called doughnut granuloma, consists of a dense fibrin ring surrounded by a central lipid vacuole. These granulomas are not specific for Q fever since they have also been seen in Hodgkin's disease and infectious mononucleosis. Two weeks of antibiotic therapy with a tetracycline compound is usually sufficient. Most cases of hepatitis represent the acute form of the disease, although an occasional patient with hepatitis can have the serological profile of chronic Q fever—these patients should be treated for longer than 2 weeks. A number of patients with Q fever hepatitis remain febrile despite therapy with antibiotics. For these individuals treatment with prednisone 0.5 mg/kg has resulted in defervescence within 2 to 15 days (Crespo *et al.* 1999). Once defervescence has occurred the dose of steroids is tapered over the next month.

Neurological manifestations

Severe headache is the most common neurological manifestation of Q fever. Aseptic meningitis and/or encephalitis is rare (Marrie and Raoult 1992).

Two recent studies from the United Kingdom report a very high incidence of neurological manifestations of Q fever infection. In a study from Plymouth, Reilly *et al.* (1990) reported an incidence of neurological complications in 22% of 103 patients with Q fever. Forty-six of the patients had acute Q fever, 5 had chronic Q fever, and 52 had remote infections. Six of the 45 patients with acute Q fever had residual neurological impairment, including weakness, recurrent meningismus, blurred vision, residual paraesthesis, and sensory loss involving the left leg. In the study from the West Midlands (Smith *et al.* 1993), 23 of 101 patients reported neurological symptoms. Eight complained of hallucinations—in six these were visual, in one auditory, and in one olfactory. Six patients described symptoms compatible with an expressive dysphasia. Three had hemifacial pain suggestive of trigeminal neuralgia. Diplopia and dysarthria were described by one patient each, and one patient had a visual-field disturbance. These deficits lasted for only a few days. The rate of neurological involvement in these two studies is so much higher than that reported from any other country in the world that it raises the possibility that a neurotrophic strain of *C. burnetii* was circulating in the United Kingdom.

Rarely, Q fever meningoencephalitis may be accompanied by seizures and coma. Other neurological manifestations of Q fever include behavioural disturbances, cerebellar signs and symptoms, cranial nerve palsies, extrapyramidal disease, and the MillerFisher syndrome.

Q fever in the immunocompromised host

Raoult and co-workers (1993) found that 10% of 500 HIV-positive individuals had IgG antibodies at a titre of ≥1; 25 to *C. burnetii*, twice the rate in healthy blood donors. They also found that 5 of 68 (7.3%) of patients hospitalized with Q fever from 1987 to 1989 in Marseilles were HIV positive. They went on to estimate that in HIV-positive individuals the number of cases of Q fever was 13 times higher than that in the general population. The same investigators reviewed all cases of chronic Q fever in France from 1982 to 1990 (Brouqui *et al.* 1993) and they found that 20% of these 84 patients were immunocompromised.

Q fever in pregnancy

Coxiella burnetii was isolated from the placenta of a woman who became pregnant 2 years after an episode of acute Q fever. This suggests that re-activation of Q fever occurs during human pregnancy as it does in other animals (Syrucek *et al.* 1958). In this same study three women who had Q fever during pregnancy had normal children and *C. burnetii* was isolated from the placenta of two of them. The third had her pregnancy interrupted because of rubella and *C. burnetii* was isolated from her placenta. The fifth woman's child had hypospadias—*C. burnetii* was isolated from her placenta.

A 21 year old Israeli woman had Q fever at 21 weeks of pregnancy (Reichmann *et al.* 1988). Her course was complicated by thrombocytopenia and labour was induced at 28 weeks—the baby was normal.

Marrie reported two cases of Q fever in pregnancy (Marrie 1993). One of these cases was subclinical—her husband developed Q fever pneumonia following exposure to parturient cats. At this point she was 36 weeks into her pregnancy but she had never had any symptoms of infection. However, serological testing demonstrated a fourfold rise in antibody titre and *C. burnetii* was isolated from her placenta. The second patient had Q fever pneumonia at 12 weeks of gestation. She was treated with antibiotics and recovered from her pneumonia; however, she went on to deliver at 31 weeks' gestation. Her infant weighed 1550 g and required 1 month in the neonatal intensive care unit. When examined at one year of age, his head circumference was in the tenth percentile, weight was between the tenth and twenty-fifth percentile and developmental milestones and physical examination was normal. *Coxiella burnetii* was isolated from her placenta.

There is now good evidence that patients with Q fever during pregnancy should receive at least 5 weeks treatment with cotrimoxazole (320 mg of trimethoprim and 1,600 mg sulfamethoxazole daily) (Carcopino *et al.* 2007). These investigators studied 53 women whose pregnancies were complicated by Q fever. Sixteen women received co-trimoxazole treatment for 5 weeks whereas 37 did not. The obstetric complications were significantly higher in the latter group at 81.1% versus 43.8% for the co-trimoxazole group. Infection in the first trimester was associated with a higher rate of complications. Long term treatment with co-trimoxazole protected against maternal chronic Q fever, placental infection and obstetric complications especially intrauterine death. After delivery patients with chronic Q fever serologic profiles were treated with a combination of doxycycline, 200 mg daily, and hydroxychlorquine 600 mg daily for one year.

Q fever in infancy and other manifestations of Q fever

Q fever may occur in infancy where it has caused pneumonia, febrile seizures, pyrexia of unknown origin, malaise, and meningeal irritation. Haematological manifestations of Q fever include bone marrow necrosis haemophagocytosis, haemolytic anaemia, lymphadenopathy mimicking lymphoma, transient hypoplastic anaemia, reactive thrombocytosis, thrombocytopenia, and splenic rupture. Optic neuritis and erythema nodosum have also been reported in association with Q fever.

Post Q fever fatigue syndrome

Prolonged fatigue can follow Q fever and consists of a constellation of symptoms including fatigue, headaches, sweats, arthralgia, myalgias, blurred vision, muscle fasciculations and enlarged and painful lymph nodes (Marmion *et al.* 1996). Persistence of *C. burnetii* in the host and resultant cytokine dysfunction may be key factors in this syndrome (Harris *et al.* 2000; Pentilla *et al.* 1998).

Epidemiology

Coxiella burnetii has been a remarkably successful pathogen. It has spread to most countries in the world. When Kaplan and Bertagna reviewed the literature up to 1955 they found that Q fever was present in 51 countries on 5 continents. At that time they noted that Ireland, The Netherlands, New Zealand, and Poland did not have Q fever. In the interim, Q fever has been demonstrated in Ireland, The Netherlands, and Poland. New Zealand still remains free of Q fever.

Transmission

Aerosols are the most important means of transmission to man. A dose-response effect is evident. For example, guinea-pigs exposed to 10^4 infectious dose units had an incubation period of 6 days whereas those exposed to 10 units had an incubation of 10 days (Tiggert and Benennon 1956). Human volunteers who inhaled 1 infectious unit had an incubation period of 16 days, whereas those who were exposed to 1,500 infectious units had an incubation period of 10 days. We have observed that individuals who cleaned up the products of conception of their infected parturient cats had the shortest incubation period for Q fever and the most severe illness. In this group the incubation period ranged from 7 to 30 days, according to the intensity of the exposure.

Indirect exposure to contaminated aerosols was also important as British residents who lived along a road over which farm vehicles travelled developed Q fever as a result of exposure to contaminated straw, manure, or dust from the farm vehicles (Salmon et al. 1981). Four hundred and fifteen residents of a Swiss valley who lived along a road over which sheep travelled to and from mountain pastures developed Q fever (Dupuis et al. 1987).

A number of recent outbreaks indicate the importance of indirect exposure to C. burnetii. In an outbreak of Q fever in a truck-repair plant, 16 of 32 employees were infected (Marrie et al. 1989). One of the employees had a cat which had given birth to kittens 2 weeks prior to the outbreak. The cat refused to let the kittens suckle and the employee, after donning his work clothes, fed the kittens from a bottle and then went to work. The attack rate for the employees who worked upstairs where the cat owner worked was 67%, compared with 25% for those who worked downstairs. The cat and the kittens had antibodies to C. burnetii. The contaminated clothing of the cat's owner may have served as a vehicle whereby C. burnetii was introduced into the truck repair plant. An outbreak described by Marmion and Stoker (1956) involved 10 of 30 people who performed a play in a village church. The only source of Q fever was indirect contact with sheep through a shepherd who had a role in the play and who came to the rehearsals in his working clothes, accompanied by his sheepdog. Twenty four samples of dust from the shepherd's clothing and others who came into contact with the two known infected flocks of sheep were obtained with a suction device. Coxiella burnetii was isolated from one specimen of dust collected from the shepherd's clothing. Contaminated clothing from the Rocky Mountain Laboratory in Montana, a Q fever research facility, led to cases of Q fever among laundry workers (Oliphant et al. 1949).

In Baddeck, Nova Scotia a parturient cat with vaginal bleeding for 3 weeks after delivery led to an outbreak of Q fever affecting 2.8% of the population of the town (Marrie et al. 1988b). Sixteen people who attended a birthday party became ill with Q fever. At 3 p.m. on the day of the party the hostess' cat gave birth to kittens in the bedroom closet. The hostess shut the closet and bedroom doors and prepared for the party which began at 6 p.m. None of the guests entered the bedroom; however, all spent time in the kitchen which adjoined the bedroom. Coxiella burnetii was isolated from the cat's uterus (Marrie et al. 1988a). Even activity as tame as playing poker can be a risk factor for Q fever if an infected parturient cat gives birth during the course of the poker game (Langley et al. 1988).

Q fever became a reportable disease in the Netherlands in 1978 and an average of 17 cases per year were reported (Schimmer et al. 2009). An outbreak began in 2007 and continued through May 2009 with 168, 1,000 and 345 cases for 2007, 2008 and the first few months of 2009 respectively (Schimmer et al. 2009). In many instances the clusters of cases are related to small ruminant farms and in others not so. Pneumonia is the predominant manifestation but there are cases of hepatitis as well. Goats and to a lesser extent sheep are involved. The average number of goats per farm is 900 of which 20% aborted and there are about 400 sheep per farm with a 5% abortion rate (Schimmer et al. 2009). A vaccination program is underway. One small study showed that the outbreak involves multiple genotypes (Klassen et al. 2009).

Outbreaks of Q fever that have occurred in institutions, illustrate how infectious are the aerosols of C. burnetii. Prior to the recognition that sheep were infected with C. burnetii they were often transported to a research institute that, in many instances, was part of a hospital. Several large outbreaks of Q fever have occurred as a result of the use of infected pregnant sheep in research (Hall et al. 1982). In these outbreaks most of the people who became ill (63–70%) did not have direct contact with the sheep but worked the route along which the sheep were transported to the laboratory.

Several authors have suggested that ingestion of raw (presumably contaminated milk) is a risk factor for acquisition of Q fever. Coxiella burnetii was not killed by pasteurization techniques used in the 1940s and 1950s (Wentworth 1955); however, current pasteurization techniques are effective. A study carried out at the Idaho State Penitentiary showed that seroconversion to C. burnetii could occur after ingestion of raw contaminated milk, but clinical disease did not (Benson et al. 1963). This observation correlates with findings from a study in which cats experimentally infected via the oral route did not become ill, whereas cats infected via the subcutaneous route became ill and lethargic (Gillespie and Baker 1952). In one study 11 Portuguese volunteers ingested food contaminated with C. burnetii but only two developed complement fixing antibodies (Anon. 1950). In another study reported from Milwaukee, 34 human volunteers consumed unpasteurized raw milk naturally infected with C. burnetii. None became ill and none developed antibodies that could be detected by the complement fixation test, the capillary agglutination, or the radioisotope precipitation test (Krumbiegel and Wisniewski 1970).

Percutaneous transmission has been demonstrated experimentally; 29 Portuguese volunteers who were infected intradermally developed signs of disease (Anon. 1950). A 24 year old male who crushed ticks between his fingers while hiking in the mountains in Montana became ill with Q fever 16 days later (Eklund et al. 1947). There is one report of transmission of Q fever via a blood transfusion (Anon. 1977).

Coxiella burnetii has been isolated from human placenta and one study, at least, demonstrated immunological evidence of human fetal infection with C. burnetii (Fiset et al. 1975). However, it is unlikely that vertical transmission has much of a role in the epidemiology of Q fever in man.

Person to person transmission is very uncommon, although there have been instances where the evidence is suggestive (Mann et al. 1986). There are two reports of the transmission of C. burnetii to attendants during autopsies (Harman 1949; Gerth and Leidig 1982), but while these cases are cited as instances of person to person transmission, it is possible that aerosols generated during the autopsy could have resulted in the infection. Because of the rarity of person to person transmission of Q fever there is no need to isolate patients hospitalized with this illness, but precautions should be taken during autopsy of patients with presumed or documented Q fever infection.

Epizoology

There is an extensive wildlife reservoir of *C. burnetii*, as reviewed above. Since many species of ticks are known to be infected with *C. burnetii*, it was assumed that ticks infected wild and domestic animals. Other possible routes of infection from wild animals to domestic animals are by contamination of the environment by infected products of conception (aerosols from these products could infect domestic animals and man), ingestion of contaminated grass, or ingestion of contaminated animals, such as mice, by cats. A seasonal variation in the prevalence of antibodies among deer was evident in one study—antibody prevalence peaked in mid-winter (January), was lowest in late spring just prior to parturition in May, and increased thereafter (Enright *et al.* 1971).

Prevention and control

Outbreaks of Q fever in laboratory workers in the 1940s led to the production of a formalin-inactivated whole-cell vaccine. This vaccine seemed to be protective, although no formal trials were carried out. A formalin-killed, ether-extracted 10% suspension of *C. burnetii*-infected yolk sac had a complement fixation antigen titre of 1:8 and seemed to be effective (Ormsbee and Marmion 1991).

Early vaccines were accompanied by occasional severe reactions in the form of an indolent, indurated mass at the vaccination site or the formation of a sterile abscess which pointed and discharged and sometimes formed a chronic draining sinus requiring excision. Reactions were associated with frequent vaccination and the possession of antibody before inoculation. This led to a pre-vaccination screening programme to detect pre-existing cellular immunity or hypersensitivity. A small dose of diluted Q fever vaccine was inoculated intradermally and those who reacted in 5–7 days with erythema at the inoculation site were excluded from vaccination.

After Stoker and Fiset (1956) described phase variation in *C. burnetii*, it was recognized that antibody against phase I antigen had protective effects in immunized mice and guinea-pigs. The next development was the observation that phase I antigen, like bacterial lipopolysaccharide, could be extracted from *C. burnetii* with phenol-water mixtures, dimethylsulphoxide, formamide or trichloroacetic acid; the extracts had haptenic, antigenic and, in some instances, immunogenic activity. Following this, methods were devised to purify *Coxiella* cells from yolk sac protein and lipid.

The use of formalin-inactivated, low-dose phase I highly purified *C. burnetii* suspensions together with pre-vaccination serotesting and skin testing facilitated the prophylactic use of the vaccine in laboratory workers and eventually in industrial groups. Between 1966 and 1968 vaccine trials with a purified Henzerling phase I vaccine were carried out by Hornick *et al.* (1991). Doses ranging from 1 to 30 μg were given subcutaneously. Three to ten months later subjects were challenged with a *C. burnetii* aerosol. Protection ranged from 71% for the 1 μg dose to 89–100% for the 30 μg dose.

In Australia, Marmion and co-workers (1984), in response to an increase in the prevalence of Q fever in abattoirs following the introduction of feral goats into the slaughtering programme, produced a formalin-inactivated Henzerling strain of *C. burnetii* vaccine from infected yolk sac by low–high salt extraction. They went on to perform a trial involving abattoir workers in South Australia. The vaccine was effective. While the yearly rates of Q fever among the unvaccinated workers fluctuated, a typical result in the trial was three cases of Q fever among 2,716 vaccinated workers compared with 52 cases among 2,012 unvaccinated workers. Common reactions included fever, headache, and local tenderness.

Measurement of antibody by traditional serological tests (such as the complement fixation test) after vaccination does not accurately reflect protection. Only 56–64% of vaccine recipients in the South Australia trials had measurable antibody by these tests at 20–60 months after vaccination. Eighty-four percent had measurable antibody 0.6–3 months post-vaccination. The implication is that cell-mediated immunity is important in providing protection from infection and that a positive cell-mediated immune response can be produced by vaccination even though a humoral immune response cannot be detected. The finding that a single microgram dose of whole-cell *C. burnetii* vaccine induces a lymphoproliferative response in 80–90% of vaccines tends to substantiate this.

Fries *et al.* (1993) reported their results of an evaluation of the safety and immunogenicity of a chloroform-methanol residue (CMR) vaccine for Q fever. They immunized 35 healthy adults with a single CMR subcutaneous dose of 30, 60, 120, or 240 μg. No adverse reactions were seen at the 30 or 60 μg doses. However, 7 of the 10, 240 μg recipients reported erythema and/or induration at the inoculation site. Two subjects reported malaise and one had low-grade fever. Serum IgM responses, best detected with phase II antigen, developed in 30, 60, 73, and 90% of recipients with the 30, 60, 120, and 240 μg doses, respectively results were encouraged enough to proceed with field trials.

A *C. burnetii* vaccine suitable for easy mass inoculation of those at risk is not yet available. Presently, vaccination should be limited to individuals, such as veterinarians and abattoir workers, who are at high risk of acquiring Q fever.

Vaccination of animals

A phase I formalin-inactivated vaccine was administered to 1400 Holstein-Friesian dairy calves and heifers. Only 1% of vaccinated cows shed *C. burnetii*, whereas 39 of 164 (24%) of non-vaccinated cows shed *C. burnetii* (Biberstein *et al.* 1977). Four immunized cows were challenged with 4×10^8 infected guinea-pig doses via the subcutaneous route. These cows had normal full-term calves, whereas two non-vaccinated cows aborted late in pregnancy and *C. burnetii* was isolated from the tissue of the fetuses. While organisms were recovered from the milk, colostrum, and placenta of both vaccinated and unvaccinated cows, the number of organisms recovered from unvaccinated cows was 1,000 times greater than that from vaccinated cows (Behymer *et al.* 1976). Similar results were obtained when a whole-cell, phase I Henzerling strain vaccine or a chloroform method residue vaccine was used in ewes (Brooks *et al.* 1986).

Other preventative measures

Use of only seronegative and PCR negative (vaginal mucus) sheep in research facilities should prevent outbreaks of Q fever in most institutions. Pregnant sheep should not be transported through hospitals. Research facilities should be designed so that outside access to the animal quarters is direct, with contact confined to the animal quarters. The care of animals in such facilities should conform to nationally accepted standards.

Consumption of pasteurized milk only will serve to eliminate the few cases that may be transmitted in this manner.

In Cyprus the incidence of *C. burnetii* infection among goats and sheep was reduced by a programme in which aborted material was destroyed, affected dams isolated, and the premises disinfected (Polydorou 1985). Control of ectoparasites on cattle, sheep, and goats may also be important in the control of Q fever.

Blood donations should not be accepted from those living in an area where there is an outbreak of Q fever both during the outbreak and for up to 4 weeks following cessation of the outbreak.

References

Abinanti, F. R. and Marmion, B. P. (1957). Protective or neutralizing antibody in Q fever. *Am. J. Hyg.*, **66**: 173–95.

Akporiaye, E. T. and Baca, O. G. (1983). Superoxide anion production and superoxide dismutase and catalase activities in *Cornelia burnetii*. *J. Bacteriol.*, **154**: 520–23.

Anon. (1950). Experimental Q fever in man. *BMJ*, **1**: 1000.

Anon. (1977). Comment on Q fever transmitted by blood transfusion—United States. *Can Dis. Wkly. Rep.*, **3**: 210.

Babudieri, B. (1959). Q fever: A zoonosis. *Ad. Vet. Sci.*, **5**: 81–82.

Baca, O. G., Roman M. J., Glew, R. H., Christner, R. F., Buhler, J. E. *et al.* (1993). Acid phosphatase activity in *Coxiella burnetii*: a possible virulence factor. *Infect. Immun.*, **61**: 4232–39.

Baca, O. G. (1991). Pathogenesis of rickettsial infection: emphasis on Q fever. *Euro. J. Epidemiol.*, **7**: 222–28.

Bamberg, W. M., Pape, W. J., Beebe, J. L. *et al.* (2007). Outbreak of Q fever associated with a horse-boarding ranch, Colorado, 2005. *Vector-Borne Zoon. Dis.*, **7**: 49–55.

Behymer, D. E., Biberstein, E. L., Riemann, H. P. *et al.* (1976). Q fever (*Coxiella burnetii*) investigations in dairy cattle: challenge of immunity after vaccination. *Am. J. Vet. Res.*, **37**: 631–34.

Bell, J. F., Luoto, L., Casey, M., and Lackmand, D. B. (1964). Serologic and skin test response after Q fever vaccination by the intracutaneous route. *J. Immunol.*, **93**: 403–8.

Benson, W. W., Brock, D. W., and Mather, J. (1963). Serologic analysis of a penitentiary group using raw milk from a Q fever infected herd. *Pub. Heal. Rep.*, **78**: 707–10.

Biberstein, E. L., Riemann, H. P., Franti, C. E. *et al.* (1977). Vaccination of diary cattle against Q fever (*Coxiella burnetii*): results of field trials. *Am. J. Vet. Res.*, **38**: 189–93.

Biggs, B. A., Douglas, J. G., Grant, I. W., and Crompton, G. K. (1984). Prolonged Q fever associated with inappropriate secretion of anti-diuretic hormone. *J. Infect.*, **8**: 61–63.

Brooks, D. L., Ermel, R. W., Franti, C. E. *et al.* (1986). Q fever vaccination of sheep. Challenge of immunity in ewes. *J. Vet. Res.*, **47**: 1235–38.

Brouqui, P., Dupont, H. T., Drancourt, M. *et al.* (1993). Chronic Q fever: Ninety-two cases from France; including 27 cases without endocarditis. *Arch. Intern. Med.*, **153**: 642–49.

Brouqui, P., Marrie, T., and Raoult, D. (2007). *Coxiella.* In: P. R. Murray, E. J. Barron, J. H. Jorgensen, M. L. Landry and M. A. Pfaller (eds.) *Manual of Clinical Microbiology*, (9th edn.), Chapter 68, pp. 1062–69. Washington DC: ASM Press.

Burnet, F. M. and Freeman, M. (1937). Experimental studies on the virus of Q fever. *Med. J. Aus.*, **2**: 299–305.

Capo, C., Lindberg, F. P., Meconi, S. *et al.* (1999). Subversion of monocyte functions by *Coxiella burnetii*: impairment of the cross-talk between alpha v beta 3 integrin and CR3. *J. Immun.*, **163**: 6078–85.

Carcopino, X., Raoult, D., Bretelle, F., Boubli, L., and Stein, A. (2007). Managing Q fever during pregnancy: the benefits of long term cotrimoxazole therapy. *Clin. Infect. Dis.*, **45**: 548–55.

Christie, A. B. (1974). *Infectious diseases, epidemiology and clinical practice*, pp. 876–91. Edinburgh: Churchill Livingston.

Clark, W. H., Lennette, E. H., Railsback, O. C, and Romer, M. S. (1951). Q fever in California. VII. Clinical features in one hundred and eighty cases. *Arch. Intern. Med.*, **88**:155–67.

Crespo, M., Sopena, B., Bordon, J., de la Fuente, J., Bubianes, M., *et al.* (1999). Steroids treatment of granulomatous hepatitis complicating *Coxiella burnetii* acute infection. *Infect.*, **27**: 132–33.

Dellacasagrande, J., Ghigo, E., Raoult, D., Capo, C., and Mege, J. (2002). IFN-induced apoptosis and microbicidal activity in monocytes harboring the intracellular bacterium *Coxiella burnetii* require membrane TNF and homotypic cell adherence. *J. Immun.*, **169**: 6309–15.

Derrick, E. H. (1937). 'Q' fever, new fever entity: clinical features, diagnosis and laboratory investigation. *Med. J. Aus.*, **2**: 281–99.

Derrick, E. H. (1939). Rickettsia burnetii: the cause of 'Q' fever. *Med. J. Aus.*, **1**: 14.

Tissot Dupont, H. T., Raoult, D., Brouqui, P. *et al.*(1992). Epidemiologic features and clinical presentation of acute Q fever in hospitalized patients: 323 French cases. *Am. J. Med.*, **93**: 427–34.

Dupuis, G., Peter, O., Pedroni, D., and Petite, J. (1985). Aspects cliniques observées lors d'une épidémie de 415 cas de fièvre Q. *Schweizer. Medizinis. Wochens.*, **115**: 814–18.

Dupuis, G., Petite, J., Peter, O., and Vouilloz, M. (1987). An important outbreak of human Q fever in Swiss Alpine Valley. *Inter. J. Epidemiol.*, **16**: 282–87.

Eklund, C. M., Parker, R. R, and Lackman, D. B. (1947). Case of O fever probably contracted by exposure to ticks in nature. *Pub. Heal. Rep.*, **62**: 1413–16.

Enright, J. B., Franti, C. E., Behymer, D. E., Longhurst, W. M., Dutson, V. J., and Wright, M. E. (1971). *Coxiella burnetii* in a wildlife-livestock environment. Distribution of Q fever in wild mammals. *Am. J. Epidemiol.*, **94**: 79–90.

Field, P. R., Hunt, J. G., and Murphy, M. A. (1983). Detection and persistence of specific IgM antibody to *Coxiella burnetii* by enzyme-linked immunosorbent assay: a comparison with immunofluorescence and complement fixation tests. *J. Infect. Dis.*, **148**: 477–87.

Fiset, P., Ormsbee, R. A., Silberman, R., Peacock, M., and Spielman, S. H. (1969). A microagglutination technique for detection and measurement of rickettsial antibodies. *Acta Virol.*, **13**: 60–66.

Fiset, P., Wisseman Jr., C. L. and El-Bataine, Y. (1975). Immunologic evidence of human fetal infection with *Coxiella burnetii*. *Am. J. Epidemiol.*, **101**: 65.

Fournier, P. E., Marrie, T. J., and D. Raoult, D. (1998). Diagnosis of Q fever. *J. Clin. Micro.*, **36**: 1823–34.

Fries, L. F., Waag, D. M., and Williams, J. C. (1993). Safety and immunogenicity in human volunteers of a chloroform-methanol residue vaccine for Q fever. *Infect. Immun.*, **61**: 1251–58.

George, J. and Marrie, T. J. (1987). Serological evidence of *Coxiella burnetii* infection in horses in Atlantic Canada. *Canad. Vet. J.*, **28**: 425–26.

Gerth, H-J. and Leidig, U. (1982). Reimenschneider Th. Q-fieber-epidemie in einem Institute fur Humanpathologie. *Deuts. Medizin. Wochensc.*, **107**: 1391–95.

Ghigo, E., Capo, C., Amirayan, N., Raoult, D., and Mege, J. (2000). The 75-kD tumour necrosis factor (TNF) receptor is specifically up-regulated in monocytes during Q fever endocarditis. *Clin. Experim. Immun.*, **121**: 295–301.

Ghigo, E., Capo, C., Raoult, D., and Mege, J. L. (2001). Il-10 stimulates *Coxiella burnetii* replication in human monocytes through TNF down-modulation: Role in microbicidal defect of Q fever. *Infect. Immun.*, **69**: 2345–52.

Gillespie, J. H. and Baker, J. A. (1952). Experimental Q fever in cats. *Am. J. Vet. Res.*, **13**: 91–94.

Glazunova, D., Roux, V., and Freylikman, O. (2005). *Coxiella burnetii* genotyping. *Emerg. Infect. Dis.*, **11**: 1211–17.

Gordon, J. D., MacKeen, A. D., Marrie, T. J., Fraser, D. B. (1984). The radiographic features of epidemic and sporadic Q fever pneumonia. *J. Can. Assoc. Radio.*, **35**: 293–96.

Grist, N. R. (1959). The persistence of Q fever infection in a dairy herd. *Vet. Rec.*, **71**: 839–41.

Hacksteadt, T., Peacock, N. G., Hitchcock, P. J., and Cole, R. L. (1985). Lipopolysaccharide variation in *Coxiella burnetii*; intrastrain heterogenicity in structure and antigenicicty. *Infect. Immun.*, **48**: 359–65.

Hall, C. J., Richmond, S. J., Caul, E. O., Pearce, N. H., and Silver, I. A. (1982). Laboratory outbreak of Q fever acquired from sheep. *Lancet*, **1**: 1004–1006.

Harman, J. B. (1949). Q fever in Great Britain; clinical account of eight cases. *Lancet*, **2**: 1028.

Harris, R. J., Storm, P. A., Lloyd, A., Arens, M., and Marmion, B. P. (2000). Long-term persistence of Coxiella burnetii in the host after primary Q fever. *Epidemiol. Infect.*, **124**: 543–49.

Hendrix, L. R., Mallavia, L. P., and Samuel, J. E. (1993). Cloning and sequencing of *Coxiella burnetii* outer membrane protein gene *com*1. *Infect. Immun.*, **61**: 470–77.

Hofmann, C. E. R. and Heaton, J. W. (1982). Q fever hepatitis. Clinical manifestations and pathological findings. *Gastroenterol.*, **83**: 474–79.

Hornibrook, J. W. (1940). An institutional outbreak of pneumonitis. 1. Epidemiologic and clinical studies. *Pub. Heal. Rep.*, **55**: 1936–44.

Huebner, R. J. (1947). Report of an outbreak of Q fever at the National Institute of Health. II. Epidemiological features. *Am. J. Pub. Heal.*, **37**: 431–40.

Huebner, R. J., Jellison, W. L., Beck, M. D., Parker, R. R., and Shepard, G. G. (1948). Q fever studies in Southern California. I. Recovery of *Rickettsia burnetii* from raw milk. *Pub. Heal. Rep.*, **63**: 214–22.

Huebner, R. J., Hottle, G. A., and Robinson, E. B. (1948). Action of streptomycin in experimental infection with Q fever. *Pub. Heal. Rep.*, **63**: 357–62.

Hunt, J. G., Field, P. R., and Murphy, A. M. (1983). Immunoglobulin responses to *Coxiella burnetii* (Q fever): Single-serum diagnosis of acute infection using an immunofluorescence technique. *Infect. Immun.*, **39**: 977–81.

Janigan, D. T. and Marrie, T. J. (1983). An inflammatory pseudotumor of the lung in Q fever pneumonia. *N. Engl. J. Med*, **30**: 86–88.

Kaplan, M. M. and Bertagna, P. (1955). The geographical distribution of Q fever. *Bull. World Health Organ.*, **13**: 829–60.

Klassen, C. H. W., Nabwers-Fassen, M. H., Tilb, J. J. H. C., Hamans, M. A. W. M., and Horrevorts, A. M. (2009). Multigenotype Q fever outbreak, the Netherlands. *Emerg. Infect. Dis.*, **15**: 613–14.

Krumbiegel, E. R. and Wisniewski, H. J. (1970). Q fever in Milwaukee. II. Consumption of infected raw milk by human volunteers. *Arch. Environ. Heal.*, 21, 63–65.

Lang, G. H. (1990). *Coxiellosis in animals*. In: T. J. Marrie (ed.) *Q fever the disease*, pp. 23–48. Boca Raton, FLA: CRC Press.

Langley, J. M., Marrie, T. J., Covert, A. A., Waag, D. M., and Williams, J. C. (1988). Poker players pneumonia—an urban outbreak of Q fever following exposure to a parturient cat. *N. Engl. J. Med.*, **319**: 354–56.

Laughlin, T., Waag, D., Williams, J., and Marrie, T. J. (1991). Q fever: from deer to dog to man. *Lancet*, **337**: 676–77.

Lennette, E. H., Clark, W. H., and Dean, B. H. (1949). Sheep and goats and the epidemiology of Q fever in Northern California. *Am. J. Trop. Med.*, **29**: 527–41.

Lennette, E. H. and Welsh, H. H. (1951). Q fever in California. X. Recovery of *Coxiella burnetii* from the air of premises harbouring infected goats. *Am. J. Hyg.*, **54**: 44.

Levy, P. Y., Drancourt, M., Etienne, J. *et al.* (1991). Comparison of different antibiotic regimens for therapy of 32 cases of Q fever endocarditis. *Antimicrob. Agents Chemother.*, **35**: 533–37.

Luoto, L. and Huebner, R. J. (1950). Q fever studies in Southern California. IX. Isolation of Q fever organisms from parturient placentas of naturally infected cows. *Pub. Heal. Rep.*, **65**: 541–44.

McCaul, T. F. (1991). *The developmental cycle of Coxiella burnetii*. In: J. G. Williams and H. A. Thompson (eds.) *Q fever: the disease*, pp. 224–58. Boca Raton, FLA: CRC Press.

McDade, J. E. (1990). *Historical aspects of Q fever*. In: J. G. Williams and H. A. Thompson (eds.) *Q fever: the disease*, Vol. 1, pp. 5–21. Boca Raton, FLA: CRC Press.

Mallavia, L. P., Samuel, J. E., and Frazier, M. E. (1991). The genetics of Coxiella burnetii: Etiological agent of Q fever and chronic endocarditis. In: J. G. Williams and H. A. Thompson (eds.) *Q fever: the disease*, pp. 259–85. Boca Raton, FLA: CRC Press.

Mann, J. S., Douglas, J. S., Inglis, J. M., and Leitch, A. G. (1986). Q fever: person to person transmission within a family. *Thorax*, **41**: 974–75.

Marecki, N., Becker, F., Baca, O. G., and Paretsky, D. (1978). Changes in liver and L-cell plasma membranes during infection with *Coxiella burnetii*. *Infect. Immun.*, **19**: 272–80.

Marmion, B. P., Ormsbee, R. A., Kyrkou, M. *et al.* (1984). Vaccine prophylaxis of abattoir-associated Q fever. *Lancet*, **2**: 1411–14.

Marmion, B. P. and Stoker, M. G. P. (1956). The varying epidemiology of Q fever in the South East region of Great Britain. II. In two rural areas. *J. Hyg.*, **54**: 547–61.

Marmion, B. P., Shannon, M., Meddocks, I., Storm, P., and Pentilla, I. (1996). Protracted debility and fatigue after acute Q fever. *Lancet*, **347**: 977–78.

Marrie, T. J. (1993). Q fever in pregnancy: Report of two cases. *Infect. Dis. Clin. Pract.*, **2**: 207–209.

Marrie, T. J. and Raoult, D. (1992). Rickettsial infections of the central nervous system. *Semin. Neurol.*, **12**: 213–24.

Marrie, T. J., van Buren, J., Fraser, J. *et al.*(1985). Seroepidemiology of Q fever among domestic animals in Nova Scotia. *Am. J. Pub. Heal.*, **75**: 763–66.

Marrie, T. J., Durant, H., Williams, J. G., Mintz, E., and Waag, D. M. (1988a). Exposure to parturient cats is a risk factor for acquisition of Q fever in Maritime Canada. *J. Infect. Dis.*, **158**: 101–108.

Marrie, T. J., MacDonald, A., Durant, H., Yates, L., and McCormick, L. (1988b). An outbreak of Q fever probably due to contact with a parturient cat. *Chest*, **93**: 98–103.

Marrie, T. J., Langille, D., Papukna, V., and Yates, L. (1989). An outbreak of Q fever in a truck repair plant. *Epidemiology and Infection*, **102**: 119–27.

Marrie, T. J., Embil, J., and Yates, L. (1993). Seroepidemiology of *Coxiella burnetii* among wildlife in Nova Scotia. *Am. J. Trop. Med. Hyg.*, **49**: 613–15.

Marrie, T. J. (2002). *Coxiella burnetii (Q Fever)*. In: V. L. Yu, R. Weber and D. Raoult (eds.) *Antimicrobial Therapy and Vaccines, Volume I: Microbes*, pp. 869–74. LLC, New York, NY: Apple Trees, Productions.

Maurin, M., Benoliel, A. M., Bongrand, P., and Raoult, D. (1992). Phagolysomal alkalinization and the bactericidal effect of antibiotics: The *Coxiella burnetii* paradigm. *J. Infect. Dis.*, **166**: 1097–102.

McCaughey, C., Murray, L. J., McKenna, J. P. *et al.* (2009). *Coxiella burnetii* (Q fever) seroprevalence in cattle. *Epidemiol. Infect.* E publication, June 2009; 1–7.

McQusiton, J. H., Childs, J. E. (2002). Q fever in humans and animals in the United States. *Vector Borne Zoon. Dis.*, **2**: 179–91.

Michael, F., Minnick, R., Heinzen, A., Dowthrait, R., Mallavia, L. P. *et al.* (1990). Analysis of QpRS specific sequences from *Coxiella burnetii*. *Ann. NY Acad. Sci.*, **5990**: 514–23.

Minnick, M. F., Heinzen, R. A., Reschke, D. K., Frazier, M. E. *et al.* (1991). A plasmid-encoded surface protein found in chronic disease isolates of *Coxiella burneti*. *Infect. Immun.*, **59**: 4735–39.

Nelder, M. P., Lloyd, J. E., Loftus, A. D., and Reeves, W. K. (2008). *Coxiella burnetii* in wild-caught filth flies. *Emerg. Infect. Dis.*, **14**: 1002–1004.

Oliphant, J. W., Gordon, D. A., Meis, A., and Parker, R. R. (1949). Q fever in laundry workers, presumably transmitted from contaminated clothing. *Am. J. Hyg.*, **49**: 76–82.

Omsland, A., Howe, D., Cockrell, D. C., Omsland, A., Hansen, B. *et al.* (2009). Host cell-free growth of the Q fever bacterium *Coxiella burnetii*. *Proc. Nat. Acad. Sci. USA*, **106**: 4430–33.

Ormsbee, R. A. and Marmion, B. P. (1991). *Prevention of Coxiella burnetii infection: vaccines and guidelines for those at risk.* In: J. G. Williams and H. A. Thompson (eds.) *Q fever: the disease*, pp. 225–40. Boca Raton, FLA: CRC Press.

Ormsbee, R. A. (1952). The growth of *Coxiella burnetii* in embryonated eggs. *The J. Bacteriol.*, **63**: 73.

Palmer, N. C., Kierstead, M., Key, D. W., Williams, J. G., Peacock, M. G. *et al.* (1983). Placentitis and abortion in sheep and goats in Ontario caused by *Coxiella burnetii*. *Can. Vet. J.*, **24**: 60–61.

Palmer, S. R. and Young, S. E. J. (1982). Q fever endocarditis in England and Wales, 1975–81. *Lancet,* **ii**: 1148–49.

Penttila, I. A., Harris, R. J., Storm, P., Haynes, D., Worswick, D.A. *et al.* (1998). Cytokine dysregulation in the post-Q fever fatigue syndrome. *Quart. J. Med.*, **91**: 549–60.

Philip, G. B. (1948). Comments on the nature of the Q fever organism. *Pub. Heal. Rep.*, **63**: 58.

Polydorou, K. (1985). Q fever in Cyprus—recent progress. *Brit. Vet. J.*, **141**: 427–30.

Raoult, D., Etienne, J., Massip, P. *et al.* (1987). Q fever endocarditis in the south of France. *J. Infect. Dis.*, **155**: 570–73.

Raoult, D., Drancourt, M., and Vestris, G. (1990). Bactericidal effect of Doxycycline associated with lysosomotropic agents on *Coxiella burnetii* in P388D1 cells. *Antimicrob. Agents and Chemother.*, **34**: 1512–14.

Raoult, D., Torres, H., and Drancourt, M. (1991). Shell-vial assay: Evaluation of a new technique for determining antibiotic susceptibility, tested in 13 isolates of *Coxiella burnetii*. *Antimicrob. Agents and Chemother.*, **35**: 2070–77.

Raoult, D., Levy, P. Y., Dupont, H. T. *et al.* (1993). Q fever and HIV infection. *AIDS*, **7**: 81–86.

Raoult, D., Laurent, J. C., and Mutillod, M. (1994). Monoclonal antibodies to *Coxiella burnetii* for antigenic detection in cell cultures and in paraffin-embedded tissues. *Am. J. Clin. Pathol.*, **101**: 318–20.

Raoult, D., Houpikian, P., Tissot Dupont, H., Riss, J. M., Arditi-Djiane, J., *et al.* (1999). Treatment of Q fever endocarditis. Comparison of 2 regimens containing doxycycline and ofloxacin or hydroxychlorquine. *Arch. Intern. Med.*, **159**: 167–73.

Reichmann, N., Raz, R., Keysary, A., Goldwasser, R., and Faltau, E. (1988). Chronic Q fever and severe thrombocytopenia in a pregnant woman. *Am. J. Med.*, **85**: 253–54.

Reilly, S., Northwood, J. L., and Caul, E. O. (1990). Q fever in Plymouth, 1972–88. A review with particular reference to neurological manifestations. *Epidemiol. Infect.*, **105**: 91–108.

Ren, Q., Robertson, S. J., Howe, D., Barrows, L. F. and Heinzen, R. A. (2003). Comparative DNA microarray analysis of host cell transcriptional responses to infection by *Coxiella burnetii* or *Chlamydia trachomatis*. *Ann. NY Acad. Sci.*, **990**: 701–13.

Robbins, F. C. and Regan, G. A. (1946). Q fever in the Mediterranean area: report of its occurrence in allied troops. I. Clinical features of the disease. *Am. J. Hyg.*, **44**: 6–22.

Robbins, F. C., Gauld, R. L., and Warner, F. B. (1946). Q fever in the Mediterranean area: reported of its occurrence in allied troops. II. Epidemiology. *Am. J. Hyg.*, **44**: 23–50.

Rodolakis, A., Berri, M., Hechard, C., Caudron, C., Souriau, A., *et al.* (2007). Comparison of *Coxiella burnetii* shedding in milk of dairy bovine, caprine and ovine herds. *J. Dairy Sci.*, **90**: 5352–60.

Rodolakis, A. (2009). Q fever in dairy animals. *Ann. NY Acad. Sci.*, **1166**: 90–93.

Rolain, J. M., Boulos, A., Mallet, M. N., and Raoult, D. (2005). Correlation between ratio of serum doxycycline concentration to MIC and rapid decline of antibody levels during treatment of Q fever endocarditis. *Antimicrob. Agents and Chemother.*, **49**: 2673–76.

Salmon, M. M., Howells, B., Glencross, E. J. G., Evans, A. D., and Palmer, S. R. (1981). Q fever in an urban area. *Lancet,* **1**: 1004.

Samuel, J. E., Frazier, M. E., and Mallavia, L. P. (1985). Correlation of plasmid type and disease caused by *Coxiella burnetii*. *Infect. Immun.*, **49**: 775–77.

Sanders, D. M., Parker, J. E., Walker, W. W., Bucholz, M. W., Blount, K., *et al.* (2008). Field collection and genetic classification of tick-borne rickettsiae and rickettsiae-like pathogens from South Texas: *Coxiella burnetii* isolated from field-collected *Amblyomma cajennese*. *Ann. NY Acad. Sci.*, **1149**: 208–11.

Sawyer, L. A., Fishbein, D. B., and McDade, J. E. (1987). Q fever: current concepts. *Rev. Infect. Dis.*, **9**: 935–46.

Schimmer, B., Dijkstra, F., Velleme, P. *et al.* (2009). Sustained intensive transmission of Q fever in the Netherlands. *Eurosurveillance*, **14**: 1–3.

Schramek, S. and Mayer, H. (1982). Different sugar compositions of lipopolysaccharides isolated from phase I and pure phase II cells of *Coxiella burnetii*. *Infect. Immun.*, **38**: 53–57.

Seshadri, R., Paulsen, I. T., Eisen, J. A. *et al.* (2003). Complete genome sequence of the Q-fever pathogen *Coxiella burnetii*. *Proc. Nat. Acad. Sci.*, **100**: 5455–60.

Shepard, C. C. (1947). An outbreak of Q fever in a Chicago packing house. *Am. J. Hyg.*, **46**: 185–92.

Sidwell, R. W., Thorpe, B. D., and Gebhardt, L. P. (1964a). Studies of latent Q fever infections. I. Effects of whole body X irradiation upon latently infected guinea pigs, white mice and deer mice. *Am. J. Hyg.*, **79**: 113–24.

Sidwell, R. W., Thorpe, B. D., and Gebhardt, L. P. (1964b): Studies of latent Q fever infections. II. Effects of multiple cortisone injections. *Am. J. Hyg.*, **79**: 320–27.

Smith, D. L., Ayers, J. G., Blair, I. *et al.* (1993). A large Q fever outbreak in the West Midlands: clinical aspects. *Respirat. Med.*, **87**: 509–16.

Somma-Moreira, R. E., Caffarena, R. M., Somma, S., Pérez, G., and Monteiro, M. (1987). Analysis of Q fever in Uruguay. *Rev. Infect. Dis.*, **9**: 386–87.

Spelman, D. W. (1981). Q fever: a study of 111 consecutive cases. *Med. J. Aus.*, **1**: 547–53.

Spicknall, C. G., Huebner, R. J., Finger, J. A., and Blocker, W. P. (1947). Report of an outbreak of Q fever at the National Institute of Health. I. Clinical features. *Ann. Intern. Med.*, **27**: 28–40.

Stein, A. and Raoult, D. (1992a). Phenotypic and genotypic heterogenicity of eight new human *Coxiella burnetii* isolates. *Acta Virologia*, **36**: 7–12.

Stein, A. and Raoult, D. (1992b). Detection of *Coxiella burnetii* by DNA amplification using polymerase chain reaction. *J. Clin. Microbiol.*, **30**: 2462–66.

Stoenner, H. G. and Lachman, D. E. (1960). The biological properties of *Coxiella burnetii* isolated from rodents collected in Utah. *Am. J. Hyg.*, **71**: 775–79.

Stoker, M. G. P. and Fiset, P. (1956). Phase variation of the nine mile and other strains of *Rickettsia burnetii Canadian*. *J. Microbiol.*, **2**: 310–21.

Syrucek, L., Sobeslavsky, O., and Gutvirth, L. (1958). Isolation of *Coxiella burnetii* from human placentas. *J. Hyg., Epidemiol., Microbiol. Immunol.*, **2**: 29–35.

Thiele, D., Willems, H., Kopf, G., and Krauss, H. (1993). Polymorphism in DNA restriction patterns of *Coxiella burnetii* isolates investigated by pulsed field gel electrophoresis and image analysis. *Europ. J. Epidemiol.*, **9**: 419–25.

Tiggert, W. D. and Benenson, A. S. (1956). Studies on Q fever in man. *Trans. Assoc. Am. Physic.*, **69**: 98–104.

Tissot-Dupont, H., Thirion, X., and Raoult, D. (1994). Q fever serology: cutoff determination for microimmunofluorescence. *Clin. Diagn. Lab. Immunol.*, **1**: 189–96.

Topping, N. H., Shepard, C. C., and Irons, J. V. (1947). Q fever in the United States. I. Epidemiologic studies of an outbreak of among stock handlers and slaughterhouse workers. *J. Am. Med. Assoc.*, **33:** 813–15.

Turck, W. P., Howitt, G., Turnberg, L. A. *et al.* (1976). Chronic Q fever. *Quart. J. Med.*, **45:** 193–217.

Velasco, F. P., Enciso, M. V. B., Lama, Z. G., and Porras, M. C. (1996). Clinical presentation of acute Q fever in Lanzarote (Canary Islands): A 2-year prospective study. *Scandin. J. Infect. Dis.*, **28:** 533–34.

Viciana, P., Pachon, J., Cuello, J. A., Palomino, J., Jimenez-Mejias, M. E. *et al.* (1992). *Fever of indeterminate duration in the community. A seven year study in the South of Spain.* Abstract no 683. 32nd Interscience Conference on Antimicrobial Agents and Chemotherapy, 11–14 October. Washington DC: American Society for Microbiology.

Vodkin, M. H. and Williams, J. C. (1988). A heat shock operon in *Coxiella burnetii* produces a major antigen homologous to a protein in both mycobacteria and *Escherichia coll. J. Bacteriol.*, **170:** 1227–34.

Waag, D., Chulay, J., Marrie, T., England, M., and Williams, J. (1995). Validation of an enzyme immunoassay for serodiagnosis of acute Q fever. *Euro. J. Clin. Microbiol. Infect. Dis.*, **14:** 421–27.

Webster, J. P., Lloyd, G., and Macdonald, D.W. (1995). Q fever (Coxiella burnetii) reservoir in wild brown rat (*Rattus norvegicus*)populations in the UK. *Parasitol.*, **110:** 31–35.

Weiss, E., Williams, J. C., and Thompson, H. A. (1991). The place of *Coxiella burnetii* in the microbial world. In: J. C. Williams and H. A. Thompson (eds.) *Q fever: The biology of Coxiella burnetii*, pp. 2–19. Boca Raton, FLA: CRC Press.

Welsh, H. H., Lennette, E. H., Abinanti, R. F., and Winn, J. F. (1958). Air-borne transmission of Q fever: The role of the parturition in the generation of infective aerosols. *Ann. NY Acad. Sci.*, **70:** 528–40.

Wentworth, B. B. (1955). Historical review of the literature on Q fever. *Bacteriolog. Rev.*, **19:** 129–49.

Yeaman, M. R., Mitscher, L. A., and Baca, O. G. (1987). *In vitro* susceptibility of *Coxiella* burnetii for antibiotics, including several quinolones. *Antimicrob. Agents and Chemother.*, **31:** 1079–84.

CHAPTER 19a

Other bacterial diseases

Diseases caused by corynebacteria and related organisms

Aruni De Zoysa

Summary

The genus *Corynebacterium* contains the species *Corynebacterium diphtheriae* and the non-diphtherial corynebacteria. *C. diphtheriae* is the major human pathogen in this genus, but several species of nondiphtheria corynebacteria appear to be emerging as important pathogens.

Zoonotic corynebacteria rarely cause disease in humans, but recent reports have indicated that the frequency and severity of infection associated with *Corynebacterium ulcerans* has increased in many countries. In the past most human *C. ulcerans* infections have occurred through close contact with farm animals or by consumption of unpasteurized dairy products. However, recently, there have been cases of human infection following close contact with household pets. *Rhodococcus equi* appears to be emerging as an important pathogen in immunocompromised patients, especially those with acquired immunodeficiency syndrome (AIDS). Human infections caused by *Corynebacterium pseudotuberculosis* is still a very rare occurrence.

Antibiotics in combination with surgery and vaccination are the treatment of choice for human infection. Control of human infection is best achieved by raising awareness in those at risk (e.g. domestic pet owners, sheep shearers, the immunocompromised), clinicians involved in treating these groups and by vaccination. Reducing prevalence in the animal population could be achieved by improving hygiene in farms and husbandry practices, reducing minor injuries (e.g. cuts and abrasions) during routine procedures, and by vaccination.

History

The genus *Corynebacterium* is derived from the Greek words *koryne*, meaning club, and *bacterion*, meaning little rod. The genus *Corynebacterium* was first proposed by Lehmann and Neumann in 1896 (Skerman *et al.* 1980) to include the diphtheria bacillus and other morphologically similar organisms. *Corynebacterium* species are found in soil and water, and reside on the skin and mucous membranes of humans and animals.

C. pseudotuberculosis (previously known as *Corynebacterium. ovis*) was also called the Preisz-Nocard bacillus in honour of the researchers who first isolated the organism in the early 1890s (Lipsky *et al.* 1982). *C. pseudotuberculosis* was originally identified as the causative microorganism of caseous lymphadenitis (CLA) in sheep and goats, but this bacterium has also been isolated from horses, cattle, camels, swine, buffaloes and humans (Dorella *et al.* 2006). Human infection caused by *C. pseudotuberculosis* was first reported in 1966 (Lopez *et al.* 1966).

C. ulcerans was first isolated in 1926 from human throat lesions (Gilbert and Stewart 1926). The organism has been recovered from cattle, wild animals and recently from domestic cats and dogs (Hommez *et al.* 1999; Fox *et al.* 1974; De Zoysa *et al.* 2005; Lartigue *et al.* 2005). *C. ulcerans* can produce diphtheria toxin which is immunologically identical to that of *C. diphtheriae* (Lipsky *et al.* 1982) and may cause human infections mimicking cutaneous and classical respiratory diphtheria.

Corynebacterium kutscheri was first described by Kutscher in 1894 (Noble and Smith 1990). It has since been described as a commensal bacterium in mice, rats, and voles and has been identified in the oral cavity, oesophagus, colon, rectum, and submaxillary lymph nodes of these rodents (Bonsfield and Cally 1978). It can cause pulmonary infection in mice and rats (Giddens *et al.* 1968). Human infection caused by *C. kutscheri* has been reported. However in some cases a definitive identification was not established (Holmes and Korman 2007).

Corynebacterium bovis was first isolated in 1916 by Evans who named the organsim *Bacillus abortus var. lipolyticus* (Evans 1916). Bergey *et al.* (1923) renamed the organism *C. bovis*. It is a commensal of the bovine udder and can cause bovine mastitis and may contaminate milk (Smith 1966). Only nine human cases have been reported (Achermann *et al.* 2009; Dalal *et al.* 2008; Bolton *et al.* 1975; Vale and Scott 1977).

Arcanobacterium pyogenes, formerly classified as *Corynebacterium pyogenes,* and *Actinomyces pyogenes* was first described by Lucet in 1983 (Noble and Smith 1990). *A. pyogenes* is a well known animal pathogen causing a variety of pyogenic infections in many species (Smith 1966). Few zoonotic cases of human infections with *A. pyogenes* have been reported (Gahrn-Hansen and Frederiksen 1992).

Rhodococcus equi formerly classified as *Corynebacterium equi* was first isolated from foals in 1923. Infection in a human caused by *R. equi* was first reported in 1967 in a 29 year old man with plasma cell hepatitis receiving immunosuppressants. Since then *R. equi* has become an important opportunistic pathogen in immunocompromised patients, mainly those with AIDS (Fierer *et al.* 1987; Mandarino *et al.* 1994; Cardoso *et al.* 1996; Martin-Dávila *et al.* 1998).

The agents

C. ulcerans, C. pseudotuberculosis, C. bovis, and C. kutscheri are zoonotic corynebacteria that are known to cause clinical disease to varying extents in humans and their animal hosts. For the purpose of this review, *Rhodococcus equi,* formerly classified as *Corynebacterium equi,* and *Arcanobacterium pyogenes*, initially classified as *Corynebacterium pyogenes,* have also been included.

C. diphtheriae is the major human pathogen within the genus *Corynebacterium* and is the causative agent of diphtheria. Though *C. diphtheriae* is traditionally considered a non-zoonotic pathogen the organism has occasionally been isolated from equine wound infections, the udder and teats of cows, and equids, and canids (Henricson *et al.* 2000). *C. diphtheriae* can, when lysogenised by certain bacteriophages, produce diphtheria toxin which is the major virulence determinant.

The uncertain taxonomic status of *C. ulcerans* was resolved by Riegel *et al.* (1995). On the basis of DNA-DNA homology and rRNA gene sequences, they demonstrated that *C. ulcerans* is a distinct species. Phylogenetically *C. ulcerans* together with *C. pseudotuberculosis* is the closest relative of *C. diphtheriae* (Pascual *et al.* 1995; Ruimy *et al.* 1995). *C. ulcerans* can also harbour the diphtheria toxin. When lysogenic for a tox+ carrying phage, the organism produces two exotoxins in varying proportions (Petrie *et al.* 1934; Carne and Onon 1982). One is identical to *C. diphtheriae* toxin and is neutralized by diphtheria anti-toxin. The other is identical to *C. pseudotuberculosis* toxin Phospholipase D (PLD) which is unaffected by diphtheria antitoxin. The majority of the strains isolated from humans produce diphtheria toxin.

Over 10% of the *C. pseudotuberculosis* isolates produce the diphtheria toxin (Maximescu *et al.* 1974). However, there have not been any clinical cases of diphtheria attributed to infection with *C. pseudotuberculosis* (MacGregor 2000). PLD is the main virulence factor of *C. pseudotuberculosis*. PLD facilitates the persistence and spread of the organism within the host. The organism also possesses a toxic lipid coat on the surface which protects it from hydrolytic enzymes in the host and allows it to persist inside host cells. The *fag*BCD operon is another known virulence factor in *C. pseudotuberculosis* (Billington *et al.* 2002).

A. pyogenes produces several virulence factors that may contribute to its pathogenicity. These include, a haemolysin (Pyolysin PLO), neuraminidases and collagen binding proteins for adhesion and colonizing host tissue (Jost *et al.* 1999, 2001, 2002; Pietrocola *et al.* 2007).

The hosts and transmission

Zoonotic corynebacteria that have been known to cause the most economic losses are *C. pseudotuberculosis, A. pyogenes and R. equi. C. pseudotuberculosis* is the etiological agent of CLA in sheep and goats worldwide (Williamson 2001). The organism has also been isolated from horses with lymphanginitis and from cattle, camels, swine, and buffaloes, with pigeon fever (Yeruham *et al.* 2004; Selim 2001; Peel *et al.* 1997). Most human cases have been related to occupational exposure (Peel *et al.* 1997). CLA causes significant economic losses to sheep and goat producers in the world. External CLA is characterized by abscess formation in superficial lymph nodes and subcutaneous tissues. The abscesses can also develop in the lungs, kidneys, liver and the spleen characterizing visceral CLA.

Infections in humans caused by *C. pseudotuberculosis* are very rare. Human infections have been recorded in farm workers and vets exposed to infected animals, usually manifesting as lymphadenitis (Goldberger *et al.* 1981; Richards and Hurse 1985; House *et al.* 1986; Peel *et al.* 1997; Mills *et al.* 1997). Most of the reported episodes of human infection with *C. pseudotuberculosis* have been reported from Australia (Peel *et al.* 1997), where the patients have had extensive contact with animals (especially sheep), except for one case of eosinophilic pneumonia after exposure to *C. pseudotuberculosis* in a laboratory (Keslin *et al.* 1979).

Transmission among sheep and goats mainly occur through contamination of superficial wounds, which can appear during shearing, castration, and ear tagging (Dorella *et al.* 2006). Bacteria may be present in faeces of infected sheep which leads to a reservoir being present in soil. In cattle, transmission may occur through houseflies (Yeruham *et al.* 1996).

C. ulcerans causes mastitis in cattle and goats. Cattle are a known reservoir for *C. ulcerans* and may shed the organism for months to years. The organism has been isolated from other wild animals and domestic pets (Hommez *et al.* 1999; Fox *et al.* 1974; De Zoysa *et al.* 2005; Lartigue *et al.* 2005; Hogg *et al.* 2009). Toxigenic strains of *C. ulcerans* have been associated with classical and cutaneous diphtheria, pharyngitis, sinusitis, and extrapharygeal disease (Ahmad, *et al.* 2000; Hart 1984; Barrett 1986; Pers 1987; Kisely *et al.* 1994), and it has been recommended that the public health response to human infection with *C. ulcerans* should be the same as for *C. diphtheriae*. Usually human infections are acquired through contact with farm animals or by ingestion of unpasteurized dairy products (Bostock *et al.* 1984; Hart 1984; Barrett *et al.* 1986). Previously it was thought that person-to-person spread of toxigenic *C. ulcerans* did not occur (Meers 1979) but in 1996 *C. ulcerans* was isolated from siblings, and in 1998, the organism was isolated from a father and son (Bonnet and Begg 1999; White *et al.* 2001). Recently domestic animals have been identified as possible sources of human *C. ulcerans* infection. De Zoysa *et al.* (2005) reported the isolation of toxigenic *C. ulcerans* from domestic cats with bilateral nasal discharge in the UK, and Hogg *et al.* (2009) reported a fatal human case of diphtheria resulting from a possible zoonotic transmission of toxigenic *C. ulcerans* from a dog in the UK.

C. kutscheri causes latent infection in healthy rats and mice, but can cause severe illness in immunocompromised or nutritionally deficient rodents. Illness is characterized by bacteremia with septic emboli and end-organ disease in lungs of rats and kidneys and liver of mice (Amao *et al.* 2002; Pierce-Chase *et al.* 1964). Three cases of human infection have been reported, a case of chorioamnionitis and funisitis, septic arthritis, and soft tissue infection (Fitter *et al.* 1979; Messina *et al.* 1989; Natasha *et al.* 2007). It has been suggested that the organism may transmit via aerosol droplet, faecal-oral or by direct contact. Experimentally it has been shown that mice can shed the organism in faeces for up to 5 months (Amao *et al.* 2008).

C. bovis is a commensal of the bovine udder and may cause bovine mastitis, and in severe cases may result in loss of the udder or even death of the animal. The mode of transmission to humans is unclear; the organism appears to be a sporadic opportunistic agent of human disease (Bernard *et al.* 2002). To date, eight human cases with *C. bovis* have been reported, including ventriculojugular shunt nephritis, line-related sepsis, meningitis, leg ulcers, otitis media, epidural abscess, and endocarditis (Bolton *et al.* 1975; Dalal *et al.* 2008; Vale and Scott 1977).

A. pyogenes, initially classified as *Corynebacterium pyogenes*, is a common inhabitant of the upper respiratory and genital tracts of cattle sheep, swine, and many other species (Billington *et al.* 2002; Azawi and Azar 2003; Gröhn *et al.* 2004; Ertaş *et al.* 2005). It is one of the most important bacterial pathogens of cattle, causing liver abscesses, mastitis, infertility, abortion, and postpartum urine infections (Lechtenberg *et al.* 1988; Hillerton and Bramley 1989; Semambo 1991; Ruder *et al.* 1981). Contact of teats with a contaminated environment such as milking apparatus may cause the spread of mastitis. *A pyogenes* may also be transmitted by biting flies. It is also an opportunistic pathogen associated with suppurative or granulomatous lesions in domestic animals and avian species (Timoney *et al.* 1988; Brinton *et al.* 1993).

Human infections due to *A. pyogenes* are very rare. Human disease has been reported in people living in rural areas with underlying diseases such as cancer or diabetes (Plamondon *et al.* 2007). Types of human infections reported have been abdominal abscesses, otitis media, septic arthritis, endocarditis, and pneumonia (Plamondon *et al.* 2007; Levy *et al.* 2009). Cases have also been reported after organ and hematopoietic stem cell transplantation and patients with liver disease (Chen *et al.* 2009).

R. equi, previously known as *Corynebacterium equi*, is one of the most important causes of zoonotic infections in grazing animals, mainly horses and foals. It causes chronic suppurative bronchopneumonia, lymphadenitis and ulcerative enteritis in foals up to six months and the organism is considered as one of the most significant pathogens in the equine breeding industry (Hébert *et al.* 2010). The organism has also been isolated from cats and dogs (Jang *et al.* 1975; Farias *et al.* 2007; Cantor *et al.* 1998). *R. equi* is an important opportunistic pathogen in immunocompromised patients, especially those with AIDS. Infection with *R. equi* is associated with significant mortality. The organism is a soil inhabitant and exposure to soil contaminated with manure is the most likely route of both animal and human infection. Exposure is usually through inhalation, but may occur via ingestion or direct inoculation.

Epidemiology

C. ulcerans

C. ulcerans has been isolated from a wide range of domestic and wild animals. Diphtheria-like illness caused by toxigenic *C. ulcerans* appears to be increasingly recognized in many industrialized countries including the UK, France, Germany, Japan, Italy, and the USA (Hogg *et al.* 2009; Elden *et al.* 2007; Bonmarin *et al.* 2009; Sing *et al.* 2005; Hatanaka *et al.* 2003; von Hunolstein *et al.* 2003; Tiwari *et al.* 2008). In the UK, between 1986 and 2007, a total of 56 clinical isolates of toxigenic *C. ulcerans* were submitted to the WHO Streptococcus and Diphtheria Reference Unit, Health Protection Agency for identification. Amongst the 56 isolates, seven were from cases of classical diphtheria, and more than three deaths in the UK have been attributed to such infection (Tiwari *et al.* 2008).

Previous reports have usually linked human *C. ulcerans* infections to consumption of unpasteurized milk to having close contact with infected farm animals (Hart 1984; Higgs *et al.* 1967) but more recently a lack of association with farming or ingestion of raw milk products has been a notable feature. Toxigenic *C. ulcerans* have now been isolated from domestic cats with bilateral nasal discharge and dogs with rhinorrhoea (Taylor *et al.* 2002; Lartigue *et al.* 2005) and cases have now been recognized of human infection believed to have been contracted from contact with domestic cats and dogs (Hogg *et al.* 2009; Bonmarin *et al.* 2009; Lartigue *et al.* 2005; Hatanaka *et al.* 2003).

C. pseudotuberculosis

Epidemiological studies have shown a high prevalence of CLA in adult sheep (26%) in Australia (Paton *et al.* 2003) and in Canada (21%) (Arsenault *et al.* 2003). A study carried out in the UK showed that 45% of the farmers interviewed had seen abscesses on their sheep, possibly due to CLA, but only a few farmers had determined the cause of the abscesses (Binns *et al.* 2002). CLA remains a veterinary concern throughout the world.

Most of the reported episodes of human infection with *C. pseudotuberculosis* have been reported from Australia (Peel *et al.* 1997) where the patients have had extensive contact with sheep. To date, approximately 25 cases of human infection caused by *C. pseudotuberculosis* have been reported (Liu *et al.* 2005; Mills *et al.* 1997; Peel *et al.* 1997). Infected humans presented with lymphadenitis, abscesses and constitutional symptoms (Peel *et al.* 1997). A case of human necrotizing granulomatous lymphadentis in a boy following contact with infected animals, and a case of eye infection due to an ocular implant have also been reported (Mills *et al.* 1997; Liu *et al.* 2005).

R. equi

R. equi primarily causes zoonotic infections in horses and foals. Between 1967 and 1982 only 12 cases were reported (Lipsky *et al.* 1982). However with the AIDS epidemic the number of human infections has greatly increased (Weinstock and Brown 2002). The mortality rate among HIV infected patients is approximately 50–55% compared with 11% among immunocompetent patients.

A. pyogenes

Human infections due to *A. pyogenes* are very rare in the UK, however in other countries it may be a cause of significant morbidity. Between 1966 and 2007 approximately 13 cases of human infection have been reported, as reviewed by Plamondon *et al.* (2007). Most cases had an underlying illness such as cancer or diabetes and were also exposed to farm animals.

A. pyogenes is an important bacterial pathogen of cattle, causing liver abscesses, mastitis, abortion and infertility (Lechtenberg *et al.* 1988; Hillerton *et al.* 1989; Semambo *et al.* 1991). While not a major cause of mastitis the incidence of *A. pyogenes* mastitis within a herd can be high as 18% (Jones and Ward 1989). In a study carried out in the East of Turkey, it was reported that *A. pyogenes* was isolated from 40 out of 100 cattle with kidney abscesses at a local abattoir (Ertas *et al.* 2005).

Treatment, prevention and control

The mainstay of treatment for clinical diphtheria caused by toxigenic *C. ulcerans* is equine diphtheria anti-toxin (DAT). DAT is promptly administered to the patient, after testing for sensitivity to DAT. Antibiotics are not substitutes for DAT. The antibiotics of choice for diphtheria-like illness caused by *C. ulcerans* are erythromycin and penicillin. Tiwari (2008) reported a strain of *C. ulcerans* which was resistant to erythromycin and clindomycin but susceptible to penicillin, vancomycin, ciprofloxacin, and cephalosporins. This highlights the importance of testing strains of this organism for susceptibility to antimicrobials used for treatment. In the UK, there is no licensed erythromycin product for use in domestic pets. Hogg *et al.* (2009) reported the use of spiramycin in combination with metronidazole for eliminating *C. ulcerans* infection in dogs. Cattle have classically been considered as the main reservoir of *C. ulcerans* and infection can be prevented by eliminating consumption of unpasteurized milk and milk products and also by raising awareness amongst those at risk such as domestic pet owners.

C. pseudotuberculosis infection in humans can be prevented by covering cuts and abrasions when handling animals and also by raising awareness amongst sheep shearers, butchers and clinicians.

Surgical excision of the affected lymph glands in human cases of lymphadenitis is the mainstay of management, and antibiotic treatment is additional. The use of a combined toxoid vaccine against caseous lymphadenitis in sheep may result in a decrease in the number of human cases of this zoonoses (Peel *et al.* 1997; Paton *et al.* 1995).

Treatment of *R. equi* infection in humans requires prolonged combination antibiotic therapy, and sometimes surgical therapy. Combination antibiotic therapy may decrease the risk of developing resistance. The use of a carbapenem such as meropenem and a glycopeptide such as vancomycin and use of macrolides in combination with rifampicin are good choices (Tse *et al.* 2008; Prescott 1991). Increasing awareness of *R. equi* infection among those with weakened immune systems, and taking precautions such as reducing dust levels on farms and covering wounds may help to avoid transmission of *R. equi*. Experimentally it has been shown that the combination of clarithromycin and rifampicin is superior to azithromycin-rifampicin and erythromycin-rifampicin for treatment of pneumonia caused by *R. equi* in foals (Giguere *et al.* 2004). Control measures for *A. pyogenes* infection include fly control programmes, maintaining cows in clean and dry calving areas and removing affected cows from the herd. Once infected, the prognosis is poor as antibiotic therapy is often ineffective.

References

Achermann, Y., Trampuz, A., Moro, F., Wüst, J. and Vogt, M. (2009). *Corynebacterium bovis* shoulder prosthetic joint infection: the first reported case. *Diagn. Microbiol. Infect. Dis.*, **64:** 213–15.

Ahmad, N., Gainsborough, N. and Paul, J. (2000). An unusual case of diphtheria and its complications. *Hosp. Med.*, **61:** 436–37.

Amao, H., Akimoto, T., Komukai, Y., Sawada, T., Saito, M. *et al.* (2002). Detection of *Corynebacterium kutscheri* from the oral cavity of rats. *Experi. Anim.*, **5:** 99–102.

Amao, H., Moriguchi, N., Komukai, Y., Kawasumi, H., Takahashi, K. *et al.* (2008). Detection of *Corynebacterium kutscheri* in the faeces of subclinically infected mice. *Laborat. Anim.*, **42:** 376–82.

Arsenault, J., Girard, C., Dubreuil, P. *et al.* (2003). Prevalence of and carcass condemnation from maedi-visna, paratuberculosis and caseous lymphadenitis in culled sheep from Quebec, Canada. *Prev. Vet. Med.*, **59:** 67–81.

Azawi, O.I. and Azar, Z.A. (2003). Bacteriological and histopathological studies in repeat breeder cows. *Iraqi J. Vet. Sci.*, **16:** 49–50.

Barrett, N.J. (1986). Communicable disease associated with milk and dairy products in England and Wales: 1983–1984. *J. Infect.*, **12:** 265–72.

Bergey, D.H., Harrison, F.C., Breed, R.S., Hammer, B.W. and Huntoon, F.M. (eds.) (1923). Bergey's manual of determinative bacteriology, Baltimore: Williams & Wilkens.

Bernard, K.A., Munro, C., Wiebe, D. and Ongsansoy, E. (2002). Characteristics of rare or recently described corynebacterium species recovered from human clinical material in Canada. *J. Clin. Microbiol.*, **40:** 4375–81.

Billington, S.J., Esmay, P.A., Songer, J.G. and Jost, B.H. (2002). Identification and role in virulence of putative iron acquisition genes from *Corynebacterium pseudotuberculosis. FEMS Microbiol. Lett.*, 208: 41–45.

Binns, S.H., Bairley, M. and Green, L.E. (2002). Postal survey of ovine caseous lymphadenitis in the United Kingdom between 1990 and 1999. *Vet. Rec.*, **150:** 263–68.

Bolton, W.K., Sande, M.A., Normansell, D.E., Sturgill, B.C. and Westervelt Jr., F.B., (1975). Ventriculojugular shunt nephritis with *Corynebacterium bovis*. Successful therapy with antibiotics. *Am. J. Med.*, **59:** 417–23.

Bonmarin, I., Guiso, N., Le Flèche-Matéos, A., Patey, O., Grimont, P.A.D. et al. (2009). Diphtheria: A zoonotic disease in France. Vaccine, 27: 4196–4200.

Bonsfield, I.J. and Cally, A.G. (1978). Coryneform bacteria. London: Academic Press.

Bostock, A.D., Gilbert, F.R., Lewis, D. and Smith, D.C.M. (1984). Corynebacterium ulcerans infection associated with untreated milk. J. Infect., 9: 286–88.

Brinton, M.K., Schellberg, L.C., Johnson, J.B., Frank, R.K., Halvorson, D.A. et al. (1993). Description of osteomyelitis lesions associated with Actinomyces pyogenes infection in the proximal tibia of adult male turkeys. Avian Dis., 37: 259–62.

Cantor, G.H., Byrne, B.A., Hines, S.A. and Richards III, H.M. (1998). VapA-negative Rhododoccus equi in a dog with necrotizing pyogranulomatous hepatitis, osteomyelitis, and myositis. J. Vet. Diagn. Investig., 10: 297–300.

Cardoso, F.L.L., Machado, M.S., Souza, M.J. and Cunha, R. (1996). Rhodococcus equi mastoiditis in a patient with AIDS. Clin. Infect. Dis., 22: 713.

Carne, H.R. and Onon, E.O. (1982). The exotoxins of Corynebacterium ulcerans. J. Hyg., 88: 173–91.

Chen, X., Xu, F., Xia, J., Cheng, Y. and Yang, Y. (2009). Bacteremia due to Rhodococcus equi: a case report and review of the literature. J. Zheji. Uni. Sci. B, 10: 933–36.

Dalal, A., Urban, C., Ahluwalia, M. and Rubin, D. (2008). Corynebacterium bovis line related septicaemia: a case report and review of the literature. Scandin. J. Infect. Dis., 40: 575–77.

De Zoysa, A., Hawkey, P.M., Engler, K. et al. (2005). Characterization of toxigenic Corynebacterium ulcerans strains isolated from humans and domestic cats in the United Kingdom. J. Clin. Microbiol., 43: 4377–81.

Dorella, F.A., Pacheco, L.G., Oliveira, S.C., Miyoshi, A. and Azevedo, V. (2006). Corynebacterium pseudotuberculosis: microbiology, biochemical properties, pathogenesis and molecular studies of virulence. Vet. Res., 37: 201–18.

Elden, S., Colle, L., Efstratiou, A. and Doshi, N. (2007). Laboratory-confirmed case of toxigenic Corynebacterium ulcerans in the United Kingdom. Euro Surveill., 12: E070329.3.

Ertaş, H.B., Kiliç, A., Özbey, G. and Muz, A. (2005). Isolation of Arcanobacterium (Actinomyces) pyogenes from abscessed cattle kidney and identification by PCR. Turk. J. Vet. Anim. Sci., 29: 455–59.

Evans, A.C. (1961). The bacteria of milk freshly drawn from normal udders. J. Infect. Dis., 18: 437–76.

Farias, M.R., Takai, S., Ribeiro, M.G., Fabris, V.E. and Franco, S.R.V.S. (2007). Cutaneous pyogranuloma in a cat caused by virulent Rhodococcus equi containing an 87 kb type I plasmid. Aus. Vet. J., 85: 29–31.

Fierer, J., Wolf, P., Seed, L., Gay, T., Noonan, K. et al. (1987). Non-pulmonary Rhodococcus equi infections in patients with acquired immune deficiency syndrome (AIDS). J. Clin. Path., 40: 556–58.

Fitter, W.F., De Sa, D.J. and Richardson, H. (1979). Chorioamnionitis and funisitis due to Corynebacterium kutscheri. Arch. Dis. Childh., 55: 710–12.

Fox, J.G. and Frost, W.W. (1974). Corynebacterium ulcerans mastitis in a bonnet macaque (Macaca radiata). Lab. Anim. Sci., 24: 820–22.

Gahrn-Hansen, B. and Frederiksen, W. (1992). Human infections with Actinomyces pyogenes (Corynebacterium pyogenes). Diagn. Microbiol. Infect. Dis., 15: 349–54.

Giddens Jr., W.E., Keahey, K.K., Carter, G.R. and Whitehair, C.K. (1968). Pneumonia in rats due to infection with Corynebacterium kutscheri. Pathol. Vet., 5: 227–37.

Giguere, S., Jacks, S., Roberts, G. D., Hernandez, J., Long, M.T. et al. (2004). Retrospective comparison of azithromycin, clarithromycin, and erythromycin for the treatment of foals with Rhodococcus equi pneumonia. J. Vet. Intern. Med., 18: 568–73.

Gilbert, A.M. and Stewart, M.S. (1926). Corynebacterium ulcerans: a pathogenic microorganism resembling C. diphtheriae. J. Lab. Clin. Med., 12: 756–61.

Goldberger, A.C., Lipsky, B.A. and Plorde, J.J. (1981). Suppurative granulomatous lymphadenitis caused by Corynebacterium ovis (pseudotuberculosis). Am. J. Clin. Pathol., 76: 486–90.

Gröhn, Y.T., Wilson, D.J., González, R.N. et al. (2004). Effect of pathogen specific clinical mastitis on milk yield in dairy cows. J. Dairy Sci., 87: 3358–74.

Hart, R.J. (1984). Corynebacterium ulcerans in humans and cattle in North devon. J. Hyg. Lond., 92: 161–64.

Hatanaka, A., Tsunoda, A., Okamoto, M. et al. (2003). Corynebacterium ulcerans diphtheria in Japan. Emerg. Infect. Dis., 9: 752–53.

Hébert, L., Cauchard, J., Doligez, P., Quitard, L., Laugier, C. et al. (2010). Viability of Rhodococcus equi. Curr. Microbiol., 60: 38–41.

Henricson, B., Segarra, M., Garvin, J. et al. (2000). Toxigenic Corynebacterium diphtheriae associated with an equine wound infection. J. Vet. Diagn., 12: 253–57.

Higgs, T.M., Smith, A., Cleverly, L.M. and Neave, F.K. (1967). Corynebacterium ulcerans infections in a dairy herd. Vet. Rec., 81: 43–45.

Hillerton, J.E. and Bramley, A.J. (1989). Infection following challenge of the lactating and dry udder of dairy cows with Actinomyces pyogenes and Peptostreptococcus indolicus. Brit. Vet. J., 145: 148–59.

Hogg, R.A., Wessels, J., Hart, A. et al. (2009). Possible zoonotic transmission of Toxigenic Corynebacterium ulcerans from companion animals in a human case of fatal diphtheria. Vet. Rec., 165: 691–92.

Holmes, N.E. and Korman, T.M. (2007). Corynebacterium kutscheri infection of skin and soft tissue following rat bite. J. Clin. Microbiol., 45: 3468–69.

Hommez, J., Devriese, L.A., Vaneechoutte, M., Riegel, P., Butaye, P. et al. (1999). Identification of nonlipophilic corynebacteria isolated from Dairy Cows with Mastitis. J. Clin. Microbiol., 37: 954–57.

House, R.W., Schousboe, M., Allen, J.P. and Grant, C.C. (1986). Corynebacterium ovis (pseudotuberculosis) lymphadenitis in a sheep farmer a new occupational disease in New Zealand. N. Zealand Med. J., 99: 659–62.

Jang, S.S., Lock, A. and Biberstein, E.L. (1975). A cat with Corynebacterium equi lymphadenitis clinically simulating lymphosarcoma. Cornell Vet., 65: 232–39.

Jones, G.F. and Ward, G.E. (1989). Cause, occurrence, and clinical signs of mastitis and anorexia in cows in a Wisconsin study. J. Am. Vet. Med. Assoc., 195: 1108–13.

Jost, B.H., Songer, J.G. and Billington, S.J. (1999). An Arcanobacterium (Anctinomyces) pyogenes mutant deficient in production of the pore-forming cytolysin pyolysin has reduced virulence. Infect. Immun., 67: 1723–28.

Jost, B.H., Songer, J.G. and Billington, S.J. (2001). Cloning, expression and characterization of a neuraminidase gene from Arcanobacterium pyogenes. Infect. Immun., 69: 4430–37.

Jost, B.H., Songer, J.G. and Billington, S.J. (2002). Identification of a second Arcanobacterium pyogenes neuraminidase and involvement of neuraminidase a activity in host cell adhesion. Infect. Immun., 70: 1106–12.

Keslin, M.H., McCoy, E.L., McCusker, J.J. and Lutch, J.S. (1979). Corynebacterium pseudotuberculosis. A new cause of infectious and eosinophilic pneumonia. Am. J. Med., 67: 228–31.

Kisely, S.R., Price, S. and Ward, T. (1994). 'Corynebacterium ulcerans' a potential cause of diphtheria. Commun. Dis. Rep. - CDR Review, 4: R63–64.

Lartigue, M.F., Monnet, X., Le Fleche, A. et al. (2005). Corynebacterium ulcerans in an immunocompromised patient with diphtheria and her dog. J. Clin. Microbiol., 43: 999–1001.

Lechtenberg, K.F., Nagaraja, T.G., Leipold, H.W. and Chengappa, M.M. (1988). Bacteriologic and histologic studies of hepatic abscesses in cattle. *Am. J. Vet. Res.*, **49**: 58–62.

Levy, C.E., Pedro, R.J., Nowakonski, A.V. *et al.* (2009). *Arcanobacterium pyogenes* sepsis in farmer, Brazil. *Emerg. Infect. Dis.*, **15**: 1131–32.

Lipsky, B.A., Goldberger, A.C., Tompkins, L.S. and Plorde, J.J. (1982). Infections caused by nondiphtheria corynebacteria. *Rev. Infect. Dis.*, **4**: 1220–35.

Liu, D.T., Chan, W.M., Fan, D.S. and Lam, D.S. (2005). An infected hydrogel buckle with *Corynebacterium pseudotuberculosis. Brit. J. Ophthalmol.*, **89**: 245–46.

Lopez, J.F., Wong, F.M. and Quesada, M.S. (1966). *Corynebacterium pseudotuberculosis*- first case of human infection. *Am. J. Clin. Path.*, **46**: 562.

MacGregor, R.R. (2000). Gram positive bacilli. In: G.L. Mandell, J.E. Bennett, and R. Dolin (eds.). *Principles and Practice of Infectious Diseases, (5th edn.)* pp. 2190–208. NY, USA: Churchhill Livingstone.

Mandarino, E., Rachlis, A., Towers, M. and Simor, A.E. (1994). Prostatic abscess due to *Rhodococcus equi* in a patient with acquired immunodeficiency syndrome. *Clin. Microbiol. Newslett.*, **16**: 14–16.

Martin-Dávila, P., Quereda, C., Rodriguez, H. *et al.* (1998). Thyroid abscess due to *Rhodococcus equi* in a patient infected with the human immunodeficiency virus. *Euro. J. Clin. Microbiol. Infect. Dis.*, **17**: 55–57.

Maximescu, P., Oprisan, A., Pop, A. and Potorac, E. (1974). Further studies on *Corynebacterium* species capable of producing diphtheria toxin (*C. diphtheriae, C. ulcerans, C. ovis*). *J. Gen. Microbiol.*, **82**: 49–56.

Meers, P.D. (1979). A case of classical diphtheria and other infections due to *Corynebacterium ulcerans. J. Infect.*, **1**: 139–42.

Messina, O.D., Maldonado-Cocco, J.A., Pescio, A., Farinati, A. and Garcia-Morteo, O. (1989). *Corynebacterium kutsch*eri septic arthritis. *Arthritis Rheumat.*, **32**: 1053.

Mills, A.E., Mitchell, R.D. and Lim, E.K. (1997). *Corynebacterium pseudotuberculosis* is a cause of human necrotising granulomatous lymphadenitis. *Pathol.*, **29**: 231–33.

Noble, W.C. and Smith, E.R. (1990). Other Corynebacterial and coryneform infections. In: G.R. Smith and C.S.F. Easman (eds.) Topley and Wilson's Principles of Bacteriology, Virology and Immunity, pp. 75–79. NY, USA: Oxford University Press, Inc.

Pascual, C., Lawson, P.A., Farrow, J.A., Gimenez, M.N. and Collins, M.D. (1995). Phylogenetic analysis of the genus *Corynebacterium* based on 16S rRNA gene sequences. *Intern. J. System. Bacterio.*, **45**: 724–28.

Paton, M.W., Sutherland, S.S., Rose, I.R., Hart, R.A., Mercy, A.R. *et al.* (1995). The spread of *Corynebacterium pseudotuberculosis* infection to unvaccinated and vaccinated sheep. *Aus. Vet. J.*, **72**: 266–69.

Paton, M.W., Walker, S.B., Rose, I.R. and Watt, G.F. (2003). Prevalence of caseous lymphadenitis and usage of caseous lymphadenitis vaccines in sheep flocks. *Aus. Vet. J.*, **81**: 91–95.

Peel, M.M., Palmer, G.G., Stacpoole, A.M. and Kerr, T.G. (1997). Human lymphadenitis due to *Corynebacterium pseudotuberculosis*: report of ten cases from Australia and review. *Clin. Infect. Dis.*, **24**: 185–91.

Pers, C. (1987). Infection due to '*Corynebacterium ulcerans*' producing diphtheria toxin- a case report from Denmark. *Acta Pathol. Microbiol. Immunol. Scandin. - Section B.*, **95**: 361–62.

Petrie, G.F. and McLean, D. (1934). The inter-relations of *Corynebacterium ovis, Corynebacterium diphtheriae*, and certain diphtheria strains derived from the human nasopharynx. *J. Pathol. Bacteriol.*, **39**: 635–63.

Pierce-Chase, C.H., Fauve, R.M. and Dubos, R. (1964). Corynebacterial *pseudotuberculosis* in mice: I. Comparative susceptibility of mouse strains to experimental infection with *Corynebacterium kutscheri. J. Experim. Med.*, **12**: 267–81.

Pietrocola, G., Valtulina, V., Rindi, S., Jost, B.H. and Speziale, P. (2007). Functional and structural properties of CbpA, a collagen binding protein from *Arcanobacterium pyogenes. Microbiol.*, **153**: 3380–89.

Plamondon, M., Martinez, G., Raynal, L., Touchette, M. and Valiquette, L. (2007). A fatal case of *Arcanobacterium pyogenes* endocarditis in a man with no identified animal contact: case report and review of the literature. *Euro. J. Clin. Microbiol. Infect. Dis.*, **26**: 663–66.

Prescott, J.F. (1991). *Rhodococcus equi*: an animal and human pathogen. *Clin. Microbiol. Rev.*, **4**: 20–34.

Richards, M. and Hurse, A. (1985). *Corynebacterium pseudotuberculosis* abscesses in a young butcher. *Aus. N. Zealand J. Med.*, **15**: 85–86.

Riegel, P., Ruimy, R., de Briel, D. *et al.* (1995). Taxonomy of *Corynebacterium diphtheriae* and related taxa with recognition of *Corynebactreium ulcerans* sp. Nov. nom. Rev. *FEMS Microbiol. Lett.*, **126**: 271–76.

Ruder, C.A., Sasser, R.G., Williams, R.J., Ely, J.K., Bull, R.C. *et al.* (1981). Uterine infections in the postpartum cow. II. Possible synergistic effect of *Fusobacterium necrophorum* and *Corynebacterium pyogenes. Theriogeno.*, **15**: 573–80.

Ruimy, R., Riegel, P., Boiron, H., Monteil, H. and Christen, R. (1995). Phylogeny of the genus *Corynebacterium* deduced from analyses of small-subunit ribosomal DNA sequences. *Inter. J. System. Bacteriol.*, **45**: 740–46.

Selim, A.S. (2001). Oedematous skin disease of buffalo in Egypt. *J. Vet. Med. Series B- Infect. Dis. Vet. Pub. Heal.*, **48**: 241–58.

Semambo, D.K.N., Ayliffe, T.R., Boyd, J.S. and Taylor, D.J. (1991). Early abortion in cattle induced by experiment intrauterine infection with pure cultures of *Actinomyces pyogenes. Vet. Rec.*, **129**: 1216.

Sing, A., Bierschenk, S. and Heesemann, J. (2005). Classical diphtheria caused by *Corynebacterium ulcerans* in Germany: amino acid *sequence differences between diphtheria toxins from Corynebacterium diphtheriae* and *C. ulcerans. Clin. Infect. Dis.*, **40**: 325–26.

Skerman, V.B.D., McGowan, V. and Sneath, P.H.A. (eds.) (1980). Approved lists of bacterial names. *Inter. J. System. Bacteriol.*, **30**: 225–420.

Smith, J.E. (1966). *Corynebacterium* species as animal pathogens. *J. Appl. Microbiol.*, **29**: 119–30.

Taylor, D.J., Efstratiou, A. and Reilly, W.J. (2002). Diphtheria toxin production by *Corynebacterium ulcerans* from cats. *Vet. Rec.*, **150**: 355.

Timoney, J., Gillespie, J., Scott, F. and Barlough, J. (1988). *The genus Actinomycesagan and Bruner's microbiology and infectious diseases of domestic animals*, pp. 264–67. New York: Cornell University Press.

Tiwari, T.S., Golaz, A., Yu, D.T. *et al.* (2008). Investigations of 2 cases of diphtheria-like illness due to Toxigenic *Corynebacterium ulcerans. Clin. Infect. Dis.*, **46**: 395–401.

Tse, K.C., Tang, S.C., Chan, T.M. and Ian, K.N. (2008). *Rhodococcus* lung abscess complicating kidney transplantation: successful management by combination antibiotic therapy. *Trans. Infect. Dis.*, **10**: 44–47.

Vale, J.A. and Scott, G.W. (1977). *Corynebacterium bovis* as a cause of human disease. *Lancet*, **2**: 682–84.

von Hunolstein, C., Alfarone, G. and Scopetti, F. *et al.* (2003). Molecular epidemiology and characteristics of *Corynebacterium diphtheria* and *Corynebacterium ulcerans* strains isolated in Italy during the 1990s. *J. Medical Microbiol.*, **52**: 181–88.

Weinstock, D.M. and Brown, A.E. (2002). *Rhodococcus equi*: an emerging pathogen. *Clin. Infect. Dis.*, **34**: 1379–85.

Williamson, L.H. (2001). Caseous lymphadenitis in small ruminants. *Vet. Clin. N. Am. Food Anim. Pract.*, **17**: 359–71.

Yeruham, I., Braverman, Y., Shpigel, N.Y., Chizov-Ginzburg, A., Saran, A. *et al.* (1996). Mastitis in dairy cattle caused by *Corynebacterium pseudotuberculosis* and the feasibility of transmission by houseflies. *Vet. Quart.*, **18**: 87–89.

Yeruham, I., Friedman, S., Perl, S., Elad, D., Berkovich, Y. *et al.* (2004). A herd level analysis of a *Corynebacterium pseudotuberculosis* outbreak in a diary cattle herd. *Vet. Dermat.*, **15**: 315–20.

CHAPTER 19b

Other bacterial diseases

Anaplasmosis, ehrlichiosis and neorickettsiosis

Richard Birtles

Summary

In 2001, taxonomic reorganization of the bacterial genera *Anaplasma*, *Ehrlichia*, *Cowdria* and *Neorickettsia* resulted in the transfer of numerous species between these taxa, and the renaming of the transferred species to reflect their new taxonomic position (Dumler *et al.* 2001). Among the members of these genera, there are four species of established zoonotic importance (Table 19b.1), which are therefore the subject of this chapter. Two of these species were affected by the changes outlined above.

Although these four species possess markedly different ecologies, they share the fundamental biological character of being obligate intracellular bacteria that reside within vacuoles of eukaryotic cells. This lifestyle underlies their fastidious nature in the laboratory and hence our limited knowledge of their biology and pathogenicity. Nonetheless, despite this shortfall, all four are associated with diseases of established or emerging importance:

◆ *E. chaffeensis* provokes human monocytic ehrlichiosis (HME),

◆ *E. ewingii* causes human ewingii ehrlichiosis (HEE),

◆ *A. phagocytophilum* causes human granulocytic anaplasmosis (HGA),

◆ *N. sennetsu* is the agent of sennetsu neorickettsiosis.

The first three pathogens are transmitted by hard (ixodid) ticks and are encountered across the temperate zones of the northern hemisphere (and maybe beyond), although the vast majority of human infections caused by them are currently reported in the USA. There, HME and HGA are second only to Lyme disease (caused by *Borrelia burgdorferi*) in terms of public health significance. Furthermore, given that there is evidence of increasing

Table 19b.1 Renaming of transferred species

Former name	Current name
Ehrlichia chaffeensis	*Ehrlichia chaffeensis*
Ehrlichia ewingii	*Ehrlichia ewingii*
Ehrlichia phagocytophila	*Anaplasma phagocytophilum*
Ehrlichia sennetsu	*Neorickettsia sennetsu*

population sizes and changing distributions for ixodid species (Scharlemann *et al.* 2008), it is not unreasonable to predict that the infections they transmit will present an increased medical burden in the future. *N. sennetsu* remains an enigmatic pathogen; case reports remain scarce, but serological surveys suggest high levels of exposure. The widespread consumption of raw fish across east Asia presents specific infection risks to this region, and an increased awareness that sennetsu neorickettsiosis is among the infections that can be acquired from this source is required before its public health importance can be accurately assessed.

History

E. chaffeensis and *E. ewingii* can still be considered as recent discoveries, having both been first described in the last 20 years. HME was first recognized in the USA in the mid 1980s (Maeda *et al.* 1987), and *E. chaffeensis* was demonstrated to be its aetiological agent a few years later after being isolated from a HME patient (Anderson *et al.* 1991). *E. ewingii* was first described in 1992, when it was implicated in canine granulocytic ehrlichiosis (Anderson *et al.* 1992), but it was not recognized as a zoonotic pathogen until 1999, when PCR was used to detect DNA from the species in the blood of four patients from Missouri, USA with suspected ehrlichiosis (Buller *et al.* 1999). In the USA, national collation of reports of *E. chaffeensis* infections has been ongoing for several years. These figures reveal that there was an almost four-fold rise in the number of cases between 2004 to 2008 culminating in almost 1,200 reports. In 2009, this number declined, although about 800 cases were still reported (Centers for Disease Control and Prevention (CDC) 2010). Conversely, reports of *E. ewingii* remain rare; only 15 cases were collated during 2008 and 2009 (CDC 2010).

A. phagocytophilum was first implicated as a human pathogen in 1994 (Bakken *et al.* 1994; Chen *et al.* 1994). However, prior to this date, it had long been recognized as a veterinary pathogen, associated with pasture fever and tick-borne pyaemia in livestock primarily in Northern Europe (Woldehiwet 2010). The first reported cases of HGA were in patients living in Midwestern USA, and, despite *A. phagocytophilum* having a distribution stretching across most of the temperate regions of the northern hemisphere, the vast majority of subsequent cases have also been from the USA. Like *Ehrlichia* infections, those caused by *A. phagocytophilum* are reportable in the USA, and the collation of data has shown that between

2004 and 2009, over 4,500 HGA cases were reported nationally (CDC 2010). Elsewhere in the world, HGA was first reported in Slovenia in 1997 (Petrovec *et al.* 1997), and a handful of further cases have been encountered in that country (Lotric-Furlan *et al.* 2004). Occasional case reports have demonstrated the presence of HGA in numerous other countries.

The earliest reports of an illness compatible with sennetsu neorickettsiosis, associated with the consumption of raw fish on Kyushu, the most south-westerly of the four main islands that comprise Japan, date from the 1800s (Misao and Katsuta 1956; Rikihisa 1991). However, demonstration of the pathogenic role *N. sennetsu* was not obtained until far more recently, with its recovery in mice from the samples collected from a patient with a typical clinical history and mononucleosis in the 1950s (Misao and Kobayashi 1954). This achievement provoked a flurry of activity in which the isolate was further characterized and its physiology explored, but further cases were not reported and the disease apparently vanished. However, more recently, serological evidence of exposure to *N. sennetsu* among febrile Malaysian patients was reported (Ristic 1990) together with the acquisition of an isolate from the blood of one patient (Weiss *et al.* 1990). Very recently, PCR-based demonstration of *N. sennetsu* infection in a febrile patient from Laos was reported, together with evidence of a high prevalence of anti-*N. sennetsu* antibodies in a sample of over 1,000 blood donors and febrile patients from the country (Newton *et al.* 2009).

Ecology

E. chaffeensis

The primary natural reservoir of *E. chaffeensis* is the white-tailed deer (*Odocoileus virginianus*). Experimental inoculations of white-tailed deer have shown them to be susceptible to infection and capable of transmitting *E. chaffeensis* to its natural vector, the lone star tick (*Amblyomma americanum*). In deer, infections are chronic and characterized by bacteraemia and sequestration of bacteria in lymph nodes and bone marrow for at least several months (Davidson *et al.* 2001). The range of the white-tailed deer extends across most of the USA, northwards into Canada and south, through Central America as far as Peru. Serological surveys for *E. chaffeensis* antibodies in cervids in numerous states in the USA have revealed a generally high seroprevalence, with typically at least 25% (and sometimes a far higher proportion) of animals having evidence of exposure. PCR-based surveys for *E. chaffeensis* DNA in deer tissues are generally concordant with serosurveys (Yabsley 2010). Low infection prevalences in deer tend only to be encountered on the periphery of the range of *Am. americanum*. Other mammals have also been implicated in the natural maintenance of *E. chaffeensis* in the USA, and, given the broad host range of *Am. americanum*, the exploitation of diverse vertebrates by the pathogen is feasible. Raccoons (*Procyon lotor*) and possums (*Didelphis virginiana*) feed all three life stages of *Am. americanum*, and serosurveys of these species have indicated that both are naturally exposed to *E. chaffeensis*. However, experimental infections of raccoons resulted in only short-lived infections (Yabsley *et al.* 2008). Serological or PCR-based evidence of natural infections have also been reported for coyotes (*Canis latrans*) and captive and free-ranging lemur species. Rodents do not appear to play a role as a reservoir for *E. chaffeensis* (Yabsley 2010).

Am. americanum is a three-host tick with a catholic feeding behaviour, although white-tailed deer are the most important hosts for all three life stages. Larvae and nymphs will, however, also feed on other small and medium sized mammals and birds, and, within its natural range, *Am. americanum* is the tick most commonly found on humans (Merten and Durden 2000). The distribution of *Am. americanum* is considerably more limited than that of white-tailed deer, and most cases of HME occur where the population densities of *Am. americanum* are highest, in the south-central, south-eastern and, increasingly, eastern USA. Although *E. chaffeensis* cases have been reported in most US states, not all are thought to be autochthonous and doubts have been raised about the accuracy of diagnosis in some cases (Paddock and Childs 2003). Survey of ticks has demonstrated the widespread presence of *E. chaffeensis* at varying prevalences, typically under 10%, but rising to almost 30% in some locations (Yabsley 2010). Although some circumstantial evidence for the role of ticks other than *Am. americanum* in the transmission of *E. chaffeensis*, further studies are required to confirm their involvement.

There is now clear evidence that *E. chaffeensis*, or at least closely related organisms, are present outside of the USA. A study in China (Gao *et al.* 2001) reported the presence of DNA from an *E. chaffeensis*-like organism in the blood of febrile, tick-bitten patients, and the same diagnostic approach was used to identify infection in a Venezuelan child (Martinez *et al.* 2008). In Cameroon, DNA from an organism indistinguishable from *E. chaffeensis* was detected in the blood of 12/118 patients with fever of unknown origin (Ndip *et al.* 2009). Numerous reports have presented serological evidence of infection in most regions of the world, but in the absence of other diagnostic evidence, these must be treated with a degree of caution. Serological and PCR-based surveys of wildlife and livestock have indicated the existence of an *E. chaffeensis*-like agent in many parts of the world including East Asia and South America, and PCR-based surveys of various ticks in Asia, Africa and South America have also demonstrated the presence of such organisms (Yabsley 2010).

E. ewingii

Both dogs and deer have been implicated as important reservoir hosts for *E. ewingii*. A survey of 88 dogs, most with suspected acute ehrlichiosis, but some apparently healthy, revealed the presence of *E. ewingii* DNA in the blood of 20 dogs (18 of which were sick and two of which were healthy), and provoked the suggestion that dogs serve as a reservoir for the pathogen (Liddell *et al.* 2003). The presence of *E. ewingii* DNA has been demonstrated in the blood of white-tailed deer, and naïve fawns inoculated with blood drawn from infected deer were susceptible to the pathogen and remained bacteraemic for 68 days (Yabsley *et al.* 2002). Like *E. chaffeensis*, *E. ewingii* is transmitted by *Am. americanum*. An early study demonstrated that this tick, but not other species, was capable of experimental transmission of *E. ewingii* from infected to naïve dogs (Anziani *et al.* 1990). *E. ewingii* DNA has been detected in host-seeking *Am. americanum* ticks in several states in the USA at a prevalence of infection of up to 5% (in adults), but more often somewhat lower (Wolf *et al.* 2000).

A. phagocytophilum

A. phagocytophilum is a generalist species, capable of exploiting numerous mammal species as reservoir hosts and multiple ixodid tick species as vectors, and is encountered throughout the temperate regions of the northern hemisphere, from the western coast of north America, across Europe, North Africa and Asia, and as far east as Siberia and Japan. Early interest in *A. phagocytophilum* related to its aetiological role in infections of livestock in northern Europe, including sheep and cattle (MacLeod and Gordon 1933; Woldehiwet 2010). It was first recognized in North America as a parasite of voles (Tyzzer 1938), then as a veterinary pathogen in horses (Gribble 1969) and subsequently in dogs (Madewell and Grimble 1982). *A. phagocytophilum* infections in deer in the UK were first described in 1965 (McDiarmid 1965). The demonstration of *A. phagocytophilum* as a human pathogen in the early 1990s, resulted in renewed efforts to define the transmission network of the bacterium. In the USA, the importance of rodents in this network is well established (Telford *et al.* 1996; Foley *et al.* 2008), although other species including deer (Massung *et al.* 2005), foxes (Gabriel *et al.* 2009), and maybe even reptiles (Nieto *et al.* 2009) are also thought to be involved. In Europe, a similarly wide range of wildlife species have been implicated as reservoir hosts including rodents, insectivores, cervids, and even bears (Vichova *et al.* 2010; Woldehiwet 2010). Rodents and cervids also appear to be key reservoir hosts for *A. phagocytophilum* in Asia (e.g. Kawahara *et al.* 2006; Zhan *et al.* 2009). There is currently no evidence to indicate that birds are involved in the natural maintenance of *A. phagocytophilum*.

Several *Ixodes* species have been implicated in the transmission of *A. phagocytophilum* including, in North America, *Ixodes scapularis* (Pancholi *et al.* 1995), *Ixodes pacificus* (Barlough *et al.* 1997), and *Ixodes spinipalpis* (Holden *et al.* 2003, Zeidner *et al.* 2000), in Europe and North Africa, *Ixodes ricinus* (MacLeod and Gordon 1933), *Ixodes trianguliceps* (Bown *et al.* 2003), and *Ixodes ventalloi* (Santos *et al.* 2003), and in Asia, *Ixodes persulcatus* (Cao *et al.* 2000), and *Ixodes ovatus* (Ohashi *et al.* 2005). It is likely that other *Ixodes* species are also competent vectors for the pathogen, and there is some evidence than ticks from other genera may also fulfil this role; *A. phagocytophilum* DNA has been detected in questing members of the genera *Haemaphysalis* (Barandika *et al.* 2008; Kim *et al.* 2003; Yoshimoto *et al.* 2010), *Dermacentor* (Baldridge *et al.* 2009; Cao *et al.* 2006; Holden *et al.* 2003), *Hyalomma* and *Rhipicephalus* (Barandika *et al.* 2008; Sarih *et al.* 2005; Toledo *et al.* 2009). Furthermore, the vector competence of *Dermacentor albipictus* has been demonstrated in an experimental study (Baldridge *et al.* 2009). However, *A. phagocytophilum* does not appear to be transmitted by *Am. americanum*, the vector of *E. chaffeensis* and *E. ewingii* (Ewing *et al.* 1997).

The extent to which ticks are able to maintain *A. phagocytophilum* trans-ovarially, and the relative importance of this transmission mode for the natural persistence of the species, remains uncertain. Early studies on *I. ricinus* found no evidence for trans-ovarial transmission (MacLeod and Gordon 1933) and subsequently, consensus agreed with these findings. However, conflicting evidence has occasionally been published; for example, a report of the natural transmission of infection to sentinel mice by an *I. spinipalpis* larvum (Burkot *et al.* 2001), and, perhaps more compelling, experimental evidence for infection in a small proportion of experimentally-reared *D. albipictus* larvae (Baldridge *et al.* 2009).

There is increasing evidence that although *A. phagocytophilum* can be considered a generalist, within the species are subpopulations, or ecotypes, adapted to specific host and vectors. An ecotype specifically adapted to exploiting white-tailed deer rather than

other mammals has been encountered in the USA (Massung *et al.* 2002; Massung *et al.* 2005) and studied in some depth (Massung *et al.* 2003; Massung *et al.* 2007). Evidence for other host-restricted *A. phagocytophilum* ecotypes in the USA has also emerged (Foley *et al.* 2009). Furthermore, the existence of different ecotypes circulating in distinct yet coexisting transmission cycles has been described in the UK (Bown *et al.* 2009). Interestingly, the basis of this distinction appears to be the adaptation of *A. phagocytophilum* ecotypes to specific vector species rather than their reservoirs (Bown *et al.* 2009).

N. sennetsu

Very little is known about the ecology of *Neorickettsia sennetsu*. Its natural cycle is unknown but is thought to involve infection of fish-associated trematodes. Human infection results from the consumption of uncooked fish that are parasitized by infected trematodes. An organism referred to as the SF agent has been identified in *Stellantchasmus falcatus* flukes parasitizing gray mullet (*Mugil cephalus*)(Wen *et al.* 1996), but this organism does not appear to be the same as the human-infecting *N. sennetsu*. The recent rediscovery of sennetsu neorickettsiosis in Laos (Newton *et al.* 2009) provoked exploration of possible sources of infection, with *N. sennetsu* DNA being detected in a gill tissue samples from a climbing perch (*Anabas testudineus*).

Microbiology and pathogenesis

All these pathogens are obligate intracellular Gram-negative bacteria belonging to the order Rickettsiales within the α subclass of the proteobacteria. *E. chaffeensis* and *N. sennetsu* have a tropism for monocytes, whereas *E. ewingii* and *A. phagocytophilum* parasitize neutrophils. Given the role of these cell types at the frontline of innate antimicrobial defence, it is remarkable that bacteria have evolved to exploit such potentially toxic targets. The unique molecular and cellular mechanisms that underlie this exploitation have begun to be unravelled, and themes common to *Ehrlichia* and *Anaplasma* have emerged. Both genera of bacteria possess cell walls that lack peptidoglycan and lipopolysaccharide (LPS), and the absence of these molecules strips the bacteria of two of the key triggers of host immunity. Without these two pathogen-associated molecular patterns (PAMPs), the bacteria cannot be effectively recognized by Toll-like receptors and other monocytic and granulocytic cell surface molecules, thereby facilitating their survival inside the host (Rikihisa 2010). Arthropod innate immunity is also responsive to PAMPs, hence the lack of peptidoglycan and LPS in *Ehrlichia* and *Anaplasma* species is likely to also facilitate exploitation of their tick vectors.

Differential recognition of cell surface receptors is likely to underlie the different cell tropisms of *E. chaffeensis* and *A. phagocytophilum*. Receptors for *A. phagocytophilum* on the neutrophil cell surface have been identified, and binding to these, and maybe other as yet unrecognized molecules, is thought to provoke endocytosis (Carlyon and Fikrig 2006; Rikihisa 2010). Both *Ehrlichia* and *Anaplasma* species remain within the phagosome but inhibit its fusion with lysosomes or NAPDH oxidase components, thereby preventing its acidification and creating an intracellular niche in which to replicate (Carlyon and Fikrig 2006; Rikihisa 2010). Exploration of the influence of intracellular infection on host cell physiology has revealed significant changes in iron metabolism and inhibition of interferon gamma signalling pathways (Rikihisa 2010). The exploitation of neutrophils and monocytes is extended by prolonging their lifespan through the inhibition/delay of apoptosis (Carlyon and Fikrig 2006; Rikihisa 2010). Both *E. chaffeensis* and *A. phagocytophilum* upregulate production of several proinflammatory cytokines including IL-1β and IL-8, which may result in the recruitment of additional neutrophils and monocytes to the site of infection (Carlyon and Fikrig 2006; Rikihisa 2010). *A. phagocytophilum* and *E. chaffeensis* possess type 4 secretion systems (T4SS) that bring about host cell subversion via the export of bacterial effector molecules, and, in both species, upregulation of T4SS is associated with intracellular growth (Rikihisa 2010). T4SS effector molecules are beginning to be identified; *A. phagocytophilum* delivers at least two proteins via its T4SS, AnkA and Ats1 (Niu *et al.* 2010). Whereas AnkA migrates to the neutrophil nucleus, Ats1 travels to, and enters mitochondria, where it is thought to act by reducing the sensitivity of mitochondria to respond to apoptosis-inducing factors, leading to the inhibition of host cell apoptosis (Niu *et al.* 2010).

Exploitation of reservoir hosts by *A. phagocytophilum* is characterized by chronic infection. During this time the bacteria must circumvent host immunity. Work outlined above has explored how *A. phagocytophilum* subverts innate immunity during the acute phase of infection, but, in order to chronically persist, it must also counter acquired humoral responses; antibodies are produced in abundance by infected hosts, but appear to be ineffective in curtailing infection. The basis for this failure appears to be the ability of *A. phagocytophilum* to express a multitude of antigenic variants during the course of infection, thus, although variants dominating during the first weeks of infection will eventually be countered by specific antibodies, other variants will replace those lost, thereby facilitating persistence. *A. phagocytophilum* possesses a number of immunogenic surface proteins, but one, termed P44 (MSP2), is immunodominant (Dumler *et al.* 1995). Exploration of the *A. phagocytophilum* genome has revealed that it contains more than 100 well dispersed *msp2* pseudogenes characterized by conserved sequences flanking a hypervariable region (Caspersen *et al.* 2002; Zhi *et al.* 1999), and these pseudogenes are inserted into a unique *msp2* expression site by gene combinatorial conversion mechanisms (Zhi *et al.* 1999; Barbet *et al.* 2003). Some experimental evidence for the sequential expression of different pseudogenes during the course of prolonged infection has been obtained (Barbet *et al.* 2003; Granquist *et al.* 2008; Wang *et al.* 2004).

As well as possessing a wide diversity of mechanisms for interaction with their reservoir hosts, *Ehrlichia* and *Anaplasma* species must also exploit ticks to complete their natural cycles. Very little is known about the mechanisms that underlie this exploitation. However, studies have revealed that *A. phagocytophilum* persists within the secretory salivary acini of tick salivary glands (Telford *et al.* 1996), and that tick feeding stimulates the replication and migration of the bacteria from the salivary glands to the mammalian host (Hodzic *et al.* 2001). Studies suggest that transmission of *A. phagocytophilum* occurs between 24 and 48 hours after tick attachment (Katavolos *et al.* 1998), and acquisition of *A. phagocytophilum* by uninfected *I. scapularis* larva begins within two days of tick attachment on *A. phagocytophilum*-infected mice (Hodzic *et al.* 1998). Once in the tick, *A. phagocytophilum* moves across the gut wall and infects the salivary glands, a migration that occurs as early as 24 hours after engorgement (Sukumaran *et al.* 2006).

During tick engorgement, *A. phagocytophilum* is thought to induce expression of salivary gland proteins to facilitate its transmission. One such protein, Salp16, has been characterized and its essential role in *A. phagocytophilum* survival demonstrated (Sukumaran *et al.* 2006), although the mechanism underlying this interaction remains to be elucidated. Very recently, it has been shown that *A. phagocytophilum* also interacts with α1,3-fucose to facilitate its acquisition by ticks (Pedra *et al.* 2010).

Comparative genomics of *A. phagocytophilum*, *E. chaffeensis* and *N. sennetsu* has been reported following the sequencing of complete genomes for each and for a number of close relatives (Dunning Hotopp *et al.* 2006). All three species have single, circular genomes, but differ quite markedly in size. The *N. sennetsu* genome is only 860 kilobases, whereas that of *E. chaffeensis* is 1.18 megabases and that of *A. phagocytophilum* is almost 1.5 megabases. These differences are, in part, due to a remarkably large expansion of immunodominant outer membrane proteins that is thought to facilitate antigen variation in *Anaplasma* and *Ehrlichia* species. Unlike their near-neighbours within the Rickettsiales, these two genera have also retained the ability to make vitamins, enzyme co-factors and nucleotides for themselves. That *N. sennetsu* possesses a far less expansive inventory of genes suggests that the complexity of its natural cycle is less than those of *A. phagocytophilum* and *E. chaffeensis*, which involve mammalian hosts and arthropod vectors (Dunning Hotopp *et al.* 2006).

Disease in humans

E. chaffeensis, *E. ewingii* and *A. phagocytophilum* infections can be transmitted to humans through the bite of a single tick. Onset of symptoms occurs between one week and three weeks after being bitten. All infections range dramatically in severity, from asymptomatic seroconversion to a severe febrile illness and even organ failure and death. Most patients present with non-specific symptoms such as headache, fever, malaise, and myalgia, eliminating the possibility of a reliable clinical diagnosis. However, identifying risk factors can help steer a clinician towards a diagnosis; thus, it is important to establish if a patient has had a recent tick bite, or even if he/she has been pursuing outdoor activity in tick-infested areas at the time of the year when questing ticks are most prevalent. Another potentially useful indicator is the presentation of a similar illness in other family members or even pet dogs (Thomas *et al.* 2009); temporal and geographical clusters of HME have been reported (Standaert *et al.* 1995; Yevich *et al.* 1995). However, as many people do not realise they have been bitten by ticks, a patient's ignorance of tick bite should not exclude diagnosis of HME or HGA.

A recent meta-analysis of HME and HGA symptoms, signs and clinical laboratory findings indicated that fever was the most common symptom, occurring in over 90% of patients, and that over 75% of patients reported headaches and malaise. Myalgia occurred in 77% of HGA patients, but only 57% of those with HME. Other relatively common symptoms included nausea, vomiting, diarrhoea, cough, and arthralgias. A rash appeared on 31% of HME patients, but only 6% of HGA patients (Dumler *et al.* 2007). Common clinical laboratory findings include leukopenia (62% HME, 49% HGA), thrombocytopenia (71% HME and HGA), and elevated serum aspartate aminotransferase or alanine aminotransferase levels (83% HME, 71% HGA) (Dumler *et al.* 2007). Thus, the key to diagnosing HME or HGA is the identification of fever and thrombocytopenia, leukopenia and elevated serum aminotransferase levels in a patient with a history of tick bite or who is likely to have been exposed to tick bite in areas where these diseases are extant. 42% of HME patients and between 33 and 50% of HGA patients are hospitalized, primarily to rule out more sinister differentials (Dumler *et al.* 2007). Complications are not very common, although between 7–17% of patients may develop serious, life threatening syndromes; HME patients can develop fulminant toxic shock, particularly those with underlying immunocompromise, and HGA infection can progress to involve the central nervous system, with peripheral neuropathies, including brachial plexopathy, demyelinating polyneuropathy and facial palsy being the most common presentations (Dumler *et al.* 2007). Deaths are extremely rare.

Most commonly, patients with sennetsu neorickettsiosis experience sudden-onset chills and a fever of 38–39°C, which lasts for approximately two weeks. Other manifestations include headache, malaise, myalgias, arthromyalgia, pharyngitis and generalized lymphadenopathy (Tachibana 1986). The most recent case report relates to a patient from Laos (Newton *et al.* 2009), who presented with a two week history of fever, headache and weakness, and who, on admission, was pale, jaundiced and febrile, with palpable inguinal and cervical lymph nodes and hepato-splenomegaly. He was anaemic but had normal peripheral white cell count except relative and absolute lymphocytosis and raised liver enzymes. Treatment with ofloxacin led to rapid resolution of all symptoms and the patient was discharged five days after admission.

Diagnosis

Given the non-specific clinical presentation of *Anaplasma* and *Ehrlichia* infections, laboratory confirmation of aetiology is essential. The simplest and cheapest means of providing this confirmation is the microscopic examination of Giemsa or Wright-stained peripheral blood smears. Inclusions of bacteria, termed morulae, stain purple within neutrophils (*A. phagocytophilum* or *E. ewingii*) or monocytes (*E. chaffeensis*). This approach is most sensitive during the first week of infection, but is considerably better for diagnosing *A. phagocytophilum* infections than those caused by *E. chaffeensis*; only about 10% of HME patients have visible intra-monocytic morulae, compared to between 25–75% of HGA patients (Dumler *et al.* 2007). PCR-based methods, performed using blood held on anticoagulant, are now the diagnostic test of choice, particularly when samples are taken soon after the patient has first presented. A variety of assays have been described and their sensitivity is relatively high, ranging from 60–85% for *E. chaffeensis* infection and 65–90% for *A. phagocytophilum* infection (Dumler *et al.* 2007). This difference may be due to *A. phagocytophilum* provoking more intense bacteraemia, although it may also reflect more sensitive assays; for example, PCR targeting conserved sections of p44 pseudogenes, which exist in excess of 100 copies per genome, is likely to significantly enhance the sensitivity of *A. phagocytophilum*-specific assays (Courtney *et al.* 2004). PCR is currently the only definitive test for *E. ewingii* infection. The sensitivity of both blood smear analysis and PCR-based assays for all three pathogens is adversely affected by antecedent antibiotic treatment, thus, if possible, blood samples should be collected before initiation of therapy (Dumler *et al.* 2007).

Proof of ongoing infection is unequivocally obtained by *in vitro* cultivation of bacteria. This is possible for *E. chaffeensis* and *A. phagocytophilum*, but not for *E. ewingii*, which, to date, has resisted all isolation attempts. However, the obligate intracellular nature of these pathogens requires that they are co-cultured with appropriate eukaryotic cell lines and thus the routine use of this approach is limited to a relatively small number of reference laboratories that have the relevant facilities and expertise. *E. chaffeensis* and *A. phagocytophilum* grow in a variety of cell lines, but *E. chaffeensis* is most often isolated by inoculation of monocytes into the DH82 canine histiocytic cell line (Standaert *et al.* 2000). Typically, co-cultures must be incubated for up to six weeks before infected cells are detected (Dumler *et al.* 2007). *A. phagocytophilum* is most frequently isolated by inoculation of leukocytes into HL60, a human promyelocytic leukaemia cell line (Goodman *et al.* 1996). Again, patience is required as infected cells may not become apparent for several weeks after inoculation (Dumler *et al.* 2007). Alternative cell lines, specifically those derived from *Ixodes* ticks, are now being increasingly used for the cultivation of *A. phagocytophilum* strains (Munderloh *et al.* 1994).

Serodiagnosis is the most frequently used approach to laboratory confirmation of *E. chaffeensis* and *A. phagocytophilum* infections (but not for *E. ewingii* as, in the absence of isolates, suitable antigen cannot be produced). Although of no use for identifying acute-phase infections, serology has proven an extremely sensitive means of confirming aetiology at two weeks or more after onset of symptoms (Walls *et al.* 1999). Infections are confirmed using the classical criteria of a four-fold increase in antibody titre or a seroconversion to a titre of 128 or higher. However, a task force aimed at developing a consensus approach to diagnosis of HME has also proposed that a single titre of 64 or greater is highly suggestive of infection, and a single titre of greater than 256 is indicative of infection (Walker *et al.* 2000). Nonetheless, as IgG antibodies can persist for many months, antibody titres must be considered in the context of the patient's clinical history (Thomas *et al.* 2009). Immunofluorescence assays, incorporating whole cell antigens, are the most commonly used format for serodiagnosis, and have a sensitivity rate of about 90% for HME and between 80–100% for HGA (Dumler *et al.* 2007). The specificity of serodiagnosis of HGA has been estimated to be between 83–100% (Dumler *et al.* 2007), although cross-reactivity between *E. chaffeensis*, *E. ewingii* and *A. phagocytophilum* antibodies can occur (Buller *et al.* 1999; Dumler *et al.* 2007). Furthermore, sera from patients with Rocky Mountain spotted fever, Q fever, brucellosis, Lyme disease and Epstein Barr virus infection, together with those with autoimmune conditions, may provoke false positive serological test results (Dumler *et al.* 2007), re-emphasizing the importance of a polyphasic diagnostic approach, combining, if possible, a variety of laboratory methods and clinical examination.

The recent case of sennetsu neorickettsiosis was diagnosed using PCR-based assays to amplify *N. sennetsu* DNA fragments from buffy coat (Newton *et al.* 2009). This study also used a micro-immunofluoresence assay and Western blotting to screen patients with fever of unknown origin and/or jaundice for *N. sennetsu* antibodies. The antigen for both assays was whole cell *N. sennetsu* Miyayama strain (ATCC VR367). Western blotting revealed an apparent *N. sennetsu*-specific antigen of about 25 kilodaltons size (Newton *et al.* 2009).

Treatment, prevention and control

The two antibiotics most commonly prescribed for the treatment of *Ehrlichia* and *Anaplasma* infections are doxycycline and tetracycline. Doxycycline is probably considered the drug of choice as it has a less frequent dosage. Although prolonged or repeated exposure to this antibiotic increases the risk of dental staining, its limited use has negligible effect. Indeed, the Committee on Infectious Diseases of the American Academy of Pediatrics promotes the use of doxycycline for the treatment of ehrlichiosis in children of all ages (Dumler *et al.* 2007). The recommended dosage for doxycycline is 100 milligrams for adults, and 2.2 milligrams per kilogram for children, given orally every 12 hours for between 5 and 14 days. Tetracycline is orally administered every six hours at a dosage of 500 milligrams per day for adults or 25 milligrams to 50 milligrams per kilogram per day for children. Clinical response to treatment is usually dramatic, with marked resolution of symptoms with 48 hours and full recovery within a few days. Prophylactic antibiotic treatment for those bitten by ticks is not recommended because most people who get bitten by ticks do not develop an *Ehrlichia* or *Anaplasma* infection.

The best way for preventing HME or HGA is to avoid tick bites. However, this does not preclude outdoor activities; wearing protective clothing such as boots or solid shoes, long trousers tucked into socks and long-sleeves shirts, or using repellent sprays will markedly reduce the risk of tick bite. Although the rapid removal of ticks from the skin does not necessarily exclude the chance of infection, being aware of tick bite, and informing the clinician of this if symptoms should develop, will greatly facilitate accurate diagnosis of *Ehrlichia* and *Anaplasma* infections, hence the prescription of an appropriate treatment regimen.

In cell culture, *N. sennetsu* is sensitive to doxycycline, ciprofloxacin and rifampicin (Brouqui and Raoult 1990) although the relative efficacies of these antibiotics for the treatment of infections remains untested. A recent case report described apparently successful treatment with ofloxacin (Newton *et al.* 2009).

N. sennetsu infections are closely linked with the consumption of uncooked fish, and thus are considered preventable by appropriate cooking. However, raw fish form part of the staple diet of many in Eastern and South Eastern Asia, as demonstrated by the widespread human *Opisthorchis* and *Clonorchis* liver fluke infections, which are also acquired from this source (Sripa 2008).

References

Anderson, B.E., Dawson, J.E., Jones, D.C. and Wilson, K.H. (1991). *Ehrlichia chaffeensis*, a new species associated with human ehrlichiosis. *J. Clin. Microbiol.*, **29**: 2838–42.

Anderson, B.E., Greene, C.E., Jones, D.C. and Dawson, J.E. (1992). *Ehrlichia ewingii* sp. nov., the etiologic agent of canine granulocytic ehrlichiosis. *Inter. J. System. Bacteriol.*, **42**: 299–302.

Anziani, O.S., Ewing, S.A. and Barker, R.W. (1990). Experimental transmission of a granulocytic form of the tribe Ehrlichieae by *Dermacentor variabilis* and *Amblyomma americanum* to dogs. *Am. J. Vet. Res.*, **51**: 929–31.

Bakken, J.S., Dumler, J.S., Chen, S.M., Eckman, M.R., Van Etta, L.L. *et al.* (1994). Human granulocytic ehrlichiosis in the upper Midwest United States. A new species emerging? *J. Am. Med. Assoc.*, **272**: 212–18.

Baldridge, G.D., Scoles, G.A., Burkhardt, N.Y., Schloeder, B., Kurtti, T.J. *et al.* (2009). Transovarial transmission of *Francisella*-like endosymbionts and *Anaplasma phagocytophilum* variants in *Dermacentor albipictus* (Acari: Ixodidae). *J. Med. Entomol.*, **46**: 625–32.

Barandika, J.F., Hurtado, A., García-Sanmartín, J., Juste, R.A., Anda, P. *et al.* (2008). Prevalence of tick-borne zoonotic bacteria in questing adult ticks from northern Spain. *Vector Borne Zoon. Dis.*, **8**: 829–35.

Barbet, A.F., Meeus, P.F., Bélanger, M. *et al.* (2003). Expression of multiple outer membrane protein sequence variants from a single genomic locus of *Anaplasma phagocytophilum*. *Infect. Immun.*, **71**: 1706–18.

Barlough, J.E., Madigan, J.E., Kramer, V.L. *et al.* (1996). *Ehrlichia phagocytophila* genogroup rickettsiae in ixodid ticks from California collected in 1995 and 1996. *J. Clin. Microbiol.*, **35**: 2018–21.

Bown, K.J., Begon, M., Bennett, M., Woldehiwet, Z. and Ogden, N.H. (2003). Seasonal dynamics of *Anaplasma phagocytophila* in a rodent-tick (*Ixodes trianguliceps*) system, United Kingdom. *Emerg. Infect. Dis.*, **9**: 63–70.

Bown, K.J., Lambin, X., Ogden, N.H. *et al.* (2009). Delineating *Anaplasma phagocytophilum* ecotypes in coexisting, discrete enzootic cycles. *Emerg. Infect. Dis.*, **15**: 1948–54.

Brouqui, P. and Raoult, D. (1990). In vitro susceptibility of *Ehrlichia sennetsu* to antibiotics. *Antimicrob. Agents and Chemother.*, **34**: 1593–96.

Buller, R.S., Arens, M., Hmiel, S.P. *et al.* (1999). *Ehrlichia ewingii*, a newly recognized agent of human ehrlichiosis. *N. Engl. J. Med.*, **341**: 148–55.

Burkot, T.R., Maupin, G.O., Schneider, B.S. *et al.* (2001). Use of a sentinel host system to study the questing behavior of *Ixodes spinipalpis* and its role in the transmission of *Borrelia bissettii*, human granulocytic ehrlichiosis, and *Babesia microti*. *Am. J. Trop. Med. Hyg.*, **65**: 293–99.

Carlyon, J.A. and Fikrig, E. (2006). Mechanisms of evasion of neutrophil killing by *Anaplasma phagocytophilum*. *Curr. Opin. Hematol.*, **13**: 28–33.

Cao, W.C., Zhan, L., He, J. *et al.* (2006). Natural *Anaplasma phagocytophilum* infection of ticks and rodents from a forest area of Jilin Province, China. *Am. J. Trop. Med. Hyg.*, **75**: 664–68.

Cao, W.C., Zhao, Q.M., Zhang, P.H. *et al.* (2000). Granulocytic ehrlichiae in *Ixodes persulcatus* ticks from an area in China where Lyme disease is endemic. *J. Clin. Microbiol.*, **38**: 4208–10.

Caspersen, K., Park, J.H., Patil, S. and Dumler, J.S. (2002). Genetic variability and stability of *Anaplasma phagocytophila msp2* (*p44*). *Infect. Immun.*, **70**: 1230–34.

Centers for Disease Control and Prevention (2010). Notifiable diseases and mortality tables. *Morb. Mort. Wkly. Rep.*, **59**: 1461.

Chen, S.M., Dumler, J.S., Bakken, J.S. and Walker, D.H. (1994). Identification of a granulocytotropic *Ehrlichia* species as the etiologic agent of human disease. *J. Clin. Microbiol.*, **32**: 589–95.

Courtney, J.W., Kostelnik, L.M., Zeidner, N.S. and Massung, R.F (2004). Multiplex real-time PCR for detection of *Anaplasma phagocytophilum* and *Borrelia burgdorferi*. *J. Clin. Microbiol.*, **42**: 3164–68.

Davidson, W.R., Lockhart, J.M., Stallknecht, D.E., Howerth, E.W., Dawson, J.E. *et al.* (2001). Persistent *Ehrlichia chaffeensis* infection in white-tailed deer. *J. Wildlife Dis.*, **37**: 538–46.

Dumler, J.S., Asanovich, K.M., Bakken, J.S., Richter, P., Kimsey, R. *et al.* (1995). Serologic cross-reactions among *Ehrlichia equi*, *Ehrlichia phagocytophila*, and human granulocytic *Ehrlichia*. *J. Clin. Microbiol.*, **33**: 1098–103.

Dumler, J.S., Barbet, A.F., Bekker, C.P. *et al.* (2001). Reorganization of genera in the families *Rickettsiaceae* and *Anaplasmataceae* in the order Rickettsiales: unification of some species of *Ehrlichia* with *Anaplasma*, *Cowdria* with *Ehrlichia* and *Ehrlichia* with *Neorickettsia*, descriptions of six new species combinations and designation of *Ehrlichia equi* and 'HGE agent' as subjective synonyms of *Ehrlichia phagocytophila*. *Inter. J. System. Evolut. Microbiol.*, **51**: 2145–65.

Dumler, J.S., Madigan, J.E., Pusterla, N. and Bakken, J.S. (2007). Ehrlichioses in humans: epidemiology, clinical presentation, diagnosis, and treatment. *Clin. Infect. Dis.*, **45**: S45–51.

Dunning Hotopp, J.C., Lin, M., Madupu, R. *et al.* (2006). Comparative genomics of emerging human ehrlichiosis agents. *PLoS Genetics*, **2**: e21.

Ewing, S.A., Dawson, J.E., Mathew, J.S., Barker, R.W., Pratt, K.W. *et al.* (1997). Attempted transmission of human granulocytotropic ehrlichia (HGE) by *Amblyomma americanum* and *Amblyomma maculatum*. *Vet. Parasitol.*, **70**: 183–90.

Foley, J.E., Nieto, N.C., Adjemian, J., Dabritz, H. and Brown, R.N. (2008). *Anaplasma phagocytophilum* infection in small mammal hosts of *Ixodes* ticks, western United States. *Emerg. Infect. Dis.*, **14**: 1147–50.

Foley, J.E., Nieto, N.C., Massung, R., Barbet, A., Madigan, J. *et al.* (2009). Distinct ecologically relevant strains of *Anaplasma phagocytophilum*. *Emerg. Infect. Dis.*, **15**: 842–43.

Gabriel, M.W., Brown, R.N., Foley, J.E., Higley, J.M. and Botzler, R.G. (2009). Ecology of *Anaplasma phagocytophilum* infection in gray foxes (*Urocyon cinereoargenteus*) in northwestern California. *J. Wildlife Dis.*, **45**: 344–54.

Gao, D., Cao, W. and Zhang, X. (2001). Investigations on human ehrlichial infections in people in the Daxingan Mountains. *Chinese J. Epidemiol.*, **22**: 137–41.

Goodman, J.L., Nelson, C., Vitale, B. *et al.* (1996). Direct cultivation of the causative agent of human granulocytic ehrlichiosis. *N. Engl. J. Med.*, **334**: 209–15.

Granquist, E.G., Stuen, S., Lundgren, A.M., Bråten, M. and Barbet, A.F. (2008). Outer membrane protein sequence variation in lambs experimentally infected with *Anaplasma phagocytophilum*. *Infect. Immun.*, **76**: 120–26.

Gribble, D.H. (1969). Equine ehrlichiosis. *J. Am. Vet. Med. Assoc.*, **155**: 462–69.

Hodzic, E., Borjesson, D.L., Feng, S. and Barthold, S.W. (2001). Acquisition dynamics of Borrelia burgdorferi and the agent of human granulocytic ehrlichiosis at the host-vector interface. *Vector Borne Zoon. Dis.*, **1**: 149–58.

Holden, K., Boothby, J.T., Anand, S. and Massung, R.F. (2003). Detection of *Borrelia burgdorferi*, *Ehrlichia chaffeensis* and *Anaplasma phagocytophilum* in ticks (Acari: Ixodidae) from a coastal region of California. *J. Med. Entomol.*, **40**: 534–39.

Katavolos, P., Armstrong, P.M., Dawson, J.E. and Telford, S.R. 3rd. (1998). Duration of tick attachment required for transmission of granulocytic ehrlichiosis. *J. Infect. Dis.*, **177**: 1422–25.

Kawahara, M., Rikihisa, Y., Lin, Q. *et al.* (2006). Novel genetic variants of *Anaplasma phagocytophilum*, *Anaplasma bovis*, *Anaplasma centrale*, and a novel *Ehrlichia* sp. in wild deer and ticks on two major islands in Japan. *Appl. Environ. Microbiol.*, **72**: 1102–9.

Kim, C.M., Kim, M.S., Park, M.S., Park, J.H. and Chae, J.S. (2003). Identification of *Ehrlichia chaffeensis*, *Anaplasma phagocytophilum*, and *A. bovis* in *Haemaphysalis longicornis* and *Ixodes persulcatus* ticks from Korea. *Vector Borne Zoon. Dis.*, **3**: 17–26.

Liddell, A.M., Stockham, S.L., Scott, M.A. *et al.* (2003). Predominance of *Ehrlichia ewingii* in Missouri dogs. *J. Clin. Microbiol.*, **41**: 4617–22.

Lotric-Furlan, S., Petrovec, M., Avsic-Zupanc, T. and Strle, F. (2004). Comparison of patients fulfilling criteria for confirmed and probable human granulocytic ehrlichiosis. *Scandan. J. Infect. Dis.*, **36**: 817–22.

MacLeod, J. and Gordon, W.S. (1933). Studies on tick-borne fever of sheep. I. Transmission by the tick *Ixodes ricinus* with a description of the disease produced. *Parasit.*, **25**: 273–83.

Madewell, B.R. and Gribble, D.H. (1982). Infection in two dogs with an agent resembling *Ehrlichia equi*. *J. Am. Vet. Med. Assoc.*, **180**: 512–14.

Maeda, K., Markowitz, N., Hawley, R.C., Ristic, M., Cox, D. *et al.* (1987). Human infection with *Ehrlichia canis*, a leukocytic rickettsia. *N. Engl. J. Med.*, **316**: 853–56.

Martínez, M.C., Gutiérrez, C.N., Monger, F. *et al.* (2008). *Ehrlichia chaffeensis* in child, Venezuela. *Emerg. Infect. Dis.*, **14**: 519–20.

Massung, R.F., Courtney, J.W., Hiratzka, S.L., Pitzer, V.E., Smith, G. *et al.* (2005). *Anaplasma phagocytophilum* in white-tailed deer. *Emerg. Infect. Dis.*, **11**: 1604–6.

Massung, R.F., Mauel, M.J., Owens, J.H. *et al.* (2002). Genetic variants of *Ehrlichia phagocytophila*, Rhode Island, and Connecticut. *Emerg. Infect. Dis.*, **8**: 467–72.

Massung, R.F., Priestley, R.A., Miller, N.J., Mather, T.N., and Levin, M.L. (2003). Inability of a variant strain of *Anaplasma phagocytophilum* to infect mice. *J. Infect. Dis.*, **188**: 1757–63.

Massung, R.F., Levin, M.L., Munderloh, U.G. *et al.* (2007). Isolation and propagation of the Ap-Variant 1 strain of *Anaplasma phagocytophilum* in a tick cell line. *J. Clin. Microbiol.*, **45**: 2138–43.

McDiarmid, A. (1965). Modern trends in animal health and husbandry. Some infectious diseases of free-living wildlife. *Brit. Vet. J.*, **121**: 245–57.

Merten, H.A. and Durden, L.A. (2000). A state-by-state survey of ticks recorded from humans in the United States. *J. Vector Ecol.*, **25**: 102–13.

Misao, T. and Katsuta, K. (1965). Epidemiology of infectious mononucleosis. *Jap. J. Clin. Experim. Med.*, **33**: 73–82.

Misao, T. and Kobayashi, Y. (1954). Studies on infectious mononucleosis I. Isolation of etiologic agent from blood, bone marrow and lymph node of a patients with infectious mononucleosis by using mice. *Tokyo Med. J.*, **71**: 683–86.

Munderloh, U.G., Liu, Y., Wang, M., Chen, C. and Kurtti, T. (1994). Establishment, maintenance and description of cell lines from the tick *Ixodes scapularis*. *J. Parasitol.*, **80**: 533–43.

Ndip, L.M., Labruna, M., Ndip, R.N., Walker, D.H. and McBride, J.W. (2009). Molecular and clinical evidence of *Ehrlichia chaffeensis* infection in Cameroonian patients with undifferentiated febrile illness. *Ann. Trop. Med. Parasitol.*, **103**: 719–25.

Newton, P.N., Rolain, J.M., Rasachak, B. *et al.* (2009). Sennetsu neorickettsiosis: a probable fish-borne cause of fever rediscovered in Laos. *Am. J. Trop. Med. Hyg.*, **81**: 190–94.

Nieto, N.C., Foley, J.E., Bettaso, J. and Lane, R.S. (2009). Reptile infection with *Anaplasma phagocytophilum*, the causative agent of granulocytic anaplasmosis. *J. Parasitol.*, **95**: 1165–70.

Niu, H., Kozjak-Pavlovic, V., Rudel, T. and Rikihisa, Y. (2010). *Anaplasma phagocytophilum* Ats-1 is imported into host cell mitochondria and interferes with apoptosis induction. *PLoS Patho.*, **6**: e1000774.

Ohashi, N., Inayoshi, M., Kitamura, K. *et al.* (2005). *Anaplasma phagocytophilum*-infected ticks, Japan. *Emerg. Infect. Dis.*, **11**: 1780–83.

Paddock, C.D. and Childs, J.E. (2003). *Ehrlichia chaffeensis*: a prototypical emerging pathogen. *Clin. Microbiol. Rev.*, **16**: 37–64.

Pancholi, P., Kolbert, C.P., Mitchell, P.D. *et al.* (1995). *Ixodes dammini* as a potential vector of human granulocytic ehrlichiosis. *J. Infect. Dis.*, **172**: 1007–12.

Pedra, J.H., Narasimhan, S., Rendi, D. *et al.* (2010). Fucosylation enhances colonisation of ticks by *Anaplasma phagocytophilum*. *Cell. Microbiol.*, epub ahead of print.

Rikihisa, Y. (1991). The tribe *Ehrlichieae* and ehrlichial diseases. *Clin. Microbiol. Rev.*, **4**: 286–308.

Rikihisa, Y. (2010). Molecular events involved in cellular invasion by *Ehrlichia chaffeensis* and *Anaplasma phagocytophilum*. *Vet. Parasitol.*, **167**: 155–66.

Ristic, M. (1990). Current strategies in research on ehrlichiosis. In: J.C. Williams and I. Kakoma (eds.) *Ehrlichiosis: a vector-borne disease of animals and humans*, pp. 1369–53. Boston, USA: Kluwer Academic Publishers.

Santos, A.S., Santos-Silva, M.M., Almeida, V.C., Bacellar, F. and Dumler, J.S. (2004). Detection of *Anaplasma phagocytophilum* DNA in *Ixodes* ticks (Acari: Ixodidae) from Madeira Island and Setubal District, mainland Portugal. *Emerg. Infect. Dis.*, **10**: 1643–48.

Sarih, M., M'Ghirbi, Y., Bouattour, A., Gern, L., Baranton, G. *et al.* (2005). Detection and identification of *Ehrlichia* spp. in ticks collected in Tunisia and Morocco. *J. Clin. Microbiol.*, **43**: 1127–32.

Sripa, B. (2008). Concerted action is needed to tackle liver fluke infections in Asia. *PLoS Neglect. Trop. Dis.*, **2**: e232.

Scharlemann, J.P., Johnson, P.J., Smith, A.A., Macdonald, D.W. and Randolph, S.E. (2008). Trends in ixodid tick abundance and distribution in Great Britain. *Med. Vet. Entomol.*, **22**: 238–47.

Standaert, S.M., Dawson, J.E., Schaffner, W. *et al.* (1995). Ehrlichiosis in a golf-oriented retirement community. *N. Engl. J. Med.*, **333**: 420–25.

Standaert, S.M., Yu, T., Scott, M.A. *et al.* (2000). Primary isolation of *Ehrlichia chaffeensis* from patients with febrile illnesses: clinical and molecular characteristics. *J. Infect. Dis.*, **181**: 1082–88.

Sukumaran, B., Narasimhan, S., Anderson, J.F. *et al.* (2006). An *Ixodes scapularis* protein required for survival of *Anaplasma phagocytophilum* in tick salivary glands. *J. Experim. Med.*, **203**: 1507–17.

Tachibana, N. (1986). Sennetsu fever: the disease, diagnosis and treatment. In: L. Leive (ed.) *Microbiology*, pp. 205–08. Washington DC, USA: American Society of Microbiology.

Telford III, S.R., Dawson, J.E., Katavolos, P., Warner, C.K., Kolbert, C.P. *et al.* (1996). Perpetuation of the agent of human granulocytic ehrlichiosis in a deer tick-rodent cycle. *Proc. Nat. Acad. Sci. USA*, **93**: 6209–14.

Thomas, R.J., Dumler, J.S. and Carlyon, J.A. (2009). Current management of human granulocytic anaplasmosis, human monocytic ehrlichiosis and *Ehrlichia ewingii* ehrlichiosis. *Expert. Rev. Anti-Infect. Ther.*, 7: 709–22.

Toledo, A., Olmeda, A.S., Escudero, R. *et al.* (2009). Tick-borne zoonotic bacteria in ticks collected from central Spain. *Am. J. Trop. Med. Hyg.*, **81**: 67–74.

Tyzzer, E.E. (1938). *Cytœcetes microti* n.g. n.sp. a parasite developing in granulocytes and infective for small rodents. *Parasitol.*, **30**: 242–57.

Víchová, B., Majláthová, V., Nováková, M., Straka, M. and Pet'ko, B. (2009). First molecular detection of *Anaplasma phagocytophilum* in European Brown Bear (*Ursus arctos*). *Vector Borne Zoon. Dis.*, epub ahead of print.

Walker, D.H. and the Task Force on Consensus Approach for Ehrlichiosis. (2000). Diagnosing Human Ehrlichioses: Current Status and Recommendations. *Am. Soc. Microbiol. News*, **66**: 287–90.

Walls, J.J., Aguero-Rosenfeld, M., Bakken, J.S. *et al.* (1999). Inter- and intra-laboratory comparison of *Ehrlichia equi* and human granulocytic ehrlichiosis (HGE) agent strains for serodiagnosis of HGE by the immunofluorescent-antibody test. *J. Clin. Microbiol.*, **37**: 2968–73.

Wang, X., Rikihisa, Y., Lai, T.H., Kumagai, Y., Zhi, N. *et al.* (2004). Rapid sequential changeover of expressed p44 genes during the acute phase of *Anaplasma phagocytophilum* infection in horses. *Infect. Immun.*, **72**: 6852–59.

Weiss, E., Dasch, G.A., Williams, J.C. and Kang, Y-H. (1990). Biological properties of the genus Ehrlichia: substrate utilization and energy metabolism. In: **J.C.** Williams and I. Kakoma (eds.) *Ehrlichiosis: a vector-borne disease of animals and humans*, pp. 59–67. Boston, USA: Kluwer Academic Publishers.

Wen, B., Rikihisa, Y., Yamamoto, S., Kawabata, N. and Fuerst, P.A. (1996). Characterization of the SF agent, an *Ehrlichia* sp. isolated from the fluke Stellantchasmus falcatus, by 16S rRNA base sequence, serological, and morphological analyses. *Inter. J. System. Bacteriol.*, **46**: 149–54.

Woldehiwet, Z. (2010). The natural history of *Anaplasma phagocytophilum*. *Vet. Parasitol.*, **167**: 108–22.

Wolf, L., McPherson, T., Harrison, B., Engber, B., Anderson, A. *et al.* (2000). Prevalence of *Ehrlichia ewingii* in *Amblyomma americanum* in North Carolina. *J. Clin. Microbiol.*, **38**: 2795.

Yabsley, M.J., Varela, A.S., Tate, C.M. *et al.* (2002). *Ehrlichia ewingii* infection in white-tailed deer (*Odocoileus virginianus*). *Emerg. Infect. Dis.*, **8**: 668–71.

Yabsley, M.J., Murphy, S.M., Luttrell, M.P. *et al.* (2008). Experimental and field studies on the suitability of raccoons (*Procyon lotor*) as hosts for tick-borne pathogens. *Vector Borne Zoon. Dis.*, **8**: 491–503.

Yabsley, M.J. (2010). Natural history of *Ehrlichia chaffeensis*: vertebrate hosts and tick vectors from the United States and evidence for endemic transmission in other countries. *Vet. Parasitol.*, **167**: 136–48.

Yevich, S.J., Sánchez, J.L., DeFraites, R.F. *et al.* (1995). Seroepidemiology of infections due to spotted fever group rickettsiae and *Ehrlichia* species in military personnel exposed in areas of the United States where such infections are endemic. *J. Infect. Dis.*, **171**: 1266–73.

Yoshimoto, K., Matsuyama, Y., Matsuda, H. *et al.* (2010). Detection of *Anaplasma bovis* and *Anaplasma phagocytophilum* DNA from *Haemaphysalis megaspinosa* in Hokkaido, Japan. *Vet. Parasitol.*, **168**: 170–72.

Zeidner, N.S., Burkot, T.R., Massung, R. *et al.* (2000). Transmission of the agent of human granulocytic ehrlichiosis by *Ixodes spinipalpis* ticks: evidence of an enzootic cycle of dual infection with *Borrelia burgdorferi* in Northern Colorado. *J. Infect. Dis.*, **182**: 616–19.

Zhan, L., Cao, W.C., Chu, C.Y. *et al.* (2009). Tick-borne agents in rodents, China, 2004–2006. *Emerg. Infect. Dis.*, **15**: 1904–8.

Zhi, N., Ohashi, N. and Rikihisa, Y. (1999). Multiple p44 genes encoding major outer membrane proteins are expressed in the human granulocytic ehrlichiosis agent. *J. Biolog. Chem.*, **274**: 17828–36.

CHAPTER 19c

Other bacterial diseases

Pasteurellosis

Daniel Rh. Thomas

Summary

Pasteurellosis is a zoonoses that occurs worldwide, caused by bacteria of the genus *Pasteurella,* and other related organisms. Pasteurellosis reported in humans is most frequently caused by the species *Pasteurella multocida.* In humans, cutaneous infection is most common, but more severe outcomes have been reported, particularly in those with underlying chronic disease. Infection in animals is usually subclinical, but may give rise to a range of clinical symptoms, depending on the host species. Disease in animals usually occurs as a consequence of stress such as overcrowding, chilling, transportation, or as a result of a concurrent infection. In animals, pasteurellosis is known as: shipping fever or pneumonia, transport or transit fever, stockyard pneumonia, bovine pneumonic pasteurellosis, haemorrhagic septicaemia, or avian, bird or fowl cholera. The pasteurella bacterium is commonly present in the mouth and gastrointestinal tract of a wide range of mammals. Transmission to humans occurs after bites, scratches, or licks from infected animals, most frequently from dogs or cats, although infection has been associated with other animals including: cows, pigs, hamsters, and rabbits. However, not all patients report a history of direct animal contact. Infection may be prevented through the avoidance of animal bites and the prompt hygienic care of wounds. Health professionals should be aware of the risk of pasterurellosis in immunocompromised patients exposed to companion animals.

History

There is some dispute in the literature as to whether Troussaint was the first to isolate *P. multocida* in 1879 in France (Rimler and Rhoades 1989), or whether it was Pasteur in 1880 and 1881 who also successfully isolated a bacterium from blood and organs of birds infected with fowl cholera (Mutters *et al.* 1989). The first name that was given to this organism was *Micrococcus gallicidus* by Burrill in 1883; Zopf called it *M. cholerae gallinarum* in 1885, and Trevisan changed the name to *Bacterium cholerae-gallinarum* (Frederiksen 1989a). The generic name *Pasteurella* was subsequently suggested by Trevisan in 1887 who wanted to commemorate Pasteur's work on the earlier elucidation of the type species (Mutters *et al.* 1989). The first published case of human pasteurellosis appears to have been that described by Debre in 1919, although some authors believe that it was Brugnatelli in 1913 (Frederiksen 1989b). In 2001, the complete genome of a common avian clone of *P. multocida* was sequenced, providing the foundation for future research into the epidemiology, evolution, and mechanisms of pathogenesis of the organism (May *et al.* 2001).

The agent

Taxonomy and molecular biology

The genus *Pasteurella,* family *Pasteurellaceae,* are classically aerobic and facultatively anaerobic, fermentative, Gram-negative, small non-motile coccoid, ovoid, or rod-shaped organisms that do not produce spores (Mutters *et al.* 1989).

The family Pasteurellaceae includes the genera *Haemophilus* and *Actinobacillus,* and genomic sequencing provides evidence that *P. multocida* is a close relative of *Haemophilus influenzae,* diverging around 270 million years ago (May *et al.* 2001). DNA hybridization separates the *Pasteurella species into two groups: Pasteurella sensu strico,* and other *Pasteurella*-related species (Zurlo 2010). *However, t*he ongoing identification of new species and the reclassification of previously described strains mean that the interpretation of published data is difficult (Bisgaard 1993).

Christensen *et al.* (2007) have proposed guidelines for the description of genera, species and subspecies of the *Pasteurellaceae* based on both genotypic and phenotypic methods.

Pasteurella sensu stricto

According to Zurlo (2010) this group now comprises:

- *P. multocida* subspecies *multocida,*
- *P. multocida* subspecies *septicum,*
- *P. multocida* subspecies gallicida, *P. canis, P. dagmatis, P. stomatis,* and *Avibacterium gallinarum.*

The first two have been described in mammals, man, and birds, and the third from birds alone, for example:

- *P. canis* biotype I (formerly biotype 6 of *P. multocida),* found in dogs and humans following bites or scratches from these animals,
- *P. canis* biotype 2 (formerly Bisgaard's taxon 13) is found in calves,
- *P. dagmatis* (previously *P. pneumotropica* biotype Henriksen, *Pasteurella* 'gas' or *Pasteurella* new species 1) is found in both animals, particularly dogs and cats, and humans.

◆ *P. stomatis,* usually found in dogs, cats, and human injuries caused by these animals' bites.

◆ The other recognized species *A. gallinarum,* the avian respiratory pathogen, is found particularly in chickens.

Several serological classification systems have been devised to correlate specific strains of *P. multocida* with host specificity, virulence, or disease, Carter's classification in the 1950s and 1960s grouped *P. multocida* into five serotypes based on polysaccharide antigens determined by a passive or indirect haemagglutination test; A, B, D and E are all capsular types, whereas C, a component of the normal flora of the respiratory tract of dogs and cats, is a non-capsulated strain.

Other Pasteurella-related species

The species that have been excluded from *Pasteurella sensu stricto* include:

◆ *P. aerogenes,* isolated from pigs and man,

◆ *P. bettyae, P. caballi,* found in horses in the USA and Sweden, and from an infected wound of a Danish veterinary surgeon,

◆ *P. pneumotropica, P. trehalosi,* and *Mannheimia haemolytica* (previously *Pasteurella haemolytica*), reported from cattle, sheep, goats, and man.

Disease mechanisms

The virulence and multifunctional pathogenicity of members of the Pasteurellaceae has been reviewed by Nicolet (1990). Boyce and Adler (2006) review virulence mechanisms in *P. multocida.*

Growth and survival requirements

Pasteurella grow between 30 and 40°C. They may show bipolar staining, particularly as fresh isolates stained with Romanowsky stains such as Wright or Geimsa. *Pasteurella multocida* and *M. haemolytica* are glucose positive, sucrose positive, urease negative, and H_2S negative. Certain strains produce capsules of varying size and are believed by some to be more virulent than the non-capsulated strains.

Initial isolation from clinical specimens is usually made on enriched agar media supplemented with 5% inactivated serum or bovine, horse, or sheep blood in air or air plus five per cent carbon dioxide. Cultures can be maintained and colonial variants selected on BBL-trypticase soy, Difco-tryptose, Gibcodextrose starch or other comparable agars, with or without serum supplement. Several selective media have been developed to recover *Pasteurella* from specimens that are grossly contaminated (Rimler and Rhoades 1989). Alternatively, virulent strains of *P. multocida* can be recovered by subcutaneous inoculation of mice and cultures subsequently made from liver, spleen, and heart, but such methods are not appropriate for large numbers of specimens. The growth requirements for *P. multocida* have been the subject of numerous studies (Rimler and Rhoades 1989).

The hosts

Animal

Pasteurella multocida is found in the nasopharynx and gastrointestinal tract of many wild and domesticated animals. The bacterium is part of the normal oral and pharyngeal flora of dogs, cats, wild and domestic ruminants, horses, swine, rabbits, opossums, rodents, birds, and reptiles. Carriage rates are variable and may range from 3.5% in buffalo to 90% in cats (Jones and Lockton 1987). Cats have the highest rate of oropharyngeal colonization by *P. multocida* (50–90%), followed by dogs (50–66%), pigs (51%), and rats (14%). A recent study found a 90% carriage rate in Ohio cats which was independent of the cat's age, breed, food type, gingival scale, lifestyle and sex (Freshwater 2008). The range of susceptible mammals and birds is now known to be very wide and the organism has been frequently isolated from the nasopharyngeal region of healthy animals. *P. multocida* in particular is so widespread amongst terrestrial and aquatic mammals and birds (well over 100 different species have been identified) that it would probably be unwise to exclude any mammal or bird species as possible hosts (Biberstein 1981; Rimler and Rhoades 1989).

P. multocida causes severe economic loss amongst farmed poultry, pig, sheep and cattle populations, and epizootics associated with high rates of morbidity and mortality in free-ranging animal populations, including waterfowl, fallow deer, chamois, elk, American bison, bighorn sheep and pronghorn. Wild birds may be a source of infection in commercial poultry, although it is possible that wild mammals may be exposed via domestic herds sharing the same pastures. A review of the epidemiology of fowl cholera is provided by Christensen and Bisgaard (2000).

P. multocida is associated with several different clinical entities, such as haemorrhagic septicaemia (HS) and bronchopneumonia of cattle, and more rarely meningitis, localized infections, abortions, mastitis, and arthritis; septicaemia in birds; HS, pneumonia, and atrophic rhinitis in pigs; rhinitis, pneumonia, and septicaemia in rabbits; pneumonia and HS in sheep; less frequently mastitis, localized infections, abortions, and meningitis or meningoencephalitis in cattle; and possibly atrophic rhinitis and pneumonia in goats.

P. multocida also occurs as wound infections in dogs and cats and the subspecies *septica* has been associated with infections of the central nervous system (CNS) in cats. It has often been identified as a secondary invader in animals, rather than the sole cause of the above symptoms and signs. Disease may result from invasion of commensal organisms during periods of stress or following infections with viruses, mycoplasmas, or rickettsias.

Pasteurella pneumotropica is a major cause of pasteurellosis in laboratory rodents, including rats, mice, hamsters, and guinea-pigs. Mice and rabbits suffer enzootic pneumonia; septicaemia, genital infections, abscesses, and mastitis have all been reported in rodents. Laboratory rodents may carry the organism on the oropharyngeal mucous membranes.

Pasteurella dagmatis and *P. stomatis* are mainly found in the nasopharynx of dogs and cats, *P. canis* biotype 1 is found in dogs, and biotype 2 has been isolated from the lungs of calves with pneumonia and from sheep, and *P. aerogenes* in the respiratory and gastrointestinal tract of wild and domestic pigs.

Mannheimia haemolytica (formerly *Pasteurella haemolytica*) is found commonly in ruminants and has been identified as the causative agent of: enzootic pneumonia of and systemic infections in sheep; septicaemia of lambs; pneumonia or bovine respiratory disease complex (*BRDC*) in cattle, in association with *P. multocida;* and less frequently meningitis and arthritis in lambs; atypical pneumonia in sheep and pneumonia in goats; mastitis in ewes and cows; and rarely septicaemia of newborn calves. Infections may also occur in pigs. *M. haemolytica* is commonly found in the nasal cavity of healthy cattle, sheep, and goats.

Human

In contrast to *Haemophilus* spp., *Pasteurella* spp. are not commensals of humans although some strains may be present as a transient part of the normal flora. *Pasteurella multocida, M. haemolytica,* and *P. pneumotropica (P. dagmatis)* have been found in the respiratory tract of healthy people.

   Pasteurella multocida is the most commonly reported zoonotic infection in this group, resulting usually from infected dog and cat bites. *P. multocida* subsp. *multocida* appears to predominate in systemic pasteurellosis, whereas *P. multocida* subsp. *septica* is usually isolated from soft tissue infections. *P. canis* and *P. stomatis* are usually of canine origin, wheras *P. multocida* subsp. *septica* is usually feline and *P.multocida* subsp. *multocida* may originate from dogs or cats. *M. haemolytica* has also been associated with dog-bite wounds. *Pasteurella pneumotropica (P. dagmatis)* has been reported as causing wound infections and very rarely septicaemia, meningitis, respiratory tract, and bone and joint infections. *Pasteurella dagmatis, P. stomatis,* and *P. canis* biotype 1 infections have all been associated with dog bites and other animal wounds; sometimes more than one species may be isolated from a single wound. *Pasteurella dagmatis* and *P. canis* may also be found in patients with chronic respiratory tract disease, but infrequently. *Pasteurella dagmatis* may also result in systemic infections following animal bites. *Pasteurella aerogenes* wound infections usually associated with pig bites are rarely seen in man.

Incubation period

In a typical infection, acute onset of pain, erythema and swelling frequently ocurrs within hours of a bite. Onset of local symptoms within three to six hours strongly suggests *P. multocida* infection. Further symptoms usually occur within 24 to 48 hours from the bite. When the incubation period is greater than 24 hours, differential diagnosis should include stapylococcal or streptococcal infections (Westling *et al.* 2000).

Symptoms and signs, and pathology

Infections may range from trivial sepsis to severe abscesses that may be accompanied by septicaemia. A typical infection results in a diffuse cellulitis at the site of the lesion accompanied by pain and swelling. Lymphangitis occurs in about 20% of cases and regional lymphadenitis in 10%. Local complications such as osteomyelitis, tenosynositis and arthritis may cause prolonged disability. Septic arthritis particularly affects the knee joint. Other organisms such as *Staphylococcus aureus* and *Pseudomonas aeruginosa* may also be isolated from the infected sites. Conjunctivitis or endophthalmitis may occur following animal scratches or bites to the cornea.

   The respiratory tract is the second most common site of infection for pasteurella, where it may present as chronic otitis media, sinusitis, epiglottitis, pneumonia, tracheobronchitis, lung abscess, or empyema. Pneumonia is the most common manifestation of respiratory infection and patients may acutely or insidiously present with cough, shortness of breath, fever, chills, and pleuritic chest pain. Many patients also report fatigue, anorexia or abdominal pain. Those who develop respiratory infection from pasteurella tend to be elderly and have underlying chronic lower respiratory tract disease, and the route of infection appears to be through inhalation.

   The organism may also be opportunistic and affect immunocompromised patients, causing pneumonia in patients with HIV/AIDS and immunoglobulin A deficiency.

Pasteurella causes osteomyelitis, intra-abdominal infections, septic arthritis, sepsis, and meningitis. Meningitis occurred in a patient with chronic purulent otorrhoea whose dog frequently licked his ear. Pasterurella peritonitis occurred in a home dialysis patient whose dialysis tubing was bitten by a pet golden hamster (Campos *et al.* 2000). Other similar cases have occurred as a result of a cat biting the dialysis tubing.

   Prosthetic infections with pasteurella are rare but have been reported, including a case of aortic endograft infection following a rabbit bite. *P. multocida* septicemia can affect immunocompromised patients, such as liver cirrhosis, HIV, diabetes mellitus, malignancy, and long-term steroid use. Pasteurella infected arthritis has been reported in patients with gout. Nectrotizing fasciitis, a potentially fatal soft tissue infection, has been reported in an immunocompromised patient with gout, following a dog licking the limbs with gout tophi (Chang *et al.* 2007).

Diagnosis

Early diagnosis is important, especially in the young and elderly, as well as in immunosuppressed patients including pregnant women. Clinical features are varied and mostly non-specific. A history of animal contact must be sought. A possible pitfall in the subsequent identification of the causative *Pasteurella* spp. with the (API) system has recently been highlighted. *Haemophilus influenzae* and *H. parainfluenzae* may be misidentified as *P. pneumotropica,* or less frequently as *P. multocida* or *P. haemolytica.* Hamilton-Miller (1993) suggests that isolates identified as one of these species using the API system should be tested for X and V dependency. *Pasteurella* spp. should grow well on the nutrient agar required for this test whereas *Haemophilus* spp. grow only around the appropriate supplements. Various technologies have been used to genotype *P. multocida*: restriction endonuclease analysis (REA), ribotyping, pulsed gel electrophoresis (PFGE), repetitive extragenic palindromic_PCR (REP-PCR), enterobacterial repetitive intergenic consensus-polymerase chain reaction (ERIC-PCR), and multi-locus enzyme electrophoresis (MLEE), with PFGE regarded as the 'gold standard' (Chang *et al.* 2007). Genotyping can assist in providing evidence of a causal link between a sporadic case and a companion animal. Guidance on the standardization of diagnostic methods for identifying Pasteurella species and morphologically similar bacteria in humans has recently been produced (HPA 2007). Diagnostic and typing options for detecting *Pasteurella multocida* in animals have been reviewed by Dziva *et al.* (2008).

Treatment

The majority of wound infections will heal following local treatment with or without systemic antibiotics. *Pasteurella* are highly susceptible to penicillin and ampicillin. The role of antibiotics in the prophylaxis of infections in bite or scratch wounds is controversial. *Pasteurella multocida* and other *Pasteurella* spp. account for only some of the resulting infections, and other micro-organisms especially *S. aureus* should also be considered. Most infections will heal on local treatment only, but those with lowered resistance (on steroids for example), those with wounds involving the hands or face, immunocompromised, or diabetic patients may require prophylactic antibiotics. The evaluation, management, and treatment of animal bites have been reviewed by Weber and Hansen (1991). Freshwater (2008) found high susceptibility to benzylpenicillin, amoxicillin-clavulanate, cefazolin and azithromycin in 409

P. multocida isolates from domestic cats and concluded that use of penicillins (and deriviatives) is still suitable for treating cat bite wounds.

Prognosis

The disease is effectively self-limiting but septicaemia and other serious symptoms may occur.

Epidemiology

Transmission

Transmission is primarily via bites or scratches from dogs and cats, and less frequently from other animals. Animal bites are common. In the USA an estimated 4.5 million animal bites occur each year of which 19% seek medical attention (Gilchrist *et al.* 2010) and the annual incidence of dog and cat bites has been reported as 300 bites per 100,000 population (Sacks *et al.* 1996). In Denmark in the 1970s there were an estimated 10,000 dog bites annually. In England and Wales in the 1980s there were an estimated 209,000 dog bites of man that resulted in presentation at hospital each year (Young 1988). In France there were an estimated 17 million cats and dogs with 500,000 animal bites each year. Cat bites may occur less frequently, although some believe that they more often result in infection which may be due either to the nature of cat bites in that their sharp teeth penetrate more deeply, or due to the pathogenicity or virulence of the responsible organism (Weber and Hansen 1991). Dog bites tend to more frequently occur in young males whereas cat bites disproportionally affect adult females (Wright 1990). Although most bite wounds are trivial and most victims do not seek medical attention, they result in significant medical costs. In the USA dog bites account for 70–93% of animal bites, cat bites 3–15%, and wild animals less than 1%. The risk of acquiring infection from a penetrating dog bite is between 2–29%.

Human infections caused by *Pasteurella aerogenes* have resulted from pig bite wounds on the lower lateral part of the thigh, an occupational risk in the Danish pig farming industry (Ejlertsen *et al.* 1996). Two cases of human *Pasteurella caballi* infection have been reported; one in a Danish veterinary surgeon, the other in France due to a horse bite (Escande *et al.* 1997). Human infection has been reported following bites from other animals. A seven year old girl developed a wound infection with *P. multocida* and *Neisseria weaveri* following a tiger bite at a privately owned animal reserve (Capitini *et al.* 2002). No reports exist of direct transmission from poultry, but the possibility for such transmission cannot be excluded (Christensen and Bisgaard 2000).

Other routes of transmission have also been described; *P. multocida* infections may be acquired from animals by their licking on mucosal surfaces or on injured skin (Rollof *et al.* 1992). Cases of *P. multocida* meningitis and ear infections have been associated with dog and cat licks to the faces and ears, and of endocarditis via the licking of leg ulcers by a dog (Hombal and Dincsoy 1992).

Pasteurella peritonitis may occur as a result of pet cats or rodents biting or licking dialysis tubing. Humans may also become infected from the respiratory aerosol of infected cattle, sheep, pigs, poultry, and cats.

More than 70% of cases of *P. multocida* pneumonia occur in patients without a history of animal bite suggesting transmission by direct contact or by aerosol. Non-zoonotic transmission is unlikely, but may also occur amongst patients with respiratory tract disease. Vertical transmission has also been reported (Nakawan *et al.* 2009). Stojek and Dutkiewicz (2004) have postulated a role for ticks in the transmission of certain pasteurella species.

Populations at risk

Anyone coming into contact with animals is at risk of pasteurellosis. The number of people exposed to companion animals is increasing. According to the American Pet Products Associations 2009/2010 National Pet Owners Survey, 62% of households in the USA own a pet, which equates to 71.4 millions homes, and represents an increase since 1988—the first year the survey was conducted, when 56% of households in the USA owned a pet. The 2009/2010 National Pet Owners Survey estimates that 77.5 million dogs and 93.6 million cats are owned by households in the USA (American Pet Products Association 2010). Dogs and cats are also the most popular pets in the UK. In 2010, 23% of UK households owned a dog and 19% owned a cat, representing a total of 8 million dogs and 8 million cats (PFMA 2010). A recent UK survey found that dogs are more common in families that have older children (6–19 years), and that dog owners have increased contact with dogs other than their own (Westgarth *et al.* 2007).

Occupational groups at risk from animal bites or other injuries, and infections arising from indirect contact with animals, include: veterinary surgeons, laboratory workers, and farmers.

Petting zoos present a theoretical risk of pasteurellosis.

Certain chronic disease groups are at risk of complications of pastereulla infection. These include: immunocompromised patients, patients receiving peritoneal dialysis, and patients with chronic respiratory disease. *P. multocida* wound infection is a potential complication for people with dog or cat contact postoperatively.

Incidence of human disease

Despite the frequency of exposure, pasteurellosis is a relatively uncommon disease in humans. In the United Kingdom there are around 400 laboratory confirmed cases a year, of which about 70% are due to *P. multocida* (Health Protection Agency (HPA) 2010). A recent retrospective survey in Israel identified 77 hospital *P. multocida* cases between 2000 and 2005, giving an annual incidence of 0.2 per 100,000 population (Nseir *et al.* 2009). The mortality rate was 2.6% and those who died were all over 65 years of age, had diabetes mellitis or cirrhosis, and were bacteraemic. In Sweden an analysis of *Pasteurella* strains identified between 1989 and 1992 revealed that of the 159 isolates 95 were *P. multocida* subspecies *multocida*, 21 subspecies *septica*, 28 *P. canis* biotype 1, 10 *P. stomatis*, and five *P. dagmatis* (Hoist *et al.* 1992). Ninety-four per cent of infections were wounds; there were five cases of septicaemia, and three of meningitis. In a 12 year study of *Pasteurella* infections in England, Wales, and Ireland reported by laboratories from 1975 to 1986, 3699 cases were identified (Young 1988) of which 93% were *P. multocida*. Skin infections were identified in 3185 cases (86%); 9% were respiratory tract infections, 2.4% septicaemias, and less than 1% each were abdominal infections, meningitis, bone and joint, eye, and urinary tract infections.

Although pig bites are a significant occupational risk in Denmark, only 7 cases of *P. aerogenes* were reported between 1976 and 1994 (Ejlertsen *et al.* 1996).

Pasteurellosis is very rarely fatal. Between 1993 and 2009, five patients in the UK with severe infection died (HPA 2010).

Pregnancy-associated cases

Reviews and case reports of infections in pregnancy include that by Rollof *et al.* (1992) who reported on two cases of severe infections that occurred in the second trimester of pregnancy in previously healthy women, one of whom suffered meningitis and the other had cellulitis and deep abscess formation. The fetuses were not apparently affected. Both women had contact with cats and dogs; neither had been bitten, but they had been licked by their pets from which *P. multocida* and *P. stomatis* were subsequently isolated. Waldor *et al.* (1992) reported a case of *in utero* infection in the first trimester of pregnancy. Following treatment the 31 year old mother from the United States recovered rapidly from the bacteraemia but the 12 week old fetus was spontaneously aborted. *Pasteurella multocida* was isolated from the woman's blood and vagina, and also from her two cats and dog. The authors cited five previous cases of suspected or proven pasteurella bacteraemia during pregnancy recorded in the literature. All occurred in the third trimester; three fetuses died, as did one mother due to disseminated intravascular coagulation. Three of the women had been bitten/scratched by cats and one other had been in contact with pets. Wong *et al.* (1992) also reported on a case of *P. multocida* infection in a 21 year old female in Scandinavia with a twin pregnancy. The woman developed chorio-amnionitis at 27 weeks gestation after prolonged rupture of membranes. One twin in a separate sac suffered infection and died shortly after birth; the other twin was not infected. Infection is believed to have been caused by ascending infection from asymptomatic colonization of the vaginal tract. In Finland a 37 year old pregnant woman gave birth normally at 37 weeks following ruptured membranes but the infant died the next day of fulminant bacterial pneumonia (Andersson *et al.* 1994). The mother became feverous postpartum but recovered after antibiotic treatment. *Pasteurella multocida* subspecies *septica* was isolated from her cervix and the infants nasopharynx, and lung post-mortem. Swabs from the tonsils of the family's cat were also positive for the same organism although the mother did not recall any bites or scratches in the weeks preceding delivery. The mode of transmission to the child was uncertain; it may have occurred *in utero* through subclinical chorio-amnionitis, or in the vagina during delivery from an ascending infection of the mother. In 1994, Thorsen *et al.* described a case of *P. aerogenes* infection in a stillborn baby and its mother at 31 weeks gestation in Denmark. During an uncomplicated pregnancy the mother had worked on a pig farm but the organism was not subsequently isolated from some of the sows housed there. The authors suggested a relationship between the isolation of the bacterium and sudden fetal death, and that transmission may have occurred haematogenously or from the lower genital tract to the uterus and fetus.

Prevention and control

Vaccination for some forms of pasteurellosis in livestock are available (Donachie 1992). Elimination of stray dogs and cats can reduce the chances of bites and therefore prevent some cases. Education and training for pet owners in the appropriate handling and training of companion animals may help reduce injuries. Guidelines covering education of children and information for pet owners on how to avoid animal bites has been produced in the USA and an educational intervention for UK schoolchildren was shown to be effective. Generally, children should be taught to treat dogs with respect, avoid direct eye contact, and not tease them (Morgan and Palmer 2007). Wounds, particularly bites, should be thoroughly cleansed. Those working with animals should have a high index of suspicion, particularly if immunocompromised or pregnant.

Postoperative instructions for patients should include thorough hand washing and the avoidance of wound contact by pet animals. For patients on peritoneal dialysis, caution should be taken to avoid contact between their household pets and the dialysis tubing and catheter (Campos *et al.* 2000). Carnivorous animals are naturally attracted to human body fluid and should be excluded from the room where dialysis is performed. With the increasing use of pet-assisted therapy in hospitals and community-care facilities, patients and carers who handle animals should pay particular attention to hand hygiene. This is also the case for those patients using helper dogs to assist them in their daily activities. Health professionals caring for certain patient groups, including those undergoing continuous ambulatory peritoneal dialysis, must consider carefully the risks and benefits of close contact with companion animals.

Acknowledgements

This chapter is an update of the first edition chapter written by Nicola Barrett. Isabel Puscas assisted with the literature search.

References

American Pet Products Association (2010). Industry Statistics and Trends. http://www.americanpetproducts.org/press_industrytrends.asp.

Andersson, S. *et al.* (1994). Fatal congenital pneumonia caused by cat-derived *Pasteurella multocida*. *Paediat. Infect. Dis. J.*, **13**: 74–75.

Biberstein, E.L. (1981). *Haemaphilus—Pasteurella—Actinobacillus*: their significance in veterinary medicine. In: M. Kilian, W. Frederiksen and E. L. Biberstein (eds.) *Haemophilus, Pasteurella* and *Actinobacillus*, pp. 61–73. London: Academic Press.

Bisgaard, M. (1993). Ecology and significance of *Pasteurellaceae* in animals. Zentralblatt fur Bakteriologie. *Inter. J. Med. Microbiol., Virol., Parasit. Infect. Dis.*, **279**: 7–26.

Boyce, J.D. and Adler, B. (2006). How does *Pasteurella multocida* respond to the host environment? *Curr. Opin. Microbiol.*, **9**: 117–22.

Campos, A., Taylor, J.H. and Campbell, M. (2000). Hamster bite peritonitis: *Pasteurella pneumotropica* peritonitis in a dialysis patient. *Pediatr. Nephrol.*, **15**: 31–32.

Capitini, C.M., Herrero, I.A., Patel, R., Ishitani, M.B. and Boyce, T.G. (2002). Wound infection with *Neisseria weaveri* and a novel subspecies of *Pasteurella multocida* in a child who sustained a tiger bite. *Clin. Infect. Dis.*, **34**: 74–76.

Chang, K., Siu, L.K., Chen, Y.H. *et al.* (2007). Fatal *Pasteurella multocida* septicemia and necrotizing fasciitis related with wound licked by a domestic dog. *Scandin. J. Infect. Dis.*, **39**: 167–92.

Christensen, J.P. and Bisgaard, M. (2000). Fowl Cholera. *Rev. Sci tech. Off. Int. Epiz.*, **19**: 626–37.

Christensen, H., Kuhnert, P., Busse, H-J., Frederiksen, W.C. and Bisgaard, M. (2007). Proposed minimal standards for the description of genera, species and subspecies of the *Pasteurellaceae*. *Inter. J. System. Evolut. Microbiol.*, **57**: 166–78.

Dire, D.J. (1992) Emergency management of dog and cat bite wounds. *Emergency Medicine Clin. N. Am.*, **10**(4): 719–36.

Donachie, W. (1992). Prevention of pasteurellosis. *Brit. Vet. J.*, **148**: 93–95.

Dziva, F., Muhairwa, A.P., Bisgaard, M. and Christensen, H. (2008). Diagnostic and typing options for investigating diseases associated with *Pasteurella multocida*. *Vet. Microbiol.*, **128**: 1–22.

Ejlertsen, T., Gahrn-Hansen, B., Sogaard, P., Heltberg, O. and Frederikiksen, W. (1996). *Pasteurella aerogenes* isolated from ulcers or wounds in humans with occupational exposure to pigs: A report of 7 Danish cases. *Scand. J. Infect. Dis.*, **28**: 567–70.

Escande, F., Vallee, E. and Aubart, F. (1997). *Pasteurella caballi* infection following a horse bite. *Zbl. Bakt.*, **285**: 440–44.

Frederiksen, W. (1989a). A note on the name *Pasteurella multocida*. In: C. Adlarn and J.M. Rutter (eds.) Pasteurella and pasteurellosis, pp. 35–36. London: Academic Press.

Frederiksen, W. (1989b). Pasteurellosis of man. In: C. Adlam and J. M. Rutter (eds.) Pasteurella and pasteurellosis, pp. 303–20. London: Academic Press.

Freshwater, A. (2008). Why your housecat's trite little bite could cause you quite a fright: A study of domestic felines on the occurrence and antibioyic susceptibility of *Pasteurella multocida*. *Zoon. Pub. Heal.*, **55**: 507–13.

Gilchrist, J., Sacks, J.J., White, D. and Kresnow, M-J. (2010). Dog bites: still a problem? *Injury Prev.*, **14**: 296–301.

Hamilton-Miller, J.M.T. (1993). A possible pitfall in the identification of *Pasteurella* spp. with the API system. *J. Med. Microbiol.*, **39**: 78–79.

Hoist, E., Roliof, J., Larsson, L. and Nielsen, J.P. (1992). Characterization and distribution of *Pasteurella* species recovered from infected humans. *J. Clin. Microbiol.*, **30**: 2984–87.

Hombal, S.M. and Dincsoy, H.P. (1992). *Pasteurella multocida* endocarditis. *Clin. Microbiol. Infect. Dis.*, **98**: 565–68.

Health Protection Agency (2007). Identification of Pasteurella species and morphologically similar bacteria. National Standard Method BSOP ID 13 Issue 2.1. http://www.hpa-standardmethods.org.uk/pdf_sops.asp.

Health Protection Agency (2010). General Information on *Pasteurella* infections. http://www.hpa.org.uk/HPA/Topics/InfectiousDiseases/InfectionsAZ/1203409654990/</.

Jones, A.G.H. and Lockton, J.A. (1987). Fatal *Pasteurella multocida* septicaemia following a cat bite in a man without liver disease. *J. Infect.*, **15**: 229–35.

May, B.J., Zhang, Q., Li, L.L., Paustian, M.L., Whittam, T.S., and Kapur, V. (2001). Complete genomic sequence of *Pasteurella multocida*, Pm70. *Proc. Natl. Acad. Sci. USA*, **98**: 3460–65.

Morgan, M., and Palmer, J. (2007). Dog bites. *BMJ*, 334: 413–17.

Mutters, R., Ihm, P., Pohl, S., Frederiksen, W. and Mannheim, W. (1985). Reclassification of the genus *Pasteurella* Trevisan 1887 on the basis of deoxyribonucleic acid homology, with proposals for the new species *Pasteurella dagmatis, Pasteurella canis, Pasteurella stomatis, Pasteurella anatis,* and *Pasteurella langaa*. *Inter. J. System. Bacteriol.*, **35**: 309–22.

Mutters, R., Mannheim, W. and Bisgaard, M. (1989). Taxonomy of the group. In: C. Adlam and J.M. Rutter (eds.) Pasteurella and pasteurellosis, pp. 3–34. London: Academic Press.

Nakawan, N., Nakawan, N., Atta, T. and Chokephaibulkit, K. (2009). Neonatal pasteurellosis; a review of reported cases. *Arch. Dis. Child. Fetal Neonat. Ed.*, **94**: F373–76.

Nicolet, J. (1990). Overview of the virulence attributes of the HAP-group of bacteria. *Can. J. Vet. Res.*, **54**: S12–15.

Nseir, W., Giladi, M., Moroz, I., Moses, A.E., Banenson, S., *et al.* (2009). A retrospective six-year national survey of P.multocide infections in *Israel. Scandan. J. Infect. Dis.*, **41**: 445–49.

PFMA. Pet Food Manufacturers Association. (2010). Pet ownership trends. http://www.pfma.org.uk/statistics/pet-statistics.htm.

Rimler, R.B. and Rhoades, K.R. (1989). *Pasteurella multocida*. In: C. Adlarn and J. M. Rutter (eds.) Pasteurella and pasteurellosis, pp. 37–73. London: Academic Press.

Rollof, J., Johansson, H. and Hoist, E. (1992). Severe *Pasteurella multocida* infections in pregnant women. *Scandin. J. Infect. Dis.*, **24**: 453–56.

Sacks, J. J., Kresnow, M. and Houston, B. (1996). Dog bites: how big a problem? *Inj. Prev.*, 2: 52–54.

Stojek, N.M. and Dutkiewicz, J. (2004). Studies on the occurrence of gram-negative bacteria in ticks: *Ixodes ricinus* as a potential vector of *Pasteurella*. *Ann. Agric. Environ. Med.*, **11**: 319–22.

Waldor, M., Roberts, D. and Kazanjian, P. (1992). *In utero* infection due to *Pasteurella multocida* in the first trimester of pregnancy: case report and review. *Clin. Infect. Dis.*, **14**: 497–500.

Weber, D.J. and Hansen, A.R. (1991). Infections resulting from animal bites. *Infect. Dis. Clin. N. Am.*, **5**: 663–80.

Wong, C.P., Cimolai, N., Dimmick, J.E. and Martin, T.R. (1992). *Pasteurella multocida* chorioamnionitis from vaginal transmission. *Acta Obstet. Gynecol. Scandin.*, **71**: 384–87.

Weiss, H.B., Friedman, D.I., Coben, J.H. (1998). Incidence of dog bite injuries treated in emergency departments. *JAMA*, 279: 51–53.

Westgarth. C., Pinchbeck, G.L., Bradshaw, J.W.S., Dawson, S., Gaskell, R.M. *et al.* (2007). Factors associated with dog ownership and contact with dogs in a UK community. *BMC Vet. Res.*, **3**: 5.

Westling, K., Bygdeman, S., Engkvist, O. and Jorup-Ronstrom, C. (2000). *Pasteurella multocida* infection colliwing cat bites in humans. *J. Infect.*, **40**: 97–103.

Wright, J.C. (1990). Reported cat bites in Dallas: characteristics of the cats, the victims and the attack events. *Pub. Heal. Rep.*, **105**(4): 420–24.

Young, S.E.J. (1988). *Pasteurella* infections 1975–86. *PHLS Microbiol. Digest.*, 5: 4–5.

Zurlo, J. (2010). *Pasteurella* species. In: G.L. Mandell, J.E. Bennett and R. Dolin (eds.) Mandell, Douglas and Bennett's principles and practice of infectious disease (7th edn.), pp. 2939–42. Philadelphia: Churchill Livingstone Elsevier.

CHAPTER 19d

Other bacterial diseases

Rat-bite fevers

Roland L. Salmon

Summary

Rat-bite fever is an uncommon but well described clinical syndrome. Resulting from a systemic infection following a rat bite, such an illness had been recognized in India for over 2,300 years (Elliott 2007). With the advent of modern microbiology it was found to be caused by two different pathogens that are commonly found in the oropharynx of rodents—*Streptobacillus moniliformis* and *Spirillum minus*. Although *Streptobacillus moniliformis* may be found worldwide, it is said to be found more commonly in North America and Europe whereas *Spirillum minus* is more common in Asia. *Spirillum minus* is said by some to be absent in the USA (Centers for Disease Control (CDC) 2005) but in fact, historically, there are several case reports (Pritchard 1990). Common differences in the characteristic clinical features are summarized in Table 19d.1. The two organisms are then discussed separately.

Streptobacillary fever

Infection with *Streptobacillus moniliformis,* gives rise to Rat-Bite fever also known as Streptobacillary Fever, and, when epidemic, Epidemic Arthritic Erythema (Haverhill Fever). It occurs worldwide. Only three outbreaks have been described. It is either caused by the bite of, or similar close contact with, a rat or other infected rodent, or, when epidemic, by the ingestion of water or milk contaminated by rats. Control requires limiting human contact with rats, traditionally by prevention of rat infestation although, of

Table 19d.1 Characteristic clinical features of Rat-Bite fevers, by causative organism

Streptobacillus moniliformis	Spirillum minus
Incubation 1–4 days	Incubation 7–21 days
Original wound heals or is inapparent	Wound inflamed and may reopen
Arthritis common	Arthritis is rare
Lymphadenopathy is rare	Lymphadenopathy
Typical rash, particularly on hands and feet	Often no rash

recent years, in developed countries, the keeping of rats as pets has played an important role.

History

Streptobacillus moniliformis was first so named in France in 1925, following its isolation from the blood of a laboratory worker and became recognized as one of the two causes of Rat-Bite fever. (The other is *Spirillum minis*.) In fact published descriptions of disease following a rat bite due to an organism called *Streptothrix muris ratti* were made in Germany in 1914 and the USA in 1916, and this organism is likely to have been *Streptobacillus moniliformis* (Elliott 2007). At the same time as the description in France, an epidemic form of the disease, Haverhill Fever, was recognized during an outbreak in the USA that occurred in January 1926 in Haverhill, Massachusetts (Parker and Hudson 1926; Place and Sutton 1934) which was ascribed to milk. Place and Sutton's account also refers to a similar but much larger outbreak that had occurred the year before in Chester, Pennsylvania, USA that was communicated to them personally by Armstrong and Wood, the State Epidemiologists. In 1983, the only other outbreak ever published occurred among pupils and staff at a boarding school in England. The investigators, having considered unpasteurized milk, eventually concluded that the cause of contamination was probably rat urine in a private water supply from a spring (McEvoy *et al.* 1987; Shanson *et al.* 1983). Accounts of sporadic cases occur but are infrequent in the world literature. Elliott has reviewed the English language literature and identified 65 detailed case reports from 1938 to 2005 (Elliott 2007). Graves and Janda have analysed retrospectively data collected on *Streptobacillus moniliformis* cultures performed by the Microbial Diseases Laboratory of the California State Health Department, USA, between 1970 and 1998, and found 41 cases in all (Graves and Janda 2001).

The agent

Streptobacillus moniliformis is a pleomorphic Gram-negative bacterium which may occur as short coccobacillary forms as well as chains and intertwining wavy filaments. Previously believed to be related to the actinobacilli it is now thought to have more in common with the Mycoplasmates (Costas and Owen 1987). It is a facultative anaerobe and slow growing on blood, serum, or other bodily fluid. The optimal condition for isolation is culturing blood and body fluid on blood or tryptose soy agar enriched with 20%

rabbit serum and incubated in a microaerophilic atmosphere with 5–10% CO_2 and humidification. Cultures should be held for at least 5 days (Martin and Martin in Topley and Wilson 1998; CDC 2005). The optimal growth temperature is 35–37 degrees C and optimal pH 7.4–7.6. *Streptobacillus moniliformis* is inhibited by 'Liquoid' (sodium polyanethol sulphonate) present in many commercial blood culture media systems such as BACTEC™(BD, Sparks, Maryland, USA) and BacT/Alert™ (Biomerieux, Durham, North Carolina, USA) (Wang and Wong 2007). It is killed at 55° C in 30 minutes or less. Growth in broth produces characteristic 'puff-ball' colony formation (Graves and Janda 2001). Cell wall deficient L-Forms may arise spontaneously and give rise to a typical 'fried-egg' appearance of colonies in older cultures. As unfavourable outcomes have occurred when diagnosis was delayed, in part because the difficulty of rapidly isolating or identifying *Streptobacillus moniliformis,* if *Streptobacillus moniliformis* infection is suspected, in the absence of a positive culture, identification of pleomorphic Gram-negative bacilli in appropriate specimens might support a diagnosis (Washburn 2000; CDC 2005). Historically fatty acid profiles obtained by gas-liquid chromatography, together with characteristic growth were used for rapid identification (Rowbotham 1983) but this has been superseded by PCR based on the 16S rRNA gene sequence (Boot *et al.* 2002).

Hosts

Animal

Streptobacillus moniliformis is carried in the nasopharynx or excreted in the urine of healthy rats (Strangeways 1933). It may be carried in other rodents where, as in the case of mice, it may also give rise to disease, notably septicaemia or arthropathy, which may be fatal. Human cases have been ascribed to exposure to a ferret, a mouse, squirrels, a gerbil and a dog (Elliott 2007). Increasingly humans are exposed to rats as pets in domestic settings or occupationally in pet shops (Downing 2001; Graves and Janda 2001; Grant *et al.* 2004; CDC 2005; Schachter 2006; Matheson 2007).

Human

Incubation period

The incubation in the original Haverhill outbreak described was 1–4 days (Parker and Hudson 1926) and is rarely longer than 10 days.

Symptoms and signs

These are sometimes differentiated, as clinical entities between sporadic cases, usually with a history of animal exposure, and epidemic cases. It has been suggested that septic arthritis should be separately considered as a third clinical entity (Wang and Wong 2007). However, accounts of the various forms of streptobacillary fever overlap and the account of the original Haverhill outbreak identifies two patients in which organisms were recovered from their swollen knees. Typically, therefore, there is fever followed after a median of 2 days by a symmetrical erythematous, usually maculopapular, rash affecting the palms of the hands, the feet, shins, and ankles, and in about half the cases, the face. Petechial haemhorrages and haemorrhagic vesicles may develop on the hands and feet (Place and Sutton 1934; Elliott 2007). Asymmetrical arthralgia, and also arthritis, affecting usually more than one joint, occurs in most cases ('Epidemic Arthritic Erythema'). In the Haverhill outbreak wrists and elbows were most frequently involved, followed by knees (Place and Sutton 1934) and in the UK outbreak, knees followed by ankles (McEvoy *et al.* 1987).

Diagnosis

Diagnosis is usually by culture of blood, synovial fluid or lymph nodes. Strains may be distinguished by the electrophoretic profiles of cellular proteins (Costas and Owen 1987).

The list of potential differential diagnoses is lengthy including the many bacterial and viral infections that may give rise to fever and rash (e.g. Epstein Barr Virus, Coxackie Virus, hantaviruses, Rocky Mountain Spotted Fever, meningococcal disease, streptococcal disease, Lyme Disease, leptospirosis, gonorrhoea) as well as auto-immune mediated and reactive arthritides such as Rheumatoid Arthritis and Reiter's syndrome (Matheson *et al.* 2008; Wang and Wong 2007). A careful history that identifies a relevant animal exposure may be key.

Treatment

Penicillin, erythromycin and tetracycline have all been used with evidence of success (Shanson *et al.* 1983). The currently recommended treatment is intravenous penicillin, 1.2 million units/day for 5 to 7 days, followed by oral penicillin or ampicillin, 500mgs, four times a day, for a further seven days, if improvement is observed. Oral tetracycline (500mgs four times a day) or intramuscular streptomycin (7.5mgs per kilogram body weight), twice daily, are alternatives (CDC 2005).

The occurrence of endocarditis requires dual therapy with both penicillin G, at higher doses than in uncomplicated infections, and streptomycin or gentamicin (Elliott 2007). In septic arthritis, antibiotics than penetrate the inflamed synovium are desirable. This argues against the use of aminoglycosides and it has been suggested that further studies to determine an optimal regime are required. (Wang and Wong 2007).

Finally, the L-Form of *S.moniliformis* is not penicillin sensitive (although it is sensitive to tetracycline). This has given rise to a suggestion that penicillin may encourage the development of L-forms and thereby prolong the course of the illness (Roughgarden 1965). In practice, however, this does not seem to have been an important consideration and some consider that the L-form is, in fact, not pathogenic (Elliott 2007).

Prognosis

The duration of illness ranges from 2–32 days (median 16 days). At least one relapse occurs in about half the cases and more than one relapse in 17%. Mortality has been absent in epidemics of Haverhill Fever but severe complications, including endocarditis, pneumonia, metastatic abscesses, and anaemia have been described in sporadic cases. This was largely before the advent of antibiotic treatment (Roughgarden 1965; Taber and Feigen 1979). Thus Rat-Bite Fever is said to have a case fatality rate of 7–10% when left untreated (Washburn 2000) with a disproportionately higher mortality in infants and patients with endocarditis. Recently two fatal cases were identified, after their death, by the CDC's Unexplained Deaths and Critical Illnesses (UNEX) Project. Both were previously healthy women, aged 52 and 19 years respectively (CDC 2005).

Pathology and pathogenesis

A combination of the infrequency of sporadic cases of streptobacillary fever, their generally good response to treatment and the absence of fatalities in Haverhill Fever, means that information on pathogenesis is scanty.

Post mortem examination of a recent fatal case showed findings suggestive of systemic infection including disseminated intravascular coagulopathy and inflammatory cell infiltrates in the liver, heart, and lungs (CDC 2005). Endocarditis is also well described (Balakrishnan *et al.* 2006).

Epidemiology

Occurrence

Sporadic cases occur worldwide. In a case series from California, males and females were affected with approximately equal frequency, ages ranged from 6 weeks to 92 years, the mean age was just under 19 years and the median age was just over 10 years. Sixty eight per cent were children less than 16 years of age (Graves and Janda 2001). In the series based on the published literature, 77% of patients reported were male and ages ranged from 2 months to 87 years (Elliott 2007). In the two case series only 46% (Graves and Janda 2001) and 66% (Elliott 2007) respectively, gave a specific history of being bitten by a rat.

Three outbreaks have been described (Parker and Hudson 1926; Place and Sutton 1934; McEvoy *et al.* 1987). These include the first to be described which was at Haverhill, Massachussetts, which gave the epidemic form of the disease its name of 'Haverhill Fever' (Parker and Hudson 1926). Eighty six cases, aged from 8 months to 54 years, occurred. They comprised 51 females and 35 males. Except for two patients, they were drawn from 39 families, comprising 231 persons (attack rate 36%). Their onsets occurred between 2–29 January 1926, peaking on 16 January. They were largely among a population of Lithuanian, Italian, Polish or Jewish extraction, in a circumscribed district, 1,500 by 500 metres, of Haverhill, then a manufacturing city with a population of 35,000. Of the cases 97% had a fever and 93% a rash. *Streptococcus moniliformis* was isolated from the blood of 11 cases. Suspicion fell on one small on-farm dairy that supplied, directly or indirectly, every case and whose entire milk supply was distributed to the small area of the city that corresponded to the residences of the cases. Once the milk from the dairy was pasteurized, only one further case occurred who gave a history of, nevertheless, having drunk the milk unpasteurized. By contrast the water supply to the area was the same city reservoir that supplied the whole town.

Suspicion of the milk was further emphasized by the experience of an outbreak in Chester, Pennsylvania, in May and June 1925 of which the Haverhill investigators were aware and an account of which they included in their own published account (Place and Sutton 1934). Here 400 cases were discovered of which 92% received their milk from the same bottling plant in the city. About 20% of persons who received milk from this plant had the disease compared with 0.5% of the population of Chester as a whole.

In the most recent outbreak which was at a boarding school (McEvoy 1987), the school was situated on a 100-acre site in a rural area near a market town in England. Within the grounds are extensive gardens, stables, and a farm which, at the time, provided the school with unpasteurized milk. There were about 700 people on the site, including 500 schoolgirls, aged 8–19 years, of which 370 were boarders and 130 attended daily.

The first case of fever was reported on 11 February 1983, and a further 24 cases presented the next day. Cases continued to occur in children and staff members, with a peak on 14 February, when

86 people became ill. The onset of the last known cases was 21 February by which time a total of 304 cases had occurred.

Analysis of these 304 cases by day of onset of symptoms suggested a common source for the outbreak, with exposure probably continuing over several days in early February. It is likely that the earliest cases, which were recognized retrospectively, had occurred on 6–8 February. All cases had lived on or visited the site of the school, and there were no reported cases of secondary transmission.

A random sample of 230 pupils was interviewed in greater detail. There were significant associations between the development of illness and the consumption of cold milk (Relative Risk = 3.3, p = 0.02) and cold water (Relative Risk = 10, p=6 x 10^{-5}) at the school. No other exposures were associated with illness.

Milk and water consumption were examined further, with data collected from the whole at risk population. Although both milk and water drinking remained significantly associated with the development of illness, water was associated independently of milk, but milk was not associated independently of water.

The major source of supply to the school was mains chlorinated water. However, water was also supplied by a spring. In addition, the sewage system had been transferred from the old filter-bed method to the mains system 2 weeks before the onset of the outbreak. The filter-bed and cesspit were situated on high ground above the spring. Inspection of this area revealed the presence of rats. Moreover, water could have filtered back into the spring pond, where rats were also seen. The spring water fed a well in an old courtyard. The well water passed through a chlorine-dosing unit and calorifiers to a pressurized storage unit in the school basement, where it was then used to feed the hot water system. Inspection revealed no domestic hot water return to the calorifiers. It was reported to be impossible to raise the water temperature above 50°C. Despite the presence of the chorine-dosing unit there was no evidence of chlorine in the water feeding the calorifiers. An inspection of the raw milk supplied from the school farm, by contrast, showed no evidence that the milk could have been contaminated with rat urine.

S.moniliformis was isolated from the blood cultures of 4 boarders who had returned home and were subsequently admitted to hospital (Shanson *et al.* 1983). The organism was not cultured from the samples of milk or water or from rats trapped in the school grounds after 16 February.

The attack rate was 49% (304/700). The duration of illness ranged from 2 to 32 days (median 16 days). All cases had fever and 95% had a rash. The distribution of the rash, unlike the joint involvement (which affected 97%), tended to be symmetrical.

Over half had 2 or more joints involved and a third 3 or more joints. Altogether, 56% of patients experienced one recurrence, 11% two recurrences, and 6% had three.

The conclusion that water was the vehicle of infection was strongly supported by epidemiological evidence and by circumstantial evidence that opportunity existed for the consumption of water from a spring infected with rats.

The hot water supply was probably contaminated intermittently between 5–12 February. During the first 2 weeks of February, operations on the building site involved digging around the foundations and the weather was exceptionally stormy. These factors may have disturbed the local rat population, causing it to contaminate the spring pond. The mains water supply was shut off for frequent short spells during this period, and drinking water could have been drawn from the hot taps.

There was evidence that the 'hot' water was cool, and heavy demands on the supply would have caused the temperature to fall further. A higher attack rate which was observed among the boarders (54% v 20% in day pupils) can be explained by their greater exposure to contaminated water. The total absence of cases outside the school suggests that the mains water was not contaminated.

Sources and transmission

Up to 50% of rats carry the organism as do, rarely, other rodents (Strangeways 1933). Sporadic cases usually occur following rat bites ('Rat-Bite Fever') but may occur following living or working in a rat infested building. Increasingly humans are exposed to rats as pets in domestic settings or occupationally in pet shops (Downing 2001; Graves and Janda 2001; Grant *et al.* 2004; Centers for Disease Control 2005; Schachter 2006; Matheson 2007). In California between 1970 and 1998, exposure to pet rats was reported in 54% of cases where animal exposure was recorded with exposure to rats in school, presumably largely in laboratories, contributing a further 14% of exposures (Graves and Janda 2001). Outbreaks may result from the contamination by rats of milk (Parker and Hudson 1926; Place and Sutton 1934) or water (McEvoy 1987).

Communicability

Person to person transmission does not occur.

Prevention and control

Preventing the infestation by rats of human dwellings and workplaces is the key to control. Nevertheless a number of recent cases have arisen as a result of keeping or supplying rats as companion animals. It is important, therefore, that those who keep rats as companion animals or those who supply them are aware of the diagnosis as prevention of severe disease can be greatly assisted by early recognition and treatment. The CDC advise protective gloves when handling rats or cleaning their cages. They advise further that children under 5 years of age should be supervized by adults to prevent bites and hand to mouth contact and that, in the event of a rat bite, the wound should be promptly cleaned and disinfected. The efficacy of antimicrobial prophylaxis is unknown (CDC 2005).

Disease clusters must prompt the systematic search for a common source.

Spirillary fever

History

Spirillary Fever was first described in a rat in Bombay (Mumbai), India, by Henry Van Dyke Carter, a distinguished physician and pathologist who was the original illustrator of Gray's 'Anatomy', in 1888 (Hiatt and Hiatt 1995). *Spirillum minus* became recognized, with *Streptobacillus moniliformis* as one of the two causes of Rat-Bite fever. Accounts of cases have been rare and although they occur worldwide (Pritchard 1990) it has been suggested that they are more common in Asia (Booth and Katz 2002; CDC 2005).

The agent

Spirillum minus is a minute (0.2 microns wide by 2–5 microns in length) spirillar bacterium which has 2–3 rigid spirals of 0.8–1.0 micron wavelength and one or more flagella attached at each pole. It may be stained with methylene blue and with Giemsa. Its true taxonomic place is unknown (Skirrow 1990). It is aerobic and can be cultured only *in vivo* in mice and guinea pigs (Pritchard 1990).

Hosts

Animal

Spirillum minus is found in rats, mice and guinea pigs and does not seem to be pathogenic in animals.

Human

Incubation period

The incubation period is generally 7–21 days but may extend to months (Pritchard 1990).

Symptoms and signs

These can be differentiated clinically from Streptobacillary Fever (Holmgren 1970). Redness and swelling are visible at the wound site initially. This may be healed before the onset of systemic disease but *Spirillum minus* is characterized by re-opening and eventual ulceration of the wound even after it has initially healed. Systemic disease is heralded by paroxysmal fever accompanied by lymphadenopathy and dark-red eruptions on the skin. Myalgia and arthralgia, more pronounced on the side of the body affected by the bite, occur. Arthritis seldom occurs.

Diagnosis

The organism is present in the local lesion or lymph nodes but may occassionally be demonstrated, with difficulty, by dark field microscopy. Subcutaneous inoculation of fluid or lymph nodes in guinea pigs is followed by a chancre and enlargement of regional lymph nodes. In both of these sites *Spirillum minus* may be demonstrated (Pritchard 1990). Unlike Streptobacillary Fever, leucocytosis is usually absent in Spirillosis (Holmgren 1970).

Treatment

Parenteral penicillin is the drug of choice although may cause a Jarisch-Herxheimer reaction. Erythromycin or chloramphenicol may all be used in patients allergic to penicillin. Sulphonamides are ineffective.

Prognosis

Attacks last 3–4 days but, in the absence of treatment can recur, usually at a regular interval, for months or even years. Case fatality rate is 2–10% (Pritchard 1990).

Epidemiology

Sporadic cases occur worldwide. Outbreaks are not described. Wild rats, living in close proximity to man, were examined in Vancouver in 1950 and 14% carried *Spirillum minus*. (Pritchard 1990). Carriage rates in London in the 1980s in trapped rats were 25% (Martin 2005). Carriage by laboratory rats, mice and guinea pigs is also described. Disease is exclusively transmitted to humans by the bite of an infected animal in contrast to *Streptobacillus moniliformis* where transmission by the contamination of milk or water by the urine of infected animals is described.

Person to person transmission does not occur.

Prevention and control

Preventing the infestation by rats of human dwellings and workplaces is the key to control. As with *Streptobacillus moniliformis,* the taking of general precautions to avoid being bitten when handling rats, including those kept in laboratories or as pets, is important. Meticulous local wound care of any bites that do occur is also necessary. The efficacy of antimicrobial prophylaxis is unknown but is sometimes suggested (Pritchard 1990).

References

Balakrishnan, N., Menon, T., Shanmugasundaram, S., and Alagesan, R. (2006). *Streptobacillus moniliformis* endocarditis. *Emerg. Infect. Dis.*, **12**(6):1037–38.

Boot, R., Oosterhuis, A., Thuis, H. C. (2002). PCR for the detection of Streptobacillus moniliformis. *Lab. Anim.*, **36**(2): 200–208.

Booth, C. M., Katz, K. C., and Brunton, J. (2002). Fever and a rat bite. *Can. J. Infect. Dis.*, **13**(4): 269–72.

Centers for Disease Control and Prevention (2005). Fatal rat-bite fever—Florida and Washington, 2003. *Morb. Mortal. Wkly. Rep.*, **53**(51): 1198–1202.

Costas, M., Owen, R. J. (1987). Numerical analysis of electrophoretic protein patterns of *Streptobacillus moniliformis* strains from human, murine and avian infections. *J. Med. Micro.*, **23**: 303–11.

Downing, N. D., Dewnany, G. D., and Radford, P. J. (2001). A rare and serious consequence of a rat bite. *Ann. R. Coll. Surg. Engl.*, **83**(4): 279–80.

Elliott, S. P. (2007). Rat bite fever and *Streptobacillus moniliformis*. *Clin. Microbiol. Rev.*, 20(1): 1322.

Graves, M. H., and Janda, J. M. (2001). Rat-bite fever (*Streptobacillus moniliformis*): a potential emerging disease. *Int. J. Infect. Dis.*, **5**(3): 151–55.

Grant, C., Simmons, G., Sinclair, S., Bassett, R., Ruscoe, Q., et al. (2004). Outbreak case reports. *N. Zealand Pub. Heal. Surveill. Rep.*, **2**(2): 6–7.

Hiatt, J. R., and Hiatt, N. (1995). The forgotten first career of Doctor Henry Van Dyke Carter. *J. Am. Coll. Surg.*, **181**(5): 464–66.

Holmgren, E. B. and Tunevall, G. (1970). Case Report - Rat Bite Fever. *Scand. J. Infect. Dis.*, **2**: 71–74.

Martin, S. A. (2005). *Spirillum minus* and *Streptobacillus moniliformis*. In: S. P. Borriello et al. (eds.) Topley and Wilson's Microbiology and Microbial Infections, (10th edn.), Vol. 2, pp. 1908–12. London: Hodder Arnold.

Matheson, K., Langley, J. M., Lang, B., Mailman, T. (2008). Polyarthritis, fever and a rash in a young girl. *Can. J. Infect. Dis. Med. Microbiol.*, **1**: 73–74.

McEvoy, M. B., Noah, N. D., and Pilsworth, R. (1987). Outbreak of fever caused by *Streptobacillus moniliformis*. *Lancet* ii: 1361–63.

Parker, F., and Hudson, N. P. (1926). The etiology of Haverhill fever. *Am. J. Pathol.*, **2**: 357–59.

Place, E. H., and Sutton, L. E. (1934). Erythema Arthriticum Epidemicum (Haverhill Fever). *Arch. Intern. Med.*, **54**(5): 659–84.

Pritchard, D. G. (1990). Spirochaetal and leptospiral diseases: In: M. T. Parker and L. H. Collier (eds.) Topley and Wilson's Principles of Bacteriology, Virology and Immunity, (8th edn.), Vol. III, pp. 618–9. London: Edward Arnold.

Roughgarden, J. W. (1965). Antimicrobial therapy of rat-bite fever. *Arch. Intern. Med.*, **39**: 116.

Rowbotham, T. J. (1983). Rapid identification of Streptobacillus moniliformis. *Lancet*, **322**: 567.

Schachter, M. E., Wilcox, L., Rau, N., Yamamura, D., Brown, S., et al. (2006). Rat-bite fever, Canada. *Emerg. Infect. Dis.*, **12**(8): 1301–02.

Shanson, D. C., Gazzard, B. G., et al. (1983). *Streptobacillus moniliformis* isolated from blood in four cases of Haverhill fever; first outbreak in Britain. *Lancet*, **ii**: 92–94.

Skirrow, M. B. (1990). *Campylobacter, Helicobacter* and other motile curved gram-negative rods: In: M. T. Parker and B. I. Duerden (eds.) Topley and Wilson's Principles of Bacteriology, Virology and Immunity, (8th edn.), Vol. II, pp. 545–7. London: Edward Arnold.

Strangeways, W. I. (1933). Rats as carriers of *Streptobacillus moniliformis*. *J. Pathol. Bacteriol.*, **37**: 45–51.

Taber, L. H., and Feigen, R. D. (1979). Spirochetal infections. *Pediatr. Clin. N. Am.*, **26**: 337.

Wang, T. K., and Wong, S. S. (2007). *Streptobacillus moniliformis* septic arthritis: a clinical entity distinct from rat-bite fever? *BMC Infect. Dis.*, **7**: 56.

Washburn, R. G. (2005). Streptobacillus moniformis (rat-bite fever). In: G. L. Mandell, J. E. Bennett and R. Dolin (eds.) Mandell, Douglas and Bennett's Principles and Practice of Infectious Diseases, (6th edn.), Vol. II, pp. 2708–10. Philadelphia: Elsevier.

CHAPTER 19e

Other bacterial diseases

Streptococcosis

Marina Morgan

Summary

Many pyogenic (β-haemolytic) streptococci of clinical significance have animal connections. In the last edition of this book two species of streptococci were considered of major zoonotic interest, namely *Streptococcus suis* and *S. zooepidemicus*. Since then, numerous sporadic zoonoses due to other streptococci have been reported, and a newly recognized fish pathogen with zoonotic potential termed *S. iniae* has emerged. Changes in nomenclature make the terminology confusing. For example, the organism known as *S. zooepidemicus*—now termed *S. dysgalactiae* subsp. *zooepidemicus*—still causes pharyngitis in humans, complicated rarely by glomerulonephritis after ingestion of unpasteurized milk. Pigs remain the primary hosts of *S. suis* with human disease mainly affecting those who have contact with pigs or handle pork.

Once a sporadic disease, several major epidemics associated with high mortality have been reported in China. The major change in reports of zoonotic streptococcal infections has been the emergence of severe skin and soft tissue infections, and an increasing prevalence of toxic shock, especially due to *S. suis* (Tang *et al.* 2006), group C (Keiser 1992) and group G β-haemolytic streptococci (Barnham *et al.* 2002). Penicillin remains the mainstay of treatment for most infections, although some strains of group C and G streptococci are tolerant (minimum bactericidal concentration difficult or impossible to achieve *in vivo*) (Portnoy *et al.* 1981; Rolston and LeFrock 1984) and occasionally strains with increased minimum inhibitory concentrations (MIC) for penicillin are reported.

Agents preventing exotoxin formation, such as clindamycin and occasionally human intravenous immunoglobulin, may be used in overwhelming infection where circulating exotoxins need to be neutralized in order to damp down the massive release of cytokines generated by their production (Darenberg *et al.* 2003). Prevention of human disease focuses on maintaining good hygienic practice when dealing with live animals or handling raw meat or fish products, covering skin lesions, thorough cooking of meats and pasteurization of milk.

Introduction

Streptococci are Gram-positive (i.e. blue-staining) spheres arranged in chains. The name is derived from *strepto* (Greek for twisted chain or pliant) and *kokkos* (Greek for berry/kernel); the most pathogenic streptococci are termed 'pyogenic' (pus-forming). Most are β-haemolytic, i.e. colonies surrounded by a zone of β-haemolysis (complete) when cultured on agar containing blood, the haemolytic activity occasionally affected by the nature of the animal blood used. As part of the lacto-bacteria group, streptococci produce lactic acid from the fermentation of carbohydrates, being incapable of respiratory metabolism. Since streptococci are facultative anaerobes, they grow well in anaerobic conditions. Streptococcal growth is inhibited by acid conditions so growth may be optimized by buffering broth cultures, as in Todd Hewitt medium.

History

Streptococci were first described by Billroth in 1874, and five years later Pasteur isolated streptococci from the blood of a woman with puerperal sepsis. *Streptococcus pyogenes*, the type species, was first described in 1884 by Rosenbach. Throughout history *S. pyogenes* has been responsible for tonsillitis, sepsis in childbirth (puerperal sepsis), cellulitis (inflammation of skin and superficial soft tissues) and deeper soft tissue infections such as necrotizing fasciitis and myositis. In the last 20 years, *S. pyogenes* has increasingly been recognized as causing streptococcal toxic shock syndrome (STSS).

Although other β-haemolytic streptococci can produce similar illnesses, including tonsillitis, soft tissue infections and more rarely, toxic shock in animals and man, streptococcal zoonoses are comparatively unusual because of host and tissue specificity. Most streptococci exist happily as part of the normal flora of animals and man, often in the oropharynx or gut.

Serological differentiation of the β-haemolytic streptococci depends on the nature of the carbohydrate components of the cell wall. The Lancefield typing scheme, first described in 1933, is based on the capillary precipitin reaction between the group specific carbohydrate cell wall antigens (extracted by hot acids) and hyperimmune rabbit antisera (Lancefield and Hare 1935). Nowadays commercial kits are available for 'grouping' of streptococci, using various methodologies. The most predominant method utilizes agglutination of antibody-coated particles, the defining group-specific antigens denoted by letters. There are now 20 serogroups of β-haemolytic streptococci, divided according to the original Lancefield typing scheme: A to V (excluding I and J). The most common human infections are generally caused by groups A–F.

In older reports the streptococcal species was rarely identified beyond the serogroup, and some were probably misidentified. Due to advances in molecular methodology, streptococcal taxonomy has changed in recent years making the comparative evaluation and interpretation of older reports of streptococcal zoonoses difficult.

Lancefield groups may contain one or more species, but confusion in differentiation easily arises when some species possess more than one group antigen, technically having features in common with other streptococci and so may be misidentified. One classic and confusing example of overlapping group antigens is *S. dysgalactiae* subsp. *equisimilis*, which may possess Lancefield group A, C, G or L carbohydrate antigens, and is one of the so-called 'large colony' types of streptococci. Equally, many of the so-called 'small colony' strains of the *S. anginosus* group possess similar antigens but, as they are rarely associated with zoonoses, they will not be considered further in this chapter.

Biochemical tests are used in addition to 'grouping' and helps further differentiate the various strains. Finally, modern molecular techniques have enabled a much better understanding of the diversity and genetic relationship of the streptococci.

In order to simplify this complex taxonomy for better understanding, Table 19e.1 may be helpful, referring to the streptococci by their old names and modern equivalents.

Zoonotic streptococci

Group A streptococci

The agent

The type species for the haemolytic streptococci is *Streptococcus pyogenes*, the classical 'group A β-haemolytic streptococcus.' *S. pyogenes* is not, however, alone in carrying the group A antigen, as some strains of Group C streptococci such as *S. equisimilis* may also possess it.

Table 19e.1 Streptococci by old names and modern equivalent

Major Lancefield group	Type species	Subtypes
A	*S. pyogenes*	
B	*S. agalactiae* (mastitis in cattle)	
C	*S. dysgalactiae* subsp. (large colony formers)	subsp. *dysgalactiae*–very few zoonoses subsp. *Equisimilis*
	S. equi	subsp. *equi* causes strangles in horses subsp. *zooepidemicus* (formerly *S. zooepidemicus*)
E (some also P, U, V)	*S. porcinus*	
G		*S. equisimilis* subsp. *equisimilis* *S. canis*
S, R & T	*S. suis* (pneumonia in pigs)	*S. suis* 2 most pathogenic
Ungroupable	*S. iniae*	

Disease in animals

Historically, *S. pyogenes* mastitis followed contamination by the hands of human milkers. Although companion animals have long been recognized as the source of many childhood zoonoses, including tonsillitis (Copperman 1982), *S. pyogenes* is rarely isolated from asymptomatic animals (Wilson *et al.* 1995). Whilst the prevalence of *S. pyogenes* in dogs and cats is reported as 2.8% (Crowder *et al.* 1978), simultaneous Group A streptococcus (GAS) infection in animal and owner is apparently exceedingly rare (Falck 1997). Furthermore, those GAS strains colonizing companion animals are probably acquired from close contact with their owners; for example, licking or sharing sleeping areas and is effectively a 'humanosis' rather than a zoonoses. GAS infections tend to manifest clinically as conjunctivitis, the animals then acting as reservoirs for secondary human infection.

Disease in man

S. pyogenes colonizes the throat of 25–30% of otherwise asymptomatic, healthy humans, especially children, in whom the major manifestation of infection is tonsillitis. Cellulitis and the more severe skin and soft tissue infections such as necrotizing fasciitis and myositis, when associated with toxic shock syndrome, have an associated mortality as high as 80%.

Cows occasionally suffer mastitis with *S. pyogenes*. Among many historical outbreaks due to contaminated milk, Gollege (1932) reported an outbreak in a farming family where two cows were infected, but infections were confined only to the family as a result of pasteurization of the milk before sale. Infected cows may excrete *S. pyogenes* for up to 13 months (Bendixen and Minett 1937). Outbreaks may occur in meat processing (Barnham and Neilson 1987) as minor skin wounds, with contamination of knives and work surfaces facilitating horizontal spread between workers.

S. pyogenes infection may occasionally recur inexplicably within families despite control measures and companion animals may be a hidden reservoir. Extensive swabbing of 61 dogs, cats, rabbits and guinea pigs from 46 households suffering with recurrent infections found two families who owned a dog and a cat each of which were suffering with conjunctivitis (Falck 1997). After simultaneous penicillin therapy of all the family members and their pets no further infections were noted in either humans or animals (Falck 1997). Recurrent *S. pyogenes* pharyngitis was finally cleared only when the family and the dog were treated concomitantly with penicillin (Mayer and van Ore 1983). Another report implicated the family cat as the reservoir (Roos *et al.* 1988). Hence, an animal reservoir should be considered in otherwise unexplained recurrent human infection.

Group C streptococci

Six β-haemolytic species or subspecies possess the group C antigen (Facklam 2002). Most are β-haemolytic on sheep blood agar. Commonly found in domestic animals, guinea pigs, and birds, the four most common are *S. dysgalactiae*, *S. equi*, *S. equisimilis*, and *S. equi* subsp. *zooepidemicus* (formerly *S. zooepidemicus*), of which the latter currently has the most zoonotic potential.

Since *S. equi* and *S. zooepidemicus* are so similar, they are now referred to as *S. equi* subsp. *equi* and *S. equi* subsp. *zooepidemicus* respectively. Since *S. dysgalactiae* and *S. equisimilis* are closely related they are now termed *S. dysgalactiae* subsp. *dysgalactiae* and *S. dysgalactiae* subsp. *equisimilis* respectively.

Streptococcus equi subspecies equi

S. equi subsp. *equi* is a β-haemolytic streptococcus expressing a group C antigen, and found mainly in horses.

Disease in animals

S. equi subsp. *equi* causes a suppurative lymphadenitis and nasal discharge of horses which is highly contagious. Swelling of the lymph nodes occasionally compromises the airway, hence the common name 'strangles.' Once thought exclusive to horses, a case of canine strangles has been reported in a British dog (Ladlaw *et al.* 2006).

Disease in man

Many authorities have stated firmly that *S. equi* subsp. *equi* is not a zoonoses, although there is one report of 'human strangles' occurring in a 56 year old horse handler presenting with massive facial swelling and a cheek abscess from which *S. equi* subsp. *equi* and *Bacteroides* spp. were isolated. The suspected portal of entry was carious teeth (Breiman and Silverblatt 1986). A recent hospital outbreak of *S. dysgalactiae* subsp. *equisimilis* in Brazil was suggested to arise from horses grazing nearby, but despite identical strains being carried in their faeces, the link remained unproven (Torres *et al.* 2007).

Streptococcus equi subspecies zooepidemicus

S. equi subsp. *zooepidemicus* (*S. zooepidemicus* in earlier papers) is the commonest zoonotic pathogen amongst the group C streptococci and commensal in many animals, especially in the equine upper respiratory tract.

Disease in animals

S. equi subsp. *zooepidemicus* is a common commensal and opportunistic pathogen. Previously known as *S. zooepidemicus* and a cause of bovine mastitis, equine respiratory infection, poultry infection, *S. equi* subsp. *zooepidemicus* causes abortions and wound infections in younger horses, and endemic cervical lymphadenopathy with draining abscesses in guinea pigs.

Disease in man

Transmission of *S. equi* subsp. *zooepidemicus* to man is mainly associated with contact with horses or consumption of contaminated dairy products. It causes acute pharyngitis, and may spread to the lungs causing pneumonia, and via the bloodstream causing meningitis, endocarditis, and septic arthritis. *S. equi* subsp. *zooepidemicus* was not isolated from any human throat swabs in studies by Lewis and Balfour (1999), Turner *et al.* (1997), and Duca *et al.* (1969). In an outbreak of *S. equi* subsp. *zooepidemicus* in Helsinki in 2003 following the consumption of unpasteurized fresh goat cheese, six people developed septicaemia with a further case of purulent septic arthritis. The median age of the patients was 70 years and none died. Strains indistinguishable by pulsed field gel electrophoresis and ribotyping were isolated from the human throat swabs, goat cheese samples, milk tank and vaginal samples of one goat (Kuusi *et al.* 2006).

Several outbreaks of acute glomerulonephritis have occurred after consumption of unpasteurized milk. The first outbreak affected 85 people in Romania (Duca *et al.* 1969) and the second began with mild upper respiratory tract infections affecting five of six members of a dairy farming family in Yorkshire (Barnham *et al.* 1983). In the latter, the farmer and two of the three children developed malaise, oedema, abdominal pain, haematuria, and hypertension—all signs and symptoms of acute glomerulonephritis. A recent outbreak of human nephritis in Brazil attributed to *S. equi* subsp. *zooepidemicus*, 3 of 133 confirmed cases died, 7 required haemodialysis and 96 were hospitalized (Balter *et al.* 2000). Rare disease presentations include septicaemia as the first manifestation of Hairy Cell Leukaemia (Oever *et al.* 2009).

Streptococcous dysgalactiae subspecies dysgalactiae

Unlike other group C streptococci, *S. dysgalactiae* subsp. *dysgalactiae* is α-haemolytic, showing partial haemolysis and greenish discoloration on agar containing horse blood. Almost exclusively an animal pathogen, it is a well-recognized cause of bovine mastitis. The first report of isolation in dogs was from newborn Great Dane puppies which died of septicaemia within 72 hours (Vela *et al.* 2006).

Disease in man

Human infections due to *S. dysgalactiae* subsp. *dysgalactiae* are very rare, although a case of bacteraemia in a 48 year old female Chinese chef with a history of mastectomy developed two days after a puncture wound acquired whilst cleaning raw tilapia and shrimps (Koh *et al.* 2009).

Group G streptococci

Group G β-hemolytic streptococci (GGS) may be easily overlooked or misdiagnosed as *S. pyogenes* since up to 67% are sensitive to bacitracin. There are two types of GGS, *S. equisimilis* subsp. *equisimilis*, the GGS most commonly affecting humans, and *S. canis* (usually found in cattle and dogs). Similarities between GGS and *S. pyogenes* extend to the production of a streptolysin antigenically similar to that of *S. pyogenes*. Named streptolysin S (SL-S), this is one of the most potent cytotoxins known and probably responsible for much of the tissue destruction observed in animal and human infections (Humar *et al.* 2002).

Streptococcous equisimilis subspecies equisimilis

S. equisimilis subsp. *equisimilis* may possess Lancefield group A, C, G or L carbohydrate antigens. *S. equisimilis* subsp. *equisimilis* produces streptokinase and streptolysin O, and infection produces an increase in the antistreptolysin O titre (ASOT), a serological test used commonly to diagnose recent *S. pyogenes* infection.

Disease in animals

S. equisimilis subsp. *equisimilis* is a commensal of the mucous membranes of horses and swine. Occasionally isolated from aborted equine placentas, the organisms may be responsible for a strangles-like illness in horses (Preziusio *et al.* 2010). Suppurative erosive arthritis in swine, and pharyngitis in humans and horses has been reported (Turner *et al.* 1997).

Disease in man

Despite commonly colonizing humans in throat, nose and genital swabs, actual infections with *S. equisimilis* subsp. *equisimilis* are rare. Cases of endocarditis, pneumonia and cellulitis (Carmeli *et al.* 1995) have been reported with a recent recognition of its importance as a cause of vertebral osteomyelitis (Kumar *et al.* 2005).

S. equisimilis subsp. *equisimilis* commonly cause skin and soft tissue infections (SSTI) and increasingly streptococcal toxic shock syndrome (STSS).

GGS human infection is usually associated with other co-morbidities, including malignancy and defective lymphatic circulation. During a two year survey of Atlanta and San Franciscan residents with invasive group G streptococcal isolates, 87% had underlying disease (Broyles *et al.* 2009).

Streptococcus canis

Lancefield group G streptococcus *S. canis* (Devriese *et al.* 1986), is a β-haemolytic opportunistic pathogen colonizing wounds or bites and carried by dogs, foxes, cattle, rodents, mink and rabbits. Despite apparent penicillin sensitivity on plate sensitivity testing, both group C and group G streptococci may exhibit 'tolerance', i.e. the MIC is far lower than the bactericidal concentration achievable *in vivo* (Rolston and LeFrock 1984).

Disease in animals

S. canis colonizes dogs and cats and can cause neonatal septicaemia in puppies. GGS mastitis in cattle is rare, with an anecdotal report of a dog licking cows' teats as a source of the infection (Tikofsky and Zadoks 2005). However, an outbreak in a New York herd in 1999 involved 46/90 (51%) cows infected with *S. canis*. The outbreak was finally brought under control after culling many infected cows, amoxicillin treatment, and the introduction of scrupulous hand hygiene. The infection was believed to originate from a farm cat that was afflicted with chronic *S. canis* sinusitis and enjoyed free access to the milking quarters. Milk from affected cattle and nasal secretions from the cat produced identical isolates (Tikofsky and Zadoks 2005). On the basis of ribotyping the authors conclude that *S. canis* was spread by secretions from the cat with sinusitis to one of the cows, and then horizontally through the herd because of poor milking hygiene.

Disease in man

The true prevalence of human disease is unknown because of lack of full identification in many laboratories. A cluster of *S. canis* ulcer infections occurred in three dog owners. The first, a 53 year old male with diabetic neuropathy suffered *S. canis* infection on a non-healing foot ulcer which needed extensive debridement. The second patient, an 80 year old female, had a gangrenous toe infected with *S. canis* and *Pasteurella canis*. The third patient, a 75 year old male had recurrent *S. canis* septicaemia from a pressure sore (Lam *et al.* 2007). Recurrent septicaemia is not uncommon in GGS infections. A 75 year old female was treated apparently successfully with penicillin for fever and swelling of the right thigh following a dog bite. She was readmitted with recurrent septicaemia three weeks later. Transoesophageal echocardiogram excluded endocarditis and after another prolonged course of antibiotics she returned home. Isolates from her and her dog were identical (Takeda *et al.* 2001).

Whether the apparent susceptibility of patients with rheumatoid arthritis to streptococcal infection is due to concomitant steroid or other immunosuppressive therapy is unclear. A 65 year old Japanese female with rheumatoid arthritis was handling raw fish, making tempura. Small burns on her fingers acquired during deep frying the fish were thought to be the entry site for the streptococci that produced a toxic shock syndrome. Post mortem examination revealed a necrotizing arteritis, septic pulmonary emboli, splenic abscesses, intestinal arteritis and abscesses in the kidneys and muscle (Hirose *et al.* 1997).

Streptococcus iniae

S. iniae is a fish pathogen with newly recognized zoonotic potential having already caused several outbreaks. *S. iniae* is β-haemolytic on sheep blood agar, but is not groupable with Lancefield antigens. Isolates are non-motile and sensitive to vancomycin. Most strains grow at 10°C but not 45°C and few grow in 6.5% sodium chloride.

Of two highly related clones only one has caused invasive disease, suggesting that an as yet unidentified virulence factor exists (Weinstein *et al.* 1997).

Disease in animals

S. iniae causes subcutaneous abscesses in freshwater dolphins in aquaria and necrotic infection of the caudal peduncle of farmed fish. Outbreaks of invasive disease in aquaculture affect fish farms in countries worldwide, including Japan, Taiwan, Israel and North America (Weinstein *et al.* 1997).

Disease in man

Four cases of bacteraemia were identified in Toronto in 1995, three of whom suffered severe cellulitis, with one case of meningitis, endocarditis and septic arthritis. Three patients had prepared tilapias prior to infection and all had broken skin. During one year, nine further cases were found, all of whom had handled live or freshly killed tilapia imported from the USA (Weinstein *et al.* 1997). The most likely mode of entry to the body was via trauma to the hands from residual fins or scales (Koh *et al.* 2009) with 8/9 bacteraemic patients reporting having injured their hands whilst processing the fish within 24 hours prior to infection. Numerous other reports of *S. iniae* infection have emerged (Weinstein *et al.* 1997; Lau *et al.* 2003). Common risk factors are old age, and pre-existing co-morbidities such as diabetes mellitus.

Some authors have speculated that many of these infections are overlooked or misidentified, especially since six clinical isolates in the Canadian surveillance had initially been identified as *S. uberis* (non-pathogenic for man) (Weinstein *et al.* 1997).

Streptococcus suis type 2 (group R)

Since its discovery in piglets nearly fifty years ago (de Moor 1963), *S. suis* has caused only sporadic cases of zoonotic infection, but latterly has been responsible for major epidemics in humans. Facultatively anaerobic and α- or non-haemolytic, not all isolates are pathogenic. Virulence varies with the serotype of *S. suis*. Initially designated as Lancefield group R streptococci, *S. suis* now belongs to the Lancefield S, R and T groups.

The agent

In many ways *S. suis* is the porcine equivalent of *S. agalactiae*, the β-haemolytic streptococcus of Group B (GBS) that affects human babies. Adult sows are asymptomatic carriers, with ~80% carriage rate in some pig herds and, like human GBS infections, mothers can infect their infant offspring by vertical transmission. Transmission to humans is via damaged skin or the consumption of undercooked pork.

S. suis colonies are small, 0.5–1.0mm in diameter, and often slightly mucoid. *S. suis* is a facultative anaerobe, unable to grow in 6.5% sodium chloride, and may be α-haemolytic on sheep blood agar and β-haemolytic on horse blood agar and may therefore be misidentified (Tramontana *et al.* 2008). Phenotypically, *S. suis* can resemble *S. gordoniae*, *S. sanguinis* and *S. parasanguinis* (Facklam *et al.* 2002).

S. suis comprises 35 serotypes based on capsular polysaccharides. Serotypes are of variable virulence, some causing severe infections such as meningitis and septicaemia. *S. suis* types 1 and 2 are the predominant causes of infection. Serotypes 32 and 34 have now been recognized as distant from other serotypes and are termed *S. orisratti*.

S. suis type 2, the most pathogenic, is a hardy organism, resistant to many environmental conditions and survives 10 minutes at 60°C, or 2 hours at 50°C. The organism may survive six weeks on carcasses held at 10°C, one month in dust and three months in faeces at 0°C (Lun *et al.* 2007).

A surprising feature of the recent *S. suis* outbreak in China has been the high incidence of toxic shock syndrome (Chan *et al.* 2007). Whereas streptococcal toxic shock syndrome due to *S. pyogenes* is due mainly to superantigens inducing an intense inflammatory response by massively activating T-cells and releasing cytokines, *S. suis* type 2 is thought to produce toxic shock due to the presence of a unique 89kb fragment in the genome. This encodes a two-component signal transduction system (SalK-SalR) necessary for full virulence. Other potential virulence factors identified include muraminidase-released precursor, extracellular factor and 'suilysin'—a thiol-activated haemolysin originally derived from a Netherlands strain.

Multilocus sequence typing of *S. suis* showed the 2005 epidemic Chinese strains are grouped into a sequence type (ST) termed ST7 on the basis of the presence of seven housekeeping genes. Whole genome sequencing of the representative strain of the 2005 epidemic identified a potential pathogenicity island (PAI) named 89K. This may function as a new specific virulence marker for the Chinese *S. suis*-2 clones (Chen *et al.* 2007) since the virulent strains carrying 89K are ST7.

Disease in animals

S. suis type 2 is a pathogen for man and pigs. The domestic pig (*Sus scrofa domestica*) is a major reservoir although there are three reports of infections from wild boar, including a case of a poacher who contracted meningitis (Halaby *et al.* 2000).

The major site of carriage in swine is the palatine tonsils. Infection produces polyarthritis, meningitis and septicaemia in suckling pigs. Piglets are the most susceptible to infection, especially if bred in poor housing with poor ventilation.

Meningitis is common in older, weaned pigs, who present with depression, anorexia, trembling, incoordination, and with other features of nervous system dysfunction such as opisthotonous, fits, blindness, ear infections, deafness and vestibular dysfunction. Pneumonia, endocarditis and abortions have been reported and occasionally other animals may be affected. The most pathogenic type is *S. suis* type 2 (Gottschalk *et al.* 2007) and about 10% of infected pigs at slaughter have evidence of endocarditis with subacute bacteraemia in many more (Robertson and Blackmore 1989).

Epidemiology

The first human infections were reported in 1968 in Denmark (Arends and Zanen 1988). Apart from the 1996 and 2005 Chinese outbreaks, most human cases are sporadic and relatively uncommon. Although the majority of reported cases have occurred in China (69%) and Thailand (11%), there have been sporadic human cases in other countries, with 8% occurring in the Netherlands (Yang *et al.* 2009). No person to person spread has been reported (Lun *et al.* 2007). In one survey in New Zealand some 21% of New Zealand pig farmers had antibodies to *S. suis* type 2, and it has been estimated that the incidence of subclinical infections could be as high as 30% annually (Robertson and Blackmore 1989). 10% of meat inspectors and 9% of dairy farmers, most of them also kept pigs, were also seropositive (Robertson and Blackmore 1989).

Breton *et al.* (1986) reported *S. suis* 2 in 8.1% (28/347) of pig herds destined for slaughter in Ontario. A carriage rate of 9.4% was found in slaughtermen. They concluded that the eviscerators removing the larynx and lungs from carcasses were at significantly higher risk (p<0.05) of exposure to *S. suis* than other abattoir workers.

Furthermore, 80% of *S. suis* isolated from hands and knives of workers were from the lung evisceration station (Breton *et al.* 1986).

The most serious outbreaks have occurred in China. In Jiangsu province (1998 and 1999), and more recently in Sichuan province (2005), serious epidemics with a particularly high mortality were reported. Serotype 2 strains responsible for the Chinese Jiangsu outbreak (1998) killed 14/25 people affected. During June–Aug 2005 an outbreak of *S. suis* serotype 2 occurred during which 204 cases occurred and 38 died (Tang *et al.* 2006).

Disease in humans

The classical presentation of meningitis or septicaemia in humans mirror the presentations of illness in pigs. *S. suis* meningitis is associated with a high incidence of hearing loss on recovery, together with ataxia, which very occasionally persists. The prevalence of deafness in human survivors of *S. suis* infection may be due to a special affinity of *S. suis* for the meninges, especially the cochlear division of the eighth cranial nerve. In a large series of cases, 72.5% had meningitis (Jiang *et al.* 2006), often accompanied by ataxia, coma, petechiae, articular pain, ecchymoses, rashes and rhabdomyolysis. One percent had endocarditis, 0.8% pneumonia and 0.3% peritonitis. More than 80% of those with septicaemia and shock died, 42% having diarrhoea, 77% vomiting, and 93% cutaneous haemorrhages. In the largest Chinese outbreak involving 215 cases, 62% with toxic shock syndrome died (Yu *et al.* 2006). Toxic shock syndrome is now emerging as a common presentation of *S. suis* infection, associated with a high mortality.

Of 204 cases in another study, 198 were farmers, 5 were butchers and one was a veterinary surgeon (Tang *et al.* 2006); some had broken skin, with cuts on their hands and feet, and all had had direct contact with ill or dead pigs. More than 25% (59 of those affected) suffered with toxic shock, 104 with meningitis and 41 others were mainly suffering with septicaemia. Fatal cases all began acutely with malaise, fever, headache, diarrhoea, hyperpyrexia, hypotension, an erythematous blanching rash affecting the extremities and usually a leucocytosis. Of those with toxic shock, 83% developed acute respiratory distress syndrome (ARDS), and 50% became comatose (Tang *et al.* 2006).

The first reported case of *S. suis* meningitis in Hawaii affected a 34 year old Tongan coconut tree trimmer. Despite having slaughtered pigs by hand in readiness for a celebration, he had no skin lesions likely to be entry sites. Despite treatment with ceftriaxone, he needed readmission twice after discharge because of hearing loss, nystagmus and dizziness, all of which eventually resolved completely with steroid therapy (Fittipaldi *et al.* 2009).

Treatment

Penicillin resistance is uncommon. Intravenous gentamicin and penicillin was successful in a series of eight patients with septicaemia (Tramontana *et al.* 2008), in which the isolates were phenotypically similar to *S. parasanguis*, and were initially misidentified by conventional methodology but later confirmed by 16s rRNA sequencing. The patients recovered after two weeks of intravenous therapy followed by two weeks of oral amoxycillin.

In severe cases, high dose ceftriaxone has been ineffective, and combination therapy, such as amoxicillin plus ceftriaxone and gentamicin. Once septic shock has developed, there appears to be a limited effect of any antimicrobial (Lun *et al.* 2007). Several authors recommend prolonged therapy since relapse after 2 and 4 weeks of therapy (Gottschalk *et al.* 2007).

Prevention and control of streptococcal zoonoses

S. pyogenes, *S. iniae*, *S. suis* and *S. canis* can all enter the skin via traumatic scratches or breaks. Measures, such as wearing protective clothing when dealing with pig carcasses, and ensuring maximal hygiene when butchering or gutting fish are essential. Avoiding consumption of raw milk products would prevent *S. equi* subsp. *zooepidemicus* acquisition and thorough cooking of pork may prevent some infections. The World Health Organization recommend that pork should reach 70°C internal temperature or until juices run clear (Lun *et al.* 2007). Pasteurization of milk probably prevents many infections that would otherwise occur.

Despite research attempts, there are no vaccines yet available to prevent acquisition of infection. Good animal husbandry and hygiene remain the major methods of protection against infection.

References

Arends, J.P. and Zanen, H.C. (1988). Meningitis caused by *Streptococcus suis* in humans. *Rev. Infect. Dis.*, **10**: 131–77.

Balter, S.A., Benin, S.W.L., Pinto, L.M. *et al.* (2000). Epidemic nephritis in Nova Serrana, Brazil. *Lancet*, **355**: 1776–80.

Barnham, M. and Neilson, D.J. (1987). Group L β-hemolytic streptococcal infection in meat handlers: another streptococcal zoonosis? *Epidemiol. Infect.*, **99**: 257–64.

Barnham, M., Thornton, T.J. and Lange, K. (1983). Nephritis caused by *Streptococcus zooepidemicus* (Lancefield group C). *Lancet*, **1**: 945–48.

Barnham, M.R., Weightman, N.C., Anderson, A.W. and Tanna, A. (2002). Streptococcal toxic shock syndrome: a description of 14 cases from North Yorkshire, UK. *Clin. Microbiol. Infect.*, **8**: 174–81.

Bendixen, H.C. and Minett, F.C. (1938). Excretion of *Streptococcus pyogenes* in the milk of naturally infected cows. *J. Hyg.*, **3**: 374–83.

Breiman, R.F. and Silverblatt, F.J. (1986). Systemic *Streptococcus equi* infection in a horse handler - a case of human strangles. *West. J. Med.*, **145**: 385–86.

Breton, J., Mitchell, W.R. and Rosendal, S. (1986). *Streptococcus suis* in slaughter pigs and abattoir workers. *Can. J. Vet. Res.*, **50**: 338–41.

Broyles, L.N., Van Benenden, C., Beall, B. *et al.* (2009). Population-based study of invasive disease due to β-haemolytic streptococci of groups other than A and B. *Clin. Infect. Dis.*, **48**: 706–12.

Carmeli, Y., Schapiro, J.M., Neeman, D., Yinnon, A.M. and Alkan, M. (1995). Streptococcal group C bacteraemia. Survey in Israel and analytic review. *Arch. Intern. Med.*, **155**: 1170–76.

Chen, C., Tang, J., Dong, W. *et al.* (2007). A glimpse of streptococcal toxic shock syndrome from comparative genomics of *S. suis* 2 Chinese isolates. *PLoS One*, **2**: e315.

Copperman, S.M. (1982). Cherchez le chien: household pets as reservoirs of persistent or recurrent streptococcal sore throat in children. *NY State J. Med.*, **82**: 1685–87.

Crowder, H.R., Dorn, C.R. and Smith, R.E. (1978). Group A streptococcus in pets and group A streptococcal disease in man. *Intern. J. Zoon.*, **5**: 45–54.

Darenberg, J., Ihendyane, N., Sjölin, J. *et al.* (2003). Intravenous immunoglobulin G therapy in streptococcal toxic shock syndrome: a European randomized, double-blind, placebo-controlled trial. *Clin. Infect. Dis.*, **37**: 333–40.

de Moor, C.E. (1963). Septicaemic infections in pigs caused by haemolytic streptococci of new Lancefield groups designated R, S and T. *Antonie van Leeuwen.*, **29**: 272–80.

Devriese, L.A., Hommez, J., Kilpper-Balz, R. and Schleifer, K.H. (1986). *Streptococcus canis* sp. nov.: a species of group G streptococci from animals. *Intern. J. System. Bacteriol.*, **36**: 422–25.

Duca, E., Teodorovici, G., Radu, C. *et al.* (1969). A new nephritogenic streptococcus. *J. Hyg.*, **67**: 691–98.

Facklam, R. (2002). What happened to the streptococci: overview of taxonomic and nomenclature changes. *Clin. Microbiol. Rev.*, **15**: 613–30.

Falck, G. (1997). Group A Streptococci in household pets' eyes—a source of infection in humans? *Scandin. J. Infect. Dis.*, **29**: 469–71.

Fittipaldi, N., Collis, T., Prothero, B. and Gotschalk, M. (2009). *Streptococcus suis* meningitis, Hawaii. *Emerg. Infect. Dis.*, **15**: 2067–69.

Golledge, S.V. (1932). Streptococcus infection in man caused through the medium of milk from infected udders. *Vet. Rec.*, **44**: 1499–501.

Gottschalk, M., Segura, M. and Xu, J. (2007). *Streptococcus suis* infections in humans: the Chinese experience and the situation in North America. *Ani. Heal. Res. Rev.*, **8**: 29–45.

Halaby, T., Hoitsma, E., Hupperts, R., Spanjaard, L., Luirink, M. *et al.* (2000). *Streptococcus suis* meningitis, a poacher's risk. *Euro. J. Clin. Microbiol. Infect. Dis.*, **19**: 943–45.

Hirose, T., Tagi, K., Honda, H., Shibuya, H. and Okazaki, E. (1997). Toxic shock-like syndrome caused by non-group A β-hemolytic streptococci. *Arch. Intern. Med.*, **157**: 1891–94.

Humar, D., Datta, V., Bast, D.J., Beall, B., de Azavedo, C.S. *et al.* (2002). Streptolysin S and necrotising infections produced by Group G streptococcus. *Lancet*, **359**: 124–29.

Jiang, N., Yang, X.X., Tang, R.Z. *et al.* (2006). Clinical characteristics of 48 cases with infection of *Streptococcus suis* serotype 2. *Chin. J. Infect. Dis.*, **24**: 179–82.

Keiser, P. (1992). Toxic streptococcus syndrome associated with Group C streptococcus. *Arch. Intern. Med.*, **152**: 882–84.

Koh, T.H., Sng, L.H., Yuen, S.M. *et al.* (2009). Streptococcal cellulitis following preparation of fresh raw seafood. *Zoon. Pub. Heal.*, **56**: 206–8.

Kumar, A., Sandoe, J. and Kumar, N. (2005). Three cases of vertebral osteomyelitis caused by *Streptococcus dysgalactiae* subsp. *equisimilis*. *J. Med. Microbiol.*, **54**: 1103–5.

Kuusi, M., Lahti, E., Virolainaen, A. *et al.* (2006). An outbreak of *Streptococcus equi* subsp. *zooepidemicus* associated with consumption of fresh goat cheese. *BMC Infect. Dis.*, **6**: 36–37.

Ladlaw, J., Scase, T. and Waller, A. (2006). Canine strangles reveals a new host susceptible to infection with *Streptococus equi*. *J. Clin. Microbiol.*, **44**: 2664–65.

Lam, M.M., Clarridge, J.E., Young, E.J. and Mixuki, S. (2007). The other group G streptococcus: increased detection of *Streptococcus canis* ulcer infections in dog owners. *J. Clin. Microbiol.*, **45**: 2327–29.

Lancefield, R.C. and Hare, R. (1935). The serological differentiation of pathogenic and non-pathogenic strains of hemolytic streptococci from parturient women. *J. Experim. Med.*, **61**: 335–49.

Lau, S.K.P., Woo, P.Y.C., Tse, H., Leung, K.W., Wong, S.S.Y. *et al.* (2003). Invasive *Streptococcus iniae* infections outside North America. *J. Clin. Microbiol.*, **41**: 1004–9.

Lewis, R.F.M. and Balfour, A.E. (1999). Group C streptococci isolated from throat swabs: a laboratory and clinical study. *J. Clin. Path.*, **52**: 264–66.

Lun, Z.R., Wang Q.P., Chen, X.G. and Zhu, X.Q. (2007). *Streptococcus suis*: an emerging zoonotic pathogen. *Lancet Infect. Dis.*, **7**: 201–9.

Mayer, G. and Van Ore, S. (1983). Recurrent pharyngitis in a family of four. Household pet as reservoir of group A streptococci. *Postgrad. Med.*, **74:** 277–79.

Oever, J.t., Herbers, A.H.E., Verhoef, L.H.M. and van den Wall Bake, A.W.L. (2009). *Streptococcus equi* subspecies *zooepidemicus* bacteremia as first manifestation of Hairy Cell Leukemia. *Infect. Dis. Clin. Pract.*, **17:** 407–8.

Portnoy, D., Prentis, J. and Richards, G.K. (1981). Penicillin tolerance of human isolates of group C streptococci. *Antimicrob. Agents and Chemother.*, **20:** 235–38.

Preziusio, S., Laus, F., Tejeda, A.R., Calente, C. and Cuteri, V. (2010). Detection of *Streptococcus dysgalactiae* subsp. *equisimilis* in equine nasopharyngeal swabs by PCR. *J. Vet. Sci.*, **11:** 67–72.

Robertson, I.D. and Blackmore, D.K. (1989). Occupational exposure to *Streptococcus suis* type 2. *Epidemiol. Infect.*, **103:** 157–64.

Rolston, K.V. and Le Frock, J.L. (1984). In vitro susceptibility of group G streptococci with regard to tolerance. *Am. J. Med.*, **77:** 72.

Roos, K., Lind, L. and Holm, S.E. (1988). Beta-hemolytic streptococci group A in a cat, as a possible source of repeated tonsillitis in a family. *Lancet*, **2:** 1972.

Takeda, N., Kikuchi, K., Asani, R. *et al.* (2001). Recurrent septicaemia caused by *Streptococcus canis* after a dog bite. *Scandin. J. Infect. Dis.*, **33:** 937–38.

Tang, J., Wang, C., Feng, Y. *et al.* (2006). Streptococcal toxic shock syndrome caused by *Streptococcus suis* serotype 2. *PLoS Med.*, **3:** e151.

Tarradas, C., Luque, I., de Andrés, D. *et al.* (2001). Epidemiological relationship of human and swine *Streptococcus suis* isolates. *J. Vet. Med.*, **48:** 347–55.

Tikofsky, L.L. and Zadoks, R.N. (2005). Cross-infection between cats and cows: origin and control of *Streptococcus canis* mastitis in a dairy herd. *J. Dairy Sci.*, **88:** 2707–13.

Torres, R.S.L.A., de Paula, C.C., Pilonetto, M., Fontana, C.K., Minozzo, J.C.I. *et al.* (2007). An outbreak of *Streptococcus dysgalactiae* subsp. *equisimilis* in a hospital in the south of Brazil. *Brazil. J. Microbiol.*, **38:** 417–20.

Tramontana, A.R., Graham, M., Sinickas, V. and Bak, N. (2008). An Australian case of *Streptococcus suis* toxic shock syndrome associated with occupational exposure to animal carcasses. *Med. J. Aus.*, **188:** 538–39.

Turner, J.C., Hayden, G.F., Lobo, M.C., Ramirez, C.E. and Murren, D. (1997). Epidemiological evidence of Lancefield Group C streptococci as a cause of pharyngitis in college students. *J. Clin. Microbiol.*, **35:** 1–4.

Vela, A.I., Falsen, E., Simarro, I. *et al.* (2006). Neonatal mortality in puppies due to bacteremia by *Streptococcus dysgalactiae* subsp. *dysgalactiae*. *J. Clin. Microbiol.*, **44:** 666–68.

Weinstein, M.R., Litt, M., Kertesz, D.A. *et al.* (1997). Invasive infections due to a fish pathogen, *Streptococcus iniae*. *N. Engl. J. Med.*, **337:** 589–94.

Wilson, K.S., Maroney, S.A. and Gander, R.M. (1995). The family pet as an unlikely source of group A β-hemolytic streptococcal infection in humans. *Ped. Infect. Dis.*, **14:** 372–75.

Yang, Q.P., Liu W.P., Guo, L.X. *et al.* (2009). Autopsy report of four cases who died from *Streptococcus suis* infection with a review of the literature. *Euro. J. Clin. Microbiol. Infect. Dis.*, **28:** 447–53.

Yu, H., Jing, H., Chen, Z. *et al.* (2006). Human *Streptococcus suis* outbreak, Sichuan, China. *Emerg. Infect. Dis.*, **12:** 914–20.

CHAPTER 19f

Other bacterial diseases

Cat-scratch disease

Michel Drancourt

Summary

Cat-scratch disease (CSD) is a worldwide zoonoses caused by infection with the bacterium, *Bartonella henselae*. The formal description of the disease by Debré in 1950 (Debré *et al.* 1950) corresponds to the most frequently diagnosed form of the disease. Cats are the main reservoir for *B. henselae* and transmission is via Ctniocephalides felis. Humans usually become infected after being scratched or bitten by a cat and it is most frequently seen in children and young adults.

CSD is a self-limiting illness which often begins with a small papule developing at the site of cat scratch or bite within 3–14 days of the infection. Nearby lymph nodes, usually neck, axillary or groin, become swollen and can persist for several months. It may take up to 7 weeks for the enlarged lymph nodes to appear and individuals may not recall any cat scratch or bite. In healthy cases antibiotics are not indicated.

About 5–10% of patients may develop other forms of CSD including eye infection characterized by conjunctivitis and swollen lymph nodes, rash, liver and spleen enlargement, and more rarely encephalitis. Immunosuppressed patients may develop more severe disease, such as bacillary angiomatosis.

General advice for preventing CSD includes avoiding rough play with cats, particularly kittens. Cat scratches and bites should be washed immediately with water and soap and cats should not be allowed to lick open wounds.

History

Cat-scratch disease has been observed in France and the USA since 1931. Its initial description was published in 1950 by two French groups (Debré *et al.* 1950; Mollaret *et al.* 1950). In the absence of a proven aetiological agent, the diagnosis of cat-scratch disease has relied upon four diagnostic criteria:

1   Contact with a cat or dog and the presence of cutaneous scratch lesions or conjunctivitis;

2   Cutaneous hypersensitivity after experimental subcutaneous inoculation of filtered cat-scratch disease adenopathy;

3   The absence of other documented aetiology;

4   Pathological aspects, including necrotic granuloma, infiltrate with inflammatory cells and micro-abscesses.

In 1983, Wear *et al.* reported the presence of bacilli in the walls of capillaries in 34/39 cat-scratch disease adenopathies after Warthin-Starry staining. They noted that these bacteria were Gram-negative after Brown-Hopps-Gram staining, and were located into vacuoles in the cytoplasm of infected macrophages and histiocytes. The same observations were made in cutaneous lesions (Margileth *et al.* 1984), and isolation of an unidentified Gram-negative bacterium on brain-heart axenic medium was reported in 1988 from 10/19 cat-scratch disease adenopathies (English *et al.* 1988). Only one of these 10 isolates was subcultured on blood-agar medium leading to the hypothesis of a defective phase unable to grow on blood-agar. The molecular identification led to the creation of a new bacterial genus, *Afipia* and the isolate was named *Afipia felis* (Brenner *et al.* 1991).

In 1988, bacilli were observed after Warthin-Starry staining in cat-scratch disease cutaneous lesions in AIDS patients (Hall *et al.* 1988; Le Boit *et al.* 1988). Also, a new clinical and pathological entity, named bacillary angiomatosis, characterized by cutaneous lesions mimicking lesions of Kaposi's sarcoma, was described in AIDS patients (Stoler *et al.* 1983; Cockerell *et al.* 1987; Berger *et al.* 1989). Some patients had contact with cats, and the lesions were characterized by capillary angiogenesis with cuboid endothelial cells, and the presence of Warthin-Starry staining bacilli in capillary walls (Berger *et al.* 1989). Kemper *et al.* (1990) proposed that bacillary angiomatosis was part of cat-scratch disease in immuno-compromised patients including AIDS patients. Because of common Warthin-Starry tinctorial affinity, the same morphology using electron microscopy, and the occurrence of bacillary angiomatosis after contact with cats, it was hypothesis that *A. felis* was the common aetiological agent of both diseases.

In 1990, however, Relman *et al.* (1990) published the identification of a new bacterium in the cutaneous lesions of patients with bacillary angiomatosis, using the university identification methods showing 16S rRNA gene homology of 98.3% with *Rochaliaea Quintana*. This new bacterium, different from *A. felis* was then isolated from the blood of AIDS patients with fever and bacteraemia, visceral peliosis, and visceral bacillary angiomatosis (Perkocha *et al.* 1990). It was named *Rochalimaea henselae* (Regnery *et al.* 1992a). Both *R. henselae* and *R. quintana* were recently included in the genus *Bartonella* (Brenner *et al.* 1993).

At that stage, *A. felis* was regarded as the unique aetiological agent of cat-scratch disease, and *B. henselae* the unique aetiological agent of bacillary angiomatosis. However, a serological study published in 1992 (Regnery et al. 1992c) found 88% seropositivity for *B. henselae* and 25% seropositivity for *A. felis* among 41 American patients diagnosed as cat-scratch disease. *B. henselae* was later isolated from the adenopathies of cat-scratch disease patients (Dolan et al. 1993), and a specific 16S rDNA sequence was obtained after PCT amplification using adenopathies (Perkins et al. 1992; Anderson et al. 1994a) and the material used in the past as skin test antigen (Anderson et al. 1993). Consequently, the concept shifted towards *B. henselae* as a unique aetiological agent for both bacillary angiomatosis and cat-scratch disease.

B. quintana was isolated from the blood of a patient with bacillary agniomatosis (Maruin et al. 1994) and from the chronically inflamed lymph nodes of a patient who had contact with cats (Raoult et al. 1994) and it appears that both *B. henselae*, in the USA and *B. quintana* in the USA and in Europe, are the aetiological agents for bacillary angiomatosis and possibly of cat-scratch disease.

The agent

Further developments of powerful serology and molecular tools for the diagnosis of *B. henselae* infection, expanded the clinical spectrum of CSD beyond the classical lymph node infection.

Microbiology

Bartonella (previously referred to as *Rochalimea* and *Grahamella*) are Gram-negative organisms belonging to the alpha sub-group of Proteobacteria, living in close association with mammals. *B. henselae* is one of the eight *Bartonella* species acknowledged as human pathogens, along with *Bartonella bacilliformis* (Carrion disease; Oroya fever and *verruga peruana*), *Bartonella quintana* (trench fever; bacteremia; endocarditis; uveitis; bacillary angiomatosis), *Bartonella elizabethae* (endocarditis), *Bartonella vinsonii* (bacteremia and endocarditis), *Bartonella grahamii* (uveitis), *Bartonella koehlerae* (endocarditis) and *Bartonella waschoensis* (myocarditis). In the pre-genomic area, sequencing rpoB and gltA were shown to be the most discriminant tools for delineating *Bartonella* species (La Scola et al. 2003). Analysing the 1.9 Mb genome of *B. henselae* indicated that *B. henselae* was closely related to *Bartonella quintana*; that *B. quintana* was a reduced-genome derivative of *B. henselae* which genome uniquely encodes for filamentous hemagglutinin; and that both genomes were reduced versions of the *Brucella melitensis* chromosome I (Alsmark et al. 2004). 16S rDNA sequencing discriminated two genotypes which also appeared to be two distinct serotypes, i.e. Marseille (also refered as genotype II) and Houston-1 (genotype I) (Drancourt et al. 1996). Genotyping *B. henselae* DNA from clinical specimens using the Multispacer Sequence Typing (MST) found 16 genotypes and a diversity comparable to that of cats' isolates; 78.7% belonged to genotypes Marseille and Houston-1 (Li et al. 2007). Multiple-locus variable-number tandem repeat analysis (MLVA) also pointed out to the same genotype in patient and patient's cat (Monteil et al. 2007).

Pathogenesis

B. henselae infection has been linked to cat and cat fleas in patients with classical CSD (Giladi et al. 1999), endocarditis (Raoult et al. 1996) and bacillary angiomatosis-peliosis in HIV-infected patients (Koelher et al. 1997) (Fig. 19F.1). *B. henselae* bacteremia has been documented with prevalence as high as 40% in kittens

< one-year-old (Chomel et al. 1995; Chomel et al. 2006) and *B. henselae* was shown to reside within cat erythrocytes (Rolain et al. 2001). Also, the cat flea *Ctenocephalides felis* has been shown to harbour *B. henselae* and be a vector of transmission of *B. henselae* between cats and for CSD (Chomel et al. 1996). The cat is regarded therefore as the reservoir for *B. henselae* even as long as 800 years ago (La et al. 2004). *B. henselae* can be identified from a few other felids including African lions and a cheetah. Identification of strains specific to these wild felids led to the concept of a *B. henselae* group including various subspecies (Chomel et al. 2006). Cats also host *Bartonella koehlerae*, *Bartonella clarridgeiae* and *Bartonella bovis*. Cats may also host *B. quintana*, once regarded as a strict human *Bartonella* species; *B. quintana* has been diagnosed in a few patients presenting with CSD (Raoult et al. 1994; Drancourt et al. 1996). Alternative vectors such as ticks are under investigation (Breitschwerdt et al. 2007).

After inoculation, *B. henselae* invades endothelial and red blood cells (Dehio 2001). The natural history of *B. henselae* infection partially depends on the host immune status. In immunocompetent individuals *B. henselae* is responsible for a localized suppurative infection (CSD) an endovascular infection (endocarditis) and an inflammatory response without infection (encephalitis). In immunocompromised patients *B. henselae* is responsible for multifocal proliferation of endothelial cells (bacillary angiomatosis and hepatic peliosis). It is hypothesized that CSD is the primary infection resulting in endocarditis in patients with heart valve lesions (Gouriet et al. 2007). The same could be true for uveitis (Terrada et al. 2009).

Hosts

Cats

In most instances cats implicated are healthy.

The human

The most frequently diagnosed form of CSD presents as progressively enlarged regional lymphadenopathy in the territory of a cat scratch (axillary, head and neck, inguinal). The lymph node is usually painful and tender and may suppurate (Carithers 1985). CSD is typically a benign and self-limited illness lasting 6 to 12 weeks. Some patients report a primary inoculation papule or pustule developing at the site of inoculation 3–10 days after a cat scratch or bite. Low-grade fever and malaise accompany lymphadenopathy in up to 50% of patients; headache, anorexia, weight loss, nausea and vomiting and sore throat may develop.

In less of 20% of patients, other clinical signs and symptoms may develop.

In some children, the clinical presentation with high grade fever, enlarged liver and spleen mimics lymphoma.

Neurological involvements include aseptic meningitis and neuroretinitis (Wong et al. 1995). Other ocular manifestations include Parinaud oculoglandular syndrome (Wong et al. 1995; Bass et al. 1997), stellar retinitis (Reed et al. 1998) and uveitis (Drancourt et al. 2004; Drancourt et al. 2008; Terrada et al. 2009). HLA B-27 persons may be more susceptible to developing CSD uveitis (Drancourt et al. 2004), in France and *B. henselae* is the most frequent bacterial pathogen diagnosed in the course of uveitis (Drancourt et al. 2008).

Musculoskeletal manifestations include myalgia, arthritis, arthralgia, tendinitis, osteomyelitis, and neuralgia could be observed in about one-tenth of patients, typically older than 20 years

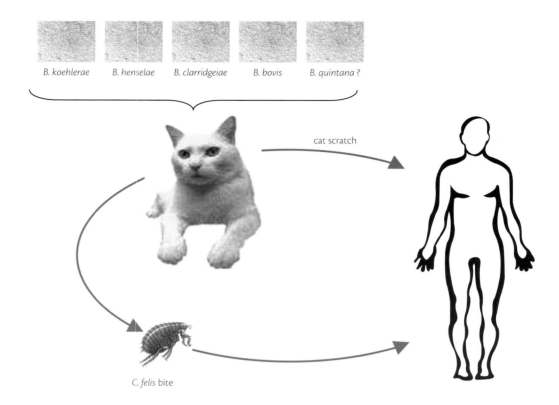

B. koehlerae   B. henselae   B. clarridgeiae   B. bovis   B. quintana ?

cat scratch

Fig. 19f.1 Epidemiology of cat-scratch disease

C. felis bite

(Maman *et al.* 2007). Arthritis is observed in medium and large joints. Osteomyelitis is a classical, but rare manifestation of CSD.

Blood culture-negative endocarditis is diagnosed in patients with previous valve anomaly (Drancourt *et al.* 1996; Casalta *et al.* 2009). It refers to patients presenting with clinical features of infective endocarditis for whom the conventional blood culture remains sterile within a few days.

In immunocompromised patients including untreated HIV-infected patients and patients receiving immunosuppressive drugs, *B. henselae* causes bacillary angiomatosis presenting as cutaneous and mucous blood vessels tumours (Relman *et al.* 1990). It is also responsible for fever and bacteraemia (Slater *et al.* 1990) and hepatic peliosis (Perkocha *et al.* 1990; Relman *et al.* 1991).

Laboratory diagnosis

Routine direct diagnosis of CSD is based on the molecular detection of specific *B. henselae* sequences in the material. The use of specific real-time PCR is superior to the use of 16S rDNA-based detection system for the detection of *B. henselae* DNA in lymph node tissue (Angelakis *et al.* 2009). In our laboratory, real-time PCR targets the 16S-23S rDNA ITS spacer (Raoult *et al.* 2006) and the pap31 gene (Angelakis *et al.* 2009).

Microscopic detection can be done by using the argentic Warthin-Starry staining which detects bacteria-like black spots in tissues and immunodetection using either polyclonal or monoclonal antibody can be also used for the specific detection of *B. henselae* in lymph node tissue and endo-ocular fluid (Terrada *et al.* 2009).

Specimens are inoculated onto blood-agar and cultured cell lines for the tentative isolation and culture of *B. henselae*. In our experience however, such isolation is rare and primary isolation can take

up to 4 weeks; therefore, isolation cannot be used as a reliable routine technique for the direct diagnosis of *B. henselae* infection (La Scola and Raoult 1999). The routine identification of isolates is done by using direct immunofluorescence, MALDI-TOF mass spectrometry (Fournier *et al.* 2009) or sequencing (La Scola *et al.* 2003; Raoult *et al.* 2006; Angelakis *et al.* 2009).

Because of the fastidious nature of *B. henselae*, antibiotic susceptibility profile is not a routine test (Rolain *et al.* 2004). Such tests demonstrated that *B. henselae* was susceptible to most antibiotics including the betalactamines, the aminoglycosides, chloramphenicol, tetracyclines, macrolides, rifampin, quinolones and cotrimoxazole (Rolain *et al.* 2004). It has been further demonstrated that only aminoglycosides were bactericidal against *B. henselae* (Musso *et al.* 1995), but this was not the case for *B. henselae* organisms in erythrocytes (Rolain *et al.* 2004). Because of the facultative intracellular location of *B. henselae* in the course of human infection, these in-vitro results do not necessarily correlate with clinical experience, and current recommendations for treating *B. henselae* infections are based on scarce clinical evidence.

Serology is usually based on ELISA with Micro-immunofluorescence as the reference method. Multiplexed methods have been developed in order to test for several microbes at once, and this format has been developed for the indirect diagnosis of blood-culture negative endocarditis including *B. henselae* (Gouriet *et al.* 2008). Because of extensive cross-reaction between *B. henselae* and other *Bartonella* species (as well as with *Chlamydia pneumoniae* and *Coxiella burnetii*), Western-blot demonstrating extensive reaction is necessary for serological confirmation of *B. henselae* endocarditis (Casalta *et al.* 2009).

Co-infection with *B. henselae* and the tuberculosis agent *Mycobacterium tuberculosis* as well as CSD in the course of lymphoma, have been reported (Rolain *et al.* 2006). Such cases emphasize the necessity of histopathological examination of enlarged lymph nodes in addition to their complete microbiological investigation.

Treatment and prognosis

CSD is a self-limited infection which typically does not respond to antibiotic treatment (Rolain *et al.* 2004). Therefore, the current recommendation is no antibiotic treatment for conventional CSD in immunocompetent patients (Rolain *et al.* 2004).

A favourable effect of doxycycline (200 mg a day, oral route) combined with rifampin (600 mg a day, oral route) has been observed for patients with CSD uveitis and encephalitis but optimal duration of treatment remains to be determined (Wong *et al.* 1995).

Gentamycin (3 mg/kg/day) for 14 days is the cornerstone of antibiotic treatment for *B. henselae* endocarditis when combined with doxycyclin (200 mg a day, oral route) for 6 weeks (Raoult 2007). It is useful to monitor the serum level of both antibiotics in order to adapt the daily dosage due to huge variations in the concentration between individuals.

In immunocompromized patients, erythromycin decreases within hours of administration the bacillary angiomatosis cutaneous lesions, due to its action on protein synthesis. It is administrated by oral route at 500 mg a day for 3 months (Rolain *et al.* 2004). The same regimen is prescribed for treating peliosis (Rolain *et al.* 2004).

Prevention and control

Cats are the only known reservoir. The only prevention strategy is to minimize risk of cat scratchs, avoid contact with cats, especially if immunocompromised. Scratches and bites should be washed immediately.

References

Alsmark, C.M., Frank, A.C., Karlberg, E.O. *et al.* (2004). The louse-borne human pathogen *Bartonella quintana* is a genomic derivative of the zoonotic agent *Bartonella henselae*. *Proc. Nat. Acad. Sci. USA.*, **101**: 9716–21.

Anderson, B., Kelly, C., Threlkel, R., Edwards, K. (1993). Detection of *Rochlimae henselae* in cat-scratch disease skin test antigens. *J. Infect. Dis.*, **168**: 1034–36.

Anderson, B. *et al.* (1994a). Detection of *Rochalimaea henselae* DNA in specimens from cat scratch disease patients by PCR. *J. Clin. Microb.*, **32**: 942–48.

Angelakis, E., Roux, V., Raoult, D. and Rolain, J.M. (2009). Real-time PCR strategy and detection of bacterial agents of lymphadenitis. *Euro. J. Clin. Microbiol. Infect. Dis.*, **28**: 1363–68.

Bass, J.W., Vincent, J.M. and Person, D.A. (1997). The expanding spectrum of *Bartonella* infections: II. *Cat-scratch disease. Pediatr. Infect. Dis. Jour.*, **16**: 163–79.

Berger, T.G., Tappero, J.W., Kaymen, A., LeBoit, P.E. (1989). Bacillary (epitheloid) angiomatosis and concurrent Kaposi's sarcoma in acquired immunodeficiency syndrome. *Arch. Dermatol.*, **125**: 1543–77.

Breitschwerdt, E.B., Maggi, R.G., Duncan, A.W., Nicholson, W.L., Hegarty, B.C. *et al.* (2007). *Bartonella* species in blood of immunocompetent persons with animal and arthropod contact. *Emerg. Infect. Dis.*, **13**: 938–41.

Brenner, D.J., Hollis, D.G., Mos, C. *et al.* (1991). Proposal of *Afipia* gen. nov., with *Afipia felis* sp. Nov (formerly the cat-scratch disease bacillus). *Afipia clevelandensis* sp. Nov (formerly the Cleveland clinic foundation strain). *Afipia broomae* sp.nov., and three unnamed genospecies. *J. Clin. Microbiol.*, **29**: 2450–60.

Brenner, D.J., O'Connor, S.P., Winkler, H.H., Steigerwalk, A.G. (1993). Proposals to unify the genera *Bartonella* and *Rochalimaea*, with

description of Bartonella Quintana, comb, nov., Bartonella vinsonii comb. Nov., Bartonella henselae comb, nov., and Bartonella elizabethae comb.nov., and to remove the family Bartonellacease from the other Rickettsiales. *Intern. System. Bacterial.*, **4**: 777–86.

Carithers, H.A. (1985). Cat scratch disease: An overview based on a study of 1,200 patients. *Am. J. Dis. Child.*, **139**: 1124–33.

Casalta, J.P., Gouriet, F., Richet, H., Thuny, F., Habib, G. and Raoult, D. (2009). Prevalence of *Coxiella burnetii* and *Bartonella* species as cases of infective endocarditis in Marseilles (1994–2007). *Clin. Microbiol. Infect.*, **15**: 152–53.

Chomel, B.B., Abbott, R.C., Kasten, R.W. *et al.* (1995). *Bartonella henselae* prevalence in domestic cats in California: risk factors and association between bacteremia and antibody titers. *J. Clin. Microbiol.*, **33**: 2445–50.

Chomel, B.B., Boulouis, H.J., Maruyama, S. and Breitschwerdt, E.B. (2006). *Bartonella* spp. in pets and effect on human health. *Emerg. Infect. Dis.*, **12**: 389–94.

Chomel, B.B., Kasten, R.W., Floyd-Hawkins, K. *et al.* (1996). Experimental transmission of *Bartonella henselae* by the cat flea. *J. Clin. Microbiol.*, **34**: 1952–56.

Chomel, B.B., Kasten, R.W., Henn, J.B. and Molia, S. (2006). *Bartonella* infection in domestic cats and wild felids. *Ann. NY Acad. Sci.*, **1078**: 410–55.

Cockerell, C.J., Whitlow, M.A., Webster, G.F. and Friedman-Kien, A.E. (1987). Epietheloid angiomatosis: a distinct vascular disorder in patients with the acquired immunodeficiency syndrome or AIDS-related complex. *Lancet*, **ii**: 654–56.

Debré, R., Lamy, M., Jammet, M.L., Costil, L. and Mozziconacci, P. (1950). La maladie des griffes du chat. *Sem. Hôpitaux de Paris*, **26**: 1895–904.

Dehio, C. (2001). *Bartonella* interactions with endothelial cells and erythrocytes. *Trends in Microbiol.*, **9**: 279–85.

Dolan, M.J., Wong, M.T., Regnery, R.L., Jorgensen, J.H., Garcia, M. *et al.* (1993). Syndrome of *Rochalimaea henselae* adenitis suggesting cat scratch disease. *Ann. Intern. Med.*, **118**: 331–36.

Drancourt, M., Berger, P., Terrada, C., Bodaghi, B., Conrath, J., Raoult, D. *et al.* (2008). High prevalence of fastidious bacteria in 1520 cases of uveitis of unknown etiology. *Medicine (Baltimore)*, **87**: 167–76.

Drancourt, M., Birtles, R., Chaumentin, G., Vandenesch, F., Etienne, J. and Raoult, D. (1996). New serotype of *Bartonella henselae* in endocarditis and cat-scratch disease. *Lancet*, **347**: 441–43.

Drancourt, M., Bodaghi, B., Lepidi, H., Le Hoang, P. and Raoult, D. (2004). Intraocular detection of *Bartonella henselae* in a patient with HLA-B27 uveitis. *J. Clin. Microbiol.*, **42**: 1822–25.

Drancourt, M., Moal, V., Brunet, P., Dussol, B., Berland, Y. and Raoult, D. (1996). *Bartonella (Rochalimaea) quintana* infection in a seronegative hemodialyzed patient. *J. Clin. Microbiol.*, **34**: 1158–60.

English, C.K., Wear, D.J., Margileth, A.M., Lissner, C.R. and Walsh, G.P. (1988). Cat-scratch disease: isolation and culture of the bacterial agent. *JAMA*, **259**: 1347–52.

Fournier, P.E., Couderc, C., Buffet, S., Flaudrops, C. and Raoult, D. (2009). Rapid and cost-effective identification of *Bartonella* species using mass spectrometry. *J. Med. Microbiol.*, **58**: 1154–59.

Giladi, M. and Avidor, B. (1999). Images in clinical medicine. *Cat scratch disease. N. Engl. J. Med.*, **340**: 108.

Gouriet, F., Lepidi, H., Habib, G., Collart, F. and Raoult, D. (2007). From cat scratch disease to endocarditis, the possible natural history of *Bartonella henselae* infection. *BMC Infect. Dis.*, **7**: 30.

Gouriet, F., Samson, L., Delaage, M. *et al.* (2008). Multiplexed whole bacterial antigen microarray, a new format for the automation of serodiagnosis: the culture-negative endocarditis paradigm. *Clin. Microbiol. Infect.*, **14**: 1112–18.

Hall, A. V., Roberts, C.M., Maurice, P.D., McLean, K.A. and Shousha, S. (1988). Cat-scratch disease in patients with AIDS: atypical skin manifestations. *Lancet* ii: 453–54.

Koehler, J.E., Sanchez, M.A., Garrido, C.S. *et al.* (1997). Molecular epidemiology of bartonella infections in patients with bacillary angiomatosis-peliosis. *N. Engl. J. Med.*, **337**: 1876–83.

Kemper, C.A., Lombard, C.M., Deresinski, S.C. and Tompkins, L.S. (1990). Visceral bacillary epitheloid angiomatosis: possible manifestations of disseminated cat scratch disease in the immunocompromised host: a report of two cases. *Am. J. Med.*, **89**: 216–22.

La, V.D., Clavel, B., Lepetz, S., Aboudharam, G., Raoult, D. *et al.* (2004). Molecular detection of *Bartonella henselae* DNA in the dental pulp of 800-year-old French cats. *Clin. Infect. Dis.*, **39**: 391–94.

La, V.D., Tran-Hung, L., Aboudharam, G., Raoult, D. and Drancourt, M. (2005). *Bartonella* quintana in domestic cat. *Emerg. Infect. Dis.*, **11**: 1287–89.

La Scola, B. and Raoult, D. (1999). Culture of *Bartonella quintana* and *Bartonella henselae* from human samples: a 5-year experience (1993 to 1998). *J. Clin. Microbiol.*, **37**: 1899–905.

La Scola, B., Zeaiter, Z., Khamis, A. and Raoult, D. (2003). Gene-sequence-based criteria for species definition in bacteriology: the *Bartonella* paradigm. *Trends in Microbiol.*, **11**: 318–21.

LeBoit, P.E. *et al.* (1988). Epitheloid haemangioma-like vascular proliferation in AIDS : manfiestation of cat scratch disease bacillus infection. *Lancet.*, i: 960–63.

Li, W., Raoult, D. and Fournier, P.E. (2007). Genetic diversity of *Bartonella henselae* in human infection detected with multispacer typing. *Emerg. Infect. Dis.*, **13**: 1178–83.

Maman, E., Bickels, J., Ephros, M. *et al.* (2007). Musculoskeletal manifestations of cat scratch disease. *Clin. Infect. Dis.*, **45**: 1535–40.

Margileth, A.M., Wear, D.J., English, C.K. (1987). Systemic cat scratch disease: report of 23 patients with prolonged or recurrent severe bacterial infection. *J. Infect. Dis.*, **155**: 390–402.

Maurin, M., Roux, V., Stein, A., Ferrier, F., Biraben, R., *et al.* (1994). Isolation and characterisation by immunofluorescence, SDS-PAGE, m Western-blot, RFLP-PCR, 16S rRNA sequencing and pulsed-field gel electrophoresis of *Rochalimaea Quintana* from a patient with bacillary angiomatosis. *J. Clin. Microbiol.*, **32**: 1166–71.

Mollaret, P., Reilly, J., Bastin, R. and Rournier, P. (1950). Sur une adenopathie regionale subaigue et spontanement curable avec intrsdermoreaction et lesions ganglionnaires particulieres. *Bull. Memb. Soc. Med. Hopitaux de Paris*, **66**: 424.

Monteil, M., Durand, B., Bouchouicha, R. *et al.* (2007). Development of discriminatory multiple-locus variable-number tandem repeat analysis for *Bartonella henselae*. *Microbiol.*, **153**: 1141–48.

Musso, D., Drancourt, M. and Raoult, D. (1995). Lack of bactericidal effect of antibiotics except aminoglycosides on *Bartonella (Rochalimaea) henselae*. *J. Antimicrob. Chemother.*, **36**: 101–8.

Perkins, B.A., Swaminathan, B.S., Jackson, L.A., Brenner, D.J., Wenger, J.D., Regnry, R.L. (1992). Pathogenesis of cat-scratch disease. *N. Engl. J. Med.*, **327**: 1599–600.

Perkocha, L.A., Geaghan, S.M., Yen, T.S. *et al.* (1990). Clinical and pathological features of bacillary peliosis hepatis in association with human immunodeficiency virus infection. *N. Engl. J. Med.*, **323**: 1581–86.

Raoult, D. (2007). From Cat scratch disease to *Bartonella henselae* infection. *Clin. Infect. Dis.*, **45**: 1541–42.

Raoult, D., Drancourt, M., Carta, A. and Gastaut, J.A. (1994). *Bartonella (Rochalimaea) quintana* isolation in patient with chronic adenopathy, lymphopenia, and a cat. *Lancet*, **343**: 977.

Raoult, D., Fournier, P.E., Drancourt, M. *et al.* (1996). Diagnosis of 22 new cases of *Bartonella* endocarditis. *Ann. Intern. Med.*, **125**: 646–52.

Raoult, D., Roblot, F., Rolain, J.M. *et al.* (2006). First isolation of *Bartonella alsatica* from a valve of a patient with endocarditis. *J. Clin. Microbiol.*, **44**: 278–79.

Reed, J.B., Scales, D.K., Wong, M.T., Lattuada Jr., C.P., Dolan, M.J. *et al.* (1998). *Bartonella henselae* neuroretinitis in cat scratch disease. Diagnosis, management, and sequelae. *Ophthalmol.*, **105**: 459–66.

Regenery, R.L., Anderson, B.E., Clarridge, J.E., Rodriquez-Barradas, M.C., *et al.* (1992a). Characterisation of a novel *Rochalimaea* species, *R.henseale* sp. Nov. isolated from blood of a febrile, human immunodeficiency virus-positive patient. *J. Clin. Microbiol.*, **30**: 265–74.

Regnery, R.L., Olson, J.G., Perkins, B.A. and Bibb, W. (1992). Serological response to *Rochalimaea henselae* antigen in suspected cat scratch disease. *Lancet*, **339**: 1443–45.

Relman, D.A., Falkow, S., LeBoit, P.E., *et al.* (1991). The organism causing bacillary angiomatosis, peliosis hepatis, and fever and bacteremia in immunocompromised patients. *N. Engl. J. Med.*, **324**: 1514.

Relman, D.A., Loutit, J.S., Schmidt, T.M., Falkow, S. and Tompkins, L.S. (1990). The agent of bacillary angiomatosis. An approach to the identification of uncultured pathogens. *N. Engl. J. Med.*, **323**: 1573–80.

Rolain, J.M., Brouqui, P., Koehler, J.E., Maguina, C., Dolan, M.J. and Raoult, D. (2004). Recommendations for treatment of human infections caused by *Bartonella* species. *Antimicrob. Agents and Chemother.*, **48**: 1921–33.

Rolain, J.M., La Scola, B., Liang, Z., Davoust, B. and Raoult, D. (2001). Immunofluorescent detection of intraerythrocytic *Bartonella henselae* in naturally infected cats. *J. Clin. Microbiol.*, **39**: 2978–80.

Rolain, J.M., Lepidi, H., Zanaret, M. *et al.* (2006). Lymph node biopsy specimens and diagnosis of cat-scratch disease. *Emerg. Infect. Dis.*, **12**: 1338–44.

Slater, L.N., Welch, D.F., Hensel, D. and Coody, D.W. (1990). A newly recognized fastidious gram-negative pathogen as a cause of fever and bacteremia. *N. Engl. J. Med.*, **323**: 1587–93.

Stoler, M.H., Bonfiglio, T.A., Steigbigel, R.T. and Pereira, M. (1983). An atypical subcutaneous infection associated with acquired immune deficiency syndrome. *Am. J. Clin. Pathol.*, **80**: 714–18.

Terrada, C., Bodaghi, B., Conrath, J., Raoult, D. and Drancourt, M. (2009). Uveitis: an emerging clinical form of *Bartonella* infection. *Clin. Microbiol. Infect.*, **15**: 132–3.

Wong, M.T., Dolan, M.J., Lattuada Jr., C.P. *et al.* (1995). Neuroretinitis, aseptic meningitis, and lymphadenitis associated with *Bartonella (Rochalimaea) henselae* infection in immunocompetent patients and patients infected with human immunodeficiency virus type 1. *Clin. Infect. Dis.*, **21**: 352–60.

CHAPTER 19g

Other bacterial diseases

Erysipeloid

Robert M. Smith

Summary

Erysipeloid is an acute bacterial infection usually causing acute localized cellulitis as a secondary infection of traumatised skin. It is caused by *Erysipelothrix rhusiopathiae* (insidiosa), a non-sporulating Gram-positive rod-shaped bacterium, ubiquitous in the environment. It is the cause of swine erysipelas and also a pathogen or commensal in a variety of wild and domestic birds, animal and marine species. Human infection primarily associated with occupational exposure to infected or contaminated animals or handling animal products and therefore is commoner in farmers, butchers and abattoir workers and fisherman.

Risk factors for the rare human invasive *E. rhusiopathiae* infection include conditions that affect the host immune response, such as alcoholism, cancer and diabetes. Treatment is with penicillin.

Erysipelas can affect animals of all ages but is recognized more frequently in juveniles. Swine exhibit similar stages to the disease in man. Clinical manifestations in swine vary from the classical rhomboid urticaria (diamond skin), the condition of greatest prevalence and economic importance, to sepsis, polyarthritis, pneumonia and death.

Prevention is largely a matter of good hygiene, herd management and by raising awareness in those at risk (especially butchers, farmers and fishermen); ensuring that clinicians are aware of *E. rhusiopathiae* as a possible cause of occupational skin lesions and bacterial endocarditis is important.

History

Erysipelothrix rhusiopathiae (erysipelas; erythros = red, pella = skin), literally 'erysipelas thread of red disease') is synonymous with *Erysipelothrix insidiosa*. The human condition is also known as *erysipeloid, Rosenbach's erysipeloid, erysipelotrichosis, fish handler's disease* and *erythema migrans*, and the animal disease as *sheep joint ill, swine erysipelas, diamonds, diamond skin disease and fish rose.*

Recognized for more than a hundred years as the agent of swine erysipelas and as the cause of human erysipeloid, the organism was first isolated from mice in 1878 (Koch 1880) and subsequently from a pig with 'rouget du porc' (Pasteur and Thuillier 1883). It was identified as the agent of swine erysipelas and as a zoonoses by Loeffler in 1886 who isolated the organism from cutaneous blood vessels in a pig that had died of swine erysipelas. The first attributable description of human disease was by Koch in 1880. Pathogenicity in man was first demonstrated in 1884 by Rosenbach, hence 'Erysipeloid of Rosenbach'. Rosenbach used the term 'erysipeloid' to differentiate the lesions of *E. rhusiopathiae* infection from erysipelas caused by Group A streptococci (Robson *et al.* 1998).

From the earliest reports, human disease has been associated with occupational and environmental exposures, and that those engaged in occupational or recreational activities involving contact with animals or animal products are at greatest risk (Heptonstall *et al.* 2000). People in occupations where animal contact occurs frequently, farmers, fishermen, butchers, abattoir workers and veterinary surgeons are most likely to be affected (Brooke and Riley 1999). The common nomenclature for human infections largely reflects this occupational diversity 'seal finger', 'whale finger', 'pork finger', and 'crayfish disease'. Infection occurs from direct contact with infected animals, their secretions, wastes or organic matter contaminated with any of these (Wood 1975). It also affects those involved in fishing and associated occupations and '*Fish handler's disease*' used to be common among fishermen, cleaners, and porters, who were often infected through skin abrasions caused by the spines or bones of fish, especially mucilaginous species such as skate, or by splinters from the wooden boxes in which they were carried (Spencer 1959). In 1926 Klauder reported 'about a thousand' cases among commercial fisherman on the eastern seaboard of America. During the Second World War a number of outbreaks occurred in Norwegian fish processing factories with over 200 human cases reported from a single fish factory with a further 235 cases reported among fish producers and trawlermen in Aberdeen (Procter and Richardson 1954). Some of these infections may have been due to the presence of *Erysipelothrix* in putrefying fish due to inadequate freezing facilities exacerbated by delays in ships returning to port because fishing boats were required to sail to and from the fishing grounds in convoy during wartime.

In 1934, McGinnes and Spindle, investigating 210 cases of erysipeloid in a bone button factory in the USA, showed that infection was highest amongst those workers who sustained traumatic injury whilst working in the warm moist environment needed to keep the bone workable.

'*Seal Finger*' and '*Whale Finger*' were caused by infection of the abrasions and other superficial injuries caused mainly by wire ropes, flensing knives and bone fragments (Hillenbrand 1953).

Infection has always been considered less common in freshwater fish but in 1930, 200 cases were identified in workers preparing Golden Perch in a processing plant in Odessa.

In pigs, the disease was not considered to be economically important until 1928 when a series of epizootics were recorded in South Dakota and spread to other major pig producing regions of the USA.

Microbiology

The genus *Erysipelothrix* comprises *E. rhusiopathiae* and *E. tonsillarum*, with a possible further as yet unnamed species (Brooke and Riley 1999). Members of the genus are all Gram-positive non-sporing thin rods. *E. rhusiopathiae* is a commensal of wild and domestic animals, birds, fish and shellfish and marine mammals.

Twenty three serovars of E.rhusiopathiae are recognized (To and Nagai 2007). Type 1 is also divided into two subtypes, 1a and 1b. Serotypes 1 and 2 are the principal agents of acute swine erysipelas and the most frequently isolated serovars; this feature is important in the immunization of swine since only a few strains of serotype 3 produce effective bacterins against swine erysipelas (Wood and Harrington 1978). *E. rhusiopathiae* serovars 1 and 2 are the most frequently isolated serovars from cases of swine erysipelas and are represented in most commercial swine erysipelas vaccines. On culture, two distinct colony morphologies have been reported: one, a small, moist convex growth with smooth margins, and the other, a larger growth with a flattened surface and serrated margins (Shimoji 2000). Electron microscopy has associated the smooth margin variant with a short rod form of the bacterium and the serrated margin variant with a longer filamentous form of the bacterium (Dunbar and Clarridge 2000). It is a facultatively anaerobic, non-spore-forming, non-capsulated and non-acid-fast bacterium.

The mechanism of pathogenicity of *E. rhusiopathiae* in animals is not clearly understood, but there is evidence of neuraminidase involvement. This enzyme is produced by all strains of *E. rhusiopathiae* so far tested, and cleaves α-glycosidic linkages in neuraminic acid, a reactive mucopolysaccharide found on the surfaces of body cells. In low or avirulent strains neuraminidase activity is lower. Pathological activity associated with the enzyme probably results from its presence in large amounts as it is not itself a toxin; this is thought to be the case with the septicaemia characteristic of acute swine erysipelas. Neuraminidase activity can be associated with a number of aspects of the pathogenesis of the disease such as increased permeability of cell walls, formation of excess fibrin from fibrinogen and stimulation of erythrocyte agglutination leading to haemolysis. It has also been shown that neuraminidase mediates cleavage of terminal scialic acid residues of glycoproteins, oligosaccharides, and glycolipids, potentially providing a mechanism for *E. rhusiopathiae* attachment and invasion of the vascular epithelium (Vendetti *et al.* 1990).

Epidemiology

Man is an accidental host of *Erysipelothrix rhusiopathiae* acquiring the infection from infected animals, their fomites or the environment. Human erysipeloid is a largely occupational disease of slaughterhouse workers, agricultural workers and those in the meat handling and fishing industries. It is not notifiable in most countries including the UK. In the USA, erysipeloid was listed as a specific occupational disease under worker's compensation laws in the states of Arizona, Colorado, Iowa, Kansas and New Mexico (Morgis *et al.* 1967). Worldwide, few human cases are reported annually and it has been suggested that the frequency of human infection has been declining, probably due to technological changes in relevant industries and reductions in occupational exposures (Brooke and Riley 1999). No population based survey of human erysipeloid has been undertaken. Few specific studies of animal populations have been reported in the literature.

In the UK swine erysipelas is mainly sporadic but in some central European countries, Asia, Canada and Central and South America it can cause epidemics with serious economic consequences. In some countries swine can only be raised profitably where systematic vaccination is practised. Outbreaks of disease tend to occur in valleys and low lying areas, especially in the summer months, although with considerable regional variations in morbidity and mortality. The reasons for this variability are uncertain but it has been suggested they may be due to differences in virulence of the organism. Acute forms of the disease tend to be rare in western Europe, and in the USA, where disease tends to occur in 4 to 5 year cycles. In the UK the disease in sheep occurs mainly in lowland flocks involved in fat lamb production where replacement ewes are often purchased annually. In such flocks this may be due to the presence of carrier ewes or to the presence of the organism in the soil. Some reported outbreaks have been associated with the spreading of pig slurry on pasture grazed by lambs but reliable evidence has generally proved elusive (Jones 1977).

A seasonal increase in warm weather has been reported in both animals and man (Barber 1948; King 1946) but Penny and Guise (1986) in a review of animal condemnation statistics in the United Kingdom demonstrated no seasonal associations between the periods 1960–72 and 1973–84. They point out that during this time major changes occurred in pig husbandry and feeding practices in the UK, with fewer pigs being raised outdoors or in yards but generally managed more intensively indoors on part slatted floors which make faecal spread of disease less likely. Other factors such as reduction in the number of skin parasites and the virtual elimination of the pig louse, both of which are possible vectors of swine erysipelas, may also have contributed to a reduction in the numbers of animal cases.

The hosts

Animals

Infections have been reported worldwide in over 50 animal species; in farmed turkeys, chickens, ducks and emus. In sheep and lambs it usually presents as polyarthritis but can cause septicaemia. Post dipping lameness caused by *E. rhusiopathiae* is seen in sheep of all ages. The disease is characterized by cellulitis at the coronary band and interdigital area 2–7 days after dipping. Most cases resolve after a few days but parenteral penicillin therapy is usually recommended because in some cases bacteraemic spread results in swelling and painful non-suppurative arthritis in one or more joints about 2–3 weeks after dipping. Response to treatment at this stage is usually poor. The source of infection is faeces-contaminated dip, in which *E. rhusiopathiae* can multiply rapidly. Sheep should be dagged if required before dipping and run over slats or stones prior to dipping to remove excess soil and faecal material from the feet.

Dip-compatible bacteriostats should be added to dip when it is to stand overnight.

Infections in lambs and calves typically occur through the umbilicus in the immediate post-partum period, resulting in polyarthritis. At other times young lambs develop an acute lameness from about two weeks of age. At this age it is virtually impossible to distinguish erysipelas arthritis from the far commoner problem caused by *Streptococcus dysgalactiae*. It is therefore important to obtain an accurate diagnosis as to the cause of the lameness.

In other domestic animal species, including turkeys and other fowl species (chickens, ducks, emus, parrots, peacocks and pheasants), infection causes a bacteraemia associated with profound weakness, and cyanosis, erythema and haemorrhage of the comb and snood. This condition is commonly known as 'blue comb'. The organism is usually isolated from the liver or spleen. Vertical transmission of *E. rhusiopathiae* has not been described and erysipelas in parent stock appears to have no adverse effects on the quality of hatching eggs in terms of embryo mortality (Mazaheri *et al.* 2006).

In pigs, *E. rhusiopathiae* is subclinically carried in the pharynx and shed in the faeces, urine and oronasal secretions in up to 30%. The organism can also be isolated from faeces, soil and water in the environment. As well as serving as subclinical sources of disease for humans, pigs develop *E. rhusiopathiae*-induced disease. As in humans, infection in pigs ranges in severity from a cutaneous condition known as 'diamond skin disease' (diamond-shaped lesions, reddish-purple or more diffuse oedema and erythema) to bacteraemia with fever, prostration, anorexia, vomiting and reluctance to walk. The case fatality rate in this acute systemic form of the disease is very high. Pigs can also develop chronic endocarditis and arthritis following *E. rhusiopathiae* infection. In many countries, pigs are routinely vaccinated against *E. rhusiopathiae*, although as the prevalence of disease decreases, vaccination coverage also tends to decrease.

Cetaceans are the most susceptible of marine mammals to erysipelas and the disease has been reported in *Tursiops truncatus*, *Tursiops aduncus*, *Stenella plagiodon*, *Grampus griseus* and *Lagenorhynchus obliquidens* (Suer and Vedros 1988). There are only scattered reports of erysipelas infection in pinnipeds; Svenkerud *et al.* (1951) described cutaneous lesions in hooded seals, harp seals and ringed seals which resembled swine erysipelas and presented as haemorrhagic infiltrations in the subcutaneous blubber. Wild pinnipeds and cetaceans are exposed to *E. rhusiopathiae* in their natural environment and they probably acquire the organism from the fish in their diet (Suer and Vedros 1988). In a Swedish study (Stenstrom *et al.* 1992), *E. rhusiopathiae* was isolated from the mucoid slime of 60% of the cod and 30% of the herring tested. There is also a report of a pet goldfish as a likely source of infection (Simionescu *et al.* 2003).

Humans

Human infection with *E. rhusiopathiae* occurs worldwide but is rare. The Centers for Disease Control (CDC) in Atlanta receives an average of one case per year and the Health Protection Agency (HPA) in England receives less than five reports annually. Reporting of infection caused by *E. rhusiopathiae* is not required by health agencies so it is unclear as to whether the incidence is increasing or decreasing (Reboli and Farrar 1989). Infection usually arises from skin scratches or puncture wounds with infective material or contamination of a pre-existing lesion although penetration of intact skin (McGinnes and Spindle 1934) and infection following ingestion of contaminated food products has been reported (Berg 1984). Person-to-person spread has not been documented. Transmission usually reflects occupational activities with use of contaminated tools such as knives, needles, fish hooks, or traumatic injury from crustacean exoskeleton, fish spines and bone splinters.

The most common manifestation of human disease is erysipeloid, a localized cellulitis (Durham *et al.* 2004) usually developing within 2 to 7 days around the site of inoculation, commonly on the hands or arms of people handling animals or animal products. This can heal without antimicrobial treatment (Nelson 1955). Systemic *E. rhusiopathiae* infection in man is rare but the bacterium has the potential to cause more unusual clinical syndromes including bacterial meningitis (Kim *et al.* 2007) and endognenous endophthalmitis (Elvy *et al.* 2008).

Pathogenesis

Erysipeloid: this is the most common manifestation; a mild cutaneous form usually localized around the arms, hands and fingers reflecting occupational acquisition. The incubation period is usually less than 4 days, but can be up to 7 days post infection. Most of these infections run a self-limiting course of about 3 weeks duration, the cutaneous rash fading with central clearing. The peripheral edge of the rash advances slowly and is usually slightly elevated. These lesions are characteristically violaceous and disproportionately painful with an intense itching or burning sensation (Wood 1975), oedematous and non-suppuring. Localized arthritis can also be present. Dissemination to remote sites may also occur and many patients will have fever, headache and malaise, and a proportion will report systemic symptoms such as arthralgia and myalgia (Garcia-Restoy *et al.* 1991; Totemchokchyakarn *et al.* 1996).

A *systemic* form with septicaemia, more frequently associated with endocarditis and often presenting with fever and malaise is rare in non-immunosuppressed patients. Endocarditis most commonly affects native, left-sided heart valves. Bacteraemia in the absence of endocarditis is recognized (Shumak *et al.* 1987; Garcia-Restoy *et al.* 1991; Fakoya *et al.* 1995) but careful cardiac examination including echocardiogram should be performed in all patients with positive blood cultures (Mahavanakul *et al.* 2007). Septic arthritis may occur in previously normal or damaged joints (Dunbar and Clarridge 2000) and typically presents as a chronic monoarthritis affecting large joints such as the knee or elbow. Brouqui and Raoult (2001) reported 44 cases of *E. rhusiopathiae* endocarditis most frequently left-sided, in which valve replacement was required in 53% of the patients. The mortality rate was 38% for these patients, almost twice that for other aetiologies. The endocarditis was associated with a history of alcohol abuse; otherwise risk factors were the same as those for cutaneous infections. Approximately one third of these cases will have the concurrent erysipeloid skin lesion and occasionally a purpuric, petechial rash accompanied by thrombocytopaenia.

Diagnosis

The diagnosis should be considered in a patient with a subacute cellulitis that typically involves the fingers. The definitive diagnosis is obtained when the organism is isolated from a biopsy specimen or from blood. Clinicians caring for patients with cellulitis involving the hands or fingers should enquire about the patient's occupation, especially about contact with pigs, sheep and fish. Erysipeloid with co-existing orf has been reported (Connor and Green 1995), and there have been occasional reports of septicaemic *Erysipelothrix* infection in people who have consumed undercooked pork. If blood culture is negative, an aspirate from the centre or leading edge of the cellulitis should be obtained in an attempt to isolate the organism.

Direct and indirect fluorescent antibody tests will also confirm the identification of *E. rhusiopathiae* in tissue, broth and human infection; however it is not as sensitive as culture. There are no serological tests routinely available to demonstrate antibodies to *E. rhusiopathiae*. The API Coryne system (BioMérieux) was extensively investigated by Soto *et al.* (1994) and appears to be a reliable alternative to biochemical methods.

Two PCR methods are available for the detection of *Erysipelothrix* species in pigs and are reported to be very sensitive. A PCR method was used in Australia to investigate 'crayfish poisoning', however the value of this test in the human clinical situation is uncertain (Brooke and Riley 1999). It is likely that a combination of culture and molecular techniques will continue to be used for diagnosis for some time to come.

Treatment

Most strains are sensitive to penicillin, erythromycin, ceftriaxone and ciprofloxacin (Fidalgo *et al.* 2002). Susceptibility to chloramphenicol and tetracyclines is variable. Most strains are resistant to the aminoglycosides, sulphonamides, vancomycin and gentamycin frequently used empirically for Gram-positive bacterial infections. Resistance to the latter two agents is important because the combination of these two agents is a frequently used empiric regimen for endocarditis.

Vaccination in man is not viable because clinical disease conveys little or no immunity (Procter and Richardson 1954), with relapse or re-infection possible.

Prevention and control

Changes in manufacturing processes have reduced occupational exposures to animal products carrying *E. rhusiopathiae*, such as the use of plastic rather than bone buttons, and the use of plastic instead of wooden fish boxes. Continued reductions in human exposures are likely to maintain the current low levels of reported erysipeloid and of *E. rhusiopathiae* endocarditis.

Control of erysipelas in swine and poultry includes good biosecurity, containment and control, with vaccine use where the disease is enzootic. With the progressive move towards confinement housing of pigs, long-term soil contamination becomes less of a concern, but the organism may still be present even in small quantities of faeces on the floors of indoor pig housing facilities.

Avoidance of human infection is primarily through awareness of occupational risks and implementation of good hygiene practices (hand washing with disinfectants and covering skin wounds or abrasions) especially when handling diseased pigs or turkeys or for those working in the fishing and fish processing industries, or dealing with cetacean strandings. Adequate hand washing with

disinfectant soap, protective gloves (chain mail gloves where knives are used) and prompt treatment of superficial cuts and abrasions are important. The control of rodent populations in meat and fish processing plants is also important.

References

Barber, M. (1948). Discussion on swine erysipelas infection *(Erysipelothrix rhusiopathiae)*, in man and animals. *Proc. R. Soc. Med.*, **41:** 328–30.

Berg, R. A. (1984). *Erysipelothrix rhusiopathiae. South. Med. J.* **77**(12): 1614.

Brooke, C. J., and Riley, T. V. (1999). *Erysipelothrix rhusiopathiae*; bacteriology, epidemiology and clinical manifestations of an occupational pathogen. *J. Med. Microbiol.*, **48:** 789–99.

Brouqui, P., and Raoult, D. (2001). Endocarditis due to rare and fastidious bacteria. *Clin. Micro. Rev.*, **14**(1): 177–207.

Connor, M. P., and Green, A. D. (1995). Erysipeloid infection in a sheep farmer with coexisting orf. *J. Infect.*, **30**(2): 161–63.

Dunbar, S.A., and Clarridge III, J. E. (2000). Potential errors in recognition of *Erysipelothrix rhusiopathiae. J. Clin. Microbiol.*, **38:** 180–81.

Durham, H. L., Mushatt, D. M., Kemmerley, S. A., and Dalovisio, J. R., (2004). online at http://www.medscape.com/viewarticle/466333.

Elvy, J., Hanspal, I., and Simcock, P. (2008). A case of *Erysipelothrix rhusiopathiae* causing bilateral endogenous endophthalmitis. *J. Clin. Pathol.*, **61:** 1223–24.

Fakoya, A., Bendall, R. P., Churchill, D. R., *et al.* (1995). *Erysipelothrix rhusiopathiae* bacteraemia in a patient without endocarditis. *J. Infect.*, **30:** 180–81.

Fidalgo, S. G., Longbottom, C. J., and Riley, T. V. (2002). Susceptibility of *Erysipelothrix rhusiopathiae* to antimicrobial agents and home disinfectants. *Pathol.*, **34:** 462–65.

Garcia-Restoy, E., Espejo, E., Bella, F., and Llebot, J. (1991). Bacteraemia due to *Erysipelothrix rhusiopathiae* in immunocompromised hosts without endocarditis. *Rev. Infect. Dis.*, **13:** 1252–53.

Heptonstall, J., Cockcroft, A., and Smith, R. M. M.(2000). Occupation and Infectious Diseases. In: P.J. Baxter, P. H. Adams, A. Cockcroft, T-C. Aw and J. M. Harrington (eds.) Hunter's Diseases of Occupations (9th edn.). London: Edward Arnold.

Hillenbrand, F. K. M. (1953). Whale finger and seal finger; their relation to erysipeloid. *Lancet*, (i): 680–81.

Jones, T. D. (1977). Aspects of the epidemiology and control of *Erysipelothrix insidiosa* polyarthritis in lambs. *Vet. Ann.*, 88–98.

Kim, S. R., Kwon, M. J., Lee, J. H., and Lee, N. Y.(2007). Chronic meningitis caused by *Erysipelothrix rhusiopathiae. J. Med. Microbiol.*, **56:** 1405–6.

King, P.F. (1946). Erysipeloid. *Lancet*, i 251: 196–98.

Klauder, J. V.(1926). Erysipeloid and swine erysipelas in man. *J. Am. Vet. Med. Assoc.*, **86:** 536–41.

Koch, R. (1880). Investigations into the aetiology of traumatic infective diseases. London: New Sydenham Society.

Loeffler, F. A. (1886). Experimentelle Untersuchungen uber Schweinerothlauf. Arb. kais. Gesundheit. *Sante*, **1:** 46–55.

Mahavanakul, W., Limmathurotsakul, D., Teerawattanasuk, N., and Peacock, S. (2007). Invasive Erysipelothrix rhusiopathiae infection in Northeast Thailand. *Southeast Asian J. Trop. Med. Pub. Heal.*, **38**(3): 478–81.

Mazaheri, A., Philipp, H. C., Bonsack, H., and Voss, M. (2006). Investigations of the vertical transmission of *Erysipelothrix rhusiopathiae* in laying hens. *Avian Dis.*, **50**(2): 306–8.

McGinnes, G. F., and Spindle, F. (1934). Erysipeloid condition among workers in a bone button factory due to the bacillus of swine erysipelas. *Am. J. Pub. Heal.*, **24:** 32–35.

Morgis, G. G., Beauregard, L. P., and Shoub, E. P. (1967). State Compensatory Provisions for Occupational Diseases. *US Bur. Mines Bull. 623*. Washington: Government Printing Office.

Nelson, E. (1955). Five hundred cases of erysipeloid. *Rocky Mt. Med. J.*, **52:** 40–42.

Pasteur, L. and Thuillier, L. (1883). Pathologie experimentale: la vaccination du rouget des porcs a l'aide du virus mortel attenue de cette maladie. *Compte Rendus Hebdom. Seances l'Acad. Siences*, **97**: 1163–69.

Penny, R. H. C., and Guise, H. J. (1986). Swine erysipelas is a seasonal disease: fact or fiction? *Vet. Ann.*, **1986**: 129–33.

Procter, D. M. and Richardson, I. M. (1954). A report on 235 cases of erysipeloid in Aberdeen. *Bri. J. Indust. Med.,* **11**: 175–79.

Reboli, A. C., and Farrar, W. E. (1989). *Erysipelothrix rhusiopathiae*: an occupational pathogen. *Clin. Microbiol. Rev,.* **2** (4): 354–59.

Robson, J. M., McDougall, R., van der Valk, S., *et al.* (1998). *Erysipelothrix rhusiopathiae*: an uncommon but ever present zoonosis. *Pathol.,* **30**: 391–94.

Rosenbach, A. J. F. (1884). *Microorganismen bei den Wundinfektionskrankheiten des Menschen*. Wiesbaden, Bergmann.

Shimoji, Y. (2000). Pathogenicity of Erysipelothrix rhusiopathiae: virulence factors and protective immunity. *Microbes Infect.*, **2**: 965–72.

Shumak, S. L., McDonald, S., Baer, P., and Cowan, D. H. (1987). Erysipelothrix septicaemia in an immunocompromised host. *CMAJ*, **136**: 273–74.

Simionescu, R., Grover, S., Shekar, R., and West, B. C. (2003). Necrotizing faciitis caused by *Erysipelothrix rhusiopathiae*. *South Med. J.*, **96**: 937–39.

Soto, A., Zapardiel, J., and Soriano, F. (1994). Evaluation of API Coryne system for identifying coryneform bacteria. *J. Clin. Pathol.,* **47**: 756–59.

Spencer, R. (1959). The sanitation of fish boxes. I. The quantitative and qualitative bacteriology of commercial wooden fish boxes. *J. Appl. Bacteriol.,* **22**: 73–84.

Stenstrom, I. M., Norrung, V., Ternstrom, A., and Molin, G. (1992). Occurrence of different serotypes of *Erysipelothrix rhusiopathiae* in retail pork and fish. *Acta Vet. Scand.*, **33**: 169–73.

Suer, L. D., and Vedros, N. A. (1988). *Erysipelothrix rhusiopathiae*.I. Isolation and characterization from pinnipeds and bite/abrasion wounds in humans. *Dis. Aquat. Organ.*, **5**: 1–5.

Svenkerud, R. R., Rosted, A. F., and Thorshaug, K. A. (1951). Lesion in seals reminding greatly of swine erysipelas. *Nord Veterinaermed.*, **3**: 147–69.

Taylor, D. J. (ed.) (1983). Pig Diseases, (3rd edn.). Glasgow: Farming Press Books.

To, H., and Nagai, S. (2007). Genetic and antigenic diversity of the surface protective antigen proteins of *Erysipelothrix rhusiopathiae*. *Clin. Vacc. Immunol.*, **14**(7): 813–20.

Totemchokchyakarn, K., Janwityanujit, S., Sathapatayavongs, B., and Puavilai, S. (1996). *Erysipelothrix rhusiopathiae* septicaemia in systemic lupus erythematosis. *Int. J. Dermatol.*, **35**: 818–20.

Vendetti, M., Gelfusa, V., and Tarasi, A. *et al.* (1990). Antimicrobial susceptibilities of *Erysipelothrix rhusiopathiae*. *Antimicrob. Agents Chemother.*, **34**: 2038–40.

Wood, R. L. (1974). Isolation of pathogenic *Erysipelothrix rhusiopathiae* from feces of apparently healthy swine. *Am. J. Vet. Res.*, **35**: 41–43.

Wood, R. L. (1975). *Erysipelothrix* infection. In: W.T. Hubbert, W.F. McCullough, and P.R. Schnurrenberger (eds.) Diseases Transmitted from Animals to Man, (6th ed.), pp. 271–81. Springfield, Ill.: Charles C Thomas.

Wood, R. L., and Harrington Jr., R. (1978). Serotypes of *Erysipelothrix rhusiopathiae* isolated from swine and from soil and from manure of swine pens in the United States. *Am. J. Vet. Res.*, **39**: 1833–40.

Other bacterial diseases

Staphylococcal zoonoses

Susan Dawson

Summary

Staphylococcal species are common commensals of the skin and mucous membranes of humans and animals but only in very recent years has zoonotic infections been recognized. They can also be associated with infection and disease, especially coagulase positive organisms. *Staphylococcus aureus* is relatively frequently carried by humans in the nasal passages and is a cause of infections in people including bacteraemias in hospitalized patients. More recently some strains of *Staphylococcus aureus* have acquired a resistance gene (*mec*A) which renders them resistant to meticillin (meticillin-resistant *Staphylococcus aureus*, MRSA). MRSA isolates are of major importance in healthcare situations as well as increasingly in the community. Animals can also be carriers of *Staphylococcus aureus* although less frequently than humans and MRSA can be carried or infect several different host species. For companion animals such as dogs and cats, the most frequently isolated MRSA strains are similar to the common local human healthcare strains; thus for the UK, EMRSA-15 and -16. This suggests a reverse zoonoses with spill over from the human population into their companion animals. In horses the situation is different, with some horses carrying or infected with human epidemic strains but others infected with strains less frequently seen in people. For food-producing animals the picture is different again with a particular strain, ST398, which appears to circulate endemically in animal populations, such as pigs, and can spill over into the human population where it can cause carriage as well as infection and disease. The transmission appears to be by direct contact with animals rather than through the food-chain.

Where risk factors for infection with MRSA have been studied in animals they appear similar to some of the risks for human infection. Therefore, for control of MRSA in animals measures such as improved hygiene and good antibacterial stewardship are important.

History

Staphylococcus are non-sporulating Gram-positive aerobic organisms which are common commensals in humans and animals. They also have the potential to become opportunistic pathogens, and in some situations they are associated with infection and disease. They can be divided into coagulase-negative and coagulase-positive organisms, the latter of which are more commonly associated with clinical signs. In humans, *Staphylococcus epidermis* (coagulase negative) and *Staphylococcus aureus* (coagulase positive) are common commensals, with other staphylococcal species found more frequently on different animal hosts (Nagase *et al.* 2002). *Staphylococcus aureus* is frequently carried by humans, with approximately one third of healthy people being nasal carriers. Some Staphylococcus strains have acquired resistance to meticillin (MRSA) and these have become of major importance to human healthcare.

MRSA

Meticillin-resistant (previously methicillin) *Staphylococcus aureus* (MRSA) is an important cause of healthcare associated infections and increasingly of community associated infections. MRSA was identified in 1961, shortly after the introduction of the antimicrobial methicillin into clinical use (Jevons *et al.* 1961). MRSA was first reported from a case of mastitis in a dairy cow in 1972 (Devriese *et al.* 1972), and it has subsequently been reported with increasing frequency in several domestic species. MRSA is capable of causing a variety of infections in both humans and animals, ranging from mild skin pyoderma to fatal pneumonia or bacteraemia.

Meticillin-resistance (MR) is mediated by the production of an altered penicillin-binding protein (PBP2a), to which β-lactams have poor affinity. The penicillin-binding protein is the target molecule for β-lactam antimicrobials such as penicillins and cephalosporins (Brown and Reynolds 1980) and thus the bacteria containing the altered molecule have resistance to this group of antimicrobials. Meticillin-resistance can occur in a number of species of *Staphylococcus*, but its presence in *S. aureus* predominates as a clinical concern, largely due to the pathogenic potential of this species.

MRSA is of little concern to healthy people. Indeed approximately 20–30% of people are colonized with meticillin sensitive *S. aureus* (MSSA) although probably less than 1% of the general population carry MRSA. However, in healthcare workers the carriage rates may be 5–10%. Veterinary personnel have also been shown to have higher carriage rates than the general population.

Levels of MRSA infections have been high over recent years, especially in hospitalized patients; risk factors for MRSA infection include skin or mucosal barrier defects, a compromised immune system, undergoing extensive surgery and length of in-patient stay. In the UK, the majority of human infections are hospital acquired

(HA) epidemic (E) strains 15 and 16 (Johnson *et al.* 2001). EMRSA-15 is also prevalent elsewhere in Europe. The prevalence of MRSA infections, often measured as bacteraemia rates, varies greatly between countries, from <1% in Scandinavia and the Netherlands to >40% in southern and western Europe (Tiemersma *et al.* 2004). In some areas the prevalence rates are reducing following implementation of control measures (Thompson *et al.* 2009).

Community acquired MRSA (CA-MRSA) are usually isolated from people with no healthcare contact nor any of the other identified risk factors (Cookson 2000). The strains found in the community differ from HA-MRSA (Herold *et al.* 1998). CA-MRSA can be severe and life-threatening and infections are usually sporadic although once these strains enter a hospital they can also circulate within that setting (Patel *et al.* 2007). Antibiotic resistance is less marked but the toxin gene Panton Valentine Leucocidin (PVL) is more often found in CA-MRSA and is associated with severe disease.

In addition to resistance to β-lactams, MRSA are often resistant to other antimicrobials such as fluoroquinolones, tetracyclines, and potentiated sulphonamides. Antimicrobial susceptibility patterns were used to identify epidemic strains, before the availability of molecular typing methods. The definition for epidemic MRSA strains (EMRSA) in the UK, are those which have caused infection in two or more patients, in two or more hospitals (Duckworth *et al.* 1998). There are two healthcare-associated epidemic clones EMRSA-15 and EMRSA-16 in UK hospitals, accounting for >95% of the bacteraemias caused by MRSA (Johnson *et al.* 2001). There are differences in the antimicrobial susceptibility of clones, with the dominant clone EMRSA-15 largely resistant to β-lactams, fluoroquinolones and macrolides, whilst EMRSA-16 can be resistant to further antimicrobials. EMRSA-15 is also problematic in Europe, where it is termed the Barnim epidemic clone. It is difficult to compare the epidemiology of epidemic strains of MRSA, as different countries have different designations for strains. Such designations are now increasingly based upon the molecular typing technique used. Molecular typing has shown that strains from healthcare-associated (HA) infections and community-associated (CA) infections represent largely distinct genetic clones, although they differ between geographic locations.

Molecular typing techniques

Currently there are a number of molecular typing techniques or 'tools', which are used to determine the strain type and epidemiology of *S. aureus*, including MSSA and MRSA. The most common method and widely regarded as the gold standard for strain typing of MRSA, is macro-restriction pulsed-field gel electrophoresis (PFGE) (Murchan *et al.* 2003). This method has good discrimination, repeatability and is useful in helping to determine sources of infection at a local level, so is an excellent tool for outbreak investigations. Furthermore, a standardized method (Murchan *et al.* 2003) has been devised to allow comparisons of strains between laboratories, but PFGE still has limitations when investigating global epidemiology.

A useful tool for studying both the population structure and evolution of *S. aureus*, and tracking of strains is multi-locus sequence typing (MLST), which involves PCR amplification of seven house-keeping genes and determination of their sequence. The sequence is then submitted to a database (http://saureus.mlst.net/), where an allele number is assigned for each loci. A sequence type is designated from the allelic profile, which belongs to a clonal complex, including the founder or 'ancestor' strain that gave rise to all subsequent strains within that complex (Enright *et al.* 2000). The advantage of sequenced based techniques is that they are objective, portable and allow the comparison of strains on a global scale. The cost of DNA sequencing has reduced in recent years, however the sequencing of seven loci is still costly, as well as time consuming, therefore MLST would be unlikely to be used routinely in the clinical setting.

A further sequence based method is *spa* gene typing. This involves the amplification and sequencing of the short sequence repeat region of the protein A gene to determine the number and organization of small DNA repeats, rather than direct comparison of sequences (Shopsin *et al.* 1999). The interpretation of these results has been made easier by the introduction of Ridom Staph type software (Ridom GmbH, Würzburg, Germany), which assigns a *spa* gene type (http://spaserver.ridom.de) and also e-genomics (http://tool.e-genomics.com/). The *spa* gene has a relatively high degree of polymorphism, but is stable enough to allow the grouping of epidemiologically related strains (Shopsin and Kreisworth 2001). Furthermore, if used in combination with another polymorphic gene, such as *clfB* (encoding clumping factor B), the discriminatory power of *spa* gene typing can be increased (Kuhn *et al.* 2007). As this method only requires the sequencing of one loci, it is relatively inexpensive, quick, and has good inter-laboratory reproducibility (Aires-de-Sousa *et al.* 2006). There is, furthermore, good congruence between assigned *spa* gene types, MLST sequence types (ST) and PFGE strain types (Hallin *et al.* 2007).

Another method used specifically for MRSA is typing of the staphylococcal cassette chromosome or SCC*mec*, in which the alternative penicillin-binding protein (PBP2a) gene, *mecA*, is encoded. By PCR amplification of genes within the SCC*mec* it is possible to determine SCC*mec* types I–VI and some subtypes, such as those found in SCC*mec* II and IV (Oliveira and de Lencastre 2002; Zhang *et al.* 2005; Oliveira *et al.* 2006; Milheirco *et al.* 2007). Such typing of isolates is extremely important in complementing other typing methods in studying MRSA epidemiology, and can differentiate between strains of the same sequence type.

Variable-number tandem repeat (VNTR) typing has been developed for use in *S. aureus*, which makes use of the tandem repeats associated with minisatellites within bacterial genomes and is PCR based. This method is a useful tool for investigating population structure and allows for strain differentiation, with greater discrimination than MLST (Hardy *et al.* 2004). In addition, gene and whole genome microarrays, are now being used to characterize *S. aureus*. Such technology can assist in strain typing, investigate evolution of strains and determine pathogenic potential (Saunders *et al.* 2004; Lindsay *et al.* 2006).

Thus, molecular typing techniques should serve a number of purposes, to allow investigation of strains locally in outbreak situations, where methods are required which can detect genetic microvariation, but which are also able to investigate global spread and evolution of strains, and therefore detect genetic macrovariation (Koreen *et al.* 2004).

MRSA in animals

MRSA and other MR-staphylococci have been isolated from healthy and diseased individuals from many animal species.

The epidemiology of colonization and infection, however, is variable between MRSA strains, animal species and geographic location. This may reflect differences in species of staphylococci found in animal and human populations, animal–human interactions, antimicrobial usage and exposure, and species susceptibility. As well as the implications of such infections for animal health and welfare, there is much concern as to the role such animal infections play in terms of public health. It is likely that there is two-way transmission of MRSA, with animals vulnerable to reverse zoonotic infections or acting as reservoirs of infection for humans. Clearance of the organism from in-contact pets may therefore need to be included in treatment regimen for humans. Furthermore, faecal transmission of MRSA is becoming recognized as a risk for re-colonization in people (Klotz et al. 2005). Despite the fact that contact with animal faeces may be a public health concern, there are very few reports of faeces being examined for the presence of MRSA in animals.

MRSA and other meticillin resistant staphylococcal species have been isolated from dogs, cats, rabbits, birds, horses and livestock. Animals can be carriers of MRSA or can be infected with associated disease and they have the potential to act as reservoirs for colonization of in-contact humans. In domestic animals the most common sites for infection are post-operative infections of bone and soft tissue, and also skin, joints, mammary glands (dairy cows) and the lungs or thoracic cavity (Baptiste et al. 2005; Devriese and Hommez 1975; Hartmann et al. 1997; Leonard et al. 2006; Owen et al. 2004; Rankin et al. 2005; Weese et al. 2006a).

Companion animals

MRSA is an emerging worldwide problem in companion animals (Shimuzu et al. 1997; Pak et al. 1999; Seguin et al. 1999; Tomlin et al. 1999; O'Mahony et al. 2005; Weese 2005; Baptiste et al. 2005; Cuny et al. 2006; Kwon et al. 2006; Strommenger et al. 2006). Not only does it pose an infection risk to animals but, if animals act as a reservoir for colonization and infection within the community, it may also constitute a risk to owners and other in-contact humans. The true prevalence of MRSA colonization and infection in companion animals is largely unknown. Few studies have been conducted, with most carried out within veterinary premises, and the prevalence of MRSA carriage in the community is not known. One Slovenian study which sampled 200 dogs in the community did not isolate any MRSA (Vengust et al. 2006). A cross-sectional study of dogs attending (although not hospitalized) UK veterinary practices found a prevalence of 0.8% nasal carriage in dogs.

More work has been carried out in veterinary hospitals or by collection of samples submitted to diagnostic laboratories. A small referral hospital based study in the UK found that MRSA was carried by up to 10% of dogs referred to the hospital without MRSA infections (Loeffler et al. 2005). Another study, however, failed to isolate MRSA from dogs attending a separate referral hospital over a two month period, during which time two dogs were found to have clinical MRSA infection. This study, furthermore failed to isolate MRSA from dogs sampled in the community (Baptiste et al. 2005). In Ireland, MRSA was recovered from 25 animals (14 dogs, eight horses, one cat, one rabbit and a seal) and from 10 in-contact veterinary personnel (O'Mahony et al. 2005). A further study examined all the clinical submissions from a German small animal hospital over a 20 month period, for the presence of MRSA and MSSA. Of 869 samples, 61 were positive for S. aureus of which,

44.3% of these isolates were MRSA. Similar proportions of samples were positive for MRSA in dogs (3.0%) and cats (2.7%), with MRSA also isolated from a bird, rabbit, guinea pig, turtle and bat. This study reported on average 1.35 clinical MRSA infections per month in the hospital, which had an annual caseload of approximately 30,000 small animals (Walther et al. 2008).

In contrast, US studies have identified meticillin-resistance in staphylococci at much higher frequency. MR-staphylococci have been isolated from 15% of healthy cats and 38% of dogs with recurrent pyoderma; MR rates for S. aureus was 35%, 17% for S. pseudintermedius and 40% for S. schleiferi (Morris et al. 2006). This high prevalence, however, has been reported from one tertiary referral centre, situated within a community with a high concentration of human healthcare and pharmaceutical industry workers, which may be a risk factor. In another US study, 20% of 1,772 clinical samples from dogs demonstrated in vitro resistance to oxacillin. These comprised 15.6% of the S. pseudintermedius, 46.6% of the S. schleiferi and 23.5% of the S. aureus isolates (Jones et al. 2007). A 6 month surveillance study in the USA, which recruited 27 veterinary teaching hospitals, reported 65 animals with S. aureus infection, of which 13% of these isolates (nine cases) were demonstrated to be MRSA. Of the MRSA positive cases, four were dogs, four horses and one was a cat. Macro-restriction PFGE performed upon 63 isolates, demonstrated 58 different patterns, and that the MRSA strains were different. This study concluded that such infections were likely to be community-acquired, rather than hospital-acquired, as no specific strain was associated with individual hospitals (Middleton et al. 2005).

In the UK isolates from small animals have largely been identical or closely related to EMRSA-15 (Loeffler et al. 2005; Moodley et al. 2006; Baptiste et al. 2005), currently the predominant epidemic health care associated MRSA strain in humans within the UK. In Ireland MRSA from non-equine companion animals were all found to be closely related to each other and the main epidemic human strain, which is similar to the UK EMRSA-15 (O'Mahony et al. 2005). Furthermore, MLST performed on EMRSA-15 canine isolates have been identified as sequence type ST22. German MRSA isolates from small animals were also found to be ST22 by MLST, with SCCmecIV and were spa gene type t032 and negative for panton-valentine leukocidin (PVL) (Strommenger et al. 2006). A further German study also found MRSA isolates from dogs and cats to be identical or closely related to the Barnim epidemic clone by PFGE, of which some were confirmed as ST22-MRSA-IV. However, two isolates from dogs were found to be ST239, as single locus variant of ST8 and belonging to CC8 (Walther et al. 2008). In contrast, one isolate from a British hospital visit dog proved to be a unique strain of unknown origin and unrelated to strains previously identified from the hospital and in-contact humans (Enoch et al. 2005). In the Netherlands, PFGE analysis of two MRSA and four MR-S. haemolyticus isolates from dogs revealed that they all had distinct clonal identities with only one showing homology to a human epidemic MRSA clonal group (van Duijkeren et al. 2004).

The situation in American and Canadian small animals is somewhat different. The predominant community-associated strain Canadian epidemic MRSA-2 (USA100) is most common in animals with clinical infections and household contacts (Weese 2005; Weese et al. 2006b). In one study of 15 feline MRSA isolates from 46 cats, all bar one were highly related and possessed SCCmec type II, which are commonly found in human isolates (Morris et al. 2006a).

These were negative for PVL, but more recently PVL-positive Canadian epidemic MRSA-10 (USA-300) has been isolated from small animals in both Canada and the USA, along with other reports of PVL positive MRSA isolates from companion animals (Rankin et al. 2005). There is one report of a PVL-positive ST8-MRSA-IVa in a household cat with a skin infection (Vitale et al. 2006).

Horses

Again, the prevalence of MRSA and MR-CNS carriage in non-infected horses, has yet to be fully established and most studies have utilized convenience sampling of large groups of horses at a limited number of locations. Surveys of clinically normal horses in the community from the UK and mainland Europe have not identified MRSA in nasal sampling (Baptiste et al. 2005; Busscher et al. 2006; Vengust et al. 2006), and a recent large cross-sectional study of 677 horses in the UK showed a low prevalence of MRSA carriage of 0.6% (Maddox et al. 2009). Reports from North America are more varied, one Canadian study of 497 clinically normal horses failed to detect any MRSA carriage (Burton et al. 2008), whilst another examining horses from both Canada and the USA identified a higher overall prevalence of 4.7% (Weese et al. 2005b). This second study used a targeted approach to sampling; a prevalence of 12% for nasal carriage of MRSA was found on yards where previous MRSA cases had been identified, but no carriage was identified on yards without any previous MRSA cases. Prevalence on the individual yards concerned ranged considerably, from zero to 45%. A relatively high prevalence for MR-CNS carriage, ranging from 22.5% to 42%, was identified by some of these studies (Busscher et al. 2006; Vengust et al. 2006).

The reported prevalence of MRSA carriage in hospitalized horses is generally higher, with figures of 2.3% and 16% documented for hospitals in Canada and the UK (Baptiste et al. 2005; Weese et al. 2006c). Surveillance undertaken during an outbreak of clinical disease in a Dutch equine hospital revealed a very high prevalence of 42% for nasal MRSA carriage (van Duijkeren et al. 2009).

Few studies have differentiated nosocomial colonization from animals colonized at admission. One study that did determine the rate of community-associated colonization in horses found that it was 27 per 1,000 admissions and that the nosocomial colonization rate was 23 per 1,000 admissions (Weese et al. 2006c). Horses colonized at admission were significantly more likely to develop clinical MRSA infections, although the incidence of nosocomial MRSA infection was lower than colonization at 1.8 per 1,000 admissions. A study at an Austrian equine hospital found a higher mean incidence of infection with MRSA, of 4.8 cases per 1,000 equine admissions, over a two year period (Cuny et al. 2006). Prevalence estimates for nasal carriage of MRSA of 9.3% and 10.9% have been reported for horses on admission to equine hospitals in Belgium and the Netherlands (van den Eede et al. 2009; van Duijkeren et al. 2009) and 2.7% for a Canadian hospital (Weese et al. 2006c). However, such horses may not be representative of the wider equine population, as they are likely to have received prior veterinary attention, antimicrobial treatment or hospitalization (especially when admitted to a secondary or tertiary referral hospital).

MRSA infections in horses have been identified, but currently only as relatively sporadic cases compared to the situation within human medicine. However, there has been a steady rise in the number of infections reported, and clusters of infection have been seen in some equine hospitals (Seguin et al. 1999; van Duijkeren

et al. 2009; Weese et al. 2005b). The majority of these have been soft tissue infections; mainly of wounds, post-surgical incisions and intravenous catheter sites. Risk factors for MRSA infection in horses have proven difficult to establish (due to the rarity of clinical disease), although horses with colonization detected at admission to a veterinary hospital have been identified as more likely to subsequently develop a clinical infection (Weese et al. 2006c). One study has identified factors associated with a poor prognosis in infected horses, such as intravenous catheterization and dissemination of infection to other sites (Anderson et al. 2009). Risk factors for colonization (rather than infection), have been better described. Previous colonization of associated animals, previous antimicrobial treatment and admission to a neonatal care unit have been identified as significant (Weese and Lefebvre 2007).

The MRSA strain types found in horses appear to be largely restricted to the horse, and less commonly encountered in humans and other animals (Baptiste et al. 2005; Cuny et al. 2006; Moodley et al. 2006; O'Mahony et al. 2005; Weese et al. 2005b). In contrast to the situation in dogs and cats, the majority of MRSA types from horses either represent less commonly encountered human strains, or strains usually confined to horses and in-contact personnel. Equine isolates recovered from a number of countries appear by MLST to be mostly either sequence type 8 or ST254 (both belonging to clonal complex 8), not reflective of the prevalent human types (Cuny et al. 2006; Cuny et al. 2008; O'Mahony et al. 2005; Walther et al. 2008). These strains possess variants of SCCmec IV and this type has predominated in reports from horses. MRSA carrying SCCmec types other than type IV appear to be rare in the horse. The sequence type common in food producing animals in some countries, ST398, is currently increasing in prominence amongst reports of MRSA in horses (Cuny et al. 2008; Hermans et al. 2008; Loeffler et al. 2009; van den Eede et al. 2009).

Food-producing animals

Food-producing animals pose a potential risk of infection to humans both through direct contact and through food products. MRSA have been isolated from several different species and in some hosts in certain geographical locations endemic infection is present.

In the Netherlands, where human healthcare MRSA cases are rare, patients were identified with what was initially classified as an untypable MRSA infection and it was noted that these patients were from pig farms (Voss et al. 2005). Samples were taken from the pigs and environment at the farms belonging to the original cases and infection was found. Subsequently studies on pig farms across the Netherlands found high prevalence with 39% (209/540) of pigs positive for MRSA in the nares (de Neeling et al. 2007). The strain has now been identified as ST 398. A number of other European countries including Belgium, Germany, Austria, and Denmark have also identified this strain, ST 398, in pigs as well as other species such as cattle, especially calves, dogs, and horses (Witte et al. 2007; Guardabassi et al. 2007). ST 398 has also been found outside Europe in the USA, Canada, China, and Singapore (Khanna et al. 2008; Smith et al. 2008; Sergio et al. 2007; Yu et al. 2008). It is suggested that livestock act as a reservoir of infection for ST 398 and spill over can occur into the human population usually following direct contact with the animals. ST 398 continues to be isolated from humans and often there is a known contact with farming or livestock. However, cases of ST 398 have occurred in

Scotland where no known livestock contact was identified. Two horses were found to be positive for ST 398 in England one of which had travelled from Spain through France but the other had resided solely in the UK (Loeffler *et al.* 2009). Sampling of pig breeding herds was carried out across Europe in 2008 and no MRSA ST 398 was found on UK farms.

These MRSA from livestock (ST 398) although untypable using sma1 PFGE, can be examined by using different typing methods and protocols. Staphylococcal protein A (spa) typing suggests a clonal structure as the strains belong to specific spa types (the predominant types t011 or t108) and MLST identifies them as ST 398 or single locus variants of ST 398 (ST752 and ST 753) (Armand-Lefevre *et al.* 2005; Huijsdens *et al.* 2009). They contain one of two SCCmec-types, either a SCCmec-type IV or V. ST 398 do not usually contain virulence genes such as pvl and do not always have resistance to a large number of antibacterials. However, they are usually resistant to tetracyclines and it has been suggested that this may be associated with the relatively frequent use of these antibacterials in farming and in particular porcine practice.

S. aureus is a common cause of bovine mastitis for which antibacterials are commonly prescribed for treatment. However, MRSA have been relatively rarely reported from bovine milk samples; they have been isolated from both normal and mastitic milk samples, and also cheese samples in Italy, Germany, Switzerland, and Korea (Monecke *et al.* 2007; Normano *et al.* 2007). More recently, higher levels of MRSA have been reported from areas where ST 398 is circulating in livestock (Fessier *et al.* 2010).

MRSA has also been found in poultry flocks in several different countries. A high proportion of the MRSA isolated from poultry flocks in the Netherlands also belong to the ST 398 lineage. In one study 35% of flocks tested, via sampling of broilers arriving at slaughterhouses, were positive for MRSA (Mulders *et al.* 2010).

MRSA has also been isolated from meat samples at abattoirs, including poultry meat in Korea and Japan (Kwon *et al.* 2006; Lee 2003). It is thought that in the latter cases meat samples were contaminated by human handlers and meat is not seen as a high risk for MRSA infection. There is currently no evidence to suggest MRSA is a frequent contaminant of UK produced or imported food products or that it poses a risk to consumers. As there is no evidence to suggest that MRSA is more heat tolerant than other *S. aureus*, cooking would be expected to destroy any MRSA if it was present on raw meat. Therefore the 4Cs principles endorsed by the Foods Standards Agency to reduce food-borne illness are relevant for ensuring that MRSA on raw meat does not pose a health risk:

Clean your hands properly and keep them clean;

Cook food properly;

Chill food properly and

Avoid Cross-contamination.

Transmission of MRSA between animals and humans

MRSA colonization may be an occupational risk for veterinary staff, farmers and people working with animals. For veterinary personnel MRSA has been isolated from the nares of 7% of vets and 12% of nurses sampled at a North American veterinary congress (Hanselman *et al.* 2006) and 10% of vets and nurses sampled at a British veterinary congress. At the American meeting, working in large animal practice was significantly associated with colonization. The pattern of colonization reflected the strains most commonly seen in animals; Canadian epidemic MRSA-2 was isolated from 11 small animal but only two large animal personnel, whereas Canadian epidemic CMRSA-5 was only isolated from large animal clinicians (Hanselman *et al.* 2006). Another study at an equine meeting isolated MRSA from 10% of the participants (Anderson *et al.* 2008). Contact with an MRSA patient increased the risk of MRSA colonization, whereas hand washing between patients and farms was protective. At a UK equine veterinary conference the prevalence of MRSA was 8% in the staff attending with approximately half the strains typical of equine associated strains, which are less common in the human population. Prevalence of MRSA can be higher amongst veterinary staff if they are sampled in their working environment in particular where they have been dealing with MRSA cases. There is a report describing skin infection in three and nasal colonization in 10 veterinary staff treating a foal with Canadian epidemic MRSA-5 (Weese *et al.* 2006a).

In households owning companion animals there may also be sharing of staphylococcal species including MRSA with MRSA colonized animals acting as reservoirs for re-colonization of in-contact humans (Scott *et al.* 1988; Cefai *et al.* 1994; Manion 2003; Vitale *et al.* 2006; van Duijkeren *et al.* 2005). Concurrent human-animal colonization occurs in 20% of *S. aureus* positive households (Hanselman *et al.* 2006). MRSA has also been isolated from up to 11% of owners in contact with infected companion animals, compared to 5% and 0% in contact with MSSA infected animals (Loeffler *et al.* 2009b). In another reported case, identical PVL-positive MRSA strains were isolated from three humans and one dog in a household (van Duijkeren *et al.* 2005). MRSA colonization has also been found in 1/1 cats and 16/88 humans in-contact with eight dogs and three cats with MRSA infections (Weese *et al.* 2006d).

For farmers and others working with food-producing animals there is evidence of transmission of MRSA between humans and animals (Aubry-Damon *et al.* 2004; Huijsdens *et al.* 2006; van Belkum *et al.* 2008). ST 398 was first recognized in humans from pig farms in the Netherlands and a high proportion of pig farmers in the Netherlands were found to be nasal carriers of ST 398 (Wulf *et al.* 2006). In a study of bovine mastitis isolates identical strains were also found from people working with the cows (Fessier *et al.* 2010). An increased risk of MRSA infection was found for workers in Dutch poultry slaughterhouses with 5.6% prevalence compared to an estimated 0.1% prevalence in the general Dutch population and the risk increased where there was direct contact with live poultry (Mulders *et al.* 2010). Following zoonotic spread of ST 398 transmission between people can then occur (Hartmeyer *et al.* 2010).

Prevention and control

To reduce the potential for MRSA as a zoonotic problem hygiene and good animal management are critical as well as antibiotic stewardship. Companion animals may be at risk of transmission from humans and so the risk may be increased in pets of healthcare workers or those with regular contact with a healthcare setting. Routine testing and decolonization of animals is not recommended as prevalence rates appear to be low. However, where a household is colonized with a pvl-positive MRSA strain, and is being decontaminated, the pets within the household may need to be included in any decolonization programme. In veterinary premises, hygiene protocols should be carried out by all staff to reduce the likelihood of transmission of MRSA (and other potential pathogens).

Hygiene on farms and good animal management are crucial for infectious disease control. Antibacterials should not be prescribed in place of good animal management. Appropriate use of antibacterials is crucial to maintain their efficacy for both animals and humans and prescribing guidelines are available from various veterinary organizations.

References

Aires-de-Sousa, M., Boye, K., de Lencastre, H., Deplano, A., Enright, M.C., et al. (2006). High interlaboratory reproducibility of DNA sequence-based typing of bacteria in a multicenter study. *J. Clin. Microbiol.*, 44(2): 619–21.

Anderson, M.E.C., Lefebvre, S.L., Rankin, S.C., Aceto, H., Morley, P.S., et al. (2009). Retrospective multicentre study of methicillin-resistant Staphylococcus aureus infections in 115 horses. *Equine Vet. J.*, 41: 401–5.

Anderson, M.E.C., Lefebvre, S.L. and Weese, J.S. (2008). Evaluation of prevalence and risk factors for methicillin-resistant Staphylococcus aureus colonization in veterinary personnel attending an international equine veterinary conference. *Vet. Microbiol.*, 129: 410–17.

Armand-Lefevre, L., Ruimy, R. and Andermont, A. (2005). Clonal comparison of *Staphylococcus aureus* isolates from healthy pig farmers, human controls, and pigs. *Emerg. Infect. Dis.*, 11: 711–14.

Aubry-Damon, H., Grenet, K., Sall-Ndiaye, P., et al. (2004). Antimicrobial resistance in commensal flora of pig farmers. *Emerg. Infect. Dis.*, 10: 873–79.

Baptiste, K.E., Williams, K., Willams, N.J., Wattret, A., Clegg, P.D., et al. (2005). Methicillin resistant Staphylococci in Companion Animals. *Emerg. Infect. Dis.*, 11: 1942–44.

Brown, D.F.J. and Reynolds, P.E. (1980). Intrinsic Resistance to Beta-Lactam Antibiotics in Staphylococcus-Aureus. *Febs Letters*, 122: 275–78.

Burton, S., Reid-Smith, R., McClure, J.T. and Weese, J.S. (2008). Staphylococcus aureus colonization in healthy horses in Atlantic Canada. *Can. Vet. J.*, 49: 797–99.

Busscher, J.F., van Duijkeren, E. and van Oldruitenborgh-Oosterbaan, M.M.S. (2006). The prevalence of methicillin-resistant staphylococci in healthy horses in the Netherlands. *Vet. Microbiol.*, 113: 131–36.

Cefai, C., Ashurst, S. and Owens, C. (1994). Human carriage of methicillin-resistant *Staphylococcus areus* linked with pet dog. *Lancet*, 344: 539–40.

Cookson, B.D. (2000). Methicillin-resistant *Staphylococcus aureus* in the community: New battlefronts, or are the battles lost? *Infect. Cont. Hosp. Epidemiol.*, 21: 398–403.

Cuny, C., Kuemmerle, J., Stanek, C., Willey, B.M., Strommenger, B., et al. (2006). Emergence of MRSA infections in horses in a veterinary hospital: strain characterisation and comparison with MRSA from humans. *Euro Surveill.*, 11: 44–47.

Cuny, C., Strommenger, B., Witte, W. and Stanek, C. (2008). Clusters of Infections in Horses with MRSA ST1, ST254, and ST398 in a Veterinary Hospital. *Microbial Drug Resist.*, 14: 307–10.

Devriese, L.A. and Hommez, J. (1975). Epidemiology of Methicillin-Resistant Staphylococcus-Aureus in Dairy Herds. *Res. Vet. Sci.*, 19: 23–27.

Devriese, L.A., Vandamme, L.R. and Fameree, L. (1972). Methicillin (Cloxacillin)-Resistant Staphylococcus-Aureus Strains Isolated From Bovine Mastitis Cases. *Zentral. Fur Veterinar. Riehe B.*, 19: 598.

Duckworth, G., Cookson, B., Humphreys, H. and Heathcock, R. (1998). Revised guidelines for the control of MRSA infection in hospitals. *J. Hosp. Infect.*, 39: 253–90.

Enoch, D.A., Karas, J.A., Stater, J.D., Emery, M.M., Kearns, A.M., et al. (2005). MRSA carriage in a pet therapy dog. *J. Hosp. Infect.*, 60: 186–88.

Enright, M.C., Day, N.P.J., Davies, C.E., Peacock, S.J. and Spratt, B.G. (2000). Multilocus sequence typing for characterization of

methicillin-resistant and methicillin-susceptible clones of Staphylococcus aureus. *J. Clin. Microbiol.*, 38: 1008–15.

Fessier, A., Scott, C., Kadlec, K., Enricht, R., Monecke, S. and Schwarz, S. (2010). Characterisation of methicillin-resistant Staphylococcus aurues ST398 from cases of bovine mastitis. *J. Antimicrobial Chemother.*, 65: 619–25.

Guardabassi, L., Stegger, M. and Skov, R. (2007). Retrospective detection of methicillin-resistant and susceptible *Staphylococcus aureus* ST398 in Danish slaughter pigs. *Vet. Microbiol.*, 122: 384–86.

Hallin, M., Deplano, A., Denis, O., De Mendonca, R., De Ryck, R., et al. (2007). Validation of pulsed-field gel electrophoresis and spa typing for long-term, nationwide epidemiological surveillance studies of Staphylococcus aureus infections. *J. Clin. Microbiol.*, 45: 127–33.

Hanselman, B.A., Kruth, S.A., Rousseau, J., Low, D.E., Willey, B.M., et al. (2006). Methicillin-resistant Staphylococcus aureus colonization in veterinary personnel. *Emerg. Infect. Dis.*, 12: 1933–38.

Hardy, K.J., Ussery, D.W., Oppenheim, B.A. and Hawkey, P.M., (2004). Distribution and characterization of staphylococcal interspersed repeat units (SIRUs) and potential use for strain differentiation. *Microbiol.*, 150: 4045–52.

Hartmann, F.A., Trostle, S.S. and Klohnen, A.A.O. (1997). Isolation of methicillin-resistant Staphylococcus aureus from a postoperative wound infection in a horse. *J. Am. Vet. Med. Assoc.*, 211: 590–92.

Hermans, K., Lipinska, U., Denis, O., Deplano, A., Struelens, M.J., et al. (2008). MRSA clone ST398-SCCmec IV as a cause of infections in an equine clinic. *Vlaams Diergen. Tijdschr.*, 77: 429–33.

Herold, B.C., Immergluck, L.C., Maranan, M.C., Lauderdale, D.S., Gaskin, R.E., et al. (1998). Community-acquired methicillin-resistant Staphylococcus aureus in children with no identified predisposing risk. *JAMA*, 279: 593–98.

Hartmeyer, G.N., Gahrn-Hansen, B., Skov, R.L. and Kolmos, H.J. (2010). Pig-associated methicillin-resistant Staphylococcus aureus: family transmission and severe pneumonia in a newborn. *Scandan. J. Infect. Dis.*, 42: 318–20.

Huijsdens, X.W., van Dijke, B.J., Splaburg, E., et al. (2006). Community-acquired MRSA and pig-farming. *Ann. Clin. Microbiol. Antimicrob.*, 5: 26–29.

Huijsdens, X.W., Bosch,. T, van Santen-Verheuvel, M.G., Spalburg, E., Pluister, G.N., et al. (2009). Molecular characterisation of PFGE non-typable methicillin-resistant Staphylococcus aureus in the Netherlands 2007. *Euro. Surveill.*, 14: 19335.

Jevons, M.P., Rolinson, G.N. and Knox, R. (1961). Celbenin-resistant staphylococci. *BMJ.*, 1: 124.

Johnson, A.P., Aucken, H.M., Cavendish, S., Ganner, M., Wale, M.C.J., et al. (2001). Dominance of EMRSA-15 and-16 among MRSA causing nosocomial bacteraemia in the UK: analysis of isolates from the European Antimicrobial Resistance Surveillance System (EARSS). *J. Antimicrob. Chemother.*, 48: 143–44.

Jones, R.D., Kania, S.A., Rohrbach, B.W., Frank, L.A., Bemis, D.A. (2007). Prevalence of oxacillin- and multidrug-resistant staphylococci in clinical samples from dogs: 1,772 samples (2001–2005). *J. Am. Vet. Med. Assoc.*, 230: 221–27.

Khanna, T., Friendship, R., Dewey, C., Weese, J.S. (2008). Methicillin resistant Staphylococcus aureus colonization in pigs and pig farmers. *Vet. Microbiol.*, 128: 298–303.

Klotz, M., Zimmerman, S., Opper, S., Heeg, K. and Mutters, R. (2005). Possible risk for re-colonization with methicillin-resistant *Staphylococcus aureus* (MRSA) by faecal transmission. *Int. J. Hyg. Environ. Health.*, 208: 401–5.

Koreen, L., Ramaswamy, S.V., Graviss, E.A., Naidich, S., Musser, J.M. and Kreisworth, B.N. (2004). *spa* typing method for discriminating among *Staphylococcus aureus* isolates: implications for use of a single marker to detect genetic micro- and macrovariation. *J. Clin. Microbiol.*, 42: 792–99.

Kuhn, G., Francioli, P. and Blanc, D.S. (2007). Double-locus sequence typing using *clfB* and *spa*, a fast and simple method for epidemiological typing of methicillin-resistant *Staphylococcus aureus*. *J. Clin. Microbiol.*, **45**: 54–62.

Kwon, N.H., Park, K.T., Jung, W.K., Youn, H.Y., Lee, Y., *et al.* (2006). Characteristics of methicillin-resistant *Staphylococcus aureus* isolated from chicken meat and hospitalized dogs in Korea and their epidemiological relatedness. *Vet. Microbiol.*, **117**: 304–12.

Lee, J.H. (2003). Methicillin- (oxacillin) resistant *Staphylococcus aureus* strains isolated from major food animals and their potential transmission to humans. *Appl. Environ. Microbiol.*, **69**: 6489–94.

Leonard, F.C., Abbott, Y., Rossney, A., Quinn, P.J., O'Mahony, R., *et al.* (2006). Methicillin-resistant Staphylococcus aureus isolated from a veterinary surgeon and five dogs in one practice. *Vet. Rec.*, **158**: 155–59.

Lindsay, J.A., Moore, C.E., Day, N.P., Peacock, S.J., Witney, A.A., *et al.* (2006). Microarrays reveal that each of the ten dominant lineages of *Staphylococcus aureus* has a unique combination of surface-associated and regulatory genes. *J. Bacteriol.*, **188**: 669–76.

Loeffler, A., Boag, A.K., Sung, J., Lindsay, J.A., Guardabassi, L., *et al.* (2005). Prevalence of methicillin-resistant Staphylococcus aureus among staff and pets in a small animal referral hospital in the UK. *J. Antimicrob. Chemother.*, **56**: 692–97.

Loeffler, A., Kearns, A.M., Ellington, M.J., Smith, L.J., Unt, V.E., *et al.* (2009). First isolation of MRSA ST398 from UK animals: a new challenge for infection control teams? *J. Hosp. Infect.*, **72**: 269–71.

Maddox, T.W., Clegg, P., Wedley, A., Pinchbeck, G.L., Ryvar, R., *et al.* (2009). Prevalence and Antimicrobial Resistance of Meticillin-Resistant Staphylococi obtained from Horses in Great Britain. In: *Methicillin-resistant Staphylococci in Animals: Veterinary and Public Health Implications*, pp 30–31. London: Conference Proceedings, American Society for Microbiology.

Manian, F.A. (2003). Asymptomatic nasal carriage of mupirocin-resistant, methicillin-resistant *Staphylococcus aureus* (MRSA) in a pet dog associated with MRSA infection in household contacts. *Clin. Infect. Dis.*, **36**: E26–28.

Middleton, J.R., Fales, W.H., Luby, C.D., Oaks, J.L., Sanchez, S., *et al.* (2005). Surveillance of *Staphylococcus aureus* in veterinary teaching hospitals. *J. Clin. Microbiol.*, **43**: 2916–19.

Milheirico, C., Oliveira, D.C. and de Lencastre, H. (2007). Multiplex PCR strategy for subtyping the staphylococcal cassette chromosome *mec* type IV in methicillin-resistant *Staphylococcus aureus*: 'SCC*mec* IV multiplex'. *J. Antimicrob. Chemother.*, **60**: 42–48.

Moodley, A., Stegger, M., Bagcigil, A.F., Baptiste, K.E., Loeffler, A., *et al.* (2006). *spa* typing of methicillin-resistant Staphylococcus aureus isolated from domestic animals and veterinary staff in the UK and Ireland. *J. Antimicrob. Chemother.*, **58**: 1118–23.

Monecke, S., Kuhnert, P., Hotzel, H., *et al.* (2007). Microarray based study on virulence-associated genes and resistance determinants of *Staphylococcus aureus* isolates from cattle. *Vet. Microbiol.*, **125**: 128–40.

Morris, D.O., Rook, K.A., Shofer, F.S. and Rankin, S.C. (2006). Screening of Staphylococcus aureus, Staphylococcus intermedius, and Staphylococcus schleiferi isolates obtained from small companion animals for antimicrobial resistance: a retrospective review of 749 isolates (2003–04). *Vet. Dermatol.*, **17**: 332–37.

Mulders, M.N., Haenen, A.P., Geenen, P.L., Vesseur, P.C., Poldervaart, E.S., *et al.* (2010). Prevalence of livestock-associated MRSA in broiler flocks and risk factors for slaughterhouse personnel in The Netherlands. *Epidemiol. Infect.*, **138**: 743–55.

Murchan, S., Kaufmann, M.E., Deplano, A., de Ryck, R., Struelens, M., *et al.* (2003). Harmonization of pulsed-field gel electrophoresis protocols for epidemiological typing of strains of methicillin-resistant *Staphylococcus aureus*: a single approach developed by consensus in 10 European laboratories and its application for tracing the spread of related strains. *J. Clin. Microbiol.*, **41**: 1574–85.

Nagase, N., Sasaki, A., Yamashita, K., Shimizu, A., Wakita, Y., *et al.* (2002). Isolation and species distribution of Staphylococci from animal and human skin. *J. Vet. Med. Sci.*, **64**: 245–50.

De Neeling, A.J., van den Broek, M.J.M., Spalburg, E.C., *et al.* (2007). High prevalence of methicillin resistant *Staphylococcus aureus* in pigs. *Vet. Microbiol.*, **122**: 366–72.

Normanno, G., Corrente, M., la Salandra, G., *et al.* (2007). Methicillin-resistant *Staphylococcus aureus* (MRSA) in foods of animal origin product in Italy. *Intern. J. Food Microbiol.*, **117**: 219–22.

Oliveria, D.C. and de Lencastre, H. (2002). Multiplex PCR strategy for rapid identification of structural types and variants of the *mec* element in methicillin-resistant *Staphylococcus aureus*. *Antimicrob. Agents and Chemother.*, **46**: 2155–61.

Oliveira, D.C., Mihheirco, C. and de Lencastre, H. (2006). Redefining a structural variant of staphylococcal cassette chromosome *mec*, SSC*mec* type VI. *Antimicrob. Agents and Chemother.*, **50**: 3457–59.

O'Mahony, R., Abbott, Y., Leonard, F.C., Markey, B.K., Quinn, P.J., *et al.* (2005). Methicillin-resistant Staphylococcus aureus (MRSA) isolated from animals and veterinary personnel in Ireland. *Vet. Microbiol.*, **109**: 285–96.

Owen, M.R., Moores, A.P. and Coe, R.J. (2004). Management of MRSA septic arthritis in a dog using a gentamicin-impregnated collagen sponge. *J. Small Anim. Pract.*, **45**: 609–12.

Pak, S.I., Han, H.R., Shimizu, A. (1999). Characterization of methicillin-resistant *Staphylococcus aureus* isolated from dogs in Korea. *J. Vet. Med. Sci.*, **61**: 1013–18.

Patel, M., Kumar, R.A., Stamm, A.M., Hoesley, C.J., Moser, S.A., *et al.* (2007). USA300 genotype community-associated methicillin-resistant *Staphylococcus aureus* as a cause of surgical site infections. *J. Clin. Microbiol.*, **45**: 3431–33.

Rankin, S., Roberts, S., O'Shea, K., Maloney, D., Lorenzo, M. *et al.* (2005). Panton valentine leukocidin (PVL) toxin positive MRSA strains isolated from companion animals. *Vet. Microbiol.*, **108**: 145–48.

Saunders, N.A., Underwood, A., Kearns, A.M. and Hallas, G. (2004). A virulence-associated gene microarray: a tool for investigation of the evolution and pathogenic potential of *Staphylococcus aureus*. *Microbiol.*, **150**: 3763–71.

Scott, G.M., Thomson, R., Malonelee, J., Ridgway, G.L. (1988). Cross-infection between animals and man: possible feline transmission of *Staphylococcus aureus* infections in humans? *J. Hosp. Infect.*, **12**: 29–34.

Seguin, J.C., Walker, R.D., Caron, J.P., Kloos, W.E., George, C.G., *et al.* (1999). Methicillin-resistant Staphylococcus aureus outbreak in a veterinary teaching hospital: Potential human-to-animal transmission. *J. Clin. Microbiol.* **37**: 1459–63.

Sergio, D.M., Koh, T.H., Hsu, L.Y., Ogden, B.E., Goh, A.L., *et al.* (2007). Investigation of meticillin-resistant Staphylococcus aureus in pigs used for research. *J. Med. Microbiol.*, **56**: 1107–9.

Shimuzu, A., Kawano, J., Yamamoto, C., Kakutani, O., Anzai, T., *et al.* (1997). Genetic analysis of equine methicillin-resistant *Staphylococcus aureus* by pulsed-field gel electrophoresis. *J. Vet. Med. Sci.*, **59**: 935–37.

Shopsin, B., Gomez, M., Montgomery, O., Smith, S.O., Smith, D.H., *et al.* (1999). Evaluation of protein A gene polymorphic region DNA sequence for typing of *Staphylococcus aureus* strains. *J. Clin. Microbiol.*, **37**: 3556–63.

Shopsin, B. and Kreisworth, B.N. (2001). Molecular epidemiology of methicillin-resistant *Staphylococcus aureus*. *Emerg. Infect. Dis.*, **7**: 323–26.

Smith, T.C., Male, M.J., Harper, A.L., Kroeger, J.S., Tinkler, G.P., *et al.* (2008). Methicillin-resistant Staphylococcus aureus (MRSA) strain ST398 is present in midwestern U.S. swine and swine workers. *PLoS One.*, **4**(1): e4258.

Strommenger, B., Kehrenberg, C., Kettlitz, C., Cuny, C., Verspohl, J., *et al.* (2006). Molecular characterization of methicillin-resistant Staphylococcus aureus strains from pet animals and their relationship to human isolates. *J. Antimicrob. Chemother.*, **57**: 461–65.

Thompson, D.S., Workman, R. and Strutt, M. (2009). Decline in the rates of meticillin-resistant Staphylococcus aureus acquisition and bacteraemia in a general intensive care unit between 1996 and 2008. *J. Hosp. Infect.*, **71**: 314–19.

Tiemersma, E.W., Bronzwaer, S.L.A.M., Lyytikainen, O., Degener, J.E., Schrijnemakers, P., *et al.* (2004). Methicillin-resistant *Staphylococcus aureus* in Europe, 1999–2002. *Emerg. Infect. Dis.,* **10:** 1627–34.

Tomlin, J., Pead, M.J., Lloyd, D.H., Howell, S., Hartmann, F., *et al.* (1999). Methicillin-resistant *Staphylococcus aureus* infections in 11 dogs. *Vet. Rec.,* **144:** 60–64.

van Belkum, A., Melles, D.C., Peeters, J.K., van Leeuwen, W.B., van Duijkeren, E., *et al.* (2008). Methicillin-resistant and -susceptible Staphylococcus aureus sequence type 398 in pigs and humans. *Emerg. Infect. Dis.,* **14:** 479–83.

van den Eede, A., Martens, A., Lipinska, U., Struelens, M., Deplano, A., *et al.* (2009). High occurrence of methicillin-resistant Staphylococcus aureus ST398 in equine nasal samples. *Vet. Microbiol.,* **133:** 138–44.

van Duijkeren, E., Box, A.T.A., Heck, M.E.O.C., Wannet, W.J.B., Fluit, A.C. (2004). Methicillin-resistant staphylococci isolated from animals. *Vet. Microbiol.,* **103:** 91–97.

van Duijkeren, E., Wolfhagen, M.J.H.M., Heck, M.E.O.C., Wannet, W.J.B. (2005). Transmission of a Panton-Valentine leucocidin-positive, methicillin-resistant *Staphylococcus aureus* strain between humans and a dog. *J. Clin. Microbiol.,* **43:** 6209–11.

van Duijkeren, E., Moleman, M., Sloet van Oldruitenborgh-Oosterbaan, M., Multem, J., Troelstra, A., *et al.* (2009). Methicillin-resistant *Staphylococcus aureus* in horses and horse personnel: An investigation of several outbreaks. *Vet. Microbiol.,* doi:10.1016/j.vetmic.2009.08.09.

Vengust, M., Anderson, M.E.C., Rousseau, J. and Weese, J.S. (2006). Methicillin-resistant staphylococcal colonization in clinically normal dogs and horses in the community. *Letters in Appl. Microbiol.,* **43:** 602–6.

Vitale, C.B., Gross, T.L., Weese, J.S. (2006). Methicillin-resistant *Staphylococcus aureus* in cat and owner. *Emerg. Infect. Dis.,* **12:** 1998–2000.

Voss, A., Loeffen, F., Bakker, J. *et al.* (2005). Methicillin-resistant *Staphylococcus aureus* in Pig Farming. *Emerg. Infect. Dis.,* **11:** 1965–66.

Walther, B., Wieler, L.H., Friedrich, A.W., Hanssen, A.M., Kohn, B., *et al.* (2008). Methicillin-resistant Staphylococcus aureus (MRSA) isolated from small and exotic animals at a university hospital during routine microbiological examinations. *Vet. Microbiol.,* **127:** 171–78.

Weese, J.S. (2005). Methicillin resistant Staphylococcus aureus: an emerging pathogen in small animals. *J. Am. Anim. Hosp. Assoc.,* **41:** 150–57.

Weese, J.S. and Lefebvre, S.L. (2007). Risk factors for methicillin-resistant Staphylococcus aureus colonization in horses admitted to a veterinary teaching hospital. *Can. Vet. J.,* **48:** 921–26.

Weese, J.S., Rousseau, J., Traub-Dargatz, J.L., Willey, B.M., McGeer, A.J., *et al.* (2005a). Community-associated methicillin-resistant Staphylococcus aureus in horses and humans who work with horses. *J. Am. Vet. Med. Assoc.,* **226:** 580–83.

Weese, J.S., Archambault, M., Willey, B.M., Hearn, P., Kreiswirth, B.N., *et al.* (2005b). Methicillin-resistant Staphylococcus aureus in horses and horse personnel, 2000–2002. *Emerg. Infect. Dis.,* **11:** 430–35.

Weese, J.S., Caldwell, F., Willey, B.M., Kreiswirth, B.N., McGeer, A., *et al.* (2006a). An outbreak of methicillin-resistant Staphylococcus aureus skin infections resulting from horse to human transmission in a veterinary hospital. *Vet. Microbiol.,* **114:** 160–64.

Weese, J.S., Dick, H., Willey, B.M., McGeer, A., Kreiswirth, B.N., *et al.* . (2006b). Suspected transmission of methicillin-resistant Staphylococcus aureus between domestic pets and humans in veterinary clinics and in the household. *Vet. Microbiol.,* **115:** 148–55.

Weese, J.S., Rousseau, J., Willey, B.M., Archambault, M., McGeer, A. *et al.* (2006c). Methicillin-resistant Staphylococcus aureus in horses at a veterinary teaching hospital: frequency, characterization, and association with clinical disease. *J. Vet. Int. Med.,* **20:** 182–86.

Weese, J.S., Dick, H., Willey, B.M. (2006d). Suspected transmission of methicillin-resistant Staphylococcus aureus between domestic pets and humans in veterinary clinics and in the household. *Vet. Microbiol.,* **115:** 148–55.

Witte, W., Strommenger, B., Stanek, C., *et al.* (2007). Methicillin-resistant *Staphylococcus aureus* ST398 in humans and animals in central Europe. *Emerg. Infect. Dis.,* **13:** 255–58.

Wulf, M., van Nes, A., Eikelenboom-Boskamp, A., de Vries, J., Melchers, W., Klaassen, C., Voss, A. (2006). Methicilin-resistant Staphylococcus aureus in veterinary doctors and students in the Netherlands. *Emerg. Infect. Dis.,* **12:** 1939–41.

Yu, F., Chen, Z., Liu, C., Zhang, X., Lin, X., Chi, S., *et al.* (2008). Prevalence of Staphylococcus aureus carrying Panton-Valentine leukocidin genes among isolates from hospitalised patients in China. *Clin. Microbiol. Infect.,* **14:** 381–84.

Zhang, K., McClure, J-A., Elsayed, S., Louie, T. and Conly, J.M. (2005). Novel multiplex PCR assay for characterization and concomitant subtyping of staphylococcal cassette chromosome *mec* types I to V in methicillin-resistant *Staphylococcus aureus*. *J. Clin. Microbiol.,* **43:** 5026–33.

CHAPTER 20

Leptospirosis

Robert M. Smith and Wendy J. Zochowski

Summary

Leptospirosis is one of the most widespread and important zoonotic pathogens and is of global medical and veterinary importance. Clinical disease ranges from mild self-limiting influenza-like illness to fulminating hepato-renal failure.

It is caused by bacterial spirochaetes of the genus Leptospira, family *Leptospiraceae*. Pathogenic *Leptospira interrogans* strains, of which there are over 250 serovars in 24 serogroups, are morphologically identical in that they are thin, helical highly motile Gram-negative bacteria, hooked at one or both ends.

Natural hosts of pathogenic strains, generally referred to as serovars, may cause infection in man and include wild animals (rodents), livestock (cattle and pigs) and pets (dogs). Most, if not all mammals may become long-term carriers (maintenance hosts). Leptospires become located in the renal tubules and excreted in the urine of infected reservoir animals, humans becoming infected through broken skin, mucous membranes and the conjunctivae.

Leptospirosis is most commonly found in tropical or sub-tropical countries in both urban and rural settings. It causes major economic losses, to the highly intensive cattle and pig industries in developed countries, primarily through their effects on reproduction. It is still an important occupational disease risk for people working in agriculture or those living in unsanitary conditions. It is increasingly recognized as a recreational and travel-associated disease.

History

Adolf Weil (1886) is usually credited with the first description of severe icteric clinical human leptospirosis, ('Weil's disease'). Earlier descriptions of clinical human disease are found in a comprehensive literature review by Faine (1994). These include:

- Descriptions by Willman in 1803 of probable leptospirosis whilst working with the British Medical Mission in Syria.

- Outbreak of 'févre jaune' in Napoleon's troops at Heliopolis in 1800 during the siege of Cairo, and of a similar disease in Egypt in 1851.

- References to epidemic jaundice and bilious typhoid which are likely to be related to leptospirosis have appeared in literature from many older cultures and both Hippocrates and Galen postulated about it.

Nomenclature for the disease is often colourful and synonyms (Table 20.1) often include occupational or geographical affiliations. Other synonyms can be found in Torten and Marshall (1994).

Human leptospirosis was described 30 years prior to discovery of the aetiologic agent, first discovered in 1914–15 by Inada and co-workers in Japan where Weil's disease was common amongst coal miners. Noguchi, working on organisms isolated from jaundiced patients, found them to be morphologically similar to a saprophytic spirochaete isolated at the same time in the USA by Wolbach and Binger from stagnant water which they named *Spirochaeta biflexa*. Inada named his isolate *Spirochaeta icterohaemorrhagia* and Noguchi, who found it morphologically dissimilar to all known spirochaete genera, proposed in 1917 a new genus, *Leptospira*.

Independently, and about the same time, the German workers Hubener and Reiter and Ulenhuth and Fromme demonstrated the spirochaete when transmitting the disease to guinea-pigs. The association between animals and risk had been known for several decades before the bacterium was identified as a cause of illness but the first account of a leptospire isolated from renal tubules in a patient who died, was credited to Stimpson in 1907; he named it *Spirochaeta interrogans* due partly to the hooked ends which gave the appearance of a question mark.

Table 20.1 Leptospiral synonyms

Synonym	Affiliation
Cane cutter's disease	Occupation
Cattle-associated leptospirosis	Maintenance host
Rice harvest jaundice	China/occupation
Fort Bragg fever	Location
Autumnal fever	Japan/season
Swineherd's disease	Europe/occupation
Sewerman's disease	USA/occupation
Weil's disease	Individual
Pulmonary haemorrhagic disease	Clinical presentation

Rapid progress in research was made during and after the 1914–18 war with increases in cases arising from trench warfare. With this, came the recognition of further disease entities with a leptospiral origin, in particular anicteric forms; agglutination-lysis, active immunization, serological differentiation of strains and recognition of their association with different forms of the disease (extensively reviewed by Faine 1994).

Leptospirosis in animals was described as a separate clinical identity in 1850, some 30 years prior to Weil's description of the disease. In 1898 an epidemic was reported in dogs in Stuttgart, but it was not until some years later that it was realized that the disease in dogs and man arose from morphologically identical organisms. Subsequently the disease was recognized in cattle in 1935, and in pigs in 1939, so that by the 1950s, leptospirosis in domestic animals had been established as a disease of major significance in both veterinary medicine and public health.

The first recorded case of leptospirosis in the UK involved a Thames waterman who had fallen into the river. Throughout the 1920s and 1930s many cases were recorded in dock-side fish workers in Aberdeen and in coal miners, particularly in Scotland and South Wales, and throughout the country in sewer workers. Between 1933 and 1948 these three occupational groups accounted for almost half the total number of cases reported in the UK. From 1980, only 4% of all cases were attributable to fish workers or those employed in sewage disposal or refuse collection, with no cases reported in coal miners. These changes largely reflect the improvements seen in the health and safety measures adopted by these industries together with the decline in employment in coal mining and fishing industries.

In contrast, farm workers represented less than 5% of the total cases identified between 1933 and 1948, but subsequently this occupational group contributed nearly 50% of the total UK reports. A more recent decline, especially in human infection with *L. borgpetersenii* serovar Hardjo since the 1990s probably reflects the state of the UK livestock farming industry. The most likely reason for the increase in infection in farm workers was the increase in serovar Hardjo in cattle herds after 1968; whilst serovar Hardjo had been detected in field voles in 1958, these animals are unlikely to have been entirely responsible for the increase in human infection with this serovar. The principal reason for the increase in infection in cattle herds was the importation of *Brucella*-free dairy cattle following the 1968 Foot and Mouth epidemic. Farm workers at greatest risk of acquiring serovar Hardjo infection were those associated with dairy herds.

Recent trends in the use of inland waterways for a variety of recreational activities such as canoeing, windsurfing or the swimming section of triathlon competitions may have contributed to recently observed changes in the aetiology of the disease.

The agent

Leptospires are thin, helical, highly motile, Gram-negative organisms which are often hooked at one or both ends with paired axial flagellae enabling them to burrow into tissue. In suitable liquid environments, they spin constantly about their long axis. They range in length from about 10 to 20μm, with an amplitude of about 0.5μm. Under adverse nutritional conditions they may become elongated, whilst under high salt concentrations, ageing culture or in tissues, they may develop into coccoid forms of about 1.5 to 2μm (Faine *et al.* 1999).

The major structural components comprise an outer envelope surrounding a cell wall and two polar endoflagellae (one originating subterminally at each end) enabling them to burrow into tissue.

Traditional classification is based on antigenic differences in the lipopolysaccharide envelope that surrounds the cell wall. Serologic detection of these differences is based on identifying serovars within each species. Based on this system, the genus *Leptospira* contains two species, the pathogenic *Leptospira interrogans* with at least 250 serovars and the non-pathogenic, free-living *Leptospira biflexa*, which contains at least 60 serovars.

Taxonomy and classification

Leptospires were traditionally classified by serology as belonging to two species within the family *Leptospiraceae*, *Leptospira interrogans* and *Leptospira biflexa* comprising pathogenic and saprophytic strains isolated from the environment, respectively.

The two species may be differentiated by their growth requirements and biochemical reactions. Both *L. interrogans* and *L. biflexa* were divided into numerous serovars defined by agglutination after cross-absorption with homologous antigens. Within the species *L. interrogans*, over 250 serovars have been validly published. Serovars which are antigenically related have been assigned to serogroups of which 24 are recognized and are based on differences in the outer protein envelope of the bacteria. Over 60 serovars of *L. biflexa* have been validated. Unlike *L. interrogans*, they can grow at low ambient temperatures.

Genotypic classification

Leptospires have now been classified using genetic typing methodology—DNA-DNA homology of at least 70% and up to 5% divergence in DNA relatedness; guanine + cytosine (G+C) content; 16S rRNA gene sequencing data and pulsed field electrophoresis (PFGE). Currently thirteen species have been described in the family *Leptospiraceae* (Brenner *et al.* 1999; Pèrolat *et al.* 1998; Levett *et al.* 2006); names for the four documented genomospecies have been proposed, (submitted to IJSEM) and a further three species await validation. These species may be further divided to include pathogenic, those demonstrating intermediate pathogenicity and saprophytic species. The pathogenic species include *Leptospira interrogans*, *L. borgpetersenii*, *L. kirschneri*, *L. noguchii*, *L. weillii*, *L. santarosai*, *L. alexanderi*. Intermediate species include *L. meyeri*, *L. inadai*, *L. broomii*, *L. fainei*. Proposed names for the genomospecies are *L. alstonii*, *L. vanthielii*, *L. terpstrae*, *L. yanagawae* (International Leptospirosis Society Meeting, Quito 2007; IJSEM 2008).

The molecular classification of leptospires does not equate with the previous classification of *L. interrogans* and *L. biflexa*. Both pathogenic and non-pathogenic serovars can occur within the same genomospecies. Serovars previously assigned to one serogroup may now occur in different genomospecies. The more familiar serological classification of leptospires into serogroups has been retained as an aid in epidemiological studies.

Molecular biology

The genus Leptospira is characterized by a guanine plus cytosine (G + C) ratio of 35–41 mol% in its chromosomal DNA, depending on species. The *Leptospira* genome has an approximate size of 5000kb comprising two chromosomes of 4400kb and 350kb respectively. Leptospires contain two sets of 16S and 23S rRNA genes, but only one 5S rRNA gene, the rRNA genes are widely spaced (Levett

2001) The 5S rRNA gene is highly conserved among the pathogenic leptospires.

Survival of leptospires

Outside the animal host, leptospiral survival is favoured by warm, moist conditions at neutral pH (Table 20.2); circumstances which may contribute to the observed seasonal pattern of human infections. They are susceptible to low concentrations of chlorine and are rapidly killed by temperatures in excess of 40°C. The anaerobic conditions and low pH found in raw sewage explain their short survival time compared with that in aerated sewage. They have a very short survival time in undiluted cows' milk, which explains the minimal risk posed by unpasteurized milk, but can survive for some time in substrates saturated with urine, fresh water, damp soils, swamps, vegetation, in mud even if the reservoir host has been removed, culture media, and the tissues of live or dead animals. Salt water kills off the organism but it may be present in brackish waters in tidal parts of rivers and estuaries. This likelihood increases going upstream and is greatest in canals, ponds or areas of slowly draining water, presenting a risk to users of river and lake banks and reservoir edges. Faine (1994) suggested that pathogenic leptospires may continue to grow and multiply under suitable environmental conditions. Survival in experimentally infected slurry for at least 138 days and in untreated abattoir sewage for up to 18 hours has been observed.

The hosts

Rodents and domestic mammals, such as cattle, pigs, and dogs serve as major reservoir hosts (Table 20.3). Infected animals may excrete leptospires intermittently or regularly for months, years, or for their lifetime. Vaccinated animals may still shed infectious organisms in their urine. A significant and interesting feature of leptospirosis is the limited range of serovars which naturally infect certain host species; under laboratory conditions, the range of leptospiral serovars causing infection is somewhat greater. The relationship between host and bacterial species is complex and not fully understood, but natural infection in animal species is generally limited to only a few strains. Strain typing is a useful epidemiologic tool because establishing the causative serogroup or serovar is

the first step towards identifying reservoirs and generating control strategies (McBride *et al.* 2005).

Epidemiology

Leptospirosis is a major, yet under recognized threat to public health. In 1999, the World Health Organization (WHO) estimated that there are more than 500,000 cases worldwide each year. The majority of reported cases have severe manifestations for which mortality exceeds 10%. Studies in Thailand show that leptospirosis may represent up to 20% of febrile illness of unknown origin (Wuthiekanum *et al.* 2007). In developing countries the burden of endemic leptospirosis is thought to be very significant for people living in rural areas involved in both arable and livestock farming and in urban settlements with poor or inappropriate sanitation (slums). Epidemics in urban settings are associated with high rainfall, whilst rural epidemics are also associated with harvest.

Leptospirosis is highly prevalent in the Asia Pacific region, where, unlike developed countries, human cases arise mainly from occupational exposure, travel to endemic areas, recreational activities or importation of wild and domestic animals. In the developing countries of the region, leptospirosis is largely a water-borne disease. Data collection and surveillance systems vary significantly among the countries and areas of the region, so that data are often incomplete and an accurate assessment of the true burden of the disease is still unavailable (Victoriano *et al.* 2009).

Table 20.3 Host species—serovar relationships

Animal species	Common serovars	Less common serovars
Dogs	Canicola Icterohaemorrhagiae Grippotyphosa Pomona	Bratislava
Cats	Seldom infected	
Cattle, Deer	Hardjo Pomona Grippotyphosa Icterohaemorrhagiae	Australis Autumnalis Bataviae Bratislava Canicola Hebdomadis Kremastos Sejroe Tarassovi
Pigs	Bratislava Canicola Icterohaemorrhagiae Pomona Tarassovi	Grippotyphosa Sejroe
Sheep	Bratislava Grippotyphosa Hardjo Pomona	
Horses	Bratislava Canicola Icterohaemorrhagiae Pomona Sejroe	

Table 20.2 Survival of leptospires

Medium	Time
Tap water pH 7	28 days
Tap water pH 5	2 days
Sea water	18–20 hours
Raw sewage	12–14 hours
Aerated sewage	2–3 days
Diluted cows' milk	60 days
Undiluted cows' milk	30 minutes
Diluted cows' urine	35 days
Damp soil	35 days
Urine saturated soil	6 months

Major outbreaks of the disease due to flooding have been reported in Orissa (1999), Jakarta (2003) and Mumbai (2005). It remains an ongoing and significant problem in many densely populated, flood-prone low lying areas. In India, the disease has been found more commonly associated with natural disasters during the monsoon period, when epidemics become more likely. Cases of leptospirosis in Puerto Rico increased in 1966 after a hurricane (Sanders *et al.* 1999). When rainfall from a heavy storm exceeds the capacity of soil to absorb the moisture, a subsequent outbreak or increase in the number of cases of leptospirosis is usually associated with leptospires previously shed by reservoir hosts and have accumulated in warm moist soils during drier periods, being discharged into watercourses from contaminated soils.

In Europe, there has been a shift from leptospirosis as an occupational disease to one where recreational activities, especially water sports and travel are major risk factors, especially among the growing number of participants in adventure travel and water sports in exotic locations (Sejvar *et al.* 2003; van Crevel *et al.* 1994). The risk of exposure whilst travelling is not restricted to tropical regions, infection may also be contracted in European countries, with France a commonly identified travel destination, having one of the highest reported incidences of leptospirosis in Western Europe; travellers to France with an interest in water sports or fishing should be aware of this association (Nardone *et al.* 2004).

Some recent outbreaks

- 1984, Italy: waterborne outbreak from a contaminated water fountain,

- 1995, Nicaragua: spread through a large population due to widespread flooding. Acute febrile illness and pulmonary hemorrhage,

- 1997, Costa Rica: US citizens white water rafting,

- 1998, USA: Swimming as part of a triathlon in lake Springfield, Illinois; 74 of 639 triathletes in races in Wisconsin and Illinois,

- 1999, Philippine floods, Manila,

- 2000, Borneo, Malaysia: Eco Challenge; 68 of 304 athletes participating in a 2-week adventure sport race,

- 2004, Hawaii: Outbreak after flooding of a university campus,

- 2006, Thailand, Nan Province, after flooding in August,

- 2007, Oahu: Outbreak associated with flooding of a university campus.

Freshwater recreational exposures, whether at home or abroad are the major route of exposure for the majority of cases acquired in developed countries.

In New Zealand, the majority of cases occur among livestock farm workers and meat processing workers (Crump *et al.* 2001). In the UK, leptospirosis has been in decline as an occupational infection, with a concomitant increase in recreationally-acquired disease. It is a notifiable disease to public health authorities in the UK and reportable to the Health and Safety Executive (HSE) under the Reporting of Injuries Diseases and Dangerous Occurrences Regulations (RIDDOR).

Signs and symptoms

Leptospirosis in animals

Leptospirosis is unusual in that several potential hosts can share the same environment yet carry different serovars. Venereal transmission has been suspected in rodents as marked increases in prevalence occur with the onset of sexual maturity. In arid climates such as the Russian Steppes where mammal population densities are low, it may be the major mode of spread. Leptospires have been demonstrated in semen from cattle and pigs, raising the possibility of transmission during both natural and artificial insemination. Transplacental spread is common in rodents and in farm animals and may result in abortion, stillbirth or infected, weak offspring.

Leptospirosis in humans

Leptospires are transmitted in the urine of chronically infected carrier animals. Infection occurs when spirochaetes in contaminated water or soil enter microabrasions in healthy intact skin or intact mucous membranes or conjunctiva. They may also cross the nasal mucosa and pass through the lungs (from inhalation of aerosolized body fluids). The incubation period is approximately 10 days (range 4–19 days). In temperate climates, peak incidence occurs during the late summer and autumn months when leptospires survive for longer in the environment and water exposures may be more common.

Most reported cases occur in men, probably due to greater occupational and recreational exposures.

Clinical presentations

Clinical manifestations include fever, malaise, myalgia, meningism and conjunctivitis as well as anorexia, abdominal pain, nausea and vomiting. Initial signs of serious infection can include jaundice, haemorrhage, and hepatosplenomegaly. The most severe form of leptospirosis, known as Weil's Syndrome, presents with hepatic and renal failure or massive pulmonary haemorrhage. There is no serotype-specific presentation of infection and each serotype can cause mild or severe disease depending on host factors. Patient factors such as older age and multiple underlying medical problems are often associated with more severe clinical illness and increased mortality (WHO 2003).

During the incubation period, leptospires actively replicate in the liver; they subsequently disseminate throughout the body, infecting multiple tissues. The main lesion in all forms of leptospirosis is damage to the walls of small blood vessels, leading to leakage. Other lesions follow as secondary effects. Virulence factors are thought to result in damage to the endothelial lining of small blood vessels. Some research has suggested that the vascular damage could be associated with an autoimmune mediated vasculitis (Chakurkar *et al.* 2008).

Patients who have recovered from severe leptospirosis commonly remain seropositive for variable periods of time, with respect to IgM, IgG and agglutinating antibodies. After severe infection with some serovars, a significant proportion of cases will have high MAT titres (≥800) for several years. Marked differences occur in both the magnitude and duration of agglutinating antibodies directed against different serogroups (Cumberland *et al.* 1999). Those in high risk occupations may maintain a high titre either as a result of an initial severe infection or through constant exposure and subclinical infection. In endemic areas where vocational exposures are commonplace, many individuals may maintain a raised titre due to constant low levels of exposure.

Signs and symptoms of leptospirosis

- Incubation period usually 5–15 days, but may range from 2–30 days.

- Many cases may have mild or subclinical infections, onset usually characterized by non-specific symptoms including fever, chills, headache, nausea, vomiting, and transient rash.

- Disease usually follows a biphasic clinical course (bacteraemic or septicaemic phase), followed by immune-mediated phase, (but may present as a single progressive illness). Overall duration of symptoms for both phases of disease varies from less than one week to several months.

- Septicaemic phase (3–7 days): fever, chills, headache, myalgia in calf and lumbar regions (80% cases), conjunctival suffusion (40% cases), nausea, transient rash, severe myalgias.

- Immune-mediated phase (variable, 1 week to several weeks): return of fever, aseptic meningitis, uveitis, jaundice, adenopathy, evidence of renal disease, muscle tenderness, purpuric rash.

- Around 10% of cases occur as severe fulminant disease, including jaundice and renal dysfunction (Weil's disease), haemorrhagic pneumonitis, cardiac arrythmias, and circulatory collapse. Weil's disease may develop after the acute phase as the second phase of illness or as progressive disease.

Laboratory diagnosis

Culture is difficult and time consuming. Isolation of leptospires from blood and CSF may be attempted during leptospiraemia in the first week of illness. Leptospires will survive in aerobic commercial blood culture systems at room temperature until inoculated into semi-solid EMJH medium containing 0.4–2% rabbit serum and 5-fluorouracil. Incubation of cultures should be continued for 20 weeks(Faine *et al.* 1999; Levett 2001).

The demonstration of leptospires by immunochemical staining methods is more suited to diagnostic laboratories; however, these tests depend on the number of organisms present and lack the sensitivity of culture. The immunochemical methods that have been used for diagnosis include immunofluorescence, PAP, avidin-biotin, and immunogold techniques. Whilst these methods have not proved as sensitive as culture, immunofluorescence has been used widely, particularly in the diagnosis of foetal leptospirosis. It has the advantage of giving better contrast between the leptospires and the tissue background than the other methods. This is particularly important since leptospires are very small and filamentous, which makes them difficult to differentiate from some connective tissue elements and cilia. Immunofluorescence has the disadvantage that the production of good-quality polyclonal antisera requires long inoculation regimes in rabbits.

Darkfield microscopy of body fluids has been widely used and can be a useful tool in the hands of an experienced diagnostician, but many tissue artifacts can be mistakenly identified as leptospires. Leptospires do not stain satisfactorily with the aniline dyes and silver staining techniques lack sensitivity and specificity.

Serological tests

Antibodies are detected in the blood 5 to 7 days after the onset of symptoms, though their detection may be depressed by the early administration of antibiotics.

The standard reference method for the diagnosis of leptospirosis is the microscopic agglutination test (MAT), where patient sera are reacted with suspensions of live or formalized leptospires. Agglutinating antibodies can be of both IgM and IgG classes and are detectable from about day 7 after onset of symptoms. Panels of antigens should include representative strains of all serogroups plus locally isolated serovars. The latter may be more antigenically reactive than reference strains. The MAT is a serogroup specific test.

In the early stages of infection it is not usually possible to determine the infecting serovars because of the presence of antigenic cross-reactions. Generally, samples taken at a later stage in the course of the illness/convalescent period are required to confirm the probable infecting serogroup/serovars. Antibodies may remain detectable by MAT for several years.

The MAT requires expertise to perform and interpret and the continued maintenance of a panel of live strains is technically demanding and biohazardous, therefore this procedure is usually restricted to reference laboratories. The MAT may be applied to sera from both humans and animals.

In the diagnosis of chronic leptospirosis in animals, the MAT is best used as a herd or flock test, rather than as a test for an individual animal. A minimum of 10 animals or 10% of the herd, whichever is the greater, should be tested to obtain useful information. Increasing the sample size and sampling a number of different cohorts markedly improves disease investigation and assessments of vaccination needs. A retrospective diagnosis of leptospirosis may be made when the majority of affected animals have titres of 1:1000 or greater. The herd test approach is not very useful for the diagnosis of serovar Hardjo-associated abortion in endemically infected cattle herds or for serovar Bratislava infection in pig herds, because of the insidious and chronic nature of herd infections and the very low levels of antibody which may be found in post abortion sera.

The complexities of the MAT have lead to a number of other methodologies being used to develop rapid screening tests to detect Leptospira antibodies. These include:

- Indirect ELISA,
- IgM dot-ELISA dipstick,
- Dot immunoblot assay,
- Microcapsule,
- Agglutination test,
- Indirect haemagglutination test,
- Latex agglutination test,
- Lateral flow.

IgM detection is more sensitive than the MAT where the sample is taken early in the acute phase of the illness, but false negative serology may be found in samples taken before the 5–7 day of illness. Screening tests are capable of detecting IgM antibody with a higher sensitivity during the second week of illness (see Table 20.4). A high IgM titre in a single serum sample as detected by ELISA or

Table 20.4 Sensitivity & specificity of rapid screening tests applied to human serum

Method	Sensitivity (%)	Specificity (%)
ELISA	86.5–90 [1,3]	94–97
Dot ELISA dip-stick	92.5–98 [1,2]	90.6–98.9 [1,2]
IgM Dip-stick	93.2 [1]	89.6 [1]
IHA	54–92.2 [1,2,3]	94.4–95.8 [1,2,3]

[1] Bajani *et al.* 2003; [2] Levett *et al.* 2001; [3] Zochowski *et al.* 2001

similar test, or a four-fold rise in titre, is consistent with current or recent leptospirosis, though IgM class antibodies may remain detectable for several months or years following infection. Weak serological reactions may represent either very early or late phase of the immune response or non-specific reactions. Low titres or a delayed response may be noted in severe cases, in immunocompromised individuals, or when high doses of antibiotics were administered in the early phase of the disease.

All positive screening test results should be confirmed, by the MAT ideally, or by a different methodology. Indication of infecting serogroup/var is only possible serologically, by the MAT.

DNA hybridization has been applied to the detection of leptospiral DNA in clinical material by both dot blot and *in situ* hybridization. However the sensitivity of these techniques was found to be lower than that for PCR and consequently their use has been limited.

PCR assays for leptospiral DNA have been published but only two have been evaluated in clinical studies (Brown *et al.* 1995; Merien *et al.* 1995). Both have limitations: the primers described by Merien *et al.* were genus specific amplifying DNA from both pathogenic and saprophytic leptospires; those evaluated by Brown required the use of a second primer set to amplify all pathogenic species. Further developments in PCR technology have resulted in Real Time PCR platforms—PCR chemistry with fluorescent probe detection of amplified product. Both TaqMan and SYBR green chemistries have been utilized (Smythe *et al.* 2003; Levett *et al.* 2005; Merien *et al.* 2005; Slack *et al.* 2007) in assays which amplified DNA from all the pathogenic leptospira species. Leptospira DNA has been amplified from blood, CSF and serum by PCR. The use of Real Time PCR methodology has the potential to facilitate the rapid diagnosis of acute leptospirosis during the early acute phase of illness, complementing IgM-antibody detection assays. Further development with Real Time PCR may result in pathogenic species identification by melt curve analysis.

Treatment

For many decades the efficacy of antibiotics in the treatment of leptospirosis has been disputed, because few controlled studies have been conducted. Three controlled randomized studies concluded that penicillin and doxycycline therapies reduced the duration of illness and prevented or reduced the duration of leptospiuria (McClain *et al.* 1984; Watt *et al.* 1988; Edwards *et al.* 1988). Effective antibiotic treatment should be administered within the first 7–10 days after infection (Watt *et al.* 1988; Faine *et al.* 1999; Sehgal *et al.* 2000). Penicillin is the antibiotic of choice; erythromycin may be given to the allergic patient. Doxycycline has reduced the severity and duration of illness in anicteric leptospirosis, and is also effective as a short term prophylactic (Seghal *et al.* 2000; Takafuji *et al.* 1984). In the hamster model doxycycline was found to be effective *in vivo* early in the course of the disease, clearing leptospires from target organs in 3 days (Truccolo *et al.* 2002). Doxycycline is contraindicated in children and pregnancy. Third generation cephalosporins appear to be effective, but limited clinical experience is available. Jarisch-Herxheimer reactions have been reported following the commencement of penicillin therapy; the effects are temporary and should not contraindicate its use. (Guidugli *et al.* 2003).

Most patients with leptospirosis will recover in 2–6 weeks, if not jaundiced. The death rate in jaundiced patients depends on the facilities available to treat liver and renal failure and on the early commencement of penicillin treatment. Patients who survive the renal and myocardial failure of severe leptospirosis usually recover completely in 6–12 weeks. Convalescence may be protracted (up to 6 months) and up to 10% of patients complain of persisting headaches and uveitis for some years (Faine *et al.* 1999). A density of 10^4 leptospires per ml of blood is a critical threshold for the vital prognosis of a patient (Truccolo *et al.* 2001).

Animals

Treatment regimes for leptospirosis in domestic animals are similar. Streptomycin or tetracycline may be used in acute leptospirosis. A single dose of Streptomycin (and its dihydro-analogue), when given at a dose of 25 mg/kg bodyweight, will markedly reduce the number of organisms an infected animal is excreting, but, with certain serovars, it will not give a microbiological cure. Long acting oxytetracycline or amoxicillin may be substituted for streptomycin to treat chronic infection. Streptomycin is not available in the USA.

Treatment of acute leptospirosis in dogs is analogous to that in man; benzylpenicillin combined with streptomycin is recommended. Doxycycline and ampicillin may also be used. Elimination of the carrier state with treatment is uncertain (Faine 1999).

In animals the prognosis is very good, provided they have not become jaundiced. Animals which abort due to leptospiral infection are extremely unlikely to abort again due to the same serovar in a later pregnancy.

Control and prevention

General advice – environmental control

- ◆ Measures to reduce rodent populations in close contact with human activities,
- ◆ Care with clearing rubbish,
- ◆ Preventing rodent access to buildings (both human and animal housing),
- ◆ Immunize and treat infected animals,
- ◆ Vaccinate dogs annually against leptospirosis,
- ◆ Always wash hands after handling all animals,
- ◆ Avoid contact with urine, faeces or saliva from infected dogs and other animals.

People at high risk of infection including travellers need to be educated about their risk of exposure. Greater awareness through education of health professionals, employers and the general public has informed safer practices in both workplace and recreational settings. This also includes leptospirosis in the differential diagnosis of fever in the returning traveller, especially from tropical countries. Urban wildlife control and reducing rodent populations, especially in urban areas where large populations are linked to areas of degraded environment with poor housing or sanitation, and removing rubbish, especially food waste is important. Increasing rat populations in sewer systems results in increased containment pressures, so that defects in the sewerage infrastructure together with poor environmental quality above ground increases the potential for increased rat population densities.

Simple measures that can easily be undertaken by individuals to reduce their risk of acquiring infection, especially in low prevalence countries include:

◆ Covering cuts, abrasions, and blisters with waterproof dressings before exposure to surface waters,

◆ Not swimming or wading in water that might be contaminated with animal urine,

◆ Protective clothing should be worn by those exposed to contaminated water or soil because of their job or recreational activities,

◆ Wearing protective footwear and gloves during exposure to surface waters and potentially contaminated environments,

◆ Showering promptly after immersion in surface waters.

For adults with short-term, high-risk exposure to leptospirosis, doxycycline provides effective prophylaxis when administered weekly as a single oral dose of 200 mg but in general, chemoprophylaxis with antibiotics for people with an infected dog in the household is not recommended.

Large scale immunization of domestic livestock will prevent clinical disease in animals and the subsequent risk of abortion; it will also reduce the risk of acquisition of the disease by humans, however most vaccines will not eradicate the disease from an endemically infected herd. Local serovars may change as a consequence of changes in farming practices and it has been demonstrated in the laboratory that vaccines have the potential to accelerate the development of new strains. Current animal vaccines have a limited effectiveness of 1–2 years and the economics of farming may influence a farmer's decision as to whether or not to immunize his livestock.

There is no human vaccine licensed for use in the UK although vaccines are available in a few European countries. Human vaccines have been used in a few high risk countries with varied success, but vaccines produced in rabbit serum may cause serious side-effects.

References

Bajani, M. D., Ashford, D. A., Bragg, S. L., *et al.* (2003). Evaluation of four commercially available rapid serologic tests for diagnosis of leptospirosis. *J. Clin. Microbiol.,* **41**(2): 803–9.

Brenner, D. J., Kaufmann, A. F., Sulzer, K. R., *et al.* (1999). Further determination of DNA relatedness between serogroups and serovars in the family Leptospiraceae with a proposal for Leptospira alexanderi sp. nov. and four new Leptospira genomospecies. *Int. J. Syst. Bacteriol.,* **49**: 839–58.

Brown, P. D., Gravekamp, C., Carrington, D. G., *et al.* (1995). Evaluation of polymerase chain reaction for early diagnosis of leptospirosis. *J. Med. Microbiol.,* **43**: 110–14.

Chakurkar, G., Vaideeswar, P., Pandit, S. P., *et al.* (2008). Cardiovascular lesions in leptospirosis: an autopsy study. *J. Infect. Dis.,* **56**(3): 197–203.

Crump, J. A., Murdoch, D. R., and Baker, M. G. (2001). Emerging infectious diseases in an island ecosystem: The New Zealand perspective. *Emerg. Inf. Dis.,* **7**: 767–72.

Cumberland, P., Everard, C. O., and Levett, P. N. (1999). Assessment of the efficacy of an IgM-ELISA and microscopic agglutination test (MAT) in the diagnosis of acute leptospirosis. *Am. J. Trop. Med. Hyg.,* **61**: 731–34.

Edwards, C. N., Nicholson, G. D., Hassell, T. A., Everard, C. O., and Callender, J. (1988). Penicillin therapy in icteric leptospirosis. *Am. J. Trop. Med. Hyg.,* **39**: 388–90.

Faine, S., Adler, B., Bolin, C., and Perolat, P. (1999). Leptospira and leptospirosis. (2nd edn). Melbourne: Med Sci.

Faine, S. (1994). Leptospira and leptospirosis. Boca Raton (FL): CRC Press.

Guidugli, F., Castro, A. A., and Atallah, A. N. (2003). Antibiotics for treating leptospirosis [review]. Cochrane Database Syst Rev. (The Cochrane Library). Issue 3. Oxford: Update Software.

Inada, R., Ido, Y., *et al.* (1916). Etiology, mode of infection and specific therapy of Weil's disease. *J. Exp. Med.,* **23**: 377–402.

International Leptospirosis Society (2007). 5th Scientific Meeting of the International Leptospirosis Society. Quito, Ecuador.

IJSEM. (2008). International Committee on Systematics of Prokaryotes. Subcommittee on the taxonomy of *Leptospiraceae.* **58**: 1049–50.

Levett, P. N. (2001). Leptospirosis. Clin. *Microbiol. Rev.,* **14**: 296–326.

Levett, P. N., Morey, R. E., Galloway, R. L., Turner, D. E., Steigerwalt, A. G., *et al.* (2005). Detection of pathogenic leptospires by real-time quantitative PCR. *J. Med. Microbiol.,* **54**: 45–49.

Levett, P. N., Morey, R. E., Galloway, R. L., and Steigerwalt, A. G. (2006). Leptospira broomii sp. nov., isolated from humans with leptospirosis. *Int. J. Syst. Evol. Microbiol.,* **56**: 671–73.

McBride, A. J., *et al.* (2005). Leptospirosis. *Curr. Opin. Infect. Dis.,* 18: 376–86.

McClain, J. B. L., Ballou, W. R., Harrison, S. M., and Steinweg, D. L. (1984). Doxycycline therapy for leptospirosis. *Ann. Intern. Med.,* **100**: 696–98.

Merien, F., Baranton, G., Perolat, P.(1995). Comparison of polymerase chain reaction with microagglutination test and culture for diagnosis of leptospirosis. *J. Infect. Dis.,* **172**: 281–85.

Merien, F., Portnoi, D., Bourhy, P., Charavary, F., Berlioz-Arthaud, A., *et al.* (2005). A rapid and quantitative method for the detection of Leptospira species in human leptospirosis. *FEMS Microbiol. Lett.,* **249**: 139–47.

Nardone, A., Capek, I., Baranton, G., *et al.* (2004). Risk factors for leptospirosis in metropolitan France: results of a national case-control study, 1999–2000. *Clin. Infect. Dis.,* **39**(5): 751–53.

Noguchi, H. (1917). Spirochaeta icterohaemorrhagiae in American wild rats and its relation to the Japanese and European strains. *J. Exp. Med.,* **5**: 755–63.

Perolat, P., Chappel, R. J., *et al.* (1998). Leptospira fainei sp. nov., isolated from pigs in Australia. *Int J Syst Bact.,* **28**: 851–858.

Sanders, E. J., Rigau-Perez, J. G., Smits, H. L., Deseda, C. C., Vorndam, V. A. (1999). Increase of leptospirosis in Dengue-negative patients after a hurricane in Puerto Rico in 1996. *Am. J. Trop. Med. Hyg.,* **61**(3): 399–404.

Seghal, S. C., Sugnan, A. P., Murhekar, M. V., Sharma, S., and Vijayachari, P. (2000). Randomized controlled trial of doxycycline prophylaxis against leptospirosis in an endemic area. *Int. J. Antimicrob. Agents.,* **13** (4): 249–55.

Sejvar, J., Bancroft, E., Winthrop, K., *et al.* (2003). Leptospirosis in 'Eco-Challenge' Athletes, Malaysian Borneo, 2000. *Emerg. Inf. Dis.,* **9**: 702–3.

Slack, A., Symonds, M., Dohnt, M., Harris, C., Brookes, D., *et al.* (2007). Evaluation of a modified TaqMan assay detecting pathogenic Leptospira spp. Against culture and Leptospira-specific IgM enzyme-linked immunosorbant assay in a clinical environment. *Diag. Microbiol. and Infect. Dis.,* **57**: 361–66.

Smythe, L. D., Smith, I. L., Smith, G. A., *et al.* (2003). A quantitative PCR (TaqMan) assay for pathogenic Leptospira spp. *BMC Infect. Dis.*, 2: 13.

Stimson, A. M. (1907). 'Note on an organism found in yellow fever tissue'. *Pub. Health Rep.*, **22**: 541.

Takafuji, E. T., Kirkpatrich, J. W., Miller, R. N., *et al.* (1984). An efficacy trial of doxycycline chemoprophylaxis against leptospirosis. *N. Engl. J. Med.*, **310**: 497–500.

Torten, M., and Marshall, R. B. (1994). Leptospirosis. In Handbook of Zoonoses: Bacterial, Rickettsial, Chlamydial and Mycotic. pp. 245–64. Baco Raton, FLA: CRC Press.

Truccolo, J., Serais, O., Merien, F., and Perolat, P. (2001). Following the course of human leptospirosis: evidence of a critical threshold for the vital prognosis using a quantitative PCR assay. *FEMS Microbiol. Lett.* **204**(2): 317–21.

Truccolo, J., Charavay, F., Merien, F. and Perolat, P. (2002). Quantitative PCR assay to evaluate ampicillin, ofloxacin, and doxycycline for treatment of experimental leptospirosis. *Antimicrob. Agents Chemother.*, **6**: 48–53.

van Crevel, R., Speelman, P., Gravekamp, C., and Terpstra, W. J. (1994). Leptospirosis in travellers. *Clin. Infect. Dis.*, **19**: 132–34.

Victoriano, A. F. B., Smythe, L. D., Gloriani-Barzaga, N., Cavinta, L. L., *et al.* (2009). Leptospirosis in the Asia Pacific region. *BMC Infect. Dis.*, **9**: 147.

Victoriano, A. F. B., Smyth, L. D., Gloriani-Barzaga, N., *et al.* (2009). *BMC Infect. Dis.*, **9**: 147. Available online: http://www.biomedcentral. com/1471-2334/9/147.

Watt, G., Padre, L. P., Tuazon, M. L., *et al.* (1988). Placebo-controlled trial of intravenous penicillin for severe and late leptospirosis. *Lancet*, **i**: 433–35.

Weil, A. (1886). Uber eine Eigentumliche mit Milztumor, Icterus and mephritis einhergenhende acute Infektionskrankheit., *Ktsch. Arch. Klin. Med.*, **39**: 209.

Wolbach, S. B., and Binger, C. A. L. (1914). Notes on a filterable spirochete from fresh water. Spirocheta biflexa (new species). *J. Med. Res.*, 30: 23.

World Health Organisation (1999). Weekly Epidemiological Record. Leptospirosis worldwide. Geneva, 74: 237–44 Available from: http://www. who.int/docstore/wer/pdf/1999/wer7429.pdf (accessed 26 Mar 2010).

World Health Organisation leptospirosis: guidance for diagnosis, surveillance and control . Geneva : The Organisation; 2003 . Available online: http://whqlibdoc.who.int/hq/2003/WHO_CDS_CSR_ EPH_2002.23.pdf (accessed 26 Mar 2010) and ILS, Available online: http://www.leptonet.net/assets/images/LeptoGuidelines_Print_ version_19May03.pdf.

Wuthiekanum, V., Sirisukkarn, N., Daengsupa, P., Sakaraserane, P., Sangkakam, A., *et al.* (2007). Clinical diagnosis and geographic distribution of leptospirosis, Thailand. *Emerg Infect Dis* [serial on the internet]. 2007 Jan [20 February]. Available from http://www.cdc.gov/ ncidod/EID/13/1/124.htm.

Zochowski, W. J., Palmer, M. F., and Coleman, T. J. (2001). An evaluation of three commercial kits for use as screening methods for the detection of leptospiral antibodies in the UK. *J. Clin. Pathol.*, **4**: 25–30.

Online resources

Centers for Disease Control and Prevention. URL: http://wwwnc.cdc.gov/ travel/yellowbook/2010/chapter-5/leptospirosis.aspx.

Centers for Disease Control and Prevention http://www.cdc.gov/ncidod/ dbmd/diseaseinfo/leptospirosis_g.htm (accessed 26 Mar 2010).

Centers for Disease Control and Prevention. http://www.cdc.gov/nczved/ divisions/dfbmd/diseases/leptospirosis/.

European Centre for Disease Prevention and Control. URL: http://www. ecdc.europa.eu/en/healthtopics/Pages/Leptospirosis.aspx.

Health and Safety Executive.(HSE–United Kingdom): Leptospirosis–are you at risk? http://www.hse.gov.uk/pubns/indg84.pdf.

Common Zoonoses in Agriculture http://www.hse.gov.uk/pubns/ais2.pdf.

Health Protection Agency (United Kingdom): http://www.hpa.org.uk/ Topics/InfectiousDiseases/InfectionsAZ/Leptospirosis/.

International Leptospirosis Society Guidelines http://www.leptonet.net/ assets/images/LeptoGuidelines_Print_version_19May03.pdf (accessed 26 Mar 2010).

International Leptospirosis Society http://www.med.monash.edu.au/ microbiology/staff/adler/ils.html (accessed 26 Mar 2010).

Leptonet. Royal Tropical Institute, Amsterdam, The Netherlands. http:// www.leptonet.net (accessed 23 Mar 2010).

OIE; World Organisation for Animal Health. http://www.oie.int/eng/en_ index.htm.

OIE; World Organisation for Animal Health. Manual of Diagnostic Tests and Vaccines for Terrestrial Animals. Available online: http://www.oie. int/eng/normes/mmanual/A_00043.htm.

Scanning electron micrograph of Leptospira interrogans strain RGA. http:// www.eol.org/pages/973464 Public Health Image Library (Public Domain).

Scanning electron micrograph of Leptospira interrogans strain RGA. http:// www.eol.org/pages/973464 Public Health Image Library (Public Domain).

The Leptospirosis Information Center http://www.leptospirosis.org (accessed 23 Mar 2010).

World Health Organisation (2006). Informal Consultation on Global Burden of Leptospirosis: Methods of Assessment. Geneva: WHO.

CHAPTER 21

Yersiniosis and plague

Michael B. Prentice

Summary

The genus Yersinia consists of three principal pathogenic species Y.enterocolitica, Y.pseudotuberculosis and Y. pestis. Yersinia enterocolitica and Y.pseudotuberculosis are the two principal pathogens of human non-plague yersiniosis. Yersinia pestis is the sole pathogen of human plague, but there are distinct Y. pestis biovars which cause enzootic infection in rodents with little human disease. There are now ten species of Yersinia recognized as well as the three principal pathogens (Table 21.1). These are mostly rarely identified and of less pathogenic potential (Y. frederiksenii, Y. bercovieri, Y. intermedia and Y. kristensenii of this group of organisms are the most frequently isolated from humans, but still relatively rare). Yersinia ruckeri is a pathogen of fish. DNA hybridization studies indicated such close relatedness between Y. pestis and Y. pseudotuberculosis that the plague bacillus was in fact Y. pseudotuberculosis subspecies pestis. This recognition of Y. pestis as a clone within the species Y. pseudotuberculosis has been confirmed by genome sequencing, multi locus sequence typing (MLST) and other genetic analyses. However, because of the pathogenic potential of this clone compared with most Y. pseudotuberculosis strains, the designation Y. pestis has been retained to avoid diagnostic confusion.

Yersiniosis

Introduction

Disease in humans is caused mostly by Y.enterocolitica belonging to serotypes 03, 05, 27, 08 and 09 and by Y.pseudotuberculosis (Skurnik *et al.* 2002; Perry and Fetherston 2006). The clinical presentations include fever, diarrhoea, abdominal pain that may mimic appendicitis, and chronic arthritis. There are typically lesions of enteritis and mesenteric lymphadenitis. Yersiniosis occurs in all European countries, with highest prevalence in northern countries and Scandinavia, as well as Canada, the USA, Australia, and Japan. Transmission is mainly from contaminated animal products such as pork and milk, and rarely from person-to-person by the faecal-oral route. Control of yersiniosis can be achieved by careful handling and cooking of meats and by pasteurization of milk and other dairy products.

History

The discoveries of Y. enterocolitica and Y.pseudotuberculosis were not attended by the same excitement and drama as the discovery of Y.pestis, and Alexandre Yersin had nothing to do with characterizing these species. Human infection by Y.enterocolitica was first reported in 1939 by Schleifstein and Coleman. It was then called Bacterium enterocoliticum but was renamed Pasteurella X by Daniels and Goudzwaard in 1963 and finally was grouped in the genus Yersinia by Frederiksen in 1964.

Pfeiffer in 1889 first described Bacillus pseudotuberculosis, which he renamed Pasteurella pseudotuberculosis in 1929. Additionally, it was called Shigella pseudotuberculosis in 1935 until Smith and Thal placed it into the genus Yersinia in 1965.

Before 1970, there was little attention given to yersinioses in the medical literature or in public health. In 1975, there were only 84 cases of Y.enterocoloitica infection reported in the USA and about 6,000 cases in the world literature. However, during the 1980s there occurred an increased interest and recognition of this organism as an important cause of diarrhoea and the appendicitis-like syndrome. Most of the reported cases were in Scandinavia, other European countries, Canada and the USA. Yersiniosis is the third commonest zoonoses recorded in Europe.

Only in the past two decades have public health officials recognized the roles of contaminated pork, recontamination of pasteurized milk, raw vegetables, and contaminated blood in blood banks as sources of Yersinia infection.

The agent

Yersinia enterocolitica and Y.pseudotuberculosis are Gram-negative, non-lactose-fermenting, urease-positive bacilli that are motile when grown at 25°C but not at 37°C. Both organisms grow on blood, heart infusion, MacConkey, and SS agars at room temperature and at 37°C, and in buffered saline at 4°C. Colonies are often very small after incubation for 24 hours but are readily apparent at 48 hours. More than 50 serotypes and five biotypes of Y.enterocolitica have been described (Wauters 1981). Most strains from patients belong to serotypes 03, 08 and 09 and to biotypes 2, 3 and 4. Six serotypes (I–VI) and four subtypes of Y.pseudotuberculosis have been identified, with O-group I accounting for approximately 80% of human cases.

Table 21.1 *Yersinia* species other than *Y. enterocolitica*, *Y. pseudotuberculosis* and *Y. pestis*: a summary

Species	Habitat	Evidence for pathogenic potential	Distinguishing features
Y. aldovae	Fresh water [1], fish alimentary tracts of wild rodents[2]		L-rhamnose and negative reactions for fermentation of sorbose, cellobiose, melibiose, and usually sucrose
Y. aleksiciae [3]	Strains isolated from the faeces of humans, rats, moles, reindeer and pigs, and from dairy products		Split from *Y. kristensenii* by 16S rRNA and lysine decarboxylase (LDC) positivity
Y. bercovieri [4]	Strains isolated from the faeces of humans, raw vegetables and water	Secretes a heat-stable enterotoxin (YbST) [5]. Can invade cells *in vitro*.	Formerly *Y. enterocolitica* biovar 3B. Pyrazinamidase positive, L-fucose positive, acid from mucate
Y. frederiksenii [6]	Strains isolated from blood, human faeces, sewage, water, milk, soil, frogs, and small mammals		Ferment rhamnose. Multiple genomospecies groups identified with the same phenotypes [7]
Y. intermedia [8]	Strains isolated from humans, frogs, snails, water		Rhamnose-positive, melibiose-positive, raffinose-positive strains
Y. kristensenii [9]	Strains isolated from environmental samples, foods, animals and humans	Lethal for iron-overloaded mice by IP injection[10]. Some strains produce enterotoxin	Trehalose-positive, sucrose-negative
Y. massiliensis [11]	Strains isolated from freshwater in Marseille, France		Indole and inositol positive L-rhamnose-negative
Y. mollaretii [4]	Meat, raw vegetables, drinking water and environmental samples, occasionally from humans		Formerly Y. enterocolitica biovar 3A Ferments L-sorbose and either i or myo-inositol
Y. rohdei [12]	Strains isolated from faeces of humans, dogs and surface water		Positive for citrate and sucrose utilization, negative reactions indole, acetoin
Y. similis [13]	Strains from animals		Melibiose-negative, specific 16S rRNA gene sequence type and polar lipid profile otherwise as for *Y. pseudotuberculosis*
Y. ruckeri [14]	Fish, water	Fish pathogen causing red mouth disease and septicaemia in salmonid fish [15]	Forms outlying clade in phylogenetic comparison of other *Yersinia* species [16–18]

1. Bercovier, H. *et al.*
2. Fukushima, H. M. *et al.*
3. Sprague, L.D. and Neubauer, H.
4. Wauters, G. *et al.*
5. Sulakvelidze, A.
6. Ursing, J. *et al.*
7. Dolina, M. and Peduzzi, R.
8. Brenner, D. *et al.*
9. Bercovier, H. *et al.*
10. Robins-Browne, R.M. *et al.*
11. Merhej, V.
12. Aleksic, S. *et al.*
13. Sprague, L.D. *et al.*
14. Ewing, W.H. *et al.*
15. Tobback, E. *et al.*
16. Ibrahim, A. *et al.*
17. Kotetishvili, M. *et al.*
18. Chen, P. *et al.*

The virulence of the yersiniae depends on a variety of plasmid and chromosomal genes expressing factors present at various times on the outside of the bacterial cell. Following initial replication in the small intestine, the organisms invade Peyer's patches of the distal ileum via M cells (Clark *et al.* 1998; Grutzkau *et al.* 1990). Invasin, a chromosomally-specified non-fimbrial adhesin interacts with 1 integrins expressed on the apical surfaces of M Cells (Clark *et al.* 1998) to bring about invasion. The gene encoding invasin (inv) is inactivated in Y. pestis (Simonet *et al.* 1996). The 70 kb virulence plasmid pYV encodes a variety of anti-host factors (Cornelis *et al.* 1998). One of these is Yersinia adhesin A (YadA) which in Y. pseudotuberculosis interacts with extracellular matrix proteins such as fibronectin and collagen to facilitate the invasin association with integrins (Eitel and Dersch 2002). In Y. enterocolitica, YadA lacks an N-terminal region and does not bind fibronectin or facilitate uptake by the host cell (Heise and Dersch 2006). YadA also binds host complement regulators and helps confer serum resistance (Kirjavainen *et al.* 2008) with another chromosomally specified extracellular protein Ail (attachment and invasion locus) (Kirjavainen *et al.* 2008; Pierson and Falkow 1993).

The ability of Yersinia YadA to bind host cell surfaces brings host cell membranes within reach of the most celebrated of the Yersinia virulence factors—the pYV specified Type III secretion system (injectisome) (Cornelis 2006). This nanomachine reduces the effectiveness of the host innate immune response by injecting toxins (Yop proteins)(Cornelis 2002) into host macrophages, neutrophils, and dendritic cells, affecting signal transduction pathways and reducing phagocytosis and bacteria-killing reactive oxygen species (ROS) production by neutrophils (Spinner et al. 2010) and triggering apoptosis in macrophages (Mills et al. 1997). Other factors important in invasive disease include yersiniabactin, a siderophore produced by the more virulent Y. enterocolitica biovar Ib strains and some Y. pseudotuberculosis strains as well as other Enterobacteriaceae. This allows bacteria to access iron from lactoferrin and reduces production of ROS by innate immune effector cells (Paauw et al. 2009). All strains of Y. enterocolitica have multiple haem/iron uptake mechanisms and their virulence is enhanced in individuals with iron overload or in the presence of the therapeutic iron chelating agent desferrioxamine (Robins-Browne and Prpic 1985), both by access to the bound iron and by an inhibitory effect of desferrioxamine on neutrophil function (Ewald et al. 1994).

A heat stable enterotoxin similar to E.coli heat stable enterotoxin is produced by many Y. enterocolitica strains (Delor et al. 1990; Ramamurthy et al. 1997). A high percentage of Y. enterocolitica strains lacking the virulence plasmid and not belonging to biovars associated with clinical disease contain known enterotoxin genes or produce another unidentified enterotoxin detected by in vivo mouse assay (Grant et al. 1998; Ramamurthy et al. 1997). Yersinia kristensenii (Ramamurthy et al. 1997) and Y. bercovieri (Sulakvelidze et al. 1999) also contain related enterotoxin genes. The prevalence of this property in strains not commonly causing human disease makes its role in human disease uncertain. Some Y. pseudotuberculosis strains make a superantigenic toxin which may be associated with more serious systemic disease (Miyoshi-Akiyama et al. 1995; Ueshiba et al. 1998).

Genome sequence data first showed insecticidal toxin genes resembling those in Photorhabdus luminescens were present in Y. pestis (Parkhill et al. 2001), subsequently these have been found in all Yersinia species (Fuchs et al. 2008; Thomson et al. 2006). Their role in yersiniosis is uncertain, although some association with mammalian gut colonization has been observed (Tennant et al. 2005). Both Y. enterocolitica and Y. pseudotuberculosis produce lipopolysaccharide enterotoxin similar to that of other Enterobacteriaceae and Y. enterocolitica enterotoxin is important in resistance to host antimicrobial peptides (Skurnik et al. 1999).

The hosts
Animals
The natural reservoirs of Y. enterocolitica include a variety of domestic and wild species. The prominent hosts are pigs, rodents, rabbits, sheep, goats, cattle, horses, dogs, and cats. Yersinia pseudotuberculosis resides in many of the same animals, including rodents, rabbits, deer, and farm animals but has also been found extensively in birds, including turkeys, ducks, geese pigeons, pheasants, and canaries. Y. pseudotuberculosis causes serious infections in high population density conditions experienced by a wide variety of animals in zoological gardens and wildlife parks (Baskin et al. 1977; Bielli et al. 1999).

The organism are localized in the oropharyngeal cavities and lumens of the gastrointestinal tract of these animals. They are excreted into the faeces to allow faecal-oral transmission among animals. Studies of pigs in slaughterhouses suggested that the tonsils and tongues contained Y.enterocolitica more frequently than other tissues. In experimental infections of pigs, organisms persisted longer on tonsils than in faeces. Raw intestines of pigs (chitterlings) are also implicated as a source of human infection. The presence of Y.enterocolitica in unpasteurized milk suggests that bacteria reach the bloodstream from the intestine and are secreted into milk by mammary glands. Alternatively, milk could be contaminated through faecal contact or through localized mastitis due to this infection.

Generally, infections of animals by Yersinia are asymptomatic carriages that do not produce clinical illness. However, illness in household dogs has been associated with transmission of infection to humans. Sheep in Australia were shown to develop intestinal microabscesses but did not appear to be clinically ill in one study (Slee and Skilbeck 1992). On the other hand, Philbey et al. (1991) found Yersinia infection in 4% of Australian sheep with diarrhoea, ill thrift, or mortality. Intestinal lesions included acute segmental suppurative erosive enterocolitis and haemorrhagic enterocolitis. One animal had a perforation of the intestine. Lesions were less frequent and less severe in sheep with Y.enterocolitica than in animals with Y.pseudotuberculosis. Yersinia infection was associated with recent changes in husbandry of affected flocks, including changes in diet, shearing and weaning; this suggested that environmental stress could have interacted with infection to result in clinical disease. In experimental infections of sheep with Y.enterocolitica, dexamethasone treatment resulted in a higher incidence of intestinal abscesses, suggesting that stress and/or immunosuppression could promote disease (Slee and Button 1990). Other factors contributing to expressions of disease in Yersinia infection of sheep could be concomitant infection with nematodes and Coccidia, which are common in infected flocks.

Humans
Humans are accidental hosts for Yersinia bacteria, after they ingest contaminated animals products, and they play no important role in maintaining the organisms in nature and transmitting it to other humans. The alimentary tract is the portal of entry in most cases. After an incubation period of 4–7 days, infection causes mucosal ulcerations in the terminal ileum (rarely ascending colon), necrotic lesions in Peyer's patches, and enlargement of mesenteric lymph nodes. In most cases, the appendix is histologically normal or shows mild inflammation. If septicaemia develops, suppurative lesions may occur in various organ systems (e.g. lung, liver, meninges). A reactive polyarthritis develops in some patients and is more common among patients with histocompatibility antigen HLA-B27. Molecular mimicry between HLA-B27 antigen and Yersinia antigen has been postulated as a mechanism for reactive arthritis. Superantigenic activity has been found in cultures of Y.enterocolitica and could be a mechanism for reactive arthritis (Stuart and Woodward 1992).

Enterocolitis accounts for two thirds of all reported cases and is characterized by fever, diarrhoea, and abdominal pain, lasting 1–3 weeks. In serious cases, rectal bleeding and perforation of the ileum may occur. Faecal excretion of the organism may continue for weeks after symptoms have subsided. Leucocytes, and less commonly blood or mucus, may be present in the stool. Most patients with this syndrome are less than 5 years of age. Patients with mesenteric adenitis and/or terminal ileitis have fever, right lower quadrant pain and leucocytosis and this syndrome is more common in older children and adolescents; it may be clinically indistinguishable from acute appendicitis.

Reactive polyarthritis, may occur in up to 30% of adults with Y.enterocolitica infection, begins a few days to a month after onset of acute diarrhoea; it may involve the knees, ankles, toes, fingers, and wrists. In most cases, two to four joints become inflamed in rapid succession over a period of 2–14 days. Symptoms persist for more than 1 month in one third. After 12 months, most patients are symptomless, but a few will have persisting low back pain, including sacroileitis, which has been specifically related to the presence of HLA-B27. Reiter's syndrome with arthritis, urethritis, and conjunctivitis has also been reported. Like arthritis, this complications is much more likely to develop in individuals with the HLA-B27 antigen.

In more recent years, exudative pharyngitis has been documented as part of the spectrum of illnesses caused by Y.enterocolitica. In one large outbreak in the USA, 8% of patients presented with acute pharyngitis and fever, without accompanying diarrhoea. Cases of pneumonia, empyema, and lung abscess have been reported.

Yersinia enterocolitica septicaemia is uncommon and is most often reported in patients with diabetes mellitus, severe anaemia, haemochromatosis, cirrhosis, malignancy and in elderly patients. Patients with iron overload, such as thalassaemic patients who receive frequent transfusions, are at risk for septicaemia. The treatment of iron-overloaded patients with desferrioxamine has been particularly associated with Yersinia sepsis because this iron chelator enhances the growth of the organism and also appears to inhibit polymorphonuclear leucocyte defence against the infection (Chiu et al. 1986; Cantinieaux et al. 1988). Septicaemic patients may develop hepatic or splenic abscesses, osteomyelitis, wound infections, or meningitis. Endocarditis and mycotic aneurysms due to Y.enterocolitica have been reported (Applebaum et al. 1983).

Septicaemia caused by transfusion of contaminated blood has been reported (Prentice et al. 1990), linked to the ability of Y. enterocolitica to multiply at refrigerator temperature (psychotrophy). It is believed that small numbers of bacteria in blood from asymptomatic bacteraemia in the donor are amplified by growth inside the blood transfusion unit during refrigerated storage (Gibb et al. 1994). This is a very rare event, one in 500,000 to one in several million units (Anon. 1997; Leclercq et al. 2005) and it has not been possible to devise a method that can prevent it without unacceptably restricting the blood supply.

By far the most common manifestation of Y.pseudotuberculosis infection in humans is mesenteric adenitis, which causes an acute appendicitis-like syndrome with fever and right lower quadrant abdominal pain. At laparotomy, there is usually a normal appendix and enlarged mesenteric lymph nodes that may be accompanied by inflammation of the terminal ileum. The infection is usually self-limited, and patients who have undergone surgery generally begin to improve promptly after laparotomy. Erythema nodosum and polyarthritis have also been described in patients with Y. pseudotuberculosis infection. Less than 100 cases of Y.pseudotuberculosis-induced septicaemia have been described (Ljungberg et al. 1995; Paglia et al. 2005). The majority of septicaemic patients have underlying disease such as cirrhosis, haemochromatosis, diabetes mellitus or HIV-AIDS.

Diagnosis

For diagnosis, culture of stool, mesenteric lymph node, pharyngeal exudate, peritoneal fluid, or blood may yield Yersinia, depending on the clinical syndrome. Recovery of organisms from otherwise uncontaminated material such as blood, cerebrospinal fluid, or mesenteric lymph node tissue is not difficult, but isolation of yersiniae from faeces is hampered by their slow growth and by overgrowth of normal faecal flora. Yield of positive stool cultures can be increased by using cold enrichment, alkali treatment, or selective CIN agar, but these methods are not cost effective in routine diagnosis because usual enteric culturing methods can detect most clinically significant infections (Kachoris et al. 1988).

Because the virulence plasmid pYV is frequently lost from pathogenic Y. enterocolitica strains on laboratory subculture, combined biochemical identification, with biotyping following a standard schema (Wauters et al. 1987), and serotyping is required to interpret the significance of Y. enterocolitica isolation from faeces.

Agglutinating or ELISA antibody titres against O antigen types are used in retrospective diagnosis of both Y. enterocolitica (Granfors et al. 1988; Stahlberg et al. 1987) and Y. pseudotuberculosis (Stahlberg et al. 1987). Cross reactions are seen between Y. enterocolitica serogroup O:9 and Brucella, and Y. pseudotuberculosis serogroups II and IV and group B and D Salmonella, respectively, due to the similarity of their LPS structures (Caroff et al. 1984; Mair and Fox 1986). A more specific immunoblot based on SDS-PAGE-separated LPS from different strains of Yersinia has been described (Chart and Cheasty 2006). Multiple O-antigen assays are required to cover even the predominant serogroups Y. enterocolitica O:3, O5,27 and O:9 and Y. pseudotuberculosis O:1a, O:1b, O:3 and these assays are generally only available in reference laboratories. Titres fall from 6 months post infection onwards in the absence of complications such as arthritis. ELISA and Western blot tests detecting antibodies to Yop proteins, in principle expressed by all pathogenic Y. enterocolitica and Y. pseudotuberculosis, are also available (Kendrick et al. 2001; Maki-Ikola et al. 1991; Tomaso et al. 2006). Most of the reactivity in the Yop antibody assays probably relates to previous Y. enterocolitica infection and higher prevalence of seropositivity in these tests is observed in healthy asymptomatic individuals (Tomaso et al. 2006).

Enteropathogenic Yersinia generally cause self-limiting diarrhoea and trial data does not support the use of antimicrobials in adults (Pai et al. 1984) or children (Abdel-Haq et al. 2000) with uncomplicated Y. enterocolitica diarrhoea. Bacteraemia or focal infections outside the gastrointestinal tract are indications for antimicrobial therapy. Infants less than three months of age with documented Y. enterocolitica infection may require antimicrobials because of an increased likelihood of bacteraemia (Abdel-Haq et al. 2000). Y. enterocolitica strains nearly always express beta lactamases (Pham et al. 2000). Recommended therapy for bacteraemia includes ciprofloxacin and beta-lactamase stable agents such as cefotaxime, or ceftriaxone (Abdel-Haq et al. 2000; Gayraud et al. 1993). Amoxyxillin and coamoxyclav have poor efficacy in case series (Gayraud et al. 1993). Cotrimoxazole, gentamicin, and imipenem are all active in vitro. Y. pseudotuberculosis strains do not express β-lactamase but are intrinsically polymyxin resistant (Marceau et al. 2004). Human infection with Y. pseudotuberculosis is less common than for Y. enterocolitica, and there is less case data, but *in vivo* studies in mice (Lemaitre *et al.* 1991) and humans (Sato *et al.* 1988) suggest ampicillin is not clinically effective and similar drugs to those employed for Y. enterocolitica should be used, with best results from a quinolone (Lemaitre *et al.* 1991).

The other main complication of yersiniosis for which antimicrobials have been tried is reactive arthritis. Trials treating reactive arthritis (including a large proportion of cases due to Yersinia) found that three months of oral ciprofloxacin therapy does not affect outcome (Sieper *et al.* 1999; Yli-Kerttula *et al.* 2000). A trend to faster remission of symptoms in a ciprofloxacin treated group with Yersinia reactive arthritis was observed but outcome was not affected (Hoogkamp-Korstanje *et al.* 2000). Follow up 4–7 years after initial antibiotic treatment of reactive arthritis (mainly post Salmonella and Yersinia infection) demonstrated efficacy in prevention of chronic arthritis in HLA-B27 positive individuals (Yli-Kerttula *et al.* 2003). Azithromycin therapy did not affect outcome in reactive arthritis (Kvien *et al.* 2004). A Cochrane review evaluating the use of antibiotics for reactive arthritis of all kinds is in progress.

Epidemiology

Yersinia enterocolitica is a relatively infrequent cause of diarrhoea and abdominal pain in the USA but is more common in Europe, where it is the third commonest zoonoses. Infections have been documented in other parts of the world including South America, Africa and Asia but Y.enterocolitica is rarely a cause of tropical diarrhoea (Carniel *et al.* 1986). Most isolates from Canada and the USA are serotypes O:3 and O:9, with the formerly common highly pathogenic O:8 so called 'American strains' now very rarely seen (Bottone 1999). Virulent serotype O:8 strains have sporadically been isolated in Europe in countries such as Italy (Chiesa *et al.* 1991) and Germany (Schubert *et al.* 2003) with a recent marked increase reported from Poland (Rastawicki *et al.* 2009).

Children and adults and both sexes are susceptible, but children are more often affected than adults (Abdel-Haq *et al.* 2000) Transmission of infection occurs by ingestion of contaminated food or water and less commonly, by direct contact with infected animals or patients (Fig. 21.1). Butchers in Finland are at increased risk of infection (Merilahti-Palo *et al.* 1991).

Transmission of infection from animals to humans has been suggested through household dogs. In northern European countries, Y.enterocolitica is frequently acquired by ingestion of incompletely cooked pork (Tauxe *et al.* 1987). The ability of this organism to grow at 4°C means that refrigerated meats can be sources of infection. The organisms have been isolated from lakes, streams and drinking water. Epidemics of food-borne disease have occurred in the USA, including one due to contaminated chocolate milk in New York (Black *et al.* 1978), one associated with pasteurized milk in Tennessee, one due to bean sprouts in Pennsylvania, and others in Atlanta and Baltimore associated with consumption or household preparation of raw pig intestine (chitterlings) (Jones 2003; Lee *et al.* 1990). Person to person spread of yersiniosis is rare, but Toivanen *et al.* (1973) reported nosocomial spread of infection in a Finnish hospital. Transfusion associated Y. enterocolitica septicaemia has been a rare but often fatal event recognized for over 30 years (Stenhouse and Milner 1982) with no easy route to eradication.

Infection due to Y. pseudotuberculosis is the rarest of the yersinioses in humans (Long *et al.* 2010; Van Noyen *et al.* 1995).

Although this infection has a worldwide distribution, more cases have been reported from Europe than other continents.

The majority of infections have been recorded in children aged 5–15 years, usually in winter months. Most cases are sporadic, but there have been well documented outbreaks associated with iceberg lettuce (Jalava *et al.* 2004; Nuorti *et al.* 2004) and grated carrots (Rimhanen-Finne *et al.* 2009) in Finland and homogenized milk in British Columbia, Canada (Nowgesic *et al.* 1999). Transmission of this infection is presumed to occur by ingestion of organisms from contact with an infected animal, or common source of contamination within a family, such as food or water.

The epizoology of yersiniosis is based on faecal oral transmission among individual animals in a flock or to members of distant species that ingest faecally contaminated food, water, or soil. Yersinia enterocolitica of serotypes 03 and 09 were cultured from more than 50% of pork tongue in butcher shops on Belgium during all seasons of the year, indicating widespread infection of pigs in Belgium year round (Wauters 1979). Pigs also constitute the major reservoir in other European countries and Japan but not in Australia (Slee and Skilbeck 1992). The pigs are healthy carriers. Recently in Finland (Laukkanen *et al.* 2008; Niskanen *et al.* 2002) Russia, and Latvia (Martinez *et al.* 2009), a potential reservoir of Y. pseudotuberculosis in pigs has also been identified, in the same sites that Y. enterocolitica has been found to colonize these animals.

In Australia, sheep and goats are the most commonly infected animals. Both Y.enterocolitica and Y.pseudotuberculosis are transmitted among sheep in the cool, damp weather of the winter and spring, under experimental conditions (Slee and Skilbeck 1992). Under natural field conditions, Y.enterocolitica was excreted year round. Infection occurred mostly in young lambs, with older sheep showing

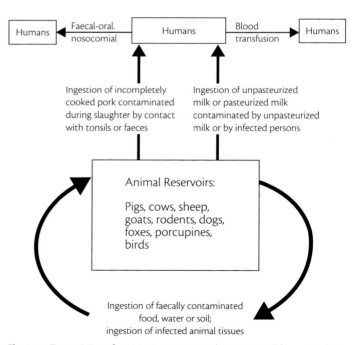

Fig. 21.1 Transmission of yersiniosis among animal reservoirs and from animals to humans and from humans to animals. Wide arrows indicate common transmission, medium arrows indicate occasional transmission, and thin arrows indicate rare transmission.

immune protection. No cross immunity was shown between Y.enterocolitica and Y.pseudotuberculosis because animals previously infected by one species could be infected by the other.

In the USA, Yersinia enterocolitica 08 that has caused large food-borne outbreaks was not found in a survey of domestic animals (Shayegani and Parsons 1987). However, the pathogenic serotype was found in some wild animals, including a fox and porcupine.

Y. enterocolitica O:3 and O:5 strains are now prevalent in pigs in the USA (Bhaduri and Wesley 2006).

Prevention and control

Public Health measures to control Yersinia infection should focus on the animal reservoirs in any particular location. Y. enterocolitica animal vaccines are not available. Y. pseudotuberculosis whole cell killed vaccines are produced commercially to prevent loss of valuable deer and zoo animals (Pseudovac in Europe and Yersiniavax® in New Zealand) rather than to control human disease. A live attenuated oral Y. pseudotuberculosis vaccine (strain IP32680) has recently been reported as suitable for animal use (Quintard et al. 2010). Attenuated strains of Y. enterocolitica are under investigation for use as carrier organisms for heterotopic oral vaccines in humans (Autenrieth and Autenrieth 2007)

Complete cooking of meats and proper pasteurization of dairy products should render potentially contaminated foods safe for consumption. Nevertheless, other approaches to reducing the frequency of contamination of uncooked foods deserve consideration. Kapperud (1991) suggested a method of reducing faecal contamination of meat by circumanal incision (using a bung cutter) and removal of intestines, with enclosure of the anus and rectum in a plastic bag. Denmark, Norway, and Sweden implemented the plastic bag technique from 1990–1995 onwards and reduced but did not eliminate human yersiniosis. Pig herds free from pathogenic Y. enterocolitica O:3 have now been established in Norway (Nesbakken et al. 2007), and have been suggested to be the next stage in increasing the general safety of pig meat, as they also have no Salmonella, Toxoplasma and Trichinella, but remain carriers of Campylobacter. Christiansen (1987) also advised that meat should not be refrigerated for prolonged periods before consumption because of the unique ability of Yersinia to multiply at 4°C. Consumption of uncooked meats, like chitterlings in the USA, or other raw pork foodstuffs in Belgium and Germany, should be avoided.

Transfusion associated yersiniosis could be reduced by screening donors for histories of recent diarrhoea or fever. However, some of the donors involved in these contaminated transfusions were reported to be asymptomatic. It is not practical in blood banks to culture all blood before it is transfused. Antibody testing is insufficiently sensitive and specific. Leucodepletion is now practiced in most blood transfusion centres (primarily to prevent non-haemolytic febrile transfusion reactions and alloimmunization to HLA antigens) and this reduces (Gong et al. 1994) but does not eliminate (Leclercq et al. 2005) the risk of Yersinia blood contamination.

Plague

Introduction

Plague is a disease of animals and humans caused by one bacterial species, Y.pestis. The most common clinical form in humans is acute febrile lymphadenitis, called bubonic plague. Less common forms include septicaemic, pneumonic and meningeal plague. Mortality is high in untreated plague, but early antibiotic treatment reduced mortality significantly. The major animal reservoirs are rodents, principally urban and domestic rats as well as squirrels and prairie dogs and field mice, and less commonly rabbits, cats, and other carnivores. Transmission among animals and from animals to man occurs mainly by flea bites and less commonly by ingestion, by inhalation of infected respiratory tract secretions, and by handling infected animals tissues. Plague is endemic in several countries of Africa, Asia, and South America and in the southwestern USA, but is absent from Europe, Canada, Australia, and Japan. Control of plague requires avoidance of human contact with infected animals, selectively trapping and killing animals, and applying insecticidal dusts. From the 1980s onward, the majority of human cases have been in Africa, with the island of Madagascar reporting most cases.

History

Plague is a disease of antiquity that has persisted to modern times. Epidemic bubonic plague was vividly described in biblical and medieval times. This disease was estimated to have killed one quarter of Europe's population in the Middle Ages. The present pandemic of plague began in China in the 1860s and spread to Hong Kong in the 1890s. The genus is called Yersinia because Alexandre Yersin (1863–1943) went to Hong Kong in 1894 and successfully isolated the causative organism in pure culture. This pandemic was subsequently spread by rats transported on ships to California and port cities of South America, Africa and Asia. Transmission by flea bites was suggested by Ogata in 1897. Efficiency of Xenopsylla cheopis fleas for transmission of plague by blockage of swallowing was shown by Bacot and Martin in 1914. Urban plague transmitted by rats was brought under control in most affected cities, but the infection was transferred to sylvatic rodents, which allowed it to become entrenched in rural areas of these countries. In the first half of this century, India was severely affected by plague epidemics and suffered more than 10 million deaths. In 1948, streptomycin was shown to reduce sharply the case fatality rate in humans. In the 1960s and 1970s, Vietnam became the leading country for plague; during the war it reported more than 10,000 cases a year (Butler 2009). Before 1970, Y.pestis was called by its earlier name, Pasteurella pestis.

Vaccines using either attenuated strains or killed cultures of Y.pestis, were developed by Haffkine in India, the USA Army, and the Pasteur Institute. Vaccines were used widely in the Second World War. During the Vietnam war, more than 10 million Vietnamese people were vaccinated with the attenuated EV76 strain of Y.pestis. Neither killed vaccines or live attenuated EV76-based vaccines are currently available in most parts of the world.

The agent

Yersinia pestis is a Gram-negative bipolar-staining bacillus that belongs to the bacterial family Enterobacteriaceae. It grows aerobically on most culture media, including blood agar and MacConkey agar. It does not ferment lactose and forms small colonies on MacConkey agar after 24 hour incubation at 35°C. On triple-sugar-iron agar, Y.pestis produces an alkaline slant and acid butt. It is non-motile and negative for citrate utilization, urease and indole.

A plethora of genetic information is available on Yersinia pestis because it was one of the first bacteria for which a genome sequence was obtained (Parkhill *et al.* 2001), and multiple strains of the organism have now been sequenced (Chain *et al.* 2006; Deng *et al.* 2002; Eppinger *et al.* 2010; Liang *et al.* 2010; Song *et al.* 2004).

Like the other yersiniae, the plague bacillus possesses the virulence plasmid pYV/pCD1 which encodes a Type III secretion system with neutralizing effects on host macrophages. Unlike the other yersiniae, the pYV specified Yad adhesin and chromosomal invasin are inactivated, and there are two additional plasmids pPst and pFra which encode properties essential for the flea transmission lifecycle. Yersinia pestis is a clone derived from Y. pseudotuberculosis in the recent evolutionary past (9,000–40,000 years) (Achtman *et al.* 1999). Phylogeographic data suggests that the origin of all current pandemic Y. pestis strains was in central Asia (Achtman *et al.* 2004; Li *et al.* 2009). The genetic basis of the key functional changes involved in the evolution of an arthropod-borne system pathogen (Y. pestis) from an enteric pathogen (Y. pseudotuberculosis) has been the subject of several reviews (Brubaker 2004; Prentice and Rahalison 2007; Wren 2003; Zhou and Yang 2009). The complex choreography of Y. pestis effectors acting on the immune system throughout the course of mammalian infection has recently been reviewed (Li and Yang 2008; Smiley 2008).

The hosts

Fleas

The classical (and very effective) flea vector is Xenopsylla cheopis (Bacot and Martin 1914), the Oriental rat flea, but many other fleas can transmit plague (Gage and Kosoy 2005). Following ingestion in a blood meal Y. pestis multiplies and forms biofilm-embedded aggregates in the flea midgut and spine-filled proventriculus (a valve connecting the oesophagus to the midgut). In X. cheopis and some other fleas, bacterial growth in biofilm blocks the proventriculus preventing blood passage from the foregut to the midgut, causing the flea to starve. Blockage occurs 2 weeks after infection and blocked fleas die within a few days but make persistent attempts to feed, regurgitating oesophageal contents and inoculating Y. pestis and biofilm into each bite site. Biofilm synthesis requires the chromosomal hms locus (Hinnebusch *et al.* 1996; Jarrett *et al.* 2004). The ability to colonize and multiply in the flea midgut also requires the phospholipase D encoded by the ymt gene on the pFra plasmid (Hinnebusch *et al.* 2002). Y. pseudotuberculosis is orally toxic for X. cheopis, causing diarrhoea, presumably due to insect toxins inactivated in Y. pestis (Erickson *et al.* 2007). The relatively high bacterial load required to infect the flea, combined with the small volume of the blood meal, imposes a requirement for high numbers of circulating bacteria per unit volume of mammalian blood to maintain the transmission cycle (Lorange *et al.* 2005).

Historically, blockage was thought to be required for efficient transmission of infection by fleas, but recent experiments show flea vectors (Eisen *et al.* 2006), including X. cheopis (Eisen *et al.* 2009), are infectious within a day after a blood meal containing Y. pestis, and may be infectious without ever becoming blocked. The possible previous underestimation of duration of infectivity of the vector has important implications for mathematical models of the transmission dynamics of plague epizootics and analyses of historical plague outbreaks.

Animals

Throughout the world, the urban and domestic rats Rattus rattus and R. norvegicus are the most important reservoirs, of the plague bacillus. In sylvatic foci of plague, such as occur in the USA, the important reservoirs are the ground squirrel, rock squirrel, and prairie dog. Rabbits and domestic cats are occasionally infected and can bring disease to man. Each endemic area has its own prominent host species. For example, in Brazil, the most numerous infected animal is the field mouse, Zygodontomys pixuna.

Y.pestis dissemination from the initial fleabite in the mammalian host is dependent on plasminogen activator Pla, encoded by the small pPst plasmid. This surface protease also degrades complement and adheres to the cell matrix laminin (Sodeinde *et al.* 1992; Welkos *et al.* 1997). It is essential for primary pneumonic plague (Lathem *et al.* 2007) and for bubo formation (Sebbane *et al.* 2006). After entry into the host, Y. pestis is taken up by neutrophils and macrophages. While most of the bacteria taken up by neutrophils are killed (Laws *et al.* 2010; Spinner *et al.* 2008), those inside macrophages survive (Cavanaugh and Randall 1959; Lukaszewski *et al.* 2005; Pujol *et al.* 2009) and are transported to the regional lymph nodes and spleen (Titball *et al.* 2003). During the course of infection, bacteria escape from macrophages (Lukaszewski *et al.* 2005) and replicate extracellularly as the pYV-specified Type III secretion system (injectisome) and pFra-specified fimbrial capsule forming proteins Caf or fraction 1 (F1) antigen prevent their further phagocytosis (Du *et al.* 2002). In the absence of Yad in Y. pestis the chromosomally encoded Ail adhesin (Felek and Krukonis 2009) binds the host immune effector cell as a preliminary for injectisome action. The type III effector LcrV is present in large amounts in infected foci and has an anti-inflammatory action, stimulating IL-10 production (Brubaker 2003). Similarly, Y. pestis lipopolysaccharide (LPS) is modified on entering the host to minimize stimulation of the host Toll-like receptor 4 (TLR-4) (Rebeil *et al.* 2004), reducing the potentially protective host inflammatory response (Montminy *et al.* 2006) and prolonging survival with high grade bacteraemia (and therefore the infective window for fleas). The chromosomal yersiniabactin locus is essential for the pathogenesis of both bubonic and pneumonic plague in mice (Bearden *et al.* 1997; Fetherston *et al.* 2010). The involved lymph nodes show polymorphonuclear leucocytes, destruction of normal architecture, haemorrhagic necrosis and extracellular bacteria.

Conventionally, disease in animals is thought to occur in enzootic (maintenance) cycles that cause little apparent host mortality because transmission occurs by resident fleas between partially resistant rodents (enzootic or maintenance hosts). Obvious outbreaks with die-offs (epizootics) may occur as a result of disease spread from enzootic hosts to highly susceptible animals, (epizootic or amplifying hosts), or by increased spread within the enzootic host population (Gage and Kosoy 2005; Wimsatt and Biggins 2009). The precipitating cause for an epizootic may ultimately be related to environmental factors (Kausrud *et al.* 2007).

In the central Asian regions where plague originally emerged, there are enzootic Y. pestis strains (originally called Yersinia pestoides) which are localized in distribution, showing no evidence of pandemic spread. They do not cause human disease because they are attenuated in many mammalian species, including guinea pigs and primates (while possessing the Y. pestis-specific plasmids and virulence factors), but are virulent in rodents (Anisimov *et al.* 2004;

Song *et al.* 2004). These are now termed *Yersinia pestis* subspecies altaica, caucasica, hissarica, ulegeica, and talassica, and usually have some phenotypic features more typical of *Y. pseudotuberculosis* than *Y. pestis*, such as fermentation of rhamnose and melibiose and expression of aspartase (Bearden *et al.* 2009). An atypical *Y. pestis* strain from Africa (strain Angola) shares some of these features of pestoides strains, and single nucleotide polymorphism (SNP) phylogenetic analysis places it very distantly from pandemic *Y. pestis* strains, and closer to a common origin with the pestoides strains. It is non-lethal for guinea pigs, and lethal by subcutaneous injection and aerosol for mice but its virulence for humans is uncertain (Eppinger *et al.* 2010).

Humans

The most common presentation is bubonic plague. During an incubation period of 2–8 days following the bite of an infected flea, bacteria proliferate in the regional lymph nodes. Patients are typically affected by the sudden onset of fever, chills, weakness, and headache. Usually at the same time, after a few hours or on the next day, patients notice the bubo, which is signalled by intense pain in one anatomic region of lymph nodes, usually the groin, axilla, or neck. A swelling evolves in this area, which is so tender that the patients typically avoid any motion that would provoke discomfort.

The buboes of patients with plague are oval swellings that vary from 1 to 10 cm in length and elevate the overlying skin, which may appear stretched or erythematous. They may appear either as smooth, uniform, egg shaped masses or as an irregular cluster of several nodes with intervening and surrounding oedema. There is warmth of the overlying skin and an underlying, firm, non-fluctuant mass. Around the lymph nodes there is usually considerable oedema, which can be either gelatinous or pitting in nature. Although infections other than plague can produce acute lymphadenitis, plague is virtually unique for the suddenness of onset of the fever and bubo, the rapid development of intense inflammation in the bubo, and the fulminant clinical course that can produce death as quickly as 2–4 days after the onset of symptoms.

Body temperature is elevated, in the range of 38.5–40.0°C, blood pressures are characteristically low, in the range of 100/60 mmHg, due to extreme vasodilation. Lower pressures that are unobtainable may occur if shock ensues. The liver and spleen are often palpable and tender (Crook and Tempest 1992).

The majority of patients with bubonic plague do not have skin lesions, however, about one quarter of the patients in Vietnam did show varied skin findings. The most common were pustules, vesicles, eschars, or papules near the bubo or in the anatomic region of skin that is lymphatically drained by the affected lymph nodes, presumably representing sites of the flea bites. Rarely, these skin lesions progress to extensive cellulitis or abscesses. Ulceration, however, may lead to a large plague carbuncle.

Another kind of skin lesion in plague is purpura, which is a result of the systemic disease. The purpuric lesions may become necrotic, resulting in gangrene of distal extremities, the probable basis of the epithet 'Black Death' attributed to plague through the ages. These purpuric lesions contain blood vessels affected by vasculitis and occlusion by fibrin thrombi, resulting in haemorrhage and necrosis.

A distinctive feature of plague, in addition to the bubo, is the propensity of the disease to overwhelm patients with a massive growth of bacteria in the blood. In the early acute states of bubonic plague, all patients probably have intermittent bacteraemia. Single blood cultures obtained at the time of hospital admission in Vietnamese patients were positive in 27% of cases. A hallmark of moribund patients with plague is high density bacteraemia, so that a blood smear revealing characteristic bacilli has been used as a prognostic indicator in this disease. Occasionally in the pathogeniesis of plague infection, bacteria are inoculated and proliferate in the body without producing a bubo. Patients may become ill with fever and actually die with bacteraemia but without detectable lymphadenitis (Hull *et al.* 1987). This syndrome has been termed 'septicaemic plague' to denote plague without a bubo.

One of the feared complications of bubonic plague is secondary pneumonia. The infection reaches the lungs by haematogenous spread of bacteria from the bubo. In addition to the high mortality, plague pneumonia is highly contagious by airborne transmission. It presents in the setting of fever and lymphadenopathy as cough, chest pain and often haemoptysis. Radiographically there is patchy bronchopneumonia, cavities, or confluent consolidation (Centres for Disease Control (CDC) 1992). The sputum is usually purulent and contains plague bacilli.

Primary inhalation pneumonia is rare now but is a potential threat following exposure to a patient with plague who has a cough. Recent cases in the USA were exposed to sick domestic cats that had pneumonia or submandibular abscess (Gage *et al.* 2000). Public health consideration has been given to the scenario of an outbreak of primary pneumonic plague in non-plague endemic regions (or an urban area where plague is rarely seen), representing a deliberate release of aerosolized *Y. pestis* bacteria in a bioterrorist attack (Inglesby *et al.* 2000). Plague pneumonia is invariably fatal when antibiotic therapy is delayed more than 1 day after the onset of illness.

Plague meningitis is a rarer complication and typically occurs more than 1 week following inadequately treated bubonic plague. It results from haematogenous spread from a bubo and carries a high mortality rate compared with that of uncomplicated bubonic plague. There appears to be an association between buboes located in the axilla and the development of meningitis. Less commonly, plague meningitis presents as a primary infection of the meninges without antecedent lymphadenitis. Plague meningitis is characterized by fever, headache, meningismus, and pleocytosis with predominance of polymorphonuclear leucocytes. Bacteria are frequently demonstrable with a Gram-stain of spinal fluid sediment, and endotoxin has been demonstrated in spinal fluid.

Plague can produce pharyngitis that may resemble acute tonsillitis. The anterior cervical lymph nodes are usually inflamed, and *Y. pestis* may be recovered from a throat culture or by aspiration of a cervical bubo. This is a rare clinical form of plague that is presumed to follow the inhalation or ingestion of plague bacilli.

Plague presents sometimes with prominent gastrointestinal symptoms of nausea, vomiting, diarrhea, and abdominal pain. These symptoms may precede the bubo or in septicaemic plague, occur without a bubo and commonly result in diagnostic delay.

Diagnosis

A bacteriological diagnosis is readily made in most patients by smear and culture of a bubo aspirate. The aspirate is obtained by inserting a 20 gauge needle on a 10 ml syringe containing 1 ml of sterile saline into the bubo and withdrawing it several times until the saline becomes blood tinged. Because the bubo does not contain liquid pus, it may be necessary to inject some of the saline and immediately re-aspirate it. Drops of the aspirate should be placed on to microscopic slides and air dried for both Gram- and Wayson's stains. The Gram-stain will reveal polymorphonuclear leucocytes and Gram-negative coccobacilli and bacilli ranging from 1 to 2 um in length. In Wayson's stain, Yersinia pestis appears as light blue bacilli with dark blue polar bodies, and the remainder of the slide has a contrasting pink counterstain. Smears of blood, sputum, or spinal fluid can be handled similarly (Butler *et al.* 1976).

The aspirate, blood and other appropriate fluid should be inoculated on to blood and MacConkey agar plates and into infusion broth. CIN agar can be used for non-sterile samples such as sputum. Because of the scarcity of laboratory facilities in countries and regions where Y. pestis is commonest in humans, and the significance of Yersinia pestis isolation in a non-endemic area, the World Health Organization (WHO) recommends an initial presumptive diagnosis followed by reference laboratory confirmation (WHO 2006). In the USA, national diagnostic facilities for plague have existed since 1999 in the federal Laboratory Response Network (LRN) (http://www.bt.cdc.gov/lrn/). Y. pestis is defined as a 'select agent' in the USA by the Public Health Security and Bioterrorism Preparedness and Response Act of 2002, and this act and the Patriot Act of 2001, apply to all USA laboratories working with Y. pestis. Reference laboratory tests include direct immunofluorescence for F1 antigen, specific PCR for the F1 capsular antigen, the pesticin gene, and the plasminogen activator gene, and specific bacteriophage lysis. PCR can also be applied to diagnostic specimens, as can direct immunofluorescence for F1 antigen (produced in large amounts by Y. pestis) by slide microscopy. An immunochromatographic test strip for F1 antigen detection in patient specimens has been assessed in endemic areas (Chanteau *et al.* 2003; WHO 2008a). This is effective for laboratory and near patient use, but is not currently commercially available. Other commercial rapid diagnostic kits for agents including Y. pestis have been described, but none is widely used for primary or reference laboratory identification. Retrospective serological diagnosis may be made by rising titres of haemagglutinating antibody to F1 antigen. ELISA tests for anti-F1 IgG and IgM antibodies are also available.

Treatment

Early treatment of patients with antibiotics is life saving. Untreated plague has an estimated mortality rate of greater than 50%. Historically, streptomycin was the parenteral treatment of choice for plague. In view of the side effect profile of streptomycin and its current limited availability, gentamicin is now recommended instead (Butler 2009; Inglesby *et al.* 2000). Gentamicin was safe and effective in clinical trials of plague therapy in Tanzania and Madagascar (Mwengee *et al.* 2006; WHO 2006), and in retrospective case review in the US (Boulanger *et al.* 2004; WHO 2006). Tetracyclines are an effective oral alternative, but are not recommended in children under 7 because of tooth discoloration. Doxycycline is the tetracycline of choice, at an oral dose of 100 mg bd . Ten days therapy is recommended for plague.

Poor response to penicillins has been seen in some clinical cases (Boulanger *et al.* 2004): β-lactams and macrolides are not generally recommended as first line therapy. Chloramphenicol is recommended alone or in combination for focal plague complications (meningitis, endophthalmitis, myocarditis) because of its tissue penetration properties. Quinolones are effective *in vitro* and in

animal models, and recommended in guidelines for possible bioterrorism-associated pneumonic plague (Inglesby *et al.* 2000).

A wild-type Y. pestis strain resistant to multiple antimicrobials was first reported from Madagascar in 1997 (Galimand *et al.* 1997) and subsequently a different strain resistant to the first-line antibiotic streptomycin was also identified (Guiyoule *et al.* 2001). Both plasmids responsible for these resistance patterns were self-transferrable to other bacteria, and one was substantially identical to a plasmid seen in numerous multidrug resistant enterobacterial strains isolated from retail meat in the USA (Welch *et al.* 2007). Fortunately, no other Y. pestis strains with multiple antimicrobial resistance have subsequently been isolated in Madagascar (Chanteau *et al.* 2004).

The buboes usually recede without need of local therapy. Occasionally, however, they may enlarge or become fluctuant during the first week of treatment, requiring incision and drainage. The aspirated fluid should be cultured for evidence of superinfection with other bacteria, but this material is usually sterile.

Epidemiology

Plague occurs worldwide, with most of the human cases reported from developing countries of Asia and Africa. Between 1989 and 2003, 38,359 cases of plague were reported to the WHO. More than 80% of these cases were in Africa, and the percentage of all cases in Africa increased over this time period, most in East Africa and the island of Madagascar. Recent pneumonic plague outbreaks were recorded in Uganda, Democratic Republic of the Congo, and China.

In North America, enzootic plague is present in the western side of the continent from southwestern Canada to Mexico, following introduction via the port of San Francisco in 1900 (Adjemian *et al.* 2007). Most human cases in the US occur in two regions: the 'Four Corners' (northern New Mexico, northern Arizona, and southern Colorado), and further west in California, southern Oregon, and western Nevada (http://www.cdc.gov/ncidod/dvbid/plague/epi. htm). 107 cases of plague were reported in the USA 1990–2005, a median of seven cases annually, most cases occurring from May to October when people are outdoors and rodents and their fleas are most plentiful. The last person to person transmission of plague in the USA occurred in 1925 (Kool 2005). Infection is most often acquired by fleabite in or around the home. Infection can also occur following handling living or dead small mammals (rabbits, hares, and prairie dogs), or larger carnivores (wildcats, coyotes, or mountain lions). Dogs and cats may bring plague-infected fleas into the home and infected cats may transmit pneumonic plague to humans (Fig. 21.2) (Gage *et al.* 2000).

In the epizoology of urban plague, the domestic black rat R. rattus has probably been the most important host historically. It climbs well, inhabits ships as well as houses, and is a good host for the efficient plague flea vector X. cheopis. Plague in other than urban setting, however, has taken on many complex variations. The classic theory of plague reservoirs requires one or more relatively resistant small mammal species, which service as the enzootic reservoir species, and one or more relatively susceptible species, which serve as the epizootic hosts and may be involved in the so called rate die offs or ratfalls. In urban plague, the same species of rats can be both the enzootic andepizootic species, whereas tin rural or sylvatic plague, there are usually two or more separate species. For example in India, Baltazard and Bahmanyar (1960a)

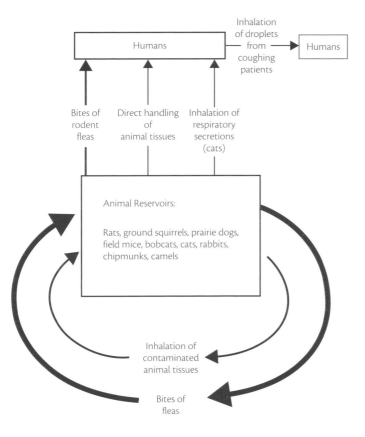

Fig. 21.2 Transmission of plague among animal reservoirs and from animals to humans and from humans to humans. Wide arrows indicate common transmission, medium arrows indicate occasional transmission, and thin arrows indicate rare transmission.

Issacson *et al.* (1981) in South Africa examined the susceptibility of Mastomys to experimental plague infection and found that M. natalensis was relatively resistant to fatal infection, as shown by a 50% death rate after a dose of 19 x 10⁵ bacteria given subcutaneously. By contrast, another species, called Mastomys coucha, which differs from other species by having diploid chromosomes of numbers 32 and 36, was susceptible to death when inoculated with only 1.9 x 10² bacteria. This suggests that genetically determined differences among species of rodents could allow the same genus to provide a relatively resistant enzootic reservoir and a more susceptible epizootic reservoir for plague infection. In Tanzania, a serosurvey of rodents in the active focus of Lushoto District in the 1980s revealed that several species were infected (Kilonzo *et al.* 1992). The most numerous seropositive species were R.rattus and M.natalensis.

Some of the fluctuations in plague occurrence have been related to changing populations of the rodent reservoirs. In Indian cities, Seal (1960) described replacement of R.rattus by B.bengalensis at the same time that human plague diminished. Although both rodents were good hosts for Y.pestis, R. rattus was more heavily parasitized with the efficient flea vector X.cheopis than were the bandicoot rats. The virtual elimination of plague infection from India after 1950 was an astonishing event and could have other explanations. One possibility is that insecticide spraying to control mosquitoes as vectors of malaria also had a controlling effect on the fleas that transmitted plague. In 1994 two plague outbreaks in the North West of India (bubonic plague in Maharashtra State and pneumonic plague in Gujarat State) were clinically diagnosed almost simultaneously, causing local and international concern and major social and economic disruption (Ramalingaswami 1995). Definite bacteriological diagnosis was not possible until well after the outbreaks were controlled, because of culture contamination, and some molecular tests (ribotyping) suggested the isolates were unusual, but they were subsequently confirmed to be Y. pestis (Shivaji *et al.* 2000). Occasional further outbreaks of plague have since been reported from India, but it remains rare in that country.

Another part of the epizoology of plague is the relationship of the potential flea vectors to their mammalian hosts. Generally, the flea species that are narrowly adapted to a particular host are so poorly adapted to man that they only have transient existences on man, but this can, of course, be long enough for a few bites and the transmission of the plague. The human flea Pulex irritans is not an efficient plague vector and rarely, if ever has been shown to transmit plague from man to man. Recently, however, the density of P. irritans and the P. irritans flea index has been noted to be higher in villages in Tanzania with a higher incidence of plague (Laudisoit *et al.* 2007).

The proliferation of fleas on rodents is believed to be crucial for the propagation of plague epizootics, as quantified by the flea index (the average number of fleas per rodent). When the flea index is high, that is, exceeding one, the chances for an epizootic among rodents are great. The multiplication of fleas on rodents is highly seasonal, being greatest in the warm and dry times when epidemics are most likely to occur. In Vietnam, the rainy season curtailed sharply the transmission of plague and concomitantly reduced flea indices (Olsen 1960).

Although rodent fleas are specific for their host species and, thus, are rarely exchanged, the intermingling of different rodent species and their fleas has been observed in the field and might

found that the field gerbil Tatera indica was resistant to plague and served as the enzootic reservoir. The domestic rats were 'liaison rodents', carrying plague from gerbils to man. In Java, the resistant field species was R.exulans and again the domestic rats were merely liaisons to man (Balazard and Bahmanuar 1960b). In the sylvatic plague that occurs in the USA, the ecology of plague does not neatly fit this pattern. Although the colonizing rodents, ground squirrels, and prairie dogs have frequently brought plague to man, the resistant enzootic species has been difficult to define. Kartman *et al.* (1958) suggested that the meadow vole was responsible for enzooticity in California. More recently in New Mexico and Arizona, the carnivorous coyotes and bobcats, as well as rabbits, were shown to be infected with plague, but the modes of transmission among these animals remain to be delineated.

In Vietnam, the brown street rate R.norvegicus was an important plague reservoir, in addition to R.rattus. The house shrew S.murinus also carried plague and appeared to be an important host for carrying infection to man (Cavanaugh *et al.* 1968; 1969).

In Africa, the wild rodent complex Mastomys natalensis has been demonstrated to be an important reservoir for the maintenance of both plague and the virus of Lassa fever by Green *et al.* (1978).

explain the migration of plague from an urban focus to a sylvatic focus and vice versa. The wild rodent flea M.telchinum was found on the urban rat R.norvegicus in San Francisco in 1938 (Kartman *et al.* 1958). Furthermore, rodent fleas have been found on dogs. Fleas of domestic dogs and cats have been implicated in the transmission of plague to man in the USA (von Reyn *et al.* 1977), but infection of these fleas with Y.pestis has only rarely been identified. Dogs in Tanzania were frequently seropositive for plague and carried approximately eight fleas per dog (Kilonzo *et al.* 1993). However, it is not known whether dogs played any role in the transmission of infection or they were simply a 'dead end' transmission following the ingestion of infected rodents.

Prevention and control

Plague is a notifiable disease in all countries with Public Health systems. In 2007 the second edition of the International Health Regulations (IHR) came into force (WHO 2008b) requiring the reporting to the WHO of any disease event which could cause a serious public health impact or spread rapidly internationally. For plague, this means reporting of all cases of pneumonic plague, or any suspected case of plague in a non-plague endemic area (WHO 2008a). The first edition of the IHR required reporting of any case of plague by all national authorities.

Patients with uncomplicated infections who are promptly treated present no health hazards to other persons. Those with cough or other signs of pneumonia must be placed in strict respiratory isolation for at least 48 hours after the institution of antibiotic therapy or until the sputum culture is negative after the institution of antibiotic therapy. Droplet precautions (including wearing disposable surgical masks) are recommended for those in close contact with suspected pneumonic plague patients—see Kool (2005) for the rationale for this. The bubo aspirate and blood must be handled with gloves and with care to avoid the formation of aerosols of these infected fluids. Laboratory workers who process the cultures should be alerted to exercise Category 3 precautions.

A formalin killed vaccine from the USA (which was not protective against primary pneumonic plague), was formerly used for travellers to endemic areas and laboratory workers, but is not currently available. A live attenuated vaccine EV76 is used in countries of the Former Soviet Union (Anisimov *et al.* 2004), but has significant side effects. A subunit vaccine composed of recombinant F1 and V proteins, which may protect against primary pneumonic plague, has gone through phase II clinical trials in humans, but is not yet licensed (Williamson 2009). The last large-scale use of plague vaccines was in American military personnel in Vietnam in 1965–75 and in Vietnamese civilians during the same years. Persons living in endemic areas should provide themselves with as much personal protection against rodents and fleas as possible, including living in rat proofed houses, wearing shoes and garments to cover the legs, and applying insecticide dusts to house when plague is anticipated.

Once an epidemic of plague has been identified by confirming the infection in several human case in one locality, the explosive epidemic potential of plague requires emergency action on the part of public health authorities. The first step is to ensure that medical facilities, personnel and antibiotics are available in the locality for treating human cases. This medical treatment will save lives but will have no significant impact on prevention because nearly all human cases result from bites of infected rodent fleas.

The next step is to prevent human cases by interrupting transmission of infection from the animal reservoirs caused by flea bites. Before embarking on any strategic plan, local health authorities should report the epidemic to the central health authorities. The WHO should be notified and would likely respond by offering advice and help. The interested reader should consult publications from the WHO regarding plague diagnosis and control (Dennis *et al.* 1999; WHO 2006).

Acknowledgement

This chapter includes sections based on the contribution of Professor Thomas C. Butler in the First Edition of this volume.

References

Abdel-Haq, N. M., Asmar, B. I., Abuhammour, W. M., and Brown, W. J. (2000). Yersinia enterocolitica infection in children. *Pediatr. Infect. Dis. J.,* **19**: 954–58.

Achtman, M., Zurth, K., Morelli, G., Torrea, G., Guiyoule, A., et al. (1999). Yersinia pestis, the cause of plague, is a recently emerged clone of Yersinia pseudotuberculosis. *Proc. Natl. Acad. Sci. USA.,* **96**: 14043–48.

Achtman, M., Morelli, G., Zhu, P., et al. (2004). Microevolution and history of the plague bacillus, Yersinia pestis. *Proc. Natl. Acad. Sci. USA.,* **101**: 17837–42.

Adjemian, J. Z., Foley, P., Gage, K. L., and Foley, J. E. (2007). Initiation and spread of traveling waves of plague, Yersinia pestis, in the Western United States. *Am. J. Trop. Med. Hyg.,* **76**: 365–75.

Aleksic, S., et al. (1987). Yersinia rodhei sp. nov. isolated from human and dog feces and surface water. *Inter. J. System. Bacteriol.,* **37**(4): 327–32.

Anisimov, A. P., Lindler, L. E., and Pier, G. B. (2004). Intraspecific diversity of Yersinia pestis. *Clin. Microbiol. Rev.,* **17**: 434–64.

Anon. (1997). Red blood cell transfusions contaminated with Yersinia enterocolitica—United States 1991–1996 and initiation of a national study to detect bacteria-associated transfusion reactions. MMWR, **46**: 553–55.

Autenrieth, S. E., and Autenrieth, I. B. (2007). Yersinia enterocolitica: Subversion of adaptive immunity and implications for vaccine development. *Int. J. Med. Microbiol.,* **29**(1–2):69–77.

Bacot, A., and Martin, C. (1914). Observations on the mechanism of the transmission of plague by fleas. *J. Hyg.,* **13**: 423–39.

Baltazard, M., and Bahmanyar, M. (1960a). Recherches sur la peste en Inde. *Bull. Wor. Heal. Organ.,* **23**: 169–215.

Baskin, G. B., Montali, R. J., Bush, M., Quan, T. J., and Smith, E. (1977). Yersiniosis in captive exotic mammals. *J. Am. Vet. Med. Assoc.,* **171**: 908–912.

Bearden, S. W., Fetherston, J. D., and Perry, R. D. (1997). Genetic organization of the yersiniabactin biosynthetic region and construction of avirulent mutants in Yersinia pestis. *Infect. Immun.,* **65**: 1659–68.

Bearden, S. W., Sexton, C., Pare, J., Fowler, J. M., Arvidson, C. G., et al. (2009). Attenuated enzootic (pestoides) isolates of Yersinia pestis express active aspartase. *Microbiol.,* **155**: 198–209.

Bercovier, H., et al. (1980). Y. kristensenii, a new species of Enterobacteriaceae composed of sucrose negative strains. *Curr. Microbiol.,* **4**: 219–24.

Bercovier, H., et al. (1984).Yersinia aldovae (formerly Yersinia enterocolitica-like group X2): A new species of Enterobacteriaceae isolated from aquatic ecosystems. *Inter. J. System. Bacteriol.,* **34**(2): 166–75.

Bhaduri, S., & Wesley, I. (2006). Isolation and characterization of Yersinia enterocolitica from swine feces recovered during the National Animal Health Monitoring System Swine 2000 study. *J. Food Prot.,* **69**: 2107–12.

Bielli, M., Lauzi, S., Pratelli, A., Martini, M., Dall'Ara, P., et al. (1999). Pseudotuberculosis in marmosets, tamarins, and Goeldi's monkeys (Callithrichidae/Callimiconidae) housed at a European zoo. *J. Zoo. Wildl. Med.,* **30**: 532–36.

Black, R. E., *et al.* (1978). Epidemic Yersinia enterocolitica infection due to contaminated chocolate milk. *N. Engl. J. Med.*, **298**: 76–79.

Bottone, E. J. (1999). Yersinia enterocolitica: overview and epidemiologic correlates. *Microbes Infect.*, **1**: 323–33.

Boulanger, L. L., Ettestad, P., Fogarty, J. D., Dennis, D. T., Romig, D., *et al.* (2004). Gentamicin and tetracyclines for the treatment of human plague: review of 75 cases in new Mexico, 1985–1999. *Clin. Infect. Dis.*, **38**: 663–69.

Brubaker, R. R. (2003). Interleukin-10 and inhibition of innate immunity to Yersiniae: roles of Yops and LcrV (V antigen). *Infect. Immun.*, **71**: 3673–81.

Brenner, D., *et al.* (1980). *Y. intermedia: a new species of Enterobacteriaceae composed of rhamnose-positive, melibiose-positive, raffinose-positive strains. Curr. Microbiol.*, **4**: 207–12.

Brubaker, R. R. (2004). The Recent Emergence of Plague: A Process of Felonious Evolution. *Microb. Ecol.*, **47**: 293–99.

Butler, T., *et al.* (1976). Yersinia pestis in Vietnam. II. Quantitative blood cultures and detection of endotoxin in the cerebrospinal fluid of patients with meningitis. *J. Infect. Dis.*, **133**: 493–99.

Butler, T. (2009). Plague into the 21st Century. *Clin. Infect. Dis.*, **49**: 736–42.

Cantinieaux, B., *et al.* (1988). Imparied neutrophil defense against Yersinia enterocolitica in patients with iron overload who are undergoing dialysis. *J. Lab. Clin. Med.*, **111**: 524–28.

Caroff, M., Bundle, D. R., and Perry, M. B. (1984). Structure of the O-chain of the phenol-phase soluble cellular lipopolysaccharide of Yersinia enterocolitica serotype O:9. *Eur. J. Biochem.*, **139**: 195–200.

Carniel, E., *et al.* (1986). Infrequent detection of Yersinia enterocolitica in childhood diarrhoea in Bangladesh. *Am. J. Trop. Med. Hyg.*, **35**: 370–71.

Cavanaugh, D. C. and Randall, R. (1959). Role of Multiplication of Pasteurella-Pestis in Mononuclear Phagocytes in the Pathogenesis of Flea-Borne Plague. *J. Immunol.*, **83**: 348–63.

Cavanaugh, D. C., *et al.* (1968). Some observations on the current plague outbreak in the Republic of Vietnam. *Am. J. Pub. Heal.*, **58**: 742–52.

Cavanaugh, D. C., Ryan, P. F., and Marshall, J. D. (1969). The role of commensal rodents and their ectoparasites in the ecology and transmission of plague in Southeast Asia. *Bull. Wildl. Dis. Assoc.*, **5**: 187–94.

Chain, P. S., Hu, P., Malfatti, S. A., Radnedge, L., Larimer, F., *et al.* (2006). Complete Genome Sequence of Yersinia pestis Strains Antiqua and Nepal516: Evidence of Gene Reduction in an Emerging Pathogen. *J. Bacteriol.*, **188**: 4453–63.

Chanteau, S., Rahalison, L., Ralafiarisoa, L., Foulon, J., Ratsitorahina, M., *et al.* (2003). Development and testing of a rapid diagnostic test for bubonic and pneumonic plague. *Lancet*, **361**: 211–16.

Chanteau, S., Madagascar, G., Carniel, E. C. S., Duchemin, J. B., Duplantier, J. M., *et al.* (2004). Atlas sur la Peste à Madagascar, pp. 53.

Chart, H., and Cheasty, T. (2006). The serodiagnosis of human infections with Yersinia enterocolitica and Yersinia pseudotuberculosis. *FEMS Immunol. Med. Microbiol.* **47**: 391–97.

Chen, P., *et al.* (2010).*Genomic characterization of the Yersinia genus. Genome Biol.*, **11**(1): R1.

Chiesa, C., Pacifico, L., Guiyoule, A., Ravagnan, G., and Mollaret, H. H. (1991). Phenotypic characterization and virulence of O8 Yersinia strains isolated in Europe. *Contrib. Microbiol. Immunol.*, **12**: 182–91.

Chiu, H. Y., *et al.* (1986). Infection with Yersinia enterocolitica in patients with iron overload. BMJ, 292: 97.

Clark, M. A., Hirst, B. H., and Jepson, M. A. (1998). M-cell surface beta1 integrin expression and invasin-mediated targeting of Yersinia pseudotuberculosis to mouse Peyer's patch M cells. *Infect. Immun.*, **66**: 1237–43.

Cornelis, G. R., Boland, A., Boyd, A. P., Geuijen, C., Iriarte, M., *et al.* (1998). The virulence plasmid of Yersinia, an antihost genome. *Microbiol. Mol. Biol. Rev.*, **62**: 1315–52.

Cornelis, G. R. (2002). The Yersinia Ysc-Yop 'type III' weaponry. *Nat. Rev. Mol. Cell. Biol.*, **3**: 742–52.

Cornelis, G. R. (2006). The type III secretion injectisome. *Nat. Rev. Microbiol.*, **4**: 811–25.

Crook, L. D., and Tempest, B. (1992). Plague. A clinical review of 27 cases. *Arch. Intern. Med.*, **152**: 1253–56.

Delor, I., Kaeckenbeeck, A., Wauters, G., and Cornelis, G. R. (1990). Nucleotide sequence of yst, the Yersinia enterocolitica gene encoding the heat-stable enterotoxin, and prevalence of the gene among pathogenic and nonpathogenic yersiniae. *Infect. Immun.*, **58**: 2983–88.

Deng, W., Burland, V., Plunkett III, G., *et al.* (2002). Genome sequence of Yersinia pestis KIM. *J. Bacteriol.* **184**: 4601–11.

Dennis, D. T., Gage, D., Gratz, N., Poland, J. D., and Tikhomirov, E. (1999). Plague manual: epidemiology, distribution, surveillance and control. Geneva: World Health Organization.

Dolina, M., and Peduzzi, R. (1993). *Population genetics of human, animal, and environmental Yersinia strains. Appl. Environ. Microbiol.*, **59**(2): 442–50.

Du, Y., Rosqvist, R., and Forsberg, A. (2002). Role of fraction 1 antigen of Yersinia pestis in inhibition of phagocytosis. *Infect. Immun.*, **70**: 1453–60.

Eisen, R. J., Bearden, S. W., Wilder, A. P., Montenieri, J. A., Antolin, M. F., *et al.* (2006). Early-phase transmission of Yersinia pestis by unblocked fleas as a mechanism explaining rapidly spreading plague epizootics. *Proc. Natl. Acad. Sci. USA*, **103**: 15380–85.

Eisen, R. J., Wilder, A. P., Bearden, S. W., Montenieri, J. A., and Gage, K. L. (2009). Early-Phase Transmission of Yersinia pestis by Unblocked Xenopsylla cheopis (Siphonaptera: Pulicidae) Is as Efficient as Transmission by Blocked Fleas. *J. Med. Entomol.*, **44**: 678–82.

Eitel, J., and Dersch, P. (2002). The YadA protein of Yersinia pseudotuberculosis mediates high-efficiency uptake into human cells under environmental conditions in which invasin is repressed. *Infect. Immun.*, **70**: 4880–91.

Eppinger, M., Worsham, P. L., Nikolich, M. P., Riley, D. R., Sebastian, Y., *et al.* (2010). Genome Sequence of the Deep-Rooted Yersinia pestis Strain Angola Reveals New Insights into the Evolution and Pangenome of the Plague Bacterium. *J. Bacteriol.*, **192**: 1685–99.

Erickson, D., Waterfield, N., Vadyvaloo, V., Long, D., Fischer, E., *et al.* (2007). Acute oral toxicity of Yersinia pseudotuberculosis to fleas: implications for the evolution of vector-borne transmission of plague. *Cell Microbiol.*, **9**: 2658–66.

Ewald, J. H., Heesemann Jr., R. H., & Autenrieth, I. B. (1994). Interaction of Polymorphonuclear Leukocytes with Yersinia enterocolitica: Role of the Yersinia Virulence Plasmid and Modulation by the Iron-Chelator Desferrioxamine B. *J. Infect. Dis.*, **170**: 140–50.

Ewing, W. H., *et al.* (1978). Yersinia ruckeri sp. nov., the Redmouth (RM) Bacterium. *Int. J. Syst. Bacteriol.*, **28**(1): 37–44.

Felek, S., and Krukonis, E. S. (2009). The Yersinia pestis Ail Protein Mediates Binding and Yop Delivery to Host Cells Required for Plague Virulence. *Infect. Immun.*, **77**: 825–36.

Fetherston, J. D., Kirillina, O., Bobrov, A. G., Paulley, J. T., and Perry, R. D. (2010). The yersiniabactin transport system is critical for the pathogenesis of bubonic and pneumonic plague. *Infect. Immun.*, **78**(5):2045–52.

Fuchs, T., Bresolin, G., Marcinowski, L., Schachtner, J., and Scherer, S. (2008). Insecticidal genes of Yersinia spp.: taxonomical distribution, contribution to toxicity towards Manduca sexta and Galleria mellonella, and evolution. *BMC Microbiol.*, **8**: 214.

Fukushima, H., Gomyoda, M., and Kaneko, S. (1990). *Mice and moles inhabiting mountainous areas of Shimane Peninsula as sources of infection with Yersinia pseudotuberculosis. J. Clin. Microbiol.*, **28**(11): 2448–55.

Gage, K. L., Dennis, D. T., Orloski, K. A., *et al.* (2000). Cases of cat-associated human plague in the Western US, 1977–1998. *Clin. Infect. Dis.*, **30**: 893–900.

Gage, K. L., and Kosoy, M. Y. (2005). Natural history of plague: perspectives from more than a century of research. *Ann. Rev. Entomol.*, **50**: 505–28.

Galimand, M., Guiyoule, A., Gerbaud, G., Rasoamanana, B., Chanteau, S., et al. (1997). Multidrug resistance in Yersinia pestis mediated by a transferable plasmid. N. Engl. J. Med., 337: 677–80.

Gayraud, M., Scavizzi, M. R., Mollaret, H. H., Guillevin, L., and Hornstein, M. J. (1993). Antibiotic treatment of Yersinia enterocolitica septicemia: a retrospective review of 43 cases. Clin. Infect. Dis., 17: 405–10.

Gibb, A. P., Martin, K. M., Davidson, G. A., Walker, B., and Murphy, W. G. (1994). Modeling the growth of Yersinia enterocolitica in donated blood. Transfus., 34: 304–10.

Gong, J., Rawal, B. D., Hogman, C. F., Vyas, G. N., Nilsson, B., et al. (1994). Complement killing of Yersinia enterocolitica and retention of the bacteria by leucocyte removal filters. Vox. Sang., 66: 166–70.

Granfors, K., Lahesmaa-Rantala, R., and Toivanen, A. (1988). IgM, IgG, and IgA Antibodies in Yersinia Infection. J. Infect. Dis., 157: 601–2.

Grant, T., Bennett-Wood, V., and Robins-Browne, R. M. (1998). Identification of virulence-associated characteristics in clinical isolates of Yersinia enterocolitica lacking classical virulence markers. Infect. Immun., 66: 1113–20.

Grutzkau, A., Hanski, C., Hahn, H., and Riecken, E. O. (1990). Involvement of M cells in the bacterial invasion of Peyer's patches: a common mechanism shared by Yersinia enterocolitica and other enteroinvasive bacteria. Gut, 31: 1011–15.

Guiyoule, A., Gerbaud, G., Buchrieser, C., Galimand, M., Rahalison, L., et al. (2001). Transferable plasmid-mediated resistance to streptomycin in a clinical isolate of Yersinia pestis. Emerg. Infect. Dis., 7: 43–48.

Heise, T. and Dersch, P. (2006). Identification of a domain in Yersinia virulence factor YadA that is crucial for extracellular matrix-specific cell adhesion and uptake. Proc. Natl. Acad. Sci. USA., 103: 3375–80.

Hinnebusch, B., Perry, R., and Schwan, T. (1996). Role of the Yersinia pestis hemin storage (hms) locus in the transmission of plague by fleas. Science, 273: 367–70.

Hinnebusch, B., Rudolph, A., Cherepanov, P., Dixon, J., Schwan, T., et al. (2002). Role of Yersinia murine toxin in survival of Yersinia pestis in the midgut of the flea vector. Sci., 296: 733–35.

Hoogkamp-Korstanje, J. A., Moesker, H., and Bruyn, G. A. (2000). Ciprofloxacin v placebo for treatment of Yersinia enterocolitica triggered reactive arthritis. Ann. Rheum. Dis., 59: 914–17.

Ibrahim, A., et al.,(1993). The phylogeny of the genus Yersinia based on 16S rDNA sequences. FEMS Microbiol. Lett., 114(2): 173–77.

Inglesby, T. V., Dennis, D. T., Henderson, D. A., et al. (2000). Plague as a biological weapon: medical and public health management. Work.ing Group on Civilian Biodefense. JAA, 283: 2281–90.

Jalava, K., Hallanvuo, S., Nakari, U. M., Ruutu, P., Kela, E., et al. (2004). Multiple Outbreaks of Yersinia pseudotuberculosis Infections in Finland. J. Clin. Microbiol., 42: 2789–91.

Jarrett, C. O., Deak, E., Isherwood, K. E., Oyston, P. C., Fischer, E. R., et al. (2004). Transmission of Yersinia pestis from an infectious biofilm in the flea vector. J. Infect. Dis., 190: 783–92.

Jones, T. F. (2003). From pig to pacifier: chitterling-associated yersiniosis outbreak among black infants. Emerg. Infect. Dis., 9:(8): 1007–9.

Kachoris, M., et al. (1988). Routine culture of stool specimens for Yersinia enterocolitica is not a cost effective procedure. J. Clin. Microbiol., 26: 582–83.

Kapperud, G. (1991). Yersinia enterocolitica in food hygiene. Intern. J. Food Microbiol., 12: 53–66.

Kartman, L., Prince, F. M., Quan, S. F., and Stark, H. E. (1958). New knowledge in the ecology of sylvatic plague. Ann. NY Acad. Sci., 70: 668–711.

Kausrud, K. L., Viljugrein, H., Frigessi, A., Begon, M., Davis, S., et al. (2007). Climatically driven synchrony of gerbil populations allows large-scale plague outbreaks. Proc. Biol. Sci., 274: 1963–69.

Kendrick, C. J., Baker, B., Morris, A. J., and O'Toole, P. W. (2001). Identification of Yersinia-infected blood donors by anti-Yop IgA immunoassay. Transfus., 41: 1365–72.

Kilonzo, B. S., Mbise, T. J., and Makundi, R. H. (1992). Plague in Lushoto district, Tanzania, 1980–1988. Trans. R. Soc. Trop. Med. Hyg., 86: 444–45.

Kirjavainen, V., Jarva, H., Biedzka-Sarek, M., Blom, A. M., Skurnik, M., et al. (2008). Yersinia enterocolitica Serum Resistance Proteins YadA and Ail Bind the Complement Regulator C4b-Binding Protein. PLoS Pathog., 4: e1000140.

Kool, J. L. (2005). Risk of person-to-person transmission of pneumonic plague. Clin. Infect. Dis., 40: 1166–72.

Kotetishvili, M., et al. (2005). Multilocus sequence typing for studying genetic relationships among Yersinia species. J. Clin. Microbiol., 43(6): 2674–84.

Kvien, T. K., Gaston, J. S., Bardin, T., et al. (2004). Three month treatment of reactive arthritis with azithromycin: a EULAR double blind, placebo controlled study. Ann. Rheum. Dis., 63: 1113–19.

Lathem, W. W., Price, P. A., Miller, V. L., and Goldman, W. E. (2007). A plasminogen-activating protease specifically controls the development of primary pneumonic plague. Sci., 315: 509–13.

Laudisoit, A., Leirs, H., Makundi, R. H., Van Dongen, S., Davis, S., et al. (2007). Plague and the human flea, Tanzania. Emerg. Infect. Dis., 13: 687–93.

Laukkanen, R., Martinez, P. O., Siekkinen, K. M., Ranta, J., Maijala, R., et al. (2008). Transmission of Yersinia pseudotuberculosis in the pork production chain from farm to slaughterhouse. Appl. Environ. Microbiol., 74: 5444–50.

Laws, T. R., Davey, M. S., Titball, R. W., and Lukaszewski, R. (2010). Neutrophils are important in early control of lung infection by Yersinia pestis. Microbes Infect., 12: 331–35.

Leclercq, A., Martin, L., Vergnes, M. L., Ounnoughene, N., Laran, J.-F., et al. (2005). Fatal Yersinia enterocolitica biotype 4 serovar O:3 sepsis after red blood cell transfusion. Transfus., 45: 814–18.

Lee, L. A., Gerber, A. R., Lonsway, D. R., et al. (1990). Yersinia enterocolitica O:3 infections in infants and children, associated with the household preparation of chitterlings. N. Engl. J. Med., 322: 984–87.

Lemaitre, B. C., Mazigh, D. A., and Scavizzi, M. R. (1991). Failure of beta-lactam antibiotics and marked efficacy of fluoroquinolones in treatment of murine Yersinia pseudotuberculosis infection. Antimicrob. Agents Chemother., 35: 1785–90.

Li, B., and Yang, R. (2008). Interaction between Yersinia pestis and the Host Immune System. Infect. Immun., 76: 1804–11.

Li, Y., Cui, Y., Hauck, Y., et al. (2009). Genotyping and phylogenetic analysis of Yersinia pestis by MLVA: insights into the worldwide expansion of Central Asia plague foci. PLoS One., 4(6): e6000.

Liang, Y., Hou, X., Wang, Y., et al. (2010). Genome Rearrangements of Completely Sequenced Strains of Yersinia pestis. J. Clin. Microbiol., 48(5):1619–23.

Ljungberg, P., Valtonen, M., Harjola, V. P., Kaukoranta-Tolvanen, S. S., and Vaara, M. (1995). Report of four cases of Yersinia pseudotuberculosis septicemia and a literature review. Eur. J. Clin. Microbiol. Infect. Dis., 14: 804–10.

Long, C., Jones, T. F., Vugia, D. J., Scheftel, J., Strockbine, N., et al. (2010). Yersinia pseudotuberculosis and Y. enterocolitica infections, FoodNet, 1996–2007. Emerg. Infect. Dis., 16: 566–67.

Lorange, E. A., Race, B. L., Sebbane, F., and Joseph Hinnebusch, B. (2005). Poor vector competence of fleas and the evolution of hypervirulence in Yersinia pestis. J. Infect. Dis., 191: 1907–12.

Lukaszewski, R. A., Kenny, D. J., Taylor, R., Rees, D. G., Hartley, M. G., et al. (2005). Pathogenesis of Yersinia pestis infection in BALB/c mice: effects on host macrophages and neutrophils. Infect. Immun., 73: 7142–50.

Mair, N. & Fox, E. (1986). Yersiniosis. London: Public Health Laboratory Service.

Maki-Ikola, O., Heesemann, J., Lahesmaa, R., Toivanen, A., and Granfors, K. (1991). Combined Use of Released Proteins and Lipopolysaccharide in Enzyme-Linked Immunosorbent Assay for Serologic Screening of Yersinia Infections. J. Infect. Dis., 163: 409–12.

Marceau, M., Sebbane, F., Ewann, F., Collyn, F., Lindner, B., *et al.* (2004). The pmrF polymyxin-resistance operon of Yersinia pseudotuberculosis is upregulated by the PhoP-PhoQ two-component system but not by PmrA-PmrB, and is not required for virulence. *Microbiol.*, **150:** 3947–57.

Martinez, P. O., Fredriksson-Ahomaa, M., Sokolova, Y., Roasto, M., Berzins, A., *et al.* (2009). Prevalence of enteropathogenic Yersinia in Estonian, Latvian, and Russian (Leningrad region) pigs. *Foodborne Pathog. Dis.*, **6:** 719–24.

Merhej, V., *et al.*, (2008). *Yersinia massiliensis sp. nov., isolated from fresh water. Int. J. Syst. Evol. Microbiol.*, **58**(4): 779–84.

Merlahti-Palo, R. *et al* (1991). Risk of Yersinia infection among butchers. Scandin. *J. Infect. Dis.*, **23:** 55–61.

Mills, S. D., Boland, A., Sory, M. P., van der Smissen, P., Kerbourch, C., *et al.* (1997). Yersinia enterocolitica induces apoptosis in macrophages by a process requiring functional type III secretion and translocation mechanisms and involving YopP, presumably acting as an effector protein. *Proc. Natl. Acad. Sci. USA*, **94:** 12638–43.

Miyoshi-Akiyama, T., Abe, A., Kato, H., Kawahara, K., Narimatsu, H., *et al.* (1995). DNA sequencing of the gene encoding a bacterial superantigen, Yersinia pseudotuberculosis-derived mitogen (YPM), and characterization of the gene product, cloned YPM. *J. Immunol.*, **154:** 5228–34.

Montminy, S. W., Khan, N., McGrath, S., *et al.* (2006). Virulence factors of Yersinia pestis are overcome by a strong lipopolysaccharide response. *Nat. Immunol.*, **7:** 1066–73.

Mwengee, W., Butler, T., Mgema, S., Mhina, G., Almasi, Y., *et al.* (2006). Treatment of plague with gentamicin or doxycycline in a randomized clinical trial in Tanzania. *Clin. Infect. Dis.*, **42:** 614–21.

Nesbakken, T., Iversen, T., and Lium, B. (2007). Pig herds free from human pathogenic Yersinia enterocolitica. *Emerg. Infect. Dis.*, **13:** 1860–64.

Niskanen, T., Fredriksson-Ahomaa, M., and Korkeala, H. (2002). Yersinia pseudotuberculosis with limited genetic diversity is a common finding in tonsils of fattening pigs. *J. Food Prot.*, **65:** 540–45.

Nowgesic, E., Fyfe, M., Hockin, J., *et al.* (1999). Outbreak of Yersinia pseudotuberculosis in British Columbia—November 1998. *Can. Commun. Dis. Rep.*, **25:** 97–100.

Nuorti, J. P., Niskanen, T., Hallanvuo, S., *et al.* (2004). A Widespread Outbreak of Yersinia pseudotuberculosis O:3 Infection from Iceberg Lettuce. *J. Infect. Dis.*, **189:** 766–74.

Paauw, A., Leverstein-van Hall, M. A., van Kessel, K. P. M., Verhoef, J., and Fluit, A. C. (2009). Yersiniabactin Reduces the Respiratory Oxidative Stress Response of Innate Immune Cells. *PLoS ONE*, **4:** e8240.

Paglia, M. G., D'Arezzo, S., Festa, A., Del Borgo, C., Loiacono, L., *et al.* (2005). Yersinia pseudotuberculosis septicemia and HIV. *Emerg. Infect. Dis.*, **11:** 1128-30.

Pai, C. H., Gillis, F., Tuomanen, E. and Marks, M. I. (1984). Placebo-controlled double-blind evaluation of trimethoprim-sulfamethoxazole treatment of Yersinia enterocolitica gastroenteritis. *J. Pediatr.*, **104:** 308–11.

Parkhill, J., Wren, B. W., Thomson, N. R., *et al.* (2001). Genome sequence of Yersinia pestis, the causative agent of plague. *Nature*, **413:** 523–27.

Perry, R. D., & Fetherston, J. D. (Eds). (2007). The Genus Yersinia: From Genomics to Function. Advances in Experimental Medicine and Biology, Vol. **603**. Springer.

Pham, J. N., Bell, S. M., Martin, L., and Carniel, E. (2000). The beta-lactamases and beta-lactam antibiotic susceptibility of Yersinia enterocolitica. *J. Antimicrob. Chemother.*, **46:** 951–57.

Philbey, A. W., Glastonbury, J. R. W., Links, I. J., and Matthews, L. M. (1991). Yersinia species isolated from sheep with enterocolitis. *Aus. Vet. J.*, **68:** 108–10.

Pierson, D. E., and Falkow, S. (1993). The ail gene of Yersinia enterocolitica has a role in the ability of the organism to survive serum killing. *Infect. Immun.*, **61:** 1846–52.

Prentice, M., Cope, D., Weinbren, M., and O'Driscoll, J. (1990). Infectious complications of blood transfusion. *BMJ.*, **300:** 678–79.

Prentice, M. B., and Rahalison, L. (2007). Plague. *The Lancet*, **369:** 1196–1207.

Pujol, C., Klein, K. A., Romanov, G. A., Palmer, L. E., Cirota, C., *et al.* (2009). Yersinia pestis Can Reside in Autophagosomes and Avoid Xenophagy in Murine Macrophages by Preventing Vacuole Acidification. *Infect. Immun.*, **77:** 2251–61.

Quintard, B., Petit, T., Ruvoen, N., Carniel, E., and Demeure, C. E. (2010). Efficacy of an oral live vaccine for veterinary use against pseudotuberculosis. Comp. *Immunol., Microbiol. Infect. Dis.*, In Press.

Ramalingaswami, V. (1995). Plague in India. *Nature Med.*, **1:** 1237–39.

Ramamurthy, T., Yoshino, K., Huang, X., Balakrish Nair, G., Carniel, E., *et al.* (1997). The novel heat-stable enterotoxin subtype gene (ystB) of Yersinia enterocolitica: nucleotide sequence and distribution of the yst genes. Microb. *Pathog.*, **23:** 189–200.

Rastawicki, W., Szych, J., Gierczynski, R., and Rokosz, N. (2009). A dramatic increase of Yersinia enterocolitica serogroup O:8 infections in Poland. Eur. J. Clin. Microbiol. *Infect. Dis.*, **28:** 535–37.

Rebeil, R., Ernst, R. K., Gowen, B. B., Miller, S. I., and Hinnebusch, B. J. (2004). Variation in lipid A structure in the pathogenic yersiniae. *Mol. Microbiol.*, **52:** 1363–73.

Rimhanen-Finne, R., Niskanen, T., Hallanvuo, S., *et al.* (2009). Yersinia pseudotuberculosis causing a large outbreak associated with carrots in Finland, 2006. *Epidemiol. Infect.*, **137:** 342–47.

Robins-Browne, R., and Prpic, J. K. (1985). Effects of iron and desferrioxamine on infections with Yersinia enterocolitica. *Infect. Immun.*, **47:** 774–79.

Robins-Browne, R.M., *et al.* (1991). *Pathogenicity of Yersinia kristensenii for mice. Infect. Immun.*, **59**(1): 162–67.

Sato, K., Ouchi, K., & Komazawa, M. (1988). Ampicillin vs. placebo for Yersinia pseudotuberculosis infection in children. *Pediatr. Infect. Dis. J.*, **7:** 686–89.

Schubert, S., Bockemuhl, J., Brendler, U., and Heesemann, J. (2003). First isolation of virulent Yersinia enterocolitica O8, biotype 1B in Germany. *Eur. J. Clin. Microbiol. Infect. Dis.*, **22:** 66–68.

Sebbane, F., Jarrett, C. O., Gardner, D., Long, D., and Hinnebusch, B. J. (2006). Role of the Yersinia pestis plasminogen activator in the incidence of distinct septicemic and bubonic forms of flea-borne plague. *Proc. Natl. Acad. Sci. USA.*, **103:** 5526–30.

Shivaji, S., Bhanu, N. V. and Aggarwal, R. K. (2000). Identification of Yersinia pestis as the causative organism of plague in India as determined by 16S rDNA sequencing and RAPD-based genomic fingerprinting. *FEMS Microbiol. Lett.*, **189:** 247–52.

Shayegani, M., and Parsons, L. M. (1987). Epidemiology and pathogenicity of Yersinia enterocolitica in New York State. *Cont. Microbiol. Immunol.*, **9:** 41–47.

Sieper, J., Fendler, C., Laitko, S. *et al.* (1999). No benefit of long-term ciprofloxacin treatment in patients with reactive arthritis and undifferentiated oligoarthritis: a three-month, multicenter, double-blind, randomized, placebo-controlled study. *Arthr. Rheum.*, **42:** 1386–96.

Simonet, M., Riot, B., Fortineau, N., and Berche, P. (1996). Invasin production by Yersinia pestis is abolished by insertion of an IS200-like element within the inv gene. *Infect. Immun.*, **64:** 375–79.

Skurnik, M., Venho, R., Bengoechea, J. A. and Moriyon, I. (1999). The lipopolysaccharide outer core of Yersinia enterocolitica serotype O:3 is required for virulence and plays a role in outer membrane integrity. *Mol. Microbiol.*, **31:** 1443–62.

Skurnik, M., Bengoechea, J. A. and Granfors, K. (Eds). (2003). The Genus Yersinia: Entering the Functional Genomic Era. Advances in Experimental Medicine and Biology, Vol 529. Springer.

Slee, K. J., and Button, C. (1990). Enteritis in sheep and goats due to Yersinia enterocolitica infection. *Aus. Vet. J.*, **67:** 396–98.

Slee, K. J., and Skilbeck, N. W. (1992). Epidemiology of Yersinia seudotuberculosis and Y. enterocolitica infections in sheep in Australia. *J. Clin. Microbiol.*, **30:** 712–15.

Smiley, S. T. (2008). Immune defense against pneumonic plague. *Immunol. Rev.,* 225: 256–71.

Sprague, L.D. and Neubauer, H. (2005)., *Yersinia aleksiciae sp. nov. Int. J. Syst. Evol. Microbiol.,* 55(2): 831–35.

Sodeinde, O. A., Subrahmanyam, Y. V., Stark, K., Quan, T., Bao, Y. *et al.* (1992). A surface protease and the invasive character of plague. *Science,* 258: 1004–7.

Song, Y., Tong, Z., Wang, J., *et al.* (2004). Complete genome sequence of Yersinia pestis strain 91 001 an isolate avirulent to humans. *DNA Res.,* 11: 179–97.

Spinner, J. L., Cundiff, J. A., and Kobayashi, S. D. (2008). Yersinia pestis Type III Secretion System-Dependent Inhibition of Human Polymorphonuclear Leukocyte Function. *Infect. Immun.,* 76: 3754–60.

Spinner, J. L., Seo, K. S., O'Loughlin, J. L., Cundiff, J. A., Minnich, S. A., *et al.* (2010). Neutrophils Are Resistant to Yersinia YopJ/P-Induced Apoptosis and Are Protected from ROS-Mediated Cell Death by the Type III Secretion System. *PLoS ONE,* 5: e9279.

Sprague, L.D., *et al.,*(2008). *Yersinia similis sp. nov. Int. J. Syst. Evol. Microbiol.,* 58(4): 952–58.

Stahlberg, T. H., Tertti, R., Wolf-Watz, H., Granfors, K., and Toivanen, A. (1987). Antibody response in Yersinia pseudotuberculosis III infection: analysis of an outbreak. *J. Infect. Dis.,* 156: 388–91.

Stenhouse, M. A., and Milner, L. V. (1982). Yersinia enterocolitica. A hazard in blood transfusion. Transfus. 22: 396–98.

Sulakvelidze, A., Kreger, A., Joseph, A., Robins-Browne, R. M., Fasano, A., *et al.* (1999). Production of enterotoxin by Yersinia bercovieri, a recently identified Yersinia enterocolitica-like species. *Infect. Immun.,* 67: 968–71.

Sulakvelidze, A. (2000). *Yersiniae other than Y. enterocolitica, Y. pseudotuberculosis, and Y. pestis: the ignored species. Microbes Infect.,* 2(5): 497–513.

Tauxe, R. V., *et al.* (1987). Yersinia enterocolitica infections and pork: the missing link. *Lancet,* 1: 1129–32.

Tennant, S. M., Skinner, N. A., Joe, A., and Robins-Browne, R. M. (2005). Homologues of Insecticidal Toxin Complex Genes in Yersinia enterocolitica Biotype 1A and Their Contribution to Virulence. *Infect. Immun.,* 73: 6860–67.

Thomson, N. R., Howard, S., Wren, B. W., *et al.* (2006). The Complete Genome Sequence and Comparative Genome Analysis of the High Pathogenicity Yersinia enterocolitica Strain 8081. *PLoS Genet.,* 2: 2039–51.

Titball, R. W., Hill, J., Lawton, D. G., and Brown, K. A. (2003). Yersinia pestis and plague. *Biochem. Soc. Trans.,* 31: 104–7.

Tobback, E., *et al.,* (2007). *Yersinia ruckeri infections in salmonid fish. J. Fish Dis.,* 30(5): 257–68.

Tomaso, H., Mooseder, G., Dahouk, S. A., Bartling, C., Scholz, H. C., *et al.* (2006). Seroprevalence of anti-Yersinia antibodies in healthy Austrians. *Eur. J. Epidemiol.,* 21: 77–81.

Ueshiba, H., Kato, H., Miyoshi-Akiyama, T., Tsubokura, M., Nagano, T., *et al.* (1998). Analysis of the superantigen-producing ability of Yersinia pseudotuberculosis strains of various serotypes isolated from patients with systemic or gastroenteric infections, wildlife animals and natural environments. *Zentralbl. Bakteriol.,* 288: 277–91.

Ursing, J., *et al.* (1980). *Y. frederiksenii: a new species of* Enterobacteriaceae *composed of rhamnose-positive strains. Curr. Microbiol.,* 4: 213–17.

Van Noyen, R., Selderslaghs, R., Bogaerts, A., Verhaegen, J., and Wauters, G. (1995). Yersinia pseudotuberculosis in stool from patients in a regional Belgian hospital. *Contrib. Microbiol. Immunol.,* 13: 19–24.

von Reyn, C. F., *et al.* (1977). Epidemiologic and clinical features of an outbreak of bubonic plague in New Mexico. *J. Infect. Dis.,* 136: 489–94.

Wauters, G., Kandolo, K., and Janssens, K. (1987). Revised biogrouping scheme of Yersinia enterocolitica. *Contr. Microbiol. Immunol.,* 9: 14–21.

Wauters, G., *et al.,* (1988). *Y. mollaretii sp. nov. and Y. bercovieri sp. nov., formerly called Yersinia enterocolitica biogroups 3A and 5B. Inter. J. System. Bacteriol.,* 38: 424–29.

Welch, T. J., Fricke, W. F., McDermott, P. F., *et al.* (2007). Multiple Antimicrobial Resistance in Plague: An Emerging Public Health Risk. PLoS ONE, 2: e309.

Welkos, S. L., Friedlander, A. M., and Davis, K. J. (1997). Studies on the role of plasminogen activator in systemic infection by virulent Yersinia pestis strain C092. *Microb. Pathog.* 23: 211–23.

WHO (2006). International meeting on preventing and controlling plague: the old calamity still has a future. *Wkly. Epidemiol. Rec.,* 28: 278–84.

Williamson, E. D. (2009). *Plague. Vaccine,* 27: D56–60.

Wimsatt, J., and Biggins, D. E. (2009). A review of plague persistence with special emphasis on fleas. *J. Vector Borne Dis.,* 46: 85–99.

World Health Organisation. (2004). Human plague in 2002 and 2003. *Wkly. Epidemiol. Rec.,* 79: 301–6.

World Health Organisation (2006). International meeting on preventing and controlling plague: the old calamity still has a future. *Wkly. Epidemiol. Rec.,* 81: 278–84.

World Health Organisation (2008a). Interregional meeting on prevention and control of plague. Madagascar: Antananarivo.

World Health Organisation (2008b). International health regulations (2005)(2nd edn.), pp. 1–75. Geneva: WHO.

Wren, B. W. (2003). The Yersiniae- a model genus to study the rapid evolution of bacterial pathogens. *Nat. Rev. Micro.,* 1: 55–64.

Yli-Kerttula, T., Luukkainen, R., Yli-Kerttula, U. *et al.* (2000). Effect of a three month course of ciprofloxacin on the outcome of reactive arthritis. *Ann. Rheum. Dis.,* 59: 565–70.

Yli-Kerttula, T., Luukkainen, R., Yli-Kerttula, U., Mottonen, T., Hakola, M., *et al.* (2003). Effect of a three month course of ciprofloxacin on the late prognosis of reactive arthritis. *Ann. Rheum. Dis.,* 62: 880–84.

Zhou, D., and Yang, R. (2009). Molecular Darwinian evolution of virulence in Yersinia pestis. *Infect. Immun.,* 77: 2242–50.

CHAPTER 22

Glanders

Sharon J. Peacock and David A. B. Dance

Summary

Glanders is a serious zoonotic disease that primarily affects equids (horses, mules, and donkeys). A disease eradication programme based on case detection and destruction of infected domestic animals has been highly successful and the number of reported glanders cases in animals worldwide is now very low. Human glanders is extremely rare and associated with occupations associated with extensive contact with equids. Glanders is caused by *Burkholderia mallei*, a Gram-negative, non-motile, facultative intracellular organism that is an obligate parasite of equids with no other known natural reservoir. *B. mallei* is transmitted by direct contact with infected animals, or indirectly via communal food and water sources that have become contaminated by an infected animal. The clinical presentation in equids can be acute or chronic and has been categorized into nasal, pulmonary, and cutaneous forms. Diagnosis is based on culturing *B. mallei* from lesions or exudates and skin or serological testing. Infected animals are usually euthanized. Optimal antimicrobial therapy for human glanders is unknown, and current advice is to adopt antimicrobial treatment guidelines for human melioidosis. There is no vaccine available for either humans or other animals. *B. mallei* is considered a potential biological weapon and is a Centers for Disease Control and Prevention (CDC) category B select agent.

History

Aristotle (384–322 BC) is credited with the first description of glanders (Sharrer 1995). *Burkholderia mallei* was first isolated by Loeffler and Schütz in 1882 (Boerner 1882). Historically, this pathogen was an important cause of morbidity and mortality in horses worldwide and was occasionally transmitted to humans or other animals. The infection is usually thought to be transmitted between animals by direct contact with other infected animals, or indirectly via communal food and water sources, such as drinking troughs, that have become contaminated by an infected animal. Occasional cases have been reported in carnivores fed on infected meat (Alibasoglu *et al.* 1986). Infections in man were usually reported in those with prolonged and extensive contact with horses, such as grooms, coachmen, veterinarians, and butchers. An eradication programme largely based on the identification and destruction of sick or infected horses, with heavy reliance on testing with mallein

(Blancou 1994; Derbyshire 2002), has been highly successful. Glanders in domestic animals was eradicated from the USA during the 1940s (Wiser *et al.* 1986) and the last reported natural human case in the USA occurred in 1940s (Howe and Miller 1947), although a case of laboratory-acquired glanders occurred in the year 2000 (Centers for Disease Control and Prevention (CDC) 2000; Srinavasan *et al.* 2001). Glanders still occurs occasionally in equids and humans in central and southeast Asia, the Middle East, parts of Africa and South America. Between 1996 and 2007, animal cases (in most instances involving one or a small number of animals) have been reported from Latvia, Belarus, Mongolia, Turkey, Brazil, Iran, Iraq, India, Pakistan, and the United Arab Emirates (Office International des Épizooties, the World Organization for Animal Health (OIE), for figures from 1996–2004; World Animal Health Information Database (WAHID) for figures from 2005–2009; Bazargani *et al.* 1996; Arun *et al.* 1999; Scholz *et al.* 2006).

Glanders has an important military history. Until the last century, this infection caused major outbreaks among horses used for military purposes, resulting in the death or necessitating the slaughter of thousands of horses (Howe 1950). *B. mallei* was used as a biological weapon during the American Civil War (Sharrer 1995), the First World War (Christopher *et al.* 1997), and the Second World War . It was reported to have been weaponized by the Soviet Union, and was claimed to have been used as a biological weapon to attack the mujaheddin in Afghanistan in the 1980s (Alibek and Handelman 1999). *B. mallei* is classified as a category B select agent by the CDC (Neubauer *et al.* 1997).

The agent

Taxonomy (classification)

Originally named 'Bacillus mallei' this bacterium has been assigned to a variety of genera over the years (e.g. *Malleomyces, Pfeifferella, Loefflerella, Actinobacillus*), and until the early 1990s resided in rRNA homology group II of the genus *Pseudomonas*. It now belongs in the genus *Burkholderia* proposed by Yabuuchi *et al.* (1992). Approximately 30 species have been assigned to the genus. Many are plant-associated inhabitants of the rhizosphere where they play a variety of roles including nitrogen fixation, provision of plant nutrients, and inhibition of pathogens, but others are obligate or opportunistic plant and animal pathogens.

Genomics

The similarity between *B. mallei* and *B. pseudomallei* that was originally recognized by Whitmore (Whitmore and Krishnaswamy 1912) has been confirmed by a variety of techniques, including DNA-DNA hybridization (Rogul *et al.* 1970), multilocus sequence typing (MLST) (Godoy *et al.* 2003), and whole genome sequencing (Nierman *et al.* 2004; Holden *et al.* 2004). *B. mallei* appears to have evolved through genomic downsizing from a single clone of *B. pseudomallei* (Godoy *et al.* 2003; Nierman *et al.* 2004; Holden *et al.* 2004).

The genome of *B. mallei* ATCC 23344 consists of two circular chromosomes containing 3,510,148 bp and 2,325,379 bp, respectively (Nierman *et al.* 2004). A total of 5,535 predicted protein-encoding ORFs have been identified (Nierman *et al.* 2004). The genome contains numerous insertion sequence (IS) elements that are probably responsible for the extensive insertion, deletion, and inversion mutations relative to the *B. pseudomallei* K96243 genome. The *B. mallei* genome also contains over 12,000 simple sequence repeats (SSRs) within the coding region of 3,752 genes and in putative promoter regions of 179 genes. Numerous examples have been identified of SSRs located within genes encoding surface or secreted proteins that may directly interact with host factors during disease (Song *et al.* 2009). Replication error-induced changes in the number of repeat units in these genes would be predicted to lead to frameshift mutations. Comparison between the published *B. mallei* ATCC 23344 genome sequence and whole genome sequence of single-colony passaged *B. mallei* ATCC 23344 isolates obtained from culture, a mouse, a horse, and two isolates from a single human patient demonstrated 49 insertions and deletions at SSRs in the five passaged strains, mostly in noncoding regions (Romero *et al.* 2006).

Microbiology

B. mallei is a facultative intracellular, Gram-negative bacillus. Very few recent clinical isolates are available to the scientific community for study, so knowledge of its characteristics is based on historical descriptions and a few archived strains, which may be laboratory adapted to varying degrees. Most strains are oxidase positive. It is aerobic but able to grow anaerobically in the presence of nitrate. It is nutritionally versatile, being able to use a wide range of organic compounds as a carbon source, and can oxidize glucose and usually mannitol, although there is strain to strain variation. It is able to grow on most laboratory media, initially forming shiny and translucent colonies which tend to become mucoid with age, although it grows less luxuriantly than *B. pseudomallei*, from which it may be distinguished by its susceptibility to aminoglycosides and lack of motility. *B. mallei* is non-flagellated, whereas *B. pseudomallei* has 2–4 polar flagella per cell. Flagellin genes are present but flagellin is not expressed (Sprague *et al.* 2002). This can be explained by the presence of a 65 kb insert that disrupts *fliP* (an essential gene for flagellum biogenesis) together with a frameshift mutation in the flagellum motor gene *mot*B that eliminates its functionality (Nierman *et al.* 2004). The optimal temperature for growth is 37°C; many strains grow poorly below 25°C but all will grow at 41°C. *B. mallei* is unable to survive in dried pus for longer than a few days, or for 24 hours when exposed to sunlight, although it can survive in tap water for at least 4 weeks (Miller *et al.* 1948; Howe 1950).

Virulence factors

Glanders has been studied using several experimental models, including horses (Lopez *et al.* 2003), although most investigators rely on hamsters or mice (Fritz *et al.* 2001).

The *B. mallei* ATCC 23344 genome contains at least two *luxI* and four *luxR* homologues (regulators of virulence factor expression based on a cell density mechanism termed quorum sensing), which when inactivated resulted in reduced bacterial virulence in mice (Ulrich *et al.* 2004a). The genome also encodes a *virAG* two-component regulatory system that is required for virulence in hamsters (Nierman *et al.* 2004). Expression profiling has demonstrated that overexpression of *virAG* resulted in transcriptional activation of approximately 60 genes (Schell *et al.* 2007).

B. mallei can survive and replicate in several eukaryotic cell lines (Harley *et al.* 1998; Ribot and Ulrich 2006; Brett *et al.* 2008). Following uptake, the bacterium escapes from endocytic vacuoles into the host cell cytoplasm where it uses actin-based motility to promote spread within and between cells (Stevens *et al.* 2005; Ribot and Ulrich 2006). An animal pathogen-like type III secretion system (T3SSAP) is essential for early vacuolar escape and survival in murine macrophages (Ribot and Ulrich 2006), and is necessary for actin-based motility (Ulrich and DeShazer 2004b). Type VI secretion (T6S) is a protein transport mechanism in Gram-negative bacteria that interacts with eukaryotic cells (Bingle *et al.* 2008). Four T6SS gene clusters have been identified in the *B. mallei* ATCC 23344 genome (Schell *et al.* 2007). The cluster 1 T6SS (T6SS-1) is part of the VirAG regulon, is essential for *B. mallei* virulence in the hamster model of glanders (Schell *et al.* 2007), and plays a critical role in growth and actin-based motility following uptake of *B. mallei* by murine macrophages (Burtnick *et al.* 2009).

B. mallei capsular polysaccharide is required for virulence in hamsters and mice (DeShazer *et al.* 2001). The structure of O-polysaccharide has been characterized, and shown to confer serum resistance *in vitro* (Burtnick *et al.* 2002). Lipopolysaccharide has also been shown to be a potent activator of Toll-like receptor-4 *in vitro* (Brett *et al.* 2007). Gene expression profiling under iron-restricted conditions *in vitro* suggests that *B. mallei* can adapt to the iron-restricted conditions in the host environment by up-regulating an iron-acquisition system and by using alternative metabolic pathways for energy production (Tuanyok *et al.* 2005). Little is known about expression of virulence determinants *in vivo*, but the use of antibody profiling as a surrogate for gene expression during experimental equine glanders demonstrated that a family of proteins that share protein domain architectures with haemagglutinins and invasins were expressed and highly immunodominant (Tiyawisutsri *et al.* 2007).

Infection in humans
Clinical features

There are few recent clinical descriptions of human glanders and knowledge depends in large part on the historical literature, together with the likelihood that it will behave similarly to human melioidosis. It is almost always seen in those in regular close contact with horses (Bernstein and Carling 1909). Initial symptoms may be non-specific, but cutaneous and subcutaneous nodules and pustules that ulcerate are said to be characteristic (Hunting 1908; Howe 1950). The disease can run an acute or chronic course, but

from infections with these serovars are often severe, resulting in substantive losses to producers. Other serovars, such as Enteritidis, Infantis, Virchow and Hadar are particularly common in poultry. These serotypes may not cause overt disease in their hosts and in contrast to infections with Typhimurium and Dublin in cattle, and Typhimurium in pigs, may not be a cause of serious economic loss to producers.

Non-typhoidal salmonellosis is traditionally regarded as a zoonoses. The transmission of organisms to humans usually occurs via consumption of contaminated foods. The most common sources of salmonella organisms associated with food poisoning are poultry and poultry products such as eggs, beef, and pork meat. Improperly prepared fruits, vegetables, dairy products, and shellfish have also been implicated as sources of *Salmonella*. Substantive international outbreaks have also been associated with products such as chocolate, peanuts and powdered infant formula preparations. Human-to-human and animal-to-human transmissions can also occur and amphibian and reptile exposures are associated with approximately 74 000 *Salmonella* infections annually in the US.

The agent

Salmonellae are Gram-negative motile bacilli that conform to the definition of the Enterobacteriaceae. The genus *Salmonella* was named after Daniel E. Salmon, an American veterinarian who first isolated *Salmonella choleraesuis* from pigs with hog cholera in 1884. Most strains are motile. Apart from a few exceptions, they produce acid and gas from glucose and mannitol, and usually also from sorbitol; they ferment sucrose or adonitol rarely, and rarely form indole. They do not hydrolyse urea or deaminate phenylalanine, usually form H_2S on triple sugar iron agar and use citrate as sole carbon source. They form lysine and ornithine decarboxylases. Salmonellae grow over a wide temperature range from 7 to 48°C, at pH 4–8 and at water activities above 0.93. Under special conditions, they may proliferate at <4°C and withstand extremes of pH <4. Over 2,500 serovars have been identified, which are closely related to each other by somatic and flagella antigens. Additionally most strains show diphasic variation of the flagella antigens (Threlfall 2005).

Classification

The *Salmonella* genus is now considered to comprise two species: *S. enterica* and *S. bongori*. There are 6 subspecies of *S. enterica*, the most important of which is *S. enterica* subsp. *enterica* (subspecies I) which includes the typhoid and paratyphoid bacilli and most of the other serotypes responsible for widespread disease in mammals (Table 23.1). Members of the other five subspecies (II–VI) are in the main parasites of cold-blooded animals or are found in the natural environment.

Nomenclature

The terminology introduced by early workers accorded specific rank to each antigenically distinguishable salmonella type. The species names given were generally descriptive of the disease or the host with which the serotype was associated, and were sometimes incorrect. Thereafter, the convention was established that each new type should be named after the place in which it was

Table 23.1 *Salmonella* species and subspecies

Salmonella enterica subsp.		
I	Enterica	1539
II	Salamae	503
IIIa	Arizonae	96
IIIb	Diarizonae	334
IV	Houtenae	71
VI	Indica	14
S. bongori		22
Total		2579

first isolated. Whereas the first published table contained some 20 serotypes, each considered to be a species, the current number is 2,579 (Popoff *et al.* 2004; Bale *et al.* 2007), an increase of 82 since 1984 (Table 20.1).

Salmonella organisms are no longer accorded specific status because more modern taxonomic techniques suggested that all serotypes of *Salmonella* probably belonged to one DNA hybridization group within which the seven subgroups are identified (Le Minor *et al.* 1982). DNA hybridization studies suggested that DNA subgroup V (*S. enterica* subsp. *bongori*) had evolved significantly from the other six subspecies (Le Minor *et al.* 1986). These observations were supported by multilocus enzyme electrophoresis (MLEE) studies. The species *S. bongori* was therefore proposed and agreed (Reeves *et al.* 1989) and subsequently confirmed by MLST http://pubmlst.org/databases.shtml.

In the latest classification only serovars of subsp. *enterica* are still named; serovars of other subspecies of *S. enterica* and of *S. bongori* are no longer named but designated by their antigenic formulae. Designations such as *Salmonella* ser. Typhimurium, *Salmonella* Typhimurium or even simply Typhimurium are convenient for use in clinical situations and indicate that the named serotype is a member of subsp. *enterica*. Subtypes of serotypes recognized by phage typing or biotyping should not be named as if they were serotypes. Thus, the names of salmonellae (e.g. 'S. Java') distinguishable from established serotypes by biotype characters has been deleted from the updated version of the Kauffmann–White scheme as published by Popoff *et al.* (2004). Nevertheless it is important to realise that for some serovars, particularly S. Paratyphi B, which caused both enteric fever and more typical gastrointestinal disease, biotype classification may be important. Thus when infections with S. Paratyphi B biotype variant Java are recognized then the initial designation of S. Paratyphi B is sometimes supplemented by the use of the 'biotype Java' designation for epidemiological investigations.

The antigens used to define the serological types of salmonellae include the O antigens—heat-stable polysaccharides that form part of the cell wall lipopolysaccharide (LPS), the H antigens—heat-labile proteins of the flagella that in salmonellae have the almost unique character of diphasic variation and surface polysaccharides that inhibit the agglutinability of the organisms by homologous O antisera, of which the Vi antigen of Typhi and Dublin are two of the most important examples.

Typing and fingerprinting of salmonella

Serotyping

Serotyping, based on antigenic variation in the 'O' and 'H' antigen structure and encapsulated in the Kauffmann-White scheme, is the basic method for the primary subdivision of salmonella organisms after preliminary speciation. The method, which has been in use since the 1930s, is internationally accepted and although several DNA- and array-based methods are being developed (Fields *et al.* 2002), serotyping still remains the internationally recognized method for the preliminary identification of subtypes within species.

Due to the common occurrence of infections caused by *Salmonella*, and due to the variety of sources of the infection in particular regarding NTS, it is in most cases not sufficient to simply perform a successful serotyping procedure in order to gain insights into the epidemiology and roots of the infections. Therefore, numerous subtyping/fingerprinting methods have been developed to dissect further the origin of salmonella isolates. Such methods may broadly be considered as phenotypic, genotypic and sequence-based. Different techniques are useful in different circumstances, depending on the reason for the investigations. In practice a combination of methods is often used.

Phenotypic subtyping

The principal phenotypic subtyping methods used are phage typing and antimicrobial susceptibility determination.

Phage typing

The underlying principle of phage typing is the host specificity of bacteriophages and on this basis several phage-typing schemes have been developed for serotypes of clinical or epidemiological importance (Threlfall *et al.* 1990).

The first phage typing scheme based on the principle of phage adaptation was that developed for the differentiation of Typhi (Craigie *et al.* 1938); in this scheme progressive adaptations were made of Vi phage II, which is specific for the Vi (capsular) antigen of Typhi. Phage typing schemes for other serotypes depend to a limited extent on phage adaptability and, for the most part, are based on patterns of lysis produced by serologically distinct phages isolated from a variety of sources. Other serotypes for which published phage typing schemes are in routine use in the UK include: Paratyphi B, Typhimurium Hadar, Enteritidis and Virchow. More than 80 phage types are now recognized in the Enteritidis scheme. For the Typhimurium scheme, 232 phage types were designated and a further 50 types have been subsequently recognized. Phage typing schemes for Enteritidis and Typhimurium use in different countries of the EU have now been rationalized as part of an international collaborative venture for salmonella surveillance (Fisher *et al.* 1994; Fisher, 1999). Thus, while apparently 'old-fashioned,' phage typing still represents a fairly robust and discriminating subtyping approach and is internationally accepted. More recently attempts have been made to develop DNA-based phage typing for Typhimurium, utilizing phage-type specific markers revealed by fluorescent amplified fragment length polymorphism fingerprinting) of isolates of Australian origin (Hu *et al.* 2002). It is possible that this method may be used for the development of a microarray-based molecular phage-typing scheme for this and other serotypes.

Antimicrobial susceptibility determination

Determination of the pattern of sensitivity to a defined panel of antimicrobial drugs (antimicrobials) can be used for subdivision within serovar or phage type. Although the antimicrobial susceptibility pattern cannot be used as definitive, such patterns can be used to define clones, such as the internationally distributed clone of S. Typhimurium definitive phage type (DT) 104 with resistance to ampicillin (A), chloramphenicol (C), streptomycin (S), sulphonamides (Su) and tetracyclines (T) (= S. Typhimurium DT 104 ACSSuT) (Threlfall 2000), or as the clone is referred to in North America, penta-resistant DT104. Nevertheless it should be realized that although antimicrobial susceptibility patterns may provide useful information at individual and population level, the same phenotypic resistance pattern may be due to different genetic mechanisms. Additionally resistance may change very rapidly, often in response to selection pressure impose by antimicrobial usage.

Genotypic subtyping

Molecular biological tools have been developed for subtyping serovars of *Salmonella* for many years. Genetic typing methods can be broadly divided into extrachromosomal analysis (plasmid profiling, restriction digest of plasmids) and chromosomal analysis (ribotyping, IS*200* typing; macrorestriction of genomic DNA visualized by PFGE typing). Plasmid profiling has been used for many years to subtype salmonellae in outbreak investigations. While technically fairly convenient, plain comparison of plasmid profiles can be misleading as plasmids of the same size may be quite different when subjected to restriction enzyme digest analysis. The use of PFGE has become the 'gold standard' for international comparison of salmonella isolates. One reason for this is the considerable progress in standardization of methods. International networks, such as PulseNet (Swaminathaan *et al.* 2006), and Enternet (Fisher 1999), have ensured reproducibility and comparability of typing data between different laboratories. Furthermore, the typing data can be stored *in silico* as reference material, or for further comparison.

Sequence-based typing

Typing schemes based on variation in particular DNA sequences have the advantage of being digital in nature. This means that the same results should be achieved wherever the test is performed and any comparison of results is simple, quantitative and absolute in nature. Sequence-based typing schemes can also be considered as classification schemes and so genetic and evolutionary inferences can be made. Current DNA- sequence-based typing methods include the detection of DNA repeats and single nucleotide polymorphisms (SNPs). Variable Number of Tandem Repeat variation (VNTR) does not penetrate into the actual DNA sequence but produces data on the copy number of short repetitive sequences of individual isolates, by determining the size of the PCR product (Lindstedt 2005). To date, VNTR is able to differentiate reliably between isolates of Typhimurium, and VNTR for the differentiation of Enteritidis is underway. MLST, which is targeted at comparing sequence diversity at multiple, conserved housekeeping genes (Maiden *et al.* 1998), has been applied to seven housekeeping genes in a collection of 26 isolates of S. Typhi collected from diverse geographical locations (Kidgell 2003). The results confirmed earlier findings from MLEE typing and conclusively demonstrated the existence of four sequence types of S. Typhi from distinct geographical areas as well as providing an estimate of the age of the organism (ca. 50,000 years old) (Kidgell *et al.* 2002). Because the genes chosen for MLST are selectively neutral, not under selective pressure, the variation detected represents the true phylogenetic relationships between strains. At present the main promise for MLST is as a replacement for serotyping. Kidgell *et al.* demonstrated that MLST can form the basis of an identification scheme for *S.* Typhi but for sub-typing, more SNPs from around the genome are needed (Holt *et al.* 2008) Typing using SNP-based methods are under development for *S.* Typhi (Baker *et al.* 2008)and for *S.* Paratyphi A (Holt *et al.* 2009). At present these methods are expensive and so the detection of SNPs remains the preserve of the research institutions for evolutionary studies and of well-funded reference laboratories for molecular epidemiology.

The availability of a large amount of genomic sequence from different strains of *Salmonella* in combination with microarray technology opens yet another perspective for typing of salmonellae. Microarrays containing all known sequences from *S. enterica* serotypes have already been prepared and used to interrogate the gene content of different serotypes. Although not currently suitable for diagnostic laboratories these methods may find utility in reference labs for defining some aspects of genetic diversity such as antimicrobial resistance. Perhaps in the era of high-throughput nucleic acid re-sequencing whole genome analysis will be the ultimate typing method—this is, however, not yet possible.

The advantages and disadvantages of the various phenotypic, genotypic and sequence-based typing methods for the differentiation of *Salmonella* for outbreak tracing have recently been reviewed by Cook *et al.* (2006).

Pathogenesis

The ability of salmonella organisms to invade, survive and replicate within eukaryotic cells is essential for successful infection. *S. enterica* usually enters the host by the oral route. Although the infectious dose varies among *Salmonella* strains, a large inoculum is thought to be necessary to overcome stomach acidity and to compete with normal intestinal flora. Large inocula are also associated with higher rates of illness and shorter incubation periods. In general, about 10^6 bacterial cells are needed to cause infection. Low gastric acidity, which is common in elderly persons and among individuals who use antacids, can decrease the infective dose to 10^3 cells, while prior vaccination can increase the number to 10^9 cells.

Invasion process

In contrast to other invasive enteric bacteria such as *Yersinia* spp. and enteropathogenic *Escherichia coli*, salmonellae require neither motility nor fimbriae to adhere to and invade eukaryotic cells. The induction of *de novo protein* synthesis is necessary for the invasion and is regulated by the microenvironment (low oxygen), growth phase, or the epithelial cell surface. Only viable, metabolically-active salmonellas can adhere to host cell surfaces. Adherence is followed almost immediately by internalization into the host cells.

After ingestion, infection with salmonellae is characterized by attachment of the bacteria by fimbriae or pili to cells lining the intestinal lumen. Salmonellae selectively attach to specialized epithelial cells (M cells) of the Peyer patches. The bacteria are then internalized by receptor-mediated endocytosis and transported within phagosomes to the lamina propria, where they are released, thereby effecting a massive efflux of electrolytes and water into the intestinal lumen. Once there, salmonellae induce an influx of macrophages (typhoidal strains) or neutrophils (non-typhoidal strains).

Virulence factors

Salmonellae possess several virulence-promoting factors which contribute to the disease process. These virulence factors are generally conserved between species, as are the mechanisms by which salmonella bacteria interact with the host cell. Such virulence factors are complex and encoded both on the organism's chromosome and on large (34–120 kd) plasmids. Ten *Salmonella* pathogenicity islands have been identified that amongst other properties contributing to virulence, mediate uptake of the bacteria into epithelial cells (type III secretion system [TTSS]), non-phagocytic cell invasion (*Salmonella* pathogenicity-island 1 [SPI-1]), and survival and replication within macrophages (*Salmonella* pathogenicity-island 2 [SPI-2], phoP/phoQ). Other putative virulence factors include outer membrane proteins, secreted proteins, Vi antigen encoding genes, virulence markers located in prophages (e.g. *sopE1*, encoded by phage SopEphi), and genes belonging to various fimbrial clusters (Hensel 2004).

The Col V plasmid and related plasmids of the FI plasmid incompatibility group have been found to possess genes coding for the production of the siderophore aerobactin, a hydroxamate iron transport compound which enhances growth of host organisms in iron-deplete media such as blood. Genes from the *Salmonella* Pathogenicity Islands (SPIs) tend to be highly conserved throughout serovars although some genes may be deleted in some strains. Other putative virulence factors are those associated with genes coding for antimicrobial drug resistance (AMR), such as *Salmonella* Genomic Island 1 (SGI1) (Boyd *at al.* 2001), although as yet an association between the presence of SGI1 and enhanced virulence has not been conclusively established.

Serovar-specific virulence plasmids

Salmonella strains belonging to a range of serovars possess plasmids of high relative molecular mass (M_I) which can be regarded as 'serovar-specific'. Serovars which harbour such plasmids include Enteritidis, Typhimurium, Dublin, Gallinarum, Pullorum, Abortusovis, Cholerae-suis, Paratyphi C, Blegdam, Rostock, Newport, and Moscow. In contrast such plasmids have not been identified in epidemiologically-important serovars such as Hadar, Infantis or Virchow, and there are phage type differences in serovars such as Typhimurium. Such plasmids range in M_I from about 45 kb in Choleraesuis to 93 kb in Typhimurium. Although for the most part serovar-specific, there are some exceptions. The closely-related serovars Rostock and Dublin harbour an identical virulence plasmid, and different virulence plasmids are found in Enteritidis and Pullorum. Such plasmids have been shown to be involved in the virulence of their host organisms for mice and chickens. Genes on the virulence region include *orfE*, *spvD*, *spvC*, *spvB*, *spvA*, *spvR*, *vagC* and *vagD* (Gulig *et al.* 1993). Six *spv* genes within a common 8 kb *Sal*I–*Xho*I fragment have now been sequenced, namely *spvR*, *spvA*, *spvB*, *spvC*, *spvD* and *spvE*. The *spvE* gene encodes a 13 kDa protein, the *spvD* gene a 25 kDa protein and the *spvC* gene a 28 kDa protein, which is located both in the outer membrane and the cytoplasm. The latter protein has a demonstrable role in virulence, as it has been shown that transposon insertion mutants in the *spvC* gene of SSP result in a significant drop in the number of Typhimurium isolated from the spleen of orally infected mice. The *spvB* gene encodes a 65 kDa protein of unknown function which is located both in the outer membrane and the cytoplasm, and the *spvA* gene a 28 kDa protein also of unknown function.

Although essential for the virulence of the host organism in certain strains of mice the role of these genes in the virulence process in humans and other animal species is not clear. Serovar-specific virulence plasmids have been shown to be necessary for intracellular survival of salmonellas in mouse phagocytes and it is possible that they may contribute to the invasive process in humans and food animals such as cattle after the initial infection and cellular attachment process.

Host properties

The severity of illness in individuals with salmonellosis is determined not only by the virulence factors of the infecting strain but also by host properties. Such properties include corticosteroid use, malignancy, diabetes, HIV infection, prior antimicrobial therapy, and immunosuppressive therapy. In developing countries sickle cell disease, malaria, schistosomiasis, bartonellosis, and pernicious anaemia have been mentioned as other co-morbidities that predispose to salmonellosis.

Epidemiology

Recent trends in incidence

Since the early 1980s the epidemiology of Salmonella infection in humans in the UK and most European countries has been dominated by two serovars, namely Enteritidis and Typhimurium (Fig. 23.1).

Salmonella Enteritidis

Enteritidis is commonly among the top three serovars from cases of human infection in many developed countries world wide. In the UK, for example, reported isolations increased 16-fold in the period 1981–94 whilst in the EU there were estimated to be 180,000 Enteritidis infections in the years 2004–2006 (EFSA 2007b). The main reservoir of S. Enteritidis is poultry, with poultry meat and contaminated eggs being important vehicles of human infection. The unprecedented epidemic of Enteritidis in the USA, UK and many several other countries in the late 1980s and early 1990s was caused by a strain of phage type (PT) 4 which spread in poultry flocks, selected by environmental pressures associated with poultry husbandry. An unusual feature of the epidemic was the transovarian spread of the strain in the avian host.

Since 1997 in the UK there has been a dramatic decline in incidence (Fig. 23.1). The reasons for this decline are multi-factorial. Several codes of practice for the control of salmonellas in chickens have been in operation in the UK since 1993. There have also been many improvements in the poultry industry in infection control and hygiene at breeding sites, and vaccination against S. Enteritidis started in breeder flocks in the UK in 1994 and in layer flocks in 1998 (Davies *et al.* 2003). Nevertheless, Enteritidis still remains the most common serotype from humans in the UK and since 2002 there have been a substantial number of outbreaks of infection caused by phage types other than PT 4 (O'Brien *et al.* 2004). In 2002–03 national surveillance databases at the Health Protection Agency (HPA) identified an increase in the incidence of infection due to a number of specific strains of *Salmonella*. Cases were widely distributed. Interlocking national and local epidemiological investigations were conducted to determine the source of these strains. These investigations demonstrated associations between infection and the consumption of foods prepared in the commercial catering and retail sectors and containing raw shell egg. The findings generated a further series of multidisciplinary food and environmental investigations coordinated by the HPA Centre for Infections and involving a number of Health Protection Units, local authorities and laboratories throughout England. Eggs imported from Spain used by caterers were implicated in local outbreaks and microbiological investigations showed that Spanish eggs were contaminated at high rates with strains of *Salmonella*. The nationally collated data from local outbreak investigations identified key interventions in catering practices.

In 2004 a Standing Multi-agency National Outbreak Control Team (comprised of the HPA, Food Standards Agency (FSA), Department of Environment, Food and Rural Affairs (Defra), Health

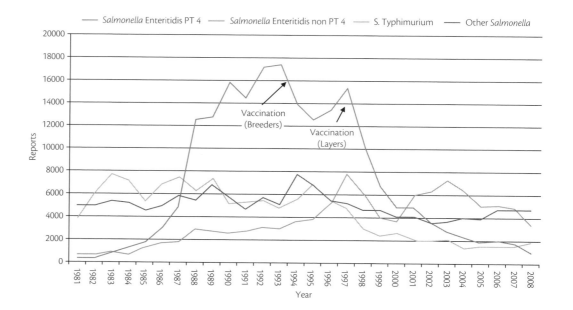

Fig. 23.1 Incidence of *Salmonella.* Humans, England and Wales, 1981–2008.

Protection [Scotland] and National Public Health Service for Wales) was convened to coordinate the development and implementation of local and national control measures. Guidance documents were produced for the catering, healthcare, retail, and wholesale sectors and discussions were held with the Spanish Government Agencies and egg producers. These actions have resulted in a sharp decline in the importation of eggs from Spain and a concomitant fall in the incidence of the outbreak strains of *Salmonella*.

Salmonella Typhimurium

Salmonella Typhimurium is one of the top three serovars isolated world wide over many decades from humans, domestic and wild animals, foodstuffs, and the environment, with cattle and poultry important sources of infection for humans (Palmer *et al.* 1986). Over the last two decades the key organism within serovar Typhimurium has been the MDR clone of S. Typhimurium DT 104 (=MDR DT 104) (see above).

Strains of MR DT104 were identified in cattle in the United Kingdom in the late 1980s. The strain was subsequently transmitted to humans through the food chain, but also became common in poultry (particularly turkeys), pigs and sheep. Throughout the 1990s, MDR DT104 spread to other parts of the world, particularly in Europe and North America where molecular epidemiological studies have contributed to the consensus that MDR DT104 represents a globally disseminated clone. Although isolations of MDR DT104 have, in general been decreasing since 1997 (Fig. 23.2), this phage type continues to be of clinical concern not only due to its rapid dissemination, but also because it has been associated with increased morbidity and mortality and because of its ability to readily acquire additional resistance to other clinically important antimicrobials such as the fluoroquinolones, trimethoprim, aminoglycosides, and cephalosporins.

Outbreaks

The free movement of people and foodstuffs between countries are effective ways of distributing disease-causing salmonella organisms internationally. To control international outbreaks there is a requirement for a mechanism whereby data and information on potential salmonella outbreaks can be disseminated rapidly to those who need to know. Within Europe this requirement was fulfilled until 2007 by the Enter-net dedicated surveillance network complimented by the Salm-gene molecular typing network (Fisher *et al.* 2005). Data on epidemiological and microbiological features on current cases, as well as background levels of infections were immediately available within the Enter-net databases. The Salm-gene network with its database of harmonized salmonella PFGE patterns from the participating European countries provided immediate, and electronically exchangeable, DNA fingerprints of outbreak strains. This prompt electronic dissemination of information regarding unusual events with international implications ensured that public health interventions could be implemented and cases of food-borne salmonella disease prevented. Examples of international salmonella outbreaks recognized by Enter-net from 2000–2007 are shown in Table 23.2.

In 2007 Enter-net was subsumed into the European Centre for Disease Prevention and Control (ECDC), and investigations of outbreaks have been coordinated by ECDC.

Contact with pets

In the UK in 2009 tetracycline-resistant S. Typhimurium DT 191a associated with pet snakes have caused over 200 infections in humans. The source of the antimicrobial-resistant strain is thought to be imported frozen mice used as food for the reptiles (Anon. 2009; Hawker *et al.* 2010). Reptiles, including snakes and turtles, have also been associated with substantive outbreaks of salmonellosis in other European countries and the USA (Bertrand *et al.* 2008; Lee *et al.* 2008; Anon. 2007). In the USA there have also been reports of the transmission of strains of S. Typhimurium and S. Virchow from pets to humans (CDC. 2001; Sato *et al.* 2000; Swanson *et al.* 2007). In Australia, ornamental fish tanks have been identified as reservoirs for MDR S. Paratyphi variant Java (Levings *et al.* 2006). Although not strictly from pets, in Canada MDR

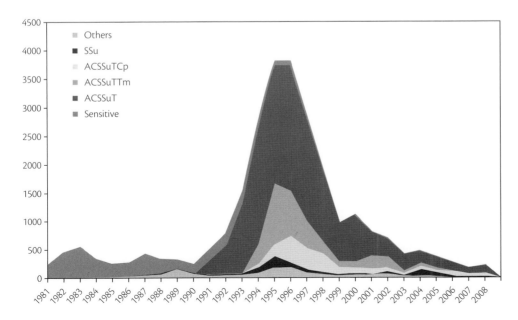

Fig. 23.2 Multi drug-resistant (MDR) S. Typhimurium DT104 isolates from Humans, England and Wales 1981–2006.
Antimicrobial resistance symbols: A, ampicillin, C, chloramphenicol, S, streptomycin, Su, sulphonamides, T, tetracyclines, Tm, trimethoprim, Cp, ciprofloxacin.

Table 23.2 Examples of international salmonella outbreaks of food-poisoning recognized through Enter-net, 2000–2007

Year	Organism	Cases	Countries involved	Vehicle implicated
2000	S. Typhimurium DT204b	392	*England and Wales*, Germany, Iceland the Netherlands, Scotland	Lettuce
2001	S. Livingstone	54	*Norway, Sweden*	Fish pie
	S. Stanley	100+	*Australia, Canada*, England and Wales, Scotland	Peanuts (China)
	S. Oranienburg	500+	Austria, Belgium, Denmark, Finland, *Germany*, the Netherlands Sweden (product in Canada, Croatia, Czech Republic	Chocolate (Germany)
	S. Typhimurium DT104	100+	Australia, Canada, England and Wales, Germany, Norway, *Sweden*	Halva (Turkey)
2002	S. Cerro	44	*Belgium*, France	Cream pastries/powder (Belgium)
2003	S. Typhimurium DT29	1100+	*Austria*, Germany	Eggs (Austria)
2004	S. Thompson	100+	Norway, Sweden, England and Wales	Lettuce (Italy)
2005	S. Stourbridge	60	Austria, England and Wales, *France*, Germany, Luxembourg, The Netherlands, Sweden, Switzerland	Unpasteurised goat's cheese (France)
	S. Typhimurium	60+	Finland, Spain, Sweden	Lettuce
	S. Hadar PT2	1,500	England and Wales, France, Spain	Cooked chicken (The Netherlands)
2006	S. 4,5,12:i:-	150+	*Luxembourg*, Germany	Pork
	S. Montevideo	60+	*England and Wales*, Scotland	Chocolate
	S. Virchow PT8	50+	*England and Wales*, Northern Ireland	Cooked chicken (Thailand)
2007	S. Typhimurium DT208	30+	Denmark, Norway	Sausage (Spain)
	S. Senftenberg	50+	*England and Wales*, Denmark, The Netherlands, USA	Basil (Israel)

Index case(s) in parentheses

S. Newport associated with pet treats has caused infections in both humans and dogs (Pitout *et al.* 2003).

Salmonella in animals

In the UK information on *Salmonella* in livestock is collated by the Veterinary Laboratories Agency. In 2007 the most common serovars in cattle were Dublin (59% of incidents) followed by Typhimurium (14%). In pigs it was Typhimurium (70% of incidents) followed by Derby (8%). In poultry it was Enteritidis (53%) followed by Typhimurium (13%) (VLA, 2008). The most common phage type in Typhimurium from cattle was DT104, and in pigs U288 (66% of incidents). In isolates of Enteritidis from poultry PT 4 predominated (47% of incidents). In the EU the most common serovar in both breeder flocks and layer flocks in 2006 was Enteritidis, but the most common serovar identified in broiler meat was Infantis. In pig meat the most common serovar in 2006 was Typhimurium, followed by Derby, and in cattle, Typhimurium predominated followed by Goldcoast (EFSA 2007b).

Prevention and control

Control of salmonella is a multifactorial process. Reduction of the occurrence of specific types in their food animal host by measures such as immunization is obviously key in reducing the overall burden of infection, as has been demonstrated with the protracted S. Enteritidis outbreaks referred to above. Reduction in the use of

antimicrobials in food-producing animals will result in a reduction in the occurrence of specific types exhibiting resistance to such antimicrobials, as exemplified by MR *S.* Typhimurium DT 104. Withdrawal of a contaminated product is also a method of control, but normally relates to products such as salads, salad vegetables and chocolate. Contamination of such products often involves organisms originating from a food production animal at some stage in the production process.

Good hygiene practices in restaurants and mass catering establishments will also contribute to salmonella control. Despite a plethora of advice and guidelines, outbreaks of infection still occur when basic hygiene practices are ignored, such as correct storage, defrosting and thorough cooking. Salmonella bacteria are killed when food is thoroughly cooked. This means cooking minced beef and similar products to at least 68°C and ensuring that all food is cooked properly. Once cooked, any food held in a buffet should be kept hotter than 60°C. Cross-contamination may be avoided by using different utensils, plates, cutting boards, and counter tops before and after cooking. Cooked food that stands at room temperature for a long time, especially poultry, is at risk. Infected persons should not be allowed to handle food or work in the kitchen before at least three negative samples have been submitted.

In the home environment basic hygiene procedures such as washing hands in hot soapy water after toileting and before handling foods are essential. Frozen foods should be thoroughly defrosted before cooking and refrigerator temperatures should be kept colder than 4°C. Raw milk and recipes involving raw or lightly-cooked eggs should be avoided. Because fruits and vegetables have now been identified as a source of salmonella, it is important that these food items be thoroughly washed in running water before they are eaten. Cutting boards for raw meat and poultry should not be used for cheese, raw vegetables and other foods that will not be cooked before being served.

Additionally infections caused by highly pathogenic salmonella bacteria are becoming increasingly associated with domestic pets, including snakes, terrapins and other reptiles as well as dogs and cats. It is essential that hand washing procedures such as outlined above are implemented after handling pets and in the case of young children, access to pets such as snakes and reptiles should be actively discouraged.

Although numbers are dropping, salmonellosis remains the second most common form of bacterial food-poisoning in the UK and in most European countries. The majority of infections are associated with contaminated food, particularly of poultry origin but also from originating from cattle and pigs, and to a lesser extent, sheep. The occurrence of resistance to 'critically important' antimicrobial drugs is increasing. Control measures such as vaccination of poultry flocks appear to have had a substantial impact on the number of infections with *Salmonella* Enteritidis. Nevertheless good hygiene practices in both catering establishments and the home remain essential for the control of infections at the local level and should be actively encouraged by health practitioners at all times.

Antimicrobial drug resistance

Antimicrobial drug resistance in *Salmonella* has increased worldwide leading to treatment failures in human and animal infectious diseases. Serious concerns about such resistance have been growing for a number of years and have been raised at both national and international levels. For *Salmonella*, of particular concern are quinolone resistance, resistance to third- and fourth-generation cephalosporins (WHO 2007), and the appearance and spread of strains exhibiting multiple resistance as a result of the acquisition of the *Salmonella* Genomic Island 1 (Boyd *et al.* 2001; Amar *et al.* 2008) (see above).

Quinolone resistance

Two fundamental types of quinolone resistance in *Salmonella* have been identified, namely chromosomally-mediated quinolone resistance and plasmid-mediated quinolone resistance (PMQR). Chromosomal resistance to quinolones, arises spontaneously under antimicrobial pressure due to point mutations that result in: (i) amino acid substitutions within the topoisomerase II (DNA gyrase) and IV subunits *gyr*A, *gyr*B, *par*C or *par*E, (ii) decreased expression of outer membrane porins or alteration of LPS, or (iii) over expression of multi-drug efflux pumps. Mutations in the *gyr*A, *gyr*B, *par*C, or *par*E genes in regions that form the fluoroquinolone binding site (termed the Quinolone Resistance-Determining Region, QRDR) change the topoisomerase structure in a way that fluoroquinolones (FQs) are unable to bind to these target sites. Single mutations affect firstly only older quinolones such as nalidixic acid in their inhibitory action. The MIC for nalidixic acid is in the range of 64–128 mg/l, whereas the MICs for FQs are generally in the range of 0.25–1.0 mg/l. This level of resistance is generally regarded as 'epidemiological'. Additional mutations are required to decrease the susceptibility to later and more recently-introduced FQs such as ciprofloxacin. These additional mutations result in the development of 'clinical resistance', with MICs of greater than 2 mg/l.

Plasmid-mediated quinolone resistance (PMQR) is mediated by genes (*qnr*) encoding proteins that protect DNA gyrase from inhibition by ciprofloxacin. One such gene, *qnr*A confers resistance to nalidixic acid (MIC; 8–16 mg/l) and epidemiological resistance to FQs (ciprofloxacin MIC: 0.25–1.0 mg/l). The basal level of quinolone resistance provided by *qnr* genes is low and strains can appear susceptible to quinolones according to the USA Clinical Laboratory Standards Institute (CLSI) guidelines. Their clinical importance lies in increasing the MIC of quinolone-resistant strains of *Salmonella* to levels that are clinically-relevant.

In the UK fluoroquinolones were licensed for veterinary use in 1993. Subsequent studies of the occurrence of resistance to quinolones in *S.* Typhimurium DT104 showed a temporal increase of quinolone-resistant isolates of MDR *S.* Typhimurium DT104 from humans, cattle, poultry, and pigs (Threlfall *et al.* 1999).

Over the five-year period 2000–2004, there has been an overall increase in cases of human infection in the EU by strains of *S.* Enteritidis exhibiting resistance to nalidixic acid and epidemiological resistance to ciprofloxacin, with the occurrence of resistance to both antimicrobials increasing from 10% to 26%. Over this period resistance remained constant at approximately 6% in *S.* Typhimurium; the highest incidence of resistance was seen in *S.* Virchow, with 68% of isolates resistant to nalidixic acid in 2002 (Meakins *et al.* 2008). From 2005–2006 to nalidixic acid/ciprofloxacin increased in both Enteritidis (135 to 15%) and Typhimurium (75 to 8%) (Table 23.3).

Ciprofloxacin resistance was commonly found in isolates of *S.* Enteritidis from broiler meat and hens from countries in southern Europe but also from certain countries in northern Europe. With the exception of certain new member states, such resistance was relatively uncommon in isolates of *S.* Typhimurium from pork, pigs and cattle. With the exception of one northern European country, there was a high incidence of quinolone resistance in *Salmonella* from turkeys (EFSA 2007b).

Foods have been implicated in several major national and international outbreaks of *S.* Typhimurium exhibiting epidemiological resistance to ciprofloxacin. Eggs contaminated with nalidixic acid-resistant *S.* Enteritidis have been linked to numerous outbreaks of salmonellosis in several European countries since 2000, although it has not been possible to precisely ascertain how many infections have been associated with contaminated eggs. Isolates with PMQR have been reported in several countries, but such strains were mostly associated with travel to countries outside of the EU (Hopkins *et al.* 2008). Of clinical concern is that the acquisition of plasmid-mediated quinolone resistance can raise the FQ MIC to clinical levels.

Cephalosporin resistance

Resistance to third- and fourth-generation cephalosporins in *Salmonella* is primarily caused by production of extended-spectrum β-lactamases (ESBLs) and/or AmpC enzymes. Both classes of enzymes confer resistance to extended-spectrum cephalosporins and to other β-lactam antimicrobials, with substrate specificity depending on the mechanism and sequential mutations involved. In particular, in different salmonella serovars ESBLs and/or AmpC

Table 23.3 Resistance to quinolones in human isolates of *Salmonella* Enteritidis and Typhimurium, European Union, 2005–2006

Serovar	2005		2006	
	Enteritidis	Typhimurium	Enteritidis	Typhimurium
Countries	15	14	15	14
Number studied	NS	NS	20148	5563
% Nal^R	13. (2–52)	7 (0–18)	15 (0–54)	8 (0–13)
% Cip^R	0.4 (0–4.)	0.6 (0–6)	0.6 (0–15)	0.7 (0–4)

Range of % shown in parentheses; NS, not stated;
Nal^R, nalidixic acid-resistant; Cip^R, ciprofloxacin-resistant
EFSA (2006, 2007a, 2007b)

enzymes have often been identified on plasmids. These plasmid-mediated resistances have frequently been found together with resistance determinants for e.g. aminoglycosides, chloramphenicol and florfenicol, sulphonamides, tetracyclines and/or trimethoprim, leading to efficient spread via co-selection. In addition, the down regulation of porins in some resistant isolates may also contribute to a decreased activity of antimicrobials that use the same entry pathway, such as FQs.

Extended-spectrum cephalosporins (ESBLs), along with fluoro-quinolones, have been classified by WHO as 'critically-important' antimicrobials (WHO 2007). ESBLs with the ability to hydrolyse and confer resistance to cefotaxime (= CTX-M) are generally regarded as having the most impact for public health.

Strains of *Salmonella enterica* with CTX-M enzymes were first reported in isolates of *S.* Typhimurium made in 1998 from cases of human infection in Greece, Hungary and Latvia. In 2000 cases of human infection in Spain in 1997 and 1998 with *S.* Virchow possessing CTX-M-were reported and in two retrospective studies of CTX-M in salmonella infections in the UK, cases of CTX-M-producing *S.* Virchow in the UK in 1997 and 1999 were identified which were associated with travel to Spain and in which the causative strain possessed CTX-M-9. Subsequently CTX-M enzymes have been identified in cases of human infection in a further 14 European countries, from food animals—poultry in five countries, and in seafood in one country outwith Europe, since 2001 salmonella organisms with CTX-M enzymes have been reported in 21 countries in five continents. The great majority of organisms have been from cases of human infection, although infections associated with imported poultry meat have been reported in Japan CTX-M-producing serovars with an international distribution within Europe included Virchow, Typhimurium, Enteritidis, and Concord. With the exception of *S.* Concord the organisms were not clonal in respect of their CTX-M types, with four CTX-M types being identified in *S.* Virchow, six in *S.* Typhimurium and three in *S.* Enteritidis. In contrast to the plethora of CTX-M-producing serovars from cases of human infection, the only serovars from food production animals in which CTX-M enzymes have been positively identified are *S.* Virchow and *S.* Java. As such *S.* Virchow with CTX-M types 2, 9, and 32 have been isolated from poultry and *S.* Java with CTX-M types 1, 2 and 9 also from poultry. Of particular note has been the rapid spread of CTX-M- producing *S.* Java in poultry in the Netherlands, with the percentage of such isolates increasing from 0% in 1999 to 20% in 2005, with a slight decline in isolations in

2006 (MARAN 2007) In almost all serovars and strains CTX-M genes have been plasmid-mediated. Other than in Europe the occurrence of salmonella strains possessing CTX-M-inactivating enzymes is low. Although such strains have emerged, and in certain cases have caused serious infections, in countries outwith Europe most CTX-M possessing salmonella strains seem to be confined to cases of human infection and, with the possible exception of China, there is no evidence of either epidemic spread or a food-animal reservoir.

Salmonella genomic island 1

SGI1 is a chromosomally-located gene cluster originally identified in the UK in MDR *S.* Typhimurium DT104 in the early 1990s (Threlfall *et al.* 1993). MDR DT104 was subsequently detected in the US in 1985 and its prevalence increased in the 1990s worldwide (Threlfall 2000). DT104 is zoonotic in origin and causes numerous infections in humans. One of the characteristics of DT104 is that it is phenotypically resistant to ampicillin (A), chloramphenicol/florfenicol (C), streptomycin (S), sulphonamides (Su), and tetracyclines (T). DT104 is also associated with enhanced ability to cause disease (virulence) SGI1 was first described in 2000 as a 43 kb chromosomal region in a Canadian isolate of DT104 and was sequenced in 2001 (Boyd *et al.* 2001). SGI1 has recently been detected in other, epidemic salmonella serovars as well as the pandemic DT104, but which has also recently been detected in other sub-species (or serovars) of *S. enterica* (e,g., Agona, Albany, Newport, Java) (Doublet *et al.* 2004), indicating that there may be a relationship between potentially enhanced virulence and MDR and the presence of this gene cluster. SGI1 seems to spread horizontally so it poses a public health risk to the future treatment of salmonella infections. Although horizontal transfer between salmonella serovars may be the mechanism by which SGI1 spreads, a biological reservoir in other organisms cannot be excluded.

Control of antimicrobial resistance

The use of antimicrobials in humans and animals is widely regarded as a major driving force in the emergence and spread of both antimicrobial resistance (AMR) and antimicrobial-resistant bacteria. The question of whether antimicrobial resistance in NTS associated with food animals is a human public health problem in developed countries has been a contentious issue since the late 1960s. In 1969 the Joint Committee on the Use of Antibiotics in Animal Husbandry and Veterinary Medicine (the Swann Committee) recommended that certain therapeutic antibiotics, at that time widely used in food animals without prescription, should be available only on prescription (Anon. 1969). The committee also recommended that therapeutic antimicrobials should not be used for the purpose of growth promotion in food-producing animals. The practice of using antimicrobials for growth promotion in food production animals has subsequently been forbidden in the EU since 2006, but such strictures have not been adopted worldwide, for example in the USA.

References

Amar, C.F.L., Arnold, C., Bankier, A., et al. (2008). Real-time PCRs and fingerprinting assays for the detection and characterization of Salmonella Genomic Island-1 encoding multi-drug resistance: Application to 445 European isolates of Salmonella, Escherichia coli, Shigella and Proteus. Microb. Drug Resist., 14: 79–92.

Anon. (1969). Report of the Joint Committee on the Use of Antibiotics in Animal Husbandry and Veterinary Medicine. HMSO: London.

Anon. (2009). Ongoing investigation into reptile-associated Salmonella infections. Heal. Protect. Rep., 3(14): 4.

Baker, S., Holt, K.E., van Roumagnac, S., et al. (2008). High-throughput genotyping of Salmonella enterica serovar Typhi allowing geographical assignment of haplotypes and pathotypes within an urban district of Jakarta, Indonesia. J. Clin. Microbiol., 46: 1741–46.

Bale, J.A., De Pinna, E., Threlfall, E.J. and Ward, L.R. (2007). Salmonella identification: serotypes and antigenic formula. Kauffmann-White Scheme 2007. Health Protection Agency, ISBN: 978-0-901144-91-1.362.

Boyd, D., Peters, G.A., Cloeckaert, A., et al. (2001). Complete nucleotide sequence of a 43-kilobase genomic island associated with the multidrug resistance region of salmonella enterica serovar Typhimurium DT104 and its identification in phage type DT120 and serovar Agona. J. Bacteriol., 183: 5725–32.

CDC (2001). Outbreaks of multidrug-resistant Salmonella Typhimurium associated with veterinary facilities: Idaho, Minnesota and Washington, 1999. Morb. Mort. Wkly. Rep., 50: 701–4.

Cooke, F.J., Threlfall, E.J. and Wain, J. (2006). Current trends in the spread and occurrence of human salmonellosis: Molecular typing and emerging antibiotic resistance. In: M. Rein, D.J. Maskell, E.J. Threlfall,(eds.) Salmonella: Molecular Biology and Pathogenesis. Norfolk UK: Horizon Bioscience, pp. 1–29.

Craigie, J., Yen, C.H. (1938). Demonstration of types of B. typhosus by means of preparations of type II Vi phage: principles and techniques. Can. Pub. Heal. J., 29: 448–63.

Crump, J.A., Luby, S.P. and Mintz, E.D. (2004). The global burden of typhoid fever. Bull. World Heal. Organ., 82: 346–53.

Davies, R. and Breslin, M. (2003). Effects of vaccination and other preventive methods for Salmonella Enteritidis on commercial laying chicken farms. Vet. Rec., 153: 673–77.

Doublet, B., Butaye, P., Imberechts, H., Boyd, D., Mulvey, M.R., et al. (2004). Salmonella Genomic island 1 multidrug resistance gene clusters in Salmonella enterica serovar Agona isolated in Belgium in 1992 to 2002. Antimicrob. Agents and Chemother., 48: 2510–17.

EFSA (2006). The Community Summary Report on Trends and Sources of Zoonoses, Zoonotic Agents and Antimicrobial resistance in the European Union in 2004. Available at: http://www.efsa.europa.eu/EFSA/efsa_locale-1178620753812_1178620772157.htm.

EFSA (2007a). The Community summary report on trends and sources of zoonoses, zoonotic agents, antimicrobial resistance and foodborne outbreaks in the European Union in 2005. EFSA J., 94: 3–288. http://www.efsa.europa.eu/EFSA/efsa_locale-1178620753812_1178620767319.htm.

EFSA (2007b). The Community summary report on trends and sources of zoonoses, zoonotic agents, antimicrobial resistance and foodborne outbreaks in the European Union in 2006. EFSA J., 130: 3–288. http://www.efsa.europa.eu/cs/BlobServer/DocumentSet/Zoon_report_2006_en,0.pdf?ssbinary=true.

Fields, P.I., Fitzgerald, C. and McQuiston, J.R. (2002). Development of DNA-based methods for the determination of serotype in Salmonella. Proc. Intern. Symp. Salmonella and Salmonellosis. Saint Brieuc, France, pp. 37–41.

Fisher, I.S.T. (1999). The Enter-net international surveillance network - how it works. Eurosurveill., 4: 52–55.

Fisher, I.S.T., Rowe, B., Bartlett, C.L.R., Gill, N.G. (1994). Salm-Net'–laboratory-based surveillance of human salmonella infections in Europe. PHLS Microbiol. Dig., 11: 181–82.

Gulig, P.A., Danbara, H., Guiney, D.G., et al. (1993). Molecular analysis of spv virulence genes of the Salmonella virulence plasmids. Mol. Microbiol., 7: 825–30.

Hawker, K.S., Lane, C., De Pinna, E., and Adak, G.C. (2010). An outbreak of Salmonella Typhimurium DT191a associated with reptile feeder mice. Epidemiol Infect, 1–8. E-pub ahead of print

Health Protection Agency (2009). Salmonella in humans (excluding S. Typhi and S. Paratyphi), 1990–2008. Available at: http://www.hpa.org.uk/webw/HPAweb&HPAwebStandard/HPAweb_C/1195733760280?p=1191942172078.

Hensel, M. (2004). Evolution of pathogenicity islands of Salmonella enterica. Inter. Med. Microbiol., 294: 95–102.

Holt, K.E., Parkhill, J., Mazzoni, P., et al. (2008). High-throughput sequencing provides insights into genome variation and evolution in Salmonella Typhi. Nature Gen., 40: 987.

Holt, K.E., Teo, Y.Y., Li, H., et al. (2009). Detecting SNPs and estimating allele frequencies in clonal bacterial populations by sequencing pooled DNA. Bioinform., 25: 2074–75.

Hopkins, K.L., Day, M. and Threlfall, E.J. (2008). Plasmid-mediated quinolone resistance in Salmonella enterica, United Kingdom. Emerg. Infect. Dis., 14: 340–42.

Hu, H., Lan, R. and Reeves, P.R. (2002). Fluorescent amplified fragment length polymorphism analysis of Salmonella enterica serovar Typhimurium reveals phage-type-specific markers and potential for microarray typing. J. Clin. Microbiol., 40: 3406–15.

Kidgell, C. (2003). Genetic variation in Salmonella enterica subspecies enterica serotype Typhi. PhD Thesis, University of London.

Kidgell, C., Riechard, U. and Wain, J. (2002). Salmonella Typhi, the causative agent of typhoid fever, is approximately 50 000 years old. Infect. Gen. Evol., 2: 39–45.

Le Minor, L., Veron, M. and Popoff, M. (1982). Proposition pour une nomenclature des Salmonella. Ann. Microbiol. (Paris), 133B: 245–54.

Le Minor, L., Popoff, M.Y., Laurent, B. and Hermant, D. (1986). Individualisation d'une septième sous-espèce de Salmonella. Ann. Microbiol. (Paris), 137B: 211–17.

Levings, R.S., Lightfoot, D., Hall, R.M. and Djordjevic, S.P. (2006). Aquariums as reservoirs for multidrug-resistant Salmonella Paratyphi B. Emerg. Infect. Dis., 12: 507–10.

Lindstedt, B.A., Heir, E., Gjernes, E. and Kapperud, G. (2002). DNA fingerprinting of Salmonella enterica subsp. enterica serovar Typhimurium with emphasis on phage type DT104 based on variable number of tandem repeat loci. J. Clin. Microbiol., 41: 1469–79.

Maiden, M.C., Bygraves, J.A., Feil, E., et al. (1998). Multilocus sequence typing: A portable approach to the identification of clones within populations of pathogenic microorganisms. Proc. Nat. Acad. Sci. USA, 95: 3140–45.

MARAN (2007). Monitoring of antimicrobial resistance and antibiotic usage in animals in The Netherlands. http://www.cvi.wur.nl.

Meakins, S., Fisher, I.S.T., Berghold, C., et al. (2008). Antimicrobial drug resistance in human nontyphoidal Salmonella isolates in Europe 2000–2004: a report from the Enter-net International Surveillance Network. Microb. Drug Resist., 14: 31–35.

O'Brien, S., Gillespie, I., Charlett, A., Adak, B., et al. (2004). National case-control study of Salmonella Enteritidis phage type 14B infections in

England and Wales implicates eggs used in the catering trade. *Eurosurveill.*, **9**: 50.

Palmer, S.R. and Rowe, B. (1986). Changing trends in salmonellosis in England and Wales. *PHLS Microbiol. Dig.*, **3**: 19–22.

Pitout, J.D., Reisbig, M.D., Mulvey, M., *et al.* (2003). Association between handling of pet treats and infection with *Salmonella enterica* serotype newport expressing the AmpC beta-lactamase, CMY-2. *J. Clin. Microbiol.*, **41**: 4578–82.

Popoff, M.Y., Bockemühl, J. and Gheesling, L.L. (2004). Supplement 2002 (no. 46) to the Kauffmann-White scheme. *Res. Microbiol.*, **155**: 568–70.

Popoff, M.Y., Bockemühl, J. and Hickman-Brenner, F.W. (1995). Supplement 1994 (no. 38) to the Kauffmann–White scheme. *Res. Microbiol.*, **146**: 799–803.

Reeves, M.W., Evins, G.M., Heiba, A.A. *et al.* (1989). Clonal nature of *Salmonella typhi* and its genetic relatedness to other salmonellae as shown by multilocus enzyme electrophoresis, and proposal of *Salmonella bongori* comb. nov. *J. Clin. Microbiol.*, **27**: 313–20.

Sato, Y., Mori, T., Koyama, T. and Nagase, H. (2000). *Salmonella* Virchow infection in an infant transmitted by household dogs. *J. Vet. Med. Sci.*, **62**: 767–69.

Swaminathaan, B., Gerner-Smidt, P., Ng, K.L., *et al.* (2006). Building PulseNet International: an interconnected system of laboratory networks to facilitate timely public health recognition and response to foodborne disease outbreaks and emerging foodborne diseases. *Foodborne Path. Dis.*, **31**: 36–50.

Swanson, S.J., Snider, C., Braden, C.R., *et al.* (2007). Multidrug-resistant *Salmonella enterica* serotype Typhimurium associated with pet rodents. *N. Engl. J. Med.*, **356**: 21–28.

Threlfall, E.J. (2000). Multiresistant *Salmonella typhimurium* DT 104: a truly international multiresistant clone. *J. Antimicrob. Chemother.*, **46**, 7–10.

Threlfall, E.J. (2005). *Salmonella*. In: S.P. Borriello, P.R. Murray, and G. Funke, *et al.* (eds.) *Topley and Wilson's Microbiology and Microbial Infections, (10th edn.) Part VI*. London: Hodder Arnold, pp. 1398–434.

Threlfall, E.J. and Frost, J.A. (1990). The identification, typing and fingerprinting of *Salmonella*: laboratory aspects and epidemiological applications. *J. Appl. Bacteriol.*, **68**: 5–16.

Threlfall, E.J., Ward, L.R. and Rowe, B. (1999). Resistance to ciprofloxacin in non-typhoidal salmonellas from humans in England and Wales - the current situation. *Clin. Microbiol. Infect.*, **5**: 130–34.

Threlfall, E.J., Frost, J.A., Ward, L.R. and Rowe, B. (1994). Epidemic in cattle of *S. typhimurium* DT 104 with chromosomally-integrated multiple drug resistance. *Vet. Rec.*, **134**: 577.

Veterinary Laboratories Agency (2009). *Salmonella in livestock production 2007*. Department for Environment, Food and Rural Affairs, Welsh Assembly Government, Planning and Countryside Agriculture Department, Scottish Executive Environment and Rural Affairs Department. ISBN 1 8995 1330 2.

WHO (2007). Report of the Second WHO Expert Meeting: Critically important antimicrobials for human medicine: Categorization for the development of risk management strategies to contain antimicrobial resistance due to non-human antimicrobial use. http://www.who.int/foodborne_disease/resistance/antimicrobials_human.pdf.

CHAPTER 24

Tularaemia

Andrew Pearson

Summary

Tularaemia is a plague-like bacterial disease of animals (particularly rodents, hares, and rabbits) and man caused by five subspecies of *Francisella*. Two subspecies predominate: *F. tularensis tularensis* in North America and *F. tularensis holarctica* throughout the northern hemisphere. *F. tularensis* occurs in persistent natural foci causing localized epidemics and sporadic cases in man.

Francisella tularensis subspecies *tularensis* was described originally as causing a more virulent form of tularaemia than was seen in Europe. More recently recognized are subpopulations of *Francisella tularensis* subspecies *tularensis* which have markedly different virulence for man. These have been designated A1a, A1b and A2. Infections resulting from type A1b have been shown to have an attributable mortality of 24% as compared to 4% for tularaemia caused by A1a types.

F. tularensis is one of the most potent bacterial pathogens affecting humans with an infective dose from 1 to 10 organisms. The incubation period is usually 3–5 days (range from 1–21 days). Onset of disease is abrupt, with fever, chills, fatigue, general body aches, and headache. When the bacteria are acquired through skin or mucous membranes, tender regional node enlargement may become conspicuous. When bacteria are inhaled, the infection will result in deep lymph node enlargement.

The clinical epidemiology of human infection is complex since it relates to one of four modes of transmission of the agent harboured in multiple hosts from diverse ecosystems. Clinical presentation of the human disease is indicative of both the mode of transmission and often the source of infection in a specific ecosystem. Tularaemia presenting as ulceroglandular disease results from either vector-borne infection from mosquito or tick bites or occurs as a result of animal contact from bites, hunting or from skinning hares or muskrats. Oropharyngeal and typhoidal infections predominate in waterborne outbreaks of *F. tularensis holarctica*. Pulmonary or influenza disease results from airborne transmission associated with either farmers moving rodent contaminated hay or laboratory acquired infection. An intentional aerosol release of *F. tularensis tularensis* would be expected to result in clinical manifestations similar to those recognized in natural respiratory tularaemia. Both vector-borne and airborne transmission of *F. tularensis* may both be associated with florid skin manifestations as a presenting symptom of tularaemia. Pulmonary or typhoidal forms of the tularaemia may occur as a complication of localized infection.

History

Historically, tularaemia-like illnesses have been recognized for more than four centuries by observers in several continents in the northern hemisphere. Isolation and transfer of a European isolate was recorded in the 1890s by veterinarians in Norway but not published until 1912, a year after the recognition of the agent causing the more virulent American form of the disease in California in 1911.

The discovery of tularaemia in the New World is attributed to McCoy (1911) who reported a plague-like illness in Californian ground squirrels (*Citellus beecheyi*) and who, with Chapin, isolated an apparently new agent (McCoy *et al.* 1912). Pure cultures of this organism, which they called *Bacterium tularensis* after the Californian county Tulare, were used to reproduce the disease in guinea-pigs. A similar agent had been observed in the 1890s in Norway by Horne (1912), who saw tiny plague-like, bipolar-staining coccobacilli in Scandinavian lemmings (*Lemmus lemmus*), and transferred the agent to guinea-pigs in which it produced an epizootic in the animal colony at the Veterinary Institute in Oslo.

However European and Russian doctors had long recognized the existence of human disease outbreaks in association with times of rodent abundance (highs). In 1532 Jacob Ziegler described how lemmings crowded together and died of epidemic disease and then caused disease among human beings '*ex quarum corruptione aer fir pestilens et ad ficit Norduegos uertigire et icteri*'. In 1653, Olaus Wormius wrote of the Norwegians' fear of lemming invasions and he described a disease which included swelling of the glands. From the early times the clergy used to read a Latin prayer of exorcism against lemmings:

> I exorcize you, pestiferous worms mice, birds or locusts, or other animals, by God the Father, …that you depart immediately from these fields, or vineyards, or waters, and dwell in them no longer, but go away to those places in which you can harm no person.

This statement in the seventeenth century represents the first written public health intervention for a tularaemia-like disease.

By the end of the nineteenth century 'lemming fever' was a well recognized clinical entity. In 1895, Collett wrote:

> It is obvious that great masses of individuals which perish incessantly during a migratory year must have an influence on sanitary conditions,

especially during the warm season of the year.... During some great prolific years definite forms of sickness have appeared in certain of the over-run districts, and the people have given these the name of 'Lemming Fever' as they presumed that they were connected with the appearance of these animals. Many of the doctors practising in the country have turned their attention to the disease and diagnosed it in their case reports.

The first case in North America for which the diagnosis was established by isolation of the organism was described by Wherry and Lamb in 1914. The next fifty years saw the description of more than a million cases, predominately in Europe and Eurasia. Subsequent scrutiny of records from the Russian literature revealed that parts of eastern Europe had widespread epidemic as well as endemic cases of tularaemia associated with farming and hunting. In Russia, 1,048 cases were reported between 1926 and 1937. Subsequently large outbreaks with 100,000 cases per year were recognized in areas of eastern Europe disrupted by the Second World War (Jusatz 1962). By the 1940s tularaemia had been reported from both the European and Asiatic parts of the former USSR; and most other countries of northern, central and eastern Europe (Jusatz 1962); and in Japan (O'Hara *et al.* 1971).

However in America the possible extent of human infection was not realized until an investigation of 'deerfly fever' by Francis in the Pahvant valley of Utah. The investigation of these early cases and outbreaks was associated with morbidity and mortality amongst the investigators and laboratory workers. In the USA between 1924 and 1950, there were 23,309 recorded cases with a 9.5% case fatality ratio before the introduction of streptomycin in 1949. Between 1960 and 1968 in North America there was a further reduction in numbers with reports of only 2,594 cases with 23 deaths. A century later the highest rate of mortality following tularaemia has been shown to be associated with the A1b subpopulation of *F. tularensis* subsp. *tularensis* found in North America.

In Western Europe the first confirmed cases of *F. tularensis holarctica* (type B) were diagnosed in Norway by Thjotta (1931 a,b) and Sweden by Olin (1942). Thjotta in Oslo described 66 cases between 1929 and 1931 and Olin and the National Bacteriology Laboratory (NBL) in Sweden recorded 757 cases between 1931 and 1951. In Czechoslovakia, there were reports of 585 cases between 1936 and 1952 and in Austria 500 cases were reported by Schafer as having occurred between 1935 and 1950.

From the 1950s the principle research resided in the cold war interest in the potential evaluation of the agent as a weapon of mass destruction and more recently as a deliberate release agent in the new era of bioterrorism (Leintenberg 2001). Since the re-emergence of a bioterrorism threat at the end of the twentieth century there has been a resurgence of research into the molecular biology and vaccine potential. This has resulted in the use of new molecular tools for both diagnosis and strain characterization: both key to ascertainment and the elucidation of emergent new foci in southern Europe and the recrudescence of old endemic foci in widespread areas of Europe (World Health Organization (WHO) 2007). It remains unclear as to the extent to which these developments have increased ascertainment or been a factor in the identification of new foci such as that described in Spain or in the elucidation of re-emergent areas of endemicity such as that seen in central and southern Sweden, Kosovo, Turkey, and China.

Despite the resurgence of interest in the disease the factors and biological mechanisms sustaining the long term maintenance in the diverse ecosystems remains an enigma as much in 2010 as it did in the nineteenth century.

The agent

Taxonomy

Francisella tularensis is one of two species in the genus *Francisella*, which is the only genus of the family Francisellacease. The two species, *F.tularensis* and *F.philomiragia*, show a 16S rRNA sequence similarity of [3]98.3%. The family is distinguished by a unique set of phenotypic characteristics including coccoidal morphology, Gram-negativity, a capability to degrade only a limited number of carbohydrates resulting in acid but no gas production, a growth requirement for cysteine, and a unique fatty acid composition (Sjostedt 2005).

Molecular biology

Francisella tulensis has a high lipid content (21% by dry weight) and contains two major phospholipids, phosphatiylethanolamine and phosphatidylglycerol. There are several unusual fatty acids, for example long chain (C20–C26) acids and 2-hydroxydexadecaanoate and 3-hydroxyoctadecanoate—which could be of diagnostic value; the non-hydroxy fatty acid composition is considered to represent a valuable taxonomic characteristic (Nichols *et al.* 1985). The antigens of *F.tularensis*, including the lipopolysaccharides, and their immunogenicity have been studies to assess their potential importance as components of vaccines (Dennis *et al.* 2001). There is an extensive literature on the molecular aspects of the host bacterial interactions of *F.tularensis* in man and animals.

Morphology and growth requirements

The different subspecies and biogroups of *F.tularensis* are morphologically indistinguishable. *In vivo*, the organism occurs as tiny coccobacilli (0.2–.07 um) surrounded by a clear area which corresponds to the capsule. It is frequently pleomorphic, ovoid, bacillary, bean-shaped, and dumb-bell and filamentous forms may occur (Eigelsbach *et al.* 1946). The organism is Gram-negative and non-motile and does not form spores. The capsule may be demonstrated by negative staining. Loss of the capsule may occur and with repeated subculture on laboratory media, but the bacteria remain viable and infective.

Cysteine is required for growth. Primary isolation from animals, birds, and man requires the use of either enriched media, inoculation into the chick embryo or preliminary animal passage: the last appears to be essential for the isolation of *F. tularensis* from water.

The hosts

Animals

Francisella species are intracellular pathogens producing fulminant acture infection in the susceptible animal hosts, chronic granulomatous infection in moderately susceptible species, or long term immunity in resistant species (WHO 2007).

Humans

The severity and type of infection and incubation period (1–14 days) in humans depends on the sub-species, the route of infection and the dose (Table 24.1). Subspecies *tularensis* can cause serious

Table 24.1 Comparison of contact and airborne outbreaks

Symptoms and signs	Contact No. cases[a]	Outbreak %	Airborne No. cases[b]	Outbreak %
Fever	38	97	343	85
Chills	23	59	285	70
Myalgia	22	56	–	–
Malaise	20	51	179	44
Diaphoresis	11	28	–	–
Headache	9	23	230	57
Nausea and/or vomiting	3	8	73	18
Lymphadenitis	31	79	65	16
Fatigue	–	–	350	86
Exanthem	–	–	142	35
Sore throat	–	–	129	32
Chest pain (pleuritic)	2	5	–	–
Cough (non productive)	2	5	–	–
Ulceration (cutaneous)	29	74	–	–
Infected ulcers/oral ulcers	–	–	81	20
Conjunctivitis	–	–	107	26
Muscle/joint pains	–	–	136	34
Symptoms of pneumonia	–	–	46	11

[a]Young et al. (1969). Vermont epidemic in 1968 of 39 symptomatic cases.
[b]Dahlstrand et al. (1971). Jantland epidemic between 1966 and 1967 of 405 serologically verified cases.

clinical manifestations and significant mortality. Before the antibiotic era, the fatality rate of type A was up to 15% overall and could be over 50% in its most severe forms. With antibiotic treatment, fatality rates are reported to be less than 2% (Dennis et al. 2001). Type B tularaemia is much less severe than type A but is frequently associated with suppurative complications. Ulceroglandular and glandular tularaemia are the most frequent forms of the disease and are acquired from insect bites, direct contact with infected animals or contaminated tools, etc. (Table 24.2). Skin abrasions will increase risk of infection. The respiratory form of tularaemia, resulting from inhalation of the organism which may be aerosolized during farming activities may present with symptoms of pneumonia including cough and chest and pain, or may occur as a complication of other forms of tularaemia due to blood borne spread. In Type A disease, pneumonia is a fulminant condition with a fatality rate of up to 60% untreated.

Localized infections may vary from a local indurated ulcer to no visible lesion, but there is usually swelling of the local lymph nodes

Table 24.2 Relationship of clinical form of tularaemia to transmission

Form	Transmission : route of acquisition
Ulceroglandular or glandular	Vector-borne or by touching infected animals or material contaminated with F. tularensis
Oculoglandular	Touching the eye with contaminated fingers or less likely by infective dust
Oropharyngeal	Ingesting contaminated food or water
Typhoid	Ingesting contaminated food or water
Respiratory	Inhalating contaminated dust, laboratory incidents and accidents, deliberate release

which may enlarge or rupture. The histology of the nymph node is a non-caseating granuloma.

Diagnosis

Protocols for diagnostic tests has been published by WHO (2007). Direct fluorescent antibody staining, using a FITC-labelled rabbit antibody directed against whole killed F.tularensis cells, is a rapid assay for identification of F.tularensis in primary specimens or for confirmation of recovered isolates (Petersen et al. 2004). Slide agglutination can be used for the rapid confirmation of recovered isolates. Immunohistochemical staining, using a monoclonal antibody directed against the LPS, can be used to visualize F.tularensis in formalin-fixed tissues. A variety of PCR methods have been developed, targeting the fopA or tul4 genes encoding the outer membrane proteins. Where possible, culture should be attempted and F.tularensis grows well on cysteine/cystine supplemented agar.

The standard serological test is either microagglutinatin or tube agglluntination for the presence of F.tularensis antibodies. ELISA tests including in combination with Western blot have also shown promise (Schmitt et al. 2005).

Treatment

This has been summarized by Dennis et al. (2001). In severe tularaemia, parenteral administration of an amino-glycoside is the first choice of treatment. Tetracyclines were once used widely and may be still be a valuable alternative for oral treatment of tularaemia. More recently, quinolones have been successfully introduced for oral treatment. Antibiotic chemoprophylaxis is indicated for post exposure for accidental exposure of laboratory personnel and should be commenced within 24 hours.

Francisella philomiragia

The organism has been isolated from the blood of nine patients, from the lung or pleura of three more, and from the peritoneum and the meninges, each in a single case. All 13 of the patients for whom records are available had suffered from a pyrexial illness; in five there was evidence of pneumonia. Only one of the patients was previously healthy, five of them had chronic granulomatous disease, two had myeloproliferative disorders, and one recurrent pleural effusions. Five other patients had recently suffered from a near-drowning incident in sea or estuarine water (Whipp et al. 2003).

Epidemiology

Global epidemiology

The epidemiology of human tularaemia is exceedingly complex and varies with subspecies, virulence and ecosystem. Our current knowledge is very much dependent on the extent of local ascertainment and reporting in particular countries and geographical regions.

The distribution of known foci, where animal epizootics, endemic and epidemic human tularaemia have been described (Figs. 24.1–24.3). Human infection has been described in most countries of the northern hemisphere between latitudes 30° and 71° N. The incidence of the disease is poorly documented because of highly variable ascertainment and reporting practices (Table 24.3). Case numbers and rates of reported tularaemia have fallen since a peak of an estimated period between the two World Wars when case numbers reached 100,000 cases per year. This reduction follows a systematic investigation of the epidemiology and recognition of the extent of occupational hazards in the former USSR by Russian epidemiologists, the introduction of streptomycin and public vaccination campaigns. Together these public health measures have reduced the number of reported cases in the former USSR between 1926 and 1942 from a period of 100,000 cases per year of *F. tularensis* subspecies *holarctica* to a few hundred per year at the present time.

In recent years there has been a resurgence of interest in tularaemia that has resulted in an increase in ascertainment and the recognition of both new and recrudescence of endemic foci. The apparent emergence of new foci causing outbreaks of tularaemia and the need to exclude deliberate release in some areas of Europe affected by civil conflicts has led the WHO to formulate and publish guidelines on the epidemiological investigation and case management of tularaemia and was a factor in WHO promoting the establishment of an International Tularaemia Society to promote the exchange of epidemiological information and scientific research.

USA

Francisella tularensis subspecies *tularensis* is the main cause of serious mortality and morbidity from tularaemia in the USA. Human infections are in the main sporadic and occur in two seasonal peaks, one in the summer, associated with tick bites, and the other in the winter attributed to hunting, mainly of rabbits (Taylor *et al.* 1991). Human infection with *Francisella tularensis* subsp. *holarctica* (type B) organisms has been much less frequently described. Parker reviewed approximately 100 such cases which had occurred from 1930–1950 when his team carried out an extensive survey

into the carriage of *F. tularensis* in water and in mud from streams where infected muskrats and beavers had been found (Parker *et al.* 1951). Between 1922 to 1966, there were 34 cases of *F.tularensis holarctica* (type B) infection actually reported in North America. Strains of this description have been isolated from muskrats where infection has been associated with water-borne epizootics, a more recent example of which occurred in Vermont among trappers who had come into contact with infected muskrats (Young *et al.* 1969).

Evidence that type B infections may be more prevalent than these reports indicate comes from two further studies. Wood examined 3,000 sera taken from Native Americans between Ontario and Manitoba and found about 12% with positive serological reactions for *F. tularensis* (Wood *et al.* 1976). In 1968 the largest recognized epidemic of American type B infection occurred in Vermont. There were 72 human infections which were in general much milder than the classic type A infections seen in North America. 74% (29 out of 39) or the infections were of the ulceroglandular type but 5 people only had systemic signs of fever, chills, myalgia, headache and general malaise. Muskrats were the source of infection with four type B organisms being isolated from 78 animals.

Europe and Asia

In Western Europe clinicians, microbiologists and veterinarians have to a large extent moulded their concept of tularaemia on the textbook accounts of the disease which are based predominately on the clinical reports and experience of treating patients who have contracted infections with *F. tularensis* type A. Recent work has shown that the organisms causing tularaemia in Asia and Europe appear to have similar characteristics as American type B bacteria (now designated *Francisella tularensis* subsp. *holarctica*). An intensive research

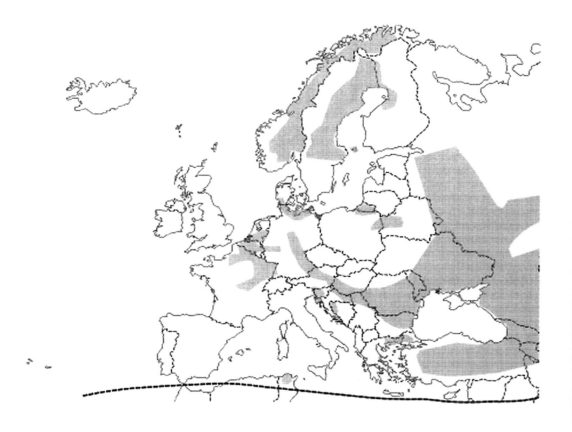

Fig. 24.1 Tularaemia foci in Europe.

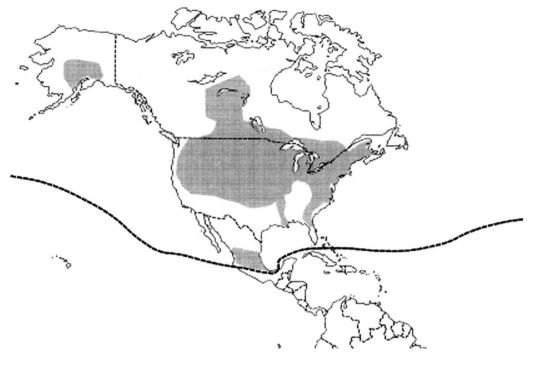

Fig. 24.2 Tularaemia foci in North America.

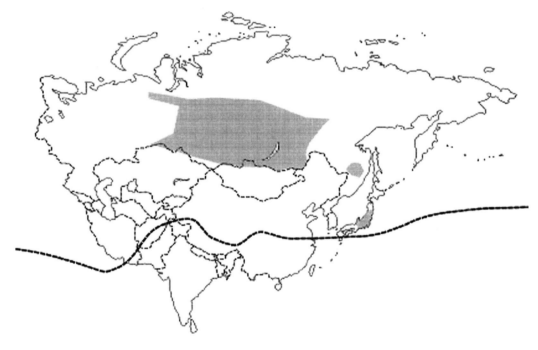

Fig. 24.3 Tularaemia foci in Asia.

effort has been made on type B infections by Russian workers during the past 40 years and in Sweden and Germany during the past two decades. It is clear from such studies that the epidemiology and clinical presentations of human tularaemia in Eurasia are more varied than in North America: in Russia and Sweden at least, rodents and ectoparasites were considered the principal reservoirs. The period of highest incidence appears to have been in the former USSR between 1940 and 1948 when it is estimated there were 100,000 cases a year (Jusatz 1962). This increase was attributed to the disruption caused by war.

The extensive Russian literature on the epidemiology indicates that four epidemic and endemic types (Table 24.4) have been recognized in Europe over the last 60 years.

The literature highlights:

◆ Contact epidemics where cases were predominately ulceroglandular through handling infected animals or carcases whilst hunting, skinning, and preparing hides and carcasses of rabbits, water rats, and other wild game and fur-bearing animals.

Table 24.3 Re-emergent and new tularaemia foci in Europe 1980–2008.

Sweden – Dalarna county	1981–2007: 379 cases. Large summer outbreaks
	1981 n = 40, 1995 n = 43, 2000 n = 49, 2003 n = 204
Örebro county	2000–2008: 362 cases mainly ulcero-transmitted by mosquitoes. glandular
	Thirty six (10%) were typhoidal/pulmonary type.
Spain – Castile and León	1997: first outbreak reported in Spain occurred during winter. Ulceroglandular type affecting women who had skinned rabbits
	2007 outbreak occurred in summer, typhoidal type in men who who had carried out activities related to the rural environment. Mode of transmission was by inhalation.
Turkey	Endemic disease in Turkey: Oropharyngeal form most common 3 water isolates from 3 epidemic areas. In Corum, Sivas and Samsun
Slovakia	1997–2008: 453 cases
Kosovo	1999 & 2001: two post-war outbreaks of 327 and 353 cases.
Serbia	1999: first epidemic. 1999–2008: 151 hospitalized cases
Italy – Pistoia,Tuscany	April 2007 & March 2008: 43 cases linked to spring water from a well

◆ Waterborne outbreaks, where 60–80% of the cases were of oropharyngeal type (angiono-bubonic) and which have been associated with consumption of water contaminated by the carcasses or excreta of infected animals.

◆ Vector-borne epidemics associated with mosquitoes and other arthropods; and airborne epidemics from inhalation of contaminated dust from rodent-infected hay.

◆ In addition, 'agricultural or mouse' associated outbreaks amongst farmers that have resulted from direct contact with mice during epizootics have been described.

The ascertaining and reporting of type *B tularensis* infection is highly variable for reason of the existence of both localized foci and restricted public reporting in some countries. Cases occur in long standing endemic foci across a wide albeit changing geographical area. In Sweden, 757 cases were recorded between 1931 and 1951, 437 cases between 1951 and 1959 rising markedly to 3,348 cases between 1960 and 1969 as a result of an airborne outbreak in Jamtland during late 1966 and the spring of 1967 and recurrent vector-borne outbreaks in Norrbotten during the summer months

between 1966 and 1973. In marked contrast to Sweden tularaemia appears to have been relatively uncommon in the rest of Scandinavia despite early recognition of the disease by Thjotta in the 1930s. Since then records exist of only a total of 66 cases in Norway up to 1974. A resurgence of interest led to the ascertainment of a further 44 cases between 1970 and 1973.

In the latter part of the twentieth century and since 2000 there appears in Sweden to have been a resurgence of activity resulting in the diagnosis of tularaemia cases that have emanated from long recognized foci in central Sweden, both in Orebro county and Dalarna. Reports from studies in both localities has provided new insights into transmission, sources and the resulting clinical presentations and pattern of disease (Tarnvick *et al.* 2004). In Örebro county (274,000 inhabitants), one of the emergent areas of tularaemia, 362 cases were reported between 2000 and 2008 (Svensson *et al.* 2009). The majority of the cases were as usual of the ulceroglandular type, vector-borne and transmitted by mosquitoes. Unusually, thirty six (10%) of the patients had typhoidal or pulmonary tularaemia. These were all sporadic cases with no geographical or time association. Cases were aged 33–90 years and 75% being men. Epidemiological investigations revealed that twenty seven of 36 typhoidal or pulmonary cases (75%) had a possible inhalation exposure from farming, grass cutting, handling horses or hay or renovating old sheds. Chest X-ray were abnormal in 20/33 cases, CT-scan in some cases revealed pathological changes not visible on ordinary X-ray, usually hilar lymph node enlargement. Of 21 patients with pathological findings on X-ray ten had no cough leading the investigators to conclude that typhoidal and pulmonary tularaemia should be considered in patients with a possible inhalation exposure who present with fever, headache, non productive cough and shivering.

This careful clinical investigation established the importance of accurate diagnosis of the clinical type of disease and suggested that pulmonary and typhoidal, although recognized before in earlier reports from Sweden is more difficult to diagnose and may be a reason for under ascertainment of pulmonary disease that occurred in this investigation in 10% of cases. Consequently the importance of the airborne route of infection may not be realized in the widespread distribution of sporadic cases that occur in summer months at the same time that vector-borne ulceroglandular tularaemia occurs in Sweden. In another Swedish study human demographic information on 379 tularaemia cases was collected in Dalarna County between 1981 and 2007. Outbreaks of predominately mosquito associated ulceroglandular infections occurred in the late summer months in 1981 (n = 40), 1995 (n = 43), 2000 (n = 49), and 2003 (n = 204). The cases had a variable but localized distribution being reported from a few villages along one river system.

Table 24.4 Classification of tularaemia foci in former USSR (from Olsufjev and Rudnev 1960)

Kind of foci	Main reservoir	Tick involved	Season of outbreaks
Meadow-field type	*Microtus arvalis*	*Dermacentor pictus*	Winter
Steppe (ravine) type	Voles, mice, hamsters, hares, etc.	Mainly Dermacentor merginatus	Autumn and winter
Forest type	Red vole (*Clethryionymous glareolus*), forest mice, hares	*Ixodes ricinis I. frianguliceps*	Tick season
Floodland-swamp type	Water rates	*Dermacentor, Rhipicephalus, Ixodes* sp.	Season of water-rat hunting
Foothill type	Water rats (voles, etc.)	*Ixodes apronophorus*	Summer
'Tungai' type	Hares, gerbils, mice, and muskrats	*Rhipicephalus pumilio*	Season of hare hunting

This apparent emergence of activity in long recognized foci in Sweden has been seen elsewhere in Europe where outbreaks and sporadic cases have been reported from Kosovo, Turkey, Georgia and China whilst new foci appear to have emerged in Spain, Kosovo, Serbia and Italy. This emerging picture of new and resurgent activity in old foci of *F. tularensis* subspecies *holarctica* has been the subject of both international and local interest from across Europe.

The first outbreak reported in Spain occurred in the winter of 1997 in Castile and León. Ulceroglandular infections occurred in women who had skinned rabbits and thereby acquired tularaemia by direct contact. The second outbreak was in the summer of 2007 with cases in the same localities but the cases a decade later were in men who had carried out activities related to the rural environment. The clinical presentation contrasted markedly from that seen in the first outbreak in that the clinical manifestations and other epidemiological features were that of the typhoidal form of tularaemia acquired by inhalation (Martin-Rodriguez *et al.* 2009).

Tularaemia outbreaks were recognized in Kosovo in 1999 and 2001 when 327 and 353 cases were confirmed as tularaemia with serological tests (Reintjes *et al.* 2002). Tularaemia cases were spread over the entire territory of Kosovo principally as a result of the war and the subsequent environmental disruption, mass population displacements and a breakdown of sanitation and hygiene. The predominant clinical presentations were glandular (79%) and ulceroglandular (21%) forms of disease and the most frequently reported sources of infection in the two outbreaks were contaminated drinking water and food. Sero-epidemilogical surveys indicated that human infections had not been prevalent before 1999. Since 2003, tularaemia cases have decreased to an estimated 100 cases per year (4/100,000 inhabitants). Investigators concluded that these two major outbreaks of tularaemia preceded the establishment of an active endemic area: the question remains as to whether in fact this was the re-emergence of an quiescient focus of tularaemia in Kosovo as has occurred in Sweden.

The first epidemic of tularaemia in South-eastern Serbia happened in 1999. During a 10 year period from 1999 to 2008, there were 151 patients who were hospitalized and diagnosed with tularaemia. Between 1997–2008 a total of 453 cases tularaemia were reported from all areas of Slovakia (incidence rate 0.71 per 100,000 population). However 95.4% of cases were in Nitra County in the west of the country (incidence rate of 4/100,000 rising in 2002 to 18/100,000 in this one region). Most frequent clinical manifestations were ulceroglandular and glandular forms—55.6%, pulmonary, oroglandular and others represented 21.2%, 18.8% and 4.4%, respectively.

Notable was the rise of pulmonary and oroglandular clinical forms over the period of investigation and surveillance. Cases occurred in all age groups but were more frequent in men (1.9:1) compared with women. Seasonal occurrence peaked in summer, month of July. More prevalent were cases transmitted from other sources—59% were from hares, 16% of which were associated with a marked decrease in the local hare population within local tularaemia foci at the time of the outbreak. Transmission of the disease resulted most frequently from manipulation with contaminated feed, litter and working in dusty environment with increased occurrence of rodents. About 12% of cases were transmitted by ticks and biting insects. The investigators concluded that there appears to be a change in predominant sources of infection and routes of transmission conditioned changes in epidemiology of

tularaemia in Slovakia as evidenced by decreased number of professional infections and a rise of cases acquired during leisure activities in summer, and infections in lower age groups.

An outbreak of 43 cases of tularaemia occurred in Tuscany in the Italian province of Pistoia during 2007 and 2008. The most frequently clinical presentation observed was a cervical lymphadenopathy and tonsillitis with sore throat being observed in a few cases. As with the majority of such oropharyngeal cases of tularaemia the outbreak was associated with the consumption of a natural source of spring water. Thirty eight cases occurred between December 2007 and March 2008. *Fransisella tularensis* subsp. *holarctica* (type B) was demonstrated in two samples of spring water collected in February and March 2008 by PCR and mice inoculation although direct culture was not achieved. Out of the 43 cases, confirmed with antibodies titres that ranged from 1:50 to 1:1,600, 34 (79%) had been exposed to this common source of spring water collected from a small cement basin at about 950 m of altitude by resident people and tourists, stored in containers and consumed at home. The outbreak was brought under control after the demolition of the cement basin and the restoration of the stream as the local source of water without the storage facility of the cement basin.

This large epidemic occurred about 20 years after two last important outbreak of Tularaemia recorded in northern and central Italy (Liguria and Tuscany regions) and confirms the potential for the recrudescence and circulation of *Fransisella tularensis* after a long period of apparent quiescence in Tuscany.

Clinical epidemiology

Transmission to man occurs in residents and travellers to endemic areas most commonly from the bites of ticks, mosquitoes and rodents or from handling infected hares or skinning carcasses in the fur trade. Water-borne outbreaks occur from drinking water from contaminated streams or wells especially at times of civil disruption and damage to supply systems and wells. Airborne outbreaks result from moving rodent-contaminated hay, when threshing corn, from laboratory accidents or might be the expected outcome of a deliberate release incident.

The clinical epidemiology of human infection appears complex since it relates to the route of transmission and the ecosystem that maintains the agent. The clinical presentation of the human disease is indicative of both the mode of transmission and often the source of infection.

Tularaemia presenting as ulceroglandular disease results from either vector-borne infection from mosquito or tick bites or occur as a result of contact lesions from skinning hares or muskrats. Oropharyhgeal and typhoidal infections predominate in waterborne outbreaks of *F. tularensis holarctica*. Pulmonary or influenza disease results from airborne transmission associated with either farmers having moved rodent contaminated hay or laboratory acquired infection. An international aerosol release of *F. tularensis* type A would be expected to result in clinical manifestations similar to those recognized in natural respiratory tularaemia. Both vector-borne and airborne transmission of *F. tularensis* may both be associated with florid skin manifestations as a presenting symptom of tularemia.

Infections caused by *F. tularensis* subspecies *tularensis* in North America most commonly causes ulceroglandular tularaemia, by contact with infected lagomorphs and rabbits or from tick bites. Cleaning contaminated carcasses may lead to an oculoglandular presentation. Rarely, eating undercooked rabbit or hare meat

Table 24.5 Epidemic types of tularaemia: prevention and control of Francisella *tularensis* subspecies *holarctica*

Origin of epidemic	Groups of the population exposed to the infection	Mode of infection	Predominant form of the disease and location of the buboes	Time of origin of the outbreak	Source of infection	The principle methods of prophylaxis and eradication of the epidemic
Type I Epidemic resulting from wounds of mucous membrane infection–contact epidemic						
The water vole fur trade. Trapping of hares and other animals susceptible to tularaemia in food-plain foci	Persons engaged in hunting and handling the carcasses	Contact with the carcass or dead body of an infected animal	The bubonic form. Buboes localized mainly in the axillary and cubital regional nodes	At the time of the spring floods and the hunting season	Water voles, hares and other animals	Prophylactic vaccination of vulnerable groups
Meat-processing factories handling sheep and hare carcasses	Workers in the carcass dressing and cutting departments	As above	As above	Any time of the year	Hares, sheep	In the event of an outbreak work should be stopped for the duration of the incubation period and until vaccination has been carried out
Rodent control work or apizootic disease surveys	Persons engaged in work of this type	As above	As above	The time of year at which the work is carried out	Murine rodents	Attention to personal prophylaxis
Hay-cutting in marshy meadows	Persons engaged in this work. The incidence is normally low.	Contact with contaminated water and other substrates	The bubonic form with buboes mainly in the inguinal region	Spring and summer (ie. the hay cutting season)	Murine rodents	
Type II Epidemic in which the infection is transmitted by an arthropod vector (Vector-borne)						
The presence of human beings in the characteristic biotopes of arthropod vectors	Random members of groups working near water, marshy ground, or bushes and trees	The bit of mosquitoes, horse flies, and other arthropod vectors	The ulcerous bubonic form. The ulcers are located mainly on exposed parts of the body if dipteran insects are responsible for the bites	From July to September. The period when arthropods are most active	The water vole and murine rodents	Protection from bites by the use of repellents and other means; prophylactic vaccination of the inhabitants of natural foci of tularaemia
Type III Epidemic in which infection is contracted orally (water and food-borne epidemic)						
Contamination of water by the discharges or corpses of disease rodents	The disease is restricted to people using water from a contaminated source. Usually a large proportion of those drawing water from one particular source contract the disease within a short space of time.	The use of contaminated water in its raw state for drinking purposes	The anginous-bubonic and the intestinal forms. An intermediate form is probably the most common, however	Summer and autumn usually. Winter outbreaks have also been recorded	Murine rodents and more rarely water voles	Sterilization of water and purification and disinfection of wells. The chlorination of piped water supplies, rodent control and prophylactic vaccination of the inhabitants of natural foci
Contamination of foodstuffs by the discharges of diseased rodents	People consuming contaminated food stuffs which have not been adequately cooked. In contract to water-borne epidemics the incidence is low	Consumption of contaminated foodstuffs	The intestinal form is the most common but the anginous-bubonic form may also be observed	Autumn and winter	Murine rodents	Protections of foodstuffs from the activities of rodents, extermination of rodents, and prophylactic vaccination of the inhabitants of natural foci
Type IV Epidemic where infection is the result of inhalation of contaminated air (aspiration epidemic)						
The threshing of stacked corn, the carting of straw and the handling of threshed grain and rodent-contaminated vegetables	The disease is confined to persons engaged in this type of work or sleeping on contaminated straw. A high incidence of disease is normally associated with epidemics of this type	Inhalation of droplets or dust contaminated by the discharges of diseased rodents	Tularaemia of the respiratory tracts and occasionally of the intestinal canal	Winter (early) spring and sometimes autumn)	Murine rodents	The use of respirators during work, the use of fir branches instead of straw for bedding, prophylactic vaccination of the inhabitants of natural foci of tularaemia and the extermination of rodents

causes a typhoidal-like illness. Any form of the disease may be complicated by pneumonia which is one of the two presenting conditions in laboratory-acquired infections, the other being the typhoid form of tularaemia. European and Asian forms of disease caused by *F. tularensis holarctica* clades have a greater diversity of clinical reports. This was originally thought to reflect the generally less virulent characteristics of *holarctica* strains. Differences between the epidemiology and clinical disease originally attracted scant attention despite the widespread geographical distribution of *F. tularensis holarctica* clades throughout the northern hemisphere with the persistence and frequent re-emergence of long established ecological foci. One hundred years after the recognition of two different types of epidemiology the molecular and ecological basis for the differences defies elicitation.

Prevention and control

The first objective is to reduce as far as possible human contact with potentially infected animal species and to avoid ticks and mosquito bites in known infected areas. This requires knowledge of the local epidemiology of tularaemia foci. When contact with potentially infected material is inevitable, specific immunisation becomes necessary. Since the Second World War, preventive measures in endemic areas have been based on the dual process of education and vaccination in selected high risk groups (Table 24.5).

Live attenuated strains of *holarctica* biotype have been used extensively as vaccines since the 1940s and have been shown to be effective (Tiggert 1962). The preferred method of vaccination was by the inhalation of dried viable vaccine. Subsequently an attenuated Russian strain (LVS) was selected for study in the USA. It was shown to be superior to a killed vaccine in immunizing activity in human subjects (Saslaw *et al.* 1961) and in experimental animals. Hornick and Eigelsback (1966) exposed human volunteers to LVS vaccine by inhalation; this led at most to a mild self-limiting illness. They were subsequently challenged by the aerial route with a virulent strain of *F.tularensis* and were shown to have substantial, though not total immunity. Burke (1977) reported that the routine sue of LVS vaccine in laboratory workers who were regularly handling *F.tularensis* led to a reduction in the number of attacks of tularaemia infection, but cases still occurred.

References

Burke, D. S. (1977). Immunisation against Tularaemia: analysis of the effectiveness of live *Francisella tularensis* vaccine in prevention of laboratory acquired Tularaemia. *J. Infect. Dis.*, **135**(1): 55–60.

Dahlstrand, S., Ringertz, O., and Zetterberg, B. (1971). Airborne tularaemia in Sweden. *Scan. J. Infect. Dis.*, **3**: 7–16.

Eigelsbach, H. T., Chambers, L. A. and Coriell, L. L. (1946). Electron microscopy of *B. tularense*. *J. Bacteriol.*, **52**: 179–85.

Horne, H. (1912). A lemming pest and a guinea pig epizootic; a contribution intended to elucidate the reasons for the mortality among lemmings during the 'lemming years', so called. *Zentral. Bakteriol. Prasiten. Infektion. Hyg., I Abt. Orig.*, **66**(2/4): 169.

Hornick, R. B. and Eigelsback, H. T. (1966). Aerogenic immunisation of man with live tularaemia vaccine. *Bacteriol. Rev.*, **30**: 532.

Jusatz, H. G. (1962). Tularaemia in Central Europe 1933–1953 II/37. In: E. Roderwaldt (ed.) *World Atlas of Infectious Disease*, Pt III (ed.), pp. 1–8. Geneva: WHO.

Martin-Rodriguez, L., Iglesias-Garcia, R., Del Ris-Martin, M., Mazon-Ramos, M. A., Arranz-Pera, M. L. (2009). Prevalence of epidemic outbreak of tularaemia in the Hospital Universitario Rio Hortega (Spain) in the year 2007. *Rev. Clin. Esp.*, **209**(7): 342–46.

McCoy, G. W. (1911). A plague like disease of rodents. *Pub. Heal. Bull., Wash. DC*, **43**: 53–71.

McCoy, G. W. and Chapin, C. W. (1912). Further observations on a plague like disease of rodents with a preliminary note of the causative agent *P. tularense*. *J. Infect. Dis.*, **10**: 61–72.

Nichols, P. D., Mayberry, W. R., Antworth, C. P. and White, D. C. (1985). Determination of monounsaturated double-bond position and geometry in the ellular fatty acids of the pathogenic bacterium *Francisella tularensis*. *J. Clin. Microbiol.*, **21**(5): 728–40.

O'Hara, S., Sato, T., and Homma, M. (1971). Serological studies on *Francisella tularensis, Francisella movicida, Yersinia philmiragia* and *Brucella abortus*. *Intern. J. System. Bacteriol.*, **2**: 336–43.

Olin, Y., Sato, T., Homma, M. (1996). Occurrence and mode of transmission of tularaemia in Sweden. *Acta Microbiol. Scandin.*, **19**: 220–47.

Olsufjev, N. G. and Rudnev, G. P. (1960). *Tularaemia*. Moscow: Publishing House for Medical Literature.

Parker, R. R. *et al.* (1951). Contamination of natural waters and mud with *Pasteurella tularensis* and tularaemia in beavers and muskrats in the northwestern US. *Bull. Nat. Instit. Heal.*, **193**: 1–161.

Petersen, J. M. *et al.* (2004). Methods for the enhanced recovery of *Francisella tularensis* cultures. *Appl. Environ. Microbiol.*, **70**: 3733–35.

Reintjes, R., Dedushaj, I., and Gjini, A. (2002). Tularaemia outbreak investigation in Kosovo: case control and environmental studies. *Emerg. Infect. Dis.*, **8**(1): 69–73.

Saslaw, S., Eigelsbach, H. T., Wilson, H. R., Prior, J. A. and Carhart, S. (1961). Tularemica vaccine study. II. Respiratory challenge. *Arch. Intern. Med.*, **107**: 702–14.

Schmitt, P. *et al.* (2005). A novel screening ELISA and a confirmatory Western blot useful for diagnosis and epidemiological studies of tularaemia. *Epidemiol. Infect.*, **133**: 757: 66.

Sjostedt, A. (2005). *Francisella*. In: G. Garrity *et al.* (eds.) *The Proteobacteria, Part B, Bergey's Manual of Systematic Bacteriology*, pp. 200–10. New York, NY: Springer.

Svensson, K., Back, E., Eliasson, H. *et al.* (2009). Landscape Epidemiology of Tularaemia Outbreaks in Sweden. *Emerg. Infect. Dis.*, **15**(12): 1937–47.

Tarnvik, A., Preibe, H. S., and Grunow, R. (2004). Tularaemia in Europe: An epidemiological overview. *Scandin. J. Infect. Dis.*, **36**: 350–55.

Taylor, J. P. *et al.* (1991). Epidemiologic characteristics of human tularaemia in the southwest central states, 1981–1987. *Am. J. Epidemiol.*, **133**: 1032–38.

Thjotta, T. (1931a). Continued investigations into occurrence of tularaemia in Norway; cases originating from the infectious carriers than the hare. *Norsk. Mag. Laegevid.*, **92**: 32–40.

Thjotta, T. (1931b). Tularaemia in Norway. *J. Infect. Dis.*, **49**: 99.

Tiggert, W. D. (1962). Soviet viable *Pasteurella tularensis* vaccines. A review of selected articles. *Bacteriolog. Rev.*, **26**: 354–73.

Whipp, M. J. *et al.* (2003). Characterisation of a *novicida*-like subspecies of *Francisella tularensis* isolated in Australia. *J. Med. Microbiol.*, **52**: 839–42.

Wood, J. B., Balteris, K., Hardy, R. H. and Pearson, A. D. (1976). Imported tularaemia. *BMJ*, **I**: 811.

World Health Organisation (2007). *WHO Guidelines on Tularaemia*. Geneva: WHO. ISBN 978 92 4 154737 6.

Young, L. S. *et al.* (1969). Tularaemia epidemic: Vermont 1968, 47 cases linked to contact with muskrats. *N. Engl. J. Med.*, **280**: 1253–60.

PART 3

Viral zoonoses

CHAPTER 25

Arenaviruses

Colin R. Howard

Summary

There are few groups of viral zoonoses that have attracted such widespread publicity as the arenaviruses, particularly during the 1960s and 1970s when Lassa emerged as a major cause of haemorrhagic disease in West Africa. More than any other zoonoses, members of the family are used extensively for the study of virus-host relationships. Thus the study of this unique group of enveloped, single-stranded RNA viruses has been pursued for two quite separate reasons. First, lymphocytic choriomeningitis virus (LCM) has been used as a model of persistent virus infections for over half a century; its study has contributed, and continues to contribute, a number of cardinal concepts to our present understanding of immunology. LCM virus remains the prototype of the *Arenaviridae* and is a common infection of laboratory mice, rats and hamsters. Once thought rare in humans there is now increasing evidence of LCM virus being implicated in renal disease and as a complication in organ transplantation. Second, certain arenaviruses cause severe haemorrhagic diseases in man, notably Lassa fever in Africa, Argentine and Bolivian haemorrhagic fevers in South America, Guaranito infection in Venezuela and Chaparé virus in Bolivia. The latter is a prime example for the need of ever-continuing vigilance for the emergence of new viral diseases; over the past few years several new arenaviruses have been reported as implicated with severe human disease and indeed the number of new arenaviruses discovered since the last edition of this book have increased the size of this virus family significantly.

In common with LCM, the natural reservoir of these infections is a limited number of rodent species (Howard 1986). Although the initial isolates from South America were at first erroneously designated as newly defined arboviruses, there is no evidence to implicate arthropod transmission for any arenavirus. However, similar methods of isolation and the necessity of trapping small animals have meant that the majority of arenaviruses have been isolated by workers in the arbovirus field. A good example of this is Guaranito virus that emerged during investigation of a dengue virus outbreak in Venezuela (Salas *et al.* 1991).

There is an interesting spectrum of pathological processes among these viruses. All the evidence so far available suggests that the morbidity of Lassa fever and South American haemorrhagic fevers due to arenavirus infection results from the direct cytopathic action
of these agents. This is in sharp contrast to the immunopathological basis of 'classic' lymphocytic choriomeningitis disease seen in adult mice infected with LCM virus and the use of this system for elucidating the phenomenon of H2-restriction of the host cytotoxic T cell response (Zinkernagel and Doherty 1979). Despite the utility of this experimental model for dissecting the nature of the immune response to virus infection and the growing interest in arenaviruses of rodents, there remains much to be done to elucidate the pathogenesis of these infections in humans.

Properties of the virus

Nomenclature and natural history

The grouping was first recognized on the basis of a serological cross reaction observed between LCM and Machupo virus the latter being found to cause Bolivian haemorrhagic fever in the 1960s. The *Arenaviridae* take their name from their sand-sprinkled appearance when viewed in the electron microscope (Latin: *arena* = sand). The members of the family are listed in Table 25.1. The various strains and isolates of LCM are now considered to be a genus within the *Arenaviridae*. A close serological relationship exists between LCM, Lassa virus and other arenaviruses from Africa. For this reason, they are loosely referred to as the 'Old World' arenaviruses, in contrast to those from the Americas, although LCM can be found world-wide (Howard and Simpson 1980). The 'New World' arenaviruses show varying degrees of serological relationships with Tacaribe virus, first isolated in Trinidad. For this reason, viruses from the Americas are frequently regarded as members of the Tacaribe complex (Fig. 25.1).

With the exception of LCM, all are referred to by names that reflect the geographical locality in which they were isolated. Various strain designations are also commonly used, in particular for LCM and arenaviruses isolated from man. Multiple isolations of non-pathogenic viruses that infect New World rodents are made less frequently, with the exception of Pichinde virus where a large number of field isolates from Columbia have been characterized.

All but one of the 24 members of the *Arenaviridae* so far described have rodents as their natural reservoir hosts. The exception is the Tacaribe virus, which was originally isolated from the fruit-bat, *Artibeus literatus*. Although rodents are divided globally into over

Table 25.1 *Arenaviridae*: host and geographic distribution

Virus	Natural Host	Human Disease	Distribution
LCM-Lassa Serocomplex (Old World)			
Ippy	*Arvicanthus spp.*	not recorded	Central African Republic
Lassa	*Mastomys natalensis*	Lassa fever	West Africa
Lujo	*Unknown*	Haemorrhagic fever	Southern Africa
Lymphocytic choriomeningitis	*Mus musculus,* *Mus domesticus*	Aseptic meningitis	Worldwide except Australasia
Mobala	*Praomys jacksoni*	infection possible	Central African Republic
Mopeia	*Mastomys natalensis*	infection possible	Mozambique Zimbabwe
Tacaribe Serocomplex (New World)			
Clade A			
Allpahuayo	*Oecomys bicolor*	not recorded	Peru
Bear Canyon	*Peromyscus californicus*	infection possible?	California, USA
Catarina	*Neotoma micropus*	Not recorded	Texas, USA
Flexal	*Neocomys spp.*	not recorded	Brazil
Paraná	*Oryzomys buccinatus*	not recorded	Paraguay
Pichinde	*Oryzomys albigularis*	not recorded	Columbia
Pirital	*Sigmodon alstoni*	not recorded	Venezuela
Tamiami	*Sigmodon hispidus*	not recorded	Florida, USA
Whitewater Arroyo	*Neotoma albigula*	Infection possible?	New Mexico, USA
Clade B			
Amapari	*Oryzomys gaedi* *Neocomys guianae*	not recorded	Brazil
Chaparé	*unknown*	Haemorrhagic fever	Bolivia
Cupixi	*Oryzomys capito*	not recorded	Brazil
Guanarito	*Zygodontomys brevicuda*	haemorrhagic fever	Venezuela
Junín	*Calomys musculinus, C. laucha, Akadon azarae*	haemorrhagic fever	Argentina
Machupo	*Calomys callosus*	haemorrhagic fever	Bolivia
Sabiá	*Unknown*	haemorrhagic fever	Brazil
Tacaribe	*Artibeus literatus (bat)*	infection possible	Trinidad
Clade C			
Latino	*Calomys callosus*	not recorded	Bolivia
Oliveros	*Bolomys obscures*	not recorded	Argentina

30 families, arenaviruses are predominantly found within two major families, the *Muridae* (e.g. mice and rats) and *Cricetidae* (e.g. voles, lemmings, gerbils). The nature of the original reservoir for LCM virus remains obscure, but it appears to be a species of the *Muridae* which evolved in the Old World and subsequently spread to most parts of the globe. There is a wide range of tropism and virulence among laboratory strains of LCM virus originally isolated from laboratory mouse colonies.

The natural reservoir of Lassa virus, *Mastomys natalensis*, is also a member of *Muridae* and, in common with the host of LCM, frequents human dwellings and food stores. In contrast, nearly all arenaviruses isolated from South America are associated with cricetid rodents whose members frequent open grasslands and woodland.

In recent years, several new arenaviruses have come to our attention. In the instance of Guanarito virus, this new form of haemorrhagic fever from Venezuela was originally mistaken as dengue (Gonzalez *et al*. 1995). A virus from Brazil dubbed Sabiá virus caused a laboratory-associated infection during investigations of a new outbreak of hitherto unrecorded febrile illness in the southern provinces. Whitewater Arroyo virus was found in the USA in 1999 and a virus distinct from Machupo caused death in Bolivia in 2004. Each instance brings into sharp relief the need for continuing vigilance of these zoonoses.

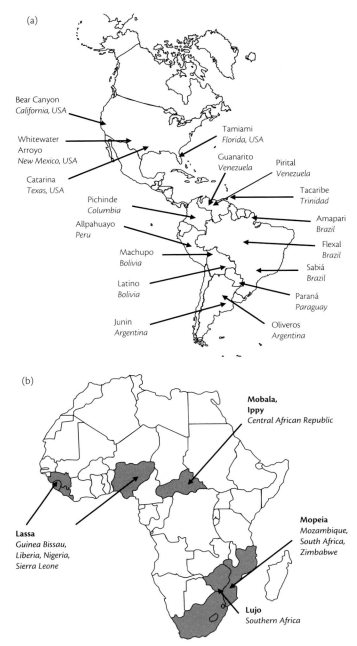

(a)

Bear Canyon
California, USA

Whitewater
Arroyo
New Mexico, USA

Catarina
Texas, USA

Pichinde
Columbia

Allpahuayo
Peru

Machupo
Bolivia

Latino
Bolivia

Junin
Argentina

Tamiami
Florida, USA

Guanarito
Venezuela

Pirital
Venezuela

Tacaribe
Trinidad

Amapari
Brazil

Flexal
Brazil

Sabiá
Brazil

Paraná
Paraguay

Oliveros
Argentina

(b)

Mobala,
Ippy
Central African Republic

Lassa
*Guinea Bissau,
Liberia, Nigeria,
Sierra Leone*

Mopeia
*Mozambique,
South Africa,
Zimbabwe*

Lujo
Southern Africa

Fig. 25.1 Geographical distribution of New (a) and Old (b) arenaviruses.

Ultrastructure of arenaviruses and infected cells

Negative-staining electron microscopy of extracellular virus shows pleomorphic particles ranging in diameter from 80 to 200 nm (Fig. 25.2).

The virus envelope is formed from the plasma membrane of infected cells. A significant thickening of both bilayers of the membrane together with an increase in the width of the electron-translucent intermediate layer is characteristic of arenavirus development. Little is known about the internal structure of the arenavirus particle, although thin sections of mature and budding viruses clearly show the ordered, and often circular, arrangements of host ribosomes that are typical of this virus group, conferring the 'sandy'

appearance from which its name is derived. Distinct well dispersed filaments 5–10 nm in diameter are released from detergent-treated virus. Two predominant size classes are present, with average lengths of 649 nm and 1300 nm respectively; these lengths do not show a close relationship with the two virus-specific L and S RNA species. Each is circular and beaded in appearance. Convoluted filamentous strands up to 15 nm in diameter can be seen in preparations of spontaneously disrupted Pichinde virus. These appear to represent globular condensations which arise from an association between neighbouring turns of the underlying helix. The basic configuration of the filaments shows a linear array of globular units up to 5 nm in diameter, probably representing single molecules of the viral polypeptide. These filaments progressively fold through a number of intermediate helical structures to produce the stable 15 nm diameter forms (Young 1987). Cryomicroscopy suggests that the nucleocapsid forms into a lattice just beneath the inner leaflet of the viral lipid layer (Neuman *et al.* 2005).

Arenaviruses replicate in experimental animals in the absence of any gross pathological effect. However, cellular necrosis may accompany virus production, not unlike that seen in virus-infected cell cultures. The variable pathological changes associated with arenavirus infections are further complicated by the occasional appearance of particles in tissue sections that react strongly with fluorescein-conjugated antisera. Granular fluorescence with convalescent serum in the perinuclear region of acutely infected Vero cells is often seen. In addition, intracytoplasmic inclusion bodies are prominent in virus-infected cells both *in vitro* and *in vivo*. These usually appear early in the replication cycle and consist largely of single ribosomes which later become condensed in an electron-dense matrix, sometimes together with fine filaments (Murphy and Whitfield 1975).

Chemical composition

Nucleic acid

The genome of arenaviruses consists of two single-stranded RNA segments of different sizes, designated L and S, with the S strand being more abundant. Analysis of RNA is complicated by the presence of ribosomal 18S and 28S RNA although these cellular RNA species are not essential for virus replication. The total ribosomal RNA content may in turn be influenced by the varying proportions of infectious to non-infectious particles present in virus stocks. Whether or not there is a role for these host RNA molecules in the establishment and maintenance of persistent infections is unclear. These are small amounts of both cell and viral low molecular weight RNA contained within virus particles, one of which codes for the Z protein required for replication (see below).

Genetic studies have shown that the S strand codes for the nucleoprotein (N) and the envelope glycoprotein precursor (GPC) in two main open reading frames located on RNA molecules of opposite polarity. The 3' half of the S RNA codes for the N protein by production of a mRNA with a nucleotide sequence complementary to the viral genome. In contrast, the GPC is expressed by the 5' half replication of the S RNA strand which is required to undergo replication before the production of a mRNA with a viral-sense sequence specific for the GPC protein. Thus expression of the genome is by synthesis of subgenomic RNA from full length templates of opposite polarities. This strategy of 'ambisense' coding for viral protein has so far been described only for the arenaviruses and some bunyaviruses. The reading frames for the two major gene

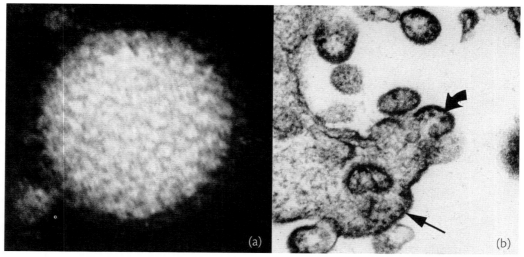

Fig. 25.2 Electron Microscopy of Arenaviruses (a) Negatively stained Lassa fever particle showing the whole surface covered in projections. Few particles are less than 100 nm, and many are twice this size (x300,000). (b) Lassa fever particles budding from a infected Vero cell. The thick arrow shows a mature particle, the thin arrow a maturing particle at the plasmalemma. Nucleocapsids and ribosomes line up immediately below the thickened membrane (thin arrow) (x39,000). Micrographs courtesy of Dr D.S. Ellis.

products are separated by a hairpin structure of approximately 20 paired nucleotides. This intergenic region may act as a control mechanism for genome expression but there is as yet no experimental evidence to support this possibility.

The L RNA strand represents about 70% of the viral genome coding for both the viral polymerase (L) and the Z protein. Re-assortment studies with virulent and avirulent strains of LCM virus have shown that lethal disease in guinea-pigs is associated with the L RNA strand. The L protein is encoded by a large open reading frame covering 70% of the L RNA strand: it is expressed via a mRNA complementary in sense to the viral genome.

Phylogenetic analysis

Genome sequencing can produce useful qualitative and quantitative comparisons between newly discovered arenavirus isolates and those already characterized. The first detailed study, reported by Bowen *et al.* (1997) used data from at least one strain of all arenaviruses recognized at that time. The resulting phylogenetic tree confirmed the distant relationship between Old World and New World arenaviruses, broadly in line with detailed antigenic analysis using monoclonal and polyclonal antibodies. Subsequent work on newer isolates coupled with the use of full length sequences shows that the New World arenaviruses are divisible into 3 lineages:

1   Clade A includes Pichinde, Tamiami, Paraná, Flexal and Whitewater Arroyo viruses,

2   Clade B encompasses the human pathogens Junín, Machupo, Sabiá, Guanarito and Chaparé viruses as well as Tacaribe and Amapari viruses,

3   Clade C the viruses Latino and Oliveros.

There seems to be much less variability among the Old World viruses with Mopeia and Mobala viruses being closely related to Lassa virus.

Nucleotide sequencing also shows extensive genetic diversity between different isolates that is not always correlated to location and/or the animal host reservoir. For example, Guanarito virus isolated from clinical cases of Venezuelan haemorrhagic fever revealed considerable heterogeneity of sequence, greater than that observed among rodent isolates (Weaver *et al.* 2000). Whether or not this is indicative of a mechanism whereby the virus evades the host immune response and is the forerunner of persistent infection in the rodent host, is unclear.

The propensity to cause serious human illness appears to have evolved quite separately among the Old World and New World arenaviruses. That the South American haemorrhagic fevers all appear confined to clade B suggests a single series of mutational events leading to a capacity to cause human disease. In contrast, Lassa virus has likely acquired its capacity to inflict serious human illness by a quite separate series of evolutionary events that are not clear from phylogenetic analysis alone.

Proteins

The arenavirus genome codes for at least five proteins; an RNA-dependent RNA polymerase and a zinc-binding (Z) protein from the L strand and three structural proteins from the smaller, S strand. Extracellular particles contain a major nucleocapsid-associated protein of molecular weight 54–68 kD with two glycoproteins in the outer viral envelope. These envelope glycoproteins are not primary gene products but arise by proteolytic cleavage of a larger, 75 kD glycoprotein precursor polypeptide (GPC) at a unique cleavage site conserved among the majority of arenaviruses. The first 59 amino acids at the N terminus of GPC act as a signal sequence for membrane insertion. Maturation and release of virus does not seem to be markedly inhibited in the presence of tunicamycin, an inhibitor of glycosylation, but glycoprotein cleavage is essential for infectivity.

The major glycoprotein species (GP2) in the molecular weight range of 34–42 kD represents the C-terminal cleavage product of the GPC envelope glycoprotein precursor. A major antigenic site has been located between amino acids 390–405, and cross-reactive monoclonal antibodies bind to epitopes in this region. The corresponding N-terminal product of GPC cleavage (GP1) is probably highly glycosylated with at least four antigenic domains. Neutralizing monoclonal antibodies to LCM virus map to two of these regions and there is less sequence homology between the GP1 than between the GP2 molecules of different arenaviruses. Once cleaved, the glycoproteins GP1 and GP2 form tetrameric structures embedded in the viral envelope. The proximal GP2 molecules forming electrovalent bonds with the underlying viral nucleocapside, possibly mediated by the Z protein.

The internal nucleocapsid-associated (N) protein accounts for much of the virus-specific protein present in purified virus and infected cells, and remains bound to the virus genome after solubilization of the virus with non-ionic detergents. Molecular cloning studies have shown a surprisingly high degree of homology between the N proteins of Old and New World arenaviruses, and this would account for the serological cross-reactions seen using certain monoclonal antibodies to the N protein. A high degree of conservation between such epidemiologically distinct viruses may indicate precise functional roles for certain areas of the N polypeptide in virus replication. Cleavage products of the N protein are a consistent feature of both virus and virus-infected cells. Cleavage is not noticeable in Vero cells; yields of arenaviruses are lower in these cells, perhaps due to reduced availability of N for packaging. A fragment of the N protein is often seen in the nuclei although the exact function of this is not clear.

A minor component with a molecular weight in excess of 150 kD is often observed in infected cells. This L protein represents the virus-specific RNA polymerase (Fuller-Pace and Southern 1989). Amino acid sequences common to the viral polymerase are present along the open reading frame coding for the L protein, which suggests the conservation of certain functional domains. A small, 12 kD viral polypeptide, the so-called Z, or zinc-binding protein is considered to play a role in controlling the replication and expression of the genome: the Z protein may also modulate interferon responses *in vivo* (Djavani *et al.* 2001).

Replication

Arenaviruses replicate in a wide variety of mammalian cells although either BHK-21 cells or monkey kidney cell lines are used for molecular studies. Maximal virus adsorption to cell surfaces is at 2 hours at 37°C. At a low multiplicity of infection (i.e. below 0.1) the latent period is approximately 6–8 hours, after which cell-associated virus increases exponentially. The titre of extracellular virus reaches a maximum 36–48 hours after infection. The passage history of any particular virus stock is probably one of the most critical factors which determines the kinetics of arenavirus replication.

Infected cells undergo only limited cytopathic changes with little or no change in the total level of host cell protein synthesis; virus yields vary in different susceptible cell types. Cell metabolism is only minimally affected and in some cells only a reduction in differentiated, or 'luxury' cell functions can be observed. Cultures of persistently infected cells are readily established, the morphology and growth kinetics of which are similar to those of uninfected cells.

Only limited information is available concerning the replication and expression of viral RNA within infected cells, although possible replication events can be predicted from the nucleotide sequences of L and S genome segments. The major feature of an ambisense coding strategy is that it allows for independent expression and regulation of the N and GPC genes from the S RNA segment. The N protein is independently expressed late in acute infection and in persistently infected cells in the absence of low levels of glycoprotein production. This is explained by the production of subgenomic mRNA from a negative polarity, virus-sense template.

A control mechanism must therefore exist which determines the fate of nascent RNA of negative polarity, destined either for encapsidation or as a template for N protein-specific mRNA. In contrast, the template for glycoprotein-specific mRNA is of complementary sense to viral RNA and as such would not be required for nascent virus production. The lack of glycoprotein late in the replicative cycle or in persistently infected cells would therefore imply selective transcriptional or translational control of this gene product.

Both viral RNA and its complementary strand contain hairpin sequences which may provide recognition points for termination of transcription by viral RNA polymerase. The nucleotide sequence in the hairpin region is of coding sense and may be transcribed, either as a discrete mRNA species or as a result of extended transcription of N or GPC messengers through this region. The postulated reading frames for viral gene products transcribed from LCM and Pichinde viral genomes would fit this hypothesis. In addition, a sequence for ribosomal 18S subunit binding is present on both mRNA molecules although the significance of this is not clear.

Diagnosis

Early diagnosis is essential but made difficult for the clinician as patients present with relatively non-specific symptoms. A history of travel to a region where arenavirus infections are common can help direct a laboratory investigation. Owing to the influenza-like nature of the early signs, other infections need to be excluded, for example yellow fever and dengue. If neurological signs are also present, then other causes of encephalitis or meningitis need to be excluded.

The diagnosis of arenavirus infections may be made by demonstration of a four-fold rise in specific antibody titre, the presence of IgM viral antibodies, or isolation of the virus. For routine isolation, the E6 clone of Vero cells is the cell line of choice, although all arenaviruses grow well in primate and rodent-derived fibroblast cell lines. However, a CPE is often difficult to see, and inoculated cultures often require examination by immunofluorescence (IF) or ELISA in order to detect the presence of viral antigens.

Both ELISA and IF tests have been used successfully for the diagnosis of human arenavirus infections. In the case of Lassa fever, infected cell substrates are used that have been treated by UV light, acetone, and cobalt irradiation to ensure safety. Drops of cell cultures dried onto glass slides can be prepared in a central laboratory and these preparations remain stable for many months. Most of the antigen detected within acetone-fixed infected cells represents cytoplasmic nucleocapsid protein. In the case of the New World arenaviruses, serological cross-reactions in the IF test (e.g. with sera from patients with Bolivian (Machupo) and Argentine (Junín) haemorrhagic fevers) are found with fixed cultures. Substrates prepared from other members of the Tacaribe complex, which includes Junín and Machupo viruses also react with sera taken from these patients during the acute phase and early convalescence. Greatest cross-reactivity can be seen between the closely-related Junín and

Machupo antigens, closely followed by Tacaribe virus-infected cells. Recent experience in Bolivia however, has shown that new arenaviruses may be missed by placing sole reliance on serology (Delgado *et al.* 2008).

The use of PCR for arenavirus diagnosis requires the rigorous testing of primer sets and the optimization of both RNA extraction and temperature cycling. Even so, an arenavirus not previously found may be missed. The use of many primer sets may lead to a loss of sensitivity and non-specific amplification, although such pitfalls can be avoided with care (Drosten *et al.* 2002). But in the final analysis virus isolation should be attempted as soon as possible by referring samples to a specialist containment laboratory.

Antigenic relationships

Monoclonal antibodies can distinguish between virus strains because they can be prepared against epitopes which go unrecognized when polyclonal antisera are used. Buchmeier *et al.* (1981) summarized the patterns of reactivity with a panel of monoclonal antibodies directed against laboratory strains of the homologous virus, and Lassa and Mopeia viruses. Reagents directed against the smaller, GP2 envelope glycoprotein cross-reacted by immunofluorescence with all substrates examined, whereas antibodies directed against the larger GP1 glycoprotein were either strain-specific or reacted with a subset only of the strains examined, presumably by binding to previously unrecognized epitopes. The observations that certain of these broadly cross-reactive antibodies also reacted with Pichinde virus suggests that epitopes on surface envelope structures among Old World and New World arenaviruses are conserved. A similar comparison has also been undertaken with monoclonal antibodies to Lassa tested against the Mopeia and Mobala viruses from Africa. Again, various degrees of cross-reactivity were observed with reagents specific for the GP2 external glycoprotein. Mobala virus from the Central African Republic, however, appears to be distinct, as several cross-reactive monoclonal antibodies originally prepared against LCM virus failed to recognize Mobala-infected substrates.

The neutralization test is highly specific for all members of the *Arenaviridae*; it is notable that the few examples of cross-reactivity were obtained with high titre animal antisera raised against Junín, Tacaribe and Machupo viruses. However, the ease with which neutralizing antibodies can be quantified varies greatly. No cross-reactions have been observed between Junín and Machupo viruses in plaque-reduction tests with human convalescent sera despite a close antigenic relationship. A similar marked specificity of neutralization has been demonstrated with LCM and Lassa sera, and both viruses are readily distinguishable from one another by this technique (however, neutralizing antibodies to Lassa virus can be detected only with great difficulty). The sensitivity of the neutralization test for LCM virus can be increased by incorporating either complement or anti-gammaglobulin into the test system.

Pathology of arenavirus infections

The mechanisms by which arenaviruses cause disease in man are not fully understood. There is no evidence that either immunopathological or allergenic processes play any part in causing disease; it appears to be more likely that disease is caused by direct damage of cells by the virus. Postmortem studies on patients who died from Junín virus infection have shown generalized lymphadenopathy, endothelial swelling in the capillaries and arterioles of almost every organ, and depletion of lymphocytes in the spleen. Virus first replicates in lymphoid tissue from whence it invades the reticuloendothelial system and those cells concerned in the immune and cellular immune responses; the host's defence mechanisms are thus impaired. Fatal illness is invariably associated with capillary damage leading to capillary fragility, haemorrhages and irreversible shock (Johnson *et al.* 1973).

Disseminated intravascular coagulation is not a typical feature. Although Lassa fever is often regarded as being hepatotropic, the extent of hepatic damage is insufficient to account for the severity of the clinical disease. Studies of Lassa virus-infected rhesus monkeys have shown that changes in vascular function may play a much greater role in pathogenesis, as a result either of viral replication in the vascular epithelium or of secondary effects of virus activity in different organs. Platelet and epithelial cell functions fail immediately before death and are accompanied by a drop in the level of prostacyclin; these functions rapidly return to normal in animals surviving infection (Fisher-Hoch *et al.* 1987). Impairment of the functions of vascular epithelium in the absence of histological changes appears to be a common feature of the final stages of viral haemorrhagic diseases in general and suggests that hypovolaemic shock may be amenable to treatment with prostacyclin.

The pathogenesis of Argentine haemorrhagic fever caused by Junín virus has been studied in experimentally infected guineapigs, this being a suitable model of human disease. There is a pronounced thrombocytopenia and leucopenia characteristic of human infections, and animals die of severe haemorrhagic lesions. Bone marrow cells are destroyed with release of proteases and acid and alkaline phosphatases into the blood; this leads to consumption of the C4 component of complement. These effects may lead in turn to progressive alterations in vascular permeability and platelet function (Rimoldi and de Bracco 1980).

The most extensive histopathological studies have been made on tissues from patients with Lassa fever (Walker and Murphy 1987). However, there are many similarities in the pathological lesions found in man following Junín and Machupo virus infections. Focal non-zonal necrosis in the liver has been described in all three conditions with hyperplasia of Kupffer cells, erythrophagocytosis and acidophilic necrosis of hepatocytes. Councilman-like bodies can be observed together with cytoplasmic vacuolations and nuclear pyknosis or lysis. As with other organs, there is little evidence of cellular inflammation. Lesions in other organs have been described, including interstitial pneumonitis, tubular necrosis in the kidney, lymphocytic infiltration of the spleen and minimal inflammation of the central nervous system and myocardium (Walker and Murphy 1987). The hepatic changes may be grouped into three categories:

1 mild to moderate infection with evidence of focal necrosis in less than 20% of hepatocytes;

2 hepatic regeneration but extensive damage probably centred on other organs

3 severe damage with multifocal necrosis involving up to 50% of hepatocytes.

These changes are consistent with a direct cytolytic action of the virus; nevertheless, the simultaneous presence of Lassa virus and specific antibodies during the later stages of the acute disease suggest that antibody-dependent cellular immune reactions may also occur. Microscopic changes in the kidneys are minimal; it is not clear whether the impairment of renal function is due to the deposition of antigen-antibody complexes.

Lymphocytic choriomeningitis

Clinical and pathological features

Until recently human infection was regarded as a rare, inapparent infection that may occasionally present as an influenza-like febrile illness, as aseptic meningitis or as severe meningoencephalomyelitis.

LCM virus may be a more important human pathogen than considered hitherto. Palacios *et al.* (2008) reported the presence of virus in patients receiving kidney and liver transplants who subsequently died of an acute febrile illness. The report follows others implicating LCM virus in fatal haemorrhagic-like illnesses following solid organ transplantation (Fischer *et al.* 2006).

The incubation period is 6–13 days. In the influenza-like illness there is fever, malaise, coryza, muscular pains and bronchitis. The meningeal form is more common; the same symptoms may remain mild and be of short duration and patients recover within a few days, but there can be more pronounced illness with severe prostration lasting 2 weeks or more. Chronic sequelae have been reported on occasion. They include headache, paralysis and personality changes. The few deaths have followed severe meningoencepalomyelitis. In one case there was mild pharyngitis and a diffuse erythematous rash followed by haemorrhages and death.

An early leucopenia followed by lymphocytosis is a constant finding. In central nervous system disease, the cerebrospinal fluid (CSF) is at increased pressure with a slight rise in protein concentration, normal or slightly reduced sugar concentration, and a moderate number of cells, mainly lymphocytes (150–400/mm^3). These changes are not, of course, restricted to LCM infections. Virus can be isolated from blood, CSF and, in fatal cases, from brain tissue.

Epidemiology

Man is usually infected through contact with rodents. Many infections have been acquired in laboratories, where LCM may be a contaminant in laboratory colonies of mice and hamsters. Hamsters kept as pet animals have also played a role in human infection. The mechanism of transmission of the virus to man is not fully understood but is likely to involve dust contaminated by urine, the contamination of food and drink, or via skin abrasions. Recent clusters of cases among transplant recipients would suggest that LCM virus may have become chronic in the otherwise asymptomatic donors. In at least one instance, donor infection could be traced back to ownership of a pet hamster infected with LCM virus (Fischer *et al.* 2006)

Lassa fever

History

Lassa virus made a dramatic appearance in Nigeria in 1969 as a lethal, highly transmissible disease. The first victim was an American nurse who was infected in a small mission station in the Lassa township in north-eastern Nigeria, whence the virus and the disease derive their names. The origin of the infection was never determined, although it is thought to have been acquired through direct contact with an infected patient in Lassa. When the nurse's condition steadily deteriorated she was flown to the Evangel Hospital in Jos, where she died the following day.

While she was in hospital she was cared for by two other American nurses, one of whom also became infected by direct contact, probably through a skin abrasion. This nurse became unwell after an 8-day incubation period and died following an illness lasting 11 days. The head nurse of the hospital, who had assisted at the post-mortem of the first patient, fell ill 7 days after the death of the second patient from who she had cared, and from whom she probably acquired the infection.

This third case was evacuated to the USA by air in the first-class cabin of a commercial airliner with two attendants and screened from economy-class passengers only by a curtain. After a severe illness under intensive care she slowly recovered. A virus, subsequently named Lassa, was isolated from her blood by workers at the Yale Arbovirus Unit. One of these virologists became ill but improved after an immune plasma transfusion donated by the third case. Five months after this infection, a laboratory technician in the Yale laboratories, who had not been working with Lassa virus, fell ill and died. The manner in which this infection was acquired has never been determined.

This trail of events not unnaturally earned for Lassa virus a formidable notoriety, which was sharply enhanced by two more devastating hospital outbreaks—one in Nigeria, the other in Liberia. A further epidemic was seen in Sierra Leone in October 1972. In sharp contrast to the previous outbreaks, this one was not confined to hospitals, although hospital staff were at considerable risk and several became infected. Most of the patients acquired their illness in the community and there was several intra-familial transmissions. This led to a revision of the initial view—formed from experience of nosocomial infections—that Lassa fever has a high mortality.

Lassa fever has since continued to occur in West Africa, usually as sporadic cases (Monath 1987). Between 1969 and 1978 there were 17 reported outbreaks affecting 386 patients in whom the mortality was 27%. Eleven of the episodes were in hospitals, where the case fatality rate reached 44%; two were laboratory infections, two were community-acquired outbreaks, and two were prolonged community outbreaks. Eight patients were flown to Europe or North America. One of them was evacuated with full isolation precautions and the remainder, of whom five were infectious, travelled on scheduled commercial flights as fare-paying passengers. Fortunately, no contact cases resulted.

Clinical features

Lassa virus causes a spectrum of disease ranging from subclinical to fulminating fatal infection. The incubation period ranges from 3 to 16 days and the illness usually begins insidiously. The disease is difficult to distinguish in the early stages from other systemic febrile illnesses, the most reliable clinical signs being a sore throat and vomiting. Between the third and sixth day of illness the symptoms suddenly worsen and there is high fever, severe prostration, chest and abdominal pains, conjunctival injection, diarrhoea, dysphagia and vomiting. Chest pain located substernally and along the costal margins, is often associated with tenderness on pressure and is exacerbated by coughing and deep inspiration. One important physical finding is a distinct pharyngitis; yellow-white exudative spots may be seen on the tonsillar pillars together with small vesicles and ulcers. The patient appears toxic, lethargic and dehydrated; the blood pressure is low and there is sometimes a bradycardia relative to the body temperature. There may be cervical lymphadenopathy, coated tongue, puffiness of the face and neck, and blurred vision. Occasionally a faint maculopapular rash may be seen during the second week of illness on the face, neck, trunk and arms. In severe cases, haemorrhages also occur. Cough is a common symptom, and light-headedness, vertigo and tinnitus appear in a few patients. Deafness has also been noted in about 20% of patients and, although it may be reversible, is more often permanent.

The fever generally lasts for 7–17 days and is variable. Convalescence begins in the second to fourth weeks, when the temperature returns to normal and the symptoms improve. Most patients complain of extreme fatigue for several weeks. Loss of hair happens occasionally and there may be brief bouts of fever.

Patients in whom the disease is fatal not uncommonly have a high sustained fever. Acutely ill patients suddenly deteriorate between days 7 and 14 with a sudden drop in blood pressure, peripheral vasoconstriction, hypovolaemia and anuria; there may be pleural effusions and ascites. In addition, coma, stupor, tremors and myoclonic twitching may occur. Death is due to shock, anoxia, respiratory insufficiency and cardiac arrest.

Epidemiology

Lassa virus has been repeatedly isolated from the multimammate rat *Mastomys natalensis* in Sierra Leone and Nigeria. This rodent is a common domestic and peridomestic species, and large populations are widely distributed in Africa south of the Sahara. During the rainy season it may desert the open fields and seek shelter indoors. Some genetic variation has been shown in *Mastomys* populations inhabiting different ecological niches; however, there appears to be no difference in the prevalence of antibody and virus in at least two of the karyotypes found in West Africa. The animals are infected at birth or during the perinatal period. Like other arenaviruses, Lassa virus produces a persistent, tolerated infection in its rodent reservoir with no ill effects and without any detectable host immune response. The animals remain infected throughout their lifetime, freely excreting Lassa virus in urine and other body fluids. The correlation between the prevalence of antibody in a community and the degree of infestation by infected rodents, however, is poor.

Studies of the ratio of clinical illness to infections have recently confirmed that Lassa fever is endemic in several regions of West Africa. It has been estimated that only 1–2% of infections are fatal, substantially less than the figures of 30–50% originally associated with the early nosocomial outbreaks. However, there may still be up to 300,000 infections per year with as many as 5,000 deaths (McCormick *et al.* 1986). The seroconversion rates among villagers in Sierra Leone vary from 4 to 22 per 100 susceptible individuals per year; up to 14% of febrile illness in such population groups is due to Lassa virus infection. These data confirm the relatively high rate of asymptomatic and mild infections in endemic areas. One reason for this may be the frequency of reinfections; although about 6% of the population lose antibody annually, rises in antibody titre are also often observed. It is not clear if reinfection results in clinical disease. A frequent finding of incomplete immunity after infection would have profound implications for the use of a vaccine.

There may be secondary spread from person to person in conditions of overcrowded housing and this is particularly important in rural hospitals. Medical attendants or relatives who provide direct personal care are most likely to contract the infection; as noted above, accidental inoculation with a sharp instrument and contact

with blood have caused infection in few cases. Airborne spread may take place, as well as mechanical transmission. Although in Sierra Leone there has been no evidence of airborne spread in hospital outbreaks, one of the 1970 outbreaks in Nigeria is believed to have been caused by airborne transmission from a woman with severe pulmonary infection.

Lassa virus infection is a common cause of spontaneous abortion in endemic areas of West Africa. Virus can easily be detected in the blood and tissues of the aborted foetuses. Pediatric infection occurs, although more frequently in male children. The acute febrile illness is accompanied by widespread oedema, abdominal distension and haemorrhaging with a case fatality rate as high as 30%.

Diagnosis

The diagnosis of Lassa fever is confirmed by isolation of the virus or demonstration of a specific serological response. Infection in the early stages can be confused clinically with a number of other infectious diseases, particularly malignant malaria (Table 25.2).

Lassa virus grows readily in Vero cell culture and virus can usually be isolated within four days. Virus can be cultured from serum, throat washings, pleural fluid and urine; it is excreted from the pharynx for up to 14 days after the onset of illness and in urine for up to 67 days after onset. Lassa infection can be diagnosed early by detection of virus-specific antigens in conjunctival cells using indirect immunofluorescence. It is important to note that virus isolation should be attempted only in laboratories equipped to provide maximum containment (Biosafety Level 4) to protect the investigator. Suspected cases should be reported immediately to local and national public health authorities.

The most sensitive serological test for the detection of Lassa antibodies is indirect immunofluorescence; antibodies can be detected by this method in the second week of illness. On occasion antibodies fail to develop in patients from whom Lassa virus has been isolated. Neutralizing antibodies are difficult to measure *in vitro*, in sharp contrast to infections by the South American arenaviruses, for reasons that are unclear.

The two most reliable prognostic markers of fatal infections are the titres of circulating virus and of aspartate aminotransferase (AST). Patients in whom the titre of virus exceeds 10^4 TCID$_{50}$/ml and with AST levels above 150 IU have a poor prognosis, and fatality rates approach 80%. In contrast, patients with virus and enzyme levels below these values have a greater than 85% chance of survival (Johnson *et al.* 1987). This demonstration of an association between

Table 25.2 Differential diagnosis of Lassa fever

Malaria
Bacterial septicaemia
Enteric fevers (typhoid, paratyphoid)
Typhus
Trypanosomiasis
Streptococcal pharyngitis
Leptospirosis
Other viral haemorrhagic fevers

the degree of viraemia and mortality is unique for virus infections and contrasts with the difficulty in predicting the outcome in patients with Argentine and Bolivian haemorrhagic fevers. Although Lassa fever can be diagnosed accurately from the presence of IgM antibodies on admission, there is no correlation between the time of appearance and the titre of specific antibodies and clinical outcome. Lassa fever is particularly severe in pregnant women. A study of 75 women in Sierra Leone showed that 11 of 14 deaths were the result of infection during the third trimester; a further 23 patients suffered abortion in the first and second trimesters.

Therapy and control

The human host is clearly restricted in its ability to clear the virus and prevent its replication in tissues, possibly because of impairment of cytotoxic T cell reactions. The poor neutralizing antibody response and the high degree of viraemia contrast sharply with those in patients with South American haemorrhagic fevers, in whom there is little viraemia and neutralizing antibodies develop rapidly during acute infection.

Although the passive administration of Lassa immune plasma may suppress viraemia and favourably alter the clinical outcome, it does not always do so, particularly if the patient has a high virus burden (McCormick *et al.* 1986). Failure may be due to the difficulty in assessing accurately the titre of viral neutralizing antibodies in the plasma, the late and non-uniform nature of this response in convalescence, and antigenic variation. The widespread occurrence of human immunodeficiency virus (HIV) infections in West Africa precludes at present the use of immune plasma from convalescent individuals in this region. Conversely, immune plasma may be of benefit in the treatment of Junín infections (Maiztegui *et al.* 1979; Enria *et al.* 1984). This may be due to the high titre of neutralizing antibodies that develops soon after the acute phase.

There has been little progress towards developing a vaccine against Lassa virus, in part due to the lack of commercial interest in developing such products and in part due to the lack of knowing what constitutes a protective immune response. Many workers believe a strong cell-mediated response is required but as this would most likely require the use of live attenuated virus, this raises questions as to possible reversion of any vaccine strain to virulence.

Greater success has been achieved with antivirals. In one study of patients with a poor prognosis treated for 10 days with intravenous ribavirin (60–70 mg/kg/per day), begun within six days after the onset of fever, showed a reduced case fatality of 5% (McCormick *et al.* 1986). In contrast, patients who began treatment seven or more days after the onset of fever had a case fatality rate of 26%. In the Sierra Leone study, viraemia of greater than $10^{3.6}$ TCID$_{50}$/ml on admission was associated with a case fatality rate of 76%. Patients with this risk factor who were treated with intravenous ribavirin within six days of the onset of fever had a case fatality rate of 9%, compared with 47% in those treated seven days or more after the onset of illness.

As with many examples of severe haemorrhagic disease, effective control requires early and strict isolation of cases coupled with rigorous disinfection and rodent control. Disinfection with 0.5% sodium hypochlorite or 0.5% phenol in detergent is recommended for surfaces and instruments. Owing to the high burden of virus replication, infection of relatives and others who have been in close contact is a distinct possibility and WHO guidelines suggest that non-casual contacts should be followed for up to 3 months for signs of illness.

The taking of body temperature thrice daily is recommended, followed by hospitalization if the body temperature exceeds 38.5°C.

Lujo virus

The emergence of Lujo virus in 2008 demonstrates how novel arenaviruses continue to emerge. The index case was a female resident of Zambia living in a semi-rural location where she kept horses, dogs and cats. She fell ill with diarrhoea and vomiting before being evacuated to a private hospital in South Africa where she died 12 days after onset of illness. Three hospital personnel—two nurses and one cleaner—also became infected, succumbing to the disease within two weeks of exposure to infection. An additional nurse was also infected but eventually recovered (Paweska *et al.* 2009).

Detailed clinical descriptions of these cases showed patients with signs typical of a viral haemorrhagic fever. The index case showed in particular a whole body rash accompanied by facial oedema, a feature frequently seen in cases with South American haemorrhagic fevers. Cerebral oedema and respiratory distress quickly followed. A marked thrombocytopenia, granulosis and elevated liver transaminases are all features common to viral haemorrhagic fevers. The single surviving case is notable in that this nurse received ribavirin within 24 hours after onset of illness, but the recovery was prolonged with levels of virus in the blood declining slowly over two months.

Phylogenetic analyses has confirmed that Lujo virus is an Old World arenavirus, although it its lineage suggests a close relationship with an ancestral virus rather than to Lassa, LCM and other Old World arenaviruses (Briese *et al.* 2009).

Argentine haemorrhagic fever (Junín virus)

Clinical and pathological features

Argentine haemorrhagic fever has been known since 1943 and Junín virus, the causative agent, was first isolated in 1958. The virus causes annual outbreaks of severe illness—with between 100 and 3,500 cases—in an area of intensive agriculture known as the wet pampas in Argentina. Mortality in some outbreaks has ranged from 10% to 20%, although the overall mortality is generally 3–15% unless supportive therapy is provided early in the course of the disease.

After an incubation period of 7–16 days, the onset of illness is insidious, with chills, headache, malaise, myalgia, retro-orbital pain and nausea; these are followed by fever, conjunctival injection and suffusion and an enanthem, exanthema and oedema of the face, neck and upper thorax. A few petechiae may be seen, mostly in the axilla. There is hypervascularity and occasional ulceration of the soft palate. Generalized lymphadenopathy is common. Tongue tremor is an early sign, and some patients present with pneumonitis. In the more severe cases the patient's condition becomes appreciably worse after a few days, with the development of hypotension, oliguria, haemorrhages from the nose and gums, haematemesis, haematuria and melaena. Oliguria may progress to anuria and pronounced neurological manifestations may develop. Laboratory findings have included leucopenia with a decrease in the number of CD4-positive cells, thrombocytopenia and urinary casts containing viral antigen. Patients recover when the fever falls, followed by diuresis and rapid improvement. Death may result from hypovolaemic shock. Subclinical infections also occur. Man-to-man transmission has not been observed.

Elevated levels of interferon can be detected in the early stages of Argentine haemorrhagic fever, and these coincide with the onset of fever and backache. Although there is no correlation between the titres of interferon and circulating virus, Levis and colleagues (1984) have suggested that at least some of the clinical signs may be directly attributable to interferon, particularly the depression of platelet and lymphocytic numbers that result from Junín virus infection of leucocytes and macrophages.

Epidemiology

Argentine haemorrhagic fever has a marked seasonal incidence, coinciding with the maize harvest between April and July, when rodent populations reach their peak. Agricultural workers, particularly those harvesting maize, are, not surprisingly, the most commonly affected.

The main reservoir hosts of Junín virus are *Calomys* field voles that live and breed in burrows under the maize fields and in the surrounding grass banks. Other rodent species may also be infected. *Calomys* spp. has a persistent viraemia and viruria, and virus is also present in considerable quantities in the saliva. The mode of transmission of Junín virus to man has not been conclusively established. The virus may be carried in the air from dust contaminated by rodent excreta or may enter by ingestion of contaminated foodstuffs.

Therapy

In contrast to Lassa fever, antibodies play a major role in recovery from Junín infection. Controlled trial of immune plasma collected from patients at least 6 months into convalescence have shown a dramatic reduction in mortality if plasma is given within the first 8 days of illness (Maiztegui *et al.* 1979). The efficacy of this therapy is directly related to the titre of neutralizing antibody in the plasma; as a result, a dose of no less than 3,000 'therapeutic units'/kg body weight has been recommended (Enria *et al.* 1984).

The late development of a neurological syndrome is seen in up to 10% of patients treated with immune plasma; it is often benign and self-limiting but points to the possible persistence of viral antigens on cells of the CNS well into convalescence. Treatment with immune plasma also restores the response of peripheral blood lymphocytes to antigenic stimuli, suggesting that the administration of plasma also results in the modulation of cellular immunity.

Of interest is the finding of Andes virus, a member of the hantavirus genus of the family Bunyaviridae, among the cohorts presenting with presumptive Argentine haemorrhagic fever but found to be serologically negative for Junín virus. Were it not for the activities of the investigators primarily working with cases of haemorrhagic disease, this new cause of acute respiratory disease would most likely have remained unrecognized.

Prophylaxis

There have been several attempts to produce a vaccine against Argentine haemorrhagic fever. The XJ-Cl$_3$ strain of virus grown in the brains of suckling mice is relatively non-pathogenic and was administered to 636 volunteers between 1968 and 1970. However, the vaccine often induced a mild febrile reaction or a subclinical infection, and its use was discontinued despite the fact that over 90% of vaccinees maintained neutralizing antibody for up to nine years.

A second vaccine was developed using a pedigree strain of Junín virus extensively passaged in cells and plaque purified. This 'candidate 1' vaccine has been administered to over 280 000 individuals in the endemic regions of Argentina with greater than 95% protection. As a result, the number of clinical cases has declined sharply to less than 100 per year. Protective efficacy has been hard to judge, however, owing to annual variations in rodent numbers and, more importantly, the prevalence of infection among the local rodent populations.

Bolivian haemorrhagic fever (Machupo virus)
Clinical features

Bolivian haemorrhagic fever was first recognized in 1959 in the Beni region in north-eastern Bolivia. The most notable outbreak affected 700 people in the San Joaquin township between late 1962 and the middle of 1964. The mortality was 18%. Originally referred to locally as 'black typhus' this disease, predominantly of males, erupted at a time of abnormally low rain fall combined with a decline in the cat population. The resulting explosion in number of *Calomys callosus* increased vastly the risk to humans: rodent trapping in half the township led to a precipitate drop in the number of new cases. The disease continued in that region more or less annually for a number of years in the form of sharply localized epidemics. Its incidence has decreased considerably since the late 1970s and human infections are now rarely reported. The mortality in individual outbreaks varied from 5% to 30%. It is worth noting that the discovery of a common morphology and serological cross-reaction between Machupo and LCM virus led to the concept of the arenavirus family.

The clinical disease is similar to Argentine haemorrhagic fever. The incubation period ranges from 7–14 days and the onset is insidious. About one-third of patients show a tendency to bleed, with petechiae on the trunk and palate, and bleeding from the gastrointestinal tract, nose, gums, and uterus. Almost half the patients develop a fine tremor of the tongue and hands, and some may have more pronounced neurological symptoms. The acute disease may last 2–3 weeks and convalescence may be protracted, generalized weakness being the most common complaint. Clinically inapparent infections are rare.

Machupo virus, the responsible agent, is readily isolated from lymph nodes and spleen taken at necropsy. Isolation of the virus from acutely ill patients has proved difficult, however, the best results being obtained from specimens taken 7–12 days after the onset of illness.

Epidemiology

The rodent reservoir of Machupo virus is *Calomys callosus*; over 60% of this species of vole caught during the San Joaquin epidemic were found to be infected. The distribution of cases in the township was associated with certain houses and *Calomys callosus* was trapped in all households where cases occurred. Transmission to man is probably by contamination of food and water or by infection through skin abrasions. Transmission from man to man is unusual but a small episode took place in 1971, well outside the endemic zone. The index case, infected in Beni, carried the infection to Cochabamba and, by direct transmission, caused five secondary cases, of which four were fatal. Abnormally low rainfall, combined with an increase in the use of insecticide, led to a rapid decline in the numbers of cats, with the result that the population of Machupo-infected rodents increased dramatically thus increasing the opportunity for human contact with contaminated soil and foodstuffs. This balance has since been restored and largely accounts for the reduction in the number of reported cases over the past two decades.

Recently a second cause of haemorrhagic disease in Bolivia has been ascribed to an unrelated arenavirus, tentatively called Chaparé virus (Delgado *et al.* 2008). Worryingly this new agent shows no serological cross-reactivity with Machupo virus; phylogenetically Chaparé virus is more closely related to Sabiá virus.

Therapy and control

There is little documented evidence that Bolivian haemorrhagic fever can be successfully treated, although laboratory studies would suggest this is possible. That animals can be partially protected against Machupo virus by immunization with Junín virus vaccine also suggests vaccination may be successful but has yet to be investigated by means of a clinical trial.

Venezuelan haemorrhagic fever (Guanarito virus)

This agent was first described in 1989, with 26 deaths being recorded among 105 cases originally suspected as being dengue infections (Salas *et al.* 1991). Most of the cases have been adults and all from the state of Portuguesa in the mid-western part of Venezuela. Lasting from 3 to 12 days, the infection is typified by fever, sore throat, nausea with vomiting, and other symptoms associated with arenavirus infections in the New World. Up to 90% of the patients showed a marked thrombocytopenia and leucopenia. Post-mortem examination of the fatal cases revealed extensive haemorrhage in the lungs and liver accompanied by cardiomegaly, splenic enlargement, and congestion of the lungs. Oedema of the kidneys was also observed, together with blood in the intestines and bladder.

The virus has since been isolated repeatedly from the cotton rat *Sigmodon alstoni*, although there have been no significant recorded cases since the original outbreak. The route of transmission remains unclear, with human-to-human spread being rare. The infections are likely to have been acquired peridomestically, however, as in the study of Salas *et al.* virus was recovered from a rodent trapped in the house of one case. The relatively high mortality of the infection parallels that seen in the early reported cases of Machupo and Junín infections; in the event of further outbreaks this level should be reduced as diagnosis improves and appropriate treatment instigated earlier in the course of the disease.

Brazilian haemorrhagic fever (Sabiá virus)

Isolated in 1990 from human cases at autopsy, Sabiá virus is thought to infect rodents in the agricultural regions surrounding Sao Paulo. The potential seriousness of this infection is highlighted by a laboratory worker at Yale University becoming critically ill after an accidental exposure to an aerosol containing Sabiá Virus. The individual developed a febrile illness accompanied by a marked leucopemia and thrombocytopenia. As is often the case with emerging haemorrhagic diseases, involvement of the liver suggests initially a case of yellow fever but this can quickly be ruled out. The recent emergence of the phylogenetically-related Chaparé virus some 1,000 km away in Bolivia is a stark reminder that distribution of these pathogenic viruses may be more extensive than is currently appreciated.

Oliveros virus

This arenavirus has been isolated from the field rodent *Bolomys obscures* trapped within the endemic region for Argentine haemorrhagic fever (Bowen *et al.* 1996). There is as yet little indication that Oliveros virus causes human disease, although approximately 25% of captured *Bolomys* rodents have been found to contain antibodies to the virus (Mills *et al.* 1996).

Whitewater Arroyo virus and other isolates from North America

The 1993 hantavirus outbreak in the 'Four Corners' region of the USA stimulated extensive studies of feral rodent populations in order to measure the extent of Sin Nombre virus distribution and the corresponding risk to rural inhabitants. During one such study, an unusually high level of arenavirus antibodies was detected among trapped pack rats (*Neotoma spp*) found in the Whitewater Arroyo of New Mexico (Kosey *et al.* 1996), similar findings were reported by Fulhorst and collaborators (1996) from trapped White-throated Woodrats (*N.albigula*). Fulhorst and colleagues showed that this new arenavirus can be passed through the urine and thus could pose a threat if excreted in recreational areas and around isolated households. Members of the Neotoma family are ubiquitous throughout the south west USA and some evidence of human infection has been obtained from three female patients presenting with acute respiratory symptoms and non-specific febrile symptoms. All three of the latter patients died within 1–8 weeks of onset: although evidence of Whitewater Arroyo virus was obtained by PCR and by virus isolation in one case, the link between Whitewater Arroyo virus and human disease has yet to be conclusively proven.

There have also been further examples of arenavirus infection among feral rodents of the USA. Infectious virus was recovered from 5 of 27 examples of the Californian mouse *Peromyscus calfornicus* caught in the Santa Ana mountains close to the Bear Canyon trailhead. Catarina virus is another arenavirus associated with the southern plains woodrat, *Neotoma micropus*, found in southern Texas (Cajimat *et al.* 2007) but there is no evidence as yet that either of these newly discovered arenaviruses causes human disease.

Summary and future directions

Unique among the viral zoonoses, the arenaviruses show a host-parasite relationship which has received intensive study. In the case of LCM virus, this has resulted in the discovery of fundamental concepts in viral immunopathogenesis and clearance. Yet much remains to be learnt, particularly from the standpoint of public health. The emergence of three new arenaviruses potentially capable of causing serious human disease since the first edition of this book illustrates vividly the need for public health microbiologists to be ever vigilant for hitherto unknown agents causing unexpected outbreaks. The epidemiology of almost all arenaviruses remains poorly understood; for example, Lassa is clearly widespread among the rural areas of West Africa, but in contrast to South America there is an inexact correlation between the distribution of infected rodents and human infections. There is also much to be learnt in terms of the susceptibility of the natural hosts to infection; a rodent of the *Calomys* family wild-caught in Venezuela, for example, may be refractory to infection whereas its cousin from elsewhere in South America can be readily infected. It is tempting to speculate that arenaviruses are instrumental in controlling rodent population numbers and that only when man radically alters the rodent habitat do zoonotic infections result. Thus there is ample scope for further studies of the natural history, epidemiology and pathology of this unique and fascinating group of viruses. By such work, we may better understand the host-parasite relationship of these agents and thus be better prepared for preventing further outbreaks of severe and debilitating human infections.

References

Bowen, M.D., Peters, C.J., Mills, J.N., and Nichol, S.T. (1996). Oliveros virus: a novel arenavirus from Argentina. *Virol.,* **217:** 362–66.

Bowen, M.D., Peters, C.J., and Nichol, S.T. (1997). Phylogenetic analysis of the Arenaviridae: patterns of virus evolution and evidence for cospeciation between arenaviruses and their rodent hosts. *Phylogen. Evol.,* **8:** 301–16.

Briese, T., Paweska, J.T., McMullan, L.K., Hutchison, S.K., Street, C., et al. (2009). Genetic detection and characterization of Lujo virus, a new hemorrhagic fever-associated arenavirus from Southern Africa. *PLoS Path.,* **4:** 1–8.

Buchmeier, M.J., Lewick, H.A., Tomori, O., and Oldstone, M.B.A. (1981). Monoclonal antibodies to lymphocytic choriomeningitis virus and Pichinde viruses: Generation, characterization and cross-reactivity with other arenaviruses. *Virol.,* **113:** 73–85.

Cajimat, M.N., Milazzo, M.L., Hess, B.D., Rood, M.P., and Fulhorst, C.F. (2007). Principal host relationships and evolutionary history of the North American arenaviruses. *Virol.,* **367:** 235–43.

Delgado, S., Erickson, B.R., Agudo, R., Blair, P.J., Vallejo, E., (2008). Chapare Virus, a Newly Discovered Arenavirus Isolated from a Fatal Hemorrhagic Fever Case in Bolivia. *PLoS Path.,* **4:** e1000047.

Djavani, M., Yin, C., Lukashevich, I.S., Rodas, J., Rai, S.K., et al. (2001). Role of the promyelocytic leukemia protein PML in the interferon sensitivity of lymphocytic choriomeningitis virus. *J. Hum. Virol.,* **4:** 103–8.

Drosten, C., Gottig, S., Schilling, S., Asper, M., Panning, M., et al. (2002). Rapid detection and quantification of RNA of Ebola and Marburg viruses, Lassa virus, Crimean-Congo hemorrhagic fever virus, Rift Valley fever virus, dengue virus, and yellow fever virus by real-time reverse transcription-PCR. *J. Clin. Microbiol.,* **40:** 2323–30.

Enria, D.A., Briggiler, A.M., et al. (1984). Importance of dose of neutralizing antibodies in treatment of Argentine haemorrhagic fever with immune plasma. *Lancet,* **2:** 25556.

Fischer, S.A., Graham, M.B., Kuehnert, M.J., Kotton, C.N., Srinivasan, A., et al. (2006). Transmission of lymphocytic choriomeningitis virus by organ transplantation. *N. Engl. J. Med.,* **354:** 2235–49.

Fisher-Hoch, S.P., Mitchell, S.W., Sasso, D.R., Lang, J.V., et al. (1987). Physiologic and immunologic disturbances associated with shock in Lassa fever in a primate model. *J. Infect. Dis.,* **155:** 465–74.

Fulhorst, C.F., Bowen, M.D., Ksiazek, T.G., Rollin, P.E., et al. (1996). Isolation and characterization of Whitewater Arroyo virus, a novel North American arenavirus. *Virol.,* **224:** 114–20.

Fuller-Pace, F., and Southern, P. (1989). Detection of virus-specific RNA-dependent RNA polymerase activity in extracts from cells infected with lymphocytic choriomeningitis virus: *In vitro* synthesis of full-length viral RNA species. *J. Virol.,* **63:** 1938–44.

Gonzalez, J-P., Sanchez, A., and Rico-Hesse, R. (1995). Molecular phylogeny of Guanarito virus, an emerging arenavirus affecting humans. *Am. J. Trop. Med. Hyg.,* **53:** 1–6.

Howard, C.R. (ed.) (1986). Arenaviruses. In: A.J. Zuckerman *Perspectives in Medical Virology, Vol. 2.* Amsterdam: Elsevier.

Howard, C.R., and Simpson, D.H.L. (1980). The biology of arenaviruses. *J. General Virol.,* **51:** 1–14.

Johnson, K.M., Webb, P.A., and Justines, G. (ed.). (1973). Biology of Tacaribe-complex virus. In: F. Lehmann-Grube *Lymphocytic choriomeningitis virus and other arenaviruses.* Verlag, Vienna: Springer, pp. 241–58.

Johnson, K.M., McCormick, J.B., Webb, P.A., Smith, E., et al. (1987). Lassa fever in Sierra Leone: clinical virology in hospitalized patients. *J. Infect. Dis.,* **155:** 45663.

Kosoy, M.Y., Elliott, L.H., Ksiazek, T.G., Fulhorst, C.F., Rollin, P.E., et al. (1996). Prevalence of antibodies to arenaviruses in rodents from the southern and western United States: evidence for an arenavirus associated with the genus Neotoma. *Am. J. Trop. Med. Hyg.,* **54:** 570–76.

Levis, S.C., Saavedra, M.C., et al. (1984). Endogenous interferon in Argentine haemorrhagic fever. *J. Infect. Dis.,* **149:** 428–33.

McCormick, J.B., King, I.J., Webb, P.A., et al. (1986). Lassa fever: effective therapy with ribavirin. *N. Engl. J. Med.,* **314:** 20–26.

Maiztegui, J.I., Fernandez, N.J., and de Damilano, A.J. (1979). Efficacy of immune plasma in treatment of Argentine haemorrhagic fever and association between treatment and a late neurological syndrome. *Lancet,* **2:** 1216–17.

Mills, J.N., Barrera-Oro, J.G., Bressler, D.S., Childs, J.E., Tesh, R.B., et al. (1996). Characterization of Oliveros virus, a new member of the Tacaribe complex (Arenaviridae: Arenavirus). *Am. J. Trop. Med. Hyg.,* **54:** 399–404.

Monath, T.P. (1987). Lassa fever—new issues raised by field studies in West Africa. *J. Infect. Dis.,* **155:** 433–36.

Murphy, F.A., and Whitfield, S.G. (1975). Morphology and morphogenesis of arenaviruses. *Bull. World Heal. Organ.,* **52:** 409–19.

Neuman, B.W., Adair, B.D., Burns, J.W., Milligan, R.A., et al. (2005). Complementarity in the supramolecular design of arenaviruses and retroviruses revealed by electron cryomicroscopy and image analysis. *J. Virol.,* **79:** 3822–30.

Paweska, J.T., Sewall, N.H., Ksiazek, T.G., Blumberg, L.H., Hale, M.J., et al. (2009). Nosocomial outbreak of novel arenavirus infection, Southern Africa. *Emerg. Infect. Dis.,* **15:** 15981602.

Rimoldi, M.T., de Bracco, M.M. (1980). *In vitro* inactivation of complement by a serum factor present in Junín virus-infected guinea pigs. *Immunol.,* **39:** 159–164.

Salas, R., Manzione, W., de Tesh, R.B., et al. (1991). Venezuela haemorrhagic fever. *Lancet,* **338:** 103336.

Walker, D.H., and Murphy, F.A. (1987). Pathology and Pathogenesis of Arenavirus Infections. *Curr. Top. Microbiol. Immunol.,* 133: 89113.

Weaver, S.C., Salas, R.A., de Manzione, N., Fulhorst, C.F., et al. (2000). Extreme genetic diversity among Pirital virus (Arenaviridae) isolates from western Venezuela. *Virol.,* **285:** 110–18.

Young, P.R. (eds.) (1987). Arenaviridae. In: M.V. Nermut, A.C. Steven *Animal virus structures.* Amsterdam: Elsevier, pp. 185–98.

Zinkernagel, R.M., and Doherty, P.C. (1979). MHC-restricted cytotoxic T-cells: studies on the biological role of polymorphic major transplantation antigens determining T-cell restriction-specificity, function and responsiveness. *Ad. Immunol.,* **27:** 151–77.

CHAPTER 26

Crimean-Congo haemorrhagic fever

R. Swanepoel and J. T. Paweska

Summary

Crimean-Congo haemorrhagic fever (CCHF) is an acute disease of humans, caused by a tick-borne virus which is widely distributed in eastern Europe, Asia and Africa. Cattle, sheep and small mammals such as hares undergo inapparent or mild infection with transient viraemia, and serve as hosts from which the tick vectors of the virus can acquire infection. Despite serological evidence that there is widespread infection of livestock in nature, infection of humans is relatively uncommon. Humans acquire infection from tick bite, or from contact with infected blood or other tissues of livestock or human patients, and the disease is characterized by febrile illness with headache, malaise, myalgia, and a petechial rash, frequently followed by a haemorrhagic state with necrotic hepatitis. The mortality rate is variable but averages about approximately 30%. Inactivated vaccine prepared from infected mouse brain was used for the protection of humans in eastern Europe and the former Soviet Union in the past, but the development of a modern vaccine is inhibited by limited potential demand. The voluminous literature on the disease has been the subject of several reviews from which the information presented here is drawn, except where indicated otherwise (Chumakov 1974; Hoogstraal 1979, 1981; Watts et al. 1989; Swanepoel 1994, 1995; Swanepoel and Burt 2004; Burt and Swanepoel 2005; Whitehouse 2004; Ergunol and Whitehouse 2007; Ergunol 2008).

History

Descriptions of a disease in eastern Europe and Asia resembling CCHF can be traced back to antiquity, but a condition given the name Crimean haemorrhagic fever was first recognized in an outbreak affecting about 200 soldiers and peasants who were exposed to ticks while harvesting crops and sleeping outdoors on the Crimean Peninsula in 1944. In the following year it was demonstrated through the inoculation of human subjects with filtered suspensions of ticks and tissues of patients, that the disease was caused by a tick-transmitted virus. However, the virus itself was only isolated in laboratory hosts, namely mice, in 1967. In 1969, it was shown that the agent of Crimean haemorrhagic fever was identical to a virus named Congo which had been isolated in 1956 from the blood of a febrile child in Stanleyville (now Kisangani) in what

was then the Belgian Congo, and since that time the two names have been used in combination.

During the three decades which followed the initial description of the disease in the Crimea, the presence of the virus came to be recognized in many east European and Asian countries, in some instances as a result of the conducting of deliberate surveys, but often as a consequence of the occurrence of nosocomial outbreaks or large epidemics, many of which were precipitated by circumstances which involved the exposure of large numbers of humans to ticks, such as the implementation of major land reclamation or resettlement schemes in Bulgaria and the Soviet Asian republics. Although an outbreak involving 90 cases of the disease occurred in Khazakstan in 1989 (Lvov 1994), large epidemics are now apparently less frequent in countries of the former Soviet Union, with the decrease being ascribed to the adoption of more intensive agricultural practices and the reduction of populations of the wild hosts of the tick vectors by hunting. More recently, outbreaks of the disease in Eurasia have resulted from the exposure of people to blood and ticks from slaughter stock imported from Africa and Asia to countries in the Near East such as Saudi Arabia, the United Arab Emirates and Oman, plus large scale exposure of war refugees to outdoor conditions in Kosovo, Albania, Macedonia and the Afghanistan-Pakistan border area (El Azazy et al. 1997; Khan et al. 1997; Papa et al. 2002a, 2002b; Scrimgeour et al. 1996; Williams et al. 2000; Avšič-Županc 2007). Occurrence of the disease has also been confirmed in Turkey and in Iran, where the presence of the virus had long been suspected on serological grounds (Karti et al. 2004; Chinikar 2007). More than 1,100 cases of CCHF have been recorded in Turkey since 2002, and it is believed that an increase in tick populations was triggered by climate change, altered grazing practices and prohibition of the hunting of wild hosts of ticks (Vatansever et al. 2007).

In Africa, only 15 cases of the disease were reported prior to 1981, eight of them laboratory infections, and only one patient had developed haemorrhagic manifestations and died. Since then, sporadic cases of haemorrhagic disease and deaths have been diagnosed regularly each year in southern Africa, probably as a result of increased awareness among clinicians, and a few cases of severe disease have also been recorded West and East Africa (Dunster et al. 2002). Contrary to earlier speculation, therefore, it is now evident that the disease which occurs in Africa is no less severe than that in Eurasia.

It is evident from surveys conducted in Africa and Eurasia that there is extensive circulation of the virus in livestock and wild vertebrates, with very high antibody prevalence rates occurring in adult livestock in some areas. In contrast, the prevalence of antibody in rural human populations is generally low, (<1–2%), but there are notable exceptions, as in northern Senegal where up to 20% of people had antibody in locations where nomadic shepherds had regular contact with sheep and slept outdoors where they were exposed to ticks. The evidence suggests that the disease of humans is probably under diagnosed in many countries due to lack of awareness and/or non-availability of appropriate medical and laboratory services, but also that there is generally a low rate of transmission of infection to humans as discussed below.

The virus

Taxonomy and molecular biology

The causative agent of CCHF is a member of the *Nairovirus* genus of the family *Bunyaviridae*, which at present contains 32 viruses arranged in seven serogroups on the basis of antigenic affinities, with CCHF virus, Hazara from Pakistan, and Khasan from the former USSR constituting one of the serogroups. All members of the genus are believed to be transmitted by either ixodid or argasid ticks, and only three are known to be pathogens of humans, namely, CCHF, Dugbe and Nairobi sheep disease viruses. Dugbe commonly causes mild infection of sheep and cattle in West Africa and is infrequently associated with benign febrile illness of humans. Nairobi sheep disease virus, which is believed to be identical to Ganjam virus of India, is a pathogen of sheep and goats in East Africa and India which occasionally causes benign illness in humans.

Nairoviruses are spherical, 90–120 nm in diameter, and have a bilipid-layer envelope from which glycoprotein spikes project. The virions contain three major structural proteins: two envelope glycoproteins G1 and G2 with molecular weights $72–84 \times 10^3$ and $30–40 \times 10^3$ Da respectively, a nucleocapsid protein N ($48–54 \times 10^3$ Da), and minor quantities of a large protein L ($>200 \times 10^3$ Da), believed to be the viral transcriptase. Hazara virus is unique in having three glycoproteins. The viruses have a three-segmented, single-stranded RNA genome which is in the negative-sense (complementary to mRNA). Each RNA segment, L (large), M (medium) and S (small), is contained in a separate nucleocapsid within the virion. The L RNA segment (molecular weight $4.1–4.9 \times 10^6$ Da) codes for the viral transcriptase, the M segment ($1.5–2.3 \times 10^6$ Da) for the G proteins, and the S segment ($0.6–0.7 \times 10^6$ Da) for the N protein. Precursors of the glycoproteins have been found in infected cells, but non-structural proteins found during the replication of viruses of other genera of the *Bunyaviridae* have not as yet been demonstrated in association with nairoviruses.

Nairoviruses attach to receptors on susceptible cells, are internalized by endocytosis, and replicate in the cytoplasm. The virions mature by budding through endoplasmic reticulum into cytoplasmic vesicles in the Golgi region, which are presumed to fuse with the plasma membrane to release virus.

Phylogenetic studies indicate that there are regional differences in virus strains, and confirm that reassortment and recombination occur in nature (Hewson *et al.* 2004; Deyde *at al.* 2006; Lukashev 2005). The epidemiological implications of these observations are not yet clear, but lower death rates occur in Turkey than elsewhere. The differences should be borne in mind in developing molecular diagnostic techniques (Duh *et al.* 2006).

Pathogenesis

The mechanisms of pathogenesis by CCHF virus are incompletely understood, but it can be surmised that there may be some initial replication in tissues at the site of inoculation, with subsequent replication of virus to high titres in macrophages/monocytes resulting in haematogenous and lymph-borne spread of infection to regional lymph nodes and certain target organs such as the liver which is a major site of virus replication. Infected cells release cytokines, chemokines and other pro-inflammatory mediators which lead to coagulation defects and fall in blood pressure with development of intractable shock and multi-organ failure (Karti *et al.* 2004; Papa *et al.* 2006; Ergunol *et al.* 2006b; Bray 2007; Doganci 2007; Fisgin *et al.* 2008; Ergunol 2008). It is postulated that release of pro-inflammatory cytokines by T-helper lymphocytes and macrophages triggers the occurrence of haemophagocytosis in bone marrow, and that endothelial damage associated with the occurrence of disseminated intravascular coagulopathy is caused by cytokine storms rather than directly by viral infection (Karti *et al.* 2004; Doganci 2007; Fisgin *et al.* 2008). Moreover, there is evidence of the formation of circulating immune complexes with activation of complement, and this would contribute to damage of the capillary bed and hence to the genesis of the skin rash and renal and pulmonary failure. Endothelial damage leads to platelet aggregation and degranulation, with activation of the intrinsic coagulation cascade. Tissue damage in organs such as the liver would result in further release of procoagulants into the bloodstream, and the impairment of the circulation through the occurrence of disseminated intravascular coagulopathy would in turn contribute to further tissue damage. Damage to the liver would limit clearance of fibrin degradation products and impair synthesis of coagulation factors to replace those consumed. Abnormalities in clinical pathology values observed in patients indicate that the occurrence of disseminated intravascular coagulopathy is probably an early and central event in the pathogenesis of the disease.

Culture of the virus

In the past, CCHF virus has been propagated and titrated most commonly by intracerebral inoculation of suckling mice. The virus is non-pathogenic for other laboratory animals, including rabbits, guinea pigs and monkeys. It can be grown in a wide variety of primary and line cell cultures, including Vero, CER, BHK_{21}, and SW13 cells, but it is poorly cytopathic and hence infectivity is titrated by plaque production or demonstration of immunofluorescence in infected cells.

Stability

Little information is available on the stability of CCHF virus, but infectivity is destroyed by low concentrations of formalin or beta-propriolactone. Being enveloped, the virus is sensitive to lipid solvents. It is labile in infected tissues after death, presumably due to a fall in pH, but infectivity is retained for a few days at ambient temperature in separated serum, and for up to three weeks at 4°C. Infectivity is stable at temperatures below −60°C, but is rapidly destroyed by boiling or autoclaving.

Infection of domestic and wild animals

Experimentally inoculated domestic ruminants and small mammals, such as little susliks, hedgehogs, hares and myomorph rodents, were found to undergo inapparent infection or mild fever and viraemia, with maximum recorded titres of infectivity ranging from $10^{2.7}$ to $10^{4.2}$ mouse intracerebral 50% lethal doses/ml ($MICLD_{50}$/ml), and with a demonstrable immune response. The virus was not abortigenic in heifers and ewes inoculated late in pregnancy (Swanepoel and Shepherd 1983–8, unpublished observations). However, when ticks of a laboratory strain of *Hyalomma truncatum* capable of causing sweating sickness, a toxicosis, were inadvertently placed on CCHF-infected sheep and cattle in the course of tick infection experiments, some of the animals became severely ill (Shepherd *et al.* 1991). Thus, animals which undergo simultaneous infection with CCHF virus and specific tick-borne pathogens of livestock in nature, constitute a source of infection for humans who treat or butcher sick animals; an observation which would explain the circumstances under which some patients have been observed to acquire infection in the former USSR and in South Africa, as discussed below.

Passerine birds and chickens were found to be refractory to infection, but they may be capable of infecting ticks despite failing to circulate detectable levels of virus, while ostriches have been shown to develop viraemic infection, as discussed under Epidemiology below.

Infection of humans

Signs and symptoms

The incubation period is generally short, ranging from one to three days (maximum nine) following infection by tick bite, and is usually five or six days (maximum 13) in persons exposed to infected blood or other tissues of livestock or human patients. There is usually very sudden onset of illness with fever, rigors, chills, severe headache, dizziness, neck pain and stiffness, sore eyes, photophobia, malaise, and myalgia with intense backache or leg pains. Nausea, sore throat and vomiting are common manifestations early in the disease and some patients experience non-localized abdominal pain and diarrhoea at this stage. Fever may be intermittent and patients may undergo sharp changes of mood over the first two days, with feelings of confusion and aggression. By the second to fourth day of illness they may exhibit lassitude, depression and somnolence, and have a flushed appearance with injected conjunctivae or chemosis. Tenderness of the abdomen localizes in the right upper quadrant, and hepatomegaly may be discernible. Tachycardia is common and patients may be slightly hypotensive. There may be lymphadenopathy, and enanthem and petechiae of the throat, tonsils, and buccal mucosa.

Patients develop a petechial rash on the trunk and limbs on day three to six of illness, and this may be followed rapidly by the appearance of large bruises and ecchymoses, especially in the anticubital fossae, upper arms, axillae and groin. Development of a haemorrhagic tendency may be evident only from the oozing of blood from injection or venipuncture sites, but epistaxis, haematemesis, haematuria, melaena, gingival bleeding and bleeding from the vagina or other orifices may commence on day four to five of illness, or even earlier. There may also be internal bleeding, including retroperitoneal and intracranial haemorrhage. Severely ill patients enter a state of hepato-renal and pulmonary failure from about day five onwards and progressively become drowsy, stuporous and comatose. Jaundice becomes apparent during the second week of illness. Deaths generally occur on days five to 14 of illness. Patients who recover usually begin to improve subjectively on day nine or 10 of illness, but asthenia, conjunctivitis, slight confusion and amnesia may continue for a month or longer (Swanepoel *et al.* 1987; Ergunol 2008).

Viraemia has been detected from the time of onset up to day 13 of illness, with highest titres occurring during the first five days. The viraemia is of greater intensity and longer duration in humans than in lower animals, with a maximum recorded titre of $10^{6.2}$ $MICLD_{50}$/ml, but is less intense than the viraemias commonly recorded in the other so-called formidable viral haemorrhagic fevers, such as Marburg, Ebola and Lassa fevers.

Clinical pathology

Changes in clinical pathology values are more marked in fatal than in non-fatal infections, and abnormalities recorded during the first few days of illness include leucocytosis or leucopenia, elevated serum aspartate transaminase (AST), alanine transaminase (ALT), gamma-glutamyl transferase, lactic dehydrogenase, alkaline phosphatase and creatine kinase levels, thrombocytopenia, prolonged activated partial thromboplastin (APTT) and thrombin times, elevated prothrombin ratio and fibrin degradation product levels, and depression of fibrinogen and haemoglobin values. Bilirubin, creatinine and urea levels increase and serum protein levels decline during the second week of illness.

Diagnosis

Specimens to be submitted for laboratory confirmation of a diagnosis of CCHF include blood from live patients and, in order to avoid performing full autopsies, heart blood and liver samples taken with a biopsy needle from deceased patients. On account of the propensity of the virus to cause laboratory infections, and the severity of the human disease, investigation of CCHF is generally undertaken in maximum security laboratories in countries which have appropriate biosafety regulations and facilities.

Virus can be isolated from blood and organ suspensions in a wide variety of primary and line cell cultures, including Vero, CER and BHK_{21} cells, and identified by immunofluorescence. Isolation and identification of virus can be achieved in 1–5 days, but cell cultures lack sensitivity and usually only detect high concentrations of virus present in the blood of severely ill patients during the first five days or so of illness. Suckling mice inoculated intracerebrally are more sensitive than cell cultures for the isolation of virus present in blood in low concentrations for up to 13 days after the onset of illness, but they take 6–9 days to succumb to the infection. Virus antigen can sometimes be demonstrated in the blood of severely ill patients with intense viraemia, or in liver suspensions, by enzyme-linked immunoassay. Viral nucleic acid can be demonstrated in serum and liver homogenates of patients by the reverse transcription-polymerase chain reaction (RT-PCR) (Burt *et al.* 1998; Duh *et al.* 2006). Observation of necrotic lesions compatible with CCHF infection in sections of liver, provides presumptive evidence in support of the diagnosis.

Antibodies, both IgG and IgM, become demonstrable by indirect immunofluorescence in a few patients from day four of illness, but most commonly become detectable from day seven onwards, and are present in the sera of all survivors of the disease by day nine at the latest. The IgM antibody activity declines to undetectable levels by the fourth month after infection, and IgG titres may begin to decline gradually at this stage, but remain demonstrable for at least five years. Recent or current infection is confirmed by demonstrating seroconversion, or a four-fold or greater increase in antibody titre in paired serum samples, or IgM antibody activity in a single sample. The antibody responses may also be demonstrated by enzyme-linked immunoassay. Patients who succumb rarely develop a demonstrable antibody response and the diagnosis is confirmed by isolation of virus from serum, or from liver specimens (Burt *et al.* 1994).

The disease must be distinguished from the other viral haemorrhagic fevers which partially overlap in distribution with CCHF: Lassa fever, Marburg disease, Ebola fever, Omsk haemorrhagic fever, Kyasanur Forest disease, and the haemorrhagic fever with renal syndrome (HFRS) group of diseases associated with hantavirus infections. Other febrile illnesses which can be acquired from contact with animal tissues within the same geographic range as CCHF include Rift Valley fever, Q fever, brucellosis and systemic anthrax, while diseases which can be acquired from ticks include Q fever and tick-borne typhus (*Rickettsia conorii* infection commonly known as tickbite fever). However, severe forms of many other common infections may resemble CCHF, including the various types of viral hepatitis, malaria and bacterial septicaemias.

Pathology

Macroscopic and microscopic lesions seen in CCHF are suggestive, but not pathognomonic of the disease. Lesions in the liver vary from disseminated foci of coagulative necrosis, mainly mid-zonal in distribution, to massive necrosis involving over 75% of hepatocytes, and a variable degree of haemorrhage, with little or no inflammatory cell response. Lesions in other organs include congestion, haemorrhage and focal necrosis in the central nervous system, kidneys and adrenals, and general depletion of lymphoid tissues. Fibrin deposits may be seen in small blood vessels in parenchymatous organs including the liver.

Treatment

Patients should be treated under conditions of barrier-nursing for the protection of medical personnel. Theoretically, therapy appropriate for disseminated intravascular coagulopathy, such as the use of heparin, could be applied early in the course of the disease, but patients rarely come to medical attention at a sufficiently early stage, and the procedure is considered to be risky so that it should only be contemplated by clinicians well versed in the treatment of haemostatic failure. Standard treatment consists of replacement of red blood cells, platelets and other coagulation factors, plus protein (albumin) and intravenous feeding as indicated by clinical pathology findings (Ergunol *et al.* 2007; Ergunol 2008).

Neutralizing antibody responses to nairovirus infections are inherently weak, and although immune plasma from recovered patients has been used in therapy, there has been no controlled trial with a uniform product of proven virus-neutralizing ability. Moreover, treatments have been initiated at various stages of illness up to and including terminal coma, so that no firm conclusions can be drawn on the efficacy of the treatment. Ribavirin inhibits virus replication in cell cultures and suckling mice (Peters and Shelokov 1990), and promising results have been obtained in limited trials on human patients with the intravenous formulation of the drug, but there have been no definitive studies. The rapid course and gastrointestinal complications to the disease render oral treatment less effective. Oral treatment for prophylaxis should only be applied very selectively to persons with severe exposure to infection, such as needle stick with confirmed infected blood, since the side effects of the treatment can cause highly inconvenient confusion if the drug is used indiscriminately during outbreaks.

The results of *in vitro* studies suggest that interferons and other immunomodulators may have a role in treatment of CCHF infection (Ergunol *et al.* 2007; Ergunol 2008).

Prognosis

The mortality rate is approximately 30% (range 20–50%), but this can be reduced considerably by careful monitoring of patients and the application of appropriate blood product replacement therapy. In southern Africa it was found that the occurrence during the first five days of illness of any of the following clinical pathology values is highly predictive of fatal outcome: leucocyte counts $\geq 10 \times 10^9$/L; platelet counts $\leq 20 \times 10^9$/L; AST ≥ 200U/L; ALT ≥ 150U/L; APTT ≥ 60 seconds; and fibrinogen ≤ 110mg/dL. Curiously, leucopenia early in the disease does not have the same poor prognostic connotation as leucocytosis, and all clinical pathology values may be grossly abnormal after day five of illness without necessarily being indicative of a poor prognosis (Swanepoel *et al.* 1989). Modifications to these predictive values have been proposed in Turkey, but the mortality rate associated with CCHF virus circulating in that country appears to be inherently lower (5%) than elsewhere (Ergunol *et al.* 2007; 2008). Elevated serum levels of pro-inflammatory cytokines, tumour necrosis factor-α and interleukin-6, are also significantly higher in patients with fatal outcome (Ergunol *et al.* 2006b; Papa *et al.* 2006). Viraemia is most intense in severe disease, and a viral load of $\geq 1 \times 10^9$ genome copies/ml as determined by quantitative RT-PCR was found to be indicative of fatal outcome (Cevik *et al.* 2007). Since an antibody response is rarely demonstrable in fatal illness, the occurrence of a detectable immune response is generally a favourable sign (Burt *et al.* 1994).

Epidemiology

Circulation of the virus in nature

The causative agent of CCHF is widely distributed in eastern Europe, Asia and Africa: the presence of the virus or antibody to it has been demonstrated in the former USSR, Albania, Serbia, Kosovo, Macedonia, Bulgaria, Greece, Turkey, Hungary, France, Portugal, Saudi Arabia, Kuwait, Dubai, Sharjah, Iraq, Iran, Afghanistan, Pakistan, India, China, Egypt, Ethiopia, Mauritania, Senegal, Burkina Faso, Benin, Nigeria, Central African Republic, Zaire, Kenya, Uganda, Tanzania, Zimbabwe, Namibia, South Africa, and Madagascar. However, the evidence for France and Portugal is based on limited serological observations and needs to be confirmed.

Although CCHF virus has been isolated from at least 31 species of ticks, including two argasids and 29 ixodids, there is no definitive evidence for most species that they are capable of serving as vectors, and in many instances virus recovered from engorged ticks may merely have been present in the bloodmeal imbibed from a viraemic host. Argasid ticks are unlikely to be vectors since the virus failed to replicate in three species inoculated intracoelomically. Members of three genera of ixodid ticks, *Hyalomma*, *Dermacentor* and *Rhipicephalus*, have been shown to be capable of transmitting infection transstadially and transovarially, but the bulk of the evidence suggests that *Hyalommas* are the principal vectors in nature, and in broad terms the known distribution of CCHF virus coincides with the world distribution of members of this genus of ticks. The prevalence of antibody to CCHF virus in the sera of wild vertebrates in southern Africa was found to be highest in large herbivores (the size of kudu antelope and greater), which are known to be the preferred hosts of adult *Hyalomma* ticks, and in small mammals up to the size of hares which are the preferred hosts of immature *Hyalommas*; wild mammals of intermediate size, which are parasitized by other genera of ticks, generally lacked evidence of infection. Virus or antibody has also been demonstrated elsewhere in the sera of small mammals of Eurasia and Africa, such as little susliks, hedgehogs, hares and certain myomorph rodents, and in some instances it has been shown that these hosts develop viraemia of sufficient intensity to infect ticks. Furthermore, it has been demonstrated that CCHF virus can be passed from infected to non-infected ticks which feed together on non-inoculated or immune mammals which fail to develop demonstrable viraemia. The phenomenon of 'non-viraemic' transmission of infection between ticks, which had been demonstrated earlier with other viruses, is believed to be mediated by factors present in tick saliva. Transovarial transmission of virus in ticks occurs with low frequency, but appears to be facilitated when virus is transmitted venereally from infected males to females.

Certain passerine birds and domestic chickens were found to be refractory to CCHF virus, while guinea fowl developed transient viraemia of low intensity following experimental inoculation, and an antibody response which was demonstrable for a few weeks only. Antibody to CCHF virus was detected in the sera of certain ground-frequenting birds in Senegal, notably the red-billed hornbill (*Tockus erythrorhyncus*), and it was shown that infection could be transferred between infected and noninfected ticks feeding on these birds through non-viraemic transmission (Zeller *et al.* 1994a; 1994b). Immature ticks of some species of *Hyalomma*, notably *H. marginatum rufipes* in Africa, utilize ground-frequenting birds as hosts, and it has long been accepted that the millions of birds which migrate annually on a north-south axis between Africa and Eurasia can serve to disseminate CCHF virus through the carriage of transovarially-infected immature ticks. The implication of the findings in Senegal is that birds may well play a significant role in infecting ticks, and that even those with a limited flight range, such as hornbills, can disseminate infected ticks locally. Antibody to CCHF virus was found in farmed ostriches (hosts to adult *Hyalomma* ticks) in South Africa, and following the occurrence of two outbreaks of the disease among workers at ostrich abattoirs it was shown that these birds develop viraemic infection similar to that in domestic ruminants (Swanepoel *et al.* 1998).

High prevalences of antibody occur in domestic ruminants in areas infested by *Hyalommas* and the virus causes inapparent infection or mild fever in cattle, sheep and goats, with viraemia of sufficient intensity to infect adult ticks. However, since transovarial transmission of infection in ticks occurs with low frequency, the role of livestock in the circulation of the virus is probably limited: infection of adult ticks followed by transovarial transmission is unlikely to sustain the virus. Hence, it is believed that the infection of immature ticks on small mammals and possibly ground-frequenting birds, constitutes an important amplifying mechanism.

Transmission of infection to humans

Sheep, goats and cattle generally acquire natural infection with CCHF virus early in life in areas with high challenge rates, and are viraemic for about a week. Hence, it is found that humans become infected when they come into contact with the viraemic blood of overtly healthy young animals in the course of performing procedures such as castrations, vaccinations, inserting ear tags or slaughtering the animals. Young ruminants are innately resistant to specific tick-borne diseases of livestock, such as anaplasmosis, babesiosis and cowdriosis, but animals which are raised under tick-free conditions and moved to infested locations later in life may acquire the tick-borne diseases at the same time that they become infected with CCHF virus; consequently humans also become infected from contact with viraemic blood in the course of treating sick animals or butchering those that die. Common source outbreaks involving more than one case of the disease can occur when several people are exposed to infected tissues. The available evidence suggests that the infection in humans is acquired through contact of viraemic blood with broken skin, and this accords with the fact that nosocomial infection in medical personnel usually results from accidental pricks with needles contaminated with the blood of patients, or similar mishaps. Infection appears to be limited to those who have contact with fresh blood or other tissues, probably because infectivity is destroyed by the fall in pH which occurs in tissues after death, and there has been no indication that CCHF virus constitutes a public health hazard in meat processed and matured according to normal health regulations. Many human infections result directly from tick bite, and it has been observed that people can also become infected from merely squashing ticks between the fingers. Some patients are unable to recall contact with blood or other tissues of livestock, or having been bitten by ticks, but live in or have visited a rural environment where such exposure to infection is possible. Town dwellers sometimes acquire infection from contact with animal tissues or tick bite while on hunting or hiking trips.

The majority of patients tend to be adult males engaged in the livestock industry, such as farmers, herdsmen, slaughtermen, and veterinarians, but this changes where women and children participate in tending livestock, or where refugee populations are exposed to the outdoors. The observation that infection of humans is relatively uncommon despite serological evidence of widespread infection occurring in livestock, may be explained by the facts that viraemia in livestock is short-lived, and of low intensity compared to that in other zoonotic diseases such as Rift Valley fever, and that humans are not the preferred hosts of *Hyalomma* ticks. The low prevalences of antibody generally found in populations at risk, and the relative paucity of evidence of inapparent infection encountered among the cohorts of cases of the disease, suggests that infection is frequently symptomatic.

Prevention and control

The control of the vectors of CCHF virus through the use of aca-ricides is impractical, particularly under the extensive or nomadic farming conditions which prevail in the arid areas where the disease is most prevalent. In South Africa, a single acaricide treatment of farmed ostriches followed by quarantine for at least 14 days is used to ensure that the birds are non-viraemic on arrival at abattoirs, and the same principle could be applied to other slaughter animals.

Stockmen, veterinarians, slaughtermen, and others involved with the livestock industry should be made aware of the disease and take practical steps to limit or evade exposure of naked skin to fresh blood and other tissues of animals, and to avoid handling and being bitten by ticks. Precautions should include the use of gloves and other protective clothing in slaughtering and treating animals, or in performing autopsies. Pyrethroid acaricides, such as permethrin, can be used at low concentration (0.05%) to kill ticks which come into contact with human clothing (Screck *et al.* 1980), and in some countries liquid or aerosol formulations are commercially available for this purpose: clothing is either dipped in the liquid and dried, or sprayed with the aerosol. Inactivated mouse brain vaccine for the prevention of human infection has been used on a limited scale in Eastern Europe and the former USSR, but the sporadic and unpredictable occurrence of the disease renders it difficult to identify target populations. A corollary to this problem is that the development of a safe and effective modern vaccine is inhibited by limited potential demand.

References

Avšič-Županc, T. (2007). Epidemiology of Crimean-Congo hemorrhagic fever in the Balkans. In: O. Ergonul and C.A. Whitehouse (eds.) *Crimean Congo Hemorrhagic Fever, a Global Perspective*, pp. 75–88. Dordrecht: Springer.

Bray, M. (2007). Comparative pathogenesis of Crimena-Congo hemorrhagic fever and Ebola hemorrhagic fever. In: O. Ergonul and C.A. Whitehouse (eds.) *Crimean Congo Hemorrhagic Fever, a Global Perspective*, pp. 221–31. Dordrecht: Springer.

Burt, F.J., Leman, P.A., and Smith, J.F. *et al.* (1998). The use of a reverse transcription-polymerase chain reaction for the detection of viral nucleic acid in the diagnosis of Crimean-Congo haemorrhagic fever. *J. Virolog. Meth.*, 70: 129–37.

Burt, F.J. and Swanepoel, R. (2005). Crimean-Congo hemorrhagic fever. In: J.L. Goodman, D. Sonenshine and D.T. Dennis (eds.) *Tickborne Infections of Humans.* Herndon: American Society for Microbiology.

Burt, F.J., Leman, P.A., Abbott, J.A. *et al.* (1994). Serodiagnosis of Crimean-Congo haemorrhagic fever. *Epidemiol. Infect.*, 113: 551–62.

Cevik, M.A., Erbay, A., Bodur, H. *et al.* (2007). Viral load as a predictor of outcome in Crimean-Congo hemorrhagic fever. *Clin. Infect. Dis.*, 45: 96–100.

Chinikar, S. (2007). Crimean-Congo hemorrhagic fever in Iran. In: O. Ergonul and C.A. Whitehouse (eds.) *Crimean Congo Hemorrhagic Fever, a Global Perspective*, pp. 89–98. Dordrecht: Springer.

Chumakov, M.P. (1974). On 30 years of investigation of Crimean hemorrhagic fever. *Trudy Instituta Polio. Virus. Entsef. Akad. Meditsin. Nauk SSSR*, 22: 5–18. [In Russian] [English translation NAMRU3-T950].

Deyde, V.M., Khristova, M.L., Rollin, P.E. *et al.* (2006). Crimean-Congo hemorrhagic fever virus genomics and global diversity. *J. Virol.*, 80: 8834–42.

Doganci, L. (2007). New insights on the bleeding disorders in Crimean-Congo hemorrhagic fever. *J. Infect.*, 55: 379–81.

Duh, D., Saksida, A., Petrovec, M. *et al.* (2006). Novel one-step real-time RT-PCR assay for rapid and specific diagnosis of Crimean-Congo hemorrhagic fever encountered in the Balkans. *J. Virolog. Meth.*, 133: 175–79.

Dunster, L., Dunster, M., Ofula, V. *et al.* (2002). First documentation of human Crimean-Congo hemorrhagic fever, Kenya. *Emerg. Infect. Dis.*, 8: 1005–6.

El Azazy, O.M. and Scrimgeour, E.M. (1997). Crimean-Congo haemorrhagic fever virus infection in the western province of Saudi Arabia. *Trans. R. Soc. Trop. Med. Hyg.*, 91: 275–78.

Ergonul, O. (2008). Treatment of Crimean-Congo hemorrhagic fever. *Antivir. Res.*, 78: 125–31.

Ergonul, O., Celikbas, A., Baykam, N. *et al.* (2006a). Analysis of risk-factors among patients with Crimean-Congo haemorrhagic fever virus infection: severity criteria revisited. *Clin. Microbiol. Infect.*, 12: 551–54.

Ergonul, O., Mirazimi, A. and Dimitrov, D.S. (2007). Treatment of Crimean-Congo hemorrhagic fever. In: O. Ergonul and C.A. Whitehouse (eds.) *Crimean Congo Hemorrhagic Fever, a Global Perspective*, pp. 245–69. Dordrecht: Springer.

Ergonul, O. and Whitehouse, C.A. (eds.) (2007). *Crimean Congo Hemorrhagic Fever, a Global Perspective*, pp. 328. Dordrecht: Springer.

Ergönül, O. (2006). Crimean-Congo haemorrhagic fever. *Lancet Infect. Dis.*, 6: 203–14.

Ergunol, O., Tuncbilek, S., Baykam, N. *et al.* (2006b). Evaluation of serum levels of interleukin (IL)-6, IL-10 and tumor necrosis factor-α in patients with Crimean-Congo hemorrhagic fever. *J. Infect. Dis.*, 193: 941–44.

Fisgin, N.T., Fisgin, T., Tanyel, E. *et al.* (2008). Crimean-Congo hemorrhagic fever: five patients with hemophagocytic syndrome. *Am. J. Hematol.*, 83: 73–76.

Hewson, R., Gyml, A., Gyml, L. *et al.* (2004). Evidence of segment reassortment in Crimean-Congo hemorrhagic fever virus. *J. Gener. Virol.*, 85: 3059–70.

Hoogstraal, H. (1979). The epidemiology of tick-borne Crimean-Congo haemorrhagic fever in Asia, Europe and Africa. *J. Med. Entomol.*, 15: 307–417.

Hoogstraal, H. (1981). Changing patterns of tick-borne diseases in modern society. *Ann. Rev. Entomol.*, 26: 75–99.

Karti, S., Odabasi, S., Korten, Z. *et al* (2004). Crimean-Congo haemorrhagic fever in Turkey. *Emerg. Infect. Dis.*, 10: 1379–84.

Khan, A.S., Maupin, G.O., Rollin, P.E. *et al.* (1997). An outbreak of Crimean-Congo hemorrhagic fever in the United Arab Emirates, 1994–1995. *Am. J. Trop. Med. Hyg.*, 57: 519–25.

Lukashev, A.N. (2005). Evidence for recombination in Crimean-Congo hemorrhagic fever virus. *J. Gener. Virol.*, 86: 2333–38.

Lvov, D.K. (1994). Arboviral zoonoses of northern Eurasia (Eastern Europe and the Commonwealth of Independent States). In: G.W. Beram (ed.) *Handbook of Zoonoses, Section B: Viral* (2nd edn.), pp. 237–60. Boca Ratan, FLA: CRC Press.

Papa, A., Bino, S., Velo, E. *et al.* (2006). Cytokine levels in Crimean-Congo hemorrhagic fever. *J. Clin. Virol.*, 36: 272–76.

Papa, A., Bosovic, B., Pavlido, V. *et al.* (2002b). Genetic detection and isolation of Crimean-Congo hemorrhagic fever virus, Kosovo, Yugoslavia. *Emerg. Infect. Dis.*, 8: 852–54.

Papa, A., Bino, S., Llagami, A. *et al.* (2002a). Crimean-Congo hemorrhagic fever in Albania, 2001. *Euro. J. Clin. Microbiol. Infect. Dis.*, 8: 603–06.

Peters, C.J. and Shelokov, A. (1990). Viral hemorrhagic fever. *Curr. Thera. Infect. Dis.*, 3: 355–60.

Screck, C.E., Snoddy, E.L. and Mount, G.A. (1980). Permethrin and repellants as clothing impregnants for protection from the lone star tick *Amblyomma americanum. J. Econ. Entom.*, 73: 436–39.

Scrimgeour, E.M., Zaki, A., Mehta, F.R. *et al.* (1996). Crimean-Congo haemorrhagic fever in Oman. *Trans. R. Soc. Trop. Med. Hyg.*, 90: 290–91.

Shepherd, A.J., Swanepoel, R., Shepherd, S.P. *et al.* (1991). Viraemic transmission of Crimean-Congo haemorrhagic fever virus to ticks. *Epidemiol. Infect.*, 106: 373–82.

Swanepoel, R., Gill, D.E., Shepherd, A.J. *et al.* (1989). The clinical pathology of Crimean-Congo hemorrhagic fever. *Rev. Infect. Dis.*, **11**: 5794–800.

Swanepoel, R. and Burt, F.J. (2004). Crimean-Congo haemorrhagic fever. In: J.A.W. Coetzer and R.C. Tustin (eds.) *Infectious Diseases of Livestock* (2nd edn.), pp. 1077–85. Cape Town, South Africa: Oxford University Press.

Swanepoel, R. (1995). Nairoviruses. In: J. S. Porterfield (ed.) *Handbook of Infectious Diseases, Vol. 3, Viruses*, pp. 285–93. London: Chapman and Hall.

Swanepoel, R. (1994). Crimean-Congo haemorrhagic fever. In: G.W. Beran (ed.) *Handbook of Zoonoses, Section B: Viral* (2nd edn.), pp. 157–70. Boca Raton, Florida: CRC Press.

Swanepoel, R., Leman P.A., Burt, F.J. *et al.* (1998). Experimental infection of ostriches with Crimean-Congo haemorrhagic fever virus. *Epidemiol. Infect.*, **121**: 427–32.

Swanepoel, R. and Shepherd, A.J. (1983–8). National Institute for Communicable Diseases, Private Bag X4, Sandringham 2131, South Africa. Unpublished observations.

Swanepoel, R., Shepherd, A.J., Leman, P.A. *et al.* (1987). Epidemiologic and clinical features of Crimean-Congo hemorrhagic fever in southern Africa. *Am. J. Trop. Med. Hyg.*, **36**: 120–32.

Vatansever, Z., Uzun, R., Estrada-Pena, A. *et al.* (2007). Crimean-Congo haemorrhagic fever in Turkey. In: O. Ergonul and C.A. Whitehouse (eds.) *Crimean Congo Hemorrhagic Fever, a Global Perspective*, pp. 59–74. Dordrecht: Springer.

Watts, D.M., Ksiazek, T.G., Linthicum, K.J. *et al.* (1989). Crimean-Congo hemorrhagic fever. In: T.P. Monath (ed.) *The Arboviruses: Epidemiology and Ecology*, Vol. II pp. 177–222. Boca Raton, Florida: CRC Press.

Whitehouse, C.A. (2004). Crimean-Congo hemorrhagic fever. *Antiv. Res.*, **64**: 145–60.

Williams, R.J., Al Busaidy, S., Mehta, F.R. *et al.* (2000). Crimean-Congo haemorrhagic fever: a seroepidemiological and tick survey in the Sultanate of Oman. *Trop. Med. Intern. Heal.*, **5**: 99–106.

Zeller, H.G., Cornet, J.P. and Camicas, J.L. (1994a). Crimean-Congo haemorrhagic fever virus infection in birds: field investigations in Senegal. *Res. Virol.*, **145**: 105–9.

Zeller, H.G., Cornet, J.P. and Camicas, J.L. (1994b). Experimental transmission of Crimean-Congo haemorrhagic fever virus by West African ground-feeding birds to *Hyalomma marginatum rufipes* ticks. *Am. J. Trop. Med. Hyg.*, **50**: 676–81.

CHAPTER 27

Foot-and-mouth disease, Vesicular stomatitis, Newcastle disease, and Swine vesicular disease

Satu Kurkela and David W. G. Brown

Summary

In this chapter we review four viral zoonoses that are an important cause of a vesicular disease in animals, but only occasionally cause human infections. These viruses represent three different taxonomical families (*Picornaviridae*, *Rhabdoviridae*, *Paramyxoviridae*). Their clinical manifestations in animals resemble each another, characterized by vesicular eruptions in skin and mucous membranes, while human manifestations are generally mild and range from skin lesions and conjunctivitis to influenza-like illness and rarely encephalitis.

Foot-and-mouth disease

Introduction

Foot-and-mouth disease (FMD) remains an economically important animal infection in many parts of the world. The virus (FMDV) is an aphthovirus in the *Picornaviridae* virus family and infects a wide range of hoofed animals. It causes severe vesicular disease particularly in cattle and pigs.

The virus spreads in a variety of ways, but aerosol transmission is important and reflects the high titres of virus excreted. Control of infection is based on control of imports of animals and animal products from infected zones including quarantine and slaughter. An inactivated vaccine is available. Human infection has been reported, but illness is rare and of little health significance.

History

A disease resembling FMD in cattle was first described in Italy in 1514 by H. Fracastorius. Another early report of probable FMD dates back to 1695 in Germany (O'Brien 1913). In 1898, Friedrich Löffler and Paul Frosch discovered that the causative agent of FMD in livestock was an infectious particle smaller than any bacteria: FMDV became the first virus to be identified from animals. Ever since its discovery, FMD has been recognized as a major animal disease with considerable economic burden. Outbreaks of FMDV in livestock have occurred practically everywhere in the world except New Zealand.

The agent

Taxonomy and molecular biology

The causative agent of FMD is FMDV, a picornavirus belonging to the genus *Aphthovirus*, which only consists of two species: FMVD and Equine rhinitis A virus.

Aphthovirus virions are 27–30 nm in diameter, and they have a round shape with icosahedral symmetry. The genome is a linear positive-polarity single-stranded RNA of approximately 8.5 kilobases in length, and contains a single long ORF with two alternative initiation sites.

After adsorption to the cell surface, the 140S virion breaks down into pentameric subunits, and the RNA is released into the cytoplasm (Baxt and Bachrach 1980). The genomic RNA is translated into a polyprotein upon virus entry into a host cell, and through autoproteolysis post-translationally cleaved to yield 4 structural capsid proteins (VP1, VP2, VP3, and VP4, also sometimes referred to as 1D, 1B, 1C, and 1A, respectively), and 10 non-structural proteins (L^{pro}, 2A^{pro}, 2B, 2C, 3A, 3B$_1$, 3B$_2$, 3B$_3$, 3C^{pro}, 3D^{pol}) (Porter 1993). Most of the proteolytic events that produce mature polypeptides from the encoded polyprotein are mediated by L^{pro}, 2A, and 3C^{pro}. In addition, L^{pro} is essentially involved in the ability of FMDV to cause disease and in permitting transmission (Mason *et al.* 1997). 3A and 3B non-structural proteins are suggested to contribute into virulence and host range of the virus (Pacheco *et al.* 2003).

FMDV replication takes place in a membrane-bound replication complex at the cell cytoplasm. During replication a negative-sense RNA intermediate is produced, which then functions as a template for the synthesis of new single-stranded positive-sense RNAs. Takes place in the final stage of the replication cycle, the encapsidation of the positive-sense viral RNA and maturation cleavage of VP0 (1AB) into VP4 and VP2.

Seven antigenically distinct FMDV serotypes are recognized: A (Allemagne), Asia 1, C, O (Oise), and South African Territories 1 (SAT1), SAT2, and SAT3. Further, each of the serotypes can have several topotypes (subtypes) featuring their own antigenic characteristics (Domingo 2003). FMDV has particularly high mutation rates, and results in very variable FMDV populations with quasispecies. Vaccination or natural infection with one serotype does not provide cross-protection to another serotype, and protection may be limited between different subtypes of one serotype (Alexandersen *et al.* 2003a).

Growth and survival

FMDV usually causes a cytopathic effect in cell cultures, which includes cell rounding and alterations in internal cellular membranes. However, establishment of a persistent infection of BHK-21 cell line has been described (De la Torre *et al.* 1985). FMDV has a short infectious cycle in cultured cells with newly formed infectious virions starting to appear 4–6 hours after infection. FMDV binds to cells in culture at both 4°C and 37°C.

FMDV is moderately stable in lower temperatures at pH range 7.0–8.5, as well as in humidities above 55–60%. Virions become unstable below pH 6.5 and above 9. FMDV can be inactivated by heat and many disinfectants, but is resistant to ether and chloroform. Drying inactivates most, but not all of FMDV, and the virus may persist in the environment for weeks or even months, especially in contaminated organic material, such as faeces, urine, or soil (Alexandersen *et al.* 2003b).

Disease mechanisms

It is apparent that the disease process of FMDV infection is mediated by virus-integrin interaction. A tripeptide sequence Arg-Gly-Asp (RGD) is a cellular recognition site present in the FMDV VP1 protein, which enables the virus to utilize specific integrins that use RGD tripeptide as a recognition sequence (at least $\alpha_v\beta_3$, $\alpha_v\beta_6$ and $\alpha_v\beta_1$) as receptors. Additionally, antibody-complex virus can infect cells through Fc receptor-mediated adsorption. Serotype O_1 has been shown to use glycosaminoglycan heparan sulphate as a co-receptor (Jackson *et al.* 1996). L^{pro} appears to play a role in the virulence of FMDV as well, influencing the replication efficiency and spread of the virus within the host (Brown *et al.* 1996), whereas alterations in the 3A protein have produced phenotypes that favour replication in certain animals over others (Knowles *et al.* 2001a).

The hosts

Clinical: animals

FMD has a broad host range including pigs, cattle, and sheep, and is considered one of the economically most important animal diseases worldwide as it causes high morbidity in livestock.

FMD is characterized by formation of vesicles typically around mouth and feet, and sometimes in snout or muzzle, teats, and genital areas. Other common clinical manifestations are fever, depression, and loss of appetite. Pain caused by vesicles in feet results in reluctance to walk and lameness. Pigs usually exhibit the most severe clinical manifestations characterized by reluctance to stand and a dog-sitting posture. In cattle, drooling of saliva and vesicles around the mouth are typical. Decreased milk production and loss of weight are common. In sheep, the overall symptoms are less prominent with more superficial skin lesions.

For adult animals, mortality is usually low. However, FMDV infection can be fatal in young animals, especially in lambs and piglets due to acute myocarditis, and typically occurs before the appearance of vesicular lesions (Alexandersen *et al.* 2003b).

Clinical: humans

Despite the extensive exposure of humans, only sporadic clinical cases have been described in the scientific literature (Armstrong *et al.* 1967; Dlugosz 1968; Hyslop 1973). Many of the earlier cases were linked with milking of animals, more recently several laboratory accidents have been reported involving e.g. skin lacerations. Also consumption of raw milk and handling of sick or diseased animals have led to infections (Hyslop 1973). FMDV serotype O is most commonly isolated from humans, but also serotype C and rarely A cause human infections (Bauer 1997).

Pathogenesis

In animals the primary site of infection is the pharyngeal area, particularly in the dorsal surface of the soft palate and the roof of the pharynx, where infection is thought to occur through non-cornified squamous epithelial cells. These cells may also be involved in persistent FMDV infection in carrier animals (Alexandersen *et al.* 2003b). FMDV is present in pharynx 1–3 days before the onset of viremia, which usually lasts for 4–5 days (Alexandersen *et al.* 2002c). Besides pharynx, infection can also occur through skin abrasions (Alexandersen *et al.* 2003b), in which case the viral replication will take place at the site of entry, in regional lymph nodes, and in epithelia of the tongue and mouth (Alexandersen 2003b).

The initial spread of virus from the pharyngeal region through regional lymph nodes and the bloodstream to epithelial cells (Alexandersen *et al.* 2001, 2002b). The secondary sites of FMDV replication are the cornified stratified squamous epithelia of the skin and mouth, as well as occasionally the myocardium (Alexandersen *et al.* 2001, 2003b), and resulting in several cycles of viral amplification and spread (Alexandersen *et al.* 2002b). Of note, FMDV can also be present in sites without visible clinical manifestations (Brown *et al.* 1995).

Practically all secretions and excretions from animals become infectious during the course of the infection, including nasal and lachrymal secretions, oral saliva, pharyngeal fluids, vesicular epithelium, milk, semen, expired breath, and to a lesser extent urine and faeces. In sheep, viremia begins 1–2 days before clinical symptoms.

Incubation

In humans, the incubation period of FMDV is usually 2–6 days (Bauer 1997). The incubation period in animals is dose-dependent: between farms it is usually within 2–14 days (Sellers 1973; Garland and Donaldson 1990) and within a single herd the incubation period is only few days for direct contact between animals (Alexandersen *et al.* 2003a).

Symptoms and signs

FMD infection in humans is frequently asymptomatic. There are several reports of FMDV isolation from upper respiratory tract or antibody response without clinical manifestations (Hyslop 1973). The incidence of asyptomatic infections is, however, impossible to estimate due to lack of seroepidemiological studies. Human clinical FMD infection resembles that observed in animals, but usually has a milder form. Symptoms can include fever, sore throat, fatigue, headache, loss of appetite, tachycardia, and enlarged lymph nodes, followed by tingling blisters of varying size in hands, feet and mouth, accompanied with excess salivation (Armstrong *et al.* 1967; Prempeh *et al.* 2001; Bauer 1997; Dlugosz 1968; Hyslop 1973). Conjunctivitis and non-vesicular stomatitis have been reported as rare manifestations (Hyslop 1973). Basic blood parameters are usually normal (Dlugosz 1968).

The zoonotic FMD needs to be clearly distinguished from the non-zoonotic hand, foot, and mouth disease (HFMD), which is mostly caused by two types of *Human enterovirus A* species of genus *Enterovirus*: Human coxackievirus A16 and Human enterovirus 71 (McMinn *et al.* 2002).

Pathology and diagnosis

Immune response to FMDV is primarily mediated by humoral response, which leads to efficient antibody protection against reinfection in a serotype-specific manner. The onset of antibody response, initially with IgM production, coincides with the clearance of viremia; in sheep this occurs at around 4–5 days after onset, and the antibody titres peak at seven days after onset (Alexandersen *et al.* 2002c). Usually IgG antibody titres remain high for months, and can be detectable for years. In cattle, IgG1 predominated over IgG2 (Salt *et al.* 1996). Good protective immunity is reached 7–14 days after infection (or vaccination).

FMVD can persist in asymptomatic animals for a long time, especially in the pharyngeal region, allowing continuous viral shedding and onward transmission through saliva and exhaled air (Sutmoller 1965). As many as 50% of sheep, for example, may become carriers of FMVD after infection (Alexandersen *et al.* 2002c). Evidence suggests that the immune status of the animal controls the level of virus replication (Alexandersen *et al.* 2002b).

The clinical manifestations of FMD can closely resemble other viral vesicular diseases in both humans and animals. Therefore clinical diagnosis of FMD should be verified with laboratory investigation by either direct detection with virus isolation, nucleic acid amplification or complement fixation test; or antibody detection with serological methods (ELISA or neutralization test). Due to the potential rapid spread of FMD, laboratory tests with a quick turnaround time are needed for its identification. ELISA antigen capture assays (Morioka *et al.* 2009) have been used as first-line test methods, and virus isolation as a confirmatory method, which also specifies the serotype. Virus isolation, however, takes several days, which is incompatible with the need for rapid diagnosis. Therefore, real time RT-PCR methods have been established for quick serotype specific diagnostics (Goris *et al.* 2009). Complexity for direct detection of FMDV may be added by low virulence of some of the FMDV strains (Alexandersen *et al.* 2003b).

ELISA methods are used for serological diagnostics of FMDV infection (Ko *et al.* 2010). Test methods which are able to distinguish between vaccine and natural FMDV immunity have been developed (Muller *et al.* 2009), and are very useful for trade markets. Some serological fielding tests are also available (Oem *et al.* 2009).

Treatment and prognosis

FMDV infection in humans is self-limited, and patients usually recover with supportive care within two weeks (Hyslop 1973). No specific antiviral treatment is available for human FMDV infection.

Epidemiology

Occurrence

According to the statistics of the World Organization for Animal Health (OIE), FMD continues to be an important animal disease. FMD affects practically all parts of Africa, especially the western and southern African countries; Middle East; China; Russia; Central, South, and South-East Asia; South America; and also a few countries in Europe, including the UK, Cyprus, and Turkey, the latter of which has reported the disease almost continuously in recent times.

During 1998–2001 a pandemic lineage of serotype O, named the Pan Asia strain, spread from Asia to parts of Africa and Europe (Knowles *et al.* 2005). The spread presumably first began from India, soon affecting a number of Middle East countries, China, and South East Asia during 1998–1999, and thereafter South Korea, Japan, Russia, Mongolia, and South Africa in 2000. In February 2001, the Pan Asia strain reached the UK, with thousands of farms affected and subsequently half a million animals slaughtered during the following months (Knowles *et al.* 2001b). Sporadic cases were also reported in Ireland, France, and the Netherlands (Knowles *et al.* 2005). This pandemic demonstrated that the Pan Asia strain of serotype O is capable of spreading into countries with strict control measures in place, and which have been free from FMDV for decades prior the spread.

Each FMDV serotype has its own geographical distribution. According to the statistics of the World Reference Laboratory for Foot-and-Mouth Disease during 2000–2006, FMDV O was found throughout South America, Africa, Middle East, South and South East Asia, and in a few European countries. FMDV A was reported throughout South America, and in parts of Africa, Middle East, and South Asia. FMDV C was found in Brazil, a few East African countries, whereas FMDV Asia 1 serotype was present exclusively, but widely in Asia. Serotypes SAT1-3 were present exclusively in Africa, except for SAT-2 which was also reported from Middle East in 2000.

Transmission in animals

FMD is one of the most highly contagious diseases in animals. FMDV has multiple routes of transmission, including direct transfer through mucosae or skin abrasions, oral transmission e.g. from contaminated food, or through respiratory tract by aerosols and droplets. In the latter case the pharynx appears to be the primary site of infection (Zhang *et al.* 2001). The virus can even be spread by the wind; some of the serotypes over hundreds of kilometres. Pigs shed large quantities of airborne virus, but at the same time, they also require a higher virus concentration to acquire the infection through the respiratory route (Alexandersen and Donaldson 2002). Thus, airborne transmission typically occurs downwind from pigs to cattle or sheep (Donaldson *et al.* 2001). Mechanical spread through, e.g. contaminated transport vehicles is not uncommon.

Transmission in humans

Veterinarians, farm workers, butchers, and laboratory workers are the occupational groups in risk for acquiring FMDV infection (Hyslop 1973). A close contact with infected animals is the most common route of infection (Prempeh *et al.* 2001). A report dating back to 1834 describes experimental infection of French veterinarians after drinking raw milk from infected cows (Hertwig 1834), and several other cases linked with consumption of unpasteurized milk have been reported (Hyslop 1973). Also, an infection through skin laceration has been described (Dlugosz 1968). FMDV can be recovered from infected humans from nose, throat, saliva, and from air expelled during coughing, sneezing, talking, and breathing (Sellers *et al.* 1970). FMDV can persist in the nose for more than 24 hours (Sellers *et al.* 1970). Person to person transmission cannot be excluded, nor transmission from humans to animals, although there are no such case reports. Viremia in humans appears to last only a few days after onset of symptoms (Armstrong *et al.* 1967).

Prevention and control

Control strategies

Long distance animal trading facilitates spread of FMDV worldwide. The OIE advises the following sanitary prophylaxis measures: protection of free zones by border animal movement control and surveillance; slaughter of infected, recovered, and FMD-susceptible contact animals; disinfection of premises and all infected material (implements, cars, clothes, etc.); destruction of cadavers, litter, and susceptible animal products in the infected area; and quarantine measures (http://www.oie.int/eng/maladies/fiches/a_A010.htm). In addition to sanitary prophylaxis, inactivated virus vaccines are available (see below).

Vaccines

FMD vaccines were one of the first animal vaccines produced. The currently available inactivated vaccines have a number of limitations (Rodriguez and Grubman 2009). Firstly, the production of inactivated vaccines is laborious, requiring growth of large volumes of virulent FMDV, inactivation, antigen concentration, and purification, also raising concerns with biosafety. Further, inactivated vaccines do not induce a long-term protection, and subsequently multiple vaccinations are needed. These vaccines are monotypic and provide no cross-protection. Production of live attenuated FMDV vaccines have failed. Therefore development of recombinant vaccines are underway. Approches are based on either recombinant protein or peptide (Taboga *et al.* 1997; Rodriguez *et al.* 2003), or empty capsid (Moraes *et al.* 2002) have been described.

There are a number of different approaches for the use of FMD vaccines, and no worldwide consensus exists. Both the disease epidemiology and economics influence the chosen strategy. In disease-free countries, only targeted vaccinations are usually implemented during outbreaks. In endemic areas an additional strategy may be prophylactic vaccinations in regular time intervals, 'ring' vaccination of selected farms, or post-outbreak vaccinations (Hutber *et al.* 2010).

Legislation

FMD free areas exercise careful control of imports of live animals and products.

Vesicular stomatitis

Introduction

There are 3 species of vesicular stomatitis virus (VSV) which are members of the genus *Vesiculovirus* in the family *Rhabdoviridae*. The virus infects a wide range of domestic and wild animals, but several vesicular diseases of the mouth and hooves are seen in horses, cattle and pigs. Mortality is low. Infection is generally through close contact, but insect vectors have also been implicated. Human infection is common in those closely exposed to infected animals. Infection generally presents as a mild flu-like illness, and is frequently not recognized.

History

First reports of vesicular stomatitis (VS) in horses and mules date back to 1884 in South Africa, although the causative agent was not identified (Theiler 1901). In the USA, VS in horses was first reported in 1916 (Teidebold *et al.* 1916), although VSV was probably present there much earlier. The first report of probable human VSV infection was described in 1917 in the USA in three individuals working with horses with symptoms compatible with VS (Burton 1917).

The agent

Taxonomy and molecular biology

VS is caused by vesicular stomatitis viruses (VSV) of the genus *Vesiculovirus* in the family *Rhabdoviridae* of the order Mononegavirales. There are three VSV species, and they cause VS in both humans and animals: VSV New Jersey, VSV Indiana, and VSV Alagoas. Of the other vesiculovirus species, Chandipura and Piry viruses are also associated with human disease.

VSV virions consist of an envelope, bullet-shaped capsid of 75 nm in diameter and 180 nm in length, with helical symmetry. The genome is a linear negative-polarity single-stranded RNA of approximately 11 kilobases in length. The genomic RNA encodes five structural proteins: the nucleoprotein (N), the phosphoprotein (P), the matrix protein (M), the glycoprotein (G), and the large polymerase protein (L). The genes are arranged in the following order: 3'-(leader), N, P, M, G, L, (trailer)-5'.

The genomic RNA is enwrapped by the N protein, forming together a helical structure. N-RNA is recognized by the VSV RNA-dependent RNA polymerase, which is composed of the L protein catalytic subunit and the P protein cofactor, and these four viral components form the VSV ribonucleoprotein (RNP) complex. The G protein is necessary for viral binding to target cells and fusing viral and cellular membranes, and thus mediates the virus entry through endocytosis into the cytoplasm (Matlin *et al.* 1982). After entry, RNP is released from the virion and serves as a template for transcription of five subgenomic mRNAs that are subsequently translated into the G, M, N, P, and L proteins. Following the translation phase, begins the genome replication during which the RNA-dependent RNA no longer functions as a transcriptase but as a replicase, and synthesizes a full-length complementary antigenome. This serves as template for synthesis of full-length genomic RNA, which in turn can be assembled into complete infectious particles together with the viral proteins (Barr *et al.* 2002). The virus exits the cell by budding through the plasma membrane. The M protein has an important role in virus assembly, budding, and cellular apoptosis (Barr *et al.* 2002).

Growth and survival

VSV can be grown in various mammalian and mosquito cell lines, as well as embryonated chicken eggs and suckling mice. VSV causes a visible cytopathic effect in mammalian cell cultures, characterized by cell rounding, and ultimately cell death. VSV can remain viable for 3-4 days in saliva and hay (Hanson 1952). VSV is stable between pH 4 and 10, and can survive for long periods at low temperatures. Thermal inactivation studies show a rapid inactivation at 56°C (Michalski *et al.* 1976). The virus can be effectively inactivated by ether and other organic solvents, as well as formalin, whereas alkaline chemicals are not very effective.

Disease mechanisms

The cell damage appears to be associated with specific inhibition of cellular gene expression, as well as dissolution of cellular cytoskeleton, leading eventually to apoptosis, which occurs simultaneously as infectious virus is produced in cultured cells (Koyama, 1995). The M protein has a role in the breakdown of the cytoskeleton by depolymerizing actin, tubulin, and vimentin (Lyles and

McKenzie 1997). Evidence suggests that the M protein also inhibits the 'Ran' nuclear guanosine triphosphatase which has a role in mediating transport of proteins into the nucleus, and mRNA out of the nucleus, which results in exclusive translation of viral mRNA (Her *et al.* 1997).

The hosts

Clinical: animals

VSV viruses infect a broad range of animals, and there are no animals known to be naturally resistant to the infection. Symptomatic VSV infection is seen in cattle, swine and horses, and cannot be clinically distinguished from FMDV infection. Many of the infections are asymptomatic. The disease is characterized by painful vesicles and lesions in tongue, oral tissues, feet, and teats (Vanleeuwen *et al.* 1995; Letchworth *et al.* 1999).

In cattle, the disease can present with maceration of mucous membranes, swelling of the nostrils and muzzle, nasal discharge, and fever. Some animals feature vesicles and swelling in teats, and lesions in feet. Recovery takes places 2–3 weeks after onset. In swine, vesicles appear on their lips, snout, coronary bands, and interdigital space, accompanied by fever and lameness. Swine usually recover within 2 weeks. Horses present with painful lesions on the lips, gums, palate, and tongue, subsequently leading to reluctance to eat or drink. Lesions are also seen in coronary bands and mammary glands. Fever and lameness are common. Horses generally recover within 3 weeks from onset.

VSV causes significant economic losses due to decreased milk and meat production, as well as quarantine and trade restrictions.

Clinical: humans

Symptomatic human infections have been reported with Alagoas, Chandipura (Bhatt and Rodrigues 1967), Piry, VSV-Indiana, and VSV-New Jersey vesiculoviruses. Dual infections have also been reported (Tesh *et al.* 1969). Studies suggest that more than half of the human VSV infections are symptomatic (Reif *et al.* 1987; Patterson *et al.* 1958).

Pathogenesis

In animals, VSV New Jersey is shown to have a greater pathogenicity than the other major serotype, VSV Indiana (Rodriguez 2002). VSV New Jersey also has a longer period of virus shedding, and more efficient virus transmission (Stallknecht 2004). Studies in swine have demonstrated the importance of G protein in the pathogenesis and virulence of VSV (Martinez *et al.* 2003). Evidence suggests that keratinocytes may be primary targets for viral replication at the early stage of the infection in skin (Scherer *et al.* 2007). Experimental studies suggest that the route of VSV infection has an influence on the clinical outcome; e.g. intranasal or intravenous inoculation leads to subclinical infection, whereas inoculation of mouth leads to formation of vesicles (Howerth *et al.* 1997). The localized nature of VSV infection is demonstrated by studies in cattle showing that after intradermal inoculation, VSV can only be recovered from lesion sites and local lymph nodes, but not from blood or internal organs (Scherer *et al.* 2007).

Incubation

The incubation period of human VSV infection is approximately 2–6 days. A case report in which the time of infection could be determined very precisely described a laboratory-acquired infection through accidental skin laceration, and reported an incubation period of 30 hours (Johnson *et al.* 1966). In animals, the incubation period can extend up to 21 days.

Symptoms and signs

Vesicular stomatitis in humans presents with influenza-like illness, which can include (sometimes biphasic) fever, malaise, myalgia, headache, retro-orbital pain, chills, sore throat, rhinorroea, vomiting, nausea, diarrhoea, and occasionally vesicles in the mucosa of mouth and pharynx (Johnson *et al.* 1966; Hanson *et al.* 1950; Patterson *et al.* 1958; Fields and Hawkins 1967; Reif *et al.* 1987). Conjunctivitis may precede other symptoms (Patterson *et al.* 1958). In children, encephalitis has been described in a few case reports (Quiroz *et al.* 1988; Letchworth *et al.* 1999). The related Chandipura virus has been associated with encephalitis in children on several occasions (Rodrigues *et al.* 1983; Chadha *et al.* 2005).

Pathology and diagnosis

The formation of skin lesions is caused by degradation of cells above the basal layer of skin. Intracellular oedema is present in the epidermis, and can extend down to basal cells. Lymph and blood vessels may be engorged, and perivascular infiltration of inflammatory cells is seen.

VSV infection in animals produces a strong antibody response, mostly against the G protein. Antibodies to the G protein both neutralize the virus, and help targeting complement, macrophages, and T cells against VSV and cells infected with VSV (Lefrancois 1984). High antibody titres usually persist for years (Rodriguez *et al.* 1990; Geleta and Holbrook 1961), and studies with mice show good protection against reinfection (Bründler *et al.* 1996). However, antibodies do not provide sufficient protection against VSV infection in cattle in natural conditions, and reinfections do occur (Rodriguez *et al.* 1990). Neutralizing monoclonal antibodies towards G protein of VSV New Jersey and Indiana serotypes do not cross-react (Lefrancois and Lyles 1982), however there is cross-reaction of non-neutralizing antibodies (Tesh *et al.* 1987). Besides serological response, the interferon system and nitric oxide also functions as a defense mechanism against VSV infection (Komatsu and Reiss 1996).

VSV antibody kinetics in humans have been poorly described. One case study on human VSV Indiana infection (Johnson *et al.* 1966) reported complement-fixing (CF) antibodies appearing at around day 13 after onset, to peak between 18 and 22 days. Neutralizing antibodies were shown to appear simultaneously with CF antibodies and are readily detectable 1 year after infection. In cattle and horses, neutralizing and CF antibodies rise quickly to high titres, and CF and IgM antibodies disappear within 2–4 months after onset (Geleta and Holbrook 1961).

Laboratory confirmation of VSV infection is important, as it is not possible to distinguish VS from FMD clinically. For direct detection of VSV, various PCR methods are available, including real time and multiplex platforms (Fernández *et al.* 2008). Virus isolation is rarely successful from humans. From animals, VSV can be isolated from throat swabs, saliva, vesicular fluid or epithelial tissue (Webb *et al.* 1987). Serological methods include ELISA methods (Katz *et al.* 1995), complement-fixation test, immunofluorescence test, and neutralization test. VSV serotypes cross-react in CF and immunofluorescence tests. ELISA methods able to discriminate between natural and vaccine immunity have been developed (Ahmad *et al.* 1993). Also serotype-specific ELISA tests are available (Lee *et al.* 2009).

Treatment and prognosis

Vesicular stomatitis in humans is a self-limited acute illness, typically with a duration of 3–5 days. No specific antiviral treatment is available.

Epidemiology

Occurrence

VSV spread to Europe during the First World War, but today it is limited to the Americas. VSV is presently endemic in Mexico, Central America, northern South America, eastern Brazil, and limited areas in the south eastern USA (e.g. state of Georgia). VSV New Jersey and VSV Indiana are the two major serotypes, of which VSV New Jersey is responsible for most of the epizootics. Most outbreaks in the USA are caused by the New Jersey serotype, whereas the Indiana serotypes mainly cause outbreaks in South America.

Transmission in animals

The reservoir of VSV is unknown. The hypotheses for reservoirs include plants, wildlife, livestock (e.g. goats and poultry), or vertical transmission within an arthropod vector. Transmission of VSV in animals usually takes place 1–5 days after infection (Letchworth et al. 1999). VSV transmission occurs efficiently from lesions and saliva, which contaminate feed and water through, as well as milking and other equipment.

Infection probably occurs through mouth abrasions and from ocular lesions. Spread of VSV is probably not dependent on arthropods but there is substantial evidence that biting arthropods play an important role in the transmission of VSV. Firstly, VSV epidemics usually occur during spring, summer, and autumn, but disappear after the first frost (Hanson 1952). The epidemics tend to occur in the presence of natural water and shade trees (Letchorth et al. 1999). Protection of animals from arthropod bites results in lower attack rates (Webb 1987). Wind patterns have been associated with outbreaks, suggesting long-distance spread of VSV with black flies, whereas high sandfly activity has been reported to coincide with antibody seroconversion in pigs (Comer et al. 1994). It is known that vesiculoviruses can naturally infect sandflies, mosquitoes, eye gnats, house flies, Simulium black flies, midges, and other non-haematophagous diptera. Also, vesiculoviruses are shown to transmit transovarially and to replicate in sandflies (Weaver et al. 1992). Additionally, vesiculoviruses are capable of spreading from infected sandflies and mosquitoes to mammals (Tesh et al. 1971).

Transmission in humans

Occupational groups at risk of acquiring VSV infection are veterinarians, researchers, and other groups coming in close contact with infected animals (Reif et al. 1987; Brody et al. 1967). In addition, symptomatic infections in laboratory workers have been reported (Hanson et al. 1950). VSV is fairly contagious, which is demonstrated by serological studies of exposed field and laboratory workers, one of which reported a 95% seroprevalence over a 7-year period (Patterson et al. 1958). High seroprevalence rates (13–90%) have been reported during epizootics or in enzootic areas (Tesh et al. 1969; Brody et al. 1967; Tesh et al. 1987). Studies suggest that such high seroprevalence rates are achieved only after continuous and long-term exposure. During an epizootic in Colorado in 1982, a seroconversion rate of only 10.5% was observed in exposed persons (Reif et al. 1987).

The likely transmission routes from animals to humans are by aerosol and through direct contact, e.g. during examination of oral cavities or otherwise direct contact with saliva of sick animals (Reif et al. 1987), and in many cases prolonged (Webb et al. 1987), close contact is required for transmission.

Prevention and control

Control strategies

The sanitary prophylaxis measures advised by OIE include restriction of animal movement accompanied by rapid laboratory diagnosis, and disinfection of trucks and fomites (http://www.oie.int/eng/maladies/fiches/a_A020.htm).

Vaccines

Vaccination against VSV infection is not widely used. Experimental attenuated and inactivated VSV vaccines have been developed, but they are not widely used due to the inability of serology to distinguish between vaccinated and naturally infected animals. Subunit vaccines allowing this differentiation have been developed, however, presently it has not been established whether they are sufficiently effective. Only a few South American countries are using commercial inactivated VSV vaccines at the moment.

Newcastle disease

Introduction

Newcastle Disease (ND) is caused by a paramyxovirus (Newcastle Disease virus; NDV). All species of bird are potentially susceptible, but the disease is most important in chickens in which mortality is highest. Clinical infections can affect the enteric, respiratory and neurological systems. In humans infection is limited to those in close contact with poultry or laboratory staff. The predominant symptoms are a self-limiting conjunctivitis and flu-like illness. An effective vaccine is available and many countries control imports of live birds and products.

History

Newcastle disease (ND) was first described in poultry independently by Doyle in Newcastle upon Tyne, England (Doyle 1927) and by Kraneveld in Java (Kraneveld 1926), Indonesia in 1926. Due to its great economic impact on the poultry industry, ND continues to be one of the most important avian viral diseases. Human NDV infections are sporadically reported.

The agent

Taxonomy and molecular biology

ND is caused by NDV (Avian Paramyxovirus 1) of the genus Avulavirus in the family *Paramyxoviridae* (subfamily *Paramyxovirinae*) of the order *Mononegavirales*. NDV strains are classified according to their pathogenicity in chickens into three major pathotypes: lentogenic (low), mesogenic, (medium) and velogenic (high) strains.

The genome of NDV is a nonsegmented, single-stranded, negative-sense RNA of approximately 15.2 kilobases in length (de Leeuw and Peeters 1999). The genomic RNA encodes the following proteins: the nucleocapsid protein (NP), phosphoprotein (P), matrix protein (M), fusion protein (F), hemagglutinin-neuraminidase protein (HN), and large polymerase protein (L). The genes are arranged in the following order: 3'-(leader), NP, P, M, F, HN, L, (trailer)-5'.

Two additional proteins, V and W, are also produced from the P gene by alternative mRNAs that are generated by RNA editing (Steward *et al.* 1993). The genomic RNA is covered by the NP protein, which together with several copies of the L protein and the P protein constitute the viral RNA-dependent RNA polymerase.

NDV enters host cells by the fusion of the viral membrane with host cell plasma membrane. The HN protein interacts with sialoglycoconjugates at the cell surface, and viral entry is mediated by the F protein, which triggers the fusion of the viral and target membranes (Eckert and Kim 2001). Early in infection, transcription of the genomic RNA results in the synthesis of a short non-translated leader RNA and six subgenomic mRNA's which are translated to produce the viral proteins. Later in infection, as viral proteins start accumulating, RNA synthesis switches from transcription to replication, resulting in the synthesis of full-length antigenomic RNA, which serves as a template for the synthesis of full-length genomic RNA.

Growth and survival

NDV causes a cytopathic effect in cell cultures, characterized by cell rounding, detachment from the surface, cytoplasm vacuolation, syncytia formation, and ultimately cell death. ND can be inactivated by treatment at 60°C in 30 min, in low pH, and by using disinfectants such as formalin or phenol (Patnayak *et al.* 2008). NDV can survive for days or even weeks in the environment, particularly in ambient temperatures and in faeces (Guan *et al.* 2009).

Disease mechanisms

NDV-induced cytopathic effects in cultured cells are caused by apoptosis (Ravindra *et al.* 2009) through activation of caspases (Elankumaran *et al.* 2006). The F protein cleavage site is critical for virulence of NDV: the less virulent strains have fewer amino acids at this site, and a leucine instead of a phenylalanine at position 117 (de Leeuw *et al.* 2005). It appears that amino acid differences in the HN protein also significantly contribute to virulence (Huang *et al.* 2004). Evidence suggests that mutations in the intergenic sequences of NDV results in attenuation of the virus in chickens, and thus may play a role in the pathogenesis of NDV (Yan and Samal 2008). V protein is also involved in the pathogenicity as inhibition of V protein expression leads to attenuation of NDV (Huang *et al.* 2003).

The hosts

Clinical: animals

NDV can cause a clinical infection in almost all birds, including poultry (chicken, turkey, goose, duck, and pigeon), and pet and free-living birds. Chicken are the most susceptible birds among poultry. The disease is characterized by respiratory, neurologic, or enteric symptoms, leading to a considerable economic burden in the poultry industry due to high morbidity and mortality, and trade restrictions. The clinical presentation depends on the NDV pathotype. The lentogenic pathotypes cause a mild respiratory disease or subclinical infection; the mesogenic pathotypes manifest with respiratory and nervous signs with moderate mortality; and the velogenic pathotypes can cause a severe gastrointestinal and neurological disease with high mortality. Clinical manifestations in birds can include nervous signs, incoordination, depression, conjunctivitis, eyelid petechiae, leg and wing paralysis, dyspnea, loss of appetite, watery diarrhoea, reduction in egg production, tremors, and uncontrolled movement of the head (Aldous *et al.* 2008; Alexander *et al.* 1997,

Al-Hilly *et al.* 1980; Borland 1972; Piacenti *et al.* 2006; Wakamatsu *et al.* 2006).

Pathogenesis

Experimental studies on pathogenesis of NDV infection have been conducted in birds. After intraconjunctival inoculation, low virulence strains appear to cause microscopic lesions only in the site of inoculation and in the respiratory system, whereas highly virulent strains also cause a marked tropism for and necrosis and apoptosis in lymphoid tissues and organs, with large amounts of virus present in e.g. cecal tonsils, bursa, spleen, thymus, bone marrow, intestines, and kidney (Kommers *et al.* 2003; Wakamatsu *et al.* 2006), followed by viral replication in brain (Wakamatsu *et al.* 2006). NDV dissemination and sites of viral replication vary depending on bird species and viral strain.

Clinical: humans
Incubation

The incubation period of human NDV infection is probably around 3–4 days, as demonstrated in a recent case report of an accidental infection of a veterinary student (Richardson *et al.* 2005). In birds, the incubation period varies between 2–15 days, but can be even longer.

Symptoms and signs

Human NDV infection typically presents with conjunctivitis and sometimes general malaise. NDV conjunctivitis can include irritation of the eye, lacrimation, redness, follicular and papillary conjunctival hypertrophy, oedema of the eye lids, and preauricular adenitis. Typically only one eye is affected (Hales and Ostler 1973; Nelson *et al.* 1952). NDV antibodies have been reported in patients with various syndromes, such as infectious mononucleosis, leprosy, systemic lupus erythematosus, multiple sclerosis, and cancer, but no causality has not been established (Powell *et al.* 1985).

Pathology and diagnosis

In human NDV conjunctivitis, the predominate inflammatory cells present in conjunctiva are mononuclear cells (Hales and Ostler 1973). In birds, histopathological abnormalities associated with NDV infection can include lymphocytic infiltration of eyelids, lymphocytic inflammation of air sacs, tracheitis, splenic hyperplasia, inflammation of brain cells, and necrotizing pancreatitis (Nakamura *et al.* 2008; Piacenti *et al.* 2006). The histopathological changes seen in NDV conjunctivitis of birds feature focal hyperplasia of the conjunctival epithelial cells with cellular infiltration in the lamina propria of the conjunctivae, or even vascular necrosis with congestion and haemorrhages (Nakamura *et al.* 2004).

Virus isolation (King 1985) or different modifications of nucleic acid amplification (Tan *et al.* 2009) can be used for direct detection of NDV. The latter can be utilized for differentiation of strains with low and high virulence. The NDV pathotype can be determined by measuring the intracerebral pathogenicity index in day-old chickens or mean death time in embryonated fowls' eggs, or determining the amino acid motif at the cleavage site of the F protein (Miller *et al.* 2010). NDV antibodies have been detected using hemagglutination inhibition tests (Heckert and Nagy 1999) or ELISA (Mohan *et al.* 2006). Velogenic and low virulence NDV strains are serologically indistinguishable.

Treatment and prognosis

ND in humans is a self-limited illness, typically with a duration of few days. No specific antiviral treatment is available.

Epidemiology

Occurrence

NDV is present practically in all parts of the world. According to the OIE statistics, during the past five years NDV outbreaks have occurred throughout Europe, Japan, southern Africa, and in Central and South America.

Transmission in animals

NDV transmission can occur through direct animal contact, contaminated feed, water, tools, transport contact, transmission by people, and in optimal conditions, airborne transmission (Li *et al.* 2009). Transmission occurs either through faecal-oral or respiratory route (Awan *et al.* 1994). Evidence suggests that NDV transmission can also occur through eggs (Chen and Wang 2002). NDV shedding can continue for several weeks after infection both through the cloaca and mouth (Li *et al.* 2009).

Transmission in humans

The human infection is typically acquired through direct inoculation of the eye, typically by accidental splashing of infectious material into the eye. Most clinical cases have been described in people with close contact with infected poultry, or in laboratory workers (Brandly 1964; Dardiri *et al.* 1962; Evans 1955; Reagan *et al.* 1956; Quinn *et al.* 1952).

Prevention and control

Control strategies

The OIE advises the following sanitary prophylaxis measures: strict isolation of outbreaks; destruction of all infected and exposed birds; thorough cleaning and disinfection of premises; proper carcass disposal; pest control in flocks; depopulation followed by 21 days before restocking; avoidance of contact with birds of unknown health status; control of human traffic; and one age group per farm ('all in-all out') breeding (http://www.oie.int/eng/maladies/fiches/a_A160.htm) .

Vaccines

Both live (attenuated) and inactivated oil adjuvant vaccines are widely used in commercial poultry (Senne *et al.* 2004). The live vaccines are produced from lentogenic or mesogenic virus strains, and are usually administered in drinking water, or by coarse spray or conjunctival instillation. In the US, also an *in ovo* vaccine is being used. The more immunogenic vaccines are more likely to cause adverse effects. The inactivated vaccines are administered intramuscularly or subcutaneously. Both live and inactivated vaccines reduce morbidity and mortality, but do not prevent infection and virus shedding (Kapczynski and King 2005). The vaccination programme should be designed according to the type of vaccine used, the immune and disease status of the birds, and the level of protection required in the local conditions (Allan *et al.* 1978). A typical vaccination programme can include the administration of live lentogenic vaccine by conjunctival instillation or coarse spray at one day of age, followed by another lentogenic vaccine at around 18–21 days, and 10 weeks of age in the drinking water, and finally an inactivated vaccine at the point of lay.

Swine vesicular disease

Introduction

Swine vesicular disease virus (SVDV) is a member of the Picornaviridae. It is closely related to the human picornavirus coxsackie B5. It causes a vesicular disease in pigs, that is difficult to distinguish from FMD. Reports of human infection are rare and the spectrum of illness similar to those reported for human enterovirus infection.

History

The highly contagious SVDV infection was originally termed 'porcine enterovirus infection'. The first outbreak was reported in Italy in 1966 (Nardelli *et al.* 1968), and the virus was detected also in Hong Kong in 1970 (Mowat *et al.* 1972). The infection was termed SVD in 1972 when it was first recognized in the UK (Dawe *et al.* 1973).

The agent

Taxonomy and molecular biology

The causative agent of SVD is SVDV, which belongs to the Human enterovirus B serotype of the genus *Enterovirus* in the family *Picornaviridae*. SVDV is antigenically very closely related to the Human coxsackievirus B5 (CVB5), but can be distinguished by cross-neutralization and immunodiffusion tests (Brown *et al.* 1973; Brown *et al.* 1976). Comparison of nucleotide sequences of SVDV and CVB5 suggests that evolution of SVDV has involved adaptation of CVB5 to pigs, genetic recombination (Zhang *et al.* 1993). Human coxsackievirus A16 and SVDV have some common non-neutralizing epitopes (Marquardt and Ohlinger 1995). The antigenic sites of SVDV are similar to those of poliovirus (Kanno *et al.* 1995). Despite the antigenic variability between SVDV isolates, all strains of SVDV are thus far considered to remain in a single serotype (Zhang *et al.* 1999).

Enterovirus virions are 28–30 nm in diameter and they have a round shape with icosahedral symmetry. The genome is a linear positive-polarity single-stranded RNA of approximately 7.4 kilobases in length, and contains 5' and 3' noncoding regions, and an open reading framing encoding the polyprotein precursor to the structural (P1) and the non-structural (P2, P3) proteins. P1 is cleaved into four structural proteins VP1, VP2, VP3, and VP4, which form the protein capsid surrounding the genomic RNA. P2 and P3 are processed to form seven non-structural proteins. The section covering FMDV in this chapter discusses Picornavirus molecular biology in more detail.

Growth and survival

SVDV is stable over a wide range of pH and can remain viable in meat products for several months or even years. SVDV can be thermoinactivated at 56°C. In presence of organic matter, sodium hydroxide combined with detergent is an effective disinfectant. Oxidizing agents, iodophores, and acids can be used in the absence of organic matter.

Disease mechanisms

SVDV uses heparan sulphate as a receptor for its binding the cell surface (Escribano-Romero *et al.* 2004), followed by conformational changes exposing N-terminal portion of VP1 (Jiménez-Clavero *et al.* 2001). Evidence suggests that SVDV is internalized through clathrin-endocytosis and transported to early endosomes (Martín-Acebes *et al.* 2009). Attenuated SVDV strains have been isolated from asymptomatic pigs (Kodama *et al.* 1980), and comparison of pathogenic and attenuated strains have allowed mapping of the genetic determinants of SVDV pathogenicity. A genomic region associated with the pathogenicity of SVDV has been mapped to the region between nucleotides corresponding to the C-terminal of VP3, the whole of VP1, and the N-terminus of 2A (Kanno *et al.* 2001).

The hosts

Clinical: animals

Clinical infections caused by SVDV have only been seen in pigs. The disease manifests with a mild fever, lameness, and vesicles on the coronary band, the bulbs of the heel, skin of the limbs, and occasionally snout, lips, tongue, and teats. Recovery takes place usually within 2–3 weeks. The clinical manifestations may be more severe in young animals. SVDV infection is not fatal to pigs, but morbidity rates can be very high, up to 100% in individual pens. Subclinical SVDV infections do occur (Burrows *et al.* 1974; Lin and Kitching 2000). SVD can be clinically indistinguishable from FMD, which makes it economically important.

Clinical: humans

The incidence of human SVDV infection is difficult to estimate due to likely underreporting, as SVDV infection is easily misdiagnosed as CVB5 infection. There are only few reports of human SVDV infections in literature, including accidental infections in laboratory, confirmed with serology and immunodiffusion tests (Garland and Mann 1974; Brown *et al.* 1976).

Pathogenesis

Studies with animals show that SVDV can enter the body either through damaged skin or through mucous membranes by ingestion; the latter requires a larger amount of virus. SVDV replication occurs at the initial site of infection, followed by spread through the lymphatic system to the blood stream. Evidence suggests that the site of viral persistence takes place in the alimentary tract (Lin and Kitching 2000).

Incubation

The incubation period of SVD in pigs is 2–7 days, and when related to eating contaminated feed, usually 2–3 days. Incubation period in humans is not known.

Symptoms and signs

Due to lack of available reports in literature, only a rough idea of human SVDV infection can be provided. The clinical picture varies from influenza-like illness, vague malaise, abdominal pain, and muscle pain to aseptic meningitis (Garland and Mann 1974; Lin and Kitching 2000). No deaths have been reported. Asymptomatic infections do occur.

Pathology and diagnosis

SVDV has strong tropism for epithelial tissues, and seems to infect both epithelial cells and cells of the basal membrane and dermis (Mulder *et al.* 1997). Usually SVDV does not persist in tissues of infected animal for more than 14 days, and the clearance is even more rapid from oral and nasal secretions (up to 7 days), and faeces (up to 1–2 days) (Burrows *et al.* 1974; Lin *et al.* 1998). However, evidence suggests that animals can in rare cases become carriers of SVDV (Lin *et al.* 1998; Lin *et al.* 2001). Production of neutralizing antibodies usually coincides with the recovery phase.

ELISA, complement fixation test, and neutralization test can be used for serology (Heckert *et al.* 1998; Ko *et al.* 2005), and virus isolation in cell cultures, nucleic acid amplification methods (Blomström *et al.* 2008), and *in situ* hybridization (Mulder *et al.* 1997) for direct detection of SVDV. Virus isolation can be attempted from vesicular fluid or epithelium, whole blood, and faecal specimens. Cross-reactions with other porcine enteroviruses occur in serological tests.

Treatment and prognosis

No antiviral treatment is available for SVDV infection. Human infection is self-limited.

Epidemiology

Occurrence

Since its discovery in 1966, SVDV has been reported in Europe, Russia, and South-East Asia. During 1970s, 1980s and 1990s, SVDV infection was seen in the following countries: Austria, Belgium Bulgaria, France, Germany, Greece, Holland, Hong Kong, Italy, Japan, Malta, Poland, Portugal, Romania, Spain, Switzerland, Taiwan, United Kingdom, and Russia (Lin and Kitching 2000). During the past ten years, SVDV has been reported almost exclusively from Italy, with the exception of Portugal, where it reappeared in 2007 (Knowles *et al.* 2007).

Transmission in animals

SVDV is very stable in the environment, and therefore highly contagious. During the viremic period of SVDV infection, practically all tissues contain virus, including epithelium vesicular fluid and blood in the pig. Large quantities of virus are found in the secretions and faeces is a major source of virus shedding. SVDV spreads by contact with infected pigs or their excretions. Pigs can acquire infection also through contaminated feed, or even through contaminated transportation vehicles. Evidence suggests that contact with environment contaminated with SVDV is equally infectious as direct contact with an infected animal (Dekker *et al.* 1995). The onward transmission occurs through skin and mucosal lesions.

Transmission in humans

SVDV transmission in humans has not been investigated, but the most likely route of transmission is inhalation of aerosols from infected pigs or contamination of skin lesions.

Prevention and control

Control strategies

The sanitary prophylaxis measures advised by OIE include the following: strict quarantine; elimination of infected and contact pigs; prohibition of feeding with ship or aircraft garbage; thorough cooking of garbage; control of movement of pigs and vehicles used for transporting pigs; thorough disinfection of premises, transport vehicles, and equipment (http://www.oie.int/eng/maladies/fiches/a_a030.htm).

Vaccines

No vaccine is available for SVD.

References

Ahmad, S., Bassiri, M., Banerjee, A. K., and Yilma, T. (1993). Immunological characterization of the VSV nucleocapsid (N) protein expressed by recombinant baculovirus in Spodoptera exigua larva: use in differential diagnosis between vaccinated and infected animals. *Virol.*, **192**(1): 207–16.

Aldous, E. W., Alexander, D. J. (2008). Newcastle disease in pheasants (Phasianus colchicus): a review. *Vet. J.*, **175**(2): 181–85.

Alexander, D. J., Manvell, R. J., Frost, K. M., *et al.* (1997). Newcastle disease outbreak in pheasants in Great Britain in May 1996. *Vet. Rec.,* **140**(1): 20–22.

Alexandersen, S., Oleksiewicz, M. B., and Donaldson, A. I. (2001). The early pathogenesis of foot-and-mouth disease in pigs infected by contact: a quantitative time-course study using TaqMan RT-PCR. *J. Gen. Virol.,* **82**(4): 747–55.

Alexandersen, S. and Donaldson, A. I. (2002a). Further studies to quantify the dose of natural aerosols of foot-and-mouth disease virus for pigs. *Epidemiol. Infect.,* **128**(2): 313–23.

Alexandersen, S., Zhang, Z., and Donaldson, A. I. (2002b). Aspects of the persistence of foot-and-mouth disease virus in animals—the carrier problem. *Microbes Infect.,* **4**(10): 1099–110.

Alexandersen, S., Zhang, Z., Reid, S. M., Hutchings, G. H. and Donaldson, A. I. (2002c). Quantities of infectious virus and viral RNA recovered from sheep and cattle experimentally infected with foot-and-mouth disease virus O UK 2001. *J. Gen. Virol.,* **83**: 1915–23.

Alexandersen, S., Quan, M., Murphy, C., Knight, J., and Zhang, Z. (2003a). Studies of quantitative parameters of virus excretion and transmission in pigs and cattle experimentally infected with foot-and-mouth disease virus. *J. Comp. Pathol.,* **129**(4): 268–82.

Alexandersen, S., Zhang, Z., Donaldson, A. I., and Garland, A. J. (2003b). The pathogenesis and diagnosis of foot-and-mouth disease. *J. Comp. Pathol.,* **129**(1): 1–36.

Al-Hilly, J. N., Khalil, H. H., Zakoo, F. I., and Hamid, A. A. (1980). An outbreak of Newcastle disease in a pheasant flock in Iraq. *Avian Pathol.,* **9**(4): 583–85.

Allan, W. H., Lancaster, J. E. and Toth, B. (1978). Newcastle disease vaccines, their production and use. Chapter 11: 93–102. In: Vaccination Programmes. Rome: Food and Agricultural Organization of the United Nations.

Armstrong, R., Davie, J., and Hedger, R. S. (1967). Foot-and-mouth disease in man. *BMJ,* **4**(5578): 529–30.

Awan, M. A., Otte, M. J., and James, A. D. (1994). The epidemiology of Newcastle disease in rural poultry: a review. *Avian Pathol.,* **23**(3): 405–23

Barr, J. N., Whelan, S. P., and Wertz, G. W. (2002). Transcriptional control of the RNA-dependent RNA polymerase of vesicular stomatitis virus. *Biochem. Biophys. Acta.,* **1577**(2): 337–53.

Bauer, K. (1997). Foot-and-mouth disease as zoonosis. *Arch. Virol. Suppl.,***13**: 95–97.

Baxt, B., and Bachrach, H. L. (1980). Early interactions of foot-and-mouth disease virus with cultured cells. *Virol.,* **104**(1): 42–55.

Blomström, A. L., Hakhverdyan, M., Reid, S. M., *et al.* (2008). A one-step reverse transcriptase loop-mediated isothermal amplification assay for simple and rapid detection of swine vesicular disease virus. *J. Virol. Meth.,***147**(1): 188–93.

Borland, E. D. (1972). Newcastle disease in pheasants, partridges and wild birds in East Anglia, 1970–1971. *Vet. Rec.,* **90**(17): 481–82

Brandly, C. A. (1964). The occupational hazard of Newcastle disease to man. *Lab. Anim. Care.,* **14**: 433–40.

Brody, J. A., Fischer, G. F., and Peralta, P. H. (1967). Vesicular stomatitis virus in Panama. Human serologic patterns in a cattle raising area. *Am. J. Epidemiol.,* **86**(1): 158–61.

Brown, C. C., Olander, H. J., and Meyer, R. F. (1995). Pathogenesis of foot-and-mouth disease in swine, studied by in-situ hybridization. *J. Comp. Pathol.,* **113**(1): 51–58.

Brown, C. C., Piccone, M. E., Mason, P. W., *et al.* (1996). Pathogenesis of wild-type and leaderless foot-and-mouth disease virus in cattle. *J. Virol.,* **70**(8): 5638–41.

Brown, F., Goodridge, D., and Burrows, R. (1976). Infection of man by swine vesicular disease virus. *J. Comp. Pathol.,* **86**(3): 409–14.

Brown, F., Talbot, P., and Burrows, R. (1973). Antigenic differences between isolates of swine vesicular disease virus and their relationship to Coxsackie B5 virus. *Nature,* **245**(5424): 315–16.

Brown, F., Wild, T. F., Rowe, L. W., Underwood, B. O., and Harris, T. J. (1976). Comparison of swine vesicular disease virus and Coxsackie B5 virus by serological and RNA hybridization methods. *J. Gen. Virol.,* **31**(2): 231–37.

Bründler, M. A., Aichele, P., Bachmann, M., *et al.* (1996). Immunity to viruses in B cell-deficient mice: influence of antibodies on virus persistence and on T cell memory. *Eur. J. Immunol.,* **26**(9): 2257–62.

Burrows, R., Mann, J. A., and Goodridge, D. (1974). Swine vesicular disease: comparative studies of viruses isolated from different countries. *J. Hyg. (Lond).,* **73**(1): 109–17.

Burton, A. C. (1917). Stomatitis contagiosa in horses. *Vet. J.,* **73**: 234–37.

Chadha, M. S., Arankalle, V. A., Jadi, R. S., Joshi, M. V., *et al.* (2005). An outbreak of Chandipura virus encephalitis in the eastern districts of Gujarat state, India. *Am. J. Trop. Med. Hyg.,* **73**(3): 566–70.

Chen, J. P., Wang, C. H. (2002). Clinical epidemiologic and experimental evidence for the transmission of Newcastle disease virus through eggs. *Avian Dis.,* **46**(2): 461–65.

Comer, J. A., Kavanaugh, D. M., Stallknecht, D. E., and Corn, J. L. (1994). Population dynamics of Lutzomyia shannoni (Diptera: Psychodidae) in relation to the epizootiology of vesicular stomatitis virus on Ossabaw Island, Georgia. *J. Med. Entomol.,* **31**(6): 850–54.

Dardiri, A. H., Yates, V. J., and Flanagan, T. D. (1962). The reaction to infection with the B1 strain of Newcastle disease virus in man. *Am. J. Vet. Res.,* **23**: 918–21.

Dawe, P. S., Forman, A. J., and Smale, C. J. (1973). A preliminary investigation of the swine vesicular disease epidemic in Britain. *Nature,* **241**(5391): 540–42.

de la Torre, J. C., Dávila, M., Sobrino, F., Ortín, J., and Domingo, E. (1985). Establishment of cell lines persistently infected with foot-and-mouth disease virus. *Virol.,* **145**(1): 24–35.

de Leeuw, O. S., Koch, G., Hartog, L., Ravenshorst, N., and Peeters, B. P. (2005). Virulence of Newcastle disease virus is determined by the cleavage site of the fusion protein and by both the stem region and globular head of the haemagglutinin-neuraminidase protein. *J. Gen. Virol.,* **86**(6): 1759–69.

de Leeuw, O., Peeters, B. (1999). Complete nucleotide sequence of Newcastle disease virus: evidence for the existence of a new genus within the subfamily Paramyxovirinae. *J. Gen. Virol.,* **80**(1): 131–36.

Dekker, A., Moonen, P., de Boer-Luijtze, E. A., and Terpstra, C. (1995). Pathogenesis of swine vesicular disease after exposure of pigs to an infected environment. *Vet. Microbiol.,* **45**(2–3): 243–50.

Dlugosz, H. (1968). Foot-and-mouth disease in man. BMJ, **1**(5586): 251–52.

Domingo, E., Escarmís, C., Baranowski, E., *et al.* (2003). Evolution of foot-and-mouth disease virus. *Virus Res.,* **91**(1): 47–63.

Donaldson, A. I., Alexandersen, S., Sorensen, J. H. and Mikkelsen, T. (2001). The relative risks of the uncontrollable (airborne) spread of foot-and-mouth disease by different species. *Vet. Rec.,* **148**(19): 602–04.

Doyle, T. M. (1927). A hitherto unrecorded disease of fowls due to a filter passing virus. *J. Comp. Pathol.,* **40**: 144–69.

Eckert, D. M., and Kim, P. S. (2001). Mechanisms of viral membrane fusion and its inhibition. *Annu. Rev. Biochem.,* **70**: 777–810.

Elankumaran, S., Rockemann, D., and Samal, S. K. (2006). Newcastle disease virus exerts oncolysis by both intrinsic and extrinsic caspase-dependent pathways of cell death. *J. Virol.,* **80**(15): 7522–34.

Escribano-Romero, E., Jimenez-Clavero, M. A., Gomes, P., *et al.* (2004). Heparan sulphate mediates swine vesicular disease virus attachment to the host cell. *J. Gen. Virol.,* **85**(3): 653–63.

Evans, A. S. (1955). Pathogenicity and immunology of Newcastle disease virus (NVD) in man. *Am. J. Pub. Heal. Nat. Heal.,* **45**(6): 742–45.

Fernández, J., Agüero, M., Romero, L., *et al.* (2008). Rapid and differential diagnosis of foot-and-mouth disease, swine vesicular disease, and vesicular stomatitis by a new multiplex RT-PCR assay. *J. Virol. Meth.,* **147**(2): 301–11.

Fields, B. N., and Hawkins, K. (1967). Human infection with the virus of vesicular stomatitis during an epizootic. *N. Engl. J. Med.,* **277**(19): 989–94.

Garland, A. J. M. and Donaldson, A. I. (1990). Foot-and-mouth disease. *Surveill.,* **17:** 6–8.

Garland, A. J., and Mann, J. A. (1974). Attempts to infect pigs with Coxsackie virus type B5. *J. Hyg.,* **73:** 85–96.

Geleta, J. N., and Holbrook, A. A. (1961). Vesicular stomatitis—patterns of complement-fixing and serum-neutralizing antibodies in serum of convalescent cattle and horses. *Am. J. Vet. Res.,* **22:** 713–19.

Goris, N., Vandenbussche, F., Herr, C., *et al.* (2009). Validation of two real-time RT-PCR methods for foot-and-mouth disease diagnosis: RNA-extraction, matrix effect, uncertainty of measurement and precision. *J. Virol. Meth.,* **160**(1–2): 157–62.

Guan, J., Chan, M., Grenier, C., *et al.* (2009). Survival of avian influenza and Newcastle disease viruses in compost and at ambient temperatures based on virus isolation and real-time reverse transcriptase PCR. *Avian Dis.,* **53**(1): 26–33.

Hales, R. H., and Ostler, H. B. (1973). Newcastle disease conjunctivitis with subepithelial infiltrates. *Br. J. Ophthalmol.,* **57**(9): 694–97.

Hanson, R. P. (1952). The natural history of vesicular stomatitis. *Bacteriol. Rev.,* **16**(3): 179–204.

Hanson, R. P., Rasmussen, A. F., Brandly, C. A., and Brown, J. W. (1950). Human infection with the virus of vesicular stomatitis. *J. Lab. Clin. Med.,* **36**(5): 754–58.

Heckert, R. A., Brocchi, E., Berlinzani, A., and Mackay, D. K. (1998). An international comparative analysis of a competitive ELISA for the detection of antibodies to swine vesicular disease virus. *J. Vet. Diag. Invest.,* **10**(3): 295–97.

Heckert, R. A., and Nagy, E. (1999). Evaluation of the hemagglutination-inhibition assay using a baculovirus-expressed hemagglutinin-neuraminidase protein for detection of Newcastle disease virus antibodies. *J. Vet. Diag. Invest.,* **11**(1): 99–102.

Her, L. S., Lund, E., and Dahlberg, J. E. (1997). Inhibition of Ran guanosine triphosphatase-dependent nuclear transport by the matrix protein of vesicular stomatitis virus. *Sci.,* **276**(5320): 1845–48.

Hertwig, C. A. (1834). Übertragung tierischer Ansteckungsstoffe auf den Menschen. *Med. Vet. Z.,* **1834:** 48.

Howerth, E. W., Stallknecht, D. E., Dorminy, M., Pisell, T., and Clarke, G. R. (1997). Experimental vesicular stomatitis in swine: effects of route of inoculation and steroid treatment. *J. Vet. Diag. Invest.,* **9**(2): 136–42.

Huang, Z., Krishnamurthy, S., Panda, A., and Samal, S. K. (2003). Newcastle disease virus V protein is associated with viral pathogenesis and functions as an alpha interferon antagonist. *J. Virol.,* **77**(16): 8676–85.

Huang, Z., Panda, A., Elankumaran, S., Govindarajan, D., Rockemann, D. D., and Samal, S. K. (2004). The hemagglutinin-neuraminidase protein of Newcastle disease virus determines tropism and virulence. *J. Virol.,* **78**(8): 4176–84.

Hutber, A. M., Kitching, R. P., Fishwick, J. C., and Bires, J. (2010). Foot-and-mouth disease: The question of implementing vaccinal control during an epidemic. *Vet. J.,* [Epub ahead of print].

Hyslop, N. S. G. (1973). Transmission of the virus of foot and mouth disease between animals and man. *Bull. World Heal. Organ.,* **49**(6): 577–85.

Jackson, T. F. M., Ellard, R. A., Ghazaleh, S. M., *et al.* (1996). Efficient infection of cells in culture by type O foot-and-mouth disease virus requires binding to cell surface heparan sulfate. *J. Virol.,* **70**(8): 5282–87.

Jiménez-Clavero, M. A., Escribano-Romero, E., Douglas, A. J., and Ley, V. (2001). The N-terminal region of the VP1 protein of swine vesicular disease virus contains a neutralization site that arises upon cell attachment and is involved in viral entry. *J. Virol.,* **75**(2): 1044–47.

Kanno, T., Inoue, T., Wang, Y., Sarai, A., and Yamaguchi, S. (1995). Identification of the location of antigenic sites of swine vesicular

disease virus with neutralization-resistant mutants. *J. Gen. Virol.,* **76**(12): 3099–106.

Kanno, T., Mackay, D., Wilsden, G., and Kitching, P. (2001). Virulence of swine vesicular disease virus is determined at two amino acids in capsid protein VP1 and 2A protease. *Virus Res.,* **80**(1–2): 101–7.

Kapczynski, D. R., and King, D. J. (2005). Protection of chickens against overt clinical disease and determination of viral shedding following vaccination with commercially available Newcastle disease virus vaccines upon challenge with highly virulent virus from the California 2002 exotic Newcastle disease outbreak. *Vaccine,* **23**(26): 3424–33.

Katz, J. B., Shafer, A. L., and Eernisse, K. A. (1995). Construction and insect larval expression of recombinant vesicular stomatitis nucleocapsid protein and its use in competitive ELISA. *J. Virol. Meth.,* **54**(2–3): 145–57.

King, D. J. (1985). Virus isolation from tracheal explant cultures and oropharyngeal swabs in attempts to detect persistent Newcastle disease virus infections in chickens. *Avian Dis.,* **29**(2): 297–311.

Knowles, N. J., Davies, P. R., Henry, T., *et al.* (2001a). Emergence in Asia of foot-and-mouth disease viruses with altered host range: characterization of alterations in the 3A protein. *J. Virol.,* **75**(3): 1551–56.

Knowles, N. J., Samuel, A. R., Davies, P. R., Kitching, R. P. and Donaldson, A. I. (2001b). Outbreak of foot-and-mouth disease virus serotype O in the UK caused by a pandemic strain. *Vet. Rec.,* **148**(9): 258–59.

Knowles, N. J., Samuel, A. R., Davies, P. R., Midgley, R. J., and Valarcher, J. F. (2005). Pandemic strain of foot-and-mouth disease virus serotype O. *Emerg. Infect. Dis.,* **11**(12): 1887–93.

Knowles, N. J., Wilsden, G., Reid, S. M., Ferris, N. P., *et al.* (2007). Reappearance of swine vesicular disease virus in Portugal. *Vet. Rec.,* **161**(2): 71.

Ko, Y. J., Choi, K. S., Nah, J. J., *et al.* (2005). Noninfectious virus-like particle antigen for detection of swine vesicular disease virus antibodies in pigs by enzyme-linked immunosorbent assay. *Clin. Diag. Lab. Immunol.,* **12**(8): 922–29.

Ko, Y. J., Lee, H. S., Jeoung, H. Y., Heo, E. J., Ko, H. R., *et al.* (2010). Use of a baculovirus-expressed structural protein for the detection of antibodies to foot-and-mouth disease virus type A by a blocking enzyme-linked immunosorbent assay. *Clin. Vaccine. Immunol.,* **17**(1): 194–98. Epub 2009 Nov 4.

Kodama, M., Saito, T., Ogawa, T., Tokuda, G., *et al.* (1980). Swine vesicular disease viruses isolated from healthy pigs in non-epizootic period. II. Vesicular formation and virus multiplication in experimentally inoculated pigs. *Natl. Inst. Anim. Heal. Q (Tokyo).,* **20**(4): 123–30.

Komatsu, T., Bi, Z., and Reiss, C. S. (1996). Interferon-gamma induced type I nitric oxide synthase activity inhibits viral replication in neurons. *J. Neuroimmunol.,* **68**(1–2): 101–8.

Kommers, G. D., King, D. J., Seal, B. S, and Brown, C. C. (2003). Pathogenesis of chicken-passaged Newcastle disease viruses isolated from chickens and wild and exotic birds. *Avian Dis.,* **47**(2): 319–29.

Koyama, A. H. (1995). Induction of apoptotic DNA fragmentation by the infection of vesicular stomatitis virus. *Virus Res.,* **37**(3): 285–90.

Kraneveld, F. C. (1926). A poultry disease in the Dutch East Indies. *Ned. Indisch. Bl. Diergeneeskd.,* **38:** 448–50.

Lee, H. S., Heo, E. J., Jeoung, H. Y., Ko, H. R., *et al.* (2009). Enzyme-linked immunosorbent assay using glycoprotein and monoclonal antibody for detecting antibodies to vesicular stomatitis virus serotype New Jersey. *Clin. Vaccine Immunol.,* **16**(5): 667–71.

Lefrancois, L. (1984). Protection against lethal viral infection by neutralizing and nonneutralizing monoclonal antibodies: distinct mechanisms of action in vivo. *J. Virol.,* **51**(1): 208–14.

Lefrancois, L., and Lyles, D. (1982). The interaction of antibody with the major surface glycoprotein of vesicular stomatitis virus. I. Analysis of neutralizing epitopes with monoclonal antibodies. *Virol.,* **121**(1): 157–67.

Letchworth, G. J., Rodriguez, L. L., Del, C., and Barrera, J. (1999). Vesicular stomatitis. *Vet. J.,* **157**(3): 239–60

Lin, F., and Kitching, R.P. (2000). Swine vesicular disease: an overview. *Vet. J.*, **160**(3): 192–201.

Lin, F., Mackay, D. K., and Knowles, N. J. (1998). The persistence of swine vesicular disease virus infection in pigs. *Epidemiol. Infect.*, **121**(2): 459–72.

Lin, F., Mackay, D. K., Knowles, N. J, and Kitching, R. P. (2001). Persistent infection is a rare sequel following infection of pigs with swine vesicular disease virus. *Epidemiol. Infect.*, **127**(1): 135–45.

Li, X., Chai, T., Wang, Z., Song, C., *et al.* (2009). Occurrence and transmission of Newcastle disease virus aerosol originating from infected chickens under experimental conditions. *Vet. Microbiol.*, **136**(3–4): 226–32.

Lyles, D. S., McKenzie, M. O. (1997). Activity of vesicular stomatitis virus M protein mutants in cell rounding is correlated with the ability to inhibit host gene expression and is not correlated with virus assembly function. *Virol.*, **229**(1): 77–89.

Marquardt, O., and Ohlinger, V. F. (1995). Differential diagnosis and genetic analysis of the antigenically related swine vesicular disease virus and coxsackie viruses. *J. Virol. Meth.*, **53**(2–3): 189–99.

Martín-Acebes, M. A., González-Magaldi, M., Vázquez-Calvo, A., Armas-Portela, R., Sobrino, F. (2009). Internalization of swine vesicular disease virus into cultured cells: a comparative study with foot-and-mouth disease virus. *J. Virol.*, **83**(9): 4216–26.

Martinez, I., Rodriguez, L. L., Jimenez, C., Pauszek, S. J., and Wertz, G. W. (2003). Vesicular stomatitis virus glycoprotein is a determinant of pathogenesis in swine, a natural host. *J. Virol.*, **77**(14): 8039–47.

Mason, P. W., Piccone, M. E., Mckenna, T. S., Chinsangaram, J., and Grubman, M. J. (1997). Evaluation of a live-attenuated foot-and-mouth disease virus as a vaccine candidate. *Virol.*, **227**(1): 96–102.

Matlin, K. S., Reggio, H., Helenius, A., and Simons, K. (1982). Pathway of vesicular stomatitis virus entry leading to infection. *J. Mol. Biol.*, **156**(3): 609–31.

McMinn, P. C. (2002). An overview of the evolution of enterovirus 71 and its clinical and public health significance. *FEMS Microbiol. Rev.*, **26**(1): 91–107.

Michalski, F., Parks, N. F., Sokol, F., and Clark, H. F. (1976). Thermal inactivation of rabies and other rhabdoviruses: stabilization by the chelating agent ethylenediaminetetraacetic acid at physiological temperatures. *Infect. Immun.*, **14**(1): 135–43.

Miller, P. J., Decanini, E. L., and Afonso, C. L. (2010). Newcastle disease: evolution of genotypes and the related diagnostic challenges. *Infect. Genet. Evol.*, **10**(1): 26–35.

Mohan, C. M., Dey, S., Rai, A., and Kataria, J. M. (2006). Recombinant haemagglutinin neuraminidase antigen-based single serum dilution ELISA for rapid serological profiling of Newcastle disease virus. *J. Virol. Meth.*,**138**(1–2): 117–22.

Moraes, M. P., Mayr, G. A., Mason, P. W., and Grubman, M. J. (2002). Early protection against homologous challenge after a single dose of replication-defective human adenovirus type 5 expressing capsid proteins of foot-and-mouth disease virus (FMDV) strain A24. *Vaccine*, **20**: 1631–39.

Morioka, K., Fukai, K., Yoshida, K., *et al.* (2009). Foot-and-mouth disease virus antigen detection enzyme-linked immunosorbent assay using multiserotype-reactive monoclonal antibodies. *J. Clin. Microbiol.*, **47**(11): 3663–68.

Mowat, G. N., Darbyshire, J. H., and Huntley, J. F. (1972). Differentiation of a vesicular disease of pigs in Hong Kong from foot-and-mouth disease. *Vet. Rec.*, **90**(22): 618–21.

Mulder, W. A., van Poelwijk, F., Moormann, R. J., *et al.* (1997). Detection of early infection of swine vesicular disease virus in porcine cells and skin sections. A comparison of immunohistochemistry and in-situ hybridization. *J. Virol. Methods.*, **68**(2): 169–75.

Muller, J. D., Wilkins, M., Foord, A. J., *et al.* (2010). Improvement of a recombinant antibody-based serological assay for foot-and-mouth disease virus. *J. Immunol. Methods*, **352**(1–2): 81–88.

Nakamura, K., Ohta, Y., Abe, Y., Imai, K., and Yamada, M. (2004). Pathogenesis of conjunctivitis caused by Newcastle disease viruses in specific-pathogen-free chickens. *Avian Pathol.*, **33**(3): 371–76.

Nakamura, K., Ohtsu, N., Nakamura, T., Yamamoto, Y., *et al.* (2008). Pathologic and immunohistochemical studies of Newcastle disease (ND) in broiler chickens vaccinated with ND: severe nonpurulent encephalitis and necrotizing pancreatitis. *Vet. Pathol.*, **45**(6): 928–33.

Nardelli, L., Lodetti, E., Gualandi, G. L., *et al.* (1968). A foot and mouth disease syndrome in pigs caused by an enterovirus. *Nature*, **219**(5160): 1275–76.

Nelson, C. B., Pomeroy, B. S., Schrall, K., Park, W. E., and Lindeman, R. J. (1952). An outbreak of conjunctivitis due to Newcastle disease virus (NDV) occurring in poultry workers. *Am. J. Pub. Heal. Nat. Heal.*, **42**(6): 672–78.

O'Brien, C. M. (1913). Foot and mouth disease in man: Aphthous fever. *Trans. R. Acad. Med. Irel.*, **31**: 31–37.

Oem, J. K., Ferris, N. P., Lee, K. N., Joo, Y. S., Hyun, B. H., and Park, J. H. (2009). Simple and rapid lateral-flow assay for the detection of foot-and-mouth disease virus. *Clin. Vaccine Immunol.*, **16**(11): 1660–64. Epub 2009 Sep 2.

Pacheco, J. M., Henry, T. M., O'Donnell, V. K., *et al.* (2003). Role of nonstructural proteins 3A and 3B in host range and pathogenicity of foot-and-mouth disease virus. *J. Virol.*, **77**(24): 13017–27.

Patterson, W. C., Mott, L. O., and Jenney, E. W. (1958). A study of vesicular stomatitis in man. *J. Am. Vet. Med. Assoc.*, **133**(1): 57–62.

Patnayak, D. P., Prasad, A. M., Malik, Y. S., *et al.* (2008). Efficacy of disinfectants and hand sanitizers against avian respiratory viruses. *Avian Dis.*, **52**(2): 199–202.

Piacenti, A. M., King, D. J., Seal, B. S., Zhang, J., and Brown, C. C. (2006). Pathogenesis of Newcastle disease in commercial and specific pathogen-free turkeys experimentally infected with isolates of different virulence. *Vet. Pathol.*, **43**(2): 168–78.

Porter, A. G. (1993). Picornavirus nonstructural proteins: emerging roles in virus replication and inhibition of host cell functions. *J. Virol.*, **67**(12): 6917–21.

Powell, J. A., Kano, K., and Milgrom, F. (1985). Antibodies to Newcastle disease virus in various human diseases. *Int. Arch. Allergy Appl. Immunol.*, **76**(4): 331–35.

Prempeh, H., Smith, R., and Müller, B. (2001). Foot and mouth disease: the human consequences. The health consequences are slight, the economic ones huge. *BMJ*, **322**(7286): 565–66.

Quinn, R. W., Hanson, R. P., Brown, J. W., and Brandly, C. A. (1952). Newcastle disease virus in man; results of studies in five cases. *J. Lab. Clin. Med.*, **40**(5): 736–43.

Quiroz, E., Moreno, N., Peralta, P. H., and Tesh, R. B. (1988). A human case of encephalitis associated with vesicular stomatitis virus (Indiana serotype) infection. *Am. J. Trop. Med. Hyg.*, **39**(3): 312–14.

Ravindra, P. V., Tiwari, A. K., Ratta, B., Chaturvedi, U., *et al.* (2009). Newcastle disease virus-induced cytopathic effect in infected cells is caused by apoptosis. *Virus Res.*, **141**(1): 13–20.

Reagan, R. L., Chang, S. C., Yancey, F. S., and Brueckner, A. L. (1956). Isolation of Newcastle disease virus from man with confirmation by electron microscopy. *J. Am. Vet. Med. Assoc.*, **129**(2): 79–80.

Reif, J. S., Webb, P. A., Monath, T. P., *et al.* (1987). Epizootic vesicular stomatitis in Colorado, 1982: infection in occupational risk groups. *Am. J. Trop. Med. Hyg.*, **36**(1): 177–82.

Richardson, J., Slemons, R., Swayne, D. E., Kapczynski, D. R., *et al.* (2005). Exotic Newcastle disease conjunctivitis in a veterinary student (abstract). Proc. N. Cent. Avian Dis. Confer., pp. 62–63.

Rodrigues, J. J., Singh, P. B., Dave, D. S., *et al.* (1983). Isolation of Chandipura virus from the blood in acute encephalopathy syndrome. *Indian J. Med. Res.,* **77**: 303–7.

Rodriguez, L. L. (2002). Emergence and re-emergence of vesicular stomatitis in the United States. *Virus Res.,* **85**(2): 211–19.

Rodriguez, L. L., Barrera, J., Kramer, E., Lubroth, J., Brown, F., and Golde, W. T. (2003). A synthetic peptide containing the consensus sequence of the G–H loop region of foot-and-mouth disease virus type-O VP1 and a promiscuous T-helper epitope induces peptide-specific antibodies but fails to protect cattle against viral challenge. *Vaccine,* **21**(25–26): 3751–56.

Rodriguez, L. L., and Grubman, M. J. (2009). Foot and mouth disease virus vaccines. *Vaccine,* 27, Suppl **4**: D90–94.

Rodriguez, L. L., Vernon, S., Morales, A. I., and Letchworth, G. J. (1990). Serological monitoring of vesicular stomatitis New Jersey virus in enzootic regions of Costa Rica. *Am. J. Trop. Med. Hyg.,* **42**(3): 272–81.

Salt, J. S., Mulcahy, G., and Kitching, R. P. (1996). Isotype-specific antibody responses to foot-and-mouth disease virus in sera and secretions of 'carrier' and 'non-carrier' cattle. *Epidemiol. Infect.,* **117**(2): 349–60.

Scherer, C. F., O'Donnell, V., Golde, W. T., Gregg, D., Estes, D. M., and Rodriguez, L. L. (2007). Vesicular stomatitis New Jersey virus (VSNJV) infects keratinocytes and is restricted to lesion sites and local lymph nodes in the bovine, a natural host. *Vet. Res.,* **38**(3): 375–90.

Sellers, R. F., and Parker, J. J. (1969). Airborne excretion of foot-and-mouth disease virus. *J. Hyg. (Lond.),* **67**(4): 671–77.

Sellers, R. F., Donaldson, A. I, and Herniman, K. A. (1970). Inhalation, persistence and dispersal of foot-and-mouth disease virus by man. *J. Hyg. (Lond.),* **68**(4): 565–73.

Sellers, R. F. and Forman, A. J. (1973). The Hampshire epidemic of foot-and-mouth disease, 1967. *J. Hyg. (Lond.),* **71**(1): 15–34.

Senne, D. A., King, D. J. and Kapczynski, D. R. (2004). Control of Newcastle disease by vaccination. *Dev. Biol.,* **119**: 165–70.

Stallknecht, D. E., Greer, J. B., Murphy, M. D., *et al.* (2004). Effect of strain and serotype of vesicular stomatitis virus on viral shedding, vesicular lesion development, and contact transmission in pigs. *Am. J. Vet. Res.,* **65**(9): 1233–39.

Steward, M., Vipond, I. B., Millar, N. S., and Emmerson, P. T. (1993). RNA editing in Newcastle disease virus. *J. Gen. Virol.,* **74** (12): 2539–47.

Sutmoller, P. and Gaggero, A. (1965). Foot-and-mouth diseases carriers. *Vet. Rec.,* **77**: 968–69.

Taboga, O., Tami, C., Carrillo, E., *et al.* (1997). A largescale evaluation of peptide vaccines against foot-and-mouth disease: lack of solid protection in cattle and isolation of escape mutants. *J. Virol.,* **71**(4): 2606–14.

Tan, S. W., Ideris, A., Omar, A. R., Yusoff, K., and Hair-Bejo, M. (2009). Detection and differentiation of velogenic and lentogenic Newcastle disease viruses using SYBR Green I real-time PCR with nucleocapsid gene-specific primers. *J. Virol. Meth.,* **160**(1–2): 149–56.

Teidebold, T. C., Mather, C. S., and Merrillat, L. A. (1916). Gangrenous glossitis of horses. *Rep. 20th Ann. Meet. US Livestock Sanit. Assoc.,* 29–42.

Tesh, R. B., Peralta, P. H., and Johnson, K. M. (1969). Ecologic studies of vesicular stomatitis virus. I. Prevalence of infection among animals and humans living in an area of endemic VSV activity. *Am. J. Epidemiol.,* **90**(3): 255–61.

Tesh, R. B., Boshell, J., Modi, G. B., Morales, A., *et al.* (1987). Natural infection of humans, animals, and phlebotomine sand flies with the Alagoas serotype of vesicular stomatitis virus in Colombia. *Am. J. Trop. Med. Hyg.,* **36**(3): 653–61.

Tesh, R. B., Chaniotis, B. N., and Johnson, K. M. (1971). Vesicular stomatitis virus, Indiana serotype: multiplication in and transmission by experimentally infected phlebotomine sandflies (Lutzomyia trapidoi). *Am. J. Epidemiol.,* **93**(6): 491–95.

Theiler, S. (1901). Eine contagi6se Stomatitis de Pferds in Sud-Afrika. *Deut. Tierarztl. Wochschr.,* **9**: 131–32.

Vanleeuwen, J. A., Rodriguez, L. L., and Waltner-Toews, D. (1995). Cow, farm, and ecologic risk factors of clinical vesicular stomatitis on Costa Rican dairy farms. *Am. J. Trop. Med. Hyg.,* **53**(4): 342–50.

Wakamatsu, N., King, D. J., Kapczynski, D. R., Seal, B. S., and Brown, C. C. (2006). Experimental pathogenesis for chickens, turkeys, and pigeons of exotic Newcastle disease virus from an outbreak in California during 2002–2003. *Vet. Pathol.,* **43**(6): 925–33.

Weaver, S. C., Tesh, R. B., and Guzman, H. (1992). Ultrastructural aspects of replication of the New Jersey serotype of vesicular stomatitis virus in a suspected sand fly vector, Lutzomyia shannoni (Diptera: Psychodidae). *Am. J. Trop. Med. Hyg.,* **46**(2): 201–10.

Webb, P. A., McLean, R. G., Smith, G. C., *et al.* (1987). Epizootic vesicular stomatitis in Colorado, 1982: some observations on the possible role of wildlife populations in an enzootic maintenance cycle. *J. Wildl. Dis.,* **23**(2): 192–98.

Webb, P. A., Monath, T. P., Reif, J. S., *et al.* (1987). Epizootic vesicular stomatitis in Colorado, 1982: epidemiologic studies along the northern Colorado front range. *Am. J. Trop. Med. Hyg.,* **36**(1): 183–88.

Yan, Y., Samal, S. K. (2008). Role of intergenic sequences in newcastle disease virus RNA transcription and pathogenesis. *J. Virol.,* **82**(3): 1323–31.

Zhang, G., Haydon, D. T., Knowles, N. J., and McCauley, J. W. (1999). Molecular evolution of swine vesicular disease virus. *J. Gen. Virol.,* **80** (3): 639–51.

Zhang, Z. D. and Kitching, R. P. (2001). The localization of persistent foot and mouth disease virus in the epithelial cells of the soft palate and pharynx. *J. Comp. Path.,* **124**(2–3): 89–94.

Zhang, G., Wilsden, G., Knowles, N. J., and McCauley, J. W. (1993). Complete nucleotide sequence of a coxsackie B5 virus and its relationship to swine vesicular disease virus. *J. Gen. Virol.,* **74**(5): 845–53.

CHAPTER 28

Hantaviruses

Antti Vaheri, James N. Mills, Christina F. Spiropoulou and Brian Hjelle

Summary

Hantaviruses (genus *Hantavirus*, family *Bunyaviridae*) are rodent- and insectivore-borne zoonotic viruses. Several hantaviruses are human pathogens, some with 10–35% mortality, and cause two diseases: haemorrhagic fever with renal syndrome (HFRS) in Eurasia, and hantavirus cardiopulmonary syndrome (HCPS) in the Americas. Hantaviruses are enveloped and have a three-segmented, single-stranded, negative-sense RNA genome. The L gene encodes an RNA-dependent RNA polymerase, the M gene encodes two glycoproteins (Gn and Gc), and the S gene encodes a nucleocapsid protein. In addition, the S genes of some hantaviruses have an NSs open reading frame that can act as an interferon antagonist. Similarities between phylogenies have suggested ancient codivergence of the viruses and their hosts to many authors, but increasing evidence for frequent, recent host switching and local adaptation has led to questioning of this model. Infected rodents establish persistent infections with little or no effect on the host. Humans are infected from aerosols of rodent excreta, direct contact of broken skin or mucous membranes with infectious virus, or rodent bite. One hantavirus, Andes virus, is unique in that it is known to be transmitted from person-to-person. HFRS and HCPS, although primarily affecting kidneys and lungs, respectively, share a number of clinical features, such as capillary leakage, TNF-α, and thrombocytopenia; notably, haemorrhages and alterations in renal function also occur in HCPS and cardiac and pulmonary involvement are not rare in HFRS. Of the four structural proteins, both in humoral and cellular immunity, the nucleocapsid protein appears to be the principal immunogen. Cytotoxic T-lymphocyte responses are seen in both HFRS and HCPS and may be important for both protective immunity and pathogenesis. Diagnosis is mainly based on detection of IgM antibodies although viral RNA (vRNA) may be readily, although not invariably, detected in blood, urine and saliva. For sero/genotyping neutralization tests/RNA sequencing are required. Formalin-inactivated vaccines have been widely used in China and Korea but not outside Asia. Hantaviruses are prime examples of emerging and re-emerging infections and, given the limited number of rodents and insectivores thus far studied, it is likely that many new hantaviruses will be detected in the near future.

History and introduction

The earliest description of a disease closely resembling haemorrhagic fever with renal syndrome (HFRS) dates back to 960 AD from the Chinese medical guide Whang-Jae-Nae-Kyung (Lee 1982). However, it was nearly 1000 years before the next descriptions of the disease were written, in 1913 in hospital records in far east Russia. HFRS has been more generally known since 1932 as nephroso-nephritis by Russians and as Songo fever by Japanese military physicians. In Europe mild HFRS-like disease was reported in 1934, simultaneously by two Swedish physicians Myhrman and Zetterholm. A large epidemic occurred in Finnish Lapland in 1942 among German and Finnish troops but HFRS received much more attention during the Korean conflict in 1951–1954, when 3200 UN soldiers contracted Korean haemorrhagic fever. It was still almost 25 years before the first etiologic agent of HFRS was discovered. In 1976 Ho-Wang Lee announced detection of what is known today as Hantaan virus in field mice (*Apodemus agrarius*), using immunofluorescence with patient sera (Lee *et al.* 1978; Lee 1982). The virus which is the prototype of the Hantavirus genus in the Bunyaviridae family was named after the Hantaan River which is near the site of discovery (Schmaljohn *et al.* 1985; Nichol *et al.* 2005). The first European hantavirus, Puumala virus was discovered a few years later from Finnish bank voles (*Myodes* [*Clethrionomys*] *glareolus*; Brummer-Korvenkontio *et al.* 1980). Other HFRS-causing pathogens were soon found: Seoul virus in 1982 from urban rats in Japan (Lee *et al.* 1982), Dobrava-Belgrade virus from yellow-necked mice (*Apodemus flavicollis*) in Slovenia and Serbia in 1992 (Avsic-Zupanc *et al.* 1992; Gligic *et al.* 1992) and Saaremaa virus from Estonian field mice (*Apodemus agrarius*) in 1997. Saaremaa virus is antigenically closely related to Dobrava-Belgrade virus but differs from it in many other respects, including its rodent host and its reduced virulence for humans (Plyusnin *et al.* 2006). Tula virus, isolated from the common vole (*Microtus arvalis*) in 1993 (Plyusnin *et al.* 1994), or a closely related virus, can apparently infect humans but seems to be apathogenic (Vapalahti *et al.* 1996). Amur-Soochong virus, a highly virulent hantavirus, was isolated from *Apodemus peninsulae* in far east Russia (Yashina *et al.* 2001) and Korea (Baek *et al.* 2006) and Thailand virus, originally recovered in 1985 from a greater bandicoot rat

(*Bandicota indica*), recently was associated with HFRS in Thailand (Pattamadilok *et al.* 2006; Nakamura *et al.* 2008).

The first recognized indigenous New World hantavirus, Prospect Hill virus, was isolated from a meadow vole (*Microtus pennsylvanicus*) in 1982 in the USA. It can infect humans (Yanagihara *et al.* 1984) but has not been associated with human disease. The real starting point for New World hantavirology occurred in the spring of 1993 when patients with acute respiratory distress syndrome (ARDS) started appearing in the Four Corners area of the southwestern USA. Patient sera reacted with hantaviruses, best with Puumala virus. The virus was soon detected in deer mice (*Peromyscus maniculatus*), perhaps the most common North American rodent (Nichol *et al.* 1993), and ultimately was named Sin Nombre (nameless), so that the exact discovery site was not identified. The disease, hantavirus pulmonary syndrome (HPS) or hantavirus cardiopulmonary syndrome (HCPS), caused by Sin Nombre virus has high case fatality, still about 35%. A plethora of related pathogenic and apathogenic hantaviruses have been discovered since 1993 in North and South America including the pathogenic Andes virus (Lopez *et al.* 1996), which has the unusual feature of being transmitted from person-to-person (Padula *et al.* 1998).

Several new hantaviruses have been detected recently in insectivores and there have been more studies on the insectivore-borne Thottapalayam virus (TPMV), which was the first insectivore-borne hantavirus to be isolated in cell culture. While the isolation of TPMV from the Asian house shrew (*Suncus murinus*), captured in India in 1964 (Carey *et al.* 1971) predates the discovery of the prototype Hantaan virus, studies on insectivore-borne hantaviruses, their epizootiology and pathogenicity to humans are still in their early stages. The International Committee on Taxonomy of Viruses currently lists only 23 hantavirus species (http://www.ictvonline.org/virusTaxonomy.asp?version=2008), but there are thousands of species of rodents and insectivores (Wilson and Reeder 2005), many of which have proved, upon examination, to host a hantavirus. Thus it is easy to predict that a large number of hantaviruses await discovery.

The virus

Morphology

Hantavirus morphology is typical of the members of the *Bunyaviridae* family with the virus particles been generally spherical (Hung *et al.* 1985). Elongated particles have been also observed (Goldsmith *et al.* 1995). Virus particle size varies from 70 to 120 nm in diameter with their surface having a characteristic square grid-like structure. The virus outside layer is composed of projections formed by the two surface glycoproteins Gn and Gc (formerly called G1 and G2, respectively), embedded in a host-cell derived lipid bilayer. Inside the bilayer are three viral genomic segments (Fig. 28.1). Inactivation of hantaviruses in samples may be achieved chemically (methanol, paraformaldehyde acetone/methanol and detergent-containing cell-lysis buffers), by ultraviolet light or by gamma cell irradiation (Kraus *et al.* 2005). Inactivation of the virus in the field can be achieved by the use of detergents (3% Lysol) or 10% bleach.

Molecular biology

Hantaviruses are enveloped RNA viruses with a three-segmented negative-sense RNA genome. The RNA segments are designated as S (small; 1600–2060 nt), M (medium; approximately 3700 nt) and L (large; 6500–7000 nt). The term 'negative-sense' refers to an RNA genome complementary to the messenger RNAs that encode the viral proteins. The naked RNA genome is not infectious. An infectious virus unit, requires the viral RNA to be encapsidated by the nucleoprotein (N), forming the nucleocapsid core associated with the large L viral polymerase protein. The S segment encodes the nucleocapsid N protein (48–49 kDa), the L segment the polymerase L protein (250 kDa) and the M segment the two glycoproteins, Gn and Gc (72 kDa and 54 kDa respectively) (Schmaljohn and Nichol 2007). Hantaviruses carried by rodents of the family Cricetidae (subfamilies Arvicolinae, Neotominae, and Sigmodontinae) have in their S segment an additional +1 open reading frame encoding the nonstructural protein NSs which can act as an interferon antagonist (Jaaskelainen *et al.* 2007).

Hantavirus replication and assembly

Hantaviruses have been shown to utilize integrins as their receptor. More specifically, hantaviruses that are pathogenic for humans utilize the β-3 integrin whereas a group of hantaviruses that are considered to be non-pathogenic utilize the β-1 integrin as their cellular receptor (Mackow and Gavrilovskaya 2001). Additional cellular receptors also have been reported for HTNV (Choi *et al.* 2008; Krautkramer and Zeier 2008). The attachment of the virus to the cell is mediated by the virus surface glycoproteins. Viral replication is initiated after virion uptake by the infected cells and release of the viral ribonucleoprotein cores into the cytoplasm. Each negative-strand virus RNA segment is transcribed by the virion associated polymerase (L) to produce a functional mRNA. The relative amounts of the mRNAs synthesized are inversely proportionally to their length. Thus, N mRNA is the most abundant and the L mRNA the least (Hutchinson *et al.* 1996). A simple explanation may be that the transcription elongation process is discontinuous with the polymerase pausing and possibly prematurely terminating at specific sites along the genome. The longer the gene, the higher the possibility for the presence of pausing sites. The length of the longer segments may itself dictate relative abundance of each mRNA, irrespective of any delay in processivity. The 5' ends of all three mRNAs are capped and contain a nontemplated guanine (G) residue. A prime and realign model has been proposed for the initiation of hantavirus RNA transcription (Garcin *et al.* 1995). The three mRNAs are transcribed in the infected cell cytoplasm in P bodies (Mir *et al.* 2008) and their translation is coupled to the transcription process.

The ratio of the individual virus proteins synthesized reflects the relative abundance of the virus mRNAs, with the N the most abundant protein. Two of the mRNAs, N and L, are translated on free ribosomes. The GPC mRNA is translated on membrane-bound polysomes. The GPC precursor molecule is cotranslationally cleaved to produce the Gn and Gc glycoproteins. Both glycoproteins are typical class 1 proteins with the N-terminus exposed at the surface of the virion and transmembrane domains anchoring the C-terminus except for short cytoplasmic tails. Four potential N-glycosylation sites are conserved among all hantavirus glycoproteins, three of which are located in Gn and one in Gc protein (Spiropoulou 2001). An additional feature also conserved in all hantaviruses is the high number of cysteine residues present in both glycoproteins (at least 57 in total).

The mechanisms by which the virus switches from the transcription to the replication mode are not known. The switch

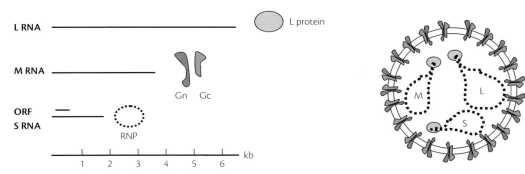

Fig. 28.1 Hantavirus structure, genes and gene products. Hantaviruses (Genus *Hantavirus* in the family *Bunyaviridae*) are enveloped viruses with a tri-segmented (L, M, S) negative-stranded RNA genome. The termini of the segments are conserved and complementary to each other. Hantaviruses carried by *Cricetidae* (but not *Muridae*) rodents have in the S segment an additional open reading frame (ORF) encoding a ~10 kDa non-structural protein (NSs) used to evade the interferon response.

from transcription to replication mode may involve increasing concentrations of N protein leading to more efficient RNA encapsidation. This model would allow the polymerase to read through the transcription termination signals and synthesize the full-length copies of the virion RNA templates.

Assembly of the virus begins once sufficient amounts of the structural proteins have been synthesized and genomic RNA has been replicated. In the endoplasmic reticulum, the two glycoproteins form heterodimers and exit to the Golgi (Spiropoulou 2001). The localization and accumulation of the two proteins in the Golgi is thought to be the reason hantavirus maturation occurs in the Golgi complex rather than at the cell surface like many other viruses (Goldsmith *et al.* 1995; Schmaljohn and Nichol 2007). The long cytoplasmic tail of Gn has been speculated to interact with the nucleocapsid cores, and promote assembly into mature virion particles; however, assembly of hantavirus virus like particles mediated by N and Gn+Gc *in vitro* has proved difficult or impossible thus far (B. Hjelle, unpublished results). In the next step, the cytoplasmic vesicles carrying the virions fuse with the plasma membrane and the mature virions are released extracellularly. In addition to Golgi maturation some of the HCPS-associated hantaviruses can also mature at the cell surface (Goldsmith *et al.* 1995; Ravkov *et al.* 1997).

Taxonomy

Following the discovery in 1993 of the New World hantaviruses that cause HPS (Nichol *et al.* 1993), the number of newly characterized hantaviruses has increased exponentially. It is often hard to distinguish between a new subtype of the same virus species or a new virus species. Some caution is appropriate, then, when reviewing the *Bunyaviridae* literature in that the mere application of a name to a particular new taxon cannot, in and of itself, be presumed to indicate that a new viral species has been discovered. In order to characterize a hantavirus as a new species based on the requirements by the International Committee on Taxonomy of Viruses (ICTV) the virus:

A) should be found in a unique primary rodent reservoir species or subspecies,

B) should show at least a 4-fold difference in two-way cross neutralization tests,

C) should exhibit at least 7% difference in amino acid identity in comparisons of the complete N, Gn and Gc of other known hantaviruses,

D) should not naturally form re-assortments with other hantavirus species.

These are of course basic guidelines with many exceptions already allowed. In general, each hantavirus is associated with one rodent host species. There are exceptions however. For example, different rodent species can be the reservoir for the same hantavirus (e.g. SEOV may be found in both *Rattus rattus* and *Rattus norvegicus*) and different hantaviruses can have the same rodent host (SNV and NYV in *Peromyscus leucopus*; BCCV and Muleshoe viruses in different subspecies of *Sigmodon hispidus*).

The old gold standard of 4-fold differences in two-way cross neutralization tests used for many years also has its limitations with regard to hantaviruses, as these viruses are often very difficult to isolate in tissue culture. Frequently multiple blind passages are necessary to get the virus to grow, and virus cross-contaminants have sometimes been an issue.

Finally, we have the last two criteria of hantavirus genetic diversity and re-assortment. As hantaviruses have tri-segmented RNA genomes, they have potential for rapid generation of genetic diversity based on their predicted high RNA polymerase error rate and the possibility of genetic reassortment (mixing of genomic RNA segments between viruses). Analysis of whole genome sequences have shown that hantaviruses have developed genetic diversity mainly by rapidly accumulating point mutations. Genetic reassortment has been seen less frequently and appears to be limited to closely related hantaviruses (Li *et al.* 1995; Rodriguez *et al.* 1998; Klempa *et al.* 2003; Rizvanov *et al.* 2004; Razzauti *et al.* 2008).

Phylogenetic analysis of the hantavirus genome reveals a complex evolutionary pattern with multiple virus lineages present in Asia, Europe and the Americas. Recently hantaviruses have also been found in Africa (Klempa *et al.* 2006). In general, there is a good correlation between viral phylogeny and the rodent phylogeny suggesting that the viruses and their rodent reservoirs have had a long association. The hantaviruses associated with Murinae, Arvicolinae, Neotominae and Sigmodontinae subfamilies form distinct phylogenetic groups (Fig. 28.2). Viral lineages correlate with the phylogeny of the reservoir and any relation to geographic location is mainly based on the distribution of the rodent host. For many years, the only recognized hantavirus with a non-rodent host was Thottapalayam virus, which had been isolated from an insectivore, the Asian house shrew *Suncus murinus*, in India in 1964. This virus was the most distinct of the hantaviruses and is quite distantly related to the rodent-associated hantaviruses (Fig. 28.2; Yadav *et al.* 2007). Recently however, there have been several additional genetically distinct hantaviruses detected in insectivores from throughout Eurasia (Arai *et al.* 2008b; Henttonen *et al.* 2008). Several authors have suggested that similarities between virus and rodent host phylogenies reflect co-divergence of the hantaviruses and their hosts. However, recent findings of insectivore-associated hantaviruses, and some analyses have suggested that these phylogenetic similarities may instead reflect more recent preferential host switching and local adaptation (Ramsden *et al.* 2009).

Virus growth

Virus isolates have been obtained from infected rodent or human samples, but usually with great difficulty; successful attempts having often involved a number of blind passages of rodent or clinical material prior to virus adaptation to tissue culture (Elliott *et al.* 1994). Once adapted to cell culture, the growth of most hantaviruses is still poor, with peak infectious titres often in the range of 10^5/ml or less, even in Type I interferon-deficient Vero E6 cells. HTNV, ANDV and TULV are among the few exceptions, as they grow to sufficiently high titre to be useful experimental systems. Human lung carcinoma cells A549 were first used for the adaptation of the prototype HTNV to tissue culture (French *et al.* 1981). Vero-E6 cells, a continuous kidney cell line from the African green monkey, are a commonly utilized cell line in which most hantaviruses propagate well without killing the cell or producing overt cell damage. Endothelial cells, the primary targets in naturally acquired hantavirus infections, are also readily infected *in vitro* with no evident cytopathic effect (Yanagihara and Silverman 1990).

The hosts

Animals

Hantaviruses establish chronic, asymptomatic infections in specific small-mammal host species. The infected host sheds large quantities of virus into the environment for extended periods, facilitating the transmission of infection to uninfected members of the population. Almost any species of mammal can become infected if it comes into contact with an infected host. This is evidenced by frequent finding of antibody in syntopic rodent species, especially under epizootic conditions (Childs *et al.* 1994), as well as other species of mammals (Mills and Childs 2001), especially those that prey on rodents including cats (Bennett *et al.* 1990; Nowotny 1994), foxes (Escutenaire and Pastoret 2002), and coyotes (Peters *et al.* 2006). Nevertheless, it appears that species other than the specific host quickly develop antibody, clear the virus infection, and do not shed large quantities of virus into the environment. Thus these are considered 'dead-end' hosts that are not of epidemiologic importance in the transmission of infection to humans or other animals (Nowotny *et al.* 1994; Peters *et al.* 2006).

The great majority of the known hantaviruses are associated with three groups of rodents (order Rodentia) in the large rodent superfamily Muroidea (Taxonomy follows Musser and Carleton 2005). These are the Old World rats and mice (family Muridae, subfamily Murinae; distributed in Europe, Africa and Asia), the New World rats and mice (family Cricetidae, subfamilies Neotominae and Sigmodontinae; distributed throughout the Americas), and the

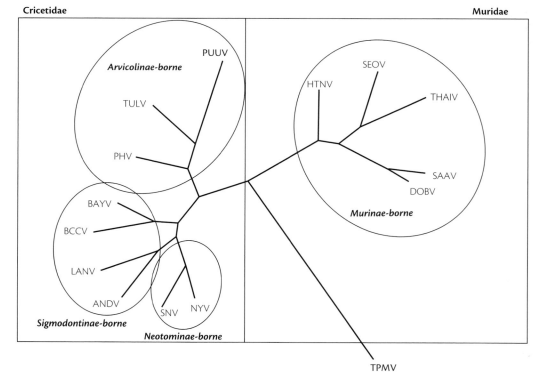

Fig. 28.2 Phylogenic tree of major hantaviruses carried by the different rodents (Family Muridae, subfamily Murinae and Family Cricetidae, subfamilies Arvicolinae, Sigmodontinae and Neotominae) and insectivores. The tree is based on the complete coding region of the S segment. HTNV, Hantaan virus; SEOV, Seoul virus; THAIV, Thailand virus; DOBV, Dobrava-Belgrade virus; SAAV, Saaremaa virus; PUUV, Puumala virus, TULV, Tula virus; PHV, Prospect Hill virus; SNV, Sin Nombre virus; NYV, New York virus; BAYV, Bayou virus; BCCV, Black Creek Canal virus; LANV, Laguna Negra virus; ANDV, Andes virus; TPMV, Thottapalayam virus. In addition to human-pathogenic viruses, two hantaviruses reported to infect humans (PHV, TULV), and a representative of insectivore-borne viruses (TPMV) is shown.
We thank Dr Tarja Sironen of Haartman Institute, University of Helsinki, for preparing this phylogenic tree.

voles and lemmings (family Cricetidae, subfamily Arvicolinae; largely circumboreal). There are several emergent characteristics of the hantavirus-host relationship:

1   Highly specific one-host-one-virus relationship,

2   Chronic, asymptomatic infection in the host,

3   Long-term (perhaps life-long) shedding of virus into the environment,

4   Association with 3 related groups of muroid rodents.

Taken together these characteristics suggest a long period of co-adaptation between the individual hosts and viruses and have led to the hypothesis of co-divergence of hantaviruses and hosts. Specifically, there would have been an ancestral hantavirus associated with an ancestral Muroid hosts before the sub-familial lineages diverged (approximately 30 million years ago) and that the now distinct viruses have co-diverged with their Muroid hosts since that time (Yates *et al.* 2002). This hypothesis is supported by molecular evidence showing a high degree of similarity between the phylogenetic structure of the host rodent and that of the viruses (Plyusnin and Morzunov 2001). Important implications of this hypothesis for hantaviruses are their extreme antiquity and their extreme potential diversity. There are approximately 500 species of New World rats and mice, 560 species of Old World rats and mice, and 150 species of voles and lemmings distributed throughout the world (Musser and Carleton 2005).

The currently recognized hantavirus hosts (Table 28.1) include 8 species of Old World rats and mice in Europe and Asia, 34 species of New World rats and mice in the Americas (all but one recognized since 1993), and 9 species of voles and lemmings in Europe, Asia, and North America. It may be of importance that the greatest pace of discovery of novel hantaviruses has been among those associated with the New World rats and mice (subfamilies Neotominae and Sigmodontinae). All of the recognized pathogenic hantaviruses from the Americas belong to this group whose center of diversity is in the American tropics, an area that receives relatively little surveillance. It is likely that only a small proportion of the pathogenic hantaviruses in the New World tropics have been identified. Hantaviruses were not recognized from the Old World rats and mice in Africa until recently when Sangassou virus was described from *Hylomyscus simus* in Guinea (Klempa *et al.* 2006). This discovery suggests that the apparent absence of hantaviruses from Africa was due to a lack of surveillance and that additional hantaviruses and human disease may be described from that continent.

A single hantavirus (Thottapalayam virus) was recognized many years ago in association with an insectivore (order Soricomorpha) (Carey *et al.* 1971). This anomalous occurrence of a hantavirus with a non-rodent host was suspected of being an unusual spillover event or cross-species jump. Recently however, several additional hantaviruses have been described in association with additional insectivore species in North America, Africa, and Asia (Arai *et al.* 2007; Song *et al.* 2007a; Song *et al.* 2007b; Arai *et al.* 2008a; Arai *et al.* 2008b). This finding challenges long held assumptions about the origin and co-divergence of hantaviruses. Questions that need to be investigated include the possible co-divergence of a clade of hantaviruses with insectivores, the question of its derivation (a spillover from the muroid lineage and subsequent radiation within the insectivores), and the potential pathogenicity of insectivore hantaviruses for humans.

Epizootiology

Infected host rodents establish persistent and asymptomatic infections that, at least in some virus-host pairings, involve the shedding of large quantities of virus into the environment in saliva and urine for extended periods, perhaps the lifetime of the rodent. However, the quantity of virus shed may be orders of magnitude greater during the first 2–8 weeks after infection (Lee *et al.* 1981; Yanagihara *et al.* 1985; Gavrilovskaya *et al.* 1990; Hutchinson *et al.* 1998; Hardestam *et al.* 2008). Host rodents for some virus-host pairs, including deer mice with SNV, are distinguished by a much more modest level of shedding, suggesting that the role for viral shedding in maintaining enzootic infections with SNV in deer mice may require some degree of modification or reconsideration (Botten *et al.* 2000; Botten *et al.* 2002). A positive association between prevalence of infection and age class of the host suggests that horizontal mechanism(s) are important means of transmission (Mills *et al.* 1997; Olsson *et al.* 2002). Indeed the demonstrated transmission of protective maternal antibody from dams to pups makes vertical transmission unlikely (Dohmae and Nishimune 1995; Botten *et al.* 2002; Kallio *et al.* 2006b). For many host species the prevalence of infection in males is consistently much higher than in females (Yahnke *et al.* 2001; Olsson *et al.* 2002; Calisher *et al.* 2007), and infected animals (especially males) are more likely to have scars or wounds than are uninfected animals (Glass *et al.* 1988; Douglass *et al.* 2001). These patterns suggest that a frequent mechanism of hantavirus transmission within rodent host populations may be via aggressive encounters, especially among males (Glass *et al.* 1988; Douglass *et al.* 2001). This hypothesis is also supported by laboratory experiments demonstrating that infection of laboratory rats with hantaviruses by the intramuscular route is 100 times more efficient than by aerosol (Nuzum *et al.* 1988). Nevertheless, for a few host species there is little or no sexual bias in infection prevalence (Childs *et al.* 1987; Childs *et al.* 1989; Korch *et al.* 1989), suggesting either more frequent fighting among females, or alternate route(s) of transmission. For example, brush mice (*Peromyscus boylii*) and western harvest mice (*Reithrodontomys megalotis*) show a much stronger sexual bias (80–90% male) than do deer mice (60% males) (Mills *et al.* 1999); prevalence of infection with Seoul virus in Norway rats may be equal among males and females (Korch *et al.* 1989). Aerosols, cross-grooming, and sexual transmission are potential alternative mechanisms. Although male bank voles are more frequently infected with Puumala virus than are females, bank voles do not defend territories and the sex bias in infection is hypothesized to be related to their greater motility and increased numbers of encounters (Olsson *et al.* 2002). Urine, faeces, and saliva from Puumala virus infected bank voles have all been shown to be infectious to naive bank voles, suggesting the possibility of aerosol transmission via any of these media. The frequency of such transmission would be related to the period of survivorship of virus in the environment. Laboratory experiments with Hantaan virus have shown that the virus remains infectious for less than 3 days on laboratory surfaces. Nevertheless, Puumala virus remained infectious for 12–15 days in bedding material at room temperature (Kallio *et al.* 2006a). Nothing is known about potential mechanisms of transmission of hantaviruses in insectivore populations.

Seasonal patterns

Incidence of HFRS and HPS cases generally follow a seasonal pattern, likely driven by responses of rodent population dynamics

Table 28.1 Major human-pathogenic hantaviruses, fatality rates of infection and rodent carriers[1]

Haemorrhagic fever with renal syndrome (HFRS): annually about 100,000 hospitalized cases

Asia

Hantaan virus (3–7%) *Apodemus agrarius mantchuricus* (striped field mouse, eastern subspecies)

[2]Seoul virus (1–2%) *Rattus rattus* (roof rat) and *Rattus norvegicus* (brown rat)

[3]Amur/Soochong virus (10%) *Apodemus peninsulae* (Korean field mouse)

Europe

Puumala virus (NE) (0.1%) *Myodes glareolus* (bank vole)

Dobrava-Belgrade virus (10%) *Apodemus flavicollis* (yellow-necked field mouse)

Saaremaa virus (mild NE-like disease) *Apodemus agrarius agrarius* (striped field mouse, western subspecies)

Hantavirus pulmonary syndrome (HPS): approximately 3700 hospitalized cases through February 2009; case fatality is highly variable but averages 30–40%

Americas

Sin Nombre virus *Peromyscus maniculatus* (North American deermouse)

New York virus *Peromyscus leucopus* (white-footed deermouse)

[4]Andes virus *Oligoryzomys longicaudatus* (long-tailed colilargo)

Bermejo virus *Oligoryzomys chacoensis* (Chacoan colilargo)

Lechiguanas virus *Oligoryzomys flavescens* (flavescent colilargo)

Maciel virus *Necromys* [*Bolomys*] *benefactus* (Argentine akodont)

Oran virus *Oligoryzomys longicaudatus* (long-tailed colilargo)

Pergamino virus *Akodon azarae* (Azara's akodont)

[3]Araraquara virus *Necromys* [*Bolomys*] *lasiurus* (hairy-tailed akodont)

Laguna Negra virus *Calomys laucha* (little laucha), *Calomys callosus* (big laucha)

Bayou virus *Oryzomys palustris* (marsh oryzomys)

[3]Anajatuba virus *Oligoryzomys fornesi* (Fornes' colilargo)

[3]Choclo virus *Oligoryzomys fulvescens costaricensis* (fulvous colilargo)

[3]Juquitiba virus *Oligoryzomys nigripes* (black-footed colilargo), *Oxymycterus nasutus* (long-nosed hocicudo)

Black Creek Canal virus *Sigmodon hispidus spadicipygus* (hispid cotton rat)

[1]Nomenclature for scientific and common names follows Wilson and Reeder 2005.

[2]Seoul virus is cosmopolitan and has been also detected in brown rats (and occasionally roof rats) on several continents, in the past in laboratory rats as well as recently in wild rats in Europe.

[3]Not officially recognized by the International Committee on Taxonomy of Viruses (ICTV).

[4]Five additional genotypes listed under Andes virus are not yet recognized by the ICTV, but are listed because of their distinct geographic distributions and host species. NE = nephropathia epidemica.

and behaviour to seasonal environmental patterns. In temperate climates host species undergo seasonal breeding, with reproduction occurring in spring and summer. This pattern results in highest population densities in the late autumn just after the cessation of breeding. Nevertheless, because the autumn population consists primarily of young, inexperienced (and therefore uninfected) individuals, the prevalence of infection in the host population is lowest at that time. The process responsible for this low prevalence has been termed the juvenile dilution effect (Mills *et al.* 1999; Tersago *et al.* 2008a). About the time that breeding begins the following spring, the overwintered population is at its lowest density, but the prevalence of infection is highest in the older, more experienced population. For host populations in Europe (Niklasson *et al.* 1995; Davis *et al.* 2005) and in the western US, the spring prevalence has been shown to be proportional to the population density the previous autumn. This phenomenon has been called delayed-density-dependent prevalence of infection (Niklasson *et al.* 1995; Mills *et al.* 1999; Madhav *et al.* 2007). This characteristic seasonal pattern of host population dynamics in temperate areas is often associated with spring/early summer peaks in numbers of human cases in the USA (Centers for Disease Control and Prevention (CDC) unpublished data), and southern South America (E. Palma *et al.* unpublished data) Host populations in the tropics may also respond to seasonal weather patterns (Teixeira *et al.* 2006) resulting in strong patterns in HCPS cases, but the important variable is more likely to be rainfall than temperature. Longitudinal studies of factors associated with hantavirus host populations in the tropics are needed.

Inter-annual patterns

Outbreaks of HFRS and HPS in human populations have been linked to increases in rodent host populations. Rodent host population dynamics, in turn, are strongly linked to environmental phenomena, although the specific environmental cues vary from place to place. Increased rainfall, especially in arid or semiarid areas is associated with increases in rodent host populations in the southwestern USA (Yates *et al.* 2002), Paraguay (Williams *et al.* 1997), and Panama (Bayard *et al.* 2004). Abrupt increases in rodent populations ('ratadas') were associated with periodic bamboo flowering events in Argentina and Chile (Murúa *et al.* 1996; Toro *et al.* 1998), and increases in bank vole populations in continental Europe are associated with mast seeding events for beech nuts and acorns (Tersago *et al.* 2008b). These environmental phenomena are all associated with climatic factors including temperature and precipitation, and it has been suggested that changes in these factors associated with global climate change may ultimately affect the incidence of human hantavirus disease (J. Mills, unpublished data).

Long-term studies of rodent host populations in Europe (Tersago *et al.* 2008b) and in the western USA (Yates *et al.* 2002) have demonstrated that rodent host population dynamics are strongly influenced by environmental conditions through bottom-up trophic processes. In the southwestern USA, El Nino Southern Oscillation (ENSO) events periodically bring unusually high quantities of rainfall to normally arid areas. After an ENSO event brought increased rainfall to the Southwest in 1997, investigators observed increased growth of vegetation and improved habitat quality and food supplies. This was followed by increased reproductive success and survivorship in deer mouse populations and abrupt increases in host population abundance in the spring of 1998 (Yates *et al.* 2002). In the spring of 1999, abundance was lower, but prevalence of SNV infection in the host population was unusually high, presumably due to increased contacts among individuals in the high density population of the previous autumn (delayed-density-dependent prevalence) (Niklasson *et al.* 1995; Madhav *et al.* 2007). Real time observation of these events allowed the prediction of high-risk conditions and targeted intervention for specific human populations in the southwestern USA (CDC 1998, 1999).

In continental Europe, a combination of high summer temperatures and low precipitation lead to mast seeding in oak and beech trees, leading to abundant food, increases in bank vole populations, and increased numbers of HFRS cases (Tersago et al. 2008b). Both direct observations of changing rodent population abundance and the use weather variables to predict human risk of HFRS in Europe show promise (Tersago et al. 2008b; Olsson et al. 2009).

In contrast, population dynamics of bank voles in Northern Europe (Finland, northern Sweden, and parts of Norway) may be driven by top-down trophic interactions. Populations of voles and lemmings undergo a 3–4 year cycle of population irruptions and crashes with up to 500-fold differences in population density between peak and crash phases. These cycles, which have been clearly linked to cycles of human HFRS incidence (Olsson et al. 2003), are hypothesized to be driven by specialist predators (Olsson et al. 2003; Hornfeldt 2004).

Anthropogenic factors

Human perturbation interacts with environmental controls to change the structure of rodent assemblages and the abundance of host populations. Human disturbance can lead the simplification of ecosystems and local extinction of specialist species, while benefiting highly fecund opportunistic species whose populations may increase to very high densities in the absence of specialist competitors (Mills 2006). These high density populations result in increased host-to-host contacts, greater prevalence of infection in the host populations, and increased frequency of contact with humans. Host populations in disturbed peridomestic environments may demonstrate a higher prevalence of infection than populations in nearby more natural habitats (Kuenzi et al. 2001). Land conversion associated with deforestation, agriculture, or ranching has been associated repeatedly with outbreaks of HPS in Central and South America (Williams et al. 1997; Bayard et al. 2004; Ruedas et al. 2004; Carroll et al. 2005; Mills 2006).

In summary, the population dynamics of hantavirus hosts, transmission of hantaviruses within host populations and, consequently, risk to human populations are influenced by multiple interacting factors. The relative importance of these factors varies among host species and location and may include environmental, anthropogenic, genetic, behavioral, and physiological factors (Mills 2005). Intensive studies of these factors in Europe and the Americas, especially environmental influences, have led to successful prediction of human risk in a few cases. Accurate and reliable predictive models will require further improvements in our understanding of host ecology.

Humans

Clinical picture and pathogenesis of HFRS and HCPS

Hantaan, Seoul and Amur-Soochong virus in Asia, and Puumala, Dobrava-Belgrade and Saaremaa viruses in Europe all cause HFRS, but the infections differ considerably in severity (Table 28.1). Dobrava-Belgrade, Amur-Soochong and Hantaan HFRS have high 3–10% mortality, Seoul infection 1–2%, and Puumala and Saaremaa viruses cause mild HFRS, often called nephropathia epidemica (NE) with only 0.1–0.2% mortality. HFRS (Lee 1982; Mustonen et al. 1994a; Mustonen et al. 1994b; Schmaljohn and Hjelle 1997; Kanerva et al. 1998; Peters et al. 1999; Vapalahti et al. 2003) has a variable incubation period, 2–6 weeks, and it begins with high fever, followed by central nervous system symptoms (headache, dizziness) and then by signs of renal insufficiency (oliguria, proteinuria, increased creatinine and later polyuria), abdominal pain, backache and haemorrhages. However, HFRS is a general infection and can manifest itself also as encephalitis, hepatitis or arthritis. About a third of NE patients experience transient visual disturbances; myopia is a pathognomonic sign. Notably, pulmonary and cardiac symptoms are quite common; at the acute stage of NE about a third of patients have pulmonary (Linderholm et al. 1997) and more than half cardiac findings (Makela et al. 2009). Thus, although HFRS and HCPS are primarily targeted at kidneys and lungs, respectively, they share a number of clinical features, such as capillary leakage, increased TNF-α, and thrombocytopenia. Notably, haemorrhages and alterations in renal function occur also in HCPS. The causes of death in HFRS include shock, (hypophyseal) haemorrhages, pulmonary oedema and acute renal insufficiency. Renal dialysis is required in about 5% of hospitalized NE patients.

The course of Puumala infection (NE) is quite variable, most infections are asymptomatic and in only 20–25% so severe that medical attention is sought. In children NE is in general quite mild (Mustonen et al. 1994b). Individuals with the HLA-B8-, DR3- and DQ2-haplotype are likely to have severe NE (Mustonen et al. 1996; Makela et al. 2002) and those carrying HLA-B27 allele mild disease (Mustonen et al. 1998). On the other hand, in patients with the HLA-B35 allele, Sin Nombre infection is often lethal (Terajima et al. 2007).

At two to six weeks, and commonly two to three weeks, the incubation periods for the infections that cause HCPS are similar to those of HFRS (Young et al. 2000; Vial et al. 2006). For SNV and the other North American viruses, asymptomatic seroconversion, as assessed in serologic surveys of healthy individuals, is quite uncommon. The case-fatality ratios of HCPS varies markedly according to virus species, but the most important etiologic agents, SNV in North America and Andes virus and its close relatives in South America, are associated with case-fatality ratios of about 35–36% (http://www.cdc.gov/ncidod/diseases/hanta/hps/noframes/epislides/episl4.htm; http://epi.minsal.cl/epi/html/bolets/reportes/Hantavirus/Hantavirus.pdf). Some less common etiologic agents for HCPS such as the Oran variant of ANDV as well as Laguna Negra virus, are clearly less pathogenic than is ANDV and SNV, and carry lower case fatality ratios. Choclo virus, carried by Oligoryzomys flavescens in Panama, carries a case fatality ratio of <10%, and causes a form of HPS without the cardiac abnormalities that must be present to be regarded as true 'HCPS'.

Regardless of which species of South American hantavirus is thought to be predominant in a particular location, it is common, perhaps universal, to detect evidence for past asymptomatic infection by hantaviruses on the basis of serosurveys results (Ferrer et al. 1998; Castillo et al. 2002; Tager Frey et al. 2003; Armien et al. 2004). Thus, while CHOCV and LANV of Panama and Paraguay, respectively, are indeed slightly less pathogenic than is the epidemiologically important ANDV, it is difficult to reconcile the known pathogenicity and significant case-fatality ratios associated with such viruses and infections with measured human population seroprevalences that reach levels of 30–40% (Ferrer et al. 1998; Armien et al. 2004).

There is considerable concordance between the nature of clinical and laboratory abnormalities and the clinical progression of HCPS in comparison to HFRS, including the nearly-universal decline in platelet counts, and elevation of serum lactate dehydrogenase. For both conditions, capillary leak is a cardinal clinical feature, involving either predominantly the pulmonary bed (HCPS) or the retroperitoneal space with secondary involvement of the pulmonary vasculature (HFRS). These distinctions are not 'pure' in that pulmonary oedema is common among patients with NE and other forms of HFRS, and SNV and especially other etiologic agents of HCPS such as BAYV, ANDV and BCCV have been long recognized as leading frequently to at least mild azotemia and proteinuria (Schmaljohn and Hjelle 1997).

Pathology and diagnostics of HFRS

In HFRS autopsy samples, oedema, haemorrhages, ischemic necrotic lesions and lymphoid cell infiltrates are commonly seen, especially in the kidneys but also at other sites such as spleen, liver and hypophysis (Kanerva *et al.* 1998; Hautala *et al.* 2002). Before rapid and specific viral diagnostics were developed, kidney biopsies were often used for diagnostic purposes in suspected Puumala virus infection (nephropathia epidemica), e.g. in Finland until about 1990 (Vaheri *et al.* 2008). The biopsy findings were not very specific, except for interstitial haemorrhages, which were seen in about a quarter of NE cases and in Northern Europe such findings were restricted to Puumala virus infected patients. Other characteristic findings in kidney biopsies were prominent expression of TNF-α and presence of lymphoid cell infiltrations, mainly CD8+ T-cells (Temonen *et al.* 1996).

Puumala hantaviruses are commonly isolated and grown in monkey kidney derived Vero E6 cells because they are defective in interferon response (Diaz *et al.* 1988). However, passages in these cells result in genetic changes and concomitant loss of capacity to infect their natural rodent host, the bank vole (Lundkvist *et al.* 1997) with which they have become highly co-adapted. The Vero E6 cell-adapted virus also has lost its capacity to infect the experimental nonhuman primate Cynomolgus macaque host (Klingstrom *et al.* 2002). In contrast, experimental infection of macaques with wild-type Puumala virus, directly from *Myodes glareolus*, results in symptoms and signs closely mimicking nephropathia epidemica in humans. Like in humans, the symptoms and signs (lethargy, anorexia, proteinuria, hematuria, IL-6, Il-10, TNF-α, C-reactive protein, creatinine, nitric oxide, viral RNA load) differ between the macaques (Klingstrom *et al.* 2002). Viral RNA and Puumala virus N protein, inflammatory cell infiltrations (mainly CD8-type T-cells like in human kidney biopsies) and tubular damage are found (Sironen *et al.* 2008). In addition to kidneys, viral markers were also seen in macaque spleen and liver tissues. Both the viral markers and T-cells appeared to co-localize in the kidneys to the sites of tissue damage, suggesting that cell-mediated immunity might be critical in the pathogenesis of hantavirus infection. In NE patients, the CD8+ T-cell response, with specificity mainly to the N protein, peaks at the onset of clinical disease, and decreases gradually within the next three weeks (Tuuminen *et al.* 2007).

Hantaviral antigen by immunocytochemistry and hantaviral RNA by *in situ* hybridization were not regularly found in NE kidney biopsies, probably because at the time of the biopsy, usually 5–8 days after onset of symptoms, Puumala virus is already disappearing and the immune response is underway. In more fulminant hantavirus infections (Dobrava, Hantaan) viral markers are more easily detected in autopsy samples than in NE patients (Poljak and Avsic-Zupanc 1994).

There are two additional potentially important findings that were made in cell cultures. Interestingly, pathogenic hantaviruses which cause either HFRS or HCPS use beta 3 integrins for entry to host cells while apathogenic hantavirus seem to employ β-1 integrins (Mackow and Gavrilovskaya 2001). Since β-3 integrins are critical adhesive receptors on platelets and endothelial cells and regulate both vascular permeability and platelet activation and adhesion, the use of these receptors by hantaviruses may be fundamental to hantavirus pathogenesis. The other finding is that while hantaviruses are not strongly cytopathic, in several models they can induce apoptosis (Kang *et al.* 1999; Markotic *et al.* 2003; Li *et al.* 2004, 2005). Yet, all in all, the pathogenesis of HFRS is not well understood.

Human HFRS-hantavirus diagnostics have been recently reviewed in detail recently (Vaheri *et al.* 2008). For diagnosis of acute hantavirus infection, μ-capture IgM enzyme immunoassay (EIA) based on recombinant full-length hantavirus nucleocapsid (N) protein is the current method of choice. In addition, rapid immunochromatographic IgM tests are available for several different HFRS-causing hantaviruses as 5-min point-of-care (POC) tests (Hujakka *et al.* 2001; Hujakka *et al.* 2003). In such tests a band is formed by binding of specific-IgM/anti-IgM-gold-conjugate complex to purified baculovirus-expressed hantavirus N protein. In more recent POC tests an optical reader is used to record the result. IgG EIAs are available for serosurveys.

In many countries several HFRS-hantaviruses coexist and hantaviral N proteins show antigenic serological cross-reactivities. For instance, in the Balkan area Puumala, Saaremaa and Dobrava-Belgrade viruses coexist and also infect humans. The cross-reactivities follow closely the phylogenetic tree of hantaviruses (Fig. 28.2) and are especially pronounced within each of the four groups (Murinae-borne, Arvicolinae-borne, Sigmodontinae-borne, Neotominae-borne). This implicates two things. Firstly, e.g. for the Balkan area at least two antigens are needed for both IgM and IgG tests: one for the vole viruses (Arvicolinae-borne) and another for the mouse/rat viruses (Murinae-borne). The second implication is that for serotyping of hantavirus infections in humans or rodents, tedious and time-consuming neutralization tests are needed, preferentially using convalescent serum taken during the first month after onset of symptoms. There are alternative possibilities: EIAs based on truncated nucleocapsid proteins that lack the cross-reactive N-terminal epitopes (Araki *et al.* 2001) or use of vesicular stomatitis virus pseudotypes bearing hantavirus envelope proteins and green fluorescent protein (GFP) which provide rapid and safe neutralization tests (Ogino *et al.* 2003).

Hantaviral RNA is found at the acute stage of HFRS in peripheral blood mononuclear cells, in blood clots, in urine, saliva and at least sometimes in cerebrospinal fluid, reflecting the fact that HFRS is a general infection (Plyusnin *et al.* 1997, 1999; Evander *et al.* 2007; Mahonen *et al.* 2007; Pettersson *et al.* 2008). No infectious virus has been detected in NE patient saliva and thus this fluid does not appear to be a medium of virus transmission (Hardestam *et al.* 2008). In general, viral RNA is more readily detected in severe HFRS (Dobrava, Hantaan) than in mild hantavirus infections (Puumala, Saaremaa). Both traditional (nested) and real-time RT-PCRs have been used. Yet, RT-PCR is not generally used for diagnostics, since serology functions so well and shipment of samples for RNA detection is far more complicated than that of IgM antibodies (Vaheri *et al.* 2008). In contrast, quantitation of the viral RNA load has predictive value for the outcome of hantaviral disease. Notably, an early high viral load predicts an unfavorable clinical course of NE and Puumala virus RNA can be demonstrated before IgM antibodies (Evander *et al.* 2007). Moreover, direct sequencing of viral RNA provides a conclusive way to genotype human hantavirus infections.

Pathology and diagnostics of HCPS

The first recognized cases of HCPS occurred in New Mexico, where the centralized Office of the Medical Investigator (OMI) for the State of New Mexico was the first institution to formally notify the state epidemiologist of the occurrence of clustered cases of the then-mysterious and oft-fatal illness (Foucar *et al.* 1994). As a result of the OMI's efforts and early involvement, it was possible to develop a detailed pathological description of the abnormalities of HCPS (Nolte *et al.* 1995; Zaki *et al.* 1995).

The gross and microscopic abnormalities in HCPS clearly revealed the lung and lymphoid organs to be the primary locus for pathological abnormalities; it was not until later, when the complete clinical/pathological spectrum of abnormalities was considered as a whole that the importance of cardiac insufficiency as the leading cause of death rose to the fore (Mertz *et al.* 2006). Lungs removed from patients who succumbed to HCPS are rubbery in consistency and commonly weigh twice that of those of other patients. Peripheral lymph nodes, the spleen, and the liver are among the organs that consistently demonstrate sometimes-florid involvement by highly atypical, immature 'immunoblastic' cell infiltrates that are among the hallmark findings of the syndrome. These cells have long been recognized as composing both T and B cells, CD4 and CD8 (Nolte *et al.* 1995; Zaki *et al.* 1995). The lungs in most cases were subject to scant to moderate infiltration by immunoblastic lymphocytes. Pleural effusions, fibrin deposition and alveolar oedema were consistently observed in the lungs. Approximately half of the livers that were examined histologically exhibited portal triaditis in a necropsy series.

Blood abnormalities in HCPS, as with several other pathological features, are highly stereotypical in nature. Specifically, clinical- and hemato-pathologists at an institution with extensive experience with SNV can usually render a highly accurate diagnosis of HCPS well in advance of the completion of specific viral serological tests, merely by examining a standard array of blood cell counts, in connection with a visual microscopic examination of the patient's blood cells (Koster *et al.* 2001). The single most sensitive abnormality of the blood is the presence of thrombocytopenia, which is nearly universal from the earliest stages, with only a tiny subset, 1% or less, of patients requiring subsequent blood sampling to detect the diminution of platelet count. By the onset of symptoms of pulmonary insufficiency, the large majority of patients also exhibit leukocytosis with profound left shift of the neutrophil series, with few or no of the toxic changes that are generally associated with bacterial sepsis or pneumonia. At least 10% of the lymphoid series in the blood of HCPS patients have immunoblastic morphology, representing immature blasts or cells with morphology mimicking that of plasma cells. Finally, patients with a significant capillary leak and pulmonary oedema also demonstrate elevated levels of blood haemoglobin or an elevated haematocrit.

For those patients who survive HCPS, the pattern of their clinical recovery demonstrates that the abnormalities of the lungs, blood/lymphoid organs, and heart are transient in nature and can be reversed rapidly if the immune system is allowed a few days to recognize and respond to the virus. This point has been especially emphasized in the wake of the first uses of extracorporeal membrane oxygenation (ECMO), which allows patients whose hearts and lungs are all but completely non-functional to survive long enough for an effective antiviral response to mature. The period of time required for even otherwise lethally-ill patients to be 'weaned' from cardiopulmonary bypass is extraordinarily brief, often amounting to a few hours, after which time even markedly diminished cardiac output returns promptly to near-normal levels, and the endotracheal tube is extracted contemporaneously or shortly thereafter. These observations reinforce the current dogma that patients with HCPS do not generally experience significantly tissue destruction either directly or indirectly through the agency of the virus, but rather a series of functional defects, perhaps exacted primarily by soluble mediators.

Investigators in Brazil have noted a high frequency of myocarditis in their autopsy series for HCPS (Saggioro *et al.* 2007), a finding that distinguishes HCPS cases associated with SNV in the North from those associated with South American ANDV-related viruses. Other than for this observation, the apparent involvement of at least some direct immunologic attack on the heart with ANDV as distinguished from purely functional cardiac depression with SNV, there are many more clinical similarities than differences between North American and South American forms of the syndrome.

Specific virologic diagnosis of HCPS can be achieved either serologically or via RT-PCR. The latter method can be conducted with either nested or real-time quantitative (qRT-PCR) technologies. Diagnosis by RT-PCR is far more sensitive when the RNA is extracted from cells, either using purified preparations of nucleated cells from anticoagulated blood, or blood clots (Hjelle *et al.* 1994). Sensitivities for RT-PCR based methods using the liquid component of blood (plasma or serum) range from ~40% (ANDV) to ~70% (SNV) so it is insufficient for routine diagnostic use. Furthermore, when samples are collected, as is often the case with HCPS, some days to weeks after the peak of the patient's illness, the virus is often already cleared from the blood compartment and can no longer be detected by RT-PCR. For those reasons, serology remains the mainstay of diagnosis even for HCPS, where RNA titers run higher in blood cells and plasma relative to some forms of HFRS.

Serologic methods in use for the etiologic agents of HCPS are primarily based upon enzyme linked immunosorbent assays (ELISA) or strip immunoblot assay (SIA), although other methods such as immunofluorescence assays (IFA) are possible as well. IgG serologic assays for SNV, LNV, ANDV and the ANDV-like Brazilian Araraquara virus have all been developed and show good sensitivity for detection of past or acute exposure (Ksiazek *et al.* 1995; Hjelle *et al.* 1997; Jenison *et al.* 1994; Padula *et al.* 2000; Figueiredo *et al.* 2009). With either ELISA or SIA, in general the investigator places viral antigens, either recombinantly-expressed or in the form of viral lysates, onto a solid matrix and exposes the antigens to the test serum sample. Any binding by specific IgG, or also IgM in the case of the SIA, is detected with an enzyme-conjugate of a goat anti-human immunoglobulin. For detection of anti-hantavirus IgM responses, mu-capture ELISA have been developed as a means to limit the incidence of false positive reactions such as those attributable to 'rheumatoid factors' and other interfering substances

(Ksiazek *et al.* 1995). To achieve this, mu-capture ELISAs usually first coat the ELISA plate with an anti-human IgM antibody that helps assure that only IgM molecules will be able to result in a signal when the test serum is added. The SIA, with current versions utilizing IgM and IgG conjugates in separate reactions, has proved very sensitive and does not suffer significant difficulties with interfering substances (Bharadwai *et al.* 2000).

Treatment and prognosis

No specific antiviral therapy is used in HFRS in Europe, although both interferon-alpha and ribavirin have been administered in trials in China and Korea with promising results (Bai *et al.* 1997; Rusnak *et al.* 2009). However, a problem is that at the time of hospitalization, virus replication is already declining and antiviral drugs would then come too late. Thus the treatment of HFRS is mainly symptomatic: maintenance of the fluid balance is important and treatment of acute renal insufficiency may necessitate kidney dialysis.

As indicated in Table 28.1, the case-fatality rate in HFRS varies extensively ranging from 0.1 to 10% depending, not only on the virus, but at least in the case of Puumala virus (PUUV) infections also on the host HLA genotype, as discussed above. PUUV infections, however, have long-term consequences that are important since PUUV infections are extremely common in several European countries and are apparently on the rise (see below). The hypophyseal damage at the acute stage of HFRS (Settergren *et al.* 1992; Hautala *et al.* 2002; Pekic *et al.* 2005) may lead to hypopituitarism, e.g. chronic fatigue, loss of weight and decreased testicle size, and need for hormone replacement therapy. More importantly, according to follow-up of hospitalized NE patients, 20% had after five years significantly increased blood pressure, cardiac pulse and proteinuria (Makela *et al.* 2000). After ten years of follow-up these long-term sequelae had largely, but not totally disappeared (Miettinen *et al.* 2006). In fact already in 1993 it was reported (Glass *et al.* 1993) that infection with rat-borne Seoul hantavirus in US residents was consistently associated with hypertensive renal disease. This finding was based on a large serological survey carried out in Baltimore.

Treatment of patients with HCPS is similar to that of most patients HFRS in that nonspecific and supportive measures are invoked and specific therapies including antiviral drugs are generally not used. ECMO, as described in a previous section, is a form of cardiopulmonary bypass that allows the patient to survive a state during which there is virtually completely shutdown of the patient's lungs and heart on a temporary (up to several days) basis. It has commonly been used in many centers to sustain term newborns who experience what would otherwise be severe pulmonary hypertension, but its use in adults has historically been far more limited. As a result, centers that encounter patients with HCPS only rarely are often not prepared to deploy ECMO. However, centers that have used the technology frequently have come to rely extensively on ECMO, where it is believed that its use has prevented the deaths of a significant fraction of patients with HCPS (Mertz *et al.* 2006; Dietl *et al.* 2008).

Human epidemiology and risk factors

Hantaviruses are globally important pathogens, but hantavirus diseases (HFRS and HCPS) are not recognized by the medical community in many countries including large areas of Europe (e.g. part of Eastern Europe) and South America, although the populations there may have a seroprevalence of several percent. The cases are missed simply because diagnostic tests are not used. A major reason for this in turn is that low-cost user-friendly diagnostic tests only recently have become available (Vaheri *et al.* 2008).

Globally most HFRS cases (an estimated 100,000) occur in China and neighbouring countries in Far East Asia. The number of HFRS cases in Russia can only be estimated. They occur mainly in European Russia (e.g. Udmurtia and Bashkiria) and may reach numbers as high as 10,000 per year. In Northern and Western Europe according to local statistics held by the national public health authorities (HFRS is a notifiable disease in most European countries), e.g. Belgium had 372 cases in 2005, Finland 3,200 cases in 2008, Germany 1,687 cases in 2007, and Sweden 2,195 cases in 2007. These high numbers are due partly to changes in climate (mild winters, more productive mast years yielding more oak and beech seeds for the rodents) but probably also to increasing recognition of HFRS by the medical community and more general use of hantaviral diagnostics.

Risk factors (Vapalahti *et al.* 1999) for acquiring HFRS include certain professions (forestry, farming, military) or outdoor activities (camping, summer cottages). Males are more likely to acquire hantavirus infection and children less likely than adults. Moreover, pediatric HFRS infections are, as a rule, mild. In the fall when frosts occur, rodents often enter human dwellings, e.g. including summer cottages, cow-houses, cellars, barns and wood and hay sheds. Humans are believed to contract the infections most frequently from inhalation of aerosols of rodent excreta and secreta (urine, faeces, saliva) and several recent studies indicate that hantaviruses are unexpectedly stable, up to ten days at room temperature (Kallio *et al.* 2006a; Hardestam *et al.* 2007) and probably longer at ambient winter temperatures. Therefore, it is important to ventilate closed spaces well before entering them. Rodent trapping (without poison) and holes in houses pose a risk. According to a recent case-control study cigarette smoking (Vapalahti *et al.* 2009) is a major risk factor for acquiring HFRS caused by PUUV.

Prevention and control

There is no specific treatment for HFRS and HPS and, in most parts of the world, there is no vaccine. Thus the most effective tool for mitigating the effects of human hantavirus disease worldwide is prevention. Except in the rare case of Andes virus in Patagonia, for which person-to-person transmission has been demonstrated (Enría *et al.* 1996; Wells *et al.* 1997; Padula *et al.* 1998), all HFRS and HPS cases arise from close contact with rodents or rodent-contaminated environments. Thus the most obvious prevention method is to avoid contact with rodents and rodent-occupied environments. Although partial control of *Rattus* species in urban and peridomestic environments may be achievable, it is neither practical nor desirable to eliminate wild rodents from nature. However, most HPS cases in the Americas probably occur in the peridomestic environment (Armstrong *et al.* 1995). Many HFRS cases, especially in northern Europe are also acquired in peridomestic habitats (Olsson *et al.* 2003). The presence of rodents in the peridomestic environment can be controlled at least partially; removal of rodents and their contamination can be done safely and the home environment can be modified to make it less attractive for rodents (CDC

2002). Rodent entry into even rustic, rural homes and cabins can be markedly reduced by simple and inexpensive modifications ('rodent-proofing') (Glass *et al.* 1997; Hoddenbach *et al.* 1997; Hopkins *et al.* 2002). Rodents found in homes or out-buildings should be removed by snap trapping, not by using live traps or glue boards which allow live rodents to continue to shed virus. Captured rodents, rodents found dead, or rodent excreta and nesting materials should be removed wearing rubber gloves and after wetting these potentially infectious materials and contaminated surfaces with a household disinfectant, dilute (5–10%) household bleach solution, or detergent. Rodent removal should always be accompanied by rodent-proofing to prevent re-infestation (Hopkins *et al.* 2002; Douglass *et al.* 2003). Environmental modification and attention to sanitation can decrease the attractiveness of peridomestic areas to rodents. Potential rodent shelter or garbage in the home environment should be removed or moved away from occupied structures and sources of food and water should be covered and protected. Particular risk has been associated with opening, occupying, and cleaning structures that have been unoccupied and infested by rodents for several weeks or months (Armstrong *et al.* 1995; Olsson *et al.* 2003; Teixeira *et al.* 2006). Such structures should be opened and allowed to air out for at least 30 minutes before entering to begin cleaning. Sweeping, vacuuming, and other activities that create aerosols should be avoided in favour of wetting contaminated surfaces with disinfectant or detergent and mopping or sponging. Several sources for detailed risk-reduction activities are available (Brummer-Korvenkontio *et al.* 1982; Hoddenbach *et al.* 1997; CDC 2002).

Several occupations have been identified as involving high-risk activities. These would include those persons who frequently handle or are exposed to wild rodents. These would include (for example) mammalogists, wildlife biologists, pest-control professionals, building and fire inspectors, soldiers, and some farm workers. Prevalence of infection was as high as 40% in Finnish mammalogists with more than 10 years experience (Vitek *et al.* 1996; Zeitz *et al.* 1997; Fritz *et al.* 2002; Fulhorst *et al.* 2007). Serosurveys of people in high-risk professions in the United States indicate that the risk of hantavirus infection in these groups is low (Mills *et al.* 1995; Murúa 1999; CDC 2002), nevertheless, special precautions, including use of high efficiency particulate air (HEPA) respirators have been recommended for handling live hantavirus host rodents in the Americas (Mills *et al.* 1995). As a minimum, those in high risk occupations should be educated concerning the risks and symptoms of hantavirus infection in their geographic areas, protective (e.g. latex or rubber) gloves should always be worn when handling host rodents whether they are alive or dead, and more stringent safety guidelines should be considered according to specific locations and circumstances.

A useful adjunct to appropriate targeting of risk-reduction activities and education is the knowledge of specific times and places of increased risk. When rodent monitoring programs identified high risk conditions in the southwestern USA following the El Nino conditions of 1997, local, State, and Federal public health authorities collaborated to produce educational programs, posters, and television and radio announcements reiterating prevention and safety messages. Although it is impossible to measure the impact of this initiative it is likely that morbidity and mortality associated with the epidemics in 1998 and 1999 were reduced. Predictive modelling efforts (now in their infancy) being pursued in the

Americas and in Europe hold promise for more accurate forecasting and more effective mitigation (Mills *et al.* in press; Tersago *et al.* 2008b).

Vaccines

The development of a safe, inexpensive and highly efficacious vaccine is a high priority to combat HFRS and HPS. However the worldwide distribution of these viruses and their high genetic diversity make development of such vaccines challenging. Early vaccine development efforts were focused in Asia due to the geographic distribution of at risk target populations. In the Republic of Korea a HTV virus vaccine, based on a formalin-inactivated HTN virus (ROK 84–105) derived from infected suckling mouse brains, has been shown to induce protective immunity in mice and humans (WHO 1991). However the protective effectiveness of the vaccine is strongly dependent on the number of doses, with the need of booster doses at 12 months in order to maintain a minimal protective antibody titre against HTV virus in humans (Cho and Howard 1999). The vaccine is produced commercially under the name Hantavax® and is licensed for use in the Republic of Korea. There are no licensed hantavirus vaccines for use outside of Asia and to date, no vaccines targeting viruses causing HPS. Schmaljohn and coworkers in the United States had developed a vaccinia-vectored recombinant vaccine against HTN involving expressing the S and M segment, which gives excellent humoral and cell-mediated immune responses in preclinical phase I and phase 2 trials (Schmaljohn *et al.* 1995). However, this vaccine did not elicit neutralizing antibodies in individuals previously vaccinated with vaccinia virus. These results terminated the vaccinia-HTNV based vaccine development and a shift was made to the development of a DNA based vaccine which ideally could elicit cross protection among major pathogenic hantaviruses. Initial trials on mice vaccinated with constructs expressing parts of the N protein have shown promising results on cross protection studies (Lindkvist *et al.* 2007). Also studies in nonhuman primates have demonstrated that DNA vaccination with a plasmid encoding the glycoproteins of ANDV and HNTV virus could elicit a long lasting immune response and neutralizing antibodies (Hooper *et al.* 2006). However further studies on mixing the M segment of HNTV and Puumala viruses have shown that a separate administration was necessary as a single immunization decreased their immunogenicity in hamsters (Spik *et al.* 2008). Recently, a non-replicating adeno vector expressing the ANDV structural proteins was shown to confer complete protection following a single dose vaccination of the Syrian hamster animal model (Safronetz *et al.* 2009). Although these results are extremely promising, pre-existing immunity to Ad5 among humans remains a substantial problem for these types of vaccines. The current literature on hantavirus vaccines leads to the conclusion that it may be necessary to prepare vaccines against multiple strains, although cross-protection may be possible among more closely related viruses.

References

Arai, S., Bennett, S.N., Sumibcay, L., Cook, J.A., *et al.* (2008a). Phylogenetically distinct hantaviruses in the masked shrew (*Sorex cinereus*) and dusky shrew (*Sorex monticolus*) in the United States. *Am. J. Trop. Med. Hyg.*, **78**: 348–51.

Arai, S., Ohdachi, S.D., Asakawa, M., Kang, H.J., *et al.* (2008b). Molecular phylogeny of a newfound hantavirus in the Japanese shrew mole (*Urotrichus talpoides*). *Proc. Nat. Acad. Sci. USA*, **105**: 16296–301.

Arai, S., Song, J.W., Sumibcay, L., Bennett, S.N., *et al.* (2007). Hantavirus in northern short-tailed shrew, United States. *Emerg. Infect. Dis.*, **13**: 1420–22.

Araki, K., Yoshimatsu, K., Ogino, M., Ebihara, H.,*et al.* (2001). Truncated hantavirus nucleocapsid proteins for serotyping Hantaan, Seoul, and Dobrava hantavirus infections. *J. Clin. Microbiol.*, **39**: 2397–404.

Armien, B., Pascale, J.M., Bayard, V., Mosca, I., *et al.* (2004). High seroprevalence of hantavirus infection on the Azuero peninsula of Panama. *Am. J. Trop. Med. Hyg.*, **70**: 682–87.

Armstrong, L.R., Zaki, S.R., Goldoft, M.J., Todd, R.L., *et al.* (1995). Hantavirus pulmonary syndrome associated with entering or cleaning rarely used, rodent-infested structures [letter]. *J. Infect. Dis.*, **172**: 1166.

Avsic-Zupanc, T., Xiao, S.Y., Stojanovic, R., Gligic, A., *et al.* (1992). Characterization of Dobrava virus: a hantavirus from Slovenia, Yugoslavia. *J. Med. Virol.*, **38**: 132–37.

Baek, L.J., Kariwa, H., Lokugamage, K., Yoshimatsu, K., *et al.* (2006). Soochong virus: an antigenically and genetically distinct hantavirus isolated from *Apodemus peninsulae* in Korea. *J. Med. Virol.*, **78**: 290–97.

Bai, J., Zhu, K., and Zhou, G. (1997). [The therapeutic effect of purified human leucocytic interferon-alpha on haemorrhagic fever with renal syndrome]. *Zhongh. Nei. Ke. Za. Zhi.*, **36**: 90–93.

Bayard, V.S., Kitsutani, P.D., Barria, E.O., Ruedas, L.A., *et al.* (2004). Outbreak of hantavirus pulmonary syndrome, Los Santos, Panama, 1999 to 2000. *Emerg. Infect. Dis.*, **10**: 1635–42.

Bennett, M., Lloyd, G., Jones, N., Brown, A., *et al.* (1990). Prevalence of antibody to hantavirus in some cat populations in Britain. *Vet. Rec.*, **127**: 548–49.

Bharadwaj, M., Nofchissey, R., Goade, D., Koster, F. and Hjelle, B. (2000). Humoral immune responses in the hantavirus cardiopulmonary syndrome. *J. Infect. Dis.*, **182**: 43–48.

Botten, J., Mirowsky, K., Kusewitt, D., Bharadwaj, M., *et al.* (2000). Experimental infection model for Sin Nombre hantavirus in the deer mouse (*Peromyscus maniculatus*). *Proc. Nat. Acad. Sci. USA*, **97**: 10578–83.

Botten, J., Mirowsky, K., Ye, C., Gottlieb, K., Saavedra, M., Ponce, L., and Hjelle, B. (2002). Shedding and intracage transmission of Sin Nombre hantavirus in the deer mouse (*Peromyscus maniculatus*) model. *J. Virol.*, **76**: 7587–94.

Brummer-Korvenkontio, M., Henttonen, H., and Vaheri, A. (1982). Hemorrhagic fever with renal syndrome in Finland: ecology and virology of nephropathia epidemica. *Scand. J. Infect. Dis.*, **36**: 88–91.

Brummer-Korvenkontio, M., Vaheri, A., Hovi, T., von Bonsdorff, C.H., *et al.* (1980). Nephropathia epidemica: Detection of antigen in bank voles and serologic diagnosis of human infection. *J. Infect. Dis.*, **141**: 131–34.

Calisher, C.H., Wagoner, K.D., Amman, B.R., Root, J.J., *et al.* (2007). Demographic factors associated with prevalence of antibody to Sin Nombre virus in deer mice in the western United States. *J. Wildl. Dis.*, **43**: 1–11.

Carey, D.E., Reuben, R., Panicker, K.N., Shope, R.E., and Myers, R.M. (1971). Thottapalayam virus: a presumptive arbovirus isolated from a shrew in India. *Indian J. Med. Res.*, **59**: 1758–60.

Carroll, D.S., Mills, J.N., Montgomery, J.M., Bausch, D.G., *et al.* (2005). Hantavirus pulmonary syndrome in central Bolivia: relationships between reservoir hosts, habitats, and viral genotypes. *Am. J. Trop. Med. Hyg.*, **72**: 54–58.

Castillo, C., Sanhueza, L., Tager, M., Munoz, S., Ossa, G., and Vial, P. (2002). Seroprevalence of antibodies against hantavirus in 10 communities of the IX Region of Chile where hantavirus infection were diagnosed. *Revista Med. Chile*, **130**: 251–58.

CDC (1998). Hantavirus pulmonary syndrome - Colorado and New Mexico, 1998. *Morb. Mort. Wkly. Rep.*, **47**: 449–52.

CDC (1999). Update: hantavirus pulmonary syndrome—United States, 1999. *Morb. Mort. Wkly. Rep.*, **48**: 521–25.

CDC (2002). Hantavirus pulmonary syndrome—United States: updated recommendations for risk reduction. *Morb. Mort. Wkly. Rep.*, **51**: 1–12.

Childs, J.E, Korch, G.W., Glass, G.E., LeDuc, J.W. and Shah, K.V. (1987). Epizootiology of hantavirus infections in Baltimore: isolation of a virus from Norway rats, and characteristics of infected rat populations. *Am. J. Epidemiol.*, **126**: 55–68.

Childs, J.E., Glass, G.E, Korch, G.W. and LeDuc, J.W. (1989). Effects of hantaviral infection on survival, growth and fertility in wild rat (*Rattus norvegicus*) populations of Baltimore, Maryland. *J. Wildl. Dis.*, **25**: 69–76.

Childs, J.E., Ksiazek, T.G., Spiropoulou, C.F., Krebs, J.W., *et al.* (1994). Serologic and genetic identification of *Peromyscus maniculatus* as the primary rodent reservoir for a new hantavirus in the southwestern United States. *J. Infect. Dis.*, **169**: 1271–80.

Cho, H. W., and Howard, C.R. (1999). Antibody responses in humans to an inactivated hantavirus vaccine (Hantavax). *Vaccine*, **17**: 2569–75.

Choi, Y., Kwon, Y.C., Kim, S.I., Park, J.M., Lee, K.H., and Ahn, B.Y. (2008). A hantavirus causing hemorrhagic fever with renal syndrome requires gC1qR/p32 for efficient cell binding and infection. *Virology*, **381**: 178–83.

Davis, S., Calvet, E., and Leirs, H. (2005). Fluctuating rodent populations and risk to humans from rodent-borne zoonoses. *Vector Borne Zoon. Dis.*, **5**: 305–14.

Diaz, M.O., Ziemin, S., Le Beau, M.M., Pitha, P., *et al.* (1988). Homozygous deletion of the alpha- and beta 1-interferon genes in human leukemia and derived cell lines. *Proc. Nat. Acad. Sci. USA*, **85**: 5259–63.

Dietl, C.A, Wernly, J.A., Pett, S.B., Yassin, S.F., *et al.* (2008). Extracorporeal membrane oxygenation support improves survival of patients with severe hantavirus cardiopulmonary syndrome. *J. Thora. Cardiov. Surg.*, **135**: 579–84.

Dohmae, K. and Nishimune, Y. (1995). Protection against hantavirus infection by dam's immunity transferred vertically to neonates. *Arch. Virol.*, **140**: 165–72.

Douglass, R.J., Kuenzi, A.J., Williams, C.Y., *et al.* (2003). Removing deer mice from buildings and the risk for human exposure to Sin Nombre virus. *Emerg. Infect. Dis.*, **9**: 390–92.

Douglass, R.J., Wilson, T., Semmens, W.J., Zanto, S.N., *et al.* (2001). Longitudinal studies of Sin Nombre virus in deer mouse dominated ecosystems of Montana. *Am. J. Trop. Med. Hyg.*, **65**: 33–41.

Elliott, L.H., Ksiazek, T.G., Rollin, P.E., Spiropoulou, C.F., *et al.* (1994). Isolation of the causative agent of hantavirus pulmonary syndrome. *Am. J. Trop. Med. Hyg.*, **51**: 102–8.

Enría, D., Padula, P., Segura, E.L., Pini, N., Edelstein, A., *et al.* (1996). Hantavirus pulmonary syndrome in Argentina - possibility of person to person transmission. *Medic. (Buenos Aires)*, **56**: 709–11.

Escutenaire, S. and Pastoret, P. (2002). Epidemiologie de l'infection par hantavirus en Belgique. *Bull. Memo. Acad. R. Med. Belgiq.*, **156**: 137–46.

Evander, M., Eriksson, I., Pettersson, L., Juto, P., Ahlm, C., *et al.* (2007). Puumala hantavirus viremia diagnosed by real-time reverse transcriptase PCR using samples from patients with hemorrhagic fever and renal syndrome. *J. Clin. Microbiol.*, **45**: 2491–97.

Ferrer, J.F., Jonsson, C.B., Esteban, E., Galligan, D., *et al.* (1998). High prevalence of hantavirus infection in Indian communities of the Paraguayan and Argentinean Gran Chaco. *Am. J. Trop. Med. Hyg.*, **59**: 438–44.

Figueiredo, L.T., Moreli, M.L., Borges, A.A., de Figueiredo, G.G., *et al.* (2009). Evaluation of an enzyme-linked immunosorbent assay based on Araraquara virus recombinant nucleocapsid protein. *Am. J. Trop. Med. Hyg.*, **81**: 273–76.

Foucar, K., Nolte, K.B., Feddersen, R.M., Hjelle, B., Jenison, S., *et al.* (1994). Outbreak of hantavirus pulmonary syndrome in the southwestern United States. Response of pathologists and other laboratorians. *Am. J. Clin. Path.*, **101** (4 Suppl 1): S1–5.

French, G.R., Foulke, R.S., Brand, O.A., Eddy, G.A., Lee, H.W., and Lee, P.W. (1981). Korean hemorrhagic fever: Propagation of the etiologic agent in a cell line of human origin. *Science*, 211: 1046–48.

Fritz, C.L., Fulhorst, C.F., Enge, B., Winthrop, K.L., Glaser, C.A., and Vugia, D.J. (2002). Exposure to rodents and rodent-borne viruses among persons with elevated occupational risk. *J. Occup. Environ. Med.*, 44: 962–67.

Fulhorst, C.F., Milazzo, M.L., Armstrong, L.R., Childs, J.E., *et al.* (2007). Hantavirus and arenavirus antibodies in persons with occupational rodent exposure. *Emerg. Infect. Dis.*, 13: 532–38.

Garcin, D., Lezzi, M., Dobbs, M., Elliott, R.M., Schmaljohn, C., Kang, C.Y., and Kolakofsky, D. (1995). The 5' ends of Hantaan virus (Bunyaviridae) RNAs suggest a prime- and-realign mechanism for the initiation of RNA synthesis. *J. Virol.*, 69: 5754–62.

Gavrilovskaya, I.N., Apekina, N.S., Bernshtein, A.D., *et al.* (1990). Pathogenesis of hemorrhagic fever with renal syndrome virus infection and mode of horizontal transmission of hantavirus in bank voles. *Arch. Virol.*, Suppl **1**: 57–62.

Glass, G.E., Childs, J.E., Korch, G.W., and LeDuc, J.W. (1988). Association of intraspecific wounding with hantaviral infection in wild rats (*Rattus norvegicus*). *Epidemiol. Infect.*, 101: 459–72.

Glass, G.E., Johnson, J.S., Hoddenbach, G.A., DiSalvo, C.L.J., *et al.* (1997). Experimental evaluation of rodent exclusion methods to reduce hantavirus transmission to humans in rural housing. *Am. J. Trop. Med. Hyg.*, 56: 359–64.

Glass, G.E., Watson, A.J., LeDuc, J.W., Kelen, G.D., Quinn, T.C., and Childs, J.E. (1993). Infection with a ratborne hantavirus in US residents is consistently associated with hypertensive renal disease. *J. Infect. Dis.*, 167: 614–20.

Gligic, A., Dimkovic, N., Xiao, S.Y., Buckle, G.J., *et al.* (1992). Belgrade virus: a new hantavirus causing severe hemorrhagic fever with renal syndrome in Yugoslavia. *J. Infect. Dis.*, 166: 113–20.

Goldsmith, C.S., Elliott, L.H., Peters, C.J., and Zaki, S.R. (1995). Ultrastructural characteristics of Sin Nombre virus, causative agent of hantavirus pulmonary syndrome. *Arch. Virol.*, 140: 2107–22.

Hardestam, J., Karlsson, M., Falk, K.I., Olsson, G., *et al.* (2008). Puumala hantavirus excretion kinetics in bank voles (*Myodes glareolus*). *Emerg. Infect. Dis.*, 14: 1209–15.

Hardestam, J., Simon, M., Hedlund, K.O., Vaheri, A., *et al.* (2007). Ex vivo stability of the rodent-borne Hantaan virus in comparison to that of arthropod-borne members of the Bunyaviridae family. *Appl. Environ. Microbiol.*, 73: 2547–51.

Hautala, T., Sironen, T., Vapalahti, O., Paakko, E., *et al.* (2002). Hypophyseal hemorrhage and panhypopituitarism during Puumala Virus Infection: magnetic resonance imaging and detection of viral antigen in the hypophysis. *Clin. Infect. Dis.*, 35: 96–101.

Henttonen, H., Buchy, P., Suputtamongkol, Y., Jittapalapong, S., *et al.* (2008). Recent discoveries of new hantaviruses widen their range and question their origins. *Ann. NY Acad. Sci.*, 1149: 84–89.

Hjelle, B., Spiropoulou, C.F., Torrez-Martinez, N., Morzunov, S., *et al.* (1994). Detection of Muerto Canyon virus RNA in peripheral blood mononuclear cells from patients with hantavirus pulmonary syndrome. *J. Infect. Dis.*, 170: 1013–17.

Hjelle, B., Jenison, S., Torrez-Martinez, N., Herring, B., *et al.* (1997). Rapid and specific detection of Sin Nombre virus antibodies in patients with hantavirus pulmonary syndrome by a strip immunoblot assay suitable for field diagnosis. *J. Clin. Microbiol.*, 35: 600–608.

Hoddenbach, G.A., Johnson, J., and Disalvo, C. (1997). *Mechanical Rodent Proofing Techniques*. National Park Service, Public Health Program. Washington, D.C.: US Department of Interior.

Hooper, J.W., Custer, D.M., Smith, J., and Wahl-Jensen, V. (2006). Hantaan/Andes virus DNA vaccine elicits a broadly cross-reactive neutralizing antibody response in nonhuman primates. *Virol.*, 347: 208–16.

Hopkins, A.S., Whitetail-Eagle, J., Corneli, A., Person, B., *et al.* (2002). Experimental evaluation of rodent exclusion methods to reduce hantavirus transmission to residents in a Native American community in New Mexico. *Vector Borne Zoon. Dis.*, 2: 61–68.

Hornfeldt, B. (2004). Long-term decline in numbers of cyclic voles in boreal Sweden: analysis and presentation of hypotheses. *Oikos*, 107: 376–92.

Hujakka, H., Koistinen, V., Eerikainen, P., Kuronen, I., *et al.* (2001). Comparison of a new immunochromatographic rapid test with a commercial EIA for the detection of Puumala virus specific IgM antibodies. *J. Clin. Virol.*, 23: 79–85.

Hujakka, H., Koistinen, V., Kuronen, I., Eerikainen, P., *et al.* (2003). Diagnostic rapid tests for acute hantavirus infections: specific tests for Hantaan, Dobrava and Puumala viruses versus a hantavirus combination test. *J. Virolog. Meth.*, 108: 117–22.

Hung, T., Chou, Z.Y., Zhao, T.X., Xia, S.M., and Hang, C.S. (1985). Morphology and morphogenesis of viruses of hemorrhagic fever with renal syndrome (HFRS). I. Some peculiar aspects of the morphogenesis of various strains of HFRS virus. *Intervirol.*, 23: 97–108.

Hutchinson, K.L., Peters, C.J., and Nichol, S.T. (1996). Sin Nombre virus mRNA synthesis. *Virol.*, 224: 139–49.

Hutchinson, K.L., Rollin, P.E., and Peters, C.J. (1998). Pathogenesis of a North American hantavirus, Black Creek Canal virus, in experimentally infected *Sigmodon hispidus*. *Am. J. Trop. Med. Hyg.*, 59: 58–65.

Jaaskelainen, K.M., Kaukinen, P., Minskaya, E.S., Plyusnina, A., *et al.* (2007). Tula and Puumala hantavirus NSs ORFs are functional and the products inhibit activation of the interferon-beta promoter. *J. Med. Virol.*, 79: 1527–36.

Jenison, S., Yamada, T., Morris, C., Anderson, B., *et al.* (1994). Characterization of human antibody responses to four corners hantavirus infections among patients with hantavirus pulmonary syndrome. *J. Virol.*, 68: 3000–3006.

Kallio, E.R., Klingstrom, J., Gustafsson, E., Manni, T., *et al.* (2006a). Prolonged survival of Puumala hantavirus outside the host: evidence for indirect transmission via the environment. *J. Gen. Virol.*, 87: 2127–34.

Kallio, E.R., Poikonen, A., Vaheri, A., Vapalahti, O., *et al.* (2006b). Maternal antibodies postpone hantavirus infection and enhance individual breeding success. *Proc. R. Soc. Biolog. Sci. Series B*, 273: 2771–76.

Kanerva, M., Mustonen, J., and Vaheri, A. (1998). Pathogenesis of Puumala and other hantavirus infections. *Rev. Med. Virol.*, 8: 67–86.

Kang, J.I., Park, S.H., Lee, P.W., and Ahn, B.Y. (1999). Apoptosis is induced by hantaviruses in cultured cells. *Virol.*, 264: 99–105.

Klempa, B., Fichet-Calvet, E., Lecompte, E., *et al.* (2006). Hantavirus in African wood mouse, Guinea. *Emer. Infect. Dis.*, 12: 838–40.

Klempa, B., Schmidt, H.A., Ulrich, R., Kaluz, S., *et al.* (2003). Genetic interaction between distinct Dobrava hantavirus subtypes in *Apodemus agrarius* and *A. flavicollis* in nature. *J. Virol.*, 77: 804–9.

Klingstrom, J., Plyusnin, A., Vaheri, A., and Lundkvist, A. (2002). Wild-type Puumala hantavirus infection induces cytokines, C-reactive protein, creatinine, and nitric oxide in cynomolgus macaques. *J. Virol.*, 76: 444–49.

Korch, G.W., Childs, J.E., Glass, G.E., Rossi, C.A. and LeDuc, J.W. (1989). Serologic evidence of hantaviral infections within small mammal communities of Baltimore, Maryland: spatial and temporal patterns and host range. *Am. J. Trop. Med. Hyg.*, 41: 230–40.

Koster, F., Foucar, K., Hjelle, B., Scott, A., Chong, Y.Y., *et al.* (2001). Rapid presumptive diagnosis of hantavirus cardiopulmonary syndrome by peripheral blood smear review. *Am. J. Clin. Path.*, 116: 665–72.

Kraus, A.A., Priemer, C., Heider, H., Kruger, D.H., and Ulrich, R. (2005). Inactivation of Hantaan virus-containing samples for subsequent investigations outside biosafety level 3 facilities. *Intervirol.*, 48: 255–61.

Krautkramer, E. and Zeier, M. (2008). Hantavirus causing hemorrhagic fever with renal syndrome enters from the apical surface and requires decay-accelerating factor (DAF/CD55). *J. Virol.*, 82: 4257–64.

Ksiazek, T.G., Peters, C.J., Rollin, P.E., Zaki, S., *et al.* (1995). Identification of a new North American hantavirus that causes acute pulmonary insufficiency. *Am. J. Trop. Med. Hyg.*, **52:** 117–23.

Kuenzi, A.J., Douglass, R.J., White, D., Bond, C.W., and Mills, J.N. (2001). Antibody to Sin Nombre virus in rodents associated with peridomestic habitats in west central Montana. *Am. J. Trop. Med. Hyg.*, **64:** 137–46.

Lee, H.W. (1982). Hemorrhagic fever with renal syndrome (HFRS). *Scan. J. Infect. Dis.*, **36:** 82–85.

Lee, H.W., Baek, L.J., and Johnson, K.M. (1982). Isolation of Hantaan virus, the etiologic agent of Korean hemorrhagic fever, from wild urban rats. *J. Infect. Dis.*, **146:** 638–44.

Lee, H.W., Lee, P.W., Baek, L.J., Song, C.K., and Seong, I.W. (1981). Intraspecific transmission of Hantaan virus, etiologic agent of Korean hemorrhagic fever, in the rodent *Apodemus agrarius*. *Am. J. Trop. Med. Hyg.*, **30:** 1106–12.

Lee, H.W., Lee, P.W., and Johnson, K.M. (1978). Isolation of the etiologic agent of Korean hemorrhagic fever. *J. Infect. Dis.*, **137:** 298–308.

Li, D., Schmaljohn, A.L., Anderson, K., and Schmaljohn, C.S. (1995). Complete nucleotide sequences of the M and S segments of two hantavirus isolates from California: evidence for reassortment in nature among viruses related to hantavirus pulmonary syndrome. *Virol.*, **206:** 973–83.

Li, X.D., Kukkonen, S., Vapalahti, O., Plyusnin, A., Lankinen, H., and Vaheri, A. (2004). Tula hantavirus infection of Vero E6 cells induces apoptosis involving caspase 8 activation. *J. Gen. Virol.*, **85:** 3261–68.

Li, X.D., Lankinen, H., Putkuri, N., Vapalahti, O., and Vaheri, A. (2005). Tula hantavirus triggers pro-apoptotic signals of ER stress in Vero E6 cells. *Virol.*, **333:** 180–89.

Linderholm, M., Sandstrom, T., Rinnstrom, O., Groth, S., *et al.* (1997). Impaired pulmonary function in patients with hemorrhagic fever with renal syndrome. *Clin. Infect. Dis.*, **25:** 1084–89.

Lindkvist, M., Lahti, K., Lilliehook, B., Holmstrom, A., Ahlm, C., and Bucht, G. (2007). Cross-reactive immune responses in mice after genetic vaccination with cDNA encoding hantavirus nucleocapsid proteins. *Vaccine*, **25:** 1690–99.

Lopez, N., Padula, P., Rossi, C., Lazaro, M.E., and Franze-Fernandez, M.T. (1996). Genetic identification of a new hantavirus causing severe pulmonary syndrome in Argentina. *Virol.*, **220:** 223–26.

Lundkvist, A., Cheng, Y., Sjolander, K.B., Niklasson, B., *et al.* (1997). Cell culture adaptation of Puumala hantavirus changes the infectivity for its natural reservoir, *Clethrionomys glareolus*, and leads to accumulation of mutants with altered genomic RNA S segment. *J. Virol.*, **71:** 9515–23.

Mackow, E.R. and Gavrilovskaya, I.N. (2001). Cellular receptors and hantavirus pathogenesis. *Curr. Top. Microbiol. Immunol.*, **256:** 91–115.

Madhav, N.K., Wagoner, K.D., Douglass, R.J., and Mills, J.N. (2007). Delayed density-dependent prevalence of Sin Nombre virus antibody in Montana deer mice (*Peromyscus maniculatus*) and implications for human disease risk. *Vector Borne Zoon. Dis.*, **7:** 353–64.

Mahonen, S.M., Sironen, T., Vapalahti, O., Paakko, E., *et al.* (2007). Puumala virus RNA in cerebrospinal fluid in a patient with uncomplicated nephropathia epidemica. *J. Clin. Virol.*, **40:** 248–51.

Makela, S., Kokkonen, L., Ala-Houhala, I., Groundstroem, K., *et al.* (2009). More than half of the patients with acute Puumala hantavirus infection have abnormal cardiac findings. *Scand. J. Infect. Dis.*, **41:** 57–62.

Makela, S., Ala-Houhala, I., Mustonen, J., Koivisto, A.M., *et al.* (2000). Renal function and blood pressure five years after Puumala virus-induced nephropathy. *Kidn. Intern.*, **58:** 1711–18.

Makela, S., Mustonen, J., la-Houhala, I., Hurme, M., *et al.* (2002). Human leukocyte antigen-B8-DR3 is a more important risk factor for severe Puumala hantavirus infection than the tumor necrosis factor-alpha (-308) G/A polymorphism. *J. Infect. Dis.*, **186:** 843–46.

Markotic, A., Hensley, L., Geisbert, T., Spik, K., and Schmaljohn, C. (2003). Hantaviruses induce cytopathic effects and apoptosis in continuous human embryonic kidney cells. *J. Gen. Virol.*, **84:** 2197–202.

Mertz, G.J., Hjelle, B., Crowley, M., Iwamoto, G., Tomicic, V., and Vial, P.A. (2006). Diagnosis and treatment of new world hantavirus infections. *Curr. Opin. Infect. Dis.*, **19:** 437–42.

Miettinen, M.H., Makela, S.M., Ala-Houhala, I.O., Huhtala, H.S., *et al.* (2006). Ten-year prognosis of Puumala hantavirus-induced acute interstitial nephritis. *Kidn. Intern.*, **69:** 2043–48.

Mills, J.N. (2005). Regulation of rodent-borne viruses in the natural host: implications for human disease. *Arch. Virol.*, **19:** 45–57.

Mills, J.N. (2006). Biodiversity loss and emerging infectious disease: an example from the rodent-borne hemorrhagic fevers. *Biodiv.*, **7:** 9–17.

Mills, J.N., Amman, B.R., and Glass, G.E. (2009). Biology of hantaviruses and their hosts in North America. *Vector-Borne Zoon. Dis.*, **9:** 1–12.

Mills, J.N. and Childs, J.E. (2001) Rodent-borne hemorrhagic fever viruses. In: E.S. Williams, and I.K. Barker (eds.) *Infectious Diseases of Wild Mammals*, pp. 254–70. Ames, IA: Iowa State University.

Mills, J.N., Ksiazek, T.G., Ellis, B.A., Rollin, P.E., *et al.* (1997). Patterns of association with host and habitat: antibody reactive with Sin Nombre virus in small mammals in the major biotic communities of the southwestern United States. *Am. J. Trop. Med. Hyg.*, **56:** 273–84.

Mills, J.N., Ksiazek, T.G., Peters, C.J., and Childs, J.E. (1999). Long-term studies of hantavirus reservoir populations in the southwestern United States: a synthesis. *Emerg. Infect. Dis.*, **5:** 135–42.

Mills, J.N., Yates, T.L., Childs, J.E., Parmenter, R.R., *et al.* (1995). Guidelines for working with rodents potentially infected with hantavirus. *J. Mammal.*, **76:** 716–22.

Mir, M.A., Duran, W.A., Hjelle, B.L., Ye, C., and Panganiban, A.T. (2008). Storage of cellular 5' mRNA caps in P bodies for viral cap-snatching. *Proc. Nat. Acad. Sci. USA*, **105:** 19294–99.

Murúa, R. (1999). Hantavirus in Chile: mammalogists as an occupational group of epidemiological risk. *Revista Chile. Hist. Natur.*, **72:** 7–12.

Murúa, R., Gonzalez, L.A., Gonzalez, M., and Jofre, C. (1996). Efectos del florecimiento del arbusto *Chusquea quila* Kunth (Poaceae) sobre la demografía de poblaciones de roedores de los bosques templados fríos del sur Chileno. *Bol. Socied. Biolog. Concepción, Chile*, **67:** 37–42.

Musser, G.G. and Carleton, M.D. (2005). Superfamily Muroidea. In: D.E. Wilson and D.M. Reeder (eds.) *Mammal species of the world, a taxonomic and geographic reference*, pp. 894–1531. Baltimore: Johns Hopkins University Press.

Mustonen, J., Brummer-Korvenkontio, M., Hedman, K., *et al.* (1994a). Nephropathia epidemica in Finland: a retrospective study of 126 cases. *Scand. J. Infect. Dis.*, **26:** 7–13.

Mustonen, J., Huttunen, N.P., Brummer-Korvenkontio, M., and Vaheri, A. (1994b). Clinical picture of nephropathia epidemica in children. *Acta Paediat.*, **83:** 526–29.

Mustonen, J., Partanen, J., Kanerva, M., Pietila, K., *et al.* (1996). Genetic susceptibility to severe course of nephropathia epidemica caused by Puumala hantavirus. *Kidn. Intern.*, **49:** 217–21.

Mustonen, J., Partanen, J., Kanerva, M., Pietila, K., *et al.* (1998). Association of HLA B27 with benign clinical course of nephropathia epidemica caused by Puumala hantavirus. *Scan. J. Immunol.*, **47:** 277–79.

Nakamura, I., Yoshimatsu, K., Lee, B.H., Okumura, M., *et al.* (2008). Development of a serotyping ELISA system for Thailand virus infection. *Arch. Virol.*, **153:** 1537–42.

Nichol, S.T., Beaty, B.J., Elliott, R.M., Goldbach, R., *et al.* (2005). Family Bunyaviridae. In: C.M. Fauquet, M.A. Mayo, *et al.* (eds.) *Virus taxonomy: eighth report of the International Committee on Taxonomy of viruses*, pp. 695–716. San Diego: Elsevier Academic Press.

Nichol, S.T., Spiropoulou, C.F., Morzunov, S., Rollin, P.E., *et al.* (1993). Genetic identification of a hantavirus associated with an outbreak of acute respiratory illness. *Sci.*, **262:** 914–17.

Niklasson, B., Hornfeldt, B., Lundkvist, A., Bjorsten, S., and LeDuc, J. (1995). Temporal dynamics of Puumala virus antibody prevalence in voles and of nephropathia epidemica incidence in humans. *Am. J. Trop. Med. Hyg.*, **53**: 134–40.

Nolte, K.B., Feddersen, R.M., Foucar, K., Zaki, S.R., et al. (1995). Hantavirus pulmonary syndrome in the United States: a pathological description of a disease caused by a new agent. *Hum. Path.*, **26**: 110–20.

Nowotny, N. (1994). The domestic cat: a possible transmitter of viruses from rodents to man. *Lancet*, **343**: 921.

Nowotny, N., Weissenboeck, H., Aberle, S., and Hinterdorfer, F. (1994). Hantavirus infection in the domestic cat. *JAMA*, **272**: 1100–1101.

Nuzum, E.O., Rossi, C.A., Stephenson, E.H., and LeDuc, J.W. (1988). Aerosol transmission of Hantaan and related viruses to laboratory rats. *Am. J. Trop. Med. Hyg.*, **38**: 636–40.

Ogino, M., Ebihara, H., Lee, B.H., Araki, K., et al. (2003). Use of vesicular stomatitis virus pseudotypes bearing Hantaan or Seoul virus envelope proteins in a rapid and safe neutralization test. *Clin. Diag. Lab. Immunol.*, **10**: 154–60.

Olsson, G.E., Dalerum, F., Hornfeldt, B., Elgh, F., Palo, T.R., Juto, P., and Ahlm, C. (2003). Human hantavirus infections, Sweden. *Emerg. Infect. Dis.*, **9**: 1395–401.

Olsson, G.E., Hjertqvist, M., Lundkvist, A., and Hornfeldt, B. (2009). Predicting high risk for human hantavirus infections, Sweden. *Emerg. Infect. Dis.*, **15**: 104–6.

Olsson, G.E., White, N., Ahlm, C., Elgh, F., Verlemyr, A.C., Juto, P., and Palo, R.T. (2002). Demographic factors associated with Hantavirus infection in bank voles (*Clethrionomys glareolus*). *Emerg. Infect. Dis.*, **8**: 924–29.

Padula, P.J., Edelstein, A., Miguel, S.D.L., et al. (1998). Hantavirus pulmonary syndrome outbreak in Argentina: molecular evidence for person-to-person transmission of Andes virus. *Virol.*, **241**: 323–30.

Padula, P.J., Rossi, C.M., Della Valle, M.O., Martínez, P.V., et al. (2000). Development and evaluation of a solid-phase enzyme immunoassay based on Andes hantavirus recombinant nucleoprotein. *J. Med. Microbiol.*, **49**: 149–55.

Pattamadilok, S., Lee, B.H., Kumperasart, S., Yoshimatsu, K., et al. (2006). Geographical distribution of hantaviruses in Thailand and potential human health significance of Thailand virus. *Am. J. Trop. Med. Hyg.*, **75**: 994–1002.

Pekic, S., Cvijovic, G., Stojanovic, M., Kendereski, A., Micic, D., and Popovic, V. (2005). Hypopituitarism as a late complication of hemorrhagic fever. *Endoc.*, **26**: 79–82.

Peters, C.J., Mills, J.N., Spiropoulou, C., Zaki, S.R., and Rollin, P.E. (2006). Hantavirus infections. In: R.L. Guerrant, D.H. Walker, and P.F. Weller (eds.) *Tropical Infectious Diseases: Principles Pathogens, and Practice*, pp. 762–80. Philadelphia: Elsevier.

Peters, C.J., Simpson, G.L., and Levy, H. (1999). Spectrum of hantavirus infection: hemorrhagic fever with renal syndrome and hantavirus pulmonary syndrome. *Ann. Rev. Med.*, **50**: 531–45.

Pettersson, L., Klingstrom, J., Hardestam, J., Lundkvist, A., et al. (2008). Hantavirus RNA in saliva from patients with hemorrhagic fever with renal syndrome. *Emerg. Infect. Dis.*, **14**: 406–11.

Plyusnin, A., Horling, J., Kanerva, M., Mustonen, J., Cheng, Y., et al. (1997). Puumala hantavirus genome in patients with nephropathia epidemica: correlation of PCR positivity with HLA haplotype and link to viral sequences in local rodents. *J. Clin. Microbiol.*, **35**: 1090–96.

Plyusnin, A. and Morzunov, S.P. (2001). Virus evolution and genetic diversity of hantaviruses and their rodent hosts. *Curr. Top. Microbiol. Immunol.*, **256**: 47–75.

Plyusnin, A., Mustonen, J., Asikainen, K., Plyusnina, A., et al. (1999). Analysis of Puumala hantavirus genome in patients with Nephropathia epidemica and rodent carriers from the sites of infection. *J. Med. Virol.*, **59**: 397–405.

Plyusnin, A., Vaheri, A., and Lundkvist, A. (2006). Saaremaa hantavirus should not be confused with its dangerous relative, Dobrava virus. *J. Clin. Microbiol.*, **44**: 1608–11.

Plyusnin, A., Vapalahti, O., Lankinen, H., Lehvaslaiho, H., et al. (1994). Tula virus: a newly detected hantavirus carried by European common voles. *J. Virol.*, **68**: 7833–39.

Poljak, M. and Avsic-Zupanc, T. (1994). Immunohistochemical detection of Hantaan virus antigen in renal tissue from patient with hemorrhagic fever with renal syndrome. *Nephr.*, **67**: 252.

Ramsden, C., Holmes, E.C., and Charleston, M.A. (2009). Hantavirus evolution in relation to its rodent and insectivore hosts: no evidence for codivergence. *Mol. Biol. Evolut.*, **26**: 143–53.

Ravkov, E.V., Nichol, S.T., and Compans, R.W. (1997). Polarized entry and release in epithelial cells of black creek canal virus, a new world hantavirus. *J. Virol.*, **71**: 1147–54.

Razzauti, M., Plyusnina, A., Henttonen, H., and Plyusnin, A. (2008). Accumulation of point mutations and reassortment of genomic RNA segments are involved in the microevolution of Puumala hantavirus in a bank vole (*Myodes glareolus*) population. *J. Gen. Virol.*, **89**: 1649–60.

Rizvanov, A.A., Khaiboullina, S.F., and St Jeor, S. (2004). Development of reassortant viruses between pathogenic hantavirus strains. *Virol.*, **327**: 225–32.

Rodriguez, L.L., Owens, J.H., Peters, C.J., and Nichol, S.T. (1998). Genetic reassortment among viruses causing hantavirus pulmonary syndrome. *Virol.*, **242**: 99–106.

Ruedas, L.A., Salazar-Bravo, J., Tinnin, D.S., Armien, B., et al. (2004). Community ecology of small mammal populations in Panama following an outbreak of hantavirus pulmonary syndrome. *J. Vector Ecol.*, **29**: 177–91.

Rusnak, J.M., Byrne, W.R., Chung, K.N., Gibbs, P.H., et al. (2009). Experience with intravenous ribavirin in the treatment of hemorrhagic fever with renal syndrome in Korea. *Antiv. Res.*, **81**: 68–76.

Safronetz, D., Hegde, N.R., Ebihara, H., Denton, M., et al. (2009). Adenovirus vectors expressing hantavirus proteins protect hamsters against lethal challenge with Andes virus. *J. Virol.*, **83**: 7285–95.

Saggioro, F.P, Rossi, M.A, Duarte, M.I, Martin, C.C., et al. (2007). Hantavirus infection induces a typical myocarditis that may be responsible for myocardial depression and shock in hantavirus pulmonary syndrome. *J. Infect. Dis.*, **195**: 1541–49. Epub 2007 Apr 5.

Schmaljohn, C.S., Chu, K.Y., Jennings, G.B., et al. (1995). Prospects for immunization to hantaviruses. *Proc. 3rd Intern. Confer. HFRS and Hantaviruses.* Helsinki, Finland. 31 May–3 June 1995, p. 52.

Schmaljohn, C.S., Hasty, S.E., Dalrymple, J.M., et al. (1985). Antigenic and genetic properties of viruses linked to hemorrhagic fever with renal syndrome. *Science*, **227**: 1041–44.

Schmaljohn, C.S. and Hjelle, B. (1997). Hantaviruses: A global disease problem. *Emerg. Infect. Dis.*, **3**: 95–104.

Schmaljohn, C.S. and Nichol, S.T. (2007). Bunyaviridae. In: B.N. Fields, D.M. Knipe and P.M. Howley (eds.) *Fields Virology*, pp. 1741–89. Philadelphia: Lippincott-Raven.

Settergren, B., Boman, J., Linderholm, M., Wistrom, J., Hagg, E., and Arvidsson, P.A. (1992). A case of nephropathia epidemica associated with panhypopituitarism and nephrotic syndrome. *Nephron*, **61**: 234–35.

Sironen, T., Klingstrom, J., Vaheri, A., Andersson, L.C., et al. (2008). Pathology of Puumala hantavirus infection in macaques. *PLoS ONE*, **3**: e3035.

Song, J.W., Gu, S.H., Bennett, S.N., Arai, S., et al. (2007a). Seewis virus, a genetically distinct hantavirus in the Eurasian common shrew (*Sorex araneus*). *Virol. J.*, **4**: 114.

Song, J.W., Kang, H.J., Song, K.J., Truong, T.T., et al. (2007b). Newfound hantavirus in Chinese mole shrew, Vietnam. *Emerg. Infect. Dis.*, **13**: 1784–87.

Spik, K.W., Badger, C., Mathiessen, I., Tjelle, T., et al. (2008). Mixing of M segment DNA vaccines to Hantaan virus and Puumala virus reduces their immunogenicity in hamsters. *Vaccine*, **26**: 5177–81.

Spiropoulou, C.F. (2001). Hantavirus maturation. *Curr. Top. Microbiol. Immunol.*, **256**: 33–46.

Täger Frey, M., Vial, P.C., Castillo, C.H., Godoy, P.M., *et al.* (2003). Hantavirus prevalence in the IX Region of Chile. *Emerg. Infect. Dis.*, **9**: 827–32.

Teixeira, K.G., Lavocat, M., Wada, M., and Elkhoury, M.R. (2006). Epidemiologia de hantavirose e da sindrome cardiopulmonar por hantavirus no Brasil no ano de 2005. *Bole. Eletron. Epidemiol.*, **6**: 1–5.

Temonen, M., Mustonen, J., Helin, H., Pasternack, A., *et al.* (1996). Cytokines, adhesion molecules, and cellular infiltration in nephropathia epidemica kidneys - an immunohistochemical study. *Clin. Immunol. Immunopath.*, **78**: 47–55.

Terajima, M., Hayasaka, D., Maeda, K., and Ennis, F.A. (2007). Immunopathogenesis of hantavirus pulmonary syndrome and hemorrhagic fever with renal syndrome: Do CD8+ T cells trigger capillary leakage in viral hemorrhagic fevers? *Immunol. Lett.*, **113**: 117–20.

Tersago, K., Schreurs, A., Linard, C., Verhagen, R., Van, D.S., and Leirs, H. (2008a). Population, environmental, and community effects on local bank vole (*Myodes glareolus*) Puumala virus infection in an area with low human incidence. *Vector Borne Zoonotic Dis.*, **8**: 235–44.

Tersago, K., Verhagen, R., Servais, A., Heyman, P., Ducoffre, G., and Leirs, H. (2008b). Hantavirus disease (nephropathia epidemica) in Belgium: effects of tree seed production and climate. *Epidemiol. Infect.*, **137**: 250–56.

Toro, J., Vega, J.D., Khan, A.S., Mills, J.N., Padula, P., *et al.* (1998). An outbreak of hantavirus pulmonary syndrome, Chile, 1997. *Emerg. Infect. Dis.*, **4**: 687–94.

Tuuminen, T., Kekalainen, E., Makela, S., Ala-Houhala, I., *et al.* (2007). Human CD8+ T cell memory generation in Puumala hantavirus infection occurs after the acute phase and is associated with boosting of EBV-specific CD8+ memory T cells. *J. Immunol.*, **179**: 1988–95.

Vaheri, A., Vapalahti, O., and Plyusnin, A. (2008). How to diagnose hantavirus infections and detect them in rodents and insectivores. *Rev. Med. Virol.*, **18**: 277–88.

Vapalahti, K., Paunio, M., Brummer-Korvenkontio, M., Vaheri, A., and Vapalahti, O. (1999). Puumala virus infections in Finland: increased occupational risk for farmers. *Am. J. Epidemiol.*, **149**: 1142–51.

Vapalahti, K., Virtala A.-M., Vaheri, A., and Vapalahti, O. (2010). Case-control study on Puumala virus infection, Finland: smoking is a major risk factor for hantavirus infection. *Epidemiol. Infect.*, **138**: 576–584.

Vapalahti, O., Lundkvist, A., Kukkonen, S.K.J., Cheng, Y., *et al.* (1996). Isolation and characterization of Tula virus, a distinct serotype in the genus *Hantavirus*, family Bunyaviridae. *J. Gen. Virol.*, **77**: 3063–67.

Vapalahti, O., Mustonen, J., Lundkvist, A., Henttonen, H., Plyusnin, A., and Vaheri, A. (2003). Hantavirus infections in Europe. *Lancet Infect. Dis.*, **3**: 653–61.

Vial, P.A., Valdivieso, F., Mertz, G., Castillo, C., *et al.* (2006). Incubation period of hantavirus cardiopulmonary syndrome. *Emerg. Infect. Dis.*, **12**: 1271–73.

Vitek, C.R., Ksiazek, T.G., Peters, C.J., Robert, F., and Breiman, R.F. (1996). Evidence against infection with hantaviruses among forest and park workers in the southwestern United States. *Clin. Infect. Dis.*, **23**: 283–85.

Wells, R.M., Estani, S.S., Yadon, Z.E., Enría, D., *et al.* (1997). An unusual hantavirus outbreak in southern Argentina: person-to-person transmission? *Emerg. Infect. Dis.*, **3**: 171–74.

WHO (1991). Working group on the development of a rapid diagnostic method and vaccine for haemorrhagic fever with renal syndrome. RS/91/GE/19 (Kor), pp. 1–9. Seoul, Republic of Korea.

Williams, R.J., Bryan, R.T., Mills, J.N., Palma, R.E., *et al.* (1997). An outbreak of hantavirus pulmonary syndrome in western Paraguay. *Am. J. Trop. Med. Hyg.*, **57**: 274–82.

Wilson, D.E. and Reeder, D.M. (2005). *Mammal Species of the World*, (3 edn.), pp. 2142. Baltimore: Johns Hopkins University Press.

Yadav, P.D., Vincent, M.J., and Nichol, S.T. (2007). Thottapalayam virus is genetically distant to the rodent-borne hantaviruses, consistent with its isolation from the Asian house shrew (*Suncus murinus*). *Virol. J.*, **4**: 80.

Yahnke, C.J., Meserve, P.L., Ksiazek, T.G., and Mills, J.N. (2001). Patterns of infection with Laguna Negra virus in wild populations of *Calomys laucha* in the central Paraguayan Chaco. *Am. J. Trop. Med. Hyg.*, **65**: 768–76.

Yanagihara, R., Amyx, H.L., and Gajdusek, D.C. (1985). Experimental infection with Puumala virus, the etiologic agent of nephropathia epidemica, in bank voles (*Clethrionomys glareolus*). *J. Virol.*, **55**: 34–38.

Yanagihara, R., Gajdusek, D.C., Gibbs Jr., C.J., and Traub, R. (1984). Prospect Hill virus: serological evidence for infection in mammalogists. *N. Engl. J. Med.*, **310**: 1325–26.

Yanagihara, R. and Silverman, D.J. (1990). Experimental infection of human vascular endothelial cells by pathogenic and nonpathogenic hantaviruses. *Arch. Virol.*, **111**: 281–86.

Yashina, L., Mishin, V., Zdanovskaya, N., Schmaljohn, C., and Ivanov, L. (2001). A newly discovered variant of a hantavirus in *Apodemus peninsulae*, far eastern Russia. *Emerg. Infect. Dis.*, **7**: 912–13.

Yates, T.L., Mills, J.N., Parmenter, C.A., Ksiazek, T.G., *et al.* (2002). The ecology and evolutionary history of an emergent disease: hantavirus pulmonary syndrome. *Biosci.*, **52**: 989–98.

Young, J.C., Hansen, G.R., Graves, T.K., Deasy, M.P., *et al.* (2000). The incubation period of hantavirus pulmonary syndrome. *Am. J. Trop. Med. Hyg.*, **62**: 714–17.

Zaki, S.R., Greer, P.W., Coffield, L.M., Goldsmith, C.S, *et al.* (1995). Hantavirus pulmonary syndrome. Pathogenesis of an emerging infectious disease. *Am. J. Path.*, **146**: 552–79.

Zeitz, P.S., Graber, J.M., Voorhees, R.A., Kioski, C., *et al.* (1997). Assessment of occupational risk for hantavirus infection in Arizona and New Mexico. *J. Occup. Environ. Med.*, **39**: 463–67.

CHAPTER 29

Herpes B virus (Cercopithecine Herpes 1)

David W. G. Brown

Summary

Herpes B virus or Cercopithecine herpes 1 as it is formally classi-fied causes a persistent infection of monkeys of the *Macaca* genus. In monkey colonies and social groups, it is transmitted by close contact and sexually. Human infection is rare with less than 50 human cases described. It has been seen in monkey handlers exposed to infected monkeys following bites, scratches and abraded skin. Infection has also been recognized in two cases following exposure through laboratory work. Following an incubation period of 9–59 days typically an ascending encephalomyelitis develops which is fatal in 80% of cases. Prevention and control of the risk of B virus is based on avoiding direct contact with infected animals by screening, following handling guidelines for monkeys used in bio-medical research and rigorous laboratory safety precautions. Treatment with acyclovir has been successful and halved mortality in recent cases. It is also recommended for prophylaxis in potential exposures.

History

B virus was first isolated in 1932 from Dr W.B. who developed a fatal acute ascending myelitis following a bite on the dorsum of the left ring and little fingers by an apparently normal rhesus monkey (*Macaca mulatto*). Three days after the bite pain and swelling were noticed at the bite site, and he was admitted to hospital after 6 days with a fever, superficial redness at the bite site and lymphangitis. Subsequently vesicles developed at the bite site followed by gener-alized abdominal cramps, nausea and vomiting. Thirteen days after the bite hyperaesthesia of the lower limbs developed and neuro-logical examination revealed generalized hyperalgesia below the umbilicus, and a flaccid paralysis with absent reflexes. The paraes-thesia progressed rapidly and the patient died of respiratory paral-ysis 16 days after the bite.

Clinical samples from this case were investigated separately by two groups: Gay and Holden (1933) reported the isolation of a herpes virus from postmortem material. They proposed the name W virus and suggested the virus was a variant of herpes simplex. In 1934 Sabin and Wright isolated a filterable agent from brain, medulla, spinal cord and spleen by intracranial and intradermal inoculation of rabbits. They named the agent B virus and suggested

it was distinct from herpes simplex. This name was universally adopted and is often used together with the descriptive term herpes virus simiae in the literature.

A second case was reported by Sabin 1949 in which an investiga-tor contracted a fatal neurological illness following contamination of a minor cut by monkey saliva. At the same time sera from macaques were shown to contain neutralizing antibodies to B virus. This, together with the exposure history of the two human cases, led to the recognition that B virus was a monkey virus. However, it was not until 1954 that Melnick and Banker isolated B virus from its natural host, when virus was cultured from the brain of a rhesus monkey in the course of studies of polio virus. Subsequent sero-logical studies showed that B virus infection was widespread in a range of macaque species. B virus infection was first linked to dis-ease in its natural hosts species when Keeble and colleagues in 1958 reported herpes-like ulcers on the lips and tongues of recently imported rhesus monkeys, from which B virus was subsequently isolated. Subsequently B virus infection was shown to be wide-spread in many macaque species. Less than 50 human cases have been reported since the original report and these all occurred fol-lowing contact with macaques species or their tissues in the course of biomedical research.

The agent

Herpes B virus, or herpes simiae as it is sometimes called is now formally classified as Cercopithecine herpes virus type 1 (Murphy *et al.* 1995). It is a herpes virus, a member of the genus simplex virus which is part of the α-herpes subfamily (Murphy *et al.* 1995).

Simplex viruses have been isolated from several primates species, and Table 29.1 lists the primate species from which simplex viruses have been isolated. B virus is closely related antigenically and genomically to other primate simplex viruses, such as human herpes simplex viruses (HSV) and simian agent 8 (SA8) in African green monkeys (Malherbe and Strickland 1970). The close relationship between the viruses in different species (HSV, SA8, B virus) reflects a common evolutionary origin. Thus the diversity of the primate simplex viruses is likely to have evolved with the individual host species following the introduction of a progenitor herpes virus into a common ancestor in the primate evolutionary line.

Table 29.1 Recognized Primate Simplex viruses by host species

Primate family	Primate species (Common name)	Indigenous alphaherpesvirus
1. Catarrhini	Macaque	B Virus (Cercopithecine Herpes 1)
Old World Monkeys	Baboon	
Apes	African Green Monkey	Herpes papio 2 (Cercopithicine herpes 16)
	Colobines	Simian Agent 8 (Cercopithecine 2)
	Orang-utan	
	Gorilla	
	Chimpanzee	Herpes simplex 1 &2 (Human Herpes virus 1 &2)
2. Platyrrhihi	Humans	
	Gibbons	
	Marmoset	
New World Monkeys	Capuchin	Herpes Virus Tamarinus (Saimirine Herpes 1)
	Squirrel	
	Aotus	
	Howler	
	Woolly	
	Spider	Spider monkey Herpevirus (Ateline Herpes 1)

The antigenic, genomic and biological characteristics of B virus have received only limited investigation (Hull 1973; Weigler 1992; Whitley 1993). These properties are very similar to the better known HSV (Roizman 1982). Electron microscopy of B virus infected tissue culture demonstrated that B virus has typical herpes virus morphology. Virions range between 100 and 200 nm in diameter and consist of an electron-dense core with iscohedral structure of 100–110 nm surrounded by the viral tegument and envelope (Reubner et al. 1975).

B virus is a double-stranded DNA virus, its genome has a molecular weight of 107×10^6 Da which corresponds to a genome size of 162 kbp. B virus DNA has a very high G + C content of 75% (Whitley 1993). The genomic structure of B virus has recently been fully determined. It is known that the B virus genome, like that of HSV, forms four isomers, which differ with respect of the orientation of large and small unique regions (Harrington et al. 1992). Sequence data for B virus in the unique small (US) region (Bennett et al. 1992; Killeen et al. 1992; Slomka et al. 1995). The genome organization in the US region shows co-linearity with equivalent HSV genes. Glycoprotein D (US6) and glycoprotein J (US5) homologues in B virus have been fully sequenced and show 69% and 57% amino acid identity with HSV-1, respectively (Bennett et al. 1992). The glycoprotein G equivalent has been characterized and shown to be similar in size to HSV-2 (593 amino acids) but shares little amino acid similarity with HSV-1 and HSV-2 (Slomka et al. 1995). Recently the

complete genome (Peretygina et al. 2003) sequence of Herpes B virus and SA8 (Tyler et al. 2005) have been described. The genome arrangements are similar to other simplex viruses with unique long and unique short regions boarded by two sets of inverted repeats. They have high G&C content 74 and 76% respectively. Both viruses contain the same range of genes as HSV with the exception of HSVy, 34.5 (RL ORF) a gene responsible for neuro-virulence in human herpes simplex.

B virus, SA8, and HSV show extensive antigenic cross-reactivity, in many test systems (Cabasso et al. 1967; Pauli and Ludwig 1977; Hutt et al. 1981; Ludwig et al. 1983; Hilliard et al. 1989). More than 50 B virus polypeptide bands have been identified by electrophoresis and immune precipitation of tissue-culture-grown virus. At least nine glycoprotein bands have been identified and the gD and gB shown to share antigenic determinants with HSV-1. Multiple other infected cell polypeptides (ICPs) produced in tissue culture infected with B virus have been shown by Western blot and immune precipitation to share antigenic determinants with HSV (Hilliard et al. 1989).

Replication

B virus grows to high titre in a range of cell lines derived from several species, including primary monkey kidney, chick embryo cell lines and vero E6 cells, which are all suitable for diagnostic isolation. In these cell lines typically B virus produces a characteristic syncytial cytopathic effect. B virus can be propagated on the chorio-allantoic membrane of embryonated eggs (Burnett et al. 1939). B virus will produce a clinical illness in mice, rabbits and New World monkeys following intradermal inoculation (Sabin and Wright 1934; Gosztonyi et al. 1992).

The reproductive cycle of B virus is short: host-cell DNA synthesis is inhibited within 4 hours after infection and infectious virus is detectable within 6 hours. Peak virus levels are found between 24 and 35 hours after infection. B virus, like other herpes viruses, causes intranuclear inclusions in cell culture.

Non-human primate infection
Epizoology

B virus has been most extensively studied in rhesus and cynomolgus monkeys, because these two species are most widely used for biomedical research. B virus probably occurs in all macaque species and it has been isolated from naturally infected rhesus (*M. mulatta*), cynomolgus (*M. fascicularis*), bonnet (*M. radiata*) monkeys and *M. cyclopis* (Endo et al. 1960; Hartley 1964; Espana 1973). B virus antibodies have been detected in most macaque species (Shah and Morrison, 1969; DiGiacano and Shah 1972; Palmer 1987) (Lee et al. 2007). B virus antibodies have also been detected in sera from a range of African primates and humans (Van Hoosier and Melnick 1961; Cabasso 1967), but these represent antibodies against the closely related SA8 and HSV viruses, since B virus specific antibody tests have only recently been developed (Katz et al. 1986; Norcott and Brown 1993).

Several studies have investigated the age of acquisition of B virus antibodies in macaques (Palmer 1987). Interpretation of the published studies is complicated because some refer to wild-caught and others to colony-held monkeys, and several factors can affect the acquisition of antibody. However, a few general points can be

Slomka, M. J., Harrington, L., Arnold, G., Norcott, J. P. N., and Brown, D. W. G. (1995). Complete nucleotide sequence of the Herpesvirus simiae glycoprotein G gene and its expression as an immunogenic fusion protein in bacteria. *J. Gen. Virol.*, **76:** 2161–68.

Tyler, S. D., Peters, G. A., and Severini, A. (2005). Complete genome sequence of cercopithecine herpesvirus 2 (SA8) and comparison with other simplexviruses. *Virol.*, **331**(2): 429–40.

Van Hoosier, G. L. and Melnick, J. L. (1961). Neutralizing antibodies in human sera to Herpesvirus simiae (B virus). *Texas Rep. Biolog. Med.*, **19:** 376–80.

Vizoso, A. D. (1975). Recovery of Herpes simiae (B virus) from both primary and latent infections in rhesus monkeys. *Br. J. Experim. Pathol.*, **56:** 485–88.

Wall, L. V. M., Zwartouw, H. T., and Kelly, D. C. (1989). Discrimination between twenty isolates of herpesvirus simiae (B virus) by restriction enzyme analysis of the viral genome. *Vir. Res.*, **12:** 283–96.

Wansbrough-Jones, M. H., Jones, M. H., Cooper, B., and Sarantis, N. (1989). Prophylaxis against B virus infection. *BMJ*, **297:** 909.

Ward, J. A., Hilliard, J. K., and Pearson, S. (2000). Herpes B-virus specific Pathogen free breeding colonies of macaques (Macaca Mulatta): diagnostic testing before and after elimination of the infection. *Comp. Med.*, **50**(3): 317–22.

Weigler, B. J. (1992). Biology of B virus in macaque and human hosts: A review. *Clin. Infect. Dis.*, **14:** 555–67.

Weigler, B. J., Roberts, J. A., Hird, D. W., Lerche, N. W., and Hilliard, J. K. (1990). A cross sectional survey for B virus antibody in a colony of group housed rhesus macaques. *Lab. Anim. Sci.*, **40:** 257–61.

Weigler, B. J., Hird, D. W., Hilliard, J. K., Lerche, N. W., *et al.* (1993). Epidemiology of cercopithecine herpesvirus 1 (B virus) infection and shedding in a large breeding cohort of rhesus macaques. *J. Infect. Dis.*, **167:** 257–63.

Wells, D. L. *et al.* (1989). Herpesvirus simiae contamination of primary rhesus monkey kidney cell cultures: CDC recommendations to minimize risks to laboratory personnel. *Diag. Microbiol. Infect. Dis.*, **12:** 333–35.

Whitley, R. J. (1993). The biology of B virus (Cercopithecine virus 1). In: B. Roizman and R. J. Whitley (eds.) The human herpesviruses, pp. 317–28. New York: Raven Press.

Zwartouw, H. T. and Boulter, E. A. (1984). Excretion of B virus in monkeys and evidence of genital infection. *Lab. Anim. Sci.*, **18:** 65–70.

Zwartouw, H. T., Macarthur, J. A., Boulter, E. A., *et al.* (1984). Transmission of B virus infection between monkeys especially in relation to breeding colonies. *Lab. Anim.*, **18:** 125–30.

Zwartouw, H. T., Humphreys, C. R., and Collins, P. (1989). Oral chemotherapy of fatal B virus (herpesvirus simiae) infection. *Antiv. Res.*, **11:** 275–83.

CHAPTER 30

Influenza

I. H. Brown, D. J. Alexander, N. Phin
and M. Zuckerman

Summary

Influenza is a highly infectious, acute illness which has affected humans and animals since ancient times. Influenza viruses form the Orthomyxoviridae family and are grouped into types A, B, and C on the basis of the antigenic nature of the internal nucleocapsid or the matrix protein. Influenza A viruses infect a large variety of animal species, including humans, pigs, horses, sea mammals, and birds, occasionally producing devastating pandemics in humans, such as in 1918 when it has been estimated that between 50–100 million deaths occurred worldwide.

There are two important viral surface glycoproteins, the haemagglutinin (HA) and neuraminidase (NA). The HA binds to sialic acid receptors on the membrane of host cells and is the primary antigen against which a host's antibody response is targeted. The NA cleaves the sialic acid bond attaching new viral particles to the cell membrane of host cells allowing their release. The NA is also the target of the neuraminidase inhibitor class of antiviral agents that include oseltamivir and zanamivir and newer agents such as peramivir. Both these glycoproteins are important antigens for inducing protective immunity in the host and therefore show the greatest variation.

Influenza A viruses are classified into 16 antigenically distinct HA (H1–16) and 9 NA subtypes (N1–9). Although viruses of relatively few subtype combinations have been isolated from mammalian species, all subtypes, in most combinations, have been isolated from birds. Each virus possesses one HA and one NA subtype (Tables 30.1 and 30.2).

Last century, the sudden emergence of antigenically different strains in humans, termed antigenic shift, occurred on three occasions, 1918 (H1N1), 1957 (H2N2) and 1968 (H3N2), resulting in pandemics. The frequent epidemics that occur between the pandemics are as a result of gradual antigenic change in the prevalent virus, termed antigenic drift. Epidemics throughout the world occur in the human population due to infection with influenza A viruses, such as H1N1 and H3N2 subtypes, or with influenza B virus. Phylogenetic studies have led to the suggestion that aquatic birds that show no signs of disease could be the source of many influenza A viruses in other species. The 1918 H1N1 pandemic strain is thought to have arisen as a result of spontaneous mutations within an avian H1N1 virus. However, most pandemic strains, such as the 1957 H2N2, 1968 H3N2 and 2009 pandemic H1N1, are considered to have emerged by genetic re-assortment of the segmented RNA genome of the virus, with the avian and human influenza A viruses infecting the same host.

Influenza viruses do not pass readily between humans and birds but transmission between humans and other animals has been demonstrated. This has led to the suggestion that the proposed re-assortment of human and avian influenza viruses takes place in an intermediate animal with subsequent infection of the human population. Pigs have been considered the leading contender for the role of intermediary because they may serve as hosts for productive infections of both avian and human viruses, and there is good evidence that they have been involved in inter-species transmission of influenza viruses; particularly the spread of H1N1 viruses to humans. Apart from public health measures related to the rapid identification of cases and isolation, the main control measures for influenza virus infection in human populations involves immunization and antiviral prophylaxis or treatment.

History

The highly infectious, acute respiratory illness now known as influenza has affected human beings since ancient times. The individual symptoms and epidemiological characteristics of the disease are sufficiently distinct that it is possible to identify a number of major epidemics in the distant past. One such epidemic was recorded by Hippocrates in 412 BC, and numerous episodes were described in the Middle Ages.

The name influenza has its origins in early fifteenth century Italy and was adopted in Europe to explain the sudden and unexpected appearance of an epidemic disease thought to be under the influence of the stars (Kaplan and Webster 1977).

The first well-recorded pandemic in humans, in which mortality was frequently high, particularly in densely populated areas, occurred in 1580 and was believed to have originated in Asia before spreading to Africa and Europe. During the following three centuries, although record keeping was irregular and reporting was often inaccurate, there were recognizable clinical accounts of a number of serious influenza pandemics. Retrospective research partially identified the virus responsible for the first pandemic of 1889 by testing for influenza antibodies in serum of people who were alive at that time (Tumova 1980).

Table 30.1 Haemagglutinin (HA) subtypes of influenza A viruses isolated from humans, pigs, horses, and birds

Subtype	Examples[a] of viruses of the subtype isolated from the specified host group			
	Humans	Pigs	Horses	Birds
H1	PR/8/34 (H1N1)	Swine/Iowa/15/30 (H1N1)	—[b]	Duck/Alberta/35/76 (H1N1)
H2	Singapore 1/57 (H2N2)	–	–	Duck/Germany/1215/73 (H2N3)
H3	Hong Kong 1/68 (H3N2)	Swine/Taiwan/70 (H3N2)	Equine/Miami/1/63 (H3N8)	Duck/Ukraine/1/63 (H3N8)
H4	–	–	–	Duck/Czechoslovakia/56 (H4N6)
H5	–	–	–	Tern/S. Africa/61 (H5N3)
H6	–	–	–	Turkey/Massachusetts/3740/65 (H6N2)
H7	–	–	Equine/Prague/1/56 (H7N7)	FPV/Dutch/27 (H7N7)
H8	–	–	–	Turkey/Ontario/6118/68 (H8N4)
H9	–	–	–	Turkey/Wisconsin/1/66 (H9N2)
H10	–	–	–	Chicken/Germany/N/49 (H10N7)
H11	–	–	–	Duck/England/56 (H11N6)
H12	–	–	–	Duck/Alberta/60/76 (H12N5)
H13	–	–	–	Gull/Maryland/704/77 (H13N6)
H14	–	–	–	Duck/Gurjev/263/82 (H14N5)
H15	–	–	–	Duck/Australia/341/83 (H15N8)

[a] The reference strains of influenza viruses, or the first isolates of the subtype from the host group.
[b] Not found in this species.

Possibly the most devastating influenza pandemic recorded occurred in 1918. It has been estimated that during this pandemic between 50–100 million deaths occurred throughout the world and that in resource rich countries, such as the USA, about 0.5% of the population died. In some parts of Alaska and the Pacific islands more than half the population was lost. In the USA alone it is estimated that life expectancy following the 1918 pandemic dropped by 12 years. There was an enormous impact on society in terms of mortality, morbidity, and economic factors. At the height of the epidemic community life in many cities was brought almost to a standstill. The repercussions of the pandemic were felt by armed forces engaged in the First World War, with some 43,000 deaths in the USA forces alone, representing about 80% of the total number of USA battle deaths in the war. The 1918 to 1919 influenza pandemic was caused by an influenza A H1N1 virus and sequence analysis of virus recovered from autopsy paraffin-embedded formalin fixed lung tissue suggested an avian source that became adapted to mammals (Reid *et al.* 2000). The virus is genetically distinct

Table 30.2 Neuraminidase (NA) subtypes of influenza A viruses isolated from humans, pigs, horses, and birds

Subtype	Examples[a] of viruses of the subtype isolated from the specified host group			
	Humans	Pigs	Horses	Birds
N1	PR/8/34 (H1N1)	Swine/Iowa/15/30 (H1N1)	—[b]	Chicken/Scotland/59 (H5N1)
N2	Singapore/1/57 (H2N2)	Swine/Taiwan/70 (H3N2)	–	Turkey/Massachusetts/3740/65 (H6N2)
N3	–	–	–	Tern/S. Africa/61 (H5N3)
N4	–	–	–	Turkey/Ontario/6118/68 (H8N4)
N5	–	–	–	Shearwater/Australia/1/72 (H6N5)
N6	–	–	–	Duck/Czechoslovakia/56 (H4N6)
N7	–	Swine/England/92 (H1N7)	Equine/Prague/1/56 (H7N7)	FPV/Dutch/27 (H7N7)
N8	–	–	Equine/Miami/1/63 (H3N8)	Duck/Ukraine/1/63 (H3N8)
N9	–	–	–	Duck/Memphis/546/74 (H11N9)

[a] The reference strains of influenza viruses, or the first isolates of the subtype from the host group.
[b] Not found in this host group.

from any of the avian or mammalian influenza virus sequences analysed from that time onwards (Basler *et al.* 2001; Reid *et al.* 2003, 2004; Taubenberger *et al.* 1997, 2003, 2005). Clinical and autopsy reports have demonstrated that the high morbidity and mortality rates were due to aggressive brochopneumonia due to secondary bacterial infections (Morens *et al.* 2010). At that time, the range of antibiotics that can now be used to effectively treat these infections were not available. In addition, there may have been an immunopathogenic cause leading to acute respiratory distress syndrome (ARDS) due to cytokine storms in some individuals. There was a high mortality rate at all ages, but especially among the 20 to 40 year age group. This may have been due to a vigorous immune response characterized by a release of pro-inflammatory cytokines or an antibody dependent enhancement of the response having been exposed to other influenza viruses in the past (Cheung *et al.* 2002).

For centuries there had been wild speculation regarding the cause of influenza, but by the end of the nineteenth century the microbiological concept of infectious disease had become accepted. Following on from this was the discovery of a bacillus in the throats of many influenza patients. This bacillus, *Haemophilus influenzae*, was for many years the leading suspect for the causative agent of influenza. The first evidence of the true viral cause came in the late 1920s when a virus was found in pigs showing disease similar to influenza in humans and successfully transmitted between pigs using filtered material. A related strain was finally isolated from a human patient in 1933 by inoculating a filtrate of throat washings into the noses of ferrets. Rapid progress followed the demonstration that influenza virus could be transmitted to ferrets and mice.

A second type of influenza virus from man was transmitted experimentally to ferrets in 1940. This virus was designated influenza B to distinguish it from the first type found, which became known as influenza A. In 1933 it was found that influenza viruses would multiply in cells lining the allantoic cavity of the developing chicken embryo. This was followed by the observation that infective allantoic fluid caused agglutination of chicken red blood cells, also referred to as haemagglutination. These developments laid the foundations for early work on influenza viruses and these techniques are still used when carrying out work with influenza viruses. The haemagglutination reaction could be inhibited by specific serum antibodies to influenza viruses, thereby a simple assay could facilitate strain differentiation and the detection of an individual's immunological response to an influenza virus infection.

The history of influenza in animals is equally confused, not least because influenza may be used as a general term for respiratory illness in animals, as it is in humans, and the wide range of infectious agents that can infect the upper respiratory tract causing influenza-like signs. However, there are many historical reports of influenza occurring simultaneously or sequentially in humans and domestic animals (Beveridge 1977) suggesting an early understanding of a possible link between the disease in animals and humans. Close correlation between human and animal influenza was made during the 1918 pandemic, and the term swine influenza was applied to a 'new' disease of pigs described at that time which produced clinical signs similar to those in humans (Dorset *et al.* 1922). Following the first isolation of influenza virus it was known that H1N1 (Hsw1N1) virus remained endemic in pig populations, particularly in the USA.

Little consideration was given to the possibility of influenza infections of other animals until 1955. In that year it was demonstrated that the causative virus of a highly pathogenic disease of chickens known as 'fowl plague', which had been isolated and described as a filterable agent as early as 1901 (Centanni and Savonuzzi, cited by Stubbs 1965), was a type A influenza virus. Several, less virulent, viruses that had been isolated from domestic poultry up to that time were also shown to be influenza A viruses. In 1956, evidence was obtained of influenza A virus infections in horses (Sovinova *et al.* 1958) and in the next two years respiratory disease in horses caused by this virus became widespread in Europe. These findings aroused the interest of many scientists working on influenza in humans, which was further concentrated by the H2N2 'Asian flu' pandemic of 1957. Since that time the World Health Organization (WHO) and World Organization for Animal Health (OIE) have coordinated work on the epidemiology of animal viruses, particularly in relation to human influenza. However, it was not until the late 1970s that the true picture of the vast reservoir of influenza viruses that exist in animals, particularly birds, had been formed.

Avian influenza (AI) infections became a major focus after bird to human transmission occurred in Hong Kong in 1997, resulting in severe infections and a number of deaths in humans. Influenza A virus infections are endemic in pigs, horses, ducks, geese, swans, shorebirds and domestic poultry. Sporadic infections have been seen in farmed mink, whales, seals, dogs, and tigers and leopards in captivity. In Europe and Asia there have been reports of small outbreaks of AI virus infections involving H5N1, H7N7 and H9N2 viruses (Keawcharoen *et al.* 2004).

In April 2009, there were reports from Mexico and Southern California of a respiratory illness caused by a novel swine influenza H1N1 virus. By June 2009, WHO had declared pandemic phase 6 as pandemic H1N1 was reported globally. This virus contained gene re-assortments from Eurasian and North American swine influenza, North American avian influenza and North American human influenza virus infections (Neumann *et al.* 2009; Dawood *et al.* 2009; Zimmer *et al.* 2009).

The agent

Taxonomy

The influenza viruses belong to the Orthomyxoviridae family of which there are five genera, influenza type A, B and C viruses, Thogoto viruses and Infectious Salmon Anaemia Virus (International Committee on Taxonomy of Viruses 2009 website http://www.ICTVdb.org/Ictv/index.htm).

Influenza viruses are grouped into types A, B, and C on the basis of the antigenic nature of the internal nucleocapsid or the matrix protein. Both these antigens are common to all viruses of the same type. Viruses of influenza A type are further divided into subtypes on the basis of the haemagglutinin (HA) and neuraminidase (NA) antigens. As of 2010, 16 HA and nine NA subtypes have been recognized; each virus possesses one HA and one NA subtype.

Influenza virus types A, B, and C infect humans, but, except for occasional reports, infections of other animals are restricted to influenza A viruses. Only influenza A viruses have been isolated from birds. Types A and B viruses both cause similar clinical disease in humans and both may be responsible for epidemics in humans. However, only influenza A viruses have produced the devastating pandemics that have made such an impact on the human population throughout recorded history.

Influenza A virus particles appear roughly spherical or filamentous, 80–120 nm in diameter. The nucleocapsid shows helical symmetry and is enclosed within a protein matrix. External to the matrix is a lipid membrane, the surface of which is covered by two types of glycoprotein projections, or spikes, with which haemagglutinin and neuraminidase activities are associated. These two surface glycopeptides, particularly the haemagglutinin, are the most important antigens stimulating protective immunity in the host. Consequently, considerable antigenic variation is seen in these polypeptides while other polypeptides are antigenically more stable.

Molecular biology

The genomes of influenza A and B viruses consist of eight unique segments of single-stranded RNA which are of negative polarity. Replication and transcription occur in the host cell nucleus. Influenza C viruses possess seven segments of RNA. The viral RNA is transcribed to complementary messenger RNA by a virus-associated polymerase complex (designated PB1, PB2, and PA). To be infectious, a single virus particle must contain each of the eight unique RNA segments. It is likely that the incorporation of RNAs into the virion is at least partly random. The random incorporation of RNA segments allows the generation of progeny viruses containing novel combinations of genes when cells are infected with two different parent viruses. This phenomenon is referred to as genetic re-assortment.

The eight influenza A viral RNA segments encode 11 proteins that include PB1, PB2, and PA polymerases, HA, nucleoprotein (NP), NA, matrix proteins (M1 and M2), and non-structural proteins (NS1 and NS2).

The three largest proteins (PB1, PB2 and PA) and one intermediate size protein (NP) are found in the RNA polymerase complex, which has transcriptase and endonuclease activities. This complex is involved in the synthesis of the three classes of virus-specific RNA molecules detected in infected cells, mRNA, virion RNA (vRNA), and complementary RNA (cRNA). PB2 functions during the initiation of viral mRNA transcription, recognizing the 5′ terminal caps of host cell mRNAs for use as viral mRNA transcription primers and is involved in the endonucleolytic cleavage of these primers. PB1 is responsible for the elongation of the primed nascent viral mRNA, template RNA and vRNA. The PA has a number of roles in replication. NP is transported into the infected cell nucleus, where it binds to and encapsidates viral RNA. NP is phosphorylated, the pattern of which is host cell dependent and may be related to viral host range restriction. NS1 has a role in virulence as it is an interferon antagonist that blocks the activation of transcription factors. It also binds to dsRNA and prevents RNase L activation thereby affecting the innate immune response to influenza virus infection. The NS1 proteins have also been associated with high levels of pro-inflammatory cytokines in the host, that may lead to more morbidity and mortality.

Influenza viruses enter the host cell via the sialic acid receptor. Endosomal entry and acidification activates the viral M2 ion channel and uncoating of the virus occurs as a result due to the disruption of the M1-viral ribonucleoprotein (RNP) complex. The HA-2 component is conformationally rearranged as a result of the pH change and leads to endosomal membrane fusion. Single vRNPs are released into the cytoplasm.

Nuclear localization signals carried by the NP protein and the importin alpha–beta mediated pathway assist the negative sense vRNA to be transported into the nucleus. These vRNAs are vRNP complexes associating heterotrimeric RNA dependent RNA polymerase (RdRp, made up of PB1, PB2, PA proteins) and nucleoprotein (NP).

An initial round of transcription produces 5′ capped and 3′ poly(A) viral mRNA exported towards the cytoplasm to be translated. Then vRNA templates are replicated into a positive sense copy RNA (cRNA).

Termination occurs by generating a poly(A) tail. After the formation of vRNPs within the nucleus, M1, NEP (Nuclear Export Protein, primary referred to as NS2) and NP catalyse its transport to the cytoplasm. M1-vRNP complexes are directed to the assembly site where both HA and NA have been accumulated. M1 interacts with cytoplasmic tails of glycoproteins, leading to assembly and budding of virions. The viral NA sialidase acts to release virions from the cell surface (Jossetab *et al.* 2008).

The HA protein is an integral membrane protein and the major surface antigen of the influenza virus virion. It is responsible for the binding of virions to host cell receptors and for fusion between the virion envelope and the host cell. Newly synthesized HA is cleaved to remove the amino-terminal hydrophobic sequence which is the signal sequence for transport to the cell membrane. Carbohydrate side-chains are added, the number and position of which vary with the virus strain. Palmitic acid is added to cysteine residues near the HA carboxy terminus. Fusion activity requires post-translational cleavage of HA by cellular proteases into the disulphide-linked fragments HA1 and HA2. This cleavage of the HA does not affect its antigenic or receptor-binding properties, but is essential for the virus to be infectious and is an important determinant in pathogenicity. HA molecules form homotrimers during maturation. The three-dimensional structure of the complete trimer has been determined, consisting of a globular head (HA1) on a stalk (HA1/2). The head contains the receptor-binding cavity as well as most of the antigenic sites of the molecule. The carboxy terminus of HA2 anchors the glycoprotein in the cell or virion membrane. The HA is subject to a high rate of mutation due to error-prone viral RNA polymerase activity. Selection for amino acid substitutions is driven at least in part by immune pressure, as the HA is the major target of the host immune response. The amino acids making up the receptor binding site are highly conserved but the remainder of the HA molecule is highly mutable. The 16 subtypes of HA recognized currently differ by at least 30% in the amino acid sequence of HA1 and are not cross-reactive serologically. Subtypes may include several variant strains which are only partially cross-reactive in serological assay.

The NA is the second major surface antigen of the virus which, like HA, is an integral membrane glycoprotein. It functions to free virus particles from host cell receptors, to enable progeny virions to escape from the cell in which they arose, and so facilitate virus spread. This activity destroys the HA receptor on the host cell preventing progeny virions reabsorbing to the host cell. The NA is specifically targeted by the NA inhibitor class of antiviral drugs, namely oseltamivir and zanamavir. By inhibiting the NA, these antivirals affect release of virions from infected cells, slowing the spread of the virus and giving time for the host immune response to act. Like HA, the NA is highly mutable, with variant selection driven by host immune pressure. The nine subtypes so far identified in nature are not cross-reactive serologically, although variants within subtypes are partially cross-reactive serologically. The NA inhibitors are effective against all 9 NA subtypes.

Pathogenicity

There are a number of molecular determinants of influenza virus pathogenicity that include the amino acid residues found at the HA cleavage-activation site, HA receptor specificity, the plasminogen binding ability of NA, specific amino acid changes in PB2 that alter the rate of RNA synthesis, the PB1-F2 ORF and the ability of PB1-F2 to induce apoptosis, and the differing ability of NS1 proteins to counteract the interferon system.

The HA plays a critical role in pathogenicity by mediating virus binding to host cells and fusing the viral and endosomal membranes for viral ribonucleoprotein release into the cytoplasm.

Host specificity is determined by preferential binding of some influenza viruses with sialic acid in the receptor binding site that is linked to galactose by an α2,6- or α2,3-linkage. The receptor binding specificity of human influenza viruses involves α2,6Gal-linkages which is matched by the α2,6Gal-linkages on human epithelial cells in the trachea.

The NS1 protein has been reported to have a number of functions including controlling the temporal synthesis of viral mRNA and viral genomic RNAs, delaying virus-induced apoptosis and avoiding host cell antiviral responses by limiting interferon induction and host T cell activation (Neumann *et al.* 2009).

Disease mechanisms

In the twentieth and twenty-first centuries there have been four major pandemics in humans, caused by viruses antigenically 'new' to the host population (antigenic shift), interspersed with both minor and major epidemics. Pandemic strains generally appear through genetic reassortment. Because vRNA is segmented, genetic reassortment can readily occur in mixed infections with different strains of influenza A viruses. This means that when two viruses infect the same cell, progeny viruses may inherit sets of RNA segments made up of combinations of segments identical to those of either of the parent viruses. This gives a theoretical possible number of 2^8 (=256) different combinations that can form a complete set of RNA segments from a concurrent infection, although in practice only a few progeny virions possess the correct gene constellation required for viability. The new subtypes of influenza viruses which appeared in humans in 1918 (Spanish influenza), 1957 (Asian influenza), 1968 (Hong Kong influenza), 1977 (Russian influenza) and 2009 (Swine influenza) had several features in common. Their appearance was sudden, they were antigenically distinct from the influenza viruses then circulating in humans, they were confined to H1, H2, and H3 subtypes and, with the exception of the 2009 pandemic virus, the first outbreaks occurred in south east Asia. Phylogenetic evidence suggested that these pandemic strains were derived from avian influenza viruses either after re-assortment or by direct transfer. There is evidence for genetic re-assortment between human and animal influenza A viruses *in vivo* (Brown *et al.* 1994; Dawood *et al.* 2009) and between human influenza viruses (Guo *et al.* 1992a). The appearance of the H2N2 and H3N2 subtypes was accompanied paralleled by the disappearance from the human population of the previously circulating subtypes, H1N1 and H2N2, respectively. This phenomenon probably occurred in 1918 when emerging H1N1 viruses replaced H3-like viruses. The reasons for the sudden disappearance of previously circulating human strains are unknown at a competition disadvantage but it is possible that the earlier strain is compared with the new strain because it has already elicited widespread immunity in the human population. This may explain the failure of the H1N1 virus to replace H3N2 on its re-emergence in 1977, as a large proportion of the population would have been infected with H1N1 prior to 1957 and retained some immunity. In 2009 H1N1 virus replaced the previously circulating H1N1 whilst the H3N2 continued circulating.

It appears that at frequent but irregular intervals between the major pandemics, variants of pandemic viruses arise which are sufficiently different antigenically to be capable of transmission within the population and thus cause an epidemic. In general, each new 'epidemic' variant appears to wane gradually in its ability to find new susceptible hosts and dies out, it is then replaced by the next epidemic variant. These variants arise due to gradual change, i.e. by mutation and selection of the original pandemic virus, and this is termed antigenic drift. Occasionally, the epidemics occurring between pandemics may be sufficiently severe and widespread to mimic a true pandemic. In 1946, an influenza A virus produced worldwide infections that were considered by some to represent a pandemic. However, epidemiological patterns were unlike those of true pandemics, and subsequent antigenic and genetic analyses revealed that the virus was a variant of the H1N1 subtype rather than a representative of antigenic shift.

The phenomenon of antigenic variation by shift and drift in influenza A viruses contrasts with influenza B viruses which show antigenic drift but not antigenic shift, resulting in regular epidemics but not explosive pandemics. Influenza C viruses do not show antigenic drift or shift, apparently only producing sporadic infections.

Two hypotheses have been proposed for the rhythm of occurrence of human influenza A viruses: an influenza circle/cycle or an influenza spiral (Shortridge 1992). The circle/cycle theory suggests there is simply a recycling of H1, H2, and H3 subtypes. The spiral theory presupposed that humans could be infected with all known HA subtypes of influenza A viruses as antibodies to the avian subtypes H4 to H13 were found in serum collected from rural dwellers in the influenza epicentre (Shortridge 1992). It is possible that the hypotheses are not mutually exclusive, as there is no reason that recycling should not occur within the spiral. The pandemic H1N1 virus of 2009 has further complicated these hypotheses since, as a direct descendant of the 1918 H1N1 strains circulated in conjunction with the 1968 H3N2 re-assortant virus as well as the 2009 swine-origin pandemic influenza virus (Shinde *et al.* 2009; Garten *et al.* 2009). It seems more likely that with 16 HAs and 9 NAs circulating in an avian reservoir that a number of events need to coincide in order for an influenza virus with pandemic potential to appear. This would involve a unique influenza virus of avian/swine descent to emerge and to reassort with a circulating human-adapted virus. In addition, the herd immunity of different age groups of the human population will vary as exposure to circulating influenza viruses change. This will also drive viral evolution.

Growth and survival requirements

Mammalian influenza A viruses replicate primarily in respiratory tract epithelial cells, whereas AI viruses replicate in both the respiratory and the intestinal tracts of birds. Viral shedding in the faeces provides the major mechanism for virus transmission from and between birds. Influenza A viruses capacity to replicate in the lungs is determined by temperature, while replication in the intestinal tract is dependent on pH. Replication of mammalian influenza A viruses is optimal at 33–35°C, reflecting the temperature found in the respiratory tract. AI viruses replicate efficiently at 40–42°C, whereas human influenza viruses do not. In contrast, some swine and equine strains possess the ability to replicate at 42°C, showing intermediate characteristics between avian and human influenza viruses. Furthermore, AI viruses replicate to high titres in the respiratory tract of pigs and can be transmitted readily to other pigs. Similarly, A1 viruses appear to have crossed the species barrier into horses and have been maintained independently of the avian population. The enterotropic avian influenza A viruses are more resistant to low pH, which enables them to pass through the pH barrier in the upper digestive tract of the host. However, a number of influenza A viruses have the potential to replicate in the intestinal tissues of some mammals such as ferrets.

The receptor specificity of the HA differs among influenza viruses and corresponds to the host receptors in the replication site from which the virus was isolated. AI viruses preferentially bind the sialic acid-α-2,3-galactose linkage, while human influenza viruses preferentially bind the sialic acid-α-2,6-galactose linkage on cell surface receptors. Both linkages are found in the epithelial cell site of virus replication lining the pig trachea, in contrast to both birds and humans. The ability of an influenza virus to replicate in avian or mammalian tissues may be genetically linked to the PB2 gene. Studies suggest that the amino acid lysine at residue 627 of the PB2 gene is a determinant of viral pathogenicity in several mammalian species by affecting viral replicative ability. In addition, the amino acid at residue 701 is another virulence determinant, whereas glycosylation of the HA gene appears to control the host range of H1 viruses. It would appear therefore that both viral and host genetic factors determine the tissue tropism of influenza viruses in mammals.

In vitro growth of influenza viruses is usually carried out in 9–11 day old embryonated fowls' eggs following inoculation of infective material into the allantoic or amniotic cavities. Incubation is carried out according to the virus host's requirements for 2–4 days, prior to the collection of allantoic/amniotic fluids. In addition, various cell systems have been used for growth, including canine kidney cells, calf kidney cells, human embryonic lung cells, chicken embryo fibroblasts, and conjunctival cells. Organ cultures from fetal and adult trachea have also been used. Whereas embryonated fowls' eggs are widely used for primary isolation and growth of influenza viruses due to their sensitivity, caution must be exercised in their wholesale application since, with human influenza viruses, genetically distinct variants are selected on passage in the allantoic cavity when compared to those of tissue culture cells, and the egg-adapted variant is not always representative of virus circulating in the human population.

High titres of virus are produced by influenza A infection in bird populations. For example, the huge numbers of ducks congregating on lakes in Canada prior to their migration south and the intestinal site of multiplication of influenza virus in these animals resulted in large doses of virus being excreted into lake water (Webster *et al.* 1978). Not only has it been shown that infections may be present at such levels to allow virus isolation from untreated samples of lake water (Hinshaw *et al.* 1979), but also that infectious virus may persist for up to 207 days at 17°C and for even longer periods at 4°C. The infectivity of influenza viruses in water is dependent on the strain of virus, salinity, pH, and temperature of the water. Pigs infected with H1N1 influenza A virus of low virulence may retain live virus in their frozen tissues for up to 3 weeks

after slaughter (Romijn *et al.* 1989). It has been postulated that the reappearance of an H1N1 influenza virus in humans in 1977 (following its disappearance in 1950), was due to reintroduction from a frozen source (Webster *et al.* 1992).

The hosts

Influenza viruses are found in a wide variety of mammalian and avian species. Pathogenicity differences among influenza viruses result in the production of a spectrum of clinical diseases that range in severity from fatal systemic disease to mild, sometimes inapparent, respiratory disease. Severity of the disease is also determined by the host species infected and in part by factors such as age, gender, virus dose, environment, and concurrent infections with other pathogens.

Incubation period and clinical signs

In humans, the incubation period varies between 1–5 days, depending on the virus strain and infective dose. Typically, the onset of clinical signs is rapid, characterized by malaise, fever, rhinorrhoea, an unproductive cough, myalgia, and headache. The illness leads rapidly to prostration which usually lasts from 3–5 days, being most severe in children and the elderly. Complications include primary viral or secondary bacterial pneumonia.

The disease in pigs and horses is similar to that in humans. After an incubation period of 1–3 days, disease signs appear suddenly in all or a large number of animals of all ages within a unit. An acute febrile, respiratory disease is characterized by fever, apathy, anorexia, coughing, sneezing, nasal discharge, conjunctivitis, a low mortality rate, and a rapid recovery. Secondary bacterial infections in both pigs and horses can often increase the severity of the illness and may result in complications such as pneumonia.

In birds the disease signs can vary considerably. Typical clinical signs of highly pathogenic AI in chickens or turkeys include decreased egg production, respiratory signs, rales, excessive lacrimation, sinusitis, cyanosis of unfeathered skin especially combs and wattles, oedema of head and face, ruffled feathers, diarrhoea, nervous disorders, and high mortality. Nonpathogenic AI viruses may replicate in the epithelial cells of the respiratory tract and the intestine of birds without inducing signs of disease, but virus may be shed at high concentrations in the faeces. Exacerbative conditions, including infection with other organisms, may result in AI viruses which are normally not pathogenic causing severe disease in infected birds.

Generally, influenza virus infections of other animals such as ruminants and sea mammals result in subclinical disease. However, H7N7, H4N5, and H3N3 influenza A viruses were associated with a high mortality in harbour seals at Cape Cod, USA in 1979 (Lang *et al.* 1981), 1982 (Stuart-Harris *et al.* 1985) and 1991 (Callan *et al.* 1995), virus being isolated from lung and brain of dead animals. Mustelids may be more susceptible to influenza infections; in addition to the historical laboratory infections of ferrets, outbreaks of severe respiratory disease with 100% morbidity and 3% mortality in commercial mink in Sweden were considered due to infections with influenza virus of H10N4 subtype. Isolates made from the mink showed close genomic homology with H10N4 viruses circulating concomitantly in avian species (Berg *et al.* 1990). In all these cases the epidemics tended to be self-limiting, and the newly introduced viruses did not appear to be maintained in sea mammals or mink.

Pathology

The respiratory pathology following infection with influenza virus is difficult to define precisely, since it is frequently complicated by the effects of secondary bacterial infection. Severe damage to the epithelium of the respiratory tract is the main feature in infections of mammals with influenza virus. The resulting damage to the epithelium facilitates secondary infection by bacterial respiratory pathogens.

In humans there is typically a rhinitis followed by tracheobronchitis and, infrequently, an interstitial pneumonitis. The disease process usually damages the respiratory tract from the nose to the small bronchi, but rarely damages alveolar cells. However, in some cases influenza A virus infection results in gross lung lesions which are patchy and randomly distributed throughout the lobes. The altered lung areas are depressed and consolidated, dark red or purple red in colour, contrasting sharply with normal lung tissue (Morens *et al.* 2010).

In typical infections of pigs the bronchi and bronchioli are dilated and filled with exudate. Bronchial and mediastinal lymph nodes are usually hyperaemic and enlarged. Histologically, there is widespread degeneration and necrosis of the epithelium in the bronchi and bronchioli. The lumen of bronchi, bronchioli, and alveoli are filled with exudate containing desquamated cells and neutrophils progressing to mainly monocytes. Furthermore, dilatation of the capillaries and infiltration of the alveolar septae with lymphocytes, histiocytes, and plasma cells occurs. Widespread interstitial pneumonia and emphysema accompany these lesions, although the severity of the former is dependent on the infecting strain (Brown *et al.* 1993a).

Significant pathological changes in other organs have not been consistently observed among infected mammals. Infections of birds with highly virulent avian viruses are characterized by haemorrhagic, necrotic, congestive, and transudative changes. Haemorrhagic changes are frequently severe in the oviducts and intestines. Encephalitis may develop in the cerebrum and cerebellum, especially in broilers. Alterations to myocardial tissues have been observed following infection with highly pathogenic strains.

Diagnosis and surveillance

Laboratory methods for detecting influenza virus and other respiratory virus infections have been revolutionized since the start of the twenty-first century. Classical techniques are still used in certain settings, such as haemagglutination inhibition, microneutralization and virus isolation. However, molecular based rapid diagnostic methods are being used around the world including reverse transcriptase and real time polymerase chain reaction (PCR) assays as well as microarrays to detect influenza virus RNA as well as type the virus; automated sequence analysis to determine whether that virus contains any antiviral resistance mutations as well as molecular epidemiological analysis using high throughput automated sequencing (Wang and Taubenberger 2010).

Clinical diagnosis of infection with influenza virus is only presumptive. The rapid confirmation of influenza requires that a respiratory sample should be tested for the presence of influenza virus RNA. Alternative classical methods that take longer periods of time to make a diagnosis include virus isolation in cell culture or testing a blood sample for influenza virus antibody, essentially demonstrating a recent infection in paired samples or a high titre antibody in a recently collected sample. Molecular diagnostic assays have revolutionized both the diagnosis and surveillance of respiratory virus infections in terms of sensitivity of detecting various infectious agents, especially influenza. Although the clinical picture includes a high temperature, myalgia and a variety of respiratory symptoms and signs, the pandemic influenza A H1N1 virus infections in 2009 demonstrated that a number of other respiratory viruses can also cause similar symptoms even when the case definition is carefully delineated. In addition to acute disease there may be subclinical infection or atypical courses of infection such as in a partially immune population.

Generally, the best material for viral RNA detection using molecular based methods such as real time PCR assays or virus isolation is nasal mucus from mammals and faecal samples from birds. These are collected using sterile swabs, which are immediately suspended in transport medium, i.e. 40% glycerol, 60% saline, to prevent them drying out. Some laboratories have used specimen tubes that contain viral lysis buffer that ensure the stability of the sample, although these samples are unhelpful if virus isolation is required. Samples should be collected as soon as possible during the acute phase of the disease. In addition, tissues from the respiratory tract of mammals and from respiratory, intestinal, and systemic organs of birds are suitable for viral RNA detection or virus isolation. Tissues may be homogenized in saline containing antibiotics and antimycotics and clarified to obtain a clear supernatant. The most suitable, easily available and reliable host system for the isolation of influenza viruses is 9–11 day old embryonated fowls' eggs.

Various cell cultures may also be used for the isolation of influenza viruses, but the Madin Darby canine kidney cell line is most frequently used for influenza isolation from humans and other mammals. Usually it is necessary to add trypsin to the growth medium, as a conditioning factor for the cleavage of the HA and the production of infectious virus.

After incubation at 35°C (mammalian influenza) or 37°C (avian influenza) for 2–4 days, the allantoic/amniotic or cell culture fluids are collected and tested for the presence of HA in the haemagglutination test using chicken red blood cells. Positive haemagglutination is presumptive for the presence of an influenza virus for mammals, but avian species are commonly infected with Newcastle disease and other paramyxoviruses. Initial identification of a virus is performed by the immunodiffusion test with specific antisera to the nucleoprotein or matrix protein of the three types of influenza virus. This confirms the isolate as an influenza virus of type A, B, or C, and distinguishes it from all other agents that exhibit haemagglutination. Further characterization of influenza A viruses is carried out to identify the antigenic nature of the surface antigens, HA and NA, in haemagglutination inhibition (HI) and neuraminidase inhibition (NI) tests, respectively, using a panel of monospecific antisera for each of the 16 HA and 9 NA types. The specific inhibition of HA and NA permits subtype identification of the influenza A virus.

Classical techniques include the use of serology for diagnosis which can be particularly useful when virus shedding is brief and is of low titre, as is often the case with respiratory viruses or when an animal or individual is no longer in the acute phase of the disease. The HI test (Palmer *et al.* 1975), may be used to diagnose influenza and offers the advantages of being relatively simple to perform, sensitive, easily adaptable, and inexpensive. The single radial immunodiffusion test is an alternative assay which is also inexpensive and simple to perform. Paired sera taken in the acute stage of illness and approximately 2–3 weeks later during convalescence are required for diagnosis, in order to demonstrate an increase in specific antibodies. In epidemic situations when influenza is suspected and paired sera are unavailable, a rapid diagnosis can often be made by examining single serum specimens from selected individuals for elevated levels of influenza antibody.

The serum of many species, particularly mammals, contains inhibitory substances that may interfere with the specificity of HI and other tests. Various treatments of sera have been suggested to remove these inhibitors, possibly the best and most widely used being incubation with receptor destroying enzyme. In addition to non-specific inhibitors of the HA, some sera contain non-viral substances that may agglutinate certain species of red blood cells used in the HI test. These substances may be removed by pre-treating the serum with erythrocytes to be used in the HI test.

Overall, molecular methods are the mainstay for the analysis of influenza virus infections in terms of rapid diagnosis, typing, determining antiviral susceptibility and for epidemiological purposes.

Treatment

The two classes of antiviral drugs used in both treatment and prophylaxis target the M2 and NA envelope proteins.

The adamantanes, amantadine and rimantadine, are M2 ion channel blockers and are effective against influenza A viruses only. These drugs date back to the early 1960s and 1990s respectively. They block the efflux of hydrogen ions due to the change in pH as they are basic compounds, and interfere with intracellular virus uncoating. They reduce the duration of fever by 24 hours and prevent 60–70% of influenza A infections if used as prophylaxis. They are associated with neuropsychiatric side effects, especially in the elderly if used in higher doses.

Amantidine-resistant influenza A virus is widespread, having first been detected in 1981. In the USA, the incidence of adamantane resistance rose to 92% in 2005. This is due to M2 gene mutations and nearly 80% of resistant viruses have a serine to asparagine mutation at codon 31. Naturally occurring influenza A viruses are essentially quasispecies of susceptible and resistant strains. The latter dominate within 3 days of starting amantadine treatment and have similar virulence to the wild type virus. The M gene of pandemic influenza H1N1 virus is similar to the M gene in the Eurasian swine virus, which confers resistance to both amantadine and rimantadine (Jefferson et al. 2006; Suzuki et al. 2003).

The NA inhibitors, oseltamivir and zanamivir, were made available in 1999 and are effective against both influenza A and B viruses. Oseltamivir (Tamiflu) is more widely used as it can be taken orally as opposed to zanamivir (Relenza) which is administered by inhalation. NA inhibitors interfere with the release of new influenza virions from infected cells, preventing the infection of new cells. Both drugs are effective in reducing the median time to alleviating influenza symptoms by up to 24 hours. The benefit of prophylaxis and treatment has been shown when these drugs are given within 48 hours of symptom onset in previously well adults. However, further analyses are awaited to demonstrate effectiveness in other clinical settings. With respect to post-exposure prophylaxis, an 80–90% reduction in influenza incidence has been reported.

Zanamivir is associated with cough, bronchospasm and death in individuals with underlying respiratory disease and is contraindicated. Oseltamivir is associated with gastrointestinal disturbances in 10% of individuals, especially nausea and vomiting.

Oseltamivir resistance has been widely reported and usually involves the histidine to tyrosine at codon 274 in N2 nomenclature or H275Y in N1 nomenclature mutation in the NA gene. In 2008, up to 99% of seasonal H1N1 isolates in the USA were oseltamivir resistant. Transmission of oseltamivir resistance has occurred in the absence of direct selective drug pressure without affecting either virulence or replicative capacity.

In general, zanamivir retains full inhibitory activity against several NA subtypes in the presence of oseltamivir resistance mutations. However, although zanamivir resistance is rare, it has been demonstrated after treating immunocompromised individuals. Most of the 2009 pandemic H1N1 isolates remained susceptible to the NA inhibitors. However, there is the potential, with the seasonal and pandemic influenza viruses co-circulating, for incorporation of the H274Y mutation leading to oseltamivir-resistant pandemic H1N1 virus infections (Hurt et al. 2006, 2009; Moscona 2005; Cooper et al. 2003; Jefferson et al. 2006, 2009; Weinstock and Zuccotti 2009; Moscona 2005, 2009; Dharan et al. 2009; Lackenby et al. 2008).

Oseltamivir and zanamivir have been made available as intravenous preparations (Gauer et al. 2010). Peramivir is another NA inhibitor that has been developed and can be given intravenously (Barroso et al. 2005). Finally, laninamivir is a long-acting NA inhibitor that is structurally related to zanamivir, but has a longer half-life.

Novel molecular targets involved in different steps in the influenza virus life cycle have been investigated (Hayden 2009). Drugs that have been studied include favipiravir that is converted into a nucleotide analogue that inhibits influenza virus RNA polymerase (Smee et al. 2009; Furuta et al. 2009). In addition, fludase is a sialidase catalytic domain/amphiregulin glycosaminoglycan binding sequence fusion protein. The mechanism of action is unique as it selectively cleaves sialic acid receptors from the host cells, so the influenza virions cannot bind (Moss et al. 2010).

Finally, another form of treatment that has a historical basis involves the use of hyperimmune plasma. This was used in the 1918 Spanish influenza pandemic and was made from blood collected from convalescent human volunteers and given to patients with severe influenza infections. Successful outcomes were reported. There were reports that in individuals with severe pandemic H1N1 infections, the IgG2 subclass deficiency could be corrected by hyperimmune plasma infusions that had been collected from individuals with pandemic H1N1 infection or from vaccinated donors (Gordon et al. 2010). This is a potential therapeutic adjunct to conventional antiviral treatment in the treatment of severe cases of pandemic H1N1 infection (Moss et al. 2010).

Antibiotics and other antibacterial agents do not affect the viral infection, but may sometimes be used to prevent complications such as bacterial co-infection. Specific control measures include the use of antiviral drugs and vaccination. General prophylactic measures in mammals and birds are based mainly on preventing the introduction of influenza viruses of wild aquatic birds into domestic pig herds and poultry flocks. Infected herds or flocks are kept warm and free from stress for a more rapid recovery.

Prognosis

In humans the effects of infection with influenza viruses in a population are most easily measured by comparing excess overall mortality with 'pneumonia-influenza' death rates, and are used to indicate the extent of an epidemic rather than the lethality of the virus. It is estimated that the 1918 pandemic resulted in 50–100 million deaths worldwide in all age groups. Subsequent pandemics in 1957 and 1968 showed dramatically increased excess mortality, but the effects compared to the 1918 pandemic were much reduced, possibly reflecting the availability of antibiotics in preventing deaths as a result of secondary bacterial infections. The combined pandemics of 1957 and 1968, in the USA, accounted for approximately 98,000 excess deaths; however, the epidemics from 1957 to 1975, excluding the pandemic years, accounted for over twice that number of excess deaths (Dowdle 1976), indicating that epidemic influenza occurring as a result of antigenic drift is a significant 'killer' disease in humans.

In most age groups, influenza infections produce high morbidity, but recovery is usually rapid and uneventful. Mortality is highest in the elderly and the very young, frequently accounting for 90% of all mortality associated with influenza virus infections. If a vaccine provided 100% protection, about 80% of influenza-related deaths could be prevented by vaccinating all people above 70 years of age (Sprenger *et al.* 1993).

In other mammals the disease usually produces a short illness, characterized by low mortality, high morbidity, and rapid recovery, but varies with the infecting strain of virus and the affected species. An H7N7 influenza A virus was associated with a high mortality in harbour seals in the USA in 1980, but was apathogenic for chickens and turkeys. A novel strain of equine influenza virus (H3N8) which emerged in horses in China in 1989 was associated with a high morbidity and relatively high mortality of up to 20%. The virus appeared to originate from birds (Guo *et al.* 1992b). The introduction of an avian-like H1N1 virus into an immunologically naive pig population resulted in a large number of disease outbreaks characterized by high morbidity but low mortality (Brown *et al.* 1993b).

Epidemiology

Most influenza viruses infecting birds produce asymptomatic disease. Outbreaks in poultry due to highly pathogenic AI viruses are rare, but when the disease does occur it may result in up to 100% mortality, often with few clinical signs preceding sudden death.

Phylogenetic studies of influenza A viruses have revealed species-specific lineages of viral genes and have demonstrated that the frequency of interspecies transmission depends on the animal species. In the early 1970s, the WHO initiated long-term global studies on the influenza viruses of mammals and birds to determine the diversity of influenza A viruses in nature and whether it was possible to isolate a future pandemic strain from them in advance of its appearance in humans.

To the present day, a large number of viruses have been isolated from a wide variety of birds and a range of terrestrial and sea mammals. These can all be grouped into 16 HA subtypes and 9 NA subtypes, suggesting there may be a limited range of antigenic subtypes in nature. However, it has been reported that phylogenetic analyses of the 1918, 1957 and 1968 pandemic viruses suggested that all evolved undetected in an intermediate mammalian host well before human infections were seen (Smith *et al.* 2009). In addition, systematic virological surveillance of swine influenza virus infections in a Hong Kong SAR abattoir, over a decade revealed a high degree of reassortment (Vijaykrishna *et al.* 2010).

Intraspecies transmission of influenza A viruses does occur, but is infrequent, and occurs most readily between host species that are closely related in which transmission is sustained. Following transmission, the influenza A virus must adapt to the new species before efficient and high level replication occurs. There is an association between efficient replication and expression of virulence.

Although a wide range of animal species are susceptible to influenza A virus infections, three groups of animals appear to be more important in terms of numbers and the epidemic/endemic nature of the disease than other animals: these are birds, pigs, and horses.

Occurrence in birds

Influenza viruses infect many avian species naturally a great variety of birds, including wild birds, captive caged birds, domestic ducks, chickens, turkeys, and other domestic poultry (Perdue and Swayne 2004).

Viruses have been isolated from species of wild bird covering all the major families of birds. This has led to the findings that non-pathogenic AI viruses are ubiquitous, particularly in aquatic birds, and that all of the different subtypes of influenza A viruses (H1 to H16 and N1 to N9) are perpetuated in aquatic birds, particularly migrating waterfowl. Furthermore, phylogenetic studies have revealed that aquatic birds are probably the source of all influenza viruses in other species.

The frequency at which viruses have been isolated from samples taken from waterfowl has varied considerably. Hinshaw *et al.* (1980) contrasted the frequent isolation of virus from ducks congregated on lakes in Alberta, Canada with the much lower isolation rates obtained from birds on migration. Some of the factors that governed whether or not waterfowl were likely to be infected and excrete virus were the age of the bird, the geographical location relative to migration, the time of year, the species, and the characteristics of a particular virus. Each year, waterfowl congregate in extremely large flocks, usually on lakes, before migratory flights are undertaken. At this stage, viruses may spread easily to susceptible birds on the crowded lakes. Isolation rates from juvenile ducks may exceed 60%. The importance of waterfowl is not only in the antigenic diversity and size of virus pools they harbour, but also the rapid dissemination of these viruses around the world due to the migratory nature of these birds.

In wild ducks, influenza viruses replicate mainly in the intestinal tract and are excreted in high concentrations in the faeces. Many birds, particularly juveniles, are infected by the virus shed into the lake water; however, viral genetic information does not persist in the individual after clearance of infectious virus, which is usually 5–7 days after infection. Certain subtypes of influenza virus predominate in wild ducks along a particular flyway, but the predominant virus differs from one flyway to another from year to year. Studies of ducks and swans from Siberia wintering in Japan have shown an influenza isolation rate during the winter months which varied from 0.5–9%, year to year.

Influenza viruses of a variety of HA and NA subtypes have also been isolated from wild waterfowl in other parts of the world, including Russia, southern China, western Europe, and Australia demonstrating the worldwide distribution of avian influenza virus gene pools in nature. Phylogenetic studies have indicated that influenza viruses from Eurasia and Australia are genetically distinct from those in North America. These studies indicated that the incidence and prevalence of influenza subtypes will vary due to physical barriers which prevent intermixing of their hosts. Studies by Sharp *et al.* (1993), suggested that whereas wild ducks perpetuated some influenza A viruses, they did not act as a reservoir for all such viruses. It has been suggested that the remainder of the influenza gene pool is maintained in shorebirds and gulls, from which the predominant isolated influenza viruses are of a different subtype to those isolated from ducks. Circumstantial evidence suggested that initial outbreaks in domestic poultry most often occurred as the result of spread from wild birds, although there were several reports of influenza viruses transmitted from pigs to turkeys. As a consequence, considerable antigenic variation has been seen in disease outbreaks in domestic poultry.

AI viruses are classified into low (LP) and high pathogenicity (HP) viruses based on virulence in chickens using an intravenous pathogenicity test. The LP viruses mostly cause respiratory or reproductive system infections with low mortality rates and do not meet the definition of an HPAI virus. The latter may produce more than 75% mortality and include any H5 and H7 AI viruses that have a haemagglutinin proteolytic cleavage site compatible with a HPAI virus. AI viruses are maintained as LPAI viruses in the wild bird reservoir. Following transfer and circulation in domestic poultry, some H5 and H7 LPAI viruses have mutated to HPAI viruses.

Influenza viruses have been isolated less frequently from feral passerine birds than from waterfowl. Studies following a highly pathogenic H7N7 outbreak in chickens in Australia concluded that there had not been significant spread to feral birds, although virulent virus was isolated from a starling found on the affected farm (Morgan and Kelly 1990). Captive, caged, and pet birds may also have a role to play in the propagation and dissemination of influenza viruses. Monitoring of such birds throughout the world has resulted in the isolation of many viruses.

It may be concluded that enormous pools of both genetically and antigenically diverse influenza viruses exist within the bird population, and provide the source of virus for the mammalian population.

In early 1997, an H5N1 influenza virus known to infect only birds caused an outbreak involving 18 people in Hong Kong, 6 of whom died. A high mortality rate had been seen in chickens infected with H5N1 influenza in three farms in Hong Kong. It was subsequently shown that individuals in close contact with the index case or with exposure to poultry in the live market were at risk of being infected (Yuen *et al.* 1998; Claas *et al.* 1998; Subbarao *et al.* 1998).

Control measures to reduce exposure included culling all poultry in Hong Kong, segregating water fowl and chickens and introducing import control measures for chickens. Although the outbreak occurred, successful controlled H5N1 virus outbreaks occurred in 9 Asian countries in 2003, causing large-scale outbreaks in poultry and at least 7 fatal cases of human infection in three countries (Sims *et al.* 2003).

Furthermore, between February and May 2003, a fowl plague outbreak due to HPAI virus of subtype H7N7 occurred in the Netherlands. This was closely related to LPAI virus isolates from wild ducks but was isolated from chickens. The same virus was detected subsequently in 89 people, most of whom developed conjunctivitis having handled affected poultry. Three of the 89 were family members whom had no direct contact demonstrating human to human transmission. Influenza-like illnesses were generally mild, but there was a fatal case of pneumonia and acute respiratory distress syndrome (Koopmans *et al.* 2004; Fouchier *et al.* 2004; Elbers *et al.* 2004).

Between November 2003 and June 2008, HPAI H5N1 viruses caused fatal human infections in 296 of 500 confirmed cases in 15 countries in Asia, Africa, the Middle East, and Europe (WHO (2009) http://www.who.int/csr/disease/avian_influenza/country/cases_table_2009_04_17/en/index.html), (Nguyen-Van-Tam *et al.* 2005; Peiris *et al.* 2004).

The HA genes of these viruses isolated from humans were consistent with those viruses that infected domestic poultry in southern China. LPAI H5N2, H4N6 and H9N3 viruses were also detected in apparently healthy geese and ducks (Webster *et al.* 2002).

HPAI H5N1 viruses isolated from domestic waterfowl in 2001 and 2003 were not the progenitors of the viruses that caused widespread outbreaks in poultry and human infections in Vietnam in 2003–2004. The latter H5N1 viruses were independently introduced into Vietnam (Jadhao *et al.* 2009).

Occurrence in pigs

H1N1 and H3N2 influenza A viruses have been widely reported in pigs, frequently associated with clinical disease. These include classical swine H1N1, avian-like H1N1, and human and avian-like H3N2 viruses (Table 30.3). Swine influenza has remained in the pig population and has been responsible for one of the most prevalent respiratory diseases in pigs.

Swine influenza is related to the movement of animals from infected to susceptible herds, clinical disease generally appears with the introduction of new pigs into a herd. Once a herd is infected, the virus is likely to persist through the production of young susceptible pigs and the introduction of new stock. Outbreaks of disease occur throughout the year but usually peak in the colder months. Infection with classical swine H1N1 influenza virus is frequently subclinical, and typical symptoms are seen often in only 25–30% of a herd. Blaskovic *et al.* (1970) showed that classical swine H1N1 influenza virus was excreted from one infected pig for over 4 months, although 7–10 days is more usual. Continuous circulation of swine influenza viruses within a herd without the apparent need for an intermediate host has been shown by the isolation of virus from a herd all the year round.

Influenza A viruses causing clinical disease reappeared in European pigs in 1976, with the introduction of classical swine H1N1 influenza virus to Italy from North America. Although usually regarded

Table 30.3 Strains of influenza A viruses endemic in pigs

Subtype	Location	comments
H1N1	North America, Europe, Asia, and South America	'Classical' virus [siv] first isolated in 1930 in USA
H1N1	Europe and Asia	'Avian-like' virus, first isolated in 1979 in Europe
H3N2	Asia, Europe, North America, South America	'Human-like' virus, first isolated in 1970 in Asia
H3N2	Asia	'Avian-like' virus, first isolated in 1978

'Human-like' H1N1 viruses often infect pigs, but do not appear to be readily transmitted from pig to pig.

as an endemic disease, influenza infections of pigs may result in epidemics when introduction of virus to an immunologically naive population occurs. Great Britain had remained free of avian-like H1N1 virus until 1992 when respiratory disease was seen spreading rapidly throughout the country as a result of infections with an H1N1 virus related to, but antigenically distinguishable from, the prototype strains of avian-like H1N1 viruses (Brown *et al.* 1993*b*).

Human H3N2 influenza A viruses related to a human strain from 1973, circulated in European pig populations long after their disappearance from the human population.

There is good evidence that genetic reassortment can occur in nature between influenza A viruses in pigs, but this has not resulted in new epidemics in the pig population in which it has occurred. Influenza A H1N2 viruses, derived from swine H1N1 and H3N2 viruses, have been isolated in Japan (Sugimura *et al.* 1980) and France (Gourreau *et al.* 1994). Phylogenetic analyses of human H3N2 viruses circulating in Italian pigs revealed that genetic reassortment had been occurring between avian and human-like viruses since 1983. The unique co-circulation of influenza A viruses within European swine may lead to pigs serving as a mixing vessel for reassortment between influenza viruses from mammalian and avian hosts, with unknown implications for both humans and pigs. Further evidence for influenza virus reassortment in the pig is provided by the isolation of an H1N7 virus from pigs in England, apparently derived from human and equine viruses, and the isolation of an H1N2 virus from pigs in Great Britain, apparently derived from human and swine viruses (Brown *et al.* 1995*a*). Unlike H1N2 viruses detected elsewhere, this H1N2 appeared to spread widely within pigs in Great Britain.

Up to 1998 in the USA, swine classical H1N1 strains were the dominant viruses circulating in pigs. Since that time, new swine H3N2 strains have been detected and resulted from a double reassortment of swine classical H1N1 with the PB1, HA, and NA segments from a human H3N2 strain, and a triple reassortment of swine classical H1N1 with the PB1, HA, and NA segments of a human H3N2 strain and the PB2 and PA segments of avian lineage. H1N2, H3N1, H2N3, H4N6, H5N1 and other subtypes have been isolated in pigs around the world as a result of inter-host reassortments of human and/or avian viruses.

Reassortant H2N3 viruses were characterized having been isolated from pigs with respiratory disease from two farms in the USA, a subtype not previously reported in swine (Ma *et al.* 2007). These H2N3 reassortant viruses contained genes derived from avian and swine influenza viruses. The virus was able to replicate in pigs, mice, and ferrets and was transmitted among pigs and ferrets.

This was an important finding as they belonged to the H2 subtype as did the 1957 human pandemic strain that disappeared in 1968. Therefore, from a public health perspective, a new generation of people would have little pre-existing immunity to this subtype. Furthermore, they were circulating in swine that could select for mammalian influenza viruses, they had receptor binding site changes associated with increased affinity for $\alpha 2,6$Gal-linked sialic acid viral receptors and could replicate and transmit in swine and ferrets.

The original source of the H2N3 virus was unclear, but it was thought that both farms used surface water collected in ponds for cleaning the barns and watering animals. Therefore, the avian virus may have infected the pigs by direct contact with the contaminated surface water.

Reassortment has also been demonstrated between avian- and human-like influenza viruses in Italian pigs.

Pigs serve as major reservoirs of H1N1 and H3N2 influenza viruses and are often involved in interspecies transmission of influenza viruses. The maintenance of these viruses in pigs and the frequent introduction of new viruses from other species could be important in the generation of pandemic strains of human influenza.

Occurrence in horses

Equine influenza virus (EIV) infection, first isolated in 1963, causes a common disease of horses throughout the world. Apart from rare reports of isolations or serological evidence of infection with other subtypes, only two subtypes of influenza A virus, H7N7 and H3N8, have been identified as infecting and causing disease in horses. It is possible that H7N7 viruses have disappeared largely from the horse population as H3N8 is apparently the only subtype currently circulating in the horse population. Equine influenza outbreaks due to infection with H3N8 virus have been seen in South Africa, India, China, Hong Kong, and Nigeria. Outbreaks in China have been due to both conventional strains of H3N8 virus, and viruses which, although they contained the same surface antigens as the other equine viruses of this subtype, had genetic features that were avian-like, indicating that the virus had been introduced from birds. In North America and Europe, two distinct groups of H3N8 (equine-2) virus have been detected. Sporadic outbreaks typically occur and may in part be due to antigenic drift, which may compromise the efficacy of the available vaccines. EIV has also jumped the species barrier and become established as a respiratory pathogen of dogs (Murcia *et al.* 2010).

In May 1993, a severe epidemic of respiratory disease spread throughout horses in China due to an H3N8 influenza A virus whose gene segments were derived entirely from classical equine-2 influenza viruses, closely related to an H3N8 equine influenza virus isolated in Sweden in 1991. These results demonstrated that European equine H3N8 influenza viruses had been transmitted to China. Swine influenza virus surveillance during 2004–2006, showed that two strains of H3N8 influenza viruses isolated from pigs in central China were of equine origin and were closely related to European equine H3N8 influenza viruses dating back to the early 1990s (Tu *et al.* 2009).

Occurrence in other species

Influenza A viruses of HA subtypes H1, H3, H4, H7, and H13 have been isolated from dead and dying seals and whales (Hinshaw *et al.* 1986). These sea mammals were probably infected from the faeces of birds, shed into the water at communal gathering sites (Shortridge 1992), as it is known that these viruses were of avian origin (Callan *et al.* 1995). Influenza viruses have been isolated from mink raised on farms. These H10N4 viruses were of avian origin (Berg *et al.* 1990), caused systemic infection and disease in the mink and spread to contacts. In all these cases the epidemics tended to be self-limiting, and the newly introduced viruses did not appear to be maintained in sea mammals or mink.

Between May and December 2007, HPAI-origin canine influenza A viruses (H3N2) spread across South Korea. The viruses shared more than 97% nucleotide sequence homology, suggesting that whole viruses were transmitted directly from birds to dogs. These viruses were also transmitted experimentally to beagles by direct contact, showing that interspecies transmission of AI viruses was possible (Song *et al.* 2009).

In January 2004, an outbreak of respiratory disease occurred in 22 racing greyhounds at a Florida racetrack in the USA. Dogs suffered a mild illness with fever and cough or died with a suppurative bronchopneumonia with pulmonary haemorrhage, a 36% case-fatality rate. From June to August 2004, respiratory disease outbreaks occurred at 14 tracks in 6 states with a combined population of ~10,000 racing greyhounds. Virological, serological, and molecular evidence for interspecies transmission of an entire equine influenza A (H3N8) virus was reported (Crawford et al. 2005). Unique amino acid substitutions in the canine virus HA, coupled with serological confirmation of infection of dogs in multiple states in the USA, were correlated with sustained circulation of the virus in the canine population.

Occurrence in humans

Influenza epidemics in humans can occur following infection with influenza A or B viruses, but pandemics result only from infection with influenza A virus. Influenza A viruses of H1, H2, and H3 subtypes have been associated with infection in humans since the mid-nineteenth century. Pandemics generally occur following antigenic shift, whereas epidemics result from antigenic drift. The 2009 pandemic H1N1 virus was an exception although it does depend on the definition of the term pandemic. Does 'pandemic' refer to a global outbreak alone or also infer high morbidity and mortality?

Antigenic shifts have resulted in new subtypes of human influenza A viruses appearing in 1918 (H1N1); in 1957, when the H2N2 subtype replaced the H1N1 subtype; in 1968, when the H3N2 virus appeared, replacing the H2N2 subtype; and in 1977 when the H1N1 virus reappeared. In the last case the reappearance of H1N1 did not result in the replacement of H3N2 viruses and both continue to circulate. Pandemic strains appear to arise at one focus and spread rapidly worldwide. Each of the new subtypes since 1957 first appeared in China and spread across all continents as a result of the available, fully susceptible world population. For example, the H1N1 virus that reappeared in May 1977 in humans in northern China, had spread to much of south east Asia by November, and by February 1978 it was already present in Europe and the USA. Within 9 months, this virus had been distributed almost worldwide (Kendal 1987).

Every few years a new antigenic variant of the prevailing subtype appears that is capable of spreading in the population and causing a significant epidemic. In temperate climates, epidemics nearly always start at the beginning of winter. They are of varying severity dependent on the infecting strain but are characterized by rapid spread, often infecting between 30–40% of the population of the affected area. Epidemic strains usually arise at one focus and spread rapidly worldwide. After their rapid start, the epidemics tend to end no less abruptly, often within several weeks at the local level, or within 3 months nationwide. The sudden cessation of epidemics, often when there are still many susceptible individuals in the population, has not been explained.

Epidemics occur worldwide in the human population due to infection with influenza A viruses of H1N1 or H3N2 subtype or with influenza B virus. Rarely, infections can occur with re-assorted influenza A viruses such as H1N2 and H3N1 although spread of such viruses appears to have been very limited.

Occurrence rates for influenza virus infection are highest in children. This is partly attributable to the increased immunity in older individuals that results from prior infections with related viruses.

Children and young adults play an important role in the dissemination of virus into the community. When adults, especially those 65 years of age or older, are exposed to influenza virus in a setting such as a nursing home, the infection rate can be as high as in younger persons, but with the potential for more severe consequences. Death rates from influenza during an epidemic are invariably high enough to affect the overall death rate and it is chiefly in the elderly that such deaths occur. Other groups at risk include people with chronic disorders of the respiratory or cardiovascular systems, children with asthma, immunosuppressed patients or those with metabolic disorders, persons infected with human immunodeficiency virus, pregnant women, regular foreign travellers and those involved in the health care of some of the aforementioned groups.

Sources

The detection of vast pools of influenza viruses of many different subtypes among animals, particularly aquatic birds gave considerable impetus to research aimed at determining where new subtypes, particularly those that cause pandemics, emerge. Many theories have been suggested, of which the most widely accepted is that by adaptation, involving genetic reassortment, virus transmission from other animals to humans occurs which results in an antigenically novel virus with the ability to infect and spread in humans. Following genetic reassortment, viruses may arise that possess the necessary genes to enable infection of humans but may have surface antigens new to the host immune system.

Genetic and biochemical studies have shown that the 1957 and 1968 pandemic viruses arose by genetic reassortment. The HA, NA and PB1 genes of the 1957 Asian H2N2 strain were from an avian virus and the remaining five genes from the preceding human H1N1 strain (Kawaoka et al. 1989). The 1968 Hong Kong H3N2 strain contained HA and PB1 genes from an avian donor and the NA and other five genes from the Asian H2N2 strain. A diagrammatic representation of the theoretical origin of influenza A viruses in humans is shown in Fig. 30.1.

The pig has been the leading contender for the role of intermediate host for reassortment of influenza A viruses. Pigs are the only mammalian species which are domesticated, reared in abundance and are susceptible to, and allow productive replication of, avian and human influenza viruses. This susceptibility is due to the presence of both $\alpha 2,3$- and $\alpha 2,6$-galactose sialic acid linkages in cells lining the pig trachea, which can result in modification of the receptor binding specificities of avian influenza viruses from $\alpha 2,3$ to $\alpha 2,6$ linkage; thereby providing a potential link from birds to humans. Furthermore, it has been shown that humans occasionally contract influenza viruses from pigs. The internal protein genes of human influenza viruses share a common ancestor with the genes of most swine influenza viruses. Also, the pig has a broader host range concerning the compatibility of the NP gene of viruses derived from other species (Scholtissek et al. 1985).

AI viruses which do not replicate in pigs can contribute genes that generate re-assortants when co-infecting pigs with a swine influenza virus. Evidence for the pig as a mixing vessel of influenza viruses of non-swine origin has been demonstrated in Europe by Castrucci et al.(1993), who detected a reassortment of human and avian viruses in Italian pigs. In addition, human and equine influenza viruses resulting in re-assortant viruses (Brown et al. 1994) or from human and swine viruses (Brown et al. 1995a) have been isolated from pigs in Great Britain.

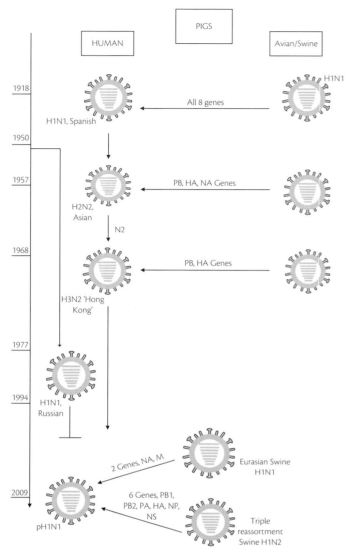

Fig. 30.1 Theoretical origin of Influenza A viruses that have circulated in humans since 1918. Phylogenetic evidence suggests that the virus causing the 1918 pandemic possessed 8 gene segments from avian strains. In 1957 the Asian pandemic virus H2N2 acquired 3 genes from avian influenza gene pool by genetic re-assortment with the circulating human strain. The 1968 Hong Kong pandemic virus H3N2 acquired 2 genes from the avian influenza gene pool. It has been suggested that the re-assortment event leading to H2N2, H3N2 pandemic strain occurred in pigs. In 1977 the Russian influenza (H1N1) strain had previously circulated before 1950 and co-circulated with H3N2 until the 2009 pandemic. The 2009 pandemic strain resulted from a re-assortment of swine strains. Ksishna, V. (2010).

Alternatively, new pandemic viruses could occur in the human population if an avian strain or a strain from another mammal became infectious for humans. Phylogenetic evidence supports this mechanism for the appearance of the Spanish influenza virus (H1N1) in 1918. Analyses of the NP gene, which is associated with host specificity, of human, swine, and avian H1N1 viruses reveals that the classical swine viruses and the contemporary human viruses probably evolved from a common avian ancestor prior to the appearance of the 1918 human pandemic strain (Gorman *et al.*

1991). Furthermore, avian-like H1N1 viruses circulating in European pigs since 1979 were implicated as the precursors of the next human pandemic virus (Ludwig *et al.* 1995). In addition, avian H1N1 viruses antigenically and genetically related to, but distinct from European avian-like swine viruses have been detected in pigs in south east Asia since 1993 (Webster *et al.* 1996).

Finally, the appearance of pandemic virus may be in fact be the re-emergence of a virus which may have caused an epidemic many years earlier. The appearance of Russian influenza (H1N1) provided support for this concept. The virus that reappeared in China in 1977 and spread subsequently to all parts of the world was identical in all of its genes to the virus which caused a human influenza epidemic in 1950 (Nakajima *et al.* 1978). Webster *et al.* (1992) suggested that this virus was most likely reintroduced to humans from a frozen source and Shoham (1993) proposed a biotic mechanism for the preservation of influenza viruses. Influenza viruses of the H3N2 subtype persist in pigs many years after their antigenic counterparts have disappeared from humans and therefore present a reservoir of virus which may in the future infect a susceptible human population. Pandemic strains may also be antigenically conserved in the avian reservoir, since counterparts of the Asian pandemic strain of 1957 circulated with increasing prevalence in wild ducks, domestic fowl, and live bird markets, coming into closer proximity to susceptible human populations.

The majority of pandemic strains have originated in China, raising the possibility that this region is an influenza epicentre (Shortridge and Stuart-Harris 1982; Shortridge 1992). In the tropical and subtropical regions of China, influenza occurs all year round. In China, influenza viruses of all subtypes are prevalent in ducks and in water frequented by ducks. The agricultural practices provide that there is close contact between domestic ducks, pigs, and humans, thereby presenting the opportunity for interspecies transmission and genetic exchange among influenza viruses, with the pig acting as an intermediary between domestic ducks and humans, as the transmission of mammalian virus strains directly to domestic poultry is unlikely to be a factor in the generation of new pandemic strains. Aquatic birds migrating or overwintering in the region might provide a source of virus for domestic ducks. Yasuda *et al.* (1991) showed that domestic ducks harbour H3 influenza viruses antigenically and genetically similar to those in pigs, suggesting they may play a role in the transfer of avian influenza viruses from feral ducks to pigs.

Transmission

Influenza viruses infect a large variety of animals, and species barriers are less important in their ecology than they were thought to be. Given the worldwide interaction between humans, pigs, birds, and other mammalian species there is a high potential for cross-species transmission of influenza viruses in nature. A proposed model of the animal reservoir of influenza A viruses is shown in Fig. 30.2.

The ability of an influenza virus to cross between species is controlled by the viral genes, and the prevalence of transmission will depend on the animal species. The theory that pandemic influenza viruses arise as a result of adaptation and/or genetic reassortment requires that viruses pass either from other animals to humans or vice versa, and that genetic reassortment then occurs by dual infection which results in progeny virus with the ability to infect and cause disease in humans, but with antigenic determinants different from recent viruses affecting the human population. It would seem reasonable to suppose that such transference between species would occur many more times than when the conditions are optimal for the emergence of pandemic viruses. While viruses do not pass to and from humans and animals with complete freedom, under some conditions such transmission does occur.

Transmission between humans and pigs

In January 1976 an H1N1 virus, identical to viruses isolated from pigs in the United States, was isolated from a soldier who had died of influenza at Fort Dix, New Jersey, USA. At least five other servicemen were shown by virus isolation to be infected, and serological evidence suggested that some 500 personnel at Fort Dix were, or had been, infected with the same virus (Hodder *et al.* 1977; Top and Russell 1977). With the 1918 pandemic in mind this stimulated a universal vaccination programme in the USA, that was eventually abandoned when it became clear that the virus had not spread any further.

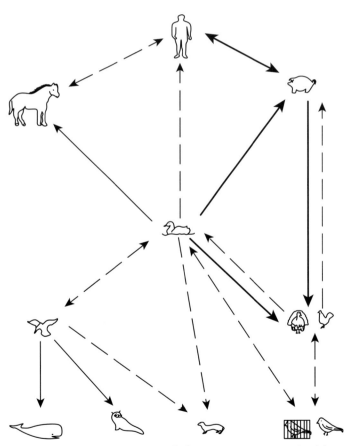

Fig. 30.2 Reservoirs and transmission of influenza A viruses. It is postulated that wild aquatic birds are the reservoir of all influenza viruses for avian and mammalian species. There is overwhelming biological, biochemical, and epidemiological evidence (—) for transmission between some species, such as pigs and humans. There is strong evidence (—) for transmission between other species, such as seabirds and sea mammals, and some evidence (---) for other transmissions, such as between horses and humans.

The Fort Dix incident cannot be regarded as evidence of zoonoses, since it was not established whether the likely source was pigs. However, there is considerable evidence that transmission from pigs to humans does occur. Kluzka *et al.* (1961) reported that humans working with pigs in Czechoslovakia had antibodies to the H1 subtype from pigs, and Schnurrenberger *et al.* (1970) reported that people in the USA who had close contact with pigs were more likely to have antibodies to classical swine H1N1 influenza virus than those who did not.

Final confirmation of the zoonotic nature of H1N1 influenza viruses from pigs came in 1976, when clinical influenza appeared in a herd of pigs on a farm in Wisconsin 2–3 days before a caretaker also became ill with influenza. Viruses isolated from the pigs and the man were shown to be both antigenically and genetically identical swine H1N1 influenza viruses (Easterday 1980). There were several reports in 1994 from North America of swine virus being isolated from humans with respiratory illness, occasionally with fatal consequences (Wentworth *et al.* 1994). All cases examined followed contact with sick pigs and were due to viruses most closely related to classical swine H1N1 influenza virus. In Europe, De Jong *et al.* (1986) reported the isolation of classical swine H1N1 influenza virus from three unrelated human cases of respiratory illness, one of which involved a 3 year old child who had apparently not been in contact with pigs, although there had been recent epizootics in pigs in the region in which she was living. Perhaps of greater significance for humans is a report of two distinct cases of infection of children in the Netherlands during 1993 with H3N2 viruses, whose genes encoding internal proteins were of avian origin (Claas *et al.* 1994). Genetically and antigenically related viruses had been detected in European pigs (Castrucci *et al.* 1993), raising the possibility of potential transmission of avian influenza virus genes to humans following genetic re-assortment in pigs.

H3N2 influenza viruses are ubiquitous in animals and endemic in most pig populations worldwide. There is no apparent evidence of pigs being infected with this subtype prior to the pandemic in humans in 1968. Indeed, the appearance of an H3N2 subtype variant strain in the pig population of a country appears to coincide with the epidemic strain infecting the human population at that time (Brown *et al.* 1995*b*).

Further evidence of the spread of influenza viruses from humans to pigs was the appearance in pigs of H1N1 viruses (or antibodies to H1N1) related to those circulating in the human population since 1977 (Nerome *et al.* 1982; Brown *et al.* 1995*b*). Genetic analysis of two strains of H1N1 virus isolated from pigs in Japan revealed that the HA and NA genes were most closely related to those of human H1N1 viruses circulating in the human population at that time. In addition, re-assortant viruses with some characteristics of human H1 viruses were isolated from pigs in England (Brown *et al.* 1995*a*).

Finally, in 2009, the triple re-assortant pandemic H1N1 virus appeared in Mexico and South California.

Transmission between humans and horses

In historical accounts of pandemics in humans, frequent reference is made to similar diseases in horses occurring either simultaneously or preceding that in humans. Beveridge (1977) noted such references in the accounts of 12 pandemics occurring during the eighteenth and nineteenth centuries.

Serological studies have revealed the presence of antibodies to equine H3 (equine-2) viruses in the sera of people born in the nineteenth century, and this has been considered as possible evidence that virus of this subtype was responsible for the pandemic of 1889–90. Experimental infection of human volunteers with H3 (equine-2) viruses has produced an influenza-like illness with virus shedding and seroconversion. There is no evidence of infection of humans with the other subtype of influenza, H7 (equine-1), which has caused widespread epizootics in horses.

There have been several isolated reports of infection of horses with subtypes H1N1, H2N2, and H3N2, usually associated with human infections. Experimental infections of horses with human-derived H3N2 virus has confirmed their susceptibility to this virus (Blaskovic et al. 1969).

Transmission between avian and mammalian species

Although there is convincing evidence that all 16 subtypes of influenza A viruses are perpetuated in the aquatic bird populations of the world, only a few of the numerous subtypes have been observed in non-avian hosts. Phylogenetic analyses have revealed that some human pandemic strains most probably emerge following re-assortment between avian and human influenza viruses, with the pig being favoured as the possible intermediate host.

The 1957 pandemic virus had the HA, NA and PB1 genes from an AI virus, while the 1968 H3 virus had two AI virus genes, the HA and PB1. Avian H3N2 viruses are readily transmitted to pigs in south east Asia.

Outbreaks of influenza in pigs in Europe since 1980 have been associated with influenza A viruses which are antigenically and genetically distinguishable from classical swine H1N1 viruses but closely related to H1N1 viruses isolated from ducks. All of the gene segments of the prototype viruses were considered to be typical of viruses of avian origin, indicating that transmission of a whole avian virus into pigs had occurred. These viruses circulated in European pigs and were reintroduced to turkeys causing economic losses.

In 1979, around the Cape Cod peninsula in North America, high mortality in the population of harbour seals was attributed to an H7N7 influenza virus which was isolated from the lungs and brains of dead seals. Antigenic and genetic analyses revealed that the virus was most closely related to viruses from avian species. During the initial studies, four people involved in postmortem examinations of the seals had developed purulent conjunctivitis within 2 days of known contamination with seal material. Although no virological studies were carried on these cases, in subsequent laboratory studies an infected seal, known to be shedding virus, sneezed directly into the eye of one of the investigators who developed conjunctivitis within 2 days. Virus identical to the seal virus was isolated from the affected eye for 4 days after this incident (Webster et al. 1981).

In March 1989 a severe outbreak of respiratory disease in horses occurred in China. An influenza virus of subtype H3N8 was isolated and was antigenically and genetically distinguishable from equine-2 (H3N8) viruses, being most closely related to avian H3N8 influenza viruses. Genetic evidence suggested that this virus was transmitted to horses without reassortment.

Transmission of avian influenza viruses to other species of mammal such as whales and mink have been reported. Genetic analysis of the viruses from whales confirmed that they had probably been introduced from birds. The potential susceptibility of mink to avian influenza viruses had been demonstrated following experimental infections.

Viruses antigenically identical to human variants of H3N2, H2N2, and H1N1 subtypes have been isolated from wild birds and domestic poultry, some have been reported to cause disease outbreaks in chickens that have shown a temporal relationship to influenza epidemics in humans.

Classical swine influenza viruses have also been isolated from ducks (Butterfield et al. 1978; Hinshaw et al. 1978), providing further supportive evidence for the natural transmission of influenza A viruses between avian and mammalian species.

There have been a number of sporadic infections with LPAI viruses in humans. For example, in 1996, a 43 year old woman in England developed self-limiting conjunctivitis. An H7N7 LPAI virus was isolated from an eye swab. She had been looking after domesticated ducks of various breeds that mixed freely with wild ducks on a small lake. An H9N2 LPAI virus was isolated from 7 children and adults in mainland China and Hong Kong in late 1998 and early 1999. The two patients in Hong Kong had developed fever and a chest infection, all recovered. In 2002, there was an H7N2 LPAI outbreak in the USA. A patient with serious underlying medical conditions developed respiratory symptoms and an H7N2 LPAI virus was isolated. Finally, an H7N3 HPAI virus was detected in samples from 2 Canadian adults with conjunctivitis, coryza, and headache.

In contrast, most human AI infections with fatal outcomes involved H5N1 infections in Asia and H7N7 HPAI viruses in the Netherlands.

Finally, in the early 2000s, an H9N2 LPAI virus infected 8 people, that appeared to be widespread in other parts of Asia (Choi et al. 2004).

Communicability

The ability of an influenza virus to spread is related to both the virus and the host involved. The age, population density, and air space may all affect transmissibility. Host-specific or host-adapted viruses have higher affinity for spread within a given host, than after transmission to a 'foreign' host. For example, the human viruses which cause epidemics and pandemics have a high capacity for spread amongst susceptible individuals. In contrast, the transfer of non-re-assorted influenza viruses derived from birds or pigs, produce only mild or inapparent infection in humans and rarely result in secondary transmission. The majority of infections of humans in the USA with classical swine H1N1 viruses have not resulted in transmission from infected to in-contact individuals (Dasco et al. 1984; Patriarca et al. 1984).

The success of interspecies transmission of influenza viruses depends on the viral gene constitution. Successful transmission between species can follow genetic reassortment, with a progeny virus containing a specific gene constitution having the ability to replicate in the new host. Re-assorted viruses may have a relatively low fitness, and will not be able to perpetuate in the new host. These observations support the potential role of the pig as a mixing vessel of influenza viruses from avian and human sources. The pig appears to have a broader host range in the compatibility of the NP gene in re-assortant viruses than both humans and birds. Furthermore, cell receptors for both avian and human viruses are present in the pig trachea and the intermediate temperature of pigs compared to humans and birds may be important since virus synthesis is influenced by temperature control.

Transmission of the H5N1 viruses to, and between, humans seems limited and that could be due to incomplete host adaptation or a dose response restriction.

In addition, close contact is required to infect other humans. The main concern is that a seasonal influenza A virus will infect an

H5N1-infected human or other mammal and a reassortant virus containing the correct combination of genes for efficient human-to-human transmission will emerge.

Prevention/control

Prevention

Generally, two control measures are available for influenza in humans: immunoprophylaxis with vaccines, especially in older adults (Monto *et al.* 2009), and chemoprophylaxis or therapy with antiviral drugs.

Since the late 1940s, the principal preventive measures against influenza have been inactivated virus vaccines. The efficacy of vaccines has varied between 60–90% and has been dependent on the closeness of the 'antigenic match' between the vaccine virus and the epidemic virus. However, even for those not completely protected, vaccination reduces the severity of the disease, thereby reducing costs and mortality (Fiore *et al.* 2009). Two basic approaches for immunization have been pursued: the use of inactivated virus preparations and the use of live, attenuated viruses.

Influenza vaccine is prepared from purified, embryonated egg grown viruses that have been rendered non-infectious. Four major innovations have been incorporated: the use of zonal centrifugation, the use of ether or other lipid solvents to disrupt the virus, the introduction of high-yield reassortants to improve yields in the chick embryo, and the development of better methods to quantitate the amount of viral antigens present in the vaccines. All of these efforts have led to inactivated vaccines that are better purified and more predictable in their reactogenicity and immunogenicity.

Each year the influenza vaccine is redefined to reflect changes in the antigenicity of circulating virus strains and contains virus strains representing influenza viruses believed likely to circulate in the forthcoming 'influenza season'. At present this involves two type A viruses, H1N1 and H3N2, and one type B virus (WHO). Recommendations for influenza vaccine composition. (Available at: www.who.int/csr/disease/influenza/vaccinerecommendations1/en/index.html.)

The exact strains of these viruses to be used are identified by an international network of laboratories that maintain surveillance for new influenza virus variants throughout the world. These laboratories are coordinated through the WHO.

The composition of the vaccine rarely causes systemic or febrile reactions. Whole virus, subvirion, and purified surface antigens are available. Depending on the age group, the response to inactivated vaccines is either a primary or booster type of immune response. Children who have not been exposed to influenza mount a primary antibody responce, and titres after the first dose of vaccine are low. After a second dose of vaccine which provides a boost, antibody titres rise in these children. Most adults, unless they are being exposed to an entirely new antigen, will mount a booster antibody response, even to strains whose antigens are marginally different. Antibodies to influenza vaccines are generally of the IgG subclass, and they react against the HA and NA of the vaccine strains. Antibody titres usually peak at 10–14 days after vaccine boost, then decline in the ensuing months. Serum antibodies appear to be very important in protecting against infection with influenza viruses. Extensive data show that the serum HI antibody titre correlates inversely with the occurrence of established infection with influenza viruses.

Most vaccinated children and young adults develop high post-vaccination HI antibody titres. These titres are protective against infection by strains similar to those in the vaccine or the related variants that emerge during outbreak periods. Elderly people and those with certain chronic diseases may develop lower post-vaccination antibody titres than healthy young adults and thus remain susceptible to influenza upper respiratory tract infection. Nevertheless, even if such people develop influenza illness, the vaccine has been shown to be effective in preventing lower respiratory tract involvement or other complications, thereby reducing the risk of hospitalization and death.

The effectiveness of influenza vaccine in preventing or attenuating illness varies, depending primarily on the age and immunocompetence of the vaccine recipient and the degree of antigenic similarity between the virus strains included in the vaccine and those circulating during the influenza season. When there is a good match between vaccine and circulating viruses, influenza vaccine has been shown to prevent illness in approximately 70% of healthy children and young adults, while preventing hospitalization for pneumonia and influenza among elderly people living in the community.

Adverse reactions to vaccination can occur locally at the vaccination site, including pain and erythema, dependent on the age group, vaccine type, and route of inoculation. Fever and systemic signs occur less frequently, in the range of 5–30%, and allergic reactions have been noted rarely, presumably to a vaccine component such as egg protein.

A live attenuated, cold-adapted (ca) re-assortant influenza virus vaccine was licensed in the USA in 2003. This vaccine relies on the use of an attenuated donor virus to confer the property of attenuation to contemporary wild-type strains by genetic re-assortment. This vaccine is very stable, owing partly to the multigenic requirement for the attenuated phenotype, and is at least as good as the inactivated vaccine in a population previously exposed to influenza virus (Fiore *et al.* 2009).

The issue with inactivated vaccines include limited global influenza vaccine manufacturing capacity, up to 6 months production time, require large supplies of chicken eggs and biological containment facilities. Plasmid (Deoxyribonucleic acid) DNA vaccines can be produced rapidly using simple bacterial fermentation procedures. DNA vaccines are a potentially powerful approach to the development of subunit vaccines (Robinson *et al.* 1993; Ulmer *et al.* 1993; Smith *et al.* 2010). Vaccination by DNA inoculation is achieved by the uptake and expression of the inoculated DNA. The protein that is expressed by host cells raises the immune response including inducing antibody and cytotoxic T-cell responses.

The antiviral drugs mentioned previously are effective when used as prophylaxis.

Control strategies

Hong Kong poultry in Hong Kong SAR are free of H5N1 due to the extensive culling programme together with a well managed surveillance programme and successful vaccination approaches (Ellis *et al.* 2004). The control programme aim is to prevent, manage or eradicate AI. In order to be effective, controls have to include biosecurity aspects to prevent the introduction or escape of the pathogen at the farm level, maintain rapid, sensitive and specific diagnostics and surveillance, managing acutely infected or convalescing animals, decreasing host susceptibility to the pathogen by immunization and educating poultry farmers and market stall holders in order to prevent transmission or spread. Increased cooperation between the veterinary and human health agencies within countries will ensure control of AI viruses and manage the public health implications.

Vaccination of people at high risk before each annual influenza season is currently the most effective measure for reducing the impact of human influenza. When vaccine and epidemic strains of virus are well matched, achieving high vaccination rates among closed populations can reduce the risk of outbreaks by inducing 'herd' immunity. This occurs when the overall number of susceptible people in a population becomes too low for virus to spread and infect a significant number of the susceptible individuals.

To maximize protection of persons at high risk, they and their close contacts should be targeted for organized vaccination programmes. Influenza vaccination is strongly recommended for any person above 6 months of age who, because of age or an underlying medical condition, is at increased risk for complications of influenza. The high-risk group consists of: persons above 65 years of age, residents of nursing homes and other chronic-care facilities, people with chronic disorders of the respiratory or cardiovascular systems, and people who have suffered chronic metabolic diseases or immunosuppression (including as a result of medication) within the past year. In addition, people who may transmit influenza to those at high risk, i.e. hospital and nursing home personnel and household members of people in high-risk groups, should also be vaccinated. Other groups may be included on individual merit, such as pregnant women, people infected with human immunodeficiency virus, and foreign travellers.

Methods and programmes

Although an influenza vaccine may contain one or more of the antigens administered in previous years, annual vaccination using the current vaccine is necessary because immunity declines within the year following vaccination. Old batches of vaccine should not be administered as the constituent virus strains are updated annually to reflect the predicted epidemic strains for the coming year.

Beginning each September, when vaccine becomes available for the forthcoming influenza season, people at high risk should be offered vaccine. Because influenza activity usually peaks between late December and early March in the northern hemisphere, people in this part of the world should be vaccinated by mid November. However, it is important to avoid administering the vaccine too far in advance of the influenza season in such places as nursing homes because antibody levels may begin to decline within a few months of vaccination. Earlier vaccination is warranted, however, in particular situations, such as the early onset of an epidemic. Unvaccinated children need two doses of vaccine, at least a month apart, and, under normal circumstances, the second dose should be given before December.

Evaluation

Each year influenza viruses isolated from epidemics are characterized antigenically in WHO influenza reference laboratories, and this information is used to evaluate the antigenic similarity with the virus strains incorporated into the current vaccine. This will provide some information on the potential efficacy of the vaccine, since the strains included in the vaccine had been selected ahead of the new 'influenza season'.

The human health aspects of managing influenza outbreaks in birds

Policy considerations

Avian influenza is primarily a disease of birds, however, certain subtypes, notably H7 and H5, can be transmitted directly to humans. Although this is rare it can cause illness in humans and H5N1 infection, in particular, is associated with a high case fatality rate. Avian viruses can be categorized into high and low pathogenicity strains, which relates to their virulence in birds. There is no evidence that virulence correlates in poultry are the same in humans. During the low path H7N2 avian influenza virus outbreak in the UK in 2008, three of the four clinical cases were admitted to hospital for a period. Outbreaks are more common than previously recognized. Table 30.4 summarizes recent avian outbreaks in UK.

There is also a risk that co-infection with an avian influenza virus and a human influenza virus could give rise, through genetic reassortment, to a hybrid virus to which there was little or no population immunity, that is capable of causing human illness and would be able spread from person to person effectively. Such a virus would meet all the prerequisites of a virus capable of causing a global pandemic. As such an important aspect of the global monitoring of influenza is detecting and investigating human disease caused by avian influenza viruses.

There are therefore three main policy aims relating to the human health aspects of avian influenza incidents:

1   Protecting the health of those exposed to the virus by way of contact with infected birds, their bedding or faecal material

2   Protecting the health of public from exposure to food stuffs that may be contaminated with an avian virus

3   Minimizing the risks of a new influenza subtype emerging by the re-assortment of an avian influenza virus and a human influenza virus

Protecting the health of those involved in an incidental exposed to the virus

EU legislation requires the rapid implementation of containment measures in affected premises when an outbreak of a highly pathogenic avian influenza, of any type, occurs (Council Directive 2005/94/EC).

These measures include movement restrictions within a prescribed area and the culling of the birds on the premises. Movement restrictions mean that there will be animal welfare issues involving contact between workers and infected birds and their bedding or faeces. The culling of the birds and the disposal of the carcasses, bedding and faecal material will also involve close contact with potentially infected material.

In 2003, a fatal human case of influenza A/H7N7 infection occurred in a veterinarian in the Netherlands involved in controlling an outbreak on a farm. The patient, and various workers and their families who became infected, had not taken measures to protect themselves from infection. This incident demonstrated the necessity of stringent protective measures for people who have close contact with sick and recently dead birds affected by any highly pathogenic avian influenza (Koopmans *et al.* 2004).

The transmission risk of low pathogenicity AI viruses to poultry handlers is the same as the risk of high pathogenicity virus

Table 30.4 Recent outbreaks of influenza in birds, with associated human cases

Date	Influenza subtype	Pathogenicity	Species affected	Number of birds involved	Human cases	Location
March 2006	H5N1	High path	Mute swans	1	0	Fife, Scotland
April 2006	H7N3	Low path	Chickens	34,500	1 (conjunctivitis)	Norfolk, England
February 2007	H5N1	High path	Turkeys	160,000	0	Suffolk, England
May 2007	H7N2	Low path	Chickens/ducks		4 (1 conjunctivitis) (1 pneumonia) (2 chest infection)	North Wales. Cheshire, England
November 2007	H5N1	High path	Turkeys/ducks	13,500	0	Suffolk, England
January 2008	H5N1	High path	Mute swans	6	0	Dorset, England
June 2008	H7N7	High path	Chickens	25,000	0	Oxfordshire, England
February 2009	H6N1	Low path	Turkeys	20,000	0	Norfolk, England

transmission and that there is no evidence that virulence correlates in poultry are the same in humans.

In order to minimize exposure to the influenza virus, workers involved in caring for the birds, the culling of the birds, and the disposal of the carcases, the bedding and faeces, are required to wear personal protective equipment (PPE). This involves the wearing of protective overalls, gloves, boots, respirators and eye protection when there is the potential for contact with the birds, their bedding or faeces. Guidance on the recommendations for the use of PPE has been developed by the European Centre for Disease Prevention and Control (ECDC).

Since the use of PPE is highly dependent on individual compliance and in acute situations it may be used by relatively inexperienced individuals, there is still a significant risk of exposure to the virus therefore prophylaxis with an antiviral is given. The neuraminidase inhibitor oseltamivir is usually used and this is given as a daily dose of 75mg for the duration of exposure and continued for 10 days after the date of last exposure. Prophylaxis should be started before exposure occurs. All individuals coming into contact with the birds, their bedding or faeces also have their health monitored and any illness is quickly investigated. The value of this monitoring was demonstrated during an outbreak of a low pathogenicity H7N3 avian influenza virus in the UK in 2006 when a conjunctivitis caused by the virus was detected in a worker (Nguyen-Van-Tam *et al.* 2006).

In addition to these measures those exposed prior to the infection being detected, for example workers on the facility, are offered post-exposure prophylaxis—oseltamivir 75mg for 10 days and undergo health monitoring while taking prophylaxis.

Protecting the health of public from exposure to food stuffs that may be contaminated

The risk to the general public from avian influenza in general and specifically from consuming meat and poultry products has been repeatedly considered to be minimal by authorities such as the ECDC, the European Food Safety Authority (EFSA), national food safety agencies within the EU and the World Health Organization International Food Safety Authorities Network.

Guidance focuses on the importance of cooking and food hygiene but this is mostly to protect against other pathogens (Campylobacter, Salmonella and E. Coli O157) that are more common, better adapted to humans and much more infectious.

The possibility of transfer of an avian influenza in or on unprocessed food or fomites such as packing or clothing and the potential for this to pose a threat to workers in the food or catering industry and those preparing food in the home is believed to be very low, as the virus remains poorly adapted to humans.

Minimizing the risks of a new influenza subtype emerging

A major concern around the handling of avian influenza incidents is the possibility of the co-infection of a worker/responder with the outbreak avian strain and a seasonal human influenza. It is theorized that such an event could lead to the creation of a new influenza subtype through genetic re-assortment which could become a pandemic strain. Low pathogenicity in poultry does not indicate a reduced tendency to transmit to humans and therefore the transmission risk of low pathogenicity AI viruses to poultry handlers is the same as the risk of high pathogenicity virus transmission.

Vaccination with seasonal influenza vaccine is therefore recommended for poultry workers, cullers, veterinarians and others who could come into contact with potentially infected birds. In the UK this operationalized by inclusion within the national influenza vaccine programme.

Vaccine is also offered to those unimmunized workers who are involved in an avian influenza response however, given that it takes between seven to ten days to mount an adequate antibody response it is difficult to see the justification for this. Proactive vaccination within the groups likely to be involved would appear to be a better strategy. It is therefore important to emphasize that other public health measures in managing an acute incident are probably of greater importance. These include preventing unnecessary exposure, use of PPE, use of Neuraminidase Inhibitors (NI) prophylaxis, and health status follow up.

References

Barroso, L., Treanor, J., Gubareva, L., *et al.* (2005). Efficacy and tolerability of the oral neuraminidase inhibitor peramivir in experimental human influenza: randomized, controlled trials for prophylaxis and treatment. *Antivir. Ther.*, **10**: 901–10.

Basler, C. F., Reid, A. H., Dybing, J. K., Janczewski, T. A., *et al.* (2001). Sequence of the 1918 pandemic influenza virus nonstructural gene (NS) segment and characterization of recombinant viruses bearing the 1918 NS genes. *Proc. Natl. Acad. Sci. USA*, **98**: 2746–51.

Berg, M., Englund, L., Abusugra, I. A., Klingeborn, A., and Linne, T. (1990). Close relationship between mink influenza (H10N4) and concomitantly circulating avian influenza viruses. *Arch. Virol.*, **113**: 61–71.

Beveridge, W. I. B. (ed.) (1977). Influenza—the last great plague. London: Heinemann.

Blaskovic, D., Jamrichova, O., Rathova, V., Skoda, R., *et al.* (1970). Experimental infection of weanling pigs with A/swine influenza virus. 2. The shedding of virus by infected animals. *Bull. Wor. Heal. Organ.*, **42**: 767–70.

Blaskovic, D., Kapitancik, B., Sabo, A., Styk, B., Vrtiak, O., and Kaplan, M. (1969). Experimental infection of horses with A/equi2/Miami/l/63 and human A2/Hong Kong/1/68 influenza viruses. The course of infection and virus recovery. *Acta Virol.*, **13**: 499–506.

Brown, I. H., Alexander, D. J., Chakraverty, P., Harris, P. A., and Manvell, R. J. (1994). Isolation of an influenza A virus of unusual subtype (H1N7) from pigs in England, and the subsequent transmission from pig to pig. *Vet. Microbiol.*, **39**: 125–34.

Brown, I. H., Chakraverty, P., Harris, P. A., and Alexander, D. J. (1995*a*). Disease outbreaks in pigs in Great Britain due to an influenza A virus of H1N2 subtype. *Vet. Rec.*, **136**: 328–29.

Brown, I. H., Done, S. H., Spencer, Y. I., Cooley, W. A., Harris, P. A., and Alexander, D. J. (1993*a*). Pathogenicity of a swine influenza H1N1 virus antigenically distinguishable from classical and European strains. *Vet. Rep.*, **132**: 598–602.

Brown, I. H., Harris, P. A., and Alexander, D. J. (1995*b*). Serological studies of influenza viruses in pigs in Great Britain 1991–2. *Epidemiol. Infect.*, **114**: 511–20.

Brown, I. H., Manvell, R. J., Alexander, D. J., Chakraverty, P., *et al.* (1993*b*). Swine influenza outbreaks in England due to a new H1N1 virus. *Vet. Rec.*, **132**: 461–62.

Butterfield, W. K., Campbell, C. H., Webster, R. G., and Shortridge, K. F. (1978). Identification of swine influenza virus (HswlNl) isolated from a duck in Hong Kong. *J. Infect. Dis.*, **138**: 686–89.

Calfee, D. P., Peng, A. W., Cass, L. M., *et al.* (1999). Safety and efficacy of intravenous zanamivir in preventing experimental human influenza A virus infection. *Antimicrob. Agents Chemother.*, **43**: 1616–20.

Callan, R. J., Early, G., Kida, H., and Hinshaw, V. S. (1995). The appearance of H3 influenza viruses in seals. *J. Gen. Virol.*, **76**: 199–203.

Castrucci, M. R., Donatelli, I., Sidoli, L., Barigazzi, G., Kawaoka, Y., and Webster, R. G. (1993). Genetic re-assortment between avian and human influenza A viruses in Italian pigs. *Virol.*, **193**: 503–6.

CDC. Swine influenza A (H1N1) infection in two children—Southern California, March–April 2009. *MMWR* **58**: 400–442.

Cheung, C. Y., Poon, L. L., Lau, A. S., Luk, W., *et al.* (2002). Peiris. Induction of pro-inflammatory cytokines in human macrophages by influenza A (H5N 1) viruses: a mechanism for the unusual severity of human disease? *Lancet*, **360**: 1831–37.

Choi, Y. K., Ozaki, H., Webby, R. J. Webster, R. G., *et al.* (2004). Continuing evolution of H9N2 influenza viruses in Southeastern China. *J. Virol.*, **78**: 8609–14.

Claas, E. C., Osterhaus, A. D., van Beek, R., *et al.* (1998). Human influenza A H5N1 virus related to a highly pathogenic avian influenza virus. *Lancet*, **351**(9101): 472–77.

Council Directive 2005/94/EC of 20 December 2005 on Community measures for the control of avian influenza and repealing Directive 92/40/EEC (OJ L 10, 14.1.2006, p. 16–65) 8ECDC Guidelines. http://www.ecdc.europa.eu/Health_topics/Avian_Influenza/pdf/Guidelines-human_exposure_HPAI.pdf.

Crawford, P. C., Dubovi, E. J., Castleman, W. L., *et al.* (2005). Transmission of equine influenza virus to dogs. *Sci.*, **310**(5747): 482–85.

Dasco, C. C., Couch, R. B., Six, H. R, Young, J. F., Quarles, J. M., and Kasel, J. A. (1984). Sporadic occurrence of zoonotic swine influenza virus infections. *J. Clin. Microbiol.*, **20**: 833–35.

Dawood, F. S., Jain, S., Finelli, L., *et al.* (2009). Novel Swine-Origin Influenza A (H1N1) Virus Investigation Team. Emergence of a novel swine-origin influenza A (H1N1) virus in humans. *N. Engl. J. Med.*, **360**: 2605–15.

De Jong, J. G *et al.* (1986). Isolation of swine influenza-like A (H1N1) viruses from man in Europe, 1986. *Lancet*, **2**(8519): 1329–30.

Dharan, N. J., Gubareva, L. V., Meyer, J. J., *et al.* (2009). Infections with oseltamivir-resistant influenza A(H1N1) virus in the United States. *JAMA*, **301**: 1034–41.

Dorset, M., McBryde, C. N., and Niles, W. B. (1922). Remarks on 'Hog Flu'. *J. Am. Vet. Med. Assoc.*, **62**: 162–71.

Dowdle, W. R. (1976). Influenza: epidemic patterns and antigenic variation. In: P. Selby (ed.) *Influenza: Virus, Vaccines, and Strategy*, pp. 17–21. London: Academic Press.

Easterday, B. C. (1980). The epidemiology and ecology of swine influenza as a zoonotic disease. *Comp. Immunol. Microbiol. Infect. Dis.*, **3**: 105–9.

Elbers, A. R. W., Fabri, T. H., *et al.* (2004). The highly pathogenic avian influenza A (H7N7) virus epidemic in the Netherlands in 2003-lessons learned from the first five outbreaks. *Avian Dis.*, **48**: 691–705.

Ellis, T. M., Leung, C. W., *et al.* (2004). Vaccination of chickens against H5N1 avian influenza in the face of an outbreak interrupts virus transmission. *Avian Pathol.*, **33**: 405–412.

European Centre for Disease Prevention and Control (2005). 'ECDC Guidelines: Minimising the risk of humans acquiring highly pathogenic avian influenza from exposure to infected birds or animals.' ECD Stockholm, December 2005

Fiore, A. E., Bridges, C. B., and Cox, N. J. (2009). Seasonal influenza vaccines. *Curr. Top. Microbiol. Immunol.*, **333**: 43–82.

Fouchier, R. A., Schneeberger, P. M., Rozendaal, F. W., *et al.* (2004). Avian influenza A virus (H7N7) associated with human conjunctivitis and a fatal case of acute respiratory distress syndrome. *Proc. Natl. Acad. Sci. SA*,**101**(5): 1356–61.

Furuta, Y., Takahashi, K., Shiraki, K., *et al.* (2009). T705 (favipravir) and related compounds: novel broad-spectrum inhibitors of RNA infections. *Antiviral. Res.* **82**: 95–102.

Garten, R. J., Davis, C. T., Russell, C. A., *et al.* (2009). Antigenic and genetic characteristics of swine-origin 2009 A(H1N1) influenza viruses circulating in humans. *Sci.*, **325**: 197–201.

Gauer, A., Bagga, B., Barman, S., *et al.* (2010). Intravenous zanamivir for oseltamivir-resistant 2009 H1N1 influenza. *N. Engl. J. Med.*, **362**: 88–89.

Gordon, C., Johnson, P., Permazei, M., *et al.* (2010). Association between severe pandemic 2009 influenza A (H1N1) virus infection and immmunoglobulin G2 subclass deficiency. *Clin. Infect. Dis.*, **50**: 672–78.

Gorman, O. T., Bean, W. J., Kawaoka, Y., Donatelli, I., Guo, Y., and Webster, R. G. (1991). Evolution of influenza A virus nucleoprotein genes: implications for the origin of H1N1 human and classical swine viruses. *J. Virol.*, **65**: 3704–14.

Gourrean, J. M., Raiser, C., Valette, M., Donglao, A. R., Labie, J., Aymard, M. (1994). Isolation of two H1N2 influence viruses from Swine in France. *Arch. Virol.*, **135**: 365–82.

Guo, Y., Wang, M., Kawaoka, Y., Gorman, O., Ito, T., Saito, T., Webster, R. G. (1992b). Characterization of a new avian-like influenza A virus from horses in China. *Virology*, **188**: 245–55.

Hayden, F. (2009). Developing new antiviral agents for influenza treatment: what does the future hold? *Clin. Infect. Dis.*, **48**(Suppl 1): S3–13.

Heilman, C. and La Montagne, J. R. (1990). Influenza: status and prospects for its prevention, therapy and control. *Pediatric. Clin. N. Am.*, **37**: 669–88.

Hinshaw, V. S., Bean, W. J., Geraci, J. R., Fiorelli, P., Early, G., and Webster, R. G. (1986). Characterization of two influenza A viruses from a pilot whale. *J. Virol.*, **58**: 655–56.

Hinshaw, V. S., Webster, R. G., and Turner, B. (1978). Novel influenza A viruses isolated from Canadian feral ducks: including strains antigenically related to swine influenza (Hsw1N1) viruses. *J. Gen. Virol.*, **41**: 115–27.

Hinshaw, V. S., Webster, R. G., and Turner, B. (1979). Water-borne transmission of influenza A viruses. *Intervir.*, **11**: 65–68.

Hinshaw, V. S., Webster, R. G., and Turner, B. (1980). The perpetuation of orthomyxoviruses and paramyxoviruses in Canadian waterfowl. *Can. J. Microbiol.*, **26**: 622–29.

Hodder, R. A., Gaydos, J. C., Allen, R. G., Top, F. H., Nowosiwsky, T., and Russell, P. K. (1977). Swine influenza A at Fort Dix, New Jersey. Extent of spread and duration of the outbreak. *J. Infect. Dis.*, **136**: 369–75.

Hurt, A. C., Ernest, J., Deng, Y. M., *et al.* (2009). Emergence and spread of oseltamivir-resistant A(H1N1) influenza viruses in Oceania, South East Asia and South Africa. *Antivir. Res.*, **83**: 90–93.

Hurt, A. C., Ho, H. T., and Barr, I. (2006). Resistance to anti-influenza drugs: adamantanes and neuraminidase inhibitors. *Expert. Rev. Anti. Infect. Ther.*, **4**: 795–805.

Hurt, A. C., Holien, J. K., Parker, M., *et al.* (2009). Zanamivir-resistant influenza viruses with a novel neuraminidase mutation. *J. Virol.*, **83**: 10366–73.

International Committee on Taxonomy of Viruses (2005). http://www.ICTVdb.org/Ictv/index.htm.

Jadhao, S. J., Nguyen, D. C., Uyeki, T. M., Shaw, M., *et al.* (2009). Genetic analysis of avian influenza A viruses isolated from domestic waterfowl in live-bird markets of Hanoi, Vietnam, preceding fatal H5N1 human infections in 2004. *Arch. Virol.*, **154**(8): 1249–61.

Jefferson, T., Demicheli, V., Di Pietrantonj, C., *et al.* (2006). Amantadine and rimantadine for influenza A in adults. *Cochr. Datab. Syst. Rev.*, **2**: CD001169.

Jefferson, T., Jones, M., Doshi, P., *et al.* (2009). Neuraminidase inhibitors for preventing and treating influenza in healthy adults: systematic review and meta-analysis. *BMJ*, **339**: b5106.

Jefferson, T. O., Demicheli, V., Di Pietrantonj, C., *et al.* (2006). Neuraminidase inhibitors for preventing and treating influenza in healthy adults. *Cochr. Datab. Syst. Rev.*, **3**: CD001265.

Jossetab, L., Frobertab, E., Rosa-Calatravaa, M. (2008). Influenza A replication and host nuclear compartments: Many changes and many questions. *J. Clin. Viro.*, **43**: 381–90.

Kaplan, M. M. and Webster, R. G. (1977). The epidemiology of influenza. *Sci. Am.*, **237**: 88–106.

Kawaoka, Y., Krauss, S. and Webster, R. G. (1989). Avian-to-human transmission of the PB1 gene of influenza A viruses in the 1957 and 1968 pandemics. *J. Virol.*, **63**: 4603–8.

Keawcharoen, J., Oraveerakul, K., Kuiken, T., Fouchier, R. A. M., *et al.* (2004). Avian influenza H5N1 in tigers and leopards. *Emerg. Infect. Dis.*, **10**: 2189–91.

Kendal, A. P. (1987). Epidemiologic implications of changes in the influenza virus genome. *Am. J. Med.*, **82**: 4–14.

Kida, H. *et al.*(1994). Potential for transmission of avian influenza viruses to pigs. *J. Gen. Virol.*, **75**: 2183–88.

Kluzka, V., Macku, M., and Mensik, J. (1961). Evidence for pig influenza virus antibodies in humans. *Ceskoslov. Pediatr.*, **16**: 408–11.

Koopmans, M., Wilbrink, B., Conyn, M., *et al.* (2004). Transmission of H7N7 avian influenza A virus to human beings during a large outbreak in commercial poultry farms in the Netherlands. *Lancet*, **363**: 587–93.

Lackenby, A., Thompson, C. I., and Democratis, J. (2008). The potential impact of neuraminidase inhibitor resistant influenza. *Curr. Opin. Infect. Dis.*, **21**: 626–38.

Lang, G., Gagnon, A., Gerani, J. R. (1981). Isolation of an influenza. A virus from Seals. *Arch. Virol.*, **68**: 189–95.

Ludwig, S., Stitz, L., Planz, O., Van, H., Fitch, W. M., and Scholtissek, C. (1995). European swine virus as a possible source for the next influenza pandemic? *Virol.*, **212**: 555–61.

Ma, W., Vincent, A., Gramer, M. R., *et al.* (2007). Identification of H2N3 influenza A viruses from swine in the United States. *Proc. Natl. Acad. Sci. USA*, **104**(52): 20949–54.

Monto, A. S., Ansaldi, F., Aspinall, R., McElhaney, J. E., *et al.* (2009). Influenza control in the 21st century: Optimizing protection of older adults. *Vaccine*, **27**(37): 5043–53.

Morens, D. M., Taubenberger, J. K, and Fauci, A. S. (2009). The persistent legacy of the 1918 influenza virus. *N. Engl. J. Med.*, **361**: 225–29.

Morens, D. M., Taubenberger, J. K., Harvey, H. A., and Memoli, M. J. (2010). The 1918 influenza pandemic: Lessons for 2009 and the future. *Crit. Care Med.*, **38**: e10–e20.

Morgan, I. R. and Kelly, A. P. (1990). Epidemiology of an avian influenza outbreak in Victoria in 1985. *Aus. Vet. J.*, **67**: 125–28.

Moscona, A. (2009). Global transmission of oseltamivir-resistant influenza. *N. Engl. J. Med.*, **360**: 953–56.

Moscona, A. (2005). Neuraminidase inhibitors for influenza. *N. Engl. J. Med.*, **353**: 1363–73.

Moscona, A. (2005). Oseltamivir resistance—disabling our influenza defenses. *N. Engl. J. Med.*, **353**: 2633–36.

Moss, R. B., Davey, R. T., Steigbigel, R. T., *et al.* (2010). Targeting pandemic influenza: a primer on influenza antivirals and drug resistance. *J. Antimicrob. Chemother.*, **65**(6): 1086–93.

Murcia, P. R., Baillie, G. J., Daly, J., Elton, D., *et al.* (2010). Intra- and interhost evolutionary dynamics of equine influenza virus. *J. Virol.*, **84**(14): 6943–54.

Nakajima, K., Desselburger, U., and Palese, P. (1978). Recent human influenza A (H1N1) viruses are closely related genetically to strains isolated in 1950. *Nature*, **274**: 334–39.

Nerome, K., Ishida, M., Oya, A., Kanai, C., Suwicha, K. (1982). Isolation of an influenza HIN1 virus from a pig. *Virol.*, **117**: 485–89.

Neumann, G., Noda, T., Kawaoka, Y. (2009). Emergence and pandemic potential of swine-origin H1N1 influenza virus. *Nature*, **459**(7249): 931–39.

Nguyen, D. C., Uyeki, T. M., Jadhao, S., *et al.* (2005). Isolation and characterization of avian influenza viruses, including highly pathogenic H5NI, from poultry in live bird markets in Hanoi, Vietnam, in 2001. *J. Virol.*, **79**: 4201–12.

Nguyen-Van-Tam, J. S., Nair, P., Acheson, P., *et al.* (2006). Outbreak of low pathogenicity H7N3 AI in UK, including associated case of human conjunctivitis. *Euro Eurosurveil.*, **11**(5).

Office International des Epizooties (OIE) (2004). Manual of standards for diagnostic tests and vaccines, 2004. Paris, France: Office International des Epizooties. pp. 1–957.

Patriarca, P. A., *et al.* (1984). Lack of significant person to person spread of swine influenza-like virus following fatal infection in an immunocompromised child. *Am. J. Epidem.*, **119**: 152–58.

Peiris, J. S., Yu, W. C., Leung, C. W., *et al.* (2004). Re-emergence of fatal human influenza A subtype H5N1 disease. *Lancet*, **363**: 617–19.

Perdue, M. L. and Swayne, D. E. (2004). Public health risk from avian influenza viruses. *Av. Dis.*, **419**: 317–27.

Pinto, L. H., Lamb, R.A. (2007). Controlling influenza virus replication by inhibiting its proton channel. *Mol. Biosyst.*, **3**: 18–23.

Reid, A. H., Fanning, T. G., Janczewski, T.A., and Taubenberger, J. K. (2000). Characterization of the 1918 'Spanish' influenza virus neuraminidase gene. *Proc. Natl. Acad. Sci. USA*, **97**(12): 6785–90.

Reid, A. H., and Taubenberger, J. K. (2003). The origin of the 1918 pandemic influenza virus: a continuing enigma. *J. Gen. Virol.*, **84**: 2285–92.

Reid, A. H., Taubenberger, J. K., and Fanning, T. G. (2004). Evidence of an absence: the genetic origins of the 1918 pandemic influenza virus. *Nat. Rev. Microbiol.*, **2**: 909–914.

Robinson, H. L., Hunt, L. A., and Webster, R. G. (1993). Protection against a lethal influenza virus challenge by immunization with a haemagglutinin-expressing plasmid DNA. *Vaccine*, 11: 957–60.

Romijn, P. C., Swallow, C., and Edwards, S. (1989). Survival of influenza virus in pig tissues after slaughter. *Vet. Rec.*, 124: 224.

Schnurrenburger, P. R., Woods, G. T., and Martin, R. J. (1970). Serologic evidence of human infection with swine influenza virus. *Am. Rev. Respir. Dis.*, 102: 356–61.

Scholtissek, C., Burger, H., Kistner, O., and Shortridge, K. F. (1985). The nucleoprotein as a possible major factor in determining host specificity of influenza H3N2 viruses. *Virol.*, 147: 287–94.

Sharp, G. B., Kawaoka, Y., Wright, S. M., Turner, B., Hinshaw, V. S., and Webster, R. G. (1993). Wild ducks are the reservoir for only a limited number of influenza A subtypes. *Epidemiol. Infect.*, 110: 161–76.

Shinde, V., Bridges, C. B., Uyeki, T. M., *et al.* (2009). Triple-reassortant swine influenza A (H1) in humans in the United States, 2005–2009. *N. Engl. J. Med.*, 360: 2616–25.

Shoham, D. (1993). Biotic abiotic mechanisms for long term preservation and reemergence of influenza type A virus genes. *Prog. Med. Virol.*, 40: 178–92.

Shortridge, K. F. (1992). Pandemic influenza: a zoonosis? *Sem. Resp. Infect.*, 7: 11–25.

Shortridge, K. F. and Stuart-Harris, C. H. (1982). An influenza epicenter? *Lancet*, 2: 812–13.

Sims, L. D., Guan, Y., Ellis, T. M., Liu, K. K., *et al.* (2003). An update on avian influenza in Hong Kong 2002. *Av. Dis.*, 47: 1083–86.

Smee, D. F., Hurst, B. L., Egawa, H., *et al.* (2009). Intracellular metabolism of favipiravir (T-705) in uninfected and influenza A (H5N1) virus-infected cells. *J. Antimicrob. Chemother.*, 64: 741–46.

Smith, G. J., Bahl, J., Vijaykrishna, D., Zhang, J., *et al.* (2009). Dating the emergence of pandemic influenza viruses. *Proc. Natl. Acad. Sci. USA*, 106: 11709–12.

Smith, L. R., Wloch, M. K., Ye, M., Reyes, L. R., *et al.* (2010). Phase 1 clinical trials of the safety and immunogenicity of adjuvanted plasmid DNA vaccines encoding influenza A virus H5 hemagglutinin. *Vaccine*, 28(13): 2565–72.

Snyder, M. H., Buckler-White, A. J., London, W. T., Tierney, E. L., and Murphy, B. R. (1987). The avian influenza virus nucleoprotein gene and a specific constellation of avian and human virus polymerase genes each specify attenuation of avian/human influenza A/Pintail/79 reassortant viruses from monkeys. *J. Vir.*, 61: 2857–63.

Song, D., Lee, C., Kang, B., Jung, K., *et al.* (2009). Experimental Infection of Dogs with Avian-Origin Canine Influenza A Virus (H3N2). *Emerg. Infect. Dis.*, 15(1): 56–85.

Sovinova, O., Tumova, B., Poutska, F., and Nemec, J. (1958). Isolation of a virus causing respiratory disease in horses. *Acta Virol.*, 2: 52–61.

Sprenger, M. W. J., Beyer, W. E. P., Kempen, B. M., Mulder, P. G. H., and Masurel, N. (1993). Risk factors for influenza mortality. In: C. Hannoun, A. P. Kendal, H. D. Klenk, and F. L. Ruben (eds.) *Options for the Control of Influenza II*, pp. 15–23. Amsterdam: Elsevier.

Stuart-Harris, C. H., Schild, G. C., Oxford, J. S. (1985). Influenza: in animals and birds. In: C. H. Stuart-Harris, G. C. Schild, J. S. Oxford, (eds.) *Influenza: The Viruses and the Disease* (2nd edn.), pp. 83–102. Maryland, Baltimore: Edward Arnold.

Stubbs, E. L. (1965). Fowl plague. In: H. E. Biester, L. H. Schwarte (eds.) *Diseases of poultry*, (5th edn.), pp. 813–22. Ames, IOWA: Iowa State University Press.

Subbarao, K., Klimov, A., Katz, J. (1998). Characterization of an avian influenza A (H5N1) virus isolated from a child with a fatal respiratory illness. *Sci.*, 279(5349): 393–96.

Sugimura, T., Yonemochi, H., Ogawa, T., Tanaka, Y., and Kumagai, T. (1980). Isolation of a recombinant influenza virus (Hsw1N2) from swine in Japan. *Arch. Virol.*, 66: 271–74.

Suzuki, H., Saito, R., Masuda, H., *et al.* (2003). Emergence of amantadine-resistant influenza A viruses: epidemiological study. *J. Infect. Chemother.*, 9: 195–200.

Taubenberger, J. K., Harvey, H. A., and Memoli, M. J. (2010). The 1918 influenza pandemic: Lessons for 2009 and the future. *Crit. Care Med.*, 38: e10–e20.

Taubenberger, J. K., Reid, A. H., Krafft, A., *et al.* (1997). Initial genetic characterization of the 1918 'Spanish' influenza virus. *Sci.*, 275: 1793–96.

Taubenberger, J. K., Reid, A. H., Lourens, R. M., *et al.* (2005). Characterization of the 1918 influenza polymerase genes. *Nature*, 437: 889–93.

Taubenberger, J. K. (2003). Fixed and frozen flu: the 1918 influenza and lessons for the future. *Avi. Dis.*, 47: 789–91.

Top, F. H. and Russell, P. K. (1977). Swine influenza A at Fort Dix, New Jersey (January–February 1976). IV. Summary and speculation. *J. Infect. Dis.*, 136(SuppL): S376–80.

Tran, T. H., Nguyen, T. L., Nguyen, T. D., *et al.* (2004). Avian influenza A (H5N1) in 10 patients in Vietnam. *N. Engl. J. Med.*, 350: 1179–88.

Tu, J., Zhou, H., Jiang, T., Li, C., *et al.* (2009). Isolation and molecular characterization of equine H3N8 influenza viruses from pigs in China. *Arch. Virol.*, 154(5): 887–90.

Ulmer, J. B., Donnelly, J. J., Parker, S. E., Rhodes, G. H., Feigner, P. L., and Dwarki, V. J. (1993). Heterologous protection against influenza by injection of DNA encoding a viral protein. *Sci.*, 259: 1745–49.

Vijaykrishna, D., Poon, L. L., Zhu, H. C., *et al.* (2010). Reassortment of pandemic H1N1/2009 influenza A virus in swine. *Sci.*, 328(5985): 1529.

Wang, R., and Taubenberger, J. K. (2010). Methods for molecular surveillance of influenza. *Expert. Rev. Anti. Infect. Ther.*, 8: 517–27.

Webster, R. G., Bean, W. J., Gorman, O. T., Chambers, T. M., and Kawaoka, Y. (1992). Evolution and ecology of influenza A viruses. *Microbiol. Rev.*, 56: 152–79.

Webster, R. G., Guan, Y., Shortridge, K. F., Rohm, C., and Kawaoka, Y. (1996). The emergence of influenza A viruses in mammalian and avian species. *Proc. Op. Cont. Influen.*, 4–9 May, Cairns, Australia, p. 40.

Webster, R. G., Geraci, J., Petursson, G., and Skirnisson, K. (1981). Conjunctivitis in human beings caused by influenza A virus of seals [letter]. *N. Engl. J. Med.*, 304: 911–81.

Webster, R. G., Hinshaw, V. S., Bean, W. J., *et al.* (1981). Characterization of an influenza A virus from seals. *Virol.*, 113: 712–24.

Webster, R. G., Guan, Y., Peiris, M., *et al.* (2002). Characterization of H5N1 influenza viruses that continue to circulate in geese in southeastern China. *J. Virol.*, 76: 118–26.

Webster, R. G., Yakhno, M. A., Hinshaw, V. S., Bean, W. J., and Murti, K. G. (1978). Intestinal influenza: replication characterization of influenza viruses in ducks. *Virol.*, 84: 268–78.

Weinstock, D. M., and Zuccotti, G. (2009). The evolution of influenza resistance and treatment. *JAMA*, 301: 1066–69.

Wentworth, D. E., *et al.* (1994). An influenza A (H1N1) virus, closely related to swine influenza virus, responsible for a fatal case of human influenza. *J. Virol.*, 68: 2051–58.

WHO INFOSAN. Five keys to safer food. http://www.who.int/foodsafety/publications/consumer/en/5keys_en.pdf.

WHO INFOSAN. Highly pathogenic H5N1 avian influenza outbreaks in poultry and in humans: Food safety implications 4 November 2005. http://www.who.int/foodsafety/fs_management/No_07_AI_Nov05_en.pdf.

WHO. Oseltamivir Resistance in Immunocompromised Hospital Patients. http://www.who.int/csr/disease/swineflu/notes/briefing_20091202/en/index.html/ (3 December 2009, date last accessed).

World Health Organization. Committee (1980). A revision of the system of nomenclature for influenza viruses: a WHO memorandum. *Bull. World Heal. Organ.*, 58: 585–91.

Yasuda, J., Shortridge, K. F., Shimizu, Y., and Kida, H. (1991). Molecular evidence for a role of domestic ducks in the introduction of avian H3 influenza viruses to pigs in Southern China, where the A/Hong Kong/68 (H3N2) strain emerged. *J. Gen. Virol.*, 72: 2007–10.

Yuen, K. Y., Chan, P. K., Peiris, M., *et al.* (1998). Clinical features and rapid viral diagnosis of human disease associated with avian influenza A H5N1 virus. *Lancet*, 351(9101): 467–71.

Zimmer, S. M., and Burke, D. S. (2009). Historical perspective—emergence of influenza A (H1N1) viruses. *N. Engl. J. Med.*, 361: 279–85.

CHAPTER 31

Marburg and Ebola viruses

G. Lloyd

Summary

Marburg and Ebola viruses cause severe and often fatal haemorrhagic disease in humans and non-human primates. They are the two established members of the family Filoviridae and have a distinctive filamentous and irregular morphology with a genome consisting of a very large (about 19 kb) single-stranded RNA of negative polarity. Features of their organization and structure at the molecular level have led to their inclusion in the taxonomic order Mononegavirales, together with the Paramyxoviruses and the Rhabdoviruses.

From its original description in 1967 to 2009, there have been eight reported outbreaks of human Marburg virus infection. The first being three simultaneous outbreaks that occurred in Europe at Marburg, Frankfurt, and Belgrade, following the importation of infected African green monkeys (*Ceropithecus aethiops*) from Uganda. The remaining outbreaks occurred in South Africa 1975; Kenya 1980 and 1987; Democratic Republic of Congo (DRC) (1988–2000); Angola (2004–5) and Uganda (2007 and 2008). These eight episodes involved 449 cases with 369 deaths, an overall fatality rate of 82.3%. All the deaths to date have occurred in the primary cases.

Between 1976 and 2009 outbreaks of human Ebola haemorrhagic fever have been identified in Zaire (1976, 1977, 1995, 2001–2, 2003 and 2007); Sudan (1976, 1979 and 2004); Uganda (2000–1 and 2007–8); Kenya (1980); Côte d'Ivoire (1994 and 1995); and the Gabon (1996 and 1997). All age groups and sexes were affected. In addition, a laboratory-derived infection occurred during the studies of the 1976 Zaire and Sudan epidemic. There is no known endemic incidence of the disease and the mortality rates are based on the limited numbers of epidemics identified. This has involved 2,292-recorded cases with 1,524 deaths, an overall case fatality rate of 66.5%.

A new strain of Ebola virus named Reston was isolated from an epizootic of dying cynomolgus monkeys shipped to the USA (1989, 1990) and Italy (1992) from the Philippines. The virus proved antigenically and genetically distinct from the African Ebola viruses. Human infections documented during the USA epizootic proved asymptomatic. There was no evidence of an epidemiological link with Africa. Therefore, unlike its African counterparts Reston Ebola Virus has proven to date to be non-pathogenic in humans. The high mortality among monkeys makes them an unlikely natural reservoirs.

However, six out of 141 slaughterhouse workers studied in the Philippines, who had daily contact with Ebola seropositive pigs, had antibodies against Reston ebolavirus. This marks the first time that Reston ebolavirus has been found in pigs and the possibility of Ebola transmission to humans from pigs to humans, has occurred (Barrette 2009; World Health Organization (WHO) 2009).

In Africa, the transmission of haemorrhagic fever caused by Ebola and Marburg has been associated with the reuse of unsterile needles and syringes, with the provision of patient care without appropriate barrier precautions preventing exposure to virus-containing blood and other body fluids and preparing bodies for funerals and burial. In addition, the killing and preparing of non-human primates for food was considered the source of SOMP outbreaks. Epidemiological studies in humans indicate that the airborne route does not readily transmit infection from person to person. By contrast, studies of Ebola and Marburg virus infections in non-human primates have suggested possible airborne spread among these species. The risk of person-to-person transmission is highest during the later stages of illness. Studies of individuals who are in contact with an infected patient during the incubation period indicate that infection risk is low.

As the natural history and reservoir of the Filoviruses are unknown, there are no specific precautions for avoiding infection from the natural environment. Non-human primates are not considered the natural reservoir of Filoviruses despite being the source of Marburg virus introduced into Europe and Ebola viruses introduced into the USA and Italy. The precautionary quarantining of non-human primates imported from Africa and Asia for a minimum of six weeks reduces the possibility of introducing a Filovirus infection. Recently, extensive studies undertaken to determine the reservoir of Filoviruses have identified in common species of fruit bat (*Rousettus aegyptiacus*) as a potential candidate (Swanepoel 1996; Towner 2007; Pourrut 2009).

Since there are no licensed vaccines or specific antiviral drugs for the treatment of Filovirus infections, early identification of infected patients or animals is essential. Prevention strategies reducing the risk of transmission in endemic and non-endemic areas rely on the introduction of strict isolation of febrile patients and rigorous use of barrier precautions. Consequently, many institutions and experts consider Filoviruses potential biological weapons (Borro 2002). Filovirus public health and biodefence research require the use of maximum-containment laboratory facilities where Filoviruses are handled under biosafety-level (BSL)-4 containment to protect laboratory workers from infection. There are only a few such facilities that exist worldwide.

History

Filovirus infections were unknown until 1967, when 31 human cases of an acute haemorrhagic fever occurred simultaneously in Marburg and Frankfurt, Federal Republic of Germany, and Belgrade, former Yugoslavia (Martini 1969). Laboratory workers, medical personnel, animal care personnel and their relatives were infected, seven of whom died. The primary cases occurred through contact with kidney tissue, blood, and cell cultures derived from Vervet or African green monkeys (*Ceropithecus aethiops*) imported from Uganda. The virus isolated from patient's blood and tissue was morphologically unique when observed by electron microscopy (see Fig. 31.1a) and antigenically unrelated to any known mammalian pathogen. This viral agent was named Marburg virus (MBG) after the city of Marburg, where most of the cases and initial work occurred. During 1975 (Zimbabwe), 1980 and 1987 (Kenya) there were sporadic fatal cases identified primarily amongst tourists. The Kenyan cases had included visits to bat infested Kitum caves in Kenya's Mount Elgon National Park (Gear *et al.* 1975; Smith *et al.* 1982; Teepe *et al.* 1983; Johnson *et al.* 1996) (Table 31.1). Apart from the 1987 case, secondary infections proved a risk to health care workers. Further epidemiological investigations in these areas has revealed no information on the origin of these infections occurred.

Between late 1998 and 2000 in Democratic Republic of the Congo the first large outbreak of this disease under natural conditions occurred, which involved 154 cases, of which 128 were fatal, representing a case fatality rate of 83%. The majority of cases occurred in young male workers at a gold mine in Durba, in the northeastern part of the country, which proved to be the epicentre of the outbreak. Cases spread to the neighbouring village of Waste. Family members involved in the close care of patients accounted for some cases, but secondary transmission appeared to be rare.

The largest Marburg outbreak in history occurred between 2004 and 2005, in Angola. It was believed to have started in Uige Province in October 2004 that resulted in 252 cases, with 227 deaths (CFR 88%) countrywide by July 2005. All cases detected in other provinces were linked to the outbreak in Uige (Towers 2006).

From June to August 2007, three confirmed cases occurred amongst mineworkers working in Kamwenge, western Uganda were identified. Of the two miners who cared for the index case who died, one also suffered a fatal illness (WHO 2007).

In July 2008, a Dutch tourist developed Marburg four days after returning to the Netherlands from a three-week holiday in Uganda. The source of the exposure has not been determined, although the woman had visited caves in Maramagambo Forest western Uganda at the southern edge of Queen Elizabeth National park, where bats were present (WHO 2008; Timen 2009).

There have been 414 primary human Marburg infections documented and an increasing number of secondary cases recorded which have originated from an increasing geographic range in Africa (Table 31.2).

In 1976, a severe and often fatal viral haemorrhagic fever occurred in simultaneous outbreaks in the equatorial provinces of

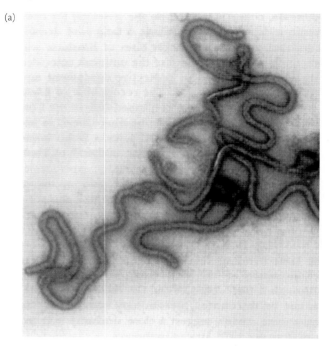

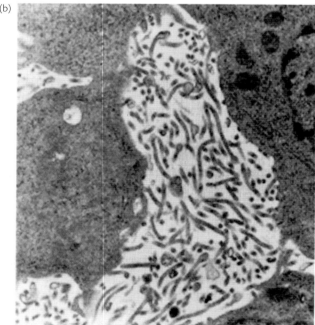

Fig. 31.1 (a) Electron micrograph, showing filamentous forms of Ebola (Reston) virus (×18 360). (b) Ebola (Sudan) virus thin section, showing virions extruding from cells into extracellular spaces (×14 040).
Courtesy of B. Dowsett

southern Sudan and northern Zaire (Table 31.2). Amongst the several hundred cases of infection identified, fatality rates of about 90 and 60% respectively occurred. Several generations of human-to-human spread contributed to the severity of the outbreak. The two virus strains isolated from patients in Sudan and Zaire where found to be morphologically identical to Marburg but

Table 31.1 Human pathogens in the order Mononegavirales

Family	Subfamily	Genus	Human pathogens
Rhabdoviridae			
		Lyssaviru	Rabies virus
Filoviridae			
		Marburg virus	Marburg virus
		Ebolavirus	Ebola virus
Paramyxoviridae			
	Paramyxovirinae		
		Rubulavirus	Mumps virus, Parainfluenzavirus 2,4
		Respirovirus	Parainfluenza virus 1,3
		Henipavirus	Hendra virus, Nipah virus
		Morbillivirus	Measles virus
		Rubulavirus	Mumps virus, Parainfluenzavirus 2,4
	Pneumovirinae		
		Pneumovirus	Respiratory syncytial virus
		Metaneumovirus	Human metapneumovirus

antigenically and biologically distinct (Bowen *et al.* 1977; WHO 1978*a, b*). The virus was named Ebola after a river in Zaire.

Numerous follow-up ecological studies have failed to discover the reservoir. During studies of the Sudanese epidemic in 1976, a non-fatal Ebola infection occurred within the UK in 1977 after a laboratory accident (Emond *et al.* 1977). Just over 6 months after the original outbreaks in Zaire, a 9 year old girl died of acute haemorrhagic fever in Tandala, northern Zaire (Heymann *et al.* 1980). A further small epidemic occurred in the same region of Sudan in 1979 when 22 (65%) of 34 infections were fatal, with transmissibility being associated with person-to-person spread (Baron *et al.* 1983). The geographic area widened when a Swiss zoologist became infected while undertaking an autopsy of a dead chimpanzee in western Côte d'Ivoire in late 1994. This resulted in her contracting a non-fatal severe Ebola illness (LeGuenno *et al.* 1995). Only after her treatment and discharge from a hospital in Switzerland was it discovered that she had suffered from an Ebola infection. A larger-scale outbreak in Kikwit, Bandundu Province, Zaire 1995 demonstrated to a worldwide audience a severe hemorrhagic illness involving some 316 cases, of which 244 died, giving a mortality rate of 77% (WHO 1995*a*). A third of the cases involved healthcare workers. The Kikwit outbreak was similar to the original episode that occurred in 1976, 1000 km to the north. As in previous outbreaks, secondary cases occurred through close personnel contact with infectious body fluids. The uncontrolled spread of infection resulted from a lack of modern medical facilities and supplies that could protect medical personnel from those patients initially affected. Unlike previous Ebola outbreaks, concern centered on the potential for community-wide spread from Kikwit, a large and densely populated area, to the larger cites of Kinshasa and Brazzaville close by. Control of the outbreak coincided with the introduction of protective equipment and barrier nursing techniques (WHO 1995*b*). The recognition of Ebola has recently extended to a confirmed case in the Côte d'Ivoire of a refugee from neighbouring Liberia in late 1995; other cases were reported to exist in his home village in Liberia (WHO 1995*c*).

During 1996–1997, two small outbreaks occurred in Gabon. These were found in the forest regions of Mayibout and Booué areas and where associated with people hunting and butchery of chimpanzees (Georges 1999). A major outbreak involving 425 cases occurring for the first time in Uganda during 2000–2001. Studies indicated that the three most import risk factors associated with its spread were associated with attendance at funerals of Ebola fever cases, having direct contact with cases and provision of medical care without adequate personal protective measures being used. The geographical spread continued during 2001–3 when Ebola outbreaks with case mortality rates reaching over 80% was recorded in Gabon and for the first time in The Democratic Republic of Congo (DRC) (Okware 2002; WHO 2003; Formenty 2003; WHO 2004). Repeat outbreaks in the DRC in 2007 and in Uganda in 2007–08 produced case fatality rates of 70% and 25% respectively.

Unexpectedly, Ebola virus has also appeared outside Africa when identified amongst cynomologus monkeys (*Macaca fasicularis*) imported into the USA in 1989 (Jahrling *et al.* 1990) and Siena, Italy in 1992 (WHO 1992). Shipments of wild-caught cynomolgus monkeys originated from the same handling facility in the Philippines, where the presence of the virus was documented. Although a truly Asian origin for these virus strains is not discounted, preliminary serological and sequencing studies, suggest a close similarity with isolates from the 1976 African outbreaks.

The agent

Taxonomy

Ebola and Marburg are members of the family Filoviridae (Kiley *et al.* 1982; Pringle 1991), named for their filamentous appearance under the electron microscope (Fig. 31.1a). Similarities of genome structure and comparable mechanisms of gene expression suggest that the filoviruses have an evolutionary origin in common with the families Paramyxoviridae (which include measles and mumps) and Rhabdoviridae (which includes rabies) (Sanchez *et al.* 1992). These three virus families are grouped into a taxonomic order (Table 31.1), the Mononegavirales (Bishop and Pringle 1995).

Progressive characterization of the filoviruses revealed substantial differences between the Marburgviruses and Ebolaviruses (Richman 1983) leading to the establishment of two genera, *Marburgvirus* and *Ebolavirus*, within the family *Filoviridae* (Feldmann 1994). The genus *Marburgvirus* contains only one species, *Lake Victoria Marburgvirus*, represented by a single virus, Lake Victoria Marburgvirus (MARV). The genus *Ebolavirus currently* contains five species: *Côte d'Ivoire ebolavirus* (Côte d'Ivoire ebolavirus, CIEBOV), *Reston ebolavirus* (Reston ebolavirus, REBOV), *Sudan ebolavirus* (Sudanebolavirus, SEBOV), '*Uganda ebolavirus*'

Table 31.2 Summary of human filovirus infections during identified outbreaks

Year	Filovirus	Source of infection	All cases deaths/total	Overall mortality rate (%)	Source	Comments
1967	Marburgvirus	Germany, Marburg	5/23	22.6	Vervet monkeys Imported from Uganda	
		Germany, Frankfurt	2/6			
		Yugoslavia, Belgrade	0/2			
1975	Marburgvirus	Zimbabwe/South Africa (Johannesburg)	1/3	33.3	Unknown	Index case infected in Zimbabwe. Secondary cases:–travelling companion and nurse
1976	Zaire ebolavirus	Northern Zaire (Yambuka)	280/318	88.1	Unknown	Index case introduced virus into hospital
1976	Sudan ebolavirus	Sudan, Maridi	116/213	53.2	Unknown	Disease amplified by transmission in large active hospital
		Sudan, Nazara	31/67			
		Sudan, Tembura	3/3			
		Sudan, Juba	1/1			Originatedin Nazara cotton factory
1976	Sudan ebolavirus	United Kingdom, Porton Down	0/1	0	Laboratory infection	Needle-stick
1977	(Zaire ebolavirus)	Zaire, Tandala	1/1	100	Unknown	Tandala
1979	Sudan ebolavirus	Southern Sudan, Yambo-Nazar District,	22/34	64.7	Unknown	Nazara, Maridi & local area
1980	Marburgvirus	Kenya, Mount Elgon	1/2	50	Unknown	Visited Kitum cave in national park
1987	Marburgvirus	Kenya, Mount Elgon, Kisumu	1/1	100	Unknown	Expatriate travelling in western Kenya. Visited Kitum cave
1988	Marburgvirus	USSR (Koltsova)	1/1	100	Laboratory infection	Associated with animal studies
1989-1990	Reston ebolavirus	US (Alice, Philadelphia, Reston)	0/4	0	Monkeys	Epizootic-imported monkeys from export facility in Philippines
1990	Reston ebolavirus	Philippines (Luzon)	0/12	0	Monkeys	Export facility
1990	Marburgvirus	USSR (Koltsovo)	0/1	0	Laboratory infection	Associated with animal studies
1992	Reston ebolavirus	Italy, Sienna	0	0	Monkeys	Epizootic-import from export facility in Philippines same as US outbreak in 1989
1994	Côte d'Ivoire ebolavirus	Côte d'Ivoire, Tai forest	0/1	0	Chimpanzees	Contracted in Scientist during post-mortem of chimpanzee repatriated to Switzerland
1994-1995	Zaire ebolavirus	Gabon (Andok, Mekouka, Minkebe, Mayela-Mbeza, Ovan, Etakangaye)	31/52	60	Unknown	
1995	Zaire ebolavirus	Zaire, Kikwit	245/317	77.3	Unknown	Confined to Bandundo region around Kikwit
1996	Zaire ebolavirus-	Gabon (Mayibout, Makokou)	21/37	57	Chimpanzees	Contact with dead primates hunted for food
1996	Zaire ebolavirus	Russia (Sergiyev Posad-6)	1/1	100	Laboratory infection	Associated with animal studies
1996-1997	Zaire ebolavirus	Gabon (Balimba, Boouee, Lastourville, Libreville, Lolo), South Africa (Johannesburg)	46/62	74.2	Chimpanzee?	Index case hunter Nurse treating imported case from Gabon to Johannesburg
1996	Reston ebolavirus	USA	0	0	Monkeys	Epizootic-Primates imported from Phillipines to quarantine facility in Texas
1996	Reston ebolavirus	Phillipines	0	0	Monkeys	Epizootic-Identified in Export facility. No human infections
1998-2000	Marburgvirus	Democratic Republic of Congo (Durba, Watsa)	128/154	83.1	Unknown	Epicentre of outbreak in young male gold workers in Durba
2000-2001	Sudan ebolavirus	Uganda (Gulu, Masindi & Mbarara Disricts)	224/425	52.7	Unknown	Spread through attending funerals, family case contact & medical centres

(Continued)

Table 31.2 (*Continued*)

Year	Filovirus	Source of infection	All cases deaths/total	Overall mortality rate (%)	Source	Comments
2001-2002	Zaire ebolavirus	Gabon (Ekata, Etakangaye, Franceville, Grand Etoumbi, Ilahounene,	53/65	82	Unknown	Community and Nosocomial spread on border region of Gabon and Congo
2001-2002	Zaire ebolavirus	Congo (Abolo, Ambomi, Entsiami, Kelle, Olloba	43/57	75.6	Unknown	
2002	Zaire ebolavirus	Congo (Olloba/Gabon(Etata))	10/11	90.9	Unknown	
2002-2003	Zaire ebolavirus	Republic of Congo (Mbomo & Kelle districts of)	129/143	89	Unknown	
2003-2004	Zaire ebolavirus	Republic of Congo (Mbomo and Mbandza villages in Mbomo district of)	29/35	83	Unknown	
2004	Zaire ebolavirus	Russia (Koltsovo)	1/1	100	Laboratory infection	Guinea pig adapted Zaire ebolavirus
2004-2005	Marburgvirus	Angola, Uige Province	227/252	90.1	Unknown	Community spread through various provinces linked to Uige
2004	Sudan ebolavirus	Sudan (Yambio)	7/17	41-.2	Unknown	Simultaneous outbreak of measles
2005	Zaire ebolavirus	Congo (Etoumbi, Mbomo)	9/11	81.9	Unknown	
2007	Marburgvirus	Uganda (Kamwenge District)	2/3	66.6	Unknown	Origins thought to be in Lead and Gold mines of area
2007	Zaire ebolavirus	Democratic Republic of Congo Kasai Occidental province	187/264	70.8	Unknown	
2007-2008	Bundibugyo ebolavirus	Uganda (Bundibugyo District)	25/149	16.8	Unknown	1st recorded occurrence of new strain
2008	Marburgvirus	Netherlands ex Uganda (Maramagambo Forest)	1/1	100	Cave in Maramagambo bats?	40 year old Dutch women,visited cave in National Park
2008	Ebola-Reston	Phillipines	6 assymptomtic cases	0	Pigs	1st known detection of Ebola-Reston in pigs. 6 assymptomtic cases amongst slaughter house workers.
2008-2009	Zaire ebolavirus	Democratic Republic of Congo	15/32	47		Outbreak in Mweka & Luebo of Kasai District
2009	Zaire ebolavirus	Germany	0/1	0	Laboratory infection	Animal vaccine studies

('Uganda ebolavirus,' 'UEBOV'), and *Zaire ebolavirus* (Zaire ebolavirus, ZEBOV) (Feldmann 2005; Mason 2008) (Table 31.3). In comparison, the genomes of members of the five ebolaviral species differ genetically by 37–41% at the nucleotide level, and all of them differ from MARV genomes by >65%. Amongst the genus Ebolavirus the three distinct species, Bundibugyo, Sudan and Zaire species have been associated with large outbreaks of Ebola haemorrhagic fever (EHF) in Africa causing death in 25–90% of all clinical cases, while Côte d'Ivoire and Reston have not.

Molecular biology

Filoviral genomes consists of a single non-segmented negative-stranded RNA about 19 kilobases in length and contain seven genes arranged linearly and that may be separated by intergenic regions. The linear arrangement of genes follows a sequence beginning with a 3′ non-coding untranslated region, the core protein genes, envelope genes, and the polymerase gene attached to the untranslated

region at the 5′ end. (Feldmann *et al.* 1993; Sanchez *et al.* 1993). Non-structural proteins are not present. Each gene is flanked by highly conserved transcription and termination sites that differ among the different Filoviruses (Weik 2002).

The genetic sequence of Marburg virus (MBG) and the available partial sequence of Ebola virus (EBO) indicate that in both cases seven structural proteins are encoded, which are expressed through transcription of monocistronic mRNA species. The first (3′) gene of the filoviral genomes, NP a major nucleoprotein (NP; M_r 94–104). The nucleocapsid is composed of RNA, L, NP, VP35, and VP30. Analysis of the NP gene shows a short putative leader sequence at the extreme 3 end followed by the complete nucleoprotein gene. The transcriptional start (3′…UUCUUCUUAUAAUU…) and termination (3′…UAAUUCUUUUU) signals of the MBG NP gene are very similar to those seen with EBO virus. The filoviral *VP35* gene is located immediately downstream of the *NP* gene. The VP35 protein is thought to be a transcriptase–polymerase component that is considered to be the P(NS) protein equivalent of paramyxo- and rhabdoviruses The VP35 and VP35-NP complexes also inhibit both dsRNA-mediated and virus-mediated induction of interferon-responsive promoters and consequently the cellular interferon innate immune response to virus infection. The filoviral matrix or membrane-associated *VP40* gene is located downstream of the *VP35* gene and is the most conserved of all filovirus genes, it encodes the matrix protein VP40 protein (M_r 32 000). The filoviral *GP* gene is a single surface glycoprotein (GP; M_r 170 000). Marburg and ebolavirus encode one and three glycoproteins from their GP genes, respectively The filoviral minor nucleoprotein *VP30* gene (VP30; M_r 32 000), located downstream of the *GP* gene, is another unique component of the filoviral genomes. It encodes a protein, VP30. The N-terminus of VP30 binds directly to single-stranded RNA, and prefers filoviral RNA over unspecific RNA (John 2007) VP30 is also a zinc-binding protein. In the absence of zinc, filovirus-genome transcription is abolished (Modrof 2003)). The *VP24* gene and its expression product is a second matrix or membrane-associated VP24 protein (M_r 24 000). Recent experiments also indicate that VP24 counteracts the interferon-response of virus-infected cells (Reid 2007). The last (5') gene of the filoviral genome is the *L* gene, which encodes the catalytic part (L protein; MARV: 2,331 amino-acid residues, 267 kD; ZEBOV: 2,212 amino-acid residues, 253 kD) of the viral RNA-dependent RNA polymerase holoenzyme, (M_r 267 000); which also contains VP35 (27, 195, 283).

In comparison to other non-structural non-segmented negative-strand (NNS) RNA viruses, filovirus transcriptional signals are very similar to those of members of the paramyxovirus and morbillivirus genera. Nucleotide sequence analysis of the 3' end, including the entire NP and L protein encoding genes of the MBG and EBO genome, has shown similar structure and organization with other NNS RNA viruses. The similarity of the filovirus NP genes and gene products to those of the paramyxoviruses imply a closer biological and phylogenetic relationship to these agents than to rhabdoviruses.

Growth and survival

Filoviruses undergo rapid, lytic replication in the cytoplasm of a wide range of host cells. The mode of entry of Filoviruses into cells occurs by binding to unidentified cell-surface receptors with their spike proteins. Although some ultrastructural studies have suggested that virions are associated with entry by endocytosis. African green monkey kidney cells, such as CV-1 and Vero derivatives, are commonly used to grow filoviruses to high titres. The filoviral nucleocapsid is released into the cytosol subsequent to fusion of the viral and cellular membrane, and complete uncoating of the filovirus genome takes place. The polymerase holoenzyme L/VP35, brought into the cell with the nucleocapsid, transcribes the filovirus genes in a sequence, synethizing the antigenome that is used as the template to synthesize the progeny genes. The filoviral messenger RNA's are abundant in infected cells and are translated into the filoviral structural proteins. The NP, VP30,VP35 and L proteins assemble with the newly synthesized genomes to form RNPs complexes. These recruit the matrix proteins VP40 and VP24 and bud from the cell's plasma membrane, acquiring the GP envelope with its surface projections by budding from the cell membranes (Noda 2006). The entire life cycle occurs in the cytoplasm of the host cell. Nucleocapsids also accumulate in the cytoplasm, forming prominent inclusion bodies.

Laboratory infection of tissue cells shows intracytoplasmic vesiculation and mitochondrial swelling followed by a breakdown of organelles and terminal rarification and condensation. These cytoplasmic changes occur simultaneously with the accumulation of viral nucleocapsid material in intracytoplasmic inclusion bodies and the large numbers of virions extracellularly (Fig. 31.1b).

The filovirus virion is bacilliform in structure and is composed of a helical nucleocapsid, consisting of a central axis (20–30 nm in diameter), surrounded by a helical capsid (40–50 nm in diameter). A host cell membrane derived lipid outer envelope, with regular 10 nm projections surrounds the nucleocapsid and completes the striking and characteristic appearance under the electron microscope (Fig. 31.1a). Although there are often structures of varying length, with loops, branches, and other irregularities, evidence exists that infectious particles consist mainly of simple linear forms about 1 μm in length.

Marburg and Ebola virus infectivity are stabilized at ambient temperature (18–20°C) but inactivated within 30 min at 60°C. Ultraviolet and gamma irradiation, lipids, solvents, β-propiolactone, hypochlorite, and phenolic disinfectants all destroy infectivity.

Disease mechanisms

The exact mechanism by which filoviruses cause such a serious illness is being unravelled. There is extensive viral replication in liver, lymphoid organs, and kidneys. Extensive visceral effusions, pulmonary interstitial oedema, and renal tubular dysfunction occurring after endothelial damage leading to hypovolaemic shock are all observations contributing to death. Severe, acute fluid loss accompanied by bleeding into the tissue and gastrointestinal tract is characteristic and leads to dehydration, electrolyte and acid-base imbalance. In primates and clinical cases studied early, lymphopenia is followed by a marked neutropenia (Fisher-Hoch *et al.* 1983). In the later stages of the infection, and in association with the thrombocytopenia, the remaining platelets are unable to aggregate in response to ADP or collagen. It has been suggested that the dysfunction of platelets and endothelia extends to other elements of the endothelial system, such as macrophages (Fisher-Hoch *et al.* 1985). In experimental monkey Ebola infections, virus has been identified in vascular endothelial cells. Humans convalescent from Marburg and Ebola infections have had virus isolated up to 3–4 months after onset in semen, in a patient with uveitis, anterior chamber fluid. There is no evidence of long-term persistence, latency or late degenerative disease in the small number of patients observed or in monkeys recovering from the disease (Fisher-Hoch *et al.* 1992a).

The hosts

Human

Incubation period

Filoviruses are transmitted through direct contact. They enter through small skin lesions or through damaged mucous membranes and initially infect target cells such as macrophages, which transport them through the body. The incubation period for Marburg virus disease is 3–9 days (Martini 1971; Bausch, 2006) and for Ebola virus about 10 days (Bwaka 1999) 5–7 days for needle transmission (Emond 1978) and 6–12 days for person-to-person spread.

Symptoms and signs

The illnesses caused by Marburg and Ebola viruses are virtually indistinguishable. Following exposure and incubation period, both infections have an abrupt onset of illness with initial non-specific symptoms such as fever, severe frontal headache, back pain malaise, and myalgia. Early signs include tachycardia, conjunctivitis, and maculopapular rashes, which develop after 5–7 days on face, buttocks, trunk or arms and later generalizes over the entire body with desquamation in survivors. Within a week to 10 days, those destined for recovery begin to improve, even though recovery from the severe debilitating effects of the disease often takes weeks. A large number of patients in both Marburg and Ebola outbreaks develop severe bleeding between the fifth and seventh days. Patients with severe infections often experience pharyngitis, severe nausea, and vomiting, progressing to haematemesis and melena. Petechiae, ecchymoses, uncontrolled bleeding from venepuncture sites and post-mortem evidence of visceral haemorrhagic effusions are characteristic of severe illness (Smith *et al.* 1978). Death usually occurs between the 7–10 days (range 1–21 days) after onset of clinical disease and is preceded by severe blood loss and shock. Convalescence is slow and marked by prostration, weight loss, and amnesia for a considerable period after the acute illness (Piot 1978; Formenty 1999). Death occurs usually after 8–16 days of infection due to shock after multi-organ failure, often brought on by secondary bacterial infections.

Clinical laboratory findings include early leucopoenia with left shift of the granulocytes accompanied by, marked thrombocytopenia, and abnormal platelet aggregation. Serum aspartate aminotransferase (AST)/alanine aminotransferase (ALT) enzyme levels are raised and characterized by a high AST/ALT ratio (10–3:1) and γ-glutamyl transpeptidase indicating liver damage. Other findings include raised levels of creatine and urea levels prior to renal failure and hypokalemia because of the diarrhea and vomiting.

As the differential diagnosis in the early acute phase is difficult, other causes need consideration. The most common causes of imported infections showing a severe, acute febrile disease are malaria and typhoid fever. Therefore, delay in differential diagnosis and treatment needs to be minimized. Alternative causes include bacterial diseases such as meningococcal septicaemia, *Yersinia pestis* infection, leptospirosis, anthrax; rickettsial diseases such as typhus and murine typhus; and viral diseases such as sandfly fever, yellow fever, chikungunya fever, Rift Valley fever, hantavirus, and Congo Crimean haemorrhagic fever.

Diagnosis

The diagnosis of Ebola or Marburg should be considered in patients showing acute, febrile illness having visited known epidemic or suspected endemic areas of rural sub-Saharan Africa and Asia, particularly when haemorrhagic signs are present. All tissues, blood, and serum collected in the acute stages of illness contain large amounts of infectious virus. Extreme care should be taken when drawing or handling blood specimens as the virus is stable for long periods at room temperature (Elliott *et al.* 1982). All needles and syringes need discarding to puncture-resistant containers with lids, and incinerated. Specimens of blood should be taken without anticoagulant. Blood or serum should be transferred to a leak proof plastic container and double wrapped in leak proof containers for transportation to a high containment laboratory. Transportation should be under appropriate biocontainment within dry or wet ice according to international transportation or national regulations (Department of Health 2007; WHO 2007) after consultation with any of the global maximum containment reference laboratories.

Inactivation of patients sera with irradiation or heating at 60°C for 30 min render them safe for undertaking immunoassay tests. Although morphologically similar, Marburg and Ebola are immunologically distinct. The immunofluorescence assay (IFA) has been the basic diagnostic test for filovirus infection and the only one that has widespread acceptance for the diagnosis of human Ebola disease (Wulff and Johnson 1979; Rollin *et al.* 1990). A rising antibody in paired serum or a high IgG titre (>64) and presence of IgM antibody, together with clinical symptoms compatible with a haemorrhagic fever, are consistent with a diagnosis. The presence of Marburg antibody is considered a specific result but Ebola virus low-titre, non-specific, false-positive serological reactions do occur. When using IFA the problem of low-titre false positives makes interpretation difficult when undertaking non-human primate and human seroepidemiological surveys. For the IFA, the antigen substrate consists of virus-infected Vero cells dried on to spot slides. Recent advances in molecular biology have expressed the nucleoprotein gene of Ebola virus in a baculovirus expression system. Thus, a large amount of non-infectious protein is a possible source of antigen for many serological tests (IFA, ELISA). There evaluation leading to an improvement in the detection capability within seroepidemiological field studies and in the screening of imported primates.

Filoviruses can be easily isolated from inoculation of fresh or stored (−70°C) specimens of blood or serum collected during the acute phase of illness into Vero monkey kidney tissue cultures cells using laboratory containment level 4 facilities. Vero cells (particularly clone E6) and MA-104 have proved to be the most sensitive and useful cells for the propagation and assay of fresh isolates and laboratory passage filovirus strains. Primary isolation using tissue culture rarely produces a specific cytoplasmic effect, thus evidence of infection is based on the appearance of cytoplasmic inclusion bodies demonstrated 2–5 days after inoculation, by immunofluoresence staining, using antipolyclonal anti-sera or virus subtype or strain-specific monoclonal antibodies. Some filovirus strains such as Ebola Sudan are difficult to grow in primary cultures and success is improved through the intraperitoneal inoculation of young guinea pigs. A monitored febrile response coincides with high levels of virus in the blood, which can be recovered in tissue culture or examined directly by the electron microscope. In each of the Filoviridae outbreaks electron microscopy has proven useful in the identification of Marburg or Ebola in body fluids and tissue, and cell culture supernatants. During the Reston epizootic, immunoelectron microscopy, when used in conjunction with standard transmission microscopy (TEM) of infected cells, provided consistent results (Geisbert and Jahrling 1990). However, the technique will not distinguish between the Filoviridae strains. Virus may also be detected in a range of specimens, including throat washings, semen and anterior eye fluid. The presence, of Ebola and Marburg in tissues of monkeys, both experimentally and during primate outbreaks, has been demonstrated by electron microscopy (Baskerville *et al.* 1985; Geisbert and Jahrling 1990); and detection of high titres in the blood of infected patients and monkeys indicated the usefulness of an antigen capture ELISA system (Ksiazek *et al.* 1992). Such a system has been of considerable use in the recent Kikwit epidemic. Immunobilized mouse monoclonal antibodies on a solid plastic surface capture Ebola antigen contained in tissue or blood specimens. Rabbit polyclonal anti-filovirus serum detects the antigen. The antigen immunoabsorbent detection assay has proved a rapid and reliable procedure for the early detection of filovirus infections and would prove useful as a method for the routine screening of imported primates.

In recent years, the use of cross-reacting and strain-specific probes for the reverse transcriptase polymerase chain reaction RT-PCR has evolved to the gold standard for Filovirus diagnosis in the field and has taken the place of previously widely used IFAs and ELISAs. Confirmatory diagnosis of RT-PCR-positive samples is usually performed by virus isolation in maximum-containment facilities (Grolla *et al.* 2005; Towner *et al.* 2004).

Currently all outbreaks of EHF and MHF, infections are confirmed by various laboratory diagnostic methods. These include virus isolation, reverse transcription-PCR (RT-PCR), including real-time quantitative RT-PCR, antigen-capture enzyme-linked immunosorbent assay (ELISA), antigen detection by immunostaining, and IgG- and IgM-ELISA using authentic virus antigens (Gibb *et al.* 2001; Ksiazek *et al.* 1992, 1999; Leroy *et al.* 2000; Towner *et al.* 2004; Zaki *et al.*1999; Saijo *et al.* 2006).

Primates

African green monkeys imported from Uganda were the identified source of the Marburg outbreak (Henderson *et al.* 1971), and cynomolgus monkeys the source ebola reston virus. Both species were imported and closely associated with medical research.

The general characteristics of primate filovirus infections amongst experimentally and naturally infected primates suggest that the incubation period varies between 4 and 20 days, during which time the virus replicates to high titre in the liver, spleen, lymph nodes, and lungs. The clinicopathological features noted include high fever, severe weight loss, anorexia, haemorrhages, and a distinctive skin rash in association with splenomegaly, marked elevation of lactate dehydrogenase, alanine aminotransferase and aspartate aminotransferase. The AST levels are constantly 2–10 times higher than that of ALT. Evidence of thrombocytopenia is a pronounced feature but anaemia is not. Both lymphocytopenia and leucocytosis are evident and dependent on the stage of the infection (Fisher-Hoch *et al.* 1983). Severe prostration with diarrhoea and bleeding leads to rapid death in almost all animals. The severity of the disease in primates depends on the filovirus infection and host involved. African green monkeys are far less susceptible to severe or fatal disease due to Ebola virus (Sudan) or Ebola (Reston) than cynomolgus monkeys. However, African green monkeys experimentally infected with Marburg virus after the 1967 outbreak all died irrespective of route of infection (Hass and Mass 1971). Marburg virus infection of rhesus monkeys is less severe or fatal, similar to Ebola (Sudan) infection. Infection by Ebola virus (Zaire) is uniformly fatal in all species so far challenged, regardless of inoculum.

Histopathological findings include severe hepatocellular necrosis, necrosis of the zona glomerulosa of the adrenal cortex, and interstitial pneumonia, all associated with the presence of intracytoplasmic amphophilic inclusion bodies. The necrotic lesions result from direct virus infection of the parenchymal cells. Little inflammatory response occurs at the site of the lesions.

Experimental pathophysiological studies have demonstrated endothelial cell and platelet dysfunction accompanied by oedema, multiple effusions, haemorrhage, and hypovolaemic shock (Fisher-Hoch *et al.* 1985). Recent studies in *Macaca fascicularis* and *Cercopithecus aethiops* suggest that the recently isolated Asian filoviruses are less pathogenic for primates than the African filoviruses (Fisher-Hoch *et al.* 1992*b*).

Treatment and prognosis

There is no licensed vaccine or effective antiviral drug treatment licensed for use in human. Therapy for Marburg and Ebola virus infection is limited to the provision of supportive measures and general nursing care. In the development of vaccines, recent advances have shown protection in animal models. Amongst the most recent promising vaccines under development are a number of recombinant based systems. The most noticeable those based vesicular stomatitis virus (VSV) that expresses a single filovirus glycoprotein (GP) in place of the VSV glycoprotein. A single dose vaccine has proved capable of protecting non-human primates against *Sudan ebolavirus* (SEBOV), *Zaire ebolavirus* (ZEBOV), *Cote d'Ivoire ebolavirus* (CIEBOV), and *Marburgvirus* (MARV) (Feldmann H *et al.* 2007; Geisbert *et al.* 2009). Recently, a two-injection filovirus vaccine regime based on an adenovirus vector expressing multiple antigens from five different filoviruses, (ZEBOV NP, ZEBOV GP, SEBOV GP, MARV Ci67 strain GP, MARV Ravn strain GP, MARV Musoke strain NP, MARV Musoke strain GP), proved successful (Pratt *et al.* 2010). All animals in these studies survived the initial filovirus challenge with a different strain or species of filovirus. However, there are a number of significant safety challenges in humans; particularly those with an altered immune status are yet to be overcome.

Intensive supportive care is currently considered most important: prevention of shock, cerebral oedema, renal failure, bacterial superinfection, hypoxia, and hypotension may be life saving. Patient care is complicated by the need for isolation and protection of medical and nursing personnel. The use of plastic patient isolators is a requirement in many countries, including the UK and Europe, despite the return to the strict barrier nursing techniques now favoured in the USA and in the recent African outbreaks in Zaire, Côte d'Ivoire, Gabon, Uganda and Angola.

Epidemiology

Epidemics

Marburg virus disease

A fulminating haemorrhagic fever caused by the Marburg virus was first recognized in August 1967 when it affected laboratory workers in three simultaneous outbreaks in Marburg and Frankfurt, Germany, and Belgrade, former Yugoslavia (Martini 1969). Altogether, there were 31 human infections, of whom 25 had primary infections acquired through contact of blood and tissues from shipments of African green monkeys (*Cercopithecus aethiops*) imported from Uganda, via London. The largest number of primary infections (20) occurred among workers of a Marburg pharmaceutical firm who prepared kidney cells for vaccine production. Among those infected, exposure was attributed to autopsies (13), cleaning of contaminated glassware (5), dissection of kidneys (1), and laboratory accident involving contaminated broken glassware (1). Personnel not in direct contact with contaminated material or who wore protective gloves or masks for work with monkeys was not infected. In Frankfurt, four further primary infections occurred in workers exposed to tissue culture.

A veterinary officer carrying out routine post-mortems was the single recorded primary case in Belgrade. Four of the secondary infections occurred in hospital personnel who came into close contact with patients. The fifth was the wife of the veterinary surgeon, who fell ill 10 days after nursing her husband at home. The sixth case involved the wife of a patient who had transmitted the disease through sexual intercourse 83 days after the illness. Seven of the primary cases were fatal, but no fatalities occurred amongst the six secondary cases.

Around 600 animals originating from four shipments reached Europe from Uganda over a 3-week period. Frankfurt received 50–60 animals from two shipments, Belgrade approximately 300 animals from three shipments, and the remainder went to Marburg. All spent between 60 and 87 days in a holding facility in Uganda before being shipped to London, Heathrow where they spent 636 hours in the animal hostel before being forwarded to Germany. Details on the Belgrade enzootic indicated that 46 of 99 animals imported from the first shipment died, and 20 and 30 from the second and third shipments, respectively. This epizootic was characterized by daily deaths of one or more animals throughout the 6-week quarantine period, suggesting ongoing transmission between animals. Epidemiological evidence of the outbreak suggested that transmission between monkeys in quarantine facilities was through direct contact with contaminated equipment. Direct contact with infected blood and tissue was considered the source for all human cases, and there was evidence of aerosol transmission. No epizootics were found in Uganda although uncorroborated information had suggested a large number of monkey deaths in colonies on the island near Lake Kyoga, north of Lake Victoria, to the east of Mount Elgon in Kenya. Ugandan monkeys were captured in this area, transported to Entebbe, where they were held for 3 days prior to shipment.

The first recognized outbreak of Marburg virus disease in Africa, and the first since the 1967 outbreak, occurred in South Africa in February 1975 (Gear *et al.* 1975) (Fig. 31.2b). The index case involved a young Australian tourist who had hitchhiked through Zimbabwe and died after admission to a Johannesburg hospital. Shortly afterwards two non-fatal secondary cases occurred, one his female travelling companion and a nurse (Table 33.1). Again, there was evidence that the virus persisted in the body; the virus was recovered from fluid aspirated from the anterior chamber of the nurse's right eye 80 days after onset of illness. In January 1980, Marburg re-appeared in Kenya (Smith *et al.* 1982). The index patient was an electrical engineer who acquired the fatal infection in western Kenya. A non-fatal secondary infection occurred 9 days later. This involved a doctor who attended the patient and had attempted mouth-to-mouth resuscitation. In 1987, an isolated case of fatal Marburg disease was again recognized in a 15 year old Danish boy who had been admitted to hospital in Kenya. Nine days prior to the onset of his disease, he also had visited Kitum Cave in Mount Elgon national park. Recent studies of colonies of *R.gypriacus* bats which inhabit these caves have demonstrated molecular and serologically positive for Marburgvirus but there role in transmission is as yet undefined (Kuzmin *et al.* 2010). Presently it is thought that the habitat of the natural host of Marburg virus is within, but not limited to, the Mount Elgon area and possibly overlaps the distribution of Ebola.

Between 1987 and 1998, the only case of Marbug reported were associated with laboratory accidents in the former Soviet Union of which one was fatal (Nikiforov *et al.* 1994) outlines the dangers associated with working with these agents in the laboratory.

However, in 1998, the largest natural outbreak of Marburg virus disease to date began in northeastern Democratic Republic of the Congo (DRC). This time, the focus of the outbreak was a town called Durba (population 16 000). A large number of men in this region work for the Kilo Moto Mining Company, which runs a number of illegal gold mines in the area. The Marburg outbreak started in November of 1998, although not reported to any international agencies until late April of 1999, following the death of the chief medical officer in the area from the disease. The outbreak had a case fatality rate of approximately 83 involving 154 cases before the declaration that the outbreak was over in 2000. The disease also spread to neighbouring villages particularly Watsa. Miners had a significantly higher risk of contracting Marburg than the general population of this area, suggesting frequent exposure to the natural reservoir of Marburg virus (Bausch 2006).

The size and extent of this outbreak was eclipsed at the beginning in 2004, when a Marburg outbreak occurred in Angola during October. Due to civil war in the country and a non-existent public health infrastructure, recognition of the outbreak was delayed until almost 6 months later, in March of 2005. The outbreak was declared over in November of 2005, after no additional cases had been reported (Towner 2006).

In 2007 three cases in young males, again associated with miners working in Lead and Gold mines in the Kamwenge District of Uganda was reported (WHO 2007). Finally in 2008, a Dutch tourist developed Marburg four days after returning to the Netherlands from a three week holiday in Uganda. To date, the source of the exposure has not been confirmed, although the woman visited Python Cave in western Uganda where bats were present (WHO 2008, 2009; Timen *et al.* 2009). The Ugandan Ministry of Health closed the cave after this case.

Ebola virus disease (Africa)

Two large simultaneous outbreaks of an acute haemorrhagic fever (subsequently named Ebola haemorrhagic fever) occurred in southern Sudan (WHO 1978*a*) and northern Zaire in 1976 (WHO 1978*b*) (Fig. 31.2b). The first outbreak was identified in southern Sudan in June, continuing through to November 1976. There were 284 cases, 67 in Nazara, 213 in Maridi, 3 in Tembura, and 1 in Juba. The focus of the epidemic was Nazara, a small town with clusters of houses scattered in dense woodland bordering the African rain-forest zone. The outbreak in Nazara originated in three employees of a cotton factory situated near the town centre. Detailed factory records for the previous 2 years did not show any

Table 31.3 Filovirus taxonomy

Order	Family	Genus	Species	Abbreviation
Mononegavirales	*Filoviridae*	*Ebolavirus*	*Sudan ebolavirus*	SEBOV
		Marburg virus	*Zaire ebolavirus*	ZEBOV
			Cote d'Ivoire ebolavirus	CIEBOV
			Reston ebolavirus	REBOV
			Bundibugyo ebolavirus	BUBOV
			Lake Victoria marburgvirus	MARV

(a) Ebola virus disease

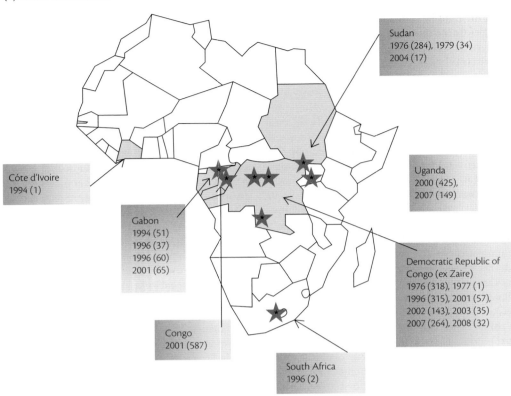

(b) Marburg virus disease

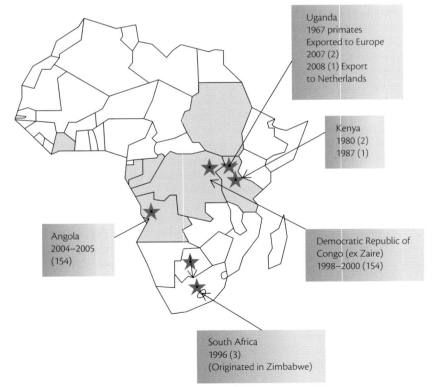

Fig. 31.2 Distribution and dates of filovirus outbreaks in Africa (a) Ebola virus disease and (b) Marburg virus disease.

fatal haemorrhagic disease in Nazara until June 1976. At that time, one or two workers started dying each week. By September, 6 factory workers and 25 of their contacts had developed the same illness, of which 21 died. Before the outbreak died out spontaneously cases were reported in two neighbouring areas. The first was in Tembura, a small town 160 km north of Nazara, where an ill woman went to be nursed by her family. Before she died, three women who cared for her also died of the same haemorrhagic disease. No other cases were discovered. Secondly, the epidemic was dramatically amplified by the larger hospital-associated outbreak (213 cases) in Maridi, following the introduction of a patient from Nazara. Maridi, a town east of Nazara, had an estimated population of 10,000 people. Ninety-three cases (46%) acquired their disease in hospital, and 105 (52%) in the community. Of the 230 staff at Maridi hospital, 72 became infected while at work and 41 died. The highest rate of infection was associated with nursing haemorrhagic patients who, at the height of the epidemic, occupied most wards. After Maridi, further cases (one from Nazara and three from Maridi) were transferred to the regional hospital in Juba. A further three patients were flown to Khartoum (1,200 km north), where two died. A nurse from Juba was the only secondary case identified as a result of these patient transfers.

Overall, there were 151 deaths (mortality rate, 53%) out of 284 cases. The outbreak in Nazara continued until October, infecting 67 people of whom 31 (46%) died, compared to 116 (54%) in Maridi. Studies on 36 families who nursed 38 primary cases indicated that of 232 contacts 30 (14%) developed disease. Similar rates of transmission were observed in subsequent generations, giving an overall secondary attack rate of 12%. Between July and October 1979, 34 cases of Ebola haemorrhagic fever recurred in the Yambio-Nazara District. Five family groups and two individuals became contracted the illness. The index case, a cotton-factory worker, transmitted the virus to several members of his family. The outbreak extended to other families through nosocomal transmission during his hospitalization and the hospitalization of subsequent cases. Mortality in this outbreak was 65% (22 deaths). It was unclear whether the cotton factory was the source of the index case of infection.

Also during September to October 1976, a large outbreak of Ebola haemorrhagic fever took place in the equatorial rain forest of northern Zaire (WHO 1978b). The index case had been touring and presented himself to the outpatient clinic at Yamkuka Mission Hospital (YMH) for treatment of acute malaria, and received an injection of chloroquine. He was admitted to hospital 10 days later with gastrointestinal bleeding and died. During the following week, nine other patients who had received treatment at the outpatient clinic of the YMH contracted Ebola haemorrhagic fever. Almost all subsequent cases had received injections or had been in close contact with other patients. The highest incidence was amongst women of 15–29 years, who had attended antenatal and outpatient clinics at this hospital and returned to their villages. After 13 of 17 staff had acquired the disease and 11 patients died, the hospital closed. The major risk factor proved to be the re-use of non-sterilized needles, which were in short supply. Between 1 September and 24 October, there were 318 known cases of Ebola haemorrhagic fever with 280 deaths, a case fatality of 88%. There were over 55 villages in the endemic area (Bumba zone), containing some 550 recorded cases. The overall secondary attack rate was calculated to be 5%, but nearer 20% in close relatives of a case. A further single fatal case

was identified in Tandala Hospital in northwestern Zaire in 1977 (Heymann et al. 1980). Studies in the Tandala region revealed two possible Ebola cases dating back to 1972, and a 7% Ebola seroprevalence rate in the local population.

In January 1995, a charcoal-maker near Kikwit, a town in Bandudu Province, 550 km east of Kinshasa, was the first fatal case of Ebola (WHO 1995a). By early March 12 members of his family had died. Simultaneously, a Shigella I dysentery epidemic was taking place and masked the early stages of the Ebola outbreak. Hospitals became sources of infection during February when an Ebola patient entered the Kikwit health centre and later transferred to the general hospital. During April, members of a resuscitating team became ill after handling a patient misdiagnosed as having typhoid. Rapid transmission of unprotected health workers and other patients occurred, many carrying the disease back into the community. Between January and June 315 cases had occurred, of which 244 died (77%). The female : male ratio was 166 : 149, which 74%(123) females and 81 per cent (121) males died. Provisional data identified 75 (26%) nurses or students and 61 (21%) housewives who contracted the disease. Two hundred and sixty-six (84%) of the cases resided within the Kikwit North and South Zones de Santé. No cases identified outside the Bandundu region.

The geographic distribution of Ebola virus widened in November 1994 when a non-fatal Ebola haemorrhagic fever case emerged for the first time in West Africa (LeGuenno et al. 1995). In the Tai National Park, Côte d'Ivoire, a 34 year old ethnologist infected herself while carrying out a post-mortem on a wild chimpanzee found dead with signs of haemorrhages. Eight days later, she was admitted to hospital in Abidjan for suspected malaria. As there was no improvement in her condition, she was repatriated by Swiss Air Ambulance and admitted to the University Hospital of Basel. As haemorrhagic fever was considered unlikely, she was treated with ciprofloxacin and deoxycyclin for suspected Gram-negative sepsis (typhoid fever), leptospirosis, or rickettsial disease. Retrospective studies isolated the Ebola virus. No clinical illness nor seroconversions were detected among 22 contact persons in the Côte d'Ivoire or 52 hospital and air-ambulance staff based in Switzerland, despite the lack of an early Ebola diagnosis. Late in 1995, a 25 year old refugee from neighbouring Liberia was admitted to the health facility of Gozon, Côte d'Ivoire, confirming the presence of Ebola virus in West Africa (Centers for Disease Control (CDC) 1995c). Patient isolation and barrier nursing prevented further spread of infection within and from the health facility. Preliminary investigation of his household contacts in the village of Plibo, Maryland County, Liberia found that two male contacts showed the signs and symptoms of early Ebola infection.

Zaire ebolavirus (ZEBOV) has repeatedly caused large outbreaks in Gabon between 1994 and 2008 (Geordes 1999: WHO 2003; Georges 1998; Pourrut, 2001), in DRC between 2001 and 2005 (Formenty 2003) and in the DRC in 1995 and 2007. In 2007, 103 people (100 adults and three children) were infected by a suspected hemorrhagic fever outbreak in the village of Kampungu, DRC. The outbreak started after the funerals of two village chiefs, and 264 people in four villages fell ill. The Congo's last major Ebola epidemic killed 245 people in 1995 in Kikwit, about 200 miles from the source of the August 2007 outbreak (WHO 2007). In 2004, it resurfaced around Gulu in Uganda (Okware 2002). Again, the disease was amplified in local hospitals and spread into several Ugandan administrative districts. There were at least 425 human cases and 224 deaths (Bitekyerezo 2002). On 30 November 2007, the Uganda Ministry of Health confirmed an outbreak of severe gastrointestinal disease caused by Ebola in the Bundibugyo District of Uganda. After confirmation of samples tested by the USA National Reference Laboratories and the CDC, the WHO confirmed the presence of a new species of *Ebolavirus* that is now named Bundibugyo. The epidemic ended on 20 February 2008. While it lasted, 149 cases of this new strain were reported, and 37 proved fatal. (Tower, 2008). The fifth ebolavirus, 'Uganda ebolavirus' ('UEBOV') was discovered during this outbreak of 2007. Ebola virus again caused an outbreak that killed 15 and infected 32 people in southern DRC in January 2009. Angola closed down part of their border with DRC to prevent the spread of Ebola after their experience with Marburgvirus in 2 004which killed 227 people.

Finally, the risks of filovirus research were demonstrated in 12 March 2009, when an unidentified 45 year old female scientist from Germany accidentally pricked her finger with a needle used to inject Ebola into laboratory mice. She was given an experimental vaccine never before used on humans. It remains unclear whether or not she was ever infected with the virus or if the experimental vaccine proved beneficial.

As in most ebolavirus-disease outbreaks, it is recognized that burial rituals and caring of and close contact with the sick contributed to the spread of filoviruses (Gear 1975). Most of these outbreaks began with people who had hunted animals in the forest or found dead animals and consumed them. The mechanism of transmission of infection in the Ebola virus outbreaks is mainly by direct contact with infected blood or tissue, by very close and prolonged contact with acutely ill patients, or by inoculation with contaminated syringes and needles. Transmission through the airborne route does not seem to be a factor in the maintenance of any of the epidemics. It is also thought that especially Zaire ebolvirus is causing epizootics among central chimpanzees (*Pan troglodytes troglodytes*) and western lowland gorillas (*Gorilla gorilla gorilla*), which may have contribute dramatically to their population decline (Karesh 2005).

Natural reservoirs

The natural reservoir of the Ebola virus is unknown despite extensive studies, but it seems to reside in the rain forests on the African continent and in the Western Pacific. Between 1976 and 1998, various mammals, birds, reptiles, amphibians, and arthropods from outbreak regions have been studied to determine the natural Fiolovirus reservoir. No *Ebolavirus* was detected apart from some genetic material found in six rodents (*Mus setulosus and Praomys*) and one shrew (*sylvisorex ollula*) collected from the Central African Republic (Peterson 2004).The virus was detected in the carcasses of gorillas, chimpanzees, and duikers during outbreaks in 2001 and 2003, which later became the source of human infections. However, the high mortality from infection in these species makes them unlikely as a natural reservoir.

Plants, arthropods, and birds have also been considered as possible reservoirs; however, bats are now considered the most likely candidate. Bats were known to reside in the cotton factory in which the Ebola index cases for the 1976 and 1979 outbreaks were employed. They have been implicated in Marburg infections in 1975 and 1980. Of 24 plant species and 19 vertebrate species experimentally inoculated with *Ebolavirus*, only bats became infected (Swanepoel 1996). The absence of clinical signs in these bats is characteristic of a reservoir species. In a 2002–2003 survey of 1,030 animals, which included 679 bats from Gabon and the DRC, 13 fruit bats were found to contain *Ebolavirus* RNA (Pourrut 2009). As of 2005, three fruit bat species (*Hypsignathus monstrosus, Epomops frangueti*, and *Myonycteris torquata*) have been identified as carrying the virus while remaining asymptomatic. Studies of Egyptian fruit bats (*Rousettus aegyptiaxcus*) inhabiting the Kitaka Cave, Uganda isolated genetically diverse Marburgvirus RNA from tissue and demonstrated virus specific antibodies (Towers 2009). To date, Gabon is the only country where bat (*Rousettus aegyptiaxcus*) proved to be the reservoirs for both Ebola and Marburg viruses. Thus, various species of bats indicate that they are potential natural host species, or reservoir, of filoviruses.

Reston ebolavirus—unlike its African counterparts—is nonpathogenic in humans. The high mortality among monkeys and its recent emergence in pigs makes them unlikely natural reservoirs.

Epizootics

Ebola virus

Several filoviruses closely related to Ebola were isolated in 1989 and early 1990 from sick or dying cynomolgus macaques in quarantine facilities located in Reston, Virginia, in Texas, and in Pennsylvania (CDC 1990a; Jahrling *et al*. 1990). Shipments to a quarantine facility in Siena, Italy in 1992 also contained animals that died with laboratory-confirmed Ebola-like virus infections (WHO 1992). The monkeys involved in each epizootic imported from the Philippines and traced to the same major export facilities. The identification of an Ebola-like virus in each facility led to the termination of all stocks, to reduce the risk of community spread. In the absence of any established link with Africa or African animals, the episode must represent evidence of Asian filoviruses. The animals being co-infected with simian haemorrhagic fever complicated the first reported epizootic in the USA; however, 223 of 1,050 exposed animals died. The natural host and geographic distribution is unknown.

Active transmission was documented at one Philippine export facility (Hayes *et al*. 1992). Antigen capture ELISA using liver homogenates revealed that 85 out of 161 (53.2%) monkeys that died within a 3 month period proved positive for filovirus antigen. The incidence was calculated to be 24.4 per 100 animals. Here captive monkeys were held in gang cages, increasing the opportunity for monkey-to-monkey transmission of virus by close contact with virus-laden blood or body secretions. The source of the infection remains unknown. Laboratory experimentation also shows the presence of high concentrations of viral antigen in pulmonary secretions, raising the possibility that the airborne route (Jaax *et al*. 1995) may spread this ebola-like virus. Parenteral inoculation with virus-contaminated blood is another possible route during the epizootics as all monkeys were tuberculin tested and given antibiotics. The common practice was to inoculate many monkeys with the same syringe and needle.

Serological evidence of filovirus exposure was found in 12 (6%) of 186 people who lived in wildlife collection areas or worked in primate facilities in Manila (Miranda *et al*. 1991). Within the export facility experiencing the epizootic, 22% of employees tested proved positive. No illness was documented in any of the positives.

In the Reston facility, five animal handlers were identified as having a high level of daily exposure to sick and dying animals. Four were found by IFA to have had serological evidence of recent infection, three seroconverting during the period of the epizootic. No filovirus illness developed. None of the 16 contacts of monkeys with Ebola-like virus imported into Italy showed any clinical or serological signs of infection.

Since the discovery of the Marburg and Ebola species of filovirus, seemingly random, sporadic fatal outbreaks of disease in humans and non-human primates have given impetus to identification of host tropisms and potential reservoirs. Domestic swine in the Philippines, experiencing unusually severe outbreaks of porcine reproductive and respiratory disease syndrome, have now been discovered to host *Reston ebolavirus* (REBOV). Although REBOV is the only member of *Filoviridae* that has not been associated with disease in humans, its emergence in the human food chain is of concern. REBOV isolates were found to be more divergent from each other than from the original virus isolated in 1989, indicating polyphyletic origins and that REBOV has been circulating since and possibly before, the initial discovery of REBOV in monkeys. The discovery of a number of seropositive abattoir workers in the Philippines having routine contact with the virus and seropositive swine has raised concern about the transmission of Ebola from animal to man (Barrette 2009).

The origin in nature and the natural history of Marburg and Ebola viruses remain unknown. It would seem that the viruses are zoonotic and transmission to humans occurs from ongoing life cycles in animals. Studies attempting to discover the source of the Marburg outbreaks in Europe or Africa, or the recent Ebola outbreak in the USA and Italy, have failed to uncover the reservoir. Whatever their source, person-to-person transmission is a means by which outbreaks and epidemics progress. This involves close contact; secondary cases have rarely exceeded 10%, indicating that transmission is not efficient. Nosocomial infection is a special case; extreme care should be taken when dealing with infected blood, secretions, tissues, and hospital waste.

Prevention and control

Prevention

Without an understanding of the natural history of the viruses, ecological controls capable of preventing the sporadic human cases that have started outbreaks and epidemics in the past are impossible. The exception would be the containment of monkeys, which might have the infections. While there is a strong suspicion that Ebola and Marburg diseases are zoonoses, the search continues for the origin and reservoir host(s) of the virus.

Control strategies

Although both Marburg and Ebola infections are rare events, they represent a dangerous nosocomial hazard. Prompt identification of active cases is essential and is dependent upon an accurate and detailed history (Department of Health and Social Security and Welsh Office 1986; CDC 1995; WHO 1995*b*). It is clear from the filovirus epidemics encountered to date that hospitals have acted as the main amplifier of the disease to the community. Therefore, it is important that physicians working in the areas where haemorrhagic fevers occur should be aware that these diseases exist and that nosocomial spread is a high possibility if not recognized early and patients placed in complete isolation under barrier nursing conditions. In non-endemic areas, it is important to maintain awareness of the current viral epidemiological developments and the threat of importation. Prevention of person-to-person spread of the virus is essential to control. Three weeks prior to illness patients at highest risk have travelled into areas where viral haemorrhagic fever (VHF) has recently occurred; had direct contact with blood, body fluids, secretions, or excretions of a person or animal with VHF; or worked in a laboratory or facility that handles the viruses. The likelihood of acquiring Ebola or Marburg is extremely low if patients do not meet any of the criteria. Contacts of such patients must be placed under surveillance and not allowed to travel. High-risk contact is associated with direct contact with blood or body fluids from acutely ill humans or animals; sexual contact with a convalescent case; or through laboratory accidents. Thus, effective surveillance of high-risk contacts and isolation of further cases ensures rapid control of an outbreak. The cause of fever in patients returning from Marburg and Ebola endemic areas is more likely to be other infectious disease (malaria or typhoid); therefore, evaluation and treatment of such infections needs urgent attention.

Patient containment

Control of outbreaks in endemic and non-endemic areas has been associated with the introduction of good hospital and laboratory infection control practices, with the isolation of febrile patients, careful handling of laboratory specimens and rigorous use of gloves and disinfectants. The containment of patients in plastic-film patient isolators (Trexlar) is favoured in the UK (Department of Health and Social Security (DHSS) and Welsh Office 1986). These are located within a room having filtered negative air pressure gradients, a separate effluent treatment plant for waste, an in-suite autoclave for solid waste, a shower, and a staff changing room. Many consider that the patient isolator reduces manual dexterity, introduces fatigue, inhibits the effectiveness of intensive care procedures, and hinders communication. Of most concern is that these isolators do not reduce the risk of injury by any sharp instruments and have no provision for resuscitation. This system is not used in endemic areas or recommended in the USA (CDC 1995) since the main risks are associated with direct inoculation of virus in blood or other material and the aerosol hazard considered low risk. Thus, it is recommended to confine patients to isolation in a single room with or without controlled filtered air. The most important consideration is staff training and supervision, the use of gloves and masks, and the mandatory use of a disinfection policy. The recommendations issued concerning the management of AIDS patients are considered adequate for containment of Filoviruses.

The repatriation to Switzerland of an acutely ill Ebola case originating in the Côte d'Ivoire in 1994 and Marburg case from Uganda to the Netherlands in 2008 demonstrates the need for vigilance, since filovirus infection was not considered or diagnosed until the patient had recovered. Had the normal barrier precautions not been undertaken, the potential for spread could have been devastating. Filovirus-infected patients should be isolated and barrier-nursed to prevent secondary infections. Handling, transportation, and testing of clinical material containing a high concentration of viruses should follow international and national guidelines.

Primate guidelines

As non-human primates are known to have introduced Marburg to Europe, and Ebola to the US and Italy, the management of transportation and quarantine facilities should ensure that personnel understand the hazards associated with handling non-human primates. Although the risk of infection is low, guidelines have been issued to minimize such risks in persons exposed to non-human primates during transport and quarantine (CDC 1990b; WHO 1990). Those at risk of infection include persons working in temporary or long-term holding facilities and persons who transport animals to these facilities (cargo handlers and inspectors). Monkeys, particularly those imported from Africa and Asia, are potential sources of a range of diseases, and severe illness or deaths in recently imported primates should be reported to health and veterinary authorities and investigated for a variety of infectious agents, including Ebola.

Captive monkeys frequently held in gang cages increase the opportunity for monkey-to-monkey transmission by virus-laden blood or body secretions. Studies of the epizootic in the USA and experimental infection studies have found high concentrations of viral antigen in pulmonary secretions, raising the possibility that filoviruses spread through the aerosol route.

Although the newly recognized Ebola virus from Asia apparently causes a fatal disease in cynomolgus macaques, initial evidence indicates that its ability to produce infection in humans may be less than that of the Ebola and Marburg viruses from Africa. However, because of the known severity of disease caused by other members of the Filoviridae, it would be premature to ignore the possibility of a possible public health threat posed by the Asian filoviruses. Four independent accounts concerning the importation of Filoviridae-infected primates into the USA and Europe from two areas of the world, Asia and Africa, increase the importance of introducing an infrastructure for the recognition, identification, and elimination polices to remove the possibility of spread.

The high degree of transmissibility among monkeys housed in confined conditions indicates the need for early identification of infected animals, both to protect the monkeys and to minimize the risk of human infection. The early detection of filovirus antigenaemia or nucleic acid would allow identification of infected animals before they become ill. Whether their elimination would prevent any outbreak has yet to be proven. At present, the potential threat from filovirus antibody-positive animals remains unclear, although there is no evidence that latent or constant infection has played any role in monkey-associated outbreaks. Improved quarantine and animal handling procedures need to be universally implemented to ensure no future outbreaks associated with wild-caught monkeys. Therefore, contact between monkeys and man should be limited and animal husbandry tightly controlled. Personnel handling animals should wear protective clothing, including rubber gloves and face respirator. All animal waste, cages, and other potentially contaminated items should be treated with appropriate disinfectants.

Finally, the increased concern for wildlife conservation and licensing of exporters/importers will further decrease the risk of filovirus spread to man.

References

Baron, R., McCormick, J., and Zubeir, O. (1983). Ebola virus disease in southern Sudan: hospital dissemination in intrafamilial spread. *Bull. World Heal. Organ.*, **61**: 997–1003.

Barrette, R. W. *et al.* (2009). Discovery of Swine as a Host for the Reston *ebolavirus. Sci.*, **325**: 204–6.

Baskerville, A., Fisher-Hoch, S. P., Neilds, G. H., and Dowsett, A. B. (1985). Ultrastructure pathology of experimental Ebola haemorrhagic fever virus infection. *J. Path.*, **147**: 199–209.

Bausch, D. G., Nichol, S. T., Muyembe-Tamfum, J. J., *et al.* (2006). Marburg hemorrhagic fever associated with multiple genetic lineages of virus. *N. Engl. J. Med.*, **355**: 909–19.

Bwaka, M. A. *et al.* (1999). EbolaHemorrhagic Fever in Kikwit, Democratic Republic of the Congo: ClinicalObservations in 103 Patients. *J. Infect. Dis.*, **179**(suppl. 1): S1–S7.

Bishop, D. H. L. and Pringle C. R. (1995). Order Mononegavirales. In: F. A. Murphy *et al.* (ed.) *Virus Taxonomy, Sixth Report of the International Committee on Taxonomy of Viruses*, pp. 265–67. Vienna: Springer-Verlag.

Bitekyerezo, M. C. *et al.* (2002). The outbreak and control of Ebola viral haemorrhagic fever in a Ugandan medical school. *Trop. Doct.*, **32**:10–15.

Borio, L. *et al.* (2002). Hemorrhagic Fever Viruses as Biological Weapons-Medical and Public Health Management. *JAMA*, **287**: 2391–2405.

Bowen, E. T. W., Platt, G. S., Lloyd, G. (1977). Viral haemorrhagic fever in southern Sudan and northern Zaire: preliminary studies on the aetiologic agent. *Lancet*, **1**: 571–73.

Bwaka, D.G. *et al.* (1999). Ebola heamoorhagic fever in Kikwit, Democratic Republic of the Congo: Clinical Observations in 103 patients. *J. Infect. Dis.*, **179**(suppl.): S1–S7.

Centers for Disease Control (1990a). Ebola virus infection in imported primates—Virginia, 1989. *MMWR*, **38**: 831–38.

Centers for Disease Control (1990b). Ebola related filovirus infection in non-human primates and interim guidelines for handling non-human primates during transit and quarantine. *MMWR*, **39**: 22–30.

Centers for Disease Control (1995c). Management of patients with suspected viral haemorrhagic fever—US. *MMWR*, **44**: 475–79.

Department of Health and Social Security and Welsh Office (1986). The control of viral haemorrhagic fevers. London: HMSO.

Department of Health (2007). Transport of Infectious Substances *Best Practice Guidance for Microbiology Laboratories*. http://www.dh.gov.uk/publications.

Elliot, L. H., McCormick, J. B., and Johnson, K. M. (1982). Inactivation of Lassa, Marburg, and Ebola viruses by Gamma irradiation. *J. Clin. Microbiol.*, **16**(4): 704–8.

Emond, R. T. D. (1978). Isolation, monitoring, and treatment of a case of Ebola infection. In: S. R. Pattyn (ed.) *Ebola virus infection*, pp. 27–32. Amersdam: Elsevier/North Holland Biomedical Press.

Emond, R. T. D., Evans, E., Bowen, E., and Lloyd, G. (1977). A case of Ebola virus infection. *BMJ*, **2**: 541–44.

Feldman, H., Klenk, H. D., and Sanchez, A. (1993). Molecular biology and evolution of filoviruses. *Arch. Virol. Suppl.*, **7**: 87–100.

Feldmann, H., Nichol, S. T., Klenk, H. D., Peters, C. J., and Sanchez, A. (1994). Characterization of Filoviruses Based on Differences in Structure and Antigenicity of the Virion Glycoprotein. *Virol.*, **199**: 469–73.

Feldmann, H. *et al.* (2007). Effective post-exposure treatment of Ebola infection. *PLoS Pathog.*, **3**(1):e2.

Fisher-Hoch, S. P., Platt, G. S., Lloyd, G., Simpson, D. I., Neils, G. H., and Barett, A. J. (1983). Haematological and biochemical monitoring of Ebola infection in rhesus monkeys: implications for patient management. *Lancet*, **2**: 1055–58.

Fisher-Hoch, S. P. *et al.* (1985). Pathophysiology of shock and haemorrhage in a fulminating viral infection (Ebola). *J. Infect. Dis.*, **152**: 887–94.

Fisher-Hoch, S. P., Perez-Oronoz, G. I., Jackson, E. L., Hermann, L. M., and Brown, B. G. (1992a). Filovirus clearance in non-human primates. *Lancet*, **340**: 451–53.

Fisher-Hoch, S. P. *et al.* (1992b). Pathogenic role of geographic origin of primate host and virus strain. *J. Infect. Dis.*, **166**(4): 753–63.

Formenty, P., Hatz, C., Le Guenno, B., Stoll, A., et al. (1999). Human Infection Due to Ebola Virus, Subtype Côte d'Ivoire: Clinical and Biologic Presentation. J. Infect. Dis., 179(suppl. 1): S48–S53.

Formenty, P. et al. (2003). Outbreak of Ebola hemorrhagic fever in the Republic of the Congo, 2003: a new strategy? Med. Trop. (Marseille), 63(3): 291–95.

Gear, J. S. S. et al. (1975). Outbreak of Marburg virus disease in Johannesburg. BMJ, 4: 489–93.

Geisbert, T. W. and Jahrling, P. B. (1990). Use of immunoelectron microscopy to show Ebola virus during the 1989 United States epizootic. J. Clin. Pathol., 43: 813–16.

Geisbert, T. W. et al. (2009). Single-Injection Vaccine Protects Nonhuman Primates against Infection with Marburg Virus and Three Species of Ebola Virus. J. Virol., 14(83): 7296–7304.

Georges, A. J., et al. (1999). Ebola hemorrhagic fever outbreaks in Gabon, 1994–1997: epidemiologic and health control issues. J. Infect. Dis., 179: S65–75.

Gibb, T. R., Norwood, D. A., Woollen, N., and Henchal, E. A. (2001). Development and evaluation of a fluorogenic 5′ nuclease assay to detect and differentiate between Ebola virus subtypes Zaire and Sudan. J. Clin. Microbiol., 39: 4125–30.

Grolla, A., Lucht, A., Dick, D., Strong, J. E., and Feldmann, H. (2005). Laboratory diagnosis of Ebola and Marburg hemorrhagic fever. Bulletin. Soc. Pathol. Exotic., 98: 205–9.

Haas, R. and Mass, G. (1971). Experimental infection of monkeys with the Marburg virus. In: G. A. Martini and R. Siegert (eds.) Marburg virus disease, pp. 136–43. Berlin: Springer-Verlag.

Hayes, C. G. et al. (1992). Outbreak of fatal illness among captive macaques in the Philippines caused by an Ebola-related filovirus. Am. J. Trop. Med. Hyg., 46: 664–71.

Henderson, B. E., Kissling, R. E., Williams, M. C., Kafuko, G. W., and Martin, M. (1971). Epidemiological studies in Uganda relating to 'Marburg agent'. In: G. A. Martini and R. Siegert (eds.) Marburg virus disease, pp. 19–23. Berlin: Springer-Verlag.

Heymann, D. L., Weisfeld, J. S., Webb, P. A., Johnson, K. M., Cairns, T., and Berquist, H. (1980). Ebola haemorrhagic fever: Tandala, Zaire, 1977–1978. J. Infect. Dis., 56: 247–70.

Jaax, M. et al. (1996). Transmission of Ebola virus (Zaire strain) to uninfected monkeys in a biocontainment laboratory. Lancet, 343: 1669–71.

Jahrling, P. B. et al. (1990). Preliminary report: isolation of Ebola virus from monkeys imported to USA. Lancet, 335: 502–5.

John, S. P., Wang, T., Steffen, S., Longhi, S., Schmaljohn, C. S., and Jonsson, C. B. (2007). The Ebola Virus VP30 is an RNA Binding Protein. J. Virol., 81: 8967–76.

Johnson, E. D., et al. (1996). Characterization of a new Marburg virus isolated from a 1987 fatal case in Kenya. Arch. Virolol., 11: 101–14.

Karesh, W., and Reed, P. (2005). Ebola and great apes in Central Africa: current status and future needs. Bull. Soc. Path. Exotic., 98: 237–38.

Kiley, M. P. et al. (1982). Filoviridae: a taxonomic home for Marburg and Ebola viruses? Intervirol., 18: 24–32.

Ksiazek, T. G., Rollin, P. E., Jahrling, P. B., Johnson, E., Dalgard, D. W., and Peters, C. J. (1992). Enzyme immunosorbent assay for Ebola virus antigens in tissues of infected primates. J. Clin. Microbiol., 30: 947–50.

Ksiazek, T. G. et al. (1999). Clinical virology of Ebola hemorrhagic fever (EHF): virus, virus antigen, and IgG and IgM antibody findings among EHF patients in Kikwit, Democratic Republic of the Congo, 1995. J. Infect. Dis., 179: S177–87.

Ksiazek, T. G., West, C. P., Rollin, P. E., Jahrling, P. B., and Peters, C. J. (1999). ELISA for the detection of antibodies to Ebola viruses. J. Infect. Dis., 179(Suppl. 1): S192–98.

Kuzmin, I. V. et al. (2010). Marburg Virus in Fruit Bat, Kenya. Emerg. Infect. Dis., 16(2): 352–54.

Le Guenno, B., Formentry, P., Wyers, M., Gounon, P., Walker, F., and Boesch, C. (1995). Isolation and partial characterisation of a new strain of Ebola virus. Lancet, 345: 1271–74.

Leroy, E. M. et al. (2000). Diagnosis of Ebola haemorrhagic fever by RT-PCR in an epidemic setting. J. Med. Virol., 60: 463–67.

Martini, G. A. (1969). Marburg agent disease in man. Trans. R. Soc. Trop. Med. Hyg., 63: 295–302.

Martini, G. A. (1971). Marburg virus disease, clinical syndrome. In: G. A. Martini and R. Siegert (eds.) Marburg virus disease, pp. 1–9. Berlin: Springer-Verlag.

Miranda, M. E. G., White, M. E., Dayrit, M. M., Hayes, C. G., Ksiazek. T. G., and Burns, J. P. (1991). Seroepidemiology study of filovirus related to Ebola in the Philippines [letter]. Lancet, 337: 425–26.

Miranda, M. E. et al. (1999). Epidemiology of Ebola (subtype Reston) virus in the Philippines, 1996. J. Infect. Dis., 179(Suppl 1): S115–19.

Mason, C. (2008). The strains of Ebola. Can. Med. J., 178: 1266–67.

Modrof, J., Becker, S., and Mühlberger, E. (2003). Ebola Virus Transcription Activator VP30 Is a Zinc-Binding Protein. J. Virol., 77: 3334–38.

Nikiforov, V. V. (1994). A case of Marburg virus laboratory infection. Zh. Mikrobiol. Epid. Immun., 3: 104–6, (Russian).

Noda, T. et al. (2006). Assembly and budding of ebolavirus. Plos Pathogens September; e99. Published online 2006 September 29. doi: 10.1371/journal.ppat.0020099.

Okware, S. I. et al. (2002). An outbreak of Ebola in Uganda. Trop. Med. Int. Heal., 7: 1068–75.

Peters, A., Sanchez, R., Swanepoel, B., and Volchkov, V. E. (2005). Family Filoviridae., In: C. M. Fauquet, M. A. Mayo, J. Maniloff, U. Desselberger, and L. A. Ball (eds.), Virus Taxonomy - Eighth Report of the International Committee on Taxonomy of Viruses. p. 645–53. San Diego, CA: Elsevier/Academic Press.

Peterson, A. T., Bauer, J. T., Mills, J. N. (2004). Ecology and geographic distribution of filovrus disease. Emerg. Infect. Dis., 10: 40–47.

Piot, P., et al. (1978). Clinical Aspects of EbolaVirus Infection in Yambuku Area, Zaire, 1976. In: S. R. Pattyn (ed.), EbolaVirus Haemorrhagic Fever, pp. 7–14. Amsterdam: Elsevier/North-Holland Biomedical Press.

Pourrut, X., et al. (2005). The natural history of Ebola virus in Africa. Microbes Infect., 7: 1005–14.

Pourrut, X., et al. (2009). Large serological survey showing cocirculation of Ebola and Marburg viruses in Gabonese bat populations, and a high seroprevalence of both viruses in Rousettus aegyptiacus. BioMed. Cen. Infect. Dis., 9: 159–69.

Pratt, W. D. et al. (2010). Protection of Nonhuman Primates against Two Species of Ebola Virus Infection with a Single Complex Adenovirus Vector. Clin. Vacc.Immun., 17: 572–58.

Pringle, C. R. (1991). Order Mononegavirales. Arch. Virol., 117: 137–40.

Reid, S. P., Valmas, C., Martinez, O., Sanchez, F. M., and Basler, C. F. (2007). Ebola virus VP24 proteins inhibit the interaction of NPI-1 subfamily karyopherin α proteins with activated STAT1. J. Virol., 81: 13469–77.

Richman, D. D., Cleveland, P. H., McCormick, J. B., and Johnson, K. M. (1983). Antigenic Analysis of Strains of Ebola Virus: Identification of Two Ebola Virus Subtypes. J. Infect. Dis., 147: 268–71.

Rollin, P. E., Ksiazek, T. G., Jahrling, P. E., Haines, M., and Peters, C. J. (1990). Detection of Ebola-like viruses by immunofluorescence. Lancet, 336: 1591.

Saijo, M., Niikura, M., Ikegami, T., Kurane, I., Kurata, T., and Morikawa, S. (2006). Laboratory Diagnostic Systems for Ebola and Marburg Hemorrhagic Fevers Developed with Recombinant Proteins. Clin. Vacc. Immunol., 13(4): 444–51.

Sanchez, A., Kiley, M. P., Klenk, H. D., and Feldman, H. (1992). Sequence analysis of the Marburg virus nucleoprotein gene: comparison to Ebola virus and other non-segmented negative stand RNA viruses. J. Gen. Virol., 73: 347–57.

Sanchez, A., Kiley, M. P., Holloway, B. P., and Asuperin, D. D. (1993). Sequence analysis of the Ebola virus genome: organisation, genetic elements, and comparison with the genome of Marburg virus. *Vir. Res.*, **29**: 215–40.

Smith, D. G., Francis, F., and Simpson, D. I. H. (1978). African haemorrhgic fever in the southern Sudan, 1976: the clinical manifestations. In: S. R. Pattyn (ed.) *Ebola virus haemorrhagic fever*, pp. 1–6. Amsterdam: Elsevier.

Smith, D. H. *et al.* (1982). Marburg-virus disease in Kenya. *Lancet*, **1**: 816–20.

Swanepoel, R., Leman, P.A., Burt, F. J. (1996). Experimental inoculation of plants and animals with Ebola virus. *Emerg. Infect. Dis.*, **2**: 321–25.

Teepe, R. G. *et al.* (1983). A probable case of Ebola virus haemorrhagic fever in Kenya. *E. Afric. Med. J.*, **60**: 718–22.

Timen, A. *et al.* (2009). Response to Imported Case of Marburg Hemorrhagic Fever, the Netherlands. *Emerg. Infect. Dis.*, **15**(8): 1171–75.

Towner, J. S. *et al.* (2004). Rapid Diagnosis of Ebola Hemorrhagic Fever by Reverse Transcription-PCR in an Outbreak Setting and Assessment of Patient Viral Load as a Predictor of Outcome. *J. Virol.*, **78**: 4330–41.

Towner, J. S. *et al.* (2007). Marburg Virus Infection Detected in a Common African Bat. *PLoS One*, **2**: article e764 [Epub Aug. 22, 2007] http://www.plosone.org.

Towner, J. S. *et al.* (2008). Newly discovered Ebola virus associated with hemorrhagic fever outbreak in Uganda. *PLos Pathogens*, **4**(11): e1000212. doi:10.1371/journal. ppat. 1000212.

Towner, J. S. *et al.* (2006). Marburgvirus genomics and association with a large hemorrhagic fever outbreak in Angola. *J. Virol.*, **80**: 6497–516.

Weik, M., Modrof, J., Klenk, H. D., Becker, S., and Mühlberger, E. (2002). Ebola Virus VP30-Mediated Transcription Is Regulated by RNA Secondary Structure Formation. *J. Virol.*, **76**: 8532–39.

World Health Organization International Commission to Sudan. (1978*a*). Ebola haemorrhagic fever in Sudan; 1976. *Bull. World Heal. Organ.*, **56**: 247–70.

World Health Organization/International Commission to Zaire (1978*b*). Ebola haemorrhagic fever in Zaire; 1976. *Bull. World Heal. Organ.*, **56**: 271–93.

World Health Organization (1990). Interim guidelines for handling nonhuman primates during transit and quarantine. *Wkly. Epidemiol. Rec.*, **65**: 45–52.

World Health Organization (1992). Viral haemorrhagic fever in imported monkeys. *Wkly. Epidemiol. Rec.*, **67**: 142–43.

World Health Organization (1995*a*). Ebola haemorrhagic fever, Zaire. *Weekly Epidemiol. Rec.*, **70**: 241–42.

World Health Organization (1995*b*). Viral haemorrhagic fevers—management of suspected cases. *Wkly. Epidemiol. Rec.*, **35**: 249–52.

World Health Organization (1995*c*). Ebola haemorrhagic fever—confirmed case in Côte d'Ivoire and suspected cases in Liberia. *Wkly. Epidemiol. Rec.*, **70**: 359.

World Health Organization (1996). Ebola haemorrhagic fever. *Wkly Epidemiol. Rec.*, **71**: 320.

World Health Organization (2003). *Outbreak(s) of Ebola haemorrhagic fever, Congo and Gabon, October 2001– July 2002 Wkly. Epidemiol. Rep.*, **78**(26): 223–25.

World Health Organization (2004). *Ebola haemorrhagic fever in the Republic of the Congo—Update 6. Wkly. Epidemiol. Rec.*, 6 January.

World Health Organization (2005). *Outbreak of Ebola haemorrhagic fever in Yambio, south Sudan, April–June 2004. Wkly Epidemiol. Rec.*, **80**: 370–75.

World Health Organization (2007). *Ebola virus haemorrhagic fever, Democratic Republic of the Congo—Update. Wkly. Epidemiol. Rec.*, **82**: 345–46.

World Health Orgaization (2007). *Guidance on regulations for the transport of infectious Substances* www.who.int/csr/resources/publications/biosafety/WHO_CDS_EPR_2007_2cc.pdf.

World Health Organization (2007). *Marburg haemorrhagic fever*, Uganda. *Wkly Epidemiol. Rec.*, **82**: 297–8.

World Health Organization (2008). *Case of Marburg Haemorrhagic Fever Imported into the Netherlands from Uganda*. 10 July.

World Health Organization (2009). *Ebola Reston in pigs and humans, Philippines. Wkly Epidemiol. Rec.*, **84**: 49–50.

Wulff, H. and Johnson, K. M. (1979). Immunoglobulin M and G responses measured by immunofluorescence in patients with Lassa or Marburg virus infections. *Bull. World Heal. Organ.*, **57**: 631–35.

Zaki, S. R. *et al.* (1999). A novel immunohistochemical assay for the detection of Ebola virus in skin: implications for diagnosis, spread, and surveillance of Ebola hemorrhagic fever. Commission de Lutte contre les Epidemies a Kikwit. *J. Infect. Dis.*, **179**(Suppl.1): S36–47.

CHAPTER 32

Mosquito-borne arboviruses

E. A. Gould

Summary

The arboviruses are all single-stranded RNA viruses, although they belong to five different viral families. Several important human pathogens belong to the mosquito-borne arboviruses including yellow fever, Japanese encephalitis and Rift Valley Fever. They cause a wide range of illnesses from unrecognized infection to severe systemic disease with hemorrhagic complications and/or encephalitis with a high mortality. A similar range of illnesses is seen in infected animals.

Arboviruses have several unique characteristics, these include; an ability to infect and be transmitted by mosquitoes, ticks, midges, sandflies, bugs, fleas, blackflies and horseflies. They infect vertebrate hosts which may amplify the virus for invertebrate vectors that feed on infected vertebrates. They have the ability to replicate in arthropods, with little pathology and in vertebrates often with significant pathology. Many arboviruses are zoonotic.

Control methods depend on the epidemiology of particular viruses, but epidemic vector control through control of insect breeding sites and the use of insecticide spraying have been successfully used in the past. Effective vaccines are available for yellow fever and Japanese encephalitis.

History

In 1881, before viruses were recognized, Carlos Finlay, a Cuban physician, proposed that yellow fever might be transmitted by mosquitoes. Despite the fact that previous alternative theories had not proven to be correct, Dr Finlay's idea was followed up (Reed 1901) and the concept that some diseases could be spread by arthropods heralded the beginning of arbovirology as we know it today. By 1930 the laboratory mouse was beginning to be used as a test animal in virology and Max Theiler reported that newborn mice inoculated intraperitoneally with Yellow Fever virus (YFV) died of encephalitis (Theiler 1930). At about the same time, Louping ill virus (LIV), which is antigenically related to YFV, was shown to be transmitted by ticks, rather than mosquitoes. This virus was also isolated using mice (Greig et al. 1931). For many years afterwards, arboviruses were preferentially isolated using newborn mice. The first classification of these viruses was based on their ability to replicate in and be transmitted by arthropods, but it was subsequently shown that some related viruses were not transmitted by arthropods. As more viruses were isolated, new tests were developed to distinguish them. Infected suckling mice were used as hosts for detecting neutralizing antibodies to the New World equine encephalitis arboviruses (Casals and Webster 1944; Lennette and Koprowski 1944) and this was soon followed by the adaptation of complement fixation tests to demonstrate that antibodies specific for rabies or poliovirus or newly isolated arboviruses did not necessarily cross-react with all the isolated viruses (Casals 1944; Casals and Webster 1944). As even more viruses were isolated and antigenic tests performed, it became clear that some were distantly related whereas others were more closely related to each other (Casals 1957). The haemagglutination test, originally developed to study influenza virus (Hirst 1941), was then modified (Casals and Brown 1954; Sabin and Buescher 1950) and adapted to the study of arboviruses. The haemagglutination-inhibition test, complement fixation test and neutralization test have proved to be exquisitely sensitive and practical tools for diagnosis and studies of virus antigenic interrelationships. Indeed, these serological procedures have stood the test of time and even though many of the taxonomic decisions made today are primarily based on sequence data, relatively few major changes have been required when compared with those based on serological studies.

General characteristics of mosquito-borne arboviruses

RNA viruses that are transmitted to vertebrate species by haematophagous (blood-feeding) arthropod vectors (including mosquitoes, ticks, sandflies, midges/gnats, bugs etc.) are known as arboviruses because they are arthropod-borne viruses. The term arbovirus reflects their ecological characteristics and is not taxonomic. Replication of the virus in the arthropod is a crucial element of the virus life cycle. However, as far as is known no significant pathological changes result from these infections, at least in the arthropods that subsequently replicate and transmit the virus to a vertebrate host. When an arthropod takes an infectious blood meal, the virus enters the midgut and infects the epithelial cells. If the virus survives transfer across the barrier of the midgut wall (Paulson et al. 1989), it enters a variety of tissues and replicates. The salivary glands of vectors competent to transmit the virus become infected, and the virus can then be transmitted to vertebrate hosts during subsequent feeding periods (Takahashi and Suzuki 1979). Transmission of the virus to vertebrate hosts may or may not result in pathology and clinical signs of infection. The time that the virus takes to infect the arthropod and to replicate and then be transmitted to a vertebrate host is known as the period of extrinsic incubation (World Health Organization (WHO) 1985). Infected female arthropods may also transmit the virus vertically (transovarially) through eggs, and infected males may transmit the virus to females during mating. Conventionally, the virus replicates in the infected vertebrate host to produce a viraemic infection that provides a source of virus for feeding haematophagous arthropods to continue the biological cycle. However, there is also evidence of virus transmission between co-feeding arthropods, in the absence of viraemia (Gould *et al.* 2003; Higgs *et al.* 2005; Jones *et al.* 1997; Labuda *et al.* 1997; Mead *et al.* 2000). The significance of non-viraemic arbovirus transmission is not yet fully understood although it clearly plays an important role in arbovirus pathogenesis, survival, dispersal and evolution. Alternatively, under some circumstances, viruses may adhere physically to the proboscis of a blood-sucking arthropod, without infecting the arthropod, and be transmitted mechanically to vertebrate hosts. Whilst this very rare form of mechanical transmission may occur, it would not be unique to arboviruses and is not a recognized method of arbovirus transmission.

More than five hundred viruses were registered in the International Catalogue of Arboviruses (Karabatsos 1985) by July 1985. This was the last issue of the Catalogue, but the number of identified arboviruses continues to increase. All recognized arboviruses are now listed within their families and genera in the VIIIth Report of the International Committee for the Taxonomy of Viruses (Fauquet *et al.* 2005). In general, individual arboviruses are primarily associated with a single family of arthropods, such as mosquitoes, ticks, midges, flies, bugs, etc. However, this is not an absolute rule, for example, whilst West Nile virus and several other closely related viruses are primarily associated with mosquito transmission, they may also infect and be transmitted by ticks (Theiler and Downs 1973). Nevertheless, the mosquito is clearly the predominant species for evolution and transmission of these viruses because phylogenetic analyses always group them in the clades occupied by mosquito-borne flaviviruses rather than tick-borne flaviviruses (Gould *et al.* 2003). The same rules apply to other arboviruses that are primarily transmitted by ticks or sandflies, i.e, some of them may also be transmissible by mosquitoes. Another complicating issue, in defining arboviruses,

is the fact that some do not have recognized arthropod vectors and may be described as having 'no known vector' (NKV) even though they are antigenically and phylogenetically clearly members of arbovirus genera (Porterfield, 1980). Whilst this could reflect the lack of evidence from environmental samples, it seems more likely that such viruses do not have arthropod vectors and thus represent either archival or descendant lineages within the genera, that have evolved this characteristic. One more complicating factor is that some genera included in the Arbovirus Catalogue clearly are not arboviruses, for example, hantaviruses and arenaviruses. Nevertheless, the history of their discovery, their genome strategies, epidemiological and/or ecological characteristics together with the specialized facilities required for their study are traditionally associated with laboratories having expertise in arbovirology, hence their inclusion in the Arbovirus Catalogue.

Classification of arboviruses

By the mid-twentieth century sufficient serological data had accumulated to enable the categorization of arboviruses into Groups A, B and C, corresponding respectively to the viruses known today as the families *Togaviridae* (genus *Alphavirus*), *Flaviviridae* (genus *Flavivirus*) *and Bunyaviridae* (genera, *Bunyavirus* and *Phlebovirus*) (Fauquet *et al.* 2005). As more viruses were isolated and defined on the basis of antigenicity, together with other biological characteristics, and sequence data, arboviruses were also recognized as being present in the additional families, *Reoviridae* (genus *Orbivirus*) and *Rhabdoviridae* (genus *Vesiculovirus*). It should be emphasized that each of these five virus families consists of genera that contain arboviruses and other genera that do not contain arboviruses. Moreover, as stated earlier, a substantial proportion of arboviruses are primarily associated with arthropods other than mosquitoes. However, this chapter focuses only on mosquito-borne arboviruses (Table 32.1) and primarily on those that cause significant disease in vertebrate species, including humans. New arboviruses are constantly being isolated and characterized. Since it takes considerable time before they are listed in the latest catalogues of viruses it is impossible to provide an absolutely up to date precise taxonomic and biological description of them. Nevertheless, the most robust current listings can be found in the VIIIth Report of the ICTV (Fauquet *et al.* 2005).

Table 32.1 Examples of mosquito-borne (and in some cases other insect species) arboviruses that are associated with disease in humans

Virus family	Virus genera	Mosquito-borne virus* examples	Principle associated mosquito vectors (and other vector species)	Typical Disease symptoms
Togaviridae	*Alphavirus*	VEEV, EEV, WEEV, MAYV, SINV, ONNV, CHIKV, RRV, SFV	*Culex* and *Aedes* species	Encephalitis Arthralgia/Polyarthritis
Flaviviridae	*Flavivirus*	YFV, DENV, JEV, WNV, SLEV, MVEV, USUV	*Culex* and *Aedes* species	Fever, Rash, Haemorrhagic fever. Encephalitis
Bunyaviridae	*Bunyavirus*	LACV, CEV, TAHV, LUMV, INKV, JCV,	*Aedes* species	Fever, Encephalitis
	Phlebovirus	RVFV	*Aedes* species Phlebotomine species	Fever, Haemorrhagic fever
Rhabdoviridae	*Vesiculovirus*	VSAV, VSIV, VSNJV, CHPV, COCV, ISFV, PIRYV, MAPV, CQIV	Phlebotomine species, blackflies *Aedes* species, *Psorophora* species	Flu-like illness Acute encephalitis

* Virus identities follow the ICTV system of nomenclature (Fauquet *et al.* 2005). In the example of vesiculoviruses, Phlebotomine species are the most commonly associated vector but some vesiculoviruses have been isolated from mosquitoes in the wild.

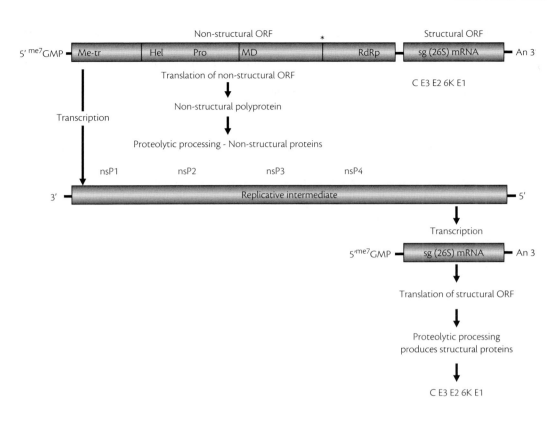

Fig. 32.1 Alphavirus genome coding strategy. Open-reading frame (ORF) represented as open box, and untranslated regions as solid black lines; sg (sub-genomic), asterisk between nsP3 and nsP4 identifies the position of the stop codon that is present in some alphaviruses and is read-through to produce the precursor nsP1,2,3,4 polyprotein, Me-tr (methyltransferase), Hel (helicase), Pro (protease), MD (macro domain - exhibits adenosine di-phosphoribose 1'-phosphate phosphatase activity), RdRp (RNA dependent RNA polymerase), C (capsid), E (envelope). Adapted from (Strauss & Strauss, 1994).

Alphaviruses: the agents, the hosts and epidemiology

Genus *Alphavirus* (Mukhopadhyay *et al.* 2006; Strauss and Strauss 1994; Weaver *et al.* 2005). Images of alphaviruses illustrating their structural details can be obtained at the following website; http://www.bio.indiana.edu/facultyresearch/faculty/Mukhopadhyay.html.

New species continue to be isolated and characterized but currently there are 29 recognized species in the genus *Alphavirus*. Virions, ~70 nm in diameter, are spherical with a lipid bilayer containing heterodimeric protein spikes composed of two glycoproteins E1 and E2. Some flaviviruses also contain a third envelope protein E3. The heterodimers are organized in a T=4 icosahedral lattice consisting of 80 trimers. The enclosed nucleocapsid core consists of 240 copies of capsid protein and a single copy of the genomic RNA. The one to one relationship between glycoprotein heterodimers and nucleocapsid proteins is important in virus assembly. The structure of the E1 glycoprotein has been resolved by crystallography. E1 is the fusion protein for virus entry into the acidic cytoplasmic endosomes. The E2 glycoprotein extends outwards from the envelope and forms the petals of the spike that cover the underlying E1 protein fusion peptide at neutral pH. The four non-structural proteins are defined as nsP1, nsP2, nsP3 and nsP4. The genomic RNA is positive stranded and serves as the mRNA for translation of the four non-structural viral proteins which are cleaved from a polyprotein precursor by the viral-encoded protease in nsP2. The non-structural proteins replicate viral RNA. The nsP1 protein is probably involved in capping of viral RNAs and initiation of negative-strand RNA synthesis. In addition to its protease function the nsP2 also provides the helicase for RNA replication. The nsP3 protein is also required for RNA replication and the nsP4 protein is believed to be the viral RNA polymerase. During RNA replication, a negative-stranded copy is produced and used as a template for the synthesis of genome-sized positive strand RNA and subgenomic 26S mRNA corresponding to the 3' third of the viral genome and encoding the viral structural proteins (Fig. 32.1).

The non-structural proteins function in the cytoplasm of infected cells in association with membrane surfaces and attachment appears to be mediated by nsP1 palmitoylation. The capsid protein assembles with the viral RNA to form the viral nucleocapsids in the cytosol. Glycoproteins are translocated via the Golgi apparatus to the plasma membrane and assembled nucleocapsids bud through these membranes, thus acquiring a lipid envelope containing the integral membrane glycoproteins, E1 and E2.

The VIIIth Edition of the International Committee for the Taxonomy of Viruses (ICTV) currently lists 29 species in the genus *Alphavirus* and family *Togaviridae* (Weaver *et al.* 2005). All arthropod-borne alphaviruses are antigenically related but most can be distinguished in cross-reactivity tests (Chanas *et al.* 1976; Clarke and Casals 1958; Karabatsos 1975; Porterfield 1961) with which they have been divided into 8 antigenic complexes: Eastern, Western, and Venezuelan equine encephalitis, Trocara, Middelburg, Ndumu, Semliki Forest and Barmah Forest. In addition, Southern elephant seal virus (SESV) has been isolated from the Seal Louse in the southern Oceans, indicating that alphaviruses can circulate in Antarctica and the non-arthropod-borne species, Salmon pancreatic disease virus (SPDV) has also been identified. These two viruses are antigenically unrelated to the other recognized alphaviruses. Based on sequence data, and with the exception of these two widely disparate viruses, the arthropod-borne alphaviruses share a minimum of about 40% amino acid identity in the more divergent structural proteins and 60% in the non-structural proteins. A phylogenetic tree based on the sequence of the envelope gene of all known alphavirus is presented in Fig. 32. 2. The tree identifies the region of the world (Old World or New World) where the viruses are known to be indigenous. Western equine encephalitis virus (WEEV) and direct descendants of this virus differ from the other alphaviruses in being recombinant viruses. It is believed that an Old World virus related to Sindbis virus (SINV) recombined with a New World virus, probably an ancestor of Eastern equine encephalitis virus (EEEV) to produce WEEV (Weaver *et al.* 1997).

Ten alphaviruses are considered to be of significant importance in terms of public health. Indeed with the recent emergence of Chikungunya fever as a major human pathogen in Asia and potentially globally (de Lamballerie *et al.* 2008), the alphavirus profile has been significantly raised (Chevillon *et al.* 2008). Alphaviruses that circulate in the Old World most commonly cause febrile illness and painful arthralgias or polyarthralgias, particularly in the small joints. A characteristic macular-papular rash often appears three to five days after illness onset. In severe cases the joints are swollen and tender, and rheumatic signs and symptoms may persist for weeks or months following the acute illness. In general, these infections are rarely fatal and only infrequently result in encephalitic disease (Lewthwaite *et al.* 2009) following infection with Old World alphaviruses such as CHIKV, or o'nyong nyong virus (ONNV) in Africa/Asia, SINV and closely related viruses (Ockelbo, Whataroa) which are widespread throughout the Old World, or Ross River virus (RRV), and Barmah Forest virus (BFV) which are confined to Australia. In contrast with these Old World diseases, the New World alphaviruses VEEV, EEEV, and WEEV present a different epidemiological and clinical picture. VEEV is divided into six distinct antigenic subtypes (Walton and Grayson 1988; Young 1972; Young and Johnson 1969). Subtypes IAB and IC are associated with major epidemics and equine epizootics during which equine mortality due to encephalitis can reach 83%. In 1995, a major outbreak in Venezuela and Colombia, was associated with the VEEV subtype IC. This epidemic resulted in roughly 100,000 human cases, with more than 300 fatal encephalitis cases (Diaz *et al.* 1997). Other recent epidemics indicate that VEEV still represents a serious public health problem (Weaver *et al.* 1996). In humans, while the overall mortality rate is low (<1%), neurological disease, including disorientation, ataxia, mental depression, and convulsions, can be detected in up to 14% of infected individuals, especially children (Johnson and Martin 1974). Neurological sequelae in humans are also common (Leon 1975). However, most human infections are either asymptomatic or present as a nonspecific febrile illness or aseptic meningitis. In rare cases, the fever and headache may progress through nausea and vomiting to somnolence or delirium and coma with seizures, impaired sensorium, and paralysis being commonly observed. The severity of neurological involvement and sequelae is greater with decreasing age. Horses are more susceptible than humans to these viruses but are considered to be dead-end hosts. Moreover, veterinary vaccines are available to reduce the risk of clinical disease. EEEV and WEEV, are widespread throughout the eastern and western regions of North America, including Canada, and also South America and Cuba. They are transmitted to horses by infected ornithophilic

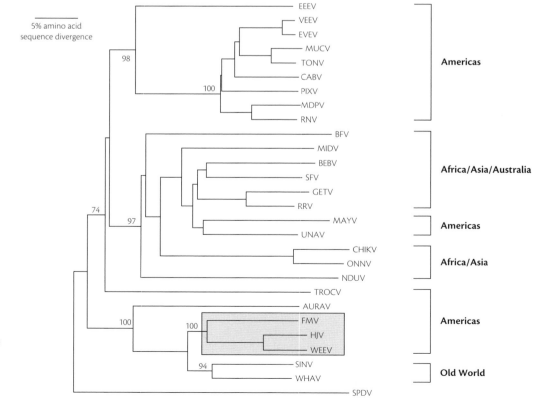

Fig. 32.2 Phylogenetic analyses of selected alphaviruses
a) Midpoint rooted tree generated using partial E1 envelope glycoprotein amino acid sequences and the neighbor joining program implemented in PAUP 4.0 (Swofford, 1998). Numbers indicate bootstrap values generated using 1,000 re-samplings. Scale indicates 5% amino acid sequence divergence. Gray box shows recombinant alphaviruses that were derived from ancestors of EEEV and SINV.

5% amino acid sequence divergence

(bird-biting) mosquitoes that thrive in wetland habitats. Highlands J virus (HJV), a close relative of WEEV, is not known to be pathogenic for humans but appears to be an important pathogen of several wild bird species. VEEV also causes encephalitic disease in horses and, occasionally, humans bitten by mosquitoes normally associated with the horses (Weaver 2005; Weaver and Barrett 2004; Weaver *et al.* 1997, 2005;). The natural life cycle of VEEV involves small mammals, particularly rodents in forest environments more frequently found in South America. Several other related alphaviruses are recognized in the Americas but in most cases they are not known to cause disease in humans or animals.

The Flaviviruses: the agents, the hosts and disease epidemiology

Currently approximately 60 species are recognized in the genus *Flavivirus* although during the past decade several new unclassified flaviviruses have been isolated from mosquitoes in different regions of the world (Cook *et al.* 2006; Crabtree *et al.* 2003; Farfan-Ale *et al.* 2009; Hoshino *et al.* 2007; Kihara *et al.* 2007; Kim *et al.* 2009; Morales-Betoulle *et al.* 2008; Sang *et al.* 2003). Recent reviews of the Genus *Flavivirus* include (Gould *et al.* 2003; Heinz 2000; Thiel *et al.* 2005). Many of these new viruses appear to be insect viruses, i.e. they do not infect vertebrates. It is possible that they will ultimately be recognized as a new genus within the family *Flaviviridae*. Other recently isolated but not yet classified flaviviruses appear to be conventional arboviruses but their natural vertebrate hosts are not necessarily recognized as yet.

Infectious (mature) flaviviruses are spherical particles (50 nm) with a relatively smooth surface and no distinct projections. They have an electron-dense core (30 nm) surrounded by a lipid membrane. The core consists of positive-polarity genomic RNA (11 kbp) and capsid (C) protein (12K). The lipid membrane incorporates an envelope glycoprotein (E, 53K) and a membrane glycoprotein (M, 8K). The immature (intracellular) virions contain a precursor membrane protein (prM, 18K), the proteolytic cleavage of which occurs in the secretory pathway, during egress of virions from infected cells.

The E glycoprotein mediates virus binding to cellular receptors and thereby directly affects virus host range, virulence, and immunological properties by inducing protective antibodies. The E-protein ectodomain (N-terminal 395 amino acids) consists of 90 homodimers folded in a 'head-to-tail' manner and orientated parallel to the membrane surface. The E protein contains three structural domains, each based on β-sheets: the central domain I, the dimerization (fusion) domain II, and receptor domain III (dI, dII, and dIII). The C-terminal 101 residues of the E protein form a stem anchor region consisting of two stem α-helices and two transmembrane α-helices that anchor the E protein into the lipid bilayer. Domain II contains a hydrophobic fusion peptide consisting of 13 residues that are highly conserved between all flaviviruses. The fusion peptide is located on the tip of domain II and plays a central role in fusion of the virion membrane to cellular endosomal membranes resulting in release of virion RNA into the cytoplasm. The E-dimers form a 'herringbone' configuration; three quasiparallel E-dimer molecules making up the main structural asymmetric unit of the shell. The fivefold symmetry axes are generated by appropriate positioning of five domain IIIs and their lateral surface is accessible to cellular receptors and neutralizing antibodies.

The M protein protrudes through holes formed between dimerization domains of E molecules. Following acid pH-dependent fusion of the E protein with cytoplasmic endosomes, the 5' and 3' untranslated regions (UTRs) of the released genomic RNA provide signals to initiate translation of the open reading frame (ORF) which is then processed by cellular signalases and viral serine protease to produce three structural (C, prM, and E) and seven nonstructural (NS1 through NS5) proteins. The N-terminal region of the NS3 protein provides the viral protease function. NS2B probably acts as a co-factor by anchoring the NS3 protein. Replication of new viral RNA requires direct interaction between the 5' and 3' UTRs resulting in the formation of double-stranded RNA replicative forms and genome circularization. Specific RNA secondary structures within the UTRs provide essential promoter and replication enhancer functions. Flavivirus RNA replication is semiconservative and asymmetric. The replicative intermediate presents a partially double-stranded RNA with nascent, and displaced, plus-sense ssRNA molecules undergoing elongation. Capping of the 5'UTR occurs on the displaced plus-strand RNA; the NS3 and NS5 proteins provide nucleoside triphosphatase and guanylyl-methyltransferase activities, respectively. The C-terminal domain of NS5 protein acts as the viral RNA polymerase and the C-terminal domain of NS3 functions as the helicase. The functions of other nonstructural proteins are less precisely identified. The NS1 glycoprotein is translocated in the endoplasmic reticulum and secreted together with virions in mammalian but not in mosquito cells. The NS2A protein associates with the NS3 helicase domain, the NS5 protein, and the 3'UTR. It may be involved in viral RNA trafficking. The NS2B protein is a membrane-anchored cofactor of the serine proteinase, NS3 and also has membrane permeability modulating activity. The hydrophobic NS4A protein in conjunction with the NS1 protein probably anchors the polymerase complex to cell membranes (Gritsun and Gould 2008; Thiel *et al.* 2005). For colour images representing the above description of the flavivirus life cycle see Gritsun and Gould (2008).

About 60% of the currently classified flaviviruses are primarily transmitted between vertebrates by mosquitoes and these viruses have been roughly divided into those associated primarily with *Aedes* spp., typified by YFV and Dengue virus (DENV) and those associated primarily with *Culex* spp., mosquitoes, typified by West Nile virus (WNV) and Japanese encephalitis virus (JEV). Indeed the entire genus shows striking relationships between epidemiology, disease association and biogeography (Gaunt *et al.* 2001). Although the flaviviruses have a wide vertebrate host range their global distribution tends to be specific for individual viruses and is largely dependent on the dispersal and/or accumulation of arthropods via associated activities such as transportation of humans, animals and commercial goods, bird migration, irrigation, deforestation or remediation projects, human demographic changes (Gould *et al.* 2003, 2006; Gould and Higgs 2009; Gould and Solomon 2008; Reiter 2008). YFV provides an excellent example of how humans have been responsible for the dispersal of viruses. In the wild, YFV circulates in the central and West African jungles and the surrounding savannah regions, and also in some of the Caribbean Islands and the South American rain forests. The virus circulates between mosquitoes and monkeys living in the canopy of the African jungles, with little evidence of disease in the simian species suggesting that this cycle has existed for a long time. In contrast, in the South American jungles, YFV causes fatal infections in non-immune howler monkeys with which the virus is most often associated, suggesting that YFV was introduced relatively recently. Indeed, this is almost certainly the case. It is the widely held opinion that YFV was introduced many times, from Africa to the New World during the trading of African slaves between these countries. These trading activities occurred for more than 400 years during which YFV became established in the New World countries of Latin America (Bloom 1993; Gould *et al.* 2003; Tabachnick, 1991). Dengue virus was also almost certainly introduced from Africa to the New World during this period of slave trading. However, after this type of trading ceased and trading routes from Asia were increasing, the introduced Dengue virus species were of Asian origin rather than African origin. By the late 1970s many Asian strains of Dengue virus had been introduced into the New World and this led to the first cases of dengue haemorrhagic fever been observed in Cuba (Guzman *et al.* 1984; Rico-Hesse *et al.* 1997). Viruses in the Japanese encephalitis virus (JEV) complex are most frequently associated with ornithophilic (bird biting) mosquitoes, in particular *Culex* spp., Their geographic distribution is therefore largely dependent upon the migratory patterns of birds. Based on phylogenetic relationships and the known geographic distribution of these viruses, it is believed that the ancestral lineage originated in Africa and evolutionary descendants of this African virus were gradually dispersed by migratory birds into Europe, Asia and Australia (Gould *et al.* 2004). Whilst WNV appears to be dispersed efficiently via migratory birds in both the Old World and the New World (Gould and Higgs 2009; Malkinson *et al.* 2002; Owen *et al.* 2006), its transition across the Oceans to the New World was almost certainly the result of accidental introduction via an aeroplane or ship. The former mode of transportation is favoured because the first outbreaks of encephalitis in birds, horses and humans appear to have occurred not too distant from the major international airport in New York (Gould *et al.* 2003; Roehrig *et al.* 2002). Another member of the JEV complex, Usutu virus (USUV), is the most recently recognized emergent virus of this group. Prior to 2001, USUV had only ever been identified in Africa. However, a sudden outbreak of encephalitis in birds in Vienna (Austria) led to the discovery of its emergence out of Africa, presumably for the first time (Weissenbock *et al.* 2002). This virus has apparently continued to disperse in Europe (Buckley *et al.* 2003, 2006; Rizzoli *et al.* 2007) and was recently identified in mosquitoes in Spain (Busquets *et al.* 2008). Other antigenically related viruses in the JEV complex, such as Murray Valley encephalitis virus, Alfuy virus and Kunjin virus are found in Australia and are assumed to be direct descendants of the African lineage that has evolved as JEV, WNV, USUV etc. In the Americas, St Louis encephalitis virus, and many related viruses such as Ilheus virus, Rocio virus and others are presumed to have been introduced from Africa during the intensive period of slave trading (Gould *et al.* 2003).

Bunyaviruses: the agent, the hosts and disease epidemiology

There have been several recent reviews of the Genus *Orthobunyavirus* (Elliott 2008; Fauquet *et al.* 2005; Nichol *et al.* 2005; Putkuri *et al.* 2007). In general, the virions of bunyaviruses are spherical or pleomorphic, 80–120 nm in diameter and display surface glycoprotein projections of 5–10 nm which are embedded in a lipid bilayered envelope approximately 5 nm thick. The viral genomes are segmented consisting of 3 unique negative or ambisense ssRNA molecules, designated L (large), M (medium) and S (small) totalling 11–19 kb. The terminal nucleotides of each segment are base-paired forming non-covalently closed, circular RNAs (and nucleocapsids). These terminal sequences are conserved amongst viruses in any one genus but are different from those in any other genus within the family. The L segment encodes the viral RNA polymerase enzyme. The M segment encodes the Gc protein which is the major target of neutralizing antibodies and acts as a ligand for cellular receptors on erythrocytes and is therefore involved in haemagglutination inhibition (Gonzalez-Scarano *et al.* 1982; Grady *et al.* 1983; Kingsford and Hill 1983) and also in viral entry, playing a critical role in fusion between the viral envelope and the cellular membrane (Pekosz *et al.* 1995; Plassmeyer *et al.* 2007). Gc undergoes a pH-dependent conformational change associated with cell-to-cell and virus-to-cell fusion (Gonzalez-Scarano 1984, 1985; Jacoby *et al.* 1993; Pekosz and Gonzalez-Scarano 1996). The M segment also encodes a Gn glycoprotein (Gonzalez-Scarano *et al.* 1982; Kingsford *et al.* 1983), which is required for targeting the Gc protein to the Golgi apparatus from the endoplasmic reticulum (Bupp *et al.* 1996). Gn probably also functions in cell-to-cell fusion (Jacoby *et al.* 1993; Plassmeyer *et al.* 2005) and may be the protein responsible for viral attachment in the mosquito midgut (Ludwig *et al.* 1991). The S segment encodes the N protein which is possibly involved in early and late RNA synthesis, and the NSs which is an interferon antagonist and acts at the level of transcription by inhibiting RNA polymerase II-mediated transcription. For detailed colour images of the general characteristics and life cycle of bunyaviruses see (Elliott 2008).

There are estimated to be more than 300 different virus species in the genus *Orthobunyavirus,* only a few of which are transmitted by mosquitoes and associated with significant human disease outbreaks. The mosquito-transmitted bunyaviruses are widespread globally but in common with other arboviruses, individual species occupy geographic niches largely dependent on their dispersal patterns and the particular mosquito vectors and vertebrate hosts with which they have established their life cycles. For example, in the California encephalitis virus serogroup which contains 12 species of antigenically related viruses, La Crosse virus (LACV) is an important cause of encephalitis in children (LeDuc 1987) in the USA. Its principal vector *Aedes triseriatus* prefers woodland habitats such as tree holes where squirrels and chipmunks serve as the vertebrate hosts, but these mosquitoes also frequently lay their eggs in small pools of water in car tyres, buckets, cans, etc in urban and rural settings and the emerging mosquitoes may then feed on humans, causing localized outbreaks. In order for this to be possible it is necessary for LACV to be passed vertically in the female mosquito to the eggs that retain the infectious virus through the next generation of mosquitoes. This form of long-term survival and transmission has been recognized for many years (Tesh and Gubler 1975). Tahyna virus (TAHV) circulates widely in central and southern Europe and also in China (Lu *et al.* 2009). TAHV usually causes a febrile flu-like illness but neurological complications are sometimes observed. Its closest relative, Snowshoe hare virus (SSHV) circulates widely in Canada and northern regions of the USA amongst a wide variety of mosquito and wild/domestic animal species. A similar virus is also found in Russia. In addition to febrile illness SSHV may cause encephalitis. Another related virus, Lumbo virus (LUMV) is found in Africa (Elliott 2008; Putkuri *et al.* 2007) and may therefore represent an early lineage of the antigenic complex. Inkoo virus (INKV) is widespread in most countries in northern Europe. It was first isolated from its principle mosquito vector *Aedes communis* in Finland in 1964 (Brummer Korvenkontio *et al.* 1973). Phylogenetic studies indicate that the closest relative to INKV is Jamestown Canyon virus, found in the US (Campbell and Huang 1999; Vapalahti *et al.* 1996). Whilst there are very few studies on the origin of these bunyaviruses, the phylogentic trees imply that they have dispersed widely across the oceans and northern land masses. Since many related bunyaviruses are found in Africa, and are not associated with significant disease in humans, Africa would appear to be a reasonable candidate for their evolutionary origins.

Phleboviruses: the agents, the hosts and disease epidemiology

The Genus *Phlebovirus in the Bunyaviridae family* (Gould and Higgs 2009; Zuckerman *et al.* 2004) contains one virus, Rift Valley fever virus (RVFV) that is a major human and animal pathogen. RVFV is primarily transmitted to animals and humans by a wide range of *Aedes* spp. mosquitoes, (Hoch *et al.* 1985; Turell *et al.* 1996) although it is also transmitted by phlebotomine species, hence its inclusion in the genus *Phlebovirus*. RVFV causes severe disease with high rates of abortion and fatal infections in livestock but appears to be relatively harmless in wild species that roam the plains in Africa. The virus was first identified in 1931 during an investigation into an epidemic on a farm in the Rift Valley of Kenya (Daubney *et al.* 1931) but it had almost certainly been responsible for outbreaks in different regions of Africa for many years before 1931. Humans that come into close contact with the blood, excreta and infected mosquitoes associated with clinically infected animals may also become infected. Most human cases are relatively mild, but some individuals develop much more severe symptoms that may present as ocular disease (0.5–2% of patients), meningoencephalitis (less than 1%), with residual neurological deficit and occasional fatalities, or haemorrhagic fever (less than 1%) with a case:fatality rate as high as 50%. RVFV is widespread throughout Africa and recently caused epidemics in the Arabian Peninsula, presumably being introduced either by infected mosquitoes or animals supplied for commercial purposes (Gould and Higgs 2009). There has been significant speculation as to whether or not this virus will continue to disperse out of Africa beyond the Arabian Peninsula. The opinion of some experts is that this is unlikely. However, others believe it would be most surprising if RVFV did not spread further.

Vesiculoviruses: the agent, the hosts and disease epidemiology

Vesiculoviruses are members of the virus family *Rhabdoviridae* (genus *Vesiculovirus*). They are primarily associated with Phlebotomine sandflies and blackflies but several vesiculoviruses (tentatively classified in the genus) have been isolated from mosquito species. Whilst in the western hemisphere the vesiculoviruses are predominantly associated with disease in ungulates, particularly cows and horses, human infections usually presenting as flu-illness are recognized in people most frequently associated with infected animals. However, Chandipura virus (CHAV), principally associated with phlebotomine sandflies, was recently shown to be the cause of a human outbreak in India that involved 329 children of which 183 died following the development of acute encephalitis (Rao *et al.* 2004). If CHAV continues to produce epidemics with high fatality rates in India (and/or elsewhere), this could raise the profile of the vesiculoviruses as human pathogens.

Orbiviruses

In general, members of the genus *Orbivirus* do not infect humans and for many orbiviruses the invertebrate vector of importance in terms of disease in animals, is the midge (*Culicoides*). Bluetongue virus of sheep and cattle, African Horse sickness virus and Epizootic haemorrhagic disease of some wild ruminants, are the most well known viruses in this genus but in general they are not associated with transmission by mosquitoes. However, some less notorious orbiviruses are vectored by mosquitoes and may infect a large variety of wild animal species but these mosquito-borne arboviruses are not generally considered to be of significant importance to animal health.

Diagnosis

Clinical diagnosis of the important mosquito virus infections can be reliable where infection is common, but definitive diagnosis requires laboratory confirmation either by virus isolation or the detection of antibody. The most widely used approaches used for diagnosis are RT-PCR tests for virus detection and detection of virus specific IgM in serum or CSF samples. A number of RT-PCR assays have been described for the clinically important viruses: JEV (Huang *et al.* 2004) Dengue (Lanciotti 2003).

Commercial assays for serological diagnosis are available (Guzman *et al.* 2004). However, serological diagnosis of DENV can be difficult to interpret because of the extensive antigenic cross reactions between Dengue serotypes and other flaviviruses.

Prevention and control

The mosquito-borne arboviruses cause a considerable amount of human morbidity and mortality worldwide. Dengue virus (DENV) in particular is an increasingly important human pathogen, comprising four serotypes (DENV-1, DENV-2, DENV-3, DENV-4) which cause epidemics in all tropical and many sub-tropical regions of the world. The number of dengue fever cases per year is estimated to exceed 50 million with approximately 2.5% of the 500,000 cases of dengue haemorrhagic fever resulting in fatal infections, and in some poorly developed areas it may reach 20% (WHO, Fact sheet N°117, March 2009). In general, other arboviruses are not as widespread, but one or two, e.g. CHIKV and WNV have become much more widely dispersed and are causing larger epidemics than appears to have been the case 50 or more years ago. This is largely due to, increasing mosquito abundance, human mobility, agricultural and commercial activities, altered utilization of land, water and forests, impacts resulting from military activities and possibly early effects of climate change (Gould and Higgs 2009). There is therefore an increasing need for more extensive arbovirus disease control strategies.

Undoubtedly, the most effective method for controlling disease due to mosquito-borne arboviruses would be to eradicate the mosquitoes. Such methods have been shown to be effective, the most well known being the control of YFV at the beginning of the twentieth century in Cuba and in specific areas of the Panama Canal where the construction engineers were working. This success is largely attributed to William Gorgas and his colleagues; see website http://www.archives.state.al.us/famous/w_gorgas.html</url|>. Whilst mosquito eradication campaigns proved to be highly successful in controlling YFV, more than a century ago, attempts to control dengue fever in Singapore and in Cuba during the past twenty years, using a similar strategy have been only partly successful in reducing DENV incidence but DENV is constantly being re-introduced into these countries from neighbouring countries where the mosquito control measures are less successfully applied, making the total eradication of the virus a seemingly impossible task.

Vaccines

The live attenuated yellow fever virus vaccine known as 17D-204 (and also 17DD) is considered to be one of the most successful virus vaccines every produced. It was originally derived as an attenuated variant of wild type YFV by extensive serial passage in mice and subsequently in chick embryo eggs. It has been in use for over 70 years and millions of doses have been used almost certainly saving many lives in Africa and Latin America. However, as described earlier, YFV has a sylvatic existence in the African and Latin American jungles and this feature of the virus provides it with a safe reservoir from where it can re-emerge amongst human populations that have failed to maintain immunity levels by vigilant implementation of immunization programmes. The vaccine is described in detail in chapter 38. Inactivated vaccines against JEV and TBEV are also available for human use and they are often recommended to westerners travelling to endemic areas such as Asia, in the case of JEV. However, these vaccines are not approved for use in all countries. China has successfully developed a series of JEV vaccines, both inactivated and live attenuated, that have been used throughout large areas of China and other regions of Asia, where JEV is known to circulate. More recently widespread campaigns have also been implemented to immunize children in India in the hope of reducing the high levels of morbidity and mortality recorded annually. Currently, there are no other widely available vaccines for human protection against the known pathogenic arboviruses. However, vaccines have been produced against a variety of arboviruses for limited use in individuals exposed to the viruses through the nature of their occupations. For example, limited quantities of inactivated human vaccines against VEEV, KFDV, and RVFV, have been produced and used in military and laboratory personnel. However, none of these vaccines has been approved for large-scale use and with the possible exception of KFDV in India, the use of these vaccines has gradually being reduced to virtually zero. Currently, several projects have been initiated to develop vaccines against DENV, WNV, JEV, VEEV and CHIKV using a variety of methods including the development of chimaeric flaviviruses that use:

1   A YFV or a DENV genetic background but containing the viral envelope and membrane protein substituted from a different pathogenic flavivirus (Monath *et al.* 2003),

2   The use of serial passage in cell cultures that are considered to be free of contaminating viruses, this method is very similar to the principle used to develop YF 17D vaccine,

3   The use of recombinant expressed flaviviral envelope proteins and

4   The use of viral DNA, engineered to have an appropriate promoter for expression of the relevant viral proteins in human cells, representing known immunogenic regions of the viral genome.

Several of these new potential human vaccines are currently undergoing clinical trials.

Several veterinary vaccines have already been developed to protect horses against a variety of arboviruses, in particular, VEEV, EEEV, and WNV. In general these vaccines are proving to be efficacious with few serious side effects in horses.

In addition to the use of virus vaccines to control infections due to mosquito-borne arboviruses, a large number of antiviral compounds are being tested for their ability to control infections that have already been initiated. At the moment no effective single antiviral therapeutic agent has been identified although several show promise and are currently undergoing clinical trials.

In conclusion, prior to the introduction of WNV into North America through New York, the global research effort on arboviruses was in relative decline when compared with malaria, hepatitis B and C, or HIV. However, the widespread dispersal of WNV throughout North America that commenced in 1999, together with the increasing epidemicity of DENV, and the recent emergence, in 2005, of CHIKV as a rapidly spreading threat to human populations throughout Asia, and potentially globally, has stimulated renewed interest in arboviruses, particularly in their rapid diagnosis, pathogenicity, modes of transmission and dispersal, their evolution and their control. Taking an optimistic viewpoint, the application of modern molecular technologies, and bioinformatics tools, combined with improved epidemiological modelling, more extensive sampling methods, a greater understanding of the disease process, and better medical support should increase our capacity to reduce the levels of human and animal suffering, due to arboviruses during the foreseeable future.

References

Bloom, K. J. (1993). *The Mississippi Valley's great yellow fever epidemic of 1878*. Baton Rouge, Louisiana: Louisiana State University Press.

Brummer Korvenkontio, M., Saikku, P., Korhonen, P. & Oker Blom, N. (1973). Arboviruses in Finland. I. Isolation of tick-borne encephalitis (TBE) virus from arthropods, vertebrates, and patients. *Am. J. Trop. Med. Hyg.,* **22:** 382–89.

Buckley, A., Dawson, A. & Gould, E. A. (2006). Detection of seroconversion to West Nile virus, Usutu virus and Sindbis virus in UK sentinel chickens. *Virol. J.,* **3:** 71.

Buckley, A., Dawson, A., Moss, S. R., Hinsley, S. A., Bellamy, P. E. & Gould, E. A. (2003). Serological evidence of *West Nile virus, Usutu virus* and *Sindbis virus* infection of birds in the UK. *J. Gen. Virol.,* **84:** 2807–17.

Bupp, K., Stillmock, K. & Gonzalez-Scarano, F. (1996). Analysis of the intracellular transport properties of recombinant La Crosse virus glycoproteins. *Virol.,* **220:** 485–90.

Busquets, N., Alba, A., Allepuz, A., Aranda, C. & Nuñez, J. I. (2008). Usutu Virus Sequences in Culex pipiens (Diptera: Culicidae), Spain. *Emerg. Infect. Dis.,* **14:** 861–62.

Campbell, W. P. & Huang, C. (1999). Sequence comparisons of medium RNA segment among 15 California serogroup viruses. *Vir. Res.,* **61:** 137–44.

Casals, J. (1944). Immunological relationship among central nervous system viruses. *J. Experim. Med.,* **79:** 341–59.

Casals, J. (1957). The arthropod-borne group of animal viruses. *Trans. NY Acad. Sci.,* **19:** 219–35.

Casals, J. & Brown, L. V. (1954). Haemagglutination with arthropod-borne viruses. *J. Experim. Med.,* **99:** 429–49.

Casals, J. & Webster, L. T. (1944). Relationship of the virus of louping ill in sheep and the virus of Russian spring-summer encephalitis in man. *J. Experim. Med.,* **79:** 45–63.

Chanas, A. C., Johnson, B. K. & Simpson, D. I. H. (1976). Antigenic Relationships of Alphaviruses by a Simple Micro-culture Cross-neutralization Method. *J. Gen. Virol.,* **32:** 295–300.

Chevillon, C., Briant, L., Renaud, F. & Devaux, C. (2008). The Chikungunya threat: an ecological and evolutionary perspective. *Trends Microbiol.,* **16:** 80–88.

Clarke, D. H. & Casals, J. (1958). Techniques for haemagglutination and haemagglutination-inhibition with arthropod-borne viruses. *Am. J. Trop. Med. Hyg.,* **7:** 561–73.

Cook, S., Bennett, S. N., Holmes, E. C., De Chesse, R., Moureau, G. & de Lamballerie, X. (2006). Isolation of a new strain of the flavivirus cell fusing agent virus in a natural mosquito population from Puerto Rico. *J. Gen. Virol.,* **87:** 7375–78.

Crabtree, M. B., Sang, R. C., Stollar, V., Dunster, L. M. & Miller, B. R. (2003). Genetic and phenotypic characterization of the newly described insect flavivirus, Kamiti River virus. *Arch. Virol.,* **148:** 1095–118.

Daubney, R., Hudson, J. R. & Garnham, P. C. (1931). Enzootic hepatitis or Rift Valley fever. An undescribed virus disease of sheep, cattle and man from East Africa. *J. Path. Bacteriol.,* **34:** 545–79.

de Lamballerie, X., Leroy, E., Charrel, R. N., Ttsetsarkin, K., Higgs, S. & Gould, E. A. (2008). Chikungunya virus adapts to tiger mosquito via evolutionary convergence: a sign of things to come? *Virol. J.,* **5:** 33.

Diaz, L. A., Cardenas, V. M., Daza, E., Bruzon, L., Alcala, A., et al. (1997). Epidemic Venezuelan equine encephalitis in La Guajira, Colombia, 1995. *J. Infect. Dis.,* **175:** 828–32.

Elliott, R. M. (2008). Bunyaviruses: General Features. In: B. W. J. Mahy & M. H. V. Van Regenmortel (eds.) *Encyclopaedia of Virology,* pp. 390–99. Oxford: Elsevier.

Farfan-Ale, J. A., Loroño-Pino, M. A., Garcia-Rejon, J. E., et al. (2009). Detection of RNA from a Novel West Nile-like Virus and High Prevalence of an Insect-specific Flavivirus in Mosquitoes in the Yucatan Peninsula of Mexico. *Am. J. Trop. Med. Hyg.,* **80:** 85–95.

Fauquet, C. M., Mayo, M. A., Maniloff, J., Desselberger, U. & Ball, L. A. (2005). *Virus Taxonomy: VIIIth Report of the ICTV.* London: Elsevier/ Academic Press.

Gaunt, M. W., Sall, A. A., de Lamballerie, X., et al. (2001). Phylogenetic relationships of flaviviruses correlate with their epidemiology, disease association and biogeography. *J. Gen. Virol.,* **82:** 1867–76.

Gonzalez-Scarano, F. (1985). La Crosse virus G1 glycoprotein undergoes a conformational change at the pH of fusion. *Virol.,* **140:** 209–16.

Gonzalez-Scarano, F., Pobjecky, N. and Nathanson, N. (1984). La Crosse bunyavirus can mediate pH-dependent fusion from without. *Virol.,* **132:** 222–25.

Gonzalez-Scarano, F., Shope, R. E., Calisher, C. H. & Nathanson, N. (1982). Characterization of monoclonal antibodies against the G1 and N proteins of LaCrosse and Tahyna, two California serogroup bunyaviruses. *Virol.,* **120:** 42–53.

Gould, E. A., de Lamballerie, X., Zanotto, P. M. and Holmes, E. C. (2003). Origins, evolution, and vector/host coadaptations within the genus Flavivirus. *Adv. Virus Res.,* **59:** 277–314.

Gould, E. A. and Higgs, S. (2009). Impact of climate change and other factors on emerging arbovirus diseases. *Trans. R. Soc. Trop. Med. Hyg.,* **103:** 109–21.

Gould, E. A., Higgs, S., Buckley, A. & Gritsun, T. S. (2006). Potential arbovirus emergence and implications for the United Kingdom. *Emerg. Infect. Dis.,* **12:** 549–55.

Gould, E. A., Moss, S. R. & Turner, S. L. (2004). Evolution and dispersal of encephalitic flaviviruses. *Arch. Virol.* Supplementum, **(18):** 65–84.

Gould, E. A. & Solomon, T. S. (2008). Pathogenic flaviviruses. *Lancet,* **371:** 500–509.

Grady, L. J., Srihongse, S., Grayson, M. A. & Deibel, R. (1983). Monoclonal antibodies against La Crosse virus. *J. Gen. Virol.,* **64:** 1699–704.

Greig, J. R., Brownlee, A., Wilson, D. R. & Gordon, W. S. (1931). The nature of louping ill. *Vet. Rec.,* **11:** 325.

Gritsun, T. S. & Gould, E. A. (2008). Tick-borne encephalitis viruses. In: B. W. J. Mahy and M. H. V. Van Regenmortel (eds,) *Encyclopaedia of Virology,* (3rd edn.), pp. 4554. Oxford: Elsevier.

Guzman, M. G., Kouri, G. P., Bravo, J., Calunga, M., et al. (1984). Dengue haemorrhagic fever in Cuba. I. Serological confirmation of clinical diagnosis. *Trans. R. Soc. Trop. Med. Hyg.,* **78:** 235–38.

Guzman, M. G., Kouri, G. (2004). Dengue diagnosis, advances and challenges. *Int. J. Infect. Dis.,* **8:** 69–80.

Heinz, F. X., Collett, M. S., Purcell, R. H., Gould, E. A., et al. (2000). Flaviviridae. In: C. F. van Regenmortel, D. H. L. Bishop et al. (eds.) *Virus Taxonomy, VIIth Report of the International Committee on Taxonomy of Viruses,* pp. 859–78. San Diego: Academic Press.

Higgs, S., Schneider, B. S., Vanlandingham, D. L., Klingler, K. A. & Gould, E. A. (2005). Nonviremic transmission of West Nile virus. *Proc. Nat. Acad. Sci. USA,* **102:** 8871–74.

Hirst, G. K. (1941). The agglutination of red cells by allantoic fluid of chick embryos infected with influenza virus. *Sci. NY,* **94:** 22–23.

Hoch, A. L., Gargan, II, T. B. & Bailey, C. L. (1985). Mechanical Transmission of Rift Valley Fever Virus by Hematophagous Diptera. *Am. J. Trop. Med. Hyg.,* **34:** 188–93.

Hoshino, K., Isawa, H., Tsuda, Y., Yano, K., et al. (2007). Genetic characterization of a new insect flavivirus isolated from Culex pipiens mosquito in Japan. *Virol.,* **359:** 405–14.

Huang, J-L., Lin, H-T., Wang, Y-M., et al. (2004). Sensitive and specific detection of strains of Japanese encephalitis virus using a one-step TaqMan RT-PCT technique. *J. Med. Virol.,* **74:** 589–96.

Jacoby, D. R., Cooke, C., Prabakaran, I., Boland, J., et al. (1993). Expression of the La Crosse M segment proteins in a recombinant vaccinia expression system mediates pH-dependent cellular fusion. *Virol.,* **193:** 993–96.

Johnson, K. M. and Martin, D. M. (1974). Venezuelan equine encephalitis. *Adv. Vet. Sci. Comp. Med.,* **18:** 79–116.

Jones, L. D., Gaunt, M., Hails, R. S., Laurenson, K., et al. (1997). Transmission of louping ill virus between infected and uninfected ticks co-feeding on mountain hares. *Med. Vet. Entom.,* **11:** 172–76.

Karabatsos, N. (1975). Antigenic relationships of group A arboviruses by plaque reduction neutralization testing. *Am. J. Trop. Med. Hyg.,* **24:** 527–32.

Karabatsos, N. (1985). International Catalogue of Arthropod-borne viruses. (3rd ed.), *San Antonio, Texas: American Society for Tropical Medicine and Hygiene,* [Suppl 1]: 137–52.

Kihara, Y., Satho, T., Eshita, Y., Sakai, K., et al. (2007). Rapid determination of viral RNA sequences in mosquitoes collected in the field. *J. Virol. Meth.,* **146:** 372–74.

Kim, D. Y., Guzman, H., Bueno, J. R., Dennett, J. A., et al. (2009). Characterization of Culex Flavivirus (Flaviviridae) strains isolated from mosquitoes in the United States and Trinidad. *Virol.,* **386:** 154–59.

Kingsford, L. & Hill, D. W. (1983). The effect of proteolytic cleavage of La Crosse virus G1 glycoprotein on antibody neutralization. *J. Gen. Virol.,* **64:** 2147–56.

Kingsford, L., Ishizawa, L. D. & Hill, D. W. (1983). Biological activities of monoclonal antibodies reactive with antigenic sites mapped on the G1 glycoprotein of La Crosse virus. *Virol.,* **129:** 443–55.

Labuda, M., Kozuch, O., Zuffova, E., Eleckova, E., et al. (1997). Tick-borne encephalitis virus transmission between ticks cofeeding on specific immune natural rodent hosts. *Virol.,* **235:** 138–43.

Lanciotti, R. S., Kerst, A. J. (2001). Nucleic acid sequence-based amplification assays for rapid detection of West Nile and St. Louis encephalitis viruses. *J. Clin. Mircrobiol.*, **39**: 4506–13.

LeDuc, J. W. (1987). Epidemiology and ecology of the California serogroup viruses. *Am. J. Trop. Med. Hyg.*, **37**: 60S–68S.

Lennette, E. H. & Koprowski, H. (1944). Neutralization Tests with Certain Neurotropic Viruses. A Comparison of the Sensitivity of the Extraneural and Intracerebral Routes of Inoculation for the Detection of Antibodies. *J. Immunol.*, **49**: 375–85.

Leon, C. A. (1975). Sequelae of Venezuelan equine encephalitis in humans: a four year follow-up. *Int. J. Epidemiol.*, **4**: 131–40.

Lewthwaite, P., Vasanthapuram, R., Osborne, J. C., *et al.* (2009). Chikungunya Virus and Central Nervous System Infections in Children, India. *Emerg. Infect. Dis.*, **15**: 329–31.

Lu, Z., Lu, X-J., Fu, S-H., Song Zhang, S., *et al.* (2009). Tahyna Virus and Human Infection, China. *Emerg. Infect. Dis.*, **15**.

Ludwig, G. V., Israel, B. A., Christensen, B. M., Yuill, T. M. & Schultz, K. T. (1991). Role of La Crosse virus glycoproteins in attachment of virus to host cells. *Virol.*, **181**: 564–71.

Malkinson, M., Banet, C., Weisman, Y., Pokamunski, S., *et al.* (2002). Introduction of West Nile virus in the Middle East by migrating white storks. *Emerg. Infect. Dis.*, **8**: 392–97.

Mead, D. G., Ramberg, F. B., Besselsen, D. G. & Mare, C. J. (2000). Transmission of Vesicular Stomatitis Virus from Infected to Noninfected Black Flies Co-Feeding on Nonviremic Deer Mice. *Sci. NY*, **287**: 485–87.

Monath, T. P., Guirakhoo, F., Nichols, R., Yoksan, S., *et al.* (2003). Chimeric live, attenuated vaccine against Japanese encephalitis (ChimeriVax-JE): phase 2 clinical trials for safety and immunogenicity, effect of vaccine dose and schedule, and memory response to challenge with inactivated Japanese encephalitis antigen. *J. Infect. Dis.*, **188**: 1213–30.

Morales-Betoulle, M. E., Pineda, M. L., Sosa, S. M., *et al.* (2008). Culex Flavivirus Isolates from Mosquitoes in Guatemala. *J. Med. Ent.*, **45**: 1187–90.

Mukhopadhyay, S., Zhang, W., Gabler, S., Chipman, P. R., *et al.* (2006). Mapping the Structure and Function of the E1 and E2 Glycoproteins in Alphaviruses. *Struct.*, **14**: 63–73.

Nichol, S. T., Beaty, B. J., Elliott, R. M., *et al.* (2005). 'Bunyaviridae'. In: C. M. Fauquet, M. A. Mayo, *et al.* (eds.) *Virus Taxonomy: Eighth Report of the International Committee on Taxonomy of Viruses*, pp. 695–716. Oxford: Elsevier Academic Press.

Owen, J., Moore, F., Panella, N., Edwards, E., Bru, R., *et al.* (2006). Migrating Birds as Dispersal Vehicles for West Nile Virus. *EcoHealth*, **3**: 79–85.

Paulson, S. L., Grimstad, P. R. & Craig, G. B. (1989). Midgut and salivary gland barriers to La Crosse virus dissemination in mosquitoes of the Aedes triseriatus group. *Med. Vet. Ent.*, **3**: 113–23.

Pekosz, A. & Gonzalez-Scarano, F. (1996). The extracellular domain of La Crosse virus G1 forms oligomers and undergoes pH-dependent conformational changes. *Virol.*, **225**: 243–47.

Pekosz, A., Griot, C., Nathanson, N. & Gonzalez-Scarano, F. (1995). Tropism of bunyaviruses: evidence for a G1 glycoprotein-mediated entry pathway common to the California serogroup. *Virol.*, **214**: 339–48.

Plassmeyer, M. L., Soldan, S. S., Stachelek, K. M., *et al.* (2005). California serogroup Gc (G1) glycoprotein is the principal determinant of pH-dependent cell fusion and entry. *Virol.*, **338**: 121–32.

Plassmeyer, M. L., Soldan, S. S., Stachelek, K. M., *et al.* (2007). Mutagenesis of the La Crosse Virus glycoprotein supports a role for Gc (1066–1087) as the fusion peptide. *Virol.*, **358**: 273–82.

Porterfield, J. S. (1961). Cross-neutralization studies with group A arthropod-borne viruses. *Bull. World Health Organ.*, **24**: 735–41.

Porterfield, J. S. (1980). Antigenic characteristics and classification of Togaviridae. In: R. W. Schlesinger (ed.) *The Togaviruses*, pp. 13–46. New York: Academic Press.

Putkuri, N., Vaheri, A. & Vapalahti, O. (2007). Prevalence and Protein Specificity of Human Antibodies to Inkoo Virus Infection. *Clin. Vacc. Immun.*, **14**: 1555–62.

Rao, B. L., Basu, A., Wairagkar, N. S., Gore, M. M., *et al.* (2004). A large outbreak of acute encephalitis with high fatality rate in children in Andhra Pradesh, India, in 2003, associated with Chandipura virus. *Lancet*, **364**: 869–74.

Reed, W. (1901). Propagation of yellow fever: observations based on recent researches. *Med. Rec.*, **60**: 209–10.

Reiter, P. (2008). Global warming and malaria: knowing the horse before hitching the cart. *Malaria Journal* **7**(Suppl 1), S3 doi:10.1186/1475-2875-1187-S1181-S1183.

Rico-Hesse, R., Harrison, L. M., Salas, R. A., *et al.* (1997). Origins of dengue type 2 viruses associated with increased pathogenicity in the Americas. *Virol.*, **230**: 244–51.

Rizzoli, A., Rosa, R., Rosso, F., Buckley, A. & Gould, E. (2007). West Nile Virus Circulation Detected in Northern Italy in Sentinel Chickens. *Vector Borne Zoon. Dis.*, **7**: 411–17.

Roehrig, J. T., Layton, M., Smith, P., Campbell, G. L., *et al.* (2002). The emergence of West Nile virus in North America: ecology, epidemiology and surveillance. In: J. S. Mackenzie, *et al.* (eds.) *Japanese encephalitis and West Nile viruses*, pp. 223–40. Berlin, Heidelberg, New York: Springer-Verlag.

Sabin, A. B. & Buescher, E. L. (1950). Unique physico-chemical properties of Japanese B encephalitis virus hemagglutinin. *Proc. Soc. Exp. Biol. Med.*, **74**: 222–30.

Sang, R. C., Gichogo, A., Gachoya, J., Dunster, M. D., *et al.* (2003). Isolation of a new flavivirus related to cell fusing agent virus (CFAV) from field-collected flood-water Aedes mosquitoes sampled from a dambo in central Kenya. *Arch. Virol.*, **148**: 1085–93.

Strauss, J. H. & Strauss, E. G. (1994). The alphaviruses: gene expression, replication, and evolution. *Microbio. Rev.*, **58**: 491–562.

Swofford, D. L. (1998). 'PAUP*. Phylogenetic Analysis Using Parsimony (*and Other Methods). Version 4.' Sunderland, Massachusetts: Sinauer Associates.

Tabachnick, W. J. (1991). Evolutionary genetics and arthropod-borne diseases. The yellow fever mosquito, *Aedes aegypti*. *Am. J. Entomol.*, **37**: 14–24.

Takahashi, M. & Suzuki, K. (1979). Japanese Encephalitis Virus in Mosquito Salivary Glands. *Am. J. Trop. Med. Hyg.*, **28**: 122–35.

Tesh, R. B. & Gubler, D. J. (1975). Laboratory studies of transovarial transmission of La Crosse and other arboviruses by Aedes albopictus and Culex fatigans. *Am. J. Trop. Med. Hyg.*, **24**: 876–80.

Theiler, M. (1930). Studies on the action of yellow fever virus in mice. *Ann. Trop. Med.*, **24**: 249–72.

Theiler, M. & Downs, W. G. (1973). *The Arthropod-borne Viruses of Vertebrates: An Account of the Rockefeller Foundation Virus Program (1951–1970)*. London: Yale University Press.

Thiel, H-J., Collett, M. S., Gould, E. A., Heinz, F. X., *et al.* (2005). Flaviviridae. In: C. M. Fauquet, M. A. Mayo, *et al.* (eds.) *Virus Taxonomy: VIIIth Report of the ICTV*, pp. 981–98. London: Elsevier/Academic Press.

Turell, M. J., Presley, S. M., Gad, A. M., Cope, S. E., *et al.* (1996). Vector competence of Egyptian mosquitoes for Rift Valley fever virus. *Am. J. Trop. Med. Hyg.*, **54**: 136–39.

Vapalahti, O., Plyusnin, A., Cheng, Y., Manni, T., *et al.* (1996). Inkoo and Tahyna, the European California serogroup bunyaviruses: sequence and phylogeny of the S RNA segment. *J. Gen. Virol.*, **77**: 1769–74.

Walton, T. E. & Grayson, M. A. (1988). Venezuelan equine encephalomyelitis. In: T. P. Monath (ed.) *The arboviruses: epidemiology and ecology*, pp. 203–31. Boca Raton, Fla: CRC Press.

Weaver, S. C. (2005). Host range, amplification and arboviral disease emergence. *Arch. Virol. Suppl.*, **19**: 33–44.

Weaver, S. C. & Barrett, A. D. (2004). Transmission cycles, host range, evolution and emergence of arboviral disease. *Nat. Rev. Microbiol.*, **2:** 789–801.

Weaver, S. C., Frey, T. K., Huang, H. V., *et al.* (2005). Togaviridae. In: C. M. Fauquet, M. A. Mayo *et al.* (eds.) *Virus Taxonomy VIIIth Report of the ICTV*, pp. 999–1008. London: Elsevier/Academic Press.

Weaver, S. C., Kang, W., Shirako, Y., Rumenapf, T., *et al.* (1997). Recombinational history and molecular evolution of western equine encephalomyelitis complex alphaviruses. *J. Virol.*, **71:** 613–23.

Weaver, S. C., Salas, R., Rico-Hesse, R., Ludwig, G. V., *et al.* (1996). Re-emergence of epidemic Venezuelan equine encephalomyelitis in South America. *Lancet,* **348:** 436–40.

Weissenbock, H., Kolodziejek, J., Url, A., Lussy, H., *et al.* (2002). Emergence of Usutu virus, an African mosquito-borne flavivirus of the Japanese encephalitis virus group, Central Europe. *Emerg. Infect. Dis.*, **8:** 652–56.

WHO (1985). Arthopod-borne and rodent-borne viral diseases; Technical Report Series, Number 719, Geneva: WHO. 1–116.

Young, N. A. (1972). Serologic differentiation of viruses of the Venezuelan encephalitis (VE) complex. In *Proc. workshop-symposium on Venezuelan encephalitis virus, scientific publication 243*, pp. 84–89. Washington DC: Pan American Health Organization.

Young, N. A. & Johnson, K. M. (1969). Antigenic variants of Venezuelan equine encephalitis virus: their geographic distribution and epidemiologic significance. *Am. J. Epidem.*, **89:** 286–307.

Zuckerman, A. J., Banatvala, J. E., Pattison, J. R., Griffiths, P. & Schoub, B. (2004). *Principles and Practice of Clinical Virology,* pp. 569–75. London: Wiley.

CHAPTER 33

Poxviruses

Hugh W. Reid and Mark P. Dagleish

Summary

The poxviruses are a large family of complex viruses infecting many species of vertebrates as well as arthropods, and members of the three genera Orthopoxvirus, Yatapoxvirus and Parapoxvirus are the cause of sporadic zoonotic infections originating from both wildlife and domestic livestock. Infections of humans are generally associated with localized lesions, regarded as inconvenient rather than life-threatening, although severe illnesses have occurred, particularly in immunologically compromised individuals.

The most celebrated of the orthopoxvirus infections is cowpox—a zoonotic infection which has been exploited to the enormous benefit of mankind as it had a pivotal role in the initiation of vaccination strategies that eventually led to the eradication of smallpox. Cowpox occurs only in Eurasia and in recent years it has become evident that infection of cattle is fortuitous and the reservoir of infection is in wild rodents. Monkeypox is another orthopoxvirus causing zoonotic infections in central and west Africa resembling smallpox and is the most serious disease in this category. While monkeypox does not readily spread between people, the potential of the virus to adapt to man is of concern and necessitates sustained surveillance in enzootic areas.

The third orthopoxvirus zoonoses of importance is buffalopox in the Indian subcontinent, which is probably a strain of vaccinia that has been maintained in buffalo for at least 30 years following the cessation of vaccination of the human population. Likewise in Brazil, in recent years widespread outbreaks of vaccinia have occurred in milkers and their cattle.

Orf virus, the most common of the parapoxviruses to cause zoonotic infection, is largely restricted to those in direct contact with domestic sheep and goats. Generally, infection is associated with a single localized macule affecting the hand which resolves without complications. Infection would appear to be prevalent in all sheep and goat populations and human orf is a relatively common occupational hazard. Sporadic parapoxvirus infections of man also occur following contact with cattle infected with pseudocowpoxvirus, and wildlife, in particular seals.

A final serious consideration with the poxvirus zoonoses is the clinical similarity of such infections with smallpox. In view of the potential for smallpox virus to be employed by bio-terrorists there can be an urgency for laboratory confirmation of unexplained zoonotic poxvirus infections. Thus there is a requirement to maintain the capacity
for rapid confirmation of poxvirus infections by molecular techniques. As representatives of the known poxviruses have all been sequenced, generic and virus specific Polymerase Chain Reactions (PCR) can readily be performed to ensure rapid confirmation of any suspect infection.

The poxviruses

The poxviruses of vertebrates are classified into eight genera within the subfamily Chordopoxviridae, three of which are associated with zoonotic infections (Table 33.1). In general, such infections in man are benign, though in immunologically compromised individuals the reaction can be severe. It is also recognized that this family of viruses is genomically labile, which permits mutation and recombination to occur, and thus they have the potential to emerge in novel disease associations (Moss 1990).

Properties

Poxviruses are large double stranded DNA viruses. A number of representative strains have been fully sequenced. The virology Poxviruses has been recently reviewed (Moss 2007).

The morphology of poxviruses is complex. They are characteristically brick-shaped, 200–400 nm in length by 150–300 nm in width. The external surface of the orthopoxviruses is ridged with tubules 10–20 nm in diameter, arranged in parallel rows, while the parapoxviruses have a single continuous helix appearing as the characteristic basketweave when examined by electron microscopy. The protein composition of poxviruses is also complex and more than 100 polypeptides have been identified in the most extensively studied representative, vaccinia virus. Within the outer membrane is an electron-dense core which, in the case of the orthopoxviruses, is biconcave with two structures known as lateral bodies present on either side. The core consists of a twisted and folded nucleoprotein fibre interconnected by DNA fibres which consist of a single double-stranded molecule. Replication occurs in the cytoplasm of infected cells and is characterized by ballooning of the cells and formation of intra-cytoplasmic inclusions. Virus is released either by budding or when the cell lyses; some particles acquire an outer membrane during this process.

The poxviruses have many common antigens and cross-reactivity between members of the orthopoxvirus and parapoxvirus genera can be shown by a variety of serological techniques. Within the

Table 33.1 Chordopoxviridae which are associated with zoonoses

Genera	Name	Natural host
Orthopoxvirus	Buffalopox virus	Water buffalo in India
	Cowpox virus	Probably a rodent in Eurasia
	Monkeypox virus	Probably squirrels in Central and West Africa
	Vaccinia virus	Probably cattle in South America
Parapoxvirus	Orf virus	Domestic sheep/goats, worldwide
	Pseudocowpox virus	Cattle, worldwide
	Papular stomatitis virus	Cattle, worldwide
	Sealpox virus	Various species of seals, Europe/America
Yatapoxvirus	Tanapox virus	Unknown in Africa
	Yaba monkey disease virus	Monkeys in Africa

orthopox genera there is also generally a high degree of cross-protection, but this provides no protection from members of the parapox genera. In general, the orthopoxviruses have a wide host range and induce good immunity in recovered animals, while the parapoxviruses have a narrow host range and produce short-lived and often incomplete immunity.

Characteristically, poxviruses cause acute infection associated with productive viral replication and shedding of virus. In the case of the orthopoxviruses this is followed by solid immunity to subsequent challenge for at least a number of years. With orthopoxviruses there is no carrier state, no latent infection occurs and hence they require a substantial population of available hosts for their survival. In contrast, infection with the parapoxviruses tends to result in incomplete protection from subsequent challenge and chronic infections also do occur. Such viruses can thus survive in much more restricted populations than the orthopoxviruses.

Orthopoxviruses

Of the virus diseases to have affected mankind, smallpox caused by the orthopoxvirus variola was probably the greatest scourge. Periodic pandemics occurred throughout Asia and Europe and invaded the Americas coincidentally with the arrival of Europeans. Infection was associated with a 20–30% mortality and those that recovered were often scarred for life. Such was the threat that up to the end of the eighteenth century variolation, in which fully virulent scab material was applied by scarification as a form of immunization, was widely practised despite causing 1–2% mortality. The observation that milkmaids often escaped the ravages of the disease and the confirmation by Jenner that cowpox could protect against subsequent challenge with smallpox virus was therefore possibly the greatest single advance in medical history. The benefit that this zoonoses has been to mankind is thus enormous, as the rapid and widespread acceptance of vaccination led to the control of smallpox in the West and ultimately to its worldwide eradication.

Cowpoxvirus

It is now realized that this virus is inappropriately named as infection in cattle is relatively uncommon and there is an alternative natural reservoir in rodents. Infection occurs only in Eurasia, suggesting a similar distribution for the reservoir host.

Infection of man is characterized generally as a single lesion which commences as a papule followed by the development of vesicles, then crusting, and the lesion will usually resolve in 4–5 weeks. In the initial phase of infection patients experience malaise, pyrexia and lymphadenopathy of the draining nodes. Recovery is normally complete and uncomplicated but the reaction may be severe: In one documented case of infection in a patient with severe endogenous eczema the reaction became generalized and had a fatal outcome.

Primary lesions are normally on the hand or lower arm, but facial lesion are also quite common. Person to person spread has not been shown to occur. Contact with animals is generally established in reported cases and in recent years the most frequent established source of infection has been the domestic cat.

In cattle, infection is considered to be rare and is characterized by pox-like lesions appearing on the teats of milking cows. Infection occurs erratically and good dairy hygiene normally ensures that only a few cases occur in an outbreak. In domestic cats the infection can be very much more severe and it is noteworthy that in the UK it is reported from only a few veterinary practices, suggesting that it may be under-reported. However, serological surveys do not suggest that infection is common in cats and it is not considered that they could represent the natural host. Almost all diagnosed cases in cats occur in animals known to be rodent hunters and most cases are reported in the autumn (Bennett et al. 1986).

In cats, visible signs of infection generally appear first as a single small bite-like lesion which frequently develops into a large abscess which may give rise to cellulitis. After 10–14 days disseminated lesions appear as erythematous macules which develop into ulcerating papules, but vesicles are only rarely observed. Scabs form over these lesions which then fall off during the next 2–3 weeks. Affected cats are pyrexic, inappetent and depressed during the acute phase of the disease but normally will recover unless there are secondary bacterial complications (Bennett et al. 1990).

There is good evidence both from the detection of antibody and viral DNA in the blood of wild-caught rodents in Great Britain that they represent the true reservoir host (Chantrey et al. 1999). In particular bank-voles (Clethrionomys glareolus) and short-tailed voles (Microtus agrestis) had a high prevalence of antibody. The fact that the distribution of these rodents across Eurasia closely reflects the distribution of cowpox adds further weight to the concept that they are the essential reservoir host. This does not preclude other rodent species, particularly wood-mice (Apodemus sylvaticus) becoming infected and amplifying the virus but such infections are probably tangential. Virus very similar to cowpox has been isolated from a gerbil (Rhombomys opimus) in Turkmenia but such rodents have a restricted range and cannot be the natural host elsewhere.

Infection has also occurred in a number of other species, mainly Felidae, held in zoological collections, but only in the Moscow Zoo outbreak was the source of infection identified. Infection had apparently been transmitted from rats fed to the carnivores, as infection was shown to be prevalent on the breeding farm from which the rats were obtained.

Clinical appearance and history of contact with infected animals can allow a presumptive diagnosis. Scab scrapings removed and processed for electron microscopic examination following negative staining can be used to identify characteristic viral particles. Although embryonated eggs traditionally have been used to isolate virus, the use of conventional tissue culture is more convenient in most laboratories. Most laboratories today will rely on detecting viral DNA by PCR (Olson *et al.* 2004) rather than conventional virological techniques and/or imaging by electronmicroscopy. A variety of serological tests can also be used to provide retrospective confirmation of orthopoxvirus infection.

There have been reports of substantial outbreaks of cowpox in Venezuela and Egypt in which a high proportion of cows and milkers have become infected. However as these reports rely on clinical diagnosis and are not substantiated by virus characterization or molecular studies it would appear likely that other poxvirus(es) are involved with vaccinia being a probable candidate, certainly in Venezuela, as similar outbreaks affecting milkers and their cattle have occurred in neighbouring Brazil.

Vaccinia

Outbreaks of vaccinia virus in dairy cattle have been reported from at least six states of Brazil resulting in infection of those involved in milking (Leite *et al.* 2008). Clinical signs generally consisted of typical pox lesions on the hands associated with headache, backache, lymphadenopathy and high fever. All isolates of virus appear genetically related and represent at least two distinct clads of virus which implies infection has originated from at least two sources. The distribution of infection appears to be increasing and to have become enzootic in this region of the New World but a reservoir of infection apart from cattle has not been reported.

As suggested above, reported outbreaks of cowpox on clinical grounds in Venezuela and Egypt may also have been due to vaccinia virus which raises the possibility that it may be emerging as a new zoonoses in other countries.

Buffalopox

Buffalopox is a disease of domestic buffalo (*Bubalus bubalis*) which has been reported from Indonesia, Russia, Egypt, Italy, Pakistan, Bangladesh, and India, where it is of economic importance in milking buffalo. Clinically the disease resembles cowpox, although lesions may be more extensive affecting the whole udder, inner thighs, head and mouth. Mastitis is a frequent sequela. However, the biological characteristics of isolates and analysis of the DNA establish that buffalopox virus is sufficiently distinct to justify classification as a separate subspecies of vaccinia (Dumbell and Richardson 1993) and would appear to be a single clade of virus (Singh *et al.* 2007).

Human infection is generally restricted to the hands, wrists, and thumbs of those milking affected buffalo and consists of 1–5 pocks. Fever and swelling of the regional lymph nodes frequently occur also, and when the scabs detach scars are usually left.

The disease in India has persisted for over 30 years following the cessation of human vaccination against smallpox, thus it is assumed that infection can be sustained in the buffalo population. Infection tends to occur in local epizootics affecting only a proportion of the animals at risk. Infected human milkers would appear to be responsible for spreading infection between herds. Cattle also sometimes become infected, but the disease is mild. Sheep also are susceptible to infection.

Diagnosis is generally made on clinical evaluation and history. But virus can either be identified directly by electron microscopy or following isolation in embryonated eggs or tissue culture. When required, molecular methodologies are replacing traditional virological diagnostic techniques.

Monkeypox

Monkeypox was identified originally as an infection in a primate colony in Copenhagen in 1958 and later in other centres in Europe and the USA. Subsequently, in 1970, outbreaks of smallpox-like disease in people inhabiting the tropical rainforest regions in Western and Central African were reported. As this was considered to potentially jeopardize the global smallpox eradication campaign, which had commenced in 1967, there followed intense investigations to establish the risk posed (Khodakewich *et al.* 1988). The potential for this virus to spread internationally was highlighted by the epidemic of infection in the USA in 2003.

The original outbreak affected primates from Asia. They suffered a severe generalized disease with papules, vesicles and pustules, which formed scabs after 7–10 days affecting the whole body, particularly on the soles of the feet and palms of the hands, with orangutans proving particularly susceptible. Subsequent investigation failed to identify any antibodies in over 1,000 sera collected from Asian primates. In contrast, in sera collected in Africa from 10 species of primate and four species of squirrel, a high prevalence of antibody was detected. This is the most serious zoonotic poxvirus infection and is regularly associated with significant mortality. It is also of greatest concern because of the possible emergence of a human-adapted form. Though normally person to person transmission is inefficient, it is possible that in an immunocompromised population, such as the HIV infected population in sub-Saharan Africa, human-to-human transmission could occur more readily and facilitate the selection of human-adapted mutants (Douglass *et al.* 1994). Selection pressure on orthopoxviruses is known to allow the emergence of variants of enhanced or diminished pathogenicity, as exemplified by myxomatosis virus in rabbit populations (Fenner and Radcliffe 1965). It is thus essential that surveillance for monkeypox infection is man is sustained to ensure that any such development is detected at an early stage.

Monkeypox virus is antigenically closely related to variola but can be distinguished by tests with adsorbed sera. Comparison of the DNA of strains derived from different regions of Africa confirmed that monkeypox was a distinct viral species and that isolates from different geographical locations were distinct clades of virus. Analysis of the DNA sequence of so-called whitepox virus isolates established that it was genetically not possible for them to have arisen through mutation from monkeypox and that these 'isolates' represented laboratory contamination with variola virus.

Human cases of monkeypox have occurred in tropical rainforest regions of Central and West Africa and have been restricted to those living in small villages where hunting is an integral activity. From the time of recognition in 1970 there appeared to have been a real increase in incidence through to 1984 and thereafter there was a decline. The reason for this decline is unclear because it has occurred during a period when the human population has become increasingly susceptible through the cessation of vaccination against smallpox (Cook 1988).

The clinical features of monkeypox cannot be differentiated from smallpox, except for the lymph node enlargement that is pronounced in monkeypox and may be generalized or confined to the nodes of the neck and inguinal region. Patients develop fever prior to developing typical pox virus lesions of papule, vesicle, peduncle, scab and desquamation, which can involve the entire body. The disease is more severe in individuals not vaccinated against smallpox, in which case the fatality rate can be over 10%.

In contrast to smallpox, monkeypox usually occurs singly or as a small cluster of infections with little evidence of person to person transmission. Most cases occur in children, particularly boys over 5 years of age, suggesting that their activities result in greater exposure. The source of infection for 70% of cases would appear to be wild animals and it is thought that several species may be involved. Examination of sera collected from wild animals in west and central Africa have identified 10 species of monkeys as being infected in addition to four species of squirrel, which are thought to be the major reservoir.

Epidemiological evidence would suggest that squirrels are the most likely source of infection for man as they tend to inhabit the secondary forest surrounding the agricultural zone where most cases appear to originate. Person to person transmission probably accounts for 30% of cases, generally following close contact, and even in a population unprotected by vaccination it has been calculated that the theoretical maximum number of transmissions from an index case would be 11 generations (Fine *et al.* 1988). The model used for these calculations assumed individuals were immunologically competent and it is possible that in a population in which a significant number were immunologically compromised, further spread and human adaptation could occur. Thus, despite the relative rarity of this infection in man and its restricted geographical distribution, monkeypox has the potential to adapt under appropriate selection pressures to give rise to variants with increased virulence and the capability to disseminate in the human population, which would have serious global repercussions.

In Africa, presumptive diagnosis will generally be reached on the basis of clinical presentation and history. However, virus can readily be demonstrated in scab material and can be recovered in tissue culture or by egg inoculation. Confirmation of the virus involved is readily achieved by use of PCR. Serological tests have also been used in retrospective diagnosis and to identify inapparent infections.

The spread of monkeypox in the US in 2003 illustrated how orthopoxvirus infection may be spread globally. In this case a consignment of rodents including giant pouched rats (*Cricetomys sp.*), rope-squirrels (*Funisciuris sp.*) and dormice (*Graphiurus sp.*) were imported from west Africa for the pet trade (Hutson *et al.* 2007). Infection spread to North American prairie dogs (*Cynomys sp.*) held by the importing traders. These infected prairie dogs acted as vectors of monkeypox resulting in 82 confirmed human cases across 11 states. Those affected were mainly from households that purchased prairie dogs and veterinary personnel that came in contact with animals when they became sick. Fortunately none of the human cases were fatal nor did free-living prairie dogs become infected. But the incident does illustrate the imperative for strict regulations of the international trade of wildlife.

Prevention

Transmission of all the poxvirus infections requires contact with infected animals or contaminated fomites and generally results following introduction through an abrasion in the skin. The handling

of raw meat from certain wild animals appears to be a risk factor in acquiring monkeypox.

Good hygienic practices and the wearing of protective gloves when handling infected animals does achieve a substantial degree of protection in most cases.

An effective vaccine is available for smallpox (Cono *et al.* 2003). It may also have some potential value for individuals at high risk of exposure to monkeypox, but the risks of vaccination need to be balanced with risk of exposure.

Yatapoxvirus

Tanapoxvirus

First isolated in 1962, tanapox virus infection is associated with a mild disease in man characterized by a febrile response with the development of one or two nodular lesions. It first appeared in the Tana River basin in Kenya, causing epidemics in 1957 and 1962. Subsequently, infection was recognized on many occasions in Zaire and it is probably enzootic in several countries in equatorial Africa (Jezek *et al.* 1985). It has also occurred in primate centres in the US where animal handlers have become infected.

The disease in man characteristically is biphasic with a pre-eruptive phase when the patient is febrile for 2–4 days, which is sometimes accompanied by severe headache. Thereafter, one or more intensely itchy macules develop, which enlarge to about 1 cm, surrounded by a large erythematous zone and ringed by swollen oedematous skin. Regional lymph nodes become enlarged. The macules contain necrotic tissue which may slough, resulting in ulceration which may increase to 2 cm in diameter. Healing, which is often slow, is associated with a permanent scar. Lesions generally appear on areas of the body which would normally be uncovered by clothing and there is no evidence of disseminated spread from human infection in any case examined.

The epidemiology of tanapox is obscure. Tanapox does spread rapidly amongst captive monkeys but it is unclear if they act as the natural reservoir. Almost all cases occur in people with close access to rivers. There is a seasonal increase in incidence coincidental with increased mosquito activity and it has been suggested that culicine mosquitoes transmit the virus mechanically. In animal handlers infection is transmitted through skin abrasions. Previous vaccination against smallpox provides no protection from infection with tanapox virus.

Diagnosis is made on the basis of history and clinical appearance. Skin scrapings or necrotic tissue from lesions contain virus particles readily detected by electron microscopy. Morphologically, the particles differ from other orthopoxviruses in that many particles are enveloped and the surface tubular arrays are much more pronounced.

Yabapox

In 1957, rhesus monkeys held at Yaba in Nigeria developed subcutaneous growths which were shown to be caused by a distinct poxvirus. These 'tumours' could be transmitted experimentally and caused the development of histiocytomas which spontaneously regressed by 6–12 weeks. Similar subcutaneous growths developed at the site of inoculation in a man who was accidentally infected and in six experimentally infected volunteers. Antibody to yabapox virus has been detected in sera from a variety of African monkeys as well as cynomolgus monkeys from Malaysia. The natural host of this virus is assumed to be primates, probably restricted to Africa, and there may be a related virus in primates of south east Asia.

Parapoxvirus

Human parapoxvirus infections are relatively common and generally produce local lesions which are an inconvenience and subsequently resolve leaving little or no residual scar. The most frequent infection is with orf virus from sheep and goats, but pseudocowpox, sealpox and unidentified sources, presumed to be transmitted from wildlife, can also be responsible for human infections. Infections are generally restricted to those who are occupationally at risk, and because infection is normally uncomplicated, often recognized by those who become infected and benefits little from treatment, parapoxvirus infections are probably markedly underreported. There is no cross-protection between the orthopoxviruses and parapoxviruses despite considerable antigenic and genomic similarity.

Orf

Orf would appear to be prevalent in all domestic sheep and goat populations and has a worldwide distribution.

Infection in sheep

Orf is associated with proliferative skin lesions, particularly around the lips of neonatal lambs, but all ages and categories of animal may be affected. Infection occurs in areas of exposed skin subjected to traumatic insult as virus will establish only in regenerated epithelium. Lesions tend to be most frequent around the lips of lambs, teats of ewes and legs and mouths of those grazing rough pasture. Lesions are characteristic of poxvirus infection—macule, vesicle, pustule and scab—but in a proportion, extensive epithelial proliferations occur and lesions may persist. Virus is shed in the scabs of lesions and infectivity can be retained for long periods provided they remain dry. Dried scabs in buildings would appear to be the principal means by which infection survives between years. However, infection would often appear to be mild or inapparent, and it is considered that such subclinical infections may also be important in the epidemiology. Immunity following infection is incomplete and reinfection can occur readily, although subsequent infections are, in general, less severe.

Vaccination of sheep is widely practiced using virus which is fully virulent. However by electively infecting ewes or lambs in the inner thigh or axilla, controlled infections which do not normally result in complications can reduce the impact of the disease and the necessity for topical treatment.

Human infection

Orf in man is most frequently diagnosed in those directly handling sheep, in particular those bottle-feeding lambs in the spring and those involved in shearing and slaughtering sheep at other times (Robinson and Peterson 1983). However, infection also can be transmitted by fomites and sometimes contact with sheep or goats is difficult to establish.

Virus infection will establish following introduction through the epidermis, thus the fingers of those feeding lambs are particularly at risk. Infection occurs only at the site of traumatized epidermis. Following an incubation period of 3–7 days the maculopustular reaction establishes, surrounded by an erythematous rim. This tends to increase in size with a weeping surface and central vesiculation and pustulation. The lesion then crusts overlying a papillomatous surface which is liable to be haemorrhagic if the crust is detached at this stage. The crust then dries and will detach after 6–8 weeks leaving no scar. Normally only a single lesion is present and spread to other areas does not usually occur (Groves et al. 1991).

Secondary bacterial infection of orf lesions can cause complications but can normally be controlled through topical antibiotic application. Lymphangitis and lymphadenitis of the draining lymphatics is a frequent complication and may be associated with flu-like symptoms. Less frequently, infection is associated with a generalized reaction including widespread maculo-papular eruption and erythema multiforme. Extensive lesions have been described also in those with burns received at the time of infection and in immunosuppressed patients, which have resulted in the development of 'giant orf' resembling pyogenic granuloma and requiring amputation of the affected digit. Patients with atopic dermatitis may also be more vulnerable to infection. Diagnosis is often made on the basis of clinical presentation and history. Virus isolation is not generally successful but characteristic parapoxvirus particles can be observed in scab or vesicular fluid collected early in the course of infection. Histological examination of biopsy material will differentiate orf infection from other proliferative skin disorders. Recovered patients will have antibody to orf virus which is most readily detected by ELISA.

As with all the other parapoxviruses, confirmation of infection by PCR of suitable scab material is a more convenient method of diagnosis and in addition provides evidence of the type of virus involved.

It should be noted that any immunity is only of short duration and reinfection occurs readily.

Infection can normally be avoided through good hygienic practices and the wearing of protective gloves when handling infected animals or raw sheep or goat products. Individuals who may be more vulnerable to infection due to immunosuppression or other factors should avoid contact with sheep or goats. It should also be recognized that the vaccine used for sheep is, in fact, fully virulent virus and operators must take great care not to autoinoculate while vaccinating.

Pseudocowpox

This is a virus disease of the teats of milking cattle which establishes as a chronic infection in herds, lesions appear periodically some 2 weeks after calving. Lesions are generally single and control can be achieved through good hygiene with respect to the milking machine teat clusters and in the preparation of teats prior to milking. Preventing damage to the teats is also essential.

The cause is a parapoxvirus of cattle which has a worldwide distribution. Though closely related to the virus of papular stomatitis, genomic analysis has established that they represent distinct viruses.

The clinical course of infection in man is essentially similar to that of orf although contact with affected cattle is the source of infection.

Bovine papular stomatitis

This is generally a mild, often inapparent infection, mainly of young cattle. Lesions appear as reddened foci developing into hyperaemic papules with central necrosis. Lesions may be present on the muzzle, nostrils, lips, tongue, buccal papillae and hard and soft palates which persist for a few days or weeks. Infection is highly contagious and most animals in a group will become infected. When infection occurs shortly after transportation and mixing, lesions may be more severe and there may also be loss of appetite and excessive salivation. The causal virus has been considered by some authors to be the same as the parapoxvirus of pseudocowpox, though genomic characterization has established them as distinct.

Human infection follows contact with clinically affected animals and the lesions are similar to those caused by other parapoxviruses of ruminants.

Sealpox

Skin lesions in a variety of species of seals have been described associated with both orthopoxvirus and parapoxvirus infection. However, those infections caused by parapoxvirus are more commonly reported and have been associated with transmission to man. Lesions have generally been observed in captive animals, most frequently in pups reared in sanctuaries, and consist of raised cutaneous swellings 1.5–2 cm in diameter which may appear proliferative, most often affecting the ventral body surface and flippers as well as around the nose and lips. The lesions may be relatively few or multiple and may become eroded and susceptible to secondary bacterial infection.

Originally, reports of affected animals involved American seals: California sealion (*Zalopkus californianus*), South American sealion (*Otaria byronia*), harbour seal (*Phoca vitulina*) and northern fur seals (*Callorhinus ursinus*), but more recently it has been observed to be widespread in European populations of grey seals (*Halichoerus grypus*).

People exposed to such infected animals have become infected through abrasions in their skin. The course of infection in man is very similar to that of other parapoxvirus infections. Protective clothing and gloves should always be worn when handling seals due to risk of this and other infections that they can carry.

Parapoxvirus of reindeer and musk ox

Outbreaks of parapoxvirus infection affecting reindeer and musk ox have occurred in which the disease has severely affected animals and been associated with considerable mortality. The virus has been shown morphologically to be a parapoxvirus. The lesions in man were reported to resemble tumours and, on initial infections, fever, enlarged lymph nodes and nausea occurred. Surgical removal was considered necessary, and in the one case that was not operated on, a 2 cm diameter proliferative growth persisted for 6 months. Infection occurred in herdsmen and in those who handled potentially contaminated clothing or were in contact with affected patients (Falk 1978). The authors of the report believe that the severity of the disease in man indicates that the virus is distinct from orf virus. However, recent genomic studies of isolates from Scandinavia indicate that both orf virus and pseudocowpox virus cause outbreaks of disease in reindeer.

Parapoxvirus infections of wildlife

Parapoxvirus infections have been identified in squirrels in Europe and the USA, and in kangaroos. Parapoxvirus-induced disease has been described in free-living deer in the US, while quite severe disease has occurred in farmed red deer in New Zealand. Infection of man does not appear to occur readily from these sources, although there is a report of three cases of parapoxvirus infection in which a wildlife source was implicated. In these cases the lesions were discrete epidermal nodules which enlarged progressively over several months. Parapoxvirus infection was confirmed by ultrastructural examination of biopsy material. Infection was considered distinct from orf and does raise the possibility that wildlife may harbour a variety of, as yet uncharacterized, parapoxviruses with zoonotic potential.

References

Bennett, M., Gaskell, C. J., Gaskell, R. M., Baxby, D., and Gruffydd-Jones, T. J. (1986). Poxvirus infection in the domestic cat: some clinical and epidemiological observations. *Vet. Rec.*, **118**: 387–90.

Bennett, M., Gaskell, G. J., Baxby, D., Gaske, R. M., Kelly, D. F., and Naidoo, J. (1990). Feline cowpox virus infection. *J. Small Anim. Pract.*, **31**: 167–73.

Chantrey, J., Meyer, H., Daxby, M., Begon, M., et al. (1999). Cowpox: reservoir hosts and geographic range. *Epidem. Infect.*, **122**: 455–60.

Cono, J, Casey, C. G., and Bell, D. M.(2003). Smallpox vaccination and adverse reactions. *Guidance for Clinicians. MMWR*, **52**: 1–28.

Cook, G. C. (1988). Human monkeypox: a viral disease with an uncertain future in Africa. *Trop. Dis. Bull.*, **85**(2): R1–R16.

Douglass, N. J., Richardson, M., and Dumbell, K. R. (1994). Evidence for recent genetic variation in monkeypox viruses. *J. Gen. Virol.*, **75**: 1303–09.

Dumbell, K. and Richardson, M. (1993). Virological investigations of specimens from buffaloes affected by buffalopox in Maharashtra State, India between 1985 and 1987. *Arch. Virol.*, **128**: 257–67.

Falk, E. S. (1978). Parapoxvirus infections of reindeer and musk ox associated with unusual human infections. *Brit. J. Dermat.*, **99**: 647–54.

Fenner, F., and Ratcliffe, F. M. (1965). Myxomatosis. London: Cambridge University Press.

Fine, P. E., Jezek, Z., Grab, B., and Dixon, H. (1988). The transmission potentials of monkeypox virus in human populations. *Int. J. Epidem.*, **17**: 43–52.

Groves, R. W., Wilson-Jones, E., and MacDonald, D. M. (1991). Human orf and milkers' nodule: A clinicopathologic study. *J. Am. Acad. Dermat.*, **25**: 706–11.

Hutson, C. L., Lee, Kemba N., Abel, J., Carroll, D. S., et al. (2007). Monkeypox Zoonotic Associations: Insights from laboratory valuation of animals associated with the multi-state US outbreak. *Am. Soc. Trop. Med. Hyg.*, **76**(4): 757–68.

Jezek, Z., Arita, I., Szczeniowski, M., Paluko, K. M., et al. (1985). Human tanapox in Zaire: clinical and epidemiological observation on cases confirmed by laboratory studies. *Bull. World Health Organ.*, **63**: 1027–35.

Kaplan, C., Healing, T. D., Evans, N., Healing, L., and Prior, A. (1980). Evidence of infection by viruses in small British field rodents. *J. Hyg.*, **84**: 285–94.

Khodakevich, L., Jezek, Z., and Messinger, D. (1988). Monkeypox virus: ecology and public health significance. *Bull. World Health Organ.*, **66**: 747–52.

Leite, J. A., Drumond, B. P., Trindate, G. S., Lobato, Z. I. P., et al. (2005). Passatempo Virus, a Vaccinia Virus Strain, Brazil. *Emerg. Infect. Dis.*, **11**: 1935–38.

Moss, B. (2007). Poxviridae: The Virus and their replication. In: B. N. Fields et al. (eds.) Virology, (5th edn.), pp. 2906–29. New York: Raven Press.

Olson, V. A., Laue, T., Laker, M. T., et al. (2004). Real-time PCR system for detection of orthopoxviruses and sumutaneous identification of smallpox virus. *J. Chn. Microbiol.*, **42**: 1940–46.

Robinson, A. J. and Petersen, G. V. (1983). Orf virus infection of workers in the meat industry. *N. Zeal. Med. J.*, **96**: 81–85.

Singh, R. K., Hasarmani, M., Balamurugan, V., Bhanuprakash, V., et al. (2007). Buffalopox: an emerging and re-emerging zoonosis. *Anim. Heal. Res. Rev.*, **8**: 105–14.

CHAPTER 34

Prion-protein-related diseases of animals and man

James Hope and Mark P. Dagleish

Summary

Scrapie, bovine spongiform encephalopathy (BSE), Creutzfeldt-Jakob disease (CJD), and related diseases of mink (transmissible mink encephalopathy), mule deer and elk (chronic wasting disease) are the founder members of a group of diseases called the transmissible degenerative (or spongiform) encephalopathies (TSE). These diseases can be transmitted by prions from affected to healthy animals by inoculation or by feeding diseased tissues. Prions are cellular proteins that can transfer metabolic and pathological phenotypes vertically from parent to progeny or horizontally between cells and animals. TSEs are characterized by the accumulation of the prion form of the mammalian prion protein (PrP^C) in the central nervous system or peripheral tissues of animals and humans. Mutations of the human PrP gene are linked to rare, familial forms of disease and prion-protein gene polymorphisms in humans and other species are linked to survival time and disease characteristics in affected individuals. Iatrogenic transmission of CJD in man has occurred, and a variant form of CJD (vCJD) is due to cross-species transmission of BSE from cattle to humans. Atypical forms of scrapie and BSE have been identified during large-scale monitoring for TSEs worldwide. This chapter outlines our current understanding of scrapie, BSE, CJD and other TSEs and highlights recent progress in defining the role in disease of the prion protein, PrP.

Prions, prion protein and transmissible spongiform encephalopathies

Definitions

Prions are cellular proteins that can transfer metabolic and pathological phenotypes vertically from parent to progeny or horizontally between cells or animals. Frequently, the conversion of a normal cellular protein into a prion form involves a conformational change that affects its degree of self-association and ability to interact with other molecules. The consequences of these molecular events can be measured by their effects on a population or on an individual organism, by the gross morphological change or damage to tissues and cells, by the metabolite flux or most directly by monitoring the change in shape and aggregation of the prion protein (Wickner *et al.* 2009).

Transmissible spongiform encephalopathies (TSEs) are diseases which are characterized by the accumulation of the prion form of the mammalian prion protein (PrP^C) in the central nervous system or peripheral tissues of animals and humans (Prusiner 1997).

Scrapie is the TSE of sheep and goats.

Creutzfeldt-Jakob disease (CJD) is the most common type of human TSE, and a novel variant (**vCJD**) is believed to be caused by the transmission of the cattle TSE.

Bovine spongiform encephalopathy (BSE) to humans.

The diseases

Scrapie

Scrapie of sheep and goats has been known in Europe for centuries and has spread to most parts of the world due to trade in livestock. It has several colloquial names—goggles, staggers, *traberkrankheit* or trotting disease, *la tremblante*—that reflect a range of clinical conditions—altered behaviour, hypersensitivity to sound or touch, loss of condition, pruritus, and associated fleece loss and skin abrasions, incoordination of the hind limbs. These signs may be diagnostic to the experienced shepherd but usually require confirmation of disease by examination of brain tissue for histopathological signs, notably gliosis and vacuolation of the brainstem particularly in the obex at the level of the dorsal motor nucleus of the vagus (Hadlow 1995). In 1998, Benestad and her colleagues in Norway recognized a neurological disorder in sheep which they termed 'Nor98' (Benestad *et al.* 2003). Subsequent investigations have shown this is an atypical form of scrapie with epidemiological, histopathological, biological and molecular characteristics distinct from those of the type described classically in veterinary textbooks: however, both classical and atypical scrapie are prion-protein-related diseases.

Classical scrapie

Classical scrapie has been reported in most breeds of sheep and goats and, within a flock or herd, it appears to occur in related animals. The within-flock/herd incidence is usually 1–2 cases/100 sheep or goats/year but there have been several instances of 40–50% of animals of a flock succumbing to the disease within a year. The scrapie status of the dam is a major risk factor for the development of disease in progeny, and introduction of a new sire into a previously clear flock/herd has been noted (anecdotally) to provoke outbreaks of clinical disease. Onset of the natural clinical disease peaks in flock/herd animals at 3.5 years, with most cases occurring in the age range of 2.5–4.5 years (Hunter *et al.* 1992). In the incubation period, the infected animal is clinically normal and indistinguishable from its uninfected flockmates. Shedding of prions into the environment via urine or faeces may occur but the lack of an *in vivo* diagnostic test for the infectious particle means that the true prevalence of infection and of the carrier status of unaffected animals within a flock are also usually unknown. The prognosis on observation of clinical signs is invariably death within a few days or months, hence in veterinary work this usually results in a recommendation to cull the affected animal from the flock/herd, and similarly to slaughter its dam and other maternally related animals.

The introduction of PrP[1] gene typing has greatly facilitated interpretation of field studies on the incidence of natural and experimental disease (Goldmann *et al.* 1994; Dawson and Del Rio Vilas 2008) and national scrapie control schemes in sheep based on elimination of PrP alleles of high susceptibility to clinical disease (VRQ2) or the expansion of relatively resistant alleles (ARR) have been highly effective in reducing the number of reported cases of classical scrapie (EFSA 2006; Dawson and Del Rio Vilas 2008). Goat scrapie is less common but the increase in intensive goat dairy farming in the last few years has become associated with animal health problems such as scrapie (Gonzalez *et al.* 2009) and a large outbreak in Cyprus has stimulated studies on the feasibility of breeding for TSE resistance in goats in the EU (EFSA 2009).

Atypical scrapie

In 1998, the molecular and histopathological spectrum of TSEs in sheep was extended by the discovery in Norway of an experimentally-transmissible, PrP-related, neurological disease of sheep that was distinguishable from classical scrapie and was therefore considered to be an 'atypical' form of scrapie (Benestad *et al.* 2003). These Nor98 cases, the prototypes of 'atypical' TSE, have little or no vacuolation and sparse staining for abnormal PrP at the obex (dorsal motor nucleus of the vagus), and in many, but not all, cases exhibit an intense cerebellar PrP^{Sc} deposition/accumulation characterized at a molecular level by a smaller and less stable protease-resistant core of PrP^{Sc}. Nor98 and other 'atypical' cases subsequently identified are more often but not uniquely, found in animals carrying alleles of the PrP gene not usually associated with classical scrapie (ARR, AHQ). For Nor98, this genotype correlation has been further refined to implicate another dimorphic codon in the PrP open reading frame, L141F (Moum *et al.* 2005; Saunders *et al.* 2006). Other 'atypical' TSE phenotypes, including those that are similar to or the same as Nor98, have now been from France (Buschmann *et al.* 2004), Germany (Buschmann *et al.* 2004), Sweden (Gavier-Widen *et al.* 2004), Ireland (Onnasch *et al.* 2004), Portugal (Orge *et al.* 2004), Belgium (De Bosschere *et al.* 2004) and the UK (Konold *et al.* 2006).

Atypical scrapie is transmissible by intra-cerebral inoculation to transgenic mice (Le Dur *et al.* 2005; Griffiths *et al.* 2010) and by both the intra-cerebral and oral route to sheep (Simmons *et al.*

---

1 This three letter acronym for the sheep prion protein gene allele is based on the amino-acid (single letter IUPAC code) at codons 136 (V/A), 154 (R/H) and 171 (commonly Q or R). The wild-type allele is ARQ and the rest of the open reading frame is highly polymorphic.

2007, 2010). Clinical disease in sheep resembles classical scrapie (Konold *et al.* 2007) although, in contrast to most forms of classical disease, little abnormal PrP has been detected in peripheral, non-neuronal tissues. Case definition of atypical scrapie (EFSA 2005) has allowed its monitoring in Europe and worldwide and its epidemiology clearly differs from that of classical scrapie (Fediaevsky *et al.* 2008). Several cases of atypical scrapie have recently been described in goats where it seems to be associated with the H154 codon (Arsac *et al.* 2007; Seuberlich *et al.* 2007).

Creutzfeldt-Jakob Disease

Creutzfeldt-Jakob disease was first described by Creutzfeldt (1920) and Jakob (1921) as a progressive dementia with clinical signs suggesting dysfunction of the cerebellum, basal ganglia, and lower motor neurones. The clinical signs are variable but most commonly the disease is associated with gradual mental deterioration leading to dementia and confusion, and a progressive impairment of motor function, including myoclonus. CJD occurs mainly in the fifth and sixth decades of life. Most patients die within 6 months of onset of clinical signs and there are no verified cases of recovery. Pathologically the lesions of the brain included variable vacuolation of the neuropil, astrocytosis and, in about 10% of CJD cases, kuru and other types of amyloid plaques. By 1968, recognition of its similarity to kuru [(a form of human prion disease first recognized in Papua New Guinea (Hadlow 1995; Gajdusek 2008)] and scrapie had stimulated the transmission of CJD to a chimpanzee by intracerebral inoculation of biopsy tissue and confirmed its classification with these diseases. Gerstmann Straussler syndrome, a progressive dementia with cerebellar amyloid plaques, is a familial variant of CJD with an extended clinical time course (Hainfellner *et al.* 1995).

Epidemiologically, these human forms of prion disease can be classified as familial, sporadic, and iatrogenic. The incidence of CJD-related disease in man is remarkably constant at 0.5–1 cases per million of population per year throughout the world. This rarity, and the heterogeneity of animal prion diseases, makes it difficult to categorically rule out a link between the two but there is no evidence of an association. The low incidence casts doubt on the role of infection in its propagation within the human population but there have been several cases of human to human transmission via cadaver-derived therapeutics or tissues—as, for example, an unfortunate consequence of corneal transplantation (Kennedy *et al.* 2001), pituitary growth hormone injection (d'Aignaux *et al.* 1999) or dura mater grafting (Yamada *et al.* 2009). Several studies of risk factors from classical CJD have been carried out, but there are no consistently observed associations with occupation or foods (EFSA 2010).

Some 13–14% of cases are familial and linked to mutations in the open reading frame (ORF) of the *PrP* gene. There have been many clinical and pathological studies on human cases of neurological disease which seem to be associated with these rare mutations of the *PrP* gene, including Jakob's original family and the first GSS case (Kovacs and Budka 2009). In some families, there is complete penetrance of the phenotype and so the mutation is regarded as the cause of the disease. Apart from iatrogenic cases induced by transplantation of infected tissues or inoculation of contaminated pharmaceuticals of human origin, there is no epidemiological evidence for horizontal transmission of the disease. A stochastic event involving conversion of the PrP protein to its disease-associated isoform or the chance mutation of a benign, ubiquitous viral-like agent are two mechanisms which have been suggested to explain the incidence of sporadic cases. There is no cure for the clinical condition although genetic counselling, where applicable, may effectively prevent transmission of disease from one generation to the next.

There is considerable clinical and pathological heterogeneity in the human prion diseases, including fatal familial insomnia (Gambetti *et al.* 1995; Parchi *et al.* 1995; Tateishi *et al.* 1995) and although genetic typing and nucleotide sequencing of the *PrP* ORF has provided some unifying concepts, other genes and epigenetic effects are implicated in this variety of phenotypes (Kovacs *et al.* 2005).

Variant Creutzfeldt-Jakob Disease

In April 1996, Will and colleagues (Will *et al.* 1996) reported a novel variant of CJD (vCJD). Ten cases, all in young adults or teenagers presented with behavioural and psychiatric disturbances and early ataxia. The duration of illness was prolonged (up to 2 years) and typical EEG changes of CJD were absent. There was extensive kuru-type, amyloid plaque formation surrounded by vacuoles. Spongiform changes were most evident in the basal ganglia and thalamus with high-density, abnormal PrP accumulation on immuno-cytochemical analysis, especially in the cerebellum.

The initial, and subsequent, focus of vCJD in Great Britain and its molecular (Collinge *et al.* 1996) and transmission (Lasmezas *et al.* 1996; Bruce *et al.* 1997) similarities to BSE immediately implicated the cattle disease as the source of vCJD infection and beef and cattle by-products were put under restriction to limit the spread of disease. Nevertheless, an estimated three million infected cattle may have entered the human food chain (Ghani *et al.* 2000) and the impact and cost of preventing a secondary, human-to-human wave of infection are still being felt in the UK in 2010. To date (March 2010), there have been 169 primary cases, and three secondary cases related to transfusion of blood products, in the UK, 25 cases in France, 5 in Spain and 11 in the rest of Europe; other cases have been reported in the USA, Canada, Saudi Arabia and Japan (www.cjd.ed.ac.uk/vcjdworld).

Bovine spongiform encephalopathy

Bovine spongiform encephalopathy (BSE) has devastated the UK cattle industry for the past twenty years. From isolated cases first reported in 1986 and some retrospectively identified in May 1985, a major epidemic was under way by 1988 which has to date claimed over 185,000 cattle within the British Isles, and several thousand more cases within Europe (www.defra.gov.uk/vla/science/sci_tse_stats).The disease produces a progressive degeneration of the central nervous system and was named because of the sponge-like appearance of BSE brain tissue when seen under the light microscope (Wells *et al.* 1987). Warning signs of the illness include changes in the behaviour and temperament of the cattle. The affected animal becomes increasingly apprehensive and has problems of movement and posture, especially of its hind limbs. The cow (or bull) has increased sensitivity to touch and sound, loss of weight and, as the disease takes hold of its nervous system, a creeping paralysis sets in. This clinical phase of BSE lasts from a fortnight to over 6 months (Konold *et al.* 2004). Although the majority of animals affected have been dairy cows, this neurological disease can occur in either sex with a modal age of onset of 4–4.5 years

(range 1.8–22 years). Most early cases of BSE occurred in cattle between the ages of 3 and 5 years in Great Britain, but as the epidemic has waned and level of exposure declined, the average age of cattle with confirmed signs of disease has increased gradually to over 13 years (EFSA 2009). This has occurred in different European countries at different times and reflects the staggered nature of the BSE epidemics that have spread throughout Europe from the UK. For most of its development time the disease gives no tell-tale sign of its presence (Wilesmith *et al.* 1988) and the inability to detect the asymptomatic carrier of BSE (or scrapie) limits refinement of the measures which can be taken to prevent infected bovine or ovine tissues from use in feed and pharmaceutical products.

The neurological lesions in BSE-affected cow brains are virtually identical to those found in scrapie-affected sheep and include the spongiform change which gives BSE its name. From its clinical and neuropathological signs, BSE was immediately suspected to belong to the scrapie family of transmissible spongiform encephalopathies. This was confirmed by biochemical studies (Hope *et al.* 1988) and by experimental transmission of BSE to mice (Fraser *et al.* 1988), cattle (Dawson *et al.* 1990), mink (Robinson *et al.* 1994), marmoset (Baker *et al.* 1993), cynomolgus macaques (Lasmezas *et al.* 1996), sheep and goats (Foster *et al.* 1993) and pigs (Wells *et al.* 2003).

The origins and control of BSE and its current status

Epidemiological analyses of BSE-affected herds identified a protein feed supplement to be the most likely source of infection (Wilesmith *et al.* 1988). During the late 1970s changes in the rendering process which salvages compounds of nutritional and commercial value from abattoir waste are thought to have led to a less efficient system for inactivating prion-infected offal and, in turn, to a contaminated protein supplement. Subsequent recycling of BSE-infected cattle waste in this process may have contributed to the persistence of the disease.

Ruminant feed legislation aimed at removing the source of infection from cattle born after 1988 was introduced in 1989–90 in the UK, and reinforced throughout Europe in October 2000. At its peak, over 1,000 cases were reported each week in Great Britain in 1993 and this has now dwindled to one or two per month in 2010. Although the feed bans have had a dramatic effect on the epidemic curve, cases of BSE continue to be confirmed in cattle born after the reinforced bans of 2000 and feeding of contaminated protein to calves is suspected as the reason for most of these 'born after the real ban' (BARB) cases (Wilesmith *et al.* 2010). Their biological and biochemical characteristics appear similar to those seen earlier in the epidemic and differ from those of atypical BSE cases that have been recognized recently (see below).

In parallel with the BSE epidemic, natural cases of transmissible spongiform encephalopathies have been also been reported for the first time in cattle-related species —greater kudu, eland, nyala and gemsbok, Arabian and scimitar-horned oryx (Kirkwood and Cunningham 1994; Cunningham *et al.* 2004)and in the cat family —puma, cheetahs (Kirkwood *et al.* 1995), and domestic cats (Pearson *et al.* 1992). Apart from some cases in the greater kudu, contaminated feed is suspected but difficult to prove because of the absence of detailed feeding records.

Experimental oral dosing of cattle with BSE-affected cattle brain homogenates has confirmed that as little as 1 milligram of brain (with ~ 10–100 mouse ic ID_{50} units) can induce disease after extended incubation periods of 8–10 years (Wells *et al.* 2007; Arnold *et al.* 2009). Larger doses (up to 100g) have been used to study oral pathogenesis of BSE in cattle in the UK (Wells *et al.* 2007) and Germany (Hoffmann *et al.* 2007) and confirmed by PrP IHC and bioassay the limited, early distribution of prions to parts of the lower alimentary tract (distil ileum, jejunum) and spread via the autonomic nervous system from the gastrointestinal tract to the central nervous system via either the coeliac and mesenteric ganglion complex, splanchnic nerves and the lumbal/caudal thoracic spinal cord or via the vagal nerve. This experimental tissue distribution of infectivity has been used to refine the list of specified risk materials from various age-cohorts of cattle banned for human consumption and has underpinned several assessments of human and animal exposure risk that have defined UK and European policy for control and management of BSE over the years (EFSA 2011).

Atypical forms of BSE

BSE surveillance testing of cattle for abnormal prion protein in Europe has allowed the identification of two further, distinct types of cattle TSE, termed H- and L-(or BASE) type BSE (Casalone *et al.* 2004; Jacobs *et al.* 2007; Biacabe *et al.* 2008; Polak *et al.* 2008). Similar cases were also detected outside Europe (Japan and USA) (Hagiwara *et al.* 2007; Clawson *et al.* 2008). About 60 atypical BSE cases have been described worldwide (from testing ~ 50 million healthy animals and fallen stock) although there is no statutory requirement to distinguish typical and atypical types of BSE in reporting and this figure is derived from research literature.

In France, a retrospective study of all the TSE-positive cattle identified through the compulsory EU surveillance programme between 2001–2007 was recently published (Biacabe *et al.* 2008). This study indicated that all BSE H and L cases detected by rapid tests were observed in animals over 8 years old in either the 'at risk' (9) or 'healthy slaughtered' surveillance target group (4). In this study, the reported frequency of H and L type TSE was respectively 1.9 and 1.7 cases per million of over 8 years old tested animals. All EU atypical cases were born before the extended or real feed ban that came into law in January 2001. Hence, as with classical BSE, exposure of these animals to feed contaminated with low titres of TSE cannot be excluded. However, the distribution of H-and L-type cases in France by year of birth differs markedly from that for classical BSE and could be interpreted to indicate that both forms of atypical BSE are sporadic diseases which arise spontaneously.

H- and L-(or BASE) type BSE have been transmitted by intracerebral challenge to inbred mice and Tg mice expressing bovine and ovine PrP. L-type BSE has also been transmitted to transgenic mice expressing alleles of the human prion protein (Beringue *et al.* 2007; Beringue *et al.* 2008; Buschmann *et al.* 2006; Capobianco *et al.* 2007; Kong *et al.* 2008). Transmission and serial passage in inbred mice and Tg VRQ mice have been interpreted to indicate that, after interspecies passage, BASE could generate classical BSE (Beringue *et al.* 2007; Capobianco *et al.* 2007). However, it should be noted that L-BSE—classical BSE phenotypic convergence has not been observed in other Tg mice, including mice expressing the ARQ allele of sheep PrP (Buschmann *et al.* 2006; Beringue *et al.* 2007). This phenomenon needs to be confirmed in an independent set of experiments but does raise the issue of a possible classical BSE re-emergence originating from atypical BSE cases.

The sensitivity and specificity of the TSE rapid screening tests are known for classical BSE but not for H- or L-type BSE. These tests use brainstem as the target tissue because this is where pathological lesions and PrPres are first detected in the CNS of cattle (Hope *et al.* 1988; Wells *et al.* 1998). Unlike classical BSE, little is known about the pathogenesis of atypical BSE and the brainstem may not be the optimal target site for the detection of H- and L-type BSE (Casalone *et al.* 2004). Consequently the BSE H- and L-type prevalence of 1–2 per million may be an under-estimation. No data are yet available on distribution of the infectivity in peripheral tissues and body fluids of cattle with H- or L-type BSE.

Small ruminant BSE

Foster and colleagues showed cattle BSE could be transmitted to ARQ/ARQ sheep and goats by feeding and intra-cerebral inoculation (Foster *et al.* 1993) and several subsequent studies have documented that there is wide-spread dissemination of prions in ARQ/ARQ sheep similar to the pathogenesis of natural cases of classical scrapie (Van Keulen *et al.* 2000). The biological and biochemical characteristics of 'BSE in small ruminants' are sufficiently distinct to allow their discrimination in 'blinded' tests although there have been concerns 'mixed' infections might pass as 'scrapie'. Historically, small ruminants were known to have been fed the same type of protein supplements implicated as the source of BSE in cattle and fear of a second wave of vCJD due to infection from sheep and goat products stimulated intensive surveillance in the EU of TSEs in sheep and goats and the application of laboratory tests aimed at at a diagnosis of 'NOT BSE' or 'BSE NOT Excluded'; the final confirmation of 'BSE in small ruminant' requires the application of bioassay in the same panels of inbred mice used to characterize vCJD and BSE (Bruce *et al.* 1997). By these stringent criteria, only two cases of BSE in SR, both in goats, have been confirmed (Eloit *et al.* 2005; Jeffrey *et al.* 2006) and current estimates of the likely prevalence of BSE in SRs in Europe is very low.

Prions

Taxonomy

Modern virus classification uses the morphology and biochemistry of virions and their mode of replication as the basis for taxonomy; for example, the nature of the virion nucleic acid—DNA or RNA—its size, symmetry, the presence or absence of a lipid envelope, genome integration, mechanism of cell entry, use of vectors, etc. Prions remain undefined in this sort of detail and so their classification has not been easy, although many structures have been described as specific for TSE-infected fractions: 14 nm particles (Cho and Greig 1975): 'nemaviruses' (Narang 1990), scrapie-associated fibrils (Merz *et al.* 1981; Merz *et al.* 1983) or prion rods (McKinley *et al.* 1986) and small, pentangular structures of 10 nm diameter (Ozel *et al.* 1996) or in tissue sections as spheres and tubes (Baringer *et al.* 1981) or tubulo-vesicular vesicular structures (TSVs) (Liberski *et al.* 1988). Only prion rods and scrapie-associated fibrils have been shown unequivocally to be different morphological forms of prion-protein (PrP) aggregates by immuno-gold electron microscopy and the orientation and packing of abnormal PrP within these structures has been exhaustively investigated by modelling, 2D-electron crystallography and X-ray fibre crystallography (Wille *et al.* 2002; Wille *et al.* 2009). Natural and synthetic prion structures recovered from brain tissue have a cross-$\tilde{\beta}$ structure characteristic of the protein fibrils of amyloid diseases and, intriguingly, while X-ray fibre diffraction patterns of these two brain PrP amyloids are similar, they differ considerably from the recombinant PrP amyloid used to induce synthetic prions in transgenic mice; the relationship between these structures and infectivity remains elusive (Wille *et al.* 2009).

Strains

Viruses, bacteria, bacteriophages, and all other conventional forms of life show phenotypic or strain variation which is encoded by their nucleic acid genomes. Strain variation is also a common feature of various TSE isolates in mice, hamsters, sheep, and goats, but while selection and mutation of murine TSE strains is documented, a coding molecule has yet to be defined. Prions and viruses share the cell's trafficking and biosynthetic systems and the perturbations they induce may share common mechanisms and appear very similar. Similarly the concepts of a 'strain' and 'mutation' have been adopted into prion biology from virology although, by definition, a prion strain lacks a nucleic genome and propagates independently of nucleic acid replication and its errors. For prions, the different effects of infection on cell integrity, host behaviour and tissue pathology are believed to be mediated by the conformation of the prion protein and its epigenetic interactions with the host. Western blotting (WB) and protease hydrolysis have provided a useful, low resolution combination of techniques for monitoring prion protein shape and several, but not all, prion 'strains' or phenotypes have been described with unique WB profiles (Somerville *et al.* 1997). However, defining a prion strain (and, by implication, its disease phenotype) solely by its WB pattern or inferring a 'mixed infection' of prion strains from seeing a mixture of protein fragments by WB is not yet possible.

Each scientific discipline—epidemiology, virology, pathology, molecular biology, biochemistry—uses its own techniques and language to categorize prions and their effects and this has led to some confusion when a lack of one or more of these types of data prevents the cross-referencing needed from a comprehensive description of prion disease phenotype. In the past few years, the discovery of apparently-novel cattle and sheep prion-protein related abnormalities by rapid surveillance testing of healthy slaughter animals in the EU has highlighted this confusion.

Historically, the two main criteria used to distinguish strains of mouse-passaged scrapie were (1) the ranking of the incubation periods they produce in mice of the three *Sinc* genotypesem—s7s7, s7p7; and p7p7; and (2) the severity and location of vacuolar degeneration induced in the brains of terminal cases of disease (Fraser 1976; Bruce *et al.* 1991). Different alleles of the PrP gene are linked to the susceptibility and disease incubation period of an animal naturally or experimentally exposed to prions (Westaway *et al.* 1987; Goldmann *et al.* 1990; Hunter *et al.* 1996) and their relative effects can change depending on the prion type or strain (Goldmann *et al.* 1994). The two mouse alleles, *Prn-i^a* and *Prn-i^b*, encode prion proteins differing in two amino acids (codons L108V and T183V) and are congruent to the *s7* and *p7* alleles of Sinc, respectively (Westaway *et al.* 1987; Moore *et al.* 1998). Ablation of the gene in transgenic mice is non-lethal and effectively protects mice from infection with prions (Bueler *et al.* 1992), and survival time, histo-pathology and the molecular characteristics of disease in mice (and other experimental models) infected with prions can be manipulated by changing the allotype, location and level of prion protein expression in exposed animals (Prusiner *et al.* 1990; Manson *et al.* 1994; Telling *et al.* 1996).

Replication

In vitro formation of PrP^{Sc} from PrP^{C} has been shown in infected cell cultures (see below) and in a cell-free system where the conversion is driven by addition of PrP^{Sc} template (Kocisko *et al.* 1994). The cell-free system mimics several aspects of the *in vivo* disease, including species and strain specificities (Bessen *et al.* 1995; Kocisko *et al.* 1995; Raymond *et al.* 1997). From these test-tube studies, two distinct models for the formation of PrP^{Sc} have evolved: in both, exogenous PrP^{Sc} forms catalytic heterodimers with PrP^{C} which results in the formation of more PrP^{Sc}; in one, these 'heterodimers' are real (Kaneko *et al.* 1995) while in the other they actually represent the growing face of a PrP^{Sc} fibril or aggregate (Caughey *et al.* 1995). This latter, 'seeded' polymerization model fits better with the kinetics of *in vitro* conversion PrP^{C} to protease-resistant PrP. This mechanism of conversion resembles a crystallization process in that it is rate-limited by nucleus formation and accelerated by seeding (Caughey *et al.* 1995).

Early studies claimed over-expression of mutant forms of human PrP (P101L-PrP) induces spontaneous brain degeneration, accumulation of protease-sensitive abnormal prion protein and apparent *de novo* synthesis of infectious particles (Hsiao *et al.* 1990, 1994); these findings were met with initial scepticism but have been reinforced by similar effects in Tg mice using different constructs (MoPrP170N, 174T (Sigurdson *et al.* 2009) and the *de novo* formation of PrP amyloid and infectious particles *in vitro* (see below, Barria *et al.* 2009) or re-folding from bacterial, recombinant PrP (Legname *et al.* 2004, 2005; Bocharova *et al.* 2006; Makarava *et al.* 2006, 2009, 2010; Benetti and Legname 2009).

Soto and colleagues have developed a protein mis-folding cyclic amplification technique (PMCA) where brain homogenates from normal and prion-infected animals are incubated together with regular sonication to create new 'nuclei' and promote an exponential increase in PrP^{Sc}; this has drastically improved the efficiency of the cell-free conversion system and animal bioassays have confirmed the serial propagation of prion infectivity and strains *in vitro* (Saborio *et al.* 2001; Castilla *et al.* 2005, 2008; Green *et al.* 2008), and the *de novo* production of prions with novel biological properties (Barria *et al.* 2009).

Although the structures and pathway of conversion between PrP^{C} and PrP^{Sc} have yet to be worked out, the atomic coordinates of a soluble, independent folding domain of the protein (residues 121–230) were defined by nuclear magnetic resonance spectroscopy more than 15 years ago (Riek *et al.* 1996). The prion-protein 'fold', a C-terminal, three-helix bundle with short, interacting β-strand segments, is highly conserved across mammalian species (Wuthrich and Riek 2001; Lysek *et al.* 2005) although the N-terminal half of the molecule (residues 23–120) containing the metal-ion binding histidine-repeat domain has a flexible, more dynamic structure. There are PrP genes and paralogues (Doppel, Dpl, and Shadoo, Sho) in most vertebrates including fish (Watts and Westaway 2007) and evolutionary descent of these mammalian prion proteins from the ZIP family of metal-ion transporters has been inferred by structural comparisons and 'interactome' analysis (Schmitt-Ulms *et al.* 2009; Watts *et al.* 2009).

Knowledge of the full structure of PrP^{C} and PrP^{Sc} may help the design of chemicals engineered to prevent the conversion process

Rohwer, R. G. (1991). The scrapie agent: 'A virus by any other name'. In: C. W. Chesebro (ed.) Current topics in Microbiology and Immunology: Transmissible Spongiform Encephalopathies, pp. 195–232. Berlin: Springer Verlag.

Russo, F., Johnson, C. J., et al. (2009). 'Pathogenic prion protein is degraded by a manganese oxide mineral found in soils.' J. Gen. Virol., 90: 275–80.

Saborio, G. P., Permanne, B., et al. (2001). 'Sensitive detection of pathological prion protein by cyclic amplification of protein misfolding.' Nature, 411: 810–13.

Safar, J. G., Kellings, K., et al. (2005). 'Search for a prion-specific nucleic acid.' J. Virol., 79: 10796–806.

Sailer, A., Bueler, H., et al. (1994). 'No Propagation of Prions in Mice Devoid of PrP.' Cell, 77: 967–68.

Saunders, G. C., Cawthraw, S. et al. (2006). 'PrP genotypes of atypical scrapie cases in Great Britain.' J. Gen. Virol., 87: 3141–49.

Sayer, N. M., Cubin, M., et al. (2004). 'Structural determinants of conformationally selective, prion-binding aptamers.' J. Biol. Chem., 279: 13102–109.

Schatzl, H. M., Dacosta, M., et al. (1995). 'Prion protein gene variation among primates.' J. Mol. Biol., 245: 362–74.

Schmitt-Ulms, G., Ehsani, S., et al. (2009). 'Evolutionary descent of prion genes from the ZIP family of metal ion transporters.' PLoS One, 4: e7208.

Schroder, H. C. and Muller, W. E. G. (2002). 'Neuroprotective effect of flupirtine in prion disease.' Drugs Today, 38: 49–58.

Scott, J. R., et al. (1991). 'Evidence for Intrinsic Control of Scrapie Pathogenesis in the Murine Visual System.' Neurosci. Lett., 133: 141–44.

Scott, J. R., Foster, J., et al. (1993). 'Conjunctival instillation of scrapie in mice can produce disease.' Vet. Microb., 34: 305–9.

Seuberlich, T., Botteron, C., et al. (2007). 'Atypical scrapie in a swiss goat and implications for transmissible spongiform encephalopathy surveillance.' J. Vet. Diag. Invest., 19: 2–8.

Sigurdson, C. J., Nilsson, K. P., et al. (2009). 'De novo generation of a transmissible spongiform encephalopathy by mouse transgenesis.' Proc. Nat. Acad. Sci. USA, 106: 304–9.

Silveira, J. R., Raymond, G. J., et al. (2005). 'The most infectious prion protein particles.' Nature, 437: 257–61.

Simmons, M. M., Konold, T., et al. (2007). 'Experimental transmission of atypical scrapie to sheep.' BMC Vet. Res., 3: 20.

Simmons, M. M., Konold, T., et al. (2010). 'The natural atypical scrapie phenotype is preserved on experimental transmission and sub-passage in PRNP homologous sheep.' BMC Vet. Res., 6: 14.

Somerville, R. A., Chong, A., et al. (1997). 'Biochemical typing of Scrapie Stains.' Scient. Corres. (Nature), 386: 564.

Somerville, R. A., Oberthur, R. C., et al. (2002). 'Characterization of thermodynamic diversity between transmissible spongiform encephalopathy agent strains and its theoretical implications.' J. Biol. Chem., 277: 11084–89.

Stahl, N., Borchelt, D. R., et al. (1987). 'Scrapie prion protein contains a phosphatidylinositol glycolipid.' Cell, 51: 229–40.

Stewart, L. A., Rydzewska, L. H., et al. (2008). 'Systematic review of therapeutic interventions in human prion disease.' Neurol., 70: 1272–81.

Tamguney, G., Miller, M. W., et al. (2009). 'Asymptomatic deer excrete infectious prions in faeces.' Nature, 461: 529–32.

Tateishi, J., Brown, P., et al. (1995). 'First experimental transmission of fatal familial insomnia.' Nature, 376: 434–35.

Tateishi, J., Kitamoto, T., et al. (2001). 'Scrapie Removal using Planova((R)) Virus Removal Filters.' Biolog., 29: 17–25.

Taylor, D. M. (1993). 'Inactivation of SE agents.' Br. Med. Bull., 49: 810–21.

Telling, G. C., Haga, T., et al. (1996). 'Interactions between wild-type and mutant prion proteins modulate neurodegeneration transgenic mice.' Genes Develop., 10: 1736–50.

Tsuboi, Y., Doh-Ura, K., et al. (2009). 'Continuous intraventricular infusion of pentosan polysulfate: clinical trial against prion diseases.' Neuropath., 29: 632–36.

Van Keulen, L. J. M., Schreuder, B. E. C., et al. (2000). 'Pathogenesis of natural scrapie in sheep.' Arch. Virol., Suppl. 16: 57–71.

Vana, K., Zuber, C., et al. (2009). 'LRP/LR as an alternative promising target in therapy of prion diseases, Alzheimer's disease and cancer.' Infect. Disord. Drug. Targ., 9: 69–80.

Wang, X., Bowers, S. L., et al. (2009). 'Cytoplasmic prion protein induces forebrain neurotoxicity.' Biochem, Biophys. Acta, 1792: 555–63.

Watts, J. C., Huo, H., et al. (2009). 'Interactome analyses identify ties of PrP and its mammalian paralogs to oligomannosidic N-glycans and endoplasmic reticulum-derived chaperones.' PLoS Pathog., 5: e1000608.

Watts, J. C. and Westaway, D. (2007). 'The prion protein family: diversity, rivalry, and dysfunction.' Biochem. Biophys. Acta, 1772: 654–72.

Wells, G. A., Hawkins, S. A., et al. (2003). 'Studies of the transmissibility of the agent of bovine spongiform encephalopathy to pigs.' J. Gen. Virol., 84: 1021–31.

Wells, G. A., Konold, T., et al. (2007). 'Bovine spongiform encephalopathy: the effect of oral exposure dose on attack rate and incubation period in cattle.' J. Gen. Virol., 88: 1363–73.

Wells, G. A. H., Hawkins, S. A. C., et al. (1998). 'Preliminary Observations on the Pathogenesis of Experimental Bovine Spongiform Encephalopathy (BSE): An Update.' Vet. Rec., 142: 103–6.

Wells, G. A. H., Scott, A. C., et al. (1987). 'A novel progressive spongiform encephalopathy in cattle.' Vet. Rec., 121: 419–20.

Westaway, D., Goodman, P. A., et al. (1987). 'Distinct prion proteins in short and long scrapie incubation period mice.' Cell, 51: 651–62.

Westergard, L., Christensen, H. M., et al. (2007). 'The cellular prion protein (PrP(C)): its physiological function and role in disease.' Biochem. Biophys. Acta, 1772: 629–44.

Wickner, R. B., Edskes, H. K., et al. (2009). 'Prion variants, species barriers, generation and propagation.' J. Biol., 8: 47.

Wilesmith, J. W., Wells, G. A. H., et al. (1988). 'BSE: Epidemiological Studies.' Vet. Rec., 123: 638–44.

Wilesmith, J. W., Ryan, J. B. M., Arnold, M. E., Stevenson, M. A. and Burke, P. J. (2010). Descriptive epidemiological features of cases of BSE born after July 31, 1996 in Great Britain. Vet. Rec., 167: 279–286.

Will, R. G., Ironside, J. W., et al. (1996). 'A new variant of Creutzfeldt-Jakob disease in the UK.' Lancet, 347: 921–25.

Wille, H., Bian, W., et al. (2009). 'Natural and synthetic prion structure from X-ray fiber diffraction.' Proc. Nat. Acad. Sci. USA, 106: 16990–95.

Wille, H., Michelitsch, M. D., et al. (2002). 'Structural studies of the scrapie prion protein by electron crystallography.' Proc. Nat. Acad. Sci. USA, 99: 3563–68.

Winklhofer, K. F., Tatzelt, J., et al. (2008). 'The two faces of protein misfolding: gain- and loss-of-function in neurodegenerative diseases.' EMBO J., 27: 336–49.

Wuertzer, C. A., Sullivan, M. A., et al. (2008). 'CNS delivery of vectored prion-specific single-chain antibodies delays disease onset.' Mol. Ther., 16: 481–86.

Wuthrich, K. and Riek, R. (2001). 'Three-dimensional structures of prion proteins.' Adv. Protein Chem., 57: 55–82.

Yamada, M., Noguchi-Shinohara, M., et al. (2009). 'Dura mater graft-associated Creutzfeldt-Jakob disease in Japan: clinicopathological and molecular characterization of the two distinct subtypes.' Neuropath., 29: 609–18.

Yoshioka, M., Murayama, Y., et al. (2007). 'Assessment of prion inactivation by combined use of Bacillus-derived protease and SDS.' Biosci. Biotechn. Biochem., 71: 2565–68.

Yunoki, M., Tanaka, H., et al. (2010). 'Infectious prion protein in the filtrate even after 15 nm filtration.' Biologicals, 38: 311–13.

Zhu, C., Li, B., et al. (2009). 'Production of Prnp -/- goats by gene targeting in adult fibroblasts.' Transgenic Res., 18: 163–71.

Zuber, C., Knackmuss, S., et al. (2008). 'Single chain Fv antibodies directed against the 37kDa/67kDa laminin receptor as therapeutic tools in prion diseases.' Mol. Immunol., 45: 144–51.

CHAPTER 35

Rabies and rabies-related lyssaviruses

Ashley C. Banyard and Anthony R. Fooks

Summary

Rabies virus is epidemic in most parts of the world. It can replicate in all warm-blooded animals in which it causes a devastating neurological illness, which almost invariably results in death. Rabies is a disease of animals and human infection is a 'spillover' event occurring most commonly following a bite from an infected dog. Infection is seen in different patterns; rabies with little or no wildlife involvement, sometimes known as urban or street rabies, or in the wildlife population with spillover into domesticated animals (sylvatic).

Eleven distinct species of lyssavirus are now recognized: species 1 is the most common strain found predominantly in terrestrial animals. Species 2–11 are detected in bat species with the exception of Mokola virus (species 3). Despite the availability of effective vaccines substantial mortality still occurs, mostly in the tropics. The majority of rabies free countries are islands which are able to remain rabies free by import controls. Effective animal vaccines are available and dog rabies is well controlled in most parts of the developed world with dog vaccination. However, rabies remains an intractable problem in many countries in Asia and Africa due to a lack of infrastructure, cost of vaccines and difficulty in controlling dog populations. In recent years progress in controlling wildlife rabies has been achieved in western Europe using vaccine in bait, which offers promise for other regions with complex epidemiology.

Introduction

Despite the availability of effective vaccines, rabies virus remains endemic across much of the globe with two thirds of the world's population living in a rabies endemic region. The ability of the virus to infect and replicate in a wide variety of hosts mean that as well as circulating in specific species, cross species transmission (CST) can also occur. From a zoonotic perspective, human infection constitutes a CST event from the infected animal reservoir. Whilst transmission of virus from infected animals into the human population is historically through the bite of an infected dog, the elimination of rabies from domestic canine populations across the developed world has highlighted other species as important transmission vectors. Several terrestrial wildlife species harbour the virus, often within distinct populations. Occasionally, transmission between different species drives the generation of different

rabies virus biotypes. Modern genetic analyses have been used to highlight mutual adaptation of virus variants and host populations. Epidemiologically, within an endemic area, disease is usually sustained within a single host species, although interactions between different species can cause a CST event to occur. This event occurs most often when clinical disease is identified.

It has long been established that whilst dogs are considered as the principal terrestrial reservoir for rabies virus, bats (Order *Chiroptera*) constitute an increasingly important reservoir of rabies and rabies-related lyssaviruses (Fooks 2004; Vos *et al.* 2007; Banyard *et al.* 2009). Indeed, ten of the defined lyssavirus species have been isolated from bats, the exception being Mokola virus (species 3). Few isolates of this virus are available for study and its epidemiology is poorly understood. Rabies virus was identified in vampire bats with records associating transmission of rabies from haematophagous bats to humans dating back as far as the sixteenth century (Blancou 1994). In the first half of the twentieth century, insectivorous and frugivorous bats were also proven to be harbouring rabies virus variants and over the past 90 years more data associating different bats species across the world with the transmission of lyssaviruses has been generated. Genetic characterization of bat derived lyssaviruses has shown that, although isolates can be grouped as the same species as terrestrial isolates, in reality the viruses remain quite distinct with several species of rabies virus variants being derived solely from bats. Certainly, isolates from different continents, whilst sharing many common characteristics at the molecular level, remain genetically diverse.

A number of reporting systems have been implemented to record individual disease outbreaks. For rabies and related lyssaviruses several organizations monitor cases of rabies and make data available to the general public, these include: RabNet (www.who.int/rabies/rabnet), the Rabies Bulletin in Europe (www.who-rabies-bulletin.org/), the Bulletin of Epidemiological Surveillance of Rabies in the Americas (www.paho.org/English/AD/DPC/VP/rabia.htm) and the Office International d'Epizooties (OIE) (www.oie.int/eng/en_index.htm) all act as reporting systems. These surveillance reports are essential in monitoring the status of countries for presence of the virus. However, rabies remains endemic in almost all continents although vaccination of dogs and wildlife, quarantine and surveillance have greatly reduced disease incidence. Currently Antarctica, as well as a number of island nations such as the United Kingdom, Japan, Barbados, Fiji, the Maldives, the Seychelles, New Zealand and Hawaii are free of classical rabies isolates. Such island nations are able, with relative ease, to remain rabies-free by the application of importation controls such as quarantine. In addition, much of Western Europe and parts of northern and southern continental Europe such as Greece, Portugal, Sweden, Norway as well as some countries within Latin America (e.g. Uruguay and Chile) are also free of terrestrial rabies. Bat lyssaviruses continue to pose a threat, albeit low, to the human population in many of these areas.

Despite the successes of island nations in controlling rabies and the elimination of canine rabies in parts of the developed world, the control of terrestrial rabies remains a challenge and the virus is still epizootic across much of Eastern Europe, Africa, Asia, and Latin America. The vast majority of human deaths from the disease occur within the developing world. Whilst figures estimated for annual human deaths within these areas are high (up to 50,000), it is widely believed that these figures are a gross underestimate of the actual number of human deaths (Fooks 2005; Fooks 2007; George Baer, personal communication). This affects our understanding of the global epidemiology of the disease and in many regions the incidence of disease is largely unknown. In some regions surveillance has identified where disease occurrence is either linked with endemic infection within the canine populations, often referred to as 'street' or 'urban' rabies, or with CST from wildlife reservoirs into domestic animals and man.

The rabies virus

Classification

Rabies virus is a member of the Order *Mononegavirales*, Family *Rhabdoviridae*, genus *lyssavirus* and contains a non-segmented negative strand genome of approximately 12 kilobases (kb) in length. As well as rabies virus, the order *Mononegavirales* includes a range of other important diseases of man including members of the Filoviridae (Ebola virus) and Paramyxoviridae (measles virus). The *Rhabdoviridae* are classified into several serologically and genetically distinct genera with the capability to infect a diverse spectrum of hosts including vertebrates, invertebrates and plants. Within this diverse family two genera are classified as being able to infect mammalian species: the *vesiculoviruses* and *lyssaviruses*. The *vesiculovirus* genus includes the viruses causing Vesicular Stomatitis virus (VSV) and bovine ephemeral fever virus (BEFV), two antigenically related viruses of economic importance in cattle. The *lyssavirus* genus includes rabies virus, the rabies-related viruses, and several other recently classified viruses that share only a distant relationship to rabies virus.

The *lyssavirus* genus was originally subdivided into four distinct serotypes and further, through genetic typing, into seven major genotypes. More recently, classification of members of the lyssavirus genus has altered from being genotypes into distinct species with the inclusion of previously unclassified rabies-related viruses. Initial characterization of the different virus isolates into the four serotypes was made by cross-immunization experiments in animals and by antigenic typing of isolates using monoclonal antibodies. Serotype 1 contained the classical rabies viruses and Australian bat lyssavirus (ABLV); serotype 2 covered isolates of Lagos bat virus (LBV); serotype 3 included Mokola virus (MOKV); and

serotype 4 included Duvenhage virus (DUVV) and both variants of the European bat lyssaviruses, -1 and -2 (EBLVs). Molecular typing then enabled these viruses to be classified into seven distinct genotypes on the basis of genetic sequence data. Genotype 1 included all isolates of classical rabies virus; genotype 2 contained LBV; genotype 3 included the MOKVs; genotype 4 included DUVVs; genotype 5 included isolates of EBLV-1; genotype 6 included EBLV-2 isolates and genotype 7 included ABLV (Tordo *et al.* 2004). With the exception of MOKV isolates all genotypes have been isolated from bats (Kuzmin *et al.* 2005). Further genetic characterization of individual isolates has then identified MOKV and LBV isolates as being distinct from the other genotypes, ultimately leading to the classification of genotypes into phylogroups where MOKV and LBV make up phylogroup 1 and the remainder of the genotypes fall into phylogroup 2 (Nadin-Davis *et al.* 2007). In addition, it is likely that MOKV isolates and LBV can be divided further using genetic characterization that reflect their geographical origins.

Isolation of several rabies-related viruses from bats across Eurasia has further altered the way that these viruses are classified. Molecular data have been used to classify several other rabies-related lyssaviruses that were originally been proposed as new members of the genus. These include; Aravan virus (ARAV), isolated in southern Kyrgystan in 1991 from a lesser mouse-eared bat (Arai *et al.* 2003); Khujand virus (KHUV) isolated from the brain material of a whiskered bat in 2003 in northern Tajikistan (Kuzmin *et al.* 2003); Irkut virus (IRKV) isolated in 2002 from a greater tube-nosed bat and West Caucasian Bat virus (WCBV) isolated in 2002 from a bent-winged bat in the Caucasus mountains (Kuzmin *et al.* 2005). Initially, these isolates were unclassified but establishment of the relationship between these new viruses and the currently defined members of the lyssavirus genus have been studied both at the molecular level as well as using more modern techniques such as antigenic cartography which seek to define the relationship between amino acid composition and antigenicity (Nel and Markotter 2007). These studies with the Eurasian lyssavirus-like isolates has further enabled the classification of the seven lyssavirus genotypes into eleven distinct species. The current classification of these viruses is detailed in Table 35.1.

Virion structure

Individual rabies virus particles were first visualized using electron microscopy in the early 1960s (Matsumoto *et al.* 1962; Davies *et al.* 1963). The virions are bullet-shaped with a 'spiky' appearance. The spikes or peplomers are 9 nanometer (nm) protrusions, spaced approximately 5nm apart within the lipid bilayer that consist of the viral glycoprotein (G). Virions have an average length of 180 (130–300) nm and diameter of 75 (60–110) nm. A number of researchers have reported differences in virion length and have attributed them to the presence of defective interfering particles (DI). These truncated forms of the virion are thought to be aberrations of virus replication whereby truncated nascent genomes lacking segments of the virus genome are generated and packaged into virions. DI particles can vary greatly in length and, as they are incapable of autonomous replication, can interfere with the replication of full-length virus by usurping proteins that they are unable to generate themselves, thus reducing the replicative ability of the full-length, non-defective virus. DI particles are often seen after multiple

Table 35.1 Lyssavirus classification

Species	Phylogroup	Virus	Distribution	Natural hosts
1	1	Rabies virus	Worldwide although a number of countries are now rabies free	Dogs, wild carnivores, Insectivorous bats, Hematophagous bats, livestock, man
2	2	Lagos Bat Virus	Nigeria, Ethiopia, Central African Republic, Senegal, Zimbabwe, South Africa	Dogs, cats, frugivorous bats
3	2	Mokola Virus	Nigeria, Central African Republic, Ethiopia, Cameroon, Zimbabwe, South Africa	Dogs, cats, shrews, rodents, man
4	1	Duvenhage virus	South Africa, Zimbabwe	Insectivorous bats, man
5	1	European bat lyssavirus-1	Denmark, Netherlands, Germany, Poland, Russia, Slovakia, France, Spain	Insectivorous bats, man
6	1	European bat lyssavirus-2	UK, Netherlands, Switzerland, Germany	Insectivorous bats, man
7	1	Australian bat lyssavirus	Australia	Insectivorous bats, frugivorous bats, man
8	1	Aravan	Southern Kyrgystan	Insectivorous bat (Lesser mouse-eared bat)
9	1	Khujand virus	Northern Tajikstan	Insectivorous bat (Whiskered bat)
10	1	Irkut virus	Eastern Siberia	Insectivorous bat (Greater tube-nosed bat)
11	2	West Caucasian Bat virus	Caucasus mountains	Insectivorous bat (Bent-winged bat)

passages in tissue culture (Holland and Villarreal 1975; Grabau and Holland 1982; Finke and Conzlemann 1999).

The minimal replicative unit for these viruses is the ribonucleo-protein complex (RNP) which consists of the RNA together with the nucleocapsid protein (N), the phosphoprotein (P) and the large polymerase protein (L). This RNP is then surrounded by the lipid containing envelope, 7.5–10nm thick, that the virus acquires from the plasma membrane of the infected cell upon exit. The matrix protein (M) plays a role in virion structure either sitting within the coiled coil, as suggested for vesicular stomatitis virus (VSV), or lining the inner surface of the virus envelope being in contact with both the RNP and the cytoplasmic tails of the glyco-protein (G) (Barge *et al.* 1993; Nakahara *et al.* 1999).

Genome structure

The lyssavirus genome consists of a single strand of negative sense RNA that can vary between 10 and 12kb in length. The negative strand genome contains 5 or more distinct open reading frames that each encode one of the viral proteins. The 3' end of the genome contains an untranslated region of 58 nucleotides that precedes the first gene, called the leader. This region shows a high degree of complementarity with the terminal 5' end of the genome where a similar region exists often referred to as the trailer region. Studies with other negative strand RNA viruses such as the paramyxovi-ruses, the filoviruses and the bornaviruses have identified distinct domains within these regions that play significant roles within the viral transcription and replication strategies (Banyard *et al.* 2005). Often referred to now as the genome and antigenome promoters (leader and trailer regions, respectively), these short untranslated regions contain all the necessary information to drive transcription to produce messenger RNA for the production of viral proteins; replication, from the genome promoter, to form a positive strand replicative intermediate; and generation of nascent negative strand genome RNA from the antigenome promoter at the 3' end of the

positive sense replicative intermediate. The exact nucleotides and viral protein complexes that interact at these regions to form viral transcriptase and replicase complexes are largely unknown although cis-acting signals for a transcriptase complex have been suggested (Conzelmann and Schnell 1994; Whelan and Wertz 1999).

Viral transcription is known to proceed from the 3' end of the genomic RNA to generate a short leader RNA followed by messen-ger RNAs encoding for each of the five viral proteins: the nucleo-protein (N), phosphoprotein (P), matrix protein (M), glycoprotein (G), and polymerase (L) (Tordo and Kouknetzoff 1993). Each of the newly generated mRNAs are capped and polyadenylated by the multifunctional polymerase (L) protein. The transcriptase com-plex generates a monocistronic mRNA from all but one of the five coding regions. The exception is the phosphoprotein (P) whereby poor Kozak consensus sequence around the primary P gene methionine leads to leaky transcription initiation and the complex initiates transcription at any of the three or four (depending on the virus isolate) in-frame initiation codons downstream of the pri-mary AUG. These amino-truncated products are of unknown function although whilst the full length P is found exclusively in the cytoplasm, truncated forms can be found in the nucleus (Takamatsu *et al.* 1998).

Each of the genes are separated by non-translated intergenic regions, which in turn are flanked by gene start and stop sequences recognized by the transcriptase. This sequence of untranslated gene signals at each of the gene boundaries leads to a transcrip-tional gradient of mRNAs being synthesized. This gradient is gen-erated as the transcriptase complex may become detached from the template at each intergenic region and, as it can only reinitiate transcription at the 3' promoter, the 3' proximal genes are gener-ated in greater quantities than each of the respective downstream genes. At some point after initiation of transcription the viral pro-teins N, P and L, acting as a transcriptase complex, switches to a replicase form whereby it is now able to ignore the gene start and stop signals and instead generate a full-length positive strand antigenome RNA. This antigenome RNA then serves as the template for the generation of nascent genome sense negative strand RNA, the nascent negative strand being generated as the replicase complex binds to the 3' end of the antigenome and synthesizes across the length of the genome. It is now recognized for several nonsegmented negative strand viruses that the protein complexes that make up the transcriptase and replicase forms contain different components. It is possible that individual proteins form different structures through the interactions with different domains to play these different roles within the viral life cycle although the mechanisms behind each of the different RNP activities remains largely unknown (Gupta *et al.* 2003). Studies using different lyssavirus isolates have attempted, to define molecular determinants of pathogenicity and N, P, M, and G have all been implicated (Mita *et al.* 2008; Pulmanausahakul *et al.* 2008; Shimizu *et al.* 2007; Takayama-Ito *et al.* 2006; Wirblich *et al.* 2008).

The mechanisms by which viral transcriptase and replicase complexes act differently at the intergenic regions as well as the stop/start gene sequences that flank them remain unknown. Whilst for a number of the negative strand viruses these regions are conserved in length if not in sequence, for rabies virus, these intergenic regions differ in length at each gene boundary. Between N and P a dinucleotide region is present whilst at both the P-M and the M-G gene boundaries a pentanucleotide is present. However, between the G and L genes some members of the lyssavirus genus contain a very long intergenic region of 423 nucleotides (Marston *et al.* 2007). Whilst some have described this long 3' non coding region as a pseudogene (Ψ) others have suggested that it is of no evolutionary significance and is unlikely to represent a remnant gene (Tordo *et al.* 1986; Ravkov *et al.* 1995). Currently, the role of this long untranslated region remains unknown although it has been postulated that it may play a role in regulating transcription of the polymerase gene (L) as the level of L gene transcription correlates with the extraordinary length of Ψ. More recent studies have indicated that this region may play a role in the neuroinvasiveness of rabies virus strains (Faber *et al.* 2004).

Pathogenesis and molecular aspects of infection and transmission

Disease transmission and human infection

The principal mechanism of human infection with rabies viruses is through the bite of an infected animal that contains virus in its saliva. The lyssaviruses are unable to infect humans through the dermal barrier unless the skin is broken. However, infection may occur at exposed mucous membranes including the conjunctivae, the nasal lining, the oral cavity, the anus and external genital organs. Infection through inhalation of aerosolized virus in bat caves has been reported (Irons *et al.* 1957; Brass 1994) and experimental studies have confirmed the possibility of infection via this route for both rabies and other lyssaviruses (Constantine 1962; Winkler 1968; Winkler *et al.* 1973; Johnson *et al.* 2006a). These studies suggest that this method is a potentially important mechanism by which virus is sustained within a colony where vast numbers of animals live in close proximity. Human infection via this route, however, remains extremely rare (Johnson *et al.* 2006).

Accidental human exposure to aerosolized virus within a laboratory has also been reported. In the incident, a veterinarian succumbed to disease whilst another laboratory worker recovered although the individual sustained substantial neurological impairment (Winkler *et al.* 1973; Tillotson *et al.* 1977).

Human-to-human transmission has also been reported albeit very rarely (Fekadu *et al.* 1996) and evidence of transplacental transmission has been suggested by a single case (Sipahioglu and Alapaut 1985). In 2004, recipients of kidneys, a liver and an arterial segment from a common donor developed fatal rabies and live virus was recovered from the recipients of the transplanted organs (Srinivasan *et al.* 2005; Burton *et al.* 2005). Several human-to-human cases of rabies transmission have also occurred through corneal transplantation (Houff *et al.* 1979; Gode and Bhide 1988; Sureau *et al.* 1981). Many cases of rabies reported annually have no origin cited as the source of infection and such cases are assumed to be as a result of transmission through minor scratches from infected animals or bites from small bat species that have gone unnoticed (Messenger *et al.* 2003). These cases underline the need for education of local populations and tourists visiting endemic areas (Fooks *et al.* 2003). Deliberate release of rabies virus remains an important and yet remote likelihood (Fooks *et al.* 2009).

Rabies virus receptors and molecular events leading to infection

The ability of rabies virus to enter cells is dependent on the ability of its glycoprotein, present on the virion surface as a trimer, to bind to cellular receptors (Gaudin *et al.* 1992). Entry of virus may occur either directly into the central nervous system (CNS) or after initial replication within muscle tissue. It has been suggested, though not proven, that rabies virus may replicate in non-neuronal tissue around the bite site. Such low level replication at the bite site in a tissue type that is not highly permissive for virus may explain long incubation periods that are occasionally observed following infection (Lafon 2005). Evidence from *in vitro* studies suggests that the virus enters motor nerves primarily through neuromuscular junctions and antigen has been detected within sensory spindles, proprioceptors and stretch receptors (Lewis *et al.* 2000; Murphy 1977).

Currently, three rabies virus receptors are proposed: the nicotinic acetylcholine receptor (nAchR), responsible for interneuronal communication within the CNS and the peripheral nerve network; neural cell adhesion molecule (NCAM), present at the nerve termini and deep within the neuromuscular junctions at the postsynaptic membranes; and to a lesser extent the neurotrophin receptor (p75NTR), which plays a role in cellular death, synaptic transmission and axonal elongation (Dechant and Barde 2002; Tuffereau *et al.* 2007). It is currently unknown to what extent each of these proposed receptors are utilized by rabies viruses and their use by other lyssaviruses also remains to be elucidated.

Once the virus has bound to a permissive receptor on the surface of a neuron or cell, entry is believed to occur either by direct fusion between the virion membrane and the plasma membrane or by receptor mediated endocytosis. In the latter case membrane fusion of the virus particle and the endosomal membrane is as a result of a lower pH environment within the endosomal compartment. Either way, the outcome of attachment and penetration into the cell is the release of the viral genetic material in the form of a ribonucleoprotein complex into the cell cytoplasm. Once released the molecular events that drive transcription and replication are initiated and the virus replicative cycle begins.

Transport of rabies virus from the axons of the peripheral nervous system to the CNS occurs by retrograde axoplasmic flow. Studies with human dorsal route ganglia neurons showed that the virus was able to move relatively quickly in a retrograde manner traveling at 50–100mm/day (Tsiang *et al.* 1991) and such fast axonal transport may be a result of the interaction of the virus phosphoprotein with actin- and microtubule-based motility networks such as dyenin LC8 (Jacob *et al.* 2000; Raux *et al.* 2000). However, more recent studies *in vivo* have suggested that mutation of the phosphoprotein LC8 binding domain has only minor effects on viral spread suggesting that other, as yet unidentified, interactions may be key to virus mobility (Mebatsion 2001; Rasalingham *et al.* 2005). Recent studies using the CVS strain of rabies virus have identified key stages of infection using the virus as a transneuronal tracer of neuronal connections. Intracellular transport of viruses from dendrites of infected neurons to the presynaptic terminals of connected neurons has been shown. The ubiquitous distribution of suitable receptor molecules within the CNS have been shown to drive the rapid movement of virus whilst peripheral infection is restricted to motor endplates and axons limiting initial propagation of virus at the periphery (Ugolini 2008).

Factors affecting incubation period

The neurotropic nature of rabies virus and other lyssaviruses generally dictates the rate of progression of disease with virus entry at a highly innervated site often leading to swift progression of virus into the CNS and the onset of clinical disease. However, as the virus is often transmitted through the bite of an infected animal, the level of innervation at the bite site may vary greatly and as a result, there is a noticeable variation in disease progression. This difference is often reflected in the length of the incubation period observed between infection and onset of clinical disease. The nature of the infecting virus particles, the dose transmitted and presence or absence of permissive receptors on peripheral nerve networks may also limit virus entry and motility (Ugolini 2008).

Historically, rabies virus infection was considered as having an incubation period of between 7 and 100 days in the sixth century (*Sun Si Miao of China*); between 9 days and 7 years in the thirteenth century (*Bernard de Gordon*); between 20 days and several years in the sixteenth century (*Fracastoro*) (Blancou 1994). Variation in the length of incubation period or prodromal period is often a reflection of the difficulty of establishing the day on which infection occurred, especially where animals are concerned. Whilst infection with rabies virus generally has an incubation period of 20–90 days, in extreme cases this period may be substantially greater, and is more variable than that noted for any other acute infection. Extremes of preclinical incubation period following rabies virus infection has been reported as being as long as 14 to 19 years although with such cases secondary exposure cannot be discounted (Fishbein 1991).

Incubation periods for the other lyssaviruses are also difficult to determine, largely due to individuals being unable to account for a possible exposure time. Cases of infection with Duvenhage virus are known to have had incubation periods of at least four weeks (Meredith *et al.* 1971; Paweska *et al.* 2006) whilst a case of European Bat lyssavirus type-1 (EBLV-1) in an adult human had a 45 day incubation period (Botvinkin *et al.* 2005). The first case of death attributed to rabies in the UK for over 100 years, that of an infection of a 55-year old bat conservationist with European Bat Lyssavirus type-2 (EBLV-2), suggested that infection may have been due to a bite 19 weeks prior to the first signs of disease although a history of previous bat bites was recorded (Fooks *et al.* 2003). For the Australian Bat Lyssaviruses a much longer incubation period was observed. A human case of ABLV in 1998 reported that infection of a 37-year old woman led to clinical disease some twenty months after the presumed exposure to virus (Hanna *et al.* 2000; Johnson *et al.* 2008a).

Factors influencing the incubation period must include the site and severity of the bite, with bites nearer the head having a shorter incubation period; degree of innervation of the bite site, highly innervated regions of the body such as the face, neck, and hands are thought to be more dangerous, presumably because of their rich nerve supply; the quantity of virus 'inoculated' with small amounts of virus possibly being transmitted through bites from bats compared to the larger volume of virus excreted in the saliva of infected dogs; the nature of the infecting virus isolate with experimental differences observed between highly neuroinvasive strains and less neuroinvasive strains and the age and immune status of the host. The incubation period in children is reported to be shorter than that in adults and is probably associated with their infant stature (Warrell 2008; World Health Organization (WHO) 2008).

Infection with rabies virus

Rabies infection of man

In regions where rabies virus is known to be circulating, when neurological symptoms of unexplained origin are observed, the possibility of a rabies virus infection should always be considered. Lack of history of a biting incident should not dismiss rabies for consideration, since such bites may have appeared trivial or have occurred many months before and been forgotten by the patient. Travellers to endemic areas should be made aware of the dangers of rabies infection as they are for other diseases such as malaria (Fooks *et al.* 2003).

Whilst infection from rabies virus was previously only associated with transmission of virus through the saliva of an infected animal, other means of infection are now recognized and care must be taken if at any stage an individual may have become exposed through 'non-bite' mechanisms such as infection of an open wound, scratches, and rarely inhalation of aerosolized virus (Vos *et al.* 2007; Johnson *et al.* 2006; Winkler *et al.* 1973). Fears surrounding potential exposure through the urine and faecal matter of an infected animal remain unresolved but are considered to be low risk mechanisms of virus transmission.

Observation of what may constitute clinical presentation characteristic of infection with a rabies virus or a related lyssavirus can be difficult. As discussed previously, incubation times can vary greatly depending on the nature of the infecting agent as well as the site of infection and the species affected. Early symptoms in rabies patients may resemble those of tetanus, typhoid, and malaria, or of viral encephalitides such as those caused by measles virus, mumps virus, herpesvirus, or enteroviruses. Furthermore, differential diagnosis can be problematic due to similarities in early clinical observations with other pathogen based and medical conditions such as transmissible spongiform encephalopathies, tetanus, listeriosis, poisoning, Aujeszky's disease and most commonly with Guillain-Barré Syndrome (Hemachudha *et al.* 2002; Solomon *et al.* 2005). Secondary infections can also mask the presence of rabies infection, occasionally leading to an incorrect diagnosis of disease (Mallewa *et al.* 2007). Even during late stage infection, highly informative technologies such as Magnetic Resonance Imaging (MRI) cannot conclusively differentiate between paralytic and furious rabies cases although such scanning may enable other sequelea to be ruled out (Laothamatas *et al.* 2008). In the absence of clinical disease that may be specifically attributed to rabies infection a 2–20 day prodromal period may occur where the victim may suffer from a number of non-specific symptoms including general malaise, weakness, and loss of appetite, fever and headaches. Paraesthesia or itching at the site of the bite is often reported during this initial prodromal phase. The disease may then progress to the clinical stage whereby acute dysfunction of the nervous system ensues leading to the symptoms that, in the public eye are responsible for the general fear attributed to infection with rabies; hydrophobia, madness and death. Approximately 80% of human cases go on to develop 'furious' rabies whilst the remaining 20% develop the paralytic, or 'dumb' form of the disease. Once clinical disease is apparent in the vast majority of cases will ultimately result in death. The few reported survivors have suffered severe neurological impairment.

Rabies infection of animals

All mammals are susceptible to infection, however, there are no species specific symptoms apart from altered behaviour as a direct result of neuronal involvement. As with human infection, a prodromal phase occurs where the infected animal may become noticeably lethargic and display signs of weakness. Domesticated animals will often become less interested in interacting with owners whilst wild animals that would normally avoid contact with man may seek out human interaction.

Similarly to human infection, rabies may manifest in a variety of different ways, although clinical progression is usually described as either a 'furious' or a 'dumb' form. However, these two distinct clinical presentations of the disease are extremes of infection and an individual animal may exhibit clinical manifestations specific for either form of disease or elements of both. It is thought that the clinical progression of disease may be linked to the primary site of viral replication within the CNS, which must be linked to the site of virus entry and the amount of virus transmitted. A number of ongoing studies are attempting to relate disease pathogenesis to involvement of different regions of the brain although currently the exact mechanism of pathogenesis within the brain is unclear (Hicks *et al.* 2009).

With furious rabies, after a brief prodrome where animals may appear more alert than normal, an acute neurological phase often occurs with signs similar to acute disease in man. Infected animals have been observed exhibiting parasthesia, with animals being seen to excessively groom or scratch areas presumed to be the site of infection. Parasthesia may progress to extremes of self-mutilation and even self-consumption of the affected region leading to severe trauma. Often animals will snap at anything within reach and will hold onto anything they are able to bite hold of with great tenacity. Neurological signs then develop progressively becoming almost continuous until death which is generally due to respiratory arrest and organ failure.

Cases of dumb rabies in dogs often initiate the cycle of clinical disease with the animal becoming lethargic and often showing a lack of coordination. This situation may rapidly worsen or remain stable for a short while before further clinical signs develop. Motor paralysis often develops initially as a 'weakness' of the hind limbs. As infection progresses the paralysis spreads affecting all limbs leaving the infected animal quadriplegic. Mandibular paralysis may also occur causing a loss of the swallowing reflex. Such ascending paralysis is commonly observed in wild as well as domestic animals. Once dumb rabies has progressed to this stage the infected animal may succumb to infection without any additional clinical signs.

Early signs of infection in dogs generally lasts for two to five days before either the development of paralytic rabies, in approximately 75% of infected animals or the aggressive form of disease, furious rabies in the remainder. Paralysis and death will often occur four to eight days after the onset of clinical disease. Although typically thought of as a disease of canines, felines can be infected and more often develop the furious form of the disease and can pose a greater threat to man as their role as a companion lap animal means that statistically they are more likely to scratch at the face and neck of their owners with claws harboring infected saliva.

Lyssavirus diagnostics and surveillance

The earliest reported experimental diagnosis of rabies virus was by the German scientist, Georg Gottfried Zinke (1804), and specific diagnostic tests have been the mainstay of case confirmation and surveillance. The majority of the traditional tests are, however, relatively slow and insensitive compared to today's techniques, and in some cases require the use of live animals. Here, we describe the techniques currently used in the diagnosis of rabies and lyssaviruses and highlight the importance of more recent molecular based technologies. Unfortunately, in countries where there is the most frequent need for robust, timely and accurate diagnostic tools, mainly across the developing world where the virus remains endemic, clinical diagnosis with or without an examination for Negri bodies is often the only diagnostic method that is attempted. However, whenever feasible clinical suspicions should be confirmed by laboratory tests. The accurate diagnosis of infection with rabies and lyssaviruses is generally confirmed by internationally standardized laboratory tests undertaken on CNS tissue removed from the brain at post mortem. Recommended regions of the brain include sites where high levels of virus antigen can be readily detected such as the hippocampus, cerebellum and the medulla oblongata. In suspect cases, it is usual for the entire head of the animal to be submitted to an approved laboratory for confirmation of infection. However, if a large number of animals are involved, brain material from individual animals may be submitted using the 'straw technique' whereby a plastic straw-like rod is passed through the occipital foramen to collect suitable material for testing (OIE 2004).

Pathological diagnosis
Autopsy

There are no gross lesions characteristic for rabies virus infection visible at autopsy. In most animals, microscopic non-specific lesions suggestive of viral encephalomyelitis with ganglioneuritis may be observed in the nerve centers, as well as histolymphocytic cuffs and gliosis. The most notable lesions are usually in the cervical spinal cord, hypothalamus and pons. The only specific lesions consist of intracytoplasmic eosinophilic inclusions termed 'Negri bodies' that are discussed below.

Histopathology

Some of the earliest diagnostic methods for the detection of rabies virus infection in post mortem material were based on histopathological examination. Specific round to oval inclusions described by Negri (1903) usually identified in the cytoplasm of undamaged nerve cells and particularly in the hippocampus were routinely used for diagnosis using both histological and immunological techniques. These 'Negri bodies', which consist of a reticulogranular matrix containing tubular structures measuring from 4 to 5μm are contiguous with maturing virus particles. However, absence of these disease markers does not exclude the disease. As will be described later, these markers of infection may be detected in almost any region of the brain, but are primarily seen in the Ammon's horn of the hippocampus, the ganglioneurones and neurones of the cerebellum, the motor area of the cerebral cortex, and in the medulla. Their frequency of occurrence, size, and shape may be influenced by the host species, the infecting virus strain, and the clinical phase.

Rabies diagnosis was previously based upon the detection of Negri bodies and the use of histological tests such as Sellers's staining techniques or Mann's fixation protocols (WHO 1996). These assays are now rarely undertaken as they have been superseded by more accurate and reliable tests and are now considered unreliable, particularly when decomposed material is submitted (McElhinney et al. 2004). However, despite histopathological techniques being discontinued for use in a diagnostic capacity, a molecular based method has been developed for the detection of species 5 and 6 lyssaviruses (Finnegan et al. 2004). This technique is a robust, highly sensitive and specific in-situ hybridization technique, and employs digoxigenin labelled riboprobes for the detection of lyssavirus RNA in mouse-infected brain tissue. Using this method, both genomic and messenger RNAs have been detected. The ability to detect messenger RNA is indicative of the presence of replicating virus. Whilst this assay is of diagnostic value, interest in such new protocols is driven by the need to investigate lyssaviruses other than the classical rabies species (Hicks et al. 2009).

Antigen detection

Detection of rabies virus antigen

Over the last ten years a number of novel techniques have been developed for diagnostic confirmation of rabies viruses in clinical specimens, yet the most commonly used test is the fluorescent antibody test (FAT) developed over 35 years ago (Dean and Abelseth 1973). This test, still recommended by the OIE and WHO as the 'Gold Standard' for diagnosis of rabies virus in clinical specimens, depends on the reaction between virus antigen in the brain and fluorescently labelled anti-rabies antibodies directed against the nucleocapsid protein. Not only is it routinely used for confirmation of the presence of antigen in brain smears but can also be used for virus isolation on passaged material as well as virus identification intra vitam from skin biopsy material. Whilst this test can give accurate (95–99%) results within hours of receipt of a fresh

clinical specimen, its sensitivity can be affected by the quality of the tissue examined, autolysis, presence of different lyssavirus antigen and the region of the brain submitted for analysis.

Use of ELISA for post mortem diagnostics

The rapid rabies enzyme immunodiagnosis (RREID) technique, based on the detection of virus nucleocapsid antigen in brain tissue, was the first technique to take rapid accurate post-mortem diagnosis out of the laboratory as it did not require microscopy and, with the aid of a special kit, could be used under field conditions. The RREID test can be used to examine partially decomposed tissue specimens for evidence of rabies virus but it cannot be used with specimens that have been fixed in formalin, and comparative studies against fluorescent antibody based tests suggested that its sensitivity may not be as effective as that of the fluorescent antibody based methods (Perrin et al. 1986; Franka et al. 2004). Despite this drawback, such methodologies have been shown to be of benefit for large scale surveillance having the potential to be automated (Bourhy et al. 1989; Perrin and Sureau 1987; Bouhry and Perrin 1996). More recently, an avidin-biotin amplified dot-blot enzyme immunoassay has shown good sensitivity and specifity in small scale trials using infected brain tissues but has not yet been tested on clinical samples such as saliva for ante-mortem diagnosis of human cases (Madhusudana et al. 2004). Use of ELISA in serological assays will be discussed later.

Virus isolation

Mouse inoculation technique

The OIE guidelines for diagnosis of the rabies virus infection primarily recommends the use of FAT on post-mortem brain material. Confirmatory virus isolation must, however, be used to support the initial diagnosis, particularly when FAT results are equivocal and where human exposure is involved. To this end the mouse inoculation test (MIT) was developed. This test relies on the detection of virus antigen in the positive FAT sample and requires processing of post-mortem tissue to generate a homogenate of brain material. As for the FAT test, regions are carefully chosen and pooled to form a homogenate, which is then inoculated intracerebrally into weanling mice. Clinical signs (positive result) may be seen as early as six to eight days for RABV although it can often take considerably longer for mice to succumb and considerable variation in the onset of clinical signs seen when using this method has been reported (Johnson et al. 2003). Mice should be observed for a period of 28 days. This in vivo test is time-consuming, expensive and involves the use of animals. The WHO recommends that it should be avoided for routine diagnosis if validated in vitro methods, such as isolation of virus on tissue culture cells, are established within the laboratory (WHO 2005).

Virus isolation in vitro

Tissue culture isolation of virus was once problematic due to the fact that lyssaviruses rarely cause cytopathic effect that can be observed using the light microscope. Some viral strains can cause the formation of large fusions of cells, termed 'syncytia', but not all strains of virus have fusogenic ability and thus infection of a cell monolayer is generally difficult to interpret.

Cell culture techniques such as the Rabies Tissue Culture Inoculation Test (RTCIT) used the fluorescently conjugated antibody developed for the FAT test to detect virus nucleocapsid in tissue culture. The test involves the inoculation of the sample into a neuroblastoma cell line that has been shown to be highly permissive for the majority of lyssaviruses. Positive results are commonly obtained within 2–4 days. The FAT is then used to confirm the presence of rabies virus antigen in either infected mice or cell monolayers. From a research perspective, these virus isolation techniques provide an opportunity to generate individual virus stocks which can be further characterized using molecular methods as described below.

Amplification of genetic material

Nucleic acid based technology

Advances in molecular techniques over the last decade have seen PCR assays replace many of the more traditional screening methods for lyssavirus diagnosis. These are now becoming more widely accepted and accessible for the diagnosis of rabies and, whilst not recommended by the WHO for routine post-mortem diagnosis of lyssaviruses, the use of the reverse transcriptase polymerase chain reaction (RT-PCR), nested or hemi-nested RT-PCR and other PCR based formats are increasingly being used. Many laboratories have now enforced strict quality control procedures and

with trained staff with demonstrable experience and expertise have applied these molecular techniques for confirmatory diagnosis and epidemiological surveys. As well as post-mortem diagnoses, RT-PCR has been used to confirm rabies infection *intra-vitam* in suspect human cases, where conventional diagnostic methods have failed and post-mortem material is not available (Smith *et al.* 2003). RT-PCR techniques can be used not only to detect rabies virus RNA in a wide variety of biological fluids and samples (e.g. saliva, cerebrospinal fluid, tears, skin biopsies and urine) but is also now used to differentiate between different species using both conventional and real time RT-PCR assays (Wakeley *et al.* 2005). Real time assays have recently been used for the rapid diagnosis and species confirmation of EBLV-2 infected Daubenton's bats in the UK (Fooks *et al.* 2004) as well as in the *intra-vitam* detection and genotyping of two human rabies cases in the UK in 2002 and 2005 (Fooks *et al.* 2003b; Solomon *et al.* 2005) and for the detection of a rabies in a quarantined puppy in UK (Fooks *et al.* 2008).

Molecular tools such as PCR and sequencing continue to enable the characterization of new virus isolates and to date a number of

Table 35.2 Available full length genome data for the lyssaviruses

Virus	Isolate	Genome length	Accession Number	Reference
Rabies virus	Pasteur strain	11932	NC_001542	Tordo *et al.* 1986; 1988
	Street Alabama Dufferin (SAD) B19	11928	RAVCGA	Conzelmann *et al.* 1990
	Nishigahara	11926	AB044824	Ito *et al.* 2001
	RC-HL	11926	AB009663	Ito *et al.* 2001
	SRV9	11928	AF499686	Yuan *et al.* 2002
	Nishigahara (Ni-CE)	11926	AB128149	Shimizu *et al.* 2006
	High egg passage (HEP)- Flury	11615	AB085828	Inoue *et al.* 2003
	Silver haired Bat rabies virus (SHBRV-18)	11923	AY705373	Faber *et al.* 2004
	Rabies virus serotype 1	11928	AY956319	Pfefferle *et al.* 2005*
	NNV-RAB-H	11928	EF437215	Desai *et al.* 2007*
	RB/E3-15	11931	EU182346	Guo *et al.* 2007*
	RV-97	11932	EF542830	Metlin *et al.* 2008
	CTN181	11923	EF64174	Liang *et al.* 2008*
	BD06	11924	EU549783	Zhang *et al.* 2008*
	8764THA	11925	EU293111	Delmas *et al.* 2008
	9001FRA	11922	EU293113	Delmas *et al.* 2008
	9147FRA	11923	EU293115	Delmas *et al.* 2008
	9704ARG	11923	EU293116	Delmas *et al.* 2008
	8743THA	11923	EU293121	Delmas *et al.* 2008
	ERA strain	11931	EF206707	Geue *et al.* 2008
	SAD Bern (Lysvulpen)	11928	EF206708	Geue *et al.* 2008
	SAD B19 (Fuchsoral)	11928	EF206709	Geue *et al.* 2008
	SAD Bern Original Var 1	11930	EF206710	Geue *et al.* 2008
	SAD Bern Original Var 2	11930	EF206711	Geue *et al.* 2008
	SAD Bern Original Var 3	11928	EF206712	Geue *et al.* 2008

(Continued)

Table 35.2 (*Continued*)

Virus	Isolate	Genome length	Accession Number	Reference
	SAD Bern Original Var 4	11928	EF206713	Geue *et al.* 2008
	SAD Bern Original Var 5	11928	EF206714	Geue *et al.* 2008
	SAD P5/88	11928	EF206715	Geue *et al.* 2008
	SAD VA1	11928	EF206716	Geue *et al.* 2008
	SAD1-3670	11931	EF206717	Geue *et al.* 2008
	SAD1-3670, Var 2	11933	EF206718	Geue *et al.* 2008
	SAG2	11928	EF206719	Geue *et al.* 2008
	SAD Beran (Sanafox)	11928	EF206720	Geue *et al.* 2008
	RVV ON-99-2	11923	EU311738	Szanto *et al.* 2008
	SAD B19-4th	11886	EU877067	Beckert *et al.* 2008*
	SAD B19-1st	11886	EU877068	Beckert *et al.* 2008*
	SAD B19-5th	11886	EU877070	Beckert *et al.* 2008*
	SAD B19-10th	11886	EU877071	Beckert *et al.* 2008*
	MRV strain	11869	DQ875050	Zhao *et al.* 2006*
	DRV strain	11863	DQ875051	Zhao *et al.* 2006*
Lagos Bat Virus	8619 NGA isolate	12006	EU293110	Delmas *et al.* 2008
	0406SEN isolate	12016	EU293108	Delmas *et al.* 2008
	KE131 isolate	12017	EU259198	Kuzmin *et al.* 2008a
Mokola Virus	86101RCA	11957	EU293118	Delmas *et al.* 2008
	8600CAM	11949	EU293117	Delmas *et al.* 2008
	Mokola virus complete genome	11940	Y09762	Le Mercier *et al.* 1997
Duvenhage virus	94286SA	11975	EU293120	Delmas *et al.* 2008
	86132SA	11976	EU293119	Delmas *et al.* 2008
European bat lyssavirus-1	RV9	11966	EF157976	Marston *et al.* 2007
	8918FRA	11971	EU293112	Delmas *et al.* 2008
	03002FRA	11966	EU293109	Delmas *et al.* 2008
European bat lyssavirus-2	RV1333	11930	EF157977	Marston *et al.* 2007
	9018HOL	11924	EU293114	Delmas *et al.* 2008
Australian bat lyssavirus	ABLV insectivorous bat isolate	11822	AF081020	Gould *et al.* 2002
	ABLV human isolate	11918	AF418014	Warrilow *et al.* 2002
Aravan virus	Aravan virus	11918	EF614259	Kuzmin *et al.* 2008b
Khujand virus	Khujand virus	11903	EF614261	Kuzmin *et al.* 2008b
Irkut virus	Irkut virus	11980	EF614260	Kuzmin *et al.* 2008b
West Caucasian bat virus	West Caucasian bat virus	12278	EF614258	Kuzmin *et al.* 2008b

* Database submission only

lyssavirus isolates have been sequenced in their entirety with at least one virus from each of the 11 species having been sequenced (Table 35.2).

Serological techniques

Detection of virus-specific antibodies is important when assessing past-exposure to infection, especially when virus can persist in a population. However, infection with rabies virus is invariably fatal and post-infective rabies antibodies are rarely detectable before death so serological techniques are superfluous in assessing the presence of virus within a population. However, the presence of virus-specific antibodies within a vaccinated population can be used to assess vaccination status and is an important tool in both monitoring individuals that receive vaccine as a requirement of their work as well as the movement of vaccinated animals between countries. Serological assays such as the rapid fluorescent focus inhibition test (RFFIT) or the fluorescent antibody virus neutralization (FAVN) test can be used to evaluate seroconversion within a vaccinated population and estimate an individual's potential likelihood of being protected from infection with a wildtype virus. Whilst this situation remains valid for rabies viruses, in recent years a number of other lyssaviruses have been isolated in bats and it seems that, within this host species, the virus may circulate in the absence of clinical disease (Serra-Cobo et al. 2002) and that animals may be serologically positive for having encountered the virus (Brookes et al. 2005; Hayman et al. 2008; Kuzmin et al. 2006).

Both the FAVN and RFFIT are OIE prescribed tests for international travel of companion animals. The principle examined with both tests is the ability of antibodies within suspect serum samples to neutralize virus. Non-neutralized virus is essentially what is detected by fluorescent antibody staining and the dilution at which the test sera was able to completely neutralize virus is quantitated. Standardized reference sera from the OIE and WHO are used as comparators that allow quantitation of virus neutralizing antibody present in samples from animals and humans. These tests are internationally accepted as the 'Gold Standard' for rabies virus serological assessment and are universally accessible. From a logistical point of view, however, use of these tests in areas where the virus remains endemic is problematic as facilities for handling live virus are frequently unavailable. This fact has been the driving force behind attempts to replace these tests with novel methodologies that do not require high security containment facilities and vaccinated staff. Recent progress has been made using novel ELISA techniques that have been shown to be suitable for the detection of rabies virus-specific antibodies in serum samples from companion animals and humans (Cliquet et al. 2004; Servat and Cliquet 2006; Servat et al. 2007; Feyssaguet et al. 2007). Recently, the companion animal ELISAs have been accepted by the OIE as a screening tool or alternative to the FAVN but await approval for use in the EU. Once fully validated these new ELISAs will overcome the problems associated with the current tests and should allow development of local and national diagnostic facilities across the developing world.

Novel diagnostic approaches

Advances in molecular biology have identified lentiviral vectors as suitable expression vectors for antigen generation for a number of viruses. Recently, this approach has been extended to members of the lyssavirus genus whereby glycoprotein genes of different lyssavirus species have been cloned into lentiviral vectors to be co-expressed with HIV/MLV gag-pol and GFP/luciferase in human epithelial cells (Wright et al. 2008). When used in neutralization assays these lyssavirus pseudotype constructs replace the use of live lyssaviruses in these tests and therefore overcome a major obstacle in transferring rabies diagnostic capabilities to the developing world, and the need for high security facilities to undertake serological work becomes redundant. The suitability of lentiviral pseudotyped lyssaviruses is currently being assessed by Rabies Reference Laboratories.

Vaccines and vaccination

Historical perspectives

Rabies vaccines that are virtually 100% effective in preventing disease have been available for over 100 years. The real constraint to

vaccination is the cost of vaccine production and delivery, awareness of the need for pre-exposure vaccination and the lack of both social and economical infrastructures in regions where the threat of human infection is highest and the virus is endemic. Although a number of vaccines developed have been associated with clinical disease and mortalities in vaccinees, primarily using nerve tissue based vaccines (NTVs), millions of lives have been saved through vaccination. Therefore the value of vaccination cannot be underestimated although it is economically prohibitive or even impractical to vaccinate local populations, especially when the regions at risk are some of the poorest populations in the world. Currently, additional cost-effective strategies for use in developing countries are required to mitigate the omnipresent risk to human health.

The first rabies vaccines developed were essentially a crude suspension of desiccated brain material and spinal cord material from an infected animal. Often live virus vaccines were prepared in sheep, rabbit or goat brains. Use of these preparations as a live virus vaccine led to many cases of vaccine associated rabies and understandably people became reluctant to be vaccinated. A further drawback to vaccines generated from infected nervous tissue was the risk of neuroallergenic responses to inoculation. Later, vaccines were inactivated using the techniques of Fermi and Semple, at first using phenol and later beta-proproprioolactone, vastly increasing the safety of the preparations (Bugyaki et al. 1959). As far back as 1973 the WHO recommended that the use of crude nerve tissue based vaccines be stopped, however, recent publications suggest that these phenol inactivated preparations may still being used in some of the poorest parts of the world where the disease remains endemic (Ayele et al. 2001; Parviz et al. 2004).

In some parts of the world vaccines of crude nervous tissue origin have now been replaced by vaccines made through growth of virus in the brains of suckling mice. These vaccines are prepared using mice aged less than 1 day to reduce the level of potential encephalitogenic substances and were shown to be considerably safer, notably reducing the number of cases of neuroallergenic side effects seen post-vaccination (Fuenzalida and Palacios 1955). However, crude nerve tissue based vaccines are thought to still be used extensively across Latin America, Africa and Asia (Briggs and Hanlon 2007). Vaccine preparations were again improved with the generation of vaccines in embryonated eggs. Vaccines like the duck embryo vaccine were used for almost 20 years across Europe and North America. Specific responses generated to the duck embryo vaccine were, however, relatively poor and low immunogenicity deemed that it required 14 to 20 doses before suitable protection was conferred to the vaccinee and thus its production was abandoned (Shaul et al. 1969; Plotkin 1980).

Current human rabies vaccines

Whilst it is believed that a number of the early NTVs and embryo based vaccines are still being used in some of the poorest parts of the developing world, modern tissue culture derived vaccines have largely replaced the use of these potentially dangerous early vaccines. The breakthrough came in the early 1960s with the development of the Human Diploid Cell Vaccine (HDCV) (Wiktor et al. 1964). This vaccine has no doubt saved millions of lives and was pushed into the global spotlight through being used in a WHO vaccine 'field-trial' to treat humans that had suffered severe bite wounds from rabid wolves (Bahmanyar et al. 1976). The ability of the HDCV to generate highly protective virus neutralizing antibody responses made it the 'vaccine of choice' for a number of years but very high production costs and low virus yield made the vaccine unaffordable in the parts of the world that needed it most.

With production costs being a pre-eminent consideration of use, further tissue culture based vaccines have been generated in an attempt to make pre-exposure vaccination affordable to the developing world, especially in regions where people live on less than US$1 per day. More recent vaccines include purified chick embryo cell vaccine (PCECV) and purified Vero rabies vaccine (PVRV). These vaccines have successfully replaced the use of controversial NTVs in several areas where the cost of administering HDCV is unaffordable, such as across Thailand. Despite their safety and antigenicity, there still remains a potential problem with successive booster injections where, as with HDCV vaccination, occasionally allergic responses, presumably to the beta-propriolactone used to inactivate the virus, have been reported. It has been suggested that individuals who have experienced such reactions should receive no further vaccination with these vaccines unless they are actually exposed to rabies virus (Nicholson 1990). PVRV vaccine is currently licensed across much of the globe including much of Europe and Latin America where it is replacing use of the suckling mouse brain vaccine that has been in use since the 1950s. However, at the global level it is recognized that several countries are still vaccinating individuals with out-dated vaccine types. Bangladesh, the Union of Myanmar, Pakistan, Peru, and Argentina have all still to convert to cell-culture based vaccines with Pakistan still reportedly using NTVs (Burki 2008). In 2008, India announced their explicit intention to phase-out and halt the use of NTVs and to replace their use with tissue-culture based vaccines for human use.

Whilst modern technological advances seek to improve vaccines, those currently available and recommended by the WHO are considered to be safe, highly immunogenic and are being used successfully across the globe (Quiambo et al. 2000; Jones et al. 2001).

Human pre-exposure immunization

The value of pre-exposure immunization is very high. However, in parts of the world where either modern, safe vaccines are not available or where medical professionals lack awareness of the current tools available to protect local populations, significant numbers of individuals continue to die annually from the disease, a large percentage of which, tragically are children. In the developed world, where resources are available to enable vaccination, pre-exposure immunization has saved many lives. It is clear that all individuals that either work with the virus or who may come into contact with infected animals (especially where the virus remains endemic) must be vaccinated.

Current recommended immunization schedules vary depending on the vaccine being used and the severity of risk. For scientists working with the viruses, it is essential that antibody titre is measured post-immunization and that an antibody titre of at least 0.5IU/ml is achieved (OIE 2004; WHO 1996). If the antibody titre of someone working routinely with the virus falls below this level then a booster injection is required although generally, boosters or antibody tests are recommended every three to five years for other risk groups such as bat workers. The discovery of a number of novel lyssaviruses, often from bat species, has prompted studies into the protection afforded by current rabies vaccines to these lyssaviruses. Whilst protection studies have been undertaken, exact protective titres are unknown (discussed further below). Recent studies using recombinant vaccinia viruses encoding the glycoprotein genes of rabies virus, Mokola virus and West Caucasian Bat Virus, either expressed individually or in pairs have shown promise as potential multivalent vaccines (Weyer et al. 2007). Development of human vaccines that protect against lyssaviruses as well as classical rabies strains are currently being developed as alternatives that could confer a cross protective response in the vaccinee (Nel 2005; Hanlon et al. 2005).

Human post exposure prophylaxis

The key to post exposure prophylaxis (PEP) following a potential transmission of lyssaviruses to an individual is timing. The risk assessment of a potential exposure to rabies and lyssaviruses must be conducted urgently. PEP should be administered rapidly following exposure. Supplies of human and equine rabies immunoglobulin are expensive, and relatively speaking in short supply, and are therefore generally given in high risk exposures. Immunoglobulins used consist of either human or equine serum that contains neutralizing antibodies directed to discrete epitopes on the rabies virus. These serum, when administered rapidly, provides passive rabies virus neutralizing antibody during the two to three day post infection 'window' where the immune system has not yet responded to the inactivated virus vaccine. As well as neutralizing infectious virus particles it is thought that RIG may also participate in the elimination of infected cells by antibody-dependent cellular cytotoxicity. In the first instance, as much RIG as is possible should be applied to the wound and any exposed mucus membranes surrounding the wound. Guideline doses are 20 IU RIG per kg bodyweight of human RIG or 40 IU RIG per kg if equine RIG is used. Any remaining RIG should be injected intramuscularly into the area around the wound site (WHO 2005). Several different regimens currently exist for the administration of RIG.

Alongside PEP, and always prior to it being administered, wound care is the principal factor that will greatly influence the possibility of survival from infection. The wound should be thoroughly washed immediately with soap and water or detergent and then, if available, it is recommended that either 70% ethanol or an aqueous solution of iodine should be used to further sterilize the affected area (WHO 2005). This immediate wound treatment serves to remove or inactivate infectious virus particles (and/or other potential pathogens) from the site before they have an opportunity to replicate or to reach the nerve endings. Importantly, the wound must never be sutured as blood flow from the wound allows for additional virus removal from the bite site.

Despite the effectiveness of PEP in practice it is rarely administered, and it is estimated that only 5% of cases actually receive PEP as recommended by the WHO. This failure is generally due to lack of availability, which is intrinsically linked to the cost of prophylactic treatment and which often far outweighs the resources available.

At the same time a suitable vaccine, usually whatever vaccine is available, should be inoculated but at a site distant to the region treated with RIG to avoid the vaccine being neutralized by complexing with the RIG. Several approaches to post exposure vaccination are used across the globe (reviewed in Briggs and Mahendra 2007). There are four basic vaccination regimens recommended for use as PEP with cell culture based rabies vaccines and their administration differs across the globe. Two intramuscular and two intradermal regimens currently exist. However, the intramuscular Essen 'four-dose' regimen is most often applied across North America and Europe (WHO 2005). Some European countries use the 'Zagreb' or '2-1-1' regimen which reduces the number of doses required compared to the Essen regimen. Intradermal vaccination regimens have been shown to be effective, although drawbacks include requirement of storage at 2–8°C post reconstitution meaning that it is often not cost effective to treat one or two individuals with these preparations as the reconstituted batch may expire. Furthermore, intradermal vaccination requires highly skilled staff. Two intradermal regimes currently exist, the 'Thai red cross' and the 'Eight site' regimen (Warrell 2008; WHO 2005). Vaccination regimens as PEP, when applied are very effective but require concomitant application of RIG. Human treatment failures where PEP has been used can generally be attributed to the incorrect PEP as the short incubation period linked to bite of the head and neck. (Arya 1999; Sriaroon *et al.* 2003; Parviz *et al.* 2004). However, the effectiveness of PEP, when administered properly, cannot be overstated.

Current rabies vaccines for use with domesticated and wild animals

With the biggest threat of infection coming from rabid dogs, the first vaccines were tested extensively in canines by Pasteur and those that followed up his initial research (Bunn 1991). Nerve tissue vaccines and vaccines developed subsequently derived through passage in embryonic chicken eggs were all developed but often either caused post-vaccinal allergic reactions that could kill the vaccinee or, with egg derived vaccines, those that were effective in adult dogs, often caused rabies in younger dogs, cats and cattle (Bunn *et al.* 1991).

Live virus vaccines were also developed and are still used in parts of the world where safer but more costly vaccines are unavailable. Passage of Pasteur's 'fixed' virus strain was continued for many years by passage in rabbit spinal cord material and mice and its common descendant is what we now term the 'Challenge virus strain' (CVS). CVS, after repeated passage in baby hamster kidney cells (BHKs) was denoted CVS-11 and was used extensively as a modified live virus vaccine in dogs although its use was confined to dogs due to concerns about safety in other animals. A number of other cell culture derived modified live vaccines have been generated using ERA, SAD and CEO strains that are used in different parts of the world (reviewed in Reculard 1996).

Genetically engineered vaccines have also been developed and used widely, in attempts to control rabies in wildlife species. Oral vaccines based on vaccinia virus expressing rabies virus glycoprotein were first produced in the early 1980s (Kieny *et al.* 1984; Pastoret *et al.* 1988). This new type of vaccine overcame fears surrounding the use of live attenuated virus vaccines and in various forms has been applied with considerable success. In 1995, after trials both in the USA and France, an oral vaccine was licensed for use against rabies in wildlife and has been successfully used to contain and eliminate rabies across much of Canada and the USA (Krebs *et al.* 2005; Slate *et al.* 2005). Oral vaccine preparations are constantly being optimized in an attempt to eliminate the virus from areas where it continues to pose a threat to the human population (Slate *et al.* 2005; Cross *et al.* 2007).

New vaccines based on using other viruses as vectors for glycoprotein sequence include those based on canarypox virus, such as the combination rabies vaccine currently licensed in the USA (Anon 2006) and a recombinant adenovirus-vectored vaccines that is showing promise as a potential canine rabies virus vaccine (Tims *et al.* 2000; Hu *et al.* 2006, 2007).

Future rabies vaccine strategies

Unfortunately, despite the number of deaths annually attributed to lyssavirus infection and the recognition that this number is likely to be vastly underestimated, rabies is not considered a priority by many governments and pharmaceutical companies whose input would be needed to try and combat the disease on a global level. The discovery of a number of novel lyssaviruses that are genetically related to classical rabies virus and are important human pathogens has increased the profile of these viruses. However, it is clear that even this emerging threat will do little to drive investment into new generation vaccines that may be needed to prevent countless further deaths. Improved oral vaccines, which are cheaper to produce and with improved bait specificity may help the current situation. Such vaccines need to be applied across much of Africa and Asia where the virus remains endemic in both domestic and wild populations (Cross *et al.* 2007). Of the few studies currently underway, those incorporating cheaper alternatives to the tools currently available such as generating vaccines in plants look promising (Girard *et al.* 2006; Lodmell *et al.* 2006; Yusibov *et al.* 2002).

Alternatives to RIG as post exposure prophylaxis are also currently being explored to overcome the expense that precludes the uses of RIG across much of the developing world. Currently, no effective antiviral strategies to combat infection with rabies or rabies-related lyssaviruses exist. Recent studies with a number of different negative strand RNA viruses have suggested that silencing virus-specific gene expression using RNA interference (RNAi) molecules to disrupt viral replication may be an effective measure in instances where antiviral agents are not available.

RNAi is the mechanism by which mRNA degradation is induced by intracellular double-stranded RNA in a targeted sequence-specific manner. This pathway is thought to be an evolutionary mechanism for protecting the host and its genome against viruses and rogue genetic elements that use double-stranded RNA (dsRNA) in their life cycles. Until recently, this intracellular process was unknown within the scientific community as the response is masked by the cellular non-sequence specific responses to generation of dsRNA moieties greater than 30 nucleotides in length that triggers the interferon pathway (Elbashir *et al.* 2001). The observation that RNAi is able to silence gene expression in a sequence specific manner has driven the application of this technology to studies with a number of viral pathogens. RNAi is a powerful tool amenable to the development of anti-viral drugs. Recent advances with this technology have shown that siRNA molecules tagged to a peptide generated from a region of the rabies glycoprotein that is known to bind acetylcholine are able to cross the blood brain barrier and inhibit viral replication in the brain (Kumar *et al.* 2007). Whilst such studies offer exciting possibilities for antiviral treatment through transvascular delivery of molecules to the CNS, a post exposure prophylaxis that can be administered in and around the 'bite site' is also of huge importance.

Global epidemiology of rabies and lyssaviruses

Rabies in Europe

The EU has made huge steps forward into the elimination of terrestrial rabies from a number of its member states over the last 20 years (OIE 2005). However, the circulation of the virus in both fox and raccoon-dog populations continues to be a major threat to domestic dog populations and hence to human health.

Historically, the disappearance of terrestrial rabies from central Europe during the first half of the twentieth century was attributed to a reduction in the number of stray animals across the continent as well as the disappearance of wolf populations through hunting and human incursion into wolf territory. This left great swathes of Central Europe largely free of rabies throughout the 1900s although wild carnivore species had become infected and so the disease remained. The disease re-emerged across much of Europe through the establishment of infection within the red fox population which through the 1940s spread rabies across the Russian-Polish border then over the following four decades through much of the rest of Europe. Rabies infection within domestic dog populations has now been controlled, largely through oral vaccination and quarantine rules set in place throughout the 1970s although the virus still exists in wildlife species, principally the red fox (*Vulpes vulpes*) and the raccoon dog (*Nyctereutes procynonoides*) (Steck and Wandeler 1980; Johnson *et al.* 2003b). Whilst the fox population has long been defined as a reservoir, it is still not clear whether the raccoon-dog population is a distinct reservoir or a spillover host. Rabies infection of other species include stoats, weasels, deer, water voles, hedgehogs, badgers, voles, stone martens and free-roaming cats, the latter of which is believed to play an important part in the epidemiology of the virus. The implications of infection within such populations are unclear as molecular and serological data for cases within these species are few.

The UK has a long history of terrestrial rabies although through the latter half of the nineteenth century and the start of the twentieth century the disease was rarely reported in wildlife species and terrestrial rabies was, through animal destruction and quarantine, finally eliminated in 1922 (Fooks *et al.* 2004). As an island nation, the UK was then able to, through very strict import regulations including the quarantine of imported dogs and cats, maintain its rabies free status. However, when cases have occurred in quarantine, such as recently with the importation of infected puppies from Sri Lanka, the disease has been identified and infected animals eliminated with no further risk of disease (Fooks *et al.* 2008).

The introduction in 1971 of vaccination of dogs and cats on arrival in quarantine has resulted in the successful maintenance of a rabies free status. The last indigenously acquired human rabies (rabies species) case occurred in Wales in 1902 with the last case of indigenous terrestrial rabies in 1922. However, since 1946 a further 25 human deaths have been recorded in the UK, all of which were the result of infection transmitted to individuals during travel abroad (Johnson *et al.* 2005; Banyard *et al.* 2010) most recently that of a young woman returning from South Africa having been previously bitten by a rabid dog (Hunter *et al.* 2010).

A further threat of rabies to the European Union comes from the identification of rabies-like viruses in the endogenous bat populations across Europe. The presence of bat rabies poses a low but serious threat to human health although infections have been reported. Four human fatalities have been attributed to EBLV infection: in Russia and the Ukraine (EBLV-1); in Finland and the UK (EBLV-2) (Lumio *et al.* 1988; King 1991; Selimov *et al.* 1989; Fooks *et al.* 2003). Furthermore, CST events into other species including Danish sheep (*Ovis aries*) and a stone marten (*Martes foina*) in Germany have also been reported although these events have only been reported for EBLV-1 (Muller *et al.* 2004; Stougaard and Ammendrup 1998; Tjornehoj *et al.* 2006) (Table 35.3). Experimentally, sheep have also been shown to be susceptible to EBLV-2 infection (Brookes *et al.* 2007). The viruses identified as being the causative agents of bats rabies within Europe were originally characterized through monoclonal antibody typing as being Duvenhage-like viruses and were grouped into serotype 4. However, more modern genetic characterization has enabled a distinction between viruses isolated and they are now defined as European Bat Lyssaviruses-1 and -2 (EBLV 1 and 2), however, both species are genetically distinct. The reservoirs for these viruses have been identified as principally being *Eptesicus serotinus* for EBLV-1 and both *Myotis dasycneme* and *Myotis daubentonii* for EBLV-2 although for both viruses infection of other bat species has been reported (Schneider and Cox 1994). Recently, in 2002 a bat conservationist died in Scotland following CST from a Daubenton's bat. The virus was characterized and typed as EBLV-2 (Fooks *et al.* 2003). Furthermore, in August 2007 a Daubenton's bat in Germany was

Table 35.3 CST cases of EBLVs to non-bat species (including humans)

Year	Country	Species affected	Virus (V) or serological (S) detection	EBLV-1 / EBLV-2 or Unknown (U)	References
1977	Ukraine	Human	V	U	Rabies Bulletin Europe, 1986
1985	Russia	Human	V	EBLV-1	Selimov *et al.* 1989; Bourhy *et al.* 1992
1985	Finland	Human	V	EBLV-2	Lumio *et al.* 1986; Roine *et al.* 1988
1998	Denmark	Sheep	V	EBLV-1	Stougaard and Ammendrup, 1998
2001	Germany	Stone marten	V	EBLV-1	Muller *et al.* 2004
2002	Denmark	Sheep	V	EBLV-1	Ronsholt, 2002
2002	Scotland	Human	V	EBLV-2	Fooks *et al.* 2003b
2002	Ukraine	Human	V	U	Botvinkin *et al.* 2006
2004	Denmark	Cat	S	EBLV-1	Tjornehoj *et al.* 2004

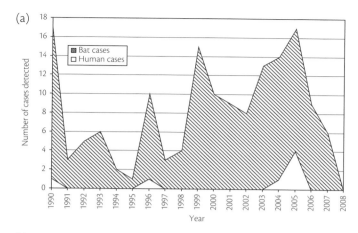

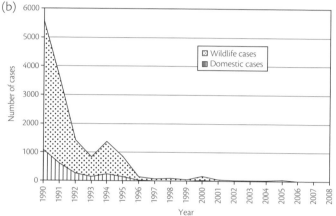

Fig. 35.1(a) Increased detection of bat rabies in Germany,1990–2008
1(b) Decline in terrestrial rabies across Germany, 1990–2008. Data sourced from www.who-rabies-bulletin.org

reported to be harbouring EBLV-2, the first isolation of the virus in this country suggesting that these viruses may have a broader geographical range than originally thought (Fig. 35.1a) (Muller *et al.* 2007; Freuling *et al.* 2008).

Oral vaccination campaigns in wildlife species have done much to reduce the incidence of rabies across Western Europe, with the decline of rabies cases in Germany giving a strong indication of the reduction in cases across the remainder of countries following vaccination programmes (Fig. 35.1b) (Brouchier *et al.* 1991). However, rabies virus still exists in regions of Eastern Europe including the Russian Federation and Belarus. Currently rabies infection in Europe is seen, from a geographical perspective, as being divided into two areas. If a line is drawn between the Baltic Sea down to the Black Sea it is clear that any future cases of rabies virus infection are more likely to occur to the east of this defined boundary, although incursions may occur where rabies still exists within areas along the boundary line such as in Turkey (Johnson *et al.* 2006b). To the East of this boundary are some of the poorest regions of Europe including the Baltic States where high numbers of rabies cases have been reported. The prevalence of the raccoon dog across parts of north-eastern Europe perpetuates the threat of the virus in these areas.

Clearly, within these areas rabies infection is not the only threat to human health and what financial resources exist may well be allocated to issues deemed to be of higher priority. New strategies are required to counter this continuing threat and the EU must focus on generating coordinated efforts between the affected countries to try and maximize the cost effectiveness of a strategy and that attempts to finally free Europe from this preventable disease. Rabies cases reported across Europe over the last decade are detailed in Fig. 35.2.

Rabies in Asia

Rabies infection in Asia continues to be vastly underreported for a wide variety of reasons; many countries do not have the infrastructure or the necessary veterinary resources to actively report cases of the disease, other regions suffer the huge problem of unknown stray dog populations that harbour the disease whilst tragically, many infected individuals are kept at home, often left to suffer, with no medical attention or PEP being available. Much of the information reported on the incidence of rabies across Central Asia comes from a small number of countries that are either willing and/or able to report such data to the WHO and the OIE with only 40% of the territory of central Asia reporting data. Again, dogs and cats are the primary domestic species affected with foxes being the most affected wildlife species.

Canine rabies of both domestic and wild populations exists across much of Asia with Afghanistan, Bangladesh, Cambodia, China, India, Indonesia, Laos, the Middle East, Nepal, Pakistan, the Philippines, Sri Lanka, most of the former Soviet Republics, Thailand, and Vietnam being endemic for canine rabies. Canine rabies therefore is the biggest threat to human health.

Across India alone, it is estimated that 20,000 people die each year as a result of canine rabies, just under two thirds of the estimated number of human lives lost to the disease annually across the whole of the Asian continent (Pradhan *et al.* 2008). In India, dogs remain as both the main reservoir for the virus and the primary transmitter to the human population, with a large proportion of cases involving children under 14 years of age. Current efforts at eliminating rabies from India are centered around

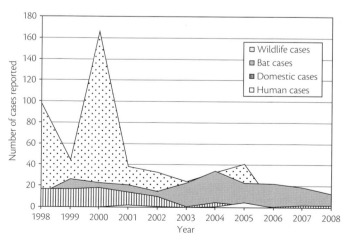

Fig. 35.2 Rabies cases across Western Europe, 1998–2008. Data sourced from www.who-rabies-bulletin.org

vaccine campaigns for domesticated dogs as well as those deemed to belong to a community (those that are not individually owned but are fed waste food and therefore continually return to a local area to be fed) and the use of oral vaccines present in bait for vaccination of wild canine populations.

In Eastern Asia, studies have shown that, the dog is the most reported reservoir. In Thailand, transmission from dogs to the human population accounts for 70–95% of rabies deaths (Kasempimolporn *et al.* 2008). Dog owners who fail to get their pets vaccinated cause additional problems in controlling rabies in domestic animals across much of Asia. Even if facilities exist for vaccination, the cost and general ignorance of the importance of such actions often leads to animals not being vaccinated. Recent studies in southern Asia have suggested through accumulated history records that as many as 78% of owned domestic dogs were not vaccinated against rabies (Singh and Sandhu 2008).

The steady increase in cases of rabies across China has also provoked public fears of the disease (Hu *et al.* 2008a). A recent study has shown that since the start of the new millennium, the incidence of rabies in southern and south western territories of China has risen dramatically (Fig. 35.3). Four defined regions have been found to be endemic for the virus and the necessary resources and infrastructure, as well as ample supply of human vaccine, are lacking in these areas. Again, as seen globally, the victims of the disease are mainly children or teenagers that have been bitten by a rabid dog and again, improper wound treatment, lack of PEP and short supplies of rabies immunoglobulin have meant that fatalities have been greater than expected. To counter this increase in cases, both local and national authorities need to act to raise awareness and provide the necessary tools to protect those at risk as well as those exposed using conventional PEP regimens (Si *et al.* 2008, Tang *et al.* 2005; Hu *et al.* 2008a).

Whilst dogs represent the greatest risk of infection with rabies across much of Asia, in the Middle East foxes, jackals and wolves also constitute important wildlife reservoirs. The red fox and the golden jackal are considered the most problematic carnivores spreading rabies virus in the Middle East although minor epidemiological roles are also thought to be played by other carnivorous mammals such as the grey wolf, the mongoose and the badger (Seimenis 2008). Several countries across the Middle East, including Iran, Israel, Oman, Saudi Arabia, Turkey, and Yemen, are experiencing an increase in cases of rabies in wildlife species with the red fox and the golden jackal carrying the greatest burden of disease (Vos 2004).

Despite the presence of bat rabies across much of Europe and the Americas, bat rabies is rarely reported from Asia, although it should be noted that bats are not generally examined unless captured following human exposure. However, a number of unclassified viruses (Aravan, West Caucasian Bat Virus, Khujand, and Irkut virus) have been isolated in and around the geopolitical areas that separates Europe, the Middle East and Asia (Arai *et al.* 2003; Kuzmin *et al.* 2003, 2005).

Rabies in Africa

Rabies has been present across much of Africa for centuries, although its history prior to 1900 is fragmentary and largely anecdotal. Characterization of viruses from Africa remains problematic due to the lack of economic infrastructure and, as a result, well equipped laboratories. Indeed, in sub-Saharan Africa, disease

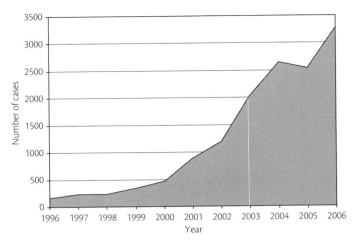

Fig. 35.3 Rabies cases in China, 1996–2006.

recognition only followed the establishment of diagnostic laboratories at the turn of the twentieth century. The origins of rabies in Africa are still questioned. However, modern phylogenetic analyses have defined a number of rabies species variants as being members of a 'cosmopolitan lineage'. This lineage includes isolates that, from molecular data are genetically related, but have been isolated from all corners of the globe. It has been suggested that that progenitors of the strains classified within this lineage were distributed widely across the globe during colonial times, giving the possibility that Europe may have served as a source of rabies for the rest of the world. Current phylogenetic analysis shows that since this period, isolates now cluster into a number of distinct clades based on geographic origin (Nadin-Davis and Bingham 2004). However, other studies suggest that the virus may have originally evolved in West Africa (Swanepoel *et al.* 1993). This hypothesis is supported by the presence of three of the four serotypes and the historical occurrence of rabies viruses in dogs which are less virulent than conventional street viruses across this region (Blancou 1988). However, it may be that rabies was introduced to West Africa some time after AD 1500 by Europeans, since nucleotide sequencing has shown similarities between European, New World, and some West African isolates (Smith and Seidel 1993). Although it is unlikely to have been the first incidence of rabies in southern Africa, the first irrefutable diagnosis was made in 1893 during an epizootic involving dogs, cats, and domestic ruminants in the vicinity of Port Elizabeth on the south east coast of South Africa (Van Sittert 2003).

The introduction of modern molecular methods and surveillance mechanisms has led to a better understanding of the problems faced across Africa (Bouhry *et al.* 2008). Today, molecular tools have divided African isolates into different phylogenetic clusters based on similarities and differences at the nucleotide level. Three main African clades are now defined that include viruses that cluster closely with one another, either in line with geographical location or associated with the nature of the host from which the viral genomic material was derived. One cluster, referred to as 'Africa 1' (Kissi *et al.* 1995) or 'Africa CD1' (Nadin-Davis *et al.* 2002) includes viruses that seem adapted to both domestic and wild members of the *Canidae* that are found widely distributed throughout Africa.

This virus lineage, however, contains two distinct clusters. Viruses from clade 1 or 'Africa 1a' have been found in Algeria, Ethiopia, Gabon, Madagascar, Morocco, Tunisia, and the Sudan (Johnson *et al.* 2004a); Clade 1b or Africa 1b contains isolates from the Central African Republic, Kenya, Mozambique, Namibia, Tanzania, Zaire, Zambia, Zimbabwe, and South Africa (Kissi *et al.* 1995; Sabeta *et al.* 2003; Mansfield *et al.* 2006a; Ngoepe *et al.* 2009).

Isolates from dog populations from West Africa form another clade, Africa 2, whilst another distinct clade, 'Africa 3' represents viruses that are circulating within mongoose populations in southern African countries including South Africa, Botswana and Zimbabwe (Johnson *et al.* 2004b). Apart from domestic dogs and cats, representatives of at least 30 different species belonging to all five families of carnivore native to southern Africa have been diagnosed with rabies (Thomson and Meredith 1993). Some species, notably the side striped jackal (*Canis adustus*), the yellow mongoose (*Cynictis penicillata*) (Nel and Rupprecht 2007), and the bat-eared fox (*Otocyon megalotis*) (Sabeta *et al.* 2007) seem to be maintaining different biotypes of the virus. Further investigation of these virus groups is needed to determine if the strong geographical segregation of these viruses truly reflects host restriction or whether this viral lineage may extend into other, as yet undefined, parts of Africa (Nel 1993; Nel and Rupprecht 2007).

Despite technological advances, the continued lack of adequately equipped regional laboratories and surveillance systems in Africa make the reporting of rabies cases, be it of human or animal occurrence, problematic. The proportion of rabies mortalities on a global scale that were reported to WHO in 1999 suggested that African cases of rabies made up only 3% of the worldwide incidence (Knobel *et al.* 2005). Continued political and economic instability across much of Africa has meant that this situation is showing few signs of improving and whilst some countries have improved capabilities, others still have no reporting or diagnostic capacity. With the domestic dog still considered to be the principal reservoir of rabies (WHO 2004), dog-associated rabies has continued to increase throughout sub-Saharan Africa. In this tropical zone, humans and animals are more widely distributed than in North Africa, and there has been a greater tendency for epidemics of dog rabies to spread over large areas and for the disease to be observed in both domestic and wild vertebrates (Blancou 1988; Nel and Rupprecht 2007). Estimates of the incidence of human rabies across Africa further suggest that the problem is much greater than previously thought. In urban and rural areas of Africa, current overall estimates of rabies incidence are 2.0 and 3.6 persons per 10^5 persons, respectively. These values highlight a shortfall in the WHO estimates of 35,000 to 50,000 rabies human mortalities globally and underpin the need for better diagnostic capabilities, reporting and surveillance within some of the poorest regions of the world.

From a conservation standpoint, rabies virus currently threatens several endangered species across the African continent. As human habitation has expanded, canine rabies has spread to wildlife species and some already endangered canids, such as the African wild dogs (*Lycaon Pictus*), the Ethiopian wolf (*Canis simensis*) and spotted hyenas (*Crocuta crocuta*) (Gascoyne *et al.* 1993) act as vectors for the disease. Certainly, the existence of Ethiopian wolves has been put under threat from the introduction of the virus, probably through the fox population (Sillero-Zubiri *et al.* 1996; Randall *et al.* 2004; Knobel *et al.* 2008).

More recently, a number of lyssaviruses of African origin have been described. Isolates of Lagos Bat virus, classified within the lyssavirus species 2, have been recovered from various countries across the African continent (Hayman *et al.* 2008; Kuzmin *et al.* 2008). These viruses, although few in number, show a high degree of genetic diversity with isolates from different regions varying (Bourhy *et al.* 1993; Johnson *et al.* 2002b; Nadin-Davis *et al.* 2002; Markotter *et al.* 2008a). Members of species 3, the Mokola viruses (MOKVs) have also been detected in a number of African countries although the majority of isolates characterized so far have been from South Africa and Zimbabwe (Nel *et al.* 2000; Markotter *et al.* 2008b). One MOKV isolate from Nigeria, West Africa, was found to be, on the limited genetic data available, distinct from the remaining isolates (Nadin-Davis *et al.* 2002; Markotter *et al.* 2008b). As with the MOKVs, members of the lyssavirus species 4, Duvenhage virus (DUVV) isolates are generally reported from South Africa and Zimbabwe. Isolates have been made from both humans and bats (Amenugal *et al.* 1997; Badrane *et al.* 2001; Johnson *et al.* 2002b; Nadin-Davis *et al.* 2002).

Rabies in the Americas

The Americas are generally divided into three major geographical areas encompassing a total of 48 defined countries, island nations and territories. North America includes the US of America and Canada; Central America includes all the mainland countries as well as the island nations of the Caribbean; South America, or Latin America includes some of the most densely populated countries of the Americas, south of Central America.

North America

The development of oral vaccine strategies to prevent sylvatic rabies in the mid 1960s and their application across much of North America greatly reduced the incidence of terrestrial rabies (Krebs *et al.* 2003). Prior to this rabies cases were rarely reported in Canada throughout the start of twentieth century until the 1940s when rabies in foxes spread into Canada causing an increase in incidence. Skunks have also played a role in the maintenance of rabies in Canada especially through the 1950s and 1960s. However, the result of extensive oral vaccination in the 1960s lead to a notable decrease in cases and over the last 15 years continued vaccination policies have meant that very few cases of rabies have been reported from Canada (Belotto *et al.* 2005).

A similar picture has been seen across the USA. Historically, the USA has a long association with rabies cases and between 1940 and 1950 over 100,000 cases were reported. Again, in the 1960s, mass vaccination campaigns and the use of oral vaccines hugely reduced the incidence of rabies in the canine population. Whilst the USA is now free of canine rabies, the incidence of rabies in wildlife species seems to be increasing across much of the country. Whilst the infection of wildlife species across the US remains a threat to the human population, surprisingly few human cases are reported annually with only four cases across the USA being reported between 2006 and the end of 2007 (Blanton *et al.* 2008).

The rabies situation in wildlife in the USA is complicated due to the presence of different terrestrial vector species as well as the presence of several bat species that harbour species 1 virus. Furthermore cases of transmission from bats to humans are often cryptic, with the interaction between infected animal and exposed individual often going unnoticed (Messenger *et al.* 2002). Most frequently reported terrestrial wildlife cases across the USA come from three different vector species; foxes, raccoons and skunks. Despite the complexity of the situation, these terrestrial species do seem to be limited in their distribution and so dispersal of virus variants may be described according to their vector species within geographically defined locations. To this end, raccoons (*Procyon lotor*) act as a major reservoir of rabies, predominantly across much of eastern US (Childs *et al.* 2001). Fox rabies exists within distinct fox populations; the red fox (*Vulpes vulpes*) and the grey fox (*Urocyon cineroargenteus*) and the Arctic fox (*Alopex lagopus*). Grey foxes maintain rabies within geographically limited populations in Arizona and Texas although oral vaccination campaigns have greatly reduced the number of fox cases reported from Texas (Sidwa *et al.* 2005). Red and Arctic fox populations maintain the virus in Alaska and can also cause incursions of disease in Canada although, again, oral vaccination programs have greatly reduced case numbers (MacInnes *et al.* 2001; Mansfield *et al.* 2006b). Rabies associated with skunks (*Mephitis mephitis, Spilogale putorius*) covers much of north central and south central USA with almost 1,500 reported cases in 2007 (Blanton *et al.* 2008).

Whilst rabies virus attributed to the infection of specific species is clearly defined, spillover into other wildlife species occurs but rarely initiates a new cycle of maintenance of virus within the new host. Transmission between animals of the same species maintains the levels of circulating virus and at the regional level may lead to continued circulation of a virus variant within a local population for decades (Blanton *et al.* 2008; Childs *et al.* 2001). The transmission of rabies virus from bats to both the human population and wildlife populations has also been reported. Historically, transmission has occurred from insectivorous bats such as the Yellow Bat (*Lasiurus intermedius*) and the Hoary bat (*Lasiurus cinereus*) (Brass 1994). The current distribution of bats species across much of the US as well as the ability for unchecked movement of bat populations makes tracking the virus difficult. Occasionally, spillover of bat variants strains of rabies occurs into wildlife species, most recently documented through the transmission from big brown bats (*Eptesicus fuscus*) to skunks in Arizona in 2001. This CST event resulted in rabies outbreaks within the skunk population in an area of Arizona that had been previously free of rabies virus infection (Leslie *et al.* 2006). Such transmission events rarely result in cycling of the bat-variant virus within the infected terrestrial population although one report suggests the probable circulation of a bat variant of rabies virus in foxes in Canada (Daoust *et al.* 1996). In this instance, it was speculated that some degree of intraspecific transmission passed the virus from bats into foxes and that adaptation of bat rabies to enable circulation within foxes may occur (Daoust *et al.* 1996).

Central and South America

Rabies remains a serious economic problem as well as being a threat to human health across much of Central and South America. In recent years there has been a sharp decrease in the number of canine cases, as a result of several mass vaccination campaigns implemented across several of the worse affected countries. Furthermore, perhaps directly linked to the reduction seen in cases of canine rabies, the number of human cases has also decreased notably although an increase in availability and application of PEP must also have assisted in reducing human fatalities.

Much of the successes seen in the reduction of cases has come since the formation of the 'Plan of Action for the Elimination of Urban Rabies from the Principal Cities of Latin America' organized by the Pan American Health Organization (PAHO). As a result, over the past 20 years an almost 90% decrease in the number of dog and human cases has been observed across the regions most greatly affected, mainly in the Spanish speaking Caribbean countries and across Latin America. In Mexico, mass parenteral vaccination of dogs over a fifteen year period resulted in more than 150 million vaccine doses being administered between 1990 and 2005. The result of this targeted campaign using modern cell culture based vaccines has been the elimination of human rabies and a 43 fold reduction in canine rabies cases across the country (Lucas *et al.* 2008). Rabies from wildlife reservoirs continues, however, to be a problem across much of Central and South America with a number of species being implicated in transmission but with the greatest number of reports involving infections of wildlife such as raccoon rabies, skunk rabies and cases involving cattle and bats (Fig. 35.4). From these data, however, it is worth emphasizing that within certain geographical regions cases linked to different wildlife species predominate with high numbers of cases of rabies in cattle and horses being reported in Brazil; cases of rabies involving skunks, raccoons and bat species are mainly reported from the USA and the problem of rabies in vampire bats being restricted to Central and South America (Belotto *et al.* 2005).

Future prospects for prevention and control

Historically, attempts to control rabies where outbreaks occur have been through slaughter, quarantine and mass vaccination of infected animals. Although such actions are still practiced, more modern approaches involving rapid identification of the source of infection, establishment of containment zones where possible and the application of oral vaccination strategies to combat further possible cases are implemented instead. In all cases a rapid, strategic plan must be implemented to minimize the potential of further spread of disease within wildlife and the likelihood of transmission to the human population. In island nations, rabies-free status is relatively easy to maintain through strict importation and quarantine programs but these must be successfully enforced to

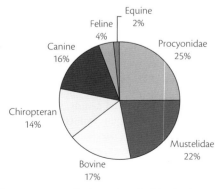

Fig. 35.4 Rabies cases reported in domestic and wild animals across the Americas (1993–2002). Adapted from Belotto *et al.*, 2005.

prevent reintroduction of the virus. Quarantine allows the animals to be assessed over a period of time within which they may develop obvious symptoms of disease. A number of island nations have successfully used quarantine to maintain a rabies-free status including Australia, New Zealand, Hawaii, Sweden, and the UK. However, recent events in a number of these countries have tested the effectiveness of the quarantine procedures in place but have successfully prevented reintroduction of the virus. Recently, in the UK, a puppy imported from Sri Lanka was placed into routine rabies quarantine and developed clinical signs of rabies, again highlighting the value of the animal control systems in place (Fooks *et al.* 2008). As well as preventing the disease from entering its own animal population, quarantine has an important role in the prevention of spread of rabies to other countries.

Canine rabies control

Controlling dog rabies across areas where the virus remains endemic is a major challenge in the global fight against the disease. The control of rabies within the domestic dog population is something that, within the developed world, has led to a dramatic reduction in the number of human cases reported. However, across much of the developing world, domestic dogs continue to act as the main reservoir for infection (Rupprecht *et al.* 2002) with transmission from wildlife into domestic dog populations often linking the virus circulating within wildlife populations to the human population. Regions where the human population lives in close proximity to populations of potentially rabid dogs would benefit from targeted vaccination campaigns. Unfortunately, the situation regarding dog rabies in such areas seems to be continuing to spiral out of control with a dramatic increase in the number of dog rabies cases being reported over the past few decades (Cleaveland 1998). A number of factors compound this situation including: the unchecked increase in dog populations in these areas; the high fluidity of human and dog movement; the lack of economic infrastructure that in turn effects the availability of both medical and veterinary services equipped to deal with rabies cases; poor public awareness through lack of educational facilities that leave much of the population unaware of simple PEP and a shortage of trained staff that can administer vaccine and PEP even where it is available.

As demonstrated across much of the developed world, the problem of dog rabies can be overcome through mass parenteral vaccination of owned dogs. However, across the developing world an inability to put mass vaccination strategies into practice often means that even where local vaccination campaigns are enforced, a temporary reduction in cases seen but the virus is soon reintroduced and the cycle of infection re-initiates. Several different studies have suggested that the level of vaccine coverage within a domestic dog population required to substantially reduce the presence of the disease range from 60 to 87% (Bogel and Joshi 1990; Perry 1995; Kayali *et al.* 2003; Kamoltham *et al.* 2003). Such high levels of vaccination coverage are immensely difficult to achieve as many dogs in such areas are considered 'community dogs' that wander between populated areas, occasionally fed waste food by different groups or individuals or are stray dogs that are not owned within a community and are often totally feral. However, where such target vaccination levels are achieved cases within populations have been shown to decrease dramatically (Cleaveland *et al.* 2003) with a sharp reduction in the number of human cases seen having

a concomitant effect on the demand for PEP. In one province of Thailand, application of awareness campaigns in concert with vaccination and administration of intradermal PEP has completely eliminated human rabies deaths over a five year period (Kamoltham *et al.* 2003).

Application of oral vaccination campaigns to combat wildlife rabies across much of North America and Western Europe has suggested a role in such elimination methods where 'community' dog populations are largely inaccessible and/or parenteral vaccination campaigns have been unsuccessful. Several types of vaccines are licensed for delivery in this manner and bait formulations have been designed to appeal to different species. Strategies to apply such oral vaccines vary with different bait formulations being attempted in different canine populations (Bishop *et al.* 2001; Harischandra *et al.* 2001; Hu *et al.* 2008b).

Unfortunately, whilst estimates suggest that if dog rabies is controlled in these areas the economic burden associated with the disease, especially through transmission to the human population, would decrease dramatically, the financial resources and economic infrastructure are generally lacking preventing the administration the type of vaccination campaigns needed to remove the threat of disease (Fishbein 1991; Meslin 1994; Kaare *et al.* 2007). Whilst the necessary tools to combat rabies within domestic dog populations exist, the application of these tools to the developing world continues to be a major challenge.

Wildlife rabies control

Wildlife rabies control in the Americas

In much the same way that canine rabies constitutes a huge economic burden across the developing world, rabies virus in wildlife populations is still problematic in much of the developed world. In North America, several different vectors are able to maintain the disease and this means that whilst much of North America is 'free' of canine rabies, the threat of spillover into the dog and human populations remain high. Attempts to control this situation using novel vaccination techniques have been partially successful in reducing the incidence of disease. However, in one species, limited success may be achieved while in another it has been totally unsuccessful. For example, oral vaccination using specific bait delivery systems to combat rabies within the raccoon population were applied to the skunk population with little success (Olson *et al.* 2000; Russell *et al.* 2005; Hanlon *et al.* 2002). Attempts to vaccinate raccoons with recombinant poxviruses virus expressing the rabies glycoprotein has also been problematic. In this instance, pre-existing antibodies generated through natural infection with raccoon-pox affected the immunostimulatory potential of the vaccine preparation (Root *et al.* 2008). Often programs such as 'trap-vaccinate-release' have been applied successfully to contain rabies in the skunk population as well as in outbreak situations (Rosatte *et al.* 2001; Engeman *et al.* 2003). In addition to the successes seen through the use of inactivated oral vaccines, several live attenuated vaccines have been developed for oral application successfully used in small scale trials with wildlife populations (Vos *et al.* 2002; Follman *et al.* 2004).

Whilst across all of the Americas terrestrial rabies is the main problem, a further threat exists in the transmission of virus from the bat population. In North America, rabies in insectivorous bats has been responsible for many human cases (Gibbons *et al.* 2002), whilst across Central and South America the threat from bat rabies is most notably associated with vampire bats and the resulting economic losses through infection of cattle (Blancou and Fooks 2008). Many different strategies have been used in an attempt to control rabies in the vampire bat populations, including early methods to destroy bat populations with smoke, fire and explosives; capture and treatment with anticoagulants such as warfarin (Linhart *et al.* 1972; Thompson *et al.* 1972). As well as applying warfarin jelly to the backs of captured bats and to previous vampire bat wounds on cattle, warfarin injected into cattle will remain in the animals blood for several days, effectively killing any bats that feed on the treated animal. This systemic treatment of cattle with anticoagulant preparations is claimed to be very effective, reducing biting rates on cattle by 85–90% (Flores-Crespo and Arellano-Sota 1991). More recently, oral vaccine preparations have been trialed in bat populations with limited success. The cost effectiveness of trying to vaccinate bat populations has, however, been questioned and as vampire bat populations continue to increase, a more destructive mechanism to reduce population sizes may be the best way to control the situation (Almeida *et al.* 2005).

Wildlife rabies control in Africa

The lack of human and financial resources available to many African countries leads to an inability to put vaccination strategies into practice. Furthermore, the continued problem of canine rabies require that co-ordinated efforts to control rabies within domestic populations be made but this rarely occurs. Exceptions to this, however, include conservation efforts to protect endangered species such as the African wild dogs (*Lycaon pictus*) from potential extinction due to the introduction of the disease into the population in the early 1990s (Gascoyne *et al.* 1993) and more recently an oral vaccine preparation has been developed to attempt to vaccinate free ranging wild dogs (Knobel *et al.* 2002; Knobel and Toit 2003; Knobel *et al.* 2008). Since then, the introduction of the virus into the Ethiopian wolf (*Canis simensis*) population in 2003 led to a internationally co-ordinated effort to save these canids from the brink of extinction with live capture and vaccination programs being implemented (Knobel *et al.* 2008).

Wildlife rabies control in Asia

It is universally accepted that wildlife rabies plays a comparatively minor role in disease maintenance across much of Asia with canine rabies remaining the major threat to human health (Wilde *et al.* 2005). Several oral vaccine preparations are available and are in use to combat rabies where it remains a problem and where wildlife vectors such as fox species and in the Middle East, jackal species, exist. Oral vaccination campaigns have recently been applied with some success across parts of the Middle East including Egypt, Israel, Jordan and Palestine (Yakobson *et al.* 2006; Rosatte *et al.* 2007). Incidence of wildlife rabies in the Middle East is often only reduced by culling stray dog populations as well as those shown to be rabid (Seimenis 2008; Vos 2004). Central Asia has a much greater incidence of wildlife rabies where several species including arctic foxes, raccoon dogs and red foxes are thought to act as vectors for the disease. Reporting cases of disease across the majority of the continent, however, remains at a very low level despite the implementation of rabies awareness campaigns. Spread of the disease seems to be confined to areas through the presence of wild vector species and limited by geological boundaries rather than by human attempts to curb the incidence of disease. Exact population densities of vector species across many Asian countries are unknown although the implementation of domestic dog vaccination in some areas has helped the situation. Russia is the only country of Central Asia that is attempting to vaccinate wild carnivore populations and, using lessons learned from global elimination campaigns, have started to use oral vaccines to reduce incidence of the disease (Gruzdev 2008).

Countries of Eastern Asia also have rabies present within wildlife species with raccoon dog populations maintaining the disease in South Korea and serological evidence existing for lyssaviruses within bat populations across several Far East Asian countries such as Cambodia (Reynes *et al.* 2004), China (Tang *et al.* 2005), Thailand (Lumlertdacha *et al.* 2005) and the Phillippines (Arguin *et al.* 2002).

Wildlife rabies control in Europe

The current status of rabies throughout the EU has vastly improved over the past decade. Successful applications of oral vaccination campaigns have now removed the threat of terrestrial rabies from much of Western Europe. The principal reservoirs of disease, red foxes and raccoon dogs have been targeted in a number of campaigns that have eliminated the virus from a number of European countries (Steck and Wandeler 1980). However, continued expansion of the EU to the East has generated new challenges and the virus remains hugely problematic across Eastern Europe and within the Baltic states. Fox and raccoon dog population increases have enhanced the problem (Zienius *et al.* 2003). Many issues remain to be solved with current oral vaccination campaigns. Bait formulations and approach to bait drops need modernizing to optimize efficiency of delivery to target species and timing of drops can profoundly affect uptake by different target species depending on breeding life cycles (Vos 2003). Innovative ideas on how to find pragmatic solutions to these problems are needed if successful elimination of the virus from the EU territory is to be witnessed in the near future.

Conclusions and future prospects

One of the biggest obstacles to successfully reducing the number of deaths attributed to rabies virus is in creating awareness of this vaccine-preventable disease. The death toll in children and young adults in areas where the virus is endemic remains high. In such areas, educating children of school age as well as informing local populations about the need to exercise extreme caution when in the presence of an animal behaving in an unusual or aggressive manner and careful wound care would greatly reduce the number deaths attributed to rabies infection. While many governments have neither the resources nor the infrastructure to provide PEP to local populations, better education and an awareness of the dangers from rabies within societies will help reduce incidence. Effective disease reporting in areas where little is known about the presence of the disease, especially in wildlife species would also be of huge value to elimination campaigns (Rupprecht *et al.* 2008).

With rabies now often falling under the banner of a 'neglected tropical disease' partnerships are being formed across the globe to try and shift the world's attention back to this devastating disease. International collaborations between expert groups have generated new focus groups such as the Partnership for Rabies Prevention (PRP) and the Alliance for Rabies Control (ARC) to try and combat the virus in areas where it remains endemic and some of the world's largest funding bodies have now recognized the need for a push towards elimination of the virus wherever possible.

References

Almeida, M. F., Martorelli, L. F. A., *et al.* (2005). Experimental rabies infection in haematophagous bats Desmodus rotundus. *Epidem. Infect.*, **133**: 523–27.

Amengual, B., Whitby, J. E., *et al.* (1997). Evolution of European bat lyssaviruses. *J. Gen. Virol.*, **78**(9): 2319–28.

Anon. (2006). Compendium of animal rabies prevention and control. *J. Am. Vet. Med. Assoc.*, **228**: 858–64.

Arai, Y. T., Kuzmin, I. V., *et al.* (2003). New lyssavirus genotype from the Lesser Mouse-eared Bat (Myotis blythi), Kyrghyzstan. *Emerg. Infect. Dis.*, **9**: 333–37.

Arguin, P. M., Murray-Lillibridge, K., *et al.* (2002). Serologic evidence of Lyssavirus infections among bats, the Philippines. *Emerg. Infect. Dis.*, **8**: 258–62.

Arya, S. C. (1999). Therapeutic failures with rabies vaccine and rabies immunoglobulin. *Clin. Infect. Dis.*, **29**: 1605.

Ayele, W., Fekadu, M., *et al.* (2001). Immunogenicity and efficacy of Fermi-type nerve tissue rabies vaccine in mice and in humans undergoing post-exposure prophylaxis for rabies in Ethiopia. *Ethiop. Med. J.*, **39**: 313–21.

Badrane, H., Bahloul, C., *et al.* (2001). Evidence of two Lyssavirus phylogroups with distinct pathogenicity and immunogenicity. *J. Virol.*, **75**: 3268–76.

Bahmanyar, M., Fayaz, A., *et al.* (1976). Successful protection of humans exposed to rabies infection. Postexposure treatment with the new human diploid cell rabies vaccine and antirabies serum. *JAMA*, **236**: 2751–54.

Banyard, A. C., Baron, M. D., Barrett, T. (2005). A role for virus promoters in determining the pathogenesis of Rinderpest virus in cattle. *J. Gen. Virol.*, **86**: 1083–92.

Banyard, A, C., Hartley, M. and Fooks, A. R. (2010). Reassessing the risk from rabies: A continuing threat to the UK? *Virus Research.* **152**: 79–84.

Banyard, A. C., Johnson, N., *et al.* (2009). Repeated isolation of a European Bat Lyssavirus from a single site in the UK: Consequences for virus transmission and maintenance within a roost. *Archives of Virology*, **154**(11): 1847–50.

Barge, A., Gaudin, Y., *et al.* (1993). Vesicular stomatitis virus M protein may be inside the ribonucleocapsid coil. *J. Virol.*, **67**: 7246–53.

Belotto, A., Leanes, L. F., *et al.* (2005). Overview of rabies in the Americas. *Virus Res.*, **111**: 5–12.

Bishop, G. (2001). Increasing dog vaccination coverage in South Africa: is oral vaccination the answer? In: B. M. F. Dodet (ed.) Rabies Control in Asia. London, pp.105–09. John Libbey and Company, Ltd.

Blancou, J. (1988). Epizootiology of rabies: Eurasia and Africa. In: J. B. Campbell (ed.) Rabies, pp. 243–65. Boston, MA: Kluwer Academic Publishers.

Blancou, J. (1994). Early methods for the surveillance and control of rabies in animals. *Rev. Sci. Tech.*, **13**: 361–72.

Blancou, J., Fooks. A. R. (2008). Rabies. In: P.C. Lefèvre *et al.* (eds.) Infectious and parasitic diseases of livestock, pp. 337–51. Paris, France: Lavoiser Publications.

Blanton, J. D., Palmer, D. (2008). Rabies surveillance in the United States during 2007. *J. Am. Vet. Med. Assoc.*, **233**: 884–97.

Bogel, K., and Joshi, D. D. (1990). Accessibility of dog populations for rabies control in Kathmandu valley, Nepal. *Bull. World Health Organ.*, **68**: 611–17.

Botvinkin, A., Selnikova, O. P., *et al.* (2005). Human rabies cases caused by a bat bite in the Ukraine. *Rabies Bull. Eur.*, **29**: 5–7.

Botvinkin, A. D., Kuzmin, I. V., *et al.* (2006). The diversity of rabies virus in Russia demonstrated by anti-nucleocapsid monoclonal antibody application and limited gene sequencing. *Dev. Biol. (Basel).*, **125**: 79–90.

Bourhy, H., Rollin, P. E., *et al.* (1989). Comparative field evaluation of the fluorescent-antibody test, virus isolation from tissue culture, and enzyme immunodiagnosis for rapid laboratory diagnosis of rabies. *J. Clin. Microbiol.*, **27**: 519–23.

Bourhy, H., Kissi, B., *et al.* (1992). Antigenic and molecular characterization of bat rabies virus in Europe. *J. Clin. Microbiol.*, **30**: 2419–26.

Bourhy, H., Kissi, B., and Tordo, N. (1993). Taxonomy and evolutionary studies on lyssaviruses with special reference to Africa. *Onderstep. J. Vet. Res.*, **60**: 277–82.

Bourhy, H., and Perrin, P. (1996). Rapid rabies enzyme immunodiagnosis (RREID) for rabies antigen detection. In: F. X. Meslin *et al.* (eds.) Laboratory Techniques in rabies, pp.105–12. Geneva: World Health Organization.

Bourhy, H., Reynes, J. M., *et al.* (2008). The origin and phylogeography of dog rabies virus. *J. Gen. Virol.*, **89**: 2673–78.

Brass, D. (1994). Rabies in bats. Ridgefield, Connecticut: Livia Press.

Briggs, D., and Hanlon, C. A. (2007). World Rabies Day: focusing attention on a neglected disease. *Vet. Rec.*, **161**: 288–89.

Briggs, D. J., and Mahendra, B. J. (2007). Public health management of humans at risk. In: A. C. Jackson, W. Wunner (eds.) Rabies, pp. 553–58. London: Elsevier/Academic Press.

Brochier, B., Kieny, M. P., *et al.* (1991). Large-scale eradication of rabies using recombinant vaccinia-rabies vaccine. *Nature*, **354**: 520–22.

Brookes, S. M., Aegerter, J. N. (2005a). European bat lyssavirus in Scottish bats. *Emerg. Infect. Dis.*, **11**: 572–78.

Brookes, S. M., Klopfleisch, R., *et al.* (2007). Susceptibility of sheep to European bat lyssavirus type-1 and -2 infection: a clinical pathogenesis study. *Vet. Microbiol.*, **125**: 210–23.

Bugyaki, L., Blockeel, S. R., and Moons, J. H. (1959). The survival of flury rabies virus under different conditions of preservation. *Rev. Pathol. Gen. Physiol. Clin.*, **59**: 981–84.

Bunn, T. O. (1991). Canine and feline vaccines, past and present. In: G. M. Baer (ed.) The Natural History of Rabies. Boston: CRC Press.

Burki, T. (2008). The global fight against rabies. *Lancet*, **372**: 1135–36.

Burton, E. C., Burns, D. K., *et al.* (2005). Rabies encephalomyelitis: clinical, neuroradiological, and pathological findings in 4 transplant recipients. *Arch. Neurol.*, **62**: 873–82.

Childs, J. E., Curns, A. T., *et al.* (2001). Rabies epizootics among raccoons vary along a North-South gradient in the Eastern United States. *Vector Borne Zoon. Dis.*, **1**: 253–67.

Cleaveland, S. (1998). Royal Society of Tropical Medicine and Hygiene Meeting at Manson House, London, 20 March 1997 - Epidemiology and control of rabies - The growing problem of rabies in Africa. *Trans. R. Soc. Trop. Med. Hyg.*, **92**: 131–34.

Cleaveland, S., Kaare, M., *et al.* (2003). A dog rabies vaccination campaign in rural Africa: impact on the incidence of dog rabies and human dog-bite injuries. *Vaccine*, **21**: 1965–73.

Cliquet, F., McElhinney, L. M., *et al.* (2004). Development of a qualitative indirect ELISA for the measurement of rabies virus-specific antibodies from vaccinated dogs and cats. *J. Virol. Meth.*, **117**: 1–8.

Constantine, D. G. (1962). Rabies transmission by nonbite route. *Public Health Rep.*, **77**: 287–89.

Conzelmann, K. K., Cox, J. H, *et al.* (1990). Molecular cloning and complete nucleotide sequence of the attenuated rabies virus SAD B19. *Virol.*, **175**: 485–99.

Conzelmann, K. K., and Schnell, M. (1994). Rescue of synthetic genomic RNA analogs of rabies virus by plasmid-encoded proteins. *J. Virol.*, **68**: 713–19.

Cross, M., Buddle, B., and Aldwell, F. (2007). The potential of oral vaccines for disease control in wildlife species. *Vet. J.*, **174**: 472–80.

Daoust, P. Y., Wandeler, A. I., and Casey, G. A. (1996). Cluster of rabies cases of probable bat origin among red foxes in Prince Edward Island, Canada. *J. Wildl. Dis.*, **32**: 403–6.

Davies, M. C., Englert, M. E., *et al.* (1963). The Electron Microscopy of Rabies Virus in Cultures of Chicken Embryo Tissues. *Virol.*, **21**: 642–51.

Dean, D. J., and Abelseth, M. K. (1973). Laboratory techniques in rabies: the fluorescent antibody test. *Monog. Series World Health Organ.*, 73–84.

Dechant, G., and Barde, Y. A. (2002). The neurotrophin receptor p75(NTR): novel functions and implications for diseases of the nervous system. *Nat. Neurosci.*, **5**: 1131–36.

Delmas, O., Holmes, E. C., *et al.* (2008). Genomic diversity and evolution of the lyssaviruses. *PLoS ONE*, **3**: e2057.

Elbashir, S. M., Harborth, J., *et al.* (2001). Duplexes of 21-nucleotide RNAs mediate RNA interference in cultured mammalian cells. *Nature*, **411**: 494–98.

Engeman, R. M., Christensen, K. L., *et al.* (2003). Population monitoring in support of a rabies vaccination program for skunks in Arizona. *J. Wildl. Dis.*, **39**: 746–50.

Faber, M., Pulmanausahakul, R., *et al.* (2004).Identification of viral genomic elements responsible for rabies virus neuroinvasiveness. *Proc. Nat. Acad. Sci. USA*, **101**: 16328–32.

Fekadu, M., Endeshaw, T., *et al.* (1996). Possible human-to-human transmission of rabies in Ethiopia. *Ethiop. Med., J,* **34**: 123–27.

Feyssaguet, M., Dacheux, L., *et al.* (2007). Multicenter comparative study of a new ELISA, PLATELIA RABIES II, for the detection and titration of anti-rabies glycoprotein antibodies and comparison with the rapid fluorescent focus inhibition test (RFFIT) on human samples from vaccinated and non-vaccinated people. *Vaccine*, **25**: 2244–51.

Finke, S., and Conzelmann, K. K. (1999). Virus promoters determine interference by defective RNAs: selective amplification of mini-RNA vectors and rescue from cDNA by a 3' copy-back ambisense rabies virus. *J. Virol.*, **73**: 3818–25.

Finnegan, C. J., Brookes, S. M., *et al.* (2004). Detection and strain differentiation of European bat lyssaviruses using in situ hybridisation. *J. Virol. Meth.*, **121**: 223–29.

Fishbein, D. B. (1991). Rabies in Humans. In: G. M. Baer (ed.) The Natural History of Rabies, pp. 519–49. Boca Raton, FLA: CRC Press.

Flores-Crespo, R., and Arellano-Sota, C. (1991). Biology and control of the vampire bat. In: G. M. Baer (ed.) The Natural History of Rabies, pp. 461–76. Boca Raton, FLA: CRC Press.

Follmann, E. H., Ritter, D. G., and Donald, W. H. (2004). Oral vaccination of captive arctic foxes with lyophilized SAG2 rabies vaccine. *J. Wildl. Dis.*, **40**: 328–34.

Fooks, A. R., Johnson, N., *et al.* (2003a). Risk factors associated with travel to rabies endemic countries. *J. Appl. Microbiol.*, **94** Suppl: 31S–36S.

Fooks, A. R., McElhinney, L. M., *et al.* (2003b). Case report: isolation of a European bat lyssavirus type 2a from a fatal human case of rabies encephalitis. *J. Med. Virol.*, **71**: 281–89.

Fooks, A. (2004a). The challenge of emerging lyssaviruses. *Expert Rev. Vacc.*, **3**: 89–92.

Fooks, A., *et al.* (2004b). Rabies in the United Kingdom. In: OIE (ed.) Historical perspective of Rabies in Europe and the Mediterranean basin, pp. 25–32. OIE, France.

Fooks, A. R. (2005). Rabies remains a 'neglected disease'. *Euro. Surveill.*, **10**: 1–2.

Fooks, A. R. (2007). Rabies - the need for a 'one medicine' approach. *Vet. Rec.*, **161**: 289–90.

Fooks, A. R., Harkess, G., *et al.* (2008). Rabies virus in a dog imported to the UK from Sri Lanka. *Vet. Rec.*, **162**: 598.

Fooks, A. R., Johnson, N., and Rupprecht, C. E. (2009). Rabies. In: A. Barrett and L. Stanberry (eds.) Vaccines for Biodefense and Emerging and Neglected Diseases, pp. 605–26. London: Elsevier Publications Ltd.

Franka, R., Svrcek, S., *et al.* (2004). Quantification of the effectiveness of laboratory diagnostics of rabies using classical and molecular-genetic methods. *Vet. Med.*, **49**: 259–67.

Freuling, C., Grossmann, E., *et al.* (2008). First isolation of EBLV-2 in Germany. *Vet. Microbiol.*, **131**: 26–34.

Fuenzalida, E., and Palacious, R. (1955). Un método mejorado en la preparación de la vacuna antirrabica. *Bol. Inst. Bact. Chile*, **8**: 3–10.

Gascoyne, S. C., King, A. A., *et al.* (1993). Aspects of rabies infection and control in the conservation of the African wild dog (Lycaon pictus) in the Serengeti region, Tanzania. *Onderstep. J. Vet. Res.*, **60**: 415–20.

Gaudin, Y., Ruigrok, R. W., *et al.* (1992). Rabies virus glycoprotein is a trimer. *Virol.*, **187**: 627–32.

Geue, L., Schares, S., *et al.* (2008). Genetic characterisation of attenuated SAD rabies virus strains used for oral vaccination of wildlife. *Vacc.*, **26**: 3227–35.

Gibbons, R. V., Holman, R. C., *et al.* (2002). Knowledge of bat rabies and human exposure among United States cavers. *Emerg. Infect. Dis.*, **8**: 532–45.

Girard, L. S., Fabis, M. J., *et al.* (2006). Expression of a human anti-rabies virus monoclonal antibody in tobacco cell culture. *Biochem. Biophys. Res. Comm.*, **345**: 602–7.

Gode, G. R., and Bhide, N. K. (1988). Two rabies deaths after corneal grafts from one donor. *Lancet*, **2**: 791.

Grabau, E. A., and Holland, J. J. (1982). Analysis of viral and defective-interfering nucleocapsids in acute and persistent infection by rhabdoviruses. *J. Gen. Virol.*, **60**: 87–97.

Gruzdev, K. N. (2008). The rabies situation in Central Asia. *Dev. Biol. (Basel)*, **131**: 37–42.

Gupta, A. K., Shaji, D., and Banerjee, A. K. (2003). Identification of a novel tripartite complex involved in replication of vesicular stomatitis virus genome RNA. *J. Virol.*, **77**: 732–38.

Hanlon, C. A., Niezgoda, M., *et al.* (2002). Oral efficacy of an attenuated rabies virus vaccine in skunks and raccoons. *J. Wildl. Dis.*, **38**: 420–27.

Hanlon, C. A., Kuzmin, I. V., *et al.* (2005). Efficacy of rabies biologics against new lyssaviruses from Eurasia. *Virus Res.*, **111**: 44–54.

Hanna, J. N., Carney, I. K., *et al.*(2000). Australian bat lyssavirus infection: a second human case, with a long incubation period. *Med. J. Aust.*, **172**: 597–99.

Harischandra, P. A. L. (2001). Dog vaccination coverage and oral rabies vaccination in Sri Lanka, an update. In: Proceedings of the Fourth International Symposium on Rabies control in Asia, Hanoi. John Libbey Eurotext, pp. 97–100.

Hayman, D. T., Fooks, A. R., *et al.* (2008). Antibodies against Lagos bat virus in megachiroptera from West Africa. *Emerg. Infect. Dis.*, **14**: 926–28.

Hemachudha, T., Laothamatas, J., and Rupprecht, C. E. (2002). Human rabies: a disease of complex neuropathogenetic mechanisms and diagnostic challenges. *Lancet* Neurol., **1**: 101–9.

Hicks, D. J., Nunez, A., *et al.* (2009). Comparative pathological study of the murine brain after experimental infection with classical rabies virus and European bat lyssaviruses. *J. Comp. Pathol.*, **140**: 113–26.

Holland, J. J., and Villarreal, L. P. (1975). Purification of defective interfering T particles of vesicular stomatitis and rabies viruses generated in vivo in brains of newborn mice. *Virology*, **67**: 438–49.

Houff, S. A., Burton, R. C., *et al.* (1979). Human-to-human transmission of rabies virus by corneal transplant. *N. Engl. J. Med.*, **300**: 603–4.

Hu, R., Zhang, S., *et al.* (2006). Prevention of rabies virus infection in dogs by a recombinant canine adenovirus type-2 encoding the rabies virus glycoprotein. *Microbes Infect.*, **8**: 1090–97.

Hu, R. L., Liu, Y., *et al.* (2007). Experimental immunization of cats with a recombinant rabies-canine adenovirus vaccine elicits a long-lasting neutralizing antibody response against rabies. *Vaccine*, **25**: 5301–7.

Hu, R., Tang, Q., *et al.* (2008a). Rabies in China: An Update. *Vector Borne Zoon. Dis.*, **11**: 29–35.

Hu, R. L., Fooks, A. R., *et al.* (2008b). Inferior rabies vaccine quality and low immunization coverage in dogs (Canis familiaris) in China. *Epidem. Infect.*, **136**: 1556–63.

Hunter, M., Johnson, N., *et al.* (2010). Immunovirological correlates in human rabies treated with therapeutic coma. *J. Med. Virol.* **82**: 1255–1265.

Inoue, K., Shoji, Y., *et al.* (2003). An improved method for recovering rabies virus from cloned cDNA. *J. Virol. Meth.*, **107**: 229–36.

Ito, N., Kakemizu, M., *et al.* (2001). A comparison of complete genome sequences of the attenuated RC-HL strain of rabies virus used for production of animal vaccine in Japan, and the parental Nishigahara strain. *Microbiol. Immunol.*, **45**: 51–58.

Jacob, Y., Badrane, H., *et al.* (2000). Cytoplasmic dynein LC8 interacts with lyssavirus phosphoprotein. *J. Virol.*, **74**: 10217–22.

Johnson, N., Mansfield, K. L., and Fooks, A. R. (2002a). Canine vaccine recipients recognize an immunodominant region of the rabies virus glycoprotein. *J. Gen. Virol.*, **83**: 2663–69.

Johnson, N., McElhinney, L. M., *et al.* (2002b). Phylogenetic comparison of the genus Lyssavirus using distal coding sequences of the glycoprotein and nucleoprotein genes. *Arch. Virol.*, **147**: 2111–23.

Johnson, N., Selden, D., *et al.* (2003a). Isolation of a European bat lyssavirus type 2 from a Daubenton's bat in the United Kingdom. *Vet. Rec.*, **152**: 383–87.

Johnson, N., Black, C., *et al.* (2003b). Rabies emergence among foxes in Turkey. *J. Wildl. Dis.*, **39**: 262–70.

Johnson, N., McElhinney, L. M., *et al.* (2004a). Molecular epidemiology of canid rabies in Sudan: evidence for a common origin of rabies with Ethiopia. *Virus Res.*, **104**: 201–5.

Johnson, N., Letshwenyo, M., *et al.* (2004b). Molecular epidemiology of rabies in Botswana: a comparison between antibody typing and nucleotide sequence phylogeny. *Vet. Microb.*, **101**: 31–38.

Johnson, N., Brookes, S. M., *et al.* (2005). Review of human rabies cases in the UK and in Germany. *Vet. Rec.*, **157**: 715.

Johnson, N., Phillpotts, R., and Fooks, A. (2006a). Airborne transmission of lyssaviruses. *J. Med.* Microb., **55**: 785–90.

Johnson, N., Un, H., *et al.* (2006b). Wildlife rabies in Western Turkey: the spread of rabies through the western provinces of Turkey. *Epidemiol. Infect.*, **134**: 369–75.

Johnson, N., Fooks, A., and McColl, K. (2008). Human rabies case with long incubation, Australia. *Emerg. Infect. Dis.*, **14**: 1950–51.

Jones, R. L., Froeschle, J. E., *et al.* (2001). Immunogenicity, safety and lot consistency in adults of a chromatographically purified Vero-cell rabies vaccine a randomized, double-blind trial with human diploid cell rabies vaccine. *Vaccine*, **19**: 4635–43.

Kaare, M., Lembo, T., *et al.* (2008). Rabies control in rural Africa: Evaluating strategies for effective domestic dog vaccination. *Vaccine*, pub. on-line.

Kamoltham, T., Singhsa, J., *et al.* (2003). Elimination of human rabies in a canine endemic province in Thailand: five-year programme. *Bull World Health Organ.*, **81**: 375–81.

Kasempimolporn, S., Jitapunkul, S., and Sitprija, V. (2008). Moving towards the elimination of rabies in Thailand. *J. Med. Assoc. Thai.*, **91**: 433–37.

Kayali, U., Mindekem, R., *et al.* (2003). Coverage of pilot parenteral vaccination campaign against canine rabies in N'Djamena, Chad. *Bull. World. Health. Organ.*, **81**: 739–44.

Kieny, M. P., Lathe, R., *et al.* (1984). Expression of rabies virus glycoprotein from a recombinant vaccinia virus. *Nature*, **312**: 163–66.

Kissi, B., Tordom, N., and Bourhy, H. (1995). Genetic polymorphism in the rabies virus nucleoprotein gene. *Virol.*, **209**: 526–37.

Knobel, D. L., DuToit, J. T., and Bingham, J. (2002). Development of a bait and baiting system for delivery of oral rabies vaccine to free-ranging African wild dogs (Lycaon pictus). *J. Wildl. Dis.*, **38**: 352–62.

Knobel, D. L., Liebenberg, A., and DuToit, J. T. (2003). Seroconversion in captive African wild dogs (Lycaon pictus) following administration of a chicken head bait/SAG-2 oral rabies vaccine combination. *Onderstep. J. Vet. Res.*, **70**: 73–77.

Knobel, D. L., Cleaveland, S., *et al.* (2005). Re-evaluating the burden of rabies in Africa and Asia. *Bull. World Health Organ.*, **83**: 360–68.

Knobel, D. L., Fooks, A. R., *et al.* (2008). Trapping and vaccination of endangered Ethiopian wolves to control an outbreak of rabies. *J. Appl. Ecol.*, **45**: 109–16.

Krebs, J. W., Williams, S. M., *et al.* (2003). Rabies among infrequently reported mammalian carnivores in the United States, 1960–2000. *J. Wildl. Dis.*, **39**: 253–61.

Krebs, J. W., Mandel, E. J., *et al.* (2005). Rabies surveillance in the United States during 2004. *J. Am. Vet. Med. Assoc.*, **227**: 1912–25.

Kumar, P., Wu, H., *et al.* (2007). Transvascular delivery of small interfering RNA to the central nervous system. *Nature*, **448**: 39–43.

Kuzmin, I. V., Orciari, L. A., *et al.* (2003). Bat lyssaviruses (Aravan and Khujand) from Central Asia: phylogenetic relationships according to N, P and G gene sequences. *Virus Res.*, **97**: 65–79.

Kuzmin, I. V., Hughes, G. J., *et al.* (2005). Phylogenetic relationships of Irkut and West Caucasian bat viruses within the Lyssavirus genus and suggested quantitative criteria based on the N gene sequence for lyssavirus genotype definition. *Virus Res.*, **111**: 28–43.

Kuzmin, I. V., Niezgoda, M., *et al.* (2006). Lyssavirus surveillance in bats, Bangladesh. *Emerg. Infect. Dis.*, **12**: 486–88.

Kuzmin, I. V., Niezgoda, M., *et al.* (2008a). Lagos bat virus in Kenya. *J. Clin. Microb.*, **46**: 1451–61.

Kuzmin, I. V., Wu, X., *et al.* (2008b). Complete genomes of Aravan, Khujand, Irkut and West Caucasian bat viruses, with special attention to the polymerase gene and non-coding regions. *Virus Res.*, **136**: 81–90.

Lafon, M. (2005). Rabies virus receptors. *J. NeuroVirol.*, **11**: 82–87.

Laothamatas, J., Wacharapluesadee, S., *et al.* (2008). Furious and paralytic rabies of canine origin: neuroimaging with virological and cytokine studies. *J. NeuroVirol.*, **14**: 119–29.

Le Mercier, P., Jacob, Y., and Tordo, N. (1997). The complete Mokola virus genome sequence: structure of the RNA-dependent RNA polymerase. *J. Gen. Virol.*, **78**(7): 1571–76.

Leslie, M. J., Messenger, S., *et al.* (2006). Bat-associated rabies virus in Skunks. *Emerg. Infect. Dis.*, **12**: 1274–77.

Lewis, P., Fu, Y., and Lentz, T. L. (2000). Rabies virus entry at the neuromuscular junction in nerve-muscle cocultures. *Muscle Nerve*, **23**: 720–30.

Linhart, S. B., *et al.* (1972). Control of vampire bats by means of an anticoagulant. *Bol. Oficina Sanit. Panam.*, **73**: 100–109.

Lodmell, D. L., Ewalt, L. C., *et al.* (2006). One-time intradermal DNA vaccination in ear pinnae one year prior to infection protects dogs against rabies virus. *Vaccine*, **24**: 412–16.

Lucas, C. H., Pino, F. V., *et al.* (2008). Rabies control in Mexico. *Dev. Biol. (Basel)*, **131**: 167–75.

Lumio, J., Hillbom, M., *et al.* (1986). Human rabies of bat origin in Europe. *Lancet*, **1**: 378.

Lumlertdacha, B., Boongird, K., *et al.* (2005). Survey for bat lyssaviruses, Thailand. *Emerg. Infect. Dis.*, **11**: 232–36.

MacInnes, C. D., Smith, S. M., *et al.* (2001). Elimination of rabies from red foxes in eastern Ontario. *J. Wildl. Dis.*, **37**: 119–32.

Madhusudana, S. N., Paul, J. P., *et al.* (2004). Rapid diagnosis of rabies in humans and animals by a dot blot enzyme immunoassay. *Int. J. Infect. Dis.*, **8**: 339–45.

Mallewa, M., Fooks, A. R., *et al.* (2007). Rabies encephalitis in malaria-endemic area, Malawi, Africa. *Emerg. Infect. Dis.*, **13**: 136–39.

Mansfield, K., McElhinney, L., *et al.* (2006a). A molecular epidemiological study of rabies epizootics in kudu (Tragelaphus strepsiceros) in Namibia. *BMC Vet. Res.*, **2**: 2.

Mansfield, K. L., Racloz, V., *et al.* (2006b). Molecular epidemiological study of Arctic rabies virus isolates from Greenland and comparison with isolates from throughout the Arctic and Baltic regions. *Virus Res.*, **116**: 1–10.

Markotter, W., Kuzmin, I., *et al.* (2008a). Phylogeny of Lagos bat virus: challenges for lyssavirus taxonomy. *Virus Res.*, **135**: 10–21.

Markotter, W., Van Eeden, C., *et al.* (2008b). Epidemiology and pathogenicity of African bat lyssaviruses. *Dev. Biol. (Basel)*, **131**: 317–25.

Marston, D. A., McElhinney, L. M., *et al.* (2007). Comparative analysis of the full genome sequence of European bat lyssavirus type 1 and type 2 with other lyssaviruses and evidence for a conserved transcription termination and polyadenylation motif in the G-L 3' non-translated region. *J. Gen. Virol.*, **88**: 1302–14.

Matsumoto, S. (1962). Electron microscopy of nerve cells infected with street rabies virus. *Virol.*, **17**: 198–202.

McElhinney, L. M., Parsons, G., *et al.* (2004). Rabies diagnosis in the presence of strychnine and carbamate. *Vet. Rec.*, **155**: 303–4.

Mebatson, T. (2001). Extensive attenuation of rabies virus by simultaneously modifying the dynein light chain binding site in the P protein and replacing Arg333 in the G protein. *J. Virol.*, **75**: 11496–502.

Meredith, C. D., Prossouw, A. P, and Koch, H. P. (1971). An unusual case of human rabies thought to be of chiropteran origin. *S. Afr. Med. J.*, **45**: 767–69.

Meslin, F. X., Fishbein, D. B., and Matter, H. C. (1994). Rationale and prospects for rabies elimination in developing countries. *Curr. Top. Microbiol. Immunol.*, **187**: 1–26.

Messenger, S. L., Smith, J. S., *et al.* (2003). Emerging pattern of rabies deaths and increased viral infectivity. *Emerg. Infect. Dis.*, **9**: 151–54.

Metlin, A., Paulin, L., *et al.* (2008). Characterization of Russian rabies virus vaccine strain RV-97. *Virus Res.*, **132**: 242–47.

Mita, T., Shimizu, K., *et al.* (2008). Amino acid at position 95 of the matrix protein is a cytopathic determinant of rabies virus. *Virus Res.*, **137**: 33–39.

Muller, T., Cox, J., *et al.* (2004). Spill-over of European bat lyssavirus type 1 into a stone marten (Martes foina) in Germany. J. *Vet. Med. B. Infect. Dis. Vet. Public Health*, **51**: 49–54.

Muller, T., Johnson, N., *et al.* (2007). Epidemiology of bat rabies in Germany. *Arch. Virol.*, **152**: 273–88.

Murphy, F. A. (1977). Rabies pathogenesis. *Arch. Virol.*, **54**: 279–97.

Nadin-Davis, S. A., Abdel-Malik, M., *et al.* (2002). Lyssavirus P gene characterisation provides insights into the phylogeny of the genus and identifies structural similarities and diversity within the encoded phosphoprotein. *Virology*, **298**: 286–305.

Nadin-Davis, S., and Bingham, J. (2004). Europe as a source of rabies for the rest of the world. In: A. A. King *et al.* (eds.) Historical perspective of rabies in Europe and the Mediterranean basin, pp. 259–80. Paris: OIE.

Nadin-Davis, S. (2007). Molecular Epidemiology. In: A. C. Jackson, W. Wunner (eds.) Rabies. London: Elsevier/Academic Press.

Nakahara, K., Ohnuma, H., *et al.* (1999). Intracellular behavior of rabies virus matrix protein (M) is determined by the viral glycoprotein (G). *Microbiol. Immunol.*, **43**: 259–70.

Nel. J. A. (1993). The bat-eared fox: a prime candidate for rabies vector? *Onderstep. J. Vet. Res.*, **60**: 395–97.

Nel, L., Jacobs, J., *et al.* (2000). New cases of Mokola virus infection in South Africa: a genotypic comparison of Southern African virus isolates. *Virus Genes*, **20**: 103–6.

Nel, L. H. (2005). Vaccines for lyssaviruses other than rabies. *Expert Rev. Vacc.*, **4**: 533–40.

Nel. L., and Markotter, W. (2007). Lyssaviruses. *Crit. Rev. Microb.*, **33**: 301–24.

Nel, L. H., and Rupprecht, C. E. (2007). Emergence of lyssaviruses in the Old World: the case of Africa. *Curr. Top. Microb. Immunol.*, **315**: 161–93.

Ngoepe, C. E., Sabeta, C., and Nel, L. (2009). The spread of canine rabies into Free State province of South Africa: A molecular epidemiological characterization. *Virus Res.*, **142**: 175–80.

Nicholson, K. G. (1990). Modern vaccines. Rabies. *Lancet*, **335**: 1201–05.

OIE (2004). Manual for diagnostic tests and vaccines for terrestrial animals (mammals, birds and bees), (5th edn.). Paris: Office International des Epizooties.

OIE (2005). Rabies in Europe. In: Developments in Biologicals, 1st International Conference, Kiev. OIE.

Olson, C. A., Mitchell, K. D., and Werner, P.A. (2000). Bait ingestion by free-ranging raccoons and nontarget species in an oral rabies vaccine field trial in Florida. *J. Wildl. Dis.*, **36**: 734–43.

Parviz, S., Chotani, R., *et al.* (2004). Rabies deaths in Pakistan: results of ineffective post-exposure treatment. *Int. J. Infect. Dis.*, **8**: 346–52.

Pastoret, P. P., Brochier, B., *et al.* (1988). First field trial of fox vaccination against rabies using a vaccinia-rabies recombinant virus. *Vet. Rec.*, **123**: 481–83.

Paweska, J. T., Blumberg, L. H., *et al.* (2006). Fatal human infection with rabies-related Duvenhage virus, South Africa. *Emerg. Infect. Dis.*, **12**: 1965–67.

Perrin, P., Rollin, P. E., and Sureau, P. (1986). A rapid rabies enzyme immuno-diagnosis (RREID): a useful and simple technique for the routine diagnosis of rabies. *J. Biol. Stand.*, **14**: 217–22.

Perrin, P., and Sureau, P. (1987). A collaborative study of an experimental kit for rapid rabies enzyme immunodiagnosis (RREID). *Bull. World Health Organ.*, **65**: 489–93.

Perry, B. D. (1995). Rabies control in the developing world: can further research help? *Vet. Rec.*, **137**: 521–22.

Plotkin, S. A. (1980). Rabies vaccination in the 1980s. *Hosp. Pract.*, **15**: 65–72.

Pradhan, H. K., Gurbuxani, J. P., *et al.* (2008). New steps in the control of canine rabies in India. *Dev. Biol. (Basel)*, **131**: 157–66.

Pulmanausahakul, R., Li, J., *et al.* (2008). The glycoprotein and the matrix protein of rabies virus affect pathogenicity by regulating viral replication and facilitating cell-to-cell spread. *J. Virol.*, **82**: 2330–38.

Quiambao, B. P., Lang, J., *et al.* (2000). Immunogenicity and effectiveness of post-exposure rabies prophylaxis with a new chromatographically purified Vero-cell rabies vaccine (CPRV): a two-stage randomised clinical trial in the Philippines. *Acta Trop.*, **75**: 39–52.

Randall, D. A., Williams, S. D., *et al.* (2004). Rabies in endangered Ethiopian wolves. *Emerg. Infect. Dis.*, **10**: 2214–17.

Rasalingam, P., Rossiter, J. P., *et al.* (2005). Comparative pathogenesis of the SAD-L16 strain of rabies virus and a mutant modifying the dynein light chain binding site of the rabies virus phosphoprotein in young mice. *Virus Res.*, **111**: 55–60.

Raux, H., Flamand, A., and Blondel, D. (2000). Interaction of the rabies virus P protein with the LC8 dynein light chain. *J. Virol.*, **74**: 10212–16.

Ravkov, E. V., Smith, J. S., and Nichol, S. T. (1995). Rabies virus glycoprotein gene contains a long 3' noncoding region which lacks pseudogene properties. *Virol.*, **206**: 718–23.

Reculard, P.(1996). Cell culture vaccine for veterinary use. In: D. D'Antona *et al.* (eds.) Laboratory techniques in rabies. Geneva, Switzerland: WHO.

Reynes, J. M., Molia, S., *et al.* (2004). Serologic evidence of lyssavirus infection in bats, Cambodia. *Emerg. Infect. Dis.*, **10**: 2231–34.

Roine, R. O., Hillbom, M., *et al.* (1988). Fatal encephalitis caused by a bat-borne rabies-related virus. *Brain*, **111**(6): 1505–16.

Ronsholt, L. (2002). A New Case of European Bat Lyssavirus (EBL) Infection in Danis Sheep. *Rabies Bull. Euro.*, **26**.

Root, J. J., McLean, R. G., *et al.* (2008). Potential effect of prior raccoonpox virus infection in raccoons on vaccinia-based rabies immunization. *BMC Immunol.*, **9**: 57.

Rosatte, R., Donovan, D., *et al.* (2001). Emergency response to raccoon rabies introduction into Ontario. *J. Wildl. Dis.*, **37**: 265–79.

Rosatte, R., Tinline, R., and Johnston, D. H. (2007). Rabies control in wild carnivores. In: A. C. Jackson and W. Wunner (eds.) Rabies, pp. 505–634. London: Elsevier/Academic press.

Rupprecht, C. E., Hanlon, C. A., and Hemachudha, T. (2002). Rabies re-examined. *Lancet* Infect. Dis., **2**: 327–43.

Rupprecht, C. E., Barrett, J., *et al.* (2008). Can rabies be eradicated? *Dev. Biol. (Basel)*, **131**: 95–121.

Russell, C. A., Smith, D. L., *et al.* (2005). Predictive spatial dynamics and strategic planning for raccoon rabies emergence in Ohio. *PLoS Biol.*, **3**: e88.

Sabeta, C. T., Bingham, J., and Nel, L. H. (2003). Molecular epidemiology of canid rabies in Zimbabwe and South Africa. *Virus Res.*, **91**: 203–11.

Sabeta, C. T., Mansfield, K. L. (2007). Molecular epidemiology of rabies in bat-eared foxes (Otocyon megalotis) in South Africa. *Virus Res.*, **129**: 1–10.

Schneider, L. G., and Cox, J. H. (1994). Bat lyssaviruses in Europe. *Curr. Top. Microb. Immunol.*, **187**: 207–18.

Seimenis, A. (2008). The rabies situation in the Middle East. *Dev. Biol. (Basel)*, **131:** 43–53.

Selimov, M. A., Tatarov, A. G., et al. (1989). Rabies-related Yuli virus; identification with a panel of monoclonal antibodies. *Acta Virol.*, **33:** 542–46.

Serra-Cobo, J., Amengual, B., et al. (2002). European bat lyssavirus infection in Spanish bat populations. *Emerg. Infect. Dis.*, **8:** 413–20.

Servat, A., Cliquet, F. (2006). Collaborative study to evaluate a new ELISA test to monitor the effectiveness of rabies vaccination in domestic carnivores. *Virus Res.*, **120:** 17–27.

Servat, A., Feyssaguet, M., et al. (2007). A quantitative indirect ELISA to monitor the effectiveness of rabies vaccination in domestic and wild carnivores. *J. Immunol. Meth.*, **318:** 1–10.

Shaul, J. F., Jacobs, C. F., and Ball, F. M. (1969). Duck embryo rabies vaccine. Anaphylactic reaction following initial injection. *J. S. C. Med. Assoc.*, **65:** 359–61.

Shimizu, K., Ito, N., et al. (2006). Sensitivity of rabies virus to type I interferon is determined by the phosphoprotein gene. *Microb. Immunol.*, **50:** 975–78.

Shimizu, K., Ito, N., et al. (2007). Involvement of nucleoprotein, phosphoprotein, and matrix protein genes of rabies virus in virulence for adult mice. *Virus Res.*, **123:** 154–60.

Si, H., Guo, Z. M., Hao, Y. T., et al. (2008). Rabies trend in China (1990–2007) and post-exposure prophylaxis in the Guangdong province. *BMC Infect. Dis.*, **8:** 113.

Sillero-Zubiri, C., King, A. A., and Macdonald, D. W. (1996). Rabies and mortality in Ethiopian wolves (Canis simensis). *J. Wildl. Dis.*, **32:** 80–86.

Singh, C. K., and Sandhu, B. S. (2008). Rabies in South Asia: epidemiological investigations and clinical perspective. *Dev. Biol. (Basel)*, **131:** 133–36.

Sipahioglu, U., and Alpaut, S. (1985). Transplacental rabies in humans. *Mikrobiyol. Bull.*, **19:** 95–99.

Slate, D., Rupprecht, C. E., et al. (2005). Status of oral rabies vaccination in wild carnivores in the United States. *Virus Res.*, **111:** 68–76.

Smith, J. S. (1981). Mouse model for abortive rabies infection of the central nervous system. *Infect. Immun.*, **31:** 297–308.

Smith, J. S., and Seidel, H. D. (1993). Rabies: a new look at an old disease. Prog. Med. *Virol.*, **40:** 82–106.

Smith, J., McElhinney, L., et al. (2003). Case report: rapid ante-mortem diagnosis of a human case of rabies imported into the UK from the Philippines. *J. Med. Virol.*, **69:** 150–55.

Solomon, T., Marston, D., et al. (2005). Paralytic rabies after a two week holiday in India. *BMJ*, **331:** 501–03.

Sriaroon, C., Daviratanasilpa, S., et al. (2003). Rabies in a Thai child treated with the eight-site post-exposure regimen without rabies immune globulin. *Vaccine*, **21:** 3525–26.

Srinivasan, A., Burton, E. C., et al. (2005). Transmission of rabies virus from an organ donor to four transplant recipients. *N. Engl. J. Med.*, **352:** 1103–11.

Steck, F., and Wandeler, A. (1980). The epidemiology of fox rabies in Europe. *Epidemiol. Rev.*, **2:** 71–96.

Stougaard, E., and Ammendrup, E. (1998). Rabies in individual countries: Denmark. *Rabies Bull. Eur.*, **22:** 6.

Sureau, P., Portnoi, D., et al. (1981). Prevention of inter-human rabies transmission after corneal graft. *C. R. Seances Acad. Sci. III*, **293:** 689–92.

Swanepoel, R., Barnard, B. J., et al. (1993). Rabies in southern Africa. *Onderstep. J. Vet. Res.*, **60:** 325–46.

Szanto, A. G., Nadin-Davis, S. A., and White, B. N. (2008). Complete genome sequence of a raccoon rabies virus isolate. *Virus Res.*, **136:** 130–39.

Takamatsu, F., Asakawa, N., et al. (1998). Studies on the rabies virus RNA polymerase: 2. Possible relationships between the two forms of the non-catalytic subunit (P protein). *Microbiol. Immunol.*, **42:** 761–71.

Takayama-Ito, M., Inoue, K., et al. (2006). A highly attenuated rabies virus HEP-Flury strain reverts to virulent by single amino acid substitution to arginine at position 333 in glycoprotein. *Virus Res.*, **119:** 208–215.

Tang, X., Luo, M., et al. (2005). Pivotal role of dogs in rabies transmission, China. *Emerg. Infect. Dis.*, **11:** 1970–72.

Thompson, R. D., Mitchell, G. C., and Burns, R. J. (1972). Vampire bat control by systemic treatment of livestock with an anticoagulant. *Sci.*, **177:** 806–8.

Thomson, G. R., and Meredith, C. D. (1993). Rabies in bat-eared foxes in South Africa. *Onderstep. J. Vet. Res.*, **60:** 399–403.

Tillotson, J. R., Axelrod, D., and Lyman, D. O. (1977). Rabies in a laboratory worker–New York. *Morb. Mortal. Wkly. Rep.*, **26:** 183–84.

Tims, T., Briggs, D. J., et al. (2000). Adult dogs receiving a rabies booster dose with a recombinant adenovirus expressing rabies virus glycoprotein develop high titers of neutralizing antibodies. *Vaccine*, **18:** 2804–7.

Tjornehoj, K., Fooks, A. R., et al. (2006). Natural and experimental infection of sheep with European bat lyssavirus type-1 of Danish bat origin. *J. Comp. Pathol.*, **134:** 190–210.

Tordo, N., Poch, O., et al. (1986). Walking along the rabies genome: is the large G-L intergenic region a remnant gene? *Proc. Nat. Acad. Sci. USA*, **83:** 3914–18.

Tordo, N., Poch, O., et al. (1988). Completion of the rabies virus genome sequence determination: highly conserved domains among the L (polymerase) proteins of unsegmented negative-strand RNA viruses. *Virol.*, **165:** 565–76.

Tordo, N., and Kouknetzoff, A. (1993). The rabies virus genome: an overview. *Onderstep. J. Vet. Res.*, **60:** 263–69.

Tordo, N., Bemansour, A., and Calisher, C. (2004). Rhabdoviridae. In: C. M. Fauquet et al. (eds.) Virus Taxonomy, VIIIth report of the ICTV, pp. 623–44. London: Elsevier/Academic Press.

Tsiang, H., Ceccaldi, P. E., and Lycke, E. (1991). Rabies virus infection and transport in human sensory dorsal root ganglia neurons. *J. Gen. Virol.*, **72(5):** 1191–94.

Tuffereau, C., Schmidt, K., et al. (2007). The rabies virus glycoprotein receptor p75NTR is not essential for rabies virus infection. *J. Virol.*, **81:** 13622–630.

Ugolini, G. (2008). Use of rabies virus as a transneuronal tracer of neuronal connections: implications for the understanding of rabies pathogenesis. *Dev. Biol. (Basel)*, **131:** 493–506.

Van Sittert, L. (2003). Class and Canicide in Little Bess: The 1893 Port Elizabeth Rabies Epidemic. *S. Afric. Hist. J.*, **48:** 1726–86.

Vos, A., Pommerening, E., et al. (2002). Safety studies of the oral rabies vaccine SAD B19 in striped skunk (Mephitis mephitis). *J. Wildl. Dis.*, **38:** 428–31.

Vos, A. (2003). Oral vaccination against rabies and the behavioural ecology of the red fox (Vulpes vulpes). *J. Vet. Med. Series B*, **50:** 477–83.

Vos, A. (2004). Wildlife rabies control in the Middle East. *Inf. Circ.*, **58:** 14–15.

Vos, A., Kaipf, I., et al. (2007). European Bat Lyssaviruses- an ecological enigma. *Acta Chiroptera.*, **9:** 283–96.

Wakeley, P. R., Johnson, N., et al. (2005). Development of a real-time, TaqMan reverse transcription-PCR assay for detection and differentiation of lyssavirus genotypes 1, 5, and 6. *J. Clin. Microbiol.*, **43:** 2786–92.

Warrell, M. J. (2008). Emerging aspects of rabies infection: with a special emphasis on children. *Curr. Opin. Infect. Dis.*, **21:** 251–57.

Warrilow, D., Smith, I. L., et al. (2002). Sequence analysis of an isolate from a fatal human infection of Australian bat lyssavirus. *Virol.*, **297:** 109–19.

Weyer, J., Rupprecht, C. E., et al. (2007). Generation and evaluation of a recombinant modified vaccinia virus Ankara vaccine for rabies. *Vaccine*, **25:** 4213–22.

Whelan, S. P., and Wertz, G. W. (1999). Regulation of RNA synthesis by the genomic termini of vesicular stomatitis virus: identification of distinct sequences essential for transcription but not replication. *J. Virol.*, **73:** 297–306.

WHO (1996). Laboratory techniques in rabies. Geneva: WHO.

WHO (2005). WHO Expert Consultation on rabies. *World Health Organ. Tech. Rep. Ser.,* **931:** 1–88.

WHO (2008). Fact sheet no. 9.

Wiktor, T. J., Fernandes, M. V., and Koprowski, H. (1964). Cultivation of Rabies Virus in Human Diploid Cell Strain Wi-38. *J. Immunol.,* **93:** 353–66.

Wilde, H., Khawplod, P., *et al.* (2005). Rabies control in South and Southeast Asia. *Vaccine,* **23:** 2284–89.

Winkler, W. G. (1968). Airborne rabies virus isolation. *Wildl. Dis.,* **4:** 37–40.

Winkler, W. G., Fashinell, T. R., *et al.* (1973). Airborne rabies transmission in a laboratory worker. *JAMA,* **226:** 1219–21.

Wirblich, C., Tan, G. S., *et al.* (2008). PPEY motif within the rabies virus (RV) matrix protein is essential for efficient virion release and RV pathogenicity. *J. Virol.,* **82:** 9730–38.

Wright, E., Temperton, N. J., *et al.* (2008). Investigating antibody neutralization of lyssaviruses using lentiviral pseudotypes: a cross-species comparison. *J. Gen. Virol.,* **89:** 2203–14.

Yakobson, B. A., King, R., *et al.* (2006). Rabies vaccination programme for red foxes (Vulpes vulpes) and golden jackals (Canis aureus) in Israel (1999–2004). *Dev. Biol. (Basel),* **125:** 133–40.

Yung, V., Favi, M., and Fernandez, J. (2002). Genetic and antigenic typing of rabies virus in Chile - Brief report. *Arch. Virol.,* **147:** 2197–205.

Yusibov, V., Hooper, D. C., *et al.* (2002). Expression in plants and immunogenicity of plant virus-based experimental rabies vaccine. *Vaccine,* **20:** 3155–64.

Zienius, D., Bagdonas, J., Dranseika, A. (2003). Epidemiological situation of rabies in Lithuania from 1990 to 2000. *Vet. Microbiol.,* **93:** 91–100.

CHAPTER 36

Rift Valley fever

R. Swanepoel and J. T. Paweska

Summary

Rift Valley fever (RVF) is an acute disease of domestic ruminants in mainland Africa and Madagascar, caused by a mosquito–borne virus and characterized by necrotic hepatitis and a haemorrhagic state. Large outbreaks of the disease in sheep, cattle and goats occur at irregular intervals of several years when exceptionally heavy rains favour the breeding of the mosquito vectors, and are distinguished by heavy mortality among newborn animals and abortion in pregnant animals. Humans become infected from contact with tissues of infected animals or from mosquito bite, and usually develop mild to moderately severe febrile illness, but severe complications, which occur in a small proportion of patients, include ocular sequelae, encephalitis and fatal haemorrhagic disease. Despite the occurrence of low case fatality rates, substantial numbers of humans may succumb to the disease during large outbreaks. Modified live and inactivated vaccines are available for use in livestock, and an inactivated vaccine was used on a limited scale in humans with occupational exposure to infection. The literature on the disease has been the subject of several extensive reviews from which the information presented here is drawn, except where indicated otherwise (Henning 1956; Weiss 1957; Easterday 1965; Peters and Meegan 1981; Shimshony and Barzilai 1983; Meegan and Bailey 1989; Swanepoel and Coetzer 2004; Flick and Bouloy 2005). In September 2000, the disease appeared in south west Saudi Arabia and adjacent Yemen, and the outbreak lasted until early 2001 (Al Hazmi *et al.* 2003; Madani *et al.* 2003; Abdo-Salem *et al.* 2006). The virus was probably introduced with infected livestock from the Horn of Africa, and it remains to be determined whether it has become endemic on the Arabian Peninsula.

History

The disease was first recognized in sheep in the Rift Valley in Kenya at the turn of the twentieth century, but the causative agent was not isolated until 1930. Over the next four decades, epizootics were recorded only in eastern and southern Africa, where they tended to occur in association with population explosions of floodwater-breeding aedine mosquitoes following heavy rains. Large outbreaks affecting sheep and cattle occurred in Kenya in 1930–31, 1968 and 1978–79, and lesser outbreaks at irregular intervals in the intervening years. A major epizootic, which caused an estimated 500,000 abortions and 100,000 deaths of sheep, occurred in South Africa in 1950–51; a second major and more widespread outbreak caused extensive losses of sheep and cattle in 1974–76, while lesser outbreaks were recorded in 1952–53, 1955–59, 1969–71 and 1981. Severe outbreaks occurred in the predominantly sheep farming areas of southern Namibia in 1955 and 1974–76. Further extensive outbreaks of the disease in southern Africa occurred in areas where cattle farming predominates, in Zimbabwe in 1955, 1957, 1969–70 and 1978, in Mozambique in 1969, and in Zambia in 1973–74, 1978 and 1985. In addition, evidence of the occurrence of the infection was recorded in many other southern and east African countries.

It was realized from the time of the original investigations in Kenya that febrile illness in humans accompanied outbreaks of disease in livestock, and that some patients experienced transient loss of visual acuity, but the occurrence of serious ocular sequelae was first recognized in the 1950–51 epizootic in South Africa. The first known human fatality was recorded in 1934 in a laboratory worker in the USA, but since the infection was complicated by thrombophlebitis and the patient died from pulmonary embolism, the potential lethality of the virus for man was overlooked until seven deaths from encephalitis and/or haemorrhagic fever with necrotic hepatitis were ascribed to RVF during the 1974–76 epizootic in South Africa. Subsequently deaths were also observed in Zimbabwe.

Prior to the 1970s, the presence of the virus was known for decades in the Sudan and certain west African countries from antibody studies, and there were periodic isolations of the virus in West Africa, where it was sometimes reported as Zinga virus, which is now known to be identical to RVF virus. In 1973 and 1976, outbreaks of RVF affecting livestock were reported in the Sudan. These epizootics were followed in 1977–78 by a major outbreak which occurred along the Nile delta and valley in Egypt, causing an unprecedented number of human infections and deaths, as well as numerous deaths and abortions in sheep and cattle and some losses in goats, water buffaloes and camels. Estimates of the number of human infections range from 18,000 to more than 200,000 with at least 598 deaths occurring from encephalitis and/or haemorrhagic fever. Thereafter, a severe epizootic was reported in 1987 in the Senegal River basin of southern Mauritania and northern Senegal. In Mauritania alone an estimated 224 human patients died of the disease, and there was a high rate of abortion in sheep and goats.

These outbreaks in North and West Africa differed in several respects from the pattern of disease which had hitherto been observed in sub-saharan Africa; in particular they occurred independently of rainfall in arid countries, apparently in association with vectors which breed in large rivers and dams.

Since the virus is capable of utilizing a wide range of mosquitoes as vectors (Turrell *et al.* 2008), the occurrence of the outbreak in Egypt raised the possibility that RVF could be introduced to the mainland of Eurasia, and extensive preventive vaccination of livestock was undertaken at the time in the Sinai Peninsula and Israel. Fears were also expressed that the virus could be transported to Saudi Arabia with animals exported from Africa for ritual slaughter on the annual Islamic pilgrimage to Mecca. In the event, only isolated outbreaks of RVF were recorded in Egypt in 1979 and 1980, and thereafter the country remained free of the disease for twelve years until it was again recognized in the Aswan Governate in May 1993. On this occasion there was not the same tendency for an explosive outbreak of the disease to occur as in 1977–78, but by October 1993 infections of humans and livestock, including sheep, cattle and water buffalo, had also been recognized in Sharqiya, Giza and El Faiyum Governates (Anon. 1993; Anon. 1994).

From late October 1997 to February 1998, a large outbreak of RVF occurred in northeastern Kenya and adjoining southern Somalia, following the occurrence of heavy rains and extensive flooding in what is essentially an arid area, and extensive outbreaks of the disease also occurred elsewhere in Kenya and Tanzania (Anon. 1998; Woods *et al.* 2002). There were heavy losses of livestock and an estimated 500 human deaths. An agent isolated from human blood was thought to be a new bunyavirus and given the name *Garissa virus*, but was later found to be *Ngari virus*, originally isolated from mosquitoes in West Africa and recently shown to be a recombinant bunyavirus (Bowen *et al.* 2001; Gerrard *et al.* 2004; Briese *et al.* 2006). Antibody to *Ngari virus* was found in people in both Kenya and Somalia, but the importance of the virus as a human pathogen remains to be determined. An outbreak of RVF was again recognized in the North Eastern Province of Kenya in November 2006 following the occurrence of heavy rains, and by the end of January 2007 it had appeared in the Coastal, Central, Rift Valley and Eastern Provinces. A total of 684 human cases of the disease were recorded, with a 20% death rate. The disease also occurred in neighbouring Somalia with 114 cases and a 45% death rate being reported. Outbreaks were recognized in Tanzania in January 2007, but investigations revealed that livestock and human disease had already occurred in late 2006, with a total of 191 cases and a 21% death rate being recorded. Following heavy rains an outbreak of RVF occurred in October–November 2007 in White Nile, Gezira and Sennar Provinces of Sudan, with 451 cases of the disease and an approximately 36% death rate being reported (Anon. 2007a; Anon. 2007b). The high death rates reported in the recent outbreaks were estimated from cases which were diagnosed mainly on clinical grounds, without reference to mild or inapparent infections. Small outbreaks of RVF were recognized in northeastern South Africa in 1999 and 2008, and also in central Madagascar in 2008.

In September, 2000, RVF broke out simultaneously in southwest Saudi Arabia and adjoining Yemen following heavy rains on the inland mountain range (Jupp *et al.* 2002; Al Hazmi *et al.* 2003; Madani *et al.* 2003; Abdo-Salem *et al.* 2006). This was the first known occurrence of outbreaks outside of the African region. The outbreaks lasted until early 2001, and resulted in 245 human deaths and the loss of thousands of sheep and goats. There was speculation that the virus may have been imported from the Horn of Africa with infected slaughter animals, possibly during the 1997–98 epidemic in East Africa. Subsequent detection of IgM antibody in sentinel sheep suggests that the virus may have become endemic on the Arabian Peninsula (Eldafil *et al.* 2006).

The Smithburn strain of RVF virus, which had been isolated from mosquitoes in Uganda in 1944 and passaged intracerebrally in mice, was subjected to further passaging in embryonated chicken eggs and mice in South Africa, and issued in the form of freeze-dried infected mouse brain for use as a partially-attenuated vaccine for livestock from 1951 onwards. In 1958, reversion was made to the use of a lower mouse passage level of the virus, and since 1971 the virus has been grown in cell cultures for the preparation of freeze-dried vaccine, recommended particularly for use in non-pregnant sheep (the virus retains abortigenic and teratogenic properties for a proportion of pregnant ewes). The same strain of virus is used at a slightly different level of mouse passage for the preparation of veterinary vaccine in Kenya when demand arises. The Smithburn virus was found to be inadequately immunogenic for cattle, and since 1975 a wild strain of virus grown in cell cultures has been used in South Africa for the preparation of a formalin-inactivated vaccine for use in cattle. An inactivated cell culture vaccine for veterinary use was also developed in Egypt in 1981. An experimental formalin-inactivated cell culture vaccine for use in humans was developed in the USA in 1962, and improvements to the vaccine were made in 1981, but it was made available for use in people with occupational exposure to infection on a very limited scale only.

The virus

Taxonomy and molecular biology

The virus has the morphological and physicochemical properties typical of a member of the *Phlebovirus* genus of the family *Bunyaviridae*. It is spherical, approximately 100 nm in diameter, and has a host cell-derived bilipid-layer envelope through which virus-coded glycoprotein spikes project. The genome comprises three segments of single-stranded RNA with a total molecular weight of 4×10^6 Da, and is in the negative-sense (complementary to mRNA), except that the small segment consists of ambisense RNA, i.e. has bi-directional coding. Each of the three RNA segments, L (large), M (medium) and S (small), is contained in a separate nucleocapsid within the virion. In common with other bunyaviruses, phlebovirus virions contain three major structural proteins: two envelope glycoproteins, G1 and G2, and a nucleocapsid protein N, plus minor quantities of viral transcriptase or L (large) protein as it is termed. The L RNA segment codes for the viral transcriptase, the M segment for the G proteins and a non-structural protein, NS_m, and the S segment for the N protein and a non-structural protein, NS_s. The glycoproteins are responsible for recognition of receptor sites on susceptible cells, manifestation of viral haemagglutinating ability, and inducing protective immune response. The N protein induces production of and reacts with complement-fixing antibody. The non-structural NS_s protein synthesized during the replication of RVF virus, enters the cell nucleus to form intranuclear inclusions which are seen histologically in infected tissues. The NS_s protein acts as a major determinant of virulence by antagonizing interferon β expression after infection (Le May *et al.* 2008).

Virus which attaches to receptors on susceptible cells is internalized by endocytosis and replication occurs in the cytoplasm. Virions mature primarily by budding through endoplasmic reticulum in the Golgi region into cytoplasmic vesicles which are presumed to fuse with the plasma membrane to release virus, but particles can also bud directly from the plasma membrane.

No significant antigenic or genetic differences have been detected between RVF isolates and laboratory passaged strains originating from widely separated countries (Battles and Dalrymple 1988; Bird *et al.* 2007a), but differences have been demonstrated in pathogenicity for laboratory rodents. However, it is uncertain whether this finding is reflected in differences in virulence for humans and livestock. Zinga virus, originally isolated in the Central African Republic in 1969 and long thought to be a distinct virus, and Lunyo virus, isolated in Uganda in 1955 and described as a variant of RVF virus, have both been found to be indistinguishable from RVF virus.

Pathogenesis

By analogy with the course of events believed to follow natural infection with other arthropod-borne viruses, it can be surmised that the pathogenesis of the disease may involve some replication of virus at the site of inoculation, conveyance of infection by lymphatic drainage to regional lymph nodes where there is further replication with spill-over of virus into the circulation to produce primary viraemia, which in turn leads to systemic infection, and that intense viraemia then results from release of virus following replication in major target organs such as the liver and spleen. Wild RVF virus, which has not been subjected to serial passaging in laboratory host systems, is described as being hepato-, viscero- or pantropic, and immunofluorescence studies in laboratory animals indicate that replication occurs in littoral macrophages of lymph nodes, most areas of the spleen except T-dependent periarteriolar sheaths, foci of adrenocortical cells, virtually all cells of the liver, most renal glomeruli and some tubules, lung tissue and scattered small vessel walls, as well as in necrotic foci in the brains of individuals which develop the encephalitic form of the disease. These sites correspond to the lymphoid necrosis in lymph nodes and spleen, hepatic necrosis and adrenal, lung and glomerular lesions seen in humans and livestock, and the brain lesions in humans (encephalitis has not been described in natural disease of ruminants). Cell damage is ascribed directly to the lytic effects of the virus, but the inflammatory response seen in human brain tissue suggests that there may also be an immunopathological element to the pathogenesis of encephalitis. The same may be true for ocular lesions. Recovery is mediated by non-specific and specific host responses, and the clearance of viraemia correlates with the appearance of neutralizing antibody. Immunity appears to be lifelong.

The mechanisms involved in the pathogenesis of the haemostatic derangement which occurs in RVF remain speculative. It is postulated that the critical lesions are vasculitis and hepatic necrosis. Destruction of the antithrombotic properties of endothelial cells is thought to trigger intravascular coagulation, and the widespread necrosis of hepatocytes and other affected cells to result in the release of procoagulants into the circulation. Severe liver damage presumably limits or abolishes production of coagulation proteins and reduces clearance of activated coagulation factors, thereby further promoting the occurrence of disseminated intravascular coagulopathy, which in turn augments tissue injury by impairing blood flow. Vasculitis and haemostatic failure result in purpura and widespread haemorrhages.

Culture of the virus

The virus can be grown in and readily produces cytopathic effect and plaques in virtually all common continuous line and primary cell cultures, including Vero and BHK21 line cells, primary calf and lamb kidney or testis cells; the only exceptions being primary macrophages and lymphoblastoid cell lines. It can be grown in embryonated chicken eggs and a variety of laboratory animals including suckling or weaned mice and hamsters inoculated by intracerebral or intraperitoneal routes. Some laboratory strains of rat are resistant, as are rabbits, guinea-pigs, chickens and African primates, but a proportion of rhesus monkeys manifests severe or fatal disease.

Stability

The virus is stable in serum and can be recovered after several months storage at 4°C or after three hours at 56°C; viraemic blood collected in an oxalate–carbol–glycerin preservative retained its infectivity after eight years of storage under a variety of conditions of refrigeration, and the virus is very stable at temperatures lower than -60°C or after freeze drying, and in aerosols at 23°C and 50 to 85% relative humidity. It is inactivated by lipid solvents, such as ether and sodium deoxycholate, and low concentrations of formalin, and infectivity is rapidly lost below pH 6.8.

Livestock disease

Newborn lambs and goat kids are extremely susceptible to the disease, and the incubation period is short, in the range of 12–36 hours. The disease is marked by the development of fever which may be biphasic, listlessness, hyperpnoea, and disinclination to move or feed. Evidence of abdominal pain can be elicited. The course is usually peracute and lambs rarely survive longer than 24–36 hours after the onset of illness; many are simply found dead. Mortality may exceed 90% in animals less than a week old. Lambs and kids older than two weeks and mature sheep and goats are significantly less susceptible to the disease. Nevertheless, following an incubation period of 24 to 72 hours, a few animals may die peracutely without exhibiting noteworthy signs of illness. Most develop an acute disease with fever of up to 42EC that lasts for 24 to 96 hours, anorexia, weakness, listlessness and hypernoea. Some animals may regurgitate ingesta, and develop melaena or foetid diarrhoea and a blood-tinged, mucopurulent nasal discharge. A few animals may be icteric. Many sheep and goats undergo inapparent infection. Reported death rates vary from 5 to 60% for sheep, with highest mortality generally occurring in pregnant animals. Non-pregnant goats were described as resistant to the disease in some outbreaks, but suffered similar mortality to sheep in other instances.

The disease in calves resembles that in lambs and sheep, with occurrence of fever, inappetence, weakness and a bloody or foetid diarrhoea, but a higher proportion of calves may develop icterus. Death generally occurs two to eight days after infection, and estimates of mortality range from less than 10% in some outbreaks to 70% in experimentally infected one week old calves. Infection is frequently inapparent in adult cattle, but some animals develop acute disease characterized by fever of 24 to 96 hours duration, anorexia, staring coat, lachrymation, salivation, nasal discharge, dysgalactia and a bloody or foetid diarrhoea. The death rate in cattle does not generally appear to exceed 5–10%, but was reported to be 30% among cattle which aborted in Egypt. Illness tended to run a prolonged course of 10 to 20 days in cattle in the Sudan in 1973, with severe icterus being a marked feature of the disease, although most animals recovered spontaneously.

Abortion appears to be the usual, if not invariable, outcome to infection in pregnant sheep, goats and cattle. Animals may abort at any stage of gestation, and the foetuses generally have an autolysed appearance. However, abortion rates vary with epidemiological circumstances, and have ranged from 15 to 100% in different outbreaks, or in separate herds and flocks in a single outbreak. Frequently, abortion may be the only overt manifestation of disease in a herd or flock. Factors which determine the pattern of disease which occurs include the immune status of the animals, the challenge rate in the particular locality (mosquito biting frequency), and timing of the outbreak relative to the livestock breeding cycle. The offspring of immune ruminants acquire protective maternal immunity through the uptake of antibody from colostrum, but it was observed in South Africa that lambs were sometimes subjected to attack by large numbers of mosquitoes as soon as they were born, and could undergo irreversible infection before colostral immunity became effective.

Viraemia is generally demonstrable in domestic ruminants at the onset of fever and may persist for up to a week, with maximum titres of infectivity recorded being $10^{10.1}$ mouse intraperitoneal 50% lethal doses/ml ($MIPLD_{50}$/ml) in lambs, $10^{8.2}$ in kids and $10^{7.5}$ in calves, with somewhat lower maximum titres being recorded in adult animals.

Inoculation of pregnant ewes with the live Smithburn vaccine virus between about five and ten weeks of gestation may result in the occurrence of a range of anomalies of the central nervous system including porencephaly, hydranencephaly and micrencephaly, as well as arthrogryposis and other defects in foetuses, and prolonged gestation and *hydrops amnii* in the ewes. Inoculation at an earlier stage of pregnancy may result in unnoticed early loss of the conceptus, while inoculation at a later stage may result in abortion, stillbirth or birth of immune or viraemic progeny. Teratology following vaccination has been recorded in the progeny of up to 15% of pregnant ewes in flocks, but on average it appears to affect less than 2% of ewes and abortion probably occurs in less than 10% of pregnant ewes.

High prevalences of antibody were found in domesticated Asian water buffaloes during the 1977–78 epizootic in Egypt, and abortion and mortality rates of 7 to 12% were recorded on some farms. Horses develop only low grade viraemia following experimental infection, but during the Egyptian epizootic there was one isolation of virus from a horse and four abortions in donkeys were ascribed to RVF, while a low prevalence of antibody to the virus was detected in the two species. No pathogenicity tests have been conducted on camels, but antibody was detected in camels in Kenya. Although there was only one isolation of RVF virus from a camel during the 1977–78 Egyptian outbreak, 56 deaths and one abortion were ascribed to the disease on the basis of circumstantial evidence. Pigs and dogs are resistant to infection, i.e. undergo inapparent infection, and birds are refractory to the virus.

Experimental RVF infection of African buffaloes (*Syncerus caffer*) in Kenya resulted in transient fever and viraemia, and one of two pregnant females aborted. It was noted on some properties involved in the 1950–51 epizootic in South Africa that abortion occurred in farmed springbok (*Antidorcas marsupialis*) and blesbok (*Damaliscus dorcas phillipsi*) antelope, but this was not confirmed to be due to RVF. A low prevalence of antibody to RVF virus was found in African buffaloes and a few species of antelopes in Zimbabwe, but no evidence of disease was recorded. RVF was confirmed as a cause of abortion in captive-bred buffaloes in north eastern South Africa in 1999 and again in 2008. Some species of wild myomorph rodents (rats and mice) exhibit transient viraemia following peripheral infection, and those that circulate the highest levels of virus succumb to the disease.

Although age and underlying illness undoubtedly influence the course of infection, it has been shown in cross-breeding experiments with inbred strains of laboratory rodent that there is a genetic basis to susceptibility to RVF, and it was postulated that the innate mechanisms involved also operate in humans and livestock to determine the manifestation of disease. It has been suggested that indigenous African breeds of livestock may be more resistant to RVF than exotic breeds, possibly through natural selection, but it was shown in limited experiments in Nigeria that local sheep were highly susceptible, and indigenous sheep, cattle and goats were severely affected in the epizootics in Egypt and West Africa.

Human disease

Signs and symptoms

The majority of RVF infections in humans are inapparent or associated with moderate to severe, non-fatal, febrile illness. After an incubation period of two to six days, the onset of the benign illness is usually very sudden and the disease is characterized by rigor, fever that persists for several days and is often biphasic, headache with retro-orbital pain and photophobia, weakness, and muscle and joint pains. Sometimes there is nausea and vomiting, abdominal pain, vertigo, epistaxis and a petechial rash. Viraemia in humans lasts for up to a week, with a maximum recorded intensity of $10^{8.6}$ mouse intracerebral 50% lethal doses/ml ($MICLD_{50}$/ml). Defervescence and symptomatic improvement occur in four to seven days in benign disease and recovery is often complete in two weeks, but in a minority of patients the disease is complicated by the development of ocular lesions at the time of the initial illness or up to four weeks later. Estimates for the incidence of ocular complications range from less than 1% to 20% of human infections, and possibly the differences stem from failure to record mild cases in populations where illiterate persons are less likely to report minor disturbances of vision. The ocular disease usually presents as a loss of acuity of central vision, sometimes with development of scotomas. The essential lesion appears to be focal retinal ischaemia, generally in the macular or paramacular area, associated with thrombotic occlusion of arterioles and capillaries, and is characterized by retinal oedema and loss of transparency caused by dense white exudate and haemorrhages. Sometimes there is severe haemorrhage and detachment of the retina. The lesions and the loss of visual acuity generally resolve over a period of months with variable residual scarring of the retina, but in instances of severe haemorrhage and detachment of the retina there may be permanent uni- or bilateral blindness.

Probably less than 1% of human patients develop the haemorrhagic and/or encephalitic forms of the disease. Underlying liver disease may predispose to the haemorrhagic form of the illness.

The haemorrhagic syndrome starts with sudden onset of febrile illness similar to the benign disease, but within two to four days there may be development of a petechial rash, purpura, ecchymoses and extensive subcutaneous haemorrhages, bleeding from needle puncture sites, epistaxis, haematemesis, diarrhoea and melaena, sore and inflamed throat, gingival bleeding, epigastric pain, hepatomegaly or hepatosplenomegaly, tenderness of the right upper quadrant of the abdomen and deep jaundice. This is followed by pneumonitis, anaemia, shock with racing pulse and low blood pressure, hepatorenal failure, coma and cardiorespiratory arrest. Factors contributing to fatal outcome in the hepatic form of the disease include anaemia, shock and hepatorenal failure, with the kidney lesions possibly being as important as shock in producing anuria. A proportion of the less severely affected patients may make a protracted recovery without sequelae.

Encephalitis may occur in combination with the haemorrhagic syndrome. Otherwise, signs of encephalitis in humans may supervene during the acute illness, or up to four weeks later and include severe headache, vertigo, confusion, disorientation, amnesia, meningismus, hallucinations, hypersalivation, grinding of teeth, choreiform movements, convulsions, hemiparesis, lethargy, decerebrate posturing, locked-in syndrome, coma and death. A proportion of patients may recover completely, but others may be left with sequelae, such as hemiparesis.

An attempt to relate the occurrence of abortion in humans to serological evidence of RVF infection in Egypt produced inconclusive results. Diagnosis of the infection in a neonatal child in Saudi Arabia in 2000 implied that there had been vertical transmission of infection, but the mother was not tested (Arishi et al. 2006).

Clinical pathology

The information available on clinical pathology findings in humans is compatible with observations made in haematological and coagulation studies on rhesus monkeys, except that leucocytosis and anaemia may be more marked in severe human disease (Peters et al. 1980; Al Hazmi et al. 2003). Rhesus monkeys may have prolonged activated partial thromboplastin times and prothrombin times even in benign infection, and in severe liver disease there may be depletion of coagulation factors II, V, VII, IX, X and XII, thrombocytopenia and platelet dysfunction, increased schistocyte counts and depletion of fibrinogen together with raised fibrin degradation product levels. Raised serum aspartate aminotransferase and alanine aminotransferase levels have been recorded even in benign disease in humans.

Diagnosis

The disease may be suspected when there is a sudden outbreak of febrile illness with headache and myalgia in humans, in association with the occurrence of abortions in domestic ruminants and deaths of young animals. Sometimes the human disease is only recognized from the occurrence of ocular complications, or haemorrhagic or encephalitic manifestations, and this is especially true in the rare instances where residents of other continents develop the illness following a visit to Africa. Frequently, outbreaks of RVF in livestock only become evident after investigations have been triggered by the recognition of the disease in humans.

Specimens to be submitted for laboratory confirmation of the diagnosis include blood from live patients, and tissue samples, particularly liver, but also spleen, kidney, lymph nodes and heart blood of deceased patients. Tissue samples should be submitted in duplicate in a viral transport medium, and in 10% buffered–formalin for histopathological examination.

Viral antigen can often be detected rapidly in blood and other tissues by a variety of immunological methods, including immunodiffusion, complement-fixation, immunofluorescence and enzyme-linked immunoassay, and viral nucleic acid can readily be detected by RT-PCR (Jupp et al. 2002; Drosten et al. 2002; Weidmann et al. 2007; Bird et al. 2007b). The virus is cytopathic and can be isolated readily in almost all cell cultures commonly used in diagnostic laboratories, and identified rapidly by immunofluorescence. Virus can also be isolated in suckling or weaned mice, or hamsters, inoculated intracerebrally or intraperitoneally, and antigen can be identified in harvested brain or liver by the immunological methods mentioned above. Definitive identification of isolates is achieved by performing neutralization tests with reference antiserum.

Antibody to RVF virus can be demonstrated in complement-fixation, enzyme-linked immunoassay, indirect immunofluorescence, haemagglutination-inhibition, or neutralization tests. Diagnosis of recent infection is confirmed by demonstrating seroconversion or a four-fold or greater rise in titre of antibody in paired serum samples, or by demonstrating IgM antibody activity in an enzyme-linked immunoassay (Paweska et al. 2005, 2007).

Benign RVF in humans must be distinguished from other febrile zoonotic diseases such as brucellosis and Q fever which can be acquired from contact with livestock carcases, while the fulminant hepatic disease must be distinguished from the so-called formidable viral haemorrhagic fevers of Africa: Lassa fever, Crimean–Congo haemorrhagic fever, Marburg disease, Ebola fever and, theoretically, the haemorrhagic fever with renal syndrome associated with hantavirus infections (there has been serological evidence of, but no virologically confirmed case of the latter syndrome in Africa).

Pathology

Histopathological lesions, particularly those in the liver, are considered to be pathognomonic, and are essentially similar in humans and domestic ruminants. The severity of the lesions varies from primary foci of coagulative necrosis, consisting of clusters of hepatocytes with acidophilic cytoplasms and pyknotic nuclei, multifocally scattered throughout the parenchyma, to massive liver destruction in which the primary foci comprising dense aggregates of cytoplasmic and nuclear debris, some fibrin and a few neutrophils and macrophages, can be discerned against a background of parenchyma reduced by nuclear pyknosis, karyorrhexis and cytolysis to scattered fragments of cytoplasm and chromatin, with only narrow rims of degenerated hepatocytes remaining reasonably intact close to portal triads. Intensely acidophilic cytoplasmic bodies which resemble the Councilman bodies of yellow fever are common, and rod-shaped or oval eosinophilic intranuclear inclusions may be seen in intact nuclei. Icterus may be evident.

Treatment

Treatment is essentially symptomatic, and supportive therapy in the haemorrhagic disease includes replacement of blood and coagulation factors. Results obtained in animal models suggest that the administration of immune plasma from recovered patients may be beneficial. The antiviral drug ribavirin inhibits virus replication in cell cultures and laboratory animals, and it was suggested that it could be used even in benign disease in order to obviate the potentially serious complications which may occur in humans. However, the drug but did not prevent the late occurrence of encephalitis in patients in Saudi Arabia, and its use is now considered contraindicated in RVF infection.

Prognosis

Despite the sudden and dramatic change perceived in the nature of the human disease in the mid-1970s, it was deduced from the 598 reported deaths and 200,000 estimated cases of disease that RVF had a case fatality rate of less than 1% in Egypt where a high prevalence of schistosomiasis may have predisposed the population to severe liver disease. The fatality rate may even have been lower in relation to total infections, since an antibody prevalence rate of approximately 30% was detected in the human population estimated at one to three million in the areas affected by the epizootic. Remarkably high estimates of approximately 5 and 14% were made for case fatality rates in two separate populations in the 1987 epizootic in Mauritania, on the basis of the proportion of IgM antibody-positive persons who actually reported illness considered to be compatible with RVF, but it can be deduced that the fatality rates in terms of total IgM antibody-positive persons are much closer to the corresponding fatality rate in Egypt. The death rates of 20–45% estimated for recent outbreaks in East Africa are based on clinically-apparent or hospitalized cases only and there is no true denominator available from seroconversion studies.

Epidemiology

Factors affecting the occurrence of epizootics

Kenya, Tanzania, Somalia, South Africa, Namibia, Mozambique, Zimbabwe, Zambia, Sudan, Egypt, Mauritania, and Senegal have experienced large outbreaks of RVF as outlined above, while lesser outbreaks, periodic isolations of virus or serological evidence of infection have been recorded in Angola, Botswana, Burkina Faso, Cameroon, Central African Republic, Chad, Gabon, Guinea, Madagascar, Malawi, Mali, Nigeria, Uganda and Democratic Republic of the Congo.

Outbreaks of RVF in eastern and southern Africa have tended to occur at irregular intervals of up to 15 years or longer, and the fate of the virus during inter-epizootic periods has long constituted a central enigma in the epidemiology of the disease. On the basis of early observations made in Uganda, Kenya and South Africa, it was accepted for decades that the virus was enzootic in indigenous forests which extend in broken fashion from East Africa to the eastern and southern coastal regions of South Africa. The virus was thought to circulate in *Eretmapodites* spp. mosquitoes and unknown vertebrates in the forests, and to spread in seasons of exceptionally heavy rainfall to livestock rearing areas where the vectors were believed to be floodwater-breeding aedine mosquitoes of the subgenera *Aedimorphus* and *Neomelaniconion*, which attach their eggs to vegetation at the edge of stagnant surface water. In contrast to other culicine mosquitoes, it is obligatory that the eggs of aedines be subjected to a period of drying as the water recedes before they will hatch on being wetted again when next the area floods. Thus, the aedine mosquitoes overwinter as eggs which can survive for long periods in dried mud, possibly for several seasons if the area remains dry.

On the inland plateau of South Africa, where sheep rearing predominates, surface water gathers after heavy rains in undrained shallow depressions (pans) and farm dams which afford ideal breeding environments for aedines. On the watershed plateau of Zimbabwe, where cattle farming predominates, aedines breed in *vleis*, low-lying grassy areas which constitute drainage channels for surrounding high ground, and which are flooded by seepage after heavy rains. *Vleis* correspond to what are termed dambos in the livestock rearing areas of central and eastern Africa. Sustained monitoring in Zimbabwe revealed that a low level of virus transmission to livestock occurred each year in the same areas where epizootics occurred. The generation of epizootics, therefore, was associated with the simultaneous intensification of virus activity over vast livestock rearing areas where it was already present, rather than lateral spread from cryptic enzootic foci: examination of satellite images and aerial photographs revealed that the enzootic areas coincided with savannah and grasslands with a high density of *vleis*, and not with canopy forests. Subsequently, RVF virus was isolated from unfed *Aedes mcintoshi* mosquitoes (= *Aedes lineatopennis* sensu lato) hatched in *dambos* on a ranch in Kenya during inter-epizootic periods in 1982 and 1984, confirming that the virus is enzootic in livestock rearing areas and indicating that it appears to be maintained by transovarial transmission in aedines. The available evidence suggests that in Zimbabwe, as in Kenya, *Aedes mcintoshi* is the most important maintenance vector of the virus while *Aedes dentatus* is probably also a maintenance vector; the same two species and possibly *Aedes unidentatus* and *Aedes juppi* are maintenance vectors on the inland plateau of South Africa.

In contrast to countries such as Zimbabwe and Kenya, or even the coastal areas of South Africa, the inland plateau of South Africa has harsh winters and prolonged droughts are not uncommon, with pans and small dams remaining dry for many years or even decades at a time, so it is possible that aedine mosquito populations could decline to the point where RVF virus activity becomes virtually undetectable or the virus entirely disappears from the area. Indeed, no outbreaks of RVF have been recorded on the interior plateau of South Africa since the major epizootic of 1974–76, although small outbreaks were recognized in a coastal bush area in northern Natal in 1981 and in the north eastern Mpumalanga and Limpopo Provinces in 1999 and 2008 (Swanepoel and Paweska 2008). This suggests either that virus activity has declined on the inland plateau to a level where considerable amplification must occur before the disease again becomes evident, or that the virus has disappeared from the area and must be reintroduced through a mechanism permitting its long range dispersal, as discussed below in relation to the appearance of the disease in Egypt in 1977.

Epizootics generally become evident in late summer after there has been an initial increase in vector populations and in circulation of the virus. Heavy rainfall and the humid conditions which prevail during epizootics favour the breeding of other biting insects besides aedine mosquitoes. Following extensive flooding of aedine breeding sites, significant numbers of livestock become infected and circulate high levels of virus in their blood during the acute stage of infection. Other culicines and anopheline mosquitoes then become infected and serve as epizootic vectors, particularly *Culex theileri* in southern Africa, and biting flies such as midges, phlebotomids, stomoxids and simulids serve as mechanical transmitters of infection. Although contagion has been demonstrated on occasion under artificial conditions, non-vectorial transmission is not considered to be important in livestock, as opposed to humans. Outbreaks generally terminate in late autumn when the onset of cold weather depresses vector activity, or when most animals are immune following natural infection, or after there has been successful intervention with vaccine.

It can be deduced, and in some instances has been demonstrated directly, that the intensity of viraemia attained in domestic ruminants, humans and many rodents is adequate for the infection of the mosquito vectors of RVF virus through the ingestion of blood-meals: estimated threshold levels of viraemia required to infect 50% of mosquitoes range from $10^{5,7}$ to $10^{8,7}$ MICLD$_{50}$/ml for the various putative vectors of southern Africa. Although extensive studies have failed to prove that the virus is maintained in natural transmission cycles in rodents, birds, or other wild vertebrates, it is felt that wild ruminants could play a role similar to their domestic counterparts in areas where they predominate. Furthermore, it is believed that the possibility that the virus is also maintained by circulation in forest mosquitoes and unidentified vertebrates, cannot be dismissed entirely and merits further investigation.

In retrospect, it can be surmised the occurrence of the massive epizootic in Egypt in 1977–78 was probably facilitated by an increase in mosquito breeding sites brought about by agricultural developments which followed the building of the Aswan dam, although it remains necessary to explain the mechanisms responsible for the introduction of the virus into the country. Various theories were advanced to account for the first known appearance of the virus in Egypt in 1977, including the long distance carriage of infected vectors at high altitude by prevailing winds associated with the inter-tropical convergence zone; a mechanism which has been invoked to explain the spread of many other arboviruses in the past. The introduction of the virus through the transportation of infected sheep and cattle on the Nile or overland from northern Sudan to markets in southern Egypt was also considered to have been a strong possibility, and the movement of slaughter animals by sea could account for the evidence of infection detected in the northern and eastern coastal areas of Egypt. Although transportation on some routes would take a long time in relation to the course of the infection, RVF virus has been shown to persist for prolonged periods in various organs of sheep, particularly the spleen for up to 21 days after infection. The same could be true for goats and cattle, or even the camels brought in by overland caravan routes. It is believed that humans slaughtering or handling the tissues of such animals could have become infected and served as the amplifying hosts for the infection of mosquitoes since the main vector in the Egyptian epizootic, *Culex pipiens*, is known to be peridomestic and anthropophilic. In at least one instance there were indications that human infections centred on a location where introduced camels were slaughtered. The incidence of the disease declined with the onset of the cool season in 1977, but it is thought that hibernation of infected adult *Culex pipiens* or other vector species, or a continued low level of biting activity by a proportion of the mosquito population, could account for the overwintering of the virus and the continuance of the epizootic into 1978.

In West Africa, the construction of the large Manantali dam on the Senegal River in Mali and the Diama dam downstream on the border between Mauritania and Senegal increased potential mosquito breeding sites in an area where the virus was already known to active, and prevailing drought conditions led to the concentration of nomadic people and their livestock in proximity to the dams.

However, virus activity has declined in the arid 'Sahelian' region since the epizootic of 1987, and RVF is thought to be enzootic in the more humid 'Guinean' areas of West Africa, where *Aedes mcintoshi*, *Aedes dalzieli* and *Aedes vexans* are considered to be potentially important vectors.

There was speculation that RVF virus may have been imported into Saudi Arabia and Yemen from Africa with slaughter animals, or carried from Africa by wind-borne mosquitoes in 2000, but there were no known epidemics in the Horn of Africa at the time. It is much more likely that infected animals were imported during the 1997–98 epidemic in East Africa, and that infection smouldered on the Arabian Peninsula until ideal circumstances for an epidemic occurred following heavy rains in 2000 (Jupp *et al.* 2002).

Factors affecting the occurrence of human infection

In contrast to the main vector in the Egyptian epizootic of 1977–78, the principal mosquito vectors of RVF virus in sub-Saharan Africa tend to be zoophilic and sylvatic, with the result that humans become infected mainly from contact with animal tissues, although there are instances where no such history can be obtained and it must be assumed that infection has resulted from mosquito bite. Occasional infections diagnosed in tourists from abroad who have visited countries in Africa fall into this category. Generally, persons who become infected are involved in the livestock industry, such as farmers who assist in dystocia of livestock, farm labourers who salvage carcases for human consumption, veterinarians and their assistants, and abattoir workers. The virus is notorious as a cause of laboratory infections, and there are numerous reports of humans becoming infected while investigating the disease in the field. The results of surveys following epizootics in southern Africa indicated that nine to 15% of farm residents became infected, with a slight preponderance of adult males, although it appeared that housewives also gained infection from handling fresh meat.

No outbreaks of the disease have been recognized in urban consumer populations and it is surmised that the fall in pH associated with the maturation of meat in abattoirs is deleterious to the virus. Moreover, highest infection rates were found in workers in the by-products sections of abattoirs in Zimbabwe and the implication is that the carcases of infected animals which reach abattoirs are generally recognized as being diseased and are condemned as unfit for human consumption, and are then sterilized in the process of preparing carcase meal which is incorporated in animal feeds.

Human infection presumably results from contact of virus with abraded skin, wounds or mucous membranes, but aerosol and intranasal infection have been demonstrated experimentally and circumstantial evidence suggests that aerosols have been involved in some human infections in the laboratory, and in the field during the Egyptian outbreak of 1977–78. Many infections in Egypt are thought to have resulted from the slaughter of infected animals outside of abattoirs, and the fact that the mosquito vector was anthropophilic is thought to explain the high incidence of infection which occurred in people of all ages and diverse occupations. Low concentrations of virus have been found in milk and body fluids such as saliva and nasal discharges of sheep and cattle, and it appears that there may have been a connection between human infection and consumption of raw milk in Mauritania. In view of the intense viraemia which occurs in humans and the fact that virus has been isolated from throat washings, it is curious that there are no confirmed records of person to person transmission of infection.

Prevention and control

Measures such as biological or chemical control of vectors, movement of livestock from low-lying areas to well drained and windswept pastures at higher altitudes, or confining of animals to mosquito-proof stables, are usually impractical or at best palliative in the face of a RVF epizootic, and immunization remains the only effective method of controlling the disease.

In addition to the modified live Smithburn strain and the formalin-inactivated vaccines referred to above, trials have been reported with small plaque variant and mutagen-derived candidate veterinary vaccines, but these have not been brought into commercial production. Promising candidate vaccines include the naturally attenuated clone 13 virus plus a genetically-engineered virus which lacks non-structural protein genes (Muller *et al.* 1995; Bird *et al.* 2008).

The Smithburn vaccine strain confers lifelong immunity in sheep and goats, and it is recommended that they should be immunized on a single occasion in the first year of life, preferably at six months of age after maternal immunity has waned. The Smithburn strain protects cattle against infection, but does not induce adequate humoral response to ensure transfer of colostral immunity to calves. Cattle and other domestic ruminants can be immunized at any age after maternal immunity has waned with inactivated vaccine, but the immunity is not durable and the animals should receive a second dose of vaccine three to six months later, plus annual boosters. It is, however, usually very difficult to persuade farmers to vaccinate livestock during long inter-epizootic periods, and the occurrence of outbreaks is difficult to predict. The result is that vaccine has almost invariably been used too late in the course of outbreaks to be fully effective. A further problem is that during outbreaks there is a chance of spreading infection with wild virus through transferring viraemic blood on needles used to inoculate different animals in succession. Nevertheless, in the past it has been practice in Kenya and South Africa to vaccinate all livestock, including pregnant ewes, with the Smithburn strain in the face of outbreaks, since it is deemed that the abortigenic and teratogenic effects of the vaccine are outweighed by the potentially severe consequences of allowing the disease to run its natural course. It is considered theoretically possible, although not proven, that live vaccine strains could revert to full virulence if passaged through hosts, as for instance through mosquitoes which become infected as a result of feeding on animals in the viraemic stage following administration of the vaccine. Hence, it is advised that only the inactivated vaccine should be used in situations where it is considered necessary to immunize animals in countries where the presence of RVF virus has not been proven.

Veterinarians and others engaged in the livestock industry should be made aware of the potential dangers of exposure to zoonotic agents in handling tissues of diseased animals, and precautions should be heightened during RVF epizootics. These should include the use of suitable protective clothing, such as an impervious gown or apron, gloves, and face mask or visor. The carcases of sick animals should not be utilized for human consumption. No registered vaccines are available for mass use on susceptible human populations, nor would their use be practicable in view of logistic problems and the essentially unpredictable occurrence and variable nature of outbreaks of the disease. A formalin-inactivated cell culture vaccine produced in the USA, was made available for use on a limited experimental basis, with the informed consent of recipients, to immunize persons such as veterinarians and laboratory workers who are regularly exposed to RVF infection, but no longer appears to be available.

Outbreaks of RVF in the Horn of Africa over the last 60 years have been shown to be related to the abnormally high and widespread rainfall caused by the El Nino in Southern Oscillation (ENSO) phenomenon. The resulting increase in green vegetation can be detected by satellite imaging (Linthicum *et al.* 1999). An RVF mapping model using climate data predicted an outbreak from December 2006–May 2007 in the Horn of Africa several months early. The predictions were confirmed by subsequent field investigations. Early warning advisory notices were given by US authorities and surveillance and outbreak response was put in place and may have saved lives (Anyamba *et al.* 2009). Increasingly, satellite imaging and prediction modelling will be used in control of such vector borne diseases.

References

Abdo-Salem, S., Gerbier, G., Bonnet, P. *et al.* (2006). Descriptive and spatial epidemiology of Rift Valley fever outbreak in Yemen 2000–2001. *Ann. NY Acad. Sci.*, **1081**: 240–42.

Al Hazmi, M., Ayoola, E.A., Abdurahman, M. *et al.* (2003). Epidemic Rift Valley fever in Saudi Arabia: a clinical study of severe illness in humans. *Clin. Infect. Dis.*, **36**: 245–52.

Anon. (1993). Rift Valley fever. *Wkly. Epidemiol. Rec.*, **68**: 300–301.

Anon. (1994). Rift Valley fever. *Wkly. Epidemiol. Rec.*, **69**: 74–75.

Anon. (1998). An outbreak of Rift Valley fever, Eastern Africa, 1997–1998. *Wkly. Epidemiol. Rec.*, **73**: 105–09.

Anon. (2007a). Outbreaks of Rift Valley fever in Kenya, Somalia and United Republic of Tanzania, December 2006–April 2007. *Wkly. Epidemiol. Rec.*, **82**: 169–78.

Anon. (2007b). Rift Valley fever, Sudan. *Wkly. Epidemiol. Rec.*, **82**: 401–2.

Arishi, H.M., Aqeel, A.Y. and Al Hazmi, M.M. (2006). Vertical transmission of fatal Rift Valley fever in a newborn. *Ann. Trop. Paediatr.*, **26**: 251–53.

Assaf, A., Chretien, J-P., Small, J. *et al.* (2009). Prediction of a Rift Valley fever outbreak. *PNAS*, **106**(3): 955–99.

Battles, J.K. and Dalrymple, J.M. (1988). Genetic variation among geographic isolates of Rift Valley fever virus. *Am. J. Trop. Med. Hyg.*, **39**: 617–31.

Bird, B.H., Khristova, M.L., Rollin, P.E., Ksiazek, T.G. and Nichol, S.T. (2007a). Complete genome analysis of 33 ecologically and biologically diverse Rift Valley fever virus strains reveals widespread virus movement and low genetic diversity due to recent common ancestry. *J. Virol.*, **81**: 2805–16.

Bird, B.H., Bawiec, D.A., Ksiazek, T.G., Shoemaker, T.R. and Nichol, S.T. (2007b). Highly sensitive and broadly reactive quantitative reverse transcription-PCR assay for high-throughput detection of Rift Valley fever virus. *J. Clin. Microb.*, **45**: 3506–13.

Bird, B.H., Albariño, C.G., Hartman, A.L., Erickson, B.R., Ksiazek, T.G. and Nichol, S.T. (2008). Rift Valley fever virus lacking the NSs and NSm genes is highly attenuated, confers protective immunity from virulent virus challenge and allows for differential identification of infected and vaccinated animals. *J. Virol.*, **82**: 2681–91.

Bowen, M.D., Trappier, S.G., Sanchez, A.J. *et al.* (2001). A reassortant bunyavirus isolated from acute hemorrhagic fever cases in Kenya and Somalia. *Virol.*, **291**: 185–90.

Briese, T., Bird, B., Kapoor, V. *et al.* (2006). Batai and Ngari viruses: M segment reassortment and association with severe febrile disease outbreaks in East Africa. *J. Virol.*, **80**: 5627–30.

Caplen, H., Peters, C.J., and Bishop, D.H.L. (1985). Mutagen directed attenuation of Rift Valley fever as a method of vaccine development. *J. Gen. Virol.*, **66**: 2271–77.

Cash, P., Robeson, G., Erlich, B.J., and Bishop, D.H.L. (1981). Biochemical characterization of Rift Valley fever virus. *Contrib. Epidemiol. Biostat.*, **3**: 1–20.

Coetzer, J.A.W. (1977). The pathology of Rift Valley fever. I. *Lesions occurring in natural cases in new-born lambs. Onderstep. J. Vet. Res.*, **44**: 205–12.

Coetzer, J.A.W. (1982). The pathology of Rift Valley fever. II. Lesions occurring in field cases in adult cattle, calves and aborted foetuses. *Onderstep. J. Vet. Res.*, **49**: 11–17.

Coetzer, J.A.W. and Barnard, B.J.H. (1977). *Hydrops amnii* in sheep associated with hydranencephaly and arthrogryposis with Wesselsbron disease and Rift Valley fever viruses as aetiological agents. *Onderstep. J. Vet. Res.*, **44**: 119–26.

Cohen, C. and Luntz, M.H. (1976). Rift–Valley–Fieber und Rickettsianretinitis einschliesslich fluoresceinangiographie. *Klinis. Monatsbl. Augenheil.*, **169**: 685–99.

Cosgriff, T.M., Morrill, J.C., Jennings, G.B., Hodgson, L.A. *et al.* (1989). Hemostatic derangement produced by Rift Valley fever virus in rhesus monkeys. *Rev. Infect. Dis.*, **11**: S807–814.

Deutman, A.F. and Klomp, H.J. (1981). Rift Valley fever retinitis. *Am. J. Ophthal.*, **92**: 38–42.

Easterday, B.C. (1965). Rift Valley fever. *Adv. Vet. Sci.*, **10**: 65–127.

Easterday, B.C., McGavran, M.H., Rooney, J.R., and Murphy, L.C. (1962). The pathogenesis of Rift Valley fever in lambs. *Am. J. Vet. Res.*, **23**: 470–78.

Easterday, B.C., Murphy, L.C., and Bennett, D.G. (1962). Experimental Rift Valley fever in calves, goats and pigs. *Am. J. Vet. Res.*, **23**: 1224–30.

Easterday, B.C., Murphy, L.C., and Bennett, D.G. (1962). Experimental Rift Valley fever in lambs and sheep. *Am. J. Vet. Res.*, **23**: 1231–40.

Eddy, G.A., Peters, C.J., Meadors, G. and Cole, F.E., Jr. (1981). Rift Valley fever vaccine for humans. *Contrib. Epidemiol. Biostat.*, **3**: 124–41.

Drosten, C., Göttig, S., Schilling, S. *et al.* (2002). Rapid detection and quantification of RNA of Ebola and Marburg viruses, Lassa virus, Crimean-Congo Hemorrhagic fever virus, Rift Valley fever virus, dengue virus, and yellow fever virus by real-time reverse transcription-PCR. *J. Clin. Microbiol.*, **40**: 2323–30.

Elfadil, A.A., Hasab-Allah, K.A. and Dafa-Allah, O.M. (2006). Factors associated with Rift Valley fever in south-west Saudi Arabia. *Rev. Scientif. Technique*, **25**: 1137–45.

Flick, R. and Bouloy, M. (2005). Rift Valley fever virus. *Curr. Mol. Med.*, **5**: 827–34.

Gerrard, S.R., Li, L., Barrett, A. *et al.* (2004). Ngari virus is a Bunyamwera virus reassortant that can be associated with large outbreaks of hemorrhagic fever in Africa. *J. Virol.*, **78**: 8922–26.

Henning, M.W. (1956). Rift Valley fever. In: *Animal Diseases in South Africa* (3rd edn.), pp. 1105–21. Cape Town: Central News Agency.

Jouan, A., Coulibaly, I., Adam, F., Philippe, B. *et al.* (1989). Analytical study of a Rift Valley fever epidemic. *Res. Virol.*, **40**: 175–86.

Jupp, P.G., Kemp, A., Grobbelaar, A. *et al.* (2002). The 2000 epidemic of Rift Valley fever in Saudi Arabia: mosquito vector studies. *Med. Vet. Entomol.*, **16**: 245–52.

Laughlin, L.W., Meegan, J.M., Strausbaugh, L.J., Morens, D.M., and Watten, H. (1979). Epidemic Rift Valley fever in Egypt: observations of the spectrum of human illness. *Trans. R. Soc. Trop. Med. Hyg.*, **73**: 630–33.

Le May, N., Mansuroglu, Z., Léger, P. *et al.* (2008). A SAP30 complex inhibits IFN-β expression in Rift Valley fever virus infected cells. *PLOS Pathogens*, **4**: e13. doi:10.1371/journal.p.pat.0040013.

Linthicum, K.J., Bailey, C.L., Davies, F.G., and Tucker, C.J. (1987). Detection of Rift Valley fever viral activity in Kenya by satellite remote sensing imagery. *Science*, **235**: 1656–59.

Linthicum, K.J., Davies, F.G., Kairo, A., and Bailey, C.L. (1985). Rift Valley fever virus (family Bunyaviridae, genus *Phlebovirus*). Isolations from Diptera collected during an inter-epizootic period in Kenya. *J. Hyg.*, **95**: 197–209.

Linthicum, K.J., Anyamba, A., Tucker, C. J. *et al.* (1991). Climate and satellite indicators to forecast Rift Valley Fever Epidemics in Kenya. *Science*, **285**: 397–400.

Madani, T.A., Al-Mazrou, Y.Y., Al-Jeffri, M.H. *et al.* (2003). Rift Valley fever epidemic in Saudi Arabia: epidemiological, clinical, and laboratory characteristics. *Clin. Infect. Dis.*, **37**: 1084–92.

Meegan, J.M. and Bailey, C.L. (1989). Rift Valley fever. In: T.P. Monath (ed.) *The Arboviruses: Epidemiology and Ecology*, Vol. IV, pp. 51–76. Boca Raton, FLA: CRC Press.

Muller, R., Saluzzo, J.F., Lopez, N., Dreier, T. *et al.* (1995). Characterization of clone 13, a naturally attenuated avirulent isolate of Rift Valley fever virus, which is altered in the small segment. *Am. J. Trop. Med. Hyg.*, **53**: 405–11.

Niklasson, B., Peters, C.J., Grandien, M., and Wood, O. (1984). Detection of human immunoglobulins G and M antibodies to Rift Valley fever virus by enzyme-linked immunosorbent assay. *J. Clin. Microb.*, **19**: 225–29.

Paweska, J.T., Burt, F.J., and Swanepoel, R. (2005). Validation of IgG-sandwich and IgM-capture ELISA for the detection of antibody to Rift Valley fever virus in humans. *J. Virol. Meth.*, **124**: 173–81.

Paweska, J.T., Janse van Vuren, P. and Swanepoel, R. (2007). Validation of an indirect ELISA based on the recombinant nucleocapsid protein of Rift Valley fever virus for the detection of IgG antibody in humans. *J. Virolog. Meth.*, **146**: 119–24.

Peters, C.J. and Anderson, G.W. (1981). Pathogenesis of Rift Valley fever. *Contrib. Epidemiol. Biostat.*, **3**: 21–41.

Peters, C.J., Jones, D., Trotter, R., Donaldson, J. *et al.* (1988). Experimental Rift Valley fever in rhesus macaques. *Arch. Virol.*, **99**: 31–44.

Peters, C.J. and Meegan, J.M. (1981). Rift Valley fever. In: G. Beran (ed.) *CRC Handbook Series in Zoonoses*, Sect. B1, pp. 403–19. Boca Raton, FLA: CRC Press.

Peters, C.J., Reynolds, J.A., Slone, T.W., Jones, D.E., and Stephen, E.L. (1986). Prophylaxis of Rift Valley fever with antiviral drugs, immune serum, interferon inducer and a macrophage activator. *Antiv. Res.*, **6**: 285–97.

Peters, C.J. and Shelokov, A. (1990). Viral hemorrhagic fever. *Curr. Ther. Infect. Dis.*, **3**: 355–60.

Rice, R.M., Erlick, B.J., Rosato, R.R., Eddy, G.A., and Mohanty, S.B. (1980). Biochemical characterization of Rift Valley fever virus. *Virol.*, **105**: 256–60.

Sellers, R.F., Pedgley, D.E., and Tucker, M.R. (1982). Rift Valley fever, Egypt—1977: disease spread by wind-borne insect vectors? *Vet. Rec.*, **110**: 73–77.

Shimshony, A. and Barzilai, R. (1983). Rift Valley fever. *Adv. Vet. Sci. Comp. Med.*, **27**: 347–425.

Shope, R.E. and Sather, G.E. (1979). Arboviruses. In: E.H. Lennette and N.J. Schmidt (ed.) *Diagnostic Procedures for Viral, Rickettsial and Chlamydial Infections* (5th edn.), pp. 767–814. Washington: American Public Health Association.

Siam, A.L., Meegan, J.M. and Gharbawi, K.F. (1980). Rift Valley fever ocular manifestation: observations during the 1977 epidemic in the Arab Republic of Egypt. *Brit. J. Ophthal.*, **64**: 366–74.

Swanepoel, R. and Coetzer, J.A.W. (2004). Rift Valley fever. In: J.A.W. Coetzer and R.C. Tustin (eds.) *Infectious Diseases of Livestock* (2nd edn.), pp. 1037–70. Cape Town: Oxford University Press Southern Africa.

Swanepoel, R. and Paweska, J.T. (2008). *National Institute for Communicable Diseases*, Sandringham, South Africa. Unpublished laboratory results.

Turrell, M.J., Linthicum, K.J., Patrican, L.A. *et al.* (2008). Vector competence of selected African mosquito (Diptera Culicidae) species for Rift Valley fever virus. *J. Med. Entom.*, **45**: 102–8.

Weidmann, M., Sanchez-Seco, M.P., Sall, A.A. *et al.* (2007). Rapid detection of important human pathogenic Phleboviruses. *J. Clin. Virol.*, **41**: 138–42.

Weiss, K.E. (1957). Rift Valley fever—a review. *Bull. Epiz. Dis. Africa*, **5**: 431–58.

Woods, C.W., Karpati, A.M., Grein, T. *et al.* (2002). An outbreak of Rift Valley fever in north-eastern Kenya, 1997–98. *Emerg. Infect. Dis.*, **8**: 138–44.

CHAPTER 37

Tick-borne encephalitides

Patricia A. Nuttall

Summary

Tick-borne encephalitides are caused by three different viruses transmitted by ticks and belonging to the Flaviviridae virus family: tick-borne encephalitis virus (Far Eastern, Siberian, and European subtypes), louping ill virus, and Powassan virus (including deer tick virus). These viruses cause encephalitis affecting humans in Eurasia and North America. In nature, they are maintained in transmission cycles involving *Ixodes* tick species and small or medium-sized wild mammals. The tick-borne flavivirus group is one of the most intensely studied groups of tick-borne pathogens.

Introduction

Many viruses transmitted by blood-feeding arthropods cause encephalitis in humans (Table 37.1). Most are transmitted by insects (mosquitoes and midges) but a significant number are tick-borne. All tick-borne encephalitides are caused by tick-borne flaviviruses in the virus family, Flaviviridae. The most important of these are the Far Eastern, Siberian, and European (or Western) subtypes of tick-borne encephalitis virus (TBEV). Louping ill virus (LIV) and Powassan virus (POWV) also cause encephalitis in humans but the disease incidence is much lower than for TBEV. LIV is more commonly associated with an encephalomyelitic disease of sheep and red grouse (*Lagopus lagopus scotica*) than with human disease. A similar disease affecting sheep is caused by the closely related Turkish encephalitis virus. Human disease has not been associated with natural infections of Langat virus (LGTV), another tick-borne flavivirus; however a few cases of encephalitis in humans were recorded following vaccination with a live attenuated LGTV-based vaccine. Three other important human pathogens belonging to the tick-borne flavivirus group are: Omsk haemorrhagic fever virus (OHFV) virus, Kyasanur forest disease virus (KFDV), and Alkhurma virus (a relative of KFDV). All of these tick-borne flaviviruses give rise to haemorrhagic rather than encephalitic disease (for reviews see Kharitonova and Leonov 1985; Lvov 1988; Banerjee 1988; Gritsun *et al.* 2003).

West Nile virus (WNV) is as a mosquito-borne flavivirus but in parts of Asia the virus is transmitted by ticks. Typically, infections are asymptomatic or cause a febrile illness in humans. However, in 1957 severe meningoencephalitis was reported during an outbreak in Israel and more cases were recorded in 1962 and 1981.

The largest outbreak of WN encephalitis to date, and the first urban outbreak of the disease, occurred in 1996 in southern Romania. The main vector was *Culex pipiens*. In 1999, WNV was identified for the first time in North America where it has rapidly spread across most of the USA. Ticks are not important in the transmission to humans of WNV.

This chapter focuses on tick-borne encephalitides caused by tick-borne flaviviruses, with emphasis on TBEV.

History

As early as the eighteenth century, descriptions suggestive of TBE were noted in church registers on the Åland islands, Finland. During the summer of 1927, Schneider, working in a hospital in Lower Austria, recognized that several patients with encephalitis showed a similar clinical picture. He discovered this condition occurred regularly, although numbers of cases varied, and that peak incidence occurred during summer months. On the basis of clinical and epidemiological observations, the condition was named 'meningitis serosa epidemica' (Schneider 1931) and later, Schneider's disease. Several other synonyms for TBE have been used (Table 37.2).

Tick-borne encephalitis was recognized clinically in the Far East of the former Soviet Union in the early 1930s. The disease was known by several names, including Russian spring–summer encephalitis (RSSE). TBEV was first isolated in 1937 as a result of an expedition to the Russian Far East headed by Professor L. A. Zil'ber (Zil'ber 1939). Within 3 months, the scientists made several groundbreaking discoveries:

i) A novel virus caused an acute panencephalitis with a clinical picture differing from that of all forms of acute central nervous system (CNS) infections known at that time.

ii) This virus differed in antigenic and biological properties from all other viruses causing human and animal encephalitides known at the time.

iii) The virus was transmitted by the taiga tick, *Ixodes persulcatus*, and probably by other ixodid ticks inhabiting the taiga zone of the Russian Far East.

iv) Blood from people who had suffered from TBE contained antibodies that specifically reacted with the virus (this discovery

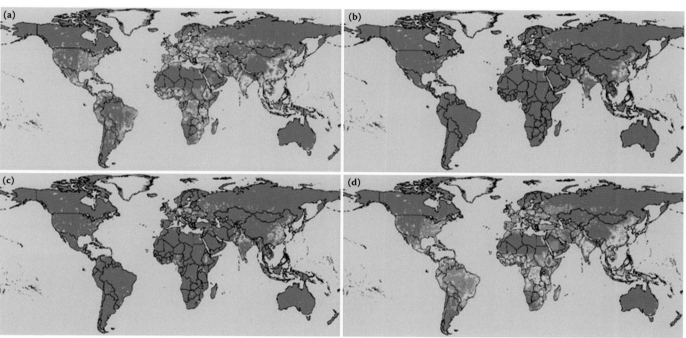

Fig. 1.2 Maps are derived for EID events caused by **a**, zoonotic pathogens from wildlife, **b**, zoonotic pathogens from non-wildlife, **c**, drug-resistant pathogens and **d**, vector-borne pathogens. The relative risk is calculated from regression coefficients and variable values in Table 1 in Jones *et al.* (2008) (omitting the variable measuring reporting effort), categorized by standard deviations from the mean and mapped on a linear scale from green (lower values) to red (higher values). Reproduced from Jones *et al.* (2008), by permission from Macmillan Publishers Ltd.

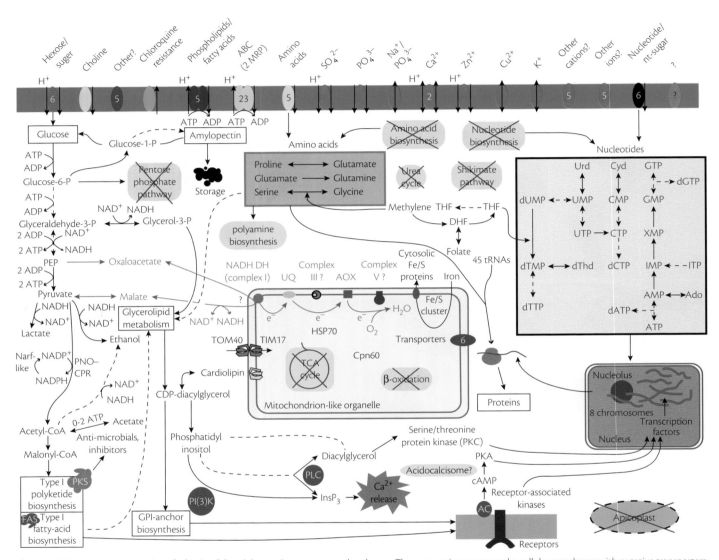

Fig. 46.4 Schematic representation of selective *C. hominis* proteins, enzymes and pathways. The green strip represents the cellular membrane with putative transporters; numbers indicate the number of genes for a given class of transporter. Solid arrows indicate pathways that are present; multistep pathways are indicated with dashed arrows. Components or pathways that are absent are crossed out. Steps or components whose exact nature is questionable are shown with question marks. Blue arrows and names indicate proposed aerobic parts of the metabolism.

Abbreviations: ABC, ATP-binding cassette; AC, adenylyl cyclase; Ado, adenosine; AOX, alternative oxidase; Cpn60, chaperone 60; Cyd, cytidine; DHF, dihydrofolate; dThd, deoxythymidine; GPI, glycosylphosphatidylinositol; Hsp70, heat-shock protein 70; InsP3, inositol phosphate; MRP, multiple-drug-resistance protein; NADH DH, NADH dehydrogenase; Narf-like, nuclear prelamin A recognition factor-like protein; PEP, phosphoenolpyruvate; PI(3)K, phosphatidylinositol 3-kinase; PKA, protein kinase A; PLC, phospholipase C; PKC, proteinkinase C; PNO–CPR, pyruvate:NADPþ oxidoreductase fused to cytochrome P450reductase domain; THF, tetrahydrofolate; TIM17, translocase of the inner mitochondrial membrane 17; TOM40, translocase of the outer mitochondrial membrane 40; UQ, ubiquinone; Urd, uridine.

Reproduced from Xu *et al.* (2004) with permission from Macmillan Publishers Ltd.

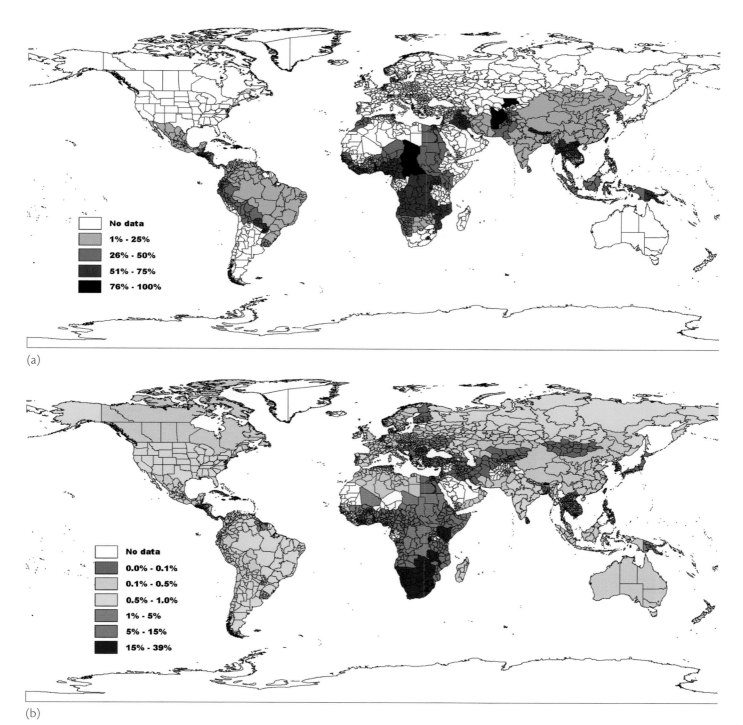

Fig. 46.6 Global indicators of high importance in the future emergence of *Cryptosporidium* as a significant human pathogen. **(a)** Percentage of the human population (by country) without access to sanitary drinking water [data from (Gleick 1998)]. **(b)** Percentage of the human population (by country) infected with Human Immunodeficiency Virus (HIV) [data from (Anonymous, 2006)].

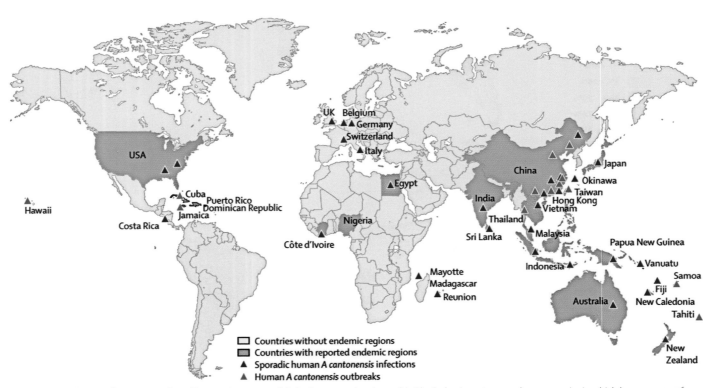

Fig. 59.3 Distribution of A. *cantonensis* and human A. *cantonensis* infections or outbreaks worldwide. Endemic regions are those countries in which human cases of angiostrongylosis or animal reservoirs of A. *cantonensis* have been identified (Red). This is not intended to imply that A. *cantonensis* is endemic throughout these entire countries. Conversely, those areas marked as Non-endemic regions may well be countries with a lack of investigation and not an absence of A. *cantonensis* infection. A region or country where sporadic A. *cantonensis* infections occurred is marked with a dark triangle, while outbreaks are marked with green triangles.

Table 37.1 Arthropod-borne viruses causing encephalitis in humans

Virus	First isolated	Geographical distribution	Natural hosts	Vector
Far Eastern tick-borne encephalitis	1937	Russia (Far East), China, Japan	mammals	ixodid ticks
European tick-borne encephalitis	1940	Europe	mammals	ixodid ticks
Siberian tick-borne encephalitis	1963	Russia (Urals, Siberia, Far East)	mammals	ixodid ticks
louping ill	1930	Europe	sheep, red grouse	ixodid ticks
Powassan[a]	1952	North America, Russia	rodents	ixodid ticks
West Nile	1937	Africa, Asia, Europe	birds	mosquitoes (ixodid and argasid ticks)
Chikungunya	1953	Africa, Asia, Europe	non-human primates	mosquitoes
Eastern equine encephalomyelitis	1933	North America	birds, horses	mosquitoes
Ilheus	1944	South America	birds	midges
Japanese encephalitis	1935	Asia	birds, pigs	mosquitoes
Kunjin	1960	Australia, Borneo	birds,	mosquitoes
La Crosse	1963	North and South America, Asia, Europe	chipmunks, squirrels	mosquitoes
Murray Valley encephalitis	(1917)[b] 1951	Australia, New Guinea	birds	mosquitoes
Rift Valley fever	1931	Africa	livestock, rodents	mosquitoes
Rocio encephalitis	1975	Brazil	birds	mosquitoes
St Louis encephalitis	1933	North and South America	rodents	mosquitoes
Semliki Forest	1942	Africa, Asia	non-human primates	mosquitoes
Venezuelan equine encephalomyelitis	1938	South and North America	rodents, birds, horses	mosquitoes, (cliff swallow bugs)
Western equine encephalomyelitis	1930	North and South America	birds, humans	mosquitoes

[a] Including deer tick virus, a variant of POWV isolated in 1996 from ixodid ticks collected in North America.

[b] The agent isolated in 1917 was lost before its identity was established.

[c] see Gubler *et al.* 2007 for phylogenetic relationships

gave rise to serological diagnosis and the first insights into the immunology of TBE) (Zil'ber 1957).

In the following years (1938–39), numerous isolates of TBEV were obtained from various geographical areas of Russia and the first evidence of their heterogeneity was reported. In 1939, Pavlovsky described the main characteristics of TBE and how the virus was maintained in nature (in 'natural foci') by transmission between *I. persulcatus* and numerous mammalian species (Pavlovsky 1966).

A less severe form of encephalitis, affecting humans residing in central Bohemia, Czech Republic, was recorded in 1948. The virus recovered from the blood of a patient and from *Ixodes ricinus* ticks was related to isolates from RSSE cases. In the following

Table 37.2 Synonyms for TBE

Bi-undulant meningoencephalitis	Forest spring encephalitis
Biphasic meningoencephalitis	Früh–Sommer–Meningo–Enzephalitis (FSME)
Central European encephalitis (CEE)	Kumlinge disease
biphasic milk fever	Russian spring–summer encephalitis (RSSE)
Far Eastern encephalitis	Schneider's disease

year, similar or milder forms of the disease, called biphasic meningoencephalitis, were observed in other central and eastern European countries. In 1951–1952, an outbreak of TBE was recorded in southern Slovakia affecting at least 600 people, and was associated with consumption of unpasteurized goat's milk. The outbreak led to extensive ecological research on TBEV in central Europe.

In Finland, a form of aseptic encephalitis affecting the inhabitants and visitors to islands in the Baltic Sea has been known for several decades. The disease was first observed in the 1940s in the small island parish of Kumlinge and became known as Kumlinge disease. The causative agent, Kumlinge virus, was isolated in 1959 and later found to be an isolate of the European subtype of TBEV. In Sweden, the first case of TBE was described in 1954; the virus was isolated in 1958 from a patient and from *I. ricinus* ticks. Owing to the seasonal occurrence of the disease, Moritsch and Krausler in 1957 coined the name 'Früh-Sommer-Meningo-Enzephalitis' (FSME). TBEV has now been isolated from most European countries although, epidemiologically, the virus is most important in central and eastern Europe.

Louping-ill virus derives its name from a disease of sheep recognized in southern Scotland for at least two centuries (reviewed by Smith and Varma 1981). 'Louping' refers to the characteristic of 'leaping' shown by sheep infected with LIV. It was an ill-defined condition until 1913 when the specific histopathological lesions of the CNS were described. Subsequent attempts to determine the cause of the condition were confounded by another common infection of sheep, tick-borne fever. However, in 1931 the aetiological agent of louping ill was established as a filterable virus transmitted by the sheep tick, *I. ricinus*. In the 1930s, louping ill was identified as a problem throughout much of the hill sheep farming areas of Scotland and northern England. Subsequently, the disease was recognized in Ireland, Wales and, in 1978, in south western England. The introduction of sheep farming to heather moorland at the end of the eighteenth century probably introduced louping ill disease to these habitats, which then became a problem for red grouse and the game industry that releases millions of birds each year for shooting. Louping ill disease also affects sheep in Norway and Spain (caused by Spanish sheep encephalitis virus); similar infections in Turkey and Greece are caused by distinct strains of TBEV European subtype. Human infection by LIV was first reported in 1934 but is rare.

Powassan virus derives its name from the town in Northern Ontario where the first fatal case of the disease was recognized (reviewed by Artsob 1988). A virus was isolated from the patient, a 5 year old boy who developed encephalitis and died in September 1958. In fact, the virus had been isolated previously from a pool of ticks collected in May 1952 in Colorado but specific identification of this virus was made subsequent to that from the fatal case in the town of Powassan. The first isolation of POWV from the Asian continent was from a pool of ticks collected in the Southern Primorskiy region of far eastern Russia in 1972 (Leonova 1997). Deer tick virus (DTV), which was first reported in 1997 from deer ticks, *Ixodes dammini*, collected in eastern North America, is so closely related to POWV that it may not warrant a separate name (Telford *et al.* 1997; Kuno *et al.* 2001).

Aetiological agent

Tick-borne flaviviruses are relatively small (about 50 nm in diameter) spherical viruses comprising a RNA genome and a lipoprotein envelope (Lindenbach *et al.* 2007; Gubler *et al.* 2007). Currently, there are 12 recognized species of tick-borne flavivirus of which two species cause encephalitis: *Tick-borne encephalitis virus* (which includes the three TBEV subtypes and LIV) and *Powassan virus* (Labuda and Nuttall 2008).

Taxonomy

Tick-borne flaviviruses belong to the *Flavivirus* genus in the virus family, Flaviviridae. Most members of this virus family are arthropod-borne viruses (arboviruses) transmitted by either mosquitoes or ticks. Medically important mosquito-borne flaviviruses include dengue, yellow fever, and Japanese encephalitis virus. The name of the virus family and genus derive from yellow fever virus (*L. flavus*, yellow), the first virus isolated from humans. The tick-borne flaviviruses are currently classified into two groups: the mammalian tick-borne virus group and the seabird tick-borne virus group. A third group, the Kadam virus group, has been proposed based on phylogenetic analysis.

Molecular biology

The viral genome is a single molecule of single-stranded RNA of approximately 11 kilobases. Unlike other tick-borne viruses, the genomic RNA of tick-borne flaviviruses is infectious and represents the only viral messenger RNA in infected cells. Within the genomic RNA is a single long open reading frame that encodes a polyprotein, comprising all the structural and nonstructural viral proteins. The coding region is flanked by relatively short untranslated regions (UTRs) at the 5' and 3' terminal ends. UTRs contain conserved structural elements that are essential for viral replication. The 5' end of the genome has a type 1 cap while the 3' end lacks a poly-A tail.

Three structural proteins and seven non-structural (NS) proteins are encoded by the genome in the order:

5'-C-prM(M)-E-NS1-NS2A-NS2B-NS3-NS4A-NS4B-NS5-3'

The characteristics of these viral proteins are summarized in Table 37.3.

The major surface glycoprotein (E) of flavivirus particles (virions) carries antigenic epitopes recognized by antibodies produced by immune hosts. These can be used in neutralization tests to distinguish between different tick-borne flaviviruses. Unlike many viruses, the flavivirus E protein does not form spikes on the surface of virions; instead, the E protein lies prone and parallel to the viral membrane, in the form of head-to-tail homodimeric rods (Rey

Table 37.3 Flavivirus structural and non-structural (NS) proteins

Protein	Molecular weight	Function
C	12–14 kDa	Core protein that complexes with the genomic RNA to form the nucleocapsid.
prM	18–19 kDa	Precursor membrane protein found in immature virus particles; proteolytically cleaved to form M.
M	8 kDa	Membrane protein found in mature virus particles.
E	50–60 kDa	Envelope protein which is anchored with M in a host-derived lipid bilayer forming the viral envelope; carries antigenic epitopes recognized by neutralizing antibodies.
NS1	40–46 kDa	Involved in viral replication and protein targeting; functionally linked to E protein.
NS2A	22–25 kDa	Hydrophobic transmembrane protein involved in generation of virus-induced membranes during virus assembly.
NS2B	12–15 kDa	Co-factor of NS3 serine protease
NS3	70 kDa	Serine protease (in complex with NS2B) for polyprotein processing, helicase/NTPase for unwinding the double-stranded replicative form of RNA, and RNA triphosphatase for capping nascent viral RNA.
NS4A	16 kDa	Integral membrane protein which induces membrane rearrangements to form the viral replication complex.
NS4B	27 kDa	Inhibits the type I interferon response and may modulate viral replication through interactions with NS3.
NS5	103–105 kDa	S-adenosyl methyltransferase and an independent RNA-dependent RNA polymerase.

et al. 1995). Conformational changes in the E protein trigger viral membrane fusion, the first step of flavivirus entry into a cell. These conformational changes occur at acidic pH, and involve conversion of the E protein dimers into trimers that adopt a hairpin-like structure during the fusion process. In virions exposed to alkaline conditions, the E dimers dissociate into monomers that interact with target membranes via the fusion peptide (a segment of the E protein) without proceeding to fusion of viral and cellular membranes (Stiasny *et al.* 2007). This conformation may be adopted when virions are secreted in alkaline tick saliva.

Infection and replication

Tick-borne flaviviruses infect vertebrate cells by receptor-mediated endocytosis; putative host cell receptors include heparin sulphate. Specificity for binding to a tick receptor(s) appears to reside in ectodomain III of the E protein. Once inside endosomes within the mammalian cell cytoplasm, the acidic environment triggers an irreversible trimerisation of the E protein that results in fusion of the viral and cell membranes. After fusion has occurred, the nucleocapsid is released into the cytosol where it disassembles releasing the infectious genomic RNA. This positive-sense RNA is translated into a single polyprotein that is processed by viral and host proteases. Replication of genomic RNA occurs on intracellular membranes. Virus assembly occurs on the surface of the endoplasmic reticulum (ER), with structural proteins and newly synthesized RNA budding into the lumen of the ER. Immature non-infectious particles (which contain E and preM proteins, lipid membrane and nucleocapsid) collect in the lumen of the ER. They are transported through the trans-Golgi network where preM is cleaved by furin (a host protease), resulting in mature, infectious particles. Mature virions are released from the mammalian host cell by exocytosis. Little is known of tick-borne flavivirus infection and replication in tick cells except that there are some striking differences from the infection of mammalian cells, in particular, the absence of gross cytopathic effects (Nuttall 2009).

Following natural tick-transmitted infections, TBEV first replicates in the skin site of inoculation (i.e. the feeding site of an infected tick) and in lymph nodes that drain the site. Studies in mice revealed that neutrophils, monocytes/macrophages and Langerhans cells, attracted to the tick feeding site, become infected (Labuda *et al.* 1996). In animals that develop viraemia, virus is carried via lymphatics to the thoracic duct and into the bloodstream. The primary viraemia seeds extraneural tissues which, in turn, support further viral replication and serve as a source for release of virus into the circulation. The level of viraemia is modulated by the rate of clearance by macrophages, and is terminated by the appearance of humoral antibodies, approximately 1 week after infection. However, key hosts of the virus in nature do not exhibit patent viraemia (see section on Vertebrate hosts below). Instead, TBEV and other tick-borne flaviviruses may be transmitted by a non-systemic route, the so-called 'red herring' hypothesis (see section on Transmission below).

Infection in humans
Incubation period
The incubation period of TBE varies between 1 and 28 days, most often 7–14 days. Approximately two out of three TBE viral infections run a subclinical course without symptoms or with mild symptoms. The incubation period following tick-borne transmission of LIV to sheep varies from 2 to 5 days; in humans, the incubation period is 4–7 days. For POWV, the reported incubation period ranges from 7 to 34 days.

Signs and symptoms
Clinical manifestations of TBE vary depending on patient susceptibility, level of care, and virus strain. They can be grouped as:

i) Mild or moderate fever with complete recovery,

ii) Subacute encephalitis with nearly complete recovery or residual symptoms that persist for a long period,

iii) Severe encephalitis resulting in disability or death,

iv) Chronic infection that slowly progresses to severe disability or death.

Typically, TBE in humans has a biphasic course. The initial stage, lasting 1–8 days, includes moderate fever, headache, and myalgia. These symptoms correspond to the viraemic phase of the disease when the virus can be isolated from systemic blood. About one-third of cases develop the second phase of the disease after an asymptomatic interval of 1–20 days, most often about 1 week. This second phase corresponds to the spread of TBEV to the CNS, resulting in meningoencephalitis of varying severity. The most serious cases of encephalitis are seen in adults, especially among persons more than 60 years old, whereas in children the disease more often runs a milder course. TBE cases with concomitant myelitis tend to have a more severe clinical course and are more likely to require intensive care. Case fatality rate of encephalitic conditions is 0.5–2% in Europe whereas 20–30% has been reported in the Far East.

Louping ill in humans (and in sheep) is biphasic, resembling the European form of TBE. After an influenza-like phase, lasting 2–11 days, there is a period of remission of 5–6 days and then the reappearance of fever and a meningoencephalitis syndrome lasting 4–10 days. At least 39 cases of infection in humans have been described, mostly affecting laboratory personnel working with the virus or people handling infected sheep. In one laboratory-acquired case, a haemorrhagic diathesis developed, and the disease closely resembled Kyasanur forest disease. Although symptomatic infections are generally fatal in sheep and red grouse, no deaths have been reported in humans (Davidson *et al.* 1991).

Powassan virus infections are characterized by a variable period of fever and non-specific symptoms, followed by neurological signs which are often severe. Approaching 40 cases of Powassan encephalitis have been reported; most were adults. During 1958–1998, of 19 recognized cases in North America, 13 were diagnosed as encephalitis, four as meningoencephalitis, and two as aseptic meningitis. Two cases terminated fatally during the acute phase of illness, and two patients died 1 and 3 years, respectively, after the onset of sequelae. Of nine cases of serologically confirmed POWV disease reported in the USA during 1999–2005, all but one patient developed encephalitis with acute onset of profound muscle weakness, confusion, and other severe neurological signs (Hinten *et al.* 2008). A case reported as Powassan encephalitis included neuropathological changes similar to those seen in the first reported case of the disease although the isolated virus was considered to be DTV (Kuno *et al.* 2001). Similarly, a fatal case of meningoencephalitis was attributed to DTV (Tavakoli *et al.* 2009). In cases reported from the Primorskiy Region in Russia, a characteristic syndrome with prominent cerebellar signs differentiates the disease from the Far Eastern form of TBE (Leonova 1997). Generally infections are described as milder than those produced by TBEV Far Eastern subtype. Because of incomplete case reports, an accurate assessment of mortality associated with Powassan encephalitis cannot be made. However, five cases (~15%) were fatal and approximately two thirds of patients demonstrate significant short- to long-term neurological sequelae (Romero and Simonsen 2008).

Diagnosis

Clinical manifestations of TBE are non-specific; hence, diagnosis relies on laboratory findings. During the initial viraemic phase of illness, virus may be detected in blood either by virus isolation or reverse transcriptase-polymerase chain reaction (RT-PCR). In practice this rarely happens because admission to hospital usually occurs in the second phase when neurological symptoms become manifest. At this stage the virus has been cleared from the blood and cerebrospinal fluid and specific antibodies are formed. Detection of specific IgM and IgG antibodies by enzyme-linked immunosorbent assay (ELISA) is therefore the method of choice for diagnosis of TBE. At onset of disease the presence of a low concentration of neutralizing antibodies in serum and a high cell count in the CSF may indicate an unfavourable course of TBE. IgM antibodies may be detectable for several months after infection; IgG antibodies persist for life and mediate immunity against reinfection. In fatal cases, TBEV can be isolated from, or detected by RT-PCR in the brain and other organs. Similar approaches are appropriate for diagnosis of louping ill and Powassan encephalitis provided that virus specific reagents are used.

Pathology

Tick-borne encephalitis presents as (myelo)meningoencephalitis with considerable mortality. Characteristic neuropathological changes include a multinodular to patchy polioencephalomyelitis accentuated in the spinal cord, brainstem, and cerebellum. Visualization of viral infection by immunohistochemistry revealed the viral neurotropism preferentially targets large neurons of anterior horns, medulla oblongata, pons, dentate nucleus, Purkinje cells, and striatum. Topographical correlation between inflammatory changes and distribution of viral antigens is poor. Immunological responses may contribute to nerve cell destruction. TBE viral antigens were immunohistochemically detectable in the brain of fatal cases that had a relatively short natural clinical course (4 to 35 days) (Gelpi et al. 2005).

Autopsy of the index case of POW encephalitis revealed inflammation in all areas of the brain, although the cerebellum and spinal cord were somewhat less affected. In sheep, LIV causes neuronal degeneration and inflammatory changes in brain-stem and cerebellum, producing a characteristic ataxic disease. In the red grouse, however, lesions localize in the forebrain. The molecular basis for the selective vulnerability of neuronal subsets to viruses remains largely unknown. The possible involvement of differences in virus-receptor interactions, particularly those involving neurotransmitter molecules, has been suggested.

Treatment

Antiviral therapy could potentially reduce morbidity and mortality from tick-borne flavivirus infections, but no effective drugs are currently available. Treatment is therefore supportive. Mechanical ventilation may be required because of apnea in which breathing is suspended through failure of respiratory muscles to contract. In the past, passive immunization has been recommended using specific IgG antibodies against TBEV as pre- or post-exposure prophylaxis (Kunz 1977). Such preparations are no longer available.

Epidemiology and ecology

Tick-borne encephalitis is endemic over a wide geographical area covering Europe, northern Asia, China, Mongolia, South Korea, and Japan. The occurrence of the disease is largely determined by the distribution and activity of the principal tick vectors, *I. persulcatus* (for Far Eastern and Siberian TBEV subtypes) and the closely related *I. ricinus* (for European TBEV subtypes). *Ixodes persulcatus* replaces *I. ricinus* in the north east of Europe, from the Baltic Sea shore and extending across northern Asia to Japan. The northern border for *I. persulcatus* extends across the forests of the central taiga. At least 30,000 natural foci of TBEV are considered to exist across the Northern Hemisphere, from Europe to Japan. These have been divided into eight zones of focal regions:

I) Central European-Mediterranean,

II) Eastern European,

III) Western Siberian,

IV) Kazakh-Central Asian,

V) Central Siberian-Transbaikalian,

VI) Khingan-Amur,

VII) Pacific,

VIII) Crimean-Caucasian.

They cover at least 27 European and 7 Asian countries. Each zone is characterized by a combination of features, both abiotic (geomorphology, climate) and biotic (tick and vertebrate host species and abundance, viral genotypes), which determine the characteristic epizootiological features of its natural foci, and by social conditions that affect the epidemiology (Korenberg and Kovalevskii 1999). Depending on the eco-epidemiological zone, the incidence of clinically expressed forms of disease is dependent on several factors (reviewed by Gritsun et al. 2003):

i) The number of exposures to infected ticks. In some endemic areas, up to 45% of the local population receives at least one tick bite per epidemic season.

ii) Infection prevalence in ticks. Infection prevalence varies in different years, and in different regions. Active foci where *I. persulcatus* is the vector may have a comparatively high infection prevalence of up to 40%. By contrast, an infection prevalence ranging from ≤ 0.1% to about 5% has been recorded for foci where *I. ricinus* is the vector. High prevalences are detected by ELISA, which is a more sensitive assay than virus isolation by animal inoculation. Long-term studies in Russia using similar techniques indicate that the virus prevalence range in *I. persulcatus* is similar to that for *I. ricinus* foci, with few exceptions (Korenberg, pers com.).

iii) Concentration of infectious virus in ticks. Most people receive bites from ticks carrying low doses of virus and only about 15% are bitten by highly infected ticks.

World-wide, 10,000 to 13,000 human cases of TBE are recorded annually, with considerable variation from year to year and from one region to another. Highest numbers of hospitalized cases are recorded for the Pre-Ural and Ural regions, and Siberia. During the 1950s and 1960s, the highest TBE occurrence was in forest workers, reaching 700–1,200 cases annually. However, following 'Perestroika' in the 1990s, the incidence of TBE increased with up to 11,000 recorded cases per year among urban dwellers who became infected when they visited local forests or even when working in their gardens. The increase resulted from fewer people being immunized against TBEV and cessation of the use of pesticides to control ticks. In Western European countries, the total number of annual cases has averaged 3,000 for the last 5 years; most infections are contracted during leisure activities. The number of reported cases of TBE from various European countries and Russia, for 1976–2007, shows an overall increase in TBE incidence during the last 30 years (Süss 2008). Little is known of the disease incidence in China; natural foci of TBEV have been reported in the Hunchun area of Jilin province, where the seroprevalence in humans was reported as 11%, and in the subtropical region of western Yunnan near the Burmese border. On Hokkaido, the northern island of Japan, a severe case of TBE was described in 1993 but this is the only reported case. Several Japanese isolates from ticks (*I. ovatus*) and dogs are related to the Far Eastern subtype of TBEV.

Although most TBEV infections of humans result from an infected tick bite, the risk of infection and resulting morbidity rate are difficult to determine as tick bites often go unnoticed. Epidemiologically, nymphs are probably the most important vector stage in the transmission of TBEV because they are more numerous than adults, tend to be less host-specific, and they are less easy to detect compared with adults. References to tick bite in the case history of patients range from 10 to 85%. In Western Europe, the estimated risk of infection varies from 1:200 to 1:900 per tick bite. Serological surveys suggest that more than 70–95% of TBEV human infections in endemic regions of Russia are sub-clinical, and indicate frequent exposure to infected ticks. One clinical case is estimated to occur for every 100 people bitten by ticks in regions of Russia endemic for TBE. TBE can affect people of all ages; however, the highest incidence usually occurs among 17–40 year olds. The highest risk groups are: agricultural and forestry workers; hikers, ramblers, and people engaged in outdoor sports that bring them into contact with tick habitats; and collectors of mushrooms and wild fruit. In addition to tick-borne infections, sporadic cases and family outbreaks of alimentary TBEV infections are observed in Slovakia almost annually, and in other countries in Central Europe and Russia where unpasteurized milk and milk products of goats, sheep and cattle are consumed.

In general, the peak incidence of human infections coincides with seasonal peaks of tick feeding activity: May and June and also September and October for *I. ricinus*, and May and June for *I. persulcatus*. Although risk maps are available for Europe (e.g. http://www.tbe-victims.info/m-6815.php), they do not provide a complete picture particularly as the disease is not notifiable in all countries. As of 2007, TBE is a notifiable disease in Austria, the Baltic States, Czech Republic, Finland, Germany, Greece, Hungary, Norway, Poland, Russia, Slovakia, Slovenia, Sweden, and Switzerland. Seasonal or annual variations in the incidence of TBE cases may vary according to changes in TBEV prevalence or merely reflect changes in human exposure (e.g. bad weather reducing

outdoor activities, socio-economic changes increasing exposure) (Sumilo *et al.* 2008). Seroprevalence cannot be used to generate risk maps because of the high level of immunization in some regions (e.g. >94% children in Austria are vaccinated against TBEV).

The only flavivirus identified in the UK is LIV (Smith and Varma 1981; Reid 1984). Infections are mainly restricted to the rough, upland grazing and unimproved pastures of the western seaboard where there is sheep farming, although the virus is also found in some areas of north east Scotland, northern and southwest England, north Wales, and Ireland. In the most common habitats there is a thick mat of vegetation and the soil remains damp throughout the summer. The increase of LIV infections of red grouse in northern England has been associated with the spread of bracken (*Pteridium aquilinum*), which provides a thick vegetation mat ideal for maintaining a microclimate suitable for ticks. Unlike TBEV infections acquired during outdoor recreational activities, LIV infections are largely an occupational health hazard confined to laboratory workers, veterinarians, farmers, and abattoir workers. In total, of 39 human cases reported, 26 resulted from laboratory exposure. Serosurveys of patients with aseptic meningitis or encephalitis of unknown aetiology identified 5/35 positive sera of patients in Ireland; examination of 775 sera from Scottish patients identified one case of LI encephalitis in a farmer and one fatal case in a slaughterman. However, 8% of sera from abattoir workers were positive despite the fact that only two clinical cases have been reported in this occupational health group.

An encephalomyelitic disease in sheep, reported in Norway, is caused by LIV-infected sheep ticks (*I. ricinus*) introduced from mainland Britain. Sheep and goat encephalomyelitis has also been reported in Spain, Greece and Turkey. Sequence analysis distinguishes British, Irish, and Spanish subtypes of LIV, and Turkish and Greek subtypes of Turkish encephalitis virus (Grard *et al.* 2007). They are thought to have emerged on the hillsides of Greece, Turkey and Spain when sheep were introduced near to wooded areas where TBEV was present.

Evidence of POWV has been documented in much of Canada, including Alberta, British Columbia, New Brunswick, Nova Scotia, Ontario, and Quebec. The highest incidence is in Ontario followed by Quebec. In the USA, POWV has been recorded in California, Connecticut, Maine, Massachusetts, New York State (highest incidence), South Dakota, Vermont, West Virginia, and Wisconsin. Additionally, serological evidence indicates the occurrence of infections in humans in Sonora, Mexico (Romero and Simonsen 2008). Risk factors include outdoor activities in endemic areas, contact with potential mammalian hosts, and possibly with exposure to family pets. During 1999–2005, nine cases of serologically confirmed POWV disease were reported in the USA. Of these nine patients, 5 (56%) were men, the median age was 69 years (range: 25–91 years), and 6 (67%) had onset during May–July. The virus is also endemic in the eastern Russian territories of Primorskiy and Khabarovsk that border the Japanese Sea. A study of 386 sera from patients in the Primorskiy region identified 15 patients with neutralizing antibodies specific for POWV. Infections of humans occur during summer and autumn. Under experimental conditions, *I. scapularis* can effectively transmit POWV to its host within 30 min of attachment (Ebel and Kramer 2004).

In certain regions, such as at higher altitudes where tick vectors are not usually active, increases in TBE incidence have been correlated with increased average monthly temperature and not with other factors that influence human exposure to infected ticks (Danielová *et al.* 2008). However, as yet there is no compelling evidence that climate change is affecting either the distribution or prevalence of tick-borne flavivirus infections (Randolph 2008; Gray *et al.* 2009; Korenberg 2009). By contrast, there is good evidence of greater human exposure to infected ticks through socioeconomic changes and higher densities of tick-feeding deer (Sumilo *et al.* 2008).

Ticks

Ticks are blood-sucking arthropods related to mites, spiders, and scorpions. They comprise two major families: the Ixodidae (ixodid or hard ticks) and the Argasidae (argasid or soft ticks). The tick hosts and vectors of encephalitic tick-borne flaviviruses are all ixodid species of the genus *Ixodes*. They are three-host ticks: the larva, nymph, and adult each feed on a different individual vertebrate host (often a wide range of species) for a period of a few days. They are absolute parasites, requiring a blood meal in order to develop to the next stage or to lay eggs. Fig. 37.1 illustrates the life cycle of *I. ricinus*. In general, immature stages (larvae and nymphs) feed on small mammals, ground-foraging birds and in some locations on lizards, while adults feed on larger species such as deer, goats, cattle, and sheep. However, in upland regions of the UK, all stages of *I. ricinus* regularly feed on sheep. Each stage of *I. ricinus* takes approximately 1 year to develop to the next, so the life cycle typically takes 3 years to complete, though it may vary from 2 to 6 years throughout the geographical range of the species. Unfed ticks can quest for several weeks but do not usually then survive from one season to the next. *Ixodes ricinus* requires a minimum relative humidity of 80–85% for development. In parts of the UK, there is a marked spring peak of feeding activity and a small autumn peak; development occurs during summer. In parts of continental Europe, the spring peak is less marked and biting activity continues through the summer and into autumn.

The developmental biology of *I. persulcatus* is very similar to that of *I. ricinus*, although the seasonal activity of *I. persulcatus* is usually shorter and the life cycle may take longer to complete (Korenberg 2000). In the Far East of Russia, *I. persulcatus* begins feeding about mid-April when the mean 24 hour temperature reaches 3–4°C, and bites humans most frequently in April/May when the mean temperature is 10–12°C; questing decreases when the temperature exceeds 18°C. Like *I. ricinus*, larvae and nymphs feed on rodents, insectivores, and birds while adults feed on hare, moose, deer, cattle, and goats. In locations within Europe where *I. ricinus* and *I. persulcatus* are sympatric, their relative roles as primary vectors of TBEV are undetermined.

One or two tick vector species play a primary role in the survival of a particular tick-borne flavivirus. Evidence that a tick species is a primary vector is based mostly on virus isolation from field-collected ticks. Since the expedition of Zil'ber and colleagues in the 1930s, repeated field studies have identified *I. persulcatus* as the principal vector of the Far Eastern TBE viral subtype and, more recently, of Siberian subtypes. The first TBEV isolates from *I. ricinus* were obtained during World War II when a TBE outbreak occurred in backup Red Army forces assembled in the forests of Leningrad oblast in spring and summer of 1942 and 1943, to break the blockade of Leningrad. Then for the first time *I. ricinus*, in addition to *I. persulcatus*, was shown to be a vector of TBEV (Petrishcheva and Levkovich 1945). Similarly, following the first

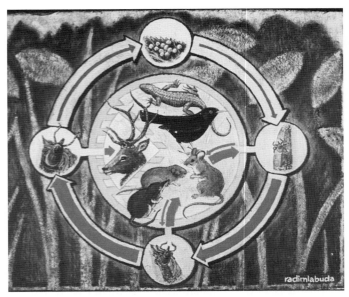

Fig. 37.1 The life cycle of *Ixodes ricinus* and transmission cycle of tick-borne encephalitis virus (dark arrow).

isolation of TBEV from *I. ricinus* ticks in the Czech Republic, numerous virus isolations have confirmed the primary role of *I. ricinus* as a vector of the European TBE viral subtype. The epizoology of LIV implicates *I. ricinus* as the sole vector of this virus (Reid 1988). In North America, most isolations of POWV have been from *I. cookei* whereas the greatest number of POWV isolates in the Primorskiy region of Russia has been recorded from *I. persulcatus* (Hoogstraal 1980; Artsob 1988).

In addition to the primary vector, all competent tick species occurring in sufficiently high numbers and having a sympatric distribution with the primary tick vector may become infected and subsequently transmit tick-borne flaviviruses. Although experimental studies have shown that numerous tick species are competent vectors of TBEV, generally their ecological roles have not been determined. For example, the vector competence of *I. hexagonus* for TBEV has been demonstrated in the laboratory, including transmission of TBEV to hedgehogs (the principal host of this tick species), and TBEV has been isolated from field-collected *I. hexagonus*. However, the importance of *I. hexagonus* in the survival of TBEV in nature is unknown. Similarly, *Ixodes arboricola*, a bird tick, and *Dermacentor reticulatus*, *Haemaphysalis concinna*, *H. inermis* and *H. punctata* are competent vectors of TBEV, and the virus has been isolated from field-collected specimens.

In contrast to TBEV, the epizootiology of LIV implicates *I. ricinus* as the exclusive vector of LIV even though *Dermacentor reticulatus* and *Haemaphysalis punctata* are present in the UK. For POWV, a few ixodid tick species have been implicated as alternative vectors to *I. cookei* (Artsob 1988). The evidence is based on virus isolations from field-collected specimens of *I. marxi* collected in Ontario and associated with red squirrels (*Tamiasciurus hudsonicus*), and from *D. andersoni* and *I. spinipalpus* in western North America. Field data indicate that the primary enzootic tick vectors and vertebrate hosts of POWV vary according to the biotope and geographical area (Hoogstraal 1966). Experimental studies have demonstrated virus transmission by *D. andersoni* and *I. pacificus*, although *I. pacificus* appears to be an inefficient vector. In Russia, POWV has been isolated from *Haemaphysalis longicornis*, *I. persulcatus*, and *D. silvarum* ticks, and also from *Aedes togoi* and *Anopheles hyrcanus* mosquitoes. However, experimental studies failed to demonstrate POWV replication following inoculation of *Aedes aegypti* and *Culex fatigans* mosquitoes. Deer tick virus, the close relative of POWV, appears to be transmitted primarily by *I. scapularis*.

Vertebrate hosts

Like ticks, vertebrate hosts play crucial roles in maintaining the transmission cycles of tick-borne flaviviruses. These roles vary depending on whether the vertebrate is a:

i) Co-feeding host. These animals are susceptible to virus infection although characteristically they produce little if any detectable viraemia (infectious virus circulating in the blood). However, they are frequently co-infested with infected and uninfected ticks, and support non-systemic transmission of the virus from the infected ticks, through their skin and probably their lymphatic system, to the uninfected co-feeding ticks (Labuda *et al.* 1997). Co-feeding virus transmission can even occur when the co-feeding host is immune (has neutralizing antibodies) to the virus. The survival of tick-borne flaviviruses in nature largely depends on the presence of these hosts. They include *Apodemus* spp. field mice and *Myodes* spp. voles (for TBEV and POWV), *Lepus timidus* mountain hare (for LIV), and *Marmota monax* groundhog (POWV).

ii) Viraemic host. Vertebrate hosts that are highly susceptible to virus infection and produce high levels of viraemia. These animals may die of the infection or develop high levels of immunity. They are unlikely to contribute to the long-term survival of the virus in nature. Examples are *Pitymys subterraneus* pine vole (TBEV European subtype) and *Lagopus scotica* red grouse (for LIV). Some species may be both viraemic hosts and co-feeding hosts, especially if they survive a short-term, high titred viraemia and then become immune and capable of supporting co-feeding transmission, e.g. *Myodes* spp. (for TBEV) and sheep (for LIV).

iii) Persistently infected host. Certain vertebrate hosts may develop persistent infections in which the virus is maintained for many months. These species may act as reservoir hosts, maintaining the virus during periods when conditions preclude active tick-borne virus transmission, e.g. winter. They include *Erinaceus europaeus* hedgehog and *Muscardinus avellanarius* doormouse (for TBEV) and *Sciurus carolinensis* grey squirrel (for POWV). However, it is unlikely their reservoir status is as significant as that of the tick vector, which can maintain a virus infection for the whole of its life cycle of several years.

iv) Refractory host. Even though a particular vertebrate host may not support virus transmission, it may still play a vital role in the eco-epidemiology of tick-borne flaviviruses. Such species feed a large proportion to the tick vector population. If they feed adult females, refractory host species will influence the size of the tick population because the female feeds only once and then lays a single large batch of eggs and dies (Fig. 37.1). Evidence suggests that ground-feeding birds are refractory to TBEV infection although they can help maintain large tick populations. For example, five pheasants (*Phasianus colchicus*) did not support experimental co-feeding of TBEV-infected and uninfected *I. ricinus* nymphs (Labuda *et al.* 1993).

In all the different roles (except that of refractory host), horizontal virus transmission occurs. The virus is transmitted either from:

1 an infected tick to a vertebrate host;

2 an infected vertebrate hosts to an uninfected tick;

3 an infected tick, through infection of a co-feeding host, to a co-feeding uninfected tick.

Of these, route (3) is probably the most important mode of transmission for the long-term survival of a tick-borne flavivirus in nature (Randolph *et al.* 1999).

The height above ground at which each tick developmental stage quests for a host is an important determinant of the vertebrate species infested. Generally larvae quest lowest to the ground, nymphs are higher in the vegetation, and adults quest highest. This is one explanation why deer often feed large numbers of adult female *Ixodes* species. Increases in deer populations are positively correlated with increases in populations of *I. persulcatus*, *I. ricinus*, and *I. scapularis*.

Transmission

Tick-borne flaviviruses rely on two different types of host for their survival: invertebrates (ticks) and vertebrates (small-/medium-sized mammals). They cannot survive solely in either ticks or in their vertebrate hosts. Ticks act as both biological virus vectors (the virus must infect and replicate within the tick before it is transmitted) and reservoir hosts in which the virus may survive for the life cycle of the tick (which can be several years). The tick (typically the larval stage) becomes infected by feeding on an infected vertebrate host. Once imbibed in the infectious bloodmeal, the virus undergoes replication within tick cells, disseminates from the gut to the salivary glands (during which time it must survive tick moulting), and is subsequently transmitted in tick saliva when the next tick stage (e.g. nymph) takes a blood meal (Nuttall *et al.* 1994). The natural vertebrate host (especially the co-feeding host; see section on Vertebrate Hosts) amplifies the virus infection by acting as a source of virus for many ticks. A typical transmission cycle for TBEV (European subtype) is indicated by the dark coloured arrows in Fig. 37.1. Since vertical transmission is comparatively rare (see below), larvae are probably more important as acquirers of the virus than as transmitters, although amplification of vertically acquired infections may occur during co-feeding of infected and uninfected larvae. Humans are not normally a source of infection for ticks and consequently they represent dead-end hosts in that their infection is not usually passed on to a new host.

Despite the vector potential of many ixodid ticks for TBEV, only two primary vector species are apparent (*I. persulcatus* and *I. ricinus*). The reasons for this have not been fully defined. Obviously, virus and tick must be sympatric in their distribution. However, this is not the complete story as many competent tick vectors are found within the geographical range of TBEV. One important factor is the contribution to the transmission cycle made by co-feeding of larvae and nymphs on small mammals. For this to happen, larvae and nymphs need to feed at the same time and on the same hosts. Such coincident feeding is characteristic of *I. ricinus*, but not of other sympatric species possibly explaining why they are not significant vectors of TBEV (Randolph 2008). However, the relative contribution of co-feeding transmission between adults and nymphs, as they feed together on medium- and large-sized vertebrate hosts (e.g. hedgehogs, hares, deer), needs further consideration (Korenberg and Kovalevskii 1994).

Another possible reason for the limited number of primary vectors species of tick-borne flaviviruses concerns vector capacity; thus, the efficiency and effectiveness of virus transmission may be greatly enhanced by the actions of tick saliva on the vertebrate host (Nuttall and Labuda 2008). Each parasitic stage of the tick life cycle must take a blood meal in order to progress to the next stage (Fig. 37.1). Blood-feeding is a complex process that takes several days to complete (ranging from 2–3 days for larvae to 5–6 days for adult females). Not surprisingly, the process of tick blood-feeding provokes the vertebrate host's protective mechanisms including coagulation to prevent blood loss, inflammation to stimulate grooming, and wound healing to repair damage at the skin site of tick feeding. For the tick to overcome the host's protective mechanisms, it synthesizes >100 pharmacologically active compounds (mostly proteins) in its salivary glands and secretes these compounds in its saliva during feeding (Titus *et al.* 1990). The net effect is that the skin site where the tick feeds is chemically controlled by the tick. This controlling effect is beneficial for many (if not all) pathogens transmitted by ticks, giving rise to so-called 'saliva-assisted transmission'. Experimental induction of saliva-assisted transmission with TBEV mimics natural non-systemic transmission of TBEV between co-feeding ticks. The possible mechanism of transmission is explained in the 'red herring' hypothesis and involves manipulations of skin dendritic cells (Langerhans cells) and lymphocytes by tick saliva ingredients (Nuttall and Labuda 2003). Intriguingly, there is growing evidence that tick-borne pathogens exploit specific components in the saliva of their vector species. If this specificity occurs between tick-borne flaviviruses and their tick vector species, it may help explain why there are such a limited number of primary vector species.

Although TBEV can be transmitted vertically from one tick generation to the next, there is no evidence of vertical transmission for LIV and POWV (Nuttall and Labuda 1994). The significance of vertical transmission is undetermined. Experimental studies showed persistence of TBEV in *I. persulcatus* for 26 months through three tick generations suggesting that vertical transmission may act as a reservoir mechanism. However, the frequency of vertical transmission generally appears to be low, although models suggest even a low level of vertical transmission can be significant, especially if amplified by virus transmission between co-feeding infected and uninfected larvae.

Although ticks are the primary route of transmission of tick-borne flaviviruses, virus transmission can occur through an oral route. Experimental studies have demonstrated TBEV in the milk of goats, sheep, and cattle for up to 8 days after infection, and in red-backed voles *Myodes rutilus* (Grešiková and Calisher 1988; Bakhvalova *et al.* 2009). LIV has not been reported in naturally infected goats; however, during experimental studies five kids acquired the infection after ingesting infected milk and all developed severe disease. Similarly, secretion of POWV in goats' milk has been demonstrated experimentally. Predation can also be a route of transmission. For example, predation of TBEV-infected small mammals by raptors led to infection, and rodents feeding on infected ticks may become infected. Infection of red grouse feeding on LIV-infected *I. ricinus* may account for the majority of infections of these game birds in their first season (Gilbert *et al.* 2004).

Prevention and control

Preventative measures were reviewed by Smorodintsev (1944) and are still relevant today, depending on the situation:

1   Regular examination of forest dwellers (twice a day) to detect and remove ticks. (Experiments revealed that no infection of mice occurred when the ticks sucked blood for 2–4 hours, but a latent or clinical form of encephalitis appeared when the ticks fed for 2–4 days.)

2   Protection of forest workers by adequate coveralls which shut out crawling ticks.

3   Application of repellents to clothing.

4   Efficient construction of military barracks and adequate preparation of the ground (removal of grass, treatment of vegetation with acaricides).

5   Drainage and forest clearance (as ticks cannot survive in dry conditions).

6   Eradication of rodents and tick control of domestic animals.

7   Vaccination of forest workers.

Protective clothing is effective, ideally light-coloured for easier detection of ticks. This may be undesirable during hot weather and reliance should then be placed on a thorough search of the body, at least daily, after exposure to tick-infested habitat. Ticks that have attached to the skin should be removed carefully using tweezers or forceps to grasp the mouthparts that are buried in the skin. Tick mouthparts have backward pointing barbs so the action of removal should be like removing a fishing hook from a fish. Several tick repellents are available but they will not prevent infection once an infected tick is attached.

As there is no treatment available for tick-borne flaviviral encephalitides, the only successful prevention apart from avoiding tick bites is active immunization. A commercial vaccine is available for TBE and for LI, but not for POW encephalitis. The International Scientific Working Group on Tick-Borne Encephalitis recommends vaccination for both children and adults residing in or travelling to endemic areas (Kunze 2008). Vaccination of laboratory personnel is strongly recommended and in some countries is mandatory for anyone working with TBEV.

The most common vaccine used in Europe is FSME-Immun prepared by Baxter Vaccine AG. This vaccine is a suspension of purified viral antigen derived from TBEV grown in chick embryo cells and inactivated with formalin. Three doses given intramuscularly provide a protective effect persisting for at least 3 years. A protective rate of more than 97% is achieved after the third dose. A booster dose is recommended at 3–5 year intervals thereafter. Cases of TBE after full immunization are rare and adverse reactions are usually mild. The LI vaccine is also a cell culture grown virus preparation inactivated with formalin. It is marketed by Intervet/Shering-Plough Animal Health for immunization of sheep. Control of LI in sheep also includes acaricide treatment (by dipping or application of pour-ons) of animals to control tick infestations.

Vaccination with commercially available vaccines is not sufficiently fast-acting to provide protection after a tick bite. Furthermore, it poses a theoretical risk of exacerbation of disease through antibody-mediated enhancement of virus infection. Hence no vaccination or other specific measure is currently recommended for someone receiving a tick bite who has not been vaccinated (Bröker and Kollaritsch 2008).

Acknowledgements

I am greatly indebted to Professor Ed Korenberg for his insightful comments and for sharing his vast knowledge and experience of the ecology and epidemiology of tick-borne encephalitis viruses.

References

Artsob, H. (1988). Powassan encephalitis. In: T. P. Monath (ed.) *The arboviruses: epidemiology and ecology, Vol. IV*, pp. 29–49. Baco Raton, FLA: CRC Press.

Bakhvalova, V., Potapova, O., Panov, V. V. and Morozova, O. V. (2009). Vertical transmission of tick-borne encephalitis virus between generations of adapted reservoir small rodents. *Virus Res.*, **140**: 172–78.

Banerjee, K. (1988). Kyasanur forest disease. In: T. P. Monath (ed.) *The arboviruses: epidemiology and ecology*, Vol. III, pp. 93–116. Boca Raton, FLA: CRC Press.

Bröker, M. and Kollaritsch, H. (2008). After a tick bite in a tick-borne encephalitis virus endemic area: current positions about post-exposure treatment. *Vaccine*, **26**: 863–68.

Danielová, V., Kliegrová, S., Daniel, M. and Benes, C. (2008). Influence of climate warming on tickborne encephalitis expansion to higher altitudes over the last decade (1997–2006) in the Highland Region (Czech Republic). *Cent. Euro. J. Publ. Heal.*, **16**: 4–11.

Davidson, M. M., Williams, H. and Macleod, J. A. J. (1991). Louping ill in man: A forgotten disease. *J. Infect.*, **23**: 241–49.

Ebel, G. and Kramer, L. D. (2004). Short report: duration of tick attachment required for transmission of Powassan virus by deer ticks. *Am. J. Trop. Med. Hyg.*, **71**: 268–71.

Gelpi, E., Preusser, M., Garzuly, F., Holzmann, H., *et al.* (2005). Visualization of Central European tick-borne encephalitis infection in fatal human cases. *J. Neuropath. Experim. Neurol.*, **64**: 506–12.

Gilbert, L., Jones, L. D., Laurenson, M. K., Gould, E. A., *et al.* (2004). Ticks need not bite their red grouse hosts to infect them with louping ill virus. *Proc. R. Soc. Lond. Ser. B: Biolog. Sci.*, **271**: S202–205.

Grard, G., Moureau, G., *et al.* (2007). Genetic characterization of tick-borne flaviviruses: New insights into evolution, pathogenetic determinants and taxonomy. *Virol.*, **361**: 80–92.

Gray, J. S., Dautel, H., Estrada-Pena, A., *et al.* (2009). Effects of climate change on ticks and tick-borne diseases in Europe. *Interdis. Persp. Infect. Dis.*, 10.1155/2009/593232.

Gritsun, T. S., Nuttall, P. A. and Gould, E. A. (2003). Tick-borne flaviviruses. *Adv. Virus Res.*, **61**: 318–71.

Grešíková, M. and Calisher, C. H. (1988). Tick-borne encephalitis. In: T. P. Monath (ed.) *The arboviruses: epidemiology and ecology*, Vol. IV, pp. 177–202. Boca Raton, FLA: CRC Press.

Gubler, D., Kuno, G. and Markoff, L. (2007). Flaviviruses. In: D. M. Knipe and P. M. Howley (eds.) *Fields' Virology*, Vol. 1, pp. 1153–253. Philadelphia, PA: Lippincott William & Wilkins.

Hinten, S. R., Beckett, G. A., *et al.* (2008). Increased recognition of Powassan encephalitis in the United States, 1999–2005. *Vector-Borne and Zoon. Dis.*, **8**: 733–40.

Hoogstraal, H. (1966). Ticks in relation to human diseases caused by viruses. *Ann. Rev. Entomo.*, **11**: 261–308.

Hoogstraal, H. (1980). Established and emerging concepts regarding tick-associated viruses, and unanswered questions. In: J. Vesenjak-Hirjan *et al.* (eds.) *Arboviruses in the Mediterranean countries.* Zentrbl. Bakt. Mikro. Hyg. I. Abt., Suppl. 9. pp. 49–62. Stottgart: Gustav Fischer Verlag.

Kharitonova, N. N. and Leonov, Y. A. (1985). The agent and epizootiology. In: P. M. P. Chumakov (ed.) *Omsk Haemorrhagic Fever*. New Delhi: Science (Nanka) Publishers.

Korenberg, E. I. and Kovalevskii, Yu. V. (1994). A model for relationships among the tick-borne encephalitis virus, its main vectors, and hosts. *Adv. Dis. Vector Res.*, **10**: 65–92.

Korenberg, E. I. (2000). Seasonal population dynamics of Ixodes ticks and tick-borne encephalitis virus. *Experimental and Applied Acarology*, **24**: 665–81.

Korenberg, E. I. (2009). Recent epidemiology of tick-borne encephalitis: an effect of climate change? *Adv. Virus Res.*, **74**: 123–144.

Korenberg, E. I. and Kovalevskii, Y. V. (1999). Main features of tick-borne encephalitis eco-epidemiology in Russia. *Zentralb. Bakteriol.*, **289**: 525–39.

Kuno, G., Artsob, H., Karabatsos, N., Tsuchiya, K. R. and Chang, G. J. (2001). Genomic sequencing of deer tick virus and phylogeny of powassan-related viruses of North America. *Am. J. Trop. Med. Hyg.*, **65**: 671–76.

Kunze, U. (2008). Combating tick-borne encephalitis: vaccination rates on the rise. *Vaccine*, **26**: 6738–40.

Labuda, M., Nuttall, P. A., Kožuch, O., Elecková, E., *et al.* (1993). Non-viraemic transmission of tick-borne encephalitis virus: a mechanism for arbovirus survival in nature. *Experientia*, **49**: 802–5.

Labuda, M., Austyn, J. M., Zuffová, E., Kozuch, O., and Nuttall, P. A. (1996). Importance of localised skin infection in tick-borne encephalitis virus transmission. *Virol.*, **219**: 357–66.

Labuda, M., Kožuch, O., Zuffová, E., Elecková, E., *et al.* (1997). Tick-borne encephalitis virus transmission between ticks cofeeding on specific immune natural rodent hosts. *Virology*, **235**: 138–43.

Labuda, M. and Nuttall, P. A. (2008). Viruses transmitted by ticks. In: A. S. Bowman and P. A. Nuttall (eds.) *Ticks: Biology, Disease and Control*, pp. 253–80. Cambridge: Cambridge University Press.

Leonova, G. H. (1997). *Tick-Borne Encephalitis in Primorye*. Dal'nauka, Valdivostok, p. 189 (in Russian).

Lindenbach, B. D. *et al.* (2007). Flaviviridae: the viruses and their replication. In D. M. Knipe and P. M. Howley (eds.) *Fields' Virology*, pp. 991–1041. Philadelphia: Lippincott Williams & Wilkins.

Lvov, D. K. (1988). Omsk haemorrhagic fever. In: T. P. Monath (ed.) *The arboviruses: epidemiology and ecology*, Vol. III, pp. 205–16. Boca Raton, Florida: CRC Press, Inc.

Nuttall, P. A. (2009). Molecular characterization of tick-virus interactions. *Frontiers in Bioscience*, **14**: 2466–83.

Nuttall, P. A. and Labuda, M. (1994). Tick-borne encephalitis subgroup. In: D. E. Sonenshine and T. N. Mather (eds.) *Ecological Dynamics of Tick-borne Zoonoses*, pp. 351–91. Oxford: Oxford University Press.

Nuttall, P. A. and Labuda, M. (2003). Dynamics of infection in tick vectors and at the tick-host interface. *Adv. Virus Res.*, **60**: 233–72.

Nuttall, P. A. and Labuda, M. (2008). Saliva-assisted transmission of tick-borne pathogens. In: A. S. Bowman and P. A. Nuttall (eds.) *Ticks: Biology, Disease and Control*, pp. 205–19. Cambridge: Cambridge University Press.

Nuttall, P. A., Jones, L. D., Labuda, M., and Kaufman, W. R. (1994). Adaptations of arboviruses to ticks. *J. Med. Entomol.*, **31**: 1–9.

Pavlovsky, E. N. (1966). *Natural nidality of transmissible diseases*. Moscow: Peace Publishers.

Petrishcheva, P. A. and Levkovich, E. N. (1945). Spontaneous infection of I. ricinus and I. persulcatus ticks by tick-borne encephalitis in Leningrad oblast. In: A. E. Pesis, N. S. Molchanov, and V. L. Portnykh (eds.) *Spring-Summer Encephalitis in Leningrad oblast: Collected Works of Volkhov Front Medics*, pp. 71–74. (in Russian). Leningrad: Lenoblsovet.

Randolph, S. E. (2008). Dynamics of tick-borne disease systems: minor role of recent climate change. *Rev. Scientif. Technique (Intern. Off. Epizoo.)*, **27**: 367–81.

Randolph, S. E. (2008). The impact of tick ecology on pathogen transmission dynamics. In: A. S. Bowman and P. A. Nuttall (eds.) *Ticks: Biology, Disease and Control*, pp. 40–72. Cambridge: Cambridge University Press.

Randolph, S. E., Miklisova, D., Lysy, J., Rogers, D., Labuda, M. (1999). Incidence from coincidence: patterns of tick infestations on rodents facilitate transmission of tick-borne encephalitis virus. *Parasitol.*, **118**: 177–86.

Reid, H. W. (1984). Epidemiology of louping-ill. In: M. A. Mayo and K. A. Harrap (eds.) *Vectors in virus biology*, pp. 161–78. London: Academic Press.

Reid, H. W. (1988). Louping-ill. In: T. P. Monath (ed.) *The arboviruses: epidemiology and ecology*, Vol. III, pp. 117–35. Boca Raton, FLA: CRC Press.

Rey, F. A., Heinz, F. X., Mandl, C. W., Kunz, C, and Harrison, S. C. (1995). The envelope glycoprotein from tick-borne encephalitis virus at 2A resolution. *Nature*, **375**: 291–98.

Romero, J. R. and Simonsen, K. A. (2008). Powassan encephalitis and Colorado Tick Fever. *Infect. Dis. Clin. N. Am.*, **22**: 545–59.

Schneider, H. (1931). Über epidemische akute 'Meningitis serosa' Wien. *Klin. Wschr*, **44**: 350–52.

Smith, C. E. G. and Varma, M. G. R. (1981). Louping ill. In: J. H. Steele (ed. in chief) *CRC Handbook Series in Zoonoses*, Section B: Viral zoonoses, (ed. G. W. Beran), Vol. I, pp. 191–200. Boca Raton, FLA: CRC Press.

Stiasny, K., Kossl, C., Lepault, J., Rey, F. A. and Heinz, F. X. (2007). Characterization of a structural intermediate of flavivirus membrane fusion. *PLoSP*, **3**: e20.

Smorodintsev, A. (1944). Tick-borne encephalitis. *Am. Rev. Sov. Med.*, **1**: 400–408.

Sumilo, D., Bormane, A., *et al.* (2008). Socio-economic factors in the differential upsurge of tick-borne encephalitis in Central and Eastern Europe. *Re. Med. Virol.*, **18**: 81–95.

Süss, J. (2008). Tick-borne encephalitis in Europe and beyond—the epidemiological situation as of 2007. *Eurosurveill.*, **13**: 4–6.

Tavakoli, N. P., Wang, H., *et al.* (2009). Fatal case of deer tick virus encephalitis. *N. Engl. J. Med.*, **360**: 2099–107.

Titus, R. G. and Ribeiro, J. M. C. (1990). The role of vector saliva in transmission of arthropod-borne disease. *Parasitol. Today*, **6**: 157–60.

Telford, S. R. (1997). A new tick-borne encephalitis-like virus infecting New England deer ticks, *Ixodes Dammini. Emerg. Infect. Dis.*, **3**: 165–70.

Zil'ber, L. A. (1937). Spring (spring-summer) epidemic tick-borne encephalitis. *Arkhiv. Biol. Nauk.*, **56**: 9–37. (in Russian).

Zil'ber, L. A. (1957). On the history of studies on far-eastern tick-borne encephalitis. *Vopr. Virusol.*, **6**: 323–34. (in Russian).

CHAPTER 38

Yellow fever

Thomas P. Monath and J. Erin Staples

Summary

Yellow fever is an acute mosquito-borne flavivirus infection characterized in its full-blown form by fever, jaundice, albuminuria, and haemorrhage. Two forms are distinguished: *urban* yellow fever in which the virus is spread from person to person by peridomestic *Aedes aegypti* mosquitoes and *jungle (sylvan)* yellow fever transmitted by tree-hole breeding mosquitoes between non-human primates and sometimes humans. Yellow fever is endemic and epidemic in tropical areas of the Americas and Africa but has never appeared in Asia or the Pacific region. Prevention and control are effected principally through yellow fever vaccination.

History

The earliest probable account of the disease was during an epidemic in the Yucatan Peninsula in 1648. In Africa, the disease was first recognized during an epidemic in 1778. During the eighteenth and nineteenth centuries, urban yellow fever was a major threat to human health in the Americas and Africa, and it invaded Europe on numerous occasions. For many years the disease was attributed to the spread of airborne miasmas. Although mosquitoes were suspected to be implicated in transmission as early as 1848, it was Carlos Finlay, a Cuban physician, who in 1881 promulgated the theory of mosquito transmission. Spurred by Finlay's suggestion, Walter Reed and his colleagues conducted studies in Cuba in 1900–1901 that proved transmission by *Aedes aegypti* mosquitoes, demonstrated that an extrinsic incubation period in the mosquito was required prior to transmission by bite, and showed that the disease was caused by a filtrable virus. Isolation of the virus proved an elusive goal until 1927, when Rockefeller Foundation scientists in Ghana and Nigeria isolated the agent by passage of human blood to rhesus macaques. The virus, recovered from a patient named Asibi, is the parent of the attenuated 17D strain now used as a vaccine.

For many years, *Ae. aegypti* was thought to be the only vector, and humans the only host for yellow fever virus. In 1932, 'jungle yellow fever' was described in an area of Colombia free from *Ae. aegypti*, and by 1938, yellow fever transmission by tree-hole breeding *Haemagogus* mosquitoes was documented. Field studies in South America and east Africa during the 1930s and 1940s unravelled many complexities of yellow fever as a zoonotic disease, demonstrating the role of sylvatic vectors in virus transmission between non-human primates and spillover of the infection to the urban cycle involving *Ae. aegypti* and humans. Research on virus survival across the long tropical dry season and on the recrudescence of epizootics/epidemics continued for several decades. In 1977, workers at the Pasteur Institute in Dakar obtained field evidence for transovarial transmission of the virus in the sylvatic vector *Ae. furcifer-taylori*. Subsequent field and experimental studies have implicated vertical transmission in vector mosquitoes as a viral maintenance mechanism.

In the Americas, control of urban yellow fever centred on the elimination of *Ae. aegypti*. Successful vector eradication programmes were undertaken in Cuba, Panama, Brazil, and other areas. Only 3 relatively small *Ae. aegypti*-borne outbreaks have occurred in South America since the early 1940s (the most recent in 2008 in Paraguay). However, control efforts were never seriously undertaken in Africa, where *Ae. aegypti*-borne epidemic continue to occur. Efforts to develop a vaccine began in the 1930s in Senegal and the USA, and were spurred on by the recognition of yellow fever as a zoonotic disease. Field trials of the French neurotropic vaccine began in 1934 in west Africa and of the 17D vaccine in 1937 in Brazil. These vaccines came into widespread use in the 1940s. Where vaccine coverage has been low, however, yellow fever epidemics continue to occur. The greatest impact of the disease is currently in Africa, but recent changes in the ecology and distribution of *Ae. aegypti* and in human demographics in the Americas raise the spectre of future urban outbreaks in densely populated coastal areas where routine immunization is not carried out.

Aetiological agent

Taxonomy

Yellow fever virus is the prototype of the family Flaviviridae, a group of 75 viruses that includes a number of other important arthropod-borne diseases, such as dengue, West Nile neuroinvasive disease, St Louis encephalitis, Japanese encephalitis, and tick-borne encephalitis. By the neutralization test, yellow fever virus is antigenically distinct, but appears to be more closely related to Banzi, Wesselsbron, Bouboui, Zika, and Uganda S viruses than to other flaviviruses. Cross-protection between yellow fever and other flaviviruses can be demonstrated in animals. Prior immunization with Wesselsbron, Zika, and dengue viruses causes a significant reduction in viraemias in monkeys challenged with virulent yellow fever virus. Cross-protection may explain certain epidemiological events, including a lower incidence of clinical yellow fever infections in adult African populations with a background of heterologous flavivirus immunity. Immunity to dengue may be a barrier to the introduction of yellow fever into Asia.

Molecular biology and basis for virulence

Yellow fever is a single-strand, positive polarity, RNA-containing virus of small size (35–45 nm in diameter), consisting of a nucleocapsid approximately 30 nm in diameter, surrounded by a lipid bilayer envelope. Replication occurs in the cytoplasm, and mature virus particles accumulate in endoplasmic reticulum and are released by host cell lysis. After adsorption, entry, and uncoating, the genome is translated to yield viral replicases and serves as a template for transcription of minus-strand complementary RNA. In turn, progeny plus-strand RNAs are synthesized. These serve as mRNA for translation of viral proteins and incorporation into new virions. For reviews of flavivirus structure and replication see (Lindenbach and Rice 2006) and (Heinz and Allison 2006).

The linear yellow fever genome has been completely sequenced and shown to contain 10,862 nucleotides with a single long open reading frame encoding, in order, the three structural proteins (C, capsid; M, membrane, and E, envelope) and seven non-structural proteins, designated NS1, NS2a, NS2b, NS3, NS4a, NS4b, and NS5. The gene products result from proteolytic processing of a polyprotein precursor. The E glycoprotein, a dimeric molecule composed of a 170 Å-long curved rod that is anchored to the viral membrane at its basal end, is involved in attachment of virus to cell receptors, and contains functional antigenic determinants, including those for haemagglutination and neutralization. Epitopes are clustered in three spatially distinct domains (domains A, B, and C) on the glycoprotein rod and biological activity (e.g. neutralization) is dependent on the native conformation of the protein. The NS1 glycoprotein, while not incorporated in the mature virion, is expressed on the surface of infected cells and elicits complement-fixing antibodies that may play a role in protection against yellow fever infection. As for protein E, most NS1 epitopes are conformation-dependent. The functions of the other non-structural proteins are less well understood. NS3 functions as a protease in post-translational processing, and NS5 as the RNA polymerase.

Attenuation by serial passage led to the development of the yellow fever 17D vaccine. Nucleotide sequencing of the virulent, parental Asibi virus and 17D vaccine provided clues to the molecular basis of virulence (Hahn et al. 1987), but the large number of mutations and their localization in many parts of the genome complicate interpretation of these comparative data. Sixty-seven nucleotide and 31 amino acid differences distributed across the genome were noted between vaccine and parental Asibi virus. Subsequent analyses of other vaccine strains derived from the 17D lineage and additional wild-type yellow fever viruses have significantly reduced the mutations that may explain attenuation. Thirteen non-conservative amino acid substitutions are specific to the vaccine strains, five of which occur in the E gene. Five of the changes in the E gene occur at sites (amino acids 52, 173, 200, 305, and 380) that are conserved in virulent yellow fever viruses from both Africa and South America isolated many years apart. Thus these mutations are likely to be implicated in yellow fever virulence.

Yellow fever virus exhibits two distinct virulence factors reflecting its capability to induce encephalitis (neurotropism) and hepatitis (viscerotropism). The attenuated 17D virus has lost its capacity to cause hepatitis, while retaining a reduced degree of neurotropism, particularly for the immature brain. Rarely have fatal cases of human encephalitis due to 17D virus been reported. In one fatal case, sequencing of the E glycoprotein and comparison with other substrains of 17D vaccines revealed a single amino acid change at position 303 that could be correlated with the increased neurovirulence of the virus recovered from brain tissue (Jennings et al. 1994). Presumably this mutation arose during replication of the vaccine in the human host. Interestingly, this mutation is spatially close to two other mutations distinguishing wild-type from vaccine virus, suggesting that this region, which lies in antigenic domain B, may represent an important locus defining neurovirulence. The B domain contains an RGD sequence and is believed to represent part of the cell receptor binding site for flaviviruses.

Yellow fever virus produces a fatal viscerotropic disease in rhesus macaques and some other monkeys, and, with adaptation by passage in golden hamsters (McArthur et al. 2003). The molecular changes associated with viscerotropism and lethality for hamsters was shown to depend on one or more of 7 mutations during adaptation, 6 of which were in the E protein.

Role of yellow fever proteins in the immune response

The E protein plays the dominant role in the genesis of neutralizing antibodies and the induction of protective immunity. The prM protein also contains neutralizing and protective domains. prM is part of immature virions and is proteolytically cleaved in the trans-Golgi region to generate M protein in mature virions. If this cleavage is incomplete, prM protein in the virion can serve as a target for neutralizing protective antibodies.

The non-structural glycoprotein NS1 is expressed on the surface of infected cells and is also secreted into the circulation of the infected host as 'soluble complement fixing' (SCF) antigen. Although antibodies to NS1 do not react with the virion and exhibit no neutralizing activity, they confer protection against yellow fever virus infection in experimental animals. This phenomenon is dependent on the Fc portion of antibodies and appears to be due to complement-mediated cytotoxicity, although other mechanisms may contribute as well.

The immunological role of the other non-structural proteins appears to be limited to cellular immunity. Studies with dengue and other flaviviruses have demonstrated epitopes for CD4+ and CD8+ T-lymphocytes on NS1, NS3, NS4A, and NS4B as well as on the E glycoprotein.

Yellow fever 17D is one of the most powerful vaccines with respect to immunogenicity and durability of the immune response. This is in part attributable to the ability of the vaccine virus to elicit innate immune responses that drive the adaptive immune response and leads to the development of vaccine virus-specific memory T cells (Wrammert et al. 2009). 17D virus activates multiple Toll-like receptors in dendritic cells and induces genes that regulate innate immunity (Querec et al. 2007, 2009).

Diversity of yellow fever virus strains: molecular epidemiology

By nucleotide sequencing, seven distinct genotypes have been distinguished, two in South America and five in Africa (Mutebi *et al.*, 2001, 2004). All seven genotypes belong to the same serotype defined by neutralization, although minor antigenic differences have been shown between strains of yellow fever virus, and virus strains from tropical America and Africa by cross-absorption. The yellow fever virus genome has been relatively conserved, presumably because of restrictions imposed by host range. African strains, belonging to five genotypes contain nucleotide substitutions varied from 0 to 25.8% and amino acid substitutions from 0 to 9.1%. The five African genotypes are: West African type I (western areas of the region, e.g. Nigeria); genotype II (virus strains from the East, e.g. Senegal, Guinea Bissau); the East/Central Africa genotype (Central African Republic, Ethiopia, Sudan, Zaire, Uganda); East Africa genotype (Uganda, Kenya); and the Angola genotype (represented by a single strain from the 1971 outbreak). The Central African, East African, and Angolan genotypes are notably different from the West African genotypes (7% amino acid differences, consistent with their ecological separation, due to utilization of different mosquito vectors. Only two genotypes (I and II) are found in South America. Genotype I occurs in Brazil, whereas the (apparently older) genotype II circulates in the western part of the continent (Peru, Bolivia, and a strain from western Brazil (Rondonia) divergent by 0–4.6% at the amino acid sequence level (Vasconcelos *et al.* 2004).

Growth *in vitro* and host range

Yellow fever virus can be propagated in a wide variety of primary and continuous cell cultures, including monkey kidney (MA-104, Vero, LLC-MK2), rabbit kidney (MA-111), baby hamster kidney (BHK), and porcine kidney (PS-2 and PK-15) cell lines, as well as in primary chick and duck embryo fibroblast monolayers, in which the virus causes cytopathic effects and plaque formation. Mosquito cells, particularly the *Ae. pseudo-scutellaris* (AP61) cell line, are highly sensitive for primary isolation of wild-type yellow fever virus. Intrathoracic inoculation of *Toxorhynchites* or *Ae. aegypti* mosquitoes may be used for primary isolation or virus titration. After an appropriate incubation period, mosquitoes can be examined directly by immunofluorescence or subpassaged to a susceptible host such as suckling mice.

In vertebrate hosts, wild-type yellow fever virus produces both neurotropic and viscerotropic patterns of infection. Viscerotropism reflects the pathogenesis of yellow fever virus in human or non-human primates, in which disease is characterized by hepatic pathology. The European hedgehog (*Erinaceus europaeus*), Sudanese hedgehog (*E. pruneri*), the golden hamster (infected by virus adapted by serial liver passage (Tesh *et al.* 2001) and mice lacking the interferon-a/b receptor (Meier *et al.* 2009) are the only non-primate species that develop viscerotropic infections (hepatitis). Infant mice are susceptible to neurotropic infection (encephalitis) after peripheral or intracerebral inoculation, whereas older mice and guinea-pigs develop encephalitis only after intracerebral inoculation. Monkeys develop encephalitis after intracerebral inoculation of wild-type virus but die of acute visceral yellow fever. Adaptation of wild-type virus by brain passage in mice reduces viscerotropism, and was the basis for development of the French neurotropic vaccine.

The host range for wild vertebrate species is described below.

The hosts

Intermediate and reservoir hosts and vectors

Maintenance of yellow fever virus in nature depends upon cyclic transmission between vertebrate hosts and mosquito vectors (Fig. 38.1). In both Africa and tropical America, monkeys are the principal wild vertebrate hosts and aedine mosquitoes are the principal vectors. Humans are also important intermediate hosts in situations where *Ae. aegypti* is responsible for transmission (urban yellow fever) or where interhuman transmission is sustained by sylvatic vectors. For a more detailed summary of the role of vertebrate hosts and vectors in yellow fever ecology, see Monath (1988).

Tropical America

In South America, tamarins, marmosets, howling monkeys (*Alouatta* spp.), spider monkeys (*Ateles* sp.), squirrel monkeys (*Saimiri* sp.), and owl monkeys (*Aotus* sp.) are effective viraemic hosts and may develop fatal infections. Monkey deaths in nature (particularly of howling monkeys) are an early sign of a yellow fever epizootic in progress. In contrast, capuchin monkeys (*Cebus* sp.), widow monkeys (*Callicebus* sp.), and wooly monkeys (*Lagothrix* sp.), are susceptible to viraemic infection but usually do not develop clinical signs. In non-human primates, viraemias at levels above the threshold for vector infection generally last several days.

Although South American marsupials have been suspected to play a role in virus transmission, they have not been clearly implicated by field studies. Experimental infection of *Didelphis marsupialis* with some yellow fever strains resulted in viraemic infections, but titres were generally low. Infection of *Marmosa cinerae* and *Metachirus nudicaudatus*, however, resulted in prolonged viraemias sufficient to infect *Haemagogus* mosquitoes. Further studies of the role of these vertebrates in yellow fever ecology are warranted. Rodents, ungulates, birds, reptiles, and amphibia are not efficient viraemic hosts. Most carnivores have been found refractory to experimental infection, an exception being the kinkajou (*Potos flavus*), but no evidence exists for a role in natural virus cycles.

Haemagogus mosquitoes (principally *Hg. janthinomys*) are the principal vectors of jungle yellow fever in tropical America. *Haemagogus* spp. breed in tree holes and feed in the forest canopy during the midday hours, but they also bite humans in forest clearings and even inside houses near the forest. In some circumstances, these mosquitoes exist in relatively high densities in neotropical forests, with documented biting rates as high as 140 per man-hour in the canopy. Vertical transmission of yellow fever virus by *Haemagogus equinus* has been demonstrated experimentally and provides a logical mechanism for maintenance of the virus during prolonged dry seasons, when adult mosquito populations are low or absent. *Sabethes chloropterus*, a drought-resistant vector species, may also play a role in virus maintenance across the dry season.

Aedes aegypti was responsible for frequent urban epidemics in the Americas through the 1930s. This highly anthropophilic mosquito reaches high densities in densely populated areas, breeds in man-made receptacles indoors and out, and has biting habits, including interrupted feeding, that favour virus transmission. In large cities in tropical America, endemic interhuman transmission of yellow fever was maintained by this mosquito in the past. Anti-*Ae. aegypti* campaigns in Latin America between the 1930s and the early 1970s led to eradication from most countries surrounding the

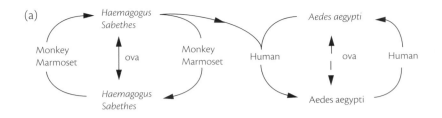

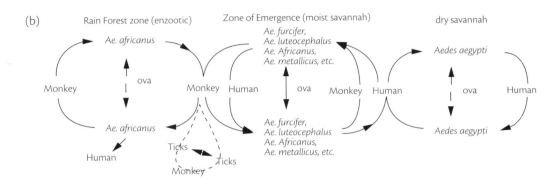

Fig. 38.1 Transmission cycles of yellow fever virus in South America (a) and Africa (b) Yellow fever virus has an enzootic maintenance cycle involving tree-hole breeding mosquito vectors and non-human primates. In tropical America, human yellow fever cases derive from contact with forest mosquito (*Haemagogus* spp.) vectors, and no urban (*Ae. aegypti*-borne) yellow fever has occurred for over 50 years. In Africa, sylvatic vectors are responsible for monkey–monkey and interhuman virus transmission, and there is frequent involvement of *Ae. aegypti* in urban areas and in the dry savannah vegetational zone. The maintenance mechanism for virus survival across the prolonged dry season (when adult mosquitoes are absent or reduced) is believed to involve vertical passage of virus in mosquito ova. Alternate mechanisms may occur, including survival of drought-resistant adult mosquitoes or secondary cycles of transmission involving ticks.

Amazon Basin. Beginning in the late 1970s, however, *Ae. aegypti* re-invaded many areas of Brazil, Paraguay, Bolivia, Peru, Ecuador, and Colombia, so that infested towns and villages are again at risk of virus incursions from the jungle yellow fever cycle (Fig. 38.2). The threat of urbanization of yellow fever in South American cities and potential for spread to the Caribbean, Central America, and the US, have significantly increased in the past decade. Spillover of jungle yellow fever to the urban (*Ae. aegypti*-borne) cycle occurred most recently in 2008 in the environs of Asuncion, Paraguay.

Africa

Non-human primates also serve as principal vertebrate hosts for yellow fever viruses in Africa. In some areas of Africa, monkey populations have been reduced and their range restricted due to human modification of their habitat. Thus, humans play an increasingly important role in the transmission cycle of yellow fever in Africa.

All species of cercopithecid and colobid monkeys, baboons, and lemurs appear to be effective viraemic hosts, circulating virus for several days at sufficient titres to infect vectors. Galagos do not play a major role in yellow fever transmission cycles. Infection rarely causes illness or death in African primates, indicating a balanced parasite-host relationship, and supporting the notion that yellow fever virus evolved in the continent.

Experimental studies have shown the Sudanese hedgehog to be susceptible to viraemia and hepatitis, but this creature has not been implicated in natural virus transmission. Other insectivores are refractory to infection. Most rodents and carnivores tested are also resistant. Yellow fever virus was isolated from an insectivorous bat

(*Epomophorus* sp.) in Ethiopia, but the role of bats in natural transmission cycles has not been confirmed.

In the equatorial forests of Africa, *Ae. africanus* mosquitoes are responsible for year-round virus transmission. Tree holes serve as oviposition sites, and biting activity is largely in the canopy, although in some areas *Ae. africanus* may also breed and bite at ground level around human habitations. The level of viral activity in the enzootic high-forest zone is generally low, reflected by low immunity rates in human and monkey populations and absence of large epidemics. This is largely due to the extreme dilution of vectors and hosts in a continuous, uniformly favourable forest environment.

The *zone of emergence* of yellow fever in Africa is a term used to refer to the savannahforest mosaic and Guinean and southern Sudan savannah vegetational zones, including riverine (gallery) forests, which support concentrated populations of monkeys and vector mosquitoes (Germain *et al.* 1981). In the moist savannah zones, yellow fever virus transmission intensifies during the rainy season and wanes during the dry season when vector populations decline. During the dry season, vertical transmission ensures virus survival in the *egg* stage. The principal species involved in virus transmission in West Africa are *Ae. africanus*, *Ae. furcifer*, and *Ae. luteocephalus*. It is not unusual for these species to penetrate into villages and even to bite indoors. Endemic transmission occurs annually and human immunity rates are high. Intense epidemics may occur at the limits of the zone, where viral activity may subside for intervals of several years or more and reappear during periods of increased or prolonged rainfall. In such fringe areas, the prevalence of human immunity is low in the younger age groups

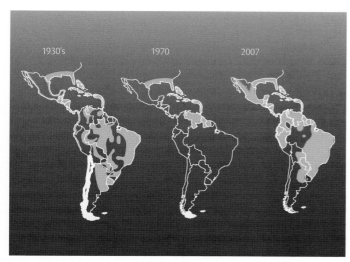

Fig. 38.2 Distribution of *Aedes aegypti* in the Americas (shaded areas). Re-invasion of the South American continent by *Ae. aegypti* occurred in the late 1970s and 1980s due to collapse of vector control programmes, the increase in breeding sites due to urbanization, and other factors, raising the risk of renewed urban outbreaks of yellow fever.

Figure kindly provided by Dr D. J. Gubler.

and children sustain the highest incidence of disease. Other vector species which play a secondary or accessory role in the zone of emergence are: *Ae. opok*, *Ae. neoafricanus*, *Ae. vittatus*, and *Ae. metallicus*. In East Africa, *Ae. simpsoni gr.* mosquitoes have been responsible for interhuman transmission; this species complex is not anthropophilic in West Africa.

In areas of Africa subject to extreme drying, e.g. in the dry northern Sudan and Sahel savannah zones of western Africa, yellow fever occurs in intermittent epidemic form, and human immunity patterns indicate a low incidence of infection during interepidemic periods. In these areas, domestic water storage is intensively practiced, often with clay water storage jars being buried in the ground so that they cannot be cleaned or emptied. These receptacles are permanent breeding sites for domestic *Ae. aegypti*. Vector densities are high, and introduction of yellow fever virus into such an area (usually by a viraemic human) may result in an explosive outbreak. In 1987, for example, yellow fever was introduced into large towns of western Nigeria from a remote area undergoing a sylvatic outbreak. An explosive *Ae. aegypti*-borne epidemic followed and continued for over 5 years. *Aedes aegypti* density as measured by the Breteau index (number of infested breeding sites/100 houses) provides an estimate of the risk of urban yellow fever. An index of 5 is considered to constitute a low risk, and an index of 50 or greater a high risk of transmission. During the Nigerian epidemic in 1987, Breteau indices exceeded 600 in some affected localities.

Experimental studies show variation among geographical populations of *Ae. aegypti* in their vector competence for yellow fever virus. West African *Ae. aegypti* strains involved in epidemic transmission have proved to be biologically poor vectors; in this region high vector density compensated for low susceptibility, permitting reproduction of the epidemic. It has been suggested that low vector competence may select virus strains that elicit high viraemias and that may have high human virulence (Miller *et al.* 1989).

Yellow fever virus has been isolated from ticks (*Amblyomma variegatum*) in the Central African Republic, raising the possibility that alternate vectors play a role in dispersal or maintenance of the virus. Yellow fever virus is also transovarially transmitted in *Amblyomma* ticks.

Yellow fever virus has been isolated from other arthropods, including *Ae. dentatus*, *Coquillettidia fuscopennata*, and phlebotomine flies. In some areas (e.g. northern Nigeria and northern Kenya), *Mansonia africana* mosquitoes have been suspected to play a role in transmission. These observations are probably peripheral to the ecology of yellow fever, but are worthy of further study.

Humans

Clinical infection varies from a mild undifferentiated febrile illness to a fulminating fatal disease with pathognomonic features. The incubation period is usually 3–6 days, with a median of 4.3 days (Johansson *et al.* 2010). Abortive infections are not recognizable except in the setting of an epidemic. In its mildest form, yellow fever is a self-limited infection characterized by sudden onset of fever and headache without other symptoms. In other patients, fever and headache are more severe and accompanied by myalgia, albuminuria, and bradycardia in relation to the height of fever (Faget's sign). In such cases, the illness lasts several days, with uneventful recovery. Severe yellow fever, present in roughly 15% of symptomatic individuals, begins abruptly with fever to 40°C, chills, severe headache, lumbosacral pain, and generalized muscle aches. The patient appears toxic, the conjunctiva congested, the face and neck flushed, the tongue reddened at the tip and edges, and the heart rate slow despite fever. Anorexia, nausea and vomiting, and minor gingival haemorrhages or epistaxes are common. This syndrome lasts approximately 3 days and is named the *period of infection*, since yellow fever virus is present in the blood. A *period of remission* follows, with defervescence and mitigation of symptoms, lasting up to 24 hours. Fever and symptoms then recur with more intense vomiting, epigastric pain, prostration, and the appearance of jaundice (*period of intoxication*). Viraemia is generally absent, and antibodies appear during this phase. A bleeding diathesis may be evident, with haematemesis (black vomit), melena, metorrhagia, petechiae, ecchymoses, and oozing blood from the gingival membranes and needle-puncture sites. Bleeding is occasionally life-threatening. Dehydration results from vomiting and increased insensible losses. Renal dysfunction is marked by a sudden increase in albuminuria and by diminishing urine output. Physical findings include scleral and dermal icterus, haemorrhages, and epigastric tenderness without hepatic enlargement. Oedema and ascites are not present. The patient recovers either rapidly after a period of intoxication of 3–4 days or over a protracted course of up to 2 weeks. Death occurs during the second week and is heralded by intensifying jaundice, haemorrhage, rising pulse, shock, oliguria, and azotaemia. Hypothermia, agitated delirium, intractable hiccup, stupor, and coma are terminal signs. The case fatality rate in patients who develop jaundice is 20–50%.

Convalescence is often prolonged, with aesthenia lasting several weeks. Late death, occurring at the end of convalescence or even weeks after complete recovery from the acute illness, is a rare phenomenon attributed to yellow fever myocardial damage and cardiac arrythmia. Secondary bacterial infections, such as pneumonia or parotitis, may complicate recovery. The duration of icterus in surviving cases is poorly established, but jaundice has been observed for up to 3 months after recovery from serologically documented yellow fever.

Leucopenia (white cell counts as low as 1.5×10^9 cells/1) occurs during the first week of illness. Differential counts show an absolute neutropenia and lymphopenia. Leucocytosis often occurs during the terminal stage of the disease. Prolongation of the clotting, prothrombin, and partial thromboplastin times, decreased platelet count and presence of fibrin-split products may be found. Hyperbilirubinaemia may be present as early as the third day, with a peak on the sixth to eighth day at average levels of 9–10 mg/dl, but in fatal cases it may reach 48 mg/dL. Serum glutamic oxaloacetic, and pyruvic transaminase levels are markedly elevated in icteric patients, with elevation on the second day and peak values between days 5 and 10 of the illness. Elevations of serum transaminase levels have been documented to persist for at least 2 months after onset. The alkaline phosphatase level is generally normal. Hypoglycaemia has been noted in patients with severe hepatic damage. Plasma protein (especially gamma globulin) concentration may fall during the acute illness. During the period of infection, the urine may contain a small amount of albumin, which then increases during the period of intoxication, reaching levels of up to 5 g/1 (rarely up to 40 g/1). The cerebrospinal fluid is clear and does not contain cells, but may be under increased pressure and may contain elevated protein.

The pathogenesis of yellow fever in humans remains poorly understood (Monath and Barrett, 2006; Monath, 2008). It is likely that profound activation of the immune response ('cytokine storm') is a factor and it is of interest that immune clearance of the virus appears to coincide with the terminal pathophysiological events.

Diagnosis

Mild yellow fever cannot be clinically distinguished from a wide array of other infections. Cases of yellow fever with jaundice must be differentiated from viral hepatitis (particularly hepatitis E), falciparum malaria, leptospirosis, Congo–Crimean haemorrhagic fever, Rift Valley fever, typhoid, Q fever, typhus, and surgical, drug-induced, and toxic causes of jaundice. The other viral haemorrhagic fevers, which usually present without jaundice, include dengue haemorrhagic fever, Lassa fever, Marburg and Ebola virus diseases, and Bolivian, Argentinian, and Venezuelan haemorrhagic fevers.

Specific diagnosis is made by detection of the virus in blood, demonstration of a specific antibody response or histopathology. The virus may be isolated from serum during the first 3 or 4 days of illness; however the virus has been found in the blood up to 17 days after illness onset. During epidemics, patients with fever and generalized, non-specific symptoms may provide useful specimens for virus isolation attempts. Proper handling and cold transport of specimens is essential to avoid bacterial contamination and to preserve virus for culture. Virus isolation from clinical specimens can be made by intracerebral inoculation of infant mice, by intrathoracic inoculation of *Toxorhynchites* mosquitoes, or by use of cell cultures, the most sensitive being AP61 mosquito cells. Type-specific monoclonal antibodies may be used for viral identification by immunofluorescence. The polymerase chain reaction is increasingly used and provides a sensitive means of detection of virus in blood and tissue specimens. Virus may be occasionally isolated from postmortem liver specimens, or viral antigen detected by ELISA. Serological diagnosis includes demonstrating specific IgM in early sera or a rise in titer of specific antibodies in paired acute and convalescent sera. Serological cross-reactions occur with other flaviviruses so positive results should be confirmed with a more specific test, such as plaque reduction neutralization test. Immunohistochemical staining of formalin-fixed material may detect yellow fever viral antigen on histopathologic specimens.

Pathology

Gross pathological lesions include bile staining of tissues; cardiac enlargement; swelling and congestion of the kidneys; haemorrhages or petechiae of the mucous membranes, stomach, duodenum, renal capsule, and urinary bladder; and presence of bloody pleural and peritoneal effusions. The liver is usually normal in size, red or yellow in colour, and shows obliteration of normal lobular pattern and a greasy consistency.

Histopathological changes in the liver include coagulative necrosis of hepatocytes in the midzone of the liver lobule, sparing cells bordering the central vein. Eosinophilic degeneration of hepatocytes results in the formation of Councilman bodies and intranuclear esoinophilic granular inclusions (Torres bodies). Multi- and microvacuolar fatty changes are nearly always present, especially after the eighth day of illness. An inflammatory response is absent or mild, and the reticulin framework is preserved, so that healing is complete in surviving cases. Typical changes are seen in biopsy specimens taken as early as the third day of illness, while interpretation of necropsy material obtained after the tenth day is often difficult. It should be emphasized that biopsy during life is contraindicated as a diagnostic procedure, due to the high risk of haemorrhage. Deaths have resulted from this procedure.

Renal glomerular changes are insignificant compared to the marked acute tubular necrosis and fatty change. The myocardial fibres show cloudy swelling, degeneration, and fatty infiltration. The brain may show oedema and petechial haemorrhages. Lymphocytic elements in the spleen and lymph nodes are depleted, and large mononuclear or histocytic cells accumulate in the splenic follicles.

Treatment

Because medical services are rudimentary in areas where the disease occurs, most patients with yellow fever have not benefited from the intensive care required for management of this complex disease. Nevertheless, in cases of vaccine associated viscerotropic adverse events, which mimic wild-type yellow fever, intensive care interventions have not changed the inexorable course of the disease.

Approaches to the management of patients are summarized in Monath (1987, 2008). The patient should be hospitalized and closely monitored. Isolation is not required, but precautions should be taken with sharp objects potentially contaminated with infectious blood, and a bed net or screened room should be used to limit access to vector mosquitoes. Temperature, pulse, blood pressure, respiratory rate, fluid intake, urine output, and other gastrointestinal losses should be closely monitored. Analgesics (acetaminophen) may be used to reduce headache and myalgia. Antiemetics (piperazine, phenothiazines) may be used sparingly to control nausea and vomiting, but should be avoided if hepatic dysfunction worsens or stupor appears. Patients who enter the period of intoxication should be frequently evaluated for cardiovascular status, renal function, and electrolyte and acid-base balance. Oxygen should be administered, nutrition maintained, and 10–20% glucose solution given intravenously with care to avoid fluid overload. Nasogastric suction should be used to monitor haemorrhage and to prevent gastric distension and aspiration. Although no studies have been performed, it would seem logical to reduce the risk of gastric haemorrhage by suppressing gastric acid with parenteral H$_2$-receptor antagonists. If severe bleeding occurs, fresh-frozen plasma or fresh whole blood may be required to maintain adequate blood volume. In cases with strong laboratory evidence for disseminated intravascular coagulation, the use of heparin may be considered. In those with signs of progressive acute renal failure, haemodialysis may be required. Secondary bacterial infections or concurrent infections (including malaria) should be treated by the usual appropriate means. Antiviral chemotherapy with ribavirin or α-interferon have not proved useful in preclinical studies.

There is no clear indication for treatment with antibodies (or pooled gamma globulin) or immunosuppressive agents. Passive antibody and interferon are only useful during the first 24 hours after infection, and are thus relevant to an inadvertent needle stick injury of unvaccinated medical staff (Monath 2008). Research is needed on the role of cytokines in the pathogenesis of shock in yellow fever, and may lead to specific means of intervention. Of interest is a retrospective analysis of patients with vaccine associated viscerotropic disease suggesting that use of stress dose corticosteroids was associated with significantly lower mortality (Vellozi *et al.* 2006). No antiviral drugs are currently available, although there is active research on other flaviviruses that may ultimately yield an active compound.

Epidemiology

Transmission and communicability

Yellow fever virus is acquired by the bite of an infected mosquito, and is not transmissible by contact with infected individuals. Inanimate sharp objects contaminated with blood pose a theoretical risk of accidental infection in the hospital setting. Laboratory infections have occurred, some possibly by the aerosol route. However, droplet or aerosol transmission between humans does not occur.

Distribution and incidence

Yellow fever occurs in tropical South America and sub-Saharan Africa (Fig. 38.3), where virus activity may be focal and intermittent. The distribution of reported human cases gives an incomplete picture of the natural circulation of yellow fever virus. Vaccination, inadequate reporting systems, low human population density, and other factors may result in an apparent absence of disease from areas with a high level of zoonotic viral transmission. The geographic boundaries of endemic yellow fever are incompletely known (and subject to change due to expanding/contracting epizootics). A new assessment of these boundaries is currently underway by the World Health Organization (WHO) and a group of experts, and the result will be a change in some aspects of the map in 2009 (Fig. 38.3). This re-assessment will assist in decisions for vaccination of travellers.

The annual number of officially reported yellow fever cases is between 50 and 300 in tropical America, and between 5 and 5,000 in Africa (Fig. 38.4). However, the true morbidity may greatly exceed the reported number of cases, as shown by investigations of various epidemics, especially in Africa. In South America, the incidence of jungle yellow fever is highest in the Amazon region of Brazil and in areas of eastern Bolivia, Peru, Ecuador, and Colombia which encircle the Amazon Basin. The disease occurs principally during months with peak rainfall, humidity, and temperature—January to March in the Amazon Basin. Occasionally, epizootic waves and attendant human cases have swept outside the traditional enzootic zone in eastern Panama, Central America, Paraguay, northern Argentina, and south eastern Brazil (Minas Gerais, Sao Paulo, Parana, and Santa Catarina states). Between 1987 and 2006, 3,487 cases and 1,955 deaths were reported from South America (WHO, 2005, 2006, 2008).

Human cases occur in rural areas, among persons living near and working in the forest. The opening of forested areas to agricultural exploitation, oil exploration, and road construction has led to an influx of unvaccinated persons, with ensuing epidemics. It is estimated that 1 in 10 cases of jungle yellow fever are recognized and reported in tropical America. A system of viscerotomy (collection

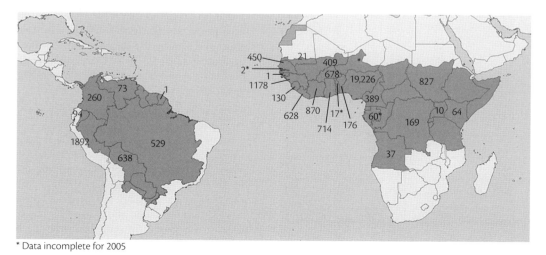

* Data incomplete for 2005

Fig. 38.3 Approximate regions of enzootic-endemic yellow fever risk (shaded). The number of human cases of yellow fever officially notified to the WHO during the interval 1987–2006 is shown by country.

and pathological examination of liver samples from suspect fatal cases) has been used successfully for surveillance.

In Africa, sporadic cases are less often recognized, due to confusion with other diseases and the lack of organized surveillance, although the latter is currently improving. It is likely that endemic yellow fever actually constitutes an important public health problem in many parts of Africa. In Nigeria, for example, the annual incidence of endemic disease with jaundice was estimated to be 1.1–2.4 cases per 1,000, and of the incidence of yellow fever death at 0.2–0.5 per 1,000, rates below the threshold of detection of medical surveillance but constituting a significant health problem (Monath and Nasidi 1993). Epidemics have occurred at irregular intervals, principally in West Africa and in the southern Sudan. These outbreaks have sometimes involved large areas and affected hundreds of thousands of people. The epidemic in Nigeria, which began in 1986, ultimately spread throughout the country, to Cameroun and Niger (DeCock *et al.* 1988; Nasidi *et al.* 1989). Between 1987 and 2006, 26,044 cases and 5,655 deaths were officially reported from Africa (WHO 2005, 2006, 2008), but the true morbidity was undoubtedly many times higher. Investigations in one region documented an incidence of human infection of 20%. Approximately 3% of the affected population developed clinical disease (jaundice). In 1993, a yellow fever epidemic occurred in Kenya for the first time in history and for the first time in East Africa in 27 years.

In Africa, epidemics spread by tree-hole breeding mosquitoes peak during the late rainy season and early dry season. Where domestic *Ae. aegypti* is present, transmission may occur at any time of year, but is enhanced during the rainy season, when artificial containers around houses provide additional breeding sites.

Age, gender, and occupation

In tropical America, jungle yellow fever principally affects young adult males, the male-female case ratio being 10:1, reflecting the higher incidence of exposure of males to *Haemagogus* vectors during wood-cutting and forest-clearing activities in the forest. In Africa, background immunity is the principal factor determining the age distribution of cases. In outbreaks affecting immunologically virgin populations (e.g. in Ethiopia, 1960–62), all ages were equally affected, whereas in West Africa, where endemic flavivirus

and yellow fever transmission occurs, the highest rates in epidemics are in immunologically susceptible children. An excess of cases in males has been observed in some African outbreaks, possibly indicating greater exposure of males to sylvatic vectors.

Inapparent infection

Inapparent, abortive, or clinically mild infections with yellow fever are frequent. In endemic areas of West Africa subject to yearly wet season recrudescence and amplification of yellow fever, the mean annual incidence of infection may be as high as 1.7% and the prevalence of immunity in young adults in such areas reaches 20–40%. The ratio of inapparent to apparent yellow fever infection has not been definitely established. In one study, a low ratio (2:1) was found in children who sustained primary yellow fever infections, whereas individuals with serological patterns indicating yellow fever infection after prior exposure to one or more heterologous flaviviruses (of which Zika virus was the most prominent), an inapparent:apparent infection ratio of 22:1 was found (Monath *et al.* 1980).

Prevention and control

Vaccines

Travellers to endemic areas and persons working with yellow fever virus or vaccine in the laboratory should be immunized. The decision to vaccinate a traveller should take into account the following factors:

a) The risk of exposure to yellow fever virus during travel. This risk is dependent on the locations visited (with respect to yellow fever geography), potential exposure to vectors, duration of stay, time of visit, etc. The risk of acquiring yellow fever during travel has been estimated as 5 per 100,000 in South America and 50 per 100,000 in Africa for a 2-week stay in a non-epidemic area (Monath and Cetron 2002), but is many fold higher for travel within an area undergoing an epidemic.

b) An assessment of the individual's risk of adverse events to the vaccine (discussed below)

c) The full itinerary of the traveler and knowledge of country requirements for a certificate of yellow fever vaccination. If the risk of adverse events to the vaccine outweighs the benefit, or if a medical contraindication to vaccination exists, it is possible to exempt the traveller from regulations by writing a letter to that effect and signing the International Certificate of Vaccination or Prophylaxis (ICVP) in the designated area. However this may not guarantee that a traveller may not experience difficulties at a border.

Preventive yellow fever vaccination is a highly effective public health measure. In endemic areas of South America, yellow fever vaccination has been introduced into the expanded programme of immunization. In addition, mass immunization campaigns in many areas have achieved a high level of vaccine immunity. However, most South American countries have coastal areas outside the endemic zone where vaccination is not practiced, and these areas are at theoretical risk of introduction and urban transmission of yellow fever. In Africa, the approach in some countries has been to undertake mass immunization in response to the occurrence of disease outbreaks, whereas others have incorporated yellow fever vaccine in the expanded programme of immunization of children. WHO has

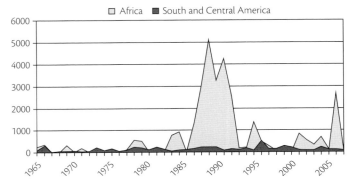

Fig. 38.4 Number of cases of yellow fever by region reported to the WHO, 1965–2006

promulgated yellow fever immunization in the 33 endemic countries in Africa since 1988, and in 2006 began, with support from the Bill and Melinda Gates Foundation and the Global Alliance of Vaccine and Immunizations, an intensified program of catch up vaccination in West Africa, the goal of which is to achieve a high level of immunity in countries at highest risk of epidemics.

Yellow fever 17D is a highly effective live viral vaccine. It is prepared from infected chicken embryos under standards developed by WHO. The 0.5 ml dose, delivered subcutaneously by syringe and needle or jet injector, results in a demonstrable immune response in over 95% of vaccinees within 7–10 days. For the purposes of international certification, immunization is valid for 10 years, but studies have shown persistence of neutralizing antibodies for 35 years or more, and immunity is probably life-long. The vaccine requires cold storage and a cold chain for delivery to remote areas.

Contraindications and precautions

Young age

Infants are at higher risk of neurotropic adverse events. The vaccine should never be administered to infants < 6 months of age. Routine immunization may be performed at 9 months of age or older. Infants > 6 and <9 months of age should be immunized if there is a significant risk of exposure.

Pregnancy and lactation

The hypothetical risk of transplacental infection and the recognition that young infants (and thus, potentially, the fetus) were susceptible to neuroinvasion by 17D virus led to the general recommendation that the vaccine not be administered during pregnancy unless clearly required, based on potential exposure to natural infection. Recommendations vary considerably. The position of the WHO is that vaccination is generally contraindicated in pregnancy, but, '…is permitted after the sixth month of pregnancy when justified epidemiologically'. The Advisory Committee on Immunization Practices (ACIP) does not specify a stage of pregnancy, but stipulates that a clear need for immunization of a pregnant woman should be established based on individual assessment of risks and benefits.

A risk to the fetus has not been established by various studies following field use of the vaccine in which pregnant women have been immunized. Therefore pregnant women who have received the vaccine inadvertently should be reassured that there is minimal risk to themselves or to the fetus, and there is no indication for abortion.

Lactation is considered a precaution to 17D vaccination in the USA because of the potential risk of transmission of 17D virus to the breastfed infant. There has been one suspect case of yellow fever vaccine-associated neurotropic disease (YEL-AND) in a one-month old infant whose mother was vaccinated with 17D and the infant was exclusively breastfeed. Testing was unable to determine if the breast milk was the mode of transmission. In addition to this case, further concern regarding the possible transmission of yellow fever vaccine virus in breast milk is based on the knowledge that West Nile virus may be transmitted via human breast milk and some tick-borne flaviviruses are secreted in milk of domesticated livestock.

Immunosuppression

Because of the theoretical risk of neuroinvasion or viscerotropic disease, the vaccine is contraindicated in patients with known immunosuppression due to HIV infection, or immunologic deficiency states (cancer chemotherapy, leukemia, lymphoma, generalized malignancy, other conditions affecting humoral and cellular immune responses, or treatment with immunosuppressive drugs, including high-dose corticosteroids). Low-dose corticosteroid treatment (20 mg prednisone or equivalent per day), short-term corticosteroids (<2 week course) or intra-articular injections of corticosteroids are not considered contraindications to vaccination.

A history of thymectomy is a significant risk factor for serious (viscerotropic) adverse events; such patients should not be vaccinated.

Adverse events

Common adverse events to 17D vaccine occur during the first few days after vaccination and are mild, well tolerated and rarely reported except in the setting of clinical trails. These are characterized by acute phase reactions (headache, myalgia, malaise) and local reactions.

Serious adverse reactions to 17D vaccine are uncommon, but have been the focus of new concern over the past decade, due both to the relatively high incidence compared to other vaccines and the severity of viscerotropic adverse events, which are highly lethal. Three types of serious adverse events are of most concern: allergic reactions (anaphylaxis), (YEL-AND) and yellow fever vaccine-associated viscerotropic disease (YEL-AVD). The overall risk of a serious adverse event following 17D vaccine is approximately 4.7 per 100,000 but is higher in the elderly (8.3 per 100,000 for persons ≥60 years) (Lindsey et al. 2008).

The risk of anaphylaxis (and other allergic adverse events) is increased in persons with allergy to eggs and gelatin. Egg allergy is a contraindication but if necessary, egg-allergic patients may undergo scratch testing with 1:10 diluted vaccine and a negative and positive (histamine) control. If the test is negative, an intradermal test is performed with 0.02 mL of 1:100 vaccine. In a subject with a positive intradermal test (a wheal 5 mm or larger), and a clear need for yellow fever vaccine, the patient may be desensitized by increasing subcutaneous doses at 15- to 20-minute intervals under the supervision of an experienced physician. In persons without egg allergy, the risk of anaphylaxis is on the order of 0.4–1.8 per 100,000 (Kelso et al. 1999; Lindsey et al. 2008).

Yellow fever vaccine-associated neurotropic disease (YEL-AND)

These events, which occur after primary vaccination at an incidence of 0.8 per 100,000 (Lindsey et al. 2008), include both acute meningoencephalitis due to neuroinvasion and direct viral injury by 17D virus, and autoimmune events, such as Guillain Barré syndrome and acute disseminated encephalomyelitis (McMahon et al. 2007). Very young age (<6 months) and advanced age are risk factors for YEL-AND. The incidence of YEL-AND in persons over 60 years is 1.8 per 100,000. Male gender may also be a risk factor. Neurological signs appear generally within two weeks after vaccination, and are generally self-limited. A useful diagnostic test is the measurement of yellow fever IgM antibodies in cerebrospinal fluid, at least in cases of non-autoimmune etiology. The case fatality ratio is low, probably <5%.

Yellow fever vaccine-associated viscerotropic disease (YEL-AVD)

This adverse event, which occurs only after primary vaccination at an incidence of 0.4 per 100,000 (Lindsey et al. 2008), is characterized by high viremia, multi-organ failure and closely resembles wild-type yellow fever (Vasconcelos *et al.* 2001; Martin *et al.* 2001). Again advanced age is associated with a higher risk (1.4 per 100,000 in individuals ≥ 60 years). A higher incidence (10 per 100,000) was reported following a mass campaign in Peru when multiple deaths due to viscerotropic disease were noted following the use of one vaccine lot of yellow fever vaccine in 2007. Thymectomy is a recognized predisposing factor, and it is suspected that other immunological dysregulation, such as systemic lupus erythematosus may increase risk of this adverse event. The case-fatality ratio is >50%. The incidence is higher in males but this may be an artifact due to a higher exposure of males to the vaccine. The onset of illness may be very rapid, with the majority falling ill within the first week. Post-mortem studies have revealed wide dissemination of yellow fever antigen in vital organs. In addition to the acquired risk factors (advanced age, thymectomy) it is likely that genetic susceptibility plays a role, possibly mutations in the 2'5' oligo adenylate synthetase or CCR5/RANTES genes. Thus a history of this adverse event in a family member warrants caution.

Preventive vector control

Areas infested with domestic *Ae. aegypti* are at risk of the introduction and interhuman spread of yellow fever. The threat of urban yellow fever (and epidemic dengue) has been the rationale for *Ae. aegypti* eradication programmes. Elimination of breeding sites (tires, artificial containers, etc.) and insecticidal treatments in the context of a well-administered programme have been successful in some areas, but have often been difficult to sustain.

Epidemic control

The occurrence of epidemic yellow fever with its high case-fatality rate, constitutes a major public health emergency. Emergency mass vaccination has generally been the principal approach to control. Such campaigns have often been initiated after the epidemic peak, because of delays in disease recognition and in mobilization of teams for mass vaccination. The effective use of mass vaccination to abort a yellow fever epidemic depends upon early recognition, epidemiological investigation, and rapid deployment of vaccination teams. After inoculation of 17D vaccine, individuals may remain susceptible to infection with wild-type virus for an undetermined period, perhaps up to a week.

Emergency vector control is aimed at rapid reduction of the adult female mosquito population. Aerial ultra-low volume (ULV) application of insecticides may be used, but because they are not effective against immature stages, the applications must be repeated to achieve suppression of biting vectors across two incubation periods in humans (12 days). The control of yellow fever epidemics involving wild vector species requires aerial treatment of large forested areas. In experimental trials, ULV application of malathion was effective against *Ae. simpsoni* breeding in plantations in Ethiopia. Ground and aerial applications of malathion rapidly suppressed populations of *Ae. africanus* in forest habitats in west Africa for a period of time sufficient to interrupt virus transmission (Bang *et al.* 1980). Aerial ULV was also used to attempt control of *Haemagogus* vectors in forested areas in eastern Panama in 1974.

References

Bang, Y. H. *et al.* (1980). Ground application of malathion thermal fogs and cold mists for the control of sylvatic vectors of yellow fever in rural communities near Enugu, Nigeria. *Mosq. News*, **40:** 541–50.

DeCock, K. M. *et al.* (1988). Epidemic yellow fever in eastern Nigeria, 1986. *Lancet*, **i:** 6303.

Germain, M. *et al.* (1981). Sylvatic yellow fever in Africa recent advances and present approach (author's transl). *Med. Tropic. (Marseille)*, **41:** 31–43.

Hahn, C. S. *et al.* (1987). Comparison of the virulent Asibi strain of yellow fever virus with the 17D vaccine strain derived from it. *Proc. Nat. Acad. Sci. USA*, **84:** 2019–23.

Heinz, F. X. and Allison, S. L. (2006). Flavivirus structure and membrane fusion. *Adv. Virus Res.*, **59:** 63–99.

Jennings, A. D. *et al.* (1994). Analysis of a yellow fever virus isolated from a fatal case of vaccine-associated human encephalitis. *J. Infect. Dis.*, **169:** 512–18.

Johannsson, M. A *et al.* (2010). Incubation periods of yellow fever virus. *Am J Trop Med Hyg*, **83:** 183–8.

Kelso, J. M. *et al.* (1999). Anaphylaxis from yellow fever vaccine. *J. Aller. Clin. Immunol.*, **103:** 698–701.

Lindenbach, B. D. and Rice, C. M. (2006). Molecular biology of flaviviruses. *Adv. Virus Res.*, **59:** 23–62.

Lindsey, N. P. *et al.* (2008). Adverse event reports following yellow fever vaccination. *Vaccine*, **26:** 6077–82.

Martin, M. *et al.* (2001). Multisystemic illness in elderly receipients of yellow fever vaccine: report of four cases. *Lancet*, **358:** 98.

McArthur, M. A. *et al.* (2003). Molecular characterization of a hamster viscerotropic strain of yellow fever virus. *J. Virol.*, **77:** 1462–68.

McMahon, A. W. *et al.* (2007). Neurologic disease associated with 17D-204 yellow fever vaccination: a report of 15 cases. *Vaccine*, **25:** 1727–34.

Meier, K. C. *et al.* (2009). A mouse model for studying viscerotropic disease caused by yellow fever virus infection. *PLoS Pathogen*, **5**(10): e1000614.

Miller, B. M. *et al.* (1989). Epidemic yellow fever caused by an incompetent mosquito vector. *Trop. Med. Parasitol.*, **40:** 396–99.

Monath, T. P. (1987). Yellow fever: a medically neglected disease. *Rev. Infect. Dis.*, **9:** 165–75.

Monath, T. P. (1988). Yellow fever. In: T. P. Monath (ed.) The arboviruses: ecology and epidemiology, vol. V, pp. 89–231. Boca Raton, FLA: CRC Press.

Monath, T. P. and Nasidi, A. (1993). Should yellow fever vaccine be included in the Expanded Program of Immunization in Africa? A cost-effectiveness analysis for Nigeria. *Am. J. of Trop. Med. Hyg.*, **48:** 274–99.

Monath, T. P. *et al.* (1980). Yellow fever in the Gambia, 1978–1979: epidemiologic aspects with observations on the occurrence of Orungo virus infections. *Am. J. Trop. Med. Hyg.*, **29:** 912–28.

Monath, T. P. (2008). Treatment of yellow fever. *Antiv. Res.*, **78:** 116–24.

Monath, T. P. and Barrett, A. D. T. (2006). Pathogenesis and pathophysiology of yellow fever. *Adv. Virus Res.*, **60:** 273–342.

Monath, T. P. and Cetron, M. (2002). Prevention of yellow fever in persons traveling to the tropics. *Clin. Infect. Dis.*, **34:** 1369–78.

Mutebi, J. P. *et al.* (2001). Phylogenetic and evolutionary relationships among yellow fever virus isolates in Africa. *J. Virol.*, **75:** 6999–7008.

Mutebi, J. P. *et al.* (2004). Genetic relationships and evolution of genotypes of yellow fever virus and other members of the yellow fever virus group within the Flavivirus genus based on the 3' noncoding region. *J. Virol.*, **78:** 9652–65.

Nasidi, A. *et al.* (1989). Urban yellow fever epidemic in western Nigeria, 1987. *Trans. R. Soc. Trop. Med. Hyg.*, **83:** 401–6.

Querec, T. *et al.* (2007). Yellow fever vaccine YF-17D activates multiple dendritic cell subsets via TLR2, 7, 8, and 9 to stimulate polyvalent immunity. *J. Experim. Med.*, **203:** 413–24.

Querec, T. D. *et al.* (2009). Systems biology approach predicts immunogenicity of the yellow fever vaccine in humans. *Nature Immunol.*, **10:** 116–25.

Tesh, R. B. *et al.* (2001). Experimental yellow fever virus infection in the Golden Hamster (*Mesocricetus auratus*). I. Virologic, biochemical, and immunologic studies. *J. Infect. Dis.*, **183:** 1431–36.

Vasconcelos, P. F. *et al.* (2004). Genetic divergence and dispersal of yellow fever virus, Brazil. *Emerg. Infect. Dis.*, **10:** 1578–84.

Vasconcelos, P. F. *et al.* (2001). Serious adverse events associated with yellow fever 17DD vaccine in Brazil: a report of two cases. *Lancet*, **358:** 91–97.

Vellozzi, C. *et al.* (2006). Yellow fever vaccine-associated viscerotropic disease (YEL-AVD) and corticosteroid therapy: eleven United States cases, 1996–2004. *Am. J. Trop. Med. Hyg.*, **75:** 333–36.

WHO (2005). Yellow fever database www.who.int/globalatlas/dataQuery.

WHO (2006). Yellow fever situation in Africa and South America, 2005. *Wkly. Epidemiol. Rec.*, **81:** 317–24.

WHO (2008). Yellow fever in Africa and South America, 2006. *Wkly. Epidemiol. Rec.*, **83:** 69–76.

Wrammert, J. *et al.* (2009). Human Immune Memory to Yellow Fever and Smallpox Vaccination. *J. Clin. Immunol.* 2008 Dec 4. [Epub ahead of print.]

CHAPTER 39

Severe Acute Respiratory Syndrome (SARS)

Merion Evans and Diana J. Bell

Summary

Severe acute respiratory syndrome (SARS) has been described by the World Health Organization (WHO) as the first serious and readily transmissible disease to emerge in the 21st century (WHO 2003a). The epidemic first appeared in southern China in late 2002 and was finally contained in July 2003 after spreading to 29 countries worldwide and infecting over 8,000 people with 774 reported deaths. The last known cases occurred in April 2004 after a laboratory acquired infection in China. The global response to the SARS epidemic, co-ordinated by WHO, led to the rapid identification of the causal agent, the development of diagnostic tests for the virus, the initiation of treatment protocols, estimation of key epidemiological factors affecting spread and the implementation of a range of public health interventions (WHO 2003a; Anderson et al. 2005).

The cause of SARS has been conclusively identified as a previously unknown coronavirus (Peiris et al. 2003a; Ksiazek et al. 2003; Drosten et al. 2003). Early reports suggested a wild animal reservoir for the virus and attention focused on the wildlife trade in southern China (Xu et al. 2004). Numerous animal reservoirs of the SARS coronavirus have since been identified (Shi and Hu 2007). Masked palm civets (*Paguma larvata*) have been most consistently identified as the intermediate host responsible for passing the virus to humans (Guan et al. 2003; Song et al. 2005; Wang et al. 2005), while the definitive hosts may be the horseshoe bat species (genus *Rhinolophus*) (Wang et al. 2006).

In humans, the illness is characterized by high fever (>38°C) usually accompanied by chills and rigors and often by myalgia and malaise. Symptoms are milder in children, while in older people respiratory symptoms may be more prominent (Donnelly et al. 2003; Xu et al. 2004). Most patients have early unilateral, interstitial infiltrates on chest X-ray progressing to more generalized, bilateral infiltrates. Diagnosis is by RT-PCR to amplify SARS-CoV nucleic acid, particularly from lower respiratory tract samples. The overall case fatality among persons with SARS is estimated to be 14–15%, but rises to over 50% in people aged 65 years and over (Donnelly et al. 2003; WHO 2003b). There is no consensus on optimal treatment for SARS and no convincing evidence for the effectiveness of either antiviral or corticosteroid therapy (Stockman et al. 2006).

SARS is spread in the majority of cases through close contact with an infected person and exposure to respiratory droplets. Health care workers are at high risk, especially if infection control procedures are not properly followed. At present, the most effective way to control SARS is to break the chain of transmission from infected to healthy people. There are three key actions necessary to achieve this: early case detection, patient isolation, and contact tracing (WHO 2003c). There are currently no vaccines against SARS, but the spike (S) protein of the SARS virus, which is involved in receptor recognition, virus attachment and entry, has been identified as the most important potential target (Du et al. 2009). In the meantime, prevention of SARS depends on the effective regulation of the often illegal wildlife trade network (Karesh et al. 2005).

History

SARS first appeared as an apparent outbreak of atypical pneumonia in Guangdong Province, southern China. The first known case occurred in Foshan city in late November 2002 and was followed by clusters of cases in several cities in the province, most notably the provincial capital, Guangzhou (Zhong et al. 2003; Zhong and Zeng 2005). On 11 February 2003, the Chinese Ministry of Health reported that the disease had affected 305 persons and caused five deaths, and that around 30% of cases had occurred in health care workers (Rosling and Rosling 2003). On 21 February 2003, an infected medical doctor travelled from Guangzhou and stayed one night at a hotel in Hong Kong. He infected numerous other guests and visitors to the hotel. Within days, the disease began spreading around the world along international air travel routes as hotel contacts seeded outbreaks in Hong Kong, Vietnam, Singapore, and Canada (Fig. 39.1) (Centers for Disease Control and Prevention (CDC) 2003). Hospital staff, unaware that this was a new, highly infectious, disease, exposed themselves to the infection without barrier protection. These initial outbreaks were characterized by rapid increases in numbers of cases, especially in health care workers and their close contacts. Subsequently, chains of secondary transmission occurred outside the hospital environment.

The response to the outbreak was extraordinary. The world was alerted to SARS by Dr Carlo Urbani, a WHO infectious disease specialist working at the French Hospital in Hanoi, Vietnam who later died from the disease. He reported several cases of severe respiratory disease in health workers treating a businessman who had recently travelled to southern China. WHO subsequently issued, on 12 March 2003, a global alert on atypical pneumonia (WHO 2003d) and on 15 March WHO named the new disease 'Severe Acute Respiratory Syndrome' (WHO 2003e). On March 17, WHO set up a series of

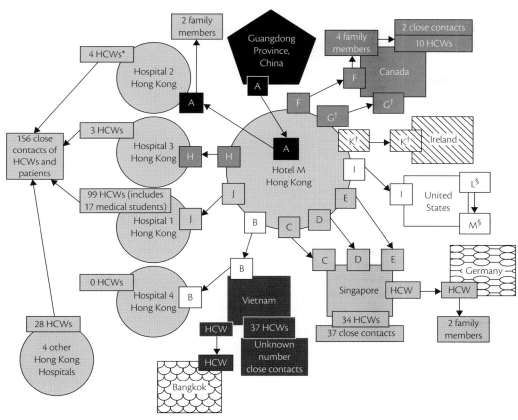

Fig. 39.1 Chain of transmission among guests at Hotel M—Hong Kong, 2003.
Reproduced from Centers for Disease Control and Prevention. (2003a), with permission.

* Health-care workers.
†All guests except G and K stayed on the 9th floor of the hotel. Guest G stayed on the 14th floor, and Guest K stayed on the 11th floor.
§Guests L and M (spouses) were not at Hotel M during the same time as index Guest A but were at the hotel during the same times as Guests G, H, and I, who were ill during this period.

laboratories worldwide to determine the aetiology of the new disease. The absence of response to antibiotics indicated a viral illness (Peiris and Guan 2005). Between 21 and 24 March, three laboratories in the USA, Germany, and Hong Kong, independently reported the isolation of a novel coronavirus (Ksiazek *et al.* 2003; Drosten *et al.* 2003; Peiris *et al.* 2003a; Peiris and Guan 2005). Three weeks later, on 16 April 2003, WHO announced that the new agent had been conclusively identified as the cause of SARS (WHO 2003f).

The diseases spread rapidly, initially in Hong Kong (Tsang *et al.* 2003), Hanoi (Vu *et al.* 2003), Toronto (Poutanen *et al.* 2003) and Singapore (Hsu *et al.* 2003), subsequently in mainland China and Taiwan (Twu *et al.* 2003). Cumulative number of SARS cases passed 4,000 on 23 April, 5,000 on 28 April, 6,000 on 2 May, 7,000 on 8 May, and 8,000 on 28 May (WHO 2003g). At the peak of the outbreak, during the beginning of May, more than 200 new cases were being reported each day. On 28 April, Vietnam became the first country to stop local transmission of SARS, followed by the Philippines on 20 May, and Singapore on 31 May (WHO 2003g). By June the number of new cases was dwindling and on 5 July 2003, WHO declared the global SARS epidemic to be over. There had been over 8,000 cases in 29 countries worldwide, and 774 deaths (Table 39.1).

The agent

The coronaviruses (family *Coronaviridae*, genus Coronavirus) are members of a large family of large, enveloped, positive-sense single-stranded RNA viruses (Siddell *et al.* 1983). The *Coronaviridae*

family has been divided into three groups on the basis of genomic sequence homology.

◆ Group 1 (canine and feline infectious peritonitis, porcine transmissible gastroenteritis and porcine respiratory viruses, human coronavirus 229E),

◆ Group 2 (rat sialodacryoadenitis viruses, bovine and murine hepatitis, human coronavirus OC43) contain mammalian viruses,

◆ Group 3 contains only avian viruses (avian infectious bronchitis, turkey coronavirus).

The SARS coronavirus was identified as a new fourth class of coronavirus subsequently referred to as SARS-CoV (Marra *et al.* 2003).

Koch's postulates were confirmed by reproducing the illness in macaques (Kuiken *et al.* 2003; Fouchier *et al.* 2003; Osterhaus *et al.* 2005). Like many emergent infectious viruses, SARS-CoV has RNA rather than DNA genomes (Holmes and Rambaut 2005). These authors dismiss earlier suggestions that SARS-CoV resulted from the recombination of different coronavirus lineages (e.g. Stavrinoides and Guttman 2004). Later genotyping of samples collected during the 2002–2003 epidemic found that two genotypes dominated during the initial phase of the epidemic in Guangdong Province (He *et al.* 2004) and that these sequences were similar to coronaviruses infecting other mammalian hosts. During the second phase of the epidemic, following rapid spread within Guangdong

Table 39.1 Summary of human SARS infections during identified outbreaks

Date	Place	Cases	Deaths	Source
Nov 2002–Jul 2003	Worldwide (29 countries)	8098	774	Unknown
Sep 2003	Singapore	1	0	Laboratory infection
Dec 2003	Taiwan	1	0	Laboratory infection
Dec 2003–Jan 2004	Guangzhou, China	4	0	Unknown
Mar–Apr 2004	Beijing, China	9	1	Laboratory infection

Province, these authors reported a new 29 nucleotide deletion in SARS-CoV which dominated during the rest of the epidemic. There was a further small outbreak in Guangdong Province, China in Dec 2003–Jan 2004 (Table 39.1) (Wang *et al.* 2005). Molecular epidemiology research suggests that the viruses responsible differ from those in the previous period, suggesting independent species-transmission events (Liang *et al.* 2004; Song *et al.* 2005).

The hosts

Animals

Following reports that early cases of SARS-CoV were among animal handlers in wildlife markets and restaurants in Guangdong Province, Guan *et al.* (2003) collected samples from a range of species and people in these locations and found SARS-like coronaviruses in two families of Canidae, namely masked palm civets (*Paguma larvata*) and raccoon dogs (*Nyctereutes procyonoides),* and antibodies to SARS-CoV in a third species, Chinese ferret badgers (*Melogale moschata*). Furthermore five of ten civet dealers sampled in these markets were found to have antibodies which cross-reacted with the SARS-CoV virus. The search for the animal origins of SARS-CoV subsequently focussed on the civet farms in southern China that produce large numbers of these animals in captivity (Bell *et al.* 2004).

SARS-CoV has since been found to infect at least 10 mammalian species in the laboratory, including mice, cynomolgus macaques, rhesus macaques, guinea pigs, golden hamsters, ferrets, African green monkeys, domestic cats and rats and there is some evidence that the latter may have played a role in the transmission of the virus (Wang *et al.* 2006). A recent review has catalogued studies on animal reservoirs of the SARS coronavirus (Shi and Hu 2008).

The clinical signs observed in these species are summarized by Wang *et al.* (2006) and by Osterhaus *et al.* (2005). Experimental work suggests a disseminated infection with SARS being isolated from several organs similar to the situation reported in humans (Bermingham 2005; Peiris 2003b). Cynomolgus macaques, ferrets and cats have been used as models in which to test intervention treatments (Osterhaus *et al.* 2005). These studies include the discovery that a drug approved for use in humans, pegylated interferon-alpha limits lung damage and SARS-CoV replication in experimentally infected macaques (Haagmans *et al.* 2004; Osterhaus *et al.* 2005).

The role of palm civets in directly transmitting SARS-CoV to humans is now well established both by field epidemiology (Wang *et al.* 2005) and by molecular epidemiology (Liang *et al.* 2004; Song *et al.* 2005; Li 2008). However, Wu *et al.* (2005) found that when palm civets were experimentally infected with two strains of SARS-CoV all showed clinical signs of lethargy and fever. As natural reservoir hosts tend not to display clinical signs of infection because they have co-evolved with their viruses, this suggests that palm civets are not the definitive host (Wang *et al.* 2006).

The more recent discovery that a high proportion of Chinese and other horseshoe bats (genus *Rhinolophus*) shed SARS-CoV like viruses strongly suggests that bats could be the natural reservoir for this group of viruses (Li *et al.* 2005; Lau *et al.* 2005). Li *et al.* (2005) reported a high SARS-CoV antibody prevalence in three species of *Rhinolophus* (horseshoe bats) wild-trapped in two locations (Guangxi and Hubei) in China. Using PCR, a complete genome sequence was determined from one faecal sample and the virus named SARS-like coronavirus isolate Rp3 (SL-CoVRp3). This showed 92% similarity to SARS-CoV Orf2 in overall nucleotide sequence identity. Partial genome sequences were also identified from another four PCR-positive bat faecal samples. The authors suggested that bats may be a natural reservoir of 'the SARS cluster of coronaviruses' and that further SARS-related coronaviruses may occur in bats. Li *et al.* (2005) also speculate that spillover from infected bats into a susceptible amplifying host, for example, the masked palm civet, could occur during contact of such species at some point within the wildlife trade chain (see also Bell *et al.* 2004). Independently, another group found SARS-like coronaviruses in horseshoe bats as well as a number of other new coronaviruses belonging to groups 1, 2 and 3 (Lau *et al.* 2005).

Janies *et al.* (2008) evaluated the hypothesis that SARS-CoV isolated from bats are the original zoonotic source for SARS-CoV by sampling from diverse hosts including chiroptera, carnivores, artiodactyls, rodents, birds and humans. The resulting phylogenies indicate that SARS-CoV was transmitted to small carnivores later than the initial SARS epidemic in humans in 2002 with isolates from small carnivores in Shenzhen markets forming a terminal clade which emerged from within the human SARS-CoV radiation. The authors found evidence for subsequent exchange of SARS-CoV between humans and carnivores and that SARS-CoV was transmitted independently from humans to farmed pigs.

Bat SARS-CoV isolates were basal to the human/carnivore clade. However, although this indicated that bats were a possible candidate for the original reservoir of SARS-CoV, the structural biology of the spike protein of Chiropteran SARS-CoV provided evidence that these viruses are unable to interact with the human variant of the SARS-CoV receptor angiotensin-converting enzyme 2 (ACE2). Janies *et al.* (2008) concluded that further sampling of coronaviruses from diverse hosts, particularly bats, carnivores and primates is needed to unravel their genomic and biochemical evolution, including that of SARS-CoV. Rats should be added to that list. Interestingly, a group 2 coronavirus was recently isolated from the first non-insectivorous bat, a vampire bat *Desmodus rotundus,* in

Brazil and its mean nucleotide identity with SARS-CoV was 66% (Brandaol *et al.* 2008).

Humans

Pathogenesis

The primary site of pathology is the respiratory tract with bilateral and patchy airspace consolidation in the lungs. Viraemia or toxaemia is also suggested by the presence of lymphopaenia and the presence of elevated serum enzymes. Quantitative studies of viral load indicate that viral load is higher in the lower respiratory tract than in the upper airways (Cheng *et al.* 2004). Viral load is low during the first four days and peaks at around day 10 of the illness (Peiris *et al.* 2003b; Cheng *et al.* 2004), in marked contrast to the early peak seen in influenza (Kaiser *et al.* 1999). This helps explain both the low transmissibility of SARS and the poor sensitivity of first generation RT-PCR diagnostic tests early in the illness.

Post mortem findings show gross consolidation of the lungs with diffuse alveolar damage with a mixed alveolar infiltrate, lung oedema, and hyaline membrane formation consistent with the pathological manifestations of acute respiratory distress syndrome.

Incubation period

The incubation period for SARS, based on analysis by WHO of individuals with well-defined single-point exposures in Singapore, Canada, and Europe, is usually 2–7 days but may be as long as 10 days (WHO 2003b). Although there have been anecdotal reports of incubation periods longer than 10 days, these have not been corroborated.

Symptoms and signs

The initial symptoms of SARS are non-specific and this combined with a relatively long incubation period make early clinical diagnosis difficult (Bermingham *et al.* 2005). The most common symptom in SARS patients is high fever (>38°C), often accompanied by chills and rigors. However, fever may be absent during the early stages of the disease and in individuals with an impaired ability to mount a fever. Other common early symptoms include myalgia and malaise. Some cases have mild respiratory symptoms though these are not prominent in the early stage of the illness. A few patients have reported diarrhoea during the febrile prodrome. After 3–7 days, a lower respiratory phase begins with the onset of a dry, non-productive cough or dyspnoea. Symptoms are milder in children (Hon *et al.* 2003) whilst in older people respiratory symptoms may be more prominent (Xu *et al.* 2004).

Radiological and laboratory findings

Chest radiographs may be normal during the febrile prodrome but are abnormal in about 75% of patients at the time of presentation. Most patients have early focal infiltrates progressing to more generalized, patchy, interstitial infiltrates. These changes are unilateral in around 40–45% of patients at presentation and bilateral in around 30%. Typically, radiological changes begin with small, unilateral, patchy shadowing and progress over 1–2 days to become bilateral and generalized with confluent infiltrates. The initial radiographic changes may be indistinguishable from those associated with bronchopneumonia. In the late stages of SARS, some chest radiographs have also shown areas of consolidation.

Lymphopaenia and thrombocytopaenia are common in SARS patients. Early in the course of disease, the absolute lymphocyte count is often decreased. Over half of patients have lymphopaenia at presentation (Booth *et al.* 2003; Lee *et al.* 2003) and up to a third have leucopaenia. At the peak of the respiratory illness, up to half of patients have leucopenia and thrombocytopenia or low-normal platelet counts. Early in the respiratory phase, elevated creatine phosphokinase levels and hepatic transaminases have been noted. Renal function remains normal in the majority of patients.

In 10%–20% of cases, the respiratory illness is severe enough to require intubation and mechanical ventilation. The overall case fatality among persons with SARS is estimated to be 14–15%, but ranges from 0% to 50% depending on age. Case fatality is less than 1% in persons aged 24 years or younger, 6% in persons aged 25 to 44 years, 15% in persons aged 45 to 64 years, and greater than 50% in persons aged 65 years and older (Donnelly *et al.* 2003; WHO 2003c). Patients with underlying disease, such as diabetes, are more likely to have a poor outcome (Booth *et al.* 2003).

Diagnosis

Considerable efforts have been made to develop molecular and serological tests to aid rapid diagnosis of SARS. The primary method of diagnosis is RT-PCR to amplify SARS-CoV nucleic acid from body fluid samples using methods developed by the WHO collaborative laboratory network (Bermingham *et al.* 2005). It is also important to take a variety of samples, particularly from the lower respiratory tract, at different stages in the illness since virus excretion is low during the early phase but increases in respiratory samples during the second week, and is highest in the lower respiratory tract (Peiris *et al.* 2003b, Bermingham *et al.* 2005). Virus load in the lower respiratory tract peaks on day 10 while that in faeces occurs slightly later at around 15–17 days (Chan *et al.* 2004). Internationally agreed WHO criteria for the confirmation of SARS include virus detection in two different clinical sample categories by RT-PCR or from serial samples on different days from the same body site.

It is also important to conduct parallel testing of samples for other infections such as human metapneumovirus, *Legionella pneumophila*, influenza and *Mycoplasma pneumoniae*, and to perform serological tests on convalescent sera to confirm SARS infection in view of the sub-optimal predictive value of molecular detection tests conducted during acute illness. It is possible to culture SARS-CoV at 33°C and 37°C in various continuous cell lines including FRhK and Ver E6 cells where it has a distinctive cytopathic effect (Bermingham *et al.* 2005).

Treatment and prognosis

There is no consensus on optimal treatment for SARS. Antibiotics are often used empirically in the early stages before diagnosis is confirmed to cover against common respiratory pathogens. Ribavirin is widely chosen because of its broad-spectrum antiviral activity against both DNA and RNA viruses. However, clinical experience in association with monitoring of viral load has failed to confirm any beneficial effect (Peiris *et al.* 2003b). Ribavirin is also associated with dose dependent side-effects including haemolytic anaemia. A systematic review of treatments for SARS found that it was not possible to determine any beneficial effects from treatment, including ribavirin, lopinavir and ritonavir, type I interferon, intravenous immunoglobulin, or corticosteroids (Stockman *et al.* 2006). Osterhaus *et al.* (2005) have proposed the need for clinical studies of the drug pegylated interferon-alpha if future outbreaks of SARS occur and suggest it may be useful in prophylactic and early-post-exposure treatment.

In southern China, corticosteroids (methylprednisolone 1–2 mg/kg/d) were widely used for treatment of SARS and reported to have positive effects in patients with critical symptoms (Zhong and Zeng 2005). However, there have been recent reports from China of around 300 survivors of the epidemic now suffering after-effects such as lung fibrosis, bone necrosis, and depression possibly as a consequence of the aggressive hormone treatment involved at the time (Promed 2009; Gomersall et al. 2004).

Epidemiology

Occurrence

The first epidemic of SARS occurred between November 2002 and July 2003. Cases occurred in 29 countries across five continents. Just over 65% of the cases occurred in mainland China, but there were also substantial outbreaks in Hong Kong, Taiwan, Canada, Singapore and Vietnam. Other affected countries mostly experienced small numbers of imported cases with little onward transmission. Since the end of the first epidemic there have been 15 further documented cases of laboratory confirmed SARS in four separate incidents (Table 39.1). Three incidents, in Singapore (WHO 2003h), Taiwan (WHO 2003i), and Beijing, China (WHO 2004), have involved laboratory acquired infection. The incidents in Singapore and Taiwan both involved a single laboratory worker. The Beijing outbreak involved two cases of laboratory-acquired infection with secondary spread to seven contacts. A fourth incident occurred in December 2003 and involved a temporal cluster of four community cases of SARS in Guangdong province, China (WHO 2003j). No source was identified although all four cases had a history of close contact with civets, including a waitress and a customer at a restaurant that kept live civets (Wang et al. 2005).

SARS is predominantly a disease of younger adults, especially health care workers. Between 24–62% of SARS cases have been in health care workers, the proportion varying by the type of case series and declining as experience in the application of hospital infection control measures has improved (Booth et al. 2003; Lee et al. 2003; Xu et al. 2004). For example, in Guangdong, the proportion of cases in health care workers was 32% in January 2003, declining to 27% in February, and 17% by March and April (Xu et al. 2004). There is a slight excess of cases in women, probably due to the predominance of female health workers. Most cases have been in people aged between 25–44 years. The median age of cases was 35 years in Guangdong province (Xu et al. 2004), 39 years in Hong Kong (Lee et al. 2003) and 45 years in Canada (Booth et al. 2003). There have been very few cases in children and in older people. However, the highest age-specific incidence is in older people and the relatively small numbers in this age group most likely reflect the younger population profile of countries such as China. This means that in countries with a substantial proportion of older people, such as many western countries, far more cases might be expected in older people if community transmission of SARS occurs. The proportion of cases with underlying disease is between 10–25% depending on the setting in which infection occurs, being higher in situations where nosocomial transmission to other patients occurred as in Canada (Booth et al. 2003). The commonest co-morbidity is diabetes or chronic heart disease.

Sources

Newly emerging viruses typically have an animal reservoir host so that their appearance in humans is generally due to cross-species transmission (Holmes and Rambaut 2005). In a detailed analysis of the early epidemiology of the SARS epidemic in Guangdong, Xu et al. (2004) showed that although a high percentage (nine out of 23; 39%) of early cases (i.e. November 2002 to January 2003) were categorized as 'food handlers' (prepared, served food or handled, killed and sold animals for food) none were animal farmers. Also early phase patients (Nov 2002–Jan 2003) were more likely to live close to a market selling and/or killing live animals than late phase patients (Feb–April 2003) whereas 'living near a poultry or livestock farm or having other types of animal contact, including domestic pets or livestock, poultry, or specific wild animals or birds, was not associated with a high risk for SARS'. Of particular interest is these authors' observation that the index patient in Guangxi (the adjacent province) was a young man who worked as a driver for a wild animal dealer who 'supplied Guangdong market with wild animals from Guangxi, other Chinese provinces, and Vietnam'.

The search for the source of SARS-CoV has since been directed away from commercial civet farms supplying Guangdong animal markets to focus on wild-caught animals originating from the region's expanding and illegal international wildlife trade (Bell et al. 2004). This has expanded the search outside China's international borders into other countries in Indochina, such as Vietnam and Lao PDR where the putative hosts (masked palm civets, raccoon dogs and Chinese ferret badgers) may have originated.

Several strands of evidence support the idea that wild-caught civets were the direct source of SARS-CoV that infected humans. SARS-CoV was isolated from a high proportion of marketplace civets during the epidemic (Guan et al. 2003). A serological comparison of antibodies to SARS-CoV in civets sourced from farms or animal markets found no evidence of these in 75 animals from farms, but 14/18 samples from an animal market showed neutralizing antibodies to SARS-CoV (Tu et al. 2005). Another study found that prevalence of IgG antibody to SARS-CoV was significantly higher among animal traders than in a control population: 72/792 (13%) of animal traders sampled in three animal markets in Guangdong Province tested positive for SARS-CoV IgG antibody compared to between 1 and 3% prevalence in three control groups (Yu et al. 2003). The prevalence of traders with IgG antibody varied between markets and was highest amongst those who reported trading primarily in masked palm civets (73%).

The high susceptibility of civets to SARS-CoV infection and their widespread presence in markets and restaurants strongly indicate an important role for palm civets in the SARS epidemic. However, the lack of widespread infection in wild or farmed civets makes them unlikely to be the natural host reservoir (Wang et al. 2006). Data obtained more recently strongly suggest that bats (particularly horseshoe bats) are the most likely reservoir of SARS-CoV (Wang et al. 2006).

Transmission and communicability

SARS is spread in the majority of cases through close contact with an infected person. Transmission occurs mainly through exposure to infected large or medium droplets expelled during coughing or sneezing, and probably also occasionally from contact with contaminated fomites (Tsang et al. 2003; Poutanen et al. 2003). SARS virus is also known to be shed in faeces and urine (Peiris *et al.* 2003b; WHO 2003k), but the role of body fluids (such as saliva, tears, urine) and of faeces in transmission of infection is less clear. In vitro laboratory tests show that the virus can survive in faeces for at least 2 days and in urine for at least 24 hours (WHO 2003k). Virus in faeces taken from patients suffering from diarrhoea, which has a lower acidity than normal stools, can survive for 4 days raising the possibility that surfaces contaminated by diarrhoea could be an important source of infection. However, the dose of virus needed to cause infection remains unknown and further studies are needed before the role of faecal-oral transmission can be determined.

On average, one SARS case generates around three secondary cases (Riley *et al.* 2003) However, certain individuals with SARS have been implicated in spreading the disease to numerous (10 or more) other individuals, and these cases have been described as 'superspreaders' (WHO 2003l; WHO 2003m). Several such individuals have been described particularly during the early phase of the SARS outbreak. They include the hotel index case in Hong Kong who triggered the worldwide dissemination of SARS (Centers for Disease Control and Prevention 2003), as well as the index case for each of the outbreaks in Vietnam and Singapore (Vu *et al.* 2003; Hsu *et al.* 2003). Superspreaders have also been described with other diseases such as Ebola (Khan *et al.* 1995). Isolation of contacts, rapid admission of cases to hospital, and improved hospital infection control have all been shown to significantly reduce the average number of new cases of SARS arising from a single source case (Riley *et al.* 2003).

Period of infectivity

The initial rapid spread of SARS in hospitals in Hanoi, Vietnam and in Hong Kong first indicated that the disease was highly contagious. Since then it has become clear that most cases of SARS occur in close contacts of patients, particularly household members, and in health care workers, other patients and visitors inadvertently exposed to a case (Tsang *et al.* 2003; Poutanen *et al.* 2003). The period of infectivity appears to be greatest after the person with SARS develops respiratory symptoms, but transmission may occur during the prodromal period (Peiris *et al.* 2003b). Persons with SARS do not appear to be infectious during the incubation period or after febrile symptoms have resolved. Anderson *et al.* (2005) concluded that the combination of peak infectiousness occurring after onset of clinical signs and the low transmissibility of the virus simplified public health measures such as isolating patients and quarantining contacts, required to control the SARS epidemic.

Transmission in hospital

Health care workers are at high risk of SARS. Most infections have occurred either before infection control procedures were instituted or where procedures have not been properly followed. Observations from Hong Kong suggest that this risk is greatest when a hospital receives its first admissions of SARS, when patients are admitted to a general ward, and when large numbers of patients are admitted over a short period of time (Chan-Yeung 2004). Nosocomial spread is less likely when patients are admitted directly to a designated ward. Ill-fitting masks, contamination during mask removal and failure to wash hands are all risk factors for acquiring infection in hospital staff (Seto *et al.* 2003; Centers for Disease Control and Prevention 2003b; Teleman *et al.* 2004).

Transmission in the community

SARS transmits readily within the household setting, although if patients are isolated early in the course of the illness, secondary transmission to other members of the household can be prevented (Riley *et al.* 2003). The main risk is to individuals providing direct care to symptomatic SARS patients (Tuan *et al.* 2007). Other instances of spread in the community are rare with the highest risk probably being in those exposed to symptomatic patients in confined areas such as taxi drivers, and airline staff and passengers. A review by WHO of 35 flights with symptomatic probable SARS cases on board identified 4 flights during which in-flight transmission may have occurred (WHO 2003o). Cases in other settings are rare though there have been reports of transmission in the banqueting room of a restaurant, in the workplace, and at a wholesale market (WHO 2003m).

In contrast to experience in hospitals, there have been very few large outbreaks in the community. One notable exception was a large and sudden cluster of over 300 cases that occurred in residents of the Amoy Gardens housing estate, a high density apartment block, in Hong Kong. Cases associated with this cluster were much more likely to present with diarrhoea and to require intensive care compared with previously documented SARS cases. This raised the possibility of transmission by a different route and infection with a high virus load such as might happen following exposure to a concentrated environmental source. Subsequent investigations have implicated airborne transmission by means of a communal air shaft (Yu *et al.* 2004).

Prevention and control
Prevention

In 2004 Chinese health experts concluded that civets were the primary source of the previous year's epidemic and planned measures to ban their consumption (Promed 20 October 2004). In late 2003 there was a large scale cull of civets in breeding farms and wildlife markets involving over 10,000 animals (Watts 2004; Anderson *et al.* 2005). In early 2004 action was taken by the Guangdong Department of Public Health and local government to try to stop the spread, specifically the implementation of a ban on the rearing, sale, transport and slaughter of small mammals, particularly civets and efforts to maintain early identification, reporting, isolation and management of the disease in humans (Zhong and Zeng 2005). The latter authors report that no new cases were found in the community between 30 January 2004 and the summer of that year and attribute this to these activities. However, the wildlife markets subsequently re-opened and remain so.

In terms of lessons from SARS-CoV, Bell *et al.* (2004) highlight a series of ecological shifts which are favourable for the emergence of this and other zoonotic diseases, particularly in SE Asia. These include:

a) The shift from subsistence hunting to the sale of captured animals into an expanding wildlife trade,

b) The extensive cross-exposure within this trade of species and species populations which would not mix under natural conditions,

c) The exploitation of new source populations and their pathogens as areas become depleted of target species,

d) The movement of these animals often over vast distances as part of the international, and often illegal wildlife trade network,

e) Their encounter with naïve human or animal consumer populations.

The scale of this wildlife trade is immense and ranks alongside drugs and arms as one of the top multi-billion illegal activities. Karesh *et al.* (2005) have proposed that since wildlife trade functions as a system of networks with major hubs, these points provide control opportunities to maximize the effects of regulatory efforts.

Control strategies

Breaking the chain of transmission

The speed with which the SARS epidemic was managed demonstrates the decisive power of high-level political commitment to bring the disease under control even in the absence of effective treatments or vaccines. At present, the most effective way to control SARS is to break the chain of transmission from infected to healthy people. There are three key actions necessary to achieve this: early case detection, patient isolation, and contact tracing (WHO 2003c; WHO 2003n). Case detection aims to identify a SARS case as soon as possible after the onset of symptoms. Once a case is identified, the next step is to ensure they are isolated promptly and managed according to strict infection control procedures. Finally, it is vital to identify all close contacts of each case and make sure they are carefully followed-up, including daily health checks and voluntary home isolation. These measures limit the daily number of contacts possible for each potentially infectious case. By shortening the amount of time that elapses between onset of illness and isolation of the patient the opportunity for the virus to spread to others is reduced, as is the average number of new cases generated by each case (the effective reproduction number) (Donnelly *et al.* 2003; Riley *et al.* 2003).

Isolation of patients

The earliest possible isolation of all suspect and probable cases of SARS in hospital is vital. A short time between the onset of symptoms and isolation of the patient reduces opportunities for transmission of infection to other people and reduces the number of contacts that require active follow-up (Riley *et al.* 2003). It also gives patients the best chance of receiving life-saving care should their condition take a critical course. In an outbreak of SARS every effort should be made to reduce the average time from onset of symptoms to isolation to less than three days.

Hospital infection control

Health care settings seem to provide an ideal setting for outbreaks of SARS, and have served to amplify and propagate the infection. The reasons are unclear but appear to be a combination of factors such as the potential for aerosol generating procedures, poor ventilation and air flow patterns, and the presence of vulnerable patients. Inadequate training or compliance with infection control, high workload, and cryptic clinical presentations can compound the problem. Meticulous infection control procedures are necessary to prevent nosocomial spread including:

- Comprehensive triage arrangements in emergency departments and clinics,
- Adequate facilities for patient isolation with appropriate air flow control,
- Scrupulous hand hygiene,
- Use of appropriate personal protective equipment,
- Avoidance of aerosol generating procedures.

SARS has clearly demonstrated that a single case admitted to an unprepared hospital can ignite a new outbreak.

Contact tracing and isolation of contacts

The case should be interviewed by a trained health worker as soon as possible after the diagnosis of SARS is made, either face-to-face or by telephone. The date of onset of symptoms should be corroborated and details of all close contacts since that date obtained. Close contacts are defined as anyone who cared for, lived with, or had direct contact with respiratory secretions or body fluids or stool of a person with SARS. All close contacts should be followed up for 10 days from the last date of contact with the case. Quarantine or home confinement of contacts was employed with considerable success to bring the outbreaks in mainland China, Hong Kong and Singapore under control.

Vaccines

A safe and effective vaccine against SARS is urgently needed. An ideal vaccine should:

a) Elicit highly potent neutralizing antibody responses against a broad spectrum of viral strains,

b) Induce protection against infection and transmission,

c) Be safe by not inducing any infection-enhancing antibodies or harmful immune or inflammatory responses (Jiang *et al.* 2005). There have been trials of inactivated SARS-CoV vaccine but there are concerns over its safety (Marshall and Enserink 2004).

The spike (S) protein of SARS-CoV is the major inducer of neutralizing antibodies. S protein also has a key role in the ability of SARS-CoV to overcome the species barrier as adaptive evolution of the S protein can contribute to the animal-to-human transmission of SARS-CoV (Zhang *et al.* 2006). The receptor binding domain in the S1 sub-unit of S protein is responsible for the virus binding to host cell receptors. The domain contains multiple conformational neutralising epitopes and these provide a potential target for recombinant protein vaccines (Jiang *et al.* 2005). Because the S protein is involved in receptor recognition as well as virus attachment and entry, it represents one of the most important targets not only for the development of vaccines but also of therapies for SARS (Du *et al.* 2009).

References

Anderson, R., Fraser, C., Ghani, A., *et al.* (2005). Epidemiology, transmission dynamics and control of SARS: the 2002–2003 epidemic. In: A. R. McLean *et al.*, SARS—A case study in emerging infections. Oxford University Press: Oxford and Oxford Scholarship Online.

Bermingham, A., Heinen, P., Iturriza-Gomara, M., *et al.* (2005). Laboratory diagnosis of SARS. In: A. R. McLean *et al.*, SARS—A case study in emerging infections. Oxford University Press: Oxford and Oxford Scholarship Online.

Booth, C. M., Matukas, L. M., *et al.* (2003). Clinical features and short-term outcomes of 144 patients with SARS in the Greater Toronto area. *JAMA*, **289:** 2801–9.

Brandaol, P. E., Scheffer, K., *et al.* (2008). A coronavirus detected in the vampire bat *Desmodus rotundus. Brazil. J. Infect. Dis.*, **12:** 466–68.

Centers for Disease Control and Prevention (2003a). Outbreak of severe acute respiratory syndrome–worldwide, 2003. *Morbid. Mortal.Wkly. Rep.*, 52: 241–48.

Centers for Disease Control and Prevention (2003b). Cluster of severe acute respiratory syndrome cases in protected health care workers–Toronto, Canada, April 2003. *Morbid. Mortal. Wkly. Rep.*, 52: 433–36.

Chan-Yeung, M. (2004). Severe acute respiratory syndrome (SARS) and healthcare workers. *Intern. J. Occupat. Environm. Heal.*, 10: 421–27.

Cheng, P. K. C., Wong, D. A., et al. (2004). Viral shedding patterns of coronavirus in patients with probable severe acute respiratory syndrome. *Lancet*, 363: 1699–1700.

Donnelly, C., Ghani, A. C., et al. (2003). Epidemiological determinants of spread of causal agent of severe acute respiratory syndrome in Hong Kong. *Lancet*, 361: 1761–66.

Drosten, C., Gunther, S., et al. (2003). Identification of a novel coronavirus in patients with severe acute respiratory syndrome. *N. Engl. J. Med.*, 348: 1967–76.

Du, L., He, Y., Zhou, Y., et al. (2009). The spike protein of SARS-CoV–a target for vaccine and therapeutic development. *Nature Rev. Microbiol.*, 7: 226–36.

Fouchier, R. A., Kuiken, T., Schutten, M., et al. (2003). Aetiology: Koch's postulates fulfilled for SARS virus. *Nature*, 423: 240.

Guan, Y., Zheng, B. J., He, Y. Q., et al. (2003). Isolation and characterisation of viruses related to the SARS coronavirus from animals in Southern China. *Science*, 302: 276–79.

Holmes, E. and Rambaud, A. (2005) Evolutionary genetics and the emergence of SARS coronavirus. In: A. R. McLean et al., SARS—A case study in emerging infections. Oxford University Press: Oxford and Oxford Scholarship Online.

Hon, K. L. E., Leung, C. W., and Cheng, W. F. T. (2003). Clinical presentations and outcome of severe acute respiratory syndrome in children. *Lancet*, 361: 1701–3.

Hsu, L-Y., Lee, C-C., Green, J. A., et al. (2003). Severe acute respiratory syndrome (SARS) in Singapore: clinical features of index patient and initial contacts. *Emerg. Infect. Dis.*, 6: 713–17.

Janies, D., Habib, F., Alexandrov, B., Hill, A., and Pol, D. (2008). Evolution of genomes, host shifts and the geographic spread of SARS–CoV and related coronaviruses. *Cladistics*, 24: 111–30.

Jiang, S., He, Y. and Liu, S. (2005). SARS vaccine development. *Emerg. Infect. Dis.*, 11: 1016–20.

Karesh, W. B., Cook, R. A., Bennett, E. L., Newcomb, J. (2005). Wildlife trade and global disease emergence. *Emerg. Infect. Dis.*, 11: 1000–1002.

Khan, A. S., Tshioko, F. K., et al. (1999). The re-emergence of Ebola haemorrhagic fever, Democratic Republic of Congo, 1995. *J. Infect. Dis.*, 179(Suppl 1): S76–86.

Ksiazek, T. G., Erdman, D. E., et al. (2003). A novel coronavirus associated with severe acute respiratory syndrome. *N. Engl. J. Med.*, 348: 1953–66.

Kuiken, T., Fouchier, R. A., et al. (2003). Newly discovered coronavirus as the primary cause of severe acute respiratory syndrome. *Lancet*, 362: 263–70.

Lee, N., Hui, D., Wu, A., et al. (2003). A major outbreak of severe acute respiratory syndrome in Hong Kong. *N. Engl. J. Med.*, 348: 1986–94.

Li, W., Shi, Z., et al. (2005). Bats are natural reservoirs of SARS-like coronavirus. *Science*, 310: 676–79.

Lau, S. K., Woo, P. C., et al. (2005). Severe acute respiratory syndrome coronavirus-like virus in Chinese horseshoe bats. *Proc. Nat. Acad. Sci. USA*, 102: 14040–45.

Liang, G., Chen, Q., Xu, J., et al. (2004). Laboratory diagnosis of four recent sporadic cases of community-acquired SARS, Guangdong Province, China. *Emerg. Infect. Dis.*, 10: 1774–81.

Marra, M. A., Jones, S. J. M., et al. (2003). The genome sequence of the SARS-associated coronavirus. *Science*, 300: 1399–1404.

Marshall, E. and Enserink, M. (2004). Caution urged on SARS vaccines. *Science*, 303: 944–46.

Peiris, J. S., Lai, S. T., et al. (2003a). Coronavirus as a possible cause of severe acute respiratory syndrome. *Lancet*, 361: 1319–25.

Peiris, J. S. M., Chu, C. M., Cheng, V. C. C., et al. (2003b). Prospective study of the clinical progression and viral load of SARS-associated coronavirus pneumonia in a community outbreak. *Lancet*, 361: 1767–72.

Peiris, J. S. M. and Guan, Y. (2005). Confronting SARS: a view from Hong Kong. In: A. R. McLean et al., SARS—A case study in emerging infections. Oxford University Press: Oxford and Oxford Scholarship Online.

Poutanen, S. M., Low, D. E., Henry, B., et al. (2003). Identification of severe acute respiratory syndrome in Canada. *N. Engl. J. Med.*, 348: 1995–2005.

Promed (2004). SARS—Worldwide–China (32): Civet Cat Ban. 20041020.2842.

Promed (2009b). SARS–China; hormone therapy, RFI. 20091225: 4344.

Riley, S., Fraser, C., Donnelly, C. A., et al. (2003). Transmission dynamics of the etiological agent of SARS in Hong Kong: impact of public health interventions. *Science*, 300: 1961–66.

Rosling, L. and Rosling, M. (2003). Pneumonia causes panic in Guangdong province. *BMJ*, 326: 416.

Seto, W. H., Tsang, D., Yung, R. W., et al. (2003). Effectiveness of precautions against droplets and contact in prevention of nosocomial transmission of severe acute respiratory syndrome (SARS). *Lancet*, 361: 1519–20.

Shi, Z. and Hu, Z. (2008). A review of studies of animal reservoirs of the SARS coronavirus. *Virus Res.*, 133: 74–87.

Siddell, S., Wege, H., ter Meulen, V. (1983). The biology of coronaviruses. *J. Gen. Virol.*, 64: 761–76.

Song, H. D., Tu, C. C., Zhang, G. W., et al. (2005). Cross-host evolution of severe acute respiratory syndrome coronavirus in palm civet and humans. *Proc. Natl. Acad. Sci. USA*, 102: 2430–35.

Teleman, M. D., Boudville, I. C., Heng, B. H., Zhu, D., Leo. Y. S. (2004). Factors associated with transmission of severe acute respiratory syndrome among health-care workers in Singapore. *Epidemiol. Infect.*, 132: 797–803.

Tsang, K. W,. Ho, P. L., Ooi, G. C., et al. (2003). A cluster of cases of severe acute respiratory syndrome in Hong Kong. *N. Engl. J. Med.*, 348: 1977–85.

Tu, C., Crameri, G., et al. (2005). Antibodies to SARS coronavirus in civets. *Emerg. Infect. Dis.*, 11: 1860–65.

Tuan, P. A., Horby, P., Dinh, P. N., et al. (2007). SARS transmission in Vietnam outside the health-care setting. *Epidemiol. Infect.*, 135: 392–401.

Twu, S-J., Chen, T-J., Chen, C-J., et al. (2003). Control measures for severe acute respiratory syndrome (SARS) in Taiwan. *Emerg. Infect. Dis.*, 6: 718–20.

Vu, T. H., Cabau, J. F., et al. (2003). SARS in North Vietnam. *N. Engl. J. Med.*, 348: 2035.

Wang, L. F., Shi, Z., Zhang, S., Field, H., et al. (2006). Review of bats and SARS. *Emerg. Infect. Dis.*, 12: 1834–40.

Wang, M., Yan, M., Xu, H., et al. (2005). SARS-CoV infection in a restaurant from a palm civet. *Emerg. Infect. Dis.*, 11: 1860–65.

Watts, J. (2004). China culls wild animals to prevent new SARS threat. *Lancet*, 363: 134.

World Health Organization. (2003a). Severe acute respiratory syndrome (SARS): status of the outbreak and lessons for the immediate future. Geneva, World Health Organsation, 20 May 2003. Available at: http://www.who.int/csr/media/sars_wha.pdf.

World Health Organization. (2003b). SARS—Update 49. SARS case fatality ratio, incubation period. 7 May 2003. Available at: http://www.who.int/csr/don/archive/disease/severe_acute_respiratory_syndrome/en/index.html.

World Health Organization. (2003c). SARS—Update 54. Outbreaks in the initial hot zones indicate that SARS can be contained. 13 May 2003. Available at: http://www.who.int/csr/don/archive/disease/severe_acute_respiratory_syndrome/en/index.html.

World Health Organization. (2003d). WHO issues a global alert about cases of atypical pneumonia. 12 March 2003. Available at: http://www.who.int/csr/don/2003_03_12/en/index.html.

World Health Organization. (2003e). WHO issues emergency travel advisory. Severe acute respiratory syndrome (SARS) spreads worldwide. 15 Mar 2003. Available at: http://www.who.int/csr/don/2003_03_15/en/index.html.

World Health Organization. (2003f). SARS—Update 31. Coronavirus never before seen in humans is the cause of SARS. 16 April 2003. Available at: http://www.who.int/csr/don/archive/disease/severe_acute_respiratory_syndrome/en/index.html.

World Health Organization. (2003g). Severe acute respiratory syndrome (SARS): over 100 days into the outbreak. *Wkly. Epidemiol. Rec.*, **78:** 217–20.

World Health Organization. (2003h). Severe acute respiratory syndrome (SARS) in Singapore. 10 December 2003. Available at: http://www.who.int/csr/don/archive/disease/severe_acute_respiratory_syndrome/en/index.html.

World Health Organization. (2003i). Severe acute respiratory syndrome (SARS) in Taiwan. 17 December 2003. Available at: http://www.who.int/csr/don/archive/disease/severe_acute_respiratory_syndrome/en/index.html.

World Health Organization. (2003j). Suspected severe acute respiratory syndrome (SARS) in southern China. 28 December 2003. Available at: http://www.who.int/csr/don/archive/disease/severe_acute_respiratory_syndrome/en/index.html.

World Health Organization. (2003k). SARS—Update 47. Studies of SARS virus survival, situation in China. 5 May 2003. Available at: http://www.who.int/csr/don/archive/disease/severe_acute_respiratory_syndrome/en/index.html.

World Health Organization. (2003l). SARS—Update 30. Status of diagnostic test, significance of superspreaders, situation in China. 15 April 2003. Available at: http://www.who.int/csr/don/archive/disease/severe_acute_respiratory_syndrome/en/index.html.

World Health Organization. (2003m). Severe acute respiratory syndrome–Singapore 2003. *Wkly. Epidemiol. Rec.*, **78:** 157–62.

World Health Organization. (2003n). Vietnam SARS-free. *Wkly. Epidemiol. Rec.*, **78:** 97–99.

World Health Organization. (2003o). SARS—Update 62. More than 8000 SARS cases reported, situation in Taiwan, data on in-flight transmission, report on Henan province, China. 22 May 2003. Available at: http://www.who.int/csr/don/archive/disease/severe_acute_respiratory_syndrome/en/index.html.

World Health Organization. (2004) China confirms SARS infection in another previously reported case; summary of cases to date–Update 5. 30 April 2004. Available at: http://www.who.int/csr/don/archive/disease/severe_acute_respiratory_syndrome/en/index.html.

Wu, D., Tu, C., Xin, C., *et al.* (2005). Civets are equally susceptible to infection by two different severe acute respiratory syndrome coronavirus isolates. *J. Virology*, **79:** 2620–25.

Xu, R. H., He, J. F., *et al.* (2004). Epidemiologic clues to SARS origin in China. *Emerg. Infect. Dis.*, **10:** 1030–37.

Yu, I. T., Li, Y., Wong, T. W., *et al.* (2004). Evidence of airborne transmission of the severe acute respiratory syndrome. *N. Engl. J. Med.*, **350:** 1731–39.

Zhang, C. Y., Wei, J. F. and He, S. H. (2006). Adaptive evolution of the spike gene of SARS coronavirus: changes in positively selected sites in different epidemic groups. *BMC Microbiol.*, **6:** 88.

Zhong, N. S., Zheng, B. J., *et al.* (2003). Epidemiology and cause of severe acute respiratory syndrome (SARS) in Guangdong, People's Republic of China, in February, 2003. *Lancet*, **362:** 1353–58.

Zhong, N. and Zeng, G. (2005). Management and prevention of SARS in China. In: A. R. McLean *et al.*, SARS—A case study in emerging infections. Oxford University Press: Oxford and Oxford Scholarship Online.

CHAPTER 40

Zoonotic paramyxoviruses

Paul A. Rota and William J. Bellini

Summary

Hendra virus (HeV), Nipah virus (NiV), and Menangle virus (MenV) are recently emergent paramyxoviruses that are responsible for zoonotic infections and represent potential threats to agriculture and humans. In particular, HeV and NiV cause fatal disease in animals and man, and outbreaks of NiV continue to occur almost annually in Southeast Asia. Molecular biologic studies have made substantial contributions to the characterization of these new paramyxoviruses by providing an accurate picture of their relative taxonomic positions, and molecular techniques were used to provide rapid diagnostic capabilities. In the outbreaks of NiV in Malaysia, Bangladesh, and India, molecular biological data quickly identified the etiologic agent present, and RT-PCR and serologic assays were used to rapidly confirm NiV infections in humans and animals. There has only been one report of human illness due to MenV and one study has detected an antibody response to a related rubulavirus, Tioman virus (TiV), in humans. It is interesting that all of these viruses share a common reservoir in large fruit bats. Because of their clear potential to cause severe disease in humans and animals, NiV and HeV have been designated as Class C Select Agents and have been the focus of intense study since their emergence.

The agents

Virology of Hendra and Nipah viruses

Classification

Analysis of the sequences of the entire genomes of both Hendra virus (HeV) and Nipah virus (NiV) provided convincing evidence that these viruses are members of a novel genus, *Henipavirus*, within the subfamily *Paramyxovirinae* (Mayo and van Regenmortel 2000). HeV and NiV share 68–92% amino acid identity in their protein coding regions and 40–67% nucleotide homology in the non-translated regions of their genomes (Harcourt *et al.* 2000, 2001). Compared to the other four genera within the *Paramyxovirinae*, the henipaviruses are more closely related to the respiroviruses and morbilliviruses than to the rubulaviruses and avulaviruses (Fig. 40.1). Of course, the recent genetic characterization of a number of novel paramyxoviruses shows that our understanding of the amount of diversity within this group of viruses is still incomplete (Bowden *et al.* 2001; Chua *et al.* 2000a, 2001b;

Franke *et al.* 2001; Lamb 1996; Murray *et al.* 1995b; Philbey *et al.* 1998). However, it is clear that the henipaviruses have the potential to cause severe disease in humans and animals and further studies to characterize the pathogenesis, epidemiology, and virology of these viruses are clearly warranted (Eaton *et al.* 2006; Halpin and Mungall 2007; Lo and Rota 2008).

Genome structure and gene function of HeV and NiV

The single stranded, negative sense RNA genomes of NiV and HeV have the same gene order, 3'-nucleoprotein (N)-phosphoprotein (P)-matrix protein (M)-fusion protein (F)-attachment protein (G)-RNA dependant RNA polymerse (L)- 5', as the respiroviruses and the morbilliviruses (Fig. 40.2). HeV and NiV retain a number of genetic features found in viruses throughout the subfamily (Harcourt *et al.* 2001, 2005), although the henipaviruses also have several unique genetic and biochemical features.

The genomes of HeV and NiV are 18,234 and 18,246 nucleotides in length, which, until the characterization of Beilong and J viruses (Jack *et al.* 2005; Li *et al.* 2006), were the largest genomes among the paramyxoviruses. In contrast, the average genome size for the other members of the *Paramyxovirinae* is approximately 15,500 nucleotides. The increased size of the HeV and NiV genomes is mostly due to the large sizes of the open-reading frame (ORF) for the P gene and the large 3' untranslated regions present in several genes (Harcourt *et al.* 2001; Wang *et al.* 2000). The functional significance of the large 3' untranslated regions has not been explored. The 'rule of six' (interaction of the nucleocapsid (N) protein with six nucleotides on the RNA genome, i.e. N phase context) states that the total length of the genomic RNA of viruses within the subfamily *Paramyxovirinae* must be evenly divisible by six in order to replicate (Calain and Roux 1993) and the sizes of the genomes of both HeV and NiV are evenly divisible by six indicating that the henipaviruses adhere to the rule of six. Additional evidence is provided by the observation that for HeV and NiV the differences in genome sizes as well as the sizes of the individual genes are evenly divisible by six (Harcourt *et al.* 2001, 2005), and by results of studies with a minigenome replication assay (Halpin *et al.* 2004).

The complete nucleotide sequence of HeV was completed in 2000 (Wang 1998; Wang *et al.* 2000) and since that time, only a few other HeV isolates have been sequenced and found to be virtually identical (Halpin *et al.* 2000; Hooper *et al.* 2000). Analysis of the

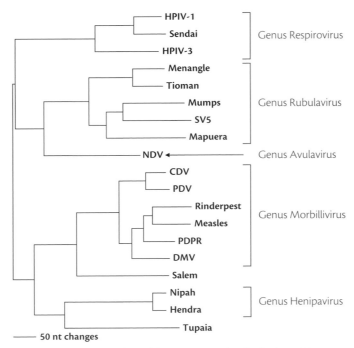

Fig. 40.1 Phylogenetic analysis of the sequences coding for the ORF of the nucleoprotein gene from viruses in the subfamily *Paramyxovirinae*. The genus name is indicated at the right. Scale representing the number of nucleotide changes is shown at the bottom left. Accession numbers used: canine distemper virus (CDV), AF014953; dolphin morbillivirus (DMV), X75961; Hendra virus, AF017149; human parainfluenza virus 1 (HPIV-1), D01070; human parainfluenza virus 3 (HPIV-3), D10025; Mapuera virus, X85128; Menangle virus, AF326114; mumps virus, D86172; measles virus, K01711; Newcastle disease virus (NDV), AF064091; Nipah virus, AF212302; peste-des-petits-ruminants virus, (PPRV), X74443; phocid distemper virus, (PDV), X75717; rinderpest virus, X68311; Salem virus; AF237881; Sendai virus, X00087; simian virus 5 (SV5), M81442; Tioman virus, AF298895 and Tupaia virus, AF079780.

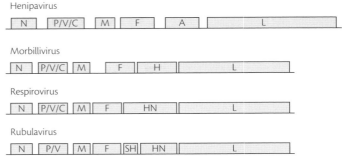

Fig. 40.2 Schematic representation of the genomes of viruses in the subfamily *Paramyxovirinae*. Genomes are single stranded, negative sense RNA shown in the 3' to 5' (left to right) orientation. Grey boxes indicate protein coding regions and solid lines indicate non-coding regions. Abbreviations for the structural genes are as follows: N, nucleoprotein; P, phosphoprotein; M, matrix protein; F, fusion protein; A, attachment protein; H, haemagglutinin protein; HN, haemagglutinin-neuraminidase; L, polymerase. The schematic genome for rubulaviruses is mumps virus and shows the position of the gene for the small hydrophobic protein (SH).

complete genomic sequences of the NiV strains associated with the outbreaks in Malaysia in 1999 (NiV-M) and Bangladesh in 2004 (NiV-B) showed that the genome of NiV-B is six nucleotides longer than NiV-M, the prototype strain of NiV, and two nucleotides shorter than HeV (Harcourt *et al.* 2005). The additional six nucleotides are inserted in the 5' non-translated region of the fusion protein (F) gene. The gene order and sizes of all the ORFs except V are conserved between NiV-B and NiV-M. The overall nucleotide homology between the genomes of NiV-B and NiV-M is 91.8% and the predicted amino acid homologies between the expressed proteins are all greater than 92% (Harcourt *et al.* 2005). The case fatality rates associated with NiV-M was lower than the case fatality rate observed in the outbreaks in Bangladesh (Chua *et al.* 2000a; Hossain *et al.* 2008). One of the major unanswered questions is whether there are differences in pathogenecity between NiV-M and NiV-B. Of course, the limited amount of sequence variation among strains could be related to their geographic distribution. The N gene sequence of a bat isolate of NiV from Cambodia (Reynes *et al.* 2005) is more closely related to the sequence of NiV-M than to the sequence of NiV-B, while sequences obtained from samples from an outbreak in India were more closely related to NiV-B (Chadha *et al.* 2006).

The genomes of paramyxoviruses contain a number of conserved cis-acting signals that regulate gene expression and replication (Lamb 2001). The cis-acting signals on the genomes of HeV and NiV including the gene start sites, gene stop sites, RNA editing sites, genomic termini and intergenic sequences are nearly identical between these viruses, and very closely related to the corresponding sequences within the genomes of respiroviruses and morbilliviruses (Harcourt *et al.* 2000, 2001; Wang 1998; Wang *et al.* 2000). The development of minigenome replication assays and reverse genetic systems for NiV (Freiberg *et al.* 2008; Halpin *et al.* 2004; Yoneda *et al.* 2006) will permit more detailed studies on the genetics and pathogenesis of the henipaviruses. NiV has been rescued from plasmid DNA and wild-type NiV and the rescued NiV showed similar percentages of mortality is a hamster infection model (Yoneda *et al.* 2006).

Proteins of HeV and NiV

The P is an essential component of the replication complex for all paramyxoviruses including HeV and NiV. The P protein of NiV contains binding domains for the N at both its amino and carboxyl termini (Chan *et al.* 2004). The coding strategy for the P gene of the henipaviruses is similar to that found in the respiroviruses and morbilliviruses. In each case, a faithful transcript of the P gene codes for the P protein, while the transcript encoding the V protein is produced by RNA editing. RNA editing refers to the insertion of non-templated guanosine (G) nucleotides into the mRNA of the P gene to permit access to additional ORFs (Thomas *et al.* 1988). The V proteins of the respiroviruses, morbilliviruses and henipaviruses share the same amino terminus as their respective P proteins which, at the editing site, are joined to a unique, carboxyl-terminal cysteine rich ORF that is unique to V. The P genes of the henipaviruses also code for a C protein, which is produced by ribosomal choice from an overlapping reading frame located near the 5' terminus of the P gene mRNA. As in the case of the morbilliviruses, the translational start site for the C protein of HeV and NiV is located downstream of the start codon for the P/V protein (Harcourt *et al.* 2000; Wang 1998). The P genes of HeV and NiV also have the capacity to code for a protein that is analogous to the W protein described for

Sendai virus; W is expressed from an mRNA with a 2 G insertion at the editing site (Vidal *et al.* 1990).

The henipaviruses produced edited transcripts at twice the frequency of other paramyxoviruses such as measles virus (MeV), Sendai virus (SeV), and Newcastle disease virus (NDV) (Bankamp *et al.* 2008; Hausmann *et al.* 1999; Kato *et al.* 1997; Mebatsion *et al.* 2003; Vanchiere *et al.* 1995) with the exception of human parainfluenza virus-3 (hPIV-3), which edits approximately half of its P gene mRNA transcripts (Galinski *et al.* 1992), and bovine parainfluenza virus (Pelet *et al.* 1991). In NiV, approximately two-thirds of all P gene transcripts were edited and 50% of all transcripts encoded for P, 25% for V, and 25% for W. The relative number of mRNA transcripts encoding P protein compared to those encoding the V and W proteins decreased over the course of the first 30 hours of infection (Kulkarni *et al.* 2009). The P, V, W, and C were detected in both infected cells and in sucrose gradient purified virions. The P protein, while localized in the cytoplasm, concentrated near the plasma membrane. The V protein was evenly distributed throughout the cytoplasm and the W protein exclusively localized to the nucleus. The C protein was distributed in the perinuclear areas in a punctuate pattern (Lo *et al.* 2009; Shaw *et al.* 2005). The V and C proteins of paramyxoviruses have been shown to affect viral replication (Horikami *et al.*, 1996; Witko *et al.* 2006). The NiV C, V, and W proteins inhibited NiV minigenome transcription and replication in a dose-dependent manner (Sleeman *et al.* 2008).

The C and V proteins of paramyxoviruses can inhibit the induction of type I IFNs and also block IFN signalling (Fontana *et al.* 2008; Lamb and Parks 2007). Several studies utilizing eukaryotic plasmid expression systems have provided insight into possible mechanisms by which NiV C, V, and W proteins block the host antiviral response. The NiV V protein inhibits IFN signal transduction by sequestering STAT1 and STAT2 in high molecular weight complexes in the cytoplasm and by inhibiting STAT1 phosphorylation (Rodriguez *et al.* 2002). The domain of V responsible for binding STAT1 resides between amino acids 100 and 160. Despite finding a STAT2 binding site on V (amino acids 230–271), STAT2 binding to V required the presence of STAT1 (Rodriguez *et al.* 2004).

Transient expression of NiV V, W, or C was able to rescue the replication of an IFN-sensitive NDV containing a GFP reporter gene in IFN-treated chicken embryo fibroblasts. The V and W proteins rescued GFP expression in a robust manner, while the level of GFP rescued by the C protein was less pronounced. Both the V and W proteins inhibited the expression of a luciferase reporter gene under the control of an IFN stimulated response element (ISRE) promoter, which demonstrated the ability to block IFN signalling (Park *et al.* 2003). The STAT1 binding domain was mapped to amino acids 50-150 of the N-terminus shared by the P, V, and W proteins (Rodriguez *et al.* 2004; Shaw *et al.* 2004). Interestingly, in spite of the shared N-terminus, P, V, and W have differential abilities to inhibit induction of ISRE promoters, with W having the most inhibitive capacity, followed by V, and then P (Shaw *et al.* 2004).

There is a nuclear localization signal (NLS) in the unique C-terminus of the NiV W protein, which requires basic residues at amino acid positions 439, 440, and 442 (Shaw *et al.* 2005). The NLS interacts with the nuclear importins, karyopherin-α3 and karyopherin-α4. While NiV V and W could inhibit an IRF-3 responsive promoter activation both by SeV infection and cytoplasmic dsRNA, only W could inhibit IRF-3 activation via dsRNA stimulation of TLR-3. The addition of a non-viral nuclear localization signal to the V protein resulted in the same inhibitory effect observed with W. This study also demonstrated that plasmid expression of the W protein in cells reduced levels of phosphorylated IRF-3, indicating a distinct mechanism of IFN evasion that was unique to W. There was a demonstrable difference in the ability of the V and W proteins to inhibit the IKK-like kinases, IKKε and TBK-1. Both V and W inhibited IKKε–mediated activation of ISG transcription, while only W was able to inhibit TBK-1-mediated activation of ISG transcription. The authors concluded that because W localizes to the nucleus, it could inhibit both pathways leading to IRF-3 activation, the TLR-3 pathway and the virus/dsRNA pathway (Shaw *et al.* 2005).

A single amino acid change at residue 125 abolished the ability of NiV V to bind STAT1 and to block IFN signalling. NiV was able to block IFN signalling in cell lines from numerous mammalian species, indicating that this ability does not constrain the virus from crossing species (Hagmaier *et al.* 2006). More recently, it has been shown that plasmid expressed NiV V; along with many other paramyxovirus V proteins bind the helicase Mda-5 via its cysteine-rich C-terminal domain, and blocks activation of the IFN-α promoter by preventing the oligomerization of Mda-5 upon binding to dsRNA (Childs *et al.* 2007, 2009). A novel interaction between NiV V and a host cell kinase Polo-like kinase 1 (PLK1) has recently been demonstrated (Ludlow *et al.* 2008). The binding site for PLK1 overlaps with the STAT1 binding region. By constructing point mutants in the shared binding region, STAT1 binding was abrogated independently of PLK1 binding to NiV V. Modifying the binding sites to STAT1 and PKL1 on the NiV P protein did not affect NiV minigenome replication, which indicates the possibility of attenuating NiV by altering the ability of viral proteins to interact with host proteins.

The genes coding for the RNA dependent RNA polymerase (L protein) of HeV and NiV have a linear domain structure that is conserved in all of the *Mononegavirales* (Poch *et al.* 1990). In domain III, all of the negative stranded RNA viruses have a predicted catalytic site with the amino acid sequence GDNQ. The sequence, QDNE, is found only in HeV, NiV and Tupaia paramyxovirus (Harcourt *et al.* 2005; Tidona *et al.* 1999). However, substitution of the E for Q did not affect the function of the L protein of NiV in a minigenome replication assay (Magoffin *et al.* 2007).

The two membrane glycoproteins of HeV and NiV, F and G, serve the same functions as the membrane glycoproteins of the morbilliviruses and respiroviruses. Both G and F are required for cell fusion and heterotypic mixtures of the G and F proteins of HeV and NiV are also fusion competent (Bossart *et al.* 2002; Tamin *et al.* 2002).

The F proteins of the *Paramyxovirinae* are type I membrane glycoproteins that facilitate the viral entry process by mediating fusion of the virion membrane with the plasma membrane of the host cell. F proteins are synthesized as inactive precursors, F_0, that are converted to biologically active subunits, F_1 and F_2, following proteolytic cleavage by a host cell protease (Lamb 2001). The fusion peptide, located at the amino terminus of the F_1 protein, is highly conserved within the *Paramyxovirinae* (Langedijk *et al.* 1997) and the fusion peptides of HeV and NiV are related to the fusion proteins of other paramyxoviruses with the exception that HeV and

NiV have leucine at the first position while almost all of the other viruses have phenylalanine (Harcourt *et al.* 2000). However, substitution of phenylalanine for leucine in the F_1 of NiV does not affect its ability to form syncytia (Moll *et al.* 2004a).

Among the paramyxoviruses, the carboxyl terminus of F_2 protein subunits contains either single basic, or multiple basic, amino acids that comprise the cleavage site between F_1 and F_2. F proteins with multiple basic amino acids are cleaved by furin-like protease during exocytosis from the host cell. F proteins of viruses with a single basic amino acid are cleaved at the cell surface by trypsin like proteases and these viruses usually require the addition of exogenous trypsin to replicate in cell culture. While HeV and NiV have a single basic residue at the cleavage site, both produce productive infections in a variety of cell lines in the absence of exogenous trypsin. In addition, the cleavage site of the F proteins of NiV and HeV do not contain a furin-like protease consensus sequence (R-X-R/K-R) found in most morbilliviruses, rubulaviruses, and pneumoviruses (Lamb and Jardetzky 2007; Langedijk *et al.* 1997), and the basic amino acids are not required for cleavage (Moll *et al.* 2004b). Cleavage of the F protein of NiV and HeV occurs by a novel mechanism involving clatherin mediated endocytosis via a tyrosine dependant signal on the cytoplasmic tail (Michalski *et al.* 2000; Vogt *et al.* 2005). The F proteins of both HeV and NiV require the endosomal protease, cathepsin L, for proteolytic processing (Pager and Dutch 2005). N glycans of the F protein of NiV are required for proper proteolytic processing and these glycans may modulate access to neutralization epitopes (Aguilar *et al.* 2006; Moll *et al.* 2004b).

Attachment and receptors

The attachment proteins of the *Paramyxoviridae* are type II membrane glycoproteins and are responsible for binding to receptors on host cells (Lamb and Jardetzky 2007; Lamb 1996, 2001). Unlike many other paramyxoviruses, neither of the henipaviruses has been shown to have erythrocyte binding or neuraminidase activities. The G proteins of the henipaviruses are most closely related the haemagglutinin neuraminidase (HN) proteins of the respiroviruses (Yu *et al.* 1998). The conservation of most of the structurally important amino acids suggests that the G proteins of HeV and NiV would have structures that are very similar to the structure proposed for the attachment proteins of other paramyxoviruses (Langedijk *et al.* 1997). EphrinB2, the membrane-bound ligand for the EphB class of receptor tyrosine kinases, specifically binds to G proteins of henipaviruses and is a functional receptor for HeV and NiV (Bonaparte *et al.* 2005) While EphrinB3 has also been shown to be a functional receptor for both viruses, the binding of NiV to EphrinB3 is much more efficient than the binding of HeV (Negrete *et al.* 2005, 2006) and the G protein of NiV has distinct binding regions for EphrinB2 and EphrinB3 (Negrete *et al.* 2006). EphrinB3 but not EphrinB2 is expressed in the brain stem, so the difference in the abilities of HeV and NiV to bind to these cellular receptors is consistent with the neuroinvasiveness of NiV (Negrete *et al.* 2005, 2006). NiV infection does not appear to down regulate cell surface expression of EphrinB2 or EphrinB3 (Sawatsky *et al.*2007).

Analysis of the crystal structures of the ephrinB2 and ephrinB3 interactions with NiV G (Bowden *et al.* 2008b; Xu *et al.* 2008) confirmed the accuracy of the functional mapping studies (Negrete *et al.* 2006), and also provided a comprehensive analysis of critical residues composing the hydrophobic binding cleft which interacts with high affinity to ephrinB2 and ephrinB3. The unbound form of NiV G contains highly processed complex-type glycans with negligible amounts of oligomannose-type glycans. Interestingly, the *N*-acetylglucosamine (GlcNAc) $\beta1\rightarrow2$Man terminal structures on NiV G were noted as a potential ligand for LSECtin, a C-type lectin expressed on sinusoidal endothelial cells of lymph nodes and the liver (Bowden *et al.* 2008a). A receptor binding activation site in the stalk region of NiV G triggers fusion by the F protein (Aguilar *et al.* 2009). This finding is consistent with the attachment and fusion proteins of paramyxoviruses (Corey and Iorio 2007, 2009; Lamb and Parks, 2007; Lee *et al.* 2008; Melanson and Iorio 2004, 2006).

As for the other paramyxoviruses, the NiV surface glycoproteins are the primary targets for neutralizing antibodies (Crameri *et al.* 2002; Guillaume *et al.* 2006; Tamin *et al.* 2002). Recombinant vaccinia viruses expressing NiV F and G proteins elicit neutralizing antibodies against NiV and protect Syrian hamsters and pigs against lethal NiV challenge (Guillaume *et al.* 2006; Tamin *et al.* 2002; Weingartl *et al.* 2006) and cats are protected from a lethal challenge by a soluble NiV G (McEachern *et al.* 2008). Antibodies to F or G also provided passive protection in the hamster challenge model (Guillaume *et al.* 2004a).

Virology of Menangle and Tioman viruses

The sequences of the complete genomes of these antigenically related viruses clearly showed that both MenV and TiV are members of the rubulaviruses (Bowden and Boyle 2005; Bowden *et al.* 2001; Chua *et al.* 2002b). Like other members of the genus, these viruses lack the SH gene that is found in mumps virus and simian virus 5. The coding strategy for the P genes is also the same as that found in the other rubulaviruses. The unedited transcript codes for the V protein while a 2 G insertion at the RNA editing site produces the transcript coding for the P protein. MenV lacks detectable neuraminidase and erythrocyte binding activity (Paton *et al.* 1999) and the HN proteins of MeV and TiV lack the hexapeptide, NRKSCS, that is proposed to be essential for neuraminidase activity (Bowden *et al.* 2001). Compared to the other rubulaviruses, TiV and MeV also have some unique genetic features in their RNA start sites and intergenic regions (Chua *et al.* 2001b; Chua *et al.* 2002b).

Epidemiology and pathogenesis

Epidemiology and pathogenesis of Hendra virus

Epidemiology

All of the outbreaks of HeV have occurred in Australia and all have involved horses with or without spillover into humans. The first incident occurred in September 1994 at a stable in Hendra, a suburb of Brisbane. An outbreak of acute respiratory disease resulted in 14 horse deaths (Murray *et al.* 1995a, 1995b; Selvey *et al.* 1995). Approximately 1 week after exposure to the index horse case, two humans who had contact with the horses developed influenza-like illness and one died after a seven day illness. The first isolate of HeV was isolated from this fatal case. The second incident in 1995 involved the death of a farmer who lived near Brisbane (O'Sullivan *et al.* 1997) and who had assisted a veterinary surgeon during treatment of horses. The patient developed meningitis shortly after he assisted in the autopsies of two horses that died of acute respiratory distress and rapid-onset neurological symptoms, respectively. Both horses were retrospectively diagnosed with HeV (Hooper *et al.* 1996). The patient recovered completely and remained symptom-free for 13 months before his fatal illness, which is believed to have resulted from persistent infection with HeV. A third fatal case of HeV infection occurred in 2008 in a veterinarian who had been treating sick horses at a veterinary clinic outside of Brisbane (PROMED-MAIL 2008). In 2004, a veterinarian working near Cairns became infected with HeV after treating a terminally ill horse. The illness was mild and the patient recovered and remains well (Hanna *et al.* 2006).

Transmission

Despite the potential for HeV to infect a wide variety of animals under experimental conditions (Williamson *et al.* 1998, 2000), horses appear to be the primary source of human HeV infection (O'Sullivan *et al.* 1997; Selvey *et al.* 1995). After the first two incidents, no evidence of infection was found in 22 other persons who reported feeding or nursing sick horses or participating in their autopsies and more than 110 other persons associated with, or living near, the affected stables (McCormack *et al.* 1999). These data indicate that transmission of infection from horses to humans is not very efficient and requires very close contact. Laboratory experiments suggest that the urine and saliva from infected horses are important in disease transmission (Williamson *et al.* 1998), whereas respiratory spread is less likely. Human-to-human transmission of HeV has not been documented, either among domestic contacts or among health care workers (McCormack *et al.* 1999; Selvey *et al.* 1995).

Pathogenesis in humans

The pathology of HeV infections and factors in disease production are incompletely characterized because of the small number of cases. Following initial infection with the virus, possibly through the oral or respiratory route or through direct inoculation of cutaneous abrasions with infectious secretions, viremia develops resulting in spread to various organs, including the central nervous system. The incubation period of acute disease is approximately 5–7 days. Autopsy of the horse trainer who died in the first HeV incident showed a severe interstitial pneumonia with both lungs congested, hemorrhagic, and edematous. Histologic examination showed focal necrotizing alveolitis, with giant cells, syncytium formation, and viral inclusions. HeV was isolated from post-mortem lung, liver, kidney, and spleen specimens (Murray *et al.* 1995b; Selvey *et al.* 1995). The farmer from Mackay who died more than one year after initial infection with HeV (O'Sullivan *et al.* 1997) showed leptomeningitis with prominent lymphocyte and plasma cell infiltration. There were discrete foci of necrosis in the neocortex, basal ganglia, brainstem, and cerebellum and multinucleate endothelial cells were observed in the brain, liver, spleen, and lungs.

Clinical manifestations

HeV infections begin with abrupt onset of an influenza-like illness, which includes myalgia, headache, lethargy, and vertigo (Hanna *et al.* 2006; Murray *et al.* 1995a, 1995b). The first patient developed nausea and vomiting on the fourth day of illness, and deteriorated rapidly in the next 2 days, requiring admission to an intensive care unit and mechanical ventilation. He died on the seventh day of illness. Laboratory results showed thrombocytopenia, increased levels of creatine phosphokinase, lactic dehydrogenase, aspartate aminotranferase, alanine aminotransferase, and glutamyltransferase, and features of dehydration and acidosis (Murray *et al.* 1995b). Chest radiographs showed diffuse alveolar shadowing.

No laboratory abnormalities were detected in the patient who survived.

The affected farmer in the second HeV incident primarily had neurologic manifestations (O'Sullivan *et al.* 1997). He initially presented with features of meningitis, including headache, drowsiness, vomiting, and neck stiffness. Thirteen months following complete recovery, the patient presented again with a 2-week history of irritable mood and low back pain, 3 episodes of focal seizures of the right arm, and an episode of generalized tonic-clonic seizures. In the following week, he continued to have a low-grade fever, focal and generalized seizures. By day 7, he developed dense right hemiplegia, signs of brainstem involvement, and depressed consciousness, requiring intubation. The patient remained unconscious and febrile until he died 25 days after admission. Cerebrospinal fluid examination showed an elevated protein level, normal glucose level, and mononuclear pleocytosis. MRI imaging of the brain showed multifocal cortical lesions sparing the subcortical white matter that became more pronounced and widespread prior to death.

Epidemiology and pathogenesis of Nipah virus

Epidemiology

The first known human infections with NiV occurred during an outbreak of severe encephalitis in Southeast Asia in 1998–1999. Two hundred sixty-five patients (40% fatal) and 11 patients (1 fatal) with laboratory-confirmed NiV disease were reported in Peninsular Malaysia and Singapore, respectively (Anon. 1999a, 1999b; Chua *et al.* 2000a; Eaton *et al.* 2006). This outbreak began in October 1998 in northern Malaysia and then spread southward in conjunction with the movement of pigs, resulting in at least three other clusters of human disease in Malaysia. In Singapore, abattoir workers who slaughtered pigs imported from outbreak-affected areas in Malaysia were exclusively affected (Chew *et al.* 2000; Paton *et al.* 1999). Adult males who were primarily involved in pig farming activities accounted for more than three-fourths of cases in Malaysia. Infections were also documented in abattoir workers (Chew *et al.* 2000; Paton *et al.* 1999), in veterinary personnel, and in military personnel involved in pig culling activities.

Since the initial outbreak, human cases of NiV encephalitis have occurred in several small outbreaks in India, 2001 (Chadha *et al.* 2006), and Bangladesh, 2001 to 2007 (Anon. 2003; Eaton *et al.* 2006; Hossain *et al.* 2008; Hsu *et al.* 2004; World Health Organization (WHO) 2001, 2004a, 2004b, 2004c). These smaller outbreaks had a marked increase of case fatality rate (CFR) which ranged from 67% to 92% and a number of epidemiologic features associated with these outbreaks differed from those of the initial outbreak. In the outbreak in Meherpur, Bangladesh in 2001, both close contacts with infected patients as well as with sick cows were associated with NiV infection, although samples from cows were not available for testing (Hsu *et al.* 2004). Eight households were affected, and of the 13 cases reported, 9 were related either by blood or by marriage to the index patient. Person-to-person contact was also a primary risk factor during the 2003 outbreak in the Nagoan district of Bangladesh, but in this instance there were no blood relationships between affected households (Hossain *et al.* 2008). In the outbreak in Faridpur, Bangladesh in 2004, person-to-person transmission was implicated, and the possibility of nosocomial transmission was demonstrated by the detection of NiV RNA on hospital surfaces (Gurley *et al.* 2007a, 2007b). Retrospective analysis of an outbreak in Siliguri, India in 2001 confirmed that nosocomial transmission resulted in the amplification of the outbreak (Chadha *et al.* 2006). Ingestion of NiV-contaminated date palm sap was reported as the primary risk factor during an outbreak in the Tangail district of Bangladesh in 2005, and this practice was potentially linked to more recent outbreaks of NiV in the Manikganj and Rajbari districts of Bangladesh (Luby *et al.* 2006; PROMED-MAIL, 2008). The increase in CFR in the Bangladesh outbreaks may be due to the inherent strain-specific differences between Malaysian and Bangladeshi strains of NiV, or the comparatively lower level of supportive care available in Bangladesh compared to Malaysia and Singapore (Harcourt *et al.* 2005).

Sequence analysis of different strains of NiV has also provided some information about the transmission patterns of the virus. Molecular biological data suggest that there were at least two introductions of NiV into pigs prior to the outbreak on 1999 (AbuBakar *et al.* 2004). Only one of these variants was associated with the explosive spread within pig farms and subsequent transmission to humans suggesting that a single spillover from the reservoir triggered the outbreak. In contrast, the sequence heterogeneity observed between samples obtained from the outbreak in Bangladesh in 2004 suggesting multiple spillovers between the reservoir and humans (Harcourt *et al.* 2005).

Transmission

During the outbreaks in Malaysia and Singapore, close contact with pigs was the primary source of human NiV infection (Mohd Nor *et al.* 2000; Parashar *et al.* 2000). In pigs, extensive infection of the upper and lower airways is seen with evidence of tracheitis, and bronchial and interstitial pneumonia and a harsh, non-productive cough was a prominent clinical feature (Chua *et al.* 2000a; Hooper and Williamson 2000). Vasculitis of small vessels in the kidney was also seen (Chua *et al.* 2000a; Hooper and Williamson 2000), and viral antigen was detected by IHC studies as focal staining in renal tubular epithelium. Therefore, exposure to respiratory secretions and possibly the urine of infectious pigs likely resulted in transmission of virus among pigs and to humans. In experimental studies, transmission among pigs occurred through both oral and in-contact exposure (Hooper and Williamson 2000). Serologic studies demonstrated evidence of infection among other species of animals in Malaysia, including dogs and cats (Chua *et al.* 2000a; Hooper and Williamson 2000). It is unclear whether humans are at risk from exposure to infected animals other than pigs, but this possibility cannot be excluded because some patients reported no direct contact with pigs (Goh *et al.* 2000; Parashar *et al.* 2000). In Bangladesh, pigs did not act as intermediate hosts of the virus, and transmission directly from bats or from fruits or commodities such as date palm syrup that were contaminated by bats may have caused the primary infections in the small outbreaks occurring there (Anon. 2004; Luby *et al.* 2006; Montgomery *et al.* 2008).

Although NiV is excreted in respiratory secretions and urine of patients (Chua *et al.*2001a), a survey of health care workers demonstrated no evidence of human-to-human transmission in Malaysia (Mounts *et al.* 2001). Transmission from patients to relatives or caregivers in contact with patients during the course of disease was strongly implicated in at least some of the cases in Bangladesh and perhaps in India (Anon. 2004; Chadha *et al.* 2006; Gurley *et al.* 2007a, 2007b; Montgomery *et al.* 2008). The risk of person-to-person transmission may be increased in settings in which standard infection control measures are not the usual practice.

Pathogenesis in humans

The incubation period among Bangladeshi patients with NiV infection who had well-defined exposure to another case, was 9 days (range, 6–11 days) (Hossain *et al.* 2008), though longer incubation periods were noted in Malaysia (Parashar *et al.* 2000). A multiorgan vasculitis associated with infection of endothelial cells was the major pathologic feature of NiV infection (Goh *et al.* 2000). Occasionally, multinucleate giant cells characteristic of paramyxovirus infections were observed in the affected vascular endothelium. Infection was most pronounced in the central nervous system, where a diffuse vasculitis characterized by segmental endothelial cell damage, mural necrosis, karyorrhexis, and infiltration with polymorphonuclear leukocytes and mononuclear cells was noted. The lesions are primarily seen in the cerebral cortex and brain stem with extension to parenchymal tissue, where extensive areas of rarefaction necrosis were seen. Eosinophilic, mainly intracytoplasmic, viral inclusions with a 'melted-tallow' appearance were seen in the affected neurons and parenchymal cells. Evidence of endothelial infection and vasculitis were also seen in other organs, including the lung, heart, spleen, and kidney (Wong *et al.* 2002). NiV has been isolated from cerebrospinal fluid, tracheal secretions, throat swab, nasal swab, and urine specimens of patients (Goh *et al.* 2000) (Parashar *et al.* 2000).

Limited data are available on the immune response to NiV infection, correlates of immune protection and disease resolution. A serum IgM response occurs shortly after onset of illness, with 50% of patients being antibody-positive on the first day of illness and 100% being antibody-positive by the third day (Ramasundrum 2000) with persistent IgM detectable up to 3 months after symptom onset. An IgG antibody response is seen in 10–29% of patients in the first 10 days of illness, and in 100% of patients after days 17–18 of illness.

Clinical manifestations

The onset of NiV disease is abrupt, usually with the development of fever. Often, patients deteriorate rapidly, requiring hospitalization 3–4 days after onset of symptoms. Severe encephalitis is the most prominent clinical manifestation. Fever, headache, dizziness, vomiting, and reduced level of consciousness are the most common features; acute respiratory failure was noted in some of the outbreaks in Bangladesh (Goh *et al.* 2000; Hossain *et al.* 2008). Several other features of neurologic involvement, particularly signs of brain-stem dysfunction, were noted in patients during the course of illness. NiV disease was fatal in up to one-third of hospitalized patients in Malaysia (Chua *et al.* 2000b; Goh *et al.* 2000). Residual neurological deficits occurred in 10%–15% of patients (Goh *et al.* 2000; Paton *et al.* 1999; Sarji *et al.* 2000). Recurrence of neurologic dysfunction was seen in some patients, including neurologic relapse with seizures and/or cognitive impairment or focal signs such as isolated cranial nerve dysfunction (Sarji *et al.* 2000). In another study, delayed progression to neurologic illness following NiV infection was not observed, but persistent fatigue and functional impairment were frequent (Sejvar *et al.* 2007). Neurologic dysfunction may persist for years after acute infection.

Reservoirs of Hendra virus and Nipah virus

Antibodies to HeV antibodies were detected in several fruit bat species primarily of the *Pteropus* genus in Queensland and the virus isolated from a fruit bat was indistinguishable from that isolated from horses and humans (Halpin *et al.* 1999, 2000).

Transmission of HeV to horses may occur through the ingestion of pasture recently contaminated by the urine or infected fetal tissue of fruit bats (Field *et al.* 2000; Halpin *et al.* 2000). Despite the ability of NiV to infect many mammalian species (dogs, cats, ferrets, pigs, horses), the absence of neutralizing antibody in non-infected hosts indicated that these were 'dead-end hosts' (Mohd *et al.* 2000). Since HeV had been detected in fruit bats, they were the logical reservoir for NiV (Halpin *et al.* 2000). Neutralizing antibodies to NiV were found primarily in *Pteropus hypomenalus* and *Pteropus vampyrus* during initial surveillance studies, but virus was not isolated (Yob *et al.* 2001). The first isolation NiV from bats was from *Pteropus hypomenalus* on Tioman Island, Malaysia (Chua *et al.* 2002a). Since then, antibodies to henipaviruses have been detected in other *Pteropus* species (*Pteropus lylei, Pteropus giganteus,*) as well as in non-*Pteropus* species (*Hipposideros larvatus, Scotophiilus kuhlii*) at much lower frequencies, in Cambodia, China, Thailand, India, Indonesia, Bangladesh, to Madagascar (Epstein *et al.* 2008; Hsu *et al.* 2004; Li *et al.* 2008; Reynes *et al.* 2005; Sendow *et al.* 2006; Wacharapluesadee *et al.* 2005). Antibodies to henipaviruses have been detected in *Eidolon helvum* in west Africa (Hayman *et al.* 2008).

Pathogenesis and epidemiology of Menangle virus and Tioman virus

Epidemiology

In 1997 a piggery in New South Wales, Australia noticed a decline in the farrowing rate of sows, which was associated with an increase in the proportion of malformed, mummified, and stillborn piglets, with occasional abortions (Philbey *et al.* 1998, 2007). The affected piglets had craniofacial and spinal abnormalities and degeneration of the brain and spinal cord. A new paramyxovirus, MenV, was isolated from the brain, heart, and lung specimens of several affected piglets. No disease was seen in postnatal pigs of any age, but a high proportion of serum specimens (>95%) collected from these animals contained high titres of antibodies that neutralized the virus. Evidence of infection with MenV was also detected in porcine sera from two other associated piggeries that received weaned pigs from the affected piggery, but not in sera from several other piggeries throughout Australia (Kirkland *et al.* 2001).

A serologic survey of persons who came into contact with the affected piglets (Chant *et al.* 1998) detected a high titre of neutralizing antibodies in two workers, one at the affected piggery and one at an associated piggery. Both workers had an influenza-like illness at the same time as the outbreak in pigs and no alternative cause for their infection was identified despite serologic testing. Thus, the illness was attributed to MenV virus infection.

Close contact with infected piglets appears to be the primary mode of transmission of MenV to humans (Chant *et al.* 1998). A large breeding colony of fruit bats roosted within 200 m of the affected piggery and sera from several bats had antibodies that neutralized MenV (Philbey *et al.* 1998). Serum samples collected from bats before the outbreak also had detectable antibodies to MenV, while all other serum samples collected from a variety of wild and domestic animals in the vicinity of the affected piggery tested negative for antibodies to the virus. Fruit bats are likely the primary reservoirs of MeV.

Both of the affected workers had a similar illnesses which were characterized by abrupt onset of fever, malaise, chills, drenching sweats, and severe headache (Chant *et al.* 1998). On the fourth day of illness, both developed a spotty, red, nonpruritic rash. Bilateral hypochondrial tenderness was present in one patient, and an abdominal ultrasound conducted 2 months after the illness showed splenomegaly and liver size at the upper limit of normal. Both patients recovered after approximately 10 days of illness.

Very little is known about Tioman virus (TiV) which was isolated from fruit bats on Tioman Island, Malaysia (Chua *et al.* 2001b). Several pigs experimentally inoculated with TiV developed pyrexia, produced neutralizing antibodies and shed virus (Yaiw *et al.* 2008). Serologic testing of 169 inhabitants of Tioman Island showed that a small percentage (3.0%) had serologic evidence of infection by TiV or a related virus (Yaiw *et al.* 2007).

Pathogenesis of Hendra and Nipah viruses in animal models

The development or characterization of animal models to study henipavirus infections is critical for understanding their pathogenesis and development of new therapeutics or vaccines. Both cats and golden hamsters have been used as small animal models and both develop fatal disease after challenge with NiV. In cats, virus is mostly present in the respiratory epithelium, while hamsters develop neurologic disease (Guillaume *et al.* 2004a, 2006; Mungall *et al.* 2006a). NiV in pigs causes a febrile respiratory illness with or without neurological signs (Middleton *et al.* 2002; Mohd Nor *et al.* 2000; Weingartl *et al.* 2005). Infection of fruit bats with NiV did produce clinical signs; some of the bats seroconverted with intermittent excretion of low levels of virus (Middleton *et al.* 2007). Golden hamsters are highly susceptible to HeV infection (Guillaume *et al.* 2009).

Diagnostics, antivirals and vaccines

Diagnostic methods

NiV is internationally classified as a biosafety level 4 (BSL-4) agent, thus clinical specimens must be handled with caution. Propagation of viruses from clinical specimens known to be infected with NiV is not recommended without appropriate containment facilities. The Centers for Disease Control and Prevention, Atlanta, GA USA (CDC) and the Australian Animal Health Laboratory, Geelong, Australia (AAHL) have adopted the approach that primary virus isolation from specimens of outbreaks not already proven to be NiV takes place at BSL-3. However, if the results of cell culture suggest the presence of these agents, cultures should be transferred to BSL-4 to conform to biosafety guidelines (Daniels *et al.* 2001).

During the initial NiV outbreak, enzyme-linked immunosorbent assays (ELISAs) specific for detecting anti-HeV IgM and IgG were used to diagnose NiV infection. A NiV-specific ELISA was eventually transferred to surveillance labs in Malaysia (Daniels *et al.* 2001). For cases in which the ELISAs gave equivocal results, negative-stained cerebrospinal fluid (CSF) specimens were subjected to transmission electron microscopy to visually confirm the presence of NiV (Chow *et al.* 2000). Immunohistochemistry was crucial in detecting NiV antigen in *ex vivo* tissues of humans, dogs, and pigs (CDC 1999a, 1999b; Chua *et al.* 2000a). Complete molecular characterization of both the Malaysian and Bangladeshi strains of NiV has enabled the development of both standard and real-time RT-PCR assays to detect viral RNA from serum, urine, and CSF (AbuBakar *et al.* 2004; Guillaume *et al.* 2004b; Wacharapluesadee and Hemachudha 2007). Recently-developed ELISAs now utilize recombinant-expressed purified NiV antigens, and a number of high-affinity monoclonal antibodies have been generated for diagnostic and prophylactic purposes (Chen *et al.* 2006; Eshaghi *et al.* 2004, 2005a; Eshaghi *et al.* 2005b; Juozapaitis *et al.* 2007; Kashiwazaki *et al.* 2004; Tan *et al.* 2004; Tanimura *et al.* 2004a, 2004b; Yu *et al.* 2006; Zhu *et al.* 2006, 2008). While serum neutralization tests (SNTs) have long been a reference standard, the next generation of SNTs will circumvent the use of live virus, and be able to differentiate between NiV and HeV specific infection (Bossart *et al.* 2007; Chen *et al.* 2007; Kaku *et al.* 2009; Tamin *et al.* 2009).

Antivirals

In Malaysia, ribavirin treatment was shown to reduce mortality rates (Chong *et al.* 2001). The interferon inducer poly(I)-poly($C_{12}U$) prevented mortality in 5 of 6 animals in a hamster model of NiV infection, while a 5-ethynyl analogue of ribavirin and several other OMP-decarboxylase inhibitors were shown to have anti-NiV activity *in vitro* (Georges-Courbot *et al.* 2006). Recent developments for NiV antivirals focus on inhibitors of fusion and receptor-binding. Peptides corresponding to the C-terminal heptad repeat of the F protein from HeV, NiV, and human parainfluenzavirus 3C have been shown to inhibit HeV and NiV infection *in vitro* (Bossart *et al.* 2005b; Porotto *et al.* 2006, 2007). Soluble versions of the G glycoprotein and Ephrin B2 have been shown to inhibit NiV envelope-mediated infection, and could be used as therapeutics (Bonaparte *et al.* 2005; Bossart *et al.* 2005a; Negrete *et al.* 2005).

Prevention and vaccination

No passive immunoprophylaxis, antiviral chemoprohylaxis, or vaccine is currently available for henipavirus infections. The principal means of preventing human infections are early recognition of disease and use of standards protective precautions to avoid exposure. Since interruption of transmission to horses or pigs from the natural reservoir of these viruses, presumably fruit bats, is difficult to prevent, early identification of infected animals and use of appropriate personal protective measures to prevent transmission are keys to reducing the risk to humans.

The G glycoprotein of NiV shared with 83.3% homology with the G protein of HeV virus, whereas the F proteins of the two viruses have 88.1% homology (Harcourt *et al.* 2000; Wang *et al.* 2001). Recombinant expressed, soluble versions of the G glycoprotein (sG) from NiV (Bossart *et al.* 2005a) were used to vaccinate cats and produced high antibody titres along with complete protection from NiV challenge (McEachern *et al.* 2008; Mungall *et al.* 2006b). Purified sG retains a number of important native structural, functional and antigenic features, making it potentially suitable as a vaccine candidate, although consistent large scale expression has been problematic. Expression of NiV F, G and M proteins leads to production VLPs (Ciancanelli and Basler 2006; Patch *et al.* 2007). Since VLPs have been able to generate a protective immune response against Ebola and Marburg viruses (Swenson *et al.* 2005) they might serve as a more efficient method of immunization against NiV. DNA vaccination with plasmids containing either NiV G or F genes stimulated considerable IgG responses in mice (Wang *et al.* 2006), while canarypox virus-based vaccine vectors expressing NiV G or F (or both) protected pigs against challenge and prevented viral shedding (Weingartl *et al.* 2006). Vaccination with these canarypox virus-based vaccines appeared to stimulate both type 1 and type 2 cytokine responses, suggesting this approach may be highly effective for the prevention of livestock infection.

References

AbuBakar, S., Chang, L.Y., Ali, A.R., Sharifah, S.H., *et al.*(2004). Isolation and molecular identification of Nipah virus from pigs. *Emerg. Infect. Dis.*, **10**(12): 2228–30.

Aguilar, H.C., Ataman, Z.A., Aspericueta, V., *et al.* (2009). A novel receptor-induced activation site in the Nipah virus attachment glycoprotein (G) involved in triggering the fusion glycoprotein (F). *J. Biol. Chem.*, **284**(3): 1628–35.

Aguilar, H.C., Matreyek, K.A., Filone, C.M., *et al.* (2006). N-glycans on Nipah virus fusion protein protect against neutralization but reduce membrane fusion and viral entry. *J. Virol.*, **80**(10): 4878–89.

Anon. (1999a). Outbreak of Hendra-like virus—Malaysia and Singapore, 1998–1999. *Morb. Mortal. Wkly. Rep.*, **48**(13): 265–69.

Anon. (1999b). Update: outbreak of Nipah virus—Malaysia and Singapore, 1999. *Morb. Mortal. Wkly. Rep.*, **48**(16): 335–37.

Anon. (2003) Outbreaks of Encephalitis Due to Nipah/Hendra-like Viruses, Western Bangladesh. *Heal. Sci. Bull. (English)*, **1**: 1–6.

Anon. (2004). Person-to-person transmission of Nipah virus during outbreak in Faridpur District, 2004. *Health Sci. Bull.*, **2**: 5–9.

Bankamp, B., Lopareva, E.N., Kremer, J.R., *et al.* (2008). Genetic variability and mRNA editing frequencies of the phosphoprotein genes of wild-type measles viruses. *Virus Res.*, **135**(2): 298–306.

Bonaparte, M.I., Dimitrov, A.S., Bossart, K.N., *et al.* (2005). Ephrin-B2 ligand is a functional receptor for Hendra virus and Nipah virus. *Proc. Natl. Acad. Sci. USA*, **102**(30): 10652–57.

Bossart, K.N., Crameri, G., Dimitrov, A.S., *et al.* (2005a). Receptor binding, fusion inhibition, and induction of cross-reactive neutralizing antibodies by a soluble G glycoprotein of Hendra virus. *J. Virol.*, **79**(11): 6690–702.

Bossart, K.N., McEachern, J.A., Hickey, A.C., *et al.* (2007). Neutralization assays for differential henipavirus serology using Bio-Plex protein array systems. *J. Virol. Meth.*, **142**(1–2): 29–40.

Bossart, K.N., Mungall, B.A., Crameri, G., Wang, L.F., Eaton, B.T. and Broder, C.C. (2005b). Inhibition of Henipavirus fusion and infection by heptad-derived peptides of the Nipah virus fusion glycoprotein. *J. Virol.*, **2**: 57.

Bossart, K.N., Wang, L.F., Flora, M.N., *et al.* (2002). Membrane fusion tropism and heterotypic functional activities of the Nipah virus and Hendra virus envelope glycoproteins. *J. Virol.*, **76**(22): 11186–98.

Bowden, T.A., Aricescu, A.R., Gilbert, R.J., *et al.* (2008a). Structural basis of Nipah and Hendra virus attachment to their cell-surface receptor ephrin-B2. *Nat. Struct. Mol. Biol.*, **15**: 567–72.

Bowden, T.A., Crispin, M., Harvey, D.J., *et al.* (2008b). Crystal structure and carbohydrate analysis of nipah virus attachment glycoprotein: a template for antiviral and vaccine design. *J. Virol.*, **82**(23): 11628–36.

Bowden, T.R. and Boyle, D.B. (2005). Completion of the full-length genome sequence of Menangle virus: characterisation of the polymerase gene and genomic 5' trailer region. *Arch. Virol.*, **150**(10): 2125–37.

Bowden, T.R., Westenberg, M., Wang, L.F., Eaton, B.T. and Boyle, D.B. (2001). Molecular characterization of Menangle virus, a novel paramyxovirus which infects pigs, fruit bats, and humans. *Virology*, **283**(2): 358–73.

Calain, P. and Roux, L. (1993). The rule of six, a basic feature for efficient replication of Sendai virus defective interfering RNA. *J. Virol.*, **67**(8): 4822–30.

CDC. (1999a). Outbreak of Hendra-like virus—Malaysia and Singapore, 1998–1999. *Morb. Mortal. Wkly. Rep.*, **48**: 265–69.

CDC. (1999b) Update: outbreak of Nipah virus—Malaysia and Singapore, 1999. *Morb. Mortal. Wkly. Rep.*, **48**: 335–37.

Chadha, M.S., Comer, J.A., Lowe, L., Rota, P.A., *et al.* (2006). Nipah virus-associated encephalitis outbreak, Siliguri, India. *Emerg. Infect. Dis.*, **12**(2): 235–40.

Chan, Y.P., Koh, C.L., Lam, S.K. and Wang, L.F. (2004). Mapping of domains responsible for nucleocapsid protein-phosphoprotein interaction of Henipaviruses. *J. Gen. Virol.*, **85**(6): 1675–84.

Chant, K., Chan, R., Smith, M., Dwyer, D.E. and Kirkland, P. (1998). Probable human infection with a newly described virus in the family Paramyxoviridae. The NSW Expert Group. *Emerg. Infect. Dis.*, **4**(2): 273–75.

Chen, J.M., Yaiw, K.C., Yu, M., Wang, L.F., *et al.* (2007). Expression of truncated phosphoproteins of Nipah virus and Hendra virus in Escherichia coli for the differentiation of henipavirus infections. *Biotechn. Lett.*, **29**(6): 871–75.

Chen, J.M., Yu, M., Morrissy, C., Zhao, Y.G., *et al.* (2006). A comparative indirect ELISA for the detection of henipavirus antibodies based on a recombinant nucleocapsid protein expressed in Escherichia coli. *J. Virol. Meth.*, **136**(1–2): 273–76.

Chew, M.H., Arguin, P.M., Shay, D.K., *et al.* (2000). Risk factors for Nipah virus infection among abattoir workers in Singapore. *J. Infect. Dis.*, **181**(5): 1760–63.

Childs, K., Stock, N., Ross, C., Andrejeva, J., *et al.* (2007). mda-5, but not RIG-I, is a common target for paramyxovirus V proteins. *Virology*, **359**(1): 190–200.

Childs, K.S., Andrejeva, J., Randall, R.E. and Goodbourn, S. (2009). Mechanism of mda-5 Inhibition by paramyxovirus V proteins. *J. Virol.*, **83**(3): 1465–73.

Chong, H.T., Kamarulzaman, A., Tan, C.T., *et al.* (2001). Treatment of acute Nipah encephalitis with ribavirin. *Ann. Neurol.*, **49**(6): 810–13.

Chow, V.T., Tambyah, P.A., Yeo, W.M., Phoon, M.C. and Howe, J. (2000). Diagnosis of nipah virus encephalitis by electron microscopy of cerebrospinal fluid. *J. Clin. Virol.*, **19**(3): 143–47.

Chua, K.B., Bellini, W.J., Rota, P.A., Harcourt, B.H., *et al.* (2000a). Nipah virus: a recently emergent deadly paramyxovirus. *Science*, **288**(5470): 1432–35.

Chua, K.B., Koh, C.L., Hooi, P.S., Wee, K.F., *et al.* (2002a). Isolation of Nipah virus from Malaysian Island flying-foxes. *Microbes Infect.*, **4**(2): 145–51.

Chua, K.B., Lam, S.K., Goh, K.J., Hooi, P.S., *et al.* (2001a). The presence of Nipah virus in respiratory secretions and urine of patients during an outbreak of Nipah virus encephalitis in Malaysia. *J. Infect.*, **42**(1): 40–43.

Chua, K.B., Lam, S.K., Tan, C.T., Hooi, P.S., *et al.* (2000b). High mortality in Nipah encephalitis is associated with presence of virus in cerebrospinal fluid. *Ann. Neurol.*, **48**(5): 802–5.

Chua, K.B., Wang, L.F., Lam, S.K., Crameri, G., *et al.* (2001b). Tioman virus, a novel paramyxovirus isolated from fruit bats in Malaysia. *Virology*, **283**(2): 215–29.

Chua, K.B., Wang, L.F., Lam, S.K. and Eaton, B.T. (2002b). Full length genome sequence of Tioman virus, a novel paramyxovirus in the genus Rubulavirus isolated from fruit bats in Malaysia. *Arch. Virol.*, **147**(7): 1323–48.

Ciancanelli, M.J. and Basler, C.F. (2006). Mutation of YMYL in the Nipah virus matrix protein abrogates budding and alters subcellular localization. *J. Virol.*, **80**(24): 12070–78.

Corey, E.A. and Iorio, R.M. (2007). Mutations in the stalk of the measles virus hemagglutinin protein decrease fusion but do not interfere with virus-specific interaction with the homologous fusion protein. *J. Virol.*, **81**(18): 9900–10.

Corey, E.A. and Iorio, R.M. (2009). Measles virus attachment proteins with impaired ability to bind CD46 interact more efficiently with the homologous fusion protein. *Virology*, **383**(1): 1–5.

Crameri, G., Wang, L.F., Morrissy, C., White, J. and Eaton, B.T. (2002). A rapid immune plaque assay for the detection of Hendra and Nipah viruses and anti-virus antibodies. *J. Virol, Meth.*, **99**(1–2): 41–51.

Daniels, P., Ksiazek, T. and Eaton, B.T. (2001). Laboratory diagnosis of Nipah and Hendra virus infections. *Microbes Infect.*, **3**(4): 289–95.

Eaton, B.T., Broder, C.C., Middleton, D. and Wang, L.F. (2006). Hendra and Nipah viruses: different and dangerous. *Nat. Rev. Microbiol.*, **4**(1): 23–35.

Epstein, J.H., Prakash, V., Smith, C.S., *et al.* (2008). Henipavirus infection in fruit bats (Pteropus giganteus), India. *Emerg. Infect. Dis.*, **14**(8): 1309–11.

Eshaghi, M., Tan, W.S., Chin, W.K. and Yusoff, K. (2005a) Purification of the extra-cellular domain of Nipah virus glycoprotein produced in Escherichia coli and possible application in diagnosis. *J. Biotechn.*, **116**(3), 221–26.

Eshaghi, M., Tan, W.S., Mohidin, T.B. and Yusoff, K. (2004). Nipah virus glycoprotein: production in baculovirus and application in diagnosis. *Virus Res.*, **106**(1): 71–76.

Eshaghi, M., Tan, W.S., Ong, S.T. and Yusoff, K. (2005b). Purification and characterization of Nipah virus nucleocapsid protein produced in insect cells. *J. Clin. Microbiol.*, **43**(7): 3172–77.

Field, H.E., Barratt, P.C., Hughes, R.J., Shield, J. and Sullivan, N.D. (2000). A fatal case of Hendra virus infection in a horse in north Queensland: clinical and epidemiological features. *Aust. Vet. J.*, **78**(4): 279–80.

Fontana, J.M., Bankamp, B. and Rota, P.A. (2008). Inhibition of interferon induction and signaling by paramyxoviruses. *Immunol. Rev.*, **225**: 46–67.

Franke, J., Essbauer, S., Ahne, W. and Blahak, S. (2001). Identification and molecular characterization of 18 paramyxoviruses isolated from snakes. *Virus Res.*, **80**(1–2): 67–74.

Freiberg, A., Dolores, L.K., Enterlein, S. and Flick, R. (2008). Establishment and characterization of plasmid-driven minigenome rescue systems for Nipah virus: RNA polymerase I- and T7-catalyzed generation of functional paramyxoviral RNA. *Virology*, **370**(1): 33–44.

Galinski, M.S., Troy, R.M. and Banerjee, A.K. (1992). RNA editing in the phosphoprotein gene of the human parainfluenza virus type 3. *Virology*, **186**(2): 543–50.

Georges-Courbot, M.C., Contamin, H., Faure, C., *et al.* (2006). Poly(I)-poly(C12U) but not ribavirin prevents death in a hamster model of Nipah virus infection. *Antimicrob. Agents Chemother.*, **50**(5): 1768–72.

Goh, K.J., Tan, C.T., Chew, N.K., Tan, P.S., *et al.* (2000). Clinical features of Nipah virus encephalitis among pig farmers in Malaysia. *N. Engl. J. Med.*, **342**(17): 1229–35.

Guillaume, V., Contamin, H., Loth, P., *et al.* (2004a). Nipah virus: vaccination and passive protection studies in a hamster model. *J. Virol.*, **78**(2): 834–40.

Guillaume, V., Contamin, H., Loth, P., *et al.* (2006). Antibody prophylaxis and therapy against Nipah virus infection in hamsters. *J. Virol.*, **80**(4): 1972–78.

Guillaume, V., Lefeuvre, A., Faure, C., *et al.* (2004b). Specific detection of Nipah virus using real-time RT-PCR (TaqMan). *J. Virol. Meth.*, **120**(2): 229–37.

Guillaume, V., Wong, K.T., Looi, R.Y., *et al.* (2009). Acute Hendra virus infection: Analysis of the pathogenesis and passive antibody protection in the hamster model. *Virology*, **387**(2): 459–65.

Gurley, E.S., Montgomery, J.M., Hossain, M.J., Bell, M., *et al.* (2007a). Person-to-person transmission of Nipah virus in a Bangladeshi community. *Emerg. Infect. Dis.*, **13**(7): 1031–37.

Gurley, E.S., Montgomery, J.M., Hossain, M.J., Islam, M.R., *et al.* (2007b). Risk of nosocomial transmission of Nipah virus in a Bangladesh hospital. *Infect. Control. Hosp. Epidemiol.*, **28**(6): 740–42.

Hagmaier, K., Stock, N., Goodbourn, S., Wang, L.F. and Randall, R. (2006). A single amino acid substitution in the V protein of Nipah virus alters its ability to block interferon signalling in cells from different species. *J. Gen. Virol.*, **87**(12): 3649–53.

Halpin, K., Bankamp, B., Harcourt, B.H., Bellini, W.J. and Rota, P.A. (2004). Nipah virus conforms to the rule of six in a minigenome replication assay. *J. Gen. Virol.*, **85**(3), 701–7.

Halpin, K. and Mungall, B.A. (2007). Recent progress in henipavirus research. Comp. Immunol. Microbiol. Infect. *Dis.*, **30**(5–6): 287–307.

Halpin, K., Young, P.L., Field, H. and Mackenzie, J.S. (1999). Newly discovered viruses of flying foxes. *Vet. Microbiol.*, **68**(1–2): 83–87.

Halpin, K., Young, P.L., Field, H.E. and Mackenzie, J.S. (2000). Isolation of Hendra virus from pteropid bats: a natural reservoir of Hendra virus. *J. Gen. Virol.*, **81**(8): 1927–32.

Hanna, J.N., McBride, W.J., Brookes, D.L., *et al.* (2006). Hendra virus infection in a veterinarian. *Med. J. Aust.*, **185**(10): 562–64.

Harcourt, B.H., Lowe, L., Tamin, A., *et al.* (2005). Genetic characterization of Nipah virus, Bangladesh, 2004. *Emerg. Infect. Dis.*, **11**(10): 1594–97.

Harcourt, B.H., Tamin, A., Halpin, K., Ksiazek, T.G., *et al.* (2001). Molecular characterization of the polymerase gene and genomic termini of Nipah virus. *Virology*, **287**(1): 192–201.

Harcourt, B.H., Tamin, A., Ksiazek, T.G., *et al.* (2000). Molecular characterization of Nipah virus, a newly emergent paramyxovirus. *Virology*, **271**(2): 334–49.

Hausmann, S., Garcin, D., Morel, A.S. and Kolakofsky, D. (1999). Two nucleotides immediately upstream of the essential A6G3 slippery sequence modulate the pattern of G insertions during Sendai virus mRNA editing. *J. Virol.*, **73**(1): 343–51.

Hayman, D.T., Suu-Ire, R., Breed, A.C., *et al.* (2008). Evidence of henipavirus infection in West African fruit bats. *PLoS ONE*, **3**(7): e2739.

Hooper, P.T., Gould, A.R., Hyatt, A.D., *et al.* (2000). Identification and molecular characterization of Hendra virus in a horse in Queensland. *Aust. Vet. J.*, **78**(4): 281–82.

Hooper, P.T., Gould, A.R., Russell, G.M., Kattenbelt, J.A. and Mitchell, G. (1996). The retrospective diagnosis of a second outbreak of equine morbillivirus infection. *Aust. Vet. J.*, **74**(3): 244–45.

Hooper, P.T. and Williamson, M.M. (2000). Hendra and Nipah virus infections. *Vet. Clin. North. Am. Equine Pract.*, **16**(3): 597–603, xi.

Horikami, S.M., Smallwood, S. and Moyer, S.A. (1996). The Sendai virus V protein interacts with the NP protein to regulate viral genome RNA replication. *Virology*, **222**(2): 383–90.

Hossain, M.J., Gurley, E.S., Montgomery, J.M., *et al.* (2008). Clinical presentation of nipah virus infection in Bangladesh. *Clin. Infect. Dis.*, **46**(7): 977–84.

Hsu, V.P., Hossain, M.J., Parashar, U.D., Ali, M.M., *et al.* (2004). Nipah virus encephalitis reemergence, Bangladesh. *Emerg. Infect. Dis.*, **10**(12): 2082–87.

Jack, P.J., Boyle, D.B., Eaton, B.T. and Wang, L.F. (2005). The complete genome sequence of J virus reveals a unique genome structure in the family Paramyxoviridae. *J. Virol.*, **79**(16): 10690–700.

Juozapaitis, M., Serva, A., Zvirbliene, A., *et al.* (2007) Generation of henipavirus nucleocapsid proteins in yeast Saccharomyces cerevisiae. *Virus Res.*, **124**(1–2): 95–102.

Kaku, Y., Noguchi, A., Marsh, G.A., *et al.* (2009). A neutralization test for specific detection of Nipah virus antibodies using pseudotyped vesicular stomatitis virus expressing green fluorescent protein. *J. Virol. Meth.*, **160**(1–2): 7–13. Epub 9 May 2009.

Kashiwazaki, Y., Na, Y.N., Tanimura, N. and Imada, T. (2004). A solid-phase blocking ELISA for detection of antibodies to Nipah virus. *J. Virol. Meth.*, **121**(2): 259–61.

Kato, A., Kiyotani, K., Sakai, Y., Yoshida, T. and Nagai, Y. (1997). The paramyxovirus, Sendai virus, V protein encodes a luxury function required for viral pathogenesis. *EMBO J.*, **16**(3): 578–87.

Kirkland, P.D., Love, R.J., Philbey, A.W., Ross, A.D., Davis, R.J. and Hart, K.G. (2001). Epidemiology and control of Menangle virus in pigs. *Aust. Vet. J.*, **79**(3): 199–206.

Kulkarni, S., Volchkova, V., Basler, C.F., Palese, P., *et al.* (2009). Nipah Virus Edits its P Gene at High Frequency to Express the V and W Proteins. *J. Virol.*, **83**: 3982–87.

Lamb, R.A. and Jardetzky, T.S. (2007). Structural basis of viral invasion: lessons from paramyxovirus F. *Curr. Opin. Struct. Biol.*, **17**(4): 427–36.

Lamb, R.A., Kolakofsky, D. (2001). Paramyxoviridae: The Viruses and Their Replication. In: D.M. Knipe, P.M. Howley, *et al.* (eds.), Fields Virology, 4th edn., Vol. 1, pp. 1305–40. Philadelphia: Lippincott Williams & Wilkins.

Lamb, R.A. and Parks, G.D. (2007). Paramyxoviridae: The Viruses and Their Replication. In: H.P. Knipe *et al.* (eds.), Fields Virology, 5th edn., Vol. 1, pp. 449–96. Philadelphia: Lippincott Williams & Wilkins.

Lamb, R.A. *et al.* (1996). Paramyxoviridae; The viruses and their replication. In: H.P. Knipe *et al.* (eds.), Fields Virology, 3th edn., Philadelphia: Lippincott Williams & Wilkins.

Langedijk, J.P., Daus, F.J. and van Oirschot, J.T. (1997). Sequence and structure alignment of Paramyxoviridae attachment proteins and discovery of enzymatic activity for a morbillivirus hemagglutinin. *J. Virol.*, **71**(8): 6155–67.

Lee, J.K., Prussia, A., Paal, T., White, L.K., Snyder, J.P. and Plemper, R.K. (2008). Functional interaction between paramyxovirus fusion and attachment proteins. *J. Biol. Chem.*, **283**(24): 16561–72.

Li, Y., Wang, J., Hickey, A.C., Zhang, Y., *et al.* (2008). Antibodies to Nipah or Nipah-like viruses in bats, China. *Emerg. Infect. Dis.*, **14**(12): 1974–76.

Li, Z., Yu, M., Zhang, H., Magoffin, D.E., *et al.* (2006). Beilong virus, a novel paramyxovirus with the largest genome of non-segmented negative-stranded RNA viruses. *Virology*, **346**(1): 219–28.

Lo, M.K., Harcourt, B.H., Mungall, B.A., *et al.* (2009). Determination of the henipavirus phosphoprotein gene mRNA editing frequencies and detection of the C, V and W proteins of Nipah virus in virus-infected cells. *J. Gen. Virol.*, **90**(2): 398–404.

Lo, M.K. and Rota, P.A. (2008). The emergence of Nipah virus, a highly pathogenic paramyxovirus. *J. Clin. Virol.*, **43**(4): 396–400. Epub Oct 2.

Luby, S.P., Rahman, M., Hossain, M.J., *et al.* (2006). Foodborne transmission of Nipah virus, Bangladesh. *Emerg. Infect. Dis.*, **12**(12): 1888–94.

Ludlow, L.E., Lo, M.K., Rodriguez, J.J., *et al.* (2008). Henipavirus V protein association with Polo-like kinase reveals functional overlap with STAT1 binding and interferon evasion. *J. Virol.*, **82**(13): 6259–71.

Magoffin, D.E., Halpin, K., Rota, P.A. and Wang, L.F. (2007). Effects of single amino acid substitutions at the E residue in the conserved GDNE motif of the Nipah virus polymerase (L) protein. *Arch. Virol.*, **152**(4): 827–32.

Mayo, M.A. and van Regenmortel, M.H. (2000). ICTV and the Virology Division News. *Arch. Virol.*, **145**(9): 1985–88.

McCormack, J.G., Allworth, A.M., Selvey, L.A. and Selleck, P.W. (1999). Transmissibility from horses to humans of a novel paramyxovirus, equine morbillivirus (EMV). *J. Infect.*, **38**(1): 22–23.

McEachern, J.A., Bingham, J., Crameri, G., Green, D.J., *et al.* (2008). A recombinant subunit vaccine formulation protects against lethal Nipah virus challenge in cats. *Vaccine*, **26**(31): 3842–52.

Mebatsion, T., de Vaan, L.T., de Haas, N., Romer-Oberdorfer, A. and Braber, M. (2003). Identification of a mutation in editing of defective Newcastle disease virus recombinants that modulates P-gene mRNA editing and restores virus replication and pathogenicity in chicken embryos. *J. Virol.*, **77**(17): 9259–65.

Melanson, V.R. and Iorio, R.M. (2004). Amino acid substitutions in the F-specific domain in the stalk of the newcastle disease virus HN protein modulate fusion and interfere with its interaction with the F protein. *J. Virol.*, **78**(23): 13053–61.

Melanson, V.R. and Iorio, R.M. (2006). Addition of N-glycans in the stalk of the Newcastle disease virus HN protein blocks its interaction with the F protein and prevents fusion. *J. Virol.*, **80**(2): 623–33.

Michalski, W.P., Crameri, G., Wang, L., Shiell, B.J. and Eaton, B. (2000). The cleavage activation and sites of glycosylation in the fusion protein of Hendra virus. *Virus Res.*, **69**(2): 83–93.

Middleton, D.J., Morrissy, C.J., van der Heide, B.M., *et al.* (2007). Experimental Nipah virus infection in pteropid bats (Pteropus poliocephalus). *J. Comp. Pathol.*, **136**(4): 266–72.

Middleton, D.J., Westbury, H.A., Morrissy, C.J., *et al.* (2002). Experimental Nipah virus infection in pigs and cats. *J. Comp. Pathol.*, **126**(2–3): 124–36.

Mohd, N.M.N., Gan, C.H. and Ong, B.L. (2000). Nipah virus infection of pigs in peninsular Malaysia. *Rev. Sci. Tech. Off. Int. Epiz.*, **19**(1): 160–65.

Mohd Nor, M.N., Gan, C.H. and Ong, B.L. (2000). Nipah virus infection of pigs in peninsular Malaysia. *Rev. Sci. Tech.*, **19**(1): 160–65.

Moll, M., Diederich, S., Klenk, H.D., Czub, M. and Maisner, A. (2004a). Ubiquitous activation of the Nipah virus fusion protein does not require a basic amino acid at the cleavage site. *J. Virol.*, **78**(18): 9705–12.

Moll, M., Kaufmann, A. and Maisner, A. (2004b). Influence of N-glycans on processing and biological activity of the nipah virus fusion protein. *J. Virol.*, **78**(13): 7274–78.

Montgomery, J.M., Hossain, M.J., Gurley, E., *et al.* (2008). Risk factors for Nipah virus encephalitis in Bangladesh. *Emerg. Infect. Dis.*, **14**(10): 1526–32.

Mounts, A.W., Kaur, H., Parashar, U.D., Ksiazek, T.G., *et al.* (2001). A cohort study of health care workers to assess nosocomial transmissibility of Nipah virus, Malaysia, 1999. *J. Infect. Dis.*, **183**(5): 810–13.

Mungall, B.A., Middleton, D., Crameri, G., *et al.* (2006a). Feline model of acute nipah virus infection and protection with a soluble glycoprotein-based subunit vaccine. *J. Virol.*, **80**(24): 12293–302.

Mungall, B.A., Middleton, D., Crameri, G., Bingham, J., *et al.* (2006b). A feline model of acute Nipah virus infection and protection with a soluble glycoprotein-based subunit vaccine. *J. Virol.*, **80**: 12293–302.

Murray, K., Rogers, R., Selvey, L., Selleck, P., *et al.* (1995a). A novel morbillivirus pneumonia of horses and its transmission to humans. *Emerg. Infect. Dis.*, **1**(1): 31–33.

Murray, K., Selleck, P., Hooper, P., Hyatt, A., *et al.* (1995b). A morbillivirus that caused fatal disease in horses and humans. *Science*, **268**(5207): 94–97.

Negrete, O.A., Levroney, E.L., Aguilar, H.C., *et al.* (2005). EphrinB2 is the entry receptor for Nipah virus, an emergent deadly paramyxovirus. *Nature*, **436**(7049): 401–5.

Negrete, O.A., Wolf, M.C., Aguilar, H.C., *et al.* (2006). Two key residues in ephrinB3 critical for its use as an alternative receptor for Nipah virus. *PLoS Pathog.*, **2**(2): e7.

O'Sullivan, J.D., Allworth, A.M., Paterson, D.L., *et al.* (1997). Fatal encephalitis due to novel paramyxovirus transmitted from horses. *Lancet*, **349**(9045): 93–95.

Pager, C.T. and Dutch, R.E. (2005). Cathepsin L is involved in proteolytic processing of the Hendra virus fusion protein. *J. Virol.*, **79**(20): 12714–20.

Parashar, U.D., Sunn, L.M., Ong, F., Mounts, A.W., *et al.* (2000). Case-control study of risk factors for human infection with a new zoonotic paramyxovirus, Nipah virus, during a 1998–1999 outbreak of severe encephalitis in Malaysia. *J. Infect. Dis.*, **181**(5): 1755–59.

Park, M.S., Shaw, M.L., Munoz-Jordan, J., *et al.* (2003). Newcastle disease virus (NDV)-based assay demonstrates interferon-antagonist activity for the NDV V protein and the Nipah virus V, W, and C proteins. *J. Virol.*, **77**(2): 1501–11.

Patch, J.R., Crameri, G., Wang, L.F., Eaton, B.T. and Broder, C.C. (2007). Quantitative analysis of Nipah virus proteins released as virus-like particles reveals central role for the matrix protein. *Virol. J.*, **4**: 1.

Paton, N.I., Leo, Y.S., Zaki, S.R., Auchus, A.P., *et al.* (1999). Outbreak of Nipah-virus infection among abattoir workers in Singapore. *Lancet*, **354**(9186): 1253–56.

Pelet, T., Curran, J. and Kolakofsky, D. (1991). The P gene of bovine parainfluenza virus 3 expresses all three reading frames from a single mRNA editing site. *EMBO J.*, **10**(2): 443–48.

Philbey, A.W., Kirkland, P.D., Ross, A.D., *et al.* (1998). An apparently new virus (family Paramyxoviridae) infectious for pigs, humans, and fruit bats. *Emerg. Infect. Dis.*, **4**(2): 269–71.

Philbey, A.W., Ross, A.D., Kirkland, P.D. and Love, R.J. (2007). Skeletal and neurological malformations in pigs congenitally infected with Menangle virus. *Aust. Vet. J.*, **85**(4): 134–40.

Poch, O., Blumberg, B.M., Bougueleret, L. and Tordo, N. (1990). Sequence comparison of five polymerases (L proteins) of unsegmented negative-strand RNA viruses: theoretical assignment of functional domains. *J. Gen. Virol.*, **71**(5): 1153–62.

Porotto, M., Carta, P., Deng, Y., Kellogg, G.E., *et al.* (2007). Molecular determinants of antiviral potency of paramyxovirus entry inhibitors. *J. Virol.*, **81**(19): 10567–74.

Porotto, M., Doctor, L., Carta, P., Fornabaio, M., *et al.* (2006). Inhibition of hendra virus fusion. *J. Virol.*, **80**(19): 9837–49.

PROMED-MAIL. (2008). Hendra virus, human, equine - Australia (07): (QLD).

PROMED-MAIL. (2008) Nipah virus, fatal - Bangladesh.

Ramasundrum, V., Tan, C.T., Chua, K.B., *et al.* (2000). Kinetics of IgM and Igg seroconversion in Nipah virus infection. *Neurol. J. Southeast Asia*, **5**: 23–28.

Reynes, J.M., Counor, D., Ong, S., Faure, C., *et al.* (2005). Nipah virus in Lyle's flying foxes, Cambodia. *Emerg. Infect. Dis.*, **11**(7): 1042–47.

Rodriguez, J.J., Cruz, C.D. and Horvath, C.M. (2004). Identification of the nuclear export signal and STAT-binding domains of the Nipah virus V protein reveals mechanisms underlying interferon evasion. *J. Virol.*, **78**(10): 5358–67.

Rodriguez, J.J., Parisien, J.P. and Horvath, C.M. (2002). Nipah virus V protein evades alpha and gamma interferons by preventing STAT1 and STAT2 activation and nuclear accumulation. *J. Virol.*, **76**(22): 11476–83.

Sarji, S.A., Abdullah, B.J., Goh, K.J., Tan, C.T. and Wong, K.T. (2000). MR imaging features of Nipah encephalitis. *Am. J. Roentgenol.*, **175**(2): 437–42.

Sawatsky, B., Grolla, A., Kuzenko, N., Weingartl, H. and Czub, M. (2007). Inhibition of henipavirus infection by Nipah virus attachment glycoprotein occurs without cell-surface downregulation of ephrin-B2 or ephrin-B3. *J. Gen. Virol.*, **88**(2): 582–91.

Sejvar, J.J., Hossain, J., Saha, S.K., Gurley, E.S., Banu, S., *et al.* (2007). Long-term neurological and functional outcome in Nipah virus infection. *Ann. Neurol.*, **62**(3): 235–42.

Selvey, L.A., Wells, R.M., McCormack, J.G., *et al.* (1995). Infection of humans and horses by a newly described morbillivirus. *Med. J. Aust.*, **162**(12): 642–45.

Sendow, I., Field, H.E., Curran, J., *et al.* (2006). Henipavirus in Pteropus vampyrus Bats, Indonesia. *Emerg. Infect. Dis.*, **12**(4): 711–12.

Shaw, M.L., Cardenas, W.B., Zamarin, D., Palese, P. and Basler, C.F. (2005). Nuclear localization of the Nipah virus W protein allows for inhibition of both virus- and toll-like receptor 3-triggered signaling pathways. *J. Virol.*, **79**(10): 6078–88.

Shaw, M.L., Garcia-Sastre, A., Palese, P. and Basler, C.F. (2004). Nipah virus V and W proteins have a common STAT1-binding domain yet inhibit STAT1 activation from the cytoplasmic and nuclear compartments, respectively. *J. Virol.*, **78**(11): 5633–41.

Sleeman, K., Bankamp, B., Hummel, K.B., Lo, M.K., *et al.* (2008). The C, V and W proteins of Nipah virus inhibit minigenome replication. *J. Gen. Virol.*, **89**(5): 1300–1308.

Swenson, D.L., Warfield, K.L., Negley, D.L., *et al.* (2005). Virus-like particles exhibit potential as a pan-filovirus vaccine for both Ebola and Marburg viral infections. *Vaccine*, **23**(23): 3033–42.

Tamin, A., Harcourt, B.H., Ksiazek, T.G., *et al.* (2002). Functional properties of the fusion and attachment glycoproteins of Nipah virus. *Virology*, **296**(1): 190–200.

Tamin, A., Harcourt, B.H., Lo, M.K., *et al.* (2009). Development of a neutralization assay for Nipah virus using pseudotype particles. *J. Virol. Meth.*, **60**(1–2): 1–6. .

Tan, W.S., Ong, S.T., Eshaghi, M., Foo, S.S. and Yusoff, K. (2004). Solubility, immunogenicity and physical properties of the nucleocapsid protein of Nipah virus produced in Escherichia coli. *J. Med. Virol.*, **73**(1): 105–12.

Tanimura, N., Imada, T., Kashiwazaki, Y., Shahirudin, S., *et al.* (2004a). Monoclonal antibody-based immunohistochemical diagnosis of Malaysian Nipah virus infection in pigs. *J. Comp. Pathol.*, **131**(2–3): 199–206.

Tanimura, N., Imada, T., Kashiwazaki, Y., *et al.* (2004b). Reactivity of anti-Nipah virus monoclonal antibodies to formalin-fixed, paraffin-embedded lung tissues from experimental Nipah and Hendra virus infections. *J. Vet. Med. Sci.*, **66**(10): 1263–66.

Thomas, S.M., Lamb, R.A. and Paterson, R.G. (1988). Two mRNAs that differ by two nontemplated nucleotides encode the amino coterminal proteins P and V of the paramyxovirus SV5. *Cell*, **54**(6): 891–902.

Tidona, C.A., Kurz, H.W., Gelderblom, H.R. and Darai, G. (1999). Isolation and molecular characterization of a novel cytopathogenic paramyxovirus from tree shrews. *Virology*, **258**(2): 425–34.

Vanchiere, J.A., Bellini, W.J. and Moyer, S.A. (1995). Hypermutation of the phosphoprotein and altered mRNA editing in the hamster neurotropic strain of measles virus. *Virology*, **207**(2): 555–61.

Vidal, S., Curran, J. and Kolakofsky, D. (1990). Editing of the Sendai virus P/C mRNA by G insertion occurs during mRNA synthesis via a virus-encoded activity. *J. Virol.*, **64**(1): 239–46.

Vogt, C., Eickmann, M., Diederich, S., Moll, M. and Maisner, A. (2005). Endocytosis of the Nipah virus glycoproteins. *J. Virol.*, **79**(6): 3865–72.

Wacharapluesadee, S. and Hemachudha, T. (2007). Duplex nested RT-PCR for detection of Nipah virus RNA from urine specimens of bats. *J. Virol. Meth.*, **141**(1): 97–101.

Wacharapluesadee, S., Lumlertdacha, B., Boongird, K., *et al.* (2005). Bat Nipah virus, Thailand. *Emerg. Infect. Dis.*, **11**(12): 1949–51.

Wang, L., Harcourt, B.H., Yu, M., Tamin, A., Rota, P.A., *et al.* (2001). Molecular biology of Hendra and Nipah viruses. *Microbes Infect.*, **3**(4): 279–87.

Wang, L.F., Michalski, W.P., Yu, M., Pritchard, L. I., *et al.* (1998). A novel P/V/C gene in a new member of the paramyxoviridae family, which causes lethal infection in humans, horses, aand other animals. *J. Virol.*, **72**: 1482–90.

Wang, L.F., Yu, M., Hansson, E., Pritchard, L.I., Shiell, B., *et al.* (2000). The exceptionally large genome of Hendra virus: support for creation of a new genus within the family Paramyxoviridae. *J. Virol.*, **74**(21): 9972–79.

Wang, X., Ge, J., Hu, S., Wang, Q., Wen, Z., Chen, H. and Bu, Z. (2006). Efficacy of DNA immunization with F and G protein genes of Nipah virus. *Ann. NY Acad. Sci.*, **1081**: 243–45.

Weingartl, H., Czub, S., Copps, J., Berhane, Y., *et al.* (2005). Invasion of the central nervous system in a porcine host by nipah virus. *J. Virol.*, **79**(12): 7528–34.

Weingartl, H.M., Berhane, Y., Caswell, J.L., Loosmore, S., *et al.* (2006). Recombinant nipah virus vaccines protect pigs against challenge. *J. Virol.*, **80**(16): 7929–38.

Williamson, M.M., Hooper, P.T., Selleck, P.W., *et al.* (1998). Transmission studies of Hendra virus (equine morbillivirus) in fruit bats, horses and cats. *Aust. Vet. J.*, **76**(12): 813–18.

Williamson, M.M., Hooper, P.T., Selleck, P.W., Westbury, H.A. and Slocombe, R.F. (2000). Experimental hendra virus infectionin pregnant guinea-pigs and fruit Bats (Pteropus poliocephalus). *J. Comp. Pathol.*, **122**(2–3): 201–7.

Witko, S.E., Kotash, C., Sidhu, M.S., Udem, S.A. and Parks, C.L. (2006). Inhibition of measles virus minireplicon-encoded reporter gene expression by V protein. *Virology*, **348**(1): 107–19.

World Health Organization (2001). Nipah virus. Fact sheet N0 262 [Web Page] 2001 Sep.

World Health Organization (2004a). Nipah-like virus in Bangladesh-update [Web page] 2004 Feb 26.

World Health Organization (2004b). Nipah-like virus in Bangladesh [Web Page] 2004 Feb 12.

World Health Organization (2004c) Nipah virus outbreak(s) in Bangladesh, January–April 2004. *Wkly. Epidemiol, Rec.*, **79**(17): 168–71.

Wong, K.T., Shieh, W.J., Kumar, S., *et al.* (2002). Nipah virus infection: pathology and pathogenesis of an emerging paramyxoviral zoonosis. *Am. J. Pathol.*, **161**(6): 2153–67.

Xu, K., Rajashankar, K.R., Chan, Y.P., Himanen, J.P., *et al.* (2008). Host cell recognition by the henipaviruses: crystal structures of the Nipah G attachment glycoprotein and its complex with ephrin-B3. *Proc. Natl. Acad. Sci. USA*, **105**(29): 9953–58.

Yaiw, K.C., Bingham, J., Crameri, G., *et al.* (2008). Tioman virus, a paramyxovirus of bat origin, causes mild disease in pigs and has a predilection for lymphoid tissues. *J. Virol.*, **82**(1): 565–68.

Yaiw, K.C., Crameri, G., Wang, L., Chong, H.T., *et al.* (2007). Serological evidence of possible human infection with Tioman virus, a newly described paramyxovirus of bat origin. *J. Infect. Dis.*, **196**(6): 884–86.

Yob, J.M., Field, H., Rashdi, A.M., Morrissy, C., *et al.* (2001). Nipah virus infection in bats (order Chiroptera) in peninsular Malaysia. *Emerg. Infect. Dis.*, **7**(3): 439–41.

Yoneda, M., Guillaume, V., Ikeda, F., Sakuma, Y., *et al.* (2006). Establishment of a Nipah virus rescue system. *Proc. Natl. Acad. Sci. USA*, **103**(44): 16508–13.

Yu, F., Khairullah, N.S., Inoue, S., Balasubramaniam, V., *et al.* (2006). Serodiagnosis using recombinant nipah virus nucleocapsid protein expressed in Escherichia coli. *J. Clin. Microbiol.*, **44**(9): 3134–38.

Yu, M., Hansson, E., Langedijk, J.P., Eaton, B.T. and Wang, L.F. (1998). The attachment protein of Hendra virus has high structural similarity but limited primary sequence homology compared with viruses in the genus Paramyxovirus. *Virology*, **251**(2): 227–33.

Zhu, Z., Bossart, K.N., Bishop, K.A., Crameri, G., *et al.* (2008). Exceptionally potent cross-reactive neutralization of Nipah and Hendra viruses by a human monoclonal antibody. *J. Infect. Dis.*, **197**(6): 846–53.

Zhu, Z., Dimitrov, A.S., Bossart, K.N., Crameri, G., *et al.* (2006). Potent neutralization of Hendra and Nipah viruses by human monoclonal antibodies. *J. Virol.*, **80**(2): 891–99.

CHAPTER 41

Hepatitis E virus

X. J. Meng[1]

Summary

Hepatitis E virus (HEV) is a small, non-enveloped, single-strand, positive-sense RNA virus of approximately 7.2 kb in size. HEV is classified in the family *Hepeviridae* consisting of four recognized major genotypes that infect humans and other animals. Genotypes 1 and 2 HEV are restricted to humans and often associated with large outbreaks and epidemics in developing countries with poor sanitation conditions, whereas genotypes 3 and 4 HEV infect humans, pigs and other animal species and are responsible for sporadic cases of hepatitis E in both developing and industrialized countries. The avian HEV associated with Hepatitis-Splenomegaly syndrome in chickens is genetically and antigenically related to mammalian HEV, and likely represents a new genus in the family. There exist three openreading frames (ORF) in HEV genome: ORF1 encodes non-structural proteins, ORF2 encodes the capsid protein, and the ORF3 encodes a small phosphoprotein. ORF2 and ORF3 are translated from a single bicistronic mRNA, and overlap each other but neither overlaps ORF1. Due to the lack of an efficient cell culture system and a practical animal model for HEV, the mechanisms of HEV replication and pathogenesis are poorly understood. The recent identification and characterization of animal strains of HEV from pigs and chickens and the demonstrated ability of cross-species infection by these animal strains raise potential public health concerns for zoonotic HEV transmission. It has been shown that the genotypes 3 and 4 HEV strains from pigs can infect humans, and vice versa. Accumulating evidence indicated that hepatitis E is a zoonotic disease, and swine and perhaps other animal species are reservoirs for HEV. A vaccine against HEV is not yet available.

Introduction

Hepatitis E accounts for a significant proportion of enterically transmitted form of viral hepatitis in humans (Purcell and Emerson 2001). The disease is an important public health problem in many developing countries of Asia and Africa, and is also endemic in many industrialized countries including the USA and several European countries (Meng 2008). Although the overall mortality of hepatitis E is less than 1% in the general population, it can reach up to 28% in infected pregnant women (Purcell and Emerson 2001). The causative agent, hepatitis E virus (HEV), is transmitted primarily via the faecal-oral route through contaminated water or food. In industrialized countries, acute cases of hepatitis E were reported in travellers returning from endemic regions although sporadic cases have also been reported in patients with no known epidemiological risk factors (Clemente-Casares *et al.* 2003). In developing countries with poor sanitation conditions, rare outbreaks of acute hepatitis E in more explosive epidemic form are generally associated with faecal contamination of drinking water (Arankalle *et al.* 1995; Purcell and Emerson 2001).

The recent discoveries of animal strains of HEV, swine hepatitis E virus (swine HEV) from pigs in 1997 (Meng *et al.* 1997) and avian hepatitis E virus (avian HEV) from chickens in 2001 (Haqshenas *et al.* 2001), and the existence of other animal species that are seropositive for IgG anti-HEV (Meng 2006; Meng and Halbur 2006; Meng *et al.* 2008), have broadened the host ranges and diversity of the virus. Accumulating evidences indicate that hepatitis E is a zoonotic disease, and domestic pigs, wild boars and maybe other animal species are reservoirs for HEV. The ubiquitous nature of the virus in domestic pigs and wild boars as well as in other animal species raises public health concern for zoonoses and food safety.

History

Human HEV

In 1980, seroepidemiological studies of waterborne epidemics of hepatitis originally thought to be caused by hepatitis A virus (HAV) in India revealed that the patients were negative for antibodies to HAV, thus providing evidence for the existence of a new form of enterically transmitted viral hepatitis which was later designated as hepatitis E (Purcell and Emerson 2001). Successful transmission of viral hepatitis E to a human volunteer via faecal-oral route with a stool sample collected from a hepatitis E patient was demonstrated in 1983, and virus-like particles were detected in the stool of the infected volunteer (Balayan *et al.* 1983). However, the causative agent, hepatitis E virus (HEV), was not identified until 1990 when its complete genome was cloned and sequenced (Tam *et al.* 1991). Thus far HEV still could not be efficiently propagated in cell culture system, and this has greatly hindered our understanding of its biology and pathogenesis.

[1] This chapter was originally published in Veterinary Microbiology journal (Meng, X.J., 2010. Hepatitis E virus: Animal reservoirs and zoonotic risk. Veterinary Microbiology, 140, 256–265) and is reproduced with the kind permission of the author and Elsevier Publishing Group.

Swine HEV

Balayan *et al.* (1990) reported an experimental infection of domestic swine with an Asian strain of human HEV, and thus providing the first experimental evidence of HEV infections in pigs. However, a retrospective study revealed that the virus infecting the pigs in that study was not a human HEV but rather a strain of swine origin (Lu *et al.* 2004). Subsequently, two independent laboratories in the US failed to reproduce HEV infections in pigs using a well-characterized genotype 1 Asian strain (Sar-55) and a genotype 2 Mexican strain (Mex-14) of human HEV (Meng 2003). Detections of HEV antibodies and RNA were also reported from pigs in Nepal in 1995, although the identity of the virus infecting the Nepalese pigs was not known (Clayson *et al.* 1995). In 1997, the first animal strain of HEV, swine HEV, was identified and characterized from pigs in the US (Meng *et al.* 1997). The authors serendipitously found out that the majority of adult pigs in the US were positive for IgG anti-HEV, suggesting that the pigs were exposed to a HEV-related agent. To identify the agent responsible for the seropositivity in pigs, a prospective study was conducted in a commercial swine farm in Illinois (Meng *et al.* 1997). Twenty piglets born to both IgG anti-HEV seronegative and seropositive sows in a swine farm were monitored for more than 5 months for evidence of HEV infection. By 21 weeks of age, 16 of the 20 piglets monitored in this prospective study had seroconverted to IgG anti-HEV, and subsequently a novel virus genetically and antigenically closely related to human HEV, designated swine HEV, was molecularly cloned and characterized from the naturally infected piglets. Koch's postulates were fulfilled as specific-pathogen-free (SPF) pigs were experimentally infected with swine HEV, and the same virus was recovered from experimentally infected pigs (Meng *et al.* 1998).

Avian HEV

Payne *et al.* (1999) reported a HEV-related virus associated with big liver and spleen disease (BLS) in chickens from Australia. The BLS disease affects commercial broiler breeder flocks and causes decreased egg production and slight increase in mortality. Based upon the sequence of a 523 bp fragment of the BLS virus (BLSV), it was found that BLSV shared approximately 62% nucleotide sequence identity with human HEV (Payne *et al.* 1999). In the USA and Canada, a disease known as Hepatitis-Splenomegaly (HS) syndrome with no known cause was also reported. Bacteria could not be routinely isolated from affected livers, and toxins or bacterins were ruled out as the cause of the HS syndrome. Haqshenas *et al.* (2001) first isolated and characterized a virus genetically and antigenically related to human HEV from bile samples of chickens with HS Syndrome in the USA States. Based upon the similar genomic organization and significant sequence identities with human and swine HEVs, the novel virus in chickens is designated as avian HEV to distinguish it from the mammalian HEV. Avian HEV shared approximately 80% nucleotide sequence identity with the Australian BLSV (Haqshenas *et al.* 2001), suggesting that BLS in Australia and HS syndrome in North America are likely caused by variant strains of the same virus.

The infectious agent

Virion properties

HEV is an icosahedral, non-enveloped, spherical virus particle with a diameter of approximately 32–34 nm in size. The open reading frame 2 (ORF2) encodes the only known structural protein, the capsid protein (Purcell and Emerson 2001). It has been demonstrated that a N-terminally truncated capsid protein containing amino acid residues 112660 can self-assemble into empty virus-like particles when expressed in baculovirus (Li *et al.* 2005a). The buoyant density of HEV virions is reportedly 1.35–1.40 g/cm^3 in CsCL, and 1.29 g/cm^3 in potassium tartrate and glycerol. HEV virion is sensitive to low-temperature storage and iodinated disinfectants (Purcell and Emerson 2001). Recently, Emerson *et al.* (2005) showed that HEV virion is more heat labile than is HAV: HAV was only 50% inactivated at 60 8C for 1 h but was almost totally inactivated at 66 8C; in contrast, HEV was about 50% inactivated at 56 8C and almost totally inactivated (96%) at 60 8C. It has been demonstrated that the *in vivo* infectivity of HEV present in commercial pig livers is completely inactivated by adequate cooking such as frying or boiling the contaminated pig livers for 5 min, however incubation of the HEV-contaminated pig liver homogenates at 56C for 1 hour did not abolish the virus infectivity (Feagins *et al.* 2008a). It is believed that HEV is resistant to inactivation by acidic and mild alkaline conditions in the intestinal tract, and thus facilitating the faecal-oral route of transmission (Purcell and Emerson 2001).

Classification

Based upon its superficial similarity in morphology and genomic organization to that of caliciviruses, HEV was originally classified in the family *Caliciviridae* (Purcell and Emerson 2001). However, subsequent studies showed that HEV does not share significant sequence homology or codon usage with caliciviruses. For example, at the 5' end of the viral genome, HEV has a Cap structure (Kabrane-Lazizi *et al.* 1999a) whereas caliciviruses contains a VPg. Therefore, HEV was officially declassified from the family *Caliciviridae*, and was placed in a new genus *Hepevirus* of the proposed family *Hepeviridae* (Emerson *et al.* 2004). Currently, there are four recognized major genotypes of HEV within the genus *Hepevirus* (Meng 2008; Okamoto, 2007): genotype 1 (primarily Burmese-like Asian strains of human HEV), genotype 2 (a Mexican strain of human HEV and recent African strains of human HEV) (Nicand *et al.* 2005), genotype 3 (human HEV strains from sporadic cases in industrialized countries, and swine HEV strains from pigs in both developing and industrialized countries), and genotype 4 (variant strains of human HEV from sporadic cases in Asia, and swine HEV strains from pigs in both developing and industrialized countries). The avian HEV from chickens is genetically very divergent from mammalian HEV strains sharing only approximately 50% nucleotide sequence identity, and thus avian HEV likely represents a yet-to-be-named separate genus within the family *Hepeviridae* (Meng *et al.* 2008) (Fig. 41.1). Despite the extensive nucleotide sequence variations between mammalian HEV and avian HEV, however, it appears that there exists a single serotype (Guo *et al.* 2006; Meng 2006).

Genome organization

The genome of mammalian HEV is a single-stranded, positive-sense, RNA molecule of approximately 7.2 kb consisting of a short 5' non-coding region (NCR), three ORFs (ORFs 1, 2 and 3), and a 3' NCR (Tam *et al.* 1991). ORF2 overlaps ORF3, but neither overlaps with ORF1. The ORF1 at the 5' end encodes non-structural polyproteins. Based upon computer predictions and analogy with other positive-strand RNA viruses, numerous functional domains

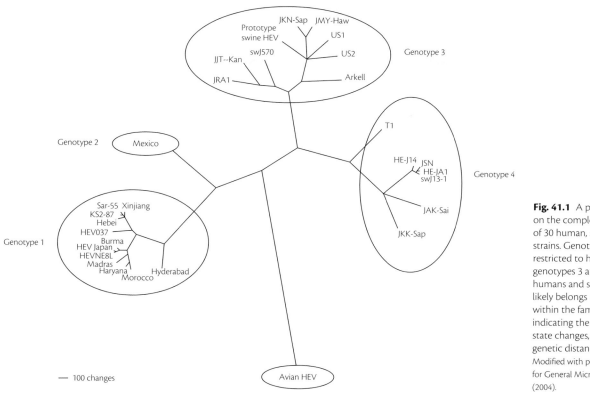

Fig. 41.1 A phylogenetic tree based on the complete genomic sequences of 30 human, swine, and avian HEV strains. Genotypes 1 and 2 HEV are restricted to humans, whereas genotypes 3 and 4 HEV infect both humans and swine. The avian HEV likely belongs to a separate genus within the family. A scale bar, indicating the number of character state changes, is proportional to the genetic distance.
Modified with permission by the Society for General Microbiology from Huang *et al.* (2004).

including methyltransferases, papain-like cysteine proteases, helicases and RNA-dependent RNA polymerases were identified in the ORF1 (Huang *et al.* 2007). The ORF2 encodes the capsid protein that contains immunogenic epitopes, induces neutralizing antibodies, and is the target for vaccine development (Meng 2008). The ORF3 encodes a small cytoskeleton-associated phosphoprotein with unknown function (Zafrullah *et al.* 1997). The N-terminus of ORF3 has a cysteine-rich region, binds to HEV RNA, and enters into a complex with the capsid protein. The C-terminal region of the ORF3 protein is a multifunctional domain, and may be involved in HEV virion morphogenesis and viral pathogenesis. Monoclonal antibodies raised against the ORF3 protein can capture HEV particles in culture supernatant and serum but not those in faeces suggesting that the ORF3 protein is present on the surface of HEV virions newly released from infected cells (Takahashi *et al.* 2008). ORF3 antigen has been used in a serological assay to detect HEV antibodies (Herremans *et al.* 2007).

Avian HEV is morphologically and genetically related to the mammalian HEV. The genome of avian HEV is only about 6.6 kb in length, which is approximately 600 bp shorter than that of mammalian HEV. Although avian HEV shares only about 50% nucleotide sequence identity with mammalian HEV across the entire genome, the genomic organization and functional motifs are relatively conserved between avian and mammalian HEV (Haqshenas *et al.* 2001; Huang *et al.* 2004). Antigenic epitopes in the capsid protein that are unique to avian HEV as well as common between mammalian HEV and avian HEV have been identified (Guo *et al.* 2006). Phylogenetic analyses indicated that avian HEV is distinct from mammalian HEV, and thus likely belongs to a

separate genus within the family (Meng 2008). Additional sequences of avian HEV isolates from different geographic regions of the world will help more definitively classify avian HEV as a separate genus (Peralta *et al.* 2008).

Replication strategy

The mechanisms of HEV replication, transcription and translation are largely unknown due to the lack of an efficient cell culture system for HEV. A bicistronic subgenomic mRNA was identified by using an *in vitro* HEV replicon system, and found to encode both ORF2 and ORF3 proteins (Graff *et al.* 2006). Subgenomic mRNAs were also detected in HEV-infected liver tissues (Purcell and Emerson 2001). The ORF3 gene contains a *cis*-reactive element and is translated from the third in-frame AUG codon in the ORF1/ORF2 intergenic region (Huang *et al.* 2007). It has been demonstrated that the ORF3 encodes a protein that is essential for virus infectivity *in vivo* (Huang *et al.* 2007), although the expression of ORF3 protein is not required for virus replication, virion assembly or infection of liver cells *in vitro* (Emerson *et al.* 2006). The translation and posttranslational processes of the ORF1 polyprotein remain largely unknown (Meng 2008). When expressed in baculovirus, the ORF1 polyprotein was reportedly processed into smaller proteins that correlate with predicted functional domains in ORF1. However, when the ORF1 polyprotein was expressed in bacterial or mammalian expression system, no processing of the ORF1 polyprotein was detected. A proline-rich hyper-variable region within the ORF1 of HEV is found to be dispensable for HEV replication both *in vitro* and *in vivo* (Pudupakam *et al.* 2009), although the biological and pathological significance of this region is not yet known.

Diseases in animals and man

Epidemiology

In humans, hepatitis E is endemic in both industrialized and developing countries worldwide. Epidemics, however, only occurs in developing countries of Asia, Africa and in Mexico. The epidemics are usually associated with HEV-contaminated drinking water, whereas the risk factors associated with endemic cases are often difficult to identify although contaminated shellfish, animal meats and direct contacts with infected animals have been linked to sporadic cases of acute hepatitis E in both developing and industrialized countries (Meng 2003, 2006; Purcell and Emerson 2001). The prevalence of IgG anti-HEV is very high in some developing countries such as Egypt with more than 70% of the general population positive for IgG anti-HEV (Stoszek et al. 2006). Surprisingly, IgG anti-HEV prevalence in some industrialized countries is much higher than expected: for example, in some regions of the USA, up to 30% of the normal blood donors were positive for IgG anti-HEV (Drobeniuc et al. 2001; Meng et al. 2002). The source of the relatively high seropositivity in individuals from industrialized countries is unknown but zoonotic transmissions through contacts with animals or consumption of contaminated animal meats are suspected (Meng 2006). The disease has a higher attack rate in young adults, although the seroprevalence is age-dependent and appears to increase with ages (Arankalle et al. 1995).

In pigs, swine HEV infection is widespread in swine farms worldwide from both developing and industrialized countries, regardless of whether HEV is endemic in the respective human populations (Meng 2003; Meng and Halbur 2006). The infection in pigs generally occurs at about 2–3 months of age. Infected pigs generally have a transient viremia lasting for 1–2 weeks, and shed viruses in faeces for about 3–7 weeks. The majority of adult pigs including sows and boars, although mostly positive for IgG anti-HEV, are free of virus shedding. Sequence analyses of swine HEV isolates identified thus far revealed that there exist at least two genotypes of swine HEV worldwide, genotypes 3 and 4, both of which are known to cause sporadic cases of hepatitis E in humans (Meng 2003; Meng and Halbur 2006). Like human HEV, the transmission route for swine HEV is presumably faecal-oral. Faeces from infected pigs contain large amount of infectious virus, and are likely the main source of virus for transmission. It is believed that pigs acquire infection through direct contact with infected pigs or through ingestion of faeces-contaminated feed or water (Bouwknegt et al. 2008). However, experimental reproduction of swine HEV infection in pigs via the oral route of inoculation has been difficult (Kasorndorkbua et al. 2004; Bouwknegt et al. 2008), even though pigs can be readily infected with swine HEV via the intravenous route of inoculation. Other route(s) of transmission cannot be ruled out. Since faeces from infected pigs contain large amounts of virus and thus, swine manure and faeces could contaminate irrigation or coastal waters, and thus leading to possible contamination of produce or shellfish (Meng and Halbur 2006). HEV strains of swine origins have been detected in sewage water, and consumption of contaminated shellfish has been implicated in sporadic cases of acute hepatitis E (Meng and Halbur 2006).

In chickens, HS syndrome associated with avian HEV infection was first reported in western Canada in 1991, but the disease has now been reported in eastern Canada and the USA (Meng et al. 2008). BLS associated with avian HEV infection has been reported from chickens in Australia, and serological evidence of avian HEV infection was also reported in the UK Kingdom and Spain (Peralta et al. 2008). Leghorn hens in cages are typically affected although the disease has also been recognized in broiler breeder hens. In the USA, avian HEV infection is enzootic in chicken flocks. A recent serosurvey of 1276 chickens of different ages and breeds from 76 different flocks in five states showed that approximately 71% chicken flocks and 30% chickens in the USA were positive for antibodies to avian HEV (Huang et al. 2002). Like human and swine HEV, the seroprevalence in chickens appears to be age-dependant: approximately 17% of young chickens of less than 18 weeks of age and 36% of adult chickens were positive for avian HEV-specific antibodies (Huang et al. 2002). Transmission of avian HEV within and between chicken flocks appears to occur readily. In a prospective study of natural avian HEV infection in a chicken flock, all 14 chickens monitored in the study were seronegative at 12 weeks of age. The first chicken became seroconverted at 13 weeks of age, and by 21 weeks of age, all 14 chickens in the flock had seroconverted (Sun et al. 2004a). Like mammalian HEVs, the transmission route for avian HEV is presumably faecal-oral, and experimental avian HEV infection has been successfully reproduced via oronasal route inoculation of SPF chickens (Billam et al. 2005), although other routes of transmission cannot be ruled out. In addition to chickens, young turkeys experimentally inoculated with avian HEV also became infected. However, attempts to experimentally infect rhesus monkeys and mice with avian HEV were unsuccessful (Meng et al. 2008). There is no known carrier or vector implicated in the transmission of avian HEV, although rodents in the chicken farms might serve as a mechanical carrier (Sun and Meng, unpublished data).

Clinical signs and pathological lesions

The histopathological lesions are similar in humans, pigs and chickens infected by different strains of HEV, although the manifestation of clinical diseases varies in different species.

In humans, not all HEV-infected individuals develop overt clinical disease. For examples, a significant proportion of individuals in many industrialized countries are seropositive for HEV antibodies, although these individuals had no known history of hepatic diseases (Drobeniuc et al. 2001; Meng et al. 2002). It is known that hepatitis E is a dose-dependant disease: patients exposed to higher doses of HEV often develop clinical symptoms of hepatitis E whereas patients exposed to lower doses of the virus generally had only subclinical infections (Purcell and Emerson 2001). The incubation period ranges from 2 weeks to 2 months. Patients generally have jaundice, anorexia, and hepatomegaly, and approximately 50% of the patients will also have abdominal pains and tenderness, nausea, vomiting and fever (Purcell and Emerson 2001). The disease in many industrialized countries is sporadic in nature, although rare outbreaks do occur in developing countries. A unique feature of HEV infection is the observed high mortality during pregnancy in women. However, under experimental conditions, pregnant sows infected with swine HEV at various stages of gestation had no clinical signs of hepatitis or elevation of liver enzymes (Meng and Halbur 2006). Similarly, pregnant rhesus monkeys experimentally infected with human HEV did not manifest more severe hepatitis than the non-pregnant monkeys either (Tsarev et al. 1995). The observed severe and fulminant hepatitis in infected pregnant women could not be experimentally reproduced in pregnant pigs or rhesus monkeys experimentally infected with HEV.

In pigs, swine HEV infection is ubiquitous essentially in all swine-producing regions worldwide (Meng 2003; Meng and Halbur 2006). Pigs naturally infected with swine HEV are asymptomatic. In a prospective study of naturally infected piglets in a farm from the USA, gross pathological lesions were not detected in the liver or 18 other tissues and organs in four pigs necropsied during early stages of swine HEV infection (Meng et al. 1997), although all four piglets had microscopic evidence of hepatitis characterized by mild to moderate multifocal and periportal lymphoplasmacytic hepatitis with mild focal hepatocellular necrosis. Similar to natural infections, pigs experimentally infected with swine HEV and a genotype 3 strain of human HEV had no clinical signs (Halbur et al. 2001), although the infected pigs did have mildly to moderately enlarged hepatic and mesenteric lymph nodes from 7 to 55 days postinoculation (DPI). Histological lesions including mild-to-moderate multifocal lymphoplasmacytic hepatitis, and focal hepatocellular necrosis were also observed.

In chickens, the morbidity and mortality of HS syndrome (or BLS) associated with avian HEV infection in the field are relatively low, although subclinical infections of avian HEV are very common in chicken flocks in the USA and perhaps in other countries as well (Huang et al. 2002; Sun et al. 2004a: Peralta et al. 2008). HS syndrome is characterized by above-normal mortality in broiler breeder hens and laying hens of 30–72 week of age, with the highest incidence occurring between 40–50 weeks of age. Prior to death, clinical sign is generally not recognized in chickens with HS syndrome. In some (but not all) cases, a drop in egg production of up to 20% was observed. Weekly mortality increases to approximately 0.3% for several weeks during the middle of the production period and may sometimes exceed 1.0%. Similar to HS syndrome, the clinical signs for BLS in Australia also vary from subclinical infection to egg drops that may reach 20% with up to 1% mortality per week over a period of 3–4 weeks (Meng et al. 2008). Affected flocks in the USA, Canada and Europe appear to have milder or subclinical infections compared to those in Australia. Dead chickens associated with avian HEV infection usually have regressive ovaries, red fluid in the abdomen, and enlarged liver and spleen. Livers are enlarged with haemorrhage and may have subcapsular hematomas. Spleens from affected birds are mild to severely enlarged. Microscopically, liver lesions varied from multifocal haemorrhage to extensive areas of necrosis and haemorrhage and infiltration of heterophils and mononuclear inflammatory cells around portal triads (Meng et al. 2008). Under experimental conditions, gross lesions characteristic of HS syndrome including subcapsular haemorrhages and slightly enlarged right intermediate lobe of the livers were reproduced in approximately one-fourth of the SPF chickens experimentally infected with avian HEV (Billam et al. 2005). Foci of lymphocytic periphlebitis and phlebitis were the characteristic histological lesions in livers. There was no significant elevation of serum levels of liver enzymes AST, albumin/globulin (A/G) ratios or bile acids. However, LDH levels behaved differently over time (Billam et al. 2005).

Hepatitis E as a zoonotic disease

Hepatitis E is now considered as a zoonotic disease, and domestic pigs and wild boars are reservoirs for HEV (Meng 2006). Pig farmers, swine veterinarians and other pig handlers in both developing and industrialized countries have been shown to be at increased risk of HEV infection. Meng et al. (2002) tested a total of 465 swine veterinarians for IgG anti-HEV prevalence using recombinant capsid antigens from swine HEV and a genotype 1 strain of human HEV. Among the 295 swine veterinarians from 8 USA from which 400 age- and geography-matched normal USA blood donors were available, approximately 23% (swine HEV antigen) or 27% (human HEV antigen) of swine veterinarians were positive for IgG anti-HEV compared to only 17% (swine HEV antigen) or 18% (human HEV antigen) in normal blood donors. Swine veterinarians in the USA were 1.51 times (swine HEV antigen, p = 0.03) and 1.46 times (human HEV antigen, $p = 0.06$) more likely to be anti-HEV positive than normal U.S. blood donors. Veterinarians who reported having needle sticks while performing procedures on pigs were about 1.9 times more likely to be seropositive than those who did not. Also, individuals from traditionally major swine States appear to be more likely seropositive than those from traditionally non-swine States: for example, subjects from Minnesota, a major swine State, are approximately 5–6 times more likely to be seropositive than those from Alabama, which is traditionally not a major swine State. Drobeniuc et al. (2001) also determined the IgG anti-HEV prevalence in 264 swine farmers and 255 control subjects in Moldova, and found that approximately 51% of swine farmers were positive for IgG anti-HEV, whereas only 25% of control subjects with no occupational exposure to swine were seropositive. Withers et al. (2002) reported that swine workers in North Carolina had a 4.5-fold higher IgG anti-HEV prevalence rate (10.9%) than the control subjects (2.4%).

Sporadic and cluster cases of acute hepatitis E due to the consumption of raw or undercooked pig livers have been reported in patients from Japan. It has been shown that approximately 2% of the pig livers sold in local grocery stores in Japan (Yazaki et al. 2003) and 11% in the USA (Feagins et al. 2007) were positive for swine HEV RNA. Most importantly, the contaminating virus in commercial pig livers sold in local grocery stores from the USA States remains fully infectious when inoculated into pigs (Feagins et al. 2007). The virus sequences recovered from pig livers in grocery stores are closely related, or identical in some cases, to the viruses recovered from human hepatitis E patients in Japan (Yazaki et al. 2003). Besides domestic pigs, IgG anti-HEV is also found to be highly prevalent in the wild boar populations (de Deus et al. 2008; Michitaka et al. 2007), and sequences of genotype 3 HEV strains have been detected from wild boars (de Deus et al. 2008; Sonoda et al. 2004; Takahashi et al. 2004). Importantly, sporadic cases of hepatitis E have been reported in patients who consumed wild boar meats (Li et al. 2005b; Masuda et al. 2003, 2005;). These data provided compelling evidence that hepatitis E is a zoonotic disease, and both domestic and wild swine are the reservoirs.

In addition to swine and chickens, IgG anti-HEV has also been detected in a number of other animal species including rodents, cattle, cats, deer, horses, and dogs (Meng 2006, 2008). Unfortunately, the source of HEV seropositivity in these animal species, with the exception of domestic and wild swine, chickens, deer and mongoose (Nakamura et al. 2006; Tei et al. 2003), could not be identified, since virus was either not recovered from these species or the recovered virus could not be sequenced to confirm its identity. Also, genotype 1 HEV sequences indistinguishable from Egyptian isolates of human HEV were reportedly detected from horses in Egypt (Saad et al. 2007), although independent confirmation of genotype 1 HEV infection in horses is still lacking. A relatively high prevalence of HEV antibody has been detected in rats, suggesting that there is a widespread infection of rats by a HEV-related agent. Rodents may play a role in HEV transmission (Kabrane-Lazizi *et al.* 1999b), as they are frequently found in contact with humans both in urban and rural settings. It has been reported that human populations with occupational exposure to wild animals have an increased risk of zoonotic infection. Karetnyi *et al.* (1999) tested 87 field workers of the Iowa Department of Natural Resources (DNR) and 332 normal blood donors for prevalence of HEV antibodies, and found that the DNR workers had higher HEV antibody prevalence than normal blood donors (P < 0.05). Transmissions of hepatitis E from a pet cat and a pet pig to its human owners have also been reported (Kuno *et al.* 2003; Renou *et al.* 2007). In Japan, a cluster of four cases of acute hepatitis E were definitively linked to the consumption of raw deer meats in two families (Tei *et al.* 2003). The HEV sequence amplified from the leftover frozen deer meat was 99.7–100% nucleotide sequence identical to the viruses recovered from the four human patients. Taken together, these evidences strongly indicate that pigs are likely not the only animal reservoirs for HEV.

Cross-species infections by HEV

It has been demonstrated that rhesus monkeys and a chimpanzee can be experimentally infected with swine HEV (Meng *et al.* 1998). The infected rhesus monkeys seroconverted to IgG anti-HEV 4 weeks postinoculation, developed viremia, shed virus in faeces, and had elevation of serum liver enzymes isocitrate dehydrogenase and alanine aminotransferase. Microscopic lesions of viral hepatitis characterized by focal necroinflammatory changes were also observed in liver biopsies. The chimpanzee inoculated with swine HEV also became infected as evidenced by the detection of swine HEV RNA in faeces of the inoculated chimpanzee, and seroconversion to IgG anti-HEV at 6 weeks postinoculation, although both rhesus monkeys and the chimpanzee infected with swine HEV remained clinically normal. Conversely, it has been shown that SPF swine experimentally inoculated with a genotype 3 human HEV (Halbur *et al.* 2001) and a genotype 4 human HEV (Feagins *et al.* 2008b) rapidly became infected as evidenced by viremia and seroconversion to IgG anti-HEV within 2 weeks postinoculation.

Besides pigs, experimental interspecies transmissions of HEV have also been reported in other animal species. Usmanov *et al.* (1994) has reported experimental infections of lambs with two human HEV isolates, and the inoculated lambs reportedly developed clinical signs of hepatitis and shed virus in faeces. Wistar rats experimentally inoculated with a human HEV also became infected (Maneerat *et al.* 1996): HEV RNA was detected in faeces and sera, and HEV antigen was detected in the liver and several other tissues of the inoculated rats. However, independent studies to confirm the rat transmission results with a genotype 1 human HEV, a genotype 3 swine HEV, a genotype 4 swine HEV, and an avian HEV were unsuccessful (Meng 2003, 2006; Sun and Meng, unpublished data). Although a HEV-related agent of rat origin can be successfully transmitted in laboratory rats, the identity of the virus could not be determined (Emerson and Purcell, personal communication). It is likely that the virus infecting the rats is genetically very different from the known strains of HEV. Like mammalian HEV, the avian HEV can also cross-species barriers and infect turkeys (Sun *et al.* 2004b). However, under experimental conditions, avian HEV failed to infect two rhesus monkeys (Huang *et al.* 2004), suggesting that chickens are likely not a reservoir for HEV, although

more studies are needed to further evaluate the zoonotic potential of avian HEV. The expanded host ranges of HEV and its ability to infect across species (Table 41.1) raise additional concern for zoonotic infection of HEV.

Diagnosis

The clinical symptoms of human hepatitis E could not be distinguished from other types of acute viral hepatitis, and thus accurate diagnosis of hepatitis E must rely on laboratory tests. HEV is a difficult virus to work with since it cannot be efficiently propagated in cell culture. Currently, the diagnosis of HEV infection is primarily based on PCR and ELISA. Commercial ELISA reagents and test kits are available in many countries.

The diagnosis of HEV infection in pigs must depend upon RT-PCR and serology, since swine HEV infection is subclinical in swine herds. The recombinant human HEV capsid antigen cross-reacted well with antibodies to swine HEV in ELISA assay, and has been used to detect anti-HEV antibody in swine (Meng *et al.* 1997, 1998, 2002). In addition, the capsid protein of a genotype 3 swine HEV has been expressed and used in an ELISA to detect anti-HEV in pigs. Unfortunately, there is no specific test that could distinguish infections by swine HEV and human HEV. Since genotypes 3 and 4 swine and human HEV are genetically indistinguishable, a differential diagnostic assay for swine HEV is not possible or necessary. Sensitive and specific RT-PCR assays have also been developed for the detection of swine HEV from infected pigs (Jothikumar *et al.* 2006; Meng and Halbur 2006), however, the specificity of the RT-PCR assays in detecting swine HEV in pigs from different geographic regions is not known. The preferred sample for RT-PCR diagnosis is faecal materials from infected pigs since viremia in pigs is transient (Meng *et al.* 1997).

A presumptive diagnosis of avian HEV infection in chickens can be made on the basis of clinical signs and characteristic pathological lesions of HS syndrome. Virus particles of 30–35 nm may be detected in bile of chickens with HS syndrome by EM. Since the majority of chickens infected by avian HEV infection are subclinical, laboratory tests are needed to make a definitive diagnosis of avian HEV infection. Embryonic chicken eggs can be experimentally infected with avian HEV via intravenous inoculation, however, virus isolation with chicken embryos is not practical due to the technical difficulty and high mortality associated with the intravenous inoculation procedure. Currently, the diagnosis of avian HEV infection is primarily based on detection of the virus RNA by

Table 41.1 Host range and cross-species infection of the hepatitis E viruses (HEV) under natural and experimental conditions

HEV strains	Natural hosts	Experimental hosts
Genotype 1	Humans	Non-human primates, rats, lambs
Genotype 2	Humans	Non-human primates
Genotype 3	Humans, pigs, deer, mongoose, horse (?)	Non-human primates, pigs
Genotype 4	Human, pigs	Non-human primates, pigs
Avian HEV	Chickens	Turkeys, chickens

RT-PCR or detection of antibodies by ELISA. A truncated version of the avian HEV capsid protein has been expressed and used in an ELISA to detect avian HEV antibodies in chickens (Huang *et al.* 2002; Sun *et al.* 2004a). Avian HEV-specific RT-PCR assays have also been developed for the detection of avian HEV infections in chickens (Sun *et al.* 2004a). However, the specificity of the RT-PCR assays in detecting avian HEV strains in chickens from different geographic regions is not known, since avian HEV strains identified from chickens in different geographic regions are genetically heterogenic.

Prevention and control

A vaccine against HEV in humans is not yet available, although the experimental recombinant HEV vaccines appear to be very promising (Shrestha *et al.* 2007). In the absence of a vaccine, preventive measures such as practice good hygiene and avoid drinking water of unknown purity or consuming raw or undercooked pig livers are necessary to minimize the risk of HEV infection. Swine HEV has the ability to infect and cause hepatitis in humans especially in high risk groups such as pig handlers, therefore, effective prevention of swine HEV infection in pigs may prevent its transmission to humans, and thus reduce the risk of pork safety concern. A simple measure to prevent HEV infection for pig handlers is to wash hands thoroughly with soap and water after handling pigs. Although swine HEV is non-pathogenic in pigs, it is not known if concurrent infections of swine HEV with other swine pathogens could have any synergistic effects. Therefore, it will still be advantageous for the swine industry to develop a vaccine against swine HEV infections in pigs. Avian HEV apparently is not a risk for zoonotic human infection. Implementation of strict biosecurity in chicken farms may limit the spread of virus, although development of a vaccine against avian HEV will help protect chickens from developing HS syndrome or BLS.

Conclusions

HEV is an important but extremely understudied human pathogen. The discoveries of swine HEV from pigs, and the demonstrated ability of swine HEV to infect across species and the recovery of viruses resembling swine HEV from human patients with acute hepatitis E raise a serious concern for zoonotic HEV infection. The discovery of avian HEV from chickens and the existence of several other animal species that are positive for HEV antibodies suggest that, in addition to pigs, there likely exist other animal reservoirs for HEV. Therefore, HEV poses a potential public health risk for zoonoses and food safety (especially for pork products). The inability to efficiently propagate HEV in cell cultures greatly hinders our understanding of the biology and pathogenesis of the virus and slows the progress of developing an affordable vaccine against HEV.

Future prospects

The existence of numerous animal species that are seropositive for IgG anti-HEV suggest that these animal species are infected by a HEV-related agent(s). Unfortunately, thus far only swine HEV from pigs and avian HEV from chickens have been fully characterized. Failure to identify HEV from these animal species based upon the known sequences of mammalian and avian HEV strains suggest that these animal species may harbour their own strains of HEV that are genetically distinct from the known strains. Future studies to genetically identify and experimentally characterize the agent(s) responsible for the seropositivity in these animal species are warranted. Additional research on the natural history and ecology of HEV will help understand the magnitude and significance of the HEV zoonotic risk. The relatively high prevalence of HEV antibody in individuals from industrialized countries suggests that the occurrence of hepatitis E in these countries may be underestimated, since sporadic cases of acute hepatitis E may go undiagnosed. Therefore, it is important to fully assess the extent and impact of HEV infections in industrialized countries. Although the current experimental vaccines appear to be promising, it will be important to evaluate the efficacies of the vaccines against the emerging strains of HEV, especially those animal strains with zoonotic potential. Development of vaccines against the animal strains of HEV may minimize the risks of zoonotic transmission and increase food safety.

References

Arankalle, V.A., Tsarev, S.A., Chadha, M.S., *et al.* (1995). Age-specific prevalence of antibodies to hepatitis A and E viruses in Pune, India, (1982) and (1992). *J. Infect. Dis.*, **171**: 447–50.

Balayan, M.S., Andjaparidze, A.G., Savinskaya, S.S., *et al.* (1983). Evidence for a virus in non-A, non-B hepatitis transmitted via the fecal-oral route. *Intervirology*, **20**: 23–31.

Balayan, M.S., Usmanov, R.K., Zamyatina, D.I., Karas, F.R., (1990). Brief report: experimental hepatitis E infection in domestic pigs. *J. Med. Virol.*, **32**: 58–59.

Billam, P., Huang, F.F., Sun, Z.F., Pierson, F.W., *et al.* (2005). Systematic pathogenesis and replication of avian hepatitis E virus in specific-pathogen-free adult chickens. *J. Virol.*, **79**: 3429–37.

Bouwknegt, M., Frankena, K., Rutjes, S.A., *et al.* (2008). Estimation of hepatitis E virus transmission among pigs due to contact-exposure. *Vet. Res.*, **39**: 40.

Clayson, E.T., Myint, K.S., Snitbhan, R., *et al.* (1995). Viremia, fecal shedding, and IgM and IgG responses in patients with hepatitis E. *J. Infect. Dis.*, **172**: 927–33.

Clemente-Casares, P., Pina, S., Buti, M., Jardi, R., *et al.* (2003). Hepatitis E virus epidemiology in industrialized countries. *Emerg. Infect. Dis.*, **9**: 448–54.

de Deus, N., Peralta, B., Pina, S., Allepuz, A., *et al.* (2008). Epidemiological study of hepatitis E virus infection in European wild boars (Sus scrofa) in Spain. *Vet. Microbiol.*, **129**: 163–70.

Drobeniuc, J., Favorov, M.O., Shapiro, C.N., Bell, B.P., Mast, E.E., Dadu, A., Culver, D., Iarovoi, P., Robertson, B.H., Margolis, H.S., (2001). Hepatitis E virus antibody prevalence among persons who work with swine. *J. Infect. Dis.*, **184**: 1594–97.

Emerson, S.U., Anderson, D., Arankalle, V.A., *et al.* (2004). Hepevirus. In: C.M. Fauquet, M.A. Mayo, *et al.* (eds.), Virus Taxonomy, VIIIth Report of the ICTV, pp. 851–55. London: Elsevier/Academic Press.

Emerson, S.U., Arankalle, V.A., Purcell, R.H., (2005). Thermal stability of hepatitis E virus. *J. Infect. Dis.*, **192**: 930–33.

Emerson, S.U., Nguyen, H., Torian, U., Purcell, R.H., (2006). ORF3 protein of hepatitis E virus is not required for replication, virion assembly, or infection of hepatoma cells in vitro. *J. Virol.*, **80**: 10457–64.

Feagins, A.R., Opriessnig, T., Guenette, D.K., Halbur, P.G., Meng, X.J., (2007). Detection and characterization of infectious Hepatitis E virus from commercial pig livers sold in local grocery stores in the USA. *J. Gen. Virol.*, **88**: 912–17.

Feagins, A.R., Opriessnig, T., Guenette, D.K., Halbur, P.G., Meng, X.J., (2008a). Inactivation of infectious hepatitis E virus present in commercial pig livers sold in local grocery stores in the United States. *Int. J. Food Microbiol.*, **123**: 32–37.

Feagins, A.R., Opriessnig, T., Huang, Y.W., Halbur, P.G., Meng, X.J., (2008b). Cross-species infection of specific-pathogen-free pigs by a genotype 4 strain of human hepatitis E virus. *J. Med. Virol.*, **80**: 1379–86.

Graff, J., Torian, U., Nguyen, H., Emerson, S.U., (2006). A bicistronic subgenomic mRNA encodes both the ORF2 and ORF3 proteins of hepatitis E virus. *J. Virol.*, **80**: 5919–26.

Guo, H., Zhou, E.M., Sun, Z.F., Meng, X.J., Halbur, P.G., (2006). Identification of B-cell epitopes in the capsid protein of avian hepatitis E virus (avian HEV) that are common to human and swine HEVs or unique to avian HEV. *J. Gen. Virol.*, **87**: 217–23.

Halbur, P.G., Kasorndorkbua, C., Gilbert, C., et al. (2001). Comparative pathogenesis of infection of pigs with hepatitis E viruses recovered from a pig and a human. *J. Clin. Microbiol.*, **39**: 918–23.

Haqshenas, G., Shivaprasad, H.L., Woolcock, P.R., Read, D.H., Meng, X.J., (2001). Genetic identification and characterization of a novel virus related to human hepatitis E virus from chickens with hepatitis-splenomegaly syndrome in the United States. *J. Gen. Virol.*, **82**: 2449–62.

Herremans, M., Bakker, J., Duizer, E., Vennema, H., Koopmans, M.P., (2007). Use of serological assays for diagnosis of hepatitis E virus genotype 1 and 3 infections in a setting of low endemicity. *Clin. Vaccine Immunol.*, **14**: 562–68.

Huang, F.F., Sun, Z.F., Emerson, S.U., Purcell, R.H., et al. (2004). Determination and analysis of the complete genomic sequence of avian hepatitis E virus (avian HEV) and attempts to infect rhesus monkeys with avian HEV. *J. Gen. Virol.*, **85**: 1609–18.

Huang, F.F., Haqshenas, G., Shivaprasad, H.L., Guenette, D.K., et al. (2002). Heterogeneity and seroprevalence of a newly identified avian hepatitis E virus from chickens in the United States. *J. Clin. Microbiol.*, **40**: 4197–202.

Huang, Y.W., Opriessnig, T., Halbur, P.G., Meng, X.J., (2007). Initiation at the third in-frame AUG codon of open reading frame 3 of the hepatitis E virus is essential for viral infectivity in vivo. *J. Virol.*, **81**: 3018–26.

Jothikumar, N., Cromeans, T.L., Robertson, B.H., Meng, X.J., Hill, V.R., (2006). A broadly reactive one-step real-time RT-PCR assay for rapid and sensitive detection of hepatitis E virus. *J. Virol. Meth.*, **131**: 65–71.

Kabrane-Lazizi, Y., Meng, X.J., Purcell, R.H., Emerson, S.U., (1999a). Evidence that the genomic RNA of hepatitis E virus is capped. *J. Virol.*, **73**: 8848–50.

Kabrane-Lazizi, Y., Fine, J.B., Elm, J., Glass, G.E., et al. (1999b). Evidence for widespread infection of wild rats with hepatitis E virus in the United States. *Am. J Trop. Med. Hyg.*, **61**: 331–35.

Karetnyi, Y.V., Gilchrist, M.J., Naides, S.J., (1999). Hepatitis E virus infection prevalence among selected populations in Iowa. *J. Clin. Virol.*, **14**: 51–55.

Kasorndorkbua, C., Guenette, D.K., Huang, F.F., Thomas, P.J., et al. (2004). Routes of transmission of swine hepatitis E virus in pigs. *J. Clin. Microbiol.*, **42**: 5047–52.

Kuno, A., Ido, K., Isoda, N., Satoh, Y., Ono, K., et al. (2003). Sporadic acute hepatitis E of a 47-year-old man whose pet cat was positive for antibody to hepatitis E virus. *Hepatol. Res.*, **26**: 237–42.

Li, T.C., Takeda, N., Miyamura, T., Matsuura, Y., et al. (2005a). Essential elements of the capsid protein for self-assembly into empty virus-like particles of hepatitis E virus. *J. Virol.*, **79**: 12999–13006.

Li, T.C., Chijiwa, K., Sera, N., Ishibashi, T., et al. (2005b). Hepatitis E virus transmission from wild boar meat. *Emerg. Infect. Dis.*, **11**: 1958–60.

Lu, L., Drobeniuc, J., Kobylnikov, N., Usmanov, R.K., et al. (2004). Complete sequence of a Kyrgyzstan swine hepatitis E virus (HEV) isolated from a piglet thought to be experimentally infected with human HEV. *J. Med. Virol.*, **74**: 556–62.

Maneerat, Y., Clayson, E.T., Myint, K.S., Young, G.D., Innis, B.L., (1996). Experimental infection of the laboratory rat with the hepatitis E virus. *J. Med. Virol.*, **48**: 121–28.

Masuda, J., Yano, K., Tamada, Y., Takii, Y., Ito, M., et al. (2005). Acute hepatitis E of a man who consumed wild boar meat prior to the onset of illness in Nagasaki. *Jpn. Hepatol. Res.*, **31**: 178–83.

Matsuda, H., Okada, K., Takahashi, K., Mishiro, S., (2003). Severe hepatitis E virus infection after ingestion of uncooked liver from a wild boar. *J. Infect. Dis.*, **188**: 944.

Meng, X.J., Purcell, R.H., Halbur, P.G., Lehman, J.R., et al. (1997). A novel virus in swine is closely related to the human hepatitis E virus. *Proc. Natl. Acad. Sci. USA*, **94**: 9860–65.

Meng, X.J., Halbur, P.G., Shapiro, M.S., et al. (1998). Genetic and experimental evidence for cross-species infection by swine hepatitis E virus. *J.Virol.*, **72**: 9714–21.

Meng, X.J., Wiseman, B., Elvinger, F., et al. (2002). Prevalence of antibodies to hepatitis E virus in veterinarians working with swine and in normal blood donors in the United States and other countries. *J. Clin. Microbiol.*, **40**: 117–22.

Meng, X.J., (2003). Swine hepatitis E virus: cross-species infection and risk in xenotransplantation. *Curr. Top. Microbiol. Immunol.*, **278**: 185–216.

Meng, X.J., (2006). Hepatitis E as a zoonosis. In: H. Thomas, A. Zuckermann, S. Lemon (eds.), Viral Hepatitis, pp. 611–23, 3rd edn. Oxford, UK: Blackwell Publishing Ltd.

Meng, X.J., Halbur, P.G., (2006). Swine hepatitis E virus. In: B. E. Straw et al. (eds.), Diseases of Swine, pp. 537–45, 9th edn. Oxford, UK: Blackwell Publishing Press.

Meng, X.J., (2008). Hepatitis E virus *(hepevirus)*. In: B.M.J. Mahy, M.H.V. van Regenmortel (eds.), Encyclopedia of Virology, Vol 5, pp. 377-83, (3rd edn.). pp. 377–83. Oxford: Elsevier.

Meng, X.J., Shivaprasad, H.L., Payne, C., (2008). Hepatitis E virus infections. In: M. Saif et al. (eds.), Diseases of Poultry, pp. 443–52, (12th edn.). Oxford: Blackwell Publishing Press.

Michitaka, K., Takahashi, K., Furukawa, S., Inoue, G., et al. (2007). Prevalence of hepatitis E virus among wild boar in the Ehime area of western Japan. *Hepatol. Res.*, **37**: 214–20.

Nakamura, M., Takahashi, K., Taira, K., Taira, M., et al. (2006). Hepatitis E virus infection in wild mongooses of Okinawa, Japan: demonstration of anti-HEV antibodies and a full-genome nucleotide sequence. *Hepatol. Res.*, **34**: 137–40.

Nicand, E., Armstrong, G.L., Enouf, V., et al. (2005). Genetic heterogeneity of hepatitis E virus in Darfur, Sudan, and neighboring Chad. *J. Med. Virol.*, **77**: 519–21.

Okamoto, H., (2007). Genetic variability and evolution of hepatitis E virus. *Virus Res.*, **127**: 216–28.

Payne, C.J., Ellis, T.M., Plant, S.L., Gregory, A.R., Wilcox, G.E., (1999). Sequence data suggests big liver and spleen disease virus (BLSV) is genetically related to hepatitis E virus. *Vet. Microbiol.*, **68**: 119–25.

Peralta, B., Biarnes, M., Ordonez, G., Porta, R., et al. (2008). Evidence of widespread infection of avian hepatitis E virus (avian HEV) in chickens from Spain. *Vet. Microbiol.*, Dec 13 (Epub ahead of print).

Pudupakam, R.S., Huang, Y.W., Opriessnig, T., Halbur, P.G., et al. (2009). Deletions of the hypervariable region (HVR) in open reading frame 1 of hepatitis E virus do not abolish virus infectivity: evidence for attenuation of HVR deletion mutants in vivo. *J. Virol.*, **83**: 384–95.

Purcell, R.H., Emerson, S.U., (2001). Hepatitis E virus. In: D. Knipe, P. Howley et al. (eds.), Fields Virology, pp. 3051–61, 4th edn. Philadelphia: Lippincott Williams and Wilkins.

Renou, C., Cadranel, J.F., Bourliere, M., et al. (2007). Possible zoonotic transmission of hepatitis E from pet pig to its owner. *Emerg. Infect. Dis.*, **13**: 1094–96.

Saad, M.D., Hussein, H.A., Bashandy, M.M., Kamel, H.H., et al. (2007). Hepatitis E virus infection in work horses in Egypt. *Infect. Genet. Evol.*, **7**: 368–73.

Shrestha, M.P., Scott, R.M., Joshi, D.M., Mammen Jr., M.P., et al. (2007). Safety and efficacy of a recombinant hepatitis E vaccine. *N. Engl. J. Med.*, **356**: 895–903.

Sonoda, H., Abe, M., Sugimoto, T., Sato, Y., et al. (2004). Prevalence of hepatitis E virus (HEV) Infection in wild boars and deer and genetic identification of a genotype 3 HEV from a boar in Japan. *J. Clin. Microbiol.*, **42:** 5371–74.

Stoszek, S.K., Engle, R.E., Abdel-Hamid, M., *et al.* (2006). Hepatitis E antibody seroconversion without disease in highly endemic rural Egyptian communities. *Trans. R. Soc. Trop. Med. Hyg.*, **100:** 89–94.

Sun, Z.F., Larsen, C.T., Dunlop, A., Huang, F.F., *et al.* (2004a). Genetic identification of avian hepatitis E virus (HEV) from healthy chicken flocks and characterization of the capsid gene of 14 avian HEV isolates from chickens with hepatitis-splenomegaly syndrome in different geographical regions of the United States. *J. Gen. Virol.*, **85:** 693–700.

Sun, Z.F., Larsen, C.T., Huang, F.F., Billam, P., *et al.* (2004b). Generation and infectivity titration of an infectious stock of avian hepatitis E virus (HEV) in chickens and cross-species infection of turkeys with avian HEV. *J. Clin. Microbiol.*, **42:** 2658–62.

Takahashi, K., Kitajima, N., Abe, N., Mishiro, S., (2004). Complete or near-complete nucleotide sequences of hepatitis E virus genome recovered from a wild boar, a deer, and four patients who ate the deer. *Virology*, **330:** 501–5.

Takahashi, M., Yamada, K., Hoshino, Y., Takahashi, H., *et al.* (2008). Monoclonal antibodies raised against the ORF3 protein of hepatitis E virus (HEV) can capture HEV particles in culture supernatant and serum but not those in feces. *Arch. Virol.*, **153:** 1703–13.

Tam, A.W., Smith, M.M., Guerra, M.E., Huang, C.C., *et al.* (1991). Hepatitis E virus (HEV): molecular cloning and sequencing of the full-length viral genome. *Virology*, **185:** 120–31.

Tei, S., Kitajima, N., Takahashi, K., Mishiro, S., (2003). Zoonotic transmission of hepatitis E virus from deer to human beings. *Lancet*, **362:** 371–73.

Tsarev, S.A., Tsareva, T.S., Emerson, S.U., Rippy, M.K., *et al.* (1995). Experimental hepatitis E in pregnant rhesus monkeys: failure to transmit hepatitis E virus (HEV) to offspring and evidence of naturally acquired antibodies to HEV. *J. Infect. Dis.*, **172:** 31–37.

Usmanov, R.K., Balaian, M.S., Dvonikova, O.V., *et al.* (1994). An experimental infection in lambs by the hepatitis E virus. *Vopr. Virusol.*, **39:** 165–68.

Withers, M.R., Correa, M.T., Morrow, M., Stebbins, M.E., *et al.* (2002). Antibody levels to hepatitis E virus in North Carolina swine workers, non-swine workers, swine, and murids. *Am. J. Trop. Med. Hyg.*, **66:** 384–88.

Yazaki, Y., Mizuo, H., Takahashi, M., Nishizawa, T., *et al.* (2003). Sporadic acute or fulminant hepatitis E in Hokkaido, Japan, may be food-borne, as suggested by the presence of hepatitis E virus in pig liver as food. *J. Gen. Virol.*, **84:** 2351–57.

Zafrullah, M., Ozdener, M.H., Panda, S.K., Jameel, S., (1997). The ORF3 protein of hepatitis E virus is a phosphoprotein that associates with the cytoskeleton. *J. Virol.*, **71:** 9045–53.

Disease mechanisms

Trypanosoma brucei ssp. trypanosomes do not just circulate in the bloodstream, but invade various tissues most importantly the CNS, where they can more effectively evade the immune system. Trypanosomes interact in various ways with cells of the immune system, the complexities of which have yet to be fully unravelled, but are key to understanding the nature and extent of pathology and thus the course of disease (Rhind and Shek 1999; Vincendeau *et al.* 1999; Mansfield 2001). Trypanosomes multiply initially at the site of the fly bite and local inflammation may result in the first sign of the disease, the chancre. From here the trypanosomes invade the bloodstream and lymphatic system, causing generalized febrile attacks. Each parasitaemic wave is associated with expression of a limited number of VSGs; trypanosomes expressing these antigens are cleared from the blood by a specific antibody response, releasing further internal antigens. Subsequent parasitaemic waves are initiated by residual trypanosomes that have switched to expression of new surface antigens (VSGs). The sequential parasitaemic waves stimulate polyclonal B cell proliferation, particularly IgM, followed by T cell-dependent production of specific antibodies, which lead to destruction of parasites by the usual routes (complement-mediated lysis, phagocytosis, cell-mediated cytotoxicity). This initial robust immune response is followed in a chronic infection by exhaustion of the immune system and immunosuppression, an effect observed on both T and B cell responses. Macrophages are thought to play a major role in destroying trypanosomes in the tissues and are activated during infection by exposure to IFN-γ produced by CD8+ T cells, and trypanosome components, notably VSG. The activated macrophages secrete many components such as nitric oxide and reactive oxygen species capable of destroying trypanosomes, and various cytokines, notably TNFα, resulting in tissue damage and systemic effects. In animal models, the catabolic effects of TNFα (cachectin) give rise to anorexia, fever and weight loss, suggesting that it alone could be responsible for much of the clinical picture of trypanosomosis.

Invasion of the CNS commences at an early stage of infection and leads to progressive damage, culminating in coma and eventual death, if the disease remains untreated. In experimental animals dye-tracer studies show that the blood-CSF barrier is compromised within a few days of infection. An early change is the breakdown of the choroid plexus allowing infiltration of trypanosomes and lymphocytes into the circumventricular regions. No toxins are known to be released from the trypanosomes themselves; rather it appears to be the interactions of the parasites with the immune system that manifest disease. In particular, the cytokine/prostaglandin network appears to play a key role in the inflammatory processes in the brain, and also may be influencing wider physiological abnormalities such as somnolence and fever. Unravelling this complex series of interactions will eventually help to clarify late stage pathogenesis.

Growth and survival requirements

Trypanosomes are obligate parasites, which have no survival stages outside their hosts. In the mammalian host, trypanosome metabolism is dependent on high levels of glucose, as found in the bloodstream and CNS, while in the fly the main energy source is proline. Trypanosomes can survive for a limited time (hours) in samples of body fluids, e.g. blood, CSF, but are easily destroyed by heat, desiccation, detergents and disinfectants. There is no record of aerosol transmission.

The hosts

General

Besides man, *T. brucei* ssp. can infect a wide variety of domestic and wild mammal species; natural infection has also been recorded in a bird (domestic hen) and a large reptile, the monitor lizard, which frequently serves as a source of blood meals for some tsetse species. In general *T. b. rhodesiense* and *T. b. brucei* are more virulent than *T. b. gambiense* and produce more rapid and severe symptoms. Animal trypanosomosis is also caused by other tsetse-transmitted trypanosome species in Africa, notably *T. vivax*, *T. congolense* and *T. simiae*, which are considered to be of far greater veterinary importance than *T. brucei* ssp., except perhaps for dogs, horses and camels (Stephen 1986; Brown *et al.* 1990). Mixed infections of two or more trypanosome species occur frequently in livestock kept in endemic zones. Outside sub-Saharan Africa, *Trypanosoma evansi* assumes great importance as a pathogen of livestock, particularly camels and horses, but also cattle and buffalo, and has occasionally caused the death of zoo carnivores fed on infected carcasses; *T. evansi* is included here, because of a single, well-documented case of human infection in an Indian farmer (Joshi *et al.* 2005).

Incubation period

The incubation period in both man and animals is highly variable due to differences in trypanosome virulence and number of organisms inoculated, besides individual and species differences in susceptibility and previous exposure to tsetse challenge. It is also difficult to assess in an endemic area where fly bite is frequent. For the most virulent strains in susceptible hosts, the incubation period is probably as little as a week, but may be several weeks or much longer; prolonged incubation periods of several years are on record for Gambian sleeping sickness. Trypanosome infection in animals may remain cryptic for years, as evidenced by the development of disease in zoo animals several years after removal from a tsetse-endemic zone.

Symptoms and signs

Generally the early symptoms of Rhodesian sleeping sickness tend to be more severe and acute than those of the Gambian form, and the early and late stages are less clearly demarcated (WHO 1998). The early stage is characterized by intermittent fever, weakness, headache, backache, joint pains, oedema, pruritis, and enlargement of the lymph glands and spleen, while the late stage is marked by neurological symptoms and endocrine disorders, e.g. amenorrhea or impotence. However, due to the early invasion of the CNS, neurological signs, such as facial ticks and mood and appetite changes, may be present at an early stage. Two of the first signs of sleeping sickness are the chancre, an indurated swelling at the site of fly bite which may be present in early cases of Rhodesian sleeping sickness, but is seldom observed for Gambian sleeping sickness, and swelling of the lymph nodes, particularly the cervical glands 'Winterbottom's sign'. The eponymous sleep disorders include nocturnal insomnia and daytime somnolence, and classically sleeping sickness manifests itself finally in coma. Cerebral involvement may also be evident from psychiatric disturbances, ranging in severity from behavioural changes, often increased aggression or violence, to frank psychosis. Late-stage patients have ended up in mental institutions or even prison for these reasons.

Some animals infected with *T. brucei* ssp. (e.g. horses, dogs) may be obviously ill, but others, particularly bovids and wild animals, may remain asymptomatic, possibly showing disease only if stressed (Brown *et al.* 1990). There is the added complication that when a mixture of trypanosome species is present, the presence of *T. brucei* ssp. may be easily missed. Early infection is characterized by intermittent parasitaemia associated with bouts of fever. Clinical features of the chronic disease include anaemia, fever, cachexia, lymphadenopathy, and oedema. *Nagana* was the Zulu name for animal trypanosomosis and means 'a state of depressed spirits', which nicely sums up the clinical picture. Lameness of the hindquarters is characteristic of infection in dogs and horses, as is corneal opacity—so-called 'white eyes'—in dogs. There may also be disorders of reproduction, particularly sterility and abortion. A similar clinical picture is observed in camels, horses and dogs with *Surra*, while *T. evansi* infection may remain cryptic in less susceptible animals such as bovids.

Diagnosis

For human patients parasite demonstration is generally required before treatment commences as drug treatment is not without risk. For animal trypanosomosis, this is not always necessary, and for example, herd treatment may be carried out after demonstration of trypanosomes in some individuals only. Much the same diagnostic methods are used for both human and animal trypanosomosis, but levels of parasitaemia may often be very low and fluctuating. Parasitaemias tend to be higher in Rhodesian sleeping sickness and therefore it is usually possible to find motile trypanosomes by simple microscopic examination of wet blood films. A trypanosome concentration method is usually necessary for demonstration of *T. b. gambiense*, the simplest being thick blood film stained with Giemsa or Field's stain; other concentration methods include mini-anion exchange columns, haematocrit (HTC) buffy coat and QBC (quantitative buffy coat technique); for animal use, HTC has the advantage that packed cell volume can be measured at the same time to provide an assessment of the degree of anaemia. If enlarged lymph glands are present, trypanosomes can often be demonstrated by gland puncture; this method has also been used for cattle. However, trypanosome numbers may be extremely low and the most reliable and sensitive means of demonstrating parasites is then by inoculation of rodents, immunosuppressed in the case of *T. b. gambiense*.

Serological tests such as the CATT (Card Agglutination Test for Trypanosomosis) (Magnus *et al.* 1978), which rely on antibody detection, are useful for preliminary screening in endemic areas of Gambian sleeping sickness, but suspects require parasitological confirmation before treatment. New diagnostic methods are constantly being sought, and an ELISA test for antigen detection, various PCR (polymerase chain reaction)-based tests and LAMP (loop-mediated isothermal amplification) tests have all been developed in recent years. The cost and ease of use of any new diagnostic test in the field are factors always to be borne in mind.

In man, CNS involvement is assessed by microscopic examination of centrifuged CSF withdrawn by lumbar puncture. If no parasites can be demonstrated, then high numbers of cells (more than 5 per ml) or high levels of protein (greater than 37mg/100ml) indi-

cate CNS involvement (WHO 1998). In exceptional cases, where trypanosomes can neither be demonstrated in the blood or CSF, diagnosis may be made on clinical grounds only.

Pathology

Much of the recent work has been carried out in animal models, which appear to share similar pathology with man; the older post-mortem data on patients who died in late stage disease was reviewed by Kristensson and Bentivoglio (1999). *Trypanosoma brucei* ssp. trypanosomes invade the intercellular fluids of various tissues, as well as the bloodstream and extracellular fluids. In the early haemolymphatic stage of sleeping sickness, the lymph nodes and spleen are enlarged and infiltrated with lymphocytes, plasma cells and monocytes (Greenwood and Whittle 1980; WHO 1998). Later the lymph nodes become shrunken and atrophied with progressive exhaustion of the immune system. Anaemia is haemolytic and large numbers of reticulocytes are present. There is also thrombocytopaenia. The intercellular spaces of various tissues are invaded, notably the heart, with resultant myocarditis and pericardial effusions. Invasion of the CNS begins with congestion of the meninges and infiltration of lymphocytes and large vesiculated cells. These are the so-called morular cells originally observed by Mott in 1905, which are plasma cells containing huge amounts of immunoglobulin. Inflammation extends into the brain tissue and blood vessels show perivascular cuffing. There is proliferation of neuroglial cells (astrocytes and microglia) associated with diffuse meningoencephalitis.

Treatment

Unfortunately, all the drugs currently used for treatment of human sleeping sickness are rather toxic and cause side effects ranging from unpleasant to severe; only one new drug—eflornithine—has been introduced in the past 60 years (Pepin 2007), although several are now in the pipeline. Early cases without CNS involvement are treated with suramin or, for Gambian sleeping sickness only, pentamidine (Lomidine). Some use has also been made of diminazene aceturate (Berenil), although this drug is not registered for human use. None of these drugs cross the blood-brain barrier to any extent and late stage cases require one or more courses of the arsenical melarsoprol (Arsobal). This drug is dissolved in propylene glycol and leakage into the tissues at the injection site causes severe irritation. Relapses following melarsoprol treatment are problematic as the patient may already be in a poor state; relapsed cases of Gambian sleeping sickness can be treated with eflornithine (DFMO; Ornidyl), but this drug is not effective against *T. b. rhodesiense*. Nifurtimox in combination with melarsoprol has produced encouraging results for treatment of late stage Gambian sleeping sickness (Bisser *et al.* 2007).

For animal trypanosomosis, three drugs are in common use for treatment of ruminants—Berenil, isometamidium (Samorin, Trypamidium) and homidium salts (Ethidium, Novidium). Of these only Berenil and Samorin are recommended for treatment of *T. brucei* ssp. infections. For horses and camels, Samorin, suramin (Naganol) or quinapyramine sulphate (Antrycide, Trypacide) are the drugs of choice and Samorin is recommended for treatment of dogs. Samorin and Trypacide Prosalt (quinapyramine sulphate together with the more insoluble chloride salt) are recommended for prevention as well as cure in cattle and horses, the effects lasting 3–6 months. There is some degree of drug resistance to all veterinary trypanocidal drugs and the small number available make this possibility a constant concern.

Prognosis

Untreated sleeping sickness is fatal, with death resulting in 3–9 months with Rhodesian sleeping sickness and possibly a matter of years with Gambian sleeping sickness. In cases without CNS involvement, prognosis is generally good; however, such cases may relapse if CNS involvement was unrecognized at the time of treatment. The state of some patients admitted with late stage disease may already be so poor that they require general nursing and supportive therapy before commencement of treatment. The most severe complication of treatment in late stage patients is so-called reactive encephalopathy, which occurs in 5–10% of cases and leads to high mortality. In the past, this syndrome was considered to be a severe side effect of arsenical treatment. However, it also occurs when other drugs are used for treatment of late stage disease. This could indicate that it is a reaction to the rapid release of trypanosomal antigens in the CNS as the trypanosomes are killed, but work in an experimental mouse model suggests the cause to be the persistence of small numbers of live trypanosomes in the brain. The latter would indicate the beneficial effect of aggressive rather than gradual drug therapy. The results of reactive encephalopathy can be ameliorated by supportive treatment with anti-inflammatory drugs.

All patients need to be followed up after treatment for at least a year to ascertain whether cure has taken place. WHO (1998) recommend follow up examinations at six monthly intervals for two years. A full parasitological and clinical examination is necessary, including lumbar puncture.

In animals the course and outcome of *T. brucei* ssp. infection is highly variable, depending on the subspecies and strain of infecting trypanosomes, the species and breed of mammalian host and its previous exposure to trypanosomes. In horses and dogs the disease may take an acute and fatal course within a few weeks. Severe chronic trypanosomosis leads to progressive debility and emaciation and death in a matter of months. Alternatively, infection may be transient. Drug therapy is generally curative, but relapses may arise from residual parasites hidden in the tissues or from drug resistance.

Epidemiology and epizootiology

Occurrence

Incidence

The number of new cases of sleeping sickness is estimated to be in the tens of thousands annually, but accurate figures are difficult to obtain as many endemic foci are located in remote and inaccessible areas, with poor health facilities (WHO 2008). It is costly to maintain surveillance in such regions, but control programmes may also fail for other reasons such as civil disturbance, war, or other economic and political problems.

Prevalence

Accurate data would need to be gathered over a period of years to gain a true picture of the prevalence of sleeping sickness in an endemic focus. As noted above, such data are hard to come by for humans, and even harder to obtain for potential animal reservoir hosts. The activity and distribution of tsetse flies varies according to wet or dry seasons, with consequent effects on transmission rates

and presumably prevalence. There may also be seasonal movements of domestic stock or wildlife. On top of this, survey work may be restricted, if not impossible, during the wet season in remote areas.

Sampling from animal species present in a focus is often unrepresentative, depending on the ease with which they can be caught. Conservation measures in some countries mean that a licence is required to sample wild animals. Some information on prevalence can be obtained from tsetse flies caught in an endemic area by examining trypanosome infection rates, together with blood meal identification.

Epidemics

Most endemic foci smoulder on with a low annual incidence and occasional flare ups (Kuzoe 1993). The usual reason for recrudescence of foci is breakdown of routine control measures. Sometimes control programmes are discontinued because the economic costs of control appear to outweigh the benefits of dealing with relatively few cases or small numbers of flies. This can be a false economy due to the high cost of controlling any ensuing epidemic. Some outbreaks result from prolonged civil disruption, when routine control measures break down and aid agencies withdraw financial and technical resources. Reliable statistics are then hard to come by. In these circumstances, people may flee their homes and seek refuge in areas where they are more at risk of tsetse bite and less likely to receive medical help. Recent epidemics in the Democratic Republic of Congo (DRC), Angola and Uganda reflect past civil strife. Government resettlement schemes or unofficial settlement adjacent to designated wildlife areas have also resulted in new outbreaks.

Risk groups

There are considered to be 60 million at risk living in the 250 or so endemic foci of sleeping sickness scattered throughout sub-Saharan Africa (Fig. 42.1). Occupational risk groups include hunters, firewood or honey gatherers and tourists to wildlife parks in endemic areas in East Africa, who may contract sporadic Rhodesian sleeping sickness from wild animal reservoirs (Jelinek *et al.* 2002). No specific occupational groups, except perhaps fishermen, are at risk for Gambian sleeping sickness, since all sectors of the population come into contact with the fly in its riverine/lakeshore habitat during daily activities such as bathing and collecting water.

Population movements may also increase risk (Ford 1971). For example, resettlement schemes may bring people into close contact with flies which previously fed on wild animal reservoir hosts. Refugees fleeing from one country may move into an endemic focus in another, as happened in the 1990s on the Sudan-Uganda-DRC border spanned by an endemic focus of Gambian sleeping sickness. Immigrants are at no greater risk of infection than the indigenous population, since exposure does not confer immunity to re-infection. Returning refugees may find their abandoned farmland overgrown with bush and infested with tsetse, giving rise to new outbreaks.

Geography

Sleeping sickness has been reported in 36 countries in sub-Saharan Africa between latitudes 14°N and 29°S (WHO 2008). The distribution of the disease is restricted by that of the tsetse fly, which needs the right conditions of humidity and temperature for survival (Leak 1999). *Palpalis*-group flies, which are the main vectors of Gambian sleeping sickness, need high humidity and are found in the forested zones of West and Central Africa, Uganda and southern Sudan; their range also extends northwards through more arid country, following the lines of fringing vegetation on river and lakeshore. *Morsitans*-group flies can tolerate drier conditions and are found throughout the wooded savannah regions.

Sources

The source of infection is always another infected mammalian host. In an epidemic, other infected humans are generally thought to be the major source of infection, although it is acknowledged that a high infection rate in domestic livestock could boost transmission, if flies take a significant proportion of feeds from both hosts. At the other end of the spectrum, sporadic infections can be contracted when man breaks into a wild animal-tsetse cycle. This occurs most frequently in East Africa, where there are large concentrations of wild animals in uninhabited bush, but this possibility cannot be ruled out in some areas of West and Central Africa with plentiful wildlife. Domestic livestock will probably become increasingly important in disease transmission, either acting as an intermediary in transferring trypanosome strains from wild animals to man, or by replacing wild animal reservoirs altogether. The single human case of *T. evansi* infection in an Indian farmer was probably contracted from infected livestock (cattle) (Joshi *et al.* 2005).

Transmission

The usual mode of transmission is via the bite of an infected tsetse fly (Fig. 42.4), as can be deduced from the restriction of the disease to the area of tsetse infestation. Trypanosomes undergo a developmental and multiplicative cycle in the fly, first in the midgut and then in the salivary glands, from whence they are conveyed to new hosts with the saliva (Hoare 1972). Flies are relatively refractory to infection, only readily becoming infected at the first blood meal after emergence from the puparium (Maudlin 1991); consequently much less than 1% of flies are found infected with *T. brucei* ssp. in the wild. The cycle takes a minimum of about two weeks to complete. With a lifespan of two to three months under favourable conditions and a requirement to feed every few days, an individual fly could infect at least 20 new hosts. It is for this reason that close man-fly contact, rather than sheer numbers of flies, is so important in the epidemiology of sleeping sickness: the classic example is of one resident infected fly at the village water hole with the potential to cause a small epidemic in the dry season when people spend more time there (Nash 1969). By contrast, large concentrations of flies feeding predominantly on wild animals may pose very little risk.

Other modes of transmission are possible, but depend on relatively high parasitaemia in the donor and a susceptible recipient, e.g. contaminative transmission by tsetse or other biting flies such as tabanids (= mode of transmission of *T. evansi*); direct transmission via fresh infected blood or raw meat (Moloo *et al.* 1973). Congenital transmission has rarely been recorded.

Communicability

The main route of sleeping sickness transmission is via the tsetse fly. Laboratory studies have shown not only that different trypanosome subspecies and strains vary in infectivity to flies, but also that the flies themselves differ in susceptibility to trypanosome infection (Maudlin 1991). In fact it appears that most flies are refractory to infection and transmission appears to be sustained by relatively few flies. The long-term stability of endemic foci is evidence that

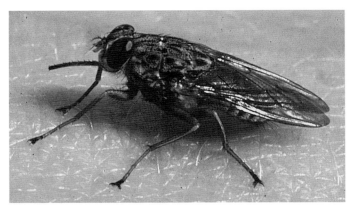

Fig. 42.4 Tsetse fly, *Glossina morsitans morsitans*, resting on hand. Photo by Tim Colborn School of Biological Sciences, University of Bristol. Used with permission.

this minimalist strategy is successful and further emphasizes the fundamental importance of the behaviour of individual flies rather than populations in transmission of the disease.

Establishment of infection in a new host following fly bite will depend on several factors: the number of trypanosomes inoculated with the saliva; the virulence of the trypanosome subspecies or strain; the level of intrinsic resistance of the host.

Prevention and control

Prevention

The risk of contracting human trypanosomosis outside the known foci of the disease is minimal, although sporadic infections could potentially be acquired in some tsetse-infested wildlife areas. Animal trypanosomosis exists throughout the tsetse belt, however, and *T. evansi* is a widespread pathogen of livestock in parts of N. Africa, the Middle East, Asia and S. America; only in very rare cases have these animal trypanosomes ever been isolated from humans.

Even in an endemic area, the risk of being bitten by an infected fly is small. The risk of infection can be lowered by avoiding tsetse fly bite, easier said than done in the African bush. All tsetse species require some degree of shade and habitats vary from light bush to dense forest and even conifer or coffee plantations. Tsetse can be found in the peridomestic environment if there is suitable cover and those species favouring a riverine habitat may also be encountered at waterholes, river crossing points and bathing places. Tsetse feed during the day and find their hosts by sight as well as smell. They are attracted to large moving objects, particularly vehicles, and also dark colour clothing. Clothing is no barrier to tsetse bite, but insect repellents might be of limited use if practical. Animals can be treated with pour-on residual insecticide, but this might not prevent fly bite and the possibility of infection.

Prophylactic drugs for human use cannot be recommended, although pentamidine was widely used in the past (Mulligan 1970). There would be too great a risk of masking early infection, giving the parasites time to invade the CNS. For animals, various drugs can be given prophylactically, but there could be toxic effects from long-term use and prophylaxis would probably be ineffectual in areas of high challenge.

Control strategies

There are two current strategies for control: control of the parasite by regular medical surveillance of the population at risk or control of the fly. The parasite is targeted by drug therapy of its human host; there have been few if any attempts to eliminate trypanosomes in reservoir hosts, other than early attempts to destroy the wild animal reservoir. Eradication of tsetse flies in Africa remains a distant hope. Despite their slow breeding cycle—each female produces only a single larva every 9 days or so—and the various measures used to combat them, tsetse fly populations remain buoyant and tsetse have actually increased in distribution in some areas. Present environmental concerns favour limited use of insecticides and low-tech methodologies that can be widely and cheaply applied at local level; for example, the use of locally-made traps or targets (Dransfield *et al.* 1991). On the larger scale, Sterile Insect Technique (SIT) was used successfully to eradicate tsetse from Zanzibar island in a four year campaign started in 1994; whether tsetse control by SIT will prove either possible or economic on the African mainland is hotly debated (Rogers and Randolph 2002).

Methods and programmes

Sleeping sickness control is usually organized at governmental level; however other organizations, such as aid agencies and missions, may be involved, especially during epidemics. For example, besides local government, several European governments, UN organizations and charities have all provided financial or technical aid for control of recent epidemics in south east Uganda, DRC and Angola. International organizations such as Organisation of African Unity (OAU) and WHO take responsibility for coordination of control measures between African countries. This is especially important where foci span borders and for communication between French- and English-speaking countries.

Control of the parasite

Case detection and treatment is possible at a number of organizational levels, with various degrees of cost-effectiveness. At one extreme, mobile teams can be used to survey endemic areas screening the whole population every year. Active surveillance like this is very costly, but also fulfils the requirement for patient follow-up to assess cure. Such programmes are necessary to cover large areas of endemic Gambian sleeping sickness. At the other extreme, patients can be left to report to their local health centre. This is so-called passive surveillance and is adequate for small outbreaks of Rhodesian sleeping sickness.

Individual governments must decide the level of resources to devote to sleeping sickness surveillance on the basis of the population at risk, the level of endemicity and their own health priorities. Present pressures on health budgets and the relatively small number of cases mean that sleeping sickness is often seen as a low priority. However, since it is simpler and less expensive to undertake regular surveillance than deal with an explosive epidemic, the risk of epidemics makes sleeping sickness a major public health problem in Africa. Epidemics cause fear in local populations, since the etiology of the disease is still mysterious, and have both social and economic consequences, such as depopulation and abandonment of farmland.

Tsetse control

Methods for controlling tsetse flies currently comprise insecticide application by knapsack sprayers or by air, trap/target technology,

bush clearance, or sterile male release (SIT). In planning an insecticide campaign, both adult flies and offspring must be considered. Females deposit their fully grown larvae on the ground in suitable sites where the soil is loose and moist; this is to facilitate rapid burrowing of the larva into the ground, where it pupates (Buxton 1955). Survival of pupae depends greatly on humidity and temperature and adult flies emerge roughly 3 weeks later. Thus, a single application of non-residual insecticide will have little effect on the tsetse population. Aerial spraying of insecticide (e.g. endosulphan) necessitates several spray cycles at weekly intervals. Effective knapsack spraying uses residual insecticides (e.g. dieldrin) applied to tsetse resting sites on foliage and branches. In the dry season tsetse populations retreat to the most favourable parts of their range making control far more cost-effective. Thorough knowledge of the distribution and habits of the tsetse species to be controlled is invaluable.

Environmental concerns have put widespread insecticide use into disfavour and promoted the development of trap and target technology (Fig. 42.5). Traps were originally used as a sampling method for tsetse populations and work on the principle that tsetse are attracted by sight to large dark objects. Whether this is in order to seek shade or a host is unclear, as one optimum but curious design is a biconical trap made of dark blue cloth. The tsetse enter at the bottom and move upwards through the trap towards the light, where they are imprisoned in a small cage and soon succumb to death by desiccation or hunger. Targets consisting of simple square sheets of the same colour cloth are also attractive and can be impregnated with insecticide (e.g. deltamethrin) to kill the flies as they land. Odour attractants (constituents of cow breath or urine) can be used in combination with traps or targets to increase the catch. These methodologies, although environmentally sound and low cost, are labour intensive. Large numbers of traps/targets need to be deployed to give adequate coverage and they require regular repair and replenishment of odour baits or insecticide. For these reasons, trap/target methodology is well suited to programmes involving community participation (Dransfield *et al.* 1991). Ideally traps or targets are constructed locally out of indigenous or cheap materials and are maintained by the community.

Bush clearance permanently destroys the habitat of tsetse and is cost effective when new farmland is gained. Sometimes, though, farming practices actually create new tsetse habitats: for example,

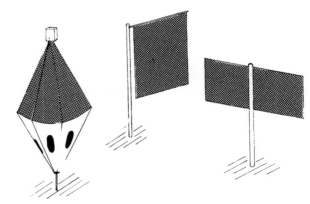

Fig. 42.5 Trap and targets for control of tsetse flies. Biconical trap (left); flies enter via holes at base and emerge into box cage at top. Insecticide-impregnated simple screen target (centre) and pivoted target (right).

the widespread introduction of *Lantana* hedges or plantations of conifers, coffee or cocoa.

Control by sterile male release or SIT depends on the fact that females mate once only and store the sperm until required. Sufficiently large numbers of sterile males in competition with wild males will thus reduce the population density over time. This technique is essentially long-term and requires high capital input initially to set up facilities for rearing and irradiating large numbers of male tsetse. The area of release needs to be isolated by geographical features or bush clearance in order to prevent re-invasion, and other techniques such as trapping or insecticides may need to be used in conjunction to push the tsetse population below recoverable levels. Hence, SIT was ideally suited to eradication of the single tsetse species on the island of Zanzibar, too far from the Tanzanian mainland for re-invasion. Multiple tsetse species and real possibilities for re-invasion, as well as high levels of capital cost, present enormous challenges for application of SIT elsewhere on the African continent.

Control of tsetse is often of both medical and veterinary concern, and this can lead to problems of communication if more than one government department or agency is involved. Sustained control programmes will be more cost-effective than emergency action in the long run. For example, regular application of insecticide by teams with knapsack sprayers or schemes to involve rural communities in making and maintaining tsetse traps are long-term, low-cost methods of control; application of insecticide from the air can rapidly and dramatically reduce transmission, but is a short-term, costly measure, unless the spraying permanently eliminates tsetse from the area.

Evaluation

The success of control programmes should be measurable by a decreasing incidence of sleeping sickness and, indeed, numbers of sleeping sickness cases have steadily dropped over the past ten years from the very high levels recorded in the 1990s. However, this was in part due to emergency interventions by international organizations to control epidemic disease. Resurgence will be prevented in the long-term by regular surveillance and fly control, difficult to maintain in countries where health resources are strained to the limits and there are other health priorities.

In principle, community participation schemes should devolve responsibility for control activities to local level thereby rendering them sustainable. In practice, without continued technical input, communities lose interest in control schemes as the problem becomes less acute.

Legislation

There is no legislation to control sleeping sickness in most endemic countries and cases are not adequately reported. Within tropical Africa it is potentially possible that movement of infected livestock between countries in the tsetse-infested zone could create new foci of disease, and disease spread has certainly happened in this way within Uganda (Hutchinson *et al.* 2003). The translocation of wildlife species from endemic to non-endemic areas is another potential risk. Infection with tsetse-transmitted trypanosomes is generally not considered to be a risk outside tropical Africa, since the chance of transmission is minimal. Cases are imported into Europe from time to time, usually in those who have visited wildlife areas.

References

Ashcroft, M.T. (1959). The importance of African wild animals as reservoirs of trypanosomiasis. *E. African Med. J.*, **36**: 289–97.

Berriman, M., Ghedin, E., Hertz-Fowler, C., et al. (2005). The genome of the African trypanosome *Trypanosoma brucei. Science*, **309**: 416–22.

Bisser, S., N'Siesi, F.X., Lejon, V., et al. (2007). Equivalence trial of Melarsoprol and nifurtimox monotherapy and combination therapy for the treatment of second-stage *Trypanosoma brucei gambiense* sleeping sickness. *J. Infect. Dis.*, **195**: 322–29.

Borst, P. and Cross, G.A.M. (1982). Molecular basis for trypanosome antigenic variation. *Cell*, **29**: 291–303.

Brown, C.G.D., Hunter, A.G. and Luckins, A.G. (1990). Protozoa. In: M.M.H. Sewell and D.W. Brocklesby (eds.) *Handbook on Animal Diseases in the Tropics*, pp. 161–226. London: Bailliere Tindall.

Brun, R. and Jenni, L. (1987). Human serum resistance of metacyclic forms of *Trypanosoma brucei brucei, T. brucei rhodesiense* and *T. brucei gambiense. Parasitology Research*, **73**: 218–23.

Buxton, P.A. (1955). *The natural history of tsetse flies. Memoir 10 London School of Hygiene and Tropical Medicine*. London: HK Lewis.

Cavalier-Smith, T. (1981). Eukaryote Kingdoms—seven or nine? *Biosystems*, **14**: 461–81.

Davies, J.N.P. (1962). The cause of sleeping sickness. Parts I and II. *E. African Med. J.*, **39**: 81–99 and 145–60.

De Greef, C., Imberechts, H., Matthyssons, G., Van Meirvenne, N. and Hamers, R. (1989). A gene expressed only in serum-resistant variants of *Trypanosoma brucei rhodesiense. Mol. Biochem. Parasit.*, **36**: 169–76.

Dransfield, R.D., Williams, B.G. and Brightwell, R. (1991). Control of tsetse flies and trypanosomiasis: myth or reality. *Parasit. Today*, **7**: 287–91.

Ford, J. (1971). *The role of the trypanosomiases in African ecology. A study of the tsetse fly problem*. Oxford: Clarendon Press.

Geigy, R., Jenni, L., Kauffmann, M., Onyango, R.J. and Weiss, N. (1975). Identification of *Trypanosoma brucei* subgroup strains isolated from game. *Acta Trop.*, **32**: 190–205.

Greenwood, B.M. and Whittle, H.C. (1980). The pathogenesis of sleeping sickness. *Trans. R. Soc. Trop. Med. Hyg.*, **74**: 716–25.

Heisch, R.B., McMahon, J.P. and Manson-Bahr, P.E.C. (1958). The isolation of *Trypanosoma rhodesiense* from a bushbuck. *BMJ*, **2**: 1203–4.

Hoare, C.A. (1972). *The Trypanosomes of Mammals*. Oxford: Blackwell Scientific Publications.

Hutchinson, O.C., Fevre, E.M., Carrington, M. and Welburn, S.C. (2003). Lessons learned from the emergence of a new *Trypanosoma brucei rhodesiense* sleeping sickness focus in Uganda. *Lancet Infect. Dis.*, **3**: 42–45.

Jelinek, T., Bisoffi, Z., Bonazzi, L., et al. (2002). Cluster of African trypanosomiasis in travelers to Tanzanian national parks. *Emerg. Infect. Dis.*, **8**: 634–35.

Joshi, P.P., Shegokar, V.R., Powar, R.M., et al. (2005). Human trypanosomiasis caused by *Trypanosoma evansi* in India: The first case report. *Am. J. Trop. Med. Hyg.*, **73**: 491–95.

Kristensson, K. and Bentivoglio, M. (1999). Pathology of African Trypanosomiasis. In: M. Dumas, B. Bouteille and A. Buguet (eds.) *Progress in Human African Trypanosomiasis, Sleeping sickness*, pp. 157–81. Paris: Springer-Verlag France.

Kuzoe, F.A.S. (1993). Current situation of African trypanosomiasis. *Acta Trop.*, **54**: 153–62.

Leak, S.G.A. (1999). *Tsetse biology and ecology. Their role in the epidemiology and control of trypanosomosis*. Oxford: CAB International.

Magnus, E., Vervoort, T. and van Meirvenne, N. (1978). A card agglutination test with stained trypanosomes (CATT) for the serological diagnosis of *Trypanosoma brucei gambiense* trypanosomiasis. *Ann. Soc. Belge Med. Tropic.*, **58**: 169–76.

Mansfield, J.M. (2001). Discussion document on pathogenesis/applied genomics. In: *Report of the Scientific Working Group on African Trypanosomiasis*, pp. 121–39. Geneva: WHO.

Maudlin, I. (1991). Transmission of African Trypanosomiasis: Interactions among tsetse immune system, symbionts and parasites. *Ad. Dis. Vector Res.*, **7:** 117–48.

Mehlitz, D., Zillmann, U., Scott, C.M. and Godfrey, D.G. (1982). Epidemiological studies on the animal reservoir of gambiense sleeping sickness. III. Characterisation of *Trypanozoon* stocks by isoenzymes and sensitivity to human serum. *Tropen. Parasit.*, **33:** 113–18.

Melville, S.E., Leech, V., Gerrard, C.S., Tait, A. and Blackwell, J.M. (1998). The molecular karyotype of the megabase chromosomes of *Trypanosoma brucei* and the assignment of chromosome markers. *Mol. Biochem. Parasit.*, **94:** 155–73.

Moloo, S.K., Losos, G.J. and Kutuza, S.B. (1973). Transmission of *Trypanosoma brucei* to cats and dogs by feeding on infected goats. *Trans. R. Soc. Trop. Med. Hyg.*, **67:** 287.

Moreira, D., López-García, P. and Vickerman, K. (2004). An updated view of kinetoplastid phylogeny using environmental sequences and a closer outgroup: proposal for a new classification of the class Kinetoplastea. *Intern. J. System. Evol. Microbiol.*, **54:** 1861–75.

Mulligan, H.W. (1970). *The African Trypanosomiases*. London: George Allen and Unwin.

Nash, T.A.M. (1969). *The tsetse fly —Africa's bane*. London: Collins.

Navarro, M. and Gull, K. (2001). A pol I transcriptional body associated with VSG mono-allelic expression in *Trypanosoma brucei. Nature*, **414:** 759–63.

Onyango, R.J., Van Hoeve, K. and De Raadt, P. (1966). The epidemiology of *Trypanosoma rhodesiense* sleeping sickness in Alego location, Central Nyanza, Kenya. I. Evidence that cattle may act as reservoir hosts of trypanosomes infective to man. *Trans. R. Soc. Trop. Med. Hyg.*, **60:** 175–82.

Opperdoes, F.R. (1985). Biochemical peculiarities of trypanosomes, African and South American. *Brit. Med. Bull.*, **41:** 130–36.

Pays, E., Vanhamme, L. and Perez-Morga, D. (2004). Antigenic variation in *Trypanosoma brucei*: facts, challenges and mysteries. *Curr. Opin. Microbiol.*, **7:** 369–74.

Pepin, J. (2007). Combination therapy for sleeping sickness: A wake-up call. *J. Infect. Dis.*, **195:** 311–13.

Rhind, S. and Shek, P. (1999). Cytokines in the pathogenesis of human African trypanosomiasis: antagonistic roles of TNF alpha and IL-10. In: M. Dumas, B. Bouteille and A. Buguet (eds.) *Progress in human African trypanosomiasis, sleeping sickness*, pp. 119–35. Paris: Springer-Verlag France.

Rickman, L.R. and Robson, J. (1970). The testing of proven *Trypanosoma brucei* and *T. rhodesiense* strains by the blood incubation infectivity test. *Bull. WHO*, **42:** 911–16.

Rogers, D.J. and Randolph, S.E. (2002). A response to the aim of eradicating tsetse from Africa. *Trends in Parasit.*, **18:** 534–36.

Simpson, L. (1990). RNA editing a novel genetic phenomenon? *Science*, **250:** 512–13.

Stephen, L.E. (1986). *Trypanosomiasis, a veterinary perspective*. Oxford: Pergamon Press.

Stuart, K.D., Schnaufer, A., Ernst, N.L. and Panigrahi, A.K. (2005). Complex management: RNA editing in trypanosomes. *Trends in Biochem. Sci.*, **30:** 97–105.

Vanhamme, L., Paturiaux-Hanocq, F., Poelvoorde, P., *et al.* (2003). Apolipoprotein L-1 is the trypanosome lytic factor of human serum. *Nature*, **422:** 83–87.

Vanhollebeke, B., Truc, P., Poelvoorde, P., *et al.* (2006). Brief report: human *Trypanosoma evansi* infection linked to a lack of apolipoprotein L-I. *N. Eng. J. Med.*, **355:** 2752–56.

Vincendeau, P., Jauberteau-Marchan, M.O., Daulouede, S. and Ayed, Z. (1999). Immunology of African Trypanosomiasis. In: M. Dumas, B. Bouteille and A. Buguet (eds.) *Progress in Human African Trypanosomiasis, Sleeping sickness*, pp. 137–56. Paris: Springer-Verlag France.

WHO (1998). *Control and surveillance of African Trypanosomiasis. Report of a WHO expert committee*. Geneva: World Health Organization.

WHO (2001). Overview and objectives, in (ed.) *Report of the Scientific Working Group on African Trypanosomiasis*, pp. 3–5. (Geneva: WHO)

WHO (2008). *African trypanosomiasis*. Available at: http://www.who.int/tdr/diseases/tryp/diseaseinfo.htm (access date June 2008).

Xong, V.H., Vanhamme, L., Chamekh, M., *et al.* (1998). A VSG expression site-associated gene confers resistance to human serum in *Trypanosoma rhodesiense. Cell*, **95:** 839–46.

CHAPTER 43

American trypanosomosis (Chagas disease)

C. J. Schofield

Summary

American trypanosomosis (more usually known as American trypanosomiasis) is due to infection with *Trypanosoma cruzi* (Protozoa, Kinetoplastidae). This is a widespread parasite of small mammals and marsupials throughout most of the Americas, roughly from the Great Lakes of North America (approx. 42°N) to southern Argentina (approx. 46°S). It is mainly transmitted by blood-sucking bugs of the subfamily Triatominae (Hemiptera, Reduviidae) which are widespread in the Americas, but rare in the Old World. Except in some research laboratories, and infected immigrants from Latin America, *T.cruzi* has not been reported from the Old World, although closely-related trypanosome species are commonly found in Old and New World bats.

Human infection with *T.cruzi* is generally known as Chagas disease, taking the name of Brasilian clinician Carlos Justiniano das Chagas who first described it from patients in central Brasil (Chagas 1909). Chagas isolated and described the parasite, correctly deduced most of its life-cycle and clinical symptoms associated with the infection, identified the insect vectors and some of the reservoir hosts, and also trialed initial attempts to control it. He was nominated at least twice for the Nobel prize in medicine (Coutinho and Dias 2000; Lewinsohn 2003).

Although difficult to treat, Chagas disease can be controlled by measures to halt transmission, primarily by eliminating domestic populations of the insect vectors, together with serological screening to avoid transmission by blood donation from infected donors. Since 1991, a series of multinational initiatives have used this approach to halt transmission over vast regions of the areas previously endemic for the human infection. Estimated prevalence of the human infection has declined from the 1990 estimate of 16–18 million people infected, to the current estimate of just over 7 million infected (OPS 2006; Schofield and Kabayo 2008). Prevalence is expected to decline further, and control strategies are now being adjusted to develop a sustainable system of disease surveillance, focal vector control, and specific treatment for any new cases (Schofield *et al.* 2006; WHO 2007). Guidance for diagnosis and treatment is also required for non-endemic countries, where recent years have seen increasing migration from Latin America such that cases of chronic Chagas disease have now been reported from amongst Latin American migrants in Europe, USA and Canada, and Japan, together with some congenital cases and transmission from infected blood donors and by organ transplant.

Introduction

Chronic Chagas disease is the principal cause of cardiomyopathy in Latin America, causing severe debility in up to 30% of those infected (Table 43.1). In some areas—particularly south of the Amazon region—the chronic disease is also associated with severe intestinal lesions leading to disfunctional dilations of the intestinal tract known as megasyndromes (eg. megaoesophagus, megacolon, and less frequently, megastomach) and sometimes also with neurological disorders although these are now less frequently seen. At its peak in the mid-1980s, the prevalence of human infection was estimated at around 24 million (Walsh 1984), suggesting an incidence of over 800,000 new cases each year in the absence of control interventions (Hayes and Schofield 1990) with an aggregate mortality rate of over 55,000 deaths per year. The early acute phase of infection can be fatal in up to 10% of cases, but more usually progresses to a chronic phase, initially asymptomatic, that leads to progressive tissue destruction, particularly of heart muscle, but also nervous tissue, mainly of the autonomous parasympathic innervation, that controls the dynamics of the hollow viscera. In 1993, the World Bank ranked Chagas disease as the most serious parasitic disease of the Americas in terms of its public health impact, with a disease burden (measured as DALYs—disability-adjusted life years) far exceeding even the combined burden of other parasitic diseases such as malaria, schistosomosis, and leishmaniosis (World Bank 1993). Since then, a series of multinational control initiatives has effectively halted transmission over vast areas of Latin America, such that current prevalence estimates have been reduced to around 7 million people infected, with a current incidence of little more than 50,000 new cases each year (OPS 2006; Dias *et al.* 2002; Schofield *et al.* 2006). Prevalence and incidence can be expected to decline further, although interruption of the current control and surveillance programmes would probably lead to a resurgence of transmission.

The causative parasite of Chagas disease, *Trypanosoma cruzi*, is mainly transmitted to humans in the faeces of blood-sucking bugs of the subfamily Triatominae (Hemiptera, Reduviidae). As the insects feed, they may defaecate the remains of their previous blood meal onto the host skin; parasites in these faeces can survive as long as they are moist, and will readily transit the mucosae of mouth, eye or nose, and in some cases may also transit abraded skin. Direct oral-route transmission of *T.cruzi* can occur by ingestion of food or

Table 43.1 Prevalence estimates for Chagas disease in Latin America

	2005 Population	Estimated number of *T.cruzi* infected individuals (OPS, 2006)
Argentina	38,747,000	1,600,000
Belize	270,000	2,000
Bolivia	9,182,000	620,000
Brazil	186,405,000	1,900,000
Chile	16,257,000	160,200
Colombia	45,600,000	436,000
Costa Rica	4,327,000	23,000
Ecuador	13,228,000	230,000
El Salvador	6,881,000	232,000
Guatemala	12,589,000	250,000
Honduras	7,205,000	220,000
Mexico	107,029,000	1,100,000
Nicaragua	5,142,000	58,600
Panama	3,232,000	21,000
Paraguay	5,899,000	150,000
Peru	27,968,000	192,000
Uruguay	3,306,000	21,700
Venezuela	26,749,000	310,000

drink contaminated with infected bug faeces, or triturated infected bugs, or by consuming undercooked meat or blood products of infected mammals. *T.cruzi* can also be transmitted by blood donation or organ transplant from infected donors, and occasionally by transplacental passage from infected mothers to the foetus (1–10% of infected mothers). Control in Latin America is therefore based primarily on eliminating domestic populations of the insect vectors, together with serological screening of blood donors to avoid the risk of transfusional transmission, and improved maternal health-care with specific treatment of infected new-borns. Vector-borne transmission does not yet occur outside the Americas (Schofield *et al.* 2009) but with migration of people from Latin America to other countries, there have been increasing reports of transmission by blood transfusion, organ transplant, and congenital transmission, in regions previously considered non-endemic for Chagas disease—particularly in North America and parts of Europe.

The agent

Trypanosoma cruzi is a widespread parasite of small mammals and marsupials throughout much of the New World, roughly from the Great Lakes of North America (approx. 42°N) to southern Argentina (approx. 46°S). It is a kinetoplastid flagellate whose bloodstream forms are typified by a large kinetoplast at the posterior end. This readily differentiates it from other trypanosomes, especially *T.rangeli* which is also a common parasite of small mammals in Latin America and can transiently infect humans (but without significant pathology). As far as is known, all mammals and marsupials are susceptible to infection with *T.cruzi*,

although birds, amphibians and reptiles are refractory. In marsupials and autochthonous mammals, *T. cruzi* appears to cause little if any pathology, and the infection in such animals tends to retain a relatively high parasitaemia. In humans however, and in mammals (such as dogs, cats, murine rodents) probably brought in recent times to the Americas, parasitaemia is reduced to subpatent levels after the initial acute phase, and the parasites mainly develop intracellularly causing pathology primarily through inflammation and progressive tissue disruption.

Since the pioneering studies of Miles *et al.* (1977), the phylogenetics of *T.cruzi* have been extensively studied, showing that different isolates of the parasite could be consistently grouped according to their isoenzymatic profiles, with zymodeme 1 (Z1) being the most widespread, zymodeme 2 (Z2) found mainly from human infections and domestic animals in the Southern Cone region (south of the Amazon basin), and zymodeme 3 (Z3) from Amazonian isolates (see: Miles and Cibulskis 1986). Subsequent studies led to a consensus of two main lineages denoted *T.cruzi* I and *T.cruzi* II (Anon,1999). Of these, *cruzi* I (Z1) appears to be the more widespread both in North and South America, and in silvatic habitats seems particularly associated with didelphid opossums. *T. cruzi* II (including Z2 and Z3) is genetically more variable (now subdivided into *cruzi* II *a-e*, and also into a series of numbered clones, according to genetic differences) and is mainly found in South America (south of Panama) (Table 43.2). A reclassification of *T.cruzi* into 6 discrete typing units (DTUs) has recently been proposed (Zingales *et al.* 2009), elevating *cruzi* II *a-e* to *cruzi* II-VI. In human infections, both *cruzi* I and *cruzi* II can be associated with chronic cardiomyopathy, but in general it is only forms of *cruzi* II that are also associated with the gastrointestinal lesions known as megasyndromes.

There is genetic and biogeographical evidence to suggest that the ancestral forms of *T.cruzi* developed originally as parasites of marsupials within the southern supercontinent, and in genetic terms, some of the closest extant relatives of *T.cruzi* are trypanosomes of kangaroos and wombats in Australia (Stevens *et al.* 2001). From these ancestral forms, the original form of *T.cruzi* may have developed as a parasite of didelphid opossums as the supercontinent divided to give rise to South America some 70mya, accompanying the didelphids along their subsequent spread northwards. This original form would probably have been directly transmitted between opossums via their anal gland secretions and/or urine (Jansen and Deane 1985; Olsen *et al.* 1964), and would be represented today by the form now referred to as *T.cruzi* I. The genetic divergence from *cruzi* I to *cruzi* II, now dated as 4-10mya (Brisse *et al.* 2003) may have resulted from the advent of triatomine insect vectors, providing the physical means to transmit the parasite to different mammalian hosts, such that the variability now seen in *cruzi* II probably represents a series of adaptations to these different host species (Schofield 2000) with recombination and genetic exchange also contributing to differentiation within this lineage (e.g. Yeo *et al.* 2005; Freitas *et al.* 2006).

In general terms, *T.cruzi* seems a rather non-specific parasite, in the sense that all mammals and marsupials seem to be susceptible to infection, and, once infected, will usually retain the infection for life. Birds, reptiles and amphibians however, are refractory to the infection as the parasite is killed by complement-mediated lysis in avian or reptilian blood. Amongst mammals, the infection tends to be most prevalent in those that construct nests or lodges which

Table 43.2 Subspecific nomenclature of *Trypanosoma cruzi*

Subspecific designation	Zymodeme (Miles *et al.* 1977, 1978)	Clonets (Zymodemes) (Tibayrenc *et al.* 1991)	DTU (Discrete Typing Units) (Zingales *et al.* 2009)	Known Distribution
T.cruzi I	Z1	1–25	TcI	North, Central and South America, human and silvatic mammal isolates (especially opossums)
T.cruzi II a	Z3	26–29	TcIV	USA, Amazon basin, human and silvatic mammal isolates
T.cruzi II b	Z2	30–34	TcII	Mainly South American, mainly human and rodent isolates
T.cruzi II c	Z3/Z1 ASAT	35–37	TcIII	USA, Amazon basin, human and silvatic mammal isolates
T.cruzi II d	Bolivian Z2 'heterozygous' (hybrid genotype)	38–39	TcV	Bolivia, associated with humans, rodents, and *T.infestans*, and human cases in other parts of the Southern Cone countries
T.cruzi II e	Paraguayan Z2 'heterozygous' (hybrid genotype)	40–43	TcVI	Bolivia and Paraguay, associated with humans and rodents

may be infested with vector species of Triatominae, so that larger mammals such as cattle and horses are less likely to be infected.

T.cruzi can also survive in a wide variety of invertebrate hosts, even artificially infected leeches and wax-moth larvae (see Schofield *et al.* 2009). It seems to survive, at least transiently, in most blood-sucking insects especially ticks and cimicid bedbugs, but tends not to develop further except in Triatominae, and no invertebrate except for triatomine bugs has ever been shown to have epidemiological significance as a vector of *T.cruzi*. In triatomine bugs, ingested bloodstream forms of the parasite (bloodstream trypomastigotes) multiply as epimastigotes in the midgut, transforming to infective (metacyclic) trypomastigotes in the hindgut (rectum) from where they can be expelled as the bug defaecates. *T.cruzi* does not survive in the haemocoele of the bugs, and so cannot penetrate the salivary glands and cannot be transmitted by the bug's bite.

The infection—Chagas disease

The course of *T.cruzi* infection in mammals is extremely variable throughout the infection, depending on type of host and parasite strain. In general, the course of human infection is marked by an initial acute phase, defined by patent parasitaemia, followed by a life-long chronic phase during which the parasites are mainly present inside the cells of various organs rather than in the bloodstream.

After infection, the parasites multiply locally at the portal of entry, sometimes causing a localized palpable lesion known as a 'chagoma'. Where the portal of entry was the eye, this may result in palpable unilateral ocular oedema known as 'Romañas sign' following the work of Argentine clinician Dr Cecilio Romaña who showed its clear association with acute Chagas disease in humans. In such cases, trypanosomes may be present in the chagoma, and, in the case of Romañas sign, in the orbital tissues, especially the ocular muscles and lachrymal glands (so that some trypanosomes may also be shed in the tears). But Romañas sign can be readily distinguished from other unilateral ocular oedemas since it is persistent (a month or more), painless, and without indications of inflammation or haematoma (thus distinguishing it from conjunctivitis

which is generally inflamed and not so persistent, a blow to the eye which is usually painful and bruised, or a wasp/bee sting which would be inflamed, painful, and of relatively short duration). In some regions, over 50% of acute *T.cruzi* infections show Romañas sign or detectable chagoma, although in other regions such signs are now rarely seen. It is possible that a high frequency of Romañas sign is indicative of an unusual parasite strain becoming locally dominant, such that frequency of the sign may decline with time as that strain becomes more adapted to humans.

The acute phase of infection generally lasts 6–8 weeks, and is defined by the presence of a patent parasitaemia (ie. parasites visible by microscopy of a fresh blood film). This phase may show few if any symptoms, although it is often accompanied by fever, usually low-grade and non-cyclic, together with malaise, headache, lymphadenopathy, and diffuse heart pains. In some cases there may be tachycardia, hepatosplenomegaly, subcutaneous nodules, or a diffuse rash resembling measles. The acute-phase can be life-threatening, with mortality in 5–10% of acute-phase patients—usually due to overwhelming myocarditis or meningoencephalitis. For those who survive, parasites are progressively cleared from the bloodstream by a strong immune response, such that *cruzi*-specific serology then tends to remain positive for the remainder of the infection. In immunocompromised patients, the acute phase can be prolonged and life-threatening. Similarly, immunosuppression of patients in the chronic phase, e.g. by HIV infection or immunosuppression during transplant, can lead to reactivation of the acute phase. During the chronic phase of infection, the parasites mainly survive as intracellular amastigote forms that multiply and transform within the host cells until the infected cell bursts, liberating trypomastigotes to infect neighbouring cells where the process is repeated. A few of these trypomastigotes will also escape to the peripheral bloodstream—insufficient to cause patent parasitaemia, but generally sufficient to infect a triatomine bug feeding from this infected host.

For most patients, the chronic phase of *T.cruzi* infection is asymptomatic, and the infection is often described as 'indeterminate'. For many, this state will persist for life, without any need for supportive treatment or modifications of their general life-style.

Nevertheless, a positive diagnosis, e.g. following screening of blood donors, can be extremely stressful because, at present, no specific treatment is offered to chronic adult patients, and there is no reliable way to predict whether or not the infection will remain asymptomatic in that patient. It is therefore important that all chronic cases, even if entirely asymptomatic, receive adequate counselling to explain possible progression of the infection, together with regular clinical check-up to monitor progress. For some, estimated at 20–40% in different studies, the chronic infection will lead to moderate or severe lesions, especially of the heart, often decades after the initial infection.

The early signs of cardiomyopathy are revealed by electrocardiography, usually mild arhythmias such as extra-systoles or first degree atrioventricular block. These can often be controlled using antiaryhthmic drugs, of which amiodarone is generally recommended and seems also to have some specific anti-trypanosome effects (Benaim et al. 2006). In some cases the aryhthmias will progress to complete right bundle branch block (often considered pathognomic for chronic symptomatic Chagas disease) with left anterior hemiblock and eventually complete atrioventricular block and consequent Stokes-Adams attacks. Repeated heart attacks, severe aryhthmias and emboli are signs of a poor prognosis, and sudden death due to cardiac arrest or ventricular fibrillation is well documented. More common however, is simple pump failure due to extensive pancarditis with muscle fibre destruction—the patient is lethargic, with cold extremities, and quite unable to work (and it is this debility that, in epidemiological terms, is mainly responsible for the high socio-economic cost of the disease). In extreme cases, destruction of the heart muscle is severe enough to lead to cardiac aneurism, especially at the apex, with the heart bursting on exercise.

Cardiomyopathy is the most common symptom of chronic symptomatic Chagas disease, seen throughout the endemic areas of Latin America. Informal polls of cardiologists in Mexico and Central America indicate that 20–25% of all cardiac pacemakers implanted are due to chronic Chagas disease, and this has been a major factor prompting large-scale initiatives designed to halt transmission of T.cruzi. In the southern part of the continent however, where strains of cruzi II predominate in human cases, chronic Chagas disease is also commonly associated with lesions of the intestinal tract collectively known as megasydromes. Most common is megaoesophagous—the oesophagous becomes dilated with solid residues due to aperistalsis and spasm of the cardiac sphincter. Patients have difficulties in swallowing, and require copious liquid to assist the passage of food. Also common in some areas,especially central Brasil and Bolivia, is megacolon, associated with persistent constipation requiring manual evacuation. More rarely, other parts of the digestive tract may be involved, including megaduodenum, megabladder, mega-gallbladder, and megastomach. In early cases, treatment by sphincter dilation has been widely used, while for later cases surgical resectioning can be successful (Dias and Coura 1997).

Pathogenesis and treatment

One of the least understood aspects of Chagas disease has been the mechanism of pathogenesis, and this has affected policies of transmission control and policies regarding specific treatment.

The strong immune response generated by immunocompetent people during the acute phase of infection, which then persists throughout the infection, has been recognized since the earliest studies of the disease, with the first immunological assays of infection being developed in 1914. However, this immunological response also led to a generalized assumption that reinfection would be both unlikely and of little relevance, because any newly-introduced parasites would meet an immune defence already maintained by the initial infection. The implication for policies of transmission control is, therefore, that even halting new transmission would do nothing for those already infected. In recent years however, this idea has become strongly challenged, first by clinical anecdote and epidemiological indications that the prognosis for chronic cases seemed to improve in areas where vector-borne transmission had been interrupted (Dias et al. 2002) and then by direct experimentation in murine models showing that the likelihood of chronic cardiopathy was significantly increased in mice that were repeatedly challenged, compared to mice that were infected only once (Bustamente et al. 2002; 2007). There is also evidence that the likelihood of transplacental (congenital) transmission by infected mothers to the foetus tends to decline when the mothers are no longer subject to repeated reinfections, e.g. following successful vector control interventions. It appears that both pathology, and likelihood of transmission, have a positive relationship with what might be termed 'parasite load'.

There were also many theories offering different explanations of the main pathogenic mechanisms, most of which tended to assume that pathology was triggered by the parasites but not otherwise directly dependent on them. The painstaking studies of Köberle for example, who carefully studied patterns of denervation in chronic infections, were generally interpreted to suggest that during the chronic phase the incipient organic damage had been done, so that specific chemotherapy against the parasite would be of little relevance. Similarly, the idea that Chagas disease was primarily an autoimmune phenomenon, i.e. a response to self-antigens that have been mimicked by the parasite, also carried the implication that specific treatment during the chronic phase would be of little relevance, because the parasite had already triggered the autoimmune response and so played little role in the development of chronic pathology. Again however, these ideas have been seriously questioned by more recent work that indicates that persistence of the parasite, together with some 'imbalance' of the immune system which may include autoimmune components, is the primary requisite for triggering and maintaining the inflammatory processes responsible for the chronic lesions. And since a key component of this process seems to be related to cellular destruction caused by the parasites themselves, these studies have led to considerable re-interest in the idea of developing new drugs, and also in offering treatment to all those infected, chronic as well as acute, as a means to inhibit development of the chronic disease.

Only two drugs are currently available for treatment of Chagas disease, both introduced some 30 years ago. Nifurtimox, a nitrofuran developed by Bayer in 1967 and marketed as Lampit®, acts by reduction of the nitro group to give nitro-anions that then react with molecular oxygen to produce toxic superoxide and peroxide radicals. Benznidazole, a nitroimidazol developed by Roche in 1972 and marketed as Rochagan® or Radanil®, appears to act differently, producing metabolites that react with macromolecules such as DNA, RNA, proteins and possibly some lipids. In both cases however, the antiparasitic activity is intimately linked with their inherent toxicity, such that adverse side effects during treatment are quite common, especially amongst older patients. Both drugs can induce malaise, headaches, and loss of concentration; nifurtimox frequently causes loss of appetite, weight-loss and in some cases anorexia, while benznidazole is more frequently associated with allergic dermatitis and in some cases peripheral neuritis. In a few cases, the reactions can be severe enough to require suspension of treatment, although intolerance to one drug is rarely associated with intolerance to the other.

Both nifurtimox and benznidazole were quickly shown to be effective in treating acute infections, with cure rates typically well above 80% (Table 43.3). However, because of side-effects and doubts about the likelihood of cure for chronic patients (see above) their potential for treating chronic infections was largely ignored. Only since the work of Viotti et al. (1994) has the benefit of specific treatment of chronic infections begun to be more widely accepted, and since the Pan American Health Organization (PAHO) expert committee meeting in 1998 (PAHO document OPS/HCP/HCT140/99) there is growing consensus that treatment should be given to all acute cases and asymptomatic chronic cases, with the aim of inhibiting the development of disease even if radical parasitological cure is not obtained. At present, most endemic countries accept the recommendation to treat all chronic infections in children below the age of 15–16 years, although current studies are suggesting that specific treatment should also be offered, at least to asymptomatic cases, up to 50 years of age (Viotti et al. 2006, 2009).

Due to lack of demand during the 1980s and 90s, the production of nifurtimox was abandoned in 1997, but restarted in 1999 in response to the usefulness of this drug in treating melarsoprol-resistant cases of gambiense sleeping sickness in West Africa. Through agreement with the World Health Organization (WHO), production has now been assured, at least until 2012, and nifurtimox is available free-of-charge through WHO Geneva and WHO-PAHO offices in Latin America. Under a technology-transfer agreement from Roche, benznidazole is now produced by Laboratorios Farmaceuticas do Estado de Pernambuco (LAFEPE) in Brasil, but can be made available at cost through WHO Geneva.

Table 43.3 Recommended treatment regimes for *T.cruzi* infection (4)

Nifurtimox (Lampit®)

Adults: 8–10 mg/Kg body weight per day, divided in two or three doses orally during 60 days

Newborns and children: 15 mg/Kg per day, same regime

Benznidazole (Rochagan®, Radanil®)

Adults: 5 mg/Kg body weight per day, divided in two or three doses orally, during 60 days (1,2,3)

Newborns and children: 10 mg/Kg body weight per day, same regime (3).

1: a 10 day treatment regime with benznidazole is suggested for *immediate* presumptive treatment, eg. following a laboratory accident, as this avoids most risk of side-effects that generally start to appear after the eighth day of treatment.

2: total dose of benznidazole should not exceed 300mg per day, irrespective of body weight. If the patient weighs more than 60kg, treatment can be extended for more than 60 days in order to complete the total required dosage.

3: some clinicians use a regime of 30 days treatment with benznidazole, but this is often insufficient—especially in cases of infection with *T.cruzi* IIb, which is the most common in central and southern Brazil.

4: following successful treatment with nifurtimox or benznidazole, seronegativisation may be seen after about 12–24 months in newborns and children, but in adults seronegativisation may require several years, even decades.

Several newer compounds are currently in development for the treatment of *T.cruzi* infections, especially sterol inhibitors such as pozaconazol and ravuconazol originally developed as fungicides, as well as cistein-protease inhibitors (cruzipain), trypanothione inhibitors, and pyrophosphate inhibitors (Urbina and Docampo 2003) although none is expected to become available for public health use for several years.

The vectors—Triatominae (Hemiptera, Reduviidae)

The Triatominae are traditionally defined as a subfamily of the Reduviidae, characterized by their blood-sucking habit and associated morphological features (such as a slim three-segmented rostrum with articulated third segment). Adults tend to be large insects, typically around 2.5 cm long, although some silvatic species reach no more than 0.5cm while the largest species, *Dipetalogaster maxima* from Baja California, has adults up to 4.5 cm long. Triatominae are hemimetabolous (exopterygote) insects, such that their developmental cycle proceeds from eggs through 5 nymphal stages to the adults. All the nymphal stages and both sexes of adult are haematophagous and potentially capable of becoming infected and transmitting *T.cruzi*. However there is no transovarial transmission of *T.cruzi*, meaning that newly hatched nymphs will not become infected until their first blood meal from an infected host. As a result, the likelihood of them being infected increases with the number of blood meals taken, so that the infection rate tends to be low in the youngest nymphs, but often increases to above 50% in the adults. Triatominae generally require at least one replete blood meal during each nymphal stage (although a series of smaller meals can be sufficient). Replete feeding typically requires 10–20 minutes, during which time the bugs will usually engorge several times their unfed weight of blood, so that the blood meal of an average-sized adult bug will typically be around 0.4ml—although adult *D. maxima* have been recorded as engorging up to 4.5ml during a single feed. At temperatures between 20–30°C, most Triatominae will try to feed every 5–15 days, and can complete their egg-to-adult development in 5–6 months with adults then living a further 3–12 months, although some of the larger species will often take 12 months to complete their developmental cycle. However, feeding activity and development is slower at cooler temperatures, and generally halts at temperatures below 15°C.

At the time of writing, 140 species of Triatominae are recognized, customarily grouped into 5 tribes with 17 genera (Schofield and Galvão 2009) (Table 43.4). Over half of these species have been shown to be naturally or experimentally infected with *T.cruzi*, and it is assumed that all may be capable of transmitting the parasite. In epidemiological terms however, relatively few of these species are of major significance, because most occupy silvatic habitats with little contact with humans. Of greatest epidemiological importance are those species that have adapted to live in close association with humans, especially those that colonize human dwellings. Of these, most important in the Southern Cone countries is *Triatoma infestans*, together with *T.brasiliensis* and *Panstrongylus megistus* in NE and central Brasil. In the Andean Pact countries, the most important is *Rhodnius prolixus* in Venezuela and parts of Colombia, together with *R.ecuadoriensis* in southern Ecuador and northern Peru. A derivative form of *R. prolixus* is also the most important domestic vector in parts of Central America, together with

Table 43.4 Tribes and genera of Triatominae *

Tribe	Genus	Number of species
Alberproseniini	*Alberprosenia*	2
Bolboderini	*Belminus*	8
	Bolbodera	1
	Microtriatoma	2
	Parabelminus	2
Cavernicolini	*Cavernicola*	2
Rhodniini	*Psammolestes*	3
	Rhodnius	16
Triatomini	*Dipetalogaster*	1
	Eratyrus	2
	Hermanlentia	1
	Linshcosteus	6
	Panstrongylus	13
	Paratriatoma	1
	Triatoma	80

* following Schofield and Galvão (2009).

T.dimidiata whose distribution also extends southwards into Colombia and Ecuador, and northwards into Mexico.

Over their wide distribution in the Americas, silvatic Triatominae can usually be found in almost any habitat offering shelter and ready access to a source of vertebrate blood. Habitats such as mature palm-tree crowns, opossum lodges, rodent burrows, rock-piles, and the more permanent nests of colonial parrots or dendro-colaptid birds (irrespective of the host currently occupying the nest) seem particularly favoured. In general terms, species of *Rhodnius* tend to be associated with palm-tree crowns, *Psammolestes* with birdnests, *Panstrongylus* with burrows (especially of ground dwelling edentates), and *Triatoma* with rockpiles and rodent burrows. Species of *Rhodnius* are mainly found in the Amazon region and neighbouring parts of the Venezuelan llanos and Brasilian caatinga and cerrado, broadly bounded by the distribution of the three main groups of *Triatoma*—the rubrofasciata group mainly of Central and North America, the dispar complex along the Andean mountains, and the infestans group of the caatinga-cerrado-chaco corridor of open vegetation to the east and south of the Amazon basin (Schofield and Galvão 2009).

Most populations of silvatic Triatominae tend to be relatively small, consisting of only a few adults and nymphs, which probably reflects some unreliability in their likelihood of encountering a suitable food source. Similarly, individual bugs from silvatic populations are often physically larger than conspecific individuals from domestic populations, which may be a reflection of their need to be able to store food for longer periods between relatively irregular blood meals. The generally low nutritional status of silvatic Triatominae is also indicated by the efficiency of the 'Noireau trap', a sticky trap containing a live mouse or similar small host, which is widely used to collect samples of bugs from silvatic habitats (e.g. Abad-Franch *et al.* 2000). By contrast, similar animal-baited traps have proved much less effective is sampling domestic triatomine populations, presumably

because the 'bait' must compete with a much wider range of other blood meal sources in a domestic habitat.

Silvatic triatomine populations are increasingly studied, because of their potential importance in recolonizing rural houses, and also for the capacity of some species to enter houses without necessarily succeeding in forming new colonies there. Bugs that fly into houses, e.g. attracted by house lights, can be a nuisance due to their relatively painful bites, and also represent a risk of transmitting *T.cruzi* even in areas where domestic bug populations do not occur. In such cases, transmission may be direct, e.g. to dogs and cats that may eat an infected bug, or it may be indirect due to the bugs contaminating food or drink. In and around the Amazon region for example, there are now several records of 'family microepidemics' where outbreaks of acute Chagas disease have been attributed to infected adult bugs contaminating fruit juice, soup, or other food-stuffs, that have then been consumed by several family members and their guests (e.g. Coura *et al.* 2002; Valente and Valente 1999). However, there are several key aspects of the biology of silvatic bugs that remain poorly understood—particularly the factors that may trigger adult bugs to fly into houses, their mechanisms of orientation, and the factors that influence whether or not they will successfully establish a new domestic colony.

Light-trap collections of silvatic bugs, and direct studies of laboratory-reared bugs, indicate that adult flight occurs only when the bugs are relatively starved, that is to say, well-fed adult bugs usually do not fly (Lehane *et al.* 1992). From this, and from the few epidemiological cases that have been studied in detail, it is suggested that flight of silvatic bugs is mainly triggered by ecological events such as flood, drought or fire, that lead to host death or flight. Bugs then become hungry, and adults may fly—presumably in search of new blood meal sources. However, little is known about their orientation mechanisms. Although it is generally assumed that bugs fly into houses attracted by light at night, such a process cannot explain how bugs move from one silvatic habitat to another. New silvatic habitats do become colonized, but it is not clear how the bugs find the new silvatic habitats. Specific odour attractants have not been clearly demonstrated, and it may be that the silvatic bugs are responding mainly to the warmth (e.g. infrared) emitted by different vertebrates.

Biology of domestic Triatominae

In houses, especially rural dwellings with cracked adobe or mud walls, domestic populations of Triatominae encounter a ready supply of blood meal sources in the form of the people and domestic animals occupying the house, together with some protection from climatic extremes and silvatic predators. As a result, they can build up very large populations, often with several thousand nymphs and adults in a single house—the 'record' is a rural house in Colombia dismantled to reveal a population of over 11,000 *R.prolixus* (Sandoval *et al.* 2000). The final population size is naturally regulated through a density-dependent mechanism mediated primarily by the bugs' access to blood meals—in a sense, more blood = more bugs (Schofield 1980). Hungry bugs, resting in cracks and crevices of the house walls and roof during the day, emerge at night to feed on the sleeping occupants. As more bugs try to feed from a single host, that host–although still asleep–tends to become more restless, disturbing the bugs from completing their meal (Schofield *et al.* 1986). Nymphs with a smaller blood meal develop more slowly, and adult females with a smaller blood meal lay fewer eggs, so that the rate of recruitment from one stage to the next tends to decline, so reducing the overall blood demand. Conversely, as bug density declines, then each bug can access more blood, so increasing their rate of development and rate of egg-laying and increasing the rate of recruitment from one stage to the next. In this way, an established domestic bug population tends to be stable, not in numbers, but in total blood demand (in the sense that an older bug has a larger blood demand than a younger bug). Studies of *T.infestans* in houses in central Brasil, and of *R.prolixus* in houses in Venezuela, both indicate that the average blood intake of the bug populations is equivalent to about 2.5ml per person per night, typically representing about 25 bites per person per night (Rabinovich *et al.* 1979; Schofield 1981). For many people, especially those on a poor diet or with other blood-sucking parasites such as intestinal hookworms, this level of chronic blood loss probably contributes significantly to chronic iron-deficiency anaemia.

As Triatominae feed, they may defaecate the remains of their previous blood meal onto the host, and, if infected, this can pose a risk of *T.cruzi* transmission. This method of transmission is inefficient compared to direct injection of, say, malaria parasites by a feeding mosquito. Studies in Venezuela suggest that on average, each successful transmission event is associated with around 1,000 feeding contacts by infected *R. prolixus* (Rabinovich *et al.* 1995) although with 25 bites per night, this is readily achieved in a few months, and helps explain why the average age of new human infections tends to be in the first few years of life. The timing of defaecation depends on bug species, such that some (such as the aptly-named *T.protracta*) may defaecate up to an hour after having left their host, while others are more likely to defaecate while still in the act of feeding and so still in contact with the host. But for each species, defaecation also seems to be a density-dependent process, in the sense that in high density bug populations where each insect takes only a small blood meal, defaecation tends to be later than in low density populations where each bug is feeding towards complete engorgement (Kirk and Schofield 1987; Trumper and Gorla 1991). Paradoxically therefore, it is in low density bug populations (i.e. those recently established, that are still growing towards their maximum) where the risk of new transmission is highest, since each bug is more likely to take a full meal and so defaecate while feeding on the host. By contrast, in high density bug populations, where each bug takes a smaller meal, defaecation tends to be retarded and generally occurs when the fed bug has returned to its resting site. The walls of heavily infested houses are thus often streaked with the characteristic faecal smears of Triatominae— white streaks representing their uric acid, together with dark brown streaks representing the undigested part of haemoglobin.

Understanding these density-dependent processes in the development and feeding behaviour of domestic Triatominae carries an important moral for the vector control strategies, suggesting that poorly-executed or partial vector control interventions can be more dangerous than no control at all. Partial control, that does not eliminate the bug population, implies that the remaining bugs will now be able to feed to a maximum, defaecating while still in contact with their hosts, and so facilitating further transmission of *T.cruzi*.

Control and surveillance

The essence of Chagas disease control in Latin America is the elimination of domestic vector populations. Prior to the current

multinational initiatives (see below) domestic vectors were estimated to account for well over 80% of all transmission (e.g. Schofield 1994) and adequate techniques for eliminating these populations had been available since the 1940s. In addition, there are further justifications for eliminating domestic Triatominae, beyond their role as Chagas disease vectors, because of the severe nuisance and chronic blood-loss associated with them.

Early attempts to control domestic Triatominae relied on the idea of improving rural houses, for example by plastering over the cracked walls where bugs were seen to be resting. By itself, house improvement is usually insufficient to eliminate a domestic triatomine population, but can reduce the likelihood that an un-infested house becomes recolonized by the bugs (Guillén *et al.* 1997). In the 1940s, attempts were also made with cyanide gas fumigation, petrol or diesel applied to house walls, and even flame-throwers, but such approaches proved impractical on an extended scale (Dias and Schofield 2004). Since then, a wide range of other techniques has been tested, including insecticides of various classes, insect growth regulators, chemosterilants, insect pathogens or predators, and various approaches at genetic control, e.g. by trying to select for heritable sub-sterility, and also by genetically-modified symbionts rendering the bugs refractory to infection with *T.cruzi*. Most have been rejected for large-scale use due to ineffectiveness or impracticability for large-scale interventions, except for indoor application of adequate insecticides, house improvement where economically feasible, and health education to promote community participation in reporting domestic infestations so they can be adequately sprayed.

Although DDT was quickly found to be ineffective against domestic Triatominae, other organochlorine insecticides such as gamma-BHC (also known as HCH or lindane) and dieldrin proved to be effective when applied at high doses (>500mg a.i./m²) and these compounds remained the main products used for domestic triatomine control until being progressively replaced by synthetic pyrethroids during the 1980s. The alpha-cyano pyrethroids proved to have several advantages, being effective at much lower doses and so proving cost-effective in spite of their higher price per kilo (Table 43.5). They were also preferred by spraymen and householders as they were easier to transport and apply, and generally did not mark the sprayed walls.

In general terms, the interventions begin by informing the householders and checking to see if the house has evidence of a current infestation. Several techniques are used for this, involving householder reports of bugs, and visual inspection of the interior house walls and furnishings (using torch and long blunt forceps) for evidence such as live bugs, bug eggs, eggshells, exuviae, and faecal streaks. In some cases, the search for live bugs is aided by spraying an aqueous dislodgant agent into cracks, usually a non-residual pyrethroid such as tetramethrin, which irritates the bugs making them more easy to see. With the aid of the householders, the house is then prepared for residual spraying, removing to the outside all children, animals, foodstuffs, kitchen utensils, bedding and clothes, and the furniture is moved to give access the walls behind. All internal surfaces are then sprayed with the recommended dose of pyrethroid (Table 43.5) including the furniture and inner roof space. Spraying is best done by well-trained operators, thus avoiding the possibility of missing areas that can serve as untreated refuges for the bugs. In most cases, peridomestic structures are also sprayed, including latrines, chicken coops and animal enclosures, since these can also harbour bugs.

Table 43.5 Recommended insecticides and dose rates for elimination of domestic Triatominae

Insecticide	Formulation*	Target application dose (mg a.i./m²)**
Deltamethrin	SC or WP	25
Lambda-cyhalothrin	WP or CS	30
Cyfluthrin	WP	50
Betacyfluthrin	SC	25
Alphamethrin	SC or WP	50
Cypermethrin	WP	125

* SC = suspension concentrate; WP = wettable powder; CS = microencapsulated; note that EC formulations (emulsifiable concentrates) are not recommended for this purpose, as they absorb too rapidly into the wall structure.

** mg a.i./m² = mg of active ingredient applied per square metre of surface.

A thorough spray with an adequate pyrethroid at the correct dose is usually sufficient to eliminate the domestic Triatominae, and can also give transient control of other domestic pests such as fleas, cockroaches, and scorpions. However, the sprayed house remains vulnerable to reinfestation by bugs coming from elsewhere. The technical response to this problem has been to try to increase the residual effect of the insecticides, for example by using longer-lasting formulations such as wettable powders (WP), suspension concentrates (SC), microencapsulated formulations (CS), or even polymerized formulations (often known as 'insecticidal paints'). But the strategic response is to eliminate the sources of 'reinvading' bugs, i.e. to extend the geographical scale of the control programme to include all the infested houses that could provide source populations for bugs to re-infest those houses already treated. This implies very large-scale coverage, often reaching national or multinational scales of intervention in the case of the most widespread domestic vectors.

The multinational initiatives

Following from a series of field trials, and large-scale campaigns in São Paulo (Wanderley 1994; Jacintho da Silva 1999) and in several states of Venezuela (Guevara de Sequeda *et al.* 1986) the government of Brasil in 1983 launched the first national campaign designed to eliminate all domestic populations of their main Chagas disease vector, *Triatoma infestans*. Although highly successful at the outset (Dias 1987) the campaign was interrupted in 1986 by re-emergence of *Aedes aegypti* in several coastal cities, with the associated threat of widespread dengue outbreaks. The national Chagas disease campaign essentially collapsed as field staff engaged in Chagas disease control were redeployed against urban *Aedes*.

Two key features of this Brasilian campaign guided development of what then became known as the Southern Cone Initiative (INCOSUR). The national campaign had shown the effectiveness of the control techniques and operational strategy, but also indicated that elimination of *T.infestans* would be unsustainable in Brasil if neighbouring countries did not carry out similar campaigns. Control interventions would also be unsustainable if interrupted by changing ministerial priorities. In essence the campaign would require a wider geographical scale together with continuous political commitment. The enlightened response was to develop a

multinational initiative designed to cover the entire geographical distribution of *T.infestans*, some 6 million km² covering parts of seven countries (Argentina, Bolivia, Brazil, Chile, Paraguay, southern Peru, and Uruguay). This initiative, coordinated by the PAHO, was launched in 1991 following resolution of the Ministers of Health at their meeting in Brasilia, with the stated objective of interrupting the transmission of Chagas disease by elimination of *T.infestans* (and suppression of other domestic vectors in the same areas) and improved screening of blood donors to reduce the risk of transfusional transmission (Schofield and Dias 1999).

Although the INCOSUR objectives have not been entirely realized, substantial progress has been made. Through large-scale indoor spraying of infested premises, the distribution of *T.infestans* has been reduced from its predicted maximum of some 6.28 million km² (Gorla 2002) to less than 1 million km². Uruguay was formally declared free of Chagas disease transmission due to *T. infestans* in 1997, Chile in 1999, Brasil in 2006, together with several provinces and departments of Argentina and Paraguay. Some progress has also been made in parts of Bolivia and southern Peru, although much remains to be done in the Chaco region of Bolivia and northwestern Argentina. Concurrently with the vector control interventions, substantial progress has also been made on improved serological screening of blood donors, with all countries of the region now achieving close to 100% screening coverage.

The Southern Cone Initiative also encouraged similar initiatives elsewhere in the endemic regions of Latin America. By 1995, detailed planning discussions were being held for two further multinational initiatives, covering the Central American and Andean Pact regions (Schofield *et al.* 1996). Both were launched by resolution of the respective Ministers of Health in 1997, with the primary targets of eliminating the main domestic vector of these regions (*Rhodnius prolixus*), suppressing secondary vectors such as *T. dimidiata* and *R.ecuadoriensis*, and also improving serological screening of blood donors. With initial support from the government of Taiwan, followed by sustained support from the Japanese International Cooperation Agency (JICA), substantial progress has been made in the Central American initiative (IPCA), such that *R.prolixus* now seems to have been eliminated from El Salvador and Guatemala, and may be close to elimination from Nicaragua and Honduras, with substantial reductions also in the rate of domestic infestation with *T.dimidiata* in these countries (Yamagata and Nakagawa 2006). Both Central America and the Andean Pact countries have also made considerable improvements in blood donor screening, with coverage close to 100% in most of the region. However, in spite of strenuous efforts by University-based research teams, much remains to be done in terms of vector control interventions in the Andean Pact countries. In Mexico also, in spite of progress in epidemiological research and surveys, and some improvements in blood donor screening, much remains to be done in terms of elimination of the domestic vector populations in most of the endemic rural areas.

For the Amazon region, encompassing parts of nine countries, the epidemiological situation is quite different. Long considered to be 'non-endemic' for Chagas disease, in spite of the presence of a very wide range of silvatic vectors, the Amazonian Chagas Initiative (AMCHA) focuses on epidemiological surveillance rather than vector control (Guhl and Schofield 2004). Vector-borne transmission of Chagas disease in the Amazon region is mainly due to silvatic bugs occasionally entering houses and causing oral-route transmission by contamination of food or drink. Domestic colonization is relatively rare (except for some populations of *T.maculata* on the northwestern fringes of the region) so that there is little scope for the type of vector control interventions widely used in the other multinational initiatives. Instead, the emphasis is on early detection and treatment of any new cases that occur. This is carried out through the primary health care networks, and also by the networks of malaria slide microscopists now trained to identify *T.cruzi* (as well as *Plasmodium*) in febrile patients. There is also increasing research on Amazonian vector species, which can help to guide the surveillance initiative to areas where additional transmission may be expected (e.g. Abad-Franch *et al.* 2009).

To complete the suite of multinational initiatives against Chagas disease, 2007 saw the launch of a further initiative focusing on the problem of Chagas disease in the so-called 'non-endemic countries'. At the time of writing, this initiative encompasses the USA, Canada, Japan, much of Europe, and Australia—all countries that have received considerable inflows of immigrants from Latin America, particularly over the last decade. The focus is on health education (clinicians as well as patients), treatment and counselling of chronic cases, serological screening (or deferral) of blood and organ donors from Latin America, and also maternal health care with serological screening during pregnancy and checks for possible transplacental transmission. The initiative, coordinated by WHO Geneva, is much-needed because of the paucity of experience with Chagas disease in the 'non-endemic' countries, and procedures, both for diagnosis and treatment, currently vary enormously between these countries. In 2007, the USA Food and Drug Administration (FDA) recommended screening all blood donors (regardless of origin) resulting in substantial expense for executive agencies such as the American Red Cross; in the UK, by contrast, potential donors of Latin American origin are deferred, but routine serological screening is not yet carried out.

The future of Chagas disease control

Throughout the twentieth century, the main focus of Chagas disease control has been on elimination of the domestic vector populations, and improved serological screening of blood donors. Much has been achieved in both fields, as shown by the marked decline in prevalence estimates, steadily reducing seropositivity rates in blood donors, and also by declining public awareness of the disease and its vectors in previously endemic areas. But abundant domestic vector populations remain in parts of Bolivia, Peru, northwestern Argentina, northeastern Brasil, Colombia, Ecuador, Venezuela, Costa Rica, and Mexico, and the technical knowledge and experience about how to eliminate them will count for little without the requisite organization and political commitment. Similarly, although most of the endemic countries have achieved substantial improvements in serological screening of blood donors, with coverage close to 100% in most areas, the quality of the screening remains variable, partly due to the range of different diagnostic approaches used, partly due to different management practices, and also to the different levels of quality control by external reference laboratories.

To a large extent, vector control operations over the last 15 years have concentrated on eliminating domestic species that appeared to have been accidentally spread from their presumed origins in association with human migration or trade. *T.infestans*, for example,

appears to have been spread from its origins in the Andean valleys of Bolivia in association with human migrations (Schofield 1988; Panzera *et al.* 2004), while *R.prolixus* appears to have spread in Central America following an escape of laboratory-reared bugs originating from Venezuela (Dujardin *et al.* 1998; Zeledón 2004). The idea of targeting such populations, apart from their vectorial importance, carries the politically-convenient hope that once elimination has been achieved then that situation will be sustained without further intervention. But this is unlikely in practice, and takes no account of local silvatic or peridomestic species that may also invade and colonize rural houses. Instead, greater emphasis is now being placed on the idea of eliminating any domestic population of Triatominae, of whatever species, and developing a sustainable system of surveillance through which any future house infestations can be detected and treated, and any new cases of infection can also be diagnosed and treated—but with the implicit assumption that these surveillance activities must be continuous, carried out through an annual routine (Schofield *et al.* 2006).

The operational approach currently being developed relies on surveillance of school-age children (Ponce and Schofield 2004). The idea is to make an annual check of children to ask if they have seen any bugs (using life-size photographs of the local vector species) and also to make a rapid serological diagnosis of any new infections amongst the children (using one of the current generation of immunochromatographic rapid tests for *T.cruzi* antigens in peripheral blood). Such periodic health checks can be integrated within similar approaches to child health, such as vaccination programmes and head-lice control. Diagnoses of seropositive children are then confirmed by a quantitative ELISA test, with specific treatment and follow-up, and the cases can be taken as evidence of possible house infestation requiring a check and possible focal intervention by vector control specialists. Similarly, absence of infection and absence of visual sightings of the bugs can be taken as evidence of no current house infestation in the catchment area of that school. But the most important aspect of this approach is to establish it as an annual routine, accepting that in Latin America, triatomine bugs can and will enter houses, and can cause occasional transmission of *T.cruzi*. For the future however, no one should be obliged to live with domestic colonies of Triatominae, and any new cases of infection can and should be diagnosed and treated.

Acknowledgements

Preparation of this chapter has benefited from international collaboration through the ECLAT network. I also thank Dr Alejandro Luquetti (Universidade de Goiania, Brasil) and Dr Pedro Albajar-Viñas (WHO, Geneva) for guidance on clinical aspects.

References

Abad-Franch F., Noireau F., Paucar C.A., *et al.* (2000). The use of live-bait traps for the study of sylvatic *Rhodnius* populations (Hemiptera: Reduviidae) in palm trees. *Trans. R. Soc. Trop. Med. Hyg.*, **94:** 629–30.

Abad-Franch F., Monteiro F., Jaramillo N., Gurgel-Gonçalves R., *et al.* (2009). Ecology, evolution, and the long-term surveillance of vector-borne Chagas disease: a multi-scale appraisal of the tribe Rhodniini (Triatominae). *Acta Trop. (special issue)*, **110:** 159–77.

Anon. (1999). Recommendations from a Satellite Meeting: International Symposium to commemorate the 90th anniversary of the discovery of

Chagas disease April 11–16 1999, Rio de Janeiro, Brazil. *Memor. Instituto Oswaldo C.*, **94**(suppl. I): 429–32.

Benaim G., Sanders J.M., Garcia-Marchán Y., Colina C., *et al.* (2006). Amiodarone has intrinsic anti-*Trypanosoma cruzi* activity and acts synergistically with posaconazole. *J. Med. Chem.*, **49**: 892–99.

Brisse S., Henriksson J., Barnabé C., Douzery E.J.P., *et al.* (2003). Evidence for genetic exchange and hybridization in *Trypanosoma cruzi* based on nucleotide sequences and molecular karyotype. *Infect. Genet. Evol.*, **2**: 173–83.

Bustamante J.M., Rivarola H.W., Fernandez A.R., *et al.* (2002). *Trypanosoma cruzi* reinfections in mice determine the severity of cardiac damage. *Int. J. Parasitol.*, **32**: 889–96.

Bustamante J.M., Novarese M., Rivarola H.W., *et al.* (2007). Reinfections and *Trypanosoma cruzi* strains can determine the prognosis of the chronic chagasic cardiopathy in mice. *Parasitol. Res.*, **100**: 1407–10.

Chagas C. (1909). Nova trypanosomiase humana. *Gaceta Medica da Bahia*, **40**: 433–40.

Coura J.R., Junqueira A.C., Fernandes O., Valente S.A., Miles M.A. (2002). Emerging Chagas disease in Amazonian Brazil. *Trends Parasitol.*, **18**: 171–76.

Coutinho M. and Dias J.C.P. (2000). The rise and fall of Chagas disease. *Persp. Sci.*, **7**: 447–85.

Dias J.C.P. (1987). Control of Chagas disease in Brazil. *Parasitol. Today*, **3**: 336–41.

Dias J.C.P. & Schofield C.J. (2004). Control of Triatominae. In: I. Maudlin, P.H. Holmes, M.A. Miles *(eds.) The Trypanosomiases*, pp. 547–63. Oxon, UK: CAB International.

Dias J.C.P., Silveira A.C., Schofield C.J. (2002). The impact of Chagas disease control in Latin America. *Memó. Instituto Oswaldo C.*, **97**: 603–12.

Dujardin J.P., Muñoz M., Chavez T., Ponce C., *et al.* (1998). The origin of *Rhodnius prolixus* in Central America. *Med. Vet. Entomol.*, **12**: 113–15.

Freitas J.M. de, Augusto-Pinto L., Pimenta J.R., *et al.* (2006). Ancestral genomes, sex, and the population structure of *Trypanosoma cruzi*. *PLoS Path.*, **2**: e24.

Guevara de Sequeda M., Villalobos López L.P., *et al.* (1986). Enfermedad de Chagas. *VII Congreso Venezolano de Salud Publica. Ponencias* vol. II. pp. 905–29.

Guhl F. & Schofield C.J. (eds.) (2004). *Proceedings of the ECLAT-AMCHA International Workshop on Chagas disease surveillance in the Amazon Region, Palmari, Brasil*, pp. 174. Bogota: Universidad de Los Andes.

Guillén G., Diaz R., Jemio A., Alfred Cassab J., *et al.* (1997). Chagas disease vector control in Tupiza, southern Bolivia. *Memor. Instituto Oswaldo.*, **92**: 1–8.

Hayes R. & Schofield C.J. (1990). Estimación de las tasas de incidencia de infecciones y parasitosis crónicas a partir de la prevalencia: la enfermedad de Chagas en America Latina. *Bolet. Ofic. Sanit. Panam.*, **108**: 308–16.

Jacintho da Silva L. (1999). *A Evolução da Doença de Chagas no Estado de Sao Paulo*, p. 159. Sao Paulo: Editora Hucitec.

Jansen A.M. & Deane M.P. (1985). *Trypanosoma cruzi* infection of mice by ingestion of food contaminated with material of the anal glands of the opossum *Didelphis marsupialis*. *XIX Reunião Annual sobre Pesquisa Basica em Doença de Chagas, Caxambu* BI–09.

Kirk M.L. & Schofield C.J. (1987). Density dependent timing of defaecation by *Rhodnius prolixus*, and its implications for the transmission of *Trypanosoma cruzi*. *Trans. R. Soc. Trop. Med. Hyg.*, **81**: 348–49.

Lehane M.J., McEwan P.K., Whitaker C.J., Schofield C.J. (1992). The role of temperature and nutritional dependence in flight initiation by *Triatoma infestans*. *Acta Trop.*, **52**: 27–38.

Lewinsohn R. (2003). *Três Epidemias Lições do Passado*, p. 318. Sao Paulo: Editora Unicamp.

Miles M.A. & Cibulskis R.E. (1986). Zymodeme characterization of *Trypanosoma cruzi*. *Parasit. Today*, **2**: 94–97.

Miles M.A., Toye P.J., Oswald S.C., Godfrey D.G. (1977). The identification by isoenzyme patterns of two distinct strain-groups of *Trypanosoma*

cruzi, circulating independently in a rural area of Brazil. *Trans. R. Soc. Trop. Med. Hyg.*, **71**: 217–25.

Miles M.A., Souza A., Povoa M., Shaw J.J., Lainson R., Toye P.J. (1978). Isozymic heterogeneity of *Trypanosoma cruzi* in the first autochthonous patients with Chagas disease in Amazonian Brazil. *Nature*, **272**: 819–21.

Olsen P.F., Shoemaker J.P., Turner H.F., Hays K.L. (1964). Incidence of *Trypanosoma cruzi* (Chagas) in wild vectors and reservoirs in east-central Alabama. *J. Parasitol.*, **50**: 599–603.

OPS (2006). *Estimación cuantitativa de la Enfermedad de Chagas en las Américas*, p. 28. OPS/HDM/CD/425-06. Washington D.C.: Pan American Health Organization.

Panzera F., Dujardin J.P., Nicolini P., Caraccio M.N., *et al.* (2004). Genomic changes of Chagas disease vector, South America. *Emerg. Infect. Dis.*, **10**: 438–46.

Ponce C. & Schofield C.J. (2004). Strategic options for the control of *Triatoma dimidiata* in Central America. *Iniciativa de los Paises Centroamericanas*, OPS Tegucigalpa Honduras. Sept 2004.

Rabinovich J.E., Leal J.A., Feliciangeli de Piñero D. (1979). Domiciliary biting frequency and blood ingestion of the Chagas disease vector *Rhodnius prolixus* Ståhl (Hemiptera: Reduviidae), in Venezuela. *Trans. R. Soc. Trop. Med. Hyg.*, **73**: 272–83.

Rabinovich J.E., Gürtler R.E., Leal J.A., Feliciangeli D. (1995). Density estimates of the domestic vector of Chagas disease, *Rhodnius prolixus* Stål (Hemiptera: Reduviidae), in rural houses in Venezuela. *Bull. World Health Organ.*, **73**: 347–57.

Sandoval C.M., Gutiérrez R., Luna S., Amaya M., Esteban L., *et al.* (2000). High density of *Rhodnius prolixus* in a rural house in Colombia. *Trans. R. Soc. Trop. Med. Hyg.*, **94**: 372–73.

Schofield C.J. (1980) Density regulation of domestic populations of *Triatoma infestans* in Brazil. *Trans. R. Soc. Trop. Med. Hyg.*, **74**: 761–69.

Schofield C.J. (1981). Chagas disease, triatomine bugs, and blood-loss. *The Lancet*, **i**: p.1316.

Schofield C.J. (1988). The biosystematics of Triatominae. In: M.W. Service, *(ed.) Biosystematics of Haematophagous Insects*, pp. 284–312. Oxford, UK: Systematics Association special volume 37, Clarendon Press.

Schofield C.J. (1994). *Triatominae - Biology & Control*, p. 80. West Sussex, UK: Eurocommunica Publications.

Schofield C.J. (2000). *Trypanosoma cruzi*–The vector-parasite paradox. *Memor. Instituto Oswaldo C.*, **95**: 535–44.

Schofield C.J. & Dias J.C.P. (1999). The Southern Cone Initiative against Chagas disease. *Adv. Parasitol.*, **42**: 1–27.

Schofield C.J. & Galvão C. (2009). Classification, evolution, and species groups within the Triatominae. *Acta Trop. (special issue)*, **110**: 88–100.

Schofield C.J. & Kabayo J.P. (2008). Trypanosomiasis vector control in Africa and Latin America. *Parasites & Vectors*, **1**: 24 (http://www.parasitesandvectors.com/content/pdf/1756-3305-1-24.pdf).

Schofield C.J., Williams N.G., Marshall T.F. (1986). Density dependent perception of bites of triatomine bugs. *Ann. Trop. Med. Parasitol.*, **80**: 351–58.

Schofield C.J., Dujardin J.P., Jurberg J. (eds.) (1996). *Proceedings of the International Workshop on Population Genetics and Control of Triatominae, Santo Domingo de los Colorados, Ecuador*, p. 116. Mexico City: INDRE.

Schofield C.J., Jannin J., Salvatella R. (2006). The future of Chagas disease control. *Trends Parasitol.*, **21**: 583–88.

Schofield C.J., Grijalva M.J., Diotaiuti L. (2009). Distribución de los vectores de la Enfermedad de Chagas en países 'no endémicos': la posibilidad de transmisión vectorial fuera de América Latina. *Enfermed. Emerg.*, **11**(supl.1): 20–27.

Stevens J., Noyes H., Schofield C.J., Gibson W. (2001). The molecular evolution of Trypanosomatidae. *Adv. Parasitol.*, **48**: 1–53.

Tibayrenc M., Kjellberg F., Ayala F.J. (1991). The clonal theory of parasitic protozoa: a taxonomic proposal applicable to other clonal organisms. *Bioscience*, **41**: 767–74.

Trumper E.V. & Gorla D.E. (1991). Density-dependent timing of defaecation by *Triatoma infestans*. *Trans. R. Soc. Trop. Med. Hyg.*, **85:** 800–802.

Valente S.A.S. & Valente V.C. (1999). Epidemiologia e transmissão da doença de Chagas na Amazonia. In: *Proceedings of the Second International Workshop on Population Genetics and Control of Triatominae, Tegucigalpa*, pp. 101–104. Mexico City: INDRE.

Walsh J.A. (1984). Estimating the burden of illness in the tropics. In: K.S. Warren & A.A.F. Mahmoud (eds.) *Tropical and Geographical Medicine*, pp. 1073–85. NY, USA: McGraw-Hill.

Wanderley D.M.V. (1994). *Perspectivas de Controle da Doença de Chagas no Estado de Sao Paulo*, Thesis, pp. 161. Brasil: Universidade de Sao Paulo.

WHO (2007). *Neglected Tropical Diseases: Innovative and Intensified Disease Management* (http://www.who.int/neglected_diseases).

Urbina J.A. & Docampo R. (2003). Specific chemotherapy of Chagas disease: controversies and advances. *Trends in Parasit.*, **19:** 495–501.

Viotti R., Vigliano C., Armenti H., Segura E. (1994). Treatment of chronic Chagas disease with benznidazole: clinical and serologic evolution of patients with long-term follow-up. *Am. Heart J.*, **127:** 151–62.

Viotti R., Vigliano C., Lococo B., Bertocchi G., *et al.* (2006). Long-term cardiac outcomes of treating chronic Chagas disease with benznidazole versus no treatment: a nonrandomized trial. *Ann. Internal Med.*, **144:** 724–34.

Viotti R., Vigliano C., Lococo B., Alvarez M.G., *et al.* (2009). Side effects of benznidazole as treatment in chronic Chagas disease: fears and realities. *Expert Rev. Anti-Infect. Ther.*, **7:** 157–63.

World Bank (1993). *World Development Report 1993. Investing in Health*, pp. 329. New York: Oxford University Press.

Yamagata Y. & Nakagawa J. (2006). Control of Chagas disease. *Adv. Parasitol.*, **61:** 129–65.

Yeo M., Acosta N., Llewellyn M., Sánchez H., *et al.* (2005). Origins of Chagas disease: *Didelphis* species are natural hosts of *Trypanosoma cruzi* I and armadillos hosts of *Trypanosoma cruzi* II, including hybrids. *Intern. J. Parasitol.*, **35:** 225–33.

Zeledón R.A. (2004). Some historical facts and recent issues related to the presence of *Rhodnius prolixus* (Stal, 1859) (Hemiptera, Reduviidae) in Central America. *Entom. Vectores*, **11:** 233–46.

Zingales B., Andrade S.G., Briones M.R., *et al.* (2009). A new consensus for *Trypanosoma cruzi* intraspecific nomenclature: second revision meeting recommends TcI to TcVI. *Memor. Instituto Oswaldo C.*, **104:** 1051-54.

CHAPTER 44

The Leishmanioses

Marina Gramiccia

Summary

Leishmanioses, a large group of parasitic diseases, range over the intertropical zones of America and Africa and extend into temperate regions of South America, southern Europe and Asia. The clinical aspects of the disease is wide ranging from a simple, self-resolving cutaneous lesion to the potentially fatal visceral leishmanioses, known as kala-azar. In numerous underdeveloped countries, leishmanioses remain a major public health problem representing one of the most neglected diseases. Among 15 well-recognized *Leishmania* species known to infect humans, 13 have definite zoonotic nature, which include agents of visceral, cutaneous and mucocutaneous forms of the disease in both the Old and New Worlds. Mammal reservoir hosts belong to the marsupalia, edentata, carnivora, hyracoidea, and rodentia, maintaining sylvatic zoonotic foci in the deserts of Africa and Asia, the forests of South and Central America, as well as synanthropic foci in the Mediterranean basin and much of South America. Although the known vectors are all phlebotomine sand flies, these have a wide range of specific habits and habitats. The complexity of this group of infections has only recently been appreciated and is still being worked out. Currently, leishmanioses show a wider geographical distribution than previously known, with increased global incidence of human disease. Environmental, demographic and human behavioural factors contribute to the changing leishmaniosis landscape, which basically include increasing risk factors for zoonotic cutaneous leishmanioses, and new scenarios associated with the zoonotic entity of visceral leishmaniosis. In comparison with the anthroponotic entities of leishmaniosis, limited progresses were made for the control of the zoonotic ones, consisting mainly in new tools developed for the control of *L. infantum* in the canine reservoir.

Introduction

Leishmanioses are protozoan diseases caused by members of the genus *Leishmania*, parasites infecting numerous mammal species, including humans, and transmitted by the bite of phlebotomine sand flies. Human leishmanioses have diverse clinical manifestations. Visceral leishmaniosis (VL), caused by *Leishmania donovani* in the Old World and *L. infantum* in both the Old and New Worlds, is the most severe form which, if left untreated, invariably leads to death. A number of different species of *Leishmania* cause cutaneous (CL) or mucocutaneous (MCL) leishmanioses which, if not fatal, are responsible for considerable morbidity of a vast number of people in endemic foci. The impact of leishmanioses on human health has been grossly underestimated for many years and it has now been classified by the World Health Organization (WHO) as one of the most neglected tropical diseases. At present, an estimated 12 million people are infected in 66 Old World and 22 New World endemic countries (72 developing and 16 developed) with an estimated yearly incidence of 1–1.5 million cases of CL forms and 500,000 cases of VL forms (Desjeux 1996). Incidence of leishmanioses is not uniformly distributed in endemic areas: about 90% of CL cases occur in 7 countries only (Afghanistan, Algeria, Brazil, Iran, Peru, Saudi Arabia, and Syria), whereas some 90% of VL cases occur in rural and suburban areas of 5 countries (Bangladesh, India, Nepal, Sudan, and Brazil). At least 60,000 people succumb to VL each year and a loss of 2.4 million disability-adjusted life years (DALYs) has been calculated (Hotez *et al.* 2004). These figures are much probably underestimated, as official data are often obtained through passive case detection.

During the last decade, it appears that the global incidence of human leishmanioses is higher than before, although it is difficult to differentiate between real and artificial increase, due to progress in diagnosis, case detection, improved reporting, and accessibility to treatment. For example, in Brazil, CL cases passed from 21,800 in 1998, to 40,000 in 2002; VL cases recorded in the same periods were 1,840 and 6,000, respectively; in Kabul, Afghanistan, CL cases were 14,200 in 1994 and 65,000 in 2002 (Desjeux 2001; 2004). Undoubtedly, human and animal leishmanioses show a wider geographical distribution than previously known. Autochthonous *Leishmania* transmission has been recently recorded in traditionally non-endemic areas, as in western Upper Nile, Sudan (Desjeux 2001), a number of U.S. states and Canada provinces (Duprey *et al.* 2006), Australia's Northern Territory (Rose *et al.* 2004), and in some parts of Europe (Gramiccia and Gradoni 2005). It is widely accepted that leishmanioses are dynamic diseases and the circumstances of transmission are continually changing in relation to environmental, demographic and human behavioural factors. Changes in the habitat of the natural host and vector, immunosuppressive conditions (e.g. HIV infection or organ transplantation-associated therapies) and the consequences of conflicts, all contribute to the changing leishmaniosis landscape.

Leishmania organism: Origin and evolution

Lesions suggestive of CL have been known in Egypt since 2000 BC and in Assyria since 650 BC. The earliest clear reference to CL is by Ibn Sina (Avicenna) who wrote of Balkh sore; actually, 10 centuries later Balkh Province in northern Afghanistan is still suffering annual outbreaks of CL caused by *Leishmania major*. As for the New World, texts from the Inca period in the fifteenth and sixteenth centuries mention the risk run by seasonal agricultural workers who returned from the Andes with skin ulcers (CL) called 'valley sickness' or 'Andean sickness'. Later, the disfigurements of the nose and mouth become known as white leprosy to the resemblance to the lesions caused by leprosy.

Evidence for VL has been found recently in ancient Egyptian mummies from the Middle Kingdom period (2050–1650BC). Clinically, this disease was probably masked for centuries by the overlapping malaria, however several decades before the discovery of the aetiological agent, Mediterranean infantile VL was known as infantile infectious splenic pseudo-leukemia.

In the first few years of the twentieth century, in a rush of discovery, it was found that this different set of diseases, oriental sore, kala-azar, infantile splenomegaly, and espundia, were all caused by indistinguishable organisms. During the same period Nicolle, working in Tunis, found dogs to be infected with similar parasites, and postulated the zoonotic origin of infantile kala-azar. The term leishmaniosis was initially applied only to the canine disease and only became widely used for the human diseases in the 1930s. Reconstruction of the history of this disease has been facilitated by the collection of DNA and amplification of nucleic acids (PCR) to identify protozoan material from paleontological fossils (Tuon *et al.* 2008). The definition of a digenetic parasite makes it difficult to consider the emergence of the current genus *Leishmania* before the emergence of two adequate hosts, one of them a winged insect vector. Considering *Leishmania* as an evolutionary form of a primitive protozoan, the first host could have been a primitive water-dwelling animal and it appeared around the Proterozoic when the Earth was covered by water with a lower concentration of oxygen. The theory of digenetic life goes back up to the Ordovician. The separation of primitive winged insects within the Diptera occurred during the Triassic, more than 200 millions of years ago (Mya). Flagellates could be transmitted to a vertebrate, thus establishing a continuing cycle between vectors and vertebrates, during the Paleocene before the appearance of placental mammals. It was after this that the current vector of *Leishmania* (*Phlebotomus*) appeared. The vector, mammal host and fossils suggest that leishmanioses may have been established during the Paleogene, around 50 Mya. While the subgenus *L.* (*Leishmania*) can be reasonably considered as originated in Paleoartic, the origin of subgenus *L.* (*Viannia*) is controversial, some authors considering that it originated independently from the Neotropic, others from the Paleoartic or Neoartic. Apart from its origin, the dissemination of *Leishmania* followed the migration of vectors and hosts together.

Leishmania life cycle and classification

Leishmania (Kinetoplastida: Trypanosomatidae) are dimorphic protozoa characterized by the intracellular presence of the kinetoplast, a network of maxi- and mini-circles of mitochondrial DNA

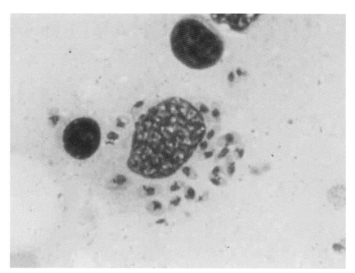

Fig. 44.1 *Leishmania* amastigote stage.

found close to the base of the flagellum. *Leishmania* shows two principal morphological stages:

- The amastigote, a round or oval body of 2.5–6.8 μ in diameter, is found in the phagolysosome of mononuclear phagocyte cells of the mammalian host (Fig. 44.1).

- The promastigote, an extracellular dividing form of 15–30 μ in length with a long anterior flagellum, is found in the gut of the phlebotomine vectors (Diptera: Psychodidae) (Fig. 44.2). Small, fast swimming and non-dividing promastigotes found in the foregut of the infected sandflies are metacyclic forms infective to the mammal. The population structure is clonal with rare genetical exchanges.

Leishmania are alternatively hosted by the sand fly and by mammals hosts. When a female sand fly takes a blood meal from a *Leishmania*-infected mammal, amastigotes are ingested and, following at least one cycle of binary division, they transform into motile promastigotes which escape through the peritrophic membrane enveloping the blood meal. The promastigotes multiply intensively inside the intestinal tract of the sand fly. This development

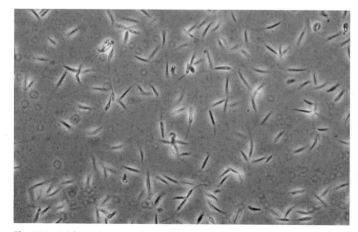

Fig. 44.2 *Leishmania* promastigote stage.

occurs in the midgut (*Leishmania* subgenus) or in the hindgut and the midgut (*Viannia* subgenus). Whatever the multiplication site, the parasites subsequently migrate to the foregut (anterior cardia area and/or pharynx and proboscis) where they change into meta-cyclic forms. The time requested to complete the parasite cycle in the sand fly is variable, depending on both *Leishmania* and phlebot-omine species, but is about 5 days on average.

Once the metacyclic promastigotes have been deposited in the mammal's dermis by the bite of the sand fly, they are rapidly phago-cytosed by cells of the mononuclear phagocyte system. The ingested parasites change into the non-motile amastigote stage. The surviv-ing amastigotes divide by mitosis within the macrophage's phagolysosome and the infection can spread in the mammalian host when heavily parasitized macrophages burst and amastigotes are ingested by other macrophages. The outcome of exposure to infection may not necessarily be overt disease and, in any case, the complex of parasite-cell biochemical interactions affects the course of the disease. The life cycle of *Leishmania* is completed when a female sand fly takes a blood meal containing *Leishmania*-infected cells. The inoculation of metacyclic promastigotes through the sand fly bite is the usual method of leishmaniosis transmission, other routes (e.g. transfusion or congenital transmission) being exceptional. The life cycle is illustrated in Fig. 44.3.

Since the creation of the genus *Leishmania* by Ross in 1903, the classification and nomenclature of the species and subspecies has for a long time and, sometime still is, a contentious matter. They show a homogeneous protozoan group mostly morphologically undistinguishable, for which the initial taxonomic criteria, like the human clinical picture and geographical distribution, were not enough for a correct taxonomical identification. Since the 1980s considerable efforts have been made to base the taxonomy of the genus *Leishmania* on scientific footings. The technique of multilocus enzyme electrophoresis (MLEE) has been applied from more than 25 years on several thousand parasite strains and still represents the current gold standard for *Leishmania* identifi-cation and taxonomy. Strains are characterized by their enzy-matic profiles and grouped into homogeneous taxonomic units, the zymodemes. Phylogenetic classification of zymodeme com-plexes reveals a parental relationship between different *Leishmania* taxa (Table 44.1).

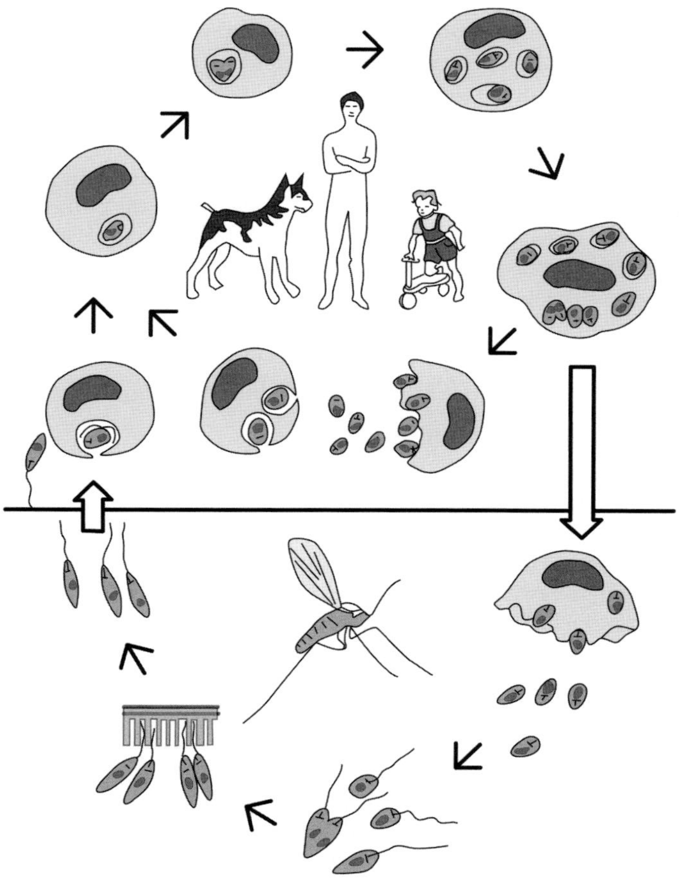

Fig. 44.3 *Leishmania* life cycle.

Table 44.1 *Leishmania* taxa including species pathogenic to humans, identified by multilocus enzyme electrophoresis

Subgenus	World distribution	Species
Leishmania Ross (1903)	Old World	**L. donovani complex** *L. donovani* Laveran and Mesnil (1903) *L. archibaldi* Castellani and Chalmers (1919)
		L. infantum complex* *L. infantum* Nicolle (1908) (syn. *L. chagasi* Cunha and Chagas (1937))
		L. tropica complex *L. tropica* Wright (1903)
		L. killicki complex** *L. killicki* Rioux, Lanotte and Pratlong (1986)
		L. aethiopica complex *L. aethiopica* Bray, Ashford and Bray (1973)
		L. major complex *L. major* Yakimoff and Shokhor (1914)
	New World	**L. mexicana complex** *L. mexicana* Biagi (1953) (syn. *L. pifanoi* Medina and Romero (1959))
		L. amazonensis complex *L. amazonensis* Lainson and Shaw 1972 (syn. *L. garnhami* Scorza *et al.* (1979)) *L. aristidesi* Lainson and Shaw (1979)
Viannia Lainson and Shaw (1987)		**L. braziliensis complex** *L. braziliensis* Viannia (1911) *L. peruviana* Velez (1913)
		L. guyanensis complex *L. guyanensis* Floch (1954) *L. panamensis* Lainson and Shaw (1972) *L. shawi* Lainson *et al.* (1989)
		L. naiffi complex *L. naiffi* Lainson and Shaw (1989)
		L. lainsoni complex *L. lainsoni* Silveira *et al.* (1987)

*This complex is also diffuse in the New World, with the local name of *L. chagasi*. It is believed that Mediterranean *L. infantum* was imported in South America by the Spanish conquerors (Tuon *et al.* 2008).

**It is believed that this complex belongs to the *L. tropica* complex.

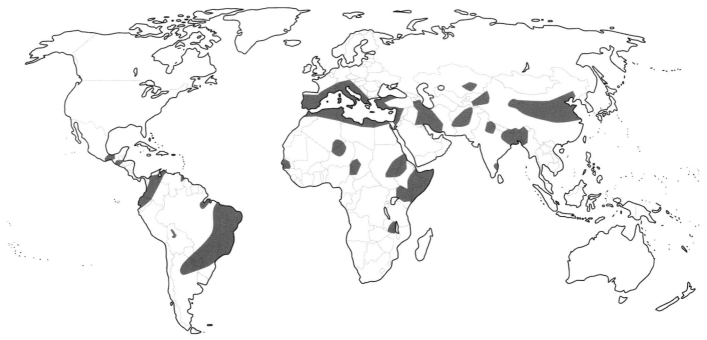

Fig. 44.4 Global distribution of Visceral Leishmanioses.

MLEE shows some limitations mainly due to the need for live parasite cultures and time-consuming procedures, therefore DNA genotyping methods have been investigated as alternative techniques, e.g. multi-locus microsatellite typing (MLMT) and PCR-restriction fragment length polymorphism (RFLP) (Schönian *et al.* 2008). Phylogenies based on nucleotide polymorphisms in different genomic targets have largely confirmed the taxonomy of the genus *Leishmania* by MLEE with some exceptions, e.g. the intra-zymodeme genetic polymorphism of *L. infantum* Montpellier (MON)-1, or the taxonomic status of the *L. donovani* complex in east Africa (Kuhls *et al.* 2007; Lukeš *et al.* 2007).

Clinical aspects

The establishment of metacyclic parasites in the dermis of the mammalian skin is facilitated by the sand fly saliva, which enhances *Leishmania* infectivity. After phagocytosis by macrophages, amastigotes have the capacity to resist intracellular digestion as a result of several parasite and host cell factors.

When the intracellular development of the amastigotes remains localized at the inoculation site, various cytokines are released and cell reactions are generated, resulting in the development of a CL localized lesion. In other instances, the parasites spread to organs rich in mononuclear phagocytes, giving rise to VL. Amastigotes may also spread to other cutaneous sites, as in diffuse CL (DCL), or to facial mucosae in the case of MCL. The localization of parasites in various tissues and organs is dependent on both intrinsic parasite tropism of a given *Leishmania* species and the immunological status of the host, resulting in the clinical expression of the disease.

Visceral leishmaniosis (VL)

Two species are usually responsible for VL: *L. donovani* in the Indian sub-continent, east-Africa and Arabic peninsula, and *L. infantum* in the Mediterranean, Middle East, central Asia and the Americas (Fig. 44.4). The incubation period is generally 2–6 months, but can range from 10 days (exceptional) to years (more common). A classical VL syndrome includes fever, asthenia, weight loss, anaemia, splenomegaly, hepatomegaly, and sometimes adenopathy. An intermittent and irregular fever is the major symptom. Splenomegaly appears early and is almost invariably present; anaemia is responsible for an extreme paleness of skin and mucosa. In India, patient skin has a greyish pigmentation which gives rise to the local name of the disease (kala-azar). If left untreated, VL is fatal in more than 90% of patients. VL caused by *L. donovani* shows frequently a dermal manifestation known as post kala-azar dermal leishmaniosis (PKDL) occurring after an apparent VL cure or recovering. Begining as depigmented maculae, the PKDL lesions can extend to the whole body, playing an important role in the sand fly transmission.

Cutaneous leishmaniosis (CL)

The world distribution of all tegumentary leishmanioses is shown in Fig. 44.5. CL consists of one or more localized skin lesions (depending on the infecting bites) without mucosal involvement nor evidence of dissemination. Lesions occur on exposed parts of the body accessible to sand fly bites. All anthropophilic *Leishmania* species, including the viscerotropic ones, can be responsible for a localized CL, which presents as a mild self-healing infection. The incubation period varies between a week and several months. The mature lesion is well defined, generally round or oval with variable dimensions ranging 0.5–10 cm in diameter. The most common clinical feature is the ulcerative lesion with sloping sides and central ulcer. A 'wet' type is typical of zoonotic CL lesions caused by *L. major*, *L. mexicana*, *L. peruviana* and *L. braziliensis*. A 'dry' type, showed as papulo-nodular lesions covered by scales, is the usual form of the anthroponotic CL caused by *L. tropica*. The clinical evolution of CL is chronic and leads to spontaneous cure in a time

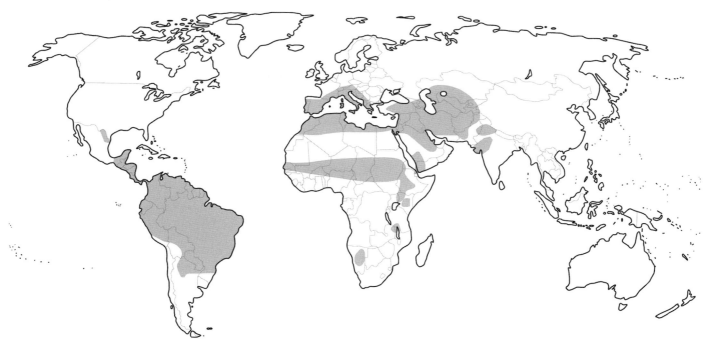

Fig. 44.5 Global distribution of Cutaneous Leishmanioses.

varying from few months (*L. major, L. mexicana, L. peruviana*) to few years (*L. aethiopica, L. infantum, L. tropica, L. guyanensis, L. panamensis*). The spontaneous cure always results in a disfiguring scar, while early treatment with pentavalent antimony salts can prevent such condition.

Other tegumentary forms

DCL is a severe form caused by a few *Leishmania* species, *L. aethiopica* in the Old World and *L. amazonensis* (rarely *L. mexicana*) in the New World, in patients who defect in cell-mediated immunity. The primary lesion is a non-ulcerated nodule rich in parasites. The nodules become numerous, disseminate to the whole body mimicking the presentation of lepromatous leprosy. The severity of DCL is shown by its resistance to anti-leishmanial drugs and it never cures spontaneously.

MCL, known also as 'espundia', is a severe clinical entity caused by *L. braziliensis* and occasionally *L. panamensis*. Following a primary CL lesion, secondary mucosal involvement occurs in a period between several weeks to many years. The mucosal involvement usually starts from the cartilaginous part of the nasal septum, which is rapidly destroyed. Mouth and lips mucosa is affected at a later stage of the disease which, in the advanced stage, leads to severe tissue necrosis and disfigurement. Death can occur following pulmonary superinfections. When treated and cured, MCL patients show disfiguring, sometimes retractile scars.

Epidemiology, transmission and geographical distribution of zoonotic forms of leishmaniosis

Leishmanioses range over the intertropical zones of America and Africa, and extend into temperate regions of South America, southern Europe and Asia. Their extension limits are latitude 45°

North and 32° South. About 30 sand fly species are proven vectors. Each parasite species circulate in natural foci of infection where susceptible phlebotomine species and mammals coexist. Few human VL cases have been reported as congenital and blood transfusion transmission. However, direct transmission by sexual contact and exchange of syringes has been incriminated to explain the high prevalence of *L. infantum*-HIV co-infection in drug users in southern Europe. In CL cases contact with the active lesion is innocuous.

There are two main epidemiological leishmanioses entities:

◆ Zoonotic leishmanioses: where domestic or wild animal reservoirs are involved in the tramsmission cycle and humans play a role of an accidental host;

◆ Anthroponotic leishmanioses: where man is the sole or principal reservoir and source of vector's infection.

Zoonotic forms of leishmaniosis

There is no consensus about the named *Leishmania* species causing disease in humans. The New World species *L. chagasi* is now widely accepted to be a synonym of *L. infantum;* some authors describe *L. archibaldi* and *L. killicki* as species distinct from the close related species *L. donovani* and *L. tropica*, respectively. Finally, the taxonomic status of the New World species *L. colombiensis* is still controversial.

Among the 15 well-recognized *Leishmania* species known to cause disease in humans, 13 have zoonotic nature (Gramiccia and Gradoni 2005). Futhermore, for the only two species considered as having an exclusive or predominant anthroponotic transmission pattern, i.e. *L donovani* and *L. tropica*, the presence of animal reservoir hosts has been indicated in several endemic settings, such as eastern Sudan for *L. donovani*, and Morocco, northern Israel and Iran for *L. tropica*.

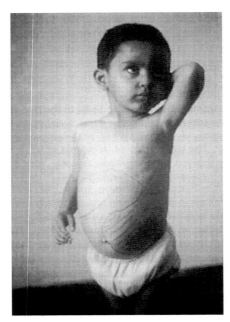

Fig. 44.6 Clinical aspect of zoonotic visceral leishmaniosis caused by *Leishmania infantum*.

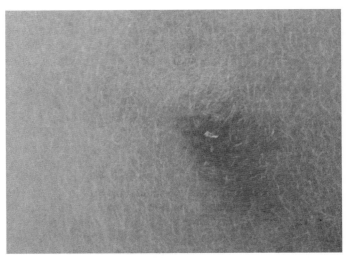

Fig. 44.7 Clinical aspect of zoonotic cutaneous leishmaniosis caused by *Leishmania infantum*.

Finally, a number of *Leishmania* species have been recorded in animal hosts but not in humans: *L. gerbilli*, *L. turanica* and *L. arabica*, from Old World rodents; *L. equatoriensis* from arboreal mammals in Ecuador; *Leishmania* sp. from red kangaroo, *Macropus rufus*.

Zoonotic visceral leishmaniosis (ZVL)

It is the most widespread entity of zoonotic leishmanioses caused by a single species complex, *L. infantum*. In the acute disease the agent multiplies in the macrophages of the reticuloendothelial system, resulting in generalized signs and symptoms like fever, splenomegaly and pancytopenia (Fig. 44.6). The disease occurs in several countries of Central and South America (especially in Brazil), Mediterranean basin, and Central Asia. Sporadic cases of localized CL due to dermotropic *L. infantum* strains are found in the same endemic areas (Fig. 44.7).

The principal vector in the New World is *Lutzomyia longipalpis* but in the Old World several species are involved, mainly belonging to the subgenus *Phlebotomus (Larroussious)*, e.g. *P. perniciosus*, *P. ariasi*, *P. neglectus*, *P. perfiliewi* and *P. kandelakii* (Fig. 44.8). Dogs are the main domestic reservoirs, and foxes, jackals and wolfs are thought to be the sylvatic ones. With the combined use of

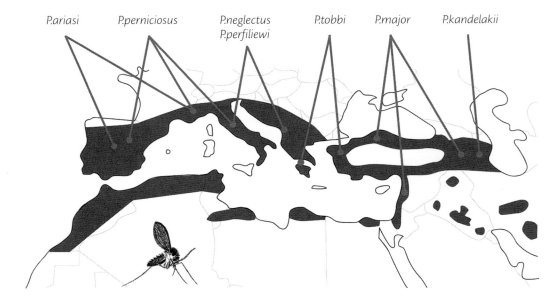

Fig. 44.8 Distribution of the main *Phlebotomus (Larroussious)* vectors in the Mediterranean basin and Middle East.

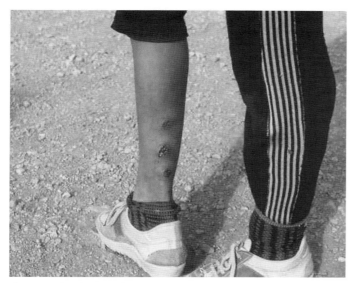

Fig. 44.9 Clinical aspect of zoonotic cutaneous leishmaniosis caused by *Leishmania major*.

serological and molecular diagnostic techniques, the prevalence rates of canine infections in different endemic settings were found to be much higher than previously thought. Asymptomatic *L. infantum* infections are common in healthy populations. Known risk factors for clinical disease are age below 2 years, malnutrition and immunosuppression (e.g. HIV patients or transplant recipients).

Zoonotic cutaneous leishmanioses (ZCL)

The main foci of ZCL are found in Africa, Asia, and in most Latin American countries. The *Leishmania* species involved are:

- In the Old World, *L. major*, *L. aethiopica* and dermotropic *L. infantum*;
- In the New World, *L. braziliensis*, *L. guyanensis*, *L. lainsoni*, *L. naiffi*, *L. panamensis*, *L. peruviana*, *L. shawi* (*Viannia* subgenus), and *L. mexicana*, *L. amazonensis*, *L. venezuelensis* and dermotropic *L. infantum* (*Leishmania* subgenus).

The usual clinical CL feature consists in localized nodulo-ulcerative lesions. Rarely, it may evolve toward a DCL, with multiple, not ulcerating nodules distributed over large areas of the skin, or to MCL, with the involvement of oronasopharyngeal mucosa and cartilages.

Old World ZCL

Leishmania major

The parasite is widely distributed in arid and savannah rodents from the Old World. In humans the parasite causes localized, self-healing CL, often presenting as multiple lesions associated with numerous bites by infected sand flies (Fig. 44.9).

Several rodents species are the reservoir hosts:

- The great gerbil *Rhombomys opimus* in central Asia, northern Afghanistan, and Iran,
- *Meriones hurrianae* in India,
- The fat sand-rat *Psammomys obesus*,

- and *M. crassus* in northern Africa and Middle East.
- *M. libycus* in the Arabian peninsula and central Asia,
- Several rodent species (e.g. *Arvicanthis* spp., *Tatera* spp., *Xerus* spp., etc) in sub-Saharan Africa.

All the proven vectors belong to the subgenus *Phlebotomus* (*Phlebotomus*): *P. papatasi*, the principal one, and the related species *P. salehi* and *P. dubosqi*. Well described stable zoonotic systems are the associations between the parasite and *P. obesus*/*P.papatasi* in north Africa and Middle East, and *R. opimus*/*P. papatasi* in central Asia, Afghanistan, and Iran. Unstable systems are the parasite associations with any *Meriones* spp./*Phlebotomus* spp. found in areas from Morocco to India, where population surges of *Meriones* may cause CL outbreaks in humans (Elfari *et al.* 2005). Migrations and fluctuations of rodent populations were the cause of several epidemic phenomena occurred in the Maghreb countries in the 1980s. Despite this widespread geographical distribution and the involvement of different rodent species, *L. major* appears genetically uniform, with large genetic groups corresponding to the Asian, Middle Eastern and African parasite populations.

L. major cases are increasingly reported from sub-Saharan African countries, e.g. Mali, Senegal, Camerun, Niger, Nigeria, and Burkina Faso, with some cases associated with HIV infection.

Leishmania aethiopica

The parasite shows a geographical distribution limited to the highlands of Ethiopia, and to similar biotopes in Kenya. Suspected human cases were also reported from Uganda and Yemen. It is a classical parasite of the Hyracoidea, such as *Procavia capensis* and *Heterohyrax brucei*, which live in a wide altitudinal range up to 4,000 m. They always require restricted habitat as large rock outcrops with deep crevices for shelter. The vectors are two highland species of the subgenus *Larroussius*, *P. longipes* and *P. pedifer*. Recently *L. aethiopica* was isolated from a squirrel (*Xerus rutilus*) and from *P. (Paraphlebotomus) sergenti* at lower altitudes in Ethiopia (Gramiccia and Gradoni 2005). The caused clinical form results in a spectrum from uncomplicated localized, to DCL (Fig. 44.10).

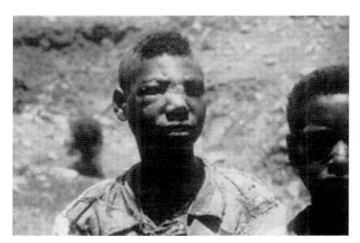

Fig. 44.10 Clinical aspect of diffuse cutaneous leishmaniosis caused by *Leishmania aethiopica*.

New World ZCL

American CL forms are originally sylvatic zoonoses. Some of them have shown a remarkable potential to adapt to human modifications of the environment and can show a synanthropic distribution, as in tropical rain forest, secondary forest or peri-urban areas.

Leishmania mexicana

This parasite is a Central American species with a geographical distribution restricted to the Mexican peninsula of Yucatan and the northern part of Guatemala, Belize, and Honduras, although strains of this species were described from Peru and Ecuador. *L. mexicana* has been found infecting various species of sylvatic ground-dwelling rodents in which produce generally small cutaneous lesions. The primary reservoir is commonly considered the tree rat *Ototylomys phyllotis*, with diverse forest rodents as secondary reservoir. The principal vector is *Lu. olmeca olmeca*, a sand fly highly attracted by rodents but also anthropophilic, biting during the day. The clinical form is a classical localized CL, although some cases of DCL have been recently described.

Leishmania amazonensis

Originally described in the Brazilian Amazon region, *L. amazonensis* shows a vast geographical distribution in different states of Brazil, Bolivia, Colombia, Ecuador, Peru, French Guiana, Panama and Venezuela. The primary reservoirs are generally considered forest rodents which develop subpatent infections. Secondary hosts are marsupial species where the parasite was isolated. The principal vector is *Lu. flaviscutellata*. The main clinical forms are localized or DCL, with frequent anergic or borderline anergic features.

Leishmania venezuelensis

This parasite was firstly described in 1980 in human cases of localized CL from Barquisimeto, Lara state, Venezuela. This species was subsequently identified in several urban centres of that state. So far vectors remain unknown, while domestic cats were suspected as the reservoir host.

Leishmania braziliensis

This species shows the widest geographical distribution among the American CL agents. *L. braziliensis* spreads from the majority of countries of South America (Argentina, Bolivia, Brazil, Colombia, Ecuador, Paraguay, Peru, and Venezuela), to Central America (Belize, Guatemala, Nicaragua, Costa Rica, Honduras, Panama) and Mexico. Until now, the life cycle(s) is not completely known due to the wide dispersion of the species that covers multiple biotopes, with different reservoir and vector interactions. The disease appears originally as a wild zoonoses of primary rain forest areas that has been adapted to the human environments resulting from deforestation and agriculture extension. Various mammals have been found infected by the parasite including carnivores, rodents, and perissodactyls. Dogs have been recently found infected in the absence of other infected mammal hosts, in Guatemala (Ryan *et al.* 2003). Although *L. braziliensis* was identified in several *Lutzomyia* species, *Lu. wellcomei* is considered the most efficient vector. The usual clinical form caused by the parasite is a localized CL, with variable evolution toward a severe MCL in 30–80% of patients (Fig. 44.11).

Leishmania guyanensis

This parasite is localized in the northern part of the Amazon Basin, especially in Guyana and some Brazilian states. The life cycle has long been elucidated, with a primary reservoir in a sylvatic

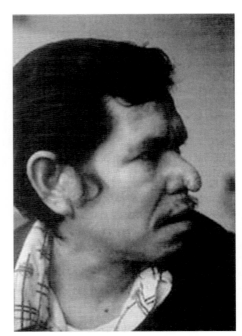

Fig. 44.11 Disfiguring mucocutaneous leishmaniosis due to *L. braziliensis*.

edentate, the sloth, and the principal vector in *Lu. umbratilis*. The clinical form is a localized CL and human exposure to *L. guyanensis* results from occasional intrusions into the forest.

Leishmania lainsoni

This species occurs in the rain forest of the northern part of the Para state of Brazil, Bolivia, and Peru. The life cycle is known since 1987, showing its reservoir in the rodent *Agouti paca* and the vector in *Lu. ubiquitalis*, a sand fly species abundant in the endemic area. The clinical form caused is a localized CL.

Leishmania naiffi

This species was firstly described in 1989 as a parasite of the armadillo *Dasypus novemcinctus* in Amazon Brazil. The uncertain taxonomical position was clarified by Thomaz-Soccol *et al.* (1993), who demonstrated *L. naiffi* as a *Viannia* parasite in an intermediate state between *L. braziliensis* and *L. guyanensis*. Although being a prevalent parasite in armadillos, it was found as a cause of human localized CL in Brazil, French Guiana, Ecuador and Peru (Pratlong *et al.* 2002).

Leishmania panamensis

This parasite is distributed in Central America countries as Panama, Costa Rica, Nicaragua, Honduras, Guatemala, and in Pacific regions of Colombia and Ecuador. Epidemiological investigations showed the reservoir in different sloths and the possible vector in *Lu. trapidoi*. As in the case of *L. guyanensis*, its life cycle is closely associated to the forest biotope. In humans, clinical forms vary from localized CL to MCL in 2–5% of patients.

Leishmania peruviana

This agent is the only non-sylvatic species responsible for American CL known prior to the conquest by Europeans. Its geographical distribution is limited to the Peruvian Andes, confined to the arid valleys of the western slopes between 1,200 and 3,000 metres altitude. The life cycle was elucidated only recently by the identification of the natural reservoir of *L. peruviana* in dogs (Llanos-Cuentas *et al.* 1999). The principal vectors are *Lu. verrucarum* and *Lu. peruensis*, even if other anthropophilic *Lutzomyia* species were found infected. The clinical form, locally called 'uta', is a typical localized ulcerative CL.

Leishmania shawi

This is a sylvatic *Leishmania* species parasitizing various arboreal mammals in the rain forest of the Para state of Brazil, and causing localized CL in humans. It was originally discovered in the monkey *Cebus apella* and then isolated from different wild mammals as monkeys (*Chiropotes satanas*), sloths (*Choloepus didactylus* and *Bradypus tridactylus*) and coatis (*Nasua nasua*). In the forest of Para state, *Lu. whitmani* was found infected by *L. shawi*.

Changing patterns of leishmanioses

Over the past few years, there have been a number of eco-epidemiological situations which resulted in changing patterns of leishmanioses transmission. Not all factors underlying such changes were identified however both climatic modifications associated to global warming and human behavioural factors probably play a major role. The distribution and seasonality of vector-borne diseases are likely to be affected by climate changes, especially in temperate zones where increased average temperatures allow extension of the breeding seasons of the endemic vector species, or the *de novo* introduction of exogenous vectors, permitting pathogen transmission in areas where low temperatures had prevented their over-wintering.

Impact of human behaviour on zoonotic CL changes

Risk factors for ZCL are strongly associated to human exposure depending by the presence of the vectors and their activity cycles. In the Old World, urbanization is a major risk factor: new human settlements or suburbs located in the outskirts of the towns, when intruded on the terrain formerly inhabited by *P. papatasi* and the rodent *P. obesus*, have led to an increased transmission of *L. major* to humans, as observed in several areas of north Africa, Middle East, and Central Asia. Also, the building of dams with new irrigation schemes and crops may cause a rapid change in the rodent reservoir populations, followed by epidemics (Desjeux 2001).

In the New World, industrial and commercial projects have produced relevant immigration of workers in the Brazilian Amazon, resulting in the construction of several suburbs on the border of the primary forest. Newly urbanized areas brought the new population in contact with the zoonotic cycle of *L. guyanensis* and the incidence of new localized CL cases rapidly increased. In the Andean countries, the development of new projects (road building, mining, tourism etc.) and the subsequent new settlements and deforestation, has frequently caused a domestication of zoonotic transmission cycles with an increase of the peri and intra-domiciliary transmission (Desjeux 2001).

The current spread of *Leishmania infantum* in the Old and New Worlds

Several re-emerging issues are associated with the zoonotic entity of VL due to *L. infantum*. Spreading of infections in different territories have been monitored and recorded by means of investigations carried out among susceptible domestic dogs, which act as suitable sentinel hosts.

Expansion of endemic foci in Europe and Central Asia

Being previously confined to coastal Mediterranean biotopes, ZVL incidence has been increased in Italy in human and dogs since 1990s (Maroli *et al.* 2008). During 2002–2009, the northward spread of the disease was monitored through human, canine and entomological surveys performed in northern continental regions at the border with France, Switzerland, Austria and Slovenia. Results showed that the most competent *L. infantum* vector, *P. perniciosus*, was widespread in these territories, associated with *P. neglectus* in the sub-Alpine and with *P. perfiliewi* in sub-Apennines territories. The large Padana valley was apparently found free from sandfly colonization, probably acting as natural barrier. CanL investigations confirmed the ongoing northward spread of ZVL, with a mean seroprevalence of 1.8% found in sub-Alpine sites, and an increase from 2 to 4% in sub-Apennines sites during the survey period. Despite the presence of a competent vector, Bolzano-South Tyrol province at the border with Austria was found still free from autochthonous CanL. Both VL and CL autochthonous human cases due to *L. infantum* have been recorded in the newly endemic regions. These findings demonstrate conclusively that northern continental Italy became focally endemic for ZVL after 1990s.

In Germany, the detection of leishmaniosis cases in humans and animals (dog, cat, horse) that never travelled abroad, has led to the hypothesis of a recent establishment of autochthonous transmission in that country (Naucke *et al.* 2008). A northward *L. infantum* expansion was suggested, although entomological surveys did not provide solid evidence for the presence of competent vector species.

The description of a novel CanL focus, with *P. perniciosus* and *P. ariasi* acting as local vectors, has been recently reported in a territory of French Pyrenees outside the traditional endemic range of leishmanioses in southern France (Dereure *et al.* 2009). During a period of 13 years, seroprevalence rates in foothill villages increased by 10 folds as a probable consequence of the 1°C increase in the mean annual temperature.

The progressive increase in CanL seroprevalence rate was also reported at elevated altitudes of 600–900m a.s.l. in the Alpujarras region of southeastern Spain, climbing from 9.2% in 1984, to 15.4% in 1991 and 20.1% in 2006 (Martin-Sanchez *et al.* 2009).

In the former USSR, ZVL was prevalent in republics of Central Asia and in the Caucasus. Due to intensive control programs, disease incidence decreased dramatically and was almost forgotten by local doctors. However, persistence of stable but sporadic foci in the Namangan and Fergana regions of Uzbekistan has been documented. In 1987–1999, nineteen VL cases were recorded in three villages of Namangan region. Clinical and epidemiological features suggested that the disease was zoonotic, with *L. infantum* as putative agent and *P. longiductus* as possible vector. Subsequent VL surveillance during 2004–2007 revealed an epidemic trend with a total of 34 human cases, of which 15 recorded in 2007. The pathogen was then identified from both Uzbek and neighbouring Tajik territories, and assigned to a distinct *L. infantum* genetic cluster different from Europe, Middle East and Africa ones. This suggests the local origin of the parasite in Uzbekistan and Tajikistan, rather than a newly introduction by human or reservoir migration. (Alam *et al.* 2009).

CanL and zoonotic VL spread in the Americas

Human VL is rarely reported in USA, occasionally diagnosed in persons returning from endemic countries. An unexpected outbreak among foxhounds recently suggested endemic transmission of the disease (Duprey *et al.* 2006). In a New York state hunt club, in the summer 1999 some foxhounds developed severe illness characterized by typical CanL signs. A serosurvey revealed a high prevalence among foxhounds (but not in other breeds) and *L. infantum* MON-1 was isolated by infected animals. Serological screenings in other states revealed a widespread infection in a vast region of eastern North America extending from Florida state northward to Ontario province, Canada, and from the Eastern coastal regions to Kansas and Oklahoma in the West, for a total of 21 US states and 2 Canadian provinces. The transmission routes in these dogs are still unclear. Some epidemiological characteristics support only partially a classical vectorial transmission, whereas suggest possible dog-to-dog transmission both vertical (transplacental and transmammary) and horizontal (by direct contacts). No cases of autochthonous human VL were reported from the affected areas.

Only 14 autochthonous human VL cases were reported in Argentina from 1925 to 1989, interspersed with *L. braziliensis* CL cases. *Lu. longipalpis*, the most competent vector of *L. infantum*, was reported only twice in Misiones province, on the border with Brazil. The risk for ZVL transmission in Argentina changed dramatically since 2000s when, despite rapid human and canine disease spreading in the neighbour Paraguay state, no preventive CanL surveys were carried out in Misiones until autochthonous human VL cases have appeared. Both CanL infections and *Lu. longipalpis* vector were found widespread following active surveys. This is the first autochthonous ZVL focus reported in Argentina, representing the southernmost focus in Latin America (Salomon *et al.* 2008).

Feline and equine leishmaniosis

Among recent reports on newly identified or unusual animal hosts recurrently found infected with different *Leishmania* species, those regarding domestic cats and equines deserve attention for the obvious implications in public health.

Leishmaniosis in cats has been described since 1912. Afterwards several scattered reports on feline *Leishmania* infections have appeared in southern America (Brazil), Europe (Portugal, Spain, France, Italy, Switzerland, Germany) and Middle East (Israel, Iran) (Gramiccia and Gradoni 2005; Maia *et al.* 2008, Nasereddin *et al.* 2008; Hatam *et al.* 2009). Recently, the seroprevalence of infection has been estimated in feline populations of southern Europe, which showed antibody titres usually lower than in CanL. Seroprevalences ranged 0.6–59.1% in different endemic settings. Five *Leishmania* species have been identified in feline cases: *L. mexicana*, *L. venezuelensis*, *L. braziliensis* and *L. amazonensis* in the New World, and *L. infantum* in both the New and Old Worlds. Polymorphic cutaneous forms are frequent, including localized nodular, ulcerative, crusty or papular lesions, or generalized dermatits, alopecia and scaling. Systemic disease was described less frequently. The first evidence of transmissibility of feline parasites to a proven vector was recently provided in Italy, suggesting that cats may represent a secondary reservoir host for *L. infantum* (Maroli *et al.* 2007).

Since early 1980s *Leishmania* infections have been reported in domestic equines from different regions of Latin America (Brazil, Venezuela, Argentina and Puerto Rico) (Gramiccia and Gradoni 2005). Epidemics due to *L. braziliensis* were described in donkeys, and sporadic cases in horses and mules. The clinical forms observed consisted of nodular or ulcerated cutaneous lesions, occasionally disseminating without visceralization. Spontaneous regression of the lesions was also reported. In the past few years, there have been sporadic cases of horse leishmaniosis in Europe caused by *L. infantum*. Like for the New World forms, infections consisted of self-resolving cutaneous lesions. Domestic equines seem to display clinical and immunological responses of resistant type, and much probably they represent an incidental host.

Diagnosis

Parasitological, molecular and serological assays are routine methods available for the diagnosis of leishmanioses. However, the direct demonstration of parasite is the only way to confirm the disease conclusively. Isolation and identification of the parasite from biopsies (skin, lymph node, bone marrow, and spleen aspirate) is performed by slide smear microscopy and/or culture in appropriate blood-agar based media. In VL, because sensitivity of standard parasitological methods may not be high enough, immunodiagnostic and molecular tests are also recommended. Serological tests include indirect immunofluorescent antibody test, ELISA, Direct Agglutination Test and Western-blot assay. More recently, immunochromatographic dipsticks using recombinant antigen k39 have been developed. Direct parasitological diagnosis is necessary for confirmation of CL (by means of scraping, punch biopsy or needle aspiration of the lesions) as neither clinical examination nor serology are adequate. Several protocols are now available for the PCR amplification of *Leishmania* DNA from biopsy material for both diagnosis of different clinical forms, and the identification of the agent.

Treatment

Indian kala-azar has been included by the WHO in the list of neglected tropical diseases targeted for elimination by 2015 (WHO 2009). Since there is no vaccine in clinical use, control relies almost exclusively on chemotherapy. Treatment depended on arsenicals and tartar emetic until the efficacy of pentavalent antimony compounds was discovered in the 1920s. Since then, treatment with pentavalent antimonial compounds represents the mainstay therapy for all forms of leishmaniosis. Following the increasing incidence of *Leishmania*-HIV co-infections and the acquired antimonial resistance in India, amphotericin B formulations have joined the antimonials as treatment choice. Alternative drugs as pentamidine and paromomycin (aminosidine) were included in the VL and CL treatment. Since 2006 the new oral agent miltefosine has been introduced especially in the areas with reported antimonial resistance. In response to concerns about preserving the currently available antileishmanials, especially in regions with anthroponotic parasite transmission, there is growing interest on combinations regimens.

In Europe, treatment of CanL in pets has followed the same historical process. Nowadays, veterinary brands include pentavalent antimony, miltefosine and aminosidine (Solano-Gallego *et al.* 2009).

Drugs

Antimonials

Two closely related pentavalent antimonials are currently used, sodium stibogluconate (Pentostam®) and meglumine antimoniate (Glucantime®). It is generally accepted that pentavalent antimonials (SbV) are the prodrug and that they should convert to trivalent antimonials (SbIII) in order to demonstrate their antileishmanial activity. Recent evidence indicates that antimonials kill leishmanias by a process of apoptosis involving thiol metabolism and trypanothione activity. SbIII inhibits trypanothione reductase *in vitro*, inducing the loss of intracellular thiolsan, a lethal imbalance in thiol homeostasis, leading to accumulation of reactive oxygen species. In spite of numerous side effects attributed to antimonials, the scarcity of reported accidents allows their continued use. Initially antimonial were given at 10mg/kg for 6–10 days with 90% cure rates, however after the first treatment failure in India twenty years ago, higher doses and prolonged schemes (up to 20mg/kg for 30 days) were gradually introduced and in parallel with the increasing rates of antimony unresponsiveness. During the last decade antimonial resistance reached epidemic dimension in Bihar, India that abandoned the antimonials use. Low rates of antimonial resistance have been reported in Sudan. This aspect is not an emerging problem in Mediterranean areas (Gradoni *et al.* 2008). Low cost is the main advantage of antimonials.

Amphotericin-B and its lipid association

Conventional amphotericin B (AmB) is a polyene antibiotic isolated in 1955 and currently used in the treatment of systemic fungal infections. Since 1960s it was used as a second-line treatment for VL. Its target is ergosterol-like sterols, which are the major membrane sterols of *Leishmania* as well as fungi. Lipid formulations of AmB improved highly antileishmanial activity and safety profile of this drug. Lipid formulations are taken selectively by the reticuloendothelial system, and exhibit a highly localized enhanced antileishmanial action. There are three lipid formulations of amphotericin B:

- Liposomal amphotericin B (AmBisome®) the only drug licensed for VL,
- Amphotericin B lipid complex (Abelcet®),
- Amphotericin B cholesterol dispersion (Amphocil®).

Currently, liposomal formulations of AmB are the first treatment choice in southern Europe endemic countries as well as in other developed countries, because of their rapid and up to 100% cure rates with 3–5 days schemes, improved convenience for the patient included immunocompromised patients, and reduction of health care costs. However, in poor countries even short courses of liposomal formulations are unaffordable, and the selection of antileishmanial treatment turns more to a question of cost than of efficacy or toxicity. Short-course treatment is now currently used, including five daily injections of 3–4mg/kg, plus a further same dose on the 10th day.

Miltefosine

It is alkilphospholipid (hexadecylphosphocoline) oral antineoplastic agent. This is the first oral administered drug for VL and the latest to enter the market. This agent is associated with high efficacy rates including cases unresponsive to antimonials. So far, miltefosine is licensed in India, Germany, and Colombia. The scheme of miltefosine is 100 mg/kg/day for 28 days in adults weighing ≥50 kg, 50mg/kg/day in adults <50 kg, and 2.5mg/kg/day in children (maximum dose: 100 mg/day). Major concerns for the wide use of miltefosine include its teratogenic potential and its long half-life (approximately 150 hours) which may facilitate the emergence of resistance. Miltefosine is strictly forbidden in women of child-bearing age who may become pregnant up to two months following drug discontinuation. In India, miltefosine is available over the counter, a fact that may expose this drug to misuse and emergence of resistance. The exact anti-leishmanial mechanism of miltefosine remains largely unknown. The intracellular accumulation of the drug appears to be the critical step for its action. It includes the following steps: binding to plasma membrane, internalization in the parasite cell and intracellular targeting and metabolism. It has been found that miltefosine induces an apoptosis like cell death in *L. donovani*, by producing numerous defects.

Alternative drugs

Paromomycin

Paromomycin (aminosidine) is an aminoglycoside with antileishmanial activity. In a phase IV study of VL in India, this drug was associated with 94.6% cure rates, similar to amphotericin B. Adverse effects were more frequent and high in the paromomycin-treated group compared with the amphotericin B-treated group; paromomycin-related adverse effects included elevated hepatic transaminases, ototoxicity, and pain at injection-site. Paromomycin is inexpensive but requires daily intramuscular injections for 21 days. Paromomycin inhibits protein synthesis and modifies membrane fluidity and permeability and *in vitro* study showed that mitochondria are the targets of the drug. Since paromomycin is an aminoglycoside, it is possible that resistance will emerge rapidly if used as monotherapy.

Pentamidine

Pentamidine is an aromatic diamine. The isethionate salt (Pentacarinat®) is the only form now available for human use and is restricted to systemic CL treatment. The drug inhibits the synthesis of parasitic DNA by blocking thymidine synthase and fixation of transfer RNA. It can be responsible for immediate and side effects which severity depends on the dose. Pentamidine is given in doses of 4mg/kg per injection for a short course of four doses on alternate days.

Combination regimens

The rational for using combination regimens with different resistance mechanisms over monotherapy relies on the expected enhanced efficacy, shorter treatment duration, less toxicity, improved compliance, reduced likelihood of emergence of resistance, and reduced costs. A combination policy for VL is supported by the fact that anti-leishmanial drugs belong to different chemical classes. Recent studies have investigated this option. In a retrospective study conducted among Sudanese patients with VL, it was found that combination of sodium stibogluconate and paromomycin administered for 17 days was associated with higher cure and survival rates compared to sodium stibogluconate. Combinations of miltefosine with amphotericin B, paromomycin or pentavalent antimonials have been evaluated in an *in vivo* model and revealed that the combinations of miltefosine with amphotericin B or paromomycin were efficacious. Recent studies indicate that a single dose of liposomal amphotericin B followed by 7–14 days of miltefosine is active against Indian VL.

Therapy in different clinical forms of leishmaniosis

VL should be treated as soon as diagnosis is completed. Treatment requires confirmed first line drugs, principally antimonials or various AmB formulations. Clinical response is slow, the patient become afebrile within 4–5 days, other clinical symptoms and biological parameters slowly regressing and evolving to normal. VL occurring in HIV-infected patients appears generally as non-responsive to the classical anti-leishmanial drugs with incomplete cure and frequent relapses. Similar poor responses are observed in VL following organ transplantation or generalized immunosuppression, such as that caused by prolonged corticosteroid therapies.

With regard to CL and MCL, most of the Old World forms consist of simple lesions in contrast with the variety of the New World forms. The drugs employed are basically the same as for VL, with different applications and regimens according to the type and character of lesions. A variety of physical treatments, such as heat-, cryo-, laser- and radiotherapy, is commonly employed for topical use in highly CL endemic countries. Topical treatment, consisting of local infiltrations of pentavalent antimonials 2 or 3 times/week, is mainly employed for the Old World CL. Systemic treatment is recommended for the New World CL and MCL, using pentavalent antimonials at similar dosages used for VL, or pentamidine with a course of 4–5 injections on alternate days.

The treatment of MCL should be as early as possible, in order to avoid extension of lesions and subsequent mutilations. The cure rate is variable according to *Leishmania* (*Viannia*) species/strain involved and the evolution of the lesions. Antimonials and AmB are the first line drugs, while oral miltefosine is still under study. Drug treatments are not efficacious in DCL conditions once established.

The first line pharmaceutical protocol for CanL is the combination of meglumine antimoniate and allopurinol, but many different therapeutic protocols are suggested (Solano-Gallego *et al.* 2009). Recently a combination of miltefosine with allopurinol was proposed as an alternative to the association antimonial-allopurinol. However, although most dogs recover clinically after therapy, complete elimination of the parasite is usually not achieved and infected dogs may relapse.

Surveillance and control

Over the past few years, international health agencies have increased efforts to improve methodologies for the surveillance and control of leishmanioses characterized by a predominant anthroponotic transmission pattern (Desjeux 2004). In the field of zoonotic leishmanioses, no significant advances were made in the CL control in both Old and New Worlds. The exophilic habit of the phlebotomine vectors and the sylvatic nature of the mammal reservoir hosts would require expensive environmental management difficult to implement and sustain, such as forest cleaning or destruction of rodent burrows around human dwellings.

On the other hand, new tools have been developed for the surveillance and control of zoonotic VL, based on the control of CanL. Culling of infected dogs is not considered an acceptable measure, for both ethical considerations and the low efficacy. Several canine

vaccine candidates are under study (Gradoni 2001); one of them has been recently registered in Brazil for veterinary use. A number of insecticide-based preparations have been specifically registered for dog protection against sand fly bites, which include deltamethrin impregnated collars and topical ('spot-on') permethrin. Laboratory and field studies have shown elevated efficacy of these preparations for both individual and mass protection. The impact of this type of control measure can be limited if not integrated with stray dog control.

Legislation

With the exception of the compulsory reporting of cases, which applies in an increasing number of countries following WHO recommendations (Desjeux 1991), legislation appears inappropriate for most of leishmanioses endemic countries. Governmental control programmes against VL are in course in Brazil, which is based on CanL control, and in the Indian sub-continent (some states of India, Nepal, and Bangladesh), which is mainly addressed to interrupt the anthroponotic transmission of *L. donovani*.

References

Alam, M.Z., Kovalenko, D.A., Kuhls, K., *et al.* (2009). Identification of the agent causing visceral leishmaniasis in Uzbeki and Tajiki foci by analysing parasite DNA extracted from patients' Giemsa-stained tissue preparations. *Parasitology*, **136**: 981–86.

Dereure, J., Vanwambeke, S.O., Malé, P., *et al.* (2009). The potential effects of global warming on changes in canine leishmaniasis in a focus outside the classical area of the disease in Southern France. *Vector Borne Zoonotic Dis.*, **9**: 687–94.

Desjeux, P. (1996). Leishmaniasis Public health aspects and control. *Clin. Dermatol.*, **14**: 417–23.

Desjeux, P. (2001). The increase in risk factors for leishmaniasis worldwide. *Trans. R. Soc. Trop. Med. Hyg.*, **95**: 239–43.

Desjeux, P. (2004). Leishmaniasis: current situation and new perspectives. *Comp. Immunol. Microbiol. Infect. Dis.*, **27**: 305–18.

Duprey, Z.H., Steurer, F.J., Roney, J.A., *et al.* (2006). Canine visceral leishmaniasis, United States and Canada, 2000–2003. *Emerging Infect. Dis.*, **12**: 440–46.

Elfari, M., Schnur, L.F., Strelkova, M.V., *et al.* (2005). Genetic and biological diversity among populations of *Leishmania major* from Central Asia, the Middle East and Africa. *Microbes Infect.*, **7**: 93–103.

Gradoni, L. (2001). An update on antileishmanial vaccine candidates and prospetcs for a canine *Leishmania* vaccine. *Vet. Parasitol.*, **100**: 87–103.

Gradoni, L., Soteriadou, K., Louzir, H., *et al.* (2008). Drug regimens for visceral leishmaniasis in Mediterranean countries. *Trop. Med. Int. Health*, **13**: 1272–76.

Gramiccia, M. and Gradoni, L. (2005). The current status of zoonotic leishmaniases and approaches to disease control. *Int. J. Parasitol.*, **35**: 1169–80.

Hatam, G.R., Adnani, S.J., Asgari, Q., *et al.* (2010). First report of natural infection in cats with *Leishmania infantum* in Iran. *Vector Borne Zoonotic Dis.*, **10**: 313–16.

Hotez, P.J., Romme, J.H.F., Buss, P., *et al.* (2004). Combating tropical infectious diseases: report of the disease control priorities in developing countries project. *Clin. Infect. Dis.*, **38**: 871–78.

Kuhls, K., Keilonat, L., Ochsenreither, S., *et al.* (2007). Multilocus microsatellite typing (MLMT) reveals genetically isolated populations between and within the main endemic regions of visceral leishmaniasis. *Microbes Infect.*, **9**: 334–43.

Llanos-Cuentas, E.A, Roncal, N., Villaseca, P., *et al.* (1999). Natural infections of *Leishmania peruviana* in animals in the Peruvian Andes. *Trans. R. Soc. Trop. Med. Hyg.*, **93**: 15–20.

Lukeš, J., Mauricio, I.L., Schönian, G., et al. (2007). Evolutionary and geographical history of the *Leishmania donovani* complex with a revision of current taxonomy. *Proc. Natl. Acad. Sci. USA*, **104:** 9375–80.

Maia, C., Nunes, M., and Campino, L. (2008). Importance of cats in zoonotic leishmaniasis in Portugal. *Vector Borne Zoonotic Dis.*, **8:** 555–59.

Maroli, M., Pennisi, M.G., Di Muccio, T., et al. (2007). Infection of sand flies by a cat naturally infected with *Leishmania infantum*. *Vet. Parasitol.*, **145:** 357–60.

Maroli, M., Rossi, L., Baldelli, R., et al. (2008). The northward spread of leishmaniasis in Italy: evidence from restrospective and ongoing studies on the canine reservoir and phlebotomine vectors. *Trop. Med. Int. Health*, **13:** 256–64.

Martin-Sanchez, J., Morales-Yuste, M., Acedo-Sànchez, C., et al. (2009). Canine leishmaniasis in Southeastern Spain. *Emerging Infect. Dis.*, **15:** 795–98.

Nasereddin, A., Salant, H. and Abdeen, Z. (2008). Feline leishmaniasis in Jerusalem: serological investigation. *Vet. Parasitol.*, **158:** 364–69.

Naucke, T.J., Menn, B., Massberg, D., et al. (2008). Sandflies and leishmaniasis in Germany. *Parasitol. Res.*, **103** (Suppl. 1): S65–68.

Pratlong, F., Deniau, M., Darie, H., et al. (2002). Human cutaneous leishmaniasis caused by *Leishmania naiffi* is wide-spread in South America. *Ann. Trop. Med. Parasitol.*, **96:** 781–85.

Ryan, P.R., Arana, B.A., Ryan, J.R., et al. (2003). The domestic dog, a potential reservoir for *Leishmania* in the Peten region of Guatemala. *Vet. Parasitol.*, **115:** 1–7.

Rose, K., Curtis, J., Baldwuin, T., et al. (2004). Cutaneous leishmaniasis in red kangaroos: isolation and characterization of the causative organisms. *Int. J. Parasitol.*, **34:** 655–64.

Salomon, O.D., Sinagra, A., Nevot, M.C., et al. (2008). First visceral leishmaniasis focus in Argentina, *Mem. Inst. Oswaldo Cruz*, **103:** 109–11.

Schönian, G., Mauricio, I., Gramiccia, M., et al. (2008). Leishmaniases in the Mediterranean in the era of molecular epidemiology. *Trends Parasitol.*, **24:** 135–42.

Solano-Gallego, L., Koutinas, A., Miró, G., et al. (2009). Directions for the diagnosis, clinical staging, treatment and prevention of canine leishmaniosis. *Vet. Parasitol.*, **165:** 1–18.

Tuon, F.F., Neto, V.A. and Amato, V.S. (2008). *Leishmania:* origin, evolution and future since the Precambrian. *FEMS Immunol. Med. Microbiol.*, **54:** 158–66.

World Health Organization. *Leishmaniasis:* burden of disease. Available at: http://www.who.int/leishmaniosis/burden/en (accessed August 2009).

CHAPTER 45

Giardia infections

R. C. Andrew Thompson

Summary

Giardia is a ubiquitous intestinal protozoan parasite of vertebrates and the most common intestinal pathogen of humans and domestic animals with a worldwide distribution including both temperate and tropical regions.

Giardia was first observed in 1681 by Antony van Leeuwenhoek in his own faeces (Dobell 1920), and the organism has intrigued biologists and clinicians ever since. However, the first detailed description of the parasite was not given until two centuries later by Lambl (1859). Koch's postulation was proven by Rendtorff in 1954 when he successfully transmitted symptomatic *Giardia* infection to human volunteers following orally administered cysts. The first symptoms of clinical giardiasis were reported in the early 1920s, although the significance of *Giardia* as a cause of diarrhoeal disease was controversial for many years (see Farthing 1994; Cox 1998), and it is only recently that the significance of *Giardia* as a cause of chronic disease in children and its association with failure to thrive, wasting and malabsorption syndromes has been fully realised (reviewed in Farthing 1994; Hall 1994; Gracey 1994; Rabbani and Islam 1994; Hesham *et al.* 2005; Savioli *et al.* 2006; Thompson 2008).

The question of *Giardia*'s role as a source of zoonotically transmitted disease again has been controversial. The World Health Organization (WHO) recommended that *Giardia* should be considered as a zoonotic agent in 1979 (Anon. 1979). Since that time, increasing circumstantial epidemiological evidence from waterborne outbreaks, the results of some cross-infection experiments and molecular characterization studies of *Giardia* isolates from humans and other animals has led most authorities to conclude that *Giardia* should be considered a zoonotic parasite (Acha and Szyfres 2003; Savioli *et al.* 2006; and reviewed in Thompson 2004). However, as discussed below, the frequency of zoonotic transmission is uncertain.

The agent

Taxonomy

Giardia is a member of the Phylum Sarcomoastigophora and the class Zoomastigophorea which also contains the medically important flagellates *Trichomonas*, *Trypanosoma* and *Leishmania*. Species of the genus are classified in the Order Diplomonadida and Family Hexamitidae. As such, they are characterized by a duplication of organelles, including two equivalent nuclei, bilateral symmetry and an oval shape (Thompson and Monis 2004). Almost all members of the Family are parasites of the intestinal tract of vertebrates and invertebrates.

The characteristics of the genus *Giardia* are clearly defined and well accepted (reviewed by Kulda and Nohynkova 1978; Thompson and Monis 2004) although the phylogenetic position of *Giardia* is a subject of much current debate (see below). The motile intestinal stage, the trophozoite, is binucleate and has a distinctive morphology with four pairs of flagellae, a pair of distinctive median bodies and characteristic ventral adhesive disc (Fig. 45.1). This latter structure is the principle distinguishing character used to delineate *Giardia* from other members of the Hexamitidae and is supported by a cytoskeleton of microtubules, microfilaments and associated fibrous structures. It is composed of a variety of structural proteins including tubulin (both α and β subunits) and closely-related giardins as well as actin, myosin and tropomyosin (reviewed in Thompson and Monis 2004; Palm and Svard 2009).

Over 50 species of *Giardia* have been described (Thompson *et al.* 1993; Thompson and Monis 2004). Descriptions of the majority of species in the genus *Giardia* were primarily on the basis of host occurrence, but the lack of distinguishing morphological features (Thompson *et al.* 1990; Majewska *et al.* 1993; Thompson and Monis 2004) and uncertainty regarding host specificity resulted in a taxonomic rationalization with most species described from domestic animals being placed in the one species, *G. duodenalis* (Filice 1952 and reviewed in Monis *et al.* 2008; Thompson and Monis 2004). Unfortunately, this apparently simple scheme failed to reflect the considerable phenotypic and genetic heterogeneity that exists within the species *G. duodenalis*. This species is the most widespread and is known to affect at least 40 species of vertebrates, including humans (Kulda and Nohynkova 1978; Thompson *et al.* 1990, 1993). Furthermore, there is now strong evidence that some genetic variants of *G. duodenalis* are host specific (see below).

The taxonomic rationalization proposed by Filice (1952) resulted in many described species of *Giardia* from mammals being included within the one species, *G. duodenalis*. Filice (1952) recognized that this might represent a temporary holding position until stronger evidence than purely host occurrence became available to better define species of *Giardia* affecting mammals. This is now possible

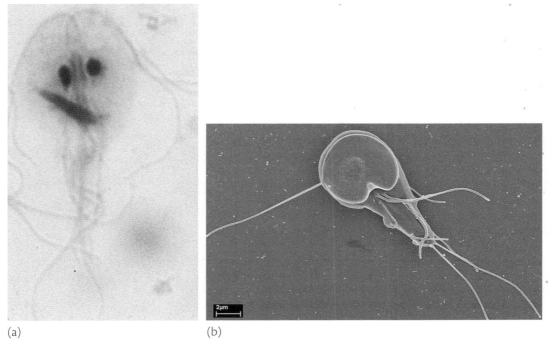

(a)   (b)

Fig. 45.1 A cultured trophozoite of *Giardia duodenalis* isolated from a human patient in Western Australia (a) stained with Giemsa (x100)—note darkly stained paired nuclei and median bodies, and flagella; and (b) scanning electron micrograph showing ventral adhesive disc anteriorly and flagella.
Courtesy of Dr Nicoletee Binz (a) and Dr Peta Clode (b).

principally through the development of appropriate molecular procedures that have demonstrated sufficient genetic diversity within the *G. duodenalis* morphological group to revise the taxonomy of *Giardia* (Thompson and Monis 2004; Monis *et al.* 2008). However, during the period after Filice's proposal, increasing evidence of phenotypic and genotypic variability resulted in an informal nomenclature being developed for the different variants/strains within *G. duodenalis* (Monis *et al.* 1998; Monis and Thompson 2003). The principal genetic groupings are known as assemblages and these have recently been proposed to warrant species status (Monis *et al.* 2008). However, within some of these assemblages/species, there is significant genetic variability which must be recognized since there is increasing evidence that it is reflected in epidemiologically important differences in host specificity and virulence (Caccio *et al.* 2005; Monis *et al.* 2008). The nomenclature of *Giardia* affecting mammals is summarized in Tables 45.1 and 45.2. In this chapter, the term 'strain' is used as a convenient means of referring to a genetic variant within a species of *Giardia*.

The nature of the differences which have been found between isolates of *G. duodenalis* have a significant influence on the epidemiology and control of giardiasis, particularly differences in host specificity, growth and development, virulence, metabolism, and drug sensitivity (Thompson 2004; Caccio *et al.* 2005; Monis *et al.* 2008).

Phylogenetic relationships

As outlined above, *Giardia* has traditionally been classified in the mastigophoran order Diplomonadida along with *Spironucleus* and *Hexamita* and has been assumed to be closely related to the trichomonads. However, the relationship of *Giardia* to other flagellates, and its phylogenetic affinities in general with respect to eukaryotes was questioned on the basis of molecular data from ribosomal DNA and proposed affinities with prokaryotes (Sogin *et al.* 1989) raising suggestions of *Giardia*'s primitive origins and that it could be a missing link between prokaryotes and eukaryotes. However, more recent molecular data shows that *Giardia* is from a lineage of early diverging eukaryotes, but like many other protistan parasites it is highly evolved and the absence of organelles and biochemical pathways is due to secondary loss (Dacks *et al.* 2008). This thus supports earlier phylogenetic analysis based on morphological characters of a range of Diplomonad protozoa, including *Giardia*, suggesting that *Giardia* is not a primitive protozoan and does not hold a pivotal position in the evolution of eukaryotes (Siddall *et al.* 1992).

As regards *G. duodenalis*, phylogenetic analysis of genetic variants has shown that they represent distinct evolutionary lineages (Monis *et al.* 1998). However, the molecular data suggests host switching/host adaptation rather than co-evolution as the basis for host specificity (Monis *et al.* 2008).

Pathogenesis

The mechanisms by which *Giardia* causes disease have been largely speculative until recently, when a complex, dynamic interplay of host and parasite factors have been demonstrated to contribute to the disease process. However, although *Giardia* infections can lead to a variety of syndromes ranging from malabsorptive diarrhoea to chronic nutritional disorders, the full range of factors involved are still unclear and much of what we know about the pathogenesis is confined to experimental infections. Parasite products, such as proteinases that break the epithelial barrier and host inflammatory and immunological

Table 45.1 Recognized species in the genus *Giardia* 1952–2007

Species	Hosts	Morphological characteristics	Trophozoite dimensions (μm)
G. duodenalis	Wide range of wild and domestic mammals including humans	Pear-shaped trophozoites with claw-shaped median bodies	12–15 long 6–8 wide
G. agilis	Amphibians	Long, narrow trophozoites with club-shaped median bodies	20–30 long 4–5 wide
G. muris	Rodents (possibly also birds and other mammals)	Rounded trophozoites with small round median bodies	9–12 long 5–7 wide
G. ardeae	Birds	Rounded trophozoites, with prominent notch in ventral disc and rudimentary caudal flagellum. Median bodies round-oval to claw-shaped.	Approx 10 long Approx 6.5 wide
G. psittaci	Birds (budgerigar, parakeet, possibly other species)	Pear-shaped trophozoites, with no ventro-lateral flange. Claw-shaped median bodies.	14/ 6
G. microti	Rodents	Trophozoites similar to *G. duodenalis*. Mature cysts contain fully differentiated trophozoites.	12–15 long 6–8 wide

responses, have all been shown to be involved (Chai *et al.* 1999; Scott *et al.* 2000, 2002; Guk *et al.* 2003; Buret 2007, 2009).

Mucosal injury is most severe in the upper small intestine, and in contrast to some early studies, it is now generally agreed that *Giardia* is not an invasive parasite (Buret 1994). *Giardia* induces enterocyte apoptosis, associated with disruption of cytoskeletal and tight junctional proteins in a strain-dependent manner (Chin *et al.* 2002). Villus atrophy, diffuse shortening of microvilli, reduced disaccharidase activity, loss of epithelial barrier function, increased permeability, impaired enterocyte function and apoptosis, have all been reported in *Giardia* infections (Buret 2007; 2009). Recent evidence also shows that *Giardia* infection can also cause hypersecretion of chloride ions (Troeger *et al.* 2007). These changes are thought to be due to a combination of parasite products, possibly a toxin, and host immune factors, particularly involving CD8+ cells (Buret 2007; 2009).

The pathophysiology of diarrhoea is multifactorial and results from electrolyte and nutrient malabsorption due to parasite-induced enterocyte injury as well as other factors (reviewed in Ortega-Perres *et al.* 2009). However, the factors leading to chronic disorders associated with *Giardia* infection are not understood but clearly the characteristics of both parasite and host will determine the outcome of such infections. The fact that symptomatic giardiasis is more likely to occur in patients who are immunocompromised, malnourished, or very young is a clear indication that host factors are important. However, in other cases, there is increasing evidence of variable virulence between strains and thus a particular strain of *Giardia* may have a greater potential to cause disease in a particular host (reviewed in Monis *et al.* 2008).

It should be emphasized that clinical signs do not always occur in humans or other animals naturally infected with *Giardia*, and it is still not clear how the changes referred to above relate to the expression of clinical disease.

Life cycle, development and host parasite relationship

Trophozoites colonize the duodenum and jejunum of their host, where they attach to the intestinal mucosa. Attachment is an essential feature of the relationship between *Giardia* and its host and a prerequisite to infection. Further, the ability to attach *in vitro* is an important indicator of viability (Meloni *et al.* 1990; Hernandez-Sanchez and Ortega-Pierres 1993; Hernández-Sánchez *et al.* 2008). Attachment is mediated by *Giardia*'s unique attachment organelle, the ventral adehesive disc. This is a rigid structure composed of microtubules and interconnected micro-ribbons (Peattie 1990). Trophozoites may detach intermittently but periods of detachment are likely to be of minimal duration since the parasite may be in danger of losing its position in the gut and being swept away as the result of peristalsis. Attachment can therefore be considered an important virulence determinant in *Giardia* infections.

The recent publication by Hernández-Sánchez *et al.* (2008) on the ability of adhesion deficient clones to initiate infection has highlighted the importance of this early process in the establishment of infection. A number of mechanisms have been proposed

Table 45.2 Genotypic groupings (assemblages) of *Giardia duodenalis* and new species designation*

Assemblage	Species	Host
Assemblage A	*G. duodenalis*	Humans and other primates, dogs, cats, livestock, rodents and other wild mammals
Assemblage B	*G. enteric*	Humans and other primates, dogs, some species of wild mammals
Assemblages C/D	*G. canis*	Dogs, other canids
Assemblage F	*G. cati*	Cats
Assemblage E	*G. bovis*	Cattle and other hoofed livestock
Assemblage G	*G. simondi*	Rats, possibly other rodents?

* Based on original taxonomic descriptions; see Thompson and Monis (2004), Monis *et al.* (2008).

to explain how *Giardia* attaches to intestinal epithelial cells but most evidence indicates that the ventral disc plays the major role in attachment and that the cytoskeletal elements of the disc are the major mediators in this process (Palm and Svard 2009). This is indicated by the fact that microtubule inhibitors, including known ß-tubulin antagonists, have been shown to inhibit adherence *in vitro* (Meloni *et al.* 1990; Edlind *et al.* 1990; Magne *et al.* 1991). It is therefore interesting that a prominent cytoskeletal protein of the ventral adhesive disc, alpha 2 giardin which is present in assemblage A (*G. duodenalis*) isolates of *G. duodenalis* is absent in assemblage B (*G. enterica*) isolates which may explain the differences emerging in the clinical consequences of infection with these two assemblages (Steuart *et al.* 2009).

In addition to the adhesive disc, it has recently been reported that a 200 kDa surface protein is involved in *G. duodenalis* adhesion to epithelial cells, and is only present in adhesion efficient *G. duodenalis* clones (Hernandez-Sanchez, *et al.* 2008). Trophozoites exhibiting deficient adhesion to epithelial cells do not express this surface antigen, and fail to establish infection in orally infected Mongolian gerbils.

Trophozoites multiply rapidly in the small intestine of their host, although the growth rate has been shown to vary between different strains of *G. duodenalis* (Binz *et al.* 1992). *Giardia* has long been considered to reproduce asexually by simple binary fission but there is increasing evidence from epidemiological and molecular genetic studies that *Giardia* is capable of sexual reproduction (Meloni *et al.* 1995 and reviewed in Monis *et al.* 2008; Lasek-Nesselquist *et al.* 2009). However, the frequency of recombination is not known, nor its impact on the epidemiology of giardiasis and the extensive genetic diversity that characterizes the forms of *Giardia* that infect mammals. The evolutionary advantage of genetic exchange to *Giardia* would be the capacity to respond to adversity, for example selection pressures imposed by regular exposure to antigiardial drugs or competition with co-habiting 'strains' in circumstances where the likelihood of mixed infections is common (Hopkins *et al.* 1999). As such, it may be a relatively rare event and further population genetic studies are required in foci of infection where the frequency of infection is high (Monis *et al.* 1999). The fact that available data indicates that the genetic assemblages of *Giardia* are conserved in terms of geographic location and host occurrence suggests that any recombination is not reflected at the assemblage and species level (Monis *et al.* 2008).

Strains of *G. duodenalis* have been shown to vary in their pH requirements, nutritional requirements and site localization in the small intestine (Binz *et al.* 1992; McInnes 1994; Thompson and Lymbery 1996). *Giardia* is an aerotolerant anaerobe that utilizes amino-acids and glucose as energy sources (Paget *et al.* 1998). Its metabolism is typically fermentative with ATP biosynthesis being supplemented with the presence of the arginine dihydrolase pathway (Minotto *et al.* 1999). *Giardia* also has limited synthetic capacity and is dependent on salvage pathways for many groups such as lipids, purines and pyrimidines. It is still not understood whether amino acid substrates are more important than glucose as basic energy requirements for *Giardia* (reviewed in Schofield and Edwards 1994) but in this respect it is interesting that evidence has shown that some strains of *G. duodenalis* are more reliant on glucose for metabolism than others (Hall *et al.* 1992).

Immunity to *Giardia* involves both innate and adaptive immune responses. However, relatively little is known about how the host specifically responds to the presence of *Giardia* and how the parasite survives host resistance mechanisms. Specifically induced secretory IgA appears to be involved in the clearance of infections, and thymus-dependent T lymphocytes appear to be important components of host immunity (Singer and Nash 2000; Langford *et al.* 2002). Cellular immunity, in the absence of antibodies, can also control infection in experimental murine models (Roxstrom-Lindquist *et al.* 2006). However, the fact that symptomatic giardiasis is more likely to occur in patients who are immunocompromised, malnourished, or very young is a clear indication that host factors are important. In other cases, there is increasing evidence that a particular strain, or isolate, of *Giardia* may have a greater potential to cause disease in a particular host. The nature and competence of immune mechanisms are likely to be central in both cases. The biological relevance of antigenic variation is uncertain (Hopkins *et al.* 1993), although a protective function seems likely (Nash *et al.* 1991; Nash 1994; Singer and Kamda 2009). In addition, it has also been suggested that *Giardia* might actively downregulate the inflammatory response (Roxstrom-Lindquist *et al.* 2005), resulting in the minimal inflammation seen histologically during infection (Oberhuber *et al.* 1997).

During the course of infection, trophozoites will encyst in the posterior small intestine. The trigger for trophozoites to encyst is not completely understood but appears to be initiated by the presence of bile salts and an interaction with cholesterol (Lauwaet and Gillin 2009; Sener *et al.* 2009). It is not clear whether all cysts are immediately infective when passed since there is evidence that some undergo a maturation period of up to seven days before becoming infective (Grant and Woo 1978; Bingham *et al.* 1979). Cysts are resistant and can survive for at least two months in suitable temperature and moisture conditions (Meyer and Jarroll 1980). Clearly, encystation is a major virulence factor as differentiation into a form that can survive in the environment and infect a new host is vital for transmission and disease progression.

Excystation follows ingestion and takes place shortly after cysts leave the stomach. The low pH of the stomach environment appears to be the major factor which initiates the excystation process (Bingham and Meyer 1979; Boucher and Gillin 1990; Lauwaet and Gillin 2009). Excystation leads to rapid colonization of the small intestine and subsequent cyst production commencing after approximatley 4–15 days. Trophozoites may also intermittently be passed in the faeces, particularly during acute infection, and could be a source of infection, especially in situations where direct transmission between individuals is likely to occur.

The hosts

Incubation/prepatent period

The first appearance of any overt symptoms usually coincides with the onset of cyst excretion. This incubation period may be short in both humans and other animals, commencing as early as three days post infection but can range up to six weeks (Rendtorff 1954; Hopkins and Juranek 1991; Lederberg *et al.* 1992; Flanagan 1992; Thompson *et al.* 2007). As few as 25 cysts appear to be required to initiate an infection (Rendtorff 1954; De Carneri *et al.* 1977). The duration of infection may vary from a few days to several months, and cyst excretion is characteristically intermittent in both humans and other animal species.

Clinical impact

Humans

The clinical signs associated with *Giardia* infections in humans vary greatly (Smith 1985; Farthing 1994; Wolfe 1990; Flanagan 1992; Thompson *et al.* 1993; Eckman 2003; Troeger *et al.* 2007; Table 45.3). There may be total latency, acute short-lasting diarrhoea or chronic syndromes associated with nutritional disorders, malabsorption, weight loss and failure to thrive.

In the majority of untreated patients, infection resolves spontaneously and symptoms usually disappear in a few weeks (Moore *et al.* 1969; Brodsky *et al.* 1974; Wolfe 1990). Occasionally, symptoms may persist for reasons that are not entirely clear (Nash *et al.* 1987; Flanagan 1992) and certain patients, such as those with hypogammaglobulinaemia, are at increased risk of chronic clinical giardiasis associated with malabsorption syndromes (Ament *et al.* 1973; Perlmutter *et al.* 1985). The pronounced variability in symptomatology that is so characteristic of *Giardia* infections is the result of a myriad of factors including host immune and nutritional status, concurrent enteric infections (e.g. with *Blastocystis*, *Hymenolepis nana*, GI nematodes) and heterogeneity in infectivity, virulence and pathogenicity of strains of *G. duodenalis* (Buret 2007; Thompson 2009a,b).

Children appear to be at most risk of contracting clinical giardiasis, particularly those from developing countries and from disadvantaged groups such as Australian Aborigines (Gracey 1983, 1994; Meloni *et al.* 1988, 1993; Islam 1990; Sawaya *et al.* 1990; Kaminsky 1991; Farthing 1994; Rabbani and Islam 1994; Hesham *et al.* 2004,

2005; Gbakima *et al.* 2007; Gonen *et al.* 2007). In such children, *Giardia* is of particular concern in the aetiology of protein calorie malnutrition, the retardation of growth and development, iron deficiency anaemia and poor cognitive function. Giardiasis is most common in children under 10 years of age (Dupont and Sullivan 1986; Speelman and Ljungstrom 1986; Meloni *et al.* 1993; Thompson, 2008). Severe forms of the disease affecting growth appear to occur most frequently in the second year of life (Farthing *et al.* 1986; Hesham *et al.* 2005). It has also been proposed that children infected with *Giardia* may be exposed to greater amounts of intestinally absorbed antigens leading to allergic disease (Di Prisco *et al.* 1993; Buret 2009).

In developed countries, high risk groups also include children in day care centres, pre-school children and inmates of nursing homes and, in these situations, levels of infection are often close to those found in developing countries (Thompson 2000, 2008; Eckmann 2003). A rising incidence in such settings has led to the designation of giardiasis as a re-emerging infectious disease in the developed world (Thompson 2000; Eckmann 2003). *Giardia* is responsible for a significant number of outbreaks of diarrhoea in day care centres, where *Giardia* infection is often identified as an epidemic either alone or in association with other intestinal pathogens (reviewed in Thompson 2000). The major factors involved in epidemics in these institutions are presence of young non-toilet-trained children, contamination of hands, communal classroom objects and lack of infection control measures (Sullivan *et al.* 1984; Thompson 2000). A proportion of each group is asymptomatic and can act as carriers of infection to relatives and the community (Pickering *et al.* 1981; Bartlett *et al.* 1985a, b; Read *et al.* 2002), together with transmission by affected children (Polis *et al.* 1986). The public health problem of transmission to the community from these centres is a significant one and needs further evaluation and control through infection control measures and education. *Giardia* is also a common cause of 'travellers' diarrhoea' and is often associated with episodes of diarrhoea contracted by tourists.

As summarized in Table 45.2, humans may be infected with different assemblages/species and strains of *Giardia* (Monis and Thompson 2003; Caccio *et al.* 2005). There is growing evidence of phenotypic differences between these two assemblages (*G. duodenalis*, *G. enterica*) including duration of infection, drug sensitivity and virulence (Thompson and Monis 2004; Monis *et al.* 2008). Of most significance are studies showing differences between assemblages and the occurrence of overt symptoms, principally diarrhoea (Read *et al.* 2002; Monis *et al.* 2008). It is considered that diarrhoea is an expression of acute infection whereas infections with no sign of diarrhoea may be associated with the development of more insidious, chronic disorders including failure to thrive. However, more controlled studies are required which also determine the sub-genotypes present since there is evidence of phenotypic variability at the sub-genotype level.

Other animals

Little attention has been given to the clinical effects of giardiasis in animals other than humans. *Giardia* is common in dogs and cats, yet is rarely associated with overt symptoms or clinical disease (Simpson *et al.* 1988; Stevenson and Hughes 1988; Robertson *et al.* 2000; Thompson 1992; Thompson and Robertson 2003; Thompson *et al.* 2008). However, it appears likely that *Giardia* infection is probably an underestimated cause of mal-absorption and diarrhoea

Table 45.3 Symptoms and signs of *Giardia* infection

Asymptomatic and/or latent
Acute or chronic:
• Nausea,
• Headache,
• Bloating,
• Anorexia,
• Cramps,
• Fever,
• Diarrhoea,
• Constipation,
• Weight loss,
• Flatulence,
• Vomiting,
• Heartburn,
• Abdominal pain,
• Fatigue/lethargy,
• Foul-smelling stool,
• Mucus in stool,
• Malabsorption syndromes,
• Protein-calorie malnutrition,
• Failure to thrive.

in many species of immature mammals (Kirkpatrick 1989). In dogs and cats, when clinical giardiasis has been reported, albeit rarely, it is usually associated with kennel or cattery situations and young animals are more likely to show symptoms of *Giardia* infection (Thompson 1992) where the effects of overcrowding, weaning and nutritional deficiencies may cause stress and exacerbate the effects of an infection. Adult dogs are usually asymptomatic carriers of *Giardia* (Barr *et al.* 1993). Overt clinical signs are rare in domestic livestock and *Giardia* infection is often asymptomatic. However, infection may be associated with the occurrence of diarrhoea, ill thrift and production losses in ruminants (Olson *et al.* 1995; O'Handley *et al.* 1999; Geurden *et al.* 2006; Thompson *et al.* 2007).

Establishing *Giardia* as a cause of disease in animals is very difficult (Thompson 1992). Concurrent infections are often present and there is increasing evidence that the clinical impact of individual parasite species may be greater under such circumstances, and since diarrhoea is the most common symptom of giardiasis in dogs and cats, a variety of nutritional factors must also be considered. The potential role of *Giardia* as a possible cause of disease in birds was highlighted with a report of infection in sick and dying nestling straw-necked ibis (*Threskiornis spinicollis*) by Forshaw *et al.* (1992). Increasingly, *Giardia* infections are being recorded in a diversity of wildlife species from throughout the world (reviewed in Thompson *et al.* 2009a). However, most attention has been given to the role of infected wildlife species as reservoirs of human infections (see below), and there is little information available on the impact of *Giardia* on wildlife health.

Diagnosis

Diagnosis of *Giardia* by traditional microscopic methods remains a reliable indicator of infection in a clinical setting despite the intermittent nature of cyst excretion in humans and other animals (Baker *et al.* 1987; Simpson *et al.* 1988; Wolfe 1990). Consequently, at least three faecal samples taken on non-consecutive days are required for reliable determination of the presence of *Giardia* since a single sample identifies only 50–75% of positive patients (Heymans *et al.* 1987; Goka *et al.* 1990; Wolfe 1990; Adam 1991). Accurate faecal examination relies on visual identification of cysts following concentration using zinc sulphate or formol-ether which may be facilitated with the use of trichrome or iron haematoxylin stains (Baker *et al.* 1987; Zajac *et al.* 2002). Other methods such as duodenal fluid aspirate, duodenal biopsy or the Entero-Test are far more invasive and costly.

There are a number of ELISA-based methods available that detect coproantigens and these work well and are increasingly used for diagnosis in both humans and companion animals, often complemented by traditional microscopy. Indirect immunofluorescence and PCR are principally epidemiological and research tools due to cost.

Treatment

A number of antigiardial drugs are available for treatment of humans and other animals with *Giardia* infections. For infections in humans, the nitroimidazoles, metronidazole, tinidazole, and furazolidone, are most commonly used, but the benzimidazole, albendazole is increasingly the drug of choice because it offers a more palatable alternative to the nitroimidazoles, particularly for children, yet multiple doses are required (Reynoldson *et al.* 1998; Savioli *et al.* 2006). Nitazoxanide has been proposed as an alternative to the conventional nitroimidazoles but more studies are required to fully evaluate its efficacy (Wright *et al.* 2003; Savioli *et al.* 2006; Gonen *et al.* 2007). Treatment failures have been reported with all the commonly used drugs but whether this is due to resistance has yet to be convincingly demonstrated (Savioli *et al.* 2006). Variability in sensitivity between strains of *G. duodenalis* may be a limiting factor in treatment.

Metronidazole has been frequently used to treat giardiasis in dogs and cats but a number of detrimental side effects have been associated with this drug, including anorexia, vomiting and signs of central nervous system toxicity (Dow *et al.* 1989; Fitch *et al.* 1992; Caylor and Cassimatis 2001). Metronidazole has also been shown to be only 67% effective in eliminating *Giardia* from infected dogs (Zimmer and Burrington 1986). Fenbendazole and its prodrug febantel appear to be a more effective and safe alternative for treating *Giardia* infections in dogs and have broader efficacy that includes enteric nematode infections (Thompson *et al.* 2008).

No drug is currently licensed for treating giardiasis in ruminants, and the need to treat infections in ruminants where environmental contamination levels are high is questionable (Geurden *et al.* 2006; O'Handley and Olson 2006). However, a number of drugs including fenbendazole have been shown to be efficacious against *Giardia* infections in calves (O'Handley and Olson 2006).

Epidemiology

Occurrence

Humans

Giardia is ubiquitous and is the most common pathogenic intestinal parasite of humans worldwide. *Giardia* is today well recognized as one of the most prevalent intestinal infections of humans in both temperate and tropical areas, with prevalence rates varying between 2–7% in Europe, USA, Canada and Australia (Schantz 1991; Eckert 1993; Thompson *et al.* 1993; Farthing 1994; Acha and Szyfres 2003; Eckmann 2003; Thompson 2000, 2009a), to over 40% in developing areas where living conditions are poor, nutritional levels are often inadequate and concurrent infections are common (Chunge *et al.* 1991; Torres *et al.* 1991; Meloni *et al.* 1993; Thompson *et al.* 1993; Farthing 1994; Hesham *et al.* 2004, 2005; Savioli *et al.* 2006; Thompson 2008). In developed countries, infections with *Giardia* are most common in children, especially in day care centres, and travellers. A rising incidence in such settings has led to the designation of giardiasis as a re-emerging infectious disease in the developed world (Thompson 2000, 2004; Eckmann 2003; Thompson and Monis 2004), and in September 2004, *Giardia* was included in WHO's 'Neglected Diseases Initiative' (Savioli *et al.* 2006).

In developing countries, particularly in Asia, Africa and Latin America, about 200 million people have symptomatic *Giardia* infections with some 500 000 new cases reported each year (WHO, 1996; Savioli *et al.* 2006). Children living in communities are most commonly infected in developing countries and among disadvantaged groups living in isolated communities such as Australian Aborigines (Thompson 2000; Thompson *et al.* 2001; Hesham *et al.* 2005; Savioli *et al.* 2006). These children are most at risk from the chronic consequences of *Giardia* infection, as well as the repeated exposure to potentially toxic drugs in some endemic regions (Thompson *et al.* 2001).

Infection varies inversely with socio-economic status and is high in regions where water supplies are poor or non-existent and sanitation and hygiene standards are inadequate (Knight 1980; Islam 1990; Anon. 1993; Meloni *et al.* 1993; Savioli *et al.* 2006). Risk factors identified as important in facilitating emergence of *Giardia* infection include high environmental faecal contamination, lack of potable water, inadequate education and housing, overcrowding and high population density, and animal reservoirs of infection.

Other animals

Giardia is the most common enteric parasite of domestic animals, including dogs, cats and livestock (Thompson 2004; Thompson and Monis 2004).

The prevalence of *Giardia* infection in dogs and cats tend to vary considerably between studies, and is often influenced by the sensitivity of the diagnostic test utilized and whether or not only a one-off faecal sample was examined, given the intermittent nature of cyst excretion. Surveys of a variety of canine populations reveal prevalences of between 10% in well cared for dogs, 36–50% in puppies and up to 100% in breeding establishments and kennels (Hahn *et al.* 1988; Kirkpatrick 1988; Leonhard *et al.* 2007).

In livestock, *Giardia* infections have been reported in cattle, sheep and cervids and most likely infects all ruminants (O'Handley and Olson 2006; Thompson *et al.* 2007). Although all ruminants are likely to be exposed to *Giardia* shortly after birth, infections are most common toward the end of the neonatal period, and in calves can be as high as 100% (O'Handley and Olson 2006; Thompson *et al.* 2007).

Sources

The sources of infection include other infected individuals and infected animals. Environmental sources are also very important and, in particular, water in certain geographical areas (Thompson 2004). Food-borne outbreaks have also been reported (Smith *et al.* 2007). Investigations of outbreaks of giardiasis and transmission patterns have been made difficult in the past by the genetic heterogeneity of *G. duodenalis* isolates and the lack of appropriate molecular markers to 'type' *Giardia* cysts and trophozoites. However, the advent of direct and retrospective molecular epidemiological studies have contributed to a much better understanding of the transmission patterns of *Giardia* (Monis and Thompson 2003; Hunter and Thompson 2005; Smith *et al.* 2006; see below).

Transmission

Faecal-oral transmission

Transmission of *Giardia* is predominantly by faecal-oral contamination and levels of infection are therefore highest under conditions of poor hygiene and sanitation, particularly in tropical and subtropical environments. Most authorities consider that direct person to person transmission is more important in this respect than water-borne, food-borne or zoonotic transmission (Pawlowski *et al.* 1987; Schantz 1991; Thompson 2004; Hunter and Thompson 2005). Other predisposing factors which may enhance the frequency of faecal-oral transmission include day care centres where conditions conducive to faecal-oral contamination are common and high prevalence rates of *Giardia* infection have often been observed (see above). Direct transmission between homosexual men is also recognized as significant in the epidemiology of *Giardia* infections (Phillips *et al.* 1981).

Water-borne transmission

Numerous cases of *Giardia* infection have been associated with contaminated water and giardiasis is the most frequently diagnosed water-borne disease in developed countries (Levine *et al.* 1990; Thompson 2004; Smith *et al.* 2006). Waterborne transmission is also a well documented cause of *Giardia* infection in travellers who usually contract infection from drinking local tap water (Hunter and Thompson 2005). Investigations of endemic water-borne giardiasis in the USA have usually found contamination of the water supply to have resulted from inadequate water treatment, ineffective filtration, or contamination with human sewage (Craun 1986, 1990; Schantz 1991; Thompson 2004). Filtration is necessary to remove *Giardia* as chlorination alone is insufficient without high concentrations of chlorine and long contact times.

The fact that human infections with *Giardia* have been traced to the consumption of water from streams in rural areas well away from urban environments has implicated a number of species of wild animals, particularly beavers and muskrats, as reservoirs of infection (Davies and Hibler 1979; Pacha *et al.* 1987; Craun 1990; Marino *et al.* 1992; Monis and Thompson 2003; Thompson 2004). However, the role of animals in waterborne transmission is controversial (Erlandsen 1994; Thompson and Boreham 1994; Wallis 1994; Thompson *et al.* 1990, 2009; Thompson 2004; Hunter and Thompson 2005). Available evidence has shown that animals usually do not serve as the original source of contamination but amplify the numbers of the originally contaminating isolate (Bemrick and Erlandsen 1988; Thompson 2004).

At the present time, it appears that zoonotic transmission does not impact significantly on the aetiology of waterborne outbreaks of *Giardia* infection (see below). To date, *Giardia* of human origin appears to be the main source of water contamination and as such may impact negatively on ecosystem health leading to infections in aquatic wildlife. Recent studies have demonstrated that filter-feeding molluscs are useful indicators of the presence of waterborne pathogens. Genotypic characterization has been utilized in a study that isolated *Giardia* cysts from clams in an estuary in North America (Graczyk *et al.* 1999). All isolates were identified as belonging to genotype assemblage A (*G. duodenalis*), highlighting contamination with faeces of mammalian origin, most probably human, that contained *G. duodenalis* cysts of public health importance. Such filter-feeding molluscan shellfish can concentrate water-borne pathogens and thus in combination with appropriate genotyping procedures can serve as biological indicators of contamination with *Giardia* cysts and can thus be used for sanitary assessment of water quality.

Food-borne transmission

Food-borne transmission, usually as a result of contamination during food preparation, is also a well recognized source of *Giardia* infection (Barnard and Jackson 1984; Petersen *et al.* 1988; Mintz *et al.* 1993; Smith *et al.* 2007). Foods associated with cyst contamination have included canned salmon, salads, sandwiches, raw vegetables and ice (Smith *et al.* 2007). The reason there are fewer reported outbreaks of *Giardia* infection involving contaminated foods is likely due to the lack of appropriate tools, or their application, in the past, the sporadic nature of such outbreaks and lack of consideration of food as a vehicle in areas of poor hygiene.

Zoonotic transmission

The significance and interpretation of the results obtained from experimental infections of animals with human isolates of *Giardia* have been controversial (reviewed by Thompson *et al.* 1990; Thompson and Monis 2004). However, with the advent of molecular epidemiological studies there is sufficient evidence to show that at least some isolates of *Giardia* are not host-specific and that humans and a variety of other animals naturally share the parasite. Therefore, as mentioned above, most authorities regard *Giardia* as a zoonotic pathogen although humans are likely to be the main reservoir of human *Giardia* infection with animals constituting an additional source of infection.

Numerous studies, primarily in developed countries, have demonstrated the occurrence of zoonotic *Giardia* assemblages in different host species highlighting the potential public health risk from domestic dogs, cats, livestock and wildlife (see below). Such data is indicative of zoonotic potential. However, data on the frequency of infection is lacking. A few molecular epidemiological studies have been undertaken in defined endemic areas which support the dog as a reservoir of human infections but this is not the case to date with livestock and wildlife as detailed below. In developing countries, studies have highlighted the key role of sanitation and personal hygiene as the major risk factor suggesting that zoonotic transmission plays at most only a minor contributing role (Hunter and Thompson 2005).

Studies of the prevalence of *Giardia* in a variety of mammals and birds (see above) underlie the fact that a potential reservoir of human infection exists. Thus treatment of *Giardia*-infected dogs and cats may be advocated, whether or not they are clinically ill, because of the potential zoonotic risk (Thompson *et al.* 2007). If both family members and their pets are found to be infected with *Giardia*, for example as reported from Canada (Cribb and Spracklin 1986), or zoo handlers and their charges (Armstrong *et al.* 1979), this must be strong circumstantial evidence of zoonotic transmission although the converse of *Giardia* infection in pets but not in their owners (Asano *et al.* 1991; Arashima *et al.* 1992; Pospisilova and Svobadova 1992) is not necessarily an indicator that humans are not susceptible to *Giardia* from their companion animals.

Livestock

Although there is clearly a definite potential for giardial contamination of ground and surface waters from livestock operations, there is no evidence that cattle represent a significant public health risk (Thompson 2004; Olson *et al.* 2004). Cattle are susceptible to infection with zoonotic genotypes of *Giardia* and it has been shown that calves infected with *Giardia* commonly shed from 10^5 to 10^6 cysts per gram of faeces (Xiao 1994; Olson *et al.* 2004; O'Handley *et al.* 1999). Thus, even a few calves infected with genotypes in assemblage A (*G. duodenalis*) could pose a significant public health risk directly to handlers or indirectly as an important reservoir for human water-borne outbreaks of giardiasis. This is of potential public health significance and may put producers, and other members of the community at risk. However, molecular epidemiological studies in several countries have shown that cattle are most commonly infected with the non-zoonotic livestock assemblage E (*G. bovis*), and although the zoonotic genotype assemblage A (*G. duodenalis*) has been reported, studies in Australia suggest that zoonotic genotypes may only be present transiently in cattle under conditions where the frequency of transmission with *G. bovis* is high and competition is thus likely to occur (Becher *et al.* 2004; Thompson 2004). In contrast, a molecular epidemiological study in Uganda where humans appear to have introduced *Giardia* into a remote

national park are also thought to have been the source of *Giardia* in a small number of cohabiting dairy cattle (Graczyk *et al.* 2002).

Dogs and cats

Numerous studies in different parts of the world have demonstrated that dogs and cats may be infected with either, or both, zoonotic and host-specific genotypes of *Giardia* (Thompson *et al.* 2007). Although these studies on the occurrence of the different genotypes of *Giardia* serve to emphasize the potential public health risk from domestic dogs and cats, data on the frequency of zoonotic transmission is lacking (Thompson 2004; Leonhard *et al.* 2007). Molecular epidemiological studies in localized endemic foci of transmission have provided evidence in support of the role of dogs in cycles of zoonotic *Giardia* transmission involving humans and domestic dogs from communities in tea growing areas of Assam, India, temple communities in Bangkok, Thailand and northern Canadian aboriginal communities (Traub *et al.* 2004; Inpankaew *et al.* 2007; Salb *et al.* 2008). In all three studies, some dogs and their owners sharing the same living area were shown to harbour isolates of *G. duodenalia* from the same assemblage. Other studies in Europe, Australia and North America have shown that zoonotic genotypes of *Giardia* may occur frequently in individual pet dogs living in urban areas (review in Leonhard *et al.* 2007; Covacin *et al.* 2010).

Some authors consider that birds may be a source of zoonotic contamination of open water with *Giardia* (Bemrick 1984). *Giardia* in a blue heron was suggested as a possible source of water-borne giardiasis in humans, but not confirmed (Georgi *et al.* 1986), although the species of *Giardia* involved was not determined. Cross infection experiments with the avian species *G. psittaci* and *G. ardeae* were taken to indicate that birds should not be considered as likely potential reservoirs of infection for mammalian hosts (Erlandsen *et al.* 1991), at least in the USA. The zoonotic significance of avian outbreaks in Australia (Forshaw *et al.* 1992) is not known but the isolates which have been characterized are quite distinct to those affecting humans (McRoberts *et al.* 1996). In addition to avian infections, aquatic birds have been shown to represent an important source of environmental contamination with *Giardia* as mechanical vehicles for cysts of zoonotic species of the parasite (Majewska *et al.* 2009).

Wildlife

The occurrence of *Giardia* in wildlife, particularly of isolates that are morphologically and/or genetically identical to *G. duodenalis*, has been the single most important factor incriminating *Giardia* as a zoonotic agent. As such, it was the association between infected animals such as beavers and water-borne outbreaks in people that led the WHO (Anon. 1979) to classify *Giardia* as a zoonotic parasite. It is therefore surprising that there is so little evidence to support the role of wildlife as a source of disease in humans, since this has dominated debate on the zoonotic transmission of *Giardia*, and in particular when water is the vehicle for such transmission (Thompson 2004; Kutz *et al.* 2009; Thompson *et al.* 2009a). Although wildlife, particularly aquatic mammals, are commonly infected with *Giardia* there is little evidence to implicate such infections as the original contaminating source in waterborne outbreaks (Thompson 2004; Appelbee *et al.* 2005). It would appear that such animals are more likely to have become infected through environmental contamination of human origin (reverse zoonoses), or less likely, domestic animal origin (Thompson *et al.* 2009a; 2010).

This has been demonstrated in presumed pristine and/or isolated environments involving wildlife species such as beavers and coyotes in North America, primates in Africa, muskoxen in the Arctic, house mice on remote islands, marsupials in Australia and marine cetaceans in various parts of the world (Graczyk *et al.* 2002; Sulaiman *et al.* 2003; Moro *et al.* 2003; Appelbee *et al.* 2005; Kutz *et al.* 2008; Dixon *et al.* 2008; Teichroeb *et al.* 2009 Thompson *et al.* 2009b, 2010). In all these cases, epidemiological evidence supports humans as the source of infection through environmental contamination, either directly or indirectly via domestic animal hosts. Some wildlife, particularly aquatic species, will thus serve to amplify the numbers of the original contaminating isolate (Monzingo and Hibbler 1987; Bemrick and Erlandsen 1988; Thompson 2004; Appelbee *et al.* 2005; Thompson *et al.* 2009a). For example, the one study that did genotype *Giardia* of beaver origin, confirmed previous suggestions that the source of *Giardia* infection in beavers was likely to be of human origin (Monzingo and Hibbler 1987; Rickard *et al.* 1999; Dixon *et al.* 2002). In this study, 12 of 113 (10.6%) beaver faecal samples from 6 of 14 different riverbank sites in southern Alberta, Canada, were positive for *Giardia*, and all those genotyped belonged to the zoonotic genotype, assemblage A (*G. duodenalis*) (Appelbee *et al.* 2002, 2005).

G. muris, *G. simondi* and *G. microti*, which are all genetically distinct, have been described from mice, rats and microtine rodents respectively (review in Thompson and Monis 2004), but there is no information on host range, prevalence of infections and geographical distribution. In all cases the hosts of these species of *Giardia* are also susceptible to zoonotic genotypes. More recently, a novel genotype of *Giardia* was described in an Australian marsupial, a bandicoot known as the quenda (*Isoodon obesulus*), and on the basis of genetic characteristics would appear to represent a distinct species that may be endemic within Australian native fauna (Adams *et al.* 2004; Thompson *et al.* 2010).

Prevention and control

With the widespread distribution of numerous species of potential animal reservoirs of infection and the fact that *Giardia* may survive for extended periods outside the host as resistant cysts in the environment, the possibility of human infection is unlikely to be eliminated. Several cases of families with affected pets and symptomless carrier relatives have been reported and highlight the need to undertake therapy in these situations in order to prevent repeated infections (Thompson *et al.* 2007). In contrast, the value of treatment in some hyperendemic communities is questionable since treatment is soon followed by re-infection (Sullivan *et al.* 1991; Thompson *et al.* 2001; Thompson 2008) and perhaps should only be considered when clinically indicated (Gilman *et al.* 1988). In many developing countries, the prevailing socioeconomic conditions make it difficult to prevent infection, especially in children (Thompson *et al.* 2001; Acha and Szyfres 2003; Hesham *et al.* 2005; Savioli *et al.* 2006; Thompson 2009).

The control of endemic gastrointestinal parasitic infections, such as those caused by *Giardia*, which are primarily transmitted in conditions of poor hygiene and sanitation calls for other primary health care activities such as health promotion and education which should encompass both hygiene aspects and nutrition, and should include appropriate evaluation procedures to determine the success of such interventions (Thompson *et al.* 2001; Hesham

et al. 2005; Thompson 2008). Intestinal parasite control programmes are regarded as highly desirable since the recipients see the beneficial effects of intervention and learn basic health care facts, and sectors of the health care services become integrated (Anon. 1987; Reynoldson *et al.* 1998; Thompson 2001; Savioli *et al.* 2006). Public health measures are also clearly required to protect water supplies against contamination by human or animal faeces. Attention to personal hygiene in high risk situations such as day care centres and residential institutions should minimize person to person transmission (Farthing 1994). Tourists should not drink tap water in places where its purity cannot be guaranteed.

The costs of not having a control programme for *Giardia* infections include those related to nutrition, growth and development, work and productivity, and medical care (Anon. 1987; Thompson 2001; Savioli *et al.* 2006). Strategies used to control giardiasis are usually based on epidemiology providing basic information on transmission, the reduction of incidence rates with control of transmission and health education, and a reduction in number of infections through therapy (Anon. 1987; Savioli *et al.* 2006).

Control measures to counter the high infection rates with *Giardia* in developing regions include those listed in Table 45.4 (Anon. 1987; Boreham 1987; Rabbani and Islam 1994; Thompson 2001; Thompson *et al.* 2001; Hesham *et al.* 2005). Practical approaches are mainly centred on sanitation control and education about indiscriminate defaecation and on personal hygiene concerning the handling of domestic animals (Anon. 1987; Savioli *et al.* 2006). The central role of health education in prevention and control programmes should be adapted for each target community with education as a primary focus in each phase of a programme including

Table 45.4 Desired results and practical approaches to controlling transmission of *Giardia*

Desired result	Practical approach
Reduction of overall prevalence in community.	Health education and non-specific hygienic approach re: faecal-oral transmission, water quality, hand-washing, sanitation, food handling,
Prevention and control of epidemics.	Quality of health education, Treatment of wastes used as fertilizer, Improved personal hygiene, Improved water quality,
Prevention of water-borne transmission.	Disinfection of local water supplies, Treatment of wastes used as fertilizer, Adequate monitoring of water supplies,
Prevention of food-borne transmission.	Effective surveillance and hygiene instruction, Screening of food handlers,
Prevention of zoonotic transmission.	Identify potential reservoir hosts, Education of pet owners and farm workers, Education of campers etc re: potential contamination of water from wildlife, Treatment of infected pets,
Reduced morbidity.	Individual chemotherapeutic treatment, Improved nutrition
Elimination of reservoirs of *Giardia* infection.	Treatment of people (e.g. in daycare, institutional settings), pets and livestock with infection who are asymptomatic cyst passers.

preparation, implementation and follow-up involving all sectors of the community and health workers (Anon. 1987; Halloran *et al.* 1989; Rabbani and Islam 1994; Hesham *et al.* 2005; Thompson *et al.* 2001; Thompson 2008).

References

Acha, P.N. and Szyfres, B. (2003). *Zoonoses and communicable diseases common to man and animals. Volume III. Parasitoses.* Scientific and Technical Publication No. 580. Washington: Pan American Health Organization.

Adam, R.D. (1991). The biology of *Giardia* spp. *Microbiol. Rev.*, **55**: 706–32.

Adams, P.J., Monis, P.T., Elliot, A.D., and Thompson, R.C.A. (2004). Cyst morphology and sequence analysis of the small subunit rDNA and *ef1_* identifies a novel *Giardia* genotype in a quenda (*Isoodon obesulus*) from Western Australia. *Infect. Genet. Evol.*, **4**: 365–70.

Ament, M.E., Ochs, H.D. and Davis, S.D. (1973). Structure and function of the gastrointestinal tract in primary immunodeficiency syndromes: a study of 39 patients. *Medicine*, **52**: 227–48.

Anon. (1979). *Parasitic Zoonoses.* Report of a WHO Expert Committee with the participation of FAO. Technical Report Series No. 637. Geneva: World Health Organization.

Anon. (1987). *Report of a WHO Expert Committee: Prevention and control of intestinal parasitic infections.* Technical Report Series No. 749. Geneva: World Health Organization.

Anon. (1993). Intestinal parasitic infections. *Wkly. Epidemiol. Rec.*, **7**: 43–44.

Anon. (1996). *The World Health Report 1996. Fighting Disease Fostering Development.* Geneva: World Health Organization.

Appelbee, A., Thorlakson, C. and Olson, M.E. (2002). Genotypic characterization of *Giardia* cysts isolated from wild beaver in southern Alberta, Canada. In: B.E. Olson, M.E. Olson and P.M. Wallis (eds.), Giardia: *The cosmopolitan parasite*, pp. 299–300. Wallingford: CAB International.

Appelbee, A.J., Thompson, R.C.A. and Olson, M.E. (2005). *Giardia* and *Cryptosporidium* in mammalian wildlife current status and future needs. *Trends Parasitol.*, **21**: 370–76.

Arashima, Y., Kumasaka, K., Kawano, K. *et al.* (1992). Studies on the giardiasis as the zoonosis. III. Prevalence of *Giardia* among the dogs and the owners in Japan. *Kansensh. Sasshi*, **66**: 1062–66. (In Japanese).

Armstrong, J., Hertzog, R.E., Hall, R.T. and Hoff, G.L. (1979). Giardiasis in apes and zoo attendants, Kansas City, Missouri. *CDC Vet. Pub. Health Notes*, January 1979.

Baker, G., Donald, B.S., Strombeck, D.R. and Gershwin, L.J. (1987). Laboratory diagnosis of *Giardia duodenalis* infection in dogs. *J. Am. Vet. Med. Ass.*, **190**: 53–56.

Barnard, R.J. and Jackson, G.J. (1984). *Giardia lamblia.* The transfer of human infections by food. In: S.L. Erlandsen and E.A. Meyer (eds.) *Giardia and giardiasis*, pp. 365–78. New York: Plenum Press.

Barr, S.C., Bowman, D.D., Heller, R.L. and Erb, H.N. (1993). Efficacy of albendazole against giardiasis in dogs. *Am. J. Vet. Res.*, **54**: 926–28.

Bartlett, A.V., Moore, M., Gary, G.W.S., Starko, K.M., *et al.* (1985a). Diarrheal illness among infants and toddlers in day care centers. I. Epidemiology and pathogens. *J. Pediat.*, **107**: 495–502.

Bartlett, A.V., Moore, M., Gary, G.W., Starko, K.M., *et al.* (1985b). Diarrheal illness among infants and toddlers in day care centers. II. Comparison with day care homes and households. *J. Pediat.*, **107**: 503–9.

Becher, K.A., Robertson, I.D., Fraser, D.M., *et al.* (2004). Molecular epidemiology of *Giardia* and *Cryptosporidium* infections in dairy calves originating from three sources in Western Australia. *Vet. Parasitol.*, **123**: 1–9.

Bemrick, W.J. (1984). Some perspectives on the transmission of giardiasis. In: S.L. Erlandsen and E.A. Meyer (eds.) *Giardia and giardiasis.* pp. 379–400. New York: Plenum Press.

Bemrick, W.J. and Erlandsen, S.L. (1988). Giardiasis - is it really a zoonosis? *Parasitol. Today*, **4**: 69–71.

Bingham, A.K. and Meyer, E.A. (1979). *Giardia* excystation can be induced *in vitro* in acidic solutions. *Nature*, **277**: 301–2.

Bingham, A.K., Jarroll, E.L., Meyer, E.A. and Radulescu, S. (1979). *Giardia* sp.: physical factors of excystation *in vitro*, and excystation *vs* eosin exclusion as determinants of viability. *Exp. Parasitol.*, **47**: 284–91.

Binz, N., Thompson, R.C.A., Lymbery, A.J. and Hobbs, R.P. (1992). Comparative studies on the growth dynamics of two genetically distinct isolates of *Giardia duodenalis in vitro. Int. J. Parasitol.*, **22**: 195–202.

Boreham, P.F.L. (1987). Transmission of *Giardia* by food and water. *Food Techn. Aust.*, **39**: 61–63.

Boucher, S.E.M. and Gillin, F.D. (1990). Excystation of *in vitro*-derived *Giardia lamblia* cysts. *Infect. Immun.*, **58**: 3516–22.

Brodsky, R.E., Spencer Jr., H.D., and Schultz, M.G. (1974). Giardiasis in American travelers to the Soviet Union. *J. Infect. Dis.*, **130**: 319–23.

Buret, A. (1994). Pathogenesis - how does *Giardia* cause disease? In: R.C.A. Thompson, J.A. Reynoldson and A.J. Lymbery (eds.) *Giardia: from molecules to disease*, pp. 293–315. Wallingford: CAB International.

Buret, A.G. (2007). Mechanisms of epithelial dysfunction in giardiasis. *Gut*, **56**: 328–35.

Buret, A.G. (2009). Pathogenic mechanisms in giardiasis and cryptosporidiosis. In: G. Ortega-Pierres, S.M. Caccio, R. Fayer, *et al.* (eds.) Giardia *and* Cryptosporidium: from molecules to disease, pp. 428–41. Wallingford: CAB International.

Caccio, S.M., Thompson, R.C., McLauchlin, J., Smith, H.V. (2005). Unravelling *Cryptosporidium* and *Giardia* epidemiology. *Trends Parasitol.*, **21**: 430–37.

Caylor, K.B., Cassimatis, M.K. (2001). Metronidazole neurotoxicosis in two cats. *J. Am. Anim. Hosp. Ass.*, **37**: 258–62.

Chai, J.Y., Guk, S.M., Han, H.K. and Yun, C.K. (1999). Role of intra-epithelial lymphocytes in mucosal immune responses of mice experimentally infected with *C. parvum. J. Parasitol.*, **85**: 234–39.

Chin, A.C., Teoh, D.A., Scott, K.G., Meddings, J.B., *et al.* (2002). Strain-dependent induction of enterocyte apoptosis by *Giardia lamblia* disrupts epithelial barrier function in a caspase-3-dependent manner. *Infect. Immun.*, **70**: 3673–80.

Chunge, R.N., Nagelkerke, N., Karumba, P.N. *et al.* (1991). Longitudinal study of young children in Kenya: intestinal parasitic infection with special reference to *Giardia lamblia*, its prevalence, incidence and duration, and its association with diarrhoea and with other parasites. *Acta Trop.*, **50**: 39–49.

Covacin, C., Aucoin, D.P., Elliot, A., and Thompson, R.C.A. (2010). Genotypic characterisation of *Giardia* from domestic dogs in the USA. *Vet. Parasit.*, (in press).

Cox, F. (1998) History of human parasitology. In: F.E.G. Cox, J.P. Kreier, and D. Wakelin (eds.) *Microbiology and Microbial Infections, Parasit.*, **5**: 3–18. London: Arnold.

Craun, G.F. (1986). Waterborne giardiasis in the United States 1965–1984. *Lancet*, **ii**: 513–14.

Craun, G.F. (1990). Waterborne giardiasis. In: E.A. Meyer (ed.) *Giardiasis*, pp. 267–93. Amsterdam: Elsevier.

Cribb, A.E. and Spracklin, D. (1986). Giardiasis in a home. *Can. Vet. J.*, **27**: 169.

Dacks, J.B., Walker, G. and Field, M.C. (2008). Implications of the new eukaryotic systematics for parasitologists. *Parasitol. Int.*, **57**: 97–104.

Davies, R.B. and Hibler, C.P. (1979). Animal reservoirs and cross-species transmission of *Giardia*. In: W. Jakubowski and J.C. Hoff (eds.) *Waterborne transmission of giardiasis*, pp. 104–26. Cincinnati: Environmental Protection Agency.

De Carneri, I., Trane, F. and Mandelli, V. (1977). *Giardia muris*: oral infection with one trophozoite and generation time in mice. *Trans. R. Soc. Trop. Med. Hyg.*, **71**: 438.

Di Prisco, M.C., Hagel, I., Lynch, N.R., Barrios, R.M., *et al.* (1993). Possible relationship between allergic disease and infection by *Giardia lamblia*. *Ann. Allergy*, **70**: 210–13.

Dixon, B.R., Bussey, J., Parrington, L., *et al.* (2002). A preliminary estimate of the prevalence of *Giardia* sp. beavers in Gatineau Park, Quebec, using flow cytometry. In: B.E. Olson, M.E. Olson and P.M. Wallis, (eds.), Giardia: *The cosmopolitan parasite*, pp. 71–79. Wallingford: CAB International.

Dixon, B.R., Parrington, L.J., Parenteau, M., Leclair, D., *et al.* (2008). *Giardia duodenalis* and *Cryptosporidium* spp. in the intestinal contents of ringed seals (*Phoca hispida*) and bearded seals (*Erignathus barbatus*) in Nunavik, Quebec, Canada. *J. Parasit.*, **94:** 1161–63.

Dobell, C. (1920). The discovery of the intestinal protozoa of man. *Proc. R. Soc. Med.*, **13:** 1–15.

Dow, S.W., Lecouteur, R.A., Poss, M.L., Beadleston, D. (1989). Central nervous system toxicosis associated with metronidazole treatment of dogs: five cases (1984–1987). *J. Am. Vet. Ass.*, **195:** 365–68.

Dupont, H.L. and Sullivan, P.S. (1986). Giardiasis: the clinical spectrum, diagnosis and therapy. *Pediat. Infect. Dis.*, **5:** 131–38.

Eckert, J. (1993). Carriers and excretors of protozoa. *Zentral. Hygiene Umweltmed.*, **194:** 173–85.

Eckmann, L. (2003). Mucosal defences against *Giardia*. *Parasite Immunol.*, **25:** 259–70.

Edlind, T.D., Hang, T.L. and Chakraborty, P.R. (1990). Activity of anthelmintic benzimidazoles against *Giardia lamblia in vitro*. *J. Infect. Dis.*, **162:** 1408–11.

Erlandsen, S.L. (1994). Biotic transmission - is giardiasis a zoonoses? In: R.C.A. Thompson, J.A. Reynoldson and A.J. Lymbery (eds.) *Giardia: from molecules to disease*, pp. 83–97. Wallingford: CAB International.

Erlandsen, S.L., Bemrick, W.J. and Jakubowski, W. (1991). Cross-species transmission of avian and mammalian *Giardia* spp.: inoculation of chicks, ducklings, budgerigars, mongolian gerbils and neonatal mice with *Giardia ardeae*, *Giardia duodenalis* (*lamblia*), *Giardia psittaci* and *Giardia muris*. *Int. J. Environ. Health Res.*, **1:** 144–52.

Farthing, M.J.G. (1994). Giardiasis as a disease. In R.C.A. Thompson, J.A. Reynoldson and A.J. Lymbery (eds.) *Giardia: from molecules to disease*, pp. 15–37. Wallingford: CAB International.

Farthing, M., Mata, L., Urrutia, J. and Kronmal, R. (1986). Natural history of *Giardia* infection of infants and children in rural Guatemala and its impact on physical growth. *Am. J. Clin. Nutrit.*, **43:** 395–405.

Filice, F.P. (1952). Studies on the cytology and life history of a *Giardia* from the laboratory rat. *Uni. Calif. Pub. Zoo.*, **57:** 53–146.

Fitch, R., Moore, M. and Roen, D. (1992). A warning to clinicians: Metronidazole neurotoxicity in a dog. *Prog. Vet. Neurol.*, **2:** 307–09.

Flanagan, P.A. (1992). *Giardia* - diagnosis, clinical course and epidemiology. *A review. Epidem. Infect.*, **109:** 1–22.

Forshaw, D., Palmer, D.G., Halse, S.A., *et al.* (1992). *Giardia* infection in straw necked ibis (*Threskiornis spinicollis*). *Vet. Rec.*, **131:** 267–68.

Gbakima, A.A., Konteh, R., Kallon, M., *et al.* (2007). Intestinal protozoa and intestinal helminthic infections in displacement camps in Sierra Leone. *Afri. J. Med. Sci.*, **36:** 1–9.

Georgi, M.E., Carlisle, M.S. and Smiley, L.E. (1986). Giardiasis in a great blue heron (*Ardea herodias*) in New York State: another potential source of waterborne giardiasis. *Am. J. Epidem.*, **123:** 916–17.

Geurden, T., Claerebout, E., Dursin, L., *et al.* (2006). The efficacy of an oral treatment with paromomycin against an experimental infection with *Giardia* in calves. *Vet. Parasit.*, **135:** 241–47.

Gilman, R.H., Marquis, G.S., Miranda, E., Vistegui, M., *et al.* (1988). Rapid reinfection by *Giardia lamblia* after treatment in a hyperendemic Third World community. *Lancet*, **i:** 343–45.

Goka, A.K.J., Rolston, D.D.K., Mathan, V.I. and Farthing, M.J.G. (1990). The relative merits of faecal and duodenal juice microscopy in the diagnosis of giardiasis. *Trans. R. Soc. Trop. Med. Hyg.*, **84:** 66–67.

Gonen, C., Yilmaz, N., Yalcin, M., Simsek, I., Gonen, O. (2007). Diagnostic yield of routine duodenal biopsies in iron deficiency anaemia: a study from Western Australia. *Euro. J. Gastroenter. Hepatol.*, **19:** 37–41.

Gracey, M. (1983). Enteric disease in young Australian Aborigines. *Aust. N. Zeal. J. Med.*, **3:** 576–79.

Gracey, M. (1994). The clinical significance of giardiasis in Australian Aboriginal children. In: R.C.A. Thompson, J.A. Reynoldson and A.J. Lymbery (eds.) *Giardia: from molecules to disease*, pp. 281–91. Wallingford: CAB International.

Graczyk, T.K., Thompson, R.C.A., Fayer, R., Adams, P., *et al.* (1999). *Giardia duodenalis* genotype A recovered from clams in the Chesapeake Bay subestruary, Rhode River. *Am. J. Trop. Med. Hyg.*, **61:** 526–29.

Graczyk, T.K., Bozso-Nizeyi, J.B., Ssebide, B., *et al.* (2002). Anthropozoonotic *Giardia duodenalis* genotype (assemblage) A infections in habitats of free-ranging human-habituated gorillas, Uganda. *J. Parasit.*, **88:** 905–9.

Grant, D.R. and Woo, P.T.K. (1978). Comparative studies of *Giardia* spp. in small mammals in southern Ontario. II. Host specificity and infectivity of stored cysts. *Can. J. Zoo.*, **56:** 1360–66.

Guk, S.M., Yong, T.S. and Chai, J.Y. (2003). Role of murine intestinal intraepithelial lymphocytes and *lamina propria* lymphocytes against primary and challenge infections with *C. parvum*. *J. Parasit.*, **89:** 270–75.

Hahn, N.E., Glaser, C.A., Hird, D.W. and Hirsch, D.C. (1988). Prevalence of *Giardia* in the feces of pups. *J. Am. Vet. Med. Ass.*, **192:** 1428–29.

Hall, A. (1994). *Giardia* infections: epidemiology and nutritional consequences. In R.C.A. Thompson, J.A. Reynoldson and A.J. Lymbery (eds.) *Giardia: from molecules to disease*, pp. 251–80. Wallingford: CAB International.

Hall, M.L., Costa, N.D., Thompson, R.C.A., *et al.* (1992). Genetic variants of *Giardia duodenalis* differ in their metabolism. *Parasit. Res.*, **78:** 712–14.

Halloran, M.E., Bundy, D.A.P. and Pollitt, E. (1989). Infectious disease and the Unesco basic education initiative. *Parasit. Today*, **5:** 359–62.

Hernandez-Sanchez, J. and Ortega-Pierres, M.G. (1993). Isolation of adhesion deficient *Giardia lamblia* clones with a reduced ability to establish infection in Mongolian gerbils. *J. Parasit.*, **79**(suppl.): 287.

Hernández-Sánchez, J., Linan, R.F., *et al.* (2008). *Giardia duodenalis*: adhesion-deficient clones have reduced ability to establish infection in Mongolian gerbils. *Experim. Parasit.*, **119:** 364–72.

Hesham, M.S., Edariah, A.B. and Norhavat, M. (2004). Intestinal parasitic infections and micronutrient deficiency: a review. *Med. J. Malay.*, **59:** 284–93.

Hesham, M.S., Azlin, M., Nor Aini, U.N., *et al.* (2005). Giardiasis as a predictor of childhood malnutrition in Orang Asli children in Malaysia. *Trans. R. Soc. Trop. Med. Hyg.*, **99:** 686–91.

Heymans, H.S.A., Aronson, D.C. and van Hooft, M.A.J. (1987). Giardiasis in childhoold: an unnecessarily expensive diagnosis. *Euro. J. Pediat.*, **146:** 401–3.

Hopkins, R.M., Thompson, R.C.A., Hobbs, R.P., *et al.* (1993). Differences in antigen expression within and between 10 isolates of *Giardia duodenalis*. *Acta Trop.*, **54:** 117–24.

Hopkins, R.M., Constantine, C.C., Groth, D.A., *et al.* (1999). DNA fingerprinting of *Giardia duodenalis* isolates using the intergenic rDNA spacer. *Parasitology*, **118:** 531–39.

Hopkins, R.S. and Juranek, D.D. (1991). Acute giardiasis: an improved clinical case definition for epidemiologic studies. *Am. J. Epidem.*, **133:** 402–7.

Hoskins, J.D. (1990). *Giardia*: a common invader. *Vet. Techn.*, **11:** 379–83.

Hunter, P.R. and Thompson, R.C.A. (2005). The zoonotic transmission of *Giardia* and *Cryptosporidium*. *Int. J. Parasitol.*, **35:** 1181–90.

Inpankaew, T., Traub, R., Thompson, R.C.A. and Sukthana, Y. (2007). Canine Parasitic zoonoses and temple communities in Thailand. *Southeast Asian J. Trop. Med. Pub. Health*, **38:** 247–55.

Islam, A. (1990). Giardiasis in developing countries, In: E.A. Meyer (ed.) *Giardiasis*, pp. 235–66. Amsterdam: Elsevier.

Kaminsky, R.G. (1991). Parasitism and diarrhoea in children from two rural communities and marginal barrio in Honduras. *Trans. R. Soc. Trop. Med. Hyg.*, **85:** 70–73.

Kirkpatrich, C.E. (1988). Epizootiology of enteroparasitic infections in pet dogs and cats presented to a veterinary teaching hospital. *Vet. Parasitol.*, **30:** 113–24.

Kirkpatrick, C.E. (1989). Giardiasis in large animals. *Comp. Contin. Ed. Pract. Vet.*, **11:** 80–84.

Knight, R. (1980). Epidemiology and transmission of giardiasis. *Trans. R. Soc. Trop. Med. Hyg.*, **74:** 433–36.

Kulda, J. and Nohynkova, E. (1978). Flagellates of the human intestine and of intestines of other species. In: J.P. Kreier (ed.) *Parasitic Protozoa* Vol. II, pp. 2–139. New York: Academic Press.

Kutz, S.J., Thompson, R.A., Polley, L., Kandola, K., *et al.* (2008). *Giardia* assemblage A: human genotype in muskoxen in the Canadian Arctic. *Parasit. Vectors*, **1:** 32.

Kutz, S.J., Thompson, R.C.A. and Polley, L. (2009). Wildlife with *Giardia*: villain or victim and vector? In: G. Ortega-Pierres, S. Caccio, R. Fayer, *et al.* (eds.) *Giardia and Cryptosporidium: From molecules to disease.* pp. 94–106. Wallingford: CAB International.

Lambl, W. (1859). Mikroskopische Untersuchungen der Darm-Excrete. *Vierteljaht. prakt. Heilk. (Prag)*, **61:** 1–58.

Langford, T.D., Housley M.P., Boes, M., *et al.* (2002). *Central importance of immunoglobulin A in host defense against Giardia spp. Infect. Immun.*, **70:** 11–88.

Lasek-Nesselquist, E., Welch, D.M., Thompson, R.C.A., *et al.* (2009). Genetic exchange within and between assemblages of *Giardia duodenalis*. *Journal of Eukary. Microbiol.*, **56:** 504–18.

Lauwaet, T. and Gillin, F.D. (2009). Signalling during *Giardia* differentiation. In: G. Ortega-Pierres, S.M. Caccio, R. Fayer, *et al.* (eds.) Giardia *and* Cryptosoridium: from molecules to disease, pp. 309–319. Wallingford: CAB International.

Lederberg, J., Shope, R.E. and Oaks, S.C. (eds.) (1992). *Emerging infections: microbial threats to health in the United States.* Washington: National Academy Press.

Leonhard, S., Pfister, K., Beelitz, P., Wielinga, C. and Thompson, R.C.A. (2007). The molecular characterisation of *Giardia* from dogs in Southern Germany. *Vet. Parasitol.*, **150:** 33–88.

Levine, W.C., Stephenson, W.T. and Craun, G.F. (1990). Waterborne disease outbreaks, 1986–1988. *Morb. Mort. Wkly. Rep.*, **39:** 1–13.

Magne, D., Favennec, L., Chochillon, C., *et al.* (1991). Role of cytoskeleton and surface lectins in *Giardia duodenalis* attachment to Caco2 cells. *Parasitol. Res.*, **77:** 659–66.

Majewska, A.C., Kasprzak, W. and Kaczmarek, E. (1993). Comparative morphometry of *Giardia* trophozoites from man and animals. *Acta Protosoologica*, **32:** 191–97.

Majewska, A.C., Graczyk, T.K., Słodkowicz-Kowalska, A., *et al.* (2009). The role of free-ranging, captive, and domestic birds of Western Poland in environmental contamination with *Cryptosporidium parvum* oocysts and *Giardia lamblia* cysts. *Parasitol. Res.*, **104:** 1093–99.

McInnes, L.M. (1994). *Phenotypic Characterisation of the Differential Sensitivity of Giardia Isolated to Drugs.* Honours Thesis, Western Australia: Murdoch University.

McRoberts, K.M., Meloni, B.P., Morgan, U.M., *et al.* (1996). Morphological and molecular characterisation of *Giardia* isolated from the straw-necked ibis (*Threskiornis spinicollis*) in Western Australia. *J. Parasitol.*, **82:** 711–18.

Meloni, B.P., Lymbery, A.J., Thompson, R.C.A. and Gracey, M. (1988). High prevalence of *Giardia lamblia* in children from a WA Aboriginal community. *Med. J. Aust.*, **149:** 715.

Meloni, B.P., Lymbery, A.J. and Thompson, R.C.A. (1995). Genetic characterization of isolates of *Giardia duodenalis* by enzyme electrophoresis: implications for reproductive biology, population structure, taxonomy and epidemiology. *J. Parasitol.*, **81:** 368–83.

Meloni, B.P., Thompson, R.C.A., Reynoldson, J.A. and Seville, P. (1990). Albendazole: a more effective antigiardial agent *in vitro* than metronidazole or tinidazole. *Trans. R. Soc. Trop. Med. Hyg.*, **84:** 375–79.

Meloni, B.P., Thompson, R.C.A., Hopkins, R.M., *et al.* (1993). The prevalence of *Giardia* and other intestinal parasites in children, dogs and cats from Aboriginal communities in the Kimberley. *Med. J. Aust.*, **158:** 157–59.

Meyer, E.A. and Jarroll, E.J. (1980). Giardiasis. *Am. J. Epidem.*, **111:** 1–12.

Minotto, L., Tutticci, E.A., Bagnara, A.S., Schofield, P.J. and Edwards M.R. (1999). Characterisation and expression of the carbamate kinase gene from *Giardia intestinalis*. *Mol. Bichem. Parasitol.*, **98:** 43–51.

Mintz, E.D., Hudson-Wragg, M., Mshar, P., *et al.* (1993). Foodborne giardiasis in a corporate office setting. *J. Infect. Dis.*, **167:** 250–53.

Monis, P. T. and Thompson, R.C.A. (2003). *Cryptosporidium* and *Giardia* zoonoses: fact or fiction? *Infect. Genet. Evol.*, **3:** 233–44.

Monis, P.T., Andrews, R.H., Mayrhofer, G., *et al.* (1998). Novel lineages of *Giardia intestinalis* identified by genetic analysis of organisms isolated from dogs in Australia. *Parasitology*, **116:** 7–19.

Monis, P.T., Andrews, R.H., Mayrhofer, G. and Ey, P.L. (1999). Molecular systematics of the parasitic protozoan *Giardia intestinalis*. *Mol. Biol. Evol.*, **16:** 1135–44.

Monis, P.T., Caccio, S.M. and Thompson, R.C.A. (2009). Variation in *Giardia*: towards a taxonomic revision of the genus. *Trends in Parasit.*, **25:** 93–100.

Monzingo, D.L., Jr. and Hibler, C.P. (1987). Prevalence of Giardia sp. in a beaver colony and the resulting environmental contamination. *J. Wildl. Dis.*, **23:** 576–85.

Moore, G.T., Cross, W.M., McGuire, D., *et al.* (1969). Epidemic giardiasis at a ski resort. *N. Engl. J. Med.*, **281:** 402–7.

Moro, D., Lawson, M.A., Hobbs, R.P. and Thompson, R.C.A. (2003). Pathogens of house mice on arid Boullanger Island and subantartic Macquarie Island, Australia. *J. Wildl. Dis.*, **39:** 762–71.

Nash, T.E. (1994). Imunology: the role of the parasite. In: R.C.A. Thompson, J.A. Reynoldson and A.J. Lymbery (eds.) *Giardia: from molecules to disease*, pp. 139–54. Wallingford: CAB International.

Nash, T.E., Merritt, J.W. and Conrad, J.T. (1991). Isolate and epitope variability in susceptibility of *Giardia lamblia* to intestinal proteases. *Infect. Immun.*, **59:** 1334–40.

Nash, T.E., Herrington, D.A., Losonsky, G.A. and Levine, M.M. (1987). Experimental human infections with *Giardia lamblia*. *J. Infect. Dis.*, **156:** 974–84.

Oberhuber, G., Kastner, N. and Stolte, M. (1997). Giardiasis: a histologic analysis of 567 cases. *Scan. J. Gastroent.*, **32:** 48–51.

O'Handley, R.M. and Olson, M.E. (2006). Giardiasis and cryptosporidiosis in ruminants. *Vet.Clin. N. Am. Food An. Pract.*, **22:** 623–43.

O'Handley, R.M., Cockwill, C., McAllister, T.A., Jelinski, M., *et al.* (1999). Duration of naturally acquired giardiasis and cryptosporidiosis in dairy calves and their association with diarrhea. *J. Am. Vet. Med. Ass.*, **214:** 391–96.

Olson, M.E., McAllister, T.A. and Deselliers, L. (1995). Effects of giardiasis on production in a domestic ruminant (lamb) model. *Am. J. Vet. Res.*, **56:** 1470–74.

Olson, M.E., O'Handley, R.M., Ralston, B.J., McAllister, T.A. and Thompson, R.C.A. (2004). Update on *Cryptosporidium* and *Giardia* infections in cattle. *Trends Parasitol.*, **20:** 185–91.

Ortega-Pierres, G., Smith, H.V., Caccio, S.M. and Thompson, R.C.A. (2009). New tools provide further insights into *Giardia* and *Cryptosporidium* biology. *Trends Parasitol.*, **25:** 410–16.

Pacha, R.E., Clark, G.W., Williams, E.A., Carter, A.M., *et al.* (1987). Small rodents and other mammals associated with mountain meadows as reservoirs of *Giardia* spp. and *Campylobacter* spp. *App. Environ. Microbiol.*, **53:** 1574–79.

Paget, T.A., Macechko, P.T. and Jarroll, E.L. (1998). Metabolic changes in *Giardia intestinalis* during differentiation. *J. Parasitol.*, **84:** 222–26.

Palm, D. and Svärd, S. (2009). *Proteomic analyses in Giardia*. In: M.G. Ortega-Pierres, S. Cacciò, R. Fayer, T. Mank, *et al.* (eds.) *Giardia and Cryptosporidium: From Molecules to Disease*. pp. 328–43. Wallingford: CAB International.

Pawlowski, Z., Kasprzak, W., Kociecka, W. and Lisowska, M. (1987). Epidemiological studies on giardiasis in Poznan Province - a review. *Wiadomosci Parazytologiczne*, **33:** 593–613.

Peattie, D.A. (1990). The giardins of *Giardia lamblia*: genes and proteins with promise. *Parasitol. Today*, **6:** 52–56.

Perlmutter, D.H., Leichtner, A.M., Goldman, H. and Winter, H.S. (1985). Chronic diarrhea associated with hypogammaglobulinemia and enteropathy in infants and children. *Digest. Dis. Sci.,* **30:** 1149–55.

Petersen, L.R., Carter, M.L. and Hadler, J.L. (1988). A food-borne outbreak of *Giardia lamblia. J. Infect. Dis.,* **157:** 846–48.

Phillips, S.C., Mildvan, D., Williams, D.C., Gelb, A.M. and White, M.C. (1981). Sexual transmission of enteric protozoa and helminths in a venereal-disease clinic population. *N. Engl. J. Med.,* **305:** 603–66.

Pickering, L.K., Evans, D.G., Du Pont, H.L., Vollet, J.J. and Evans, D.J. (1981). Diarrhea caused by *Shigella,* rotavirus, and *Giardia* in day care centers: prospective study. *J. Pediat.,* **99:** 51–56.

Polis, M.A., Tuazon, C.U., Alling, D.W. and Talmanis, E. (1986). Transmission of *Giardia lamblia* from a day care center to the community. *Am. J. Pub. Health,* **76:** 1142–44.

Pospisilova, D. and Svobodova, V. (1992). Giardiasis in dog and cat owners. *Mikrobiol. Immun.,* **41:** 106–11.

Quinn, R.W. (1971). The epidemiology of intestinal parasites of importance in the United States. *South. Med. Bull.,* **59:** 29–30.

Rabbani, G.H. and Islam, A. (1994). Giardiasis in humans: populations most at risk and prospects for control. In: R.C.A. Thompson, J.A. Reynoldson and A.J. Lymbery (eds.) *Giardia: from molecules to disease,* pp. 217–49. Wallingford: CAB International.

Read, C., Walters, J., Robertson, J.D. and Thompson, R.C.A. (2002). Correlation between genotype of *Giardia duodenalis* and diarrhoea. *Int. J. Parasitol.,* **32:** 229–31.

Rendtorff, R. (1954). The experimental transmission of human intestinal protozoan parasites. *II. Giardia lamblia cysts given in capsules. Am. J. Hyg.,* **59:** 209–20.

Reynoldson, J.A., Behnke, J.M., Gracey, M., *et al.* (1998). Efficacy of albendazole against *Giardia* and hookworm in a remote Aboriginal community in the north of Western Australia. *Acta Trop.,* **71:** 27–44.

Rickard, L.G., Siefker, C., Boyle, C.R. and Gentz, E.J. (1999). The prevalence of *Cryptosporidium* and *Giardia* spp. in fecal samples from free-ranging white-tailed deer (*Odocoileus* i) in the southeastern United States. *J. Vet. Diagn. Invest.,* **11:** 65–72.

Robertson, I.D., Irwin, P.J., Lymbery, A.J. and Thompson, R.C.A. (2000). The role of companion animals in the emergence of parasitic zoonoses. *Int. J. Parasitol.,* **30:** 1369–77.

Roxstrom-Lindquist, K., Ringqvist, E., Palm, D. and Svard, S. (2005). *Giardia lamblia*-induced changes in gene expression in differentiated Caco-2 human intestinal epithelial cells. *Infect. Immun.,* **73:** 8204–8.

Roxstrom-Lindquist, K., Palm, D., Reiner, D., Ringqvist, E. and Svärd, S.G. (2006). *Giardia immunity an update. Trends in Parasit.,* **22:** 26–31.

Salb, A.L., Barkeman, W.B., Elkin, B.T., *et al.* (2008). Parasites in dogs in two northern Canadian communities: implications for human, dog, and wildlife health. *Emerg. Infect.Dis.,* **14:** 60–63.

Savioli, L., Smith, H. and Thompson, R.C.A. (2006). *Giardia* and *Cryptosporidium* join the 'Neglected Diseases Initiative'. *Trends Parasitol.,* **22:** 203–8.

Sawaya, A.L., Amigo, H. and Sigulem, D. (1990). The risk approach in preschool children suffering malnutrition and intestinal parasitic infection in the city of Sao Paulo, Brazil. *J. Trop. Pediat.,* **36:** 184–88.

Schantz, P.M. (1991). Parasitic zoonoses in perspective. *Int. J. Parasitol.,* **21:** 161–70.

Schofield, P.J. and Edwards, M.R. (1994). Biochemistry - is *Giardia* opportunistic in its use of substrates? In: R.C.A. Thompson, J.A. Reynoldson and A.J. Lymbery (eds.) *Giardia: from molecules to disease,* pp. 171–83. Wallingford: CAB International.

Scott, K.G., Logan, M.R., Klammer, G.M., Teoh, D.A. and Buret, A.G. (2000). Jejunal brush border microvillous alterations in *G. muris*-infected mice: role of T Lymphocytes and Interleukin-6. *Infect. Immun.,* **68:** 3412–88.

Scott, K.G.-E., Meddings, J.B., Kirk, D.R., Lees-Miller, S.P. and Buret, A.G. (2002). Intestinal infection with *Giardia* spp. Reduces epithelial barrier function in a myosin light chain kinase-dependent fashion. *Gastroenterology,* **123:** 1179–90.

Sener, K., van Keulen, H. and Jarroll, E.L. (2009). Giardan: structure, synthesis, regulation and inhibition. In: G. Ortega-Pierres, S.M. Caccio, R., *et al.* (eds.) Giardia and Cryptopsoridium: from molecules to disease, pp. 382–97. Wallingford: CAB International.

Siddall, M.E., Hong, H. and Desser, S.S. (1992). Phylogenetic analysis of the diplomonadida (Wenyon, 1926) Brugerolle, 1975: evidence for heterochrony in protozoa and against *Giardia lamblia* as a 'missing link'. *J. Protozool.* **39:** 361–77.

Singer, S.M. and Nash, T.E. (2000). *T-cell-dependent control of acute Giardia lamblia infections in mice.* Infect. Immun., **68:** 170–75.

Singer, S.M. and Kamda, J. (2009). Immune response to *Giardia* infection: lessons from animal models. In: M.G. Ortega-Pierres, S. Cacciò, *et al.* (eds.), *Giardia and Cryptosporidium: From Molecules to Disease.* pp. 451–62. Wallingford: CAB International.

Simpson, J.W., Burnie, A.G., Miles, R.S., Scott, J.L. and Lindsay, D.I. (1988). Prevalence of *Giardia* and *Cryptosporidium* infection in dogs in Edinburgh. *Vet. Rec.,* **123:** 445.

Smith, P.D. (1985). Pathophysiology and immunology of giardiasis. *Ann. Rev. Med.,* **36:** 295–307.

Smith, H.V., Caccio, S.M., Tait, A., McLauchlin, J., Thompsoin, R.C.A. (2006). Tools for investigating the environmental transmission of *Cryptosporidium* and *Giardia* infections in humans. *Trends Parasitol.,* **22**(4): 160–67.

Smith, H.V., Caccio, S.M., Cook, N., Nichols, R.A.B. and Tait, A. (2007). *Cryptosporidium* and *Giardia* as foodborne zoonoses. *Vet. Parasitol.,* **149:** 29–40.

Sogin, M.L., Gunderson, J.H., Elwood, H.J., Alonso, R.A. and Peattie, D.A. (1989). Phylogenetic meaning of the kingdom concept: an unusual ribosomal RNA from *Giardia lamblia. Science,* **243:** 75–77.

Speelman, P. and Ljungström, I. (1986). Protozoal enteric infections among expatriates in Bangladesh. *Am. J. Trop. Med. Hyg.,* **35:** 1140–45.

Steuart, R.F., O'Handley, R., Lipscombe, R.J., Lock, R.A. and Thompson, R.C.A. (2008). Alpha 2 giardin is an assemblage A-specific protein of human infective *Giardia Duodenalis. Parasitol.,* **135:** 1621–27.

Stevenson, W.J. and Hughes, K.L. (1988). *Synopsis of zoonoses in Australia.* Canberra: Australian Government Publishing Service.

Sulaiman, I.M., Fayer, R., Bern, C., *et al.* (2003). Triosephosphate isomerase gene characterization and potential zoonotic transmission of *Giardia duodenalis. Emerg. Infect. Dis.,* **9:** 1444–52.

Sullivan, P.B., Marsh, M.N., Phillips, M.B. *et al.* (1991). Prevalence and treatment of giardiasis in chronic diarrhoea and malnutrition. *Arch. Dis. Childh.,* **66:** 3–6.

Sullivan, P., Woodward, W.E., Pickering, D.G. and DuPont, H.L. (1984). Longitudinal study of diarrheal disease in day care centers. *Am. J. Pub. Health,* **74:** 987–91.

Teichroeb, J.A., Kutz, S.J., Parkar, U., Thompson, R.C.A. and Sicotte, P. (2009). Ecology of the Gastrointestinal Parasites of *Colobus vellerosus* at Boabeng-Fiema, Ghana: Possible Anthropozoonotic Transmission. *Am. J. Phys. Anthrop.,* **140:** 498–507.

Thompson, R.C.A. (1992). Giardiasis, in *Zoonoses,* Proceedings 194, pp. 88–91. Sydney: Postgraduate Committee in Veterinary Science, University of Sydney.

Thompson, R.C.A. (2000). Giardiasis as a re-emerging infectious disease and its zoonotic potential. *Int. J. Parasitol.,* **30:** 1259–67.

Thompson, R.C.A. (2001). The future impact of societal and cultural factors on parasitic disease–some emerging issues. *Int. J. Parasitol.,* **31:** 949–59.

Thompson, R.C.A. (2004). The zoonotic significance and molecular epidemiology of *Giardia* and giardiasis. *Vet. Parasitol.,* **126:** 15–35.

Thompson, R.C.A. (2008). Giardiasis: modern concepts in control and management. *Ann. Nestle,* **66:** 29–35.

Thompson, R.C.A. (2009a). The impact of *Giardia* on science and society. In: G. Ortega Pierres, S.M. Caccio, R. Fayer, *et al.* (eds.) Giardia and Cryptopsoridium: from molecules to disease, pp. 1–11. Wallingford: CAB International.

Thompson, R.C.A. (2009b). *Echinococcus, Giardia* and *Cryptosporidium:* observational studies challenging accepted dogma. *Parasitology,* **136:** 1529–35.

Thompson, R.C.A. and Lymbery, A.J. (1996). Genetic variability in parasites and host-parasite interactions. *Parasitology*, **112**: S7–S22.

Thompson, R.C.A., Monis, P.T. (2004). Variation in *Giardia*: Implications for taxonomy and epidemiology. *Adv. Parasitol.*, **58**: 69–137.

Thompson, R.C.A., Lymbery, A.J. and Meloni, B.P. (1990). Genetic variation in *Giardia* Kunstler, 1882: taxonomic and epidemiological significance. *Protozool. Abs.*, **14**: 1–28.

Thompson, R.C.A., Reynoldson, J.A. and Mendis, A.H.W. (1993). *Giardia* and giardiasis. *Adv. Parasitol.*, **32**: 71–160.

Thompson, R.C.A., Reynoldson, J.A. and Lymbery, A.J. (eds.) (1994). *Giardia: From molecules to disease and beyond.* Wallingford: CAB International.

Thompson, R.C.A., Reynoldson, J.A., Garrow, S.J., McCarthy, J.S. and Behnke, J.M. (2001). Towards the eradication of hookworm in an isolated Australian community. *Lancet*, **357**: 770–71.

Thompson, R.C.A. and Robertson, I.D. (2003). Gastrointestinal parasites of dogs and cats: current issues. *Comp. Contin. Ed. Pract. Vet.*, **25**: 4–11.

Thompson, R.C.A., Traub, R.J. and Parameswaran, N. (2007). Molecular Epidemiology of Foodborne Parasitic Zoonoses. In: K.D. Murrell and B. Fried (eds.), *Food-Borne Parasitic Zoonoses*, pp. 383–415. New York: Spinger.

Thompson, R.C.A., Palmer, C.S. and O'Handley, R. (2008). The public health and clinical significance of *Giardia* and *Cryptosporidium* in domestic animals. *Vet. J.*, **177**: 18–25.

Thompson, R.C.A., Kutz, S.J., Smith, A. (2009a). Parasite zoonoses and wildlife: emerging issues. *Intern. J. Environ. Res. Pub. Health*, **6**: 678–93.

Thompson, R.C.A., Colwell, D.D., Shury, T., Appelbee, A.J., Read, C., Njiru, Z., Olson, M.E. (2009b). The molecular epidemiology of *Cryptosporidium* and *Giardia* infections in coyotes from Alberta, Canada, and observations on some cohabiting parasites. *Vet. Parasitol.*, **159**: 167–70.

Thompson, R.C.A., Smith, A., Lymbery, A.J., Averis, S., Morris, K.D. and Wayne, A.F. (2010). *Giardia* in Western Australian wildlife. *Vet. Parasi.*, **170**: 207–11.

Torres, D.M., Chieffi, P.P., Costa, W.A. and Kudzielics, E. (1991). Giardiase em creches mantidas pela prefeitura do Municipiode Sao Paulo. *Rev. Instituto Med. Trop. Sao Paulo*, **33**: 137–42.

Traub, R.J., Monis, P.T., Robertson, I., Irwin, P., *et al.* (2004). Epidemiological and molecular evidence supports the zoonotic transmission of *Giardia* among humans and dogs living in the same community. *Parasitology,* **128**: 253–62.

Troeger, H., Epple, H.J., Schneider, T., *et al.* (2007). Effect of chronic *Giardia lamblia.* infection on epithelial transport and barrier function in human duodenum. *Gut,* **56**: 316–17.

Wallis, P.M. (1994). Abiotic transmission - is water really significant? In: R.C.A. Thompson, J.A. Reynoldson and A.J. Lymbery (eds.) *Giardia: from molecules to disease*, pp. 99–122. Wallingford: CAB International.

Wolfe, M.S. (1990). Clinical symptoms and diagnosis by traditional methods. In: E.A. Meyer (ed.) *Giardiasis*, pp. 175–85. Amsterdam: Elsevier.

Wright, J.M., Dunn, L.A., Upcroft, P. and Upcroft, J.A. (2003). Efficacy of antigiardial drugs. *Exp. Opin. Drug Safety*, **2**: 529–41.

Xiao, L. (1994). *Giardia* infection in farm animals. *Parasit. Today,* **10**: 436–38.

Zimmer, J.F. and Burrington, D.B. (1986). Comparison of four protocols for the treatment of giardiasis in dogs. *J. Am. An. Hosp. Ass.*, **22**: 168–72.

CHAPTER 46

Cryptosporidiosis

Aaron R. Jex, Rachel M. Chalmers, Huw V. Smith,
Giovanni Widmer, Vincent McDonald
and Robin B. Gasser

Summary

Cryptosporidium species represent a genus of parasitic protozoa (Apicomplexa) that are transmitted *via* the faecal-oral route and commonly infect the epithelial tissues of the gastric or intestinal (or sometimes the respiratory) tract of many vertebrates, including humans. Infection occurs following the ingestion of viable and resistant oocysts, through direct host-to-host contact or in contaminated food, drinking or recreational water. Infection can be transmitted *via* anthroponotic (human-to-human, human-to-animal) or zoonotic (animal-to-human or animal-to-animal) pathways, depending upon the species of *Cryptosporidium*. Although infection can be asymptomatic, common symptoms of disease (cryptosporidiosis) include diarrhoea, colic (abdominal pain), nausea, vomiting, dehydration and/or fever. In humans, cryptosporidial infection in immunocompetent patients is usually short-lived (days to weeks) and eliminated following the stimulation of an effective immune response. However, infection in immunodeficient individuals (e.g. those with humanimmuno deficiency virus/ acquired immune deficiency syndrome (HIV/AIDS)) can be chronic and fatal (in the absence of immunotherapy), as there are few effective anti-cryptosporidial drugs and no vaccines available. The present chapter provides an account of the history, taxonomy and biology, genomics and genetics of *Cryptosporidium*, the epidemiology, pathogenesis, treatment and control of cryptosporidiosis and the advances in tools for the identification and characterization of *Cryptosporidium* species and the diagnosis of cryptosporidiosis.

History

Cryptosporidium was first described (Tyzzer 1907) in the gastric mucosa of mice (*Mus musculus*) and thus given the type species name *C. muris*. The oocyst structure and endogenous life-cycle stages of *C. muris* were described in detail in a subsequent study (Tyzzer 1910). In 1911, *C. muris* was placed within in its own family, Cryptosporidiidae (Eucoccidiorida), because, although the parasite was clearly a 'sporozoan' (now apicomplexan) and transmitted by infective oocysts, its oocysts, though containing sporozoites, lacked sporocysts (Léger 1911). In 1912, a second species, given the name *C. parvum*, was described (Tyzzer 1912) and differentiated from *C. muris* by having smaller oocysts ('parvo' meaning small) and infecting the intestine rather than the stomach of the host.

Several new species of *Cryptosporidium* [e.g. *C. croatali* from snakes (Triffit 1925), *C. vulpis* from foxes (Wetzel 1938) and *C. baikalika* from birds (Matschoulsky 1947)] were proposed in subsequent years, but have since been reclassified as species of *Sarcocystis* or gregarines (Xiao *et al.* 2004). Subsequently, it was proposed that species of *Cryptosporidium* could be defined based on their host species (Pellérdy 1965), which led to numerous new descriptions. However, this presumption is now considered to be incorrect, and many of these early descriptions are currently proposed to represent synonyms of other recognized species (for a thorough appraisal of *Cryptosporidium* taxonomy, please refer to Xiao *et al.* (2004)).

It was not until more than forty years after *C. parvum* was described that the third 'valid' *Cryptosporidium* species, *C. meleagridis*, was described (Slavin 1955). This species was isolated from the intestine of turkeys (*Meleagris gallopavo*) and was significant in that it was identified as a cause of morbidity and mortality in young turkeys (Slavin 1955). This represented the first confirmed report of *Cryptosporidium* infection resulting in disease in the host. A subsequent report of an association between *Cryptosporidium* infection and diarrhoea in a cow (Panciera *et al.* 1971) confirmed the status of members within this genus as pathogens of vertebrates rather than gastrointestinal commensals, as proposed previously (Slavin 1955).

In 1976, the first two human cases of clinical cryptosporidiosis were confirmed histologically in an otherwise healthy 3-year-old child (Nime *et al.* 1976) and in a 39-year-old immunosuppressed man (Meisel *et al.* 1976). In the early 1980s, additional cases of human cryptosporidiosis, often associated with immunocompromised people, were reported (Current *et al.* 1983), supporting the hypothesis that *Cryptosporidium* was an enteric pathogen of public health importance (O'Donoghue 1985). The rapid spread of the (HIV) and the associated AIDS pandemic (Salzberg and Dolins 1989), and the recognition that cryptosporidiosis could be fatal in severely immunocompromised individuals (Macher 1988) led to a greater awareness of the public health significance and impact of *Cryptosporidium* and cryptosporidiosis. Compounding this impact, and adding to this increased public awareness, were the waterborne outbreaks of cryptosporidiosis reported between 1984–1992 (D'Antonio *et al.* 1985; Hayes *et al.* 1989; Smith *et al.* 1989; Moore *et al.* 1993) affecting large numbers of individuals (up to 15,000) and the realization that the infectivity of *Cryptosporidium* oocysts in water was not completely ablated by common treatments, such as chlorination (Peeters *et al.* 1989; Korich *et al.* 1990).

From 1989 to 1993, two waterborne outbreaks had far-reaching impacts both on the drinking water industry and on our knowledge of *Cryptosporidium*. Following the Swindon/Oxfordshire outbreak in February and March of 1989 (Richardson *et al.* 1991), the UK government set up an 'Expert Group on *Cryptosporidium* and water supplies' to (a) review all available knowledge of *Cryptosporidium* and cryptosporidiosis, (b) fund a national research programme to broaden knowledge of *Cryptosporidium* as a waterborne pathogen, and (c) augment understanding of cryptosporidiosis and provide advice and recommendations to the government (reviewed by Smith and Rose, 1998). This shift in government policy is an example of the significant change in public concern regarding *Cryptosporidium*, and its impact in human health, in the early 1990s.

The massive waterborne outbreak of cryptosporidiosis in Milwaukee, USA, in 1993 (MacKenzie *et al.* 1994), with more than 400,000 suspected cases resulting in 100 deaths, revealed the enormity of *Cryptosporidium* as a public health threat and further emphasized the need for better diagnostic, preventative and control strategies (Gradus *et al.* 1996; Smith and Rose 1998); a recent study (Corso *et al.* 2003) estimated the total cost of this outbreak, in terms of medical expenses and lost productivity, at ~ 100 million US dollars (at the time of the outbreak). The outbreak in Milwaukee led to substantial changes in regulations governing management and, in particular, the acceptable turbidity, of municipal water supplies (US-EPA 1996). Clearly, *Cryptosporidium* is now recognized as a significant pathogen of humans and animals in both developed and developing countries globally (Medema *et al.* 2006).

The agent

Currently, based primarily on molecular data, 19 *Cryptosporidium* species and more than 44 genotypes have been reported to parasitize the epithelial cells (usually in the gastric or intestinal system) of hosts representing all classes of vertebrates (see Xiao *et al.* 2004; Xiao and Fayer 2008). Three features of the *Cryptosporidium* life-cycle facilitate the transmission of disease and may contribute to a relatively high level of environmental contamination. Firstly, the *Cryptosporidium* life-cycle is monoxenous (i.e. having a single host; see Current 1985), leading to rapid transmission, and can result in prolonged, and in some cases, chronic infection, contributing to the excretion of large numbers of oocysts into the environment. Secondly, the oocysts released are relatively thick-walled and resistant (Robertson *et al.* 1992), allowing the transmissive stage (oocyst) to persist in the environment for extended periods. Thirdly, *Cryptosporidium* species are responsible for diarrhoeal disease in a range of vertebrates (Fayer *et al.* 2000; Xiao *et al.* 2004), including humans, providing broad opportunities for transmission among susceptible host individuals. The resilience of *Cryptosporidium* oocysts in the environment, resistance to common disinfectants (Campbell *et al.* 1982; Peeters *et al.* 1989) and small size are all recognized to facilitate waterborne transmission (Smith and Grimason 2003).

Direct anthroponotic or zoonotic transmission of *Cryptosporidium* is the most common route of infection in humans, with numerous reports from day-care centres, hospitals and community (petting) farms (Cacciò *et al.* 2005; Smith and Nichols 2007). Large outbreaks of cryptosporidiosis in major urban areas

have been linked to oocyst contamination in community water supplies and recreational water facilities (Karanis *et al.* 2007). Cryptosporidial infections in immunocompetent humans are usually short-lived and are mostly eliminated within weeks by host immune responses (Theodos 1998). However, in immunocompromised people (congenital or acquired), infections can be chronic and, in the absence of effective intervention, can be fatal (e.g. Macher 1988).

Taxonomy and host specificity

Traditionally, *Cryptosporidium* species were identified based on parasite morphology and morphometrics (primarily of the oocyst), as well as host species and/or infection site within the host (Tyzzer 1910, 1912; Slavin 1955; Levine 1980; Current *et al.* 1986) and differentiated based on relative comparisons with other known species. The original descriptions of *C. muris* and *C. parvum* provide an example of this approach; both species were first recorded in mice (Tyzzer 1907, 1912), but *C. muris* had larger oocysts and infected epithelial tissues of the stomach (Tyzzer 1907, 1910), whereas *C. parvum* had smaller oocysts and infected the epithelial tissues of the intestine (Tyzzer 1912). The reliance on morphological data for specific identification resulted in the description of a large number of species and confusion or controversy regarding their taxonomy (see section on 'History'). This ambiguity impacts on our understanding of levels of host-specificity of species within this genus and on their zoonotic potential. It is now considered that neither parasite morphometry (Fall *et al.* 2003) nor host species or site of infection (see Xiao *et al.* 2004), in the absence of any additional data, provide sufficient information for the assignment of *Cryptosporidium* species (see Fayer 2008). Increasingly, these 'classical' forms of systematic data are being supported by the use of genetic data to define species within this genus (e.g. Morgan-Ryan *et al.* 2002; Xiao *et al.* 2004).

Molecular biology has provided powerful new tools for the classification of species or genetic variants (designated as 'genotypes', 'types', 'subgenotypes' or 'subtypes') within *Cryptosporidium* (see Jex *et al.* 2008b). The ability to specifically identify or genetically characterize *Cryptosporidium* isolates has revolutionized our understanding of many areas, including the biology, systematics, population genetics and epidemiology of this genus. The most commonly used genetic locus for the identification of *Cryptosporidium* species and genotypes, and the locus for which the most extensive sequence data are available, has been the small subunit (SSU) of the nuclear ribosomal RNA gene (see Xiao *et al.* 2004). Based on the analysis of SSU sequence data, as well as sequence data for the actin and the 70 kilodalton heat shock protein genes, 19 species and tens of genotypes are currently recognized (Xiao *et al.* 2004; Xiao and Fayer 2008) (see Table 46.1), and it is likely that numerous additional species and/or genotypes will be discovered. However, it should be noted that because of the presence of heterogenous copies of the ribosomal genes in *Cryptosporidium* genomes (Le Blancq *et al.* 1997), there is a possibility that SSU genotypes may overestimate diversity. In consideration of this, it is advisable that species boundaries be explored using multiple genetic markers, or large genomic datasets.

Host specificity (and hence host range) among the known species of *Cryptosporidium* is highly variable (see Table 46.1), with many species/genetic types being linked to specific hosts (Xiao *et al.* 2004). In general, it has been hypothesized that the transmission of

Table 46.1 Host group and primary (1°) infection site of presently recognized species of *Cryptosporidium*

Species	Host group	1° Infection Site	Key Refs
C. andersoni	cattle	abomasum	(Lindsay *et al.* 2000)
C. baileyi	birds	intestine, cloaca, bursa of Fabricius	(Current *et al.* 1986)
C. bovis	cattle	intestine	(Fayer *et al.* 2005)
C. canis	canids	intestine	(Fayer *et al.* 2001)
C. fayeri	marsupials	intestine[1]	(Ryan *et al.* 2008)
C. felis	cats	intestine	(Iseki 1979)
C. fragile	amphibians	intestine	(Jirku *et al.* 2008)
C. galli	birds	stomach	(Pavlásek 1999)[2]
C. hominis	humans	intestine	(Morgan-Ryan *et al.* 2002)
C. macropodum	marsupials	intestine[1]	(Power and Ryan 2008)
C. meleagridis	birds (humans)	intestine	(Slavin 1955)
C. molnari[3]	fishes	stomach	(Alvarez-Pellitero and Sitja-Bobadilla 2002)
C. muris	rodents	stomach	(Tyzzer 1910)
C. parvum[4]	mammals (humans)	intestine	(Tyzzer 1912)
C. scophthalmi[5]	fishes	intestine	(Alvarez-Pellitero *et al.* 2004)
C. serpentis	snakes	stomach	(Levine 1980)
C. suis	pigs	intestine	(Ryan *et al.* 2004b)
C. varanii[6]	reptiles	intestine	(Pavlásek *et al.* 1995)
C. wrairi	rodents	intestine	(Vetterling *et al.* 1971)

[1] Oocysts isolated from faeces only, but these species group with other intestinal species (see Xiao *et al.* 2004) upon phylogenetic analysis.

[2] Redescribed by Ryan *et al.* (2003).

[3] No molecular data available in the original report. An isolate hypothesized to be *Cryptosporidium molnari* has been sequenced by Ryan *et al.* (2004a).

[4] There is some controversy (see Šlapeta, 2006, 2007; Xiao *et al.* 2007) as to whether the currently recognized species '*C. parvum*' (based on molecular data: see Xiao and Ryan, 2004b) is the same species as originally described by Tyzzer (1912).

[5] No molecular data available for this 'species'.

[6] *Cryptosporidium saurophilum* has been proposed to represent a junior synonym of *C. varanii* (cf Pavlásek and Ryan (2008)).

a species of *Cryptosporidium* from one host to another will occur, if at all (see Xiao *et al.* 2004), between species of the same vertebrate class and that transmission of *Cryptosporidium* among the vertebrate classes is less common (see Tzipori and Ward 2002). However, at least one species, *C. meleagridis*, is capable of regularly traversing the boundary between host classes (Tzipori and Ward 2002), having been first described from turkeys (Slavin 1955) and, more recently, from other bird species (e.g. Abe and Iseki 2004; Pages-Mante *et al.* 2007) and, with significant frequency (up to ~ 1% of cases) from humans (e.g. Pedraza-Diaz *et al.* 2001; Gatei *et al.* 2006; Leoni *et al.* 2006; Jex *et al.* 2007a). The ecological gap between endothermic and ectothermic hosts seems a potential barrier to the transmission of *Cryptosporidium* infection (Graczyk *et al.* 1996c; Graczyk and Cranfield 1998; Graczyk *et al.* 1998) due to the presence or absence of key oocyst excystation stimuli (see section on Location and establishment in the host); however, this has not been experimentally tested for most known parasite or host species.

The present literature indicates that *C. parvum* is the species with the greatest number of reported hosts. The most comprehensive review of the literature to date indicates that '*C. parvum*' has been reported from more than 150 host species (Fayer *et al.* 2000), including humans and cattle. However, the specific identity of the *Cryptosporidium* isolates from many of the early studies summarized by Fayer *et al.* (2000) could not be confirmed genetically at the time they were first reported due to the unavailability of molecular tools. There have been numerous reports of molecularly distinct *Cryptosporidium* species or 'genotypes' identified in the intestines of many host species, such as cats (Xiao *et al.* 1999), dogs (Fayer *et al.* 2001), horses (Xiao *et al.* 2004), opossum (Xiao *et al.* 2002) and rabbits (Xiao *et al.* 2002), reported to be infected by '*C. parvum*'. These findings predicate further study of the actual breadth of the host range for *C. parvum* using molecular tools (see section on Diagnosis and genetic analysis).

Regardless of its host range, it is clear from the literature that *C. parvum* poses the greatest zoonotic risk to humans (see Xiao and Feng 2008), particularly in relation to cattle. The contribution that other animals may make as zoonotic reservoirs is less certain. Studies of sheep populations in Western Australia indicate that sheep may not represent a significant zoonotic source for human infection (Ryan *et al.* 2005b). However, *C. parvum* has been detected previously, by molecular based tools, in sheep in other areas (e.g. Morgan *et al.* 1998; Cacciò *et al.* 2001; Santin *et al.* 2007). In addition, direct transmission of *Cryptosporidium* to humans from lambs at a petting zoo has been supported by molecular data

(Elwin *et al.* 2001) and sheep have been implicated as the source of human infections in waterborne outbreaks in the UK (Said *et al.* 2003). Using molecular methods, *C. parvum* also has been detected in dogs (e.g. Giangaspero *et al.* 2006), goats (e.g. Cacciò *et al.* 2001) and wild ruminants (e.g. Alves *et al.* 2006), including deer (e.g. Ryan *et al.* 2005a).

At the other end of the host-specificity spectrum are *Cryptosporidium* species which appear to parasitize a single host species. The most noteworthy among these is *C. hominis*, one of the main species associated with cryptosporidiosis of humans (Morgan-Ryan *et al.* 2002). *Cryptosporidium hominis* is thought to infect humans specifically and is not commonly associated with 'host-switching' (Morgan-Ryan *et al.* 2002). Nonetheless, this species has been recorded (in rare instances) in dugong (Morgan *et al.* 2000), sheep (Giles *et al.* 2001; Giles *et al.* 2009), a goat (Giles *et al.* 2009) and cattle (Smith *et al.* 2005b), indicating that there may be some 'plasticity' even in the host-specificity of this species of parasite.

Life-cycle

Cryptosporidium is usually transmitted *via* the faecal-oral route and exhibits a monoxenous life-cycle (Fig. 46.1 and 46.2; see Fayer 2008). Briefly, a sporulated oocyst (containing four naked, infective sporozoites) is ingested by the host and excysts (for excystation stimuli, see section on Location and establishment in the host) usually in either the stomach or the intestine (depending on the species of *Cryptosporidium*; see section on Taxonomy and host specificity). Each motile sporozoite migrates, by gliding motility, along the epithelial lining of the gut (e.g. microvilli of enterocytes in the small intestine). Upon finding a suitable site for infection, the sporozoite forms an attachment zone between itself, at the apical complex, and the host cell membrane (Valigurová *et al.* 2008). This elicits the host cell membrane to envelope the sporozoite, encasing it in an epicellular parasitophorous sac (Valigurová *et al.* 2008). Although generally it is reported that this parasitophorous sac represents a dual membrane vacuole with a host-derived outer layer, which exists briefly and then disintegrates, and a parasite-derived inner layer, parasitophorous vacuolar membrane (PVM) (see Smith *et al.* 2005a), which is retained, recent scanning electron microscopy studies provide evidence suggesting that the parasitophorous sac may be entirely host-derived (Valigurová *et al.* 2008). Regardless of its origin, for simplicity, we refer herein to the parasitophorous sac as the PVM. Following the formation of the PVM, the sporozoite develops into a trophozoite. As the trophozoite develops it forms a feeder organelle, which appears to act as the interface between the developing parasite and the host cytoplasm (Marcial and Madara 1986). This results in the parasite being described as intracellular but extracytoplasmic in location (e.g. Tzipori and Griffiths 1998); however, others have suggested 'epicellular' to be a more preferable descriptive term (e.g. Valigurová *et al.* 2008). Truly intracytoplasmic invasion may occur in rare instances, but appears to be limited to the invasion of macrophages within the Peyer's patches (Marcial and Madara 1986).

Within the PVM, the trophozoite undergoes asexual reproduction (merogony or schizogony; longitudinal binary fission) to produce type 1-meronts (schizonts). Each of these type 1-meronts contains 16 merozoites, which are released from the PVM. Each merozoite infects a new enterocyte (reforming the PVM), then replicates and develops into a new type 1-meront to repeat the cycle, or enters into the reproductive phase to replicate and develop

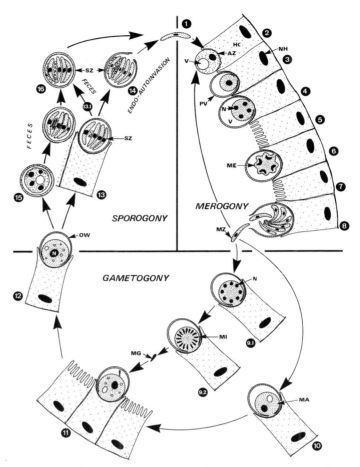

Fig. 46.1 The life-cycle of *Cryptosporidium* sp (1) Excystation of sporozoites from ingested oocysts; (2–3) Attachment to and infection of the host cell, forming the epicellular parasitophorous vacuole. (4–5) Nuclear division (2 phases); (6–8) asexual reproduction (merogony) to form the merozoites, which rupture out of the parasitophorous vacuole and infection new host cells (reforming the PVM); (9–12) Gametogony phases (sexual reproduction) in which some merozoites (9.1) form (within the PVM) multinucleated microgamonts which develop (9.2) into 16 non-flagellated microgametes and some merozoites (10) each develop into a single nucleated macrogamont, which (11) forms a macrogamete which is then fertilized by a microgamete forming (12) a zygote contained within a thin oocyst-wall. (13–14) Some of the thin-walled oocysts rupture within the host and infect new host cells (autoinfective stage), whereas in others (15–16) the oocyst wall thickens, producing a thick-walled oocysts, which is shead from the host in the faeces, infecting a new host, and thus completing the life-cycle. Abbreviations: AZ: attachment zone; HC: host cell; MA: macrogamont; ME: meront; MG: microgamete; MI: microgamont; MZ: merozoite; N: nucleas; NH: nucleus of the host cell; PV: parasitophorous vacuole; SZ: Sporozoite.
Modified from (Melhlorn, 1988). With kind permission of Springer Science+Business Media.

into type 2-meronts, each of which contain four merozoites. After infecting a host cell, each type 2-merozoite initiates the sexual reproductive cycle (gametogony) and develops either into a microgamont (containing 12–16 microgametes) or a macrogamont (maturing into a macrogamete). Microgametes (male) are released and fertilize macrogametes (female) to form zygotes, which ultimately develop into oocysts. In another asexual reproductive phase (sporogony), the oocyst sporulates to produce, internally, four naked sporozoites. Two types of oocyst are produced: thin-walled

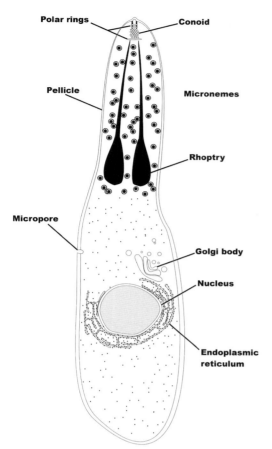

Fig. 46.2 Schematic diagram of a *Cryptosporidium* sporozoite, showing the locations of key cell surface proteins involved in attachment and invasion Based on Roberts and Janovy Jr. (2005).

oocysts remain in the alimentary tract and have the ability to sustain an autoinfection, whereas thick-walled oocysts are passed in the faeces. The thin-walled oocysts and/or type 1-meronts, which can perpetuate autoinfection, are of particular relevance in immunocompromised, immunodeficient or immunosuppressed individuals, as the likely cause of chronic cryptosporidiosis (e.g. Arenas-Pinto *et al.* 2003; Certad *et al.* 2005; Chhin *et al.* 2006).

Location and establishment in the host

Cryptosporidium mainly comprises species which infect the gastric epithelium or those which infect the intestinal epithelium (primarily the small intestine) (Xiao *et al.* 2004; Smith *et al.* 2005a). An exception to this is *C. baileyi*, which, although known to infect the intestinal tract of several bird species (Xiao *et al.* 2004), is also found in the epithelial tissues of the cloaca and the bursa of Fabricius of turkeys (Current *et al.* 1986) and the respiratory tract of chickens (Goodwin *et al.* 1990). Extra-gastrointestinal infection has been reported in immunocompromised humans (e.g. late-stage HIV/AIDS patients with CD4+ counts of < 50 cells/mm³), with chronic infection disseminating to the liver, pancreas and/or lungs (Hunter and Nichols 2002), often resulting in biliary sclerosis (e.g. Forbes *et al.* 1993), pancreatitis (e.g. Goodwin 1991) or respiratory disease (e.g. Clavel *et al.* 1996). The prevalence and

significance of extra-gastrointestinal cryptosporidiosis, particularly respiratory infection, in immunocompetent humans are not yet known, although there are some clinical data indicating that such infections are at least possible in immunocompetent children (e.g. Westrope and Acharya 2001).

The processes and stimuli which trigger the excystation of *Cryptosporidium* oocysts are still poorly understood (Smith *et al.* 2005a). Physiological cues in the gastro-intestinal environment, including salt concentrations (and particularly bile salt concentrations), pH, the presence of proteases (such as pepsin, trypsin and chymotrypsin) and their combined effects, appear to influence excystation (reviewed by Smith *et al.* 2005a). Host temperature is also hypothesized to be an important trigger for *C. parvum* (see Fayer and Leek 1984) and is likely to be important for *C. hominis* and other *Cryptosporidium* species infecting endothermic hosts. However, it seems likely that temperature is less important in ectotherms, such as reptiles and fish, which may partially explain experimental findings that oocysts isolated from endothermic hosts (both mammals and birds) are not infective to ectotherms (Graczyk *et al.* 1996a) and *vice versa* (Graczyk *et al.* 1998).

Little is known about the excystation processes and associated factors linked to extra-gastrointestinal infections (e.g. biliary, pancreatic or pulmonary cryptosporidiosis). To our knowledge, there are no reports of biliary or pancreatic cryptosporidiosis in the absence of gastrointestinal infection. Therefore, it seems likely that infection of the liver or pancreas is secondary to a gastrointestinal infection and may result from the dissemination of 'zoites of the auto-infective stage (thin-walled oocysts and/or type-1 meronts) (cf. O'Donoghue, 1995). However, there are reports, in humans, of pulmonary cryptosporidiosis in the absence of gastrointestinal infection (e.g. Clavel *et al.* 1996), which suggests that pulmonary infection can establish independently, possibly following the inhalation of aerosols contaminated with *Cryptosporidium* oocysts. Although this hypothesis requires experimental testing, it seems likely that host temperature is the stimulus for the excystation of oocysts in respiratory tract of endotherms, whereas environmental cues (e.g. bile salt concentration or pH) shown to be important in gastrointestinal infections are largely absent. Presently, we are not aware of any published reports of pulmonary cryptosporidiosis in ectotherms.

Following the excystation of oocysts (see Fig. 46.3 for morphology), sporozoites glide over the host epithelial surfaces and then attach to and infect the host cells (enterocytes). Gliding motility, sporozoite orientation and attachment are prerequisites for intracellular infection (Smith *et al.* 2005a). Currently, the interactions of parasite- and host-derived molecules involved in these processes are not completely understood; however, some of the genes and proteins involved are beginning to be identified and characterized (reviewed by Smith *et al.* 2005a; Boulter-Bitzer *et al.* 2007). The cell surface glycoprotein P23 is believed to be associated with sporozoite motility, as is the 15 kilodalton glycoprotein (GP15). The 40 and 900 kilodalton cell-surface glycoproteins GP40 and GP900, the galactose-*N*-acetylgalactosoamine (Gal/GalNAc) specific lectin (Joe *et al.* 1998), and the thombrospondin-related attachment proteins (TRAPs) are believed to be involved in the attachment of the sporozoite to the enterocytes prior to cell infection. The GP40, GP900 and the TRAPs are localized to the apical complex and/or micronemes, and presumably their role is associated with the attachment phase immediately prior to infection of the enterocyte.

The glycoprotein GP15 and the Ga1/Ga1NAc-specific lectin are distributed across the 'zoite surface and appear to be associated with initial 'zoite attachment to the epithelial cell surface and/or attachment during the gliding process. The circumsporozoite-like antigen (CSL; a 1300 kDa glycoprotein) has also been implicated in the infection process and, although its precise role and function are unclear, CSL can bind directly to an 85 kDa receptor protein on the surface of intestinal epithelial cells (Langer and Riggs 1999), suggesting that it is likely to be involved in 'zoite attachment.

Motility during sporozoite gliding and invasion is 'powered' by an intracellular actinomyosin motor (Forney *et al.* 1998), as has been found in other apicomplexans (Kappe *et al.* 1999; Sibley 2004). Upon attachment to an enterocyte, the invasion by the sporozoite is rapid (taking ~ 30 sec; Wetzel *et al.* 2005). The rhoptry of

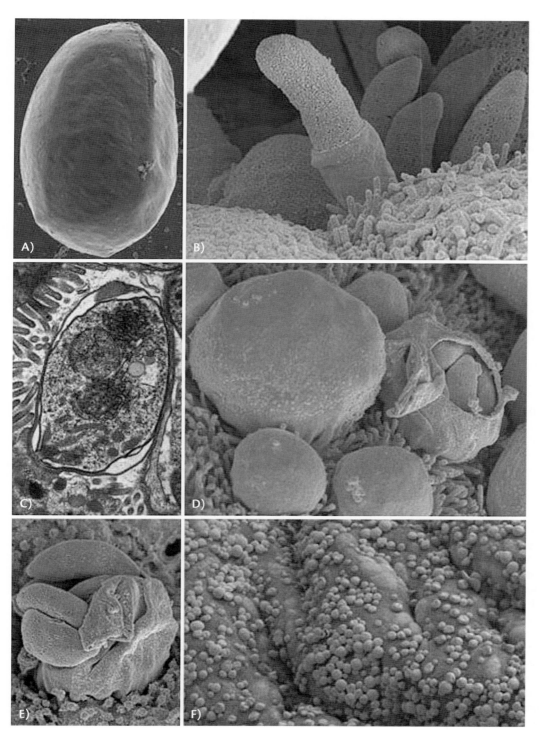

Fig. 46.3 High-resolution scanning electron micrographs representing various life-cycle stages of *Cryptosporidium*. A) *Cryptosporidium muris* oocyst showing suture line; B) *Cryptosporidium muris* sporozoite during cellular infection phase, being enveloped by the host-derived tight-fitting membrane folds; C) *Cryptosporidium muris* trophozoite developing within the parasitophorous vacuole; D) *Cryptosporidium* sp. 'toad' parasitophorous vacuoles on the gastric epithelium of the host, showing an opened vacuole containing the developing merozoites; E) *Cryptosporidium muris* merozoites budding from the residual body; F) *Cryptosporidium* sp. 'toad' parasitophorous vacuoles 'coating' the gastric epithelia of the host. Reproduced from (Valigurová *et al.*, 2008) with permission from Elsevier.

the sporozoite extends from the apical complex and is believed to initiate partial invagination of the host cell membrane, which folds over the sporozoite and envelops it (Smith *et al.* 2005a; Valigurová *et al.* 2008). Little is known about the molecules involved in the intracellular phases of the *Cryptosporidium* life-cycle due to the practical limitations in isolating these stages from infected hosts and current limitations of *in vitro* culturing methods.

Growth and survival *in vitro*

Although *Cryptosporidium* species can be maintained in animals as experimental lines, the process of maintaining these infections is costly, labourious and does not allow for the visual inspection or the isolation of any of the intracellular parasite life-cycle stages. In addition, due to the broad range in host specificities of the various species of *Cryptosporidium* (see section on Taxomony and host specificity), the maintenance of experimental infections as 'reference lines' for each known species and/or genotype is impractical. The establishment of improved *in vitro* culturing in established cell lines to allow the maintenance of a range of reference *Cryptosporidium* species is needed for further insights into the biology of this group of parasites and the efficacy of various potential chemotherapeutics through direct measurement of parasite proliferation rates before and after treatment. *In vitro* cultivation of *Cryptosporidium* has been reviewed in detail by Arrowood (2008). Due to space limitations, a brief account is given of the culturing methods and cell lines which have been used and the successes and limitations of some approaches. For detailed recommendations on methodologies and conditions for culturing *Cryptosporidium*, the reader is referred to the review by Arrowood (2008).

In vitro culturing of *Cryptosporidium* primarily involves the propagation of the intracellular developmental stages (see Fig. 46.1) in monolayers of host cell lines (Upton *et al.* 1994c). This approach has been used relatively frequently to determine the efficacy of chemotherapeutic agents (Woods *et al.* 1996) and as a surrogate system for determining *in vivo* infectivity (e.g. Rochelle *et al.* 2002; Najdrowski *et al.* 2007). *In vitro* cultivation, coupled to electron microscopic analysis, observing and capturing *Cryptosporidium* sporozoites just as they attach to the cell membrane and infect the cell have enhanced our understanding of the processes of attachment and invasion (Bhat *et al.* 2007). In addition, by facilitating the direct purification of sporozoites, *in vitro* culturing has led to the first examination of the genes expressed and/or transcribed during infection of the host cell (Jakobi and Petry 2006). Enhanced *in vitro* culturing techniques may allow examinations of the changes in the transcriptome of selected *Cryptosporidium* species during their intracellular replication and development, providing valuable data which are difficult to obtain *via* experimental infections of animals. *In vitro* culturing also facilitates some examinations of changes to the host cell during attachment and infection, as well as host evasion mechanisms (e.g. through changes to the expressional profile of beta-defensin genes (Zaalouk *et al.* 2004)) (see section on Immunology). Improved *in vitro* cell-culturing techniques, which could allow long-term laboratory maintenance of all known species of *Cryptosporidium*, would greatly facilitate our understanding of the parasite's biology and have importance in treatment and control of cryptosporidiosis by allowing detailed comparative studies to be made of human-infective and other species. This is not possible employing current technologies and cell lines. Although host-cell free cultures have been assessed for the propagation of

C. parvum (see Hijjawi *et al.* 2004), development of a cell-free *in vitro* culturing method for *C. hominis* has been unsuccessful (see Girouard *et al.* 2006), and no such methods are presently available for any other *Cryptosporidium* species.

A variety of cell lines have been explored for the cultivation of *C. parvum* following inoculation with sporozoites or excysting oocysts (see Table 46.2; Arrowood 2002). Woodmansee and Pohlenz (1983) provided the first report of the culturing of the asexual stages of the *Cryptosporidium* by successfully infecting human rectal tumour (HRT) cells cultured in the presence of foetal bovine serum (FBS). Current and Long (1983) were the first to complete the *Cryptosporidium* life-cycle *in vitro* and used oocysts from humans or calves to infect chicken embryos (chorioallantoic membrane). Shortly thereafter, *Cryptosporidium* life-cycles were completed in cultured human foetal lung (HFL), primary chicken kidney (PCK) or porcine kidney (PK-10) cells (Current and Haynes 1984). However, the results from these studies (Current and Long 1983; Current and Haynes 1984) have not been reproduced by other authors (see Arrowood 2002). In the ensuing years, a range of cell lines, including baby hamster kidney (BHK) (Naciri *et al.* 1986), HT29.74 human colon adenocarcinoma (Flanigan *et al.* 1991), Madin-Darby bovine kidney (MDBK) (Upton *et al.* 1994b; Upton *et al.* 1994a), Madin-Darby canine kidney (MDCK) (Gut *et al.* 1991; Arrowood *et al.* 1994), RL95-2 human endometrial carcinoma (Rasmussen *et al.* 1993), and Caco-2 human colon adenocarcinoma (Griffiths *et al.* 1994) cells have been tested for the *in vitro* culturing of *Cryptosporidium*. Based on published reports, perhaps the most promising of these cell lines are the human ileocaecal adenocarcinoma 8 (HCT-8; (Hijjawi *et al.* 2001b) and the VELI (rabbit chondrocyte) (Lacharme *et al.* 2004) cell lines, both of which have been used to infer the development of *C. parvum*. The life-cycle established in these *in vitro* culturing experiments (Hijjawi *et al.* 2001b; Lacharme *et al.* 2004) paralleled *in vivo* infection in relation to the epicellular location and chronology of development of the parasite, indicating that *in vitro* culture, at least superficially, reflects *in vivo* development. Furthermore, oocysts produced in VELI cells were reported to be infective to infant mice, indicating that the life-cycle of *C. parvum* can be completed effectively *in vitro* (Lacharme *et al.* 2004). Although some data are available for *C. hominis* (see Hashim *et al.* 2006), most *in vitro* studies to date have involved *C. parvum*. This information emphasizes the need for expanded culturing techniques suitable for different species and subspecific variants of *Cryptosporidium* which have been thoroughly identified and characterized using advanced molecular tools and suitable nucleic acid markers.

Diagnosis and genetic analysis

The specific diagnosis of cryptosporidiosis, including the precise identification and characterization of *Cryptosporidium* species, is central to the prevention and control of this disease and to the understanding of the intricacies of its epidemiology. A range of tools, including microscopic (following conventional staining), immunological, flow cytometric and nucleic acid–based techniques, have been utilized for the detection, characterization and/or quantitation of oocysts in biological samples (e.g. faeces, water, food or tissues; see Smith *et al.* 2006; Jex *et al.* 2008b).

Microscopic approaches for diagnosis have been based on the detection of oocysts using conventional stains, such as auramine

Table 46.2 Summary of outcomes of *in vitro* cultivation of *Cryptosporidium* species (primarily *C. parvum*) from various hosts in selected cell lines

Cell line (ATCC no.)	Oocyst source	Life-cycle stages	Infective oocysts	Key refs
HRT	Cattle	Asexual	Not detected	(Woodmansee and Pohlenz 1983)
CAM	Human, Cattle, Birds	All	Yes	(Current and Long 1983)
HFL	Human (goats)	All	Yes	(Current and Haynes 1984)
PCK	Human (goats)	All	Yes	(Current and Haynes 1984)
PK-10	Human (goats)	All	Yes	(Current and Haynes 1984)
BHK (CRL-1632)	Human (goats)	Asexual	Not reported	(Naciri et al. 1986)
HT29.74 (HTB-38)	Human	Asexual	Not reported	(Flanigan et al. 1991)
MDBK (CCL-22)	Cattle	All[1]	Yes	(Upton et al. 1994c)
MDCK (CCL-34)	Sheep, Cattle	All	Yes	(Gut et al. 1991)
RL95-2 (CRL-1671)	Cattle	All[2]	Not reported	(Rasmussen et al. 1993)
Caco-2 (HTB-37)	Human, Cattle	All[3]	Yes	(Griffiths et al. 1994)
HCT-8 (CCL-224)	Cattle	All	Yes	(Hijjawi et al. 2001a)
VELI	Sheep (lamb)	All	Yes	(Lacharme et al. 2004)

Abbreviations: ATCC (The American Type Culture Collection); HRT (human rectal tumour cells); CAM (chorioallantoic membrane); HFL (human foetal lung cells); PCK (primary chicken kidney cells); PK-10 (porcine kidney cells); BHK (baby hamster kidney cells); MDBK (Madin-Darby bovine kidney cells); MDCK (Madin-Darby canine kidney cells); RL95-2 (human endometrial carcinoma cells); HCT-8 (human colonic tumor cells); VELI (rabbit chondrocyte cell line).
Adapted from Arrowood et al. (2002).

phenol, dimethyl sulphoxide (DMSO)-carbol fuchsin, Kinyoun, safranin-methylene blue, acid fast (Ziehl-Neelsen), light green merbromide and malachite green (reviewed by Jex et al. 2008b) . Direct immunofluorescent antibody (DFA)-based detection has also been employed relatively widely (e.g. Graczyk et al. 1996b; Quílez et al. 1996; Garcia and Shimizu 1997; Johnston et al. 2003). The advantages of many of these approaches are that they are inexpensive and relatively simple to carry out; the disadvantages relate mainly to limited specificity and sensitivity (Jex et al. 2008b) and the inability to differentiate among species of *Cryptosporidium* based on the morphology of stained oocysts (Fall et al. 2003).

Methods commonly applied to environmental samples and recommended by, among others, the US Environmental Protection Agency (US-EPA 1996, 1999a, b) and the WHO (Medema et al. 2006), are those based on fluorescence and differential interference (DIC) microscopy (i.e. Method 1622 (US-EPA 1999a) and Method 1623 (US-EPA 1999b)). These techniques have been designed specifically for the detection of oocysts in water samples and rely on filteration and/or purification by immunomagnetic separation (IMS) of either small (20 litre) samples (US-EPA 1999a, b) or large (~ 1000-litre) volumes (see Anon. 1999) followed by direct labelling with the fluorogen 4'6-diamidino-2-phenyl indole (DAPI) and detection by epifluorescence and DIC microscopy. However, again, a limitation is the lack of specificity and sensitivity. Thus, although these approaches are useful for identifying oocysts to the genus level (in samples with relatively large numbers of oocysts), they do not allow specific identification or delineation. Other commonly used diagnostic tools, including agglutination assays (Pohjola et al. 1986) and enzyme-linked immunoassays available in a cartridge or dip-stick format (e.g. Garcia et al. 2003; Johnston et al. 2003; Geurden et al. 2008), flow cytometry (e.g. Vesey et al. 1994; Ferrari et al. 2000) or fluorescent *in situ* hybridization (FISH; Deere et al. 1998a, b; Vesey et al. 1998;

Smith et al. 2004a), have similar limitations (reviewed by Jex et al. 2008b).

In contrast, many of the nucleic acid-based methods developed to date provide enhanced diagnostic specificity and sensitivity, enabling the specific and genotypic detection and identification of *Cryptosporidium* (Jex et al. 2008b). Improved specificity and sensitivity have been possible largely through the use of the polymerase chain reaction (PCR; Mullis et al. 1986; Saiki et al. 1988), which enables the specific amplification of genetic loci from complex and tiny amounts of genomic DNA using a thermostable DNA polymerase. Genetic loci commonly employed in PCR-coupled methods include 'variable regions' within the nuclear ribosomal RNA, the *Cryptosporidium* oocyst wall protein (*cowp*), the 70 kilodalton heat shock protein (*hsp70*) and the 60 kilodalton glycoprotein (*gp60*) genes (reviewed by Xiao et al. 2004; Boulter-Bitzer et al. 2007; Jex and Gasser 2010).

Various PCR-coupled approaches, including microsatellite analysis, restriction fragment length polymorphism (RFLP) analysis, mutation scanning and direct DNA sequencing, have been developed for the identification and characterization of *Cryptosporidium* isolates (reviewed by Smith et al. 2006; Jex et al. 2008b; Jex and Gasser 2009). The latter two approaches used in combination (Gasser et al. 2006) have been shown to be particularly useful for genetic analysis in that they allow the accurate detection of mutations, enabling the reliable classification of *Cryptosporidium* species (Gasser et al. 2003, 2004; Jex et al. 2007b) and populations (Jex et al. 2007a; Jex and Gasser 2008; Jex et al. 2008a). There is also significant potential for PCR-coupled high resolution melt (HRM) analysis as a mutation scanning tool and, although this method requires further evaluation, it is likely to be applicable to *Cryptosporidium*, utilizing suitable genetic loci (e.g. Monis et al. 2005; Pangasa et al. 2009).

Although most nucleic acid techniques utilize the PCR-based amplification of DNA or RNA, other approaches, such as nucleic acid sequence-based amplification (NASBA; Baeumner *et al.* 2001) and loop-mediated isothermal amplification procedure (LAMP; Notomi *et al.* 2000), show promise for the specific identification of *Cryptosporidium*. Further investigation is required to evaluate the diagnostic performance of such approaches (employing suitable genetic markers). Although some of these approaches require further critical assessment, the application of established PCR-based diagnostic and analytical techniques, such as multilocus genotyping, mutation scanning, real-time PCR and HRM approaches (using suitable genetic markers), can be utilized to explore the epidemiology and population genetics of *Cryptosporidium*. Such tools also have practical utility for routine monitoring in *Cryptosporidium* reference and diagnostic centres, as well as water industries, as part of an ongoing cryptosporidiosis risk management, surveillance, prevention and/or control strategy.

Genomics and genetics

Advances in genomic and genetic technologies are providing unique insights into many fundamental areas, such as gene function, biochemical pathways, parasite-host interactions and disease, as well as population genetics, ecology and epidemiology. Such advances also support the development of new and innovative methods of diagnosis, treatment and control.

Genomics

In 1991, the sequencing of the genome of *C. parvum* commenced when Laxer and colleagues (1991), working at the Armed Forces Institute of Pathology in Washington, DC, deposited a 1,054 bp-sequence of unknown entity into the GenBank database. By 1993, the number of sequence entries was still very small (~ 20) and contained few overlapping sequences (unpublished). In 2000, the exploration of the *Cryptosporidium* genome took a dramatic turn, when the US National Institute of Allergy and Infectious Diseases (NIAID) awarded two grants to sequence the genomes of both *C. parvum* and *C. hominis*. The interest in the sequencing of the nuclear genomes of these species, no doubt, reflected changes in public awareness that occurred in the 1990's (see section on, History) and advances in the accessibility and reliability of genomic technologies. This shift in interest was not limited to the USA; a third project to sequence chromosome VI of *C. parvum* was also in progress in the UK at the same time (Bankier *et al.* 2003).

By 2004, the complete nuclear genome of *C. parvum* (see Abrahamsen *et al.* 2004) and the nearly complete genome of *C. hominis* (see Xu *et al.* 2004) were sequenced employing a shotgun approach. The assembled and annotated genome sequences for *C. parvum* and *C. hominis* can be accessed and searched on the National Center for Biotechnology Information website (http://www.ncbi.nlm.nih.gov/) or the CryptoDB database (http://cryptodb.org). CryptoDB (Heiges *et al.* 2006) has become an important resource for both fundamental and applied molecular studies. It supports queries for sequences, annotations and protein features. 'Gene pages' (Stein *et al.* 2002) provides a graphic display of genes with links to aspects of proteomics, metabolic pathways and motif search tools.

The *C. hominis* and *C. parvum* genomes (Table 46.3) each consist of 8 chromosomes and are ~ 9.1–9.2 Mbp in size, being significantly smaller than those reported for other apicomplexans, such as *Plasmodium falciparum* (~ 23 Mbp) (Gardner *et al.* 2002) and *Eimeria tenella* (~ 60 Mbp) (Shirley 1994, 2000). This size is

reflected in a smaller number of genes (~ 4,000 genes in *Cryptosporidium versus* ~ 5,300 genes in *Plasmodium*), shorter non-coding regions (~ 25–30% in *Cryptosporidium versus* ~ 47% in *Plasmodium*) and fewer introns (~ 5% in *C. parvum*; ~ 5–20% in *C. hominis*; ~ 54% in *P. falciparum*).

In addition to a 'minimalistic' genome, *Cryptosporidium* also has a reduced number of pathways for the production of simple sugars, amino acids and nucleotides (Fig. 46.4, in the colour plate section: see Abrahamsen *et al.* 2004; Xu *et al.* 2004). Both *C. hominis* and *C. parvum* lack mitochondrial and apicoplast genomes (Widmer *et al.* 2002; Abrahamsen *et al.* 2004; Xu *et al.* 2004). The absence of these organellar genomes, particularly the mitochondrial genome, has significant implications for the richness and diversity of metabolic pathways and energy production, apparently leaving these organisms reliant upon glycolysis for ATP production (Abrahamsen *et al.* 2004; Xu *et al.* 2004). Also, some nuclear genes associated with mitochondrial pathways are lacking, as are the enzymes required for ATP production *via* fatty acid and protein catabolism (Abrahamsen *et al.* 2004; Xu *et al.* 2004). Thus, energy generation appears to occur exclusively *via* simple sugars acquired from the host cell.

In addition, the genes involved in amino acid synthesis (urea and nitrogen cycles), the tricarboxylic acid (Krebs) cycle and the shikimate pathways are absent; thus, *Cryptosporidium* appears to scavenge amino acids from the host cell. This is supported by the finding that the nuclear genomes of both *C. parvum* and *C. hominis* contain numerous amino acid transporter genes hypothesized to be involved in amino acid salvaging (Abrahamsen *et al.* 2004; Xu *et al.* 2004). This feature is quite distinct from *P. falciparum* which has functional Krebs, urea and nitrogen cycles, and a functional shikimate pathway, and does not appear to import amino acids (Gardner *et al.* 2002; Abrahamsen *et al.* 2004). Although *Cryptosporidium* has lost amino acid synthesis pathways, it has 'retained' the enzymes

Table 46.3 Physical characteristics and key features of the complete nuclear genomes for *Cryptosporidium parvum* (see Abrahamsen *et al.* 2004) and *Cryptosporidium hominis* (see Xu *et al.* 2004)

Nuclear Genomes		
	C. parvum	*C. hominis*
Size (Mbp)	~ 9.1	~ 9.2
Genes	~ 4,000	~ 4,000
Introns (%)	~ 5%	~ 5-20%
Non-coding (%)	~ 25–30%	~ 25–30%

Key features
No organellar genomes.
ATP production heavily reliant upon glycolysis.
Scavenges amino acids from host (limited or no amino acid synthesis pathways).
Has enzymes necessary to convert from one amino acid to another.
Scavenges nucleotides from the host (limited or no nucleotide synthesis pathways).
Can convert purines to pyrimidines and *vice versa*.
Has a single enzyme (inosine monophosphate dehydrogenase) for converting AMP to GMP.

necessary for the conversion of the amino acids from one type to another. Because *C. parvum* and *C. hominis* also appear to lack enzymes for the synthesis of nucleosides and nucleotides, they are thought to scavenge these from the host cell, but are able to convert pyrimidines to purines and purines to pyrimidines (Abrahamsen *et al.* 2004; Striepen *et al.* 2004; Xu *et al.* 2004). However, the purine salvage/conversion pathways in *Cryptosporidium* species appear to relate only to a single pathway (inosine monophosphate dehydrogenase) for the conversion of adenosine monophosphate (AMP) to guanosine monophosphate (GMP). The 'minimal' metabolic, catabolic and anabolic systems of *Cryptosporidium* indicate a reliance on importing essential metabolites from the host cell. The differences in the biosynthetic pathways between *Cryptosporidium* and the vertebrate host are relevant to drug development. In addition, evidence supporting the acquisition during evolution of genes of bacterial origin, such as the thymidine kinase gene (Striepen *et al.* 2004), points to enzymes which could be targeted also with therapeutic agents to kill the parasite without affecting the metabolism of the host (see section on Treatment, prevention and control).

The genome of *C. parvum* has been examined also for sequences encoding cystein-rich motifs, which typify oocyst wall proteins (Ranucci *et al.* 1993). This search led to the identification of a gene family encoding proteins localized to the oocyst wall (Templeton *et al.* 2004). As the oocyst wall confers the characteristic resistance of *Cryptosporidium* oocysts to various chemical disinfectants (Korich *et al.* 1990), research on the composition and biosynthesis of this wall has important practical implications.

Although the genomes available for *C. parvum* and *C. hominis* have been of great utility in elucidating much of the detail relating to *Cryptosporidium* metabolic and synthetic systems, additional nuclear genome sequencing projects of other species of *Cryptosporidium* (e.g. *C. muris*) are needed. The availability of such data would facilitate useful comparative genomic analyses, leading to a better understanding of the evolutionary relationships among species within the genus. In addition, such analyses would aid in the identification of genes which are conserved among species as well as genes which are under positive selection (i.e. specific to *Cryptosporidium* species and genotypes). A comparison of the genome of *C. muris* (which infects the stomach and is currently being sequenced (unpublished) with those of *C. parvum* and *C. hominis* (which infect the intestine) might also lead to the identification of genes which evolve in response to the adaptation of the parasite to different host environments and provide insight into the genetic differences between species which are infective to humans and species which are usually not. Such comparative studies could be useful for identifying anti-cryptosporidial drug targets, as they may uncover genes which are not found in the host, or have significantly diverged from the their homologues in the host, but are essential for parasite survival. To date, progress in genomic and transcriptomic studies for species and genotypes of *Cryptosporidium* has been slow; however, new and exciting developments in the field of highthroughput DNA sequencing (e.g. Bennett 2004; Margulies *et al.* 2005) bring promise for unheralded advances and likely represent the future for infectious disease research.

Genetics

Feng and coworkers (2002) demonstrated the feasibility of experimentally crossing two genetically distinct lines of *C. parvum* in mice using a similar approach as employed for crossing lines of the malaria parasite, *Plasmodium falciparum* (Walliker *et al.* 1987).

Immunosuppressed mice were co-infected with two genetically and phenotypically dissimilar lines of *C. parvum*, and progeny derived from this cross. The aim of the study of *P. falciparum*, to use linkage analysis to infer the chromosomal location of genes controlling specific traits, was accomplished by 'genotyping' multiple recombinant progeny lines and determining their phenotype. Based on this information, the chromosomal location of genes controlling specific traits, such as drug resistance, was determined (Wellems *et al.* 1990; Vaidya *et al.* 1995). The experimental approach used to cross *C. parvum* (see Feng *et al.* 2002) was simpler than that employed for *P. falciparum*, because the entire development, including meiosis, takes place within the same host. Therefore, the infection of mosquitoes, which is required for the crossing of malaria parasites, is not needed. On the other hand, genetic work with *Cryptosporidium* is made difficult by a lack of clearly defined phenotypes, such as growth rate in culture, virulence or drug resistance. Moreover, for the genetic approach to reach its full potential, methods for long-term storage (cryopreservation) of live *Cryptosporidium* lines are needed. In the absence of such methods, the maintenance and characterization of multiple progeny lines of *C. parvum* is a daunting task.

In the most extensive experiment published to date, two lines of *C. parvum* were crossed and 16 clonal progeny lines derived through multiple passages of individual oocysts in mice (Tanriverdi *et al.* 2007). The lines were genotyped using 40 unlinked genetic markers randomly distributed in the genome. By tabulating the number of meiotic cross-over events, which led to the generation of the progeny lines, a first estimate of cross-over activity (10–56 kb/centiMorgan) in *Cryptosporidium* was obtained (Tanriverdi *et al.* 2007). This estimate is within the range of the cross-over frequency found in other apicomplexan protozoa, including *P. falciparum* and *Toxoplasma gondii* (see Sibley *et al.* 1992; Su *et al.* 1999). The genotyping of recombinant progeny derived from the experimental crossing of *C. parvum* lines (Tanriverdi *et al.* 2007) revealed that a fragment of chromosome V was inherited from one parental line, in contrast to the other chromosomes which were inherited from both parents. These observations may indicate the existence of genes under positive selection in this chromosome. Because of the many manipulations that were needed to derive clonal progenies, it is, however, unclear what selective pressure led to the uniparental inheritance of the chromosome V region.

Future work will focus on identifying mechanisms which select for specific genotypes. A new method, termed Linkage Group Selection, was applied to the analysis of genetic crosses between lines of *P. chabaudi chabaudi* (see Culleton *et al.* 2005), and is currently being evaluated for the analysis of recombinant *C. parvum* progeny. Using this method, chromosomal regions which are under selection are identified by genotyping uncloned progeny populations selected for the trait of interest. It is possible to map genes controlling selectable traits, such as the early production of oocysts or drug resistance. Such analyses are expected to contribute to our understanding of the genetics and biology of these parasites and their interaction with the host.

The host

Humans

In humans, *Cryptosporidium hominis* has been identified as the causative agent of cryptosporidiosis in a significant proportion of infections (e.g. Xiao and Ryan, 2004a; Cacciò, 2005; Leoni *et al.* 2006) and, with few exceptions, is considered to be a highly host-specific parasite (Morgan-Ryan *et al.* 2002). However, limited data do indicate that *C. hominis* can complete its life-cycle other hosts, including livestock (Giles *et al.* 2001; Smith *et al.* 2005b). *Cryptosporidium parvum* is also a significant cause of human cryptosporidiosis (Xiao and Ryan 2004a; Cacciò, 2005). Unlike *C. hominis*, *C. parvum* has a broad host range (Xiao *et al.* 2004), including livestock, companion animals and numerous species of wildlife, which can potentially act as zoonotic reservoirs, although cattle have been recognized specifically as being of most importance in this regard (Hunter and Thompson 2005; Smith and Nichols 2006; Xiao and Feng 2008). Additional species/genotypes (e.g. *C. meleagridis*, *C. felis*, *C. canis*, *C. muris*, *C. suis* and 'cervine and monkey' genotypes of *Cryptosporidium*) have been reported to infect people but are significantly less common (Xiao *et al.* 2001; Chalmers *et al.* 2002; Leoni *et al.* 2006) and are likely to be of lesser zoonotic importance. However, the impact of these 'less common' species/genotypes on the immunocompromised, particularly in developing countries, has not been fully examined and requires further study.

Immunocompetent individuals

Cryptosporidium is a frequent cause of acute, self-limiting gastroenteritis in humans (Kosek *et al.* 2001; Medema *et al.* 2006), although many asymptomatic infections have been detected as well (e.g. Roberts *et al.* 1989; Fafard and Lalonde 1990). In symptomatic cases, clinical signs usually commence 1 to 12 days (mean 7.2 days) after the ingestion of infective oocysts (Jokipii *et al.* 1983; Jokipii and Jokipii 1986) and can include abdominal pain, anorexia, diarrhoea, flatulence, malabsorption, malaise, mild fever, nausea, vomiting and/or weight loss (Fayer and Ungar 1986) with growing evidence that some symptomatic manifestations (e.g. vomiting) are species and/or genotype specific (e.g. Cama *et al.* 2008). Infected individuals may defaecate between two and > 20 times a day, producing watery, light-coloured, stools containing mucus (Casemore 1987). Illness usually has a mean duration of approximately one to three weeks, with a range of one to 44 days (Elsser *et al.* 1986; Jokipii and Jokipii 1986; Heijbel *et al.* 1987; Richardson *et al.* 1991). Although, chronic infections have been reported in otherwise healthy humans (Phillips *et al.* 1992; Rey *et al.* 2004), infections are usually eliminated through the stimulation of an immune response (see section on Immunity). In children, infection with *Cryptosporidium* can result in reduced growth and impaired physical fitness and sometimes impaired cognitive function, which, particularly for cryptosporidiosis in infants, can permanently impair development (Dillingham *et al.* 2002; Ricci *et al.* 2006).

Illness and oocyst excretion patterns can vary considerably among infected individuals due to host factors (including immune status; Lazar and Radulescu 1989; Goodgame *et al.* 1993) and parasite factors (such as origin and age of oocysts, the species/genotype, virulence and/or infective dose; Okhuysen *et al.* 1999; Cama *et al.* 2007). The excretion of oocysts in the faeces usually commences less than 3 to 30 days (mean = 12 days) following the ingestion of infective oocysts and usually coincides with the presence of clinical signs of disease (Jokipii and Jokipii 1986). However, oocyst excretion may continue for up to two months after the disappearance of such clinical signs (Jokipii and Jokipii 1986; Soave and Armstrong 1986). Conversely, intermittent periods with no detectable oocyst excretion in faeces have been observed in patients with clinical signs of disease (Jokipii and Jokipii 1986).

Immunocompromised individuals

Although the impact of cryptosporidiosis on immunocompetent hosts can be severe clinically, it is usually limited by the host immune response. In contrast, the disease in immunocompromised patients can be chronic and potentially fatal. In individuals with HIV/AIDS, other acquired abnormalities of T lymphocytes, congenital hypogammaglobulinaemia, severe combined immunodeficiency (SCID) syndrome, those receiving immunosuppressive treatments or those with severe malnutrition, clinical signs of cryptosporidiosis usually include frequent episodes of watery diarrhoea (six to 25 times per day, passing between one and 20 litres per day (Soave and Johnson 1998), colic (cramping and upper abdominal pains, often following meals), profound weight loss, weakness, malaise, anorexia and low-grade fever (Hunter and Nichols 2002). Infection in immunocompromised individuals can invade the mucosal layers of any region of the gastrointestinal tract, including the pharynx, oesophagus, stomach, duodenum, jejunum, ileum, appendix, colon, rectum, gall bladder, bile duct, pancreatic duct and/or the bronchial tree (e.g. Hunter and Nichols 2002). Individuals with CD4+ T-cell counts of < 150/ml invariably develop persistent infection with profound and life-threatening diarrhoea (Flanigan *et al.* 1992). Chronic infections (lasting months to years) in individuals with an acquired (Blanshard *et al.* 1992) or congenital (Hayward *et al.* 1997) immunodeficiency often spread from the intestine to the hepatobiliary and pancreatic ducts, causing cholangiohepatitis, cholecystitis, choledochitis or pancreatitis (see section on Pathogenesis). Except for individuals whose immune status can be enhanced, clinical cryptosporidiosis can be fatal (Soave and Armstrong 1986). Cryptosporidiosis in immunocompromised or immunodeficient patients is a major, life-threatening disease, causing profuse, intractable diarrhoea with severe dehydration, malabsorption, malnutrition and wasting and often being associated with infections by other opportunistic pathogens (e.g. Weber *et al.* 1993; Scaglia *et al.* 1994; Soave and Johnson 1998).

Pathogenesis

Cryptosporidium infection usually impacts most directly and severely on the gastric and/or intestinal tract (Table 46.4), depending upon the parasite species (see section on, Location and establishment in the host). Although all of the known species of *Cryptosporidium* parasitic in humans are usually 'colonizers' of the intestine (Xiao *et al.* 2004), gastric cryptosporidiosis has been reported in rare instances and is usually confined to immunocompromised individuals (cf. Hunter and Nichols 2002). In such cases, combined endoscopic and histopathological examination of the epithelial tissues reveals relatively non-specific lesions and oedema (associated with general gastritis) as well as hyperplasia of the epithelial cells and inflammation of the connective tissues of the lamina propria (Rivasi *et al.* 1999). Similar findings have been made upon histological examination of the stomach wall of nude mice (Taylor *et al.* 1999), and the abomasum in otherwise healthy cattle (Masuno *et al.* 2006) with gastric cryptosporidiosis.

Cryptosporidial infection in the intestine is well characterized and is initiated when 'zoites infect vicinal enterocytes and endogenous forms spread to the enterocytes of both the villi and crypts (Current *et al.* 1983). The extent of spread and the sites involved

Table 46.4 Key pathological changes reported to be associated with various common manifestations of human cryptosporidiosis

Infection	Salient pathological changes described	Key refs
Pulmonary	Inflammation and fibrosis of the bronchial epithelia; Loss of epithelial cilia; Thickening of the lung parenchyma; Presence of thick mucus and lesions in the bronchial sacs.	(Tarwid et al. 1985; Blagburn et al. 1987)
Gastric	Non-specific lesions and oedema; Hyperplasia of the epithelial cells; Inflammation of the lamina propria.	(Rivasi et al. 1999; Taylor et al. 1999; Masuno et al. 2006)
Intestinal	Loss of mature enterocytes; Villius atrophy; Lengthening of crypts (hyperplasia); Oedema; Loss of membrane-bound digestive enzymes; Diminished absorptive surface of the intestine.	(Inman and Takeuchi, 1979; Tzipori et al. 1981; Pearson and Logan 1983)
Pancreatic	Dilation of the pancreatic duct; Formation of hyperplasic lesions; Thickening of the epithelium.	(Cappell and Hassan 1993)

determine whether the infection is clinical or subclinical, as well as the overall intensity of the disease (Tzipori and Ward 2002). Severe and watery diarrhoea occurs mainly as a result of infection of the proximal small intestine, whereas infections confined to the distal ileum and/or the large bowel tend to be associated with intermittent diarrhoea or can be asymptomatic (Tzipori and Ward 2002). Endogenous forms of *Cryptosporidium* disrupt the microvillus border, which leads to the loss of mature enterocytes, a shortening and/or fusion of the villi and a lengthening of the crypts due to increased cell division (leading to hyperplasia) and oedema (e.g. Inman and Takeuchi 1979; Tzipori et al. 1981; Pearson and Logan 1983). This leads to the loss of membrane-bound digestive enzymes, diminishes the absorptive surface of the intestine and reduces the uptake of fluids, electrolytes and nutrients from the intestinal lumen (Argenzio et al. 1990; Adams et al. 1994; Griffiths et al. 1994). There is also a significant degree of inflammation due to local cellular infiltrates as a process of the host immune response (see section on Immunity).

Extra-gastrointestinal cryptosporidiosis, though apparently less common than gastric or intestinal infections, does occur in both immunocompetent (Westrope and Acharya 2001) and immunocompromised hosts (Bonacini 1992; Vakil et al. 1996), though more frequently in the latter. Extra-gastrointestinal infections can be divided into pulmonary cryptosporidiosis, which can occur in the absence of a gastric or intestinal infection (Clavel et al. 1996), and biliary or pancreatic cryptosporidiosis (Goodwin 1991; Forbes et al. 1993; Vakil et al. 1996; Calzetti et al. 1997), which appears to be the result of secondary colonization following an initial gastric

or intestinal infection (see section on Location and establishment in the host).

In birds, pulmonary cryptosporidiosis can be caused by *C. baileyi* infection (Blagburn et al. 1987; Lindsay et al. 1987). Examination of respiratory cryptosporidiosis in broiler chickens experimentally infected (either orally or intratracheally) with *C. baileyi* oocysts, revealed, upon necropsy, an overall 'greying and thickening' (presumably carnification) of the lung parenchyma, the presence of thick mucus and lesions in the air sacs, epithelial hyperplasia in the bronchi and a loss of cilia on the epithelial surfaces (Blagburn et al. 1987). Similar changes have been observed in turkeys with natural *C. baileyi* infection (Tarwid et al. 1985). Experimentally induced pulmonary cryptosporidiosis (*via* oral inoculation) in rat models revealed the formation of granulomata containing oocysts, as well as inflammation and fibrosis in the airways (Asaad and Sadek 2006).

Biliary or pancreatic cryptosporidiosis in humans appears to result from the systemic spread of gastric or intestinal infections (see section on Location and establishment in the host) and is considered to be more common in immunocompromised hosts (Bonacini 1992; Vakil et al. 1996), but can also occur in immunocompetent people (Verdon et al. 1998; Westrope and Acharya 2001). Ultrasonic examination of AIDS patients with biliary cryptosporidiosis has revealed a generalized dilation of the bile duct and gall bladder, an increase in the presence of pericholecystic fluid, and a thickening of the epithelium (Dolmatch et al. 1987; McCarty et al. 1989; Teixidor et al. 1991). Experimentally induced biliary cryptosporidiosis in chickens (by oral inoculation) has been reported to be associated with the formation of hyperplasic lesions within the bile duct and gall bladder as well as mononuclear leukocyte infiltration of the underlying connective tissues (Hatkin et al. 1990). Similar pathological changes have also been detected in the pancreatic ducts of AIDS patients as a result of pancreatic cryptosporidiosis (Cappell and Hassan 1993).

The pathogenesis of cryptosporidiosis appears to be associated with the effects of parasite products, such as serine and cysteine proteinases, on epithelial layers (Rosenthal 1999), and with both inflammatory and immunological responses in the host (see section on Immunity) (Savioli et al. 2006). Thickening of the epithelia of infected organs might be, in part, the result of scarring induced by the infection of the host cells during the life-cycle of the parasite (see section on Life-cycle biology), and an effect of *Cryptosporidium*-induced host cell mitosis (Wages and Ficken 1989; Hatkin et al. 1990; Masuno et al. 2006), believed to be linked to the nutrient requirements of the parasite (see section on Growth and survival *in vitro*).

The pathophysiology of diarrhoea is considered to be multifactorial, resulting from infection of enterocytes by zoites, loss of intestinal surface area for absorption due to 'carpeting' of the luminal surface by parasites, cellular destruction following schizogony and gametogony of *Cryptosporidium*, villus fusion and atrophy, and reduced enzyme synthesis in the epithelium and associated electrolyte and nutrient malabsorption (Inman and Takeuchi 1979; Tzipori et al. 1981; Pearson and Logan 1983; Buret et al. 2003). Chloride secretion in the gut due to *Cryptosporidium* enterotoxigenic insult has been proposed also as a mechanism linked to diarrhoea. Confirmation of this hypothesis appears to have been found in the form of "Substance P", a neurokinin-1 receptor antagonist which has been linked to the severity of diarrhoeal symptoms associated with cryptosporidiosis (Sonea et al. 2002; Robinson et al.

2003) and appears to directly affect both chloride ion secretion and glucose absorption (Hernandez *et al.* 2007). The attachment of *C. parvum* sporozoites to the apex of enterocytes may also contribute to the inducement of diarrhoea. Sporozoite attachment is a complex process, involving multiple parasite ligands and host receptors, and inducing reorganization of the host cell actin cytoskeleton (reviewed by Smith *et al.* 2005a) which impacts upon host cell function. Indeed, cryptosporidial infection has been demonstrated to have consequent effects on enterocyte apoptotic pathways (e.g. Chen *et al.* 1999; Ojcius *et al.* 1999), as well as enterocyte integrity and function (Argenzio *et al.* 1990).

The pathophysiology of diarrhoea as a result of cryptosporidiosis may also be linked to the loss of intestinal barrier function due to the *Cryptosporidium*-induced disruption of epithelial permeability (Savioli *et al.* 2006). Decreased intestinal barrier function appears to be due, in part, to disruptions of zonula–occludens (ZO)-1, a 220 kDa cytoperipheral protein which acts as a physical bridge between tight junction occludin and cytoskeletal F-actin (Balda and Anderson 1993; Fanning *et al.* 1998). Indeed, it has been reported that endogenous stages of *C. andersoni* induce the disruption of epithelial tight junctions and cause apoptosis in enterocytes *in vitro* (Buret *et al.* 2003). Furthermore, the administration

of 'apical epidermal growth factor' has been shown to inhibit *Cryptosporidium*-induced apoptosis and the disruption of ZO-1, and significantly reduced the percentage of cells infected in human or bovine cell lines and the impact that infection had upon the integrity of the cell layers in each culture, independent of any direct microbiocidal action (Buret *et al.* 2003). However, whether apoptotic change and the disruption of ZO-1 result in functional abnormalities of intestinal barrier function *in vivo* requires further investigation (Buret *et al.* 2003).

Immunity

The body of knowledge of the immunology of *Cryptosporidium* infection (reviewed by Gomez Morales and Pozio 2002; Riggs 2002; Deng *et al.* 2004) relates mainly to infection studies in mice, although valuable observations have come from studies of humans and large animals. The *in vitro* infection of cultured monolayers of mammalian cell lines with *C. parvum* (see Current and Haynes 1984) has also been an important tool for immunological investigations (see section on Growth and survival *in vitro*).

The innate immune response that develops rapidly after most infections is important in the establishment of immunity to *Cryptosporidium* (Fig. 46.5). Enterocytes and natural killer (NK)

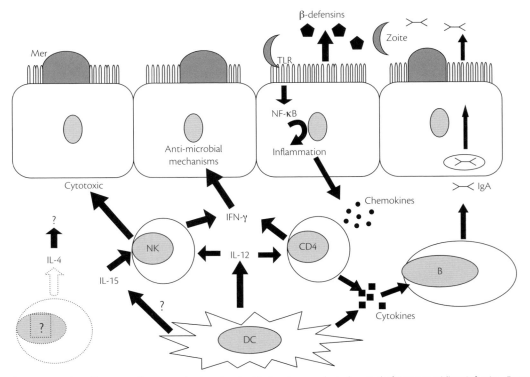

Fig. 46.5 Diagrammatic representation of immune effector mechanisms involved in host immunological control of *Cryptosporidium* infection. Extracellular sporozoites and merozoites (zoites) in the gut lumen may be inactivated by parasite-specific secretory IgA or antimicrobial peptides such as β-defensins released by epithelial cells. Sporozoites invading epithelial cells activate innate immune responses of the host cells through interaction with TLRs such as TLR4, resulting in activation of the transcription factor NF-κB. This leads to release of chemokines and an inflammatory response that attracts immune cells into the lamina propria. In the inflammatory situation DCs produce cytokines including IL-12 that activate NK cells and antigen-specific CD4+ T cells to produce the Th1 cytokine IFN-γ. The CD4+T cells are required to overcome infection and IFN-γ produced by these cells is probably a major factor in protective immunity. IFN-γ induces antimicrobial killing mechanisms by epithelial cells that prevent proliferation of meronts (mer). NK cells may develop cytotoxicity against infected cells that is enhanced by IL-15. Th2 cytokines such as IL-4 may also have a protective role although the cellular source and protective function of this cytokine is unclear. B cells activated by cytokines and contact with DCs and CD4+ T cells manufacture IgA that is transported across epithelial cells and released into the lumen.

cells have important, distinctive roles in the innate response. Following infection with *C. parvum*, enterocyte lines produce various chemokines, including Regulated upon Activation, Normal T-cell Expressed, and Secreted (RANTES) chemokines, monocyte chemotactic protein 1 (MCP-1) and interferon-inducible protein 10 (IP-10), that play an important role in initiating the intestinal inflammatory response (Lacroix-Lamonde *et al.* 2002). This activation may involve Toll-like receptors (TLR) expressed by enterocytes and other cells involved in immune responses, including dendritic cells. TLRs are sensors of infection that interact with conserved molecular structures of microbial pathogens (e.g. bacterial lipopolysaccharide or microbial DNA (Abreu *et al.* 2005)). TLR ligation with *C. parvum* sporozoites activates nuclear factor (NF)-κβ, a transcription factor involved in the expression of many inflammatory molecules, including chemokines (Chen *et al.* 2001; Chen *et al.* 2005). The parasite molecules that induce activation *via* TLRs are not known. *Cryptosporidium parvum* infection also induces the expression of the anti-microbial peptide β-defensin-2 (Zaalouk *et al.* 2004) *via* TLR ligation (Chen *et al.* 2005) and β-densin-1 and -2 are able to kill *C. parvum* sporozoites or prevent host cell invasion (Zaalouk *et al.* 2004). Enterocyte lines stimulated by pro-inflammatory cytokines, including interferon (IFN)-γ, that are expressed in the gut following *C. parvum* infection have been shown to generate other antimicrobial killing mechanisms effective against this parasite (Pollok *et al.* 2001).

NK cells are important in the early 'control' of infection caused by different types of intracellular microbial pathogens. These cells produce inflammatory cytokines, particularly IFN-γ, and may have cytolytic activity against infected cells. NK cells are activated by cytokines, including IL-12 produced by dendritic cells or macrophages stimulated by parasite antigens (Lodoen and Lanier 2006). Studies of SCID mice, which lack T and B cells but have normal NK cells, showed that *C. parvum* infection was initially maintained at a low level by an IFN-γ-dependent mechanism (McDonald and Bancroft 1994). The administration of IL-12 to neonatal SCID mice conferred resistance to infection associated with increased intestinal expression of IFN-γ (Urban *et al.* 1996). McDonald *et al.* (2000) showed, through the experimental inducement of IFN-γ production in cultured spleen cells from SCID mice by the addition of *C. parvum* antigen, that NK cells are the most likely source of IFN-γ. Another study (Dann *et al.* 2005) has indicated that NK cells from human peripheral blood treated with IL-15, a cytokine important for maturation and activation of these cells, induced cytotoxicity against enterocytes infected with *C. parvum*.

Although innate immunity has a clear role in suppressing the reproduction of *Cryptosporidium*, the elimination of infection requires an adaptive immune response. Mice lacking T cells, or the T helper (Th) CD4+ T cell subpopulation that orchestrates the adaptive immune response, were unable to eliminate cryptosporidial infection (Heine *et al.* 1984; Aguirre *et al.* 1994). Severe and often fatal cryptosporidial infections in AIDS patients have been associated with low numbers of CD4+ T cells (Blanshard *et al.* 1992). In addition, the protective immune response to *C. parvum* infection in cattle has been shown to correlate with an influx of CD4+ and cytotoxic CD8+ T cells into the intestine (Abrahamsen *et al.* 1997). However, studies of mice showed that depletion of CD8+ T cells had no effect on the intensity of cryptosporidial infection or increased susceptibility only moderately (Aguirre *et al.* 1994; McDonald and Bancroft 1994). The type of T cell receptor

(TCR) is also important in establishing immunity; transgenic mice lacking T cells with TCRαβ that are activated by peptide antigens do not suppress infection, whereas a deficiency in cells with TCRγδ that may be activated by peptide or non-peptide antigens (e.g. lipids), only increases susceptibility to infection in neonatal mice (Waters and Harp 1996).

The mechanisms by which CD4+ T cells lead to the elimination of the infection are not entirely clear but cytokines play a major part. Parasite antigen-specific CD4+ T cells from mice and humans recovering from infection produce IFN-γ (Harp *et al.* 1994; Gomez Morales *et al.* 1999). Knock-out mice lacking IFN-γ or IL-12 (the latter is important in inducing IFN-γ production by T cells) have been shown to have increased *Cryptosporidium* infection intensity as compared with wild-type mice, and infection in IFN-γ deficient mice was fatal in some studies (Mead and You 1998; Theodos 1998). The requirement of IFN-γ and IL-12 for the rapid clearance of infection is indicative that a cell-mediated or Th1 response is involved. Whether there is any involvement of a humoral/allergic (i.e. Th2-type response), involving cytokines such as IL-4, IL-5 and IL-13, is less clear. There are contradictory findings regarding the protective role of IL-4 (Aguirre *et al.* 1998; McDonald *et al.* 2004), but one investigation indicated that IL-5 was involved in immunity (Enriquez and Sterling 1993). There is little histological evidence for mastocytosis or eosinophilia linked to cryptosporidiosis, suggesting that a typical allergic response is absent (Tzipori 1988).

Cryptosporidium infection of humans and animals induces a serum and mucosal antibody response (Ungar *et al.* 1986; Peeters *et al.* 1992). Parasite-specific IgG, IgM and secretory IgA antibodies have been detected, commencing a few days after infection. Furthermore, the specific IgG response has been found to continue for long periods after the cessation of clinical signs of disease (Ungar *et al.* 1986). Some experimental studies in rodents have shown that passive transfer of secretory IgA from the bile of previously infected animals conferred passive immunity to *Cryptosporidium* in recipients (Albert *et al.* 1994). However, studies using B cell-deficient mice have indicated that B cells, and therefore antibodies, were not essential for the suppression of cryptosporidial infection (Takhi-Kilani *et al.* 1990; Chen *et al.* 2003). Also, colostrum from female mice repeatedly infected with *C. parvum* did not protect offspring from infection (Moon *et al.* 1988), and the detection of colostral antibodies in calf faeces did not appear to be associated with protective immunity (Peeters *et al.* 1992). Epidemiological studies in humans on the protective effect of breast feeding against cryptosporidiosis have provided conflicting results (Molbak *et al.* 1994; Nchito *et al.* 1998).

Although parasite-specific antibodies generated by cryptosporidial infection may not be necessary for establishment of adaptive immunity, a moderate to high degree of passive immunity has been achieved in hosts after oral administration of colostrum or colostral antibodies from cattle immunized mucosally with oocyst antigens plus adjuvant (Tzipori *et al.* 1986; Fayer *et al.* 1989a, b). This form of passive immunization in domesticated animals could help to reduce the infection levels in farm animals, which might have a favourable impact on the environment by reducing oocyst contamination and the transmission of cryptosporidiosis.

In summary, the immunological control of cryptosporidial infection comprises both innate and adaptive host responses (Fig. 46.5). Epithelial cells and NK cells may be important in innate immunity, while adaptive immunity required for elimination of the parasite is coordinated by CD4+ T cells. IFN-γ produced by both T cells and NK cells may be crucial for establishing immunity early during infection.

Epidemiology

Occurrence and distribution

Cryptosporidium is global in distribution and causes human cryptosporidiosis in both urban and rural settings in developed and developing countries (Medema *et al.* 2006). However, the application of molecular tools (allowing specific and subspecific identification and differentiation) has revealed that the distribution of cryptosporidiosis is not homogenous.

The epidemiology of this disease varies spatially and temporally (esp. seasonally). Data from some countries in temperate climatic zones show a bi-modal pattern in the distribution of cases, with a spring peak in prevalence, followed by a second peak in late-summer/early-autumn (Meinhardt *et al.* 1996). Temporal peaks in prevalence are variable in severity and timing. Changes may reflect rainfall levels, agricultural events and practices (calving or lambing; slurry or manure spreading), seasonal human behaviour (holidays or recreational activities), and changes to local health management practices, such as water quality regulations (Smerdon *et al.* 2003; Sopwith *et al.* 2005; Lake *et al.* 2007). In the UK, the spring peak has been linked to *C. parvum* and the summer/autumn peak largely to *C. hominis* (see McLauchlin *et al.* 2000). Similar patterns in the number of cases and the distribution of *Cryptosporidium* species have been reported in other temperate climates (Learmonth *et al.* 2004) and emphasize the importance of both livestock and humans as reservoirs, and water as a 'vehicle' for transmission to humans. Peaks of cryptosporidiosis have also been observed in tropical countries and appear to coincide with the rainy season (Mata 1986); however, dry weather may force the use of poor quality, contaminated water, also leading to disease outbreaks.

The use of variable molecular markers, such as in the 60 kilodalton glycoprotein (*gp60*) gene and mini- and microsatellites (see section on Diagnosis and genetic analysis), has revealed differences in subspecific population genetic structuring in various geographical regions, indicating relative differences in epidemiology in some human populations (reviewed by Jex and Gasser 2010). However, local epidemiological factors (e.g. proximity to farms and water treatment practices) may effect zoonotic transmission (e.g. Sopwith *et al.* 2005) and can impact on the genetic substructuring of *Cryptosporidium* populations in human populations at local levels. For example, *gp60* sequence data for *Cryptosporidium* isolates from Kuwait (Sulaiman *et al.* 2005) have revealed a greater representation of 'zoonotic' *C. parvum* lineages linked to sporadic human cryptosporidiosis, suggesting a larger contribution of animal sources to human infection. In the UK, where *C. hominis* accounts for similar numbers of cases as *C. parvum* (see Chalmers and Pollock 2007; Nichols 2008), zoonotic risks have been identified epidemiologically for some strains of *C. parvum* which have been found more frequently than anthroponotic lineages (Hunter *et al.* 2007). Both outbreaks and sporadic infections in countries, such as Australia (Jex *et al.* 2007a; Jex *et al.* 2008a), France (Cohen *et al.* 2006) and in some areas of the USA (Sulaiman *et al.* 2001; Zhou *et al.* 2003), indicate a greater representation of *C. hominis* and/or 'human-affiliated' *C. parvum* lineages in human populations, suggesting a more significant anthroponotic contribution to disease

transmission in these areas. These apparent geographical variations in epidemiology may arise from the sampling frame of the study but may also relate partly to differences to health and resource management practices in different regions, as evidenced by the decreased prevalence of *C. parvum* in humans in the north western part of England, linked to changes to the municipal management of water supplies (Sopwith *et al.* 2005).

Prevalence of infection

The prevalence of cryptosporidiosis is usually estimated based on routine surveillance of human populations or examination of clinical records. However, as the clinical signs of cryptosporidiosis do not allow an unequivocal diagnosis, laboratory-based testing is required (see section on Diagnosis and genetic analysis). The relative prevalence of clinical cryptosporidiosis in human populations can be influenced by seasonality of other enteropathogens (see Weber *et al.* 1993) and obscured by 'ascertainment bias' due to selective submission and testing of faecal samples and limitations of available diagnostic tools (see section on Diagnosis and genetic analysis). Despite this, some prevalence data from human populations, particularly in developed countries, are available. A study in Canada by Ratnam *et al.* (1985) examined faecal smears (submitted for routine microbiological examination) from 1,621 humans and found that *Cryptosporidium* spp. were present in ~ 1.2% (n = 19) of samples. A much larger study, conducted by 16 public health laboratories (the Public Health Laboratory Service Study Group (PHLSSG)) in England and Wales (PHLSSG 1990), over a period of two years, examined enteric pathogens in 62 421 patients with diarrhoea, and detected *Cryptosporidium* at a prevalence of ~ 2.0% (ranging from 0.5–3.9% among all laboratories), thus representing the third most common cause of diarrhoea (1295 cases), after *Campylobacter* (4775 cases) and *Salmonella* (1980 cases). In addition, this study provided some evidence of a relationship between prevalence of infection and host age. The prevalence of *Cryptosporidium* was highest in children aged 1–4 years (~ 4.9%) and slightly lower in children aged 5–14 years (~ 4.4%); there was a gradual decrease in prevalence with increasing host age (PHLSSG 1990). However, data from clinical studies (e.g. Ratnam *et al.* 1985; PHLSSG 1990) may not represent accurate estimations of the 'actual' prevalence levels of *Cryptosporidium* in human populations, as data are drawn from a 'biased' subset of patients seeking medical attention and, thus, may not be representative of the entire human population.

Much less is known about the prevalence of human cryptosporidiosis in developing countries, where often the infrastructure for large-scale epidemiological studies is lacking and where limited availability of safe drinking water (Fig. 46.6A, in the colour plate section) and adequate sanitation services mean that potential sources and causes of disease are many (Medema *et al.* 2006). The impact of cryptosporidiosis in such regions is further compounded by the high rate of HIV infection (Fig. 46.6B, in the colour plate section), and the associated high rates of AIDS due to a deficiency in the availability of effective anti-retroviral treatments in poorer nations, leading to an increased susceptibility to cryptosporidial infection (see Navin *et al.* 1999; Inungu *et al.* 2000; Hunter and Nichols 2002). In developing countries, several focal studies have indicated that the prevalence of *Cryptosporidium* in humans is highly variable and can range from ~ 4.2%–60% (Chacin-Bonilla *et al.* 1993; Javier Enriquez *et al.* 1997; Tumwine *et al.* 2003;

Steinberg *et al.* 2004; Gatei *et al.* 2006; Teixeira *et al.* 2007). A recent review of the literature available for South-east Asia (Lim *et al.* 2010) indicated, not unexpectedly, that socioeconomic wealth, specific health policy (e.g. routine testing for and reporting of *Cryptosporidium* infection) and access to modern waste disposal infrastructure, can greatly affect relative prevalence of disease (e.g. in urban *versus* rural populations), as can specific local factors which increase the likelihood of exposure (e.g. the use of human wastes as fertilizer in peri-urban farm systems). Expanded study of the prevalence and transmission of cryptosporidiosis among humans and between humans and animals in much of the developing world is urgently needed (e.g. for many countries and regions in Africa, Asia and South America; see Jex and Gasser (2010)).

Estimating the prevalence of cryptosporidiosis is challenging. Many diagnostic methods lack sensitivity, leading to false negative results in patients excreting few oocysts at the time of testing (see section on Diagnosis and genetic analysis). The recent application of sensitive and specific PCR-based methods indicates that false negative diagnoses have been made in at least half of all cases of human cryptosporidiosis using conventional, microscopic tests (Amar *et al.* 2007). 'Ascertainment bias', at all stages, from the patient through to reporting of diagnoses leads to an underestimation of the prevalence of disease. In a study of infectious intestinal diseases, undertaken in England between 1993 and 1996 using conventional (microscopic) diagnostic methods, it was estimated that for every confirmed case of cryptosporidiosis reported to national surveillance, there were 7.4 additional cases in the community (Adak *et al.* 2002). In addition, even if laboratory testing and reporting practices are the same, the annual prevalence of cryptosporidiosis may vary widely, reflecting differences in exposure and host immunity or a combination of these factors (Baxby and Hart 1986; Moodley *et al.* 1991; Iqbal *et al.* 2001). Reports from diagnostic laboratories usually reflect only the prevalence in patients exhibiting clinical signs of gastrointestinal disease and not the prevalence of the parasite in the population as a whole. All of these factors can significantly affect the estimation of the prevalence of *Cryptosporidium* infection in human populations. Thus, it is important to recognize that the estimates of the prevalence of cryptosporidiosis are skewed reflections of the actual prevalence of the disease and may not reflect the occurrence of the parasite in the community. The prevalence of *Cryptosporidium* in asymptomatic people, particularly in immunocompetent, healthy children, has been reported to range from 0 to 6.4% in developed countries (Vuorio *et al.* 1991; Pettoello-Mantovani *et al.* 1995) and from 2.3 to 7.5% in developing countries (Solorzano-Santos *et al.* 2000; Al-Braiken *et al.* 2003; Palit *et al.* 2005).

Risk groups

Reviews and analyses of case reports, surveillance data and outbreaks of cryptosporidiosis have identified the following groups to be at the greatest risk of infection by *Cryptosporidium*: neonatal, farmed animals, young children and susceptible adults, those exposed through occupational and recreational activities (e.g. veterinarians, farmers, visitors to petting farms, international travellers, infants attending day-care centres), and immunocompromised patients (see Nichols 2008). Risk factors for the acquisition of cryptosporidiosis by the human population have been identified in a limited number of reviews and case-controlled studies (Lima and Guerrant 1992; Weinstein *et al.* 1993; Anon. 1995; Robertson *et al.* 2002; Goh *et al.* 2004; Hunter *et al.* 2004). In a case-study of

sporadic cryptosporidiosis in humans in Australia, swimming in public pools and contact with a person with diarrhoea were interpreted to be important risk factors associated with infection (Robertson *et al.* 2002). According to Hunter *et al.* (2004), in England and Wales, the variables independently associated with illness were:

- Travelling outside of the UK,
- Having contact with another person with diarrhoea,
- Having direct contact with cattle,
- Helping a child (< 5 years of age) to use a toilet,
- Drinking tap water.

For *C. hominis* infection, the highly significant risk factors were: travelling abroad, and changing diapers of children (< 5 years of age) (Hunter *et al.* 2004). For *C. parvum* infection, the major risk factor associated with illness was having direct contact with farm animals (Hunter *et al.* 2004). Environmental and social factors (cf. Lim *et al.* 2010) influencing cryptosporidiosis have been identified as: socioeconomic status; presence of many individuals < 4 years of age; inhabiting regions with high estimates of *Cryptosporidium* in manure applied to land; and inhabiting areas with inadequate water treatment practices (Lake *et al.* 2007).

Despite the apparent association between increased risk of cryptosporidial infection and frequency of contact with young children (Hunter *et al.* 2004), there is presently insufficient evidence to establish whether cryptosporidiosis in humans is age-limited (e.g. as the result of acquired immunity). A study in the UK (Thomas *et al.* 1990), examining 92 cases of sporadic human cryptosporidiosis, showed that ~ 66% of cases (n = 33 of 49) were in young children (aged 1–5 years), suggesting a greater propensity for infection in this age cohort. The high prevalence of cryptosporidiosis in young children is also supported by ongoing surveillance data (Nichols 2008). However, it is possible that young children in developed countries are at a higher risk of infection than adults, due to increased rates of exposure as a result of behavioural factors (e.g. poorer hygiene). Thomas *et al.* (1990) did not show conclusive data to indicate that acquired, protective immunity developed later in life, as ~ 33% of the cases of cryptosporidiosis were in adults (n = 16 of 49). In addition, in developed countries, a significant, relative increase in cryptosporidiosis in adults is often observed in outbreaks associated with drinking water (MacKenzie *et al.* 1994; Meinhardt *et al.* 1996), suggesting a lack of acquired immunity. In contrast, studies in developing countries indicate that cryptosporidiosis is most common in children of < 1 year of age, providing circumstantial evidence of acquired immunity later in life (Pereira *et al.* 2002; Hamedi *et al.* 2005).

A number of studies (e.g. Frost *et al.* 2000; Frost *et al.* 2002) have detected serological evidence of circulating anti-*Cryptosporidium* antibodies in humans, indicating prior exposure to *Cryptosporidium*, with no evidence of patent infection. At least one study inferred a decreased susceptibility to *C. parvum* infection in humans with prior repeated, low-level exposure to this parasite (Chappell *et al.* 1999). However, few studies have examined the link between specific serum anti-*Cryptosporidium* antibody levels and immunity. A recent report (Frost *et al.* 2005) provided the first evidence of a positive link between a strong serological response to *Cryptosporidium* antigens and protective immunity, as indicated by a decrease in the severity of clinical disease. Such studies, though few, suggest the development of acquired immunity to *Cryptosporidium* in humans following sufficiently frequent, intermittent exposure to oocysts. It is possible that acquired immunity to *Cryptosporidium* (with increased host age) is not found in humans in developed countries due to a lack of sufficiently frequent exposure to viable oocysts. As such, it may be that acquired immunity is more common where exposure rates are likely to be relatively high, which is supported by the finding that, in developing countries, most *Cryptosporidium* infections occur in infants rather than in adults (Pereira *et al.* 2002; Hamedi *et al.* 2005). However, broad-scale epidemiological surveys in such regions are lacking and are thus required.

Regardless of geographical location, immunocompromised and/or severely malnourished people represent the host cohort that is most at risk to *Cryptosporidium* infection (Hunter and Nichols 2002). Cryptosporidiosis is most severe in patients with profound T-cell immunodeficiency, particularly the following groups: HIV-infected with CD4 counts of < 200/ml (and particularly < 50/ml); acute leukaemia or lymphoma patients, particularly children; and those with primary T-cell immune-deficiencies, such as SCID; and, in males, X-linked hyperimmunoglobulin M (hyper-IgM) syndrome resulting from CD40 ligand deficiency (see section on Immunity). Such patients can develop chronic diarrhoeal disease and/or atypical extra-gastrointestinal disease, such as cholangitis, cirrhosis, cholecystitis, hepatitis and pancreatitis, often resulting in death (see section on Pathology). Severe malnourishment (Sallon *et al.* 1988; Sarabia-Arce *et al.* 1990) and/or old age (Gerba *et al.* 1996; Neill *et al.* 1996) can also result in increased susceptibility to infection and increased severity of cryptosporidiosis, likely due to an immunocompromised state.

Transmission

Although *Cryptosporidium* has a monoxenous life-cycle, transmission can be direct or indirect. 'Direct' transmission (e.g. person-to-person or animal-to-person contact) is facilitated by the immediate maturity of sporozoites and infective potential of *Cryptosporidium* oocysts shed from a host (see section on Life-cycle and biology). Examples of human infection by direct transmission include animal contact on farms or person-to-person contact in households, hospitals or child day care centers (Cacciò *et al.* 2005; Smith and Nichols 2007). Direct transmission sources often contribute to sporadic infections (Hunter *et al.* 2004; Roy *et al.* 2004); however, such sources have been associated with outbreaks in institutions (e.g. hospitals or schools), particularly childcare centres (e.g. Cordell and Addiss 1994; Turabelidze *et al.* 2007).

'Indirect' transmission (e.g. *via* an environmental vehicle, such as food or water) is facilitated by factors including the resilience and longevity of the oocyst (containing the infective sporozoites) in harsh environments (Robertson *et al.* 1992) and its 'resistance' to common disinfectants (Chauret *et al.* 1998; Barbee *et al.* 1999). Large outbreaks appear to be most frequently associated with drinking or recreational water (e.g. swimming pools) (reviewed by Karanis *et al.* 2007). Other examples of 'indirect' modes of transmission which can cause outbreaks are those linked to contaminated food or beverages (e.g. Djuretic *et al.* 1997; Blackburn *et al.* 2006; Robertson 2007; Smith *et al.* 2007). However, 'indirect' transmission resulting in sporadic cryptosporidiosis has been reported also (e.g. Robertson *et al.* 2002; Goh *et al.* 2004). It is likely that any correlation between direct transmission and sporadic infections or between indirect transmission and large outbreaks

relates to greater infection opportunity in the latter over the former, due to an increased potential for oocyst dispersal.

The transmission of cryptosporidiosis is associated mainly with host-specificity (see section on Taxomomy and host specificity) and variation in infective dose (Okhuysen *et al.* 1999; Chappell *et al.* 2006). The 50% infectious dose (ID_{50}: the dosage at which 50% of a host group become infected) has been used as a tool to estimate the infectivity of *Cryptosporidium* isolates (Okhuysen *et al.* 1999; Chappell *et al.* 2006). Okhuysen *et al.* (1999) assessed the infectivity of three distinct *C. parvum*, isolates [IOWA and UCP (from cattle); TAMU (from horses)], and estimated ID_{50} levels of 87 (95% confidence interval (CI): 49–126), 1,042 (95% CI: 0–3004) and 9 (95% CI: 4–14), respectively. Recently, infectivity to humans was tested for the strain TU502 of *C. hominis*, and an ID_{50} of 10–83 oocysts was estimated (Chappell *et al.* 2006). It is possible that a proportion of humans could become ill following the ingestion of a single oocyst, a possibility consistent with experimental *C. parvum* infection (*via* oral inoculation) in immunosuppressed mice (Yang *et al.* 2000). However, as evidenced by Okhuysen *et al.* (1999), infective dose can vary substantially among isolates within a species, indicating the need for further studies using additional isolates of *Cryptosporidium*, which should be identified to the specific and subspecific levels using molecular methods (see section on Diagnosis and genetic analysis).

Cryptosporidiosis in livestock and its relevance to public health

Recently, a review of zoonotic cryptosporidiosis (Xiao and Feng 2008) emphasized the significance of cattle as a source for human infection by *Cryptosporidium*. The transmission of cryptosporidiosis from livestock to humans had been proposed many years ago (Anderson *et al.* 1982; Current *et al.* 1983), and clearly supported by results from experimental infections of human volunteers with oocysts originating from calves (DuPont *et al.* 1995; Okhuysen *et al.* 1999). The potential public health relevance of bovine cryptosporidiosis, particularly in consideration of the large numbers of oocysts excreted by infected calves (Fayer *et al.* 1998) and the associated risk of waterborne and food-borne transmission, have generated considerable interest in estimating the prevalence of *Cryptosporidium* in livestock. A recent survey of 12 dairy farms in Michigan, USA (Peng *et al.* 2003) revealed that ~ 22.6% of 248 cattle were infected with *C. parvum*, suggesting a high risk of zoonotic transmission to humans. However, this study also detected *C. andersoni* (1.6%: n = 4), which does not appear to be infective to immunocompetent humans (see section on Taxonomy and host specificity). A similar survey detected cryptosporidiosis in 35.5% of 971 cattle from the eastern USA (Santin *et al.* 2004). Using molecular tools, four distinct *Cryptospordium* species/genotypes were identified (Santin *et al.* 2004): *C. parvum* (prevalence: ~ 16.5%); *C. andersoni* (~ 1.8%); *Cryptosporidium* bovine genotype B (now *C. bovis*; see Xiao *et al.* 2004) (~ 9.4%); and *Cryptosporidium* 'deer-like' genotype (~ 5.2%), of which usually only *C. parvum* is infective to humans (see section on Taxonomy and host specifity). These studies (Peng *et al.* 2003; Santin *et al.* 2004) indicate that not all cases of bovine cryptosporidiosis are caused by a species that represent a public health risk, emphasizing the need for the application of molecular-diagnostic tools to underpin epidemiological studies (see section on Diagnosis and genetic analysis).

In addition to identifying species causing bovine cryptosporidiosis in cattle in eastern USA, Santin *et al.* (2004) studied the disease in pre-weaned (5–60 days old) and weaned (3–11 months old) calves and demonstrated strong evidence of an age-related association between host and cryptosporidiosis. The prevalence of *Cryptosporidium* in pre-weaned calves was ~ 50% (253 of 503 isolates), but decreased to ~ 20% (94 of 468) in calves following weaning (Santin *et al.* 2004). Interestingly, although 85% of the infections in pre-weaned calves related to *C. parvum*, < 1% (1 of 468) of weaned cattle were infected with this species (Santin *et al.* 2004); the dominant species in weaned calves, based on DNA sequencing, was *C. andersoni* and *C. bovis* and another genotype (similar to that reported from deer). These data suggest that young calves represent a more significant zoonotic risk than older cattle.

Because calves are likely to be infected by *C. parvum* shortly after birth (Santin *et al.* 2004), and clinical signs of disease are typically limited to a period of intense, self-limiting diarrhoea (Fayer *et al.* 1998), and given the high cost and limited effectiveness of chemotherapeutic and supportive treatment, there appears to have been little incentive for developing husbandry practices to limit bovine cryptosporidiosis. However, intensive farms (e.g. dairy and feedlots) can represent a significant source of human-infective oocyst contamination in the environment (Fayer *et al.* 1998), which is presumably exacerbated by the presence of new-born calves (Santin *et al.* 2004).

In addition to cattle, sheep have also been implicated in the transmission of *C. parvum* to humans *via* direct contact with lambs on petting farms (Elwin *et al.* 2001; Pritchard *et al.* 2007). However, a broad study of *Cryptosporidium* species and genotypes infecting older lambs (weaned; up to 12 months of age) and adult sheep (older than 12 months) in Western Australia found little evidence of infection by *C. parvum* in this species (Ryan *et al.* 2005b). This study (Ryan *et al.* 2005b) examined 1,647 sheep and detected eight distinct species of *Cryptosporidium* (total n = 43), which were identified by DNA sequencing as *C. andersoni* (n = 1), the cervine genotype of *Cryptosporidium* (n = 8), *C. hominis* (n =1), the marsupial genotype of *Cryptosporidium* (n = 4), the 'new bovine B' genotype of *Cryptosporidium* (n = 14), the pig genotype II of *Cryptosporidium* (n = 4), *C. suis* (n = 2) and an unknown genotype for which there was no prior sequence data. Although the detection of *C. hominis* in sheep was noted as an unexpected finding, the study hypothesized that sheep may not be an important source of zoonotic infection of humans (Ryan *et al.* 2005b). This contrasts the situation in the UK, where current data (McLauchlin *et al.* 2000; Smith *et al.* 2005; Mueller-Doblies *et al.* 2008) indicate that *C. parvum* is consistently the only species found in diarrhoeic faeces from neonatal lambs. Although *C. parvum* has been identified (by sequencing) in sheep elsewhere (Santin *et al.* 2007), epidemiological studies of this nature, in sheep, are limited in other geographical regions, suggesting that more research into the zoonotic potential of sheep and other small ruminants is required. In addition to sheep and cattle, the contributions that other livestock animals, such as goats and horses, might make to zoonotic infections is not yet well understood. The *Cryptosporidium parvum* TAMU isolate was originally reported to have been contracted by a human from a horse (Okhuysen *et al.* 1999), suggesting that zoonotic transmission from horses is possible. Interestingly, the *C. parvum* TAMU isolate was shown to be highly infective to humans and highly virulent in its ability to initiate prolonged disease (Okhuysen *et al.* 1999), suggesting further study of the zoonotic potential associated with small ruminants and horses may have relevance to human health.

Anthroponotic and zoonotic transmission

Historically, based on microscopic examination, human cryptosporidiosis was considered to be caused by *C. parvum*. With the development of improved molecular tools (see Jex *et al.* 2008b), refined study of the epidemiology of cryptosporidiosis in humans has become possible. Initial studies of the genetic make-up of *Cryptosporidium* using isoenzyme electrophoresis revealed the presence of two distinct '*C. parvum*' lineages, one found only in humans and one found in humans and animals (Ogunkolade *et al.* 1993; Awad-el-Kariem *et al.* 1995). Subsequent studies using PCR-based approaches employing a range of genetic loci consistently and independently supported the finding of two distinct lineages (e.g. Bonnin *et al.* 1996; Morgan *et al.* 1997), being referred to as the human (H) and the cattle (C) genotypes, respectively (Widmer *et al.* 1998). In 2002, the 'human' genotype was proposed as a distinct species (now called *C. hominis*), which was hypothesized to infect and be transmitted by humans exclusively (Morgan-Ryan *et al.* 2002). The anthroponotic transmission cycle of *C. hominis* is supported by molecular epidemiological studies (e.g. Mallon *et al.* 2003a; Hunter *et al.* 2004). However, rare observations of natural *C. hominis* infection in ruminants (Ryan *et al.* 2005b; Smith *et al.* 2005b; Giles *et al.* 2009), and reports of the experimental transmission of *C. hominis* to calves (Giles *et al.* 2001; Akiyoshi *et al.* 2002) emphasize the need for detailed study of the epidemiology of this species, assisted by the use of effective molecular tools.

Subsequent characterization of *C. parvum* using multiple genetic loci, has indicated that further, host-associated, taxonomic units may exist within this species. For example, comparative studies of *C. parvum* isolates from sporadic infections in humans and cattle from Scotland and England have discovered several 'genotypes' found exclusively in humans (Mallon *et al.* 2003b; Leoni *et al.* 2007). In addition, distinct genetic variants of *C. parvum* (as indicated by multilocus genotyping using microsatellite markers) have been linked epidemiologically to either human or animal exposures (Hunter *et al.* 2007). The genetic characterization of *C. parvum* isolates using *gp60* gene sequence data (see section on Diagnosis and genetics analysis) has allowed *C. parvum* to be divided into at least 11 genetic variants (genotypes), defined as IIa-IIk (reviewed by Jex and Gasser 2010). One of these genotypes, the one with the broadest host range, *C. parvum* IIa, has been detected in cattle, deer, dogs, humans, rodents and various ruminants other than cattle. Another genotype, *C. parvum* IIc, has been detected exclusively in humans to date (see Jex and Gasser 2010) and is hypothesized to be transmitted anthroponotically.

Molecular study has also revealed that, in rare instances, *Cryptosporidium* species other than *C. hominis* and *C. parvum* can infect humans (see section on Diagnosis and genetics analysis). Although 96–98% of cases of human cryptosporidiosis (in the UK) relate to *C. parvum* or *C. hominis* infection, rare instances of infection by *C. meleagridis* (~ 0.9%), *C. felis* (~ 0.2%), *C. andersoni* (~ 0.1%), *C. canis* (< 0.1%), *C. suis* (< 0.1%) and various genotypes (including 'cervine' and 'monkey') have been identified (Chalmers *et al.* 2002; Mallon *et al.* 2003b; Leoni *et al.* 2006). The epidemiology and pathogenicity of each of these latter species/genotypes are relatively poorly understood. These 'rare' species or genotypes (i.e. other than *C. parvum* and *C. hominis*) are found more frequently in humans in developing countries (Xiao *et al.* 2001) and some of these species have been associated with clinical cryptosporidiosis in HIV-infected people (Cama *et al.* 2007). Clearly, the zoonotic significance of such species/genotypes requires increased study, particularly in developing countries and in regions with high rates of HIV/AIDS and/or severe malnutrition.

Prevention, control and treatment

Animals

In animals, the key components for prevention and control of cryptosporidiosis include the maintenance of a 'clean' environment and the introduction of effective management strategies to minimize the potential for rapid spread from animal-to-animal and farm-to-farm (Table 46.5). The control of cryptosporidiosis in animals is not only important to their health and welfare but also to minimize environmental (including surface and ground water) contamination, and thus is significant in its impact on human health. The prevention of *Cryptosporidium* infection is challenging in intensively farmed animals due to the difficulty associated with the exclusion or elimination of the parasite from the farm environment. Although the maintenance of 'closed' flocks or herds can control the introduction of cryptosporidiosis from animals purchased from external sources (e.g. markets; Tacal *et al.* 1987), additional external factors, such as parasite transport *via* 'mechanical' means (e.g. flies; Graczyk *et al.* 1999) and parasite introduction through contaminated water or feed, can introduce infection on to a farm and are much more difficult, if not impossible, to control. Oocysts shed by wildlife and/or introduced into water supplies from wildlife, may represent another potential source of infection for herds of domestic animals. The role of wildlife as a reservoir and their involvement in the transmission of disease to livestock and humans is not yet well understood (see section on Taxonomy and host specifity) and requires further investigation using improved molecular tools (Jex *et al.* 2008b).

Because the prevention of infection in livestock herds is not always practical, control is a critical feature of any effective management strategy. However, limiting infection of neonatal animals and minimizing the risk of spread from infected to uninfected animals is a significant challenge. Numerous authors (e.g. Maldonado-Camargo *et al.* 1998; Sischo *et al.* 2000; Trotz-Williams *et al.* 2007a, b) have studied the factors linked to the prevalence of *Cryptosporidium* and the associated impact of cryptosporidiosis. Though useful to highlight potentially important factors either contributing to, or protecting against, infection and disease, such studies are usually limited to showing a statistical association (only) between any 'factor' and increased or decreased 'risk' due to unavoidable limits of the experimental designs of such surveys. Specifically, because these surveys are conducted within and among herds from multiple farms, a range of factors (e.g. housing, frequency of pen cleaning, proximity to other livestock herds, food and water source) can vary among herds or farms. All of these factors can contribute to disease prevalence, and none can be specifically isolated, making the determination of the actual impact of any single factor difficult. Thus, the guidance shown in Table 46.5 is based instead on that currently accepted for the prevention and control of calf scour in general and specifically cryptosporidiosis on farms.

Herd management practices that have appeared, in surveys in Ontario, to be associated with reduced risk from infection by *Cryptosporidium* and/or affliction with cryptosporidiosis include calving in winter rather than summer (Trotz-Williams *et al.* 2007b),

Table 46.5 Key management strategies for the prevention and control of cryptosporidiosis in livestock

Key management strategies
Prevention
Maintenance of 'closed' herds
Flies can act as transport vectors
Oocysts can be introduced from wild-life reservoirs
Provide a clean dry area for animals to give birth, and then moving to well-drained clean dry housing
Regularly move outdoor feeding areas to avoid build up of heavy contamination
Avoid spread out calving periods in suckler herds
Use an all-in, all-out calf housing process for beef herds, in pens that have been cleaned, disinfected and rested. Ammonia-based disinfectants are effective but can only be used in a building that has been de-stocked
Do not mix calves or calves of different ages between groups
Provide clean drinking water and feed, and prevent contamination
Control
Treat dehydration orally or intravenously depending on severity
Treat cryptosporidiosis with halofuginone, adhering strictly to the recommended dosage and not to treat severely dehydrated calves
Separate out animals with scours
Ensure each neonate receives an adequate initial dosage of colostrum (fresh or frozen)
Implement low population densities in each calve pen
Use non-absorptive (e.g. concrete) flooring in calve pens (rather than earth, sand or gravel)
Regularly clean calve pens (by high pressure hose)
Disinfect previously cleaned pens and/or feeding or milking apparatus using hydrogen peroxide or ammonia-based disinfectants or steam
Allow pens and instruments to dry completely after cleaning (if possible)

removing neonates from the dam within one hour of birth (Trotz-Williams *et al.* 2007b), ensuring the neonate receives an adequate initial dosage of colostrum (either fresh or frozen; Trotz-Williams *et al.* 2007a, b). Elsewhere, ensuring optimal housing for calves following birth also reduced risk (Maldonado-Camargo *et al.* 1998; Castro-Hermida *et al.* 2002; Trotz-Williams *et al.* 2007a). Additional environmental factors considered important in decreasing the risk of cryptosporidiosis in neonates included low population density for calves (Trotz-Williams *et al.* 2007b), the presence of concrete flooring, rather than earth, gravel or sand, in pens (Maldonado-Camargo *et al.* 1998; Castro-Hermida *et al.* 2002; Trotz-Williams *et al.* 2007a) and the routine cleaning of pens (Trotz-Williams *et al.* 2007a) and feeding utensils (Castro-Hermida *et al.* 2002; Trotz-Williams *et al.* 2007a).

Introducing improved hygiene measures (e.g. regular cleaning of pens and feeding apparatus with soap) are considered to be essential to a rigorous management strategy of cryptosporidiosis (Maldonado-Camargo *et al.* 1998; Castro-Hermida *et al.* 2002;

Trotz-Williams *et al.* 2007a); however, due to the robust nature of *Cryptosporidium* oocysts, care must be taken to ensure that such cleaning regimens are effective. Oocysts remain viable for long periods of time and are resistant to various disinfectants suitable for use in agricultural settings (e.g. bleach-based disinfectants) (Fayer 1995; Deng and Cliver 1999). Some ammonia-based disinfectants can kill *Cryptosporidium* oocysts (Jenkins *et al.* 1998), but release irritating fumes and can only be used after destocking. Disinfectants containing hydrogen peroxide, plus either peracetic acid or silver nitrate, have been shown to have a deleterious effect on the survival of *C. parvum* oocysts (Quilez *et al.* 2005) and are commercially available for application in a farm setting. Steam-cleaning is another supportive measure, which has been shown to be effective for killing *Cryptosporidium* oocysts on instrumentation in hospitals (Barbee *et al.* 1999), and may be suitable for decontaminating some instrumentation used in farming for feeding or milking. For concrete pen flooring, daily mechanical removal of oocysts using high pressure hosing appears to be an effective aid in controlling the spread of *Cryptosporidium* (Castro-Hermida *et al.* 2002) and is preferable to sweeping, which imposes an increased risk of cross-contamination among pens due to the mechanical transfer of oocysts on the broom bristles (Maldonado-Camargo *et al.* 1998). Importantly, the desiccation of oocysts appears to be a highly effective means of limiting parasite transmission (Anderson 1986) and further highlights the benefit of using concrete floors, over porous or absorptive materials, in pens, in order to facilitate drying.

Compared with the above management strategies, therapeutic options are somewhat limited (reviewed by Mead 2002; Armson *et al.* 2003; Zardi *et al.* 2005). The demonstrated host age stratification of *Cryptosporidium* infectious in animals (Santin *et al.* 2004) suggests that acquired immunity is possible and likely results from prior exposure to the parasite (e.g. Harp *et al.* 1990), but the effective eliciting of passive immunity is still unclear. Passive immunotherapy using colostrum from dams immunized with native or recombinant antigens of *Cryptosporidium* has been explored and shown to be protective against infection in young calves in some studies (Riggs *et al.* 1994; Perryman *et al.* 1999; Hunt *et al.* 2002), but of limited efficacy in others (Gomez Morales and Pozio 2002). 'Risk-factor' surveys indicate that neonate calves have a reduced probability of infection by *Cryptosporidium* following the ingestion of colostrum (Trotz-Williams *et al.* 2007a, b); however, the prevalence of infection in neonates, even after colostrum ingestion, is high prior to weaning (Santin *et al.* 2004), indicating that the passive transfer of immunity is limited. Overall, these data indicate that the passive transfer of immunity *via* colostrum is unlikely to be effective as a single means of defence against cryptosporidiosis in young calves.

Although various avenues have been explored for the development of a vaccine against cryptosporidiosis (Harp and Goff 1995; Harp *et al.* 1996b), none are yet commercially available (Armson *et al.* 2003). The use of a whole oocyst-based vaccines from an attenuated line of *C. parvum* (gamma-irradiated), has been revisited (Jenkins *et al.* 2004) and shown to demonstrate a protective response in calves. Other recent efforts have focused on assessing immune responses against antigens derived from oocysts or the cell surface of sporozoites (reviewed by Boulter-Bitzer *et al.* 2007). The proteins CP15 and P23, involved in 'zoite motility and/or host cell invasion (see section on Location and establishment in the host) have been expressed using recombinant methods and appear to be promising immunogens (Jenkins 2004). Although, overall, success has been limited, the availability of the complete nuclear genome sequences for *C. parvum* (see Abrahamsen *et al.* 2004) and *C. hominis* (see Xu *et al.* 2004) and developments in bioinformatic analysis capabilities may provide opportunities for identifying novel proteins as vaccine targets.

In the absence of a vaccine, supportive and chemotherapeutic treatment options have been an area of significant research. The simplest, but, at present, one of the more effective means of treating cryptosporidiosis cases in livestock is oral or intravenous rehydration of clinically affected, dehydrated animals (Garthwaite *et al.* 1994). Chemotherapy has been explored with only limited success (Armson *et al.* 2003). Numerous organic-based antimicrobial compounds, including various quinones, aminoglycosides (e.g. paramomycin and streptomycin) and folate antagonists (e.g. sulphanitran and trimethoprim), have been evaluated with mixed success (Woods *et al.* 1996; Woods and Upton 1998; Armson *et al.* 2003). Halofuginone lactate (HFL) has been used as a supportive measure to treat clinical cryptosporidiosis in calves. Studies conducted in the early 1990's (Villacorta *et al.* 1991; Peeters *et al.* 1993) indicated that administering HFL to infected calves at a dosage of 60 to 120 µg/kg body weight decreased the severity of clinical disease as well as oocyst numbers in faeces, shortly after treatment. Recent studies (Lefay *et al.* 2001; Jarvie *et al.* 2005) have provided further support of these findings, indicating that HFL is an effective chemotherapy in calves for the purpose of reducing the severity of bovine cryptosporidiosis and suggesting that HFL decreases the spread of *C. parvum* from animal-to-animal due to decreased faecal oocyst output. However, studies by Naciri *et al.* (1993) and, recently, by Klein *et al.* (2007) have suggested that, although HFL may be useful in diminishing the severity of disease symptoms, this drug only delays rather than eliminates the excretion of oocysts in faeces. In spite of the use of HFL as a supportive measure, its recommended dosage must be strictly adhered to (given its limited safety index), and severely dehydrated calves should not be treated using this compound because of its toxicity.

In addition to treatment and control regimens to limit the impact of *Cryptosporidium* infection and cryptosporidiosis on herds, management strategies are critical to limit to spread of infective *Cryptosporidium* oocysts to other farms, and, for *C. parvum*, to the human population (Anon. 2007). Manure from animals is a major contributor of *Cryptosporidium* oocysts in the environment (Dorner *et al.* 2004; Atwill *et al.* 2006), and measures also need to be implemented to reduce the risks of pollution to drinking water. Adequately controlled storage and handling of manures and slurry (e.g. from cattle yards or dairies) or leachate from bedding will assist to reduce the risk of contamination in water-ways (Hutchison *et al.* 2005). Run-off into water catchments presents a significant risk, particularly during and after heavy rainfall (Signor *et al.* 2005; Thurston-Enriquez *et al.* 2005); although the risk posed by oocysts in water run-off varies depending on the soil type and the density of vegetation in the surrounding area (Davies *et al.* 2004). In general, grazing animals should be excluded from access to water catchments and water sources through the introduction of buffer zones (Davies *et al.* 2004). Published codes of good agricultural practice and guidance should be followed to protect water supplies and crops from faecal contamination. Although there are regulations in some countries to control the risk of *Cryptosporidium* oocysts entering drinking water supplies, the WHO recommends preventative, drinking water safety plans (DWSPs) outlining the most effective means to preserve the quality of drinking water and to safeguard public health (OECD/WHO 2003). The implementation of these protocols should greatly aid in limiting the introduction of *Cryptosporidium* infection/s into herds of livestock, and have been effective in decreasing the risk of farmed animals as reservoirs for the transmission of *Cryptosporidium* to humans in the UK (Sopwith *et al.* 2005).

Humans

In humans, as in other animals, the management of *Cryptosporidium*/cryptosporidiosis, can be divided largely into prevention, control and therapy. Prevention and control (Table 46.6) are primarily focused on maintaining an environment in which the transmission of *Cryptosporidium* is minimized through active changes to personal behaviour and the environment. General guidelines for the prevention and control of person-to-person spread of common enteric pathogens are relevant to *Cryptosporidium* and include frequent washing of hands (particularly after using the toilet, changing diapers, caring for a patient with diarrhoea, or cleaning the toilet) and proper disposal of excreta and soiled materials (Anon 2004). All cases of gastroenteritis should be regarded as potentially transmissible to susceptible humans, and, thus, the afflicted should be excluded from the work place, school or other institutional settings, until oocyst shedding has ceased; this aspect is particularly relevant for food handlers and staff of healthcare facilities (Anon. 2004). Additional precautions against *Cryptosporidium* infection include handwashing prior to eating or preparing food and after contact with animals, adequate filtration/treatment of non-potable water, and thorough washing of fruit and vegetables prior to consumption.

In additional to advice on general 'hygiene' and behavioural measures, the identification of potential infection sources and considered advice on appropriate behaviour when exposed to such sources is advisable. For example, visits to open, petting or residential farms have sometimes resulted in cases of human cryptosporidiosis (e.g. Smith *et al.* 2004b), particularly in children at whom these activities are aimed (e.g. Evans and Gardner 1996; Elwin *et al.* 2001). Increased customer awareness and the availability of suitable handwashing facilities are important preventative measures, and guidance should be given both to farm managers and teachers (HSE, 2000a, b). Advice regarding the use of swimming pools is more complicated because oocysts can continue to be shed by infected persons for a considerable time (up to 2 weeks) after stools return to a normal consistency (Jokipii and Jokipii 1986). The Centre of Disease Control (CDC) recommends that the use of swimming pools be avoided during this period and that young children be taken for frequent toilet breaks and standard hygiene practices (e.g. frequent handwashing and proper changing/disposal of soiled diapers) be implemented when using public pools (Kaye 2001). In reality, this recommendation is difficult to enforce. In addition, asymptomatic carriers are known to occur (see section on Pathogenesis) and can present an epidemiological risk of infection without the infected person being aware of illness. Though improved behavioural practices can aid in reducing the risk associated with public swimming pools, improved disinfection strategies are also required.

Immunocompromised patients are at a high risk of infection with *Cryptosporidium*; general advice on the avoidance of exposure to

Table 46.6 Key management strategies for the prevention and control of cryptosporidiosis in humans

Key management strategies
Prevention
Wash hands frequently and thoroughly with soap and water (especially prior to eating or preparing food, after using the toilet, changing diapers or toileting children and after touching animals)
Implement adequate filtration/treatment of non-potable water and do not swallow recreational water
Wash fruit and vegetables in clean water prior to consumption or avoid food that might be contaminated
Dispose of excretions and soiled materials appropriately
Treat all gastrointestinal illness as potentially infective and, if cryptosporidiosis has been confirmed, minimize public contact including the use of swimming pools for two weeks after the diarrhoea has ceased
Immunocompromised people should boil or appropriately filter water prior to consumption (including water for making ice)
Control
Provide appropriate handwashing facilities in public areas
Implement recommendations for management of public swimming pools (e.g. those published by CDC or PWTAG)
Implement national guidelines for the prevention and control of person-to-person spread (e.g. by excluding confirmed cases from childcare settings, or vulnerable workplace settings, until 48 hours after the last loose stool)
Implement a 'multi-barrier' approach to water treatment (i.e. coagulation, clarification, filtration and/or disinfection)
Implement water safety plans (e.g. prohibit livestock grazing in strategic water sheds)
At a house-hold level, heat-kill infective oocysts in water by boiling
Steam clean and/or chemically disinfect instrumentation (e.g. endoscopes) and allow to dry prior to use

Cryptosporidium is available for HIV/AIDS patients (Anon 2002b) and bone-marrow transplant recipients (Anon. 2000). Current advice (e.g. in the England) is that anyone with compromised T-cell function (or low T-Cell count) should boil drinking water prior to consumption, including that used for making ice (CMO 1999). However, the precise groups of patients to whom this recommendation is directed are unclear. In a systematic review of the literature (Hunter and Nichols 2002), HIV/AIDS patients with CD4 cell counts of < 200/ml (and particularly < 50/ml), acute leukaemia or lymphoma patients (particularly children) and those with primary T-cell immunodeficiencies, such as SCID and males with hyper-IgM syndrome, have been identified as those to whom this advice should be given routinely. Severely immunocompromised patients, including those with primary immune deficiencies, HIV/AIDS, or cancer or transplant patients taking immunosuppressive drugs, are advised (e.g. in the USA) to boil their drinking water as an additional precaution (CDC/EPA 1999). Alternatively, filtration through a suitable filter (pore size of < 1 μm) is also effective at removing *Cryptosporidium* oocysts from drinking water (CDC/EPA 1999).

Adequate risk management includes strategies to limit the potential for exposure to infective oocysts by attempting to maintain as clean an environment as is practical. Such management strategies should focus particularly on 'vehicles' for *Cryptosporidium* infection which have greatest potential to facilitate mass infections. Water, and in particular drinking water, is clearly one of the most important vehicles by which *Cryptosporidium* oocysts can reach and infect human populations on a large scale. Infective oocysts in contaminated drinking and recreational water supplies (see Clancy and Hargy 2008) have resulted in numerous, large cryptosporidiosis outbreaks (Karanis *et al.* 2007) and may also account for a significant proportion of sporadic cases of disease (Goh *et al.* 2004; Hunter *et al.* 2004).

Following the protection of source water, the next step in a 'multi-barrier approach' is the optimization of the water treatment processes (Betancourt and Rose 2004), including phases of coagulation, clarification, filtration and/or disinfection, which are capable of achieving a 2 to 3-log reduction in oocyst numbers from source water (Chauret *et al.* 1999). In addition, an increased reduction in oocyst numbers can be achieved through the use of diatomaceous earth (Ongerth and Hutton 2001) or polymeric membranes (Meltzer 1993), instead of sand as the filter medium. Low-medium intensity treatment with ultraviolet light, which kills *Cryptosporidium* (Rochelle *et al.* 2005), is also a suitable enhancement. Some disinfectants, such as chlorine dioxide and ozone, have been demonstrated to have improved the efficacy of the reduction in the numbers of viable oocysts (Sivaganesan *et al.* 2003). However, when used together, ozone can form toxic by-products with chlorine dioxide (von Gunten 2003), so the use of both treatments in conjunction is contra-indicated.

In spite of the availability of these approaches, an effective water treatment approach is not always in place, even in developed countries. Where catchments or water treatment plants are at a high risk of contamination with *Cryptosporidium*, authorities may wish to implement routine testing for the detection of *Cryptosporidium* oocysts prior to water distribution. However, most of the conventional tests routinely used for the detection of oocysts in source or drinking water lack adequate sensitivity and do not allow an assessment of infectivity to humans or determination of oocyst viability (Jex *et al.* 2008b). Future strategies should include the routine use of improved molecular tests (Jex *et al.* 2008b).

In addition to preventative treatment of water, management strategies designed to limit the spread of *Cryptosporidium* infection in order to minimize the impact of an outbreak are essential. Studies have shown that *Cryptosporidium* oocysts are killed in water by pasteurization (e.g. 70°C for 15 sec: see Harp *et al.* 1996a) or by being brought to the boil (Fayer, 1994; Fayer *et al.* 1996). When an outbreak of cryptosporidiosis is declared and linked to a particular drinking water supply, the water utility may be advised by public health officials to issue a 'boil water notice' (see Harrison *et al.* 2002). Such notices provide immediate implementation of a control measure to enable the public to make an informed decision regarding their water consumption, though the effectiveness of boil water notices has been questioned (Hunter 2000).

Other measures implemented to reduce the spread of *Cryptosporidium* infection to and among humans should include decontaminating the environment of infective oocysts. For example, in hospital settings, contaminated surfaces and medical devices can play a role in the transmission of cryptosporidiosis (reviewed by Aygun *et al.* 2005). Effective disinfection of devices, such as endoscopes, prior to reuse is considered critical (Anon. 2002a).

Barbee *et al.* (1999) examined a range of chemical and physical disinfectants (e.g. hydrogen peroxide, phenol, quaternary ammonium compounds) for safe sterilization of hospital equipment and showed that three treatment methods (ethylene oxide, Sterrad 100 or steam-cleaning) could achieve a 3-log reduction in oocyst numbers on endoscopes. In addition, because desiccation will kill oocysts (Anderson 1986; Robertson *et al.* 1992), thorough drying of endoscopes and other hospital equipment following disinfection is advised (Anon. 2002a; Nelson *et al.* 2003).

However, no matter how thorough, prevention and control strategies to limit *Cryptosporidium* transmission can and do fail. When this occurs, supportive treatment is required. Basic therapy usually includes the oral and/or intravaneous rehydration of people with clinical cryptosporidiosis-induced dehydration (Eliason and Lewan 1998; Ochoa *et al.* 2004). In HIV/AIDS patients with low CD4 counts, the availability of, and adherence to, highly active anti-retroviral treatment (HAART) can control the severe complications associated with cryptosporidiosis (e.g. Miao *et al.* 2000; Zardi *et al.* 2005). However, HAART therapies are not widely available in developing countries.

As with *Cryptosporidium* infections in animals, there are presently no vaccines against cryptosporidiosis in humans, and chemotherapeutic treatments are limited (Smith and Corcoran, 2004). The necessity and feasibility of developing an anti-*Cryptosporidium* vaccine has been reviewed (see Boulter-Bitzer *et al.* 2007), and there is on-going research in this area. Anecdotal evidence suggests that repeated *Cryptosporidium* infection in humans can elicit a long-term, protective immunity against subsequent infections (Chappell *et al.* 1999; Okhuysen *et al.* 1999), suggesting that a target for a future *Cryptosporidium* vaccine may exist. However, the quest for this target has not yet been successful (see section on Treatment, prevention and control – Animals).

In the absence of an effective anti-*Cryptosporidium* vaccine, there has been considerable focus on the development of chemotherapeutic compounds (Mead 2002; Armson *et al.* 2003; Zardi *et al.* 2005). Specific treatment strategies are improving, and there are case reports describing effective reductions in oocyst excretion levels and an alleviation of clinical signs of cryptosporidiosis in immunocompromised patients upon treatment with paromomycin and/or azithromycin, following effective HAART intervention (Hommer *et al.* 2003; Denkinger *et al.* 2007; Hong *et al.* 2007). To date, some evidence indicates that nitazoxanide reduces the duration of diarrhoea associated with cryptosporidiosis in immunocompetent (Rossignol *et al.* 2001) and malnourished children (Amadi *et al.* 2002). This compound is now licensed for the treatment of cryptosporidiosis in immunocompetent children in the USA (Rossignol 2006). However, it is not licensed in Europe, and is therefore only available for use on a named-patient basis, and is not widely available in developing countries. Recent findings of the potential to reduce the symptoms of disease through targeting the proposed enterotoxin 'Substance P' (Garza *et al.* 2008; Robinson *et al.* 2008) indicates a new and promising avenue for chemotherapeutics, but, as yet, has not yielded a specific commercial outcome.

Concluding remarks

In the 100 years since Edmund Tyzzer first described *Cryptosporidium* as a 'commensalist' in the gastric glands of mice, our understanding of *Cryptosporidium*, as significant cause of disease and mortality has, without doubt, substantially improved. The life-cycle, transmission, epidemiology and control of this group of parasites has been, and continues to be, an area inspiring tremendous research efforts, yielding important research advances. Yet, despite this research, *Cryptosporidium* remains a significant cause of socio-economic loss and human suffering.

In the past twenty to thirty years, humanity has seen the rampant explosion of HIV/AIDS. Nowhere has this disease had higher impact than in the areas of the world least equipped to fight it. As HIV/AIDS has emerged as a global pandemic, *Cryptosporidium* has emerged as a global 'opportunistic' pathogen. Though spread through numerous sources, the faecal-oral transmission of this genus of parasites *via* a resilient oocyst stage provides it with tremendous potential for wide and rapid spread through susceptible animal and human populations. Certainly, this underlines the importance represented by the ability of *Cryptosporidium* species to spread 'en masse' *via* drinking and recreational water.

In the early years of the 21st century, humanity finds itself in an era of increasing climatic uncertainty. As with HIV/AIDS, it is impoverished human populations that are likely to be most immediately and most severely affected by climatic changes, as well as the effects that such changes may have on the availability of clean and safe drinking water through prolonged periods of drought and the increased salinization of aquifers. The combined impacts of HIV/AIDS, severe poverty and the lack of safe drinking water paints a foreboding picture of the potential impact of *Cryptosporidium* on human health and on the global economy in the coming years.

However, the early years of the twentieth century also find humanity in a period of unprecedented expansion in our understanding of biology at the molecular, organismal and ecological levels. Advances in genomic technologies and computer-assisted data analysis now allow the first 'whole genome' comparisons within and among parasitic species and their host. Such technologies may facilitate answers to questions, such as why some species of *Cryptosporidium* are infective to humans whereas others are not, and why some subspecific strains within a *Cryptosporidium* species are more virulent than others. With the recent availability of the human genome and the genomes of both *C. hominis* and *C. parvum*, we now have access to a vast source of potential targets for new and tailored treatments and vaccines, based on an understanding, at the molecular level, of the parasite-host interplay. Though there remain many unanswered questions regarding *Cryptosporidium* and cryptosporidiosis, and, in a broader context, in relation to other parasitic zoonoses (see other chapters in book), one cannot help but feel optimistic that, in the technology age, many of the answers to these questions are finally within our reach.

References

Abe, N. and Iseki, M. (2004). Identification of *Cryptosporidium* isolates from cockatiels by direct sequencing of the PCR-amplified small subunit ribosomal RNA gene. *Parasitol. Res.,* **92**: 523–26.

Abrahamsen, M. S., Lancto, C. A., Walcheck, B., Layton, W. and Jutila, M. A. (1997). Localization of alpha/beta and gamma/delta T lymphocytes in *Cryptosporidium parvum*-infected tissues in naive and immune calves. *Infect. Immun.,* **65**: 2428–33.

Abrahamsen, M. S. *et al.* (2004). Complete genome sequence of the apicomplexan, *Cryptosporidium parvum. Science,* **304**: 441–45.

Abreu, M. T., Fukata, M. and Arditi, M. (2005). TLR signaling in the gut in health and disease. *J. Immun.,* **174**: 4453–60.

Adak, G. K., Long, S. M. and O'Brien, S. J. (2002). Trends in indigenous foodborne disease and deaths, England and Wales: 1992 to 2000. *Gut,* **51**: 832–41.

Adams, R. B., Guerrant, R. L., Zu, S., Fang, G. and Roche, J. K. (1994). *Cryptosporidium parvum* infection of intestinal epithelium: morphologic and functional studies in an *in vitro* model. *J. Infect. Dis.,* **169**: 170–77.

Aguirre, S. A., Mason, P. H. and Perryman, L. E. (1994). Susceptibility of major histocompatibility complex (MHC) class I- and MHC class II-deficient mice to *Cryptosporidium parvum* infection. *Infect. Immun.,* **62**: 697–99.

Aguirre, S. A., Perryman, L. E., Davis, W. C. and McGuire, T. C. (1998). IL-4 protects adult C57BL/6 mice from prolonged *Cryptosporidium parvum* infection: analysis of CD4+alpha beta+IFN-gamma+ and CD4+alpha beta+IL-4+ lymphocytes in gut-associated lymphoid tissue during resolution of infection. *J. Immun.,* **161**: 1891–900.

Akiyoshi, D. E., Feng, X., Buckholt, M. A., Widmer, G. and Tzipori, S. (2002). Genetic analysis of a *Cryptosporidium parvum* human genotype 1 isolate passaged through different host species. *Infect. Immun.,* **70**: 5670–75.

Albert, M. M., Rusnak, J., Luther, M. F. and Graybill, J. R. (1994). Treatment of murine cryptosporidiosis with anticryptosporidial immune rat bile. *Am. J. Trop. Med. Hyg.,* **50**: 112–19.

Al-Braiken, F. A., Amin, A., Beeching, N. J., Hommel, M. and Hart, C. A. (2003). Detection of *Cryptosporidium* amongst diarrhoeic and asymptomatic children in Jeddah, Saudi Arabia. *Ann. Trop. Med. Parasit.,* **97**: 505–10.

Alvarez-Pellitero, P. and Sitja-Bobadilla, A. (2002). *Cryptosporidium molnari* n. sp. (Apicomplexa: Cryptosporidiidae) infecting two marine fish species, *Sparus aurata* L. and *Dicentrarchus labrax* L. *Intern. J. Parasitol.,* **32**: 1007–21.

Alvarez-Pellitero, P. *et al.* (2004). *Cryptosporidium scophthalmi* n. sp. (Apicomplexa: Cryptosporidiidae) from cultured turbot *Scophthalmus maximus*. Light and electron microscope description and histopathological study. *Dis. Aquatic Organ.,* **62**: 133–45.

Alves, M., Xiao, L., Antunes, F. and Matos, O. (2006). Distribution of *Cryptosporidium* subtypes in humans and domestic and wild ruminants in Portugal. *Parasitol. Res.,* **99**: 287–92.

Amadi, B. *et al.* (2002). Effect of nitazoxanide on morbidity and mortality in Zambian children with cryptosporidiosis: a randomised controlled trial. *Lancet,* **360**: 1375–80.

Amar, C. F. *et al.* (2007). Detection by PCR of eight groups of enteric pathogens in 4,627 faecal samples: re-examination of the English case-control Infectious Intestinal Disease Study (1993–1996). *Euro. J. Clin. Microbiol. Infect. Dis.,* **26**: 311–23.

Anderson, A. C., Donndelinger, T., Wilkins, R. M. and Smith, J. (1982). Cryptosporidiosis in a veterinary student. *JAVMA,* **180**: 408–9.

Anderson, B. C. (1986). Effect of drying on the infectivity of cryptosporidia-laden calf feces for 3- to 7-day-old mice. *Am. J. Vet. Res.,* **47**: 2272–73.

Anon. (1995). *Cryptosporidium* in water: CDC guidelines on how to protect yourself. Centers for Disease Control and Prevention. *AIDS Treatment News,* 7–8.

Anon. (1999). 'Isolation and identification of *Cryptosporidium* oocysts and *Giardia* cysts in waters' chairman Methods for examination of waters and associated materials, Standing Committee of Analysts. London: Her Majesty's Stationery Office.

Anon. (2000). Guidlines for preventing opportunistic infections among hematopoietic stem cell transplant recipients: recommendations of the CDC, the Infectious Diseases Society of America and the American Society of Blood and Marrow Transplantation. *Morbid. Mort. Wkly. Rep.,* **49**: 1–125.

Anon. (2002a). *Decontamination of endoscopes MDA DB2002(05)*, Department of Health, London. Available online at http://www.mhra.gov.uk.

Anon. (2002b). United States Public Health Service/Infectious Disease Society of America guidelines for the prevention of opportunistic infections in persons infected with human immunodeficiency virus. *Morbid. Mort. Wkly. Rep.,* **51:** 1–46.

Anon. (2004). Preventing person-to-person spread following gastrointestinal infections: guidelines for public health physicians and environmental health officers. *Comm. Dis. Pub. Health,* **7:** 362–84.

Anon. (2006). '2006 Report on the global AIDS epidemic' chairman UNAIDS, Geneva.

Anon. (2007). Compendium of measures to prevent disease associated with animals in public settings, 2007: National Association of State Public Health Veterinarians, Inc. *(NASPHV). Morbid. Mort. Wkly. Rep. Recomm. Rep.,* **56:** 1–14.

Arenas-Pinto, A. *et al.* (2003). Association between parasitic intestinal infections and acute or chronic diarrhoea in HIV-infected patients in Caracas, Venezuela. *Intern. J. STD and AIDS,* **14:** 487–92.

Argenzio, R. A. *et al.* (1990). Villous atrophy, crypt hyperplasia, cellular infiltration, and impaired glucose-Na absorption in enteric cryptosporidiosis of pigs. *Gastroenterology,* **98:** 1129–40.

Armson, A., Thompson, R. C. and Reynoldson, J. A. (2003). A review of chemotherapeutic approaches to the treatment of cryptosporidiosis. *Expert Rev. Anti-Infect. Ther.,* **1:** 297–305.

Arrowood, M. J., Xie, L. T. and Hurd, M. R. (1994). *In vitro* assays of maduramicin activity against *Cryptosporidium parvum. J. Eu. Microbiol.,* **41:** 23S.

Arrowood, M. J. (2002). *In vitro* cultivation of *Cryptosporidium* species. *Clin. Microbiol. Rev.,* **15:** 390–400.

Arrowood, M. J. (2008). *In vitro* culture. In: R. Fayer, L. Xiao (eds.) *Cryptosporidium and cryptosporidiosis,* pp. 499–525. Boca Raton, FLA: Taylor and Francis.

Asaad, N. Y. and Sadek, G. S. (2006). Pulmonary cryptosporidiosis: role of COX2 and NF-kB. *Apmis,* **114:** 682–89.

Atwill, E. R. *et al.* (2006). Environmental load of *Cryptosporidium parvum* oocysts from cattle manure in feedlots from the central and western United States. *J. Environ. Qual.,* **35:** 200–206.

Awad-el-Kariem, F. M. *et al.* (1995). Differentiation between human and animal strains of *Cryptosporidium parvum* using isoenzyme typing. *Parasitology,* **110(2):** 129–32.

Aygun, G. *et al.* (2005). Parasites in nosocomial diarrhoea: are they underestimated? *J. Hosp. Infect.,* **60:** 283–85.

Baeumner, A. J., Humiston, M. C., Montagna, R. A. and Durst, R. A. (2001). Detection of viable oocysts of *Cryptosporidium parvum* following nucleic acid sequence based amplification. *Analyt. Chem.,* **73:** 1176–80.

Balda, M. S. and Anderson, J. M. (1993). Two classes of tight junctions are revealed by Zo-1 isoforms. *Am. J. Physiol.,* **264:** C918–C24.

Bankier, A. T. *et al.* (2003). Integrated mapping, chromosomal sequencing and sequence analysis of *Cryptosporidium parvum. Genome Res.,* **13:** 1787–99.

Barbee, S. L., Weber, D. J., Sobsey, M. D. and Rutala, W. A. (1999). Inactivation of *Cryptosporidium parvum* oocyst infectivity by disinfection and sterilization processes. *Gastrointest. Endos.,* **49:** 605–11.

Baxby, D. and Hart, C. A. (1986). The incidence of cryptosporidiosis: a two-year prospective survey in a children's hospital. *J. Hyg. (London),* **96:** 107–11.

Bennett, S. (2004). Solexa Ltd. *Pharmacogen.,* **5:** 433–38.

Betancourt, W. Q. and Rose, J. B. (2004). Drinking water treatment processes for removal of *Cryptosporidium* and *Giardia. Vet. Parasitol.,* **126:** 219–34.

Bhat, N., Joe, A., Pereiraperrin, M. and Ward, H. D. (2007). *Cryptosporidium* p30, a Galactose/N-acetylgalactosamine-specific lectin, mediates infection *in vitro. J. Biol. Chem.,* **282:** 34877–87.

Blackburn, B. G. *et al.* (2006). Cryptosporidiosis associated with ozonated apple cider. *Emerg. Infect. Dis.,* **12:** 684–86.

Blagburn, B. L., Lindsay, D. S., Giambrone, J. J., Sundermann, C. A. and Hoerr, F. J. (1987). Experimental cryptosporidiosis in broiler chickens. *Poultry Sci,* **66:** 442–49.

Blanshard, C., Jackson, A. M., Shanson, D. C., Francis, N. and Gazzard, B. G. (1992). Cryptosporidiosis in HIV seropositive patients. *Quart. J. Med.,* **85:** 813–23.

Bonacini, M. (1992). Hepatobiliary complications in patients with human immunodeficiency virus infection. *Am. J. Med.,* **92:** 404–11.

Bonnin, A. *et al.* (1996). Genotyping human and bovine isolates of *Cryptosporidium parvum* by polymerase chain reaction-restriction fragment length polymorphism analysis of a repetitive DNA sequence. *FEMS Microb. Lett.,* **137:** 207–11.

Boulter-Bitzer, J. I., Lee, H. and Trevors, J. T. (2007). Molecular targets for detection and immunotherapy in *Cryptosporidium parvum. Biotechnol. Adv.,* **25:** 13–44.

Buret, A. G., Chin, A. C. and Scott, K. G. (2003). Infection of human and bovine epithelial cells with *Cryptosporidium andersoni* induces apoptosis and disrupts tight junctional ZO-1: effects of epidermal growth factor. *Intern. J. Parasitol.,* **33:** 1363–71.

Cacciò, S., Spano, F. and Pozio, E. (2001). Large sequence variation at two microsatellite loci among zoonotic (genotype C) isolates of *Cryptosporidium parvum. Intern. J. Parasitol.,* **31:** 1082–86.

Cacciò, S. M. (2005). Molecular epidemiology of human cryptosporidiosis. *Parasitologia,* **47:** 185–92.

Cacciò, S. M., Thompson, R. C., McLauchlin, J. and Smith, H. V. (2005). Unravelling *Cryptosporidium* and *Giardia* epidemiology. *Trends in Parasitol.,* **21:** 430–37.

Calzetti, C. *et al.* (1997). Pancreatitis caused by *Cryptosporidium parvum* in patients with severe immunodeficiency related to HIV infection. *Ann. Italiani Med. Interna,* **12:** 63–66.

Cama, V. A. *et al.* (2007). Differences in clinical manifestations among *Cryptosporidium* species and subtypes in HIV-infected persons. *J. Infect. Dis.,* **196:** 684–91.

Cama, V. A. *et al.* (2008). *Cryptosporidium* species and subtypes and clinical manifestations in children, Peru. *Emerg. Infect. Dis.* **14:** 1567–74.

Campbell, I., Tzipori, A. S., Hutchison, G. and Angus, K. W. (1982). Effect of disinfectants on survival of *Cryptosporidium* oocysts. *Vet. Rec.,* **111:** 414–15.

Cappell, M. S. and Hassan, T. (1993). Pancreatic disease in AIDS—a review. *J. Clin. Gastroenterol.,* **17:** 254–63.

Casemore, D. P. (1987). The antibody response to *Cryptosporidium*: development of a serological test and its use in a study of immunologically normal persons. *J. Infect.,* **14:** 125–34.

Castro-Hermida, J. A., Gonzalez-Losada, Y. A. and Ares-Mazas, E. (2002). Prevalence of and risk factors involved in the spread of neonatal bovine cryptosporidiosis in Galicia (NW Spain). *Vet. Parasitol.,* **106:** 1–10.

CDC/EPA. (1999). *Guidance for people with severely weakened immune systems,* www.gov/safewater.

Certad, G. *et al.* (2005). Cryptosporidiosis in HIV-infected Venezuelan adults is strongly associated with acute or chronic diarrhea. *Am. J. Trop. Med. Hyg.,* **73:** 54–57.

Chacin-Bonilla, L. *et al.* (1993). *Cryptosporidium* infections in a suburban community in Maracaibo, Venezuela. *Am. J. Trop. Med. Hyg.,* **49:** 63–67.

Chalmers, R. M., Elwin, K., Thomas, A. L. and Joynson, D. H. (2002). Infection with unusual types of *Cryptosporidium* is not restricted to immunocompromised patients. *J. Infect. Dis.,* **185:** 270–71.

Chalmers, R. M. and Pollock, K. G. J. (2007). Scotland 2006: reference laboratory data. *Health Protect. Wkly. Rep.,* **41:** available online.

Chappell, C. L. *et al.* (1999). Infectivity of *Cryptosporidium parvum* in healthy adults with pre-existing anti-*C. parvum* serum immunoglobulin G. *Am. J. Trop. Med. Hyg.,* **60:** 157–64.

Chappell, C. L. *et al.* (2006). *Cryptosporidium hominis*: experimental challenge of healthy adults. *Am. J. Trop. Med. Hyg.,* **75:** 851–57.

Chauret, C., Nolan, K., Chen, P., Springthorpe, S. and Sattar, S. (1998). Aging of *Cryptosporidium parvum* oocysts in river water and their susceptibility to disinfection by chlorine and monochloramine. *Can. J. Microbiol.,* **44:** 1154–60.

Chauret, C., Springthorpe, S. and Sattar, S. (1999). Fate of *Cryptosporidium* oocysts, *Giardia* cysts, and microbial indicators during wastewater treatment and anaerobic sludge digestion. *Can. J. Microbiol.,* **45:** 257–62.

Chen, W., Chadwick, V., Tie, A. and Harp, J. (2001). *Cryptosporidium parvum* in intestinal mucosal biopsies from patients with inflammatory bowel disease. *Am. J. Gastroenterology,* **96:** 3463–64.

Chen, W., Harp, J. A. and Harmsen, A. G. (2003). *Cryptosporidium parvum* infection in gene-targeted B cell-deficient mice. *J. Parasitol.,* **89:** 391–93.

Chen, X. M., Gores, G. J., Paya, C. V. and LaRusso, N. F. (1999). *Cryptosporidium parvum* induces apoptosis in biliary epithelia by a Fas/Fas ligand-dependent mechanism. *Am. J. Physiol.,* **277:** G599–608.

Chen, X. M. *et al.* (2005). Multiple TLRs are expressed in human cholangiocytes and mediate host epithelial defense responses to *Cryptosporidium parvum via* activation of NF-kappaB. *J. Immunol.,* **175:** 7447–56.

Chhin, S. *et al.* (2006). Etiology of chronic diarrhea in antiretroviral-naive patients with HIV infection admitted to Norodom Sihanouk Hospital, Phnom Penh, Cambodia. *Clin. Infect. Dis.,* **43:** 925–32.

Clancy, J. L. and Hargy, T. M. (2008). Waterborne: drinking water. In: R. Fayer, and L. Xiao (eds.) *Cryptosporidium and cryptosporidiosis,* pp. 93–106. Boca Raton, FLA: CRC Press.

Clavel, A. *et al.* (1996). Respiratory cryptosporidiosis: case series and review of the literature. *Infection,* **24:** 341–46.

CMO. (1999). *CMO's update 23 Cryptosporidium in water: clarification of the advice to the immunocompromised,* London: Department of Health. http://www.dh.gov.uk/en/Publicationsandstatistics/Lettersandcirculars/CMOupdate/DH_4003594.

Cohen, S. *et al.* (2006). Identification of Cpgp40/15 Type Ib as the predominant allele in isolates of *Cryptosporidium* spp. from a waterborne outbreak of gastroenteritis in South Burgundy, France. *J. Clin. Microbiol.,* **44:** 589–91.

Cordell, R. L. and Addiss, D. G. (1994). Cryptosporidiosis in child care settings: a review of the literature and recommendations for prevention and control. *Pediat. Infect. Dis. J.,* **13:** 310–17.

Corso, P. S. *et al.* (2003). Cost of illness in the 1993 waterborne *Cryptosporidium* outbreak, Milwaukee, Wisconsin. *Emerg. Infect. Dis.,* **9:** 426–31.

Culleton, R., Martinelli, A., Hunt, P. and Carter, R. (2005). Linkage group selection: rapid gene discovery in malaria parasites. *Genome Res.,* **15:** 92–97.

Current, W. L. and Long, P. L. (1983). Development of human and calf *Cryptosporidium* in chicken embryos. *J. Infect. Dis.,* **148:** 1108–13.

Current, W. L. *et al.* (1983). Human cryptosporidiosis in immunocompetent and immunodeficient persons. Studies of an outbreak and experimental transmission. *N. Engl. J. Med.,* **308:** 1252–57.

Current, W. L. and Haynes, T. B. (1984). Complete development of *Cryptosporidium* in cell culture. *Science,* **224:** 603–5.

Current, W. L. (1985). Cryptosporidiosis. *JAVMA.,* **187:**1334–38.

Current, W. L., Upton, S. J. and Haynes, T. B. (1986). The life cycle of *Cryptosporidium baileyi* n. sp. (Apicomplexa, Cryptosporidiidae) infecting chickens. *J. Protozool.,* **33:** 289–96.

Dann, S. M. *et al.* (2005). Interleukin-15 activates human natural killer cells to clear the intestinal protozoan *Cryptosporidium. J. Infect. Dis.,* **192:** 1294–302.

D'Antonio, R. G. *et al.* (1985). A waterborne outbreak of cryptosporidiosis in normal hosts. *Ann. Intern. Med.,* **103:** 886–88.

Davies, C. M. *et al.* (2004). Dispersion and transport of *Cryptosporidium* oocysts from fecal pats under simulated rainfall events. *Appl. Environ. Microbiol.,* **70:** 1151–59.

Deere, D. *et al.* (1998a). Evaluation of fluorochromes for flow cytometric detection of *Cryptosporidium parvum* oocysts labelled by fluorescent in situ hybridization. *Lett. Appl. Microbiol.,* **27:** 352–56.

Deere, D. *et al.* (1998b). Rapid method for fluorescent in situ ribosomal RNA labelling of *Cryptosporidium parvum. J. Appl. Microbiol.,* **85:** 807–18.

Deng, M., Rutherford, M. S. and Abrahamsen, M. S. (2004). Host intestinal epithelial response to *Cryptosporidium parvum. Adv. Drug Del. Rev.,* **56:** 869–84.

Deng, M. Q. and Cliver, D. O. (1999). *Cryptosporidium parvum* studies with dairy products. *Intern. J. Food Microbiol.,* **46:** 113–21.

Denkinger, C. M., Harigopal, P., Ruiz, P. and Dowdy, L. M. (2007). *Cryptosporidium parvum*-associated sclerosing cholangitis in a liver transplant patient. *Transp. Infect. Dis.* epub 1 JUL 2007 DOI: 10.1111/j.1399-3062.2007.00245.x.

Dillingham, R. A., Lima, A. A. and Guerrant, R. L. (2002). Cryptosporidiosis: epidemiology and impact. *Microb. Infect.,* **4:** 1059–66.

Djuretic, T., Wall, P. G. and Nichols, G. (1997). General outbreaks of infectious intestinal disease associated with milk and dairy products in England and Wales: 1992 to 1996. *Comm. Dis. Rep. CDR Rev.,* **7:** R41–45.

Dolmatch, B. L., Laing, F. C., Ferderle, M. P., Jeffrey, R. B. and Cello, J. (1987). AIDS-related cholangitis: radiographic findings in nine patients. *Radiology,* **163:** 313–16.

Dorner, S. M., Huck, P. M. and Slawson, R. M. (2004). Estimating potential environmental loadings of *Cryptosporidium* spp. and *Campylobacter* spp. from livestock in the Grand River Watershed, Ontario, Canada. *Environm. Sci. Technol.,* **38:** 3370–80.

DuPont, H. L. *et al.* (1995). The infectivity of *Cryptosporidium parvum* in healthy volunteers. *N. Engl. J. Med.,* **332:** 855–59.

Eliason, B. C. and Lewan, R. B. (1998). Gastroenteritis in children: principles of diagnosis and treatment. *Am. Fam. Physic.,* **58:** 1769–76.

Elsser, K. A., Moricz, M. and Proctor, E. M. (1986). *Cryptosporidium* infections: a laboratory survey. *Can. Med. Assoc. J.,* **135:** 211–13.

Elwin, K., Chalmers, R. M., Roberts, R., Guy, E. C. and Casemore, D. (2001). Modification of a rapid method for the identification of gene-specific polymorphisms in *Cryptosporidium parvum* and its application to clinical and epidemiological investigations. *Appl. Environ. Microbiol.,* **67:** 5581–84.

Enriquez, F. J. and Sterling, C. R. (1993). Role of CD4+ TH1- and TH2-cell-secreted cytokines in cryptosporidiosis. *Folia Parasitol. (Praha),* **40:** 307–11.

Evans, M. R. and Gardner, D. (1996). Cryptosporidiosis outbreak associated with an educational farm holiday. *Comm. Dis. Rep. CDR Rev.,* **6:** R50–51.

Fafard, J. and Lalonde, R. (1990). Long-standing symptomatic cryptosporidiosis in a normal man: clinical response to spiramycin. *J. Clin. Gastroenterol.,* **12:** 190–91.

Fall, A., Thompson, R. C., Hobbs, R. P. and Morgan-Ryan, U. (2003). Morphology is not a reliable tool for delineating species within *Cryptosporidium. J. Parasitol.,* **89:** 399–402.

Fanning, A. S., Jameson, B. J., Jesaitis, L. A. and Anderson, J. M. (1998). The tight junction protein ZO-1 establishes a link between the transmembrane protein occludin and the actin cytoskeleton. *J. Biol. Chem.,* **273:** 29745–53.

Fayer, R. and Leek, R. G. (1984). The effects of reducing conditions, medium, pH, temperature, and time on *in vitro* excystation of *Cryptosporidium. J. Protozool.,* **31:** 567–69.

Fayer, R. and Ungar, B. L. (1986). *Cryptosporidium* spp. and cryptosporidiosis. *Microbiol. Rev.,* **50:** 458–83.

Fayer, R., Andrews, C., Ungar, B. L. and Blagburn, B. (1989a). Efficacy of hyperimmune bovine colostrum for prophylaxis of cryptosporidiosis in neonatal calves. *J. Parasitol.,* **75:** 393–97.

Fayer, R., Perryman, L. E. and Riggs, M. W. (1989b). Hyperimmune bovine colostrum neutralizes *Cryptosporidium* sporozoites and protects mice against oocyst challenge. *J. Parasitol.,* **75:** 151–53.

Fayer, R. (1994). Effect of high temperature on infectivity of *Cryptosporidium parvum* oocysts in water. *Appl. Environ. Microbiol.,* **60:** 2732–35.

Fayer, R. (1995). Effect of sodium hypochlorite exposure on infectivity of *Cryptosporidium parvum* oocysts for neonatal BALB/c mice. *Appl. Environ. Microbiol.,* **61:** 844–46.

CHAPTER 47

Toxoplasmosis, sarcocystosis, isosporosis, and cyclosporosis

J. P. Dubey

Summary

Toxoplasmosis

Introduction

Toxoplasmosis is a protozoan disease caused by *Toxoplasma gondii*. It is widely prevalent in humans and animals throughout the world, especially in the western hemisphere. Virtually all warm-blooded animals can act as intermediate hosts but the life cycle is completed only in cats, the definitive host. Cats excrete the resistant stage of *T. gondii* (oocysts) in faeces, and oocysts can survive in the environment for months. Humans become infected congenitally, by ingesting undercooked infected meat, or by ingesting food and water contaminated with oocysts from cat faeces. It can cause mental retardation and loss of vision in congenitally infected children and deaths in immunosuppressed patients, especially those with Acquired immunodeficiency syndrome (AIDS). There is no vaccine to control toxoplasmosis in humans at the present time but one is available for reduction of fetal losses in sheep.

History

Toxoplasma gondii was discovered in 1908 in Tunisia in a rodent, *Ctenodoctylus gundi*, and in a laboratory rabbit in São Paulo, Brazil (Table 47.1). The name *Toxoplasma* (*toxon* = arc, *plasma* = form) is derived from the crescent shape of the tachyzoite stage, and the host, gundi. The medical importance of *T. gondii* was not discovered until late 1930s (Wolf *et al.* 1939). The development of a serological test for toxoplasmosis in 1948 led to the findings that it was a common infection of humans throughout the world (Table 47.1).

While considerable progress on the characterization of the disease in humans and animals was made between 1940 and 1960, the main routes of transmission remained a mystery. Congenital transmission occurred too rarely to explain widespread infection in humans and animals. In the 1960s it was found that organisms from tissue cysts could survive digestive enzymes and that humans can become infected by ingesting undercooked infected meat.

While congenital transmission and carnivorism partially explain transmission of *T. gondii*, these routes cannot explain the widespread *T. gondii* infection in vegetarians and in herbivores. Prevalence rates for *T. gondii* in strict vegetarians were found to be similar to those in non-vegetarians. Fresh excretions and secretions of animals which had even overwhelming infections proved essentially negative for *T. gondii* when tested in mice. Attempts to transmit *T. gondii* via arthropods were essentially unsuccessful.

The mystery of transmission was resolved when a resistant form of *T. gondii* was discovered in feline faeces and the coccidian phase of its life cycle was discovered in 1970 (Table 47.1).

The agent
Classification

Toxoplasma gondii (Nicolle and Manceaux 1908) Nicolle and Manceaux 1909 is a coccidian parasite of cats with warm-blooded animals as intermediate hosts. Coccidia are among the most important parasites of animals. Traditionally, all coccidia of veterinary importance were classified under the family Eimeriidae, Michin, 1903. Classification was based on the structure of the oocyst. Oocysts with four sporocysts, each with two sporozoites (total eight sporozoites) are classified as *Eimeria*. Oocysts containing two sporocysts, each with four sporozoites, were classified historically as *Isospora*. After the discovery of the life cycle of *T. gondii*, several other genera (*Sarcocystis*, *Besnoitia*, *Hammondia*, *Neospora*, *Frenkelia*) were found to have isosporan oocysts with two sporocysts and eight sporozoites.

Toxoplasma gondii and related genera discussed in the chapter are classified as follows:

- Phylum: Apicomplexa; Levine (1970).
- Class: Sporozoasida; Leukart (1879).
- Subclass: Coccidiasina; Leukart (1879).
- Order: Eucoccidiorida; Leger and Duboseq (1910).
- Suborder: Eimeriorina; Leger (1911).

Opinions differ regarding the further classification of *T. gondii* into families and subfamilies. It has been classified in the family Eimeriidae (Minchin 1903), Sarcocystidae (Poche 1913), or Toxoplasmatidae (Biocca 1956) by various authorities.

Structure and life cycle

There are three infectious stages of *T. gondii* (Fig. 47.1): the tachyzoites (in groups), the bradyzoites (in tissue cysts), and the sporozoites (in oocysts) (Frenkel 1973).

The tachyzoite is often crescent-shaped and is approximately $2 \times 6\ \mu m$ (Fig. 47.2). Its anterior (conoidal) end is pointed and its

Table 47.1 History of *Toxoplasma gondii* and toxoplasmosis[a]

Contributions and year	Contribution
Nicolle and Manceau (1908)	Discovered in gundi
Splendore (1908)	Discovered in rabbit
Mello (1910)	Disease described in a domestic animal (dog)
Wolf and Cowen (1937)	Congenital transmission documented
Pinkerton and Weinman (1940)	Fatal disease described in adult humans
Sabin (1942)	Disease characterized in man
Sabin and Feldman (1948)	Dye test described
Siim (1952)	Glandular toxoplasmosis described in man
Weinman and Chandler (1954)	Suggested carnivorous transmission
Hartley and Marshall (1957)	Abortions in sheep recognized
Beverley (1959)	Repeated congenital transmission observed in mice
Jacobs *et al.* (1960)	Tissue cysts characterized biologically
Hutchison (1965)	Faecal transmission recognized, nematode eggs suspected
Hutchison *et al.* (1969, 1970, 1971) ; Frenkel *et al.* (1970); Dubey *et al.* (1970a,b); Sheffield and Melton (1970); Overdulve (1970)	Coccidian phase described
Frenkel *et al.* (1970) ; Miller *et al.* (1972)	Definitive and intermediate hosts defined
Dubey and Frenkel (1972)	Five *T. gondii* types described from feline intestinal epithelium
Wallace (1969); Munday (1972)	Confirmation of the epidemiological role of cats from studies on remote islands
Luft *et al.* (1993)	Toxoplasmosis recognized in AIDS patients
Silveira *et al.* (1988)	Postnatal ocular toxoplasmosis recognized

[a] From Dubey (1993, 2005). For a complete bibliography see Dubey (1993, 2005, 2008).

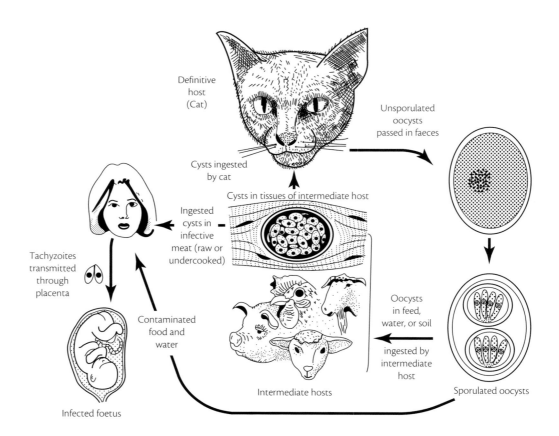

Fig. 47.1 Life cycle of *T. gondii*.

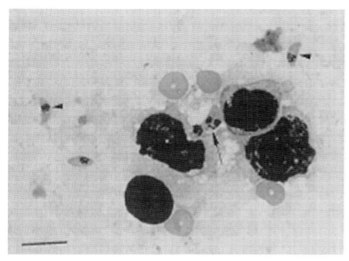

Fig. 47.2 Tachyzoites of *T. gondii*. Impression smear. Note individual crescentic (arrowheads) and dividing (arrow) tachyzoites (Giemsa; bar = 10 μm).

posterior end is round. It has a pellicle (outer covering), polar ring, conoid, rhoptries, micronemes, apicoplast, mitochondria, subpellicular microtubules, endoplasmic reticulum, Golgi apparatus, ribosomes, rough surface endoplasmic reticulum, micropore, and a well defined nucleus (Fig. 47.3). The nucleus is usually situated toward the posterior end or in the central area of the cell (Dubey 1977, 1993; Ferguson and Dubremetz 2007).

The pellicle consists of three membranes. The inner membrane complex is discontinuous at three points: the anterior end (polar ring), the lateral edge (micropore), and toward the posterior end. The polar ring is an osmiophilic thickening of the inner membrane at the anterior end of the tachyzoite. The polar ring encircles a cylindrical, truncated cone (the conoid) which consists of 6–8 fibrillar elements wound like a compressed spring. Twenty-two

subpellicular microtubules originate from the anterior end and run longitudinally almost the entire length of the cell. Terminating within the conoid are 4–10 club-shaped organelles called rhoptries (Fig. 47.3). The rhoptries are gland-like structures, often labrinthine, with an anterior narrow neck up to 2.5 μm long. Their saclike posterior end terminates anterior to the nucleus. Micronemes are rod shaped electron dense structures which occur at the anterior end of the parasite (Dubremetz and Ferguson 2007).

The functions of the conoid, rhoptries, and micronemes are not fully known but are involved in penetration and successful location within a host cell (Boothryod and Dubremetz 2008). The conoid is probably associated with the penetration of the tachyzoite through the membrane of the host cell. It can rotate, tilt, extend, and retract as the parasite searches for a host cell. *Toxoplasma gondii* can move by gliding, undulating, and rotating. Rhoptries have a secretory function associated with host cell penetration, secreting their contents through the conoid to the exterior. The microtubules probably provide the cytoskeleton.

The tachyzoite enters the host cell by active penetration of the host cell membrane. After entering the host cell the tachyzoite becomes ovoid in shape and becomes surrounded by a parasitophorous vacuole (PV). It has been suggested that the PV is derived from both the parasite and the host. Numerous intravacuolar tubules connect the parasitophorous vacuolar membrane to the parasite pellicle.

The tachyzoite multiplies asexually within the host cell by repeated endodyogeny. Endodyogeny (*endo* = inside, *dyo* = two, *geny* = progeny) is a specialized form of reproduction in which two progeny form within the parent parasite, consuming it in the process. Tachyzoites continue to divide by endodyogeny until the host cell is filled with parasites (Fig. 47.3B).

After a few divisions, *T. gondii* encysts to form tissue cysts (Fig. 47.4). Tissue cysts grow and remain intracellular as the bradyzoites (encysted *T. gondii*) divide by endodyogeny. Tissue cysts vary in size. Young tissue cysts may be as small as 5 μm and contain only two bradyzoites, while older ones may contain hundreds of organisms

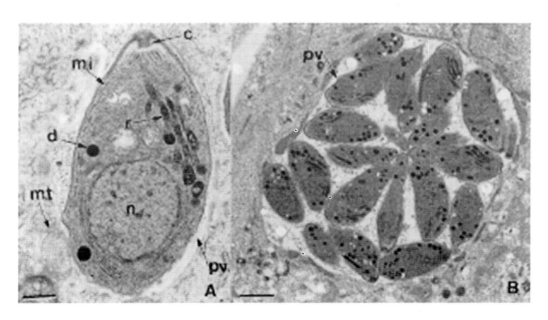

Fig. 47.3 Transmission electron micrographs of *T. gondii* tachyzoites in cell culture (A) Tachyzoite in a parasitophorous vacuole (pv) in the cytoplasm of a host cell. Note conoid (c), rhoptries (r), micronemes (mi), nucleus (n), and dense granules (d). The host cell mitochondria (mt) are closely associated with the pv (Bar = 0.5 μm). (B) Several tachyzoites in pv (Bar = 1.8 μm).

Fig. 47.4 Tissue cysts of *T. gondii* with thin cyst walls (arrows) in brain. (A) Impression smear, unstained. This tissue cyst was freed by grinding a piece of brain in a mortar with a pestle (Bar = 20 μm). (B) Impression smear. Four young tissue cysts with silver-positive cyst walls. Two tissue cysts each have two bradyzoites with terminal nuclei (arrowheads) (Silver stain, bar = 10 μm). (C) Histological section. Note bradyzoites have PAS-positive red granules that appear black in this micrograph (Periodic acid–Schiff haematoxylin; bar = 20 μm).

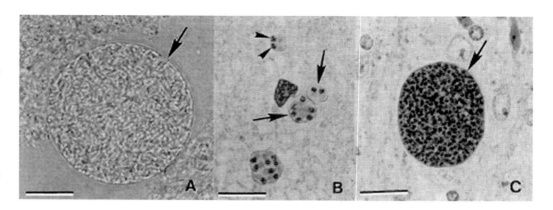

(Dubey *et al.* 1998) (Fig. 47.4). Tissue cysts in brain are often circular and rarely reach a diameter of 70 μm whereas intramuscular cysts are elongated and may be 100 μm long. Although tissue cysts may develop in visceral organs, including lungs, liver, and kidneys, they are more prevalent in the neural and muscular tissues, including the brain, eye, skeletal, and cardiac muscle. Intact tissue cysts probably do not cause any harm and can persist for the life of the host.

The tissue cyst wall is elastic, thin (< 0.5 μm) and argyrophilic (Fig. 47.4B). The bradyzoites are approximately 7 × 1.5 μm. Bradyzoites differ structurally only slightly from tachyzoites. They have a nucleus situated toward the posterior end, whereas the nucleus in tachyzoites is more centrally located. The contents of rhoptries in bradyzoites in older tissue cysts are electron dense (Fig. 46.5). Bradyzoites contain several amylopectin granules which stain red with periodic acid–Schiff (PAS) reagent (Fig. 47.4C); such material is either in discrete particles or absent in tachyzoites. Bradyzoites are more slender than are tachyzoites. Bradyzoites are less susceptible to destruction by proteolytic enzymes than are tachyzoites.

Cats excrete oocysts after ingesting tachyzoites, bradyzoites, or sporozoites. Prepatent periods (time to the shedding of oocysts after initial infection) and frequency of oocyst shedding vary according to the stage of *T. gondii* ingested. Prepatent periods are 3–10 days after ingesting tissue cysts and 18 days or more after ingesting tachyzoites or oocysts (Dubey 2005b). Intermediate prepatent periods of 11–17 days maybe associated with ingestion of transitional stages between tachyzoites and bradyzoites (Dubey 2005b). Fewer than 50% of cats shed oocysts after ingesting tachyzoites or oocysts, whereas nearly all cats shed oocysts after ingesting tissue cysts. From an epidemiological view point, cats are likely to shed oocysts after ingesting tissues of infected rodents, irrespective of their clinical status.

After the ingestion of tissue cysts by cats, the cyst wall is dissolved by the proteolytic enzymes in the stomach and small intestine. The released bradyzoites penetrate the epithelial cells of the small intestine and initiate development of numerous generations of *T. gondii* (Fig. 47.5A, B). Five morphologically distinct types (A to E) of *T. gondii* develop in intestinal epithelial cells before gametogony begins. Types A to E divide asexually by endodyogeny, endopolygeny, or schizogony (division into more than two organisms) (Dubey and Frenkel 1972; Speer and Dubey 2005).

Mature male gamonts are ovoid to ellipsoidal in shape. Each microgamete has two flagella (Fig. 47.6C). The microgametes swim to and penetrate a mature macrogamete. After penetration, oocyst wall formation begins around the fertilized gamete. When they are mature, oocysts are discharged into the intestinal lumen by the rupture of intestinal epithelial cells.

Unsporulated oocysts are subspherical to spherical and are 10 × 12 μm in diameter (Fig. 47.8A). The oocyst wall contains two colourless layers. The sporont almost fills the oocyst, and sporulation occurs outside the cat within 1–5 days, depending upon aeration and temperature.

Sporulated oocysts are subspherical to ellipsoidal and are 11 × 13 μm in diameter. Each sporulated oocyst contains two ellipsoidal sporocysts without a Stieda body. Sporocysts measure 6 × 8 μm (Fig. 47.8B). There are four sutures with lip-like thickenings in the sporocyst wall (Fig. 47.8B); these sutures open during excystation of the sporozoites. A sporocyst residuum is present. There is no oocyst residuum. Each sporocyst contains four sporozoites. The sporozoites

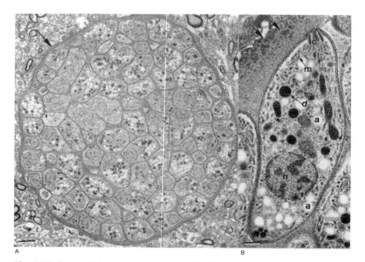

Fig. 47.5 Transmission electron micrographs of tissue cysts of *T. gondii* in brain (A) Young cyst with well-developed cyst wall (arrow). The bradyzoites are plump (dividing or preparing to divide) (Bar = 3.4 μm). (B) Longitudinally cut bradyzoite. Note electron-dense contents of rhopties (r), the subterminal nucleus (n), a conoid (c), numerous micronemes (m), and amylopectin granules (a) that appear as empty spaces here. The cyst wall (arrows) is convoluted (Bar = 0.77 μm).

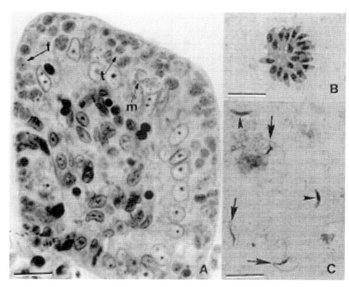

Fig. 47.6 Enteroepithelial stages of *T. gondii*, 6 days after feeding tissue cysts to a cat. (A) Histological section of a villus in small intestine. Note heavy infection of epithelial cells with *T. gondii* types (t), male gamonts (m), and numerous uninucleate female gamonts (f). Cells in the lamina propria are not infected (Haematoxylin and eosin; bar = 15 μm). (B) Impression smear. Note a type D schizont with 20 merozoites (Giemsa; bar = 10 μm). (C) Impression smear. Three biflagellate microgametes (arrows) and two free merozoites (arrowheads) (Giemsa; bar = 10 μm).

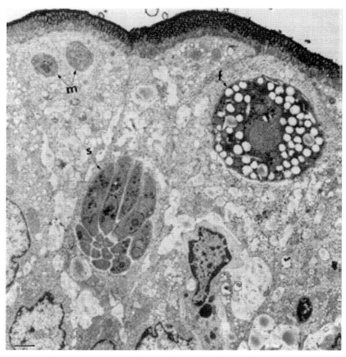

Fig. 47.7 Electron micrograph of coccidian stages of *T. gondii* in epithelial cells of ileum of a cat six days after ingesting tissue cysts. Note two merozoites (m), a female gamont (f) located just below the microvillus border, and a schizont(s) above the host cell nucleus (Bar = 2.5 μm).

are 2 × 6–8 μm in size with a subterminal to central nucleus and a few PAS-positive granules in the cytoplasm (Fig. 47.8B).

As the enteroepithelial cycle progresses, bradyzoites penetrate the lamina propria of the feline intestine and multiply as tachyzoites. Within a few hours after infection of cats, *T. gondii* may disseminate to extraintestinal tissues. *Toxoplasma gondii* persists in intestinal and extraintestinal tissues of cats for at least several months, if not for the life of the cat.

Toxoplasma gondii is biologically adapted to transmission by carnivorism in cats (Frenkel *et al.* 1970). By the oral route, bradyzoites are more infective to cats than mice and oocysts are more infective to mice and pigs than cats (Dubey 2001, 2006).

Cultivation

Toxoplasma gondii has not been grown in cell-free media. *Toxoplasma gondii* can be cultivated in laboratory animals, chick embryos, and cell cultures. Mice, hamsters, guinea-pigs, and rabbits are all susceptible but mice are generally used as hosts because they are more susceptible than the others and are not naturally infected when raised in the laboratory on commercial dry food free of cat faeces.

Tachyzoites of some strains of *T. gondii* grow in the peritoneal cavity of mice, sometimes producing ascites, and also grow in most other tissues after intraperitoneal inoculation with any of the three infectious stages of *T. gondii*. Virulent strains usually produce illness in mice and sometimes kill them within 1–2 weeks. Most strains of *T. gondii* do not kill mice.

Toxoplasma gondii tachyzoites will multiply in many cell lines in cell cultures (Fig. 47.9). Although tissue cysts can develop in cell cultures with most strains of *T. gondii*, the yield is lower than that produced by infection in mice.

Tissue cysts are obtained by injecting tachyzoites, bradyzoites, or oocysts into mice. To obtain tissue cysts from mice inoculated with a virulent strain, it is necessary to administer anti-*T. gondii* chemotherapy to prevent death from acute toxoplasmosis before tissue cysts form. Sulphadiazine is effective in controlling the acute stages of toxoplasmosis in mice. Tissue cysts are prominent in the mouse brain about 8 weeks after infection (Fig. 47.10).

Enteroepithelial stages of *T. gondii* have not yet been cultivated *in vitro*.

Oocysts can be obtained by feeding tissue cysts from infected mice to *T. gondii*-free cats.

Molecular biology

Toxoplasma gondii nucleus is haploid except during the sexual division in the intestine of the cat (Pfefferkorn 1990). Sporozoites are the results of meiosis and seem to follow classical Mendelian laws. The total haploid genome contains 14 chromosomes, 7,793 genes, with total genome size of 63,495,144 base pairs (Khan *et al.* 2007). It is an unusual parasite because of its broad host range and with only one species in the genus. Prior to the development of genetic markers, *T. gondii* isolates were grouped by their virulence to outbred mice (Dardé *et al.* 2007). Based on restriction fragment length polymorphism (RFLP), Howe and Sibley (1995) classified *T. gondii* into 3 genetic Types (I, II, III) and linked mouse virulence to genetic type. They proposed that Type I isolates were 100% lethal to mice, irrespective of the dose, and that Types II and III generally were avirulent for mice (Howe *et al.* 1996). Furthermore, until recently, *T gondii* was considered to be clonal with low genetic

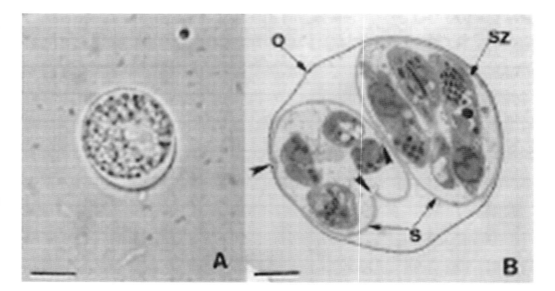

Fig. 47.8 Oocysts of *T. gondii*. (A) Unsporulated oocyst. Note sporont fills the oocyst (Unstained; bar = 6 μm). (B) Transmission electron micrograph of a sporulated oocyst. Note thin-walled oocyst (o) enclosing the two sporocysts (s) each with four sporozoites (sz). Each sporocyst has four lip-like thickenings (arrowheads) (Bar = 4.2 μm).

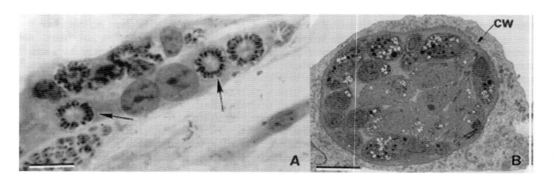

Fig. 47.9 *Toxoplasma gondii* in cell cultures (A) Tachyzoites, some groups in rosettes (arrows) (Giemsa; smear; bar = 20 μm). (B) Transmission electron micrograph of a tissue cyst. Note a well-developed cyst wall (cw) enclosing approximately 14 bradyzoites. The empty spaces in bradyzoites are amylopectin granules (Bar = 3.6 μm).

Courtesy of Dr D. S. Lindsay.

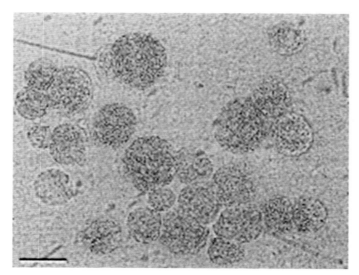

Fig. 47.10 Squash of a portion of brain of a mouse with numerous *T. gondii* tissue cysts. This mouse appeared clinically normal although it had many cysts (Unstained; bar = 50 μm).

variability, and strains isolated from asymptomatic hosts were considered avirulent. However, recent studies have indicated that most *T. gondii* isolates from asymptomatic chickens from Brazil and Colombia in South America were virulent for mice, were nonclonal, Type II was absent, and there was marked genetic variability (Dubey *et al.* 2002; Lehmann *et al.* 2006). In humans in French Guiana and Suriname, severe cases of toxoplasmosis in immunocompetent patients have been related to mouse-virulent *T. gondii* strains with atypical genotypes (Carme *et al.* 2002; Demar *et al.* 2007). Circumstantial evidence suggests that certain genetic types of *T. gondii* may be associated with clinical ocular toxoplasmosis in humans (Khan *et al.* 2006). It has been suggested that Type I isolates or recombinants of Types I and III are more likely to result in clinical toxoplasmosis, but genetic characterization has been limited essentially to isolates from patients ill with toxoplasmosis. There is very little information regarding the genetic diversity of *T. gondii* isolates circulating in the general human population. Therefore, we must be cautious in claiming a linkage between parasite genotypes and disease presentations without clear and discerning information regarding the parasite's biology in the human population and environment. In my opinion, all isolates of *T. gondii* must be considered potentially pathogenic and laboratory workers and public health persons must take appropriate precautions while handling materials potentially infected with *T. gondii* (Dubey 2009).

Host parasite relationship

Toxoplasma gondii usually parasitizes the host (both definitive and intermediate) without producing clinical signs. Only rarely does it cause severe clinical manifestations. The majority of natural infections are probably acquired by ingestion of tissue cysts in infected meat or oocysts in food or water contaminated with cat faeces. The bradyzoites from the tissue cysts or sporozoites from the oocyst penetrate the intestinal epithelial cells and multiply (Fig. 47.11A). *Toxoplasma gondii* may spread first to the mesenteric lymph nodes (Fig. 47.11B) and then to distant organs by invasion of lymph and blood. An infected host may die because of necrosis of intestine and mesenteric lymph nodes before other organs are severely damaged. Focal areas of necrosis may develop in many organs. The clinical picture is determined by the extent of injury to organs, especially vital organs such as the eye, heart, and adrenal glands. Necrosis is caused by the intracellular growth of tachyzoites. *Toxoplasma gondii* does not produce a toxin.

In those hosts which develop disease, the host may die of acute toxoplasmosis but much more often recovers with the acquisition of immunity (Frenkel 1973). In the recovering individual inflammation usually develops in sites where initially there was necrosis. By about the third week after infection, *T. gondii* tachyzoites begin to disappear from the visceral tissues and may localize in tissue cysts in neural and muscular tissues. *Toxoplasma gondii* tachyzoites may persist longer in the spinal cord and brain than in visceral tissues because immunity there is less effective than in neural organs. *Toxoplasma gondii* tachyzoites can persist in the placenta for months after the initial infection of the dam. How *T. gondii* is destroyed in immune cells is not completely known. All extracel-

lular forms of the parasite are directly affected by antibody but intracellular forms are not. It is believed that cellular factors including lymphocytes and lymphokines are more important than humoral ones in immune-mediated destruction of *T. gondii* (Frenkel 1973; Gazzinelli *et al.* 1993). Under experimental conditions, infection with avirulent strains protects the host from damage but does not prevent infection with more virulent strains. In most instances, immunity following a natural *T. gondii* infection persists for the life of the host.

Immunity does not eliminate infection. *Toxoplasma gondii* tissue cysts persist several years after acute infection. The fate of tissue cysts is not fully known. Whether bradyzoites can form new cysts directly without transforming into tachyzoites is not known but likely (Dubey 2005b). It has been proposed that tissue cysts may at times rupture during the life of the host. The released bradyzoites may be destroyed by the host's immune responses. The reaction may cause local necrosis accompanied by inflammation. Hypersensitivity plays a major role in such reactions. After such events, inflammation usually again subsides with no local renewed multiplication of *T. gondii* in the tissue; however, occasionally there may be formation of new tissue cysts.

In immunosuppressed patients, such as those given large doses of immunosuppressive agents in preparation for organ transplants and in those with AIDS, rupture of a tissue cyst may result in transformation of bradyzoites into tachyzoites and renewed multiplication (Fig. 47.12). The immunosuppressed host may die from toxoplasmosis unless treated. It is not known how corticosteroids cause relapse but it is unlikely that they directly cause rupture of the tissue cysts.

Pathogenicity of *T. gondii* is determined by the virulence of the strain and the susceptibility of the host species. *Toxoplasma gondii* strains may vary in their pathogenicity in a given host. Certain strains of mice are more susceptible than others and the severity of

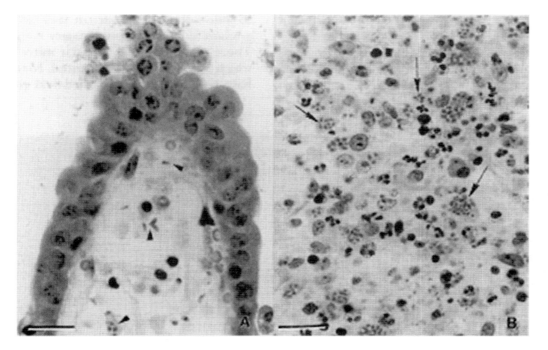

Fig. 47.11 Lesions induced by *T. gondii*. (A) Histological section of the small intestine of a mouse fed *T. gondii* oocysts. Note oedema (empty spaces), necrosis and tachyzoites (arrowheads) in the lamina propria, and desquamation of epithelial cells into the lumen (Haematoxylin and eosin; bar = 20 μm). (B) Section of mesenteric lymph node with numerous tachyzoites (arrows) destroying host cells (Haematoxylin and eosin; bar = 20 μm).

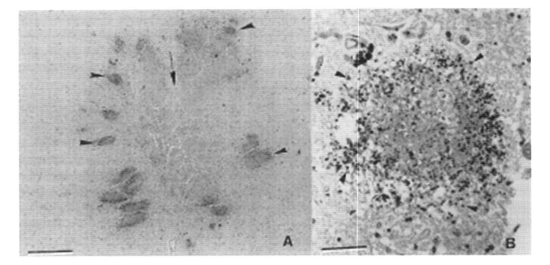

Fig. 47.12 Necrosis associated with *T. gondii* in an AIDS patient. Immunohistochemical stain with anti-*T. gondii* serum (A) Central area of necrosis (arrow) and several satellite lesions (arrowheads) (Bar = 200 μm). (B) Higher magnification of one of the satellite lesions. Note hundreds of tachyzoites (arrowheads, all black dots) at the periphery of the necrotic lesion (Bar = 20 μm).

infection in individual mice within the same strain may vary. Certain species are genetically resistant to clinical toxoplasmosis. For example, adult rats do not become ill while the young rats can die because of toxoplasmosis. Mice of any age are susceptible to clinical *T. gondii* infection. Adult dogs, like adult rats, are resistant, whereas puppies are fully susceptible. Cattle and horses are among the hosts more resistant to clinical toxoplasmosis whereas certain marsupials and New World monkeys are the most susceptible. Nothing is known concerning genetic-related susceptibility to clinical toxoplasmosis in higher mammals, including humans.

Various factors vaguely classified as stress may affect *T. gondii* infection in a host. More severe infections are found in pregnant or lactating mice than in non-lactating mice. Concomitant infection may make the host more susceptible or resistant to *T. gondii* infection.

Disease in humans and other animals

Infection in humans

Toxoplasma gondii infection is widespread among humans and its prevalence varies widely from place to place (Dubey and Beattie 1988; Dubey 2009). In the USA and the UK it is estimated that about 16–40% of people are infected, whereas in Central and South America and continental Europe estimates of infection range from 50–80%.

Most infections in humans are asymptomatic but at times the parasite can produce devastating disease. Infection may be congenitally or postnatally acquired.

Congenital infection occurs generally when a woman becomes infected during pregnancy and the severity of disease may depend upon the stage of pregnancy when the woman becomes infected (Elbez-Rubinstein *et al.* 2009) (Table 47.2). While the mother rarely has symptoms of infection, she does have a temporary parasitaemia. Focal lesions develop in the placenta and the fetus may become infected. At first there is generalized infection in the fetus. Later, infection is cleared from the visceral tissues and may localize in the central nervous system. A wide spectrum of clinical disease occurs in congenitally infected children. Mild disease may consist of slightly diminished vision only, whereas severely diseased children may have the full tetrad of signs: retinochoroiditis and hydrocephalus

Table 47.2 The relation of clinical toxoplasmosis in children to the time of infection in the mother[a]

Trimester infected	Children with toxoplasmosis (%)			
	Serious	Mild	Subclinical	Total No.
First	40	50	10	10
Second	17.7	45	37	62
Third	2.7	28.7	68.5	108
Undetermined	16.6	20.6	56.6	30

[a] From Couvreur *et al.* (1984).

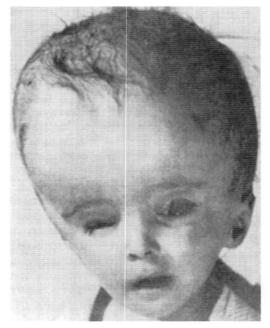

Fig. 47.13 Congenital toxoplasmosis in a child. Note hydrocephalus and microphthalmia

Courtesy of Dr R. Belfort Jr. and National Eye Institute, NIH, Bethesda, Maryland, USA.

(Fig. 47.13), convulsions and intracerebral calcification (Fig. 47.14). Of these, hydrocephalus is the least common but most dramatic lesion of toxoplasmosis. This lesion is unique to congenitally acquired toxoplasmosis in humans and has not been reported in other animals.

By far the mo`st common sequel of congenital toxoplasmosis is ocular disease (Guerina et al. 1994; McAuley et al. 1994; Remington et al. 2006). Except for the occasional involvement of an entire eye, in virtually all cases the disease is confined to the posterior chamber. *Toxoplasma gondii* proliferates in the retina and this leads to inflammation in the choroid. Therefore, the disease is correctly designated as retinochoroiditis. In humans the characteristic lesions of ocular toxoplasmosis in the acute or subacute stage of inflammation appear as yellowish-white, cotton-like patches in the fundus. The lesions may be single or multiple and may involve one or both eyes (Dutton 1989). During the acute stage, inflammatory exudate may cloud the vitreous fluid and may be so dense as to preclude visualization of the fundus by ophthalmoscope examination. As the inflammation subsides, the vitreous clears and the diseased retina and choroid can be seen through the ophthalmoscope. Retinal lesions may be single or multifocal, small, grey areas of active retinitis with minimal oedema and reaction in the vitreous humour. The punctuate lesions are usually harmless unless they are located in a macular area (Fig. 47.15). Although severe infections may be detected at birth, milder infections may go undetected until they flare up in adulthood.

The socio-economic impact of toxoplasmosis in human suffering and the cost of care of sick children, especially those with mental retardation and blindness, are enormous (Roberts and Frenkel 1990; Roberts et al. 1994). The testing of all pregnant women for *T. gondii* infection is compulsory and all pregnant women are tested serologically on their first visit to their gynaecologist. Women with *T. gondii* antibodies are not tested further. Seronegative women are tested monthly and they are treated for toxoplasmosis if they acquire *T. gondii* antibodies during pregnancy. Studies from France and Austria indicate that treatment of women during pregnancy reduces fetal damage. The cost benefits of such mass screening are being debated in many countries (Dubey and Beattie 1988; Lebech and Petersen 1992; Remington et al. 2006; Petersen 2007).

Most people infected after birth are asymptomatic (Montoya and Liesenfeld 2004; Remington et al. 2006). However, some develop a mild disease or in rare cases, a more severe systemic illness and even fatal disease, including pulmonary and multivisceral involvement, possibly from more virulent types of the organism (Carme et al. 2002; Demar et al. 2007). Once infected, people are believed to remain infected for life. Unless immunosuppression occurs and the organism reactivates, people usually remain asymptomatic. However, research is ongoing on whether chronic *T. gondii* infection has an effect on reaction time, tendency for accidents, behavior, and mental illness (Lafferty 2006; Dubey and Jones 2008).

Postnatally acquired infection may be localized or generalized (Table 47.3). Oocyst-transmitted infections may be more severe than tissue cyst-induced infections. Lymphadenitis is the most frequently observed clinical form of toxoplasmosis in humans. Although any node may be involved, the most frequently involved are the deep cervical nodes. These nodes when infected are tender, discrete but not painful, and the infections resolve spontaneously in weeks or months. Lymphadenopathy may be associated with fever, malaise, fatigue, muscle pain, sore throat, and headache. Although the condition may be benign, its diagnosis is vital in pregnant women because of the risk to the fetus.

Until recently, most of toxoplasmic retinochoroiditis was thought to be congenital (Holland 2003). Ophalmologists from Brazil first reported retinochoroiditis in multiple siblings (Silveria et al. 1988). These findings have now been amply confirmed (Burnett et al. 1998). In a largest outbreak of human toxoplasmosis epidemiologically linked to drinking water from a municipal water reservoir in Vancouver, British Columbia, Canada, 20 of 100

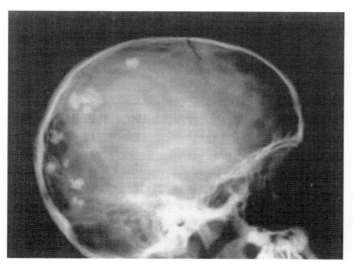

Fig. 47.14 Intracerebral calcification discovered fortuitously in a 10-year-old girl, on a dental panoramic X-ray asked for by a dentist. The girl had unilateral retinochoroiditis and an IQ of 80.
Courtesy of Dr J. Couvreur.

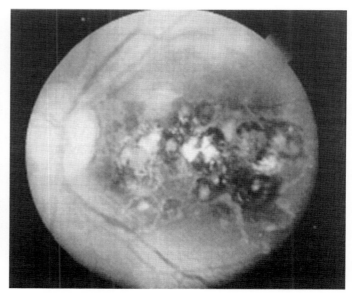

Fig. 47.15 Congenital toxoplasmosis. Retinochoroiditis in the macula of the left eye.
Courtesy of Dr R. Belfort Jr.

Table 47.3 Frequency of symptoms in people with postnatally acquired toxoplasmosis

Symptoms	Patients with symptoms (%)		
	Atlanta, USA outbreak[a] (35 patients)	Panama outbreak[b] (35 patients)	Parána outbreak[c] (155 patients)
Fever	94	90	82
Lymphadenopathy	88	77	75
Headache	88	77	87
Myalgia	63	68	80
Stiff neck	57	55	NR
Anorexia	57	NR[c]	69
Sore throat	46	NR	NR
Arthralgia	26	29	61
Rash	23	0	7
Confusion	20	NR	NR
Earache	17	NR	NR
Nausea	17	36	38
Eye pain	14	26	NR
Abdominal pain	11	55	NR

[a] From Teutsch et al. (1979).
[b] From Benenson et al. (1982).
[c] Not reported.
[d] de Moura et al. (2006).

patients had acquired retinochoroiditis (Bowie *et al.* 1997; Burnett *et al.* 1998). Lymphardenitis was found in 51 of these 100 patients (Bowie *et al.* 1997).

Toxoplasmosis ranks high in the list of diseases which lead to death of patients with AIDS; approximately 10% of AIDS patients in the USA and up to 30% in Europe are estimated to die from toxoplasmosis (Luft and Remington 1992; Luft *et al.* 1993; Rabaud *et al.* 1994). Clinically, patients may have headache, disorientation, drowsiness, hemiparesis, reflex changes, and convulsions, and many become comatose. Diagnosis is aided by serological examination. However, in immunosuppressed patients both inflammatory signs and antibody production may be suppressed, thus making the diagnosis very difficult. Although in AIDS patients any organ may be involved, including the testis, dermis, and the spinal cord, infection of the brain is most frequent. In the brain, the predominant lesion is necrosis, especially of the thalamus. In most AIDS patients, the disease is reactivation of latent *T. gondii* infection because of immunosuppressive effects of the human immunodeficiency virus infection.

By using CT scan, lesions were localized in decreasing order of frequency in cortico-medullary, white matter, basal ganglions, cortex and posterior fossa (Renold *et al.* 1992). Macroscopically, unilateral or bilateral areas of discolouration indicative of necrosis and haemorrhage were noticed. Microscopically, encephalitis involving many areas is the predominant lesion and the difference may vary depending on whether the patient has received anti-toxoplasma therapy. In untreated patients, the lesion involves

a central area of necrosis with degenerating organisms, surrounded by an inflammatory zone with oedema, perivascular infiltration of inflammatory cells and haemorrhage. *Toxoplasma gondii* are more numerous in this peripheral zone surrounding healthy and inflamed tissue. The lesion may be small or the size of a tennis ball and the contents may vary from fluid to solid. Microabscesses are more common in treated patients. In active lesions, numerous tachyzoites are found destroying host tissue. In subacute cases and treated patients, glial nodules predominate. Patients should be treated empirically for toxoplasmic encephalitis based on clinical and neurological findings and presence of *T. gondii* antibodies because a specific diagnosis may not be possible without a biopsy, which is now rarely indicated. Since the years that prophylaxis and highly active antiretroviral therapy became widely used (mid 1990s in most developed countries), the incidence and deaths associated with toxoplasmic encephalitis have declined markedly.

Transplantation of infected organs or transfusion of infected leukocytes can initiate fatal infection in a seronegative recipient receiving immunosuppressive therapy. Transplantation of non-infected organs and leukocyte transfusion can also activate latent infection in a seropositive recipient receiving immunotherapy. Ordinary blood transfusion is virtually free from danger, but transfusion of packed leukocytes and transplantation of bone marrow have caused toxoplasmosis. It seems that the danger of transplanting an organ from a seropositive donor into a seronegative recipient is greater than that of transplanting an organ from a seronegative donor into a seropositive recipient. Recipients of heart and heart lung are more likely to have symptomatic infection than kidney or liver transplant patients (Wreghitt and Joynson 2001).

Malignancies or immunosuppressive treatment of malignancies can reactivate latent toxolasmosis. Toxoplasmosis has been reported most commonly in patients treated for Hodgkin's disease. Untreated Hodgkin's disease is rarely associated with clinical toxoplasmosis. A variety of malignancies including lymphoma, leukaemia, myelomna can reactive toxoplasmosis but there are rare reports of toxoplasmosis associated with solid tumors (Wreghitt and Joynson 2001).

Infection in animals other than humans

Toxoplasma gondii is capable of causing severe disease in animals other than humans. Among livestock, great losses occur in sheep and goats. *Toxoplasma gondii* causes early embryonic death and resorption, fetal death and mummification, abortion, stillbirth, and neonatal death. Toxoplasmosis-induced abortion can occur in ewes of all ages. Infected lambs that survive the first week after birth grow normally. Abortion occurs in ewes that acquire infection during pregnancy. Therefore, ewes which have aborted should be saved for future breeding. Fatal toxoplasmosis has been reported in pigs, dogs, cats, rabbits, birds, and many species of wildlife (Dubey and Beattie 1988; Dubey 2009).

Cattle and horses are more resistant to clinical toxoplasmosis than any other species of livestock. Although both cattle and horses have been found infected with *T. gondii*, there is no documented report of clinical toxoplasmosis in horses or cattle. Toxoplasmosis is most severe in certain species of Australian marsupials and New World monkeys (Dubey and Beattie 1988). It can cause severe blindness in canaries and finches, and wallabies (Dubey 2002; Dubey and Crutchley 2008).

Recent findings of high prevalence of *T. gondii* in free-living marine mammals and mortality associated with protozoal encephalitis in sea otters in the USA has raised concerns for environmental contamination of the environment with *T. gondii* oocysts (Kreuder *et al.* 2003; Thomas *et al.* 2007; Dubey and Jones 2008).

Diagnosis

Diagnosis is made by biological, serological, histological, or molecular methods or by some combination of them. Clinical symptoms of toxoplasmosis are non-specific and toxoplasmosis in fact mimics several other infectious diseases.

Toxoplasma gondii can be isolated from patients by inoculation of laboratory animals and tissue cultures with secretions, excretions, body fluids, and tissues taken by biopsy ante-mortem or tissues with macroscopic lesions taken post-mortem.

Detection of *T. gondii* antibody in patients may aid diagnosis. There are numerous serological procedures used to detect humoral antibodies; these include the Sabin–Feldman dye test, the indirect haemaglutination assay, the indirect fluorescent antibody assay (IFA), the direct agglutination test (DAT), the latex agglutination test, the enzyme-linked immunoabsorbent assay (ELISA), and the immunoabsorbent agglutination assay test (IAAT). The IFA, IAAT, and ELISA have been modified to detect IgM antibodies. The IgM antibodies appear sooner than the IgG antibodies but IgM antibodies also disappear faster than IgG antibodies.

The result of examining one positive serum sample only establishes that the host has been infected at some time in the past. It is best to collect two samples on the same individual. A 16-fold higher antibody titre in a serum taken 2–4 weeks after the first serum was collected indicates an acute acquired infection. A high antibody titre sometimes persists for months and a rise may not be associated with clinical symptoms. As indicated earlier, most acquired infections in humans are asymptomatic.

Diagnosis can be made by finding *T. gondii* in host tissue removed by biopsy or at necropsy. A rapid diagnosis may be made by making impression smears of lesions on glass slides. After drying for 10–30 minutes, the smears are fixed in methyl alcohol and stained with Giemsa. Well-preserved *T. gondii* are crescent-shaped and stain well with any of the Romanowsky stains (Fig. 47.2). In sections, the tachyzoites usually appear as oval to round and only half the size of those in smears (Fig. 47.11). Electron microscopy can aid diagnosis. *Toxoplasma gondii* tachyzoites are always located in vacuoles and have rhoptries with honeycomb structure (Fig. 47.3). Tissue cysts are without septa and with a thin cyst wall butted against the host cell plasmalemma (Figs. 47.4, 47.5). Occasionally, tissue cysts might be found in areas with lesions. The immunohistochemical staining of parasites with *T. gondii* antiserum can aid in diagnosis (Fig. 47.12).

Using secretions, excretions, body fluids taken by biopsy it is possible to search for *T. gondii* microscopically or for toxoplasmal DNA using of the polymerase chain reaction (PCR). The PCR and other gene amplification techniques can be designed to target specific regions of the parasite genome. The most commonly used gene of *T. gondii* is B1. By gene amplification, minute quantities of DNA, representing one organism, can be detected within a few hours. The main drawbacks of these methods are the inability to differentiate between dead and live organisms and the possibility of false positives originating during sample collection and processing. It is advisable not to entirely rely on this test for making vital decisions involving the fetus.

Diagnosis of *T. gondii* infection in the pregnant women, fetus, and the newborn is difficult and may require a combination of several serological tests to estimate the duration and onset of infection and this subject was recently reviewed (Remington *et al.* 2004, 2006; Petersen 2007; Petersen and Liesenfeld 2007).

Treatment

Sulphadiazine and pyrimethamine (Daraprim®) are two drugs widely used for therapy of toxoplasmosis. These two drugs act synergistically by blocking the metabolic pathway involving *p*-taminobenzoic acid and the folic-folinic acid cycle, respectively. These drugs are usually well tolerated but sometimes thrombocytopenia or leucopenia may develop. These effects can be overcome by administering folinic acid and yeast without interfering with treatment because the vertebrate host can utilize presynthesized folinic acid while *T. gondii* cannot (Frenkel 1973). While these drugs have a beneficial action when given in the acute stage of the disease process when there is active multiplication of the parasite, they will not usually eradicate infection. It is believed that these drugs have little effect on cysts. Sulfonamides are excreted within a few hours of administration; therefore, treatment has to be administered in daily divided doses (four doses of 500 mg each) usually for several weeks or months. A loading dose (75 mg) of pyrimethamine during the first 3 days has been recommended because it is absorbed slowly and binds to tissues. From the fourth day, the dose of pyrimethamine is reduced to 25 mg, and 2–10 mg of folinic acid and 5–10 g of bakers' yeast are added (Frenkel 1973; St Georgiev 1994).

The plasma half-life of pyrimethamine is 35–139 hours. It has been administered in varying doses and schedules from daily to every 3 or 4 days. Pyrimethamine can cause nausea, headache, dysgeusia, thrombocytopaenia, and anaemia. Diagnosis and duration of treatment may have to be varied depending on the patient's age and condition (Table 47.4). For example, prenatally infected children, whether with or without clinical manifestations, should be treated for at least one year.

Spiramycin, clindamycin, atovaquone, azithromycin, roxithromycin, clarithromycin, dapsone, and several other less commonly used drugs are available for treatment of toxoplasmosis and these were reviewed by McCabe (2001). Spiramycin is relatively nontoxic to mother and the fetus. It is concentrated in placenta and binds to tissues. Thus, it is used to prevent transmission of *T. gondii* from mother to the fetus.

Clindamycin is absorbed quickly and diffuses well into the central nervous system and therefore, has been used as alternative to sulfadiazine. It is rarely used to treat the primary maternal infection in pregnancy or congenital infection because it enters foetal blood when given to pregnant women. A major side effect of clindamycin is ulcerative colitis. McCabe (2001) has discussed in detail treatment of toxoplasmosis in patients with various clinical manifestations.

Prophylactic treatment
Immunosuppressed patients
Before being given immunosuppressive treatments, patients should be serologically tested and, if devoid of *T. gondii* antibodies, be treated with pyrimethamine and sulfadiazine. This is particularly desirable in the case of patients receiving organ transplants. As it is usually impossible to carry out serologic tests on donors, they must all be considered potentially dangerous. There will, however, be

Table 47.4 Treatment schedule for toxoplasmosis [a]

I. General
Pyrimethamine + sulfadiazine: 21-day course
Pyrimethamine: 0.5 to 2 mg/kg/day
Sulfadiazine: 50 to 100 mg/kg/day in two divided doses
Folic acid (leukovorin calcium): 2 to 20 mg (or 5 to 10 g bakers' yeast) twice weekly during pyrimethamine treatment.
II. Prophylactic treatment during pregnancy
Treatment to be started as soon as prenatal diagnosis is made
Spiramnycin is 100 mg/kg/day in two divided doses, administered orally. Usually 2–4 g daily
Or
Spiramycin before the 20th week of pregnancy and thereafter pyrimethamine and sulfadiazine.
III. Congenital toxoplasmosis
Pyrimethamine: 2 mg/kg orally four times per day for 2 days, then 1 mg/kg per day for 6 months, then thrice weekly.
+ sulphadiazine: 100 mg/kg per day orally (two divided doses)
+ folinic acid: 5–10 mg orally thrice weekly
IV. Ocular toxoplasmosis
Pryimethamine 75 mg/day and sulfadiazine 2 grams daily, or Clindamycin, 300 mg orally, four times daily.
Coricosteroids: only if inflammation present
Prednisone or methylprednisone 1 to 2 mg/kg/ay in two divided doses.
Photocoagulation and cryotherapy around active retinochoroiditis lesion to kill *T. gondii* encysted at the periphery of the lesions.
V. AIDS patients
A. Acute toxoplasmic encephalitis
Primethamine 200 mg oral initially and then 75–100 mg orally four times daily
+ Sulfadiazine 1–2 grams oral, four times daily
Or
Pyrimethamine + clindamycin 60 mg orally or intravenously 6 hourly
Or
Pyrimethamine + dapsone 100 mg orally four times daily
Or
Pyrimethamine + azithromycin 1200–1500 mg orally four times daily.
Or
Pyrimethamine + clarithromycin 1 gram orally two times daily
B. Maintenance treatment
Doses of pyrimethamine and sulfadiazine reduced to half or less of those given for treating acute toxoplasmosis and the treatment continued for life
Folic acid should be given daily
C. Prophylactic treatment in AIDS patients with antibodies to *T. gondii*.
Trimethaprim–sulfamethoxazole, widely used for the prophylaxis and treatment of *Pneumocystis carinii* infections thought to reduce onset of toxoplasmic encephalitis

[a] From Dubey (2005a).

time to test the recipients, and if seronegative, they should certainly be given prophylactic treatment. This strategy appears to have been effective in reducing the incidence of latent *T. gondii* infection in patients given marrow transplants from seronegative donors. Perhaps prophylactic treatment should be given to all recipients, irrespective of their sero-status.

Prophylactic treatment of all AIDS patients with *T. gondii* antibodies is desirable. Fortunately, some drugs used to prophylactically treat *Pneumocystis* pneumonia and bacterial infections may also prevent onset of clinical toxaplasmosis. Trimethoprim (160 mg) and sulfamethoxazole (800 mg) (twice daily and two times per week) combination is often used because it is inexpensive, convenient and works against *Pneumocystis* (McCabe 2001).

Cutaneous hypersensitivity, however, can be a problem and then alternative therapies are sought. A combination of dapsone (100 mg) and pyrimethamine (25 mg) orally weekly has also been used effectively. Other combinations of pyrimethamine and sulfanomides (Fansidar, three tablets every two weeks) have also been used.

Prophylactic treatment during pregnancy

Prevention of infection of the fetus by prophylactic treatment of the mother depends on the delay which occurs between maternal infection and its transmission to the fetus. It is also hoped that if infection is already present in the fetus, treatment may limit its ill effects. Serologic surveillance to detect maternal *T. gondii* infection during pregnancy is compulsory in Austria and France and is being applied to a few other countries. Treatment is initiated as soon as possible during the prenatal incubation period. In Austria, it is by spiramycin before the twentieth week of pregnancy and thereafter by pyrimethamine and sulfonamide, and in France it is by spiramycin alone. If these measures are begun sufficiently early, they may be expected to reduce the incidence of congenital toxoplasmosis by 50 to 70%.

In places where it has been carried out with thoroughness, persistence and determination, as in France, education appears to have contributed to a reduction in the incidence of *T. gondii* infection during pregnancy. Information regarding *T. gondii* infection should be included with the general instructions given in antenatal clinics and by obstetricians and midwives dealing with individual patients. Personal instruction given by word of mouth is likely to be most effective, and should be supplemented by booklets printed in various languages and by videos in the waiting rooms of antenatal clinics.

Treatment schedules are summarized in Table 47.4.

Epidemiology

Toxoplasma gondii infection in humans is widespread and occurs throughout the world. Approximately one-half billion humans have antibodies to *T. gondii*. Infection rates in humans and others animals differ from one geographical area of a country to another. The causes of these variations are not yet known. Environmental conditions, cultural habits of the people, and animal fauna are some of the factors that may determine the level of infection with *T. gondii*. Infection is more prevalent in hot and humid areas than in dry and cold climates. Only a small proportion (less than 1%) of people acquire infection congenitally.

Women produce children with congenital infection generally once. Mothers of congenitally infected children have not been known to give birth to infected children in subsequent pregnancies.

The relative frequency of acquisition of postnatal toxoplasmosis due to eating raw meat and that due to ingestion of food contaminated by oocysts from cat faeces is not known and is difficult to investigate. *Toxoplasma gondii* infection is common in many animals used for food. Sheep, pigs, and rabbits are commonly infected throughout the world. Infection in cattle is less prevalent than in sheep or pigs. Infection is common in many species of wildlife, especially in deer and bears (Dubey 1994; Dubey and Jones 2008). *Toxoplasma gondii* tissue cysts survive in live food animals for years. As stated earlier, humans can acquire infection by eating raw or undercooked meat.

Toxoplasma gondii organisms in meat are susceptible to extremes of temperatures. Tissue cysts are killed by cooking meat to 67°C. *Toxoplasma gondii* in meat is killed by cooling to −13°C. Tissue cysts are also killed by exposure to 0.5 kGy of gamma irradiation.

Cultural habits of people may play a role in acquiring *T. gondii* infections. For example, in France the prevalence of *Toxoplasma* antibody is very high. The higher incidence in France appears to be related in part to the French habit of eating some of their meat raw. The high prevalence of *T. gondii* infection in Central and South America is in part due to high levels of contamination of the environment by oocysts (Dubey and Beattie 1988; Jones and Dubey 2010).

Oocysts are shed by domestic cats and wild felids. Widespread infection of the environment is possible because a cat may excrete millions of oocysts after ingesting one infected mouse. Oocysts are resistant to most ordinary environmental conditions and can survive in moist conditions for months and even years. Invertebrates, such as flies, cockroaches, dung beetles, and earthworms, can spread oocysts mechanically and even carry them onto food.

While only a few cats may be shedding *T. gondii* oocysts at any given time, the enormous numbers shed is important in the spread of *T. gondii*. Whether cats normally shed oocysts only once or several times during their lifetime is not known; however, under experimental conditions, cats develop good immunity to *T. gondii* against oocyst shedding but can reshed oocysts after re-inoculation of tissue cysts (Dubey 1995). Congenital infection can occur in cats and congenitally infected kittens can excrete oocysts. Infection rates of cats probably vary with the rate of infection in local avian and rodent populations because cats are thought to become infected in nature by eating these animals.

Theoretically, transmission of toxoplasmosis may be by sexual means, by ingestion of milk, saliva, or by eating of eggs. The stage most likely to be involved in these transmissions would be tachyzoites. Tachyzoites are delicate and do not survive outside the body for long. Therefore, there is practically no risk of transmission by kissing or by venereal transmission. There is little, if any, danger of *T. gondii* infection by drinking cow's milk and, in any case, milk is generally pasteurized or even boiled. However infection has followed drinking unboiled goat's milk. Raw hens' eggs, although an important source of *Salmonella* infection, are extremely unlikely to transmit *T. gondii* infection.

Transmission by transplantation is also important (Wreghitt and Hakim 1989). Toxoplasmosis may arise in two ways in people undergoing transplantation: from implantation of an organ or bone marrow from an infected donor into a non-immune immunocompromised recipient, and from induction of disease in an immunocompromised latently infected recipient. In the later case, the immunosuppressive treatment activates the latent infection of the recipient. In these cases both tachyzoites and tissue cysts might be involved, but more probably tissue cysts. In both cases the cytotoxic and immunosuppressive therapy given to the recipient is the cause of induction of the active infection and the disease.

Prevention and control
Vaccination

The objectives of use of vaccines against toxoplasmosis include reducing fetal damage, reducing the number of *T. gondii* tissue cysts in animals, and preventing the formation of oocysts in cats (Araujo 1994; Dubey 1994). All of these objectives are not currently feasible with the use of a single vaccine. At present there are no effective subunit or killed vaccines for immunization against *T. gondii* but research is under way in many laboratories.

One vaccine that contains a strain (S48) of tachyzoites that does not persist in the tissues of sheep is available in Europe and New Zealand to reduce fetal losses attributable to toxoplasmosis (Buxton 1993). Ewes vaccinated with the S48 strain vaccine retain immunity for at least 18 months (Buxton 1993). However, this vaccine does not prevent reinfection and encystment of wild strain of *T. gondii*.

Prevention

To prevent infection of human beings by *T. gondii*, hands should be washed thoroughly with soap and water after handling meat. All cutting boards, sink tops, knives, and other materials coming in contact with uncooked meat should be washed with soap and water. This is effective because the stages of *T. gondii* in meat are killed by soap and water. Meat of any animal should be cooked to 67°C before consumption, and tasting meat while cooking or seasoning home-made sausages should be avoided. Pregnant women, especially, should avoid contact with cats, soil, and raw meat. Pet cats should be fed only dry, canned, or cooked food. The cat litter box should be emptied every day, preferably not by a pregnant woman. Gloves should be worn while gardening. Vegetables should be washed thoroughly before eating because they may have been contaminated with cat faeces. Expectant mothers should be aware of the dangers of toxoplasmosis.

To prevent infection in cats, they should never be fed uncooked meat, viscera, or bones, and efforts should be made to keep cats indoors to prevent hunting. Trash cans also should be covered to prevent scavenging.

Cats should be neutered to control the feline population on farms. Dead animals should be removed promptly to prevent cannibalism by pigs and scavenging by cats. Sheep that have aborted due to toxoplasmosis usually do not have subsequent toxoplasmic abortions, and thus can be saved for future breeding. Fetal membranes and dead fetuses should be not be handled with bare hands and should be buried or incinerated to prevent infection of felids and other animals on the farm. Cats should not be allowed near pregnant sheep and goats. Grain should be kept covered to prevent oocyst contamination.

To prevent infection of zoo animals with *T. gondii*, cats, including all wild Felidae, should be housed in a building separate from other animals, particularly marsupials and New World monkeys. Cats as a rule should not be fed uncooked meat. However, if a choice has to be made, frozen meat is less likely to contain live *T. gondii* than fresh meat, and beef is less likely to contain *T. gondii* than is horse meat, pork, or mutton. Dissemination of *T. gondii* oocysts in the zoo should be prevented because of potential exposure of children. Brooms, shovels, and other equipment used to clean cat cages, and cat enclosures should be autoclaved or heated to 67°C for at least 10 minutes at regular intervals. While cleaning cages, animal caretakers should wear masks and protective clothing. Feline faeces should be removed daily to prevent sporulation of oocysts.

Sarcocystosis

Introduction and history

The *Sarcocystis* parasite was first found in the skeletal muscle of a house mouse, *Mus musculus* in Switzerland in 1843 (Table 47.5). Before 1972, many of these parasites were named based upon the finding of cysts in the muscles of a host. The true nature of these intramuscular cysts remained unknown until the discovery of the life cycle of *Sarcocystis* in 1972 (Table 47.5).

Classification

Sarcocystis species are coccidian parasites, classified in the family Sarcocystidae (Poche 1913), subfamily, Sarcocystinae (Poche 1913), and genus, *Sarcocystis* (Lankester 1882).

Structure and life cycle

Sarcocysts (in Greek *sarkos* = flesh, *kystis* = bladder) are the terminal asexual stage of development of these parasites. They are found primarily in the striated muscles of mammals, including humans (Fig. 47.16), birds, marsupials, and poikilothermic animals.

Sarcocystis has an obligatory prey-predator two host life cycle (Fig. 47.17). Asexual stages develop only in the intermediate host, which in nature is often a prey animal. Sexual stages develop only in the definitive host, which is carnivorous.

The intermediate host becomes infected by ingesting sporocysts in food or water. Sporozoites excyst from sporocysts in the small intestine and produce intravascular meronts that give rise to the encysted form (sarcocyst) in muscles. Sarcocysts become infectious only when they contain bradyzoites (Dubey 2005c).

The definitive host become infected by ingesting tissues containing mature sarcocysts. Bradyzoites liberated from the sarcocyst by digestion in the stomach and intestine transform into male (micro) and female (macro) gamonts. After fertilization of macrogamete by microgamete, a wall develops around the zygote and the oocyst is formed. The entire process of gametogony and fertilization can be completed within 24 hours, and gamonts and oocysts may be found at the same time. *Sarcocystis* species oocysts sporulate in the lamina propria (Fig. 47.18). Sporulated oocysts are generally colourless, thin-walled (< 1 μm), and contain two elongated sporocysts. Each sporocyst contains four elongated sporozoites and a residual body. The oocyst wall is thin and often ruptures. Free sporocysts, released into the intestinal lumen, are passed in the faeces.

Unlike *Toxoplasma*, there are more than 100 species of this genus (Dubey *et al.* 1989). Only certain species of *Sarcocystis* are pathogenic to intermediate hosts (Dubey *et al.* 1989). Generally species transmitted by canids are more pathogenic than those transmitted by felids. *Sarcocystis* generally does not cause illness in definitive hosts.

Sarcocystis neurona is an unusual species of the genus that does not follow the lifecycle pattern of other species outlined above. It is also one of the most pathogenic species of the genus. *Sarcocystic neurona* is the most frequent cause of a fatal equine protozoal encephalomyelitis (EPM) in horses in the Americas (Dubey *et al.* 2001). Horses are considered the aberrant host because only schizonts are found in their tissues. Unlike other species, *S. neurona* schizonts occur in neural cells, not in the vascular endothelium. Its sarcocysts occur in domestic cats, striped skunks, raccoons, sea otters, and armadillos. Opossums (*Didelphis virginianus, D. abbreventis*) are its definitive hosts. Only the sexual cycle occurs in the definitive host and it is confined to the small intestine. Encephalomyelitis associated with *S. neurona* has been reported in horses, ponies, zebras, skunks, raccoons, cats, lynx, mink and marine mammals (Pacific harbour seals and sea otters).

Sarcocystis canis is another unusual species of the genus with an unknown life cycle. Its sarcocysts, sexual phase and definitive hosts are unknown. Schizont is the only stage that is known. *Sarcocystis canis* has been found associated with fatal hepatitis in sea lions, dogs, black and grizzly bears, a horse, and a dolphin (Dubey and Speer 1991; Dubey *et al.* 2006).

Table 47.5 Historical landmarks concerning *Sarcocystis*[a]

Year	Findings	Reference
1843	Sarcocysts found in muscles of a horse	Miesher (1843)
1882	Genus *Sarcocystis* introduced	Lankaster (1982)
1943	*Sarcocystis* not transmitted from sheep to sheep, role of carnivores suspected but not proven	Scott (1943)
1972	Sexual phase cultured *in vitro*	Fayer (1972)
1972	Two-host life cycle found	Rommel and Heydorn (1972); Rommel *et al.* (1972)
1973	Vascular phase recognized and pathogenicity demonstrated	Fayer and Johnson (1975)
1975	Multiple *Sarcocystis* species within a given host recognized	Heydorn *et al.* (1975)
1975	Chemotherapy demonstrated	Fayer and Johnson (1973)
1978	Abortion due to sarcocystosis is recognized	Fayer *et al.* (1979)
1981	Protective immunity demonstrated	Dubey (1980)
1986	Vascular phase cultured *in vitro*	Speer and Dubey (1986)
2000	Unusual life cycle of *S. neurona* discovered	Dubey *et al.* (2000)

[a] From Dubey *et al.* (1989). For complete bibliography see Dubey *et al.* (1989).

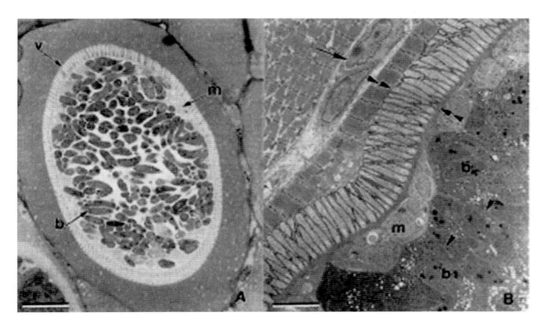

Fig. 47.16 Intramuscular *S. hominis* sarcocysts (A) Histological section of a mature sarcocyst. Note finger4ike villar protrusions on the cyst wall enclosing numerous bradyzoites (b) and a few metrocytes (m) (Toluidine blue; bar = 20 μm). (B) Transmission electron micrograph. Note villar projections on the cyst wall (double opposing arrowheads), metrocytes (m), bradyzoites (b), and septa (arrowheads). Arrow points to the host cell nucleus (Bar = 4.3 μm).

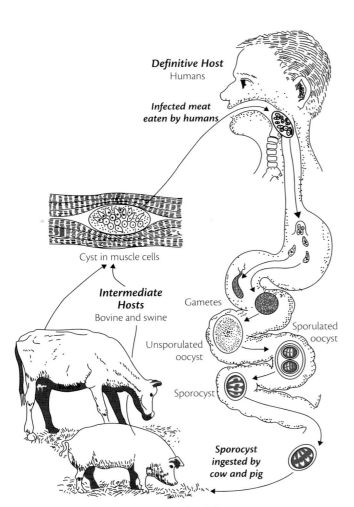

Fig. 47.17 Life cycle of *S. hominis* and *S. suihominis*

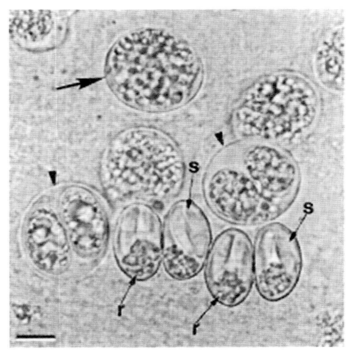

Fig. 47.18 Sporogony of *Sarcocystis* in the Intestinal lamina propria of an infected animal. Note unsporulated oocyst (arrow), two partially sporulated oocysts (arrowheads), and two fully sporulated oocysts containing sporozoites (s) and residual body (r) (Unstained; bar = 10 μm).

Sarcocystosis in humans

There are two known species of *Sarcocystis* for which humans serve as the definitive host, *S. hominis* and *S. suihominis* (Murrell *et al.* 1985). Humans also serve as accidental intermediate hosts for several unidentified species of *Sarcocystis*. Symptoms in persons with intestinal sarcocystosis are different from those persons with muscular sarcocystosis and vary with the species of *Sarcocystis* causing infection.

Intestinal sarcocystosis

Sarcocystis hominis (Railliet and Lucet 1891; Dubey 1976)

Infection with this species is acquired by ingesting uncooked beef containing *S. hominis* sarcocysts. *Sarcocystis hominis* is only mildly pathogenic for humans. Volunteers who ate raw beef developed nausea, stomach ache, and diarrhoea 3–6 hours after ingesting the beef; these symptoms lasted 24–36 hours. The volunteers excreted *S. hominis* sporocysts between 14 and 18 days after ingesting the beef (Aryeetey and Piekarski 1976; Heydorn 1977). In one report, six of seven human volunteers that ate 128–260 g of Kibbe (a preparation made from raw beef and spices) obtained from an Arabian restaurant in Saõ Paulo, Brazil, excreted *S. hominis* sporocysts 10–14 days later. Two of these volunteers became ill. One of them had abdominal pain and diarrhoea 1–3 days p.i. and the other had diarrhoea 11 days p.i. (Pena *et al.* 2001). A patient in Spain developed abdominal pain and loose stools after eating raw beef; the diagnosis was confirmed by finding *S. hominis* sporocysts in faeces (Clavel *et al.* 2001).

A *Sarcocystis* species similar to *S. hominis* named *S. dubeyi* (Huong and Uggla 1999) has been found in water buffaloes. The definitive host for *S. dubeyi* is unknown but suspected to be humans.

Sarcocystis suihominis (Tadros and Laarman 1976; Heydorn 1977)

This species, acquired by eating undercooked pork, is more pathogenic than *S. hominis*. Human volunteers developed hypersensitivity-like symptoms; nausea, vomiting, stomach ache, diarrhoea, and dyspnoea within 24 hours of ingestion of uncooked pork from naturally or experimentally infected pigs. Sporocysts were shed 11–13 days after ingesting pork (Rommel and Heydorn 1972; Piekarski *et al.* 1978; Hiepe *et al.* 1979; Kimmig *et al.* 1979; Dubey *et al.* 1989). Zho (1991) found sporocysts in stools of 123 of 414 (29.7%) persons from 3 villages in Xianguan City in China. He reported that these people ate raw pork but not raw beef.

Intestinal sarcocystosis of humans

Before the discovery of the life cycle of *Sarcocystis* and recognition of cattle and pigs as sources of human infection, *Sarcocystis* sporocysts in human faeces were referred to as *Isospora hominis*. Because of structural similarities between *S. hominis* and *S. suihominis* sporocysts, it is not possible to distinguish between them by microscopic examination. Intestinal sarcocystosis is more common in Europe than in other continents. Enteritis was associated with shedding of *Sarcocystis* sporocysts in some cases (reviewed in Dubey *et al.* 1989).

Muscular sarcocystosis of humans

Sarcocysts have been found in striated muscles of human beings, mostly as incidental findings. Judging from the published reports, sarcocysts in humans are rare (Beaver *et al.* 1979; Dubey *et al.* 1989). Most reported cases were from Asia and south east Asia. Sarcocysts were found in both in skeletal and cardiac muscles. The clinical significance of sarcocysts and their life cycles in humans are unknown. In one report, 7 of 15 USA military men developed acute illness after an army exercise in rural Malaysia (Arness *et al.* 1999).

The illness was characterized by fever, myalgias, bronchospasm, fleeting pruritic rashes, transient lymphadenopathy, and subcutaneous nodules associated with eosinophilia, elevated erythrocyte sedimentation rate, and elevated levels of muscle creatinine kinase. Sarcocysts of an unidentified *Sarcocystis* species were found in skeletal muscle biopsies of the index case. Symptoms in five other men were mild to moderate and self-limited, and one team member with laboratory abnormalities was asymptomatic. Of eight team members tested for antibody to *Sarcocystis*, six were positive; of four with the eosinophilic myositis syndrome who were tested, all were positive. The illness was considered to be sarcocystosis. Arness *et al.* (1999) also reviewed other cases of sarcocystosis after 1990.

Epidemiology and control

Poor hygiene practiced in underdeveloped countries during handling of meat from slaughter place to kitchen can be a source of *Sarcocystis* infection. In one survey in India, *S. suihominis* oocysts were found in the faeces of 14 out of 20 three to twelve year old children (Banerjee *et al.* 1994), indicating that meat was consumed raw at least by some because *S. suihominis* can only be transmitted to humans by the consumption of raw pork. In another study, 3–5 year old children from a slum area were found to consume meat scraps virtually raw, and many pigs from that area harboured *S. suihominis* sarcocysts (Solanki *et al.* 1991). In European countries where consumption of raw or undercooked meat is relatively high, humans are expected to have intestinal sarcocystosis (Dubey *et al.* 1989). To prevent intestinal infection, meat should be cooked thoroughly before human consumption.

Diagnosis

The ante-mortem diagnosis of muscular sarcocystosis can only be made at present by histological examination of muscle collected by biopsy. The finding of immature sarcocysts with metrocytes suggests recently acquired infection. The finding of mature sarcocysts only indicates past infection. The diagnosis of intestinal sarcocystosis is easily made by faecal examination. As said earlier, sporocysts or oocysts are shed fully sporulated in faeces. It is not possible to distinguish species of *Sarcocystis* based on sporocyst morphology.

Treatment

There is no treatment known for *Sarcocystis* infections of humans. The intestinal phase of *Sarcocystis* is caused by oocysts in the lamina propria of small intestine; there are no drugs that can kill oocysts *in situ*. The muscular phase is rarely diagnosed ante-mortem.

Isosporosis

Introduction and the aetiological agent

Isospora belli (Wenyon 1923), is the cause of coccidiosis in humans. It belongs to the family Eimeriidae and the genus, *Eimeria*. Most of the reported cases occurred in the tropics rather than in the temperate zone. Infection is now seen more frequently in immunocomprised patients, particularly those with AIDS (Restrepo *et al.* 1987; Dubey 1993; Michiels *et al.* 1994; Lindasy *et al.* 1997; Velàsquez *et al.* 2001; Jongwutiwes *et al.* 2007; Karanis *et al.* 2007).

CHAPTER 48

Babesiosis and malaria

F. E. G. Cox

Summary

Babesiosis and malaria are rare zoonoses that, with new developments in diagnosis and the application of molecular techniques, are becoming increasingly frequently recognized. *Babesia* species infect millions of cattle and unknown numbers of sheep, dogs, horses, and wildlife throughout the world but human infections are very uncommon. There are two distinct forms of human babesiosis. In Europe the causative agent is *Babesia divergens*, a natural parasite of cattle transmitted by the tick *Ixodes ricinus*. *B. divergens* infections in humans are extremely rare and nearly all have been recorded from asplenic or otherwise immunocompromised patients. In the USA, human babesiosis is more common than in Europe, although still very rare, and is not restricted to immunocompromised individuals. The causative agents are *Babesia microti* and *B. duncani*, common parasites of rodents, transmitted by the tick *Ixodes scapularis*. In addition there have been sporadic reports of human babesiosis from other parts of the world but in most cases the species of *Babesia* involved has not been characterized. Malaria parasites and *Babesia* both inhabit red blood cells during part of their life cycles and these stages cause the diseases, malaria and babesiosis, which are similar in many respects. The fact that humans can occasionally acquire malaria and babesiosis from animals, that both parasites appear similar when seen in blood films and that both cause similar symptoms can cause problems in diagnosis and these rare infections are, therefore, of interest to clinicians and epidemiologists.

Babesiosis

History

Babesia spp are conspicuous parasites in red blood cells in which they occur either singly or in pairs. They were recognized for the first time in 1888 and associated with a disease in cattle by Viktor Babes who thought that they were bacteria (Babes 1888). In 1893, Smith and Kilbourne realized that they were protozoa and also demonstrated their transmission by ticks thus predating the discovery of the transmission of malaria parasites by mosquitoes by several years (Smith and Kilbourne 1893). Subsequently many other animals, wild and domesticated, were shown to be infected with *Babesia* spp. (Kakoma and Melhorn 1994). The first indications that humans could be infected with *Babesia* came in 1904

when Wilson and Chowning found an organism that they named *Piroplasma hominis* in patients suffering from Rocky Mountain Spotted Fever but, although their drawings appear to show *Babesia*, whether or not these were really *Babesia* will never be known (Wilson and Chowning 1904). There then followed a number of isolated reports of human infections with *Babesia* but most, if not all, are now thought to be misidentifications of malaria parasites or blood artefacts. It was not until 1956 that the first really well documented case of human babesiosis, in a farmer in the former Yugoslavia, was reported and this was soon followed by reports of a number of other cases, nearly all in asplenic patients in Europe (Gray 2006). The importance of human babesiosis only became apparent from the mid 1960s onwards when patients suffering from febrile illness were found to be harbouring the rodent parasite *Babesia microti*, first from California and shortly afterwards from Nantucket Island, Massachusetts, USA. Since then, several hundred other cases have been recorded mainly from the USA plus increasing numbers of isolated reports from other parts of the world including Brazil, Mexico, Taiwan, China, India, Japan, Egypt, South Africa, Russia, and Europe (Gorenflot 1998; Kjemtrup and Conrad 2000; Ristic 1998; Telford and Spielman 2005).

Human babesiosis is difficult to diagnose accurately because the different species of *Babesia* are morphologically very similar and resemble malaria parasites. Thus many records, particularly earlier ones and ones from outside the recognized areas where the disease now occurs, are largely based on guess work. When only authenticated and well documented cases are considered, human babesiosis is seen to fall into two categories, the European form acquired from cattle infected with *B. divergens*, mainly in asplenic or immunocompromised individuals and which can be fatal, and the American form acquired from rodents infected with *B. microti* or a related species *B. duncani* (Gray and Weiss 2008). Phylogenetic analyses of the relationships between *Babesia* species indicate that the rodent and cattle species are distantly related and the use of molecular techniques has made it much easier to identify the occasional parasites that occur in humans (Goethert and Telford 2003). These techniques have also resulted in the recognition of a small number of *Babesia* parasites that cannot be identified as *B. divergens*, *B. microti* or *B. duncani*, for example forms from Korea that resemble ovine *Babesia*, a *B. divergens*-like parasite from the US, two forms from Japan and others from Brazil, Mexico, China, Taiwan, Egypt, and South Africa.

Cattle-derived babesiosis

The agents

The babesias, like the malaria parasites, belong to the kingdom Protozoa, phylum Sporozoa (Apicomplexa) and class Coccidea which also includes the zoonotic coccidians *Toxoplasma gondii*, *Sarcocystis* spp., *Cyclospora* spp. and *Cryptosporidium* spp. (Table 48.1). *Babesia* species are parasites of vertebrates transmitted by ticks. The form in the vertebrate host is the trophozoite or feeding stage that infects red blood cells in which it divides by binary fission to produce two to four merozoites each of which invades a new cell. These blood stages cause serious diseases in domesticated animals including cattle, horses, and dogs and the general name given is babesiosis or piroplasmosis. Over 100 species of *Babesia* have been identified in mammals mainly on the blood stages but, as there are few morphological characters to go on, this is not altogether satisfactory and new information based on molecular techniques is gradually rationalizing the number of species. The life cycles of all *Babesia* species are similar. The infection begins when sporozoites are injected via the bite of an infected tick. What happens next is unclear and it may be that there is some multiplication in cells other than red blood cells but this has been very difficult to demonstrate. However, what is clear is that there follows a phase of multiplication, usually by binary fission, within red blood cells. Eventually gametocytes are formed and these are taken up by another tick when it feeds. Within the gut of the tick, fertilization and the formation of zygotes occur followed by phases of multiplication in the intestinal cells and salivary glands resulting in the production of many sporozoites that are injected into a new host when the infected tick bites. During their life cycle, ticks pass through three stages, larva, nymph, and adult. Each stage feeds on blood but the stage that becomes infected is not the stage that is infective; if the larva is infected then the nymph is infective and if the nymph is infected then the adult is infective. In addition, in some species of ticks, infected female adults may pass the infection on to their larvae. Male ticks seldom feed so are largely irrelevant to the transmission of this disease.

The hosts

It is estimated that worldwide some 1.2 billion cattle are at risk from infection with babesiosis and actual infections with the most important pathogens, *B. bovis*, *B. divergens*, *B. major* and *B. bigemina* are very common (Ristic 1988). Human infections have been ascribed to *B. divergens* and, less reliably, to *B. bovis*. *Babesia divergens*,

Table 48.1 Outline classification of the Kingdom Protozoa. Phylum Sporozoa (Apicomplexa) showing the taxonomic positions of the genera that affect humans and the species of *Babesia* and *Plasmodium* that can be transmitted from animals to humans

KINGDOM PROTOZOA
Phylum Sporozoa
Class Coccidea
Order Eimeriida (*Cryptosporidium, Cyclospora, Isospora, Sarcocystis, Toxoplasma*)
Order Haemosporidida (*Plasmodium* spp. *P. knowlesi, P. brasilianum, P. cynomolgi, P. eylesi, P.inui, P. schwetzi, P. simium*)
Order Piroplasmida (*Babesia* spp. *B. divergens, B. microti, B. duncani*)

once thought to be the same as *B. bovis*, occurs in Europe and is transmitted by *Ixodes ricinus*, a three-host tick whose larvae, nymphs, and adults feed on different hosts that are virtually any warm blooded animals. Typically, the larvae feed on small mammals while the nymphs and larvae feed on larger ones but there is no rigidity about this pattern. *Babesia bovis* has a worldwide distribution and is transmitted by ticks belonging to the genus *Boophilus*, which feed as larvae, nymphs, and adults on the same host and are rarely found on hosts other than cattle. Transmission of *Babesia* occurs in the spring and autumn when the larvae and nymphs are most active. It is unlikely that any of the reported human infections have actually been *B. bovis* because the ticks involved seldom feed on humans. On the other hand, *I. ricinus*, the tick that transmits *B. divergens*, the species that occurs in northern Europe where most human cases have been reported, frequently feeds on humans. It is now generally accepted that human babesiosis acquired in Europe are all probably caused by *B. divergens* but that the potential for infection with other species does exist.

Since the first report in 1957, there have been further reports of human babesiosis in Europe from France, Germany, Ireland, Portugal, Spain, Sweden, the UK, the former Yugoslavia, and Russia (Gray 2006). Nearly all occurred in asplenic or otherwise immunologically compromised individuals mostly in those associated with farming, camping or other outdoor activity and most patients recalled having been bitten by ticks. Parasites isolated from humans revert to a typical *B. divergens* form when passaged back into calves. Although the vector is not known for certain, circumstantial evidence points to *I. ricinus*. In all probability, larval ticks become infected with *B. divergens* from cattle, drop off and moult into nymphs that pass the infection on to individuals, such as farmers, campers, and hikers that come in close contact with them. Not all individuals seem to be equally susceptible to infection and it is worth noting that the fatal and severe cases usually occurred in patients who were asplenic whereas none of the asymptomatic individuals found to harbour parasites had had their spleens removed.

Babesia divergens infections in cattle are relatively mild but in humans they are usually severe. After an incubation period of 1–3 weeks the patient begins to experience a range of rather vague symptoms including headaches, muscle pains and weakness and then develops a high fever, alternating sweating and chills, intestinal discomfort, vomiting and diarrhoea and haemoglobinuria. In some patients the haemoglobin level drops catastrophically, there is renal failure, loss of consciousness coma and death.

Rodent-derived babesiosis

The agents

Following an isolated case of human babesiosis from California in 1968 there were a number of other reports of rodent-derived human babesiosis from Nantucket Island Massachusetts and over the next ten years there were over 40 similar cases from the coastal strip of New England comprising islands off the Massachusetts coast, Rhode Island, and Connecticut (Kjemtrup and Conrad 2000). Since then, there have been several hundred cases of babesiosis in these areas and also in inland Connecticut. Babesiosis is now a notifiable disease in the States of Massachusetts and New York. The causative agent is a common rodent parasite, *B. microti*, transmitted by the deer tick *Ixodes scapularis* (formerly known as *I. dammini*) which feeds on small rodents and deer. Adult ticks feed on deer, *Odocoileus virginianis,* in the Autumn and lay their eggs in the following Spring. Larvae emerge in the Autumn, feed on the white footed mouse *Peromyscus leucopus,* from which they acquire their infections, then overwinter and moult into infective nymphs in the following Spring.

All the North American cases of *B. microti* in humans have occurred in the northeastern and midwestern American States but parasites that were apparently not *B. microti* were also recorded from Washington State (designated WA1-3) and California (CA1-6). The parasites isolated from these cases produce fulminating infections in hamsters, something that the East Coast and European strains never do suggesting that on the West Coast there is a completely different focus of infection. There have now been over a dozen cases which were initially attributed to *B. equi,* a parasite of horses, or *B. canis* from dogs but are now know to be caused by a novel species, *B. duncani* a species related to *B. microti* (Conrad *et al.* 2006).

The hosts

Babesia microti is also a very common parasite in small mammals throughout Europe, where the main vector is *Ixodes trianguliceps,* a tick that rarely feeds on humans. Although there have been occasional records of *B. microti* in humans in Europe none has been associated with serious disease. There have also been at least two cases of imported *B. microti,* one from the USA into the Czech Republic and one from Brazil into Poland (Gray and Weiss 2008). Elsewhere, there have been reports of human babesiosis from South America, China, Taiwan, and South Africa but there is no convincing evidence that *B. microti* has been responsible for any of these but, equally, there is no convincing evidence that it has not.

Phylogenetic analysis of rodent-derived *B. microti* isolates suggests that this species is actually a genetically diverse species complex consisting of three distinct groups or clades (Goethert and Telford 2003). Clade 1 embraces isolates from America and also from Russia and Switzerland where there have been no reports of overt human babesiosis. However, serological surveys in Germany and Switzerland suggest that subclinical *B. microti* infections in humans are not uncommon (Hunfeld *et al.* 2002). Clade 2 includes parasites from carnivores none of which is known to infect humans. Similarly, clade 3 includes isolates from areas in the USA where human babesiosis has never been identified.

Disease

After being infected from nymphs the first signs of the infection occur about 1–4 weeks later. At first the symptoms are rather vague, headaches, fever, sweating, chills, muscle pains, and malaise, accompanied by clinical signs including splenomegaly, anaemia, thrombocytopenia, haemoglobinuria and, in some cases, disseminated intravascular coagulation, and systemic organ failure. These signs and symptoms resemble those seen in patients suffering from severe malaria but without the sequestration associated with malignant tertian malaria caused by *Plasmodium falciparum* (Clark and Jacobson 1998). Parasitaemias tend to be between 1–20% but can reach 85% in individuals without spleens.

Diagnosis

Babesiosis is very difficult to diagnose clinically partly because of its rarity and partly because of vague symptomatology. Diagnosis is based on the detection of parasites in stained thin blood films but these must be interpreted with great caution because *Babesia* are virtually indistinguishable from the ring stages of malaria parasites particularly *Plasmodiumfalciparum.* Tetrads (Maltese Cross forms) are characteristic of *B. microti* but tend to be scanty in blood films. There are no records of human babesiosis from tropical countries so anyone returning from such areas should be provisionally diagnosed as having malaria. For those who have not travelled to the tropics, particular attention should be paid to individuals whose activities have taken them into contact with infected ticks, farmers, hikers, soldiers and campers for example. Most people are aware that they have been bitten by a tick and the spread of Lyme borreliosis has heightened the need to take tick bites seriously. Severe and unexplained thrombocytopenia in individuals who have been at risk is a useful indication of human babesiosis. For absolute certainty, suspected infected blood should be injected into susceptible hosts, calves or hamsters as appropriate, and the resulting infection monitored. Jirds, *Meriones unguiculatus,* can be infected with *B. divergens.* Serological tests, particularly the indirect immunofluorescent antibody test (IFAT), have proved to be useful as has the quantitative 'buffy coat' technique, devised for malaria diagnosis. The most promising diagnostic technique is the application of the polymerase chain reaction (PCR) which can detect as few as three parasites. However, it is important to point out that all these techniques, except stained blood films, are purely experimental at present.

Epidemiology

Human babesiosis is a public health problem only in restricted foci, particularly along the New England coast, and all those who camp or hike in these areas should be aware of the problem of tickborne diseases, not only babesiosis but also Lyme borreliosis particularly when the nymphs are most active in late June. Away from these endemic areas, the chances of acquiring human babesiosis are very remote. Human babesiosis is never going to be a major health problem but those who intrude into any natural life cycle do put themselves at risk.

Prevention and control

The best method of prevention is the avoidance of tick bites especially in tick-infested areas which, in the USA, are often clearly signposted because of the possible danger of Lyme borreliosis. Sensible clothing is an absolute requirement. Campers, hikers and others involved in outdoor pursuits should take particular care. Tick bites should never be ignored and anyone bitten in an endemic area should take medical advice if symptoms such as irregular fevers develop within two to three weeks of having been bitten. The removal of all ticks within 48 hours is usually sufficient to prevent infection. Individuals without spleens or undergoing immunosuppressive therapy are at particular risk. There is no evidence that those suffering from HIV/AIDS are particularly susceptible to infection with babesiosis but the possibility exists that they might well be and such individuals should be very careful about engaging in any activities that might bring them into contact with ticks particularly in places where the infection is known to be present. In the *B. microti* endemic areas in the USA efforts are being made to exclude deer from popular tourist sites largely as a precaution against Lyme borreliosis. Outside the endemic areas in the USA the chances of being bitten by an infected tick are vanishingly small but it would be just as well for immunocompromised individuals to take sensible precautions against tick bites and to be aware of the remote possibility of babesial infection if bitten.

Treatment

Human babesiosis, particularly in asplenic individuals, must be considered as an emergency. Many anti-protozoal drugs, including antimalarials, and antibiotics have been tested with limited success and the currently approved treatments are combination therapies using either the antimalarial quinine plus the antibiotic clindamycin or the antibiotic azithromycin plus the antimalarial atovaquone, the latter gradually replacing the former (Weiss 2002) but the World Health Organization (WHO) is still cautious about the use of these drugs especially in uncomplicated cases. Blood exchange transfusions followed by treatment with quinine and clindamycin have been used successfully in treating asplenic patients suffering from *B. divergens* infections.

Malaria

History

The fevers characteristic of human malaria have been known since ancient times and the Greek and Roman physicians clearly recognized the various forms of the disease and its association with marshy areas. The history of human malaria has been written about extensively many times and does not warrant further discussion here (see Garnham 1966 for an introductory history of human malaria). Although malaria-like parasites belonging to the genus *Hepatocystis* had erroneously, but not surprisingly, been recognized since 1899 malaria parasites of non-human parasites were not identified with certainty until 1907 with the independent discoveries of *Plasmodium cynomolgi*, *P. inui*, and *P. pitheci* in monkeys imported into Germany from Java (Garnham 1966). A number of reports of new species, many of them spurious, appeared throughout the 1920s and 1930s but, following the discovery of *P. knowlesi* in 1932, a framework to accommodate the various new species described in the 1930s, 1950s and 1960s was established (Garnham 1966; Collins and Aikawa 1993).

During the 1960s, there were a number of reports of accidental human infections with primate malarias and this led to intensive efforts to determine whether or not primates could act as reservoirs for human malaria because of how this might affect the malaria control and elimination schemes then in progress. In the event, it became clear that the chances of humans acquiring malaria from primates were very remote but that occasional accidental and natural infections could occur.

The agents

Like the babesias, the malaria parasites belong to the kingdom Protozoa, phylum Sporozoa (Apicomplexa) and class Coccidea (Table 48.1). Human malaria is caused by infection with one of five species of *Plasmodium*, *P. falciparum*, *P. vivax*, *P. ovale*, *P. malariae* or *P. knowlesi* of which the first four are the most important, particularly *P. falciparum* the cause of malignant tertian malaria, the most common and serious of all the forms of malaria. Together they affect over 350 million people in the tropics and sub-tropics causing deaths in excess of two million each year, particularly in children, and countless episodes of debilitating febrile disease. *P. vivax* causes benign tertian malaria, *P. ovale* causes ovale tertian malaria and *P. malariae* causes

quartan malaria. *Plasmodium* species also occur in reptiles, birds, rodents and New World and Old World monkeys, gibbons, great apes and lemurs (Garnham 1966; Collins and Aikawa 1993). All *Plasmodium* species of primates have similar life cycles and are transmitted by female blood-sucking mosquitoes belonging to the genus *Anopheles*. The infection begins when the infective stages, sporozoites, are injected through the bite of an infected mosquito and enter liver cells where a massive phase of multiplication, known as the pre-erythrocytic stage, occurs resulting in the production of thousands of merozoites. These merozoites invade red blood cells where they undergo another phase of multiplication during which they produce 8–16 merozoites every 24, 48 or 72 hours depending on the species. This phase of erythrocytic multiplication is repeated indefinitely and is responsible for periodic fevers coinciding with the liberation of merozoites and anaemia caused by the loss of red blood cells. Some merozoites, however, do not divide within the red cell but develop into male or female gametocytes which are taken up when another mosquito feeds. Within the mosquito, the male and female gametes fuse to produce a zygote which comes to lie on the outside of the gut wall where it forms an oocyst within which a third phase of multiplication occurs resulting in the formation of many sporozoites which migrate to the salivary glands of the mosquito from which they are injected when the mosquito feeds.

The malaria parasites of humans are not naturally transmissible to other animals so the malaria parasites of non-human primates have received considerable attention both in their own rights and as models for the human infections (Collins and Aikawa 1993). Of these, *P. cynomolgi*, which resembles *P. vivax*, has been the most studied and another species from macaques, *P. knowlesi*, has been widely used in laboratory studies despite the fact that it has a 24 hour periodicity and does not closely resemble any of the human species. *P. knowlesi* and *P. simium* are known to be able to infect humans naturally and *P. cynomolgi*, *P. schwetzi*, *P. brasilianum* and *P. inui* can infect humans under experimental (or accidental) conditions. The malaria parasites of rodents and birds have been extensively studied and none of them has ever been reported to infect humans.

Primate malarias transmissible to humans

Natural infections can only be acquired from infected mosquitoes but accidental and experimental infections can be acquired either from mosquitoes or from infected blood. A list of the species that have been transmitted to humans is given in Table 48.2.

Plasmodium knowlesi

The only significant zoonoses results from infection with *P. knowlesi* in Southeast Asia where its natural hosts are the macaque monkeys, *Macaca fascicularis* and *M. nemestrina*, other macaques and leaf monkeys. Other species of monkeys and higher primates can be infected experimentally. *P. knowlesi* has a 24 hour erythrocytic cycle and, probably as a result of this very rapid erythrocytic multiplication, tends to be very pathogenic especially in unnatural hosts such as rhesus monkeys which almost inevitably die with a fulminating parasitaemia as do splenectomized kra monkeys. Fevers are difficult to measure in monkeys but there is a severe anaemia reminiscent of the fatal anaemia sometimes seen in children infected with *P. falciparum*. Humans are susceptible to both blood-induced and mosquito-transmitted infection which varies

Table 48.2 Primate malarias naturally, accidentally or experimentally transmitted to humans

1.	**Natural infections**	Human equivalent	Periodicity
	P. knowlesi		24 hours
	P. simium	P. ovale	48 hours
	P. eylesi	P. vivax	48 hours
2.	**Accidental infections**		
	P. cynomolgi	P. vivax	48 hours
3.	**Experimental infections**		
	P. knowlesi		24 hours
	P. cynomolgi	P. vivax	48 hours
	P. schwetzi	P. ovale	48 hours
	P. inui	P. malariae	72 hours
	P. brasilianum	P. malariae	72 hours

from mild to life-threatening and includes the usual signs of malaria, alternating fever and chills, headaches, muscle pain and anaemia. For many years, *P. knowlesi* was used in Romania to induce fevers in patients suffering from general paralysis of the insane (GPI) but this was discontinued when the parasite became too virulent after years of blood-passage from monkey to monkey. In passing, it should be mentioned that the treatment of paralysis with malaria is not as bizarre as it seems and in Britain some 13,000 patients were therapeutically treated with *P. vivax* between 1925 and the mid 1950s (Rollin 1994). Until 1965 there had only been one authenticated case of naturally acquired human infection with *P. knowlesi*; an American surveyor working in the forests of Pahang in Malaysia who developed fever, fatigue, anorexia, and nausea and, later, sweating and rigor and who recovered naturally without treatment (Chin *et al.* 1965). He was initially diagnosed as suffering from falciparum malaria but when his blood was passaged into a monkey it developed a typical *P. knowlesi* infection. A second case, also in peninsular Malaysia, was recorded in 1971 (Yap *et al.* 1971). There were no other authenticated cases until 2004 when the application of molecular techniques identified a focus of human infections in the Kapit Division of Sarawak in Malaysian Borneo (Singh *et al.* 2004). Since then there have been increasing numbers of records from Sarawak and Sabah in Malaysian Borneo, Penang in Peninsular Malaysia, Thailand and Myanmar. In Sarawak, the natural hosts are long-tailed (*Macaca fascicularis*) and pig-tailed macaques (*M. nemestrina*) and the vector is *Anopheles latens* (formerly *A. leucosphyrus*) (Vythilingam *et al.* 2006). The incrimination of *A. latens* is important because the natural mosquito host, *A. hackeri*, lives in forest canopies and it had been thought that it was extremely unlikely that humans could become infected because this mosquito rarely feeds on any hosts other than monkeys and because contacts between monkeys, mosquitoes, and humans in the forest canopy were likely to be rare. *Anopheles latens*, on the other hand, feeds on both monkeys and humans at both canopy and ground levels. Taking into account all the epidemiological, entomological and molecular data there is overwhelming evidence that *P. knowlesi* represents a zoonoses involving macaque monkeys as reservoir hosts and *A. latens* as the

main vector in Malaysia. *Plasmodium knowlesi* in monkeys has also been recorded from the Philippines, Thailand, Vietnam, Cambodia, and Taiwan thus representing potential zoonoses in these countries and also others bordering the South China Sea. With increasing agricultural activity and intrusion into forested areas the potential for human infections could become very serious as humans, monkeys and mosquitoes come into closer contact at the forest fringes. Although *P. knowlesi* infections tend to be relatively mild, resembling those caused by *P. vivax* rather than *P. falciparum*, there have been fatal infections thus they do represent a health risk and the fact that splenectomized kra monkeys rapidly succumb to infection suggests that it would be unwise for anybody without a spleen or on immunosuppressive therapy to venture into areas such as the Malaysian forests where *P. knowlesi* is known to exist. The realisation that *P. knowlesi* is a zoonoses has necessitated reappraisal of previous records of malaria attributed to *P. malariae* in Malaysia. Retrospective examination of blood films and the application of the PCR reveal that these cases were misidentified and that they were in all probability due to *P. knowlesi* (Cox-Singh *et al.* 2008). It remains to be seen how far this is true for the rest of Southeast Asia.

Plasmodium cynomolgi

Plasmodium cynomolgi is found all over southern Asia especially in Malaysia, its natural home, and will be treated as a single entity in this chapter although it actually occurs as two sub-species, *P. c. cynomolgi* and *P. c. bastianelli*, to which humans are equally susceptible. Natural hosts include *Macaca* spp. especially *M. fascicularis* and leaf monkeys *Presbytis* spp. Experimentally, *P. cynomolgi* can be transmitted to rhesus monkeys, in which it has been extensively studied, and baboons. Many Asian species of *Anopheles* can transmit this parasite naturally and over 60 species can do so experimentally. *Plasmodium cynomolgi* can be transmitted to humans either through the bite of a mosquito or by infected blood. In 1960 there were the first reports of the accidental infection of laboratory workers and since then a number of accidental and experimental infections have been recorded. The infection, which lasts several weeks, is characterized by low parasitaemias and high fevers and an irregular 48 hour periodicity accompanied by headaches, anorexia, nausea, enlarged livers, and spleen. Because of the apparent ease with which humans can be infected, the wide range of mosquito hosts, some of which are man-biting, and the relative frequency of contact between monkeys, mosquitoes and humans, the possibility that *P. cynomolgi* might be a zoonoses is a real one although no authenticated cases have been recorded despite intensive investigations.

Plasmodium inui

Plasmodium inui is the most widely distributed malaria parasite in Asian macaques (*Macaca iris* and other *Macaca* spp.) and leaf monkeys (*Presbytis* spp.). The mosquito hosts include *A. elegans* and *A. introlatus*, neither of which bite humans, and *A. latens* (formerly *A. leucosphyrus*) which does as discussed above. Infections in monkeys are usually mild and self-limiting but are virulent in splenectomized animals. In experimental human blood-induced infections the infection is mild with fever and scanty parasites in the blood. It should be mentioned here that the parasite isolated by Romanian workers and transmitted to humans in 1934 and identified as *P. inui* was almost certainly *P. knowlesi*.

Plasmodium eylesi

Plasmodium eylesi occurs in the forests of northern Malaysia where it is a parasite of the gibbon *Hylobates lar*. The natural vector is not known but *P. eylesi* can develop in a number of anopheline mosquitoes. There have been reports that humans can be infected experimentally with sporozoites but the resulting parasitaemias are low and no signs of illness have been recorded.

Plasmodium simium

Plasmodium simium is restricted to Brazil where it infects howler monkeys, *Alouatta fusca*, particularly younger animals, and the woolly spider monkey, *Brachyteles arachnoides*. Howler monkeys live in the forest canopy where they seldom come in contact with humans. The mosquito host is thought to be *Anopheles cruzi*. It was while looking for the mosquito host that the only recorded human infection occurred. An entomological assistant working near São Paulo became ill with a periodic 48 hour fever and was found to have, in his blood, small numbers of parasites which disappeared after a week. When his blood was injected into a splenectomized *Saimiri* monkey a typical *P. simium* infection resulted. There is no doubt that this infection occurred in a tree platform where the unusual circumstances brought infected monkeys, mosquitoes and man together. This is the only authenticated record of a malaria zoonoses in the New World.

Plasmodium brasilianum

Plasmodium brasilianum occurs in tropical South America where it is a common parasite in several species of monkeys including *Alouatta* spp., *Ateles* spp., *Brachyteles* spp., *Cebus* spp. and *Saimiri* spp. The natural vector is unknown. Experimentally, *P. brasilianum* can infect an even wider range of monkeys and is very pathogenic even in its natural hosts. Early attempts to infect humans with infected blood or mosquitoes failed but subsequent attempts using *A. freeborni* as a vector were successful. Parasitaemias were low and accompanied by quartan fevers and enlarged spleens. There have been no records of naturally acquired human infections.

Plasmodium schwetzi

Plasmodium schwetzi occurs in forests in tropical Central and West Africa where it infects chimpanzees, *Pan troglodytes*, and, less frequently, gorillas, *Gorilla gorilla*. The natural vector is not known but *A. gambiae*, the main vector of human malaria in Africa, cannot be infected. Humans experimentally infected with parasitized blood develop transient febrile self-limiting infections. There have been no records of naturally acquired human infections.

Plasmodium malariae

Plasmodium malariae, a parasite of humans, occurs throughout the tropical regions of the Old World and in scattered localities in the New World and is the only species that is also recorded from non-human primates. At one time it was thought that the non-human form belonged to a different species, *P. rodhaini*, but this species is no longer recognized. *P. malariae* infects chimpanzees, *Pan troglodytes*, in tropical forests of Africa and could theoretically be transmitted to humans but there is no evidence that this has ever occurred and such transmission is unlikely given the probability that different vectors are involved in the human and in the sylvatic non-human cycles and the distances that chimpanzees maintain between themselves and humans. The discovery that the Malaysian records of *P. malariae* are actually *P. knowlesi* calls for a reappraisal of the host range of this species particularly any records from outside Africa.

Diagnosis

Although human malaria infections acquired from non-human hosts are rare, it is important that an accurate diagnosis should be made of any suspected cases. Because human and non-human parasites are so similar, the only ways to be certain that a parasite has been derived from an animal host has been the careful examination of thin blood films and the passage of infected blood into the parasite-free natural host in which a characteristic infection should occur thus fulfilling Koch's postulates. Morphological and biological criteria are gradually being replaced by molecular techniques such as those used to determine the zoonotic nature of *P. knowlesi*.

Epidemiology

The epidemiology of *P. knowlesi* in Malaysia has already been discussed. Briefly, this parasite is common in macaques up to 60% of which may be infected and many carry multiple infections with other malaria parasites. The natural life cycle occurs in the forest canopy where the most important vector is *A. hackeri* which seldom leaves the canopies and hardly ever bites humans. The discovery that *P. knowlesi* is also transmitted by *A. latens* that visits forest fringes and bites humans focuses attention on the need for more epidemiological studies in Southeast Asia and elsewhere. Apart from *P. knowlesi*, human malaria infections from animals are exceptionally rare but are known to occur thus do present some risk albeit very small. The finding in Malaysia of what was originally thought to be *P. malariae*, an infection of humans, was actually *P. knowlesi*, a parasite of monkeys, illustrates the value of the application of molecular technology in the field of epidemiology. Non-human malarias tend to be cycled between monkeys in forest canopies by zoophilic and exophilic mosquitoes thus the only people who risk becoming infected are those who intrude into such habitats. Normally, only particular high-risk groups such as explorers, biologists and surveyors are likely to be infected but, as military personnel, refugees and farmers increasingly move into areas not normally populated by humans there will always exist a slight risk particularly along the forest fringes. Splenectomy and the use of immunosuppressive drugs increase the chances of infection with unusual parasites and those individuals so affected are at even greater risk. At present, it is not known whether or not HIV infections increase susceptibility to animal malaria infections but this must be a real possibility.

Prevention and control

In areas of Southeast Asia where it is known that malaria can be acquired from monkeys the health services are well able to advise those working in particularly dangerous places to take precautions such as the use of insecticides, insect repellents, insecticide-treated bednets and prophylactic chemotherapy. Malaysia has in place well organized anti-mosquito measures designed to prevent dengue fever so is well placed to control the vector(s) of *P. knowlesi* although resistance to the most widely used insecticide, Temephos, is a potential problem. Away from Southeast Asia, the chances of being infected with a primate malaria are so rare that it is not necessary to suggest any control measures. On the other hand, those working with primate malarias should be very careful when handling infected blood and should avoid being bitten by mosquitoes.

If anyone working with these malarias does become exposed to infection any symptoms such as fever should be reported immediately and diagnosed on blood films and, if positive, expert advice should be taken and appropriate treatment begun immediately.

Treatment

All malaria parasites respond to treatment with a variety of antimalarial drugs the use of which varies from situation to situation. Until recently the most useful drug has been the 4-aminoquinoline schizonticide, chloroquine. Chloroquine resistance, which has threatened the use of this drug for human malaria in many parts of the world, does not occur naturally in non-human primates so can be used safely but with caution in cases of *P. knowlesi* and standard treatment with chloroquine and pyrimethamine is effective. So far there has been no resistance to chloroquine but this situation may not last forever so combination therapies combining artemisinin with other drugs as used in Africa are being tested. Prophylaxis is not considered necessary at the moment but the successful combination of atovaquone and proguanil is available if necessary. The only drawback is the cost which, given the small numbers of individuals likely to be affected and the relative wealth of Southeast Asian countries, should not present any problems.

References

Babes, V. (1888). Sur l'hémoglobinure bacterénne des boef. *Comp. Rendus Seances l'Acad. Sci., (Paris)*, **115**: 693–94.

Chin, W., Contacos, P.G., Coatney, R.G., and Kimbal, H.R. (1965). A naturally acquired quotidian-type malaria in man transferable to monkeys. *Science*, **149**: 865.

Clark, I.A. and Jacobson, L.S. (1998). Do babesiosis and malaria share a common disease process? *Ann. Trop. Med. Parasit.*, **92**: 483–88.

Collins, W.E. and Aikawa, M. (1993). Plasmodia of nonhuman primates. In: J.P. Kreier (ed.) *Parasitic Protozoa*, (2nd edn.), Vol. 5, pp. 105–33. San Diego: Academic Press.

Conrad, P.A., Kjemtrup, A.M., and Carreno, R.A. *et al.* (2006). Description of *Babesia duncani* n.sp. (Apicomplexa: Babesiidae) from humans and its differentiation from other piroplasms. *Int. J. Parasitol.*, **36**: 779–89.

Cox-Singh, J., Davis, T.M.E., Lee-Kim, S., Shamsui, S.S.G. *et al.* (2008). *Plasmodium knowlesi* malaria in humans is widely distributed and potentially life threatening. *Clin. Infect. Dis.*, **46**: 165–71.

Garnham, P.C.C. (1966). *Malaria Parasites and other Haemosporidia*. Oxford: Blackwell.

Goethert, H.K. and Telford III, S.R. (2003). What is *Babesia microti*? *Parasitology*, **127**: 301–9.

Gorenflot, A. (1998). Human babesiosis. *Ann. Trop. Med. Parasit.*, **92**:489–501.

Gray, J.S. (2006). Identity of the causal agents of human babesiosis in Europe. *Int. J. Med. Microbiol.*, **296** (Supplement 40): 131–36.

Gray, J.S. and Weiss, L.M. (2008). *Babesia microti*. In: N.A. Khan (ed.) *Emerging Protozoan Pathogens*, pp. 303–49. New York and Abingdon, U.K.: Taylor and Francis.

Hunfeld, K.P., Lambert, A., Kampen, H. *et al.* (2002). Seroprevanence of *Babesia microti* infections in humans exposed to ticks in Midwestern Germany. *J. Clin. Microbiol.*, **40**: 2431–36.

Kakoma, I. and Mehlhorn, H. (1994). *Babesia* of domestic animals. In: J.P. Kreier (ed.) *Parasitic Protozoa*, (2nd edn.), Vol. 7, pp. 141–216. San Diego: Academic Press.

Kjemtrup, A.M. and Conrad, P.A. (2000). Human babesiosis: an emerging tick-borne disease. *Int. J. Parasitol.*, **30**: 1323–37.

Ristic, M. (ed.) (1988). *Babesiosis of Domestic Animals and Man*. Boca Raton: CRC Press.

Rollin, H.R. (1994). The Horton Malaria Hospital, Epsom, Surrey (1925–1975). *J. Med. Biog.*, **2**: 94–97.

Singh, B., Lee, K.S., and Matusop, A. *et al.* (2004). A large focus of naturally acquired *Plasmodium knowlesi* infections in human beings. *Lancet*, **363**: 1017–24.

Smith, T. and Kilbourne, F.L. (1893). Investigations into the nature, causation and prevention of Texas or Southern cattle fever. *Bull. Bur. Anim. Ind., US Depart. Agri., Washington*, **1**: 177–304.

Telford, S.R. and Spielman, A. (2005). Babesiosis of humans. In: F.E.G. Cox, D. Wakelin, S. Gillespie and D.D. Despommier (eds.) *Topley and Wilson's Microbiology and Microbial Infections: Parasitology*, (10th edn.). London: Hodder Arnold.

Vythilingam, I., Tan, C.H., Asmad, M., Chan, S.T., Lee, K.S. and Singh, B. (2006). Natural transmission of *Plasmodium knowlesi* to humans by *Anopheles latens* in Sarawak, Malaysia. *Trans. R. Soc. Trop. Med. Hyg.*, **100**: 1087–88.

Weiss, L.M. (2002). Babesiosis in humans: a treatment review. *Expert Opin. Pharmacother.*, **3**: 1109–15.

Wilson, L.B. and Chowning, W.M. (1904). Studies in pyroplasmosis hominis ('Spotted fever' or 'tick fever' of the Rocky Mountains). *J. Infect. Dis.*, **1**: 31–57.

Yap, L.F., Cadigan, F.C., and Coatney, G.R. (1971). A presumptive case of naturally occurring *Plasmodium knowlesi* in Malaysia. *Trans. R. Soc. Trop. Med. Hyg.*, **100**: 1087–88.

CHAPTER 49

Microsporidiosis

Louis M. Weiss

Summary

History

The class or order Microsporidia was elevated in to the phylum Microspora by Sprague and Vávra (1997), and Sprague and Becnel (1998) subsequently suggested that the term Microsporidia instead be used for the phylum name. Microsporidia, i.e. *Nosema bombycis,* were first described about 150 years ago as the cause of the disease pebrine in silkworms. In 1922, there were descriptions of gram-positive spores consistent with microsporidiosis in the brain of rabbits that were being used for investigations on poliomyelitis (Wright and Craighead 1922). From 1923 to 1926, Levaditi and colleagues studied the organisms seen by Wright and Craighead, which they named *Encephalitozoon cuniculi,* recognizing them as Microsporidia and demonstrating their lack of host specificity by transmitting infections from rabbits to mice, rats and dogs (Levaditi *et al.* 1923). Microsporidia were clearly confirmed of being a cause of human disease in 1959 (Matsubayashi *et al.* 1959), when they were isolated from the cerebrospinal fluid of a 9 year old boy with encephalitis with seizures, coma, and fever lasting about 25 days. Bergquist *et al.* (1984) reported a 2 year old child with encephalitis and seizures who had *Encephalitozoon* spores in urine and Margileth *et al.* (1973) isolated the microsporidium *Anncaliia* (*Nosema*) *connori* from a 4 month old athymic male infant who died with severe diarrhoea and malabsorption. Microsporidia can produce a wide range of clinical diseases. A diarrhoeal syndrome associated with microsporidiosis and HIV infection was reported by Desportes *et al.* (1985) and the number of articles describing human disease increased rapidly after 1990. In addition to gastrointestinal tract involvement, it has been recognized that Microsporidia can infect virtually any organ system; and patients with encephalitis, ocular infection, sinusitis, myositis, and disseminated infection are well described in the literature.

General characteristics

The Microsporidia are obligate intracellular unicelluar eukaryotes containing a nucleus with a nuclear envelope, an intracytoplasmic membrane system, chromosome separation on mitotic spindles, and vesicular Golgi (Desportes-Livage 2000). While originally believed to be lacking mitochondria, it is now appreciated that they have a mitochondrial 'remnant' organelle named the mitosome (Williams *et al.* 2002). The nuclei are typical of eukaryotes, but electron-dense centriolar plaques in nuclear pores are present at the poles of division spindles in place of centrioles. In several genera, including *Vittaforma* and *Nosema,* which have been isolated from humans, the nuclei are unusual in being paired as diplokarya which are closely appressed and divide synchonously. In some genera this diplokaryotic condition is maintained throughout the life cycle but, in others, there is an alternation between unpaired and paired nuclei. In a few genera alternation of hosts is an obligate part of the life cycle but, as far as is known, these complexities do not occur in the genera infecting humans.

The Microsporidia are defined by their characteristic unicellular spores (Fig. 49.1) which are resistant to the environment (Wittner and Weiss 1999). The spore size and shape vary depending on the species. The spore coat consists of an electron-dense, proteinaceous exospore, an electron-lucent endospore composed of chitin and protein, and an inner membrane or plasmalemma (Vavra 1976). Spore coat proteins have adhesion domains that may facilitate the binding of spores to host cells or gastrointestinal track mucous (Southern *et al.* 2007). A defining characteristic of all microsporidia is an extrusion apparatus that consists of a polar filament (tube) attached to the inside of the anterior end of the spore by an anchoring disk which coils around the sporoplasm in the spore. Proteomic and genetic studies have defined some of the proteins of the polar tube and spore wall (Xu *et al.* 2006) as well as the presence of *O*-mannosylatation on these proteins (Xu *et al.* 2004). When the spore is exposed to appropriate environmental conditions it germinates and the polar filament rapidly everts, forming the hollow polar tube which forms a bridge delivering the sporoplasm into intimate contact with the host cell (Fig. 49.2) (Lom 1972; Weidner 1972). The polar tube has been described as a hypdermic needle, but the mechanism by which the polar tube interacts with the host cell membrane is not known (Foucault and Drancourt 2000). Conditions that promote germination vary widely among species, presumably reflecting the organisms' adaptation to their host and external environment (reviewed by Keohane and Weiss 1999). Interestingly, if a spore is phagocytosed by a host cell, germination occurs; and the polar tube can pierce the phagocytic vacuole, delivering the sporoplasm into the host cell cytoplasm (Franzen 2005).

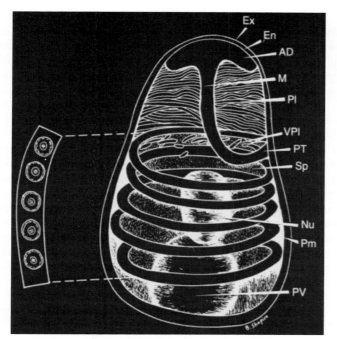

Fig. 49.1 Structure of a microsporidian spore. Depending on the species, the size of the spore can vary from 1 to 10 μm and the number of polar tubule coils can vary from a few to 30 or more. Extrusion apparatus consists of the polar tube (PT), vesiculotubular polaroplast (Vpl), lamellar polaroplast (Pl), anchoring disk (AD) and manubrium (M). This organelle is characteristic of the Microsporidia. A cross section of the coiled polar tube is illustrated. The nucleus (Nu) may be single (such as in *Encephalitozoon* spp.) or a pair of abutted nuclei termed a diplokaryon (such as in *Nosema* spp.). The endospore (En) is an inner thicker electron-lucent region. The exospore (Ex) is an outer electron-dense region. The plasma membrane (Pm) separates the spore coat from the sporoplasm (Sp), which contains ribosomes in a coiled helical array. The posterior vacuole (PV) is a membrane-bound structure.

Reproduced with permission from Wittner M, Weiss LM, eds. The Microsporidia and Microsporidiosis. Washington, DC: ASM Press; 1999.

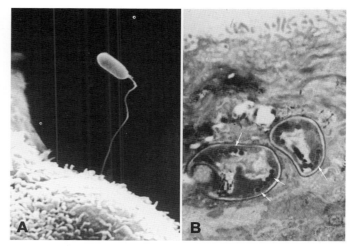

Fig. 49.2 Microsporidian polar tube **(A)** Scanning electron micrograph of a tissue culture demonstrating *Encephalitozoon intestinalis* invading a Vero cell *in vitro*. **(B)** Transmission electron micrograph of conjunctival scraping demonstrating *Encephalitozoon hellem*. Arrowheads identify polar tube coils.

(A)- Reproduced with permission from Koch NP. Diagnosis of Human Pathogenic Microsporidia. Dissertation, Berhard Nocht Institute for Tropical Medicine, Hamburg, Germany. With kind permission of N.P. Koch, C. Schmertz, and J. Schottelius.

The general features of microsporidian life cycles are as follows:

1 Spores are ingested or inhaled and then germinate, resulting in extension of the polar tube, which delivers the sporoplasm into the host cell.

2 Merogony follows, during which the injected sporoplasm develops into meronts (the proliferative stage), which multiply, depending on the species, by either binary fission or multiple fission, forming multinucleate plasmodial forms.

3 The next step is sporogony, during which meront cell membranes thicken to form sporonts.

After subsequent division the sporonts give rise to sporoblasts, which go on to form mature spores without additional multiplication. Once a host cell becomes distended with mature spores, the cell ruptures, releasing mature spores into the environment, thereby completing the life cycle. The combination of multiplication during merogony and sporogony results in a large number of spores being produced from a single infection and illustrates the enormous reproductive potential of these organisms.

Microsporidia have prokaryotic-size ribosomes (Curgy *et al.* 1980) that do not have a 5.8S ribosome subunit but do have

sequences homologous to the 5.8S region in the 23S subunit (Vossbrinck and Woese 1986). The small-subunit rRNA of many Microsporidia have been sequenced and found to be significantly shorter than both eukaryotic and prokaryotic small-subunit rRNA (Vossbrinck *et al.* 1987; Weiss and Vossbrinck 1998). These rRNA genes are in a subtelomeric location on each chromosome of *E. cuniculi* (Brugere *et al.* 2000a; Vivares and Metenier 2000) and lack the paromomycin binding site seen in protozoa and animals (Katiyar *et al.* 1995). The karyotype of several members of the phylum Microspora has been determined by pulsed-field electrophoresis. The genome size of the microsporidia varies from 2.3 to 19.5 Mb (Weiss and Vossbrinck 1999) with that of the Encephalitizoonidae being less than 3.0 Mb, making them among the smallest eukaryotic nuclear genomes so far identified (Vivares and Metenier 2000; Katinka *et al.* 2001). In the compact genomes of the Encephalitozoonidae, there are almost no introns, the gene density is high and proteins are shorter than the corresponding genes in *Saccharomyces cervisiae*. There appears to be a high degree of gene conservation among the Microsporidia (Corradi *et al.* 2007). Genome data on the Microsporidia is available at EuPathdB (http://microsporidiadb.org/micro/). Chromosomal analysis of *E. cuniculi* suggests that it is diploid (Brugere *et al.* 2000b).

Analysis of the rRNA genes of a variety of Microsporidia highlights the polyphyletic nature of the Microsporidia and brings into doubt the use of any single character for developing higher taxonomic groupings. For example, *E. hellem* and *E. cuniculi* are indistinguishable at the ultrastructural level, and *E. intestinalis* has a distinct extracellular matrix surrounding the sporoblasts and spores; based on rDNA analysis, *E. intestinalis* and *E. cuniculi* are more similar to each other than to *E. hellem* (Baker *et al.* 1995).

Microsporidia are classified by their ultrastructural features, including the size and morphology of the spores, number of coils of the polar tube, developmental life cycle, and host-parasite relationship. Overviews of the the microsporidian taxa have been reported a number of times (reviewed by Sprague *et al.* 1992). Molecular phylogenetic data indicates that the Microsporidia are related to fungi and are not 'primitive eukaryotes' (Keeling and McFadden 1998; Hirt *et al.* 1999; Weiss *et al.* 1999). Based on tubulin sequence analysis, it has been suggested that the Microsporidia are related to the fungi (Keeling and Doolittle 1996). Analysis of *hsp70* for various microsporidia provided confirmatory evidence of this relationship (Germot *et al.* 1997; Hirt *et al.* 1997). Keeling (2003), in an analysis of β-tubulin data that included additional species of Microsporidia and more fungal phyla, suggested that the Microsporidia were a sister group to the Zygomycota. Additional evidence for the relationship of Microsporidia to the fungi includes the following:

1. The *E. cuniculi* genes for thymidylate synthase and dihydrofolate reductase are separate genes (Vivares *et al.* 1996).

2. The small-subunit rRNA gene of microsporidia lacks a paromomycin binding site, similar to the fungi (Edlind *et al.* 1996).

3. The EF-1α sequence of the microsporidian *Glugea plecoglossi* has an insertion that is found only in fungi and animals, not in protozoa (Kamaishi *et al.* 1996; Edlind 1998; Hirt *et al.* 1999).

4. Microsporidia display similarities to the fungi during mitosis (e.g. closed mitosis and spindle pole bodies (Desportes 1976) and meiosis (Flegel and Pasharawipas 1995)).

5. Microsporidia have chitin in their spore wall and store trehalose, as do fungi.

6. Analyses of glutamyl-tRNA synthetase, seryl-tRNA synthetase, vacuolar ATPase, TATA box binding protein, seryl-tRNA synthetase, transcription initiation factor IIB, subunit A of vacuolar ATPase, GTP-binding protein and transcription factor IIB sequences (Hirt *et al.* 1997; Fast *et al.* 1999; Katinka *et al.* 2001) support a relationship between the Microsporidia and fungi.

7. Analysis of the *E. cuniculi* genome demonstrates that many of the *E. cuniculi* proteins are most similar to fungal homologues (Katinka *et al.* 2001).

8. The presence in *E. cuniculi* of the principal enzymes for the synthesis and degradation of trehalose confirm that this disaccharide could be the major sugar reserve in Microsporidia, as is seen in many fungi. Analysis of glycosylation pathways suggest that *O*-mannosylation (e.g. *O*-linked glycosylation with mannose), as seen in fungi, also occurs in Microsporidia. Evidence suggests that such *O*-mannosylation does indeed occur on the major polar tube protein PTP1 (Xu *et al.* 2004).

Epidemiology

Although initially regarded as rare, Microsporidia appear to be common enteric pathogens causing self-limited infections in immune competent hosts (Weber and Bryan 1994; Deplazes *et al.* 2000). Serosurveys in humans have demonstrated a high prevalence of antibodies to *E. cuniculi* and *E. hellem,* suggesting that asymptomatic infection may be common (Bergquist *et al.* 1984a,b; van Gool *et al.* 1995). *E. intestinalis* antibodies were found in 5% of pregnant French women and 8% of Dutch blood donors (van Gool *et al.* 1995). In the human immunodeficiency virus (HIV) positive Czech patients 5.3% were seropositive to *E. cuniculi* and 1.3% to *E. hellem* (Pospisilova *et al.* 1997). In Slovakia, 5.1% of slaughterhouse

workers were seropositive to *Encephalitozoon* sp (Cislakova *et al.* 1997). In a survey of blood donors in the US, 5% of donors had antibodies to *E. hellem* PTP1 antigen (L.M. Weiss, unpublished observations). Overall, these studies suggest that exposure to Microsporidia is common and that asymptomatic infection may be more common than originally suspected.

Cases of microsporidiosis have been identified from all continents except Antarctica (Morakote *et al.* 1995; van Gool *et al.* 1995; Brazil *et al.* 1996; Aoun *et al.* 1997; Bryan and Schwartz 1999; Deplazes *et al.* 2000). Human pathogenic Microsporidia have been found in municipal water supplies, tertiary sewage effluent, and ground water consistent with the concept that waterborne transmission occurs (Avery and Undeen 1987; Dowd *et al.* 1998; Cotte *et al.* 1999; Graczyk *et al.* 2007a). In addition, water contact has been found to be an independent risk factor for microsporidiosis in some studies (Enriquez *et al.* 1998; Hutin *et al.* 1998). However this has not been a consistent finding in other studies (Wuhib *et al.* 1994; Conteas *et al.* 1998a). Microsporidian spores remain viable in water for prolonged periods of time. Spores may be killed, however, by exposure to 70% ethanol, 1% formaldehyde, or 2% Lysol or by autoclaving (Waller 1979; Li and Fayer 2006). Natural transmission of most of these infections occurs when spores are ingested. However, viable spores are present in other body fluids (e.g. stool, urine, respiratory secretions) during infection, suggesting that person-to-person transmission could occur and that ocular infection may be transmitted by external autoinoculation due to contaminated fingers (Schwartz *et al.* 1993b). It has been possible to transmit *E. cuniculi* via rectal infection in rabbits, suggesting the possibility of sexual transmission (Fuentealba *et al.* 1992). *Encephalitozoon hellem* has been demonstrated in the respiratory mucosa as well as in the prostate and urogenital tract of patients, raising the possibility of respiratory and sexual transmission in humans (Schwartz *et al.* 1992c; 1994). Person-to-person transmission is supported by concurrent infections in cohabiting homosexual men (Bryan and Schwartz 1999). Transplacental transmission of *E. cuniculi* has been demonstrated in rabbits delivered by Caesarian section and reared in germ-free isolators (Hunt *et al.* 1972) and in mice similarly delivered and fostered to germ-free animals (Innes *et al.* 1962). Similar congential infections have been seen in dogs, horses, alpaca, foxes, and squirrel monkeys (Zeman and Baskin 1985), however, congenital transmission has not yet been demonstrated in humans (Hunt *et al.* 1972).

It is highly likely that the Microsporidia are zoonotic infections in humans (see Table 49.1) (Mathis *et al.* 2005). *Encephalitozoon* are found in many mammals and birds, and the onset of human infection has been associated with exposure to livestock, fowl, and pets (Yee *et al.* 1991). *Encephalitozoon hellem* infections have been described in pet birds including budgerigars (parakeets) (Black *et al.* 1997), and there is a well documented human infection in a patient from pet lovebirds (Yee *et al.* 1991). Dogs in animal shelters have been demonstrated to excrete microsporidia (Deplazes *et al.* 2000). *Encephalitozoon* were found in the stools of many animals in an epidemiologic survey in Mexico (Enriquez *et al.* 1998). *E. cuniculi* isolates from various animal species have been identified and separated based on the number of tetranucleotide repeats (5′GTTT3′) in the intergenic spacer region of their rRNA genes and these animal isolates have been found in humans (Didier *et al.* 1995b). *Enterocytozoon bieneusi* has been reported in pigs (Deplazes *et al.* 1996), dogs (del Aguila *et al.* 1999), chickens (Reetz *et al.* 2002),

Table 49.1 Microsporidia identified as pathogenic to humans

Genus and species	Reported infections	Animal hosts[‡]
Encephalitozoon		
E. cuniculi*	Hepatitis, peritonitis, encephalitis,[†] urethritis, prostatitis, nephritis, sinusitis, keratoconjunctivitis, cystitis, diarrhea,[†] cellulitis, disseminated infection	Mammals (rabbits, rodents, carnivores, primates)
E. hellem*	Keratoconjunctivitis, sinusitis, pneumonitis, nephritis, prostatitis, urethritis, cystitis, diarrhea, disseminated infection	Psittacine birds (parrots, lovebirds, budgerigars), birds (ostrich, hummingbirds, finches)
E[++]. intestinalis*	Diarrhea,[†] intestinal perforation, cholangitis, nephritis, keratoconjunctivitis	Mammals (donkeys, dogs, pigs, cows, goats, primates)
Enterocytozoon		
Ent. bieneusi	Diarrhea,[†] wasting syndrome, cholangitis, rhinitis, bronchitis	Mammals (pigs, primates, cows, dogs, cats), birds (chickens)
Trachipleistophora		
T. hominis*	Myositis, keratoconjunctivitis, sinusitis	None
T. anthropopthera	Encephalitis, disseminated infection, keratitis	None
Pleistophora sp.		
P. ronneafiei	Myositis	None
Pleistophora sp.	Myositis[†]	Fish
Anncaliia		
A[#]. vesicularum	Myositis	None
A[#]. algerae*	Keratoconjunctivitis, myositis, skin infection	Mosquitoes
A[#]. Connori	Disseminated infection	
Nosema		
N. ocularum	Keratoconjunctivitis[†]	None
Vittaforma corneae*	Keratoconjunctivitis,[†] urinary tract infection	None
Microsporidium		
M. africanus	Corneal ulcer[†]	None
M. ceylonesis	Corneal ulcer[†]	None

* Organism can be grown in tissue culture.

[†] Cases reported in immunocompetent hosts.

[‡] Animals in which organism has been found other than humans.

[#] Previously called *Brachiola*

[++] Previously called *Septata*

Adapted from Weiss LM, Microsporidiosis. In: Mandell GL, Bennett JE, Dolin R. Eds. Mandell, Douglas and Bennett's Principles and Practice of Infectious Diseases 7th Ed, Churchill Livingston, Philadelphia, 2010, p.3391–3408

pigeons (Graczyk *et al.* 2007b), falcons, and simian immunodeficiency virus (SIV)-infected rhesus monkeys (Mansfield *et al.* 1997). There is a documented case of transmission of *Ent. bieneusi* between a child and guinea pigs (Cama *et al.* 2007). Differences have also been found in the intergenic spacer region of rRNA genes of *Ent. bieneusi* and have been used to identify isolates associated with particular animals or environments (Santin and Fayer 2009). Currently all of the different isolates that have been identified are considered to be the same species. However, it is possible that there may be more than one species of *Enterocytozoon* in its mammalian and avian hosts. Enterocytozoonidae such as *Nucleospora (previously Enterocytozoon) salmonis* are pathogens found in fish (Kent *et al.* 1996). *Nosema* and *Vittaforma* infections are associated with traumatic inoculation of environmental spores of insect pathogens into the cornea (Shadduck *et al.* 1990; Silveira and Canning 1995b; Deplazes *et al.* 1998).

Surveys of pathogens seen in stool samples in Africa, Asia, South America, and Central America have demonstrated that Microsporidia are often found during careful stool examinations. In immune competent hosts, microsporidiosis usually presents as self-limited diarrhoea and both *Ent. bieneusi* and *E. intestinalis* are now appreciated to be etiologic agents of traveller's diarrhoea (Sandfort *et al.* 1994; Weber and Bryan 1994; Raynaud *et al.* 1998; Cotte *et al.* 1999; Wichro *et al.* 2005). In immune deficient hosts, such as patients with acquired immunodeficiency syndrome (AIDS) or organ transplantation, presentations have been more severe and included diarrhoea with a wasting syndrome as well as disseminated infections, depending on the species of Microsporidia. Reported prevalence rates in the studies conducted on patients with AIDS before the widespread use of active antiretroviral therapy (ART) varied between 2% and 70% depending on the symptoms of the population studied and the diagnostic techniques employed (Weber *et al.* 1994a; Weiss 1995; Kyaw *et al.* 1997; Bryan and Schwartz 1999; Deplazes *et al.* 2000). These studies suggest that asymptomatic carriage can occur in immune compromised patients. Co-infection with different Microsporidia or other enteric pathogens can occur. When combined, these studies identified 375 *Ent. bieneusi* infections among 2,400 patients with chronic diarrhoea, for a prevalence of 15% in this population. It is clear that since the institution of active antiretroviral therapy and its associated immune reconstitution the prevalence and incidence of microsporidiosis in this population has decreased.

Pathology and pathogenesis

Immunology

Infection with *E. cuniculi* in many mammals results in chronic infection with persistently high antibody titres and ongoing inflammation. In immunocompetent murine models of *E. cuniculi* infection, ascites develops and then clears. However, if corticosteroids are administered, the mice redevelop ascites, consistent with latent persistence of infection (Didier *et al.* 1994). Cell mediated immunity is important in microsporidian infection. In SCID or athymic mice, infection with *E. cuniculi* results in death, with visceral dissemination of the organism and persistent ascites (Koudela *et al.* 1993). Adoptive transfer of sensitized syngeneic T-enriched spleen cells protects athymic or SCID mice against lethal *E. cuniculi* infection (Schmidt and Shadduck 1984; Hermanek *et al.* 1993). Interferon γ and interleukin-12 are important for protective immunity against a number of microsporidia and other intracellular pathogens (Khan *et al.* 1999, 2001; Moretto *et al.* 2001, 2007). Phenotypic analysis of the spleen cells from infected animals revealed an increase in the CD8 T cell population with no significant increase in CD4 T cells. Mice deficient in CD8 cells, but not CD4 succumb to the parasitic challenge. The protective effect of CD8 T cells is mediated by their ability to produce cytokines and to reduce the parasite load by killing the infected targets in the host tissue via the perforin pathway (Khan *et al.* 1999; Moretto *et al.* 2000; Khan *et al.* 2001). Humoral immunity is not sufficient for protection against *E. cuniculi* infection, as adoptive transfer of immune B lymphocytes into either athymic or SCID mice, or passive transfer of hyperimmune serum into athymic mice does not protect these animals from death after infection. Nonetheless, maternal antibodies protect newborn rabbits from infection with *E. cuniculi* during the first 2 weeks of life (Bywater and Kellett 1979). Overall, it is probable that antibodies play a role in limiting infection in the host, although they are clearly not sufficient to prevent mortality or to cure infection. There are scant data to confirm the immune response to Microsporidia in humans. It is clear that a strong humoral response occurs during infection and that it includes antibodies that react with the spore wall and polar tube. The immunosuppressive states associated with microsporidiosis (e.g. AIDS and transplantation) are those that inhibit cell-mediated immunity. Microsporidiosis is usually seen in HIV-infected patients when there is a profound defect in cell-mediated immunity (e.g. a CD4 cell count less than 100/mm³); spontaneous cure of microsporidiosis can be induced by immune reconstitution with active antiretroviral therapy (Goguel *et al.* 1997; Conteas *et al.* 1998b; Foudraine *et al.* 1998).

Gastrointestinal tract infections

Infection of the small intestine and biliary epithelium is the most frequent presentation of microsporidiosis; with the majority of these infections being due to *Ent. bieneusi* and the remainder caused by *E. intestinalis* (Bryan and Schwartz 1999; Deplazes *et al.* 2000; Weber *et al.* 2000; Franzen and Muller 2001) (Fig. 49.3).

Granulomatous hepatitis due to *E. cuniculi* is commonly seen in mammals infected with this organism, and granulomatous hepatitis due to *Encephalitozoon* has been reported in patients with HIV infection (Terada *et al.* 1987). Hepatitis due to *Ent. bieneusi* with infection of the biliary system including the portal triad and gallbladder epithelium has been reported in SIV-infected rhesus macques (Schwartz *et al.* 1998). *Ent. bieneusi* and *E. intestinalis* infections of the biliary tract can result in sclerosing cholangitis in AIDS patients (Orenstein *et al.* 1992b; Pol *et al.* 1993). Chronic asymptomatic infection of the billiary epithelium due to *Ent. bienesui* occurs in pigs. Overall, this suggests that biliary epithelium may be a reservoir for relapse of *Ent. bieneusi* and perhaps other Microsporidia.

Genitourinary tract infection

Encephalitozoon spp. infects the genitourinary system in most mammals (Weber and Bryan 1994; Gunnarsson *et al.* 1995; Molina *et al.* 1995; Schwartz *et al.* 1996). Urinary shedding of spores is often seen in infections presenting due to symptoms related to damage in other organs. For example, in HIV-infected patients with keratitis there is usually asymptomatic infection of the urinary tract. The most frequent finding in the kidney is granulomatous interstitial nephritis composed of plasma cells and lymphocytes, which is often associated with tubular necrosis, with the lumen of the tubules containing amorphous granular material. Occasionally microabscesses and granulomas form around necrotic tubules. Spores are located in the necrotic tubes, sloughing tubular epithelial cells and occasionally in the interstitium. Glomerular involvement is rarely seen (Guerard *et al.* 1999; Gumbo *et al.* 1999a; Latib *et al.* 2001; Mohindra *et al.* 2002). Spores shed into the urine can infect other epithelial cells of the urogenital tract resulting in prostatis, necrotizing ureteritis or cystitis (Schwartz *et al.* 1996). Dissemination can occur from the urogenital epithelial cells into the adjacent mucosal macrophages, muscle, and supporting fibroblasts.

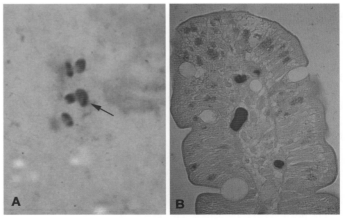

Fig. 49.3 Demonstration of microsporidia in stool and intestinal biopsy **(A)** Chromotrope 2R stain (modified trichrome stain) of a stool sample from a patient with microsporidian enteritis demonstrating microsporidian spores (arrow). **(B)** Chromotrope 2R tissue stain of a small intestinal biopsy from a patient with *Encephalitozoon intestinalis* infection. Spores are stained red and are found on both the apical and basal sides of the enterocytes.
Courtesy of D. Kotler, St Lukes-Roosevelt Hospital Center and J. M. Orenstein, George Washington University School of Medicine.

Central nervous system infection

Granulomatous encephalitis is the classic presentation of microsporidiosis in rabbits and is due to *Encephalitozoon cuniculi*. This infection has been seen in other mammals and has been reported in humans with HIV infection where it was initially mistaken for encephalitis due to *Toxoplasma gondii* (Weber *et al.* 1997). Both *E. cuniculi* type III (dog strain) and type II (rabbit strain) have been reported to cause human encephalitis (Mertens *et al.* 1997). On autopsy multiple organs were involved, but while spores were seen in the cerebral parenchyma, perivacular spaces, and macrophages they were not present in oligodendrocytes, neurons, astrocytes, or meningeal cells. Other microsporidia can also cause encephalitis and in humans there have been two case reports of encephalitis due to *Trachiplestophora anthropopthera* (Yachnis *et al.* 1996; Vavra *et al.* 1998). Both of these patients had multiple ring-enhancing lesions on computed tomography (CT) scans. On pathologic examination there was extensive necrosis with 2.0 × 2.8 μm birefringent spores located in the gray matter including astrocytes. Other organs were involved including heart, kidney, pancreas, thyroid, parathyroid, liver, bone marrow, lymph nodes, and spleen.

Ocular infection

Punctate keratopathy and conjunctivitis (e.g. superficial epithelial keratitis) has been described with Encephalitzoonidae and *Trachipliestophora anthropopthera* (Pariyakanok and Jongwutiwes 2005) (Fig. 49.4). In these infections spores are present in corneal and conjunctival epithelium, but do not invade the corneal stroma and there are few associated inflammatory cells. Ocular disease may be the presenting manifestation when there is disseminated infection (Terada *et al.* 1987; Cali *et al.* 1991b; Didier *et al.* 1991; Schwartz *et al.* 1993a). In a study of patients presenting with keratitis due to *E. hellem*, spores of this organism were present in many of these patients' sputum samples in the absence of respiratory symptoms (Schwartz *et al.* 1992c). These infections have been seen in both immune compromised and immune competent hosts. Most of these cases in immune competent patients have occurred in contact lens wearers, however, epidemic conjunctivitis in India has recently been linked to microsporidiosis (Loh *et al.* 2009; Reddy *et al.* 2009a,b). Other species of microsporidia have also been associated with ocular infection, but have involved deeper levels of the corneal stroma. These infections have often been associated with trauma, uveitis and have occurred in immune competent hosts. The species involved have been: *Vittaforma corneae*, *Microsporidium africanum*, *Microsporidium celonensis*, and *Nosema ocularum* (Joseph *et al.* 2006; Loh *et al.* 2009; Reddy *et al.* 2009a, b). Pathologic changes have included necrosis and acute inflammatory cells with some giant cells in several cases.

Musculoskeletal infection

Microsporidian myositis with inflammation has been described in humans and has included cases of *Pleistophora ronneafiei*, *Pleistophora* sp., *Trachipleistophora hominis*, *Anncaliia vesicularum*, and *Anncaliia algerae* infection (Chupp *et al.* 1993; Field *et al.* 1996; Cali *et al.* 1998; Cali and Takvorian 2003; Coyle *et al.* 2004). The *Pleistophora* sp. infections demonstrated atrophic and degenerating muscle fibers infiltrated with focal clusters of large microsporidian spores that were up to 3.4 μm in length associated with a mixed inflammatory response consisting of plasma cells,

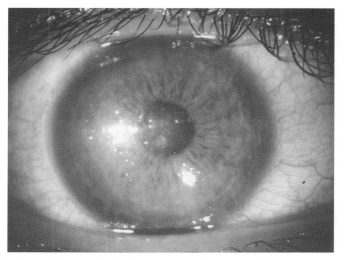

Fig. 49.4 Ocular examination of a patient with keratoconjunctivitis due to *Encephalitozoon hellem* demonstrating punctuate keratoconjunctivitis. A conjunctival scraping from this patient demonstrated spores of *E. hellem* (see Fig. 49.2B) confirmed by polymerase chain reaction testing.

lymphocytes, eosinophils, and histiocytes (Ledford *et al.* 1985; Grau *et al.* 1996; Cali and Takvorian 2003). The *T. hominis* infection occurred in a patient with AIDS and was associated with degeneration, atrophy, scarring, and intense inflammation (Cali and Takvorian 2003). The *A. vesicularum* infection occurred in an AIDS patient and was associated with cytolysis around the spores in the muscle fibers, but no cellular immune response was seen (Cali *et al.* 1998). The *A. algerae* infection occurred in a patient with rheumatoid arthritis treated with steroids and monoclonal antibody to tumor necrosis factor alpha (TNF-α) (Coyle *et al.* 2004). There was a minimal cellular response to the numerous spores present in the muscle fibers. Clinically these patients have had myalgias, weakness, elevated serum CPK and aldolase levels, and abnormal electromyography consistent with inflammatory myopathy (Ledford *et al.* 1985; Chupp *et al.* 1993; Field *et al.* 1996; Grau *et al.* 1996; Cali *et al.* 1998; Cali and Takvorian 2003).

Sinus and respiratory infection

In Encephalitozoonidae infections respiratory disease has been described with presentations including rhinitis, sinusitis, and nasal polyposis in any combination (Dunand *et al.* 1997; Gritz *et al.* 1997; Moss *et al.* 1997). Encephalitozoonidae spores have been described in the epithelial cells, neutrophils in the bronchiolar wall, cells lining the aveoli, and extracellularly in the alveolar spaces associated with trachetis and bronchiolitis (Schwartz *et al.* 1992a). All of the Encephalitozoonidae have been associated with chronic sinusitis and spores have been seen in biopsy material in the epithelium and supporting structures (Dunand *et al.* 1997; Gritz *et al.* 1997; Moss *et al.* 1997) associated with a variable inflammatory response including lymphocytes, neutrophils, macrophages, and occasional granuloma formation. There have been two reports of respiratory tract infection and one report of rinosinusitis due to *Ent. bieneusi* with spores being found in stool, brochoalveolar lavage fluid, and transbrochial biopsy specimens (Weber *et al.* 1992b; Hartskeerl *et al.* 1993; del Aguila *et al.* 1997). These cases may reflect contamination and colonization of the respiratory tract due to vomiting rather than dissemination of this organism from the gastrointestinal tract. A tongue ulcer containing *E. cuniculi* spores has been reported in a patient with disseminated microsporidiosis (Degroote *et al.* 1995).

Skin

In a child with leukemia, cellulitis was due to *A. algerae,* with spores infecting all of the cellular elements of the dermis (Visvesvara *et al.* 1999). In a second case an *Encephalitozoon* sp. was reported to be the cause of nodular skin lesions (Kester *et al.* 2000).

The agents of Microsporidia detected in humans

Enterocytozoonidae

Enterocytozoon bieneusi (Desportes *et al.* 1985) infection results in variable degrees of villous blunting and crypt hyperplasia, but is not invasive. The organism is located on the apical surface of the enterocytes of the small intestine and epithelial cells of the biliary tract and pancreas. Spores are rarely found on the basal surface or in the lamina propria and are associated with increased intraepithelial lymphocytes and epithelial immaturity and disarray (Schwartz *et al.* 1995b; 1996). Clinical manifestations include watery, nonbloody diarrhoea; nausea; diffuse abdominal pain; and fever. Infection is associated with malabsorption. Diarrhoea is self-limited in immune competent patients, but is persistent in patients with immune suppression. The most common symptom of infection is diarrhoea (Desportes-Livage *et al.* 1998; Enriquez *et al.* 1998; Raynaud *et al.* 1998; Bryan and Schwartz 1999; Rabodonirina *et al.* 2003) and the presentation classically involves chronic diarrhoea (Weber *et al.* 1992c), anorexia, weight loss, and bloating without associated fever. It is most frequently seen in AIDS patients with CD4 counts less than 50 cells/mm (Molina *et al.* 1993a; Weber *et al.* 1994a, 2000). The mortality of patients with advanced HIV disease and chronic diarrhoea with wasting has been reported to be in excess of 50% (Molina *et al.* 1993b). *Ent. bieneusi* has been identified as a cause of self-limited diarrhoea in immune competent hosts including travellers (Bryan and Weber 1993; Sandfort *et al.* 1994; Weber and Bryan 1994; Raynaud *et al.* 1998; Bryan and Schwartz 1999; Lopez-Velez *et al.* 1999; Wichro *et al.* 2005); and in epidemiologic studies has been identified in 1 to 10% of African children with diarrhoea (Orenstein *et al.* 1990; Tumwine *et al.* 2005). Although originally thought to invade only enterocytes, it has been demonstrated that *Ent. bieneusi* can also invade cholangioepithelium (Pol 1993). When present in the cholangioepithelium, this organism has been associated with sclerosing cholangitis, AIDS cholangiopathy, and cholecystitis (Beaugerie *et al.* 1992). Presentations include abdominal pain, nausea, vomiting, and fever; jaundice is rarely seen. Infections with *Ent. bieneusi* have been reported in patients with liver or heart-lung transplantation; and *Encephalitozoon* sp. infections have been reported in patients with kidney, pancreas, liver, or bone marrow transplantation (Kelkar *et al.* 1997; Guerard *et al.* 1999; Gumbo *et al.* 1999b; Latib *et al.* 2001; Sing *et al.* 2001; Mohindra *et al.* 2002; Rabodonirina *et al.* 2003).

Spores of *Ent. bieneusi* are smaller (1.0 × 1.5 μm) than those of *Encephalitozoon* spp. (1.2 × 2.2 μm) and more difficult to find in tissue sections. Other intestinal pathogens may occur simultaneously

or sequentially with the presence of this or other Microsporidia (Hewan-Lowe *et al.* 1997). A characteristic feature of *Ent. bieneusi* is the presence of electron-lucent inclusions with a lamellar structure. These inclusions are closely associated with the nuclear envelope, the endoplasmic reticulum, or both. The earliest intraepithelial stages of the parasite are rounded proliferative cells limited by a typical unit membrane in direct contact with the host cell cytoplasm. Nuclear division is not immediately followed by cytokinesis in these cells, resulting in the production of multinucleate proliferative plasmodia. After the production of multiple nuclei, the parasites form electron-dense disk-like structures that cluster in stacks of three to six, eventually forming the coiled portion of the polar tube. When these multinucleated sporagonial plasmodia divide by invagination of the plasmalemma, multiple spores are formed. In mature spores, the polar tubule has five to seven coils that appear in two rows when seen in cross sections by transmission electron microscopy.

Encephalitozoonidae

Encephalitozoonidae are widely distributed among animals (Didier *et al.* 2000) and human infection has been caused by *E. cuniculi, E. hellem,* and *E. intestinalis* (previously known as *Septata intestinalis*). The Encephalitozoonidae have the capacity to disseminate widely in their hosts, and involvement in most organs has now been documented (Orenstein *et al.* 1997; Wittner and Weiss 1999; Weber *et al.* 2000; Franzen and Muller 2001). All three organisms have been demonstrated to grow in tissue culture and rodent models exist for all of these pathogens. These organisms have been associated with gastroenteritis, keratitis, sinusitis, bronchiolitis, nephritis, cystitis/ureteritis, urethritis, prostatitis, hepatitis, fulminant hepatic failure, peritonitis, cerebritis, nodular skin lesions, corneal lesions and disseminated infection (Wittner and Weiss 1999; Weber *et al.* 2000; Franzen and Muller 2001; Zender *et al.* 1989; Mertens *et al.* 1997; Sheth *et al.* 1997; Weber *et al.* 1997; Silverstein 1998; Kester *et al.* 2000).

Encephalitozoon intestinalis

Encephalitozoon intestinalis (Cali *et al.* 1993) is commonly found in the apical and basal sides of infected intestinal enterocytes as well as in cells in the lamina propria, including fibroblasts, endothelial cells, and macrophages (Orenstein *et al.* 1992a). *E. intestinalis*-infected cells have a unique parasite-secreted fibrillar network surrounding the developing organisms so the parasitophorous vacuole appears septate. *E. intestinalis* was found in 7.8% of the stools of patients in a survey regarding the etiology of diarrhoea in Mexico (Enriquez *et al.* 1998) and has been described in travellers with chronic diarrhoea (Raynaud *et al.* 1998). The major syndrome associated with *E. intestinalis* is diarrhoea (van Gool *et al.* 1994) although it can also cause cholangitis (Cali *et al.* 1993; Willson *et al.* 1995), keratoconjunctivitis (Lowder *et al.* 1996), osteomyelitis of the mandible (Belcher *et al.* 1997), upper respiratory infections, renal failure, keratoconjunctivitis, and disseminated infection in AIDS patients (Dore *et al.* 1995; Molina *et al.* 1995; Schwartz *et al.* 1996). Elimination of this parasite by treatment with albendazole correlates with the resolution of symptoms (Weber *et al.* 1994b; Molina *et al.* 1995). Dissemination can result in necrosis of areas of the bowel, with a presentation resembling an acute abdomen (Orenstein *et al.* 1997; Soule *et al.* 1997). *E. intestinalis* spores are easier to detect than *Ent. bieneusi* spores because of their larger size, strong birefringence, and bluish color on haematoxylin and eosin staining. Sporogony is tetrasporous, and tubular appendages originate from the sporont surface and terminate in an enlarged bulb-like structure. Mature spores in cross section have a single row of four to seven coils of polar tubules.

Encephalitozoon cuniculi

Encephalitozoon cuniculi (Levaditti, Nocolau and Schoen 1923) has been associated with hepatitis (Terada *et al.* 1987), peritonitis (Schwartz *et al.* 1996), hepatic failure (Sheth *et al.* 1997), disseminated disease with fever (Mertens *et al.* 1997), renal insufficiency, and intractable cough (De Groote *et al.* 1995). Cerebral infections due to *E. cuniculi* are commonly described in many animals, but have been reported only rarely in immunocompetent humans. *Encephalitozoon* infection was demonstrated in a 3 year old boy with seizures and hepatomegaly by positive immunoglobulin G (IgG) and IgM indirect immunofluorescence assays using *E. cuniculi* (Bergquist *et al.* 1984a). Infection with *Encephalitozoon* sp. was also reported in a 9 year old Japanese boy with headache, vomiting, and spastic convulsions (Matsubayashi *et al.* 1959). Several cases of encephalitis and seizures due to *E. cuniculi* have been reported in AIDS patients (Mertens *et al.* 1997; Weber *et al.* 1997). *E. hellem* and *E. cuniculi* have similar developmental life cycles (Desportes-Livage 2000). The genus is characterized by the presence of a phagosome-like parasitophorous vacuole, unpaired nuclei, meronts which divide repeatedly by binary fission and sporonts which divide into two sporoblasts that mature into spores. No tubular appendages or fibrillar networks are produced. In cross section the mature spore has five to seven coils in single rows.

Encephalitozoon hellem

Encephalitozoon hellem (Didier *et al.* 1991) is associated with renal failure, nephritis, pneumonia, bronchitis, disseminated infection, and keratoconjunctivitis (Schwartz *et al.* 1992a; Weber *et al.* 1993; Visvesvara *et al.* 1994). Punctate keratoconjunctivitis is the most common clinical manifestation of E. hellem infection (Lowder *et al.* 1990; Rastrelli *et al.* 1994), however, occasionally punctate ketatitis can be due to either *E. cuniculi* or *E. intestinalis* (Lowder *et al.* 1996; Mertens *et al.* 1997). Clinically, patients have coarse punctate epithelial keratopathy and conjunctival inflammation resulting in redness, foreign body sensation, photophobia, excessive tearing, blurred vision, and changes in visual acuity. This is usually a superficial process restricted to the corneal epithelium and conjunctiva which rarely progresses to corneal ulceration. Infection may be either bilaterial or unilaterial. Slit-lamp examination usually demonstrates punctate epithelial opacities, granular epithelial cells with irregular fluorescein uptake, conjunctival injection, superficial corneal infiltrates, and a non-inflamed anterior chamber. Infection is often associated with disseminated disease (Lacey *et al.* 1992; Schwartz *et al.* 1992b; Weber *et al.* 1993; Degroote *et al.* 1995; Franzen *et al.* 1995) and examination of patient's urine often reveals microsporidian spores (Lacey *et al.* 1992; Schwartz *et al.* 1992b; Weber *et al.* 1993; Degroote *et al.* 1995; Franzen *et al.* 1995). *E. hellem* can also cause infection of the nasal epithelium, presenting as sinusitis (Franzen *et al.* 1996).

Other Microsporidia

Trachipleistophora hominis

Trachipleistophora hominis (Field *et al.* 1996; Hollister *et al.* 1996) is a pansporoblastic microsporidian that has been described in several patients with disseminated disease in the setting of AIDS (Field *et al.* 1996; Hollister *et al.* 1996) and can cause myositis, sinusitis, and keratoconjunctivitis. The predominant feature of all these parasites is the presence of a thick surface coat on all stages, which finally separates from the plasma membrane to become an envelope (sporophorous vesicle) enclosing the spores in groups of two to many. It is likely that the *Pleistophora sp.* described by Chupp *et al.* (1993) is also *T. hominis*, but the one seen by Ledford *et al.* (1985) may be different (Ledford *et al.* 1985; Chupp *et al.* 1993). In *T. hominis* the surface coat extends into lysed host cell cytoplasm as complex networks and merogonic and sporogonic divisions are by repeated binary fissions. The sporophorous vesicle grows to accommodate the increasing number of uninucleate sporoblasts and spores. The spores measure 4.0×2.4 µm and have about 11 coils of the polar tube.

Trachipleistophora anthropophthera

Trachipleistophora anthropophthera (Vavra *et al.* 1997) infection presents as encephalitis, myositis, and keratoconjunctivitis (Yachnis *et al.* 1996; Vavra *et al.* 1998; Pariyakanok and Jongwutiwes 2005). Morphologically it differs from *Trachipleistophora hominis* in that two types of spore are formed. One type, formed in sporophorous vesicles with varying numbers of spores, often 8, measures 3.7×2.0 µm (fixed) and has a polar tube of about 7 thick coils and 2 narrower, posterior coils (anisofilar). Spores of the second type, of which only two are formed in each sporophorous vesicle, are nearly spherical $2.2–2.5 \times 1.8–2.0$ µm. They are thin walled and have only 4–5 isofilar coils of the polar tube (Vavra *et al.* 1998). This is the first reported occurrence of a dimorphic microsporidium in mammals. Several of these patients responded clinically to albendazole.

Vittaforma corneae

Vittaforma corneae (Shadduck *et al.* 1990) can cause keratitis, urinary tract infection, disseminated infection and prostatitis (Shadduck *et al.* 1990; Deplazes *et al.* 1998). This species was isolated into culture from a corneal biopsy and was named *Nosema corneum* (Shadduck *et al.* 1990). All stages have diplokaryotic nuclei and are completely surrounded by a cisterna of host endoplasmic reticulum bearing ribosomes on the outer membrane. The cisterna divides with the parasites so that each stage is isolated in its own cisterna. Originally it was thought that sporogony was disporoblastic but Silveira and Canning (1995) demonstrated that the sporonts are multinucleate and divide to produce several linearly arranged sporoblasts (Silveira and Canning 1995b). On the basis of the multisporous sporogony and investment by host endoplasmic reticulum Silveira and Canning (1995) transferred this organism to a new genus as *Vittaforma corneae* (Silveira and Canning 1995b). Spores measure about 3.7×1.0 µm and have 5–7 coils of the polar tube.

Pleistophora ronneafiei

Pleistophora ronneafiei (Cali and Takvorian 2003) and *Pleistophora* sp. have been identified in the skeletal muscle of an HIV-negative patient as well as HIV-positive patients with myositis associated with normal creatine phosphokinase (CPK) levels (Ledford *et al.* 1985; Chupp *et al.* 1993; Grau *et al.* 1996; Cali and Takvorian 2003). In *Pleistophora* the surface coat is thicker and more uniform, the sporonts are multinucleate plasmodia and the sporophorous vesicle size is fixed by the size of the plasmodium at the onset of sporogony.

Anncaliia sp.

Anncaliia algerae (*Nosema algerae*, Vavra and Undeen 1970) infection of the skin has been seen in a patient with leukemia (Visvesvara *et al.* 1999) and in another patient with myositis who had significant elevations in CPK and muscle pain; the latter patient had rheumatoid arthritis treated with steroids and antibody to TNFα (Coyle *et al.* 2004; Vavra and Undeen 1970). *Anncaliia algerae* infection of the cornea has also been reported (Visvesvara *et al.* 1999). *Anncalia connori* (Sprague 1974) has been described from a single case in an athymic infant. Spores measuring 4.0×2.0 μm have nuclei in diplokaryotic arrangement and a polar tube with about 11 coils in a single rank. *Anncaliia vesicularum* (*Brachiola vesicularum*, Cali *et al.* 1998) was reported from a patient with AIDS and myositis. It has diplokaryotic nuclei in all stages. Prespore stages have thick surface coats with extensions of complex tubular secretions into lysed host tissue. Spores are 2.5×2.0 μm and have about 9 coils of the polar tube in 2 ranks.

Microsporidium sp. and Nosema ocularum

Microsporidium sp. and ***Nosema ocularum*** (Cali *et al.* 1991a). *Microsporidium* is used at the generic level for Microsporidia of unknown phylogenetic placement. In 1973 and 1981, two cases of corneal microsporidiosis due to *Microsporidium africanus* in Botswana (Pinnolis *et al.* 1981) and *Microsporidium ceylonesis* in Sri Lanka (Ashton and Wirasinha 1973) were described. *Microsporidium ceylonensis* spores, measuring 3.5×1.5 μm in fixed tissue were found free and in macrophages in the corneal stroma. These spores had up to 12 coils of the polar tube and there is a single nucleus lying laterally to the posterior region of the polaroplast which is lamellar (Canning and Curry, unpublished observations). Spores lie in direct contact with host cell cytoplasm. *Microsporidium africanum* (Pinnolis *et al.* 1981) spores, measured about 4.5×3.0 μm, were present mainly in the cytoplasm of histiocytes in the cornea and in direct contact with the stroma and spores had a single nucleus with 11 to 13 coils of the polar tube.

Additional cases of microsporidian keratitis have been identified in immunocompetent hosts (Wittner and Weiss 1999; Joseph *et al.* 2006). One of these organisms was classified as *N. ocularum* (Cali *et al.* 1991a), and the other, which was successfully propagated *in vitro*, was named *N. corneum* (Shadduck *et al.* 1990) (now *V. cornea*, Silveira and Canning 1995b). *Nosema ocularum* was observed in the corneal stroma of the patient, who had experienced visual problems and had a corneal ulcer but was otherwise healthy. Only spores were present, these being distributed in the host cell cytoplasm and in direct contact with it. Spores, measuring about 5.0×3.0 μm had diplokaryotic nuclei and 9–12 coils of the polar tube in a single rank. In size and number of coils of the polar tube this parasite resembles *M. africanum*. Among these immunologically normal patients with corneal infections the outcomes included: enucleation (Pinnolis *et al.* 1981), unsuccessful penetrating keratoplasty (Ashton and Wirasinha 1973), successful treatment with a corneal transplant (Cali *et al.* 1991a), and therapy with topical agents until keratoplasty (Davis *et al.* 1990).

Diagnosis

Diagnosis of gastrointestinal microsporidiosis is obtained by light microscopic examination of stool specimens using staining methods that produce differential contrast between the spores of the Microsporidia and the cells and debris in clinical samples in which Microsporidia are found. Visualization requires adequate magnification as spores range in size from 1 to 3 μm (Fig. 49.3). Chromotrope 2R, calcofluor white (fluorescent brightener 28) (Vavra *et al.* 1993), and Uvitex 2B (van Gool *et al.* 1993) are useful selective stains for Microsporidia in stool specimens and other body fluids. There are several useful chromotrope 2R-based methods. The technique of Weber *et al.* (1992a) is a modification of a standard trichrome stain using a 10-fold higher chromotrope 2R concentration and a longer staining time. Ryan *et al.* (1993) utilizes aniline blue in place of fast green and Kokoskin *et al.* (1994) use a higher temperature. Staining with chromotrope 2R results in spores which appear light pink with a belt-like stripe girding them diagonally and equatorially against a green (Weber *et al.* 1992a) or blue (Ryan *et al.* 1993) background. Microsporidian spores can also be visualized by ultraviolet (UV) microscopy using chemofluorescent optical brightening agents such as Calcofluor white M2R or Uvitex 2B which stain chitin in the spore wall. These chitin stains will also stain fungi and other faecal elements. However, microsporidian spores can be distinguished from yeast as they do not bud. In patients with proven microsporidiosis, both the chromotrope 2R and chemofluorescent brightening stains identified 100% of specimens if at least 50 high power fields were examined (van Gool *et al.* 1993; Didier *et al.* 1995a). The sensitivity of chemofluorescent brightener-based stains is slightly higher than chromotrope-based stains (especially when low numbers of spores are present in a sample). However, the specificity of the chemofluorescent stains is lower (Didier *et al.* 1995a). The limit of detecting Microsporidia by these techniques appears to be 50,000 organisms/ml (Didier *et al.* 1995a). Monoclonal antibodies to *E. hellem* (Croppo *et al.* 1998), *E. intestinalis* (Beckers *et al.* 1996), and *Ent. bieneusi* (Accoceberry *et al.* 1999; Sheoran *et al.* 2005; Singh *et al.* 2005; Zhang *et al.* 2005) have been described and can be used for immunofluorescence techniques. Detection kits for microsporidia in stool and environmental samples using antibodies to Encephalitozoonidae and *Ent. bieneusi* are commercially available (e.g. Waterborne, Inc., New Orleans, LA).

As renal involvement with shedding of spores in the urine is common in Encephalitozoonidae infections and other disseminating Microsporidia, in addition to stool specimens all patients should have urine examinations for Microsporidia. This has therapeutic implications as finding Microsporidia in the urine suggests the infection will be due to a species of Microsporidia that would respond to albendazole. Neither the chromotrope nor the chemofluorescent stain provides information on the species of Microsporidia being identified. Definitive identification of the Microsporidia causing an infection can be done using either ultrastructural examination (e.g. electron microscopy) or molecular techniques (e.g. species-specific polymerase chain reaction (PCR)). If stool examination is negative in the setting of chronic diarrhoea (more than 2 months' duration), endoscopy should be performed.

Microsporidia in body fluids other than stool (e.g. urine, cerebrospinal fluid), bile, duodenal aspirates, bronchoalveolar lavage fluid, sputum) can be visualized using Chromotrope 2R, chemofluorescent optical brightening agents, Giemsa, Brown-Hopps Gram stain, acid-fast staining, or Warthin-Starry silver staining (Weber *et al.* 2000; Field 2002). As microsporidian infections usually involve mucosa or epithelium, cytologic preparations, such as corneal swabs, are especially useful for diagnosis (Weber *et al.* 2000). On histopathological analysis spores are discernible with a modified tissue chromotrope 2R or tissue Gram stain (Brown-Hopp or Brown-Brenn) in tissue sections (Fig. 49.3). Other stains that may be useful include periodic acid-Schiff, Giemsa, and Steiner silver stains. Some Microsporidia are acid-fast stain-positive. Fresh tissue can be examined by phase contrast microscopy as unstained spores are refractile, appearing green; and birefringent. All biopsy or autopsy material should be examined by electron microscopy when microsporidiosis is suspected, as the definitive diagnosis of species is based on ultrastructural information.

Several molecular diagnostic tests have been developed for pathogenic Microsporidia. For a review of the PCR tests for microsporidiosis, see Weiss and Vossbrinck (1998). Over a hundred Microsporidia rRNA sequences are now in the GenBank database allowing the design of PCR primers to identify Microsporidia at the species level in clinical samples without the need for ultrastructural examination. Two main approaches have been employed for constructing PCR primers for Microsporidia: the use of universal pan-Microsporidia primers and of species-specific primer pairs. These PCR techniques have been applied to urine, cultures, and stool specimens (Fedorko *et al.* 1995; Katzwinkel-Wladarsch *et al.* 1997b; Ombrouck *et al.* 1997; Franzen and Muller 1999; Weiss 2000; Joseph *et al.* 2006). Biopsy specimens can also be analysed using PCR techniques, but this is best done on either unfixed frozen tissue or tissue fixed in ethanol. Currently, these molecular tests are available in reference laboratories such as the Centers for Disease Control (CDC) (Atlanta, GA, USA).

Serologic tests are useful for epidemiologic studies, but have, for the most part, not been proven useful for diagnosing microsporidiosis as infection often occurs in the setting of immune deficiency. For example, in a study of 12 AIDS patients with *Ent. bieneusi*, 2 AIDS patients with *E. intestinalis,* and 2 immunocompetent patients with *Vit. corneae*, enzyme-linked immunosorbent assay (ELISA) titers for *E. hellem, E. cuniculi,* or *Vit. corneae* were not useful for diagnosis (Didier 2000). False-negative titers were present in seven of these 14 patients.

The isolation of Microsporidia from clinical specimens is not a routine procedure, but is available in specialized research laboratories. Several of the pathogenic microsporidia including *Vittaforma corneae, E. cuniculi, E. hellem, T. hominis, T. anthropopthera, A. anncalia* and *E. intestinalis* have been cultivated *in vitro* (reviewed by Visvesvara 2002). Small animal models exist for many of these microsporidia. This has enabled these organisms to be used for screening for therapeutic agents (Beauvais *et al.* 1994; Franssen *et al.* 1995; Silveira and Canning 1995a). The most common cause of human infection is *Ent. bieneusi* and this pathogen has not been cultivated continuously *in vitro*, although limited *in vitro* cultivation has been reported (Dr Saul Tzipori, personal communication; Visvesvara *et al.* 1995; Feng *et al.* 2006). Experimental infection of SIV-infected rhesus monkeys with *Ent. bieneusi* from human tissue has been demonstrated (Katzwinkel-Wladarsch *et al.* 1997a) and serial progation has been described in immunocompromised rodents (Feng *et al.* 2006).

Treatment

For a review of drugs used against microsporidiosis in humans and animals, see Costa and Weiss (2000). Both fumagillin and albendazole

have demonstrated clinical efficacy in human infections with various Microsporidia (see Table 49.2) (Gritz *et al.* 1997; Molina *et al.* 1998, 2002; Dore *et al.* 1995; Dieterich *et al.* 1994; Corcoran *et al.* 1996; Didier 1997; Didier *et al.* 2006). Medications used without success to treat microsporidiosis are azithromycin, paromomycin (Microsporidia lack the rRNA binding site for this drug), and quinacrine. Prophylaxis with trimethoprim-sulfamethoxazole is not effective for preventing microsporidiosis, and this drug has no *in vitro* or *in vivo* activity against these organisms (Albrecht *et al.* 1995). While a few initial case reports indicated that metronidazole was effective, subsequent studies have demonstrated that this drug is not effective against clinical microsporidiosis and there is no activity seen *in vitro* (Molina *et al.* 1997; Eeftinck Schattenkerk *et al.* 1991; Beauvais *et al.* 1994; Gunnarsson *et al.* 1995). Atovaquone was reported to have some limited clinical efficacy, but it has no *in vitro* activity (Beauvais *et al.* 1994; Anwar-Bruni *et al.* 1996; Molina *et al.* 1997). Transient clinical remission of microsporidiosis has been reported with furazolidone and with nitazoxanide (1,000 mg BID) (Schwartz *et al.* 1995a; Bicart-See *et al.* 2000). Sparfloxacin and chloroquine have *in vitro* activity against Microsporidia but have not been used clinically (Beauvais *et al.* 1994). Thalidomide and octreotide have both been reported to decrease diarrhoea in some patients with microsporidiosis. However, biopsy studies demonstrate that there is no effect on parasite numbers, therefore, the effect on diarrhoea probably is due to direct effects on eneterocytes (Sharpstone *et al.* 1997).

Albendazole binds to β-tubulin and is active against all of the Encephalitozoonidae (*E. hellem, E. cuniculi, E. intestinalis*), but does not have consistent activity for treatment of infections due to *Enterocytozoon bieneusi* (Didier 1997). This is consistent with the sequence of *Encephalitozoon* β-tubulin genes which have the amino acid residues associated with sensitivity to benzimidazoles (Li *et al.* 1996), while both *Enterocytozoon* (Akiyoshi *et al.* 2007; Akiyoshi *et al.* 2009) and *Vittaforma* (Franzen and Salzberger 2008) demonstrate amino acids associated with albendazole resistance. There are numerous case reports demonstrating the efficacy of 2 to 4 weeks of albendazole 400 mg BID for infections due to Encephalitozoonidae. Treatment with albendazole (400 mg BID for 3 weeks) in a double-blind, placebo-controlled trial of eight patients with AIDS and diarrhoea due to *E. intestinalis* resulted in resolution of the diarrhoea and elimination of the organism in all eight patients, which confirms the activity of albendazole demonstrated in case reports (Weber *et al.* 1994b; Dore *et al.* 1995; Gunnarsson *et al.* 1995; Molina *et al.* 1995, 1998; Sobottka *et al.* 1995; Gritz *et al.* 1997, 1998). For *E. hellem* infections reported as chronic sinusitis, respiratory infection, and disseminated infection treatment with 400 mg of albendazole twice daily was effective therapy (Lecuit *et al.* 1994; Visvesvara *et al.* 1994). Similar efficacy was seen in a patient with disseminated *E. cuniculi* infection involving the central nervous sysyem (CNS), conjunctiva, sinuses, kidneys, and lungs (Weber *et al.* 1997). Albendazole has also been reported to be effective in cases of urethritis (Corcoran *et al.* 1996), renal failure (Aarons *et al.* 1994), and disseminated infection (Degroote *et al.* 1995). In addition to its efficacy for the Encephalitozoonidae, disseminated infection accompanied by myositis due to *T. hominis* and infection with myositis due to *Anncaliia vesicularum* have both been reported to respond to albendazole (Field *et al.* 1996; Cali *et al.* 1998). In contrast, albendazole has displayed only limited efficacy against *Ent. bieneusi* infection. In two studies examining

Table 49.2 Current treatment options for Microsporidiosis

Organism	Drug	Dosage and Duration†
All microsporidian infections	Active Antiretroviral therapy with immune restoration (an increase of CD4 count to >100 cells/μL) is associated with resolution of symptoms of enteric microsporidiosis . All patients with AIDS should be offered active antiretroviral therapy as part of the initial management of microsporidial infection. Severe dehydration, malnutrition, and wasting should be managed by fluid support and nutritional supplement. Antimotility agents can be used for diarrhea control if required.	
Enterocytozoon bieneusi	No effective commercial treatment. Fumagillin (oral) can be used as an investigational agent. *potential alternative* Nitazoxanide 1,000mg BID with food for 60 days, however, it is less effective in patients with low CD4 counts	20 mg TID (e.g. 60 mg/day)
Encephalitozoonidae infection (e.g. systemic, sinusitis, encephalitis, hepatitis)		
E. cuniculi	Albendazole	400 mg BID
E. hellem	Albendazole	400 mg BID
E. intestinalis	Albendazole	400 mg BID
Encephalitozoonidae keratoconjunctivitis	Fumagillin solution‡ (Fumadil B 3 mg/ml) Patients may also need albendazole* if systemic infection is present.	2 drops every 2 hours for 4 days then 2 drops 4 times a day§
Trachipleistophora hominis	Albendazole	400 mg BID
Anncaliia (Brachiola) vesicularum	Albendazole	400 mg BID
	± Itraconozole	400 mg QD

*Albendazole 400 mg BID.

†The duration of treatment for microsporidiosis has not been established. Relapse of infection has occurred upon stopping treatment. Patients should be maintained on treatment for at least 4 weeks, and most patients should continue on treatment until their CD4 is greater than 200 cells/μL for at least 6 months following the initiation of active antirretroviral therapy.

‡Fumadil B (fumagillin bicylohexylammonium; Mid-Continent Agrimarketing, Overland Park, KS, USA).

§Eye drops should be continued indefinitely; relapse is common on stopping treatment.

Adapted from Costa S, Weiss LM. Drug treatment of microsporidiosis. Drug Resistance Updates 2000, 3: 384–99, with permission from Elsevier.

66 patients with diarrhoea due to *Ent. bieneusi* 50% of the albendazole treated patients had some improvement in diarrhoea, but *Ent. bieneusi* persisted during treatment in all patients and there was no improvement in any patient's D-xylose absorption test (Blanshard *et al.* 1991; Dieterich *et al.* 1994; Lecuit *et al.* 1994; Sobottka *et al.* 1995; Li *et al.* 1996; Molina *et al.* 1998). Diarrhoea rapidly recurred upon discontinuing albendazole therapy in patients who reported symptom alleviation. Other studies have found that albendazole had no efficacy against *Ent. bieneusi* infection (Leder *et al.* 1998).

Fumagillin, isolated from *Aspergillus fumigatus,* was used to treat amebiasis in the 1950s, but is no longer commercially available for humans. Fumagillin is available commercially for the treatment of microsporidiosis due to *Nosema apis* in honeybees and has also been used to treat microsporidiosis in aquaculture (Kano and Fukui 1982; Higgins *et al.* 1998). Fumagillin and its analogues bind in a selective, covalent fashion to the metalloprotease methionine aminopeptidase type 2 (MetAP2). Data from the *E. cuniculi* genome project (Akiyoshi *et al.* 2009) indicates that *E. cuniculi* does not have a methionine aminopeptidase type 1 gene (MetAP1), unlike mammalian cells, which have both MetAP1 and MetAP2; therefore MetAP2 is an essential enzyme in microsporidia. The crystal structure

of *E. cuniculi* MetAP2 has recently been determined (MMDB ID: 63862, PDB ID: 3CMK) (Alvarado *et al.* 2009). Fumagillin and its analogues such as TNP-470 have significant *in vitro* and *in vivo* activity against human pathogenic Microsporidia (Molina *et al.* 1997, 2002; Didier 1997; Coyle *et al.* 1998; Didier *et al.* 2006). A dose-escalation trial of fumagillin performed on AIDS patients with diarrhoea due to *Ent. bieneusi* has demonstrated that a dose of 60 mg/day for 14 days resulted in over 80% of patients clearing this organism from their stool that was associated with resolution of diarrhoea (Molina *et al.* 2000). A subsequent randomized trial on 12 patients with either AIDS or transplantation, confirmed that 60 mg/day (given as 20 mg TID) effectively treated *Ent. bieneusi* intestinal infection with resolution of diarrhoea, clearance of spores and improvement in histology and bowel permeability (Molina *et al.* 2002). The limiting toxicity of fumagillin was thrombocytopenia, which was reversible on stopping treatment. Microsporidian infection often occurs in immunocompromised hosts, particularly in those with HIV infection and CD4 cell counts of less than 50 mm^3. Studies have demonstrated that improvement in immune function can lead to the elimination of Microsporidia and normalization of intestinal architecture (Goguel *et al.* 1997; Maggi *et al.* 2000;

Miao *et al.* 2000). Therefore, part of the primary treatment of microsporidiosis in the setting of AIDS is the institution of effective antiretroviral therapy with restoration of immune function. There has been one report of immune reconstitution syndrome in an AIDS patient with microsporidiosis who was started on antiretroviral therapy.

Prevention

There are limited data on effective preventive strategies for microsporidiosis. Microsporidian spores can survive and remain infective in the environment for prolonged periods. Experiments with *E. cuniculi* have demonstrated that they can survive for years in the environment with the correct humidity and temperature (Waller 1979). Spores are rendered noninfectious by a 30-minute exposure to most disinfectants, so the procedures used to clean most hospital rooms should be sufficient to limit infection. Spores are also killed by the commonly used methods employed for sterilization. Hand washing and general hygienic habits probably reduce the chance of contamination of the conjunctiva and cornea with microsporidian spores. The usual sanitary measures that prevent contamination of food and water with animal urine and faeces should decrease the chance for infection by water or foodborne routes, severely immune compromised patients may wish to consider using bottled or filtered water in some settings. Currently, no prophylactic agents have been identified for these organisms and infection has occurred in patients on trimethoprim-sulfamethoxazole prophylaxis (Albrecht *et al.* 1995), dapsone, pyrimethamine, itraconazole, azithromycin, and atovaquone (Beauvais *et al.* 1994; Conteas *et al.* 1998b). Several studies in AIDS patients have demonstrated that antiretroviral therapy with immune restoration can produce remission of intestinal microsporidiosis and has decreased the prevalence and incidence of infection in these patients (Goguel *et al.* 1997; Foudraine *et al.* 1998; Maggi *et al.* 2000; Miao *et al.* 2000).

References

Aarons, E.J., *et al.* (1994). Reversible renal failure caused by a microsporidian infection. *Aids*, **8**: 1119–21.

Accoceberry, I., *et al.* (1999). Production of monoclonal antibodies directed against the microsporidium Enterocytozoon bieneusi. *J. Clin. Microbiol.*, **37**: 4107–12.

Akiyoshi, D.E., *et al.* (2007). Analysis of the beta-tubulin genes from Enterocytozoon bieneusi isolates from a human and rhesus macaque. *J. Eukaryot. Microbiol.*, **54**: 38–41.

Akiyoshi, D.E., *et al.* (2009). Genomic survey of the non-cultivatable opportunistic human pathogen, *Enterocytozoon bieneusi*. *PLoS Pathog.*, **5**: e1000261.

Albrecht, H., *et al.* (1995). Does the choice of *Pneumocystis carinii* prophylaxis influence the prevalence of *Enterocytozoon bieneusi* microsporidiosis in AIDS patients? *Aids*, **9**: 302–3.

Alvarado, J.J., *et al.* (2009). Structure of a microsporidian methionine aminopeptidase type 2 complexed with fumagillin and TNP-470. *Mol. Biochem. Parasitol.*, **168**: 158–67.

Anon. (1983). WHO parasitic diseases surveillance, Antibody to *Encephalitozoon cuniculi* in man. *WHO Wkly. Epidem. Rec.*, **58**: 30.

Anwar-Bruni, D.M., *et al.* (1996). Atovaquone is effective treatment for the symptoms of gastrointestinal microsporidiosis in HIV-1-infected patients. *Aids*, **10**: 619–23.

Aoun, K., *et al.* (1997). Intestinal microsporida infections in children with primary immunologic deficiencies. *Parasite*, **4**: 386–87.

Ashton, N. and Wirasinha, P.A. (1973). Encephalitozoonosis (nosematosis) of the cornea. *Br. J. Ophthalm.*, **57**: 669–74.

Avery, S.W. and Undeen, A.H. (1987). The isolation of microsporidia and other pathogens from concentrated ditch water. *J. Am. Mosq. Control. Ass.*, **3**: 54–58.

Baker, M.D., *et al.* (1995). Small subunit ribosomal DNA phylogeny of various microsporidia with emphasis on AIDS related forms. *J. Eukaryot. Microbiol.*, **42**: 564–70.

Beaugerie, L., *et al.* (1992). Cholangiopathy associated with microsporidia infection of the common bile duct mucosa in a patient with HIV infection. *Ann. Int. Med.*, **117**: 401–2.

Beauvais, B., *et al.* (1994). In vitro model to assess effect of antimicrobial agents on *Encephalitozoon cuniculi*. *Antimicrob. Agents Chemother.*, **38**: 2440–48.

Beckers, P.J., *et al.* (1996). Encephalocytozoon intestinalis-specific monoclonal antibodies for laboratory diagnosis of microsporidiosis. *J. Clin. Microbiol.*, **34**: 282–85.

Belcher Jr., J.W., Guttenberg, S.A. and Schmookler, B.M. (1997). Microsporidiosis of the mandible in a patient with acquired immunodeficiency syndrome. *J. Oral. Maxillofac. Surg.*, **55**: 424–26.

Bergquist, N.R., *et al.* (1984a). Diagnosis of encephalitozoonosis in man by serological tests. *BMJ (Clin Res Ed)*, **288**: 902.

Bergquist, R., *et al.* (1984b). Antibody against *Encephalitozoon cuniculi* in Swedish homosexual men. *Scand. J. Infect. Dis.*, **16**: 389–91.

Bergquist, R. and Waller, T. (1984). Human microsporidiosis–does it exist? *Lakartidningen*, **81**: 1944–46.

Bicart-See, A., *et al.* (2000). Successful treatment with nitazoxanide of Enterocytozoon bieneusi microsporidiosis in a patient with AIDS. *Antimicrob. Agents Chemother.*, **44**: 167–68.

Black, S.S., *et al.* (1997). *Encephalitozoon hellem* in budgerigars (*Melopsittacus undulatus*). *Vet. Pathol.*, **34**: 189–98.

Blanshard, C., *et al.* (1991). Treatment of intestinal microsporidiosis with Albendazole. In: VII International Conference on AIDS: Science challenging AIDS, Vol. 1, Clinical Science & Trials, p. 464. Florence, Italy.

Brazil, P., *et al.* (1996). Intestinal microsporidiosis in HIV-positive patients with chronic unexplained diarrhea in Rio de Janeiro, Brazil: diagnosis, clinical presentation and follow-up. *Rev. Instituto De Med. Trop. Sao Paulo*, **38**: 97–102.

Brugere, J.F., *et al.* (2000a). *Encephalitozoon cuniculi* (Microspora) genome: physical map and evidence for telomere-associated rDNA units on all chromosomes. *Nucl. Acids Res.*, **28**: 2026–33.

Brugere, J.F., *et al.* (2000b). Occurence of subtelomeric rearrangements in the genome of the microsporidian parasite *Encephalitozoon cuniculi*, as revealed by a new fingerprinting procedure based on two-dimensional pulsed field gel electrophoresis. *Electrophoresis*, **21**: 2576–81.

Bryan, R.T. and Weber, R. (1993). Microsporidia. Emerging pathogens in immunodeficient persons. *Arch. Path. Lab. Med.*, **117**: 1243–45.

Bryan, R.T. and Schwartz, D.A. (1999). Epidemiology of microspordiosis. In: M. Wittner, L.M. Weiss (eds.), The Microsporidia and Microsporidiosis, pp. 502–16. Washington DC: ASM Press.

Bywater, J.E. and Kellett, B.S. (1979). Humoral immune response to natural infection with *Encephalitozoon cuniculi* in rabbits. *Lab. Anim.*, **13**: 293–97.

Cali, A., *et al.* (1991a). Corneal microsporidioses: characterization and identification. *J. Protozool.*, **38**: 215S–17S.

Cali, A. *et al.* (1991b). Corneal microsporidiosis in a patient with AIDS. *Am. J. Trop. Med. Hyg.*, **44**: 463–68.

Cali, A., Kotler, D.P. and Orenstein, J.M. (1993). *Septata intestinalis* N. G., N. Sp., an intestinal microsporidian associated with chronic diarrhea and dissemination in AIDS patients. *J. Eukaryot. Microbiol.*, **40**: 101–12.

Cali, A., *et al.* (1998). *Brachiola vesicularum*, n. g., n. sp., a new microsporidium associated with AIDS and myositis. *J. Eukaryot. Microbiol.*, **45**: 240–51.

Cali, A. and Takvorian, P.M. (2003). Ultrastructure and development of Pleistophora ronneafiei n. sp., a microsporidium (Protista) in the skeletal muscle of an immune-compromised individual. *J. Eukaryot. Microbiol.*, **50**: 77–85.

Cama, V.A., *et al.* (2007). Transmission of *Enterocytozoon bieneusi* between a child and guinea pigs. *J. Clin. Microbiol.*, **45**: 2708–10.

Chupp, G.L., *et al.* (1993). Myositis due to Pleistophora (Microsporidia) in a patient with AIDS. *Clin. Infect. Dis.*, **16**: 15–21.

Cislakova, L., *et al.* (1997). *Encephalitozoon cuniculi*-clinical and epidemiologic significance. Results of a preliminary serologic study in humans. *Epidem. Mikrobiol. Immuno.*, **46**: 30–33.

Conteas, C.N., *et al.* (1998a). Examination of the prevalence and seasonal variation of intestinal microsporidiosis in the stools of persons with chronic diarrhea and human immunodeficiency virus infection. *Am. J. Trop. Med. Hyg.*, **58**: 559–61.

Conteas, C.N., *et al.* (1998b). Modification of the clinical course of intestinal microsporidiosis in acquired immunodeficiency syndrome patients by immune status and anti-human immunodeficiency virus therapy. *Am. J. Trop. Med. Hyg.*, **58**: 555–58.

Corcoran, G.D., *et al.* (1996). Urethritis associated with disseminated microsporidiosis: clinical response to albendazole. *Clin. Infect. Dis.*, **22**: 592–93.

Corradi, N., *et al.* (2007). Patterns of genome evolution among the microsporidian parasites *Encephalitozoon cuniculi, Antonospora locustae* and *Enterocytozoon bieneusi*. *PLoS One*, **2**: e1277.

Costa, S.F. and Weiss, L.M. (2000). Drug treatment of microsporidiosis. *Drug Resist. Updat.*, **3**: 384–99.

Cotte, L., *et al.* (1999). Waterborne outbreak of intestinal microsporidiosis in persons with and without human immunodeficiency virus infection. *J. Infect. Dis.*, **180**: 2003–8.

Coyle, C., *et al.* (1998). TNP-470 is an effective antimicrosporidial agent. *J. Infect. Dis.*, **177**: 515–18.

Coyle, C.M., *et al.* (2004). Fatal myositis due to the microsporidian Brachiola algerae, a mosquito pathogen. *N. Engl. J. Med.*, **351**: 42–47.

Croppo, G.P., *et al.* (1998). Identification of the microsporidian *Encephalitozoon hellem* using immunoglobulin G monoclonal antibodies. *Arch. Pathol. Lab. Med.*, **122**: 182–86.

Curgy, J.J., Vavra, J. and Vivares, C. (1980). Presence of ribosomal RNAs with prokaryotic properties in Microsporidia, eukaryotic organisms. *Biol. Cell.*, **38**: 49–52.

Davis, R.M., *et al.* (1990). Corneal microsporidiosis. A case report including ultrastructural observations. *Ophthalmology*, **97**: 953–57.

De Groote, M.A., *et al.* (1995). Polymerase chain reaction and culture confirmation of disseminated Encephalitozoon cuniculi in a patient with AIDS: successful therapy with albendazole. *J. Infect. Dis.*, **171**: 1375–78.

del Aguila, C., *et al.* (1997). Identification of *Enterocytozoon bieneusi* spores in respiratory samples from an AIDS patient with a 2-year history of intestinal microsporidiosis. *J. Clin. Microbiol.*, **35**: 1862–66.

del Aguila, C., *et al.* (1999). *Enterocytozoon bieneusi* in animals: rabbits and dogs as new hosts. *J. Eukaryot. Microbiol.*, **46**: 8S–9S.

Deplazes, P., *et al.* (1996). Molecular epidemiology of *Encephalitozoon cuniculi* and first detection of Enterocytozoon bieneusi in faecal samples of pigs. *J. Eukaryot. Microbiol.*, **43**: 93S.

Deplazes, P., *et al.* (1998). Dual microsporidial infection due to *Vittaforma corneae* and *Encephalitozoon hellem* in a patient with AIDS. *Clin. Infect. Dis.*, **27**: 1521–24.

Deplazes, P., Mathis, A. and Weber, R. (2000). Epidemiology and zoonotic aspects of microsporidia of mammals and birds. *Contrib. Microbiol.*, **6**: 236–60.

Desportes-Livage, I., *et al.* (1998). Microsporidiosis in HIV-seronegative patients in Mali. *Trans. R. Soc. Trop. Med. Hyg.*, **92**: 423–24.

Desportes-Livage, I. (2000). Biology of microsporidia. *Contrib. Microbiol.*, **6**: 140–65.

Desportes, I. (1976). Ultrastructure de Stempellia mutabilis leger et Hess, microsporidie parasite de l'ephemere Ephemera vulgatta. *L. Protistol.*, **12**: 121–50.

Desportes, I. *et al.* (1985). Occurrence of a new microsporidian: *Enterocytozoon bieneusi* n. g., n. sp., in the enterocytes of a human patient with AIDS. *J. Protozool*, **32**: 250–45.

Didier, E.S. *et al.* (1991). Isolation and characterization of a new human microsporidian, Encephalitozoon hellem (n. sp.) from three AIDS patients with keratoconjunctivitis. *J. Infect. Dis.*, **163**: 617–21.

Didier, E.S., *et al.* (1994). Experimental microsporidiosis in immunocompetent and immunodeficient mice and monkeys. *Folia Parasitol.*, **41**: 1–11.

Didier, E.S., *et al.* (1995a). Comparison of three staining methods for detecting microsporidia in fluids. *J. Clin. Microbiol.*, **33**: 3138–45.

Didier, E.S., *et al.* (1995b). Identification and characterization of three *Encephalitozoon cuniculi* strains. *Parasitology*, **111**: 411–21.

Didier, E.S. (1997). Effects of albendazole, fumagillin, and TNP-470 on microsporidial replication in vitro. *Antimicrob. Agents Chemother.*, **41**: 1541–46.

Didier, E.S. (2000). Immunology of microsporidiosis. *Contrib. Microbiol.*, **6**: 193–208.

Didier, E.S., *et al.* (2000). Microsporidiosis in mammals. *Microb. Infect.*, **2**: 709–20.

Didier, P.J., *et al.* (2006). Antimicrosporidial activities of fumagillin, TNP-470, ovalicin, and ovalicin derivatives in vitro and in vivo. *Antimicrob. Agents Chemother.*, **50**: 2146–55.

Dieterich, D.T., *et al.* (1994). Treatment with Albendazole for intestinal disease due to Enterocytozoon bieneusi in patients with AIDS. *J. Infect. Dis.*, **169**: 178–83.

Dore, G.J., *et al.* (1995). Disseminated microsporidiosis due to *Septata intestinalis* in nine patients infected with the human immunodeficiency virus: response to therapy with albendazole. *Clin. Infect. Dis.*, **21**: 70–76.

Dowd, S.E., Gerba, C.P. and Pepper, I.L. (1998). Confirmation of the human-pathogenic microsporidia *Enterocytozoon bieneusi, Encephalitozoon intestinalis*, and *Vittaforma corneae* in water. *Appl. Environ. Microbiol.*, **64**: 3332–35.

Dunand, V.A., *et al.* (1997). Parasitic sinusitis and otitis in patients infected with human immunodeficiency virus: report of five cases and review. *Clin. Infect. Dis.*, **25**: 267–72.

Edlind, T. (1998). Phylogenetics of protozoan tubulin with reference to the amitochondriate eukaryotes. In: G.H. Coombs, *et al.* (eds.), Evolutionary Relationships Among Protozoa, pp. 91–108. London: Chapman & Hall.

Edlind, T.D., *et al.* (1996). Phylogenetic analysis of beta-tubulin sequences from amitochondrial protozoa. *Mol. Phylogenet. Evol.*, **5**: 359–67.

Eeftinck Schattenkerk, J.K., *et al.* (1991). Metro:idazole for microsporidium associated diarrhea in symptomatic HIV-1 infection. In: VII International Conference on AIDS, Vol. 1, pp. 464. Istituto Superiore di Sanita.

Enriquez, F.J., *et al.* (1998). Prevalence of intestinal encephalitozoonosis in Mexico. *Clin. Infect. Dis.*, **26**: 1227–29.

Fast, N.M., Logsdon Jr., J.M., and Doolittle, W.F. (1999). Phylogenetic analysis of the TATA box binding protein (TBP) gene from *Nosema locustae*: evidence for a microsporidia-fungi relationship and spliceosomal intron loss. *Mol. Biol. Evol.*, **16**: 1415–19.

Fedorko, D.P., Nelson, N.A. and Cartwright, C.P. (1995). Identification of microsporidia in stool specimens by using PCR and restriction endonucleases. *J. Clin. Microbiol.*, **33**: 1739–41.

Feng, X., *et al.* (2006). Serial propagation of the microsporidian *Enterocytozoon bieneusi* of human origin in immunocompromised rodents. *Infect. Immun.*, **74**: 4424–29.

Field, A.S., *et al.* (1996). Myositis associated with a newly described microsporidian, *Trachipleistophora hominis*, in a patient with AIDS. *J. Clin. Microbiol.*, **34**: 2803–11.

Field, A.S. (2002). Light microscopic and electron microscopic diagnosis of gastrointestinal opportunistic infections in HIV-positive patients. *Pathology*, **34**: 21–35.

Flegel, T.W. and Pasharawipas, T. (1995). A proposal for typical eukaryotic meiosis in microsporidians. *Can. J. Microbiol.*, **41**: 1–11.

Foucault, C. and Drancourt, M. (2000). Actin mediates *Encephalitozoon intestinalis* entry into the human enterocyte-like cell line, Caco-2. *Microb. Pathog.*, **28**: 51–58.

Foudraine, N.A., *et al.* (1998). Improvement of chronic diarrhoea in patients with advanced HIV-1 infection during potent antiretroviral therapy. *Aids*, **12**: 35–41.

Franssen, F.F., Lumeij, J.T. and van Knapen, F. (1995). Susceptibility of *Encephalitozoon cuniculi* to several drugs in vitro. *Antimicrob. Agents Chemother.*, **39**: 1265–68.

Franzen, C., *et al.* (1995). Immunologically confirmed disseminated, asymptomatic Encephalitozoon cuniculi infection of the gastrointestinal tract in a patient with AIDS. *Clin. Infect. Dis.*, **21**: 1480–84.

Franzen, C., *et al.* (1996). Chronic rhinosinusitis in patients with AIDS: potential role of microsporidia. *Aids*, **10**: 687–88.

Franzen, C. and Muller, A. (1999). Molecular techniques for detection, species differentiation, and phylogenetic analysis of microsporidia. *Clin. Microbiol. Rev.*, **12**: 243–85.

Franzen, C. and Muller, A. (2001). Microsporidiosis: human diseases and diagnosis. *Microb. Infect.*, **3**: 389–400.

Franzen, C. (2005). How do microsporidia invade cells? *Folia Parasitol.*, **52**: 36–40.

Franzen, C. and Salzberger, B. (2008). Analysis of the beta-tubulin gene from *Vittaforma corneae* suggests benzimidazole resistance. *Antimicrob. Agents Chemother.*, **52**: 790–93.

Fuentealba, I.C., *et al.* (1992). Hepatic lesions in rabbits infected with *Encephalitozoon cuniculi* administered per rectum. *Vet. Pathol.*, **29**: 536–40.

Germot, A., Philippe, H. and Le, G.H. (1997). Evidence for loss of mitochondria in microsporidia from a mitochondrial-type hsp70 in *Nosema locustae*. *Mol. Biochem. Parasit.*, **87**: 159–68.

Goguel, J., *et al.* (1997). Remission of AIDS-associated intestinal microsporidiosis with highly active antiretroviral therapy. *Aids*, **11**: 1658–59.

Graczyk, T.K., *et al.* (2007a). Human-virulent microsporidian spores in solid waste landfill leachate and sewage sludge, and effects of sanitization treatments on their inactivation. *Parasitol. Res.*, **101**: 569–75.

Graczyk, T.K., *et al.* (2007b). Urban feral pigeons (*Columba livia*) as a source for air- and waterborne contamination with *Enterocytozoon bieneusi* spores. *Appl. Environ. Microbiol.*, **73**: 4357–58.

Grau, A., *et al.* (1996). Myositis caused by *Pleistophora* in a patient with AIDS. *Med. Clin. (Barc).*, **107**: 779–81.

Gritz, D.C., *et al.* (1997). Ocular and sinus microsporidial infection cured with systemic albendazole. *Am. J. Ophthalm.*, **124**: 241–43.

Guerard, A., *et al.* (1999). Intestinal microsporidiosis occurring in two renal transplant recipients treated with mycophenolate mofetil. *Transplantation*, **68**: 699–707.

Gumbo, T., *et al.* (1999a). Microsporidia infection in transplant patients. *Transplantation*, **67**: 482–84.

Gumbo, T., *et al.* (1999b). Intestinal parasites in patients with diarrhea and human immunodeficiency virus infection in Zimbabwe. *Aids*, **13**: 819–21.

Gunnarsson, G., *et al.* (1995). Multiorgan microsporidiosis: report of five cases and review. *Clin. Infect. Dis.*, **21**: 37–44.

Hartskeerl, R.A., *et al.* (1993). Genetic evidence for the occurrence of extra-intestinal *Enterocytozoon bieneusi* infections. *Nucl. Acids Res.*, **21**: 4150.

Hermanek, J., *et al.* (1993). Prophylactic and therapeutic immune reconstitution of SCID mice infected with Encephalitozoon cuniculi. *Folia Parasitol.*, **40**: 287–91.

Hewan-Lowe, K., *et al.* (1997). Coinfection with *Giardia lamblia* and *Enterocytozoon bieneusi* in a patient with acquired immunodeficiency syndrome and chronic diarrhea. *Arch. Pathol. Lab. Med.*, **121**: 417–22.

Higgins, M.J., *et al.* (1998). Efficacy of the fumagillin analog TNP-470 for *Nucleospora salmonis* and *Loma salmonae* infections in chinook salmon *Oncorhynchus tshawytscha*. *Dis. Aquat. Organ.*, **34**: 45–49.

Hirt, R.P., *et al.* (1997). A mitochondrial Hsp70 orthologue in *Vairimorpha necatrix*: molecular evidence that microsporidia once contained mitochondria. *Curr. Biol.*, **7**: 995–98.

Hirt, R.P., *et al.* (1999). Microsporidia are related to Fungi: evidence from the largest subunit of RNA polymerase II and other proteins. *Proc. Natl. Acad. Sci. USA*, **96**: 580–85.

Hollister, W.S., *et al.* (1996). Development and ultrastructure of Trachipleistophora hominis n.g., n.sp. after in vitro isolation from an AIDS patient and inoculation into athymic mice. *Parasitology*, **112**: 143–54.

Hunt, R.D., King, N.W. and Foster, H.L., (1972). Encephalitozoonosis: evidence for vertical transmission. *J. Infect. Dis.*, **126**: 212–14.

Hutin, Y.J., *et al.* (1998). Risk factors for intestinal microsporidiosis in patients with human immunodeficiency virus infection: a case-control study. *J. Infect. Dis.*, **178**: 904–7.

Innes, J.R., *et al.* (1962). Occult endemic encephalitozoonosis of the central nervous system of mice (Swiss-Bagg-O'Grady strain). *J. Neuropathol. Exp. Neurol.*, **21**: 519–33.

Joseph, J., *et al.* (2006). Microsporidial keratitis in India: 16S rRNA gene-based PCR assay for diagnosis and species identification of microsporidia in clinical samples. *Invest. Ophthalm. Vis. Sci*, **47**: 4468–73.

Kamaishi, T., *et al.* (1996). Protein phylogeny of translation elongation factor EF-1 alpha suggests microsporidians are extremely ancient eukaryotes. *J. Mol. Evol.*, **42**: 257–63.

Kano, T. and Fukui, H. (1982). Studies on *Pleistophora* infection in eel, *Anguilla japonica* I. Experimental induction of microsporidiosis and fumagillin efficacy. *Fish Pathol.*, **16**: 193–200.

Katinka, M.D., *et al.* (2001). Genome sequence and gene compaction of the eukaryote parasite *Encephalitozoon cuniculi*. *Nature*, **414**: 450–53.

Katiyar, S.K., Visvesvara, G.S. and Edlind, T.D. (1995). Comparisons of ribosomal RNA sequences from amitochondrial protozoa: implications for processing, mRNA binding and paromomycin susceptibility. *Gene*, **152**: 27–33.

Katzwinkel-Wladarsch, S., *et al.* (1997). Comparison of polymerase chain reaction with light microscopy for detection of microsporida in clinical specimens. *Eur. J. Clin. Microbiol.Infect. Dis.*, **16**: 7–10.

Keeling, P.J. and Doolittle, W.F. (1996). Alpha-tubulin from early-diverging eukaryotic lineages and the evolution of the tubulin family. *Mol. Biol. Evol.*, **13**: 1297–305.

Keeling, P.J. and McFadden, G.I. (1998). Origins of microsporidia. *Trends Microbiol.*, **6**: 19–23.

Keeling, P.J. (2003). Congruent evidence from alpha-tubulin and beta-tubulin gene phylogenies for a zygomycete origin of microsporidia. *Fungal Genet. Biol.*, **38**: 298–309.

Kelkar, R., *et al.* (1997). Pulmonary microsporidial infection in a patient with CML undergoing allogeneic marrow transplant. *Bone Marr. Transp.*, **19**: 179–82.

Kent, M.L., *et al.* (1996). Taxonomy studies and diagnostic tests for myxosporean and microsporidian pathogens of salmonid fishes utilising ribosomal DNA sequence. *J. Eukaryot. Microbiol.*, **43**: 98S–99S.

Keohane, E. and Weiss, L.M. (1999). The Structure, Function, and Composition of the Microsporidian Polar Tube. In: M. Wittner and L. M. Weiss (eds.), The Microsporidia and Microsporidiosis, pp. 196–224. Washington DC: ASM Press.

Kester, K.E., Visvesara, G.S. and McEvoy, P. (2000). Organism responsible for nodular cutaneous microsporidiosis in a patient with AIDS. *Ann. Intern. Med.*, **133**: 925.

Khan, I.A., *et al.* (1999). CD8+ CTLs are essential for protective immunity against Encephalitozoon cuniculi infection. *J. Immunol.*, **162**: 6086–91.

Khan, I.A., Moretto, M. and Weiss, L.M. (2001). Immune response to *Encephalitozoon cuniculi* infection. *Microb. Infect.*, **3**: 401–5.

Koch, N.P., Schmertz, C., and Schottelius, J. (1998). *Diagnosis of Human Pathogenic Microsporidia*. Dissertation, Berhard Nocht Institute for Tropical Medicine, Hamburg, Germany.

Kokoskin, E., *et al.* (1994). Modified technique for efficient detection of microsporidia. *J. Clin. Microbiol.*, **32**: 1074–75.

Koudela, B., *et al.* (1993). The severe combined immunodeficient mouse as a model for *Encephalitozoon cuniculi* microsporidiosis. *Folia Parasitol.*, **40**: 279–86.

Kyaw, T., *et al.* (1997). The prevalence of *Enterocytozoon bieneusi* in acquired immunodeficiency syndrome (AIDS) patients from the north west of England: 1992–1995. *Br. J. Biomed. Sci.*, **54**: 186–91.

Lacey, C.J.N., *et al.* (1992). Chronic microsporidian infection of the nasal mucosae, sinuses and conjunctivae in HIV disease. *Genitour. Med.*, **68**: 179–81.

Latib, M.A., *et al.* (2001). Microsporidiosis in the graft of a renal transplant recipient. *Transpl. Int.*, **14**: 274–77.

Lecuit, M., Oksenhendler, E. and Sarfati, C. (1994). Use of albendazole for disseminated microsporidian infection in a patient with AIDS. *J. Infect. Dis.*, **19**: 332–33.

Leder, K., *et al.* (1998). Microsporidial disease in HIV-infected patients: a report of 42 patients and review of the literature. *Scand. J. Infect. Dis.*, **30**: 331–38.

Ledford, D.K., *et al.* (1985). Microsporidiosis myositis in a patient with the acquired immunodeficiency syndrome. *Ann. Intern. Med.*, **102**: 628–30.

Levaditi, C., Nicolau, S. and Schoen, R. (1923). L'agent etiologique de l'enchalite epizootique du lapin (*Encephalitozoon cuniculi*). *C. R. Soc. Biol.*, **89**: 984–86.

Li, J., *et al.* (1996). Tubulin genes from AIDS-associated microsporidia and implications for phylogeny and benzimidazole sensitivity. *Mol. Biochem. Parasitol.*, **78**: 289–95.

Li, X. and Fayer, R. (2006). Infectivity of microsporidian spores exposed to temperature extremes and chemical disinfectants. *J. Eukaryot. Microbiol.*, **53**: S77–79.

Loh, R.S., *et al.* (2009). Emerging prevalence of microsporidial keratitis in Singapore: epidemiology, clinical features, and management. *Ophthalmology*, **116**: 2348–53.

Lom, J. (1972). On the structure of the extruded microsporidian polar filament. *Z. Parasitenk.*, **38**: 200–13.

Lopez-Velez, R., *et al.* (1999). Microsporidiosis in travelers with diarrhea from the tropics. *J. Travel Med.*, **6**: 223–27.

Lowder, C.Y., *et al.* (1990). Microsporidia infection of the cornea in a man seropositive for human immunodeficiency virus. *Am. J. Ophthalmol.*, **109**: 242–44.

Lowder, C.Y., *et al.* (1996). Microsporidial keratoconjunctivitis caused by *Septata intestinalis* in a patient with acquired immunodeficiency syndrome. *Am. J. Ophthalmol.*, **121**: 715–17.

Maggi, P., *et al.* (2000). Effect of antiretroviral therapy on cryptosporidiosis and microsporidiosis in patients infected with human immunodeficiency virus type 1. *Eur. J. Clin. Microbiol. Infect. Dis.*, **19**: 213–17.

Mansfield, K.G., *et al.* (1997). Identification of an *Enterocytozoon bieneusi*-like microsporidian parasite in simian-immunodeficiency-virus-inoculated macaques with hepatobiliary disease. *Am. J. Pathol.*, **150**: 1395–405.

Margileth, A.M., *et al.* (1973). Disseminated nosematosis in an immunologically compromised infant. *Arch. Pathol.*, **95**: 145–50.

Mathis, A., Weber, R. and Deplazes, P. (2005). Zoonotic potential of the microsporidia. *Clin. Microbiol. Rev.*, **18**: 423–45.

Matsubayashi, H., *et al.* (1959). A case of Encephalitozoon-like body infection in man. *Arch. Pathol. Lab. Med.*, **67**: 181–85.

Mertens, R.B., *et al.* (1997). *Encephalitozoon cuniculi* microsporidiosis: infection of the brain, heart, kidneys, trachea, adrenal glands, and urinary bladder in a patient with AIDS. *Mod. Pathol.*, **10**: 68–77.

Miao, Y.M., *et al.* (2000). Eradication of cryptosporidia and microsporidia following successful antiretroviral therapy. *J. Acqu. Immune Defic. Syndr.*, **25**: 124–29.

Mohindra, A.R., *et al.* (2002). Disseminated microsporidiosis in a renal transplant recipient. *Transpl. Infect. Dis.*, **4**: 102–7.

Molina, J.M., *et al.* (1993a). Intestinal microsporidiosis in human immunodeficiency virus-infected patients with chronic unexplained diarrhea: prevalence and clinical and biologic features. *J. Infect. Dis.*, **167**: 217–21.

Molina, J.M., *et al.* (1995). Disseminated microsporidiosis due to *Septata intestinalis* in patients with AIDS: clinical features and response to albendazole therapy. *J. Infect. Dis.*, **171**: 245–49.

Molina, J.M., *et al.* (1997). Potential efficacy of fumagillin in intestinal microsporidiosis due to Enterocytozoon bieneusi in patients with HIV infection: results of a drug screening study. The French Microsporidiosis Study Group. *Aids*, **11**: 1603–10.

Molina, J.M., *et al.* (1998). Albendazole for treatment and prophylaxis of microsporidiosis due to *Encephalitozoon intestinalis* in patients with AIDS: a randomized double-blind controlled trial. *J. Infect. Dis.*, **177**: 1373–77.

Molina, J.M., *et al.* (2000). Trial of oral fumagillin for the treatment of intestinal microsporidiosis in patients with HIV infection. ANRS 054 Study Group. Agence Nationale de Recherche sur le SIDA. *Aids*, **14**: 1341–48.

Molina, J.M., *et al.* (2002). Fumagillin treatment of intestinal microsporidiosis. *N. Engl. J. Med.*, **346**: 1963–69.

Morakote, N., *et al.* (1995). Microsporidium and Cyclospora in human stools in Chiang Mai, Thailand. *Southeast Asian J .Trop. Med. Pub. Health*, **26**: 799–800.

Moretto, M., *et al.* (2000). Lack of CD4(+) T cells does not affect induction of CD8(+) T-cell immunity against Encephalitozoon cuniculi infection. *Infect. Immun.*, **68**: 6223–32.

Moretto, M., *et al.* (2001). Gamma delta T cell-deficient mice have a down-regulated CD8+ T cell immune response against Encephalitozoon cuniculi infection. *J. Immuno.*, **166**: 7389–97.

Moretto, M.M., *et al.* (2007). IFN-gamma-producing dendritic cells are important for priming of gut intraepithelial lymphocyte response against intracellular parasitic infection. *J. Immunol.*, **179**: 2485–92.

Moss, R.B., *et al.* (1997). Microsporidium-associated sinusitis. *Ear Nose Throat J.*, **76**: 95–101.

Ombrouck, C., *et al.* (1997). Specific PCR assay for direct detection of intestinal microsporidia *Enterocytozoon bieneusi* and *Encephalitozoon intestinalis* in faecal specimens from human immunodeficiency virus-infected patients. *J. Clin. Microbiol.*, **35**: 652–55.

Orenstein, J.M., *et al.* (1990). Intestinal microsporidiosis as a cause of diarrhea in human immunodeficiency virus-infected patients: a report of 20 cases. *Hum. Pathol.*, **21**: 475–81.

Orenstein, J.M., Dieterich, D.T. and Kotler, D.P. (1992a). Systemic dissemination by a newly recognized intestinal microsporidia species in AIDS. *Aids*, **6**: 1143–50.

Orenstein, J.M., Tenner, M. and Kotler, D.P. (1992b). Localization of infection by the microsporidian Enterocytozoon bieneusi in the gastrointestinal tract of AIDS patients with diarrhea. *Aids*, **6**: 195–97.

Orenstein, J.M., *et al.* (1997). Disseminated microsporidiosis in AIDS: are any organs spared? *Aids*, **11**: 385–86.

Pariyakanok, L. and Jongwutiwes, S. (2005). Keratitis caused by *Trachipleistophora anthropopthera*. *J. Infect.*, **51**: 325–28.

Pinnolis, M., *et al.* (1981). Nosematosis of the cornea: case report, including electron microscopic studies. *Arch. Ophthalmol.*, **99**: 1044–47.

Pol, S. (1993). Microsporidiosis and AIDS-Related Cholangitis. *Med. Sci.*, **9**: 762–63.

Pol, S., *et al.* (1993). Microsporidia infection in patients with the human immunodeficiency virus and unexplained cholangitis. *N. Engl. J. Med.*, **328**: 95–99.

Pospisilova, Z., *et al.* (1997). Parasitic opportunistic infections in Czech HIV-infected patients—a prospective study. *Cent. Eur. J. Pub. Health*, **5**: 208–13.

Rabodonirina, M., *et al.* (2003). Microsporidiosis and transplantation: a retrospective study of 23 cases. *J. Eukaryot. Microbiol.*, **50**: S583.

Rastrelli, P., Didier, E. and Yee, R. (1994). Microsporidial keratitis. *Opthalm. Clin. N. Am.*, **7**: 614–35.

Raynaud, L., *et al.* (1998). Identification of *Encephalitozoon intestinalis* in travelers with chronic diarrhea by specific PCR amplification. *J. Clin. Microbiol.*, **36**: 37–40.

Reddy, A.K., *et al.* (2009a). Polymerase Chain Reaction for the Diagnosis and Species Identification of Microsporidia in Patients with Keratitis. *Clin. Microbiol. Infect.*, Accepted article; doi:10.1111/J 1469-0691.2009.03152.x.

Reddy, A.K. (2009b). Is Microsporidial Keratitis A Seasonal Infection in India. *Clin Microbiol Infect.*, Accepted article; doi:10.1111/J 1469-0691.2009.0384.x.

Reetz, J., *et al.* (2002). First detection of the microsporidium Enterocytozoon bieneusi in non-mammalian hosts (chickens). *Int. J. Parasitol.*, **32**: 785–87.

Ryan, N.J., *et al.* (1993). A new trichrome-blue stain for detection of microsporidial species in urine, stool, and nasopharyngeal specimens. *J. Clin. Microbiol.*, **31**: 3264–69.

Sandfort, J., *et al.* (1994). *Enterocytozoon bieneusi* infection in an immunocompetent patient who had acute diarrhea and who was not infected with the human immunodeficiency virus. *Clin. Infect. Dis.*, **19**: 514–16.

Santin, M. and Fayer, R. (2009). *Enterocytozoon bieneusi* genotype nomenclature based on the internal transcribed spacer sequence: a consensus. *J. Eukaryot. Microbiol.*, **56**: 34–38.

Schmidt, E.C. and Shadduck, J.A. (1984). Mechanisms of resistance to the intracellular protozoan *Encephalitozoon cuniculi* in mice. *J. Immuno.*, **133**: 2712–19.

Schwartz, D.A., *et al.* (1992a). Disseminated microsporidiosis (*Encephalitozoon hellem*) and acquired immunodeficiency syndrome. Autopsy evidence for respiratory acquisition. *Arch. Pathol. Lab. Med.*, **116**: 660–68.

Schwartz, D.A., *et al.* (1992c). Disseminated microsporidiosis and AIDS; pathologic evidence for respiratory transmission of Encephalitozoon infection. In: VII International Conference on AIDS, Vol. 8, pp. B239. Istituto Superiore di Sanita.

Schwartz, D.A., *et al.* (1993a). Pathologic features and immunofluorescent antibody demonstration of ocular microsporidiosis (*Encephalitozoon hellem*) in seven patients with acquired immunodeficiency syndrome. *Am. J. Ophthalmol.*, **115**: 285–92.

Schwartz, D.A., *et al.* (1994). Male genital tract microsporidiosis and AIDS: prostatic abscess due to *Encephalitozoon hellem*. *J. Eukaryot. Microbiol.*, **41**: 61S.

Schwartz, D.A., *et al.* (1995a). The presence of *Enterocytozoon bieneusi* spores in the lamina propria of small bowel biopsies with no evidence of disseminated microsporidiosis. Enteric Opportunistic Infections Working Group. *Arch. Pathol. Lab. Med.*, **119**: 424–28.

Schwartz, D.A., *et al.* (1995b). The presence of *Enterocytozoon bieneusi* spores in the lamina propria of small bowel biopsies with no evidence of disseminated microsporidiosis. *Arch. Pathol. Lab. Med.*, **119**: 424–28.

Schwartz, D.A., *et al.* (1996). Pathology of microsporidiosis: emerging parasitic infections in patients with acquired immunodeficiency syndrome. *Arch. Pathol. Lab. Med.*, **120**: 173–88.

Schwartz, D.A., *et al.* (1998). Ultrastructure of atypical (teratoid) sporogonial stages of Enterocytozoon bieneusi (Microsporidia) in naturally infected rhesus monkeys (Macacca mulatta). *Arch. Pathol. Lab. Med.*, **122**: 423–29.

Shadduck, J.A., *et al.* (1990). Isolation of a microsporidian from a human patient. *J. Infect. Dis.*, **162**: 773–76.

Sharpstone, D., *et al.* (1997). Thalidomide: a novel therapy for microsporidiosis. *Gastroenterology*, **112**: 1823–29.

Sheoran, A.S., *et al.* (2005). Monoclonal antibodies against *Enterocytozoon bieneusi* of human origin. *Clin. Diagn. Lab. Immunol.*, **12**: 1109–13.

Sheth, S.G., *et al.* (1997). Fulminant hepatic failure caused by microsporidial infection in a patient with AIDS. *Aids*, **11**: 553–54.

Silveira, H. and Canning, E.U. (1995a). In vitro cultivation of the human microsporidium *Vittaforma corneae*: development and effect of albendazole. *Folia Parasitol.*, **42**: 241–50.

Silveira, H. and Canning, E.U. (1995b). *Vittaforma corneae* n. comb. for the human microsporidium *Nosema corneum* Shadduck, Meccoli, Davis & Font, 1990, based on its ultrastructure in the liver of experimentally infected athymic mice. *J. Eukaryot. Microbiol.*, **42**: 158–65.

Silverstein, B.E. (1998). Parasitic corneal infections. *Intern. Ophthalm. Clin.*, **38**: 179–82.

Sing, A., *et al.* (2001). Molecular diagnosis of an *Enterocytozoon bieneusi* human genotype C infection in a moderately immunosuppressed human immunodeficiency virus seronegative liver-transplant recipient with severe chronic diarrhea. *J. Clin. Microbiol.*, **39**: 2371–72.

Singh, I., *et al.* (2005). Sensitivity and specificity of a monoclonal antibody-based fluorescence assay for detecting *Enterocytozoon bieneusi* spores in feces of simian immunodeficiency virus-infected macaques. *Clin. Diagn. Lab. Immunol.*, **12**: 1141–44.

Sobottka, I., *et al.* (1995). Disseminated *Encephalitozoon (Septata) intestinalis* infection in a patient with AIDS: novel diagnostic approaches and autopsy-confirmed parasitological cure following treatment with albendazole. *J. Clin. Microbiol.*, **33**: 2948–52.

Soule, J.B., *et al.* (1997). A patient with acquired immunodeficiency syndrome and untreated *Encephalitozoon (Septata) intestinalis* microsporidiosis leading to small bowel perforation. Response to albendazole. *Arch. Pathol. Lab. Med.*, **121**: 880–87.

Southern, T.R., *et al.* (2007). EnP1, a microsporidian spore wall protein that enables spores to adhere to and infect host cells *in vitro*. *Eukaryot. Cell*, **6**: 1354–62.

Sprague, V. (1977). Systematics of the Microsporidia. In: L.A. Bulla and T.C. Cheng (eds.) Comparative Pathobiology, Vol. 2, pp. 1–510. NY: Plenum Press.

Sprague, V., Becnel, J.J. and Hazard, E.I. (1992). Taxonomy of phylum microspora. *Crit. Rev. Microbiol.*, **18**: 285–395.

Sprague, V.V., Becnel, J.J., (1998). Note on the Name-Author-Date Combination for the Taxon MICROSPORIDIES Balbiani, 1882, When Ranked as a Phylum. *J. Invertebr. Pathol.*, **71**: 91–94.

Terada, S., *et al.* (1987). Microsporidan hepatitis in the acquired immunodeficiency syndrome. *Ann. Intern. Med.*, **107**: 61–62.

Tumwine, J.K., *et al.* (2005). Cryptosporidiosis and microsporidiosis in ugandan children with persistent diarrhea with and without concurrent infection with the human immunodeficiency virus. *Am. J. Trop. Med. Hyg.*, **73**: 921–25.

van Gool, T., *et al.* (1993). Diagnosis of intestinal and disseminated microsporidial infections in patients with HIV by a new rapid fluorescence technique. *J. Clin. Pathol.*, **46**: 694–99.

van Gool, T., *et al.* (1994). *Septata intestinalis* frequently isolated from stool of AIDS patients with a new cultivation method. *Parasitology*, **109**: 281–89.

van Gool, T., *et al.* (1995). High prevalence of *Enterocytozoon bieneusi* infections among HIV-positive individuals with persistent diarrhoea in Harare, Zimbabwe. *Trans. R. Soc. Trop. Med. Hyg.*, **89**: 478–80.

Vavra, J. and Undeen, A.H. (1970). *Nosema algerae* n. sp. (Cnidospora, Microsporida) a pathogen in a laboratory colony of Anopheles stephensi Liston (Diptera: Culicidae). *J. Protozool.*, **17**: 240–49.

Vavra, J. (1976). Structure of the Microsporidia. In: L.A. Bulla, Jr. and T.C. Cheng (eds.) *Comparative Pathobiology*, Vol. 1, pp. 1–85. NY: Plenum Press.

Vavra, J., *et al.* (1993). Staining of microsporidian spores by optical brighteners with remarks on the use of brighteners for the diagnosis of AIDS associated human microsporidioses. *Folia Parasitol.*, **40**: 267–72.

Vavra, J., *et al.* (1998). Microsporidia of the genus Trachipleistophora—causative agents of human microsporidiosis: description of *Trachipleistophora anthropophthera* n. sp. (Protozoa: Microsporidia). *J. Eukaryot. Microbiol.*, **45**: 273–83.

Visvesvara, G.S., *et al.* (1994). Polyclonal and monoclonal antibody and PCR-amplified small-subunit rRNA identification of a microsporidian, *Encephalitozoon hellem*, isolated from an AIDS patient with disseminated infection. *J. Clin. Microbiol.*, **32**: 2760–68.

Visvesvara, G.S., *et al.* (1995b). Short-term in vitro culture and molecular analysis of the Microsporidian, Enterocytozoon bieneusi. *J. Euk. Microbiol.*, **42**: 506–510.

Visvesvara, G.S., *et al.* (1999). Isolation of *Nosema algerae* from the cornea of an immunocompetent patient. *J. Eukaryot. Microbiol.*, **46**: 10S.

Visvesvara, G.S. (2002). In vitro cultivation of microsporidia of clinical importance. *Clin. Microbiol. Rev.*, **15**: 401–13.

Vivares, C., *et al.* (1996). Chromosomal localization of five genes in *Encephalitozoon cuniculi* (Microsporidia). *J. Eukaryot. Microbiol.*, **43**: 97S.

Vivares, C.P. and Metenier, G. (2000). Towards the minimal eukaryotic parasitic genome. *Curr. Opin. Microbiol.*, **3**: 463–67.

Vossbrinck, C.R. and Woese, C.R. (1986). Eukaryotic ribosomes that lack a 5.8S RNA. *Nature,* **320**: 287–88.

Vossbrinck, C.R., *et al.* (1987). Ribosomal RNA sequence suggests microsporidia are extremely ancient eukaryotes. *Nature,* **326**: 411–44.

Waller, T. (1979). Sensitivity of *Encephalitozoon cuniculi* to various temperatures, disinfectants and drugs. *Lab. Anim.*, **13**: 227–30.

Weber, R., *et al.* (1992a). Improved light-microscopical detection of microsporidia spores in stool and duodenal aspirates. The Enteric Opportunistic Infections Working Group. *N. Engl. J. Med.*, **326**: 161–66.

Weber, R., *et al.* (1992b). Pulmonary and intestinal microsporidiosis in a patient with the acquired immunodeficiency syndrome. *Am. Rev. Respir. Dis.*, **146**: 1603–5.

Weber, R., *et al.* (1992c). Intestinal Enterocytozoon bieneusi microsporidiosis in an HIV-infected patient - diagnosis by ileo-colonoscopic biopsies and long-term follow up. *Clin. Invest.*, **70**: 1019–23.

Weber, R., *et al.* (1993). Disseminated microsporidiosis due to *Encephalitozoon hellem*: pulmonary colonization, microhematuria, and mild conjunctivitis in a patient with AIDS. *Clin. Infect. Dis.*, **17**: 415–19.

Weber, R. and Bryan, R.T. (1994). Microsporidial infections in immunodeficient and immunocompetent patients. *Clin. Infect. Dis.*, **19**: 517–21.

Weber, R., *et al.* (1994a). Human microsporidial infections. *Clin. Microbiol. Rev.*, **7**: 426–61.

Weber, R., *et al.* (1994b). Detection of *Septata intestinalis* in stool specimens and coprodiagnostic monitoring of successful treatment with albendazole. *Clin. Infect. Dis.*, **19**: 342–45.

Weber, R., *et al.* (1997). Cerebral microsporidiosis due to *Encephalitozoon cuniculi* in a patient with human immunodeficiency virus infection. *N. Engl. J. Med.*, **336**: 474–78.

Weber, R., Deplazes, P. and Schwartz, D. (2000). Diagnosis and clinical aspects of human microsporidiosis. *Contrib. Microbiol.*, **6**: 166–92.

Weidner, E. (1972). Ultrastructural study of microsporidian invasion into cells. *Z. Parasitenk.*, **40**: 227–42.

Weiss, L.M. (1995). ...and now microsporidiosis. *Ann. Intern. Med,* **123**: 954–56.

Weiss, L.M. and Vossbrinck, C.R. (1998). Microsporidiosis: molecular and diagnostic aspects. *Adv. Parasitol.*, **40**: 351–95.

Weiss, L.M., *et al.* (1999). Microsporidian molecular phylogeny: the fungal connection. *J. Eukaryot. Microbiol.*, **46**: 17S–18S.

Weiss, L.M. and Vossbrinck, C.R. (1999). Molecular Biology, Molecular Phylogeny, and Molecular Diagnostic Approaches to the Microsporidia. In: M. Wittner and L. M. Weiss (eds.) The Microsporidia and Microsporidia, pp. 129–71. Washington DC: ASM Press.

Weiss, L.M. (2000). Molecular phylogeny and diagnostic approaches to microsporidia. *Contrib. Microbiol.*, **6**: 209–35.

Weiss, L.M. (2010). Microsporidiosis. In: G.L. Mandell, J.E. Bennett, R. Dolin (eds.) Mandell, Douglas and Bennett's Principles and Practice of Infectious Diseases, (7th edn.), pp. 3391–408. Philadelphia: Churchill Livingston.

Wichro, E., *et al.* (2005). Microsporidiosis in travel-associated chronic diarrhea in immune-competent patients. *Am. J. Trop. Med. Hyg.*, **73**: 285–87.

Williams, B.A., *et al.* (2002). A mitochondrial remnant in the microsporidian *Trachipleistophora hominis. Nature,* **418**: 865–69.

Willson, R., *et al.* (1995). Human immunodeficiency virus 1-associated necrotizing cholangitis caused by infection with Septata intestinalis. *Gastroenterology,* **108**: 247–51.

Wittner, M. and Weiss, L.M. (1999). The microsporidia and microsporidiosis. Washington DC: ASM Press.

Wright, J.H. and Craighead, E.M. (1922). Infectious Motor Paralysis in Young Rabbits. *J. Exp. Med.*, **36**: 135–40.

Wuhib, T., *et al.* (1994). Cryptosporidial and microsporidial infections in human immunodeficiency virus-infected patients in northeastern Brazil. *J. Infect. Dis.*, **170**: 494–97.

Xu, Y., *et al.* (2004). Glycosylation of the major polar tube protein of *Encephalitozoon hellem*, a microsporidian parasite that infects humans. *Infect. Immun.*, **72**: 6341–50.

Xu, Y., *et al.* (2006). Identification of a new spore wall protein from *Encephalitozoon cuniculi. Infect. Immun.*, **74**: 239–47.

Yachnis, A.T., *et al.* (1996). Disseminated microsporidiosis especially infecting the brain, heart, and kidneys. Report of a newly recognized pansporoblastic species in two symptomatic AIDS patients. *Am. J. Clin. Pathol.*, **106**: 535–43.

Yee, R.W., *et al.* (1991). Resolution of microsporidial epithelial keratopathy in a patient with AIDS. *Ophthalmology,* **98**: 196–201.

Zeman, D.H. and Baskin, G.B. (1985). Encephalitozoonosis in squirrel monkeys (*Saimiri sciureus*). *Vet. Pathol.*, **22**: 24–31.

Zender, H.O., *et al.* (1989). A case of *Encephalitozoon cuniculi* peritonitis in a patient with AIDS. *Am. J. Clin. Pathol.*, **92**: 352–56.

Zhang, Q., *et al.* (2005). Production and characterization of monoclonal antibodies against *Enterocytozoon bieneusi* purified from rhesus macaques. *Infect. Immun.*, **73**: 5166–72.

CHAPTER 50

Blastocystosis

Manoj K. Puthia and Kevin S. W. Tan

Summary

History of the disease

Blastocystis, the causative agent of blastocystosis, is an intestinal protozoan commonly identified in stool specimens of patients. It is one of the most common parasites inhabiting the human intestinal tract. Clinical symptoms attributed to *Blastocystis* include recurrent watery diarrhoea, mucous diarrhoea, vomiting, abdominal cramps and flatulence. *Blastocystis* infects both children and adults and its geographical distribution appears to be global with prevalence ranging from 30 to 50% in developing countries (Stenzel and Boreham 1996).

Blastocystis was first described as a distinct organism in 1911 and the name *B. enterocola* was proposed for this organism (Alexeieff 1911). It was isolated from human faeces and the name *B. hominis* was coined (Brumpt 1912). At first, it was described as a harmless intestinal yeast and ignored for many decades. Its association with human disease was suggested by a number of reports and eventually work by Zierdt (1991) increased the awareness of *Blastocystis* infections in humans.

In spite of its description about a century ago, the exact role of *Blastocystis* as a cause of human disease is uncertain. A number of clinical and epidemiological studies implicate the parasite as a potential pathogen (Al-Tawil *et al.* 1994; El-Shazly *et al.* 2005; Garavelli *et al.* 1991; Logar *et al.* 1994) while others exonerate it as an etiology of intestinal disease (Chen *et al.* 2003; Leder *et al.* 2005; Shlim *et al.* 1995). Significant progress has been achieved on descriptions of the morphology and genetic diversity of *Blastocystis* but most aspects of its life cycle, molecular biology, and pathogenicity remain unresolved (Stenzel and Boreham 1996; Tan 2004).

Taxonomy

The taxonomic classification of *Blastocystis* is controversial. *Blastocystis* was earlier described to be a yeast or a fungus (Alexeieff 1911; O'Connor 1919), a protozoal cyst (Bensen 1909), or a degenerating cell (Swellengrebel 1917). *Blastocystis* was described as a protist on the basis of morphological and physiological features (Zierdt *et al.* 1967). These protistan features included the presence of one or more nuclei, smooth and rough endoplasmic reticulum, a Golgi complex, mitochondria-like organelles, the inability to grow on fungal medium, the ineffectiveness of antifungal drugs, and its susceptibility to some antiprotozoal drugs. Later, *Blastocystis* was classified as a sporozoan (Zierdt 1991) and finally reclassified as a sarcodine. Molecular sequencing studies of *Blastocystis* partial small-subunit rRNA (ssrRNA) showed that *Blastocystis* is not monophylectic with the yeasts, fungi, sarcodines, or sporozoans (Johnson *et al.* 1989) and it was concluded that *Blastocystis* is unrelated to yeasts. Later, the complete *Blastocystis* ssrRNA gene was sequenced and phylogenetic analysis suggested that *Blastocystis* should be classified within the Stramenopiles (also known as Heterokonta) (Silberman *et al.* 1996). Molecular phylogenetic analysis showed that *Blastocystis* is closely related to the Stramenopile *Proteromonas lacerate* (Arisue *et al.* 2002). Another study involving molecular analysis of *Blastocystis* ssrRNA, cytosolic-type 70-kDa heat shock protein, translation elongation factor 2, and the non-catalytic 'B' subunit of vacuolar ATPase confirmed that *Blastocystis* is a Stramenopile (Arisue *et al.* 2002). Stramenopiles characteristically possess flagella with mastigonemes. Interestingly, since *Blastocystis* does not have flagella and is non-motile, it was therefore placed in a newly formed Class Blastocystea in the Subphylum Opalinata, Infrakingdom Heterokonta, Subkingdom Chromobiota, and Kingdom Chromista (Cavalier-Smith 1998). In addition, elongation factor-1α (EF-1α) sequencing for phylogenetic analysis also showed that *Blastocystis* is not a fungus and suggested that it diverged before *Trypanosoma*, *Euglena*, *Dictyostelium* and other eukaryotes. Most studies in the past named *Blastocystis* species according to host origin and this may have resulted in confusion regarding specificity, cell biology and pathogenicity of the parasite. Recently, a consensus report on the terminology for *Blastocystis* genotypes was published (Stensvold *et al.* 2007). Based on this report humans can be host to *Blastocystis* from a variety of animals including mammals (subtype 1), primates (subtype 2), rodents (subtype 4), cattle and pigs (subtype 5), and birds (subtype 6 and 7) (Noel *et al.* 2005; Yan *et al.* 2007).

Speciation and genetic diversity

Blastocystis has been isolated from an extensive range of hosts that includes primates, pigs, rodents, reptiles, insects and birds (Boreham and Stenzel 1993). Morphological differences among isolates are not significant. Therefore other methods such as karyotyping and molecular phylogenetic analysis have been used to differentiate *Blastocystis* from different hosts (Tan 2004). In the past, description of new species was based on host of origin and parasite ultrastructure (Belova 1992). Others used pulsed-field gel electrophoresis for karyotyping and speciated *Blastocystis* isolated from rats (Chen *et al.* 1997b), reptiles (Teow *et al.* 1991), tortoise and rhino iguana (Singh *et al.* 1996). However, diverse intra-species karyotypes were observed and it was realized that karyotyping might not be a good method for the speciation of *Blastocystis* (Yoshikawa *et al.* 2004b). Consequently, there are arguments against assigning different species names, other than *B. hominis,* based on presumed host specificity and morphology (Tan 2004).

Recently, analysis of ssrRNA sequencing of 16 *Blastocystis* isolates from humans and other animals showed that isolates can be divided phylogenetically into seven distinct groups that are morphologically similar but genetically different (Arisue *et al.* 2003). Concurrently, other studies reported the presence of these distinct genotypes in a variety of other animal hosts (Abe *et al.* 2000a, 2003b; Noel *et al.* 2005; Yoshikawa *et al.* 2004a, 2004b). Altogether, these studies strongly suggested that *Blastocystis* is a zoonotic parasite. More recently, it was shown in an extensive ssrRNA sequence analysis that most of the 78 isolates of *Blastocystis* can be clearly grouped into seven clades referred to as groups I to VII (Noel *et al.* 2005). More importantly, *Blastocystis* isolates from both humans and animals were present in six of the seven groups. It was suggested that group I (subtype 1) comprised of zoonotic isolates of mammalian origin, group II (subtype 2) comprised of isolates of primates origin, group III (subtype 3) comprised of isolates of human origin, group IV (subtype 4) represented zoonotic isolates of rodent origin, group V (subtype 5) comprised of isolates from pigs and cattle and group VI (subtype 6) and VII (subtype 7) possibly comprised of zoonotic isolates of avian origins (Noel *et al.* 2005; Yan *et al.* 2007; Yoshikawa *et al.* 2004b). Overall, these studies suggested that *Blastocystis* is a zoonotic parasite and animal-to-animal, animal-to-human, and human-to-animal transmission can occur.

Random amplified polymorphic DNA (RAPD) analysis of 16 *Blastocystis* isolates, comprising eight isolates from symptomatic and eight asymptomatic patients, suggested a possible link between genotype with pathogenicity (Tan *et al.* 2006). However, other studies failed to show any correlation between genotype and pathogenesis of *Blastocystis* (Böhm-Gloning *et al.* 1997; Yoshikawa *et al.* 2004b). In a more recent study, correlation between the genotype and symptoms was evaluated using polymerase chain reaction (PCR) subtyping and a significant correlation between subtype 2 and the asymptomatic group was found among both paediatric and adult patients (Dogruman-Al *et al.* 2008).

The scientific basis for the control of Blastocystosis

Over the last decade, *Blastocystis* is increasingly recognized as a cause of human gastrointestinal disease. There have been reports that reveal many unexplored aspects of this protozoan's pathogenesis. *Blastocystis* is now considered to be a zoonoses and it is believed that animals such as pigs and chicken constitute large reservoirs for human infection via the faecal-oral route (Tan 2004). Many phylogenetic reports have designated *Blastocystis* as a zoonoses (Abe *et al.* 2003c; Noel *et al.* 2005; Yoshikawa *et al.* 2004a). Numerous *Blastocystis* isolates from humans are believed to be potentially

zoonotic because they have similar or fairly similar genotypes to isolates found in a variety of other animal and bird species. It has been reported that a number of genotypes from human isolates can infect chickens and rats (Hussein *et al.* 2008; Iguchi *et al.* 2007).

Blastocystis possesses a number of features that increase the likelihood of waterborne transmission and environmental contamination. These include extensive host range and low host specificity, a transmissible cyst form that is resistant to adverse environmental conditions and a lack of knowledge of specific disinfection and treatment strategies.

Blastocystis is also very common among many animal species. It was suggested that humans are host for numerous *Blastocystis* genotypes isolated from animals (Noel *et al.* 2005). It has been reported in mammals, birds, reptiles, amphibians, annelids, and arthropods. In particular, some animals showing high prevalence include laboratory rats (60%; Chen *et al.* 1997a), pigs (70–95%; Abe *et al.* 2002), and birds (50–100%; Abe *et al.* 2002; Lee and Stenzel 1999). In Brisbane, Australia, *Blastocystis* has been detected in faecal samples from 70.8% domestic dogs and 67.3% cats (Duda *et al.* 1998).

A high prevalence of *Blastocystis* infection was reported in farm animals (95% in pigs; 71% in cattle), and in zoo animals (85% in primates; 80% in pheasants; 56% in ducks) in Japan (Abe *et al.* 2002). *Blastocystis* isolates from various animals were morphologically indistinguishable from *Blastocystis* isolated from humans.

PCR-based characterization of *Blastocystis* isolates was reported from dogs and humans living in a localized endemic community in Thailand (Parkar *et al.* 2007) and provided evidence to support zoonotic transmission of *Blastocystis* infections from dogs, possums and primates. It has also been reported that people working closely with animals were at significantly higher risk of *Blastocystis* infections (Rajah Salim *et al.* 1999).

Human populations exposed to poor hygiene practices, contaminated food and water appeared to be at risk of *Blastocystis* infections (Tan 2008). Outbreaks of waterborne *Blastocystis* infections have been documented recently (Karanis *et al.* 2007; Leelayoova *et al.* 2004). *Blastocystis* cysts have been detected in Scottish and Malaysian sewage treatment facilities; and viable cysts, found in the effluent, provided evidence that *Blastocystis* infections have potential for waterborne transmission (Suresh *et al.* 2005). Evidence is growing that contaminated water and food play an important role in the transmission of *Blastocystis* to humans. Cruz Licea *et al.* (2003) detected *Blastocystis* from 41.7% of food vendors and risk analysis showed that it was associated with poor personal hygiene habits.

Microbiology of the causative agent

Blastocystis is a highly polymorphic protozoan with four major forms (vacuolar, granular, amoeboid, and cyst) reported (Stenzel and Boreham 1996; Tan *et al.* 2002). There is little information on the transition between forms and our knowledge is limited to the description of individual forms based mostly on microscopic studies. The extensive heterogeneity of various forms of *Blastocystis* has led to the misinterpretation of findings from different studies. *Blastocystis* contains typical organelles of eukaryotes and the most apparent structures in transmission electron microscopy are nuclei, Golgi apparatus and mitochondria-like organelles. It has been shown that *Blastocystis* nuclei are spherical to ovoid and a crescent-shaped chromatin mass is often observable at one end of the organelle (Tan *et al.* 2001). As *Blastocystis* is an anaerobe, the presence of mitochondria-like organelles needs to be elucidated and it was suggested that these may instead be hydrogenosomes (Boreham and Stenzel 1993; Stechmann *et al.* 2008; Tan *et al.* 2002) as a number of typical mitochondrial enzymes were not found in *Blastocystis*. Hydrogenosomes are anaerobic organelles related to mitochondria first described in trichomonads (Lindmark and Müller 1973). In a recent study, Stechmann *et al.* (2008) reported that *Blastocystis* organelles have metabolic characteristics of both anaerobic and aerobic mitochondria and of hydrogenosomes. They suggested that *Blastocystis* mitochondria-like organelles are convergently similar to organelles in the unrelated ciliate *Nyctotherus ovalis*.

Vacuolar form

The vacuolar form, also known as the vacuolated or central body form, is the most predominant form in axenized *in vitro* cultures, liquid cultures, and stool samples (Fig. 50.1A). This form varies significantly in size, ranging from 2–200 μm in diameter with average diameters of 4–15 μm (Stenzel and Boreham 1996). Vacuolar forms are spherical and contain a characteristic large vacuole surrounded by a thin rim of peripheral cytoplasm. Cellular organelles such as nucleus, mitochondria-like organelles, Golgi are located within the cytoplasmic rim. Multiple nuclei can be seen in *Blastocystis* and an average of four nuclei is common (Zierdt 1973). The plasma membrane of *Blastocystis* has pits that appear to have a role in endocytosis (Stenzel *et al.* 1989). The exact function of the central vacuole is currently unclear. It may act as a storage organelle to participate in schizogony-like reproduction (Suresh *et al.* 1994; Singh *et al.* 1995), but this is likely to due to confusion of these reproductive forms with the classical granular forms (Tan and Stenzel 2003). The central vacuole has been postulated to play a role in the deposition of apoptotic bodies during parasite programmed cell death (Tan and Nasirudeen 2005) and it may act as a repository for carbohydrates and lipids required for cell growth (Yoshikawa and Hayakawa 1996).

A surface coat or fibrillar layer of varying thickness often surrounds the organism. This surface coat is thick in freshly isolated parasites from faeces but it gradually becomes thinner with prolonged laboratory culture (Cassidy *et al.* 1994). The exact role of the surface coat is not understood but it has been suggested to play a role in trapping and degrading bacteria for nutrition (Zaman *et al.* 1997, 1999) and protecting against osmotic shock (Cassidy *et al.* 1994).

Granular form

The granular form of *Blastocystis* is morphologically identical to the vacuolar form except that granules are present in the cytoplasm or more commonly within the central vacuole (Fig. 50.1B). The size of this form ranges from 3–80 μm in diameter. Granules in the central vacuole may differ considerably in appearance and described as myelin-like inclusions, small vesicles, crystalline granules and lipid droplets (Dunn *et al.* 1989). Bacterial remnants in lysosome-like compartments in the central vacuoles were also observed (unpublished observation). The granular form is commonly observed in non-axenized or older cultures (Tan 2004).

Amoeboid form

The amoeboid form (Fig. 50.1C) is rarely observed and there are conflicting reports about its description (McClure *et al.* 1980;

Dunn *et al.* 1989). These forms have been observed in antibiotic treated cultures, old cultures or in faecal samples (Zierdt 1973). Amoeboid forms are smaller and its size ranges from 2.6–7.8 μm in diameter. Dunn *et al.* (1989) reported ameboid forms with extended pseudopodia but a central vacuole, Golgi and mitochondria were not seen. On the contrary, Tan *et al.* (2001) showed by transmission electron microscopy that this form possess a central vacuole, numerous Golgi bodies and mitochondria within the cytoplasmic extension of pseudopods suggesting that this is a highly active form. In contrast to amoebae, these pseudopodia do not seem to be involved in locomotion. It was suggested that this form may be phagocytic in nature as ingested bacteria were found within the parasite in transmission electron microscopy analysis (Boreham and Stenzel 1993).

Cyst form

An environmentally resistant cyst form (Fig. 50.1D) is the most recently reported form of *Blastocystis* (Mehlhorn 1988; Stenzel and Boreham 1991; Zaman 1998). It is considered important for faecal-oral transmission (Yoshikawa *et al.* 2004c). This form is in general much smaller and its size ranges from 2–5 μm in diameter. It is protected by a multi-layered cyst wall which is sometimes covered with a loose surface coat (Moe *et al.* 1996). Unlike vacuolar and granular forms, this form has been shown to survive in water for up to 19 days at normal temperatures (Moe *et al.* 1996). Another study has shown that *Blastocystis* cysts could survive up to 1 month at 25°C and 2 months at 4°C (Yoshikawa *et al.* 2004c). Experimental infection studies in mice (Moe *et al.* 1997), rats (Yoshikawa *et al.* 2004c) and birds (Tanizaki *et al.* 2005) have shown that the cyst form is indeed the transmissible form of *Blastocystis*.

Life cycle

Many life cycles have been proposed for *Blastocystis* (Alexeieff 1911; Boreham and Stenzel 1993; Singh *et al.* 1995; Stenzel and Boreham 1996; Tan 2004) owing to a lack of properly conducted experimental studies and the pleomorphic nature of the organism. The first life cycle was proposed by Alexeieff (1911) and it described the involvement of binary fission and autogamy. Some of the reports suggest modes of division like plasmotomy and schizogony (Singh *et al.* 1995; Zierdt 1973). Most of these observations were based on microscopic analysis. Although *Blastocystis* had been isolated from laboratory animals, the lack of a suitable animal model was considered to be a major reason for the disagreement on its life cycle (Tan 2004). Recent studies have shown successful experimental infection of *Blastocystis* in chickens (Iguchi *et al.* 2007) and rats (Iguchi *et al.* 2007; Hussein *et al.* 2008; Yoshikawa *et al.* 2004c). Rats appear to be ideal animal models for *Blastocystis* infection and this will greatly help to elucidate many aspects of its life cycle.

A life cycle proposed by Tan (2004) states that infection is initiated when cysts of *Blastocystis* are orally ingested by humans or animals. Ingested cysts develop into vacuolar forms in the large intestine and later reproduce by binary fission. Some of the vacuolar forms encyst and are passed through the faeces and the cycle is repeated. The role of the amoeboid and granular form in the life cycle of *Blastocystis* is not understood and remains to be elucidated. More recently, Tan (2008) revised the life cycle and included findings from molecular typing data suggesting that *Blastocystis* isolated from humans actually comprise human and zoonotic

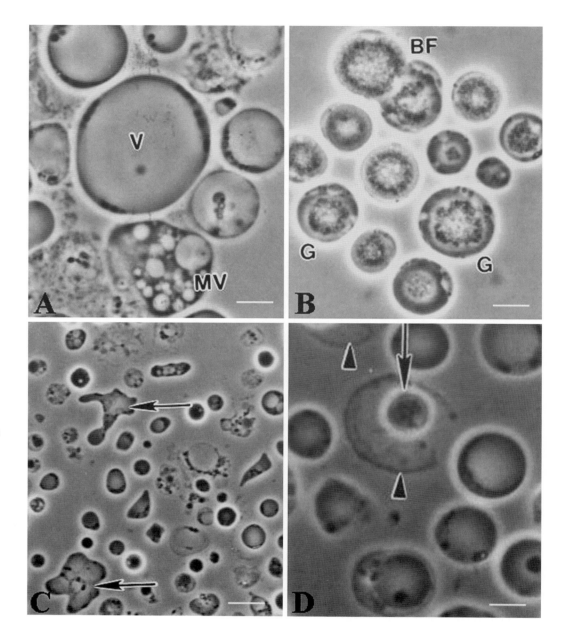

Fig. 50.1 Four morphological forms from axenic cultures of *Blastocystis* under phase-contrast microscopy. A. Vacuolar (*V*) and multivacuolar (*MV*) forms. Cells are showing extensive variations in their size. Bar = 20 μm. B. Granular forms (*G*). One of the cells appears to be dividing (*BF*). Bar = 20 μm. C. Amoeboid forms (arrow). Bar = 10 μm. D. Cyst form. Refractile cyst (arrow) with loose granular fibrillar layes (arrowhead). Bar = 5 μm. (D)- Adapted from Chen, (1999), with permission.

genotypes of varying host specificities. A modified life cycle of *Blastocystis* must take into consideration the large reservoir of this parasite in a range of animal populations with humans as potential hosts (Fig. 50.2).

Pathogenesis

There are very few *in vivo* experimental infection studies but some attempts were made to elucidate the pathogenesis of *Blastocystis* using *in vitro* models. Some studies involved the use of mammalian cell culture systems to investigate the pathogenesis of *Blastocystis* (Long *et al.* 2001; Puthia *et al.* 2006, 2008; Walderich *et al.* 1998). Live *Blastocystis* cells and parasite lysates isolated from symptomatic and asymptomatic individuals caused significant cytopathic effects on Chinese Hamster Ovary (CHO) cells. Another study

showed that *Blastocystis* reduced *Escherichia coli* or LPS-induced secretion of IL-8 and it was proposed that *Blastocystis* is capable of modulating host immune responses at initial stages of infection (Long *et al.* 2001). This suggests that *Blastocystis* may down-regulate host immune responses to improve survival in the gut. More recently, our laboratory conducted an *in vitro* study and observed that *Blastocystis* cysteine proteases can induce inter-leukin-8 production in human colonic epithelial cells and an NF-κB-dependent transcriptional process is involved (Puthia *et al.* 2008). Intestinal epithelial cell production of interleukin-8 might induce recruitment of inflammatory cells into the intestinal mucosa that can result in tissue damage and gastrointestinal disturbances. This may correlate with reports describing intestinal inflammation and oedema in patients infected with *Blastocystis* (Garavelli *et al.* 1992; Kain *et al.* 1987; Russo *et al.* 1988).

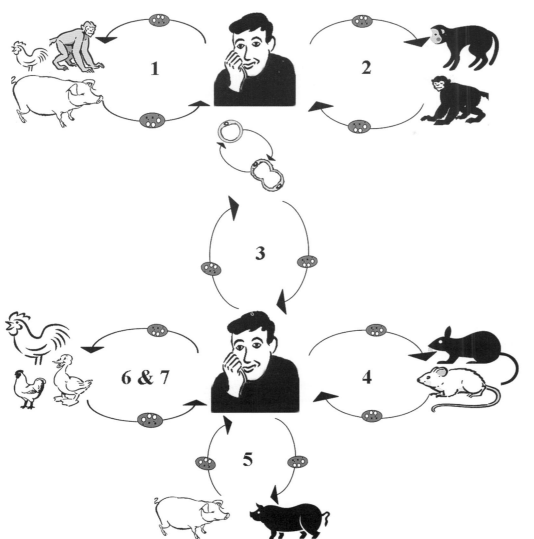

Fig. 50.2 Revised life cycle of *Blastocystis* as proposed by Tan (2008). This life cycle also suggests existence of zoonotic genotypes of *Blastocystis* (Subtypes 1–4, 6 and 7) with different host specificities. Faecal cysts of *Blastocystis* infect human and animal hosts and develop into vacuolar forms in the large intestine. Cross-infection can occur among mammalian and avian isolates of subtype 1. Subtype 2, 3 and 4 comprises primate, human and rodent isolates respectively. Subtype 5 comprise of isolates from pigs and cattle whereas subtype 6 and 7 comprise avian isolates. This proposal suggests that certain animals act as reservoirs of *Blastocystis* for human infections; and humans can be potentially infected by six or more species of *Blastocystis*.
Adapted from Tan (2008), with permission from Taylor and Francis.

Similar to many other protozoan parasites, *Blastocystis* contains predominantly cysteine proteases (Puthia *et al.* 2008; Sio *et al.* 2006) and these proteases are localized in the central vacuole of the parasite (Puthia *et al.* 2008). In gelatin SDS-PAGE analysis of parasitic lysates, high levels of protease activity was observed comprising nine protease bands of low (20–30 kDa) and high (44–75 kDa) molecular weights. It was reported that activity of these proteases was highest at neutral pH (Sio *et al.* 2006). It has been shown that *Blastocystis* lysates and conditioned medium can degrade human secretory immunoglobulin A (sIgA), the main immunoglobulin defense at mucosal surfaces (Puthia *et al.* 2005). It was observed that cysteine proteases of *B. hominis* isolate B (subtype 7) and aspartic proteases of *B. ratii* (subtype 4) were mainly responsible for IgA degradation activity. Altogether, these findings suggest that proteases of *Blastocystis* are virulence factors and these might contribute to parasite survival in the host by degrading IgA at intestinal mucosal surfaces.

Puthia *et al.* (2006) reported *Blastocystis ratti* (subtype 4) interactions with intestinal epithelial cells resulting in apoptosis of host cells and the disruption of epithelial barrier function. Importantly, it was shown that *Blastocystis* is capable of causing apoptosis in a contact-independent manner. This *in vitro* study supports the finding from other clinical reports where significantly increased intestinal permeability was observed after *Blastocystis* infections (Dagci *et al.* 2002). Inhibition of apoptosis did not rescue epithelium from permeability increase suggesting that apoptosis caused by *Blastocystis* may not play an important role in disruption of barrier function (Puthia *et al.* 2006). Induction of apoptosis of host intestinal cells seems not to be useful to a non-invasive parasite like *Blastocystis* as it might result in the loss of parasite's own colonization sites in intestine. It was suggested that *Blastocystis*-induced intestinal cell apoptosis might be a host response against some parasitic factors such as proteases that are necessary for its own life-cycle (Puthia *et al.* 2006). The cytopathic effects caused by *Blastocystis* are quite comparable to those of other pathogenic protozoans such as *Giardia intestinalis* (Chin *et al.* 2002) and thus warrants further investigation.

A number of studies have described experimental infections involving rats, mice, guinea pigs and chickens (Abou El Naga and Negm 2001; Hussein *et al.* 2008; Iguchi *et al.* 2007; Moe *et al.* 1997;

Pakandl 1992; Phillips and Zierdt 1976; Tanizaki *et al.* 2005; Yoshikawa *et al.* 2004c). In experimentally infected mice, histological examination of the cecum and colon revealed intense inflammatory cell infiltration, oedematous lamina propria, and mucosal sloughing (Moe *et al.* 1997). Lesions on the ileocecal mucosa were reported in mice experimentally infected with *Blastocystis* (Zhang *et al.* 2006). Experimentally, it has been shown that *Blastocystis* infection can be established by oral inoculation of cysts in mice (Moe *et al.* 1997) and rats (Yoshikawa *et al.* 2004c). Wistar rats were successfully infected by oral inoculation of *Blastocystis* cysts recovered from faeces of another infected rat and it was demonstrated that an oral dose of as low as ten cysts was sufficient to establish infection. These studies indicated that the faecal cyst form was responsible for faecal-oral transmission of the parasite. Clinical reports and experimental studies indicate that *Blastocystis* is not invasive but it is capable of causing gastrointestinal pathogenesis. Experimentally, it was shown that germ-free guinea pigs can be infected by oral or intracecal inoculations and heavy infections caused diarrhoea and cecal hyperemia (Phillips and Zierdt 1976). Recently, *Blastocystis* isolates from symptomatic and asymptomatic humans were experimentally tested for their infectivity in rats (Hussein *et al.* 2008). It was reported that *Blastocystis* isolates from symptomatic patients induced moderate to severe pathological changes in infected rats but isolates from asymptomatic individuals caused mild pathological changes. The authors suggested that subtype 1 was pathogenic, while subtypes 3 and 4 consisted of both pathogenic and non-pathogenic variants.

Interestingly, several reports suggest an association between *Blastocystis* infections and cutaneous lesions. The mechanism is possibly that of typical cutaneous allergic hypersensitivity where parasitic antigens induce the activation of specific clones of Th2 lymphocytes (Pasqui *et al.* 2004). Eventually, cytokine release and the consequent IgE production may lead to an allergic reaction. Moreover, it was also suggested that some *Blastocystis* virulence factors may activate the complement pathway with the production of anaphylotoxins (Valsecchi *et al.* 2004). These anaphylotoxins, upon interaction with basophils and mast cells induce histamine production which may result in cutaneous disorders.

Recent studies suggest that clinical outcome of *Blastocystis* infection is multifactorial and depends on parasite genotype, parasitic load, and host immune status (Tan 2008). In a number of cases, *Blastocystis* infections appear to be self-limiting (Babb and Wagener 1989; Doyle *et al.*1990; Markell 1995) and spontaneous elimination of infection has been reported (Sun *et al.* 1989).

Clinical features

The clinical significance of *Blastocystis* is presently ambiguous. There are many reports that either implicate or exonerate this organism as a cause of gastrointestinal disease. This parasite can be found in the intestinal tract of both healthy individuals and patients exhibiting gastrointestinal symptoms (Stenzel and Boreham 1996).

Many case reports have suggested the association of *Blastocystis* with a variety of clinical features including terminal ileitis (Tsang *et al.* 1989), colitis (Russo *et al.* 1988), ulcerative colitis (Jeddy and Farrington 1991), and infective arthritis (Lakhanpal *et al.* 1991). Interestingly, various reports associate *Blastocystis* infections with cutaneous lesions particularly urticaria (Cassano *et al.* 2005;

Giacometti *et al.* 2003; Gupta and Parsi 2006) suggesting host allergic response to some unknown parasitic factors.

Faecal leukocytes (Cohen 1985; Diaczok and Rival 1987) and rectal bleeding has been reported in *Blastocystis* infections (al-Tawil *et al.* 1994). Enlargement of liver and spleen was also reported in a study (Garavelli and Scaglione 1990). Blood analysis of a number of patients showed eosinophilia (Garavelli and Scaglione 1990; Lambert *et al.* 1992). There are reports that associated *Blastocystis* with intestinal disorders in human immunodeficiency virus (HIV) or immunocompromised patients (Ok *et al.* 1997; Cirioni *et al.* 1999; Florez *et al.* 2003; Hailemariam *et al.* 2004; Rao *et al.* 2003) suggesting that *Blastocystis* is an opportunistic organism.

Inflammation and oedema of intestinal mucosa has been reported in *Blastocystis* infections (Garavelli *et al.* 1991; Russo *et al.* 1988; Zuckerman *et al.* 1994). In *Blastocystis* infected patients, endoscopy results showed that there was no invasion of the colonic mucosa (Chen *et al.* 2003; Dawes *et al.* 1990; Kain *et al.* 1987; Zuckerman *et al.* 1990). On the other hand, (al-Tawil *et al.* 1994) reported the presence of colonic ulceration and infiltration of superficial lamina propria by *Blastocystis*. Intestinal permeability was reported to be significantly increased in *Blastocystis* patients and it was suggested that *Blastocystis* infections may damage the intestinal wall (Dagci *et al.* 2002).

Symptoms and signs

The clinical symptoms and signs associated with *Blastocystis* infections are mainly diarrhoea, abdominal pain, cramps, nausea as well as non-specific gastrointestinal signs such as bloating, vomiting, anorexia, weight loss and flatulence (Doyle *et al.* 1990; Nimri and Batchoun 1994; Qadri *et al.* 1989; Stenzel and Boreham 1996). Although most cases of *Blastocystis* are mild and chronic, profuse watery diarrhoea (Logar *et al.* 1994) and fever (Gallagher and Venglarcik1985) has also been reported in acute cases. There are reports that suggest the association of *Blastocystis* with irritable bowel syndrome (Giacometti *et al.* 1999; Yakoob *et al.* 2004), a functional bowel disorder characterized by abdominal pain and changes in bowel habits.

Interestingly, some studies have also reported symptoms like itching (Garavelli and Scaglione 1990) and joint pain (Lee *et al.* 1990). Numerous case reports have suggested association of *Blastocystis* with cutaneous disorders such as chronic urticaria (Armentia *et al.* 1993; Biedermann *et al.* 2002), angioedema (Micheloud *et al.* 2007) and palmoplantar pruritis (Kick *et al.* 2002). A recent case study of *Blastocystis* infection reported that acute urticaria was associated with amoeboid forms of *Blastocystis* subtype 3 (Katsarou-Katsari *et al.* 2008).

Numerous reports suggested that HIV and immunocompromised patients are more likely to acquire *Blastocystis*-associated intestinal disease and suggested that this parasite is opportunistic (Brites *et al.* 1997; Florez *et al.* 2003; Ok *et al.* 1997; Rao *et al.* 2003; Hailemariam *et al.* 2004). Diarrhoea and other gastrointestinal symptoms were reported in these *Blastocystis*-infected immunocompromised patients. *Blastocystis* was observed to be the most common parasite isolated from patients undergoing chemotherapy for haematological malignancies and it was suggested to be associated with diarrhoea, abdominal pain and flatulence (Tasova *et al.* 2000).

Many cases of *Blastocystis* infections appear to be asymptomatic and it is common to detect large number of *Blastocystis* in stool samples from patients without any sign of disease. It appears that absence of clinical symptoms might be due to infections with non-pathogenic genotypes of *Blastocystis*, however, whether this disease is genotype linked or not is still unresolved. In a study involving PCR-RFLP ribotyping of *Blastocystis* isolates, subtypes 1, 2 and 4 were associated with symptoms whereas subtype 3 was associated with asymptomatic infections (Kaneda *et al.* 2001). In other studies, subtype 1 was found in patients with gastrointestinal symptoms, subtype 7 was found in asymptomatic and subtypes 3 and 6 were found in both groups of patients (Hussein *et al.* 2008). On the contrary, some studies have indicated that there is no association between symptoms and *Blastocystis* genotypes (Böhm-Gloning *et al.* 1997; Yoshikawa *et al.* 2004b). In summary, studies suggest that subtype 1 might be associated with disease and subtype 3 may be non-pathogenic; however there is a need for more studies with larger sample sizes to resolve this issue. In addition, it is evident that *Blastocystis* infections can cause a variety of symptoms, not necessarily confined to the intestinal tract.

Diagnosis

Because of its uncertain pathogenesis, clinical significance is seldom given to *Blastocystis* infections. Often *Blastocystis* infections are neglected in the curriculum of medical studies and thus diagnosis of *Blastocystis* remains a challenging task for a diagnostic laboratory. Although an experienced laboratory technician can perform diagnosis in direct faecal smears, most diagnostic laboratories do not have expertise on identification of this parasite and there is a need for training to enable identification of all forms of *Blastocystis* in faecal samples. Identification of *Blastocystis* in direct faecal smears is relatively difficult as the parasite can be confused with yeast, *Cyclospora*, or fat globules.

In the past, laboratory diagnosis of *Blastocystis* was based on the identification of vacuolar and granular forms in direct faecal specimens (Katz and Taylor 2001). Direct microscopy of faecal specimens is performed by wet mounts with Lugol's iodine or permanent fixed smears with Giemsa, acid-fast, trichrome and Field's staining. Rather than the characteristic vacuolar form, the cyst form may predominate in faecal samples. Cyst forms might be difficult to identify by direct microscopy because of their small size (3–5 μm) but these can be effectively concentrated by density-gradient methods (Zaman 1996). Diagnostic labs should therefore include the faecal cyst form as an indicator of *Blastocystis* infection.

Many researchers suggest that when all other known bacterial, viral or parasitic causes of symptoms are absent and *Blastocystis* is present in large numbers it should be treated as a pathogen. More than five organisms per high power (×400) field should be considered as a heavy infection. For confirmative diagnosis in stool samples, *in vitro* culture in Jones' medium is a method of choice (Suresh and Smith 2004). It was reported that *in vitro* culture of faecal samples was six times and twice more sensitive than direct faecal smears and trichrome staining methods respectively (Termmathurapoj *et al.* 2004). However, it was also reported in this study that the *in vitro* culture method failed to detect some parasites suggesting that not all *Blastocystis* isolates can be readily cultured in laboratory. *Blastocystis* can be cultured in various mediums including Jones' medium, Boeck and Drbohlav's inspissated medium or diphasic agar slant medium with Jones' as a medium of choice for patient samples. Diphasic agar slant medium was reported to be good for the culture of *Blastocystis* from pigs, cattle and chickens (Abe 2004; Abe *et al.* 2003a). In axenized cultures, cell densities of

up to 2.5×10^7 can be achieved (Ho *et al.* 1993) and doubling time may vary from 6 to 23 hours, depending on type of medium and isolate (Boreham and Stenzel 1993). Colony growth of *Blastocystis* has been shown on solid medium and cultures were viable for up to 2 weeks (Tan *et al.* 2000).

Molecular approaches such as PCR-based diagnosis have been described for *Blastocystis*. PCR amplification using subtype specific primers is suggested to be useful for identifying and genotyping *Blastocystis* from patient samples. Knowledge of the genotype can be extremely valuable if certain *Blastocystis* genotypes are found to be more virulent than others. A recent study has demonstrated that PCR-based detection of *Blastocystis* from faecal specimens is more sensitive than *in vitro* propagation (Parkar *et al.* 2007). Recently, a sensitive and specific real-time light cycler PCR assay was developed to detect a 152 bp sequence in an uncharacterized region of the *Blastocystis* genome and 11 strains of *Blastocystis* from subtypes 1, 3, and 4 were with this method (Jones II *et al.* 2008). Using this method, *Blastocystis* was detected in stool samples that were *Blastocystis*-negative during microscopy and conventional PCR. In addition, this method showed no cross-reactivity with other common gastrointestinal pathogens.

Other methods like enzyme-linked immunosorbent assay (ELISA) and immunofluorescence detection have not been comprehensively investigated for *Blastocystis*. Although development of monoclonal antibodies against *Blastocystis* has been reported (Tan *et al.* 1996), antigenic diversity of *Blastocystis* seems to be a limiting factor in the use of immunological methods. *Blastocystis* infections have been reported to induce IgG and IgA responses in patients and detected by indirect fluorescent antibody test (IFA) and ELISA (Hussain *et al.* 1997; Kaneda *et al.* 2000; Mahmoud and Saleh 2003; Zierdt and Nagy 1993; Zierdt *et al.* 1995). ELISA titres ranged from 1:50–1:1,600 (Zierdt *et al.* 1995) and it was observed that high titres were associated with symptomatic infections of *Blastocystis* (Hussain *et al.* 1997; Mahmoud and Saleh 2003; Zierdt and Nagy 1993; Zierdt *et al.* 1995). In a recent study using ELISA, secretory IgA, serum IgA and serum IgG levels were detected in *Blastocystis* infected patients with and without clinical symptoms (Mahmoud and Saleh 2003). It was found that serum from only symptomatic patients had significantly higher antibody levels. On the other hand, Kaneda *et al.* (2000) reported asymptomatic patients with serum antibodies to *Blastocystis* and high levels were observed in chronic cases. Overall, it may be desirable to develop specific monoclonal antibodies against different genotypes and evaluate different serological assays for the diagnosis of *Blastocystis* infections.

Diagnosis of blastocystosis has been reported with the help of invasive diagnostic techniques such as endoscopy but this has not been thoroughly evaluated. *Blastocystis* colonization in the lower ileum and caecum of a patient was detected in microscopic examinations of lumen fluids aspirated during endoscopy (Matsumoto *et al.* 1987). As *Blastocystis* can be detected in faeces and no characteristic intestinal lesions are associated with infection, invasive diagnostic techniques are therefore not recommended for routine examinations.

In brief, a number of methods have been described for the diagnosis of *Blastocystis*. Direct microscopy of stained faecal smears is useful and it should be supplemented with numbers of parasites observed per high power field to help clinicians ascertain parasitic load. For confirmatory diagnosis, microscopic examination should be supplemented by *in vitro* culture and/or PCR-based methods.

Treatment and prognosis

Due to ambiguity surrounding the pathogenesis of *Blastocystis* and the non-specific nature of symptoms, the need to treat *Blastocystis* infections is controversial. In most cases, treatment with antiprotozoal drugs, in particular metronidazole, is warranted if no other cause of symptoms is observable (Cassano *et al.* 2005; Moghaddam *et al.* 2005; Nigro *et al.* 2003). Whether the mode of action of metronidazole on *Blastocystis* is similar to that described for other protozoan parasites is currently unknown. It has been shown that metronidazole induces programmed cell death in *Blastocystis* with a number of features similar to apoptosis in higher eukaryotes (Nasirudeen *et al.* 2004). In *Blastocystis* infections, various dosages of metronidazole has been recommended in different studies (Garavelli and Libanore 1990; Guirges and Al-Waili 1987; Moghaddam *et al.* 2005; Nassir *et al.* 2004; Qadri *et al.* 1989). Treatment regime ranges from 250–750 mg three times a day for 5 to 10 days, 200 mg four times per day for 7 days or 2 gm/day for 5 days. There have been reports where metronidazole has been used successfully in combination with other drugs such as paromomycin (Pasqui *et al.* 2004) and co-trimoxazole (Andiran *et al.* 2006). Some studies also reported that metronidazole was not efficacious in eliminating *Blastocystis* infection from patients (Cohen 1985; Schwartz and Houston 1992). *In vitro* studies have reported that different *Blastocystis* isolates show variable sensitivities to metronidazole (Haresh *et al.* 1999). In particular, cysts of *Blastocystis* have been shown to be resistant to high concentrations (up to 5 mg/ml) of metronidazole (Zaman and Zaki 1996). Overall, treatment failures may occur due to extensive genetic heterogeneity and differences in the susceptibility of different forms of *Blastocystis* to drugs.

In addition to metronidazole, many other drugs have been used to treat *Blastocystis* infections with high or reasonable efficacy. Among these are furazolidone, quinacrine, ornidazole, tinidazole, ketoconazole, and trimehoprim-sulfamethoxazole (Reviewed in Stenzel and Boreham 1996). Recently, a number of studies reported that the broad spectrum antiparasitic drug nitazoxanide is effective for use in *Blastocystis* infections (Cimerman *et al.* 2003; Rossignol *et al.* 2005).

There is a lack of controlled studies involving large numbers of patients and extensive studies are needed to verify the efficacy of different drugs on *Blastocystis* infections. Thus far, metronidazole seems to be the drug of choice for blastocystosis, even though there are some evidences of treatment failure. In such cases, other drugs should be employed empirically. Chemotherapy should be employed when symptoms are persistent and no other pathogen than *Blastocystis* is detected. In mild cases of *Blastocystis* infections, intervention may not be required as infection is usually self-limiting (Babb and Wagener 1989; Doyle *et al.* 1990; Markell 1995).

Epidemiology, prevention and control

Blastocystis is reported to be one of the most common protozoans found in faecal samples of both symptomatic patients and asymptomatic individuals (Cirioni *et al.* 1999; Taamasri *et al.* 2000; Windsor *et al.* 2002). *Blastocystis* has a worldwide distribution and findings of many surveys reported it to be most frequently isolated protozoan parasite (Baldo *et al.* 2004; Florez *et al.* 2003; Pegelow *et al.* 1997; Taamasri *et al.* 2000). Prevalence of *Blastocystis* infection is higher in developing countries than in developed countries

(Stenzel and Boreham 1996; Tan *et al.* 2002) and occurrence as high as 60% were reported from some developing countries (Pegelow *et al.* 1997). Occurrence of *Blastocystis* varies from country to country. A low prevalence of 0.5% has been reported among asymptomatic healthy individuals in Japan (Horiki *et al.* 1997). A moderate prevalence of 14–21% and 23% was reported in Thailand (Yaicharoen *et al.* 2005) and US (Amin 2002) respectively. A high prevalence of 40.7% and 60% was reported in Philippines (Baldo *et al.* 2004) and Indonesia (Pegelow *et al.* 1997) respectively. High incidences (36.9–44%) of *Blastocystis* were also observed in Thai military personnel (Leelayoova *et al.* 2004; Taamasri *et al.* 2002). Prevalence of *Blastocystis* may vary widely within various geographical regions of the same country. In Thailand, a prevalence of 0.8% and 45.2% was reported from Nan province (Waikagul *et al.* 2002) and Pathum Thani province (Saksirisampant *et al.* 2003) respectively. Variations in the same geographical region may represent true differences between communities or living conditions. Nevertheless, these reported variations might be due to lack of a standardized diagnostic methodology and difficulty in identifying parasitic forms other than the common vacuolar form. Recent studies have used PCR-based approaches to further elucidate genotype information which has shed light on the distribution of *Blastocystis* genotypes in humans and animals. Studies have found that *Blastocystis* subtype 3 was the most common subtype among isolates from various countries such as Turkey (Ozyurt *et al.* 2008), Greece (Menounos *et al.* 2008), Singapore (Wong *et al.* 2008), Japan, Pakistan, Bangladesh, and Germany (Yoshikawa *et al.* 2004b). In summary, studies suggest that there is no association between specific genotype and geographic origin; and due to its predominance in urbanized countries, subtype 3 is probably the subtype of human origin.

It has been observed that humans with compromised health and poor hygiene are more susceptible to *Blastocystis* infections. *Blastocystis* infections are also of special clinical interest to developed countries as millions of travellers going to developing countries are at risk of acquiring infection (Sohail and Fischer 2005). *Blastocystis* infections are more common during hot weather and during the pre-monsoonal months (Stenzel and Boreham 1996).

Based on current knowledge, it is generally accepted that *Blastocystis* is transmitted by the faecal-oral route. This assumption is strengthened by animal infection studies (Tanizaki *et al.* 2005; Yoshikawa *et al.* 2004c) and reports showing high prevalence of *Blastocystis* in population living in poor hygiene (Cruz Licea *et al.* 2003; Nimri 1993). Therefore, control measures should consist of good hygiene practices and community sanitary facilities.

Because *Blastocystis* is generally regarded as a zoonotic parasite, animals and their faecal material represent a risk for human infection. Contamination of food, water, and environment by animal faecal material should be prevented. High prevalence of *Blastocystis* has been shown in pets such as dogs and cats and it was suggested that these domestic animals could be an important source of infection to humans (Duda *et al.* 1998). Routine antiparasitic treatment practice for pet animals may be useful to eliminate the parasite. Animal handlers must take additional precautions for their personal hygiene and may go for stool examination especially if experiencing any gastrointestinal symptoms. In unhygienic and high *Blastocystis* prevalence areas, sterilization of water is recommended. Currently, the best sterilization method is to boil water as chemical methods of water sterilization have not been extensively studied for *Blastocystis*. Travellers to high prevalence areas should ensure that they consume clean water and cooked food. *Blastocystis* has been found in sewage (Suresh *et al.* 2005) and there is growing evidence for waterborne transmissions (Hakim *et al.* 2007; Karanis *et al.* 2007; Leelayoova *et al.* 2004) which makes it necessary to develop preventive measures to ensure water sanitation.

Conclusion

Accumulating evidence over the last decade suggests an association of *Blastocystis* with gastrointestinal disorders. Approximately 4 billion diarrhoea episodes occur worldwide each year which account for 4% of all deaths and 5% of days lost to disability (Sazawal *et al.* 2006). The pathophysiological basis of diarrhoea in *Blastocystis* infections can be multifactorial and may involve at least in part intestinal epithelial damage, compromised barrier function, as well as induction of proinflammatory cytokines. Although discovered almost a century ago, our knowledge on *Blastocystis* has increased tremendously only in the last decade. We now know that humans can be infected by numerous zoonotic genotypes. Laboratory rats appear to be reasonably good animal models for infection studies. There is a need to further identify and characterize *Blastocystis* virulence factors and associated genes. Most importantly, major efforts should be directed to understanding if pathogenic and non-pathogenic subtypes exist.

References

Abe, N. (2004). Molecular and phylogenetic analysis of *Blastocystis* isolates from various hosts. *Vet. Parasitol.,* 120: 235–42.

Abe, N., Nagoshi, M., Takami, K., Sawano, Y. and Yoshikawa, H. (2002). A survey of *Blastocystis* sp. in livestock, pets, and zoo animals in Japan. *Vet. Parasitol.,* 106: 203–12.

Abe, N., Wu, Z. and Yoshikawa, H. (2003a). Molecular characterization of *Blastocystis* isolates from birds by PCR with diagnostic primers and restriction fragment length polymorphism analysis of the small subunit ribosomal RNA gene. *Parasit. Res.,* 89: 393–96.

Abe, N., Wu, Z. and Yoshikawa, H. (2003b). Molecular characterization of *Blastocystis* isolates from primates. *Vet. Parasitol.,* 113: 321–25.

Abe, N., Wu, Z. and Yoshikawa, H. (2003c). Zoonotic genotypes of *Blastocystis hominis* detected in cattle and pigs by PCR with diagnostic primers and restriction fragment length polymorphism analysis of the small subunit ribosomal RNA gene. *Parasit. Res.,* 90: 124–28.

Abou El Naga, I. F. and Negm, A. Y. (2001). Morphology, histochemistry and infectivity of *Blastocystis hominis* cyst. *J. Egypt Soc. Parasit.,* 31: 627–35.

Al-Tawil, Y. S., Gilger, M. A., Gopalakrishna, G. S., *et al.* (1994). Invasive *Blastocystis hominis* infection in a child. *Arch. Pediatr. Adoles. Med.,* 148: 882–85.

Albrecht, H., Stellbrink, H. J., Koperski, K. and Greten, H. (1995). *Blastocystis hominis* in human immunodeficiency virus-related diarrhea. *Scand. J. Gastroenterol.,* 30: 909–14.

Alexeieff, A. (1911). Sur la nature des formations dites kystes de *Trichomonas intestinalis. C. R. Soc. Biol.,* 71: 296–98.

Amin, O. M. (2002). Seasonal prevalence of intestinal parasites in the United States during 2000. *Am. J. Trop. Med. Hyg.,* 66: 799–803.

Andiran, N., Acikgoz, Z. C., Turkay, S. and Andiran, F. (2006). *Blastocystis hominis*—an emerging and imitating cause of acute abdomen in children. *J. Pediatr. Surg.,* 41: 1489–91.

Arisue, N., Hashimoto, T. and Yoshikawa, H. (2003). Sequence heterogeneity of the small subunit ribosomal RNA genes among *Blastocystis* isolates. *Parasitology,* 126: 1–9.

Arisue, N., Hashimoto, T., Yoshikawa, H., Nakamura, Y., *et al.* (2002). Phylogenetic position of *Blastocystis hominis* and of stramenopiles inferred from multiple molecular sequence data. *J. Eukaryot. Microbiol.,* 49: 42–53.

Armentia, A., Mendez, J., Gomez, A., Sanchis, E., *et al.* (1993). Urticaria by *Blastocystis hominis*. Successful treatment with paromomycin. *Allergol. Immunopathol. (Madr.),* 21: 149–51.

Babb, R. R. and Wagener, S. (1989). *Blastocystis hominis*—a potential intestinal pathogen. *West J. Med.,* 151: 518–19.

Baldo, E. T., Belizario, V. Y., De Leon, W. U., Kong, H. H. and Chung, D. I. (2004). Infection status of intestinal parasites in children living in residential institutions in Metro Manila, the Philippines. *Korean J. Parasitol.,* 42: 67–70.

Barahona Rondon, L., Maguina Vargas, C., Naquira Velarde, C., *et al.* (2003). Human blastocystosis: prospective study symptomatology and associated epidemiological factors. *Rev. Gastroenter. Peru,* 23: 29–35.

Belova, L. M. (1992). A new species of *Blastocystis* anseri (Protista: Rhizopoda) from domestic geese. *Parazitologiia,* 26: 80–82.

Bensen, W. (1909). *Trichomonas intestinalis* und vaginalis des Menschen. *Arch. Protistenk.,* 18: 115–27.

Biedermann, T., Hartmann, K., Sing, A. and Przybilla, B. (2002). Hypersensitivity to non-steroidal anti-inflammatory drugs and chronic urticaria cured by treatment of *Blastocystis hominis* infection. *Br. J. Dermatol.,* 146: 1113–14.

Böhm-Gloning, B., Knobloch, J. and Walderich, B. (1997). Five subgroups of *Blastocystis hominis* from symptomatic and asymptomatic patients revealed by restriction site analysis of PCR-amplified 16S-like rDNA. *Trop. Med. Int. Health,* 2: 771–78.

Boreham, P. F. and Stenzel, D. J. (1993). *Blastocystis* in humans and animals: morphology, biology, and epizootiology. *Adv. Parasitol.,* 32: 1–70.

Brites, C., Barberino, M. G., Bastos, M. A., Sampaio Sa, M. and Silva, N. (1997). *Blastocystis hominis* as a Potential Cause of Diarrhea in AIDS Patients: a Report of Six Cases in Bahia, Brazil. *Braz. J. Infect. Dis.,* 1: 91–94.

Brumpt, E. (1912). *Blastocystis hominis* n sp. et formes voisines. *Bull. Soc. Pathol. Exot.,* 5: 725–30.

Cassano, N., Scoppio, B. M., Loviglio, M. C. and Vena, G. A. (2005). Remission of delayed pressure urticaria after eradication of *Blastocystis hominis. Acta Derm. Venereol.,* 85: 357–58.

Cassidy, M. F., Stenzel, D. J. and Boreham, P. F. (1994) Electron microscopy of surface structures of *Blastocystis* sp. from different hosts. *Parasitol. Res.,* 80: 505–11.

Cavalier-Smith, T. (1998) A revised six-kingdom system of life. *Biol. Rev. Camb. Philos. Soc.,* 73: 203–66.

Chen, T. L., Chan, C. C., Chen, H. P., Fung, C. P., Lin, C. P., *et al.* (2003). Clinical characteristics and endoscopic findings associated with *Blastocystis hominis* in healthy adults. *Am. J. Trop. Med. Hyg.,* 69: 213–16.

Chen, X. (1999). Studies on rat *Blastocystis. Department of microbiology.* Singapore: National University of Singapore.

Chen, X. Q., Singh, M., Ho, L. C., Moe, K. T., Tan, S. W. and Yap, E. H. (1997a). A survey of *Blastocystis* sp. in rodents. *Lab. Anim. Sci.,* 47: 91–94.

Chen, X. Q., Singh, M., Ho, L. C., Tan, S. W., Ng, G. C., *et al.* (1997b). Description of a *Blastocystis* species from Rattus norvegicus. *Parasitol. Res.,* 83: 313–18.

Chin, A. C., Teoh, D. A., Scott, K. G. E., Meddings, J. B., *et al.* (2002). Strain dependent induction of enterocyte apoptosis by *Giardia lamblia* disrupts epithelial barrier function in a caspase-3-dependent manner. *Infect. Immun.,* 70: 3673–80.

Cimerman, S., Ladeira, M. C. and Iuliano, W. A. (2003). Blastocystosis: nitazoxanide as a new therapeutic option. *Rev. Soc. Bras. Med. Trop.,* 36: 415–17.

Cirioni, O., Giacometti, A., Drenaggi, D., Ancarani, F. and Scalise, G. (1999). Prevalence and clinical relevance of *Blastocystis hominis* in diverse patient cohorts. *Eur. J. Epidemiol.,* 15: 389–93.

Cohen, A. N. (1985). Ketoconazole and resistant *Blastocystis hominis* infection. *Ann. Intern. Med.,* **103:** 480–81.

Cruz Licea, V., Plancarte Crespo, A., Moran Alvarez, C., *et al.* (2003). *Blastocystis hominis* among food vendors in Xochimilco markets. *Rev. Latinoam. Microbiol.,* **45:** 12–15.

Dagci, H., Ustun, S., Taner, M. S., Ersoz, G., Karacasu, F. and Budak, S. (2002). Protozoon infections and intestinal permeability. *Acta Trop.,* **81:** 1–5.

Dawes, R. F., Scott, S. D. and Tuck, A. C. (1990). *Blastocystis hominis:* an unusual cause of diarrhoea. *Br. J. Clin. Pract.,* **44:** 714–16.

Diaczok, B. J. and Rival, J. (1987). Diarrhea due to *Blastocystis hominis:* an old organism revisited. *South Med. J.,* **80:** 931–32.

Doyle, P. W., Helgason, M. M., Mathias, R. G. and Proctor, E. M. (1990). Epidemiology and pathogenicity of *Blastocystis hominis. J. Clin. Microbiol.,* **28:** 116–21.

Duda, A., Stenzel, D. J. and Boreham, P. F. (1998). Detection of *Blastocystis* sp. in domestic dogs and cats. *Vet. Parasitol.,* **76:** 9–17.

Dunn, L. A., Boreham, P. F. and Stenzel, D. J. (1989). Ultrastructural variation of *Blastocystis hominis* stocks in culture. *Intern. J. Parasitol.,* **19:** 43–56.

El-Shazly, A. M., Abdel-Magied, A. A., El-Beshbishi, S. N., *et al.* (2005). *Blastocystis hominis* among symptomatic and asymptomatic individuals in Talkha Center, Dakahlia Governorate, Egypt. *J. Egypt Soc. Parasitol.,* **35:** 653–66.

Florez, A. C., Garcia, D. A., Moncada, L. and Beltran, M. (2003). Prevalence of microsporidia and other intestinal parasites in patients with HIV infection, Bogota, 2001. *Biomedica,* **23:** 274–82.

Gallagher, P. G. and Venglarcik, J. S. (1985). *Blastocystis hominis* enteritis. *Pediatr. Infect. Dis.,* **4:** 556–57.

Garavelli, P. L. and Libanore, M. (1990). *Blastocystis* in immunodeficiency diseases. *Rev. Infect. Dis.,* **12:** 158.

Garavelli, P. L. and Scaglione, L. (1990). *Blastocystis hominis* infection in AIDS and correlated pathologies. *Minerva Med.,* **81:** 91–92.

Garavelli, P. L., Scaglione, L., Bicocchi, R. and Libanore, M. (1991). Pathogenicity of *Blastocystis hominis. Infection,* **19:** 185.

Garavelli, P. L., Scaglione, L., Merighi, A. and Libanore, M. (1992) Endoscopy of blastocystosis (Zierdt–Garavelli disease). *Ital. J. Gastroenterol.,* **24:** 206.

Giacometti, A., Cirioni, O., Antonicelli, L., D'Amato, G., Silvestri, C., *et al.* (2003). Prevalence of intestinal parasites among individuals with allergic skin diseases. *J. Parasitol.,* **89:** 490–92.

Giacometti, A., Cirioni, O., Fiorentini, A., Fortuna, M. and Scalise, G. (1999). Irritable bowel syndrome in patients with *Blastocystis hominis* infection. *Eur. J. Clin. Microbiol. Infect. Dis.,* **18:** 436–39.

Guirges, S. Y. and Al-Waili, N. S. (1987). *Blastocystis hominis:* evidence for human pathogenicity and effectiveness of metronidazole therapy. *Clin. Exp. Pharm. Physiol.,* **14:** 333–5.

Gupta, R. and Parsi, K. (2006). Chronic urticaria due to *Blastocystis hominis. Aus. J. Dermatol.,* **47:** 117–19.

Hailemariam, G., Kassu, A., Abebe, G., Abate, E., Damte, D., *et al.* (2004). Intestinal parasitic infections in HIV/AIDS and HIV seronegative individuals in a teaching hospital, Ethiopia. *Jpn. J. Infect. Dis.,* **57:** 41–43.

Hakim, S. L., Gan, C. C., Malkit, K., Azian, M. N., *et al.* (2007). Parasitic infections among Orang Asli (aborigine) in the Cameron Highlands, Malaysia. *Southeast Asian J. Trop. Med. Pub. Health,* **38:** 415–19.

Haresh, K., Suresh, K., Khairul Anus, A. and Saminathan, S. (1999). Isolate resistance of *Blastocystis hominis* to metronidazole. *Trop. Med. Intern. Health,* **4:** 274–77.

Ho, L. C., Singh, M., Suresh, G., Ng, G. C. and Yap, E. H. (1993). Axenic culture of *Blastocystis hominis* in Iscove's modified Dulbecco's medium. *Parasitol. Res.,* **79:** 614–16.

Horiki, N., Maruyama, M., Fujita, Y., Yonekura, T., *et al.* (1997). Epidemiologic survey of *Blastocystis hominis* infection in Japan. *Am. J. Trop. Med. Hyg.,* **56:** 370–74.

Hussain, R., Jaferi, W., Zuberi, S., Baqai, R., Abrar, N., *et al.* (1997). Significantly increased IgG2 subclass antibody levels to *Blastocystis hominis* in patients with irritable bowel syndrome. *Am. J. Trop. Med. Hyg.,* **56:** 301–6.

Hussein, E. M., Hussein, A. M., Eida, M. M. and Atwa, M. M. (2008). Pathophysiological variability of different genotypes of human *Blastocystis hominis* Egyptian isolates in experimentally infected rats. *Parasitol. Res.,* **102:** 853–60.

Iguchi, A., Ebisu, A., Nagata, S., Saitou, Y., Yoshikawa, H., *et al.* (2007). Infectivity of different genotypes of human *Blastocystis hominis* isolates in chickens and rats. *Parasitol. Int.,* **56:** 107–12.

Jeddy, T. A. and Farrington, G. H. (1991). *Blastocystis hominis* complicating ulcerative colitis. *J. R. Soc. Med.,* **84:** 623.

Johnson, A. M., Thanou, A., Boreham, P. F. and Baverstock, P. R. (1989). *Blastocystis hominis:* phylogenetic affinities determined by rRNA sequence comparison. *Exp. Parasitol.,* **68:** 283–88.

Jones Ii, M. S., Ganac, R. D., Hiser, G., Hudson, N. R., Le, A. and Whipps, C. M. (2008). Detection of *Blastocystis* from stool samples using real-time PCR. *Parasitol. Res.,* **103:** 551–57.

Kain, K. C., Noble, M. A., Freeman, H. J. and Barteluk, R. L. (1987). Epidemiology and clinical features associated with *Blastocystis hominis* infection. *Diagn. Microbiol. Infect. Dis.,* **8:** 235–44.

Kaneda, Y., Horiki, N., Cheng, X., Tachibana, H. and Tsutsumi, Y. (2000). Serologic response to *Blastocystis hominis* infection in asymptomatic individuals. *Tokai J. Exp. Clin. Med.,* **25:** 51–56.

Kaneda, Y., Horiki, N., Cheng, X. J., Fujita, Y., Maruyama, M. and Tachibana, H. (2001). Ribodemes of *Blastocystis hominis* isolated in Japan. *Am. J. Trop. Med. Hyg.,* **65:** 393–96.

Karanis, P., Kourenti, C. and Smith, H. (2007). Waterborne transmission of protozoan parasites: a worldwide review of outbreaks and lessons learnt. *J. Water Health,* **5:** 1–38.

Katsarou-Katsari, A., Vassalos, C. M., Tzanetou, K., Spanakos, G., *et al.* (2008). Acute urticaria associated with amoeboid forms of *Blastocystis* sp. subtype 3. *Acta Derm. Venereol.,* **88:** 80–81.

Katz, D. E. and Taylor, D. N. (2001). Parasitic infections of the gastrointestinal tract. *Gastroenterol. Clin. North Am.,* **30:** 797–815, x.

Kick, G., Rueff, F. and Przybilla, B. (2002). Palmoplantar pruritus subsiding after *Blastocystis hominis* eradication. *Acta Derm. Venereol.,* **82:** 60.

Lakhanpal, S., Cohen, S. B. and Fleischmann, R. M. (1991). Reactive arthritis from *Blastocystis hominis. Arthr. Rheum.,* **34:** 251–53.

Lambert, M., Gigi, J. and Bughin, C. (1992). Persistent diarrhoea and *Blastocystis hominis. Acta Clin. Belg.,* **47:** 129–30.

Leder, K., Hellard, M. E., Sinclair, M. I., Fairley, C. K. and Wolfe, R. (2005). No correlation between clinical symptoms and *Blastocystis hominis* in immunocompetent individuals. *J. Gastroenter. Hepatol.,* **20:** 1390–94.

Lee, M. G., Rawlins, S. C., Didier, M. and Deceulaer, K. (1990). Infective arthritis due to *Blastocystis hominis. Ann. Rheum. Dis.,* **49:** 192–93.

Lee, M. G. and Stenzel, D. J. (1999). A survey of *Blastocystis* in domestic chickens. *Parasitol. Res.,* **85:** 109–17.

Leelayoova, S., Rangsin, R., Taamasri, P., Naaglor, T., *et al.* (2004). Evidence of waterborne transmission of *Blastocystis hominis. Am. J. Trop. Med. Hyg.,* **70:** 658–62.

Logar, J., Andlovic, A. and Poljsak-Prijatelj, M. (1994). Incidence of *Blastocystis hominis* in patients with diarrhoea. *J. Infect.,* **28:** 151–54.

Long, H. Y., Handschack, A., Konig, W. and Ambrosch, A. (2001). *Blastocystis hominis* modulates immune responses and cytokine release in colonic epithelial cells. *Parasitol. Res.,* **87:** 1029–30.

Mahmoud, M. S. and Saleh, W. A. (2003). Secretory and humoral antibody responses to *Blastocystis hominis* in symptomatic and asymptomatic human infections. *J. Egypt Soc. Parasitol.,* **33:** 13–30.

Markell, E. K. (1995). Is there any reason to continue treating *Blastocystis* infections? *Clin. Infect. Dis.,* **21:** 104–5.

Matsumoto, Y., Yamada, M. and Yoshida, Y. (1987). Light-microscopical appearance and ultrastructure of *Blastocystis hominis,* an intestinal parasite of man. *Zentralbl. Bakteriol. Mikrobiol. Hyg. [A],* **264:** 379–85.

McClure, H. M., Strobert, E. A. and Healy, G. R. (1980). *Blastocystis hominis* in a pig-tailed macaque: a potential enteric pathogen for nonhuman primates. *Lab. Anim. Sci.,* **30:** 890–94.

Mehlhorn, H. (1988). *Blastocystis hominis*, Brumpt 1912: are there different stages or species? *Parasitol. Res.,* **74:** 393–95.

Menounos, P. G., Spanakos, G., Tegos, N., Vassalos, C. M., *et al.* (2008). Direct detection of *Blastocystis* sp. in human faecal samples and subtype assignment using single strand conformational polymorphism and sequencing. *Mol. Cell Probes,* **22:** 24–29.

Micheloud, D., Jensen, J., Fernandez-Cruz, E. and Carbone, J. (2007). Chronic angioedema and *Blastocystis hominis* infection. *Rev. Gastroenter. Peru,* **27:** 191–93.

Miller, S. A., Rosario, C. L., Rojas, E. and Scorza, J. V. (2003). Intestinal parasitic infection and associated symptoms in children attending day care centres in Trujillo, Venezuela. *Trop. Med. Intern. Health,* **8:** 342–47.

Moe, K. T., Singh, M., Howe, J., Ho, L. C., *et al.* (1997). Experimental *Blastocystis hominis* infection in laboratory mice. *Parasitol. Res.,* **83:** 319–25.

Moe, K. T., Singh, M., Howe, J., Ho, L. C., *et al.* (1996). Observations on the ultrastructure and viability of the cystic stage of *Blastocystis hominis* from human faeces. *Parasitol. Res.,* **82:** 439–44.

Moghaddam, D. D., Ghadirian, E. and Azami, M. (2005). *Blastocystis hominis* and the evaluation of efficacy of metronidazole and trimethoprim/sulfamethoxazole. *Parasitol. Res.,* **96:** 273–75.

Nasirudeen, A. M., Hian, Y. E., Singh, M. and Tan, K. S. (2004). Metronidazole induces programmed cell death in the protozoan parasite *Blastocystis hominis. Microbiology,* **150:** 33–43.

Nassir, E., Awad, J., Abel, A. B., Khoury, J., Shay, M. and Lejbkowicz, F. (2004). *Blastocystis hominis* as a cause of hypoalbuminemia and anasarca. *Eur. J. Clin. Microbiol. Infect. Dis.,* **23:** 399–402.

Nigro, L., Larocca, L., Massarelli, L., Patamia, I., Minniti, S., *et al.* (2003). A placebo-controlled treatment trial of *Blastocystis hominis* infection with metronidazole. *J. Travel Med.,* **10:** 128–30.

Nimri, L. and Batchoun, R. (1994). Intestinal colonization of symptomatic and asymptomatic schoolchildren with *Blastocystis hominis. J. Clin. Microbiol.,* **32:** 2865–66.

Nimri, L. F. (1993). Evidence of an epidemic of *Blastocystis hominis* infections in preschool children in northern Jordan. *J. Clin. Microbiol.,* **31:** 2706–8.

Noel, C., Dufernez, F., Gerbod, D., Edgcomb, V. P., *et al.* (2005). Molecular phylogenies of *Blastocystis* isolates from different hosts: implications for genetic diversity, identification of species, and zoonosis. *J. Clin. Microbiol.,* **43:** 348–55.

O'Connor, F. W. (1919). Intestinal protozoa found during acute intestinal conditions amongst members of the Egyptian expeditionary force, 1916–1917. *Parasitology,* **11:** 239–53.

Ok, U. Z., Cirit, M., Uner, A., Ok, E., Akcicek, F., Basci, A. and Ozcel, M. A. (1997). Cryptosporidiosis and blastocystosis in renal transplant recipients. *Nephron,* **75:** 171–74.

Ozyurt, M., Kurt, O., Molbak, K., Nielsen, H. V., *et al.* (2008). Molecular epidemiology of *Blastocystis* infections in Turkey. *Parasitol. Int.,* **57:** 300–306.

Pakandl, M. (1992). An experimental transmission of porcine strains of *Blastocystis* sp. in the laboratory mice and gerbils. *Folia Parasitol. (Praha),* **39:** 383–86.

Parkar, U., Traub, R. J., Kumar, S., Mungthin, M., Vitali, S., *et al.* (2007). Direct characterization of *Blastocystis* from faeces by PCR and evidence of zoonotic potential. *Parasitology,* **134:** 359–67.

Pasqui, A. L., Savini, E., Saletti, M., Guzzo, C., Puccetti, L. and Auteri, A. (2004). Chronic urticaria and *Blastocystis hominis* infection: a case report. *Eur. Rev. Med. Pharmacol. Sci.,* **8:** 117–20.

Pegelow, K., Gross, R., Pietrzik, K., Lukito, W., Richards, A. L. and Fryauff, D. J. (1997). Parasitological and nutritional situation of school children in the Sukaraja district, West Java, Indonesia. *Southeast Asian J. Trop. Med. Pub. Health,* **28:** 173–90.

Phillips, B. P. and Zierdt, C. H. (1976). *Blastocystis hominis*: pathogenic potential in human patients and in gnotobiotes. *Exp. Parasitol.,* **39:** 358–64.

Puthia, M. K., Lu, J. and Tan, K. S. (2008). *Blastocystis* ratti contains cysteine proteases that mediate interleukin-8 response from human intestinal epithelial cells in an NF-kappaB-dependent manner. *Eukaryot. Cell,* **7:** 435–43.

Puthia, M. K., Sio, S. W., Lu, J. and Tan, K. S. (2006). *Blastocystis* ratti induces contact-independent apoptosis, F-actin rearrangement, and barrier function disruption in IEC-6 cells. *Infect. Immun.,* **74:** 4114–23.

Puthia, M. K., Vaithilingam, A., Lu, J. and Tan, K. S. (2005). Degradation of human secretory immunoglobulin A by *Blastocystis. Parasitol. Res.,* **97:** 386–89.

Qadri, S. M., Al-Okaili, G. A. and Al-Dayel, F. (1989). Clinical significance of *Blastocystis hominis. J. Clin. Microbiol.,* **27:** 2407–09.

Rajah Salim, H., Suresh Kumar, G., Vellayan, S., Mak, J. W., *et al.* (1999). *Blastocystis* in animal handlers. *Parasitol. Res.,* **85L:** 1032–33.

Rao, K., Sekar, U., Iraivan, K. T., Abraham, G. and Soundararajan, P. (2003). *Blastocystis hominis*—an emerging cause of diarrhoea in renal transplant recipients. *J. Ass. Physic, India,* **51:** 719–21.

Rosenblatt, J. E. (1990). *Blastocystis hominis. J. Clin. Microbiol.,* **28:** 2379–80.

Rossignol, J. F., Kabil, S. M., Said, M., Samir, H. and Younis, A. M. (2005). Effect of nitazoxanide in persistent diarrhea and enteritis associated with *Blastocystis hominis. Clin. Gastroenter. Hepatol.,* **3:** 987–91.

Russo, A. R., Stone, S. L., Taplin, M. E., Snapper, H. J. and Doern, G. V. (1988). Presumptive evidence for *Blastocystis hominis* as a cause of colitis. *Arch. Intern. Med.,* **148:** 1064.

Saksirisampant, W., Nuchprayoon, S., Wiwanitkit, V., *et al.* (2003). Intestinal parasitic infestations among children in an orphanage in Pathum Thani province. *J. Med. Assoc. Thai.,* **86** Suppl 2: S263–70.

Schwartz, E. and Houston, R. (1992). Effect of co-trimoxazole on stool recovery of *Blastocystis hominis. Lancet,* **339:** 428–29.

Senay, H. and Macpherson, D. (1990). *Blastocystis hominis*: epidemiology and natural history. *J. Infect. Dis.,* **162:** 987–90.

Shilm, D. R., Hoge, C. W., Rajah, R., Rabold, J. G. and Echeverria, P. (1995). Is *Blastocystis hominis* a cause of diarrhea in travelers? A prospective controlled study in Nepal. *Clin. Infect. Dis.,* **21:** 97–101.

Silberman, J. D., Sogin, M. L., Leipe, D. D. and Clark, C. G. (1996). Human parasite finds taxonomic home. *Nature,* **380:** 398.

Singh, M., Ho, L. C., Yap, A. L., Ng, G. C., *et al.* (1996). Axenic culture of reptilian *Blastocystis* isolates in monophasic medium and speciation by karyotypic typing. *Parasitol. Res.,* **82:** 165–69.

Singh, M., Suresh, K., Ho, L. C., Ng, G. C. and Yap, E. H. (1995). Elucidation of the life cycle of the intestinal protozoan *Blastocystis hominis. Parasitol. Res.,* **81:** 446–50.

Sio, S. W., Puthia, M. K., Lee, A. S., Lu, J. and Tan, K. S. (2006). Protease activity of *Blastocystis hominis. Parasitol. Res.,* **99:** 126–30.

Sohail, M. R. and Fischer, P. R. (2005). *Blastocystis hominis* and travelers. *Travel. Med. Infect. Dis.,* **3:** 33–38.

Stechmann, A., Hamblin, K., Perez-Brocal, V., Gaston, D., *et al.* (2008). Organelles in *Blastocystis* that blur the distinction between mitochondria and hydrogenosomes. *Curr. Biol.,* **18:** 580–85.

Stensvold, C. R., Suresh, G. K., Tan, K. S., *et al.* (2007). Terminology for *Blastocystis* subtypes—a consensus. *Trends Parasitol.,* **23:** 93–96.

Stenzel, D. J. and Boreham, P. F. (1991). A cyst-like stage of *Blastocystis hominis. Int. J. Parasitol.,* **21:** 613–15.

Stenzel, D. J. and Boreham, P. F. (1996). *Blastocystis hominis* revisited. *Clin. Microbiol. Rev.,* **9:** 563–84.

Stenzel, D. J., Dunn, L. A. and Boreham, P. F. (1989). Endocytosis in cultures of *Blastocystis hominis. Int. J. Parasitol.,* **19:** 787–91.

Sun, T., Katz, S., Tanenbaum, B. and Schenone, C. (1989). Questionable clinical significance of *Blastocystis hominis* infection. *Am. J. Gastroenter.,* **84:** 1543–47.

Suresh, K., Howe, J., Ng, G. C., Ho, L. C., *et al.* (1994). A multiple fission-like mode of asexual reproduction in *Blastocystis hominis*. *Parasitol. Res.,* **80:** 523–27.

Suresh, K. & Smith, H. (2004). Comparison of methods for detecting *Blastocystis hominis*. *Eur. J. Clin. Microbiol. Infect. Dis.,* **23:** 509–11.

Suresh, K., Smith, H. V. & Tan, T. C. (2005) Viable *Blastocystis* cysts in Scottish and Malaysian sewage samples. *Appl. Environ. Microbiol.,* **71:** 5619–20.

Swellengrebel, N. H. (1917). Observations on *Blastocystis hominis*. *Parasitology,* **9:** 451–59.

Taamasri, P., Leelayoova, S., Rangsin, R., *et al.* (2002). Prevalence of *Blastocystis hominis* carriage in Thai army personnel based in Chonburi, Thailand. *Mil. Med.,* **167:** 643–46.

Taamasri, P., Mungthin, M., Rangsin, R., *et al.* (2000). Transmission of intestinal blastocystosis related to the quality of drinking water. *Southeast Asian J. Trop. Med. Pub. Health,* **31:** 112–17.

Tan, K. S. (2004). *Blastocystis* in humans and animals: new insights using modern methodologies. *Vet. Parasitol.,* **126:** 121–44.

Tan, K. S. (2008). *Blastocystis spp.* In: N.A. Khan (ed.) *Emerging Protozoan Pathogens.* London: Taylor and Francis.

Tan, K. S., Howe, J., Yap, E. H. and Singh, M. (2001). Do *Blastocystis hominis* colony forms undergo programmed cell death? *Parasitol. Res.,* **87:** 362–67.

Tan, K. S. and Nasirudeen, A. M. (2005). Protozoan programmed cell death—insights from *Blastocystis* deathstyles. *Trends Parasitol.,* **21:** 547–50.

Tan, K. S., Ng, G. C., Quek, E., Howe, J., *et al.* (2000). *Blastocystis hominis:* A simplified, high-efficiency method for clonal growth on solid agar. *Exp. Parasitol.,* **96:** 9–15.

Tan, K. S., Singh, M. and Yap, E. H. (2002). Recent advances in *Blastocystis hominis* research: hot spots in terra incognita. *Intern. J. Parasitol.,* **32:** 789–804.

Tan, K. S. & Stenzel, D. J. (2003) Multiple reproductive processes in *Blastocystis:* proceed with caution. *Trends Parasitol.,* **19:** 290–91.

Tan, S. W., Ho, L. C., Moe, K. T., Chen, X. Q., *et al.* (1996). Production and characterization of murine monoclonal antibodies to *Blastocystis hominis. Int. J. Parasitol.,* **26:** 375–81.

Tanizaki, A., Yoshikawa, H., Iwatani, S. and Kimata, I. (2005). Infectivity of *Blastocystis* isolates from chickens, quails and geese in chickens. *Parasitol. Res.,* **96:** 57–61.

Tasova, Y., Sahin, B., Koltas, S. and Paydas, S. (2000). Clinical significance and frequency of *Blastocystis hominis* in Turkish patients with hematological malignancy. *Acta Med. Okayama,* **54:** 133–36.

Teow, W. L., Zaman, V., Ng, G. C., Chan, Y. C., *et al.* (1991). A *Blastocystis* species from the sea-snake, Lapemis hardwickii (Serpentes: Hydrophiidae). *Int. J. Parasitol.,* **21:** 723–26.

Termmathurapoj, S., Leelayoova, S., Aimpun, P., *et al.* (2004). The usefulness of short-term in vitro cultivation for the detection and molecular study of *Blastocystis hominis* in stool specimens. *Parasitol. Res.,* **93:** 445–47.

Tsang, T. K., Levin, B. S. and Morse, S. R. (1989). Terminal ileitis associated with *Blastocystis hominis* infection. *Am. J. Gastroenter.,* **84:** 798–99.

Udkow, M. P. and Markell, E. K. (1993). *Blastocystis hominis:* prevalence in asymptomatic versus symptomatic hosts. *J. Infect. Dis.,* **168:** 242–44.

Valsecchi, R., Leghissa, P. and Greco, V. (2004). Cutaneous lesions in *Blastocystis hominis* infection. *Acta Derm. Venereol.,* **84:** 322–23.

Waikagul, J., Krudsood, S., Radomyos, P., *et al.* (2002). A cross-sectional study of intestinal parasitic infections among schoolchildren in Nan Province, Northern Thailand. *Southeast Asian J. Trop. Med. Pub. Health,* **33:** 218–23.

Walderich, B., Bernauer, S., Renner, M., Knobloch, J. and Burchard, G. D. (1998). Cytopathic effects of *Blastocystis hominis* on Chinese hamster ovary (CHO) and adeno carcinoma HT29 cell cultures. *Trop. Med. Int. Health,* **3:** 385–90.

Windsor, J. J., Macfarlane, L., Hughes-Thapa, G., Jones, S. K. and Whiteside, T. M. (2002). Incidence of *Blastocystis hominis* in faecal samples submitted for routine microbiological analysis. *Br. J. Biomed. Sci.,* **59:** 154–57.

Wong, K. H., Ng, G. C., Lin, R. T., *et al.* (2008). Predominance of subtype 3 among *Blastocystis* isolates from a major hospital in Singapore. *Parasitol. Res.,* **102:** 663–70.

Yaicharoen, R., Sripochang, S., Sermsart, B. and Pidetcha, P. (2005). Prevalence of *Blastocystis hominis* infection in asymptomatic individuals from Bangkok, Thailand. *Southeast Asian J. Trop. Med. Pub. Health,* **36 Suppl 4:** 17–20.

Yakoob, J., Jafri, W., Jafri, N., Khan, R., *et al.* (2004). Irritable bowel syndrome: in search of an etiology: role of *Blastocystis hominis. Am. J. Trop. Med. Hyg.,* **70:** 383–85.

Yan, Y., Su, S., Ye, J., Lai, X., Lai, R., *et al.* (2007). *Blastocystis* sp. subtype 5: a possibly zoonotic genotype. *Parasitol. Res.,* **101:** 1527–32.

Yoshikawa, H., Abe, N. and Wu, Z. (2004a). PCR-based identification of zoonotic isolates of *Blastocystis* from mammals and birds. *Microbiology,* **150:** 1147–51.

Yoshikawa, H. and Hayakawa, A. (1996). Freeze-fracture cytochemistry of membrane cholesterol in *Blastocystis hominis. Intern. J. Parasitol.,* **26:** 1111–14.

Yoshikawa, H., Wu, Z., Kimata, I., Iseki, M., *et al.* (2004b). Polymerase chain reaction-based genotype classification among human *Blastocystis hominis* populations isolated from different countries. *Parasitol. Res.,* **92:** 22–29.

Yoshikawa, H., Yoshida, K., Nakajima, A., Yamanari, K., *et al.* (2004c). Faecal-oral transmission of the cyst form of *Blastocystis hominis* in rats. *Parasitol. Res.,* **94:** 391–96.

Zaman, V. (1996). The diagnosis of *Blastocystis hominis* cysts in human faeces. *J. Infect.,* **33:** 15–16.

Zaman, V. (1998). The differential identification of *Blastocystis hominis* cysts. *Ann. Trop. Med. Parasitol.,* **92:** 233–35.

Zaman, V., Howe, J. and Ng, M. (1997). Observations on the surface coat of *Blastocystis hominis. Parasitol. Res.,* **83:** 731–33.

Zaman, V., Howe, J., Ng, M. and Goh, T. K. (1999). Scanning electron microscopy of the surface coat of *Blastocystis hominis. Parasitol. Res.,* **85:** 974–76.

Zaman, V. and Zaki, M. (1996). Resistance of *Blastocystis hominis* cysts to metronidazole. *Trop. Med. Intern. Health,* **1:** 677–78.

Zhang, H. W., Li, W., Yan, Q. Y., He, L. J. and Su, Y. P. (2006). Impact of *Blastocystis hominis* infection on ultrastructure of intestinal mucosa in mice. *Zhongguo. Ji Sheng Chong Xue Yu Ji Sheng Chong Bing Za Zhi,* **24:** 187–91.

Zierdt, C. H. (1973). Studies of *Blastocystis hominis. J. Protozool.,* **20:** 114–21.

Zierdt, C. H. (1991). *Blastocystis hominis*—past and future. *Clin. Microbiol. Rev.,* **4:** 61–79.

Zierdt, C. H. and Nagy, B. (1993), Antibody response to *Blastocystis hominis* infections. *Ann. Intern. Med.,* **118:** 985–86.

Zierdt, C. H., Rude, W. S. and Bull, B. S. (1967). Protozoan characteristics of *Blastocystis hominis. Am. J. Clin. Pathol.,* **48:** 495–501.

Zierdt, C. H., Zierdt, W. S. and Nagy, B. (1995). Enzyme-linked immunosorbent assay for detection of serum antibody to *Blastocystis hominis* in symptomatic infections. *J. Parasitol.,* **81:** 127–29.

Zuckerman, M. J., Ho, H., Hooper, L., Anderson, B. and Polly, S. M. (1990). Frequency of recovery of *Blastocystis hominis* in clinical practice. *J. Clin. Gastroenter.,* **12:** 525–32.

Zuckerman, M. J., Watts, M. T., Ho, H. and Meriano, F. V. (1994). *Blastocystis hominis* infection and intestinal injury. *Am. J. Med. Sci.,* **308:** 96–101.

CHAPTER 51

Cysticercosis and taeniosis: *Taenia solium*, *Taenia saginata* and *Taenia asiatica*

Ana Flisser, Philip S. Craig and Akira Ito

Summary

The pork and beef tapeworms, *Taenia solium* and *Taenia saginata* respectively, are taeniid cestodes and major food-borne or meat-borne zoonoses. Human tapeworms and swine cysticerci have been known since Egyptian and Greek cultures. Nevertheless their association as part of the life cycle of the same parasite was only demonstrated during the nineteenth century. Kuchenmeister fed convicts with cysticerci excised from pork meat and found adult tapeworms in the intestine after autopsy, while van Beneden fed *T. solium* eggs to pigs and found numerous cysticerci in muscles after slaughter (Grove 1990).

T. solium is the only causative agent of neurocysticercosis in humans and is, therefore, the more important of these species in public health. This chapter describes classical aspects of the morphology of the parasites as well as clinical aspects of the diseases they cause. Most importantly, detailed explanations of taxonomic aspects, specially related to the newly recognized *Taenia asiatica* are given. Furthermore, the epidemiology and transmission dynamics of the parasites, as well as intervention measures such as health education, mass drug treatment and vaccination, are described in detail. The chapter concludes with considerations on the surveillance and a discussion on prospects for the control of these cestode zoonoses.

Taxonomy

The classification of human *Taenia* is as follows:

Kingdom: Animalia,

Phylum: Platyhelminthes,

Class: Cestoidea,

Subclass: Eucestoda,

Order: Cyclophyllidea,

Family: Taeniidae,

Genus: *Taenia*,

Species: *Taenia solium* Linnaeus (1758),

Species: *Taenia saginata* Goeze (1782),

Species: *Taenia asiatica* Eom and Rim (1993).

Taeniidae are mammalian parasites with adults found in carnivores and larvae in herbivores. In the adult parasite, the scolex, which is the anchorage organ aided by suckers, usually bears 2 rows of hooks that are absent in *T. saginata*. The genital pore is irregularly alternated along the strobila with a single set of reproductive organs in each proglottid. Eggs have a radial striated appearance because of the embryophore formed by embryophoric blocks.

Adult *Taenia solium* and *Taenia saginata* are found in the human intestine. The larval stage or metacestode (cysticercus) is found in pigs (*T. solium*) and bovines (*T. saginata*).

Taenia asiatica has been recognized in Asia and the Pacific. Adult tapeworms appear to be *T. saginata* but infected people eat pork rather than beef (Huang *et al.* 1966; Kosin *et al.* 1972; Fan 1988). It has been called the Asian *Taenia* and expected to be a new species (Fan 1988; reviewed by Simanjuntak *et al.* 1997). Subsequent molecular studies revealed very small differences from *T. saginata* and it was classified as a subspecies of *T. saginata* (*T. saginata asiatica*, Fan *et al.* 1995), which used different intermediate hosts distributed in Asia and the Pacific (Fan 1988, 1995; McManus and Bowles 1994). Later, it was described as *Taenia asiatica*, an independent but sister species of *T. saginata* (Eom and Rim 1993; reviewed by Ito *et al.* 2003; Eom 2006; Hoberg 2006). Separate species are believed to be valid as *T. saginata* and *T. asiatica* are distributed sympatrically but to date no hybrids between the two have been identified which would be expected if they were subspecies or strains of the same species. However, the numbers of specimens to date examined is small (Hoberg 2006). Figure 51.1 illustrates a summary of the molecular phylogeny of taeniid cestodes (modified from Okamoto *et al.* 2007).

Molecular phylogeny

Molecular tools have been used to further characterize the 3 human *Taenia* species (McManus and Ito 2005) and their epidemiology and possible origin. Mitochondrial DNA data strongly suggest that *T. saginata* and *T. asiatica* are very closely related to each other and

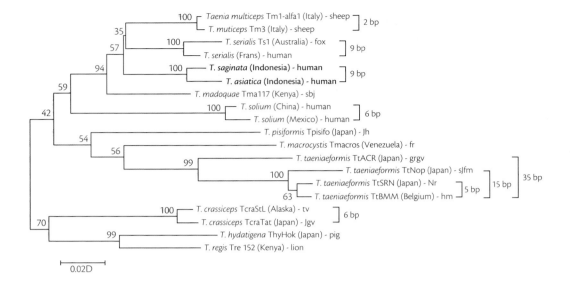

Fig. 51.1 Molecular phylogeny of genus *Taenia*.
Modified from Okamoto *et al.* (2007).

that *T. solium* is divided into two genotypes, the Asian and the American/African genotypes (Fig. 51.2). Minor diversity within the genotypes has been demonstrated in samples from Peru, Mexico and Asian countries (Nakao *et al.* 2002; Campbell *et al.* 2006; Maravilla *et al.* 2003, 2008; Sudewi *et al.* 2008). Molecular phylogenic studies (Sudewi *et al.* 2008) suggest that *T. solium* in Papua originated elsewhere in Asia rather than from nearby Bali as suggested by Gadjusek (1978).

T. saginata mitochondrial DNA analysis shows large variations (Rodriguez-Hidalgo *et al.* 2002; Myadagsuren *et al.* 2007) pointing to a higher complexity of this parasite than that of *T. solium*.

T. solium emerged in Africa several million years ago as a parasite of early hominids that probably evolved from parasites of hyaeniids (Hoberg 2001, 2006).

Detection of parasite DNA using faecal samples and multiplex PCR for identification of human *Taenia* should be used in endemic areas for *T. solium*, *T. saginata* and *T. asiatica*, because their sympatric distribution may complicate surveillance of cysticercosis control (Ananthaphruti *et al.* 2007).

Morphology

Tapeworm

Tapeworms are flat long helminths: adults measuring 1.5 to 10 m. The head or scolex, has four suckers and a rostellum, which may be armed with hooks (*T. solium*), unarmed (*T. saginata*) or have a sunken or unarmed rostellum (*T. asiatica*, Fig. 51.3). Hooks are organized as a double row crown of 22 to 32 hooks that ranges in size from 159 to 173 µm. The most conspicuous part of the tapeworm is the chain of segments that forms the strobila. It has the appearance of a ribbon and is constituted by more than a thousand proglottids (proper name for segments). Tapeworms do not have digestive organs, thus feed passively through their tegument. In contrast they have a well formed excretory system that contains numerous collecting ducts and flame cells. Proglottids develop from the neck region behind the scolex. Proximal proglottids are immature, they are followed by mature ones that contain several hundred testes and two ovary lobes per segment (Flisser *et al.* 2004a). Tapeworms are hermaphrodites; self-fertilization occurs

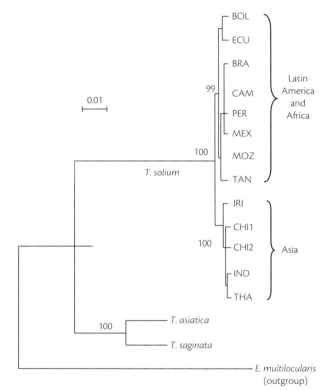

Fig. 51.2 Two genotypes of *T. solium* in the world. The neighbour-joining phylogenetic tree of taeniid tapeworms inferred from the complete nucleotide sequences of mitochondrial *cox1* gene. The scale bar represents the estimated number of nucleotide substitutions per nucleotide site. The isolates of *T. solium* were obtained from Bolivia (BOL), Brazil (BRA), Cameroon (CAM), China (CHI1 and CHI2), Ecuador (ECU), India (IND), Irian Jaya (IRI), Mexico (MEX), Mozambique (MOZ), Peru (PER), Tanzania (TAN) and Thailand (THA).
Modified from Nakao *et al.* (2002), with permission.

and eggs develop in the multi-branched sac-like uterus of gravid proglottids, at the end of the strobila, which contain between 50,000 and 80,000 eggs per gravid segment. Distal proglottids become bigger, measuring from a couple of mm to up to 2 cm long. *T. solium* has 7–14 lateral uterine branches in the proglottid whilst

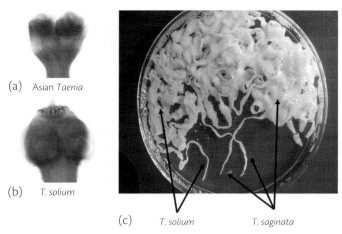

(a) Asian *Taenia*

(b) *T. solium*

(c) *T. solium*   *T. saginata*

Fig. 51.3 Three *Taenia* worms of two species were expelled from one woman in Kanchanabri, Thailand in 2004 (2 *T. solium* and 1 Asian *Taenia*) and from one Tibetan girl in 2007 (2 *T. saginata* and 1 *T. solium*). Fig. (a) and (b) show the scolex of one of the 2 *T. solium* and one Asian *Taenia* from Kanchanabri which were confirmed by DNA analysis. Fig. (a) was morphologically identified to be *T. saginata*, since there was no evidence on the distribution of Asian *Taenia* in Thailand before this study. Fig (c) shows two *T. saginata* and one *T. solium* from a Tibetan girl (Dr Li TY unpublished data). In these areas, three species have been confirmed to be occurring sympatrically.

Ananthaphruti *et al.* (2007); Li *et al.* (2006).

T. saginata has 14–32. This feature is very important for species identification when the scolex cannot be found (Eom and Rim 1993; Fan *et al.* 1995; Flisser *et al.* 2004a; Andreassen 2005).

The adult tapeworm dwells in the human small intestine. An autoradiographic analysis of the germinative tissue in evaginated cysticerci identified stem cells that proliferate continuously, differentiate and migrate to the tegument, constituting the main process by which these worms grow (Merchant *et al.* 1997). Adult *T. solium* has been established experimentally in one gibbon, one chacma baboon, many golden hamsters and, recently, in gerbils and chinchillas (Verster 1965, 1974; Cadigan *et al.* 1967; Maravilla *et al.* 1998; Flisser *et al.* 2010). Experimentally infected hamsters develop mature segments and, when rodents are immunosuppressed with steroids, long lasting gut infections (1–3 months) are attained, pre-gravid proglottids develop in hamsters and in gerbils, while gravid proglottids and mature eggs may develop in chinchillas (Maravilla *et al.* 1998; Merchant *et al.* 1998; Flisser *et al.* 2010). The inflammatory, humoral and cellular immune responses have been characterized in non immunosuppressed hamsters (Avila *et al.* 2006). Experimental infections with adult *T. saginata* have been established in immunosuppressed golden hamsters without obtaining mature or gravid proglottids (Verster 1974) but their study has not been followed.

Eggs

Eggs are spherical, range in size from 20 to 50 μm and are morphologically indistinguishable from eggs of other taeniid species. Each egg contains an embryo, which is a multi-cellular structure that has six hooks, therefore it is also named hexacanth embryo or oncosphere. When eggs are released from the definitive host, many are fully embryonated and infective whilst others are at different stages of maturation and not infective. The embryophore appears as a rigid structure that protects the oncosphere while the egg is in the environment, making eggs extremely resistant. When eggs are ingested by the intermediate host, the cementing substance that

joins embryophoric blocks is susceptible to enzymatic digestion which allows the oncosphere to be released (Laclette *et al.* 1982; Fan *et al.* 1995). Aided by their hooks and by enzymes released in vesicles, the oncospheres invade the intestinal mucosa and, after circulating, develop in the intermediate host.

Cysticercus

T. solium cysticerci have been identified in liver, brain and skeletal muscles of pigs six days after infection measuring around 0.3 mm. By 60 to 70 days after infection cysticerci are found in the skeletal muscle and the brain and have a fully developed scolex and measured between 6 to 9 mm (Yoshino 1933a, b, c). The mature cysticercus is usually spherical or oval, white or yellow, measures 0.5 and 1.5 cm and has a translucent bladder wall, through which the scolex can be seen. Young cysticerci have minimal inflammatory reaction surrounding them, while older parasites or those that are in pigs that were treated with a cestocidal drug, have an intense reaction that includes eosinophils, lymphocytes and macrophages (Flisser *et al.* 1990; Aluja and Vargas 1988; Aluja *et al.* 1998). Cysticerci have two chambers: an inner one contains the scolex and the spiral canal and is surrounded by an outer compartment that contains the vesicular fluid, usually less than 0.5 ml. When a cysticercus is ingested by the definitive host, the first event that takes place is the widening of the pore of the bladder wall for the scolex and neck to emerge, leaving the bladder wall and vesicular fluid to disintegrate in the digestive tract of the definitive host (Rabiela *et al.* 2000).

T. solium cysticerci may also establish in humans causing cysticercosis in the central nervous system, eye, striated and heart muscle and subcutaneous tissue. Two morphological types of metacestodes develop in humans: cellulose and racemose. The cellulose cysticercus is as previously described and is present in swine and in humans. This type of cysticercus is generally separated from the host tissue by a thin collagenous capsule, within which it remains alive (Escobar 1983; Aluja and Vargas 1988; Aluja *et al.* 1998). The racemose cysticercus appears either as a large, round or lobulated bladder circumscribed by a delicate wall, or resembles a cluster of grapes, it measures up to 10 or even 20 cm and may contain 60 ml fluid. Cellulose cysticerci grow and transform into racemose in spacious areas such as basal cisterns, especially optic, carotid, Sylvian and peduncular cisterns. The most important characteristics of this type of cysticercus is that usually the scolex cannot be seen, in some cases only detailed histological studies reveal its remains (Berman *et al.* 1981; Jung *et al.* 1981; Rabiela *et al.* 1989). Recent DNA analyses show that racemose and cellulose types represent genetically identical metacestodes of *T. solium* (Hinojosa-Juarez *et al.* 2008).

T. saginata cysticerci, (cysticercus bovis), is an oval bladder less than 1cm long, fluid filled and containing the invaginated scolex that does not have hooks. Cysticerci lodge in the skeletal muscle of cattle and sporadic reports of unarmed cysticerci in llamas, pronghorn, oryx, topi and other antelopes, bushbucks, gazelles, wildebeest, oryx and giraffes, have appeared in the literature (Nelson *et al.* 1965; Pawlowski and Schultz 1972; Gemmell *et al.* 1987). Intermediate hosts acquire the infection when grazing on contaminated pasture.

T. asiatica cysticerci are smaller than those of *T. saginata* measuring approximately 2–3 mm in diameter. Both metacestodes have a scolex with a round rostellum surrounded by four symmetrically placed conspicuous suckers, while *T. asiatica* has two rows of rudimentary hooklets, considered as a wart-like formation that usually do not develop into morphologically identifiable hooks. *T. asiatica* cysticerci are found in domestic pigs and wild boar

(Fan *et al.* 1995) and develop in liver but not in muscle. Most importantly, *T. asiatica* does not appear to cause cysticercosis in humans. This supports the hypothesis that it is a sister species of *T. saginata*. Both *T. saginata* and *T. asiatica* may be found sympatrically in Asia and the Pacific (Flisser *et al.* 2004a; Ito *et al.* 2008). The main features of tapeworms, cysticerci and eggs are shown in Table 51.1.

Life cycle

Life cycles of the human *Taenia* are shown in Fig. 51.4. When a person ingests raw or semi-cooked pork or beef with viable cysticerci, the scolex evaginates and attaches to the intestinal mucosa in the upper third section of the small intestine (duodenum-jejunum). Gravid proglottids are released with faeces and/or spontaneously, starting at 8–12 weeks after infection. Although some sources state that tapeworms can survive for about 25 years,

Table 51.1 Morphological characteristics of human tapeworms

	Taenia solium	Taenia saginata	Taenia asiatica
Entire body			
Length (m)	1–5	4–12	4–8
Width (mm)	7–10	12–14	9–12
Proglottids (number)	700–1,000	1000–1,500	200–1,200
Scolex			
Diameter (mm)	0.6–1.0	1.5–2.0	0.2–2.0
Suckers (number)	4	4	4
Rostellum	Present	Absent	Present, small
Hooks (number)	22–32	Absent	Vestigial***
Mature proglottid			
Testes (number)	350–600	800–1,200	300–1,200
Ovary (number of lobes)	2	2	2
Vaginal sphincter	Absent	Present	Present
Length (mm)	2.1–2.5	2.1–4.5	NR
Width (mm)	2.8–3.5	3.1–6.7	NR
Gravid proglottid			
Uterus (No of branches)	7–11	14–32	12–26
Posterior protuberance	Absent	Present	Present
Length (mm)	3.1–10	10–20	4–22
Width (mm)	3.8–8.7	6.5–9.5	3–12
Cysticercus			
Size (mm)	8–15*	6–10	0.4–3.5
Fluid contents (ml)	<0.5**	NR	NR
Hooks in scolex	Present	Absent	Rudimentary
Egg			
Size (µm)	26–34	26–34	16–45
Hooks (number)	6	6	6

* In humans racemose type cysticerci measure up to 20 cm.
** In humans racemose type cysticerci contain up to 60 ml.
*** Hooks are sunken and rudimentary
NR–not reported.

published original articles indicate that *T. saginata* can be found in the intestine of the host for approximately two years. Recent experience indicates that *T. solium* remains for shorter periods. Tapeworms release a few gravid proglottids, full of eggs, daily or 2–3 times per week (Andreassen 2005; Flisser *et al.* 2005a, 2006).

When swine or cattle ingest eggs, bile and enzymes disaggregate the embryophoric blocks and digest the oncospheral membrane. Cysticerci establish primarily in skeletal and cardiac muscle, as well as in the brain of pigs, a process that takes approximately 12 weeks. They remain viable for at least one year, when pigs are usually sent to slaughter. In cattle, cysticerci are usually calcified in adult animals, indicating that for *T. saginata* cysticercus life span is short. The main distinguishing feature of the life cycle of *T. asiatica* compared to *T. saginata* is the viscerotropic nature of cysticerci in pigs (especially to the liver), in contrast to the musculotropic cysticerci of *T. saginata* in cattle and *T. solium* in pigs. Metacestodes from beef and swine become infective to humans about 8 to 10 weeks of their development. Humans only acquire cysticercosis when they consume eggs in food handled by people infected by adult *T. solium* or through the faecal oral route (Eom and Rim 1993; Fan *et al.* 1995; Garcia *et al.* 2003a; Eom 2006).

Clinical aspects

Intestinal taeniosis

Intestinal taeniosis, caused by *T. solium* or *T. saginata*, is normally non pathogenic. It is identified because proglottids are frequently released (Craig and Ito 2007). Observations on a total of 3,100 affected people, show that by far the most frequent symptom is the discharge of proglottids (93%) (Pawlowski and Schultz 1972). This is a distinctive sign because of a sensation in the rectum followed by a crawling sensation in the perianal region and the thighs due to the discharge and movement of the proglottids. Up to 35% of tapeworm carriers felt abdominal pain and/or nausea. Weight loss only occurred in 21%, change in appetite in 17% and 15% reported headaches. In Ethiopia, 18 of 26 *T. saginata* carriers reported independent migration of segments from the anus (Tesfa-Yohannes 1990). Voluntary self-infections of humans with cysticerci of *T. saginata* reported release of 5–15 segments per day starting 10–12 weeks post infection (Craig and Ito 2007). As a result of worm migration to unusual sites or due to mechanical effects, various rare acute conditions or complications may occur, including appendicitis, invasion of the pancreatic and bile ducts, intestinal obstruction and perforation, vomiting of proglottids, or even vaginal bleeding due to a tapeworm in the uterus (reviewed in Flisser 1995; Jongwutiwes *et al.* 2004; Ahsan *et al.* 2006; Liu *et al.* 2005; Karanikas *et al.* 2007). Of greater importance in avoiding *T. solium* adult infections is that the tapeworm carrier is the main risk factor for acquiring cysticercosis (Gilman *et al.* 2000; Garcia *et al.* 2003a; Flisser and Gyorkos 2007).

Taeniosis has been diagnosed for over half a century by detecting eggs in stools under microscopy or proglottids with the naked eye (Hall *et al.* 1981). These approaches are not very sensitive because they depend on the natural release of segments and on technical expertise. Coproantigens are parasite-specific products present in host faeces that can be detected by immunologic techniques. These products are associated with adult parasite metabolism and are present independently of eggs or proglottids. In addition, they are undetectable in the faeces shortly after removal of the adult worms and therefore can indicate treatment success.

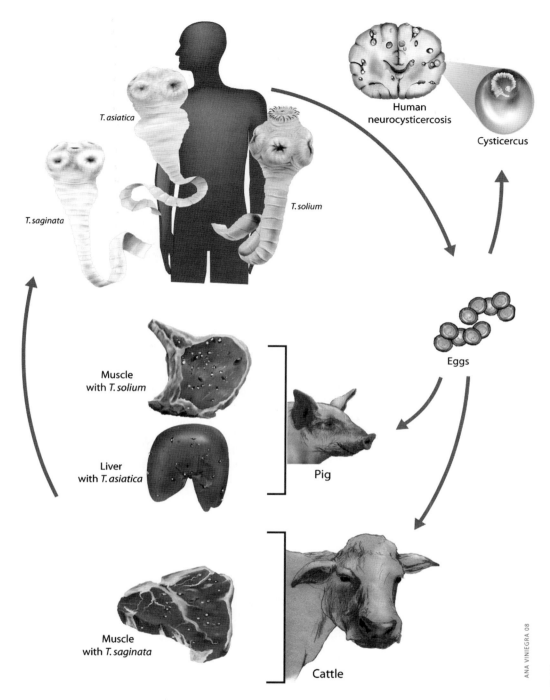

Fig. 51.4 Life cycle of human tapeworms.

Detecting human taeniosis by an enzyme-linked immunosorbent assay (ELISA), without necessarily observing eggs in the stool, represents a significant advance in diagnosis (Allan *et al.* 1992). The assay can detect as little as 35 ng protein/ml of adult parasite antigen products. The sensitivity depends on the assay format employed and the quality of the immunized rabbit serum used. A high titre rabbit serum offers a higher sensitivity. Rabbit anti-*Taenia* antiserum is not commercially available at this time so that antibody titres and avidity may vary. Coproantigen detection by ELISA have already been applied for screening of taeniosis (including *T. asiatica*) in several field studies (Flisser 2002a; Allan and Craig 2006; Wandra *et al.* 2006b; Flisser and Gyorkos 2007).

Neurocysticercosis

Neurocysticercosis (NCC) is due to the development of *T. solium* cysticerci in the human central nervous system, where parasites can be found in the parenchyma, the subarachnoid tissue, and the ventricles. Clinical manifestations are polymorphic and depend on the location, number and development or involution stages of the parasites as well as characteristics of the immune response of the host. The most important sign is epilepsy that occurs mainly when cysticerci are lodged in the brain parenchyma. Extra-parenchymal cysticerci can cause hydrocephalus due to mechanical obstruction of ventricular circulation of cerebrospinal fluid or to inflammatory reaction in basal cisterns. Symptoms usually occur after the cyst has initiated its degenerative process and are due mainly to the inflammatory response they induce or to residual scarring. In contrast, living cysticerci induce minimal inflammation, and can stay in this condition for several years because parasites evade the immune response. When the immune response becomes exacerbated it produces a cascade of immunological mechanisms that cause parasite death, but also severe damage to the neighbouring structures in the host, especially to basal blood vessels. These include dense collagen walls around cysticerci, astrocitic gliosis, microglia and capillary vessel proliferation. When cysticerci start to degenerate they have an appearance of colloidal, whitish vesicles, this stage is followed by a granulomatous one and finally parasites become calcified due to mineralization of the nodule, with surrounding intense gliosis and multinucleated giant cells, typical of a chronic inflammatory reaction to a foreign body. Parasites in different stages of involution are frequently found in the same brain, which suggests either recurrent infections, parasites with different survival abilities or different immune response in different parasites or sites in the brain (Escobar et al. 1983; Sotelo and Del Brutto 2000; Medina-Escutia et al. 2001; Saenz et al. 2006).

Diagnosis of NCC is based on two types of techniques. Imaging techniques (computed tomography, CT, and magnetic resonance, MR) allow the definition of the number, stage, location and extension of the lesions. Immunologic assays identify anticysticercus antibodies and parasite antigens. Based on these techniques and epidemiologic data, several criteria have been established for diagnosis.

1) Absolute, when there is a histological demonstration of the parasite from biopsy of a brain or spinal cord lesion, cystic lesions showing the scolex on CT or MR, and direct visualization of subretinal parasites by funduscopic examination.

2) Major, when there are lesions highly suggestive of NCC on imaging studies, positive western blot in serum for the detection of anticysticercus antibodies, resolution of intracranial cystic lesions after therapy with praziquantel or albendazole, and spontaneous resolution of small single enhancing lesions.

3) Minor, when there are lesions compatible with neurocysticercosis on imaging studies, clinical manifestations suggestive of NCC, positive ELISA for detection of anticysticercus antibodies or cysticercus antigens, and cysticercosis outside the central nervous system.

4) Epidemiologic, when there is evidence of a household contact with T. solium, individuals coming from or living in an area where cysticercosis is endemic, history of frequent travel to disease-endemic areas.

Interpretation of these criteria allows two degrees of diagnostic certainty. Definitive diagnosis is in patients who have one absolute criterion or in those who have two major plus one minor and one epidemiologic criterion. Probable diagnosis, in patients who have one major plus two minor criteria, or one major plus one minor and one epidemiologic criterion, and in those who have three minor plus one epidemiologic criterion (Del Brutto et al. 2001).

In imaging studies, a parenchymal living cysticercus generally is small, round and hypodense (CT) or hypointense (MR). When the parasite is colloidal, an external ring of inflammation appears with contrast fluid. A hyperdense (CT) or hyperintense (MR) invaginated scolex can be seen in both cases. Big living or colloidal cysticerci, up to 5 cm diameter, can be found in the subarachnoidal space or in the ventricles. Calcified parasites are round (hyperdense) and are better detected by CT (Sotelo and Del Brutto 2002, Amara et al. 2003; Arriada et al. 2003; Ito et al. 2006). For immunodiagnostic purposes currently the best technique is immunoblot using a semi-purified fraction obtained from a crude extract of cysticerci with a lentil-lectin column. Seven glycoprotein (GP) bands (with molecular masses of 50, 39–42, 24, 21, 18, 14 and 13 kDa) show 100% specificity for the detection of human cysticercosis. Sensitivity is related to the number of cysticerci in the brain and their viability: 98% sensitivity was found with three or more living cysticerci, while only 65% sensitivity was obtained with one or two parasites (Tsang et al. 1989; Wilson et al. 1991). Also immunoblot has been standardized using GP purified by preparative isoelectrofocusing, which allow successfully using them also in ELISA with almost complete sensitivity and specificity not only in humans but also in pigs and even in dogs (Ito et al. 1998, 2002, 2006; Sako et al. 2000; Sato et al. 2003, 2006).

Treatment of NCC includes cestocidal drugs (praziquantel and albendazole) to kill living parasites and surgical procedures to remove intraventricular or subarachnoidal cysticerci or to place a ventricular shunt. Drugs to control symptoms are frequently used in order to reduce inflammation (corticoids), to control convulsive crisis (antiepileptics) or to reduce pain (analgesics) (Garcia et al. 2002). Pharmacokinetic and toxicological studies performed in humans with either cestocidal drug have shown that these agents have a fast absorption and, in general, lack toxic effects. Efficacy of cestocidal treatment is measured by the reduction in the number and size of cysticerci seen in CT or MR, by clinical improvement, elimination of corticoids or anticonvulsants and by the correction of ventricular dilatation. The most frequent surgical intervention is placement of ventricular shunts to deviate the cerebrospinal fluid to the peritoneal cavity in order to control hydrocephalus. Solitary intraventricular cysticerci can by surgically removed, nowadays even by endoscopy, in order to rapidly improve the patient's health (Bergsneider et al. 2000; Del Brutto et al. 2001; Colli et al. 2002; Sotelo and Del Brutto 2002; Psarros et al. 2003; Jung et al. 2008; Suri et al. 2008).

As with T. saginata, no proven cases have been reported of human cysticercosis caused by T. asiatica, and although the possibility remains it is probably unlikely. At least one study failed to experimentally infect non-human primates (baboons) dosed orally with eggs of T. asiatica (Fall et al. 1995).

Epidemiology

The family Taeniidae comprises around 33 species of tapeworms including the 3 human species. For Taenia of non-human hosts, studies of host ecology and transmission biology are most important, while for the human Taenia species human behaviour, husbandry practices and socio-economic risk factors contribute to transmission, therefore epidemiological studies are essential.

Taenia solium

T. solium and human cysticercosis are widely distributed, with highest transmission in Latin America, India and Southeast (SE) Asia (WHO 1983; WHO/FAO/OIE 2005). Studies indicate underrecognized but significant transmission of the parasite in several countries of sub-Saharan Africa (Geerts et al. 2002), Papua, Indonesia (Gajdusek 1978; Simanjuntak et al. 1997; Margono et al. 2006; Wandra et al. 2007) and of China and SE Asia (Simanjuntak *et al.* 1997; Roman *et al.* 2000; Singh *et al.* 2002; Craig and Ito 2007; Li *et al.* 2007). Nevertheless no global burden for human cysticercosis has yet been calculated (Carabin *et al.* 2005). Epidemiologic studies estimate 5–6 million cases worldwide (Craig *et al.* 1996), including at least 400,000 symptomatic cases in Latin America (Bern *et al.* 1999), 1.5–3 million cases in sub-Saharan Africa (A. L. Willingham personal communication), and 3 million cysticercosis cases estimated for China (Li *et al.* 2007). Furthermore, due to migration there are many neurological cases in developed countries, such as USA, and also recently, tapeworm carriers in the USA and Muslim countries have expanded interest in cysticercosis proposing it as an emerging infectious disease (Schantz *et al.* 1993; Flisser *et al.* 2004a; Sorvillo *et al.* 2011). The economic impact of human and porcine cysticercosis, both in monetary burden and societal losses, is significant (Carabin *et al.* 2005; Rajkotia *et al.* 2007). There has been a formal proposal to declare NCC an international reportable disease (Roman *et al.* 2000), and *T. solium* has been included in a priority list of six human diseases (polio, mumps, rubella, dracunculiasis, lymphatic filariasis and cysticercosis) targeted for global eradication (ITFDE 1993; WHO/DFID-AHP 2006).

The epidemiology of *T. solium* taeniosis/cysticercosis is primarily linked to three main transmission features that must occur in an endemic community:

1) Keeping/raising pigs that have access to human faeces,

2) Lack of latrines or latrines accessible by pigs,

3) Eating undercooked or raw pork as part of local cuisine and/or because of poor cooking.

Human cysticercosis (including neurocysticercosis) is caused only by ingestion of the microscopic eggs or gravid proglottids. Main transmission pathways for human cysticercosis occur when eggs contaminate the hands of a tapeworm carrier which increases the chance of self-infection as up to 30% of neurocysticercosis patients report a history of taeniosis (Gilman *et al.* 2000). Eggs may contaminate persons that have contact with a tapeworm carrier, or contaminate food prepared by a carrier, or contaminate vegetables close to indiscriminate sites of human defecation, or vegetables may be contaminated by eggs via human faeces as fertilizer (the latter practice remains common in parts of China and south east Asia). Other possible routes for egg contamination in humans may occur, such as deliberate use of proglottids as traditional medicaments (for example in South Africa) (Heinz and Macnab 1965). Note therefore that absence of pork eating may not prevent occurrence of human cysticercosis in a *T. solium* endemic area or even infection in low-risk groups, as long as at least one tapeworm carrier occurs in a household or local community (Schantz *et al.* 1992, WHO/FAO/OIE 2005).

In endemic communities in Latin America prevalence of human taeniosis based on microscopy/coproantigen ELISA is usually below 3%, porcine cysticercosis seropositivity or tongue palpation prevalence range from 1–>50%, and human cysticercosis seropositivity from 3–25% (Allan *et al.* 1996a; Garcia-Noval *et al.* 1996; Rodriguez-Canul *et al.* 1999; Flisser *et al.* 2003; Garcia *et al.* 2003b; Flisser and Gyorkos 2007). The incidence of epilepsy/seizures/convulsions (the main symptom of neurocysticercosis) was 18–29 per 1,000 in Central American communities, of which 40% of cases may have detectable lesions compatible with NCC. However, there is not always a clear association between seropositivity and seizure

history and/or a CT scan positive image (Garcia-Noval *et al.* 2001, 2002). Official abattoir slaughter rates for porcine cysticercosis, while useful in identification of potential hotspots, are usually of little practical value because most pigs from poor rural endemic communities are slaughtered at home or within a village setting. For example, in one highly endemic *T. solium* area of SW China, only 1.3% of pigs slaughtered at abattoirs were positive by meat inspection (Li *et al.* 2007). In a recent study, porcine cysticercosis based on Ag-ELISA and lingual examination was mapped at household level to identify local clusters of the infection. Statistical analysis established the spatial distribution of infected pigs in Mbulu district, northern Tanzania that is expected to guide control strategies (Nogowi *et al.* 2010). Epidemiological studies in Latin America, especially in Mexico, Guatemala, Honduras, Ecuador, Bolivia and Peru, have helped to identify major risk factors for taeniosis and human and porcine cysticercosis in rural endemic communities in that region. These are summarized below.

Risk of human taeniosis

These include eating undercooked pork, living in a household with infected pigs, female, age 10–39 years, *Taenia* carriers in the household and seropositivity for anti-cysticercus antibodies (Sarti *et al.* 1988, 1992, 1997, 2000; Allan *et al.* 1996a; Rodriguez-Canul *et al.* 1999; Garcia *et al.* 2003b).

Risk of human cysticercosis

A history of taeniosis (Gilman *et al.* 2000); person older than 10 years (Garcia *et al.* 1995, 946 patients); presence of a tapeworm carrier (person who is taeniid egg positive, coproantigen positive, and/or passed proglottids) in a household/family or in a neighbouring house or housing cluster (Sarti *et al.* 1988, 1994, 2000; Diaz-Camacho *et al.* 1990; Sanchez *et al.* 1998; Garcia-Noval *et al.* 1996; Garcia *et al.* 2003b); raising pigs; presence of cysticercosis positive pigs (tongue palpation, immunoblot seropositive, or necropsy positive) in a household (Garcia *et al.* 2003b); presence in family/household of a person with a history of late-onset (>18 years of age) seizures/epilepsy; immunoblot seropositive for antibobodies against low molecular weight (<50KDa) *T. solium* metacestode glycoproteins (Garcia-Noval *et al.* 1996; Garcia *et al.* 2003b). Additionally, care should be taken regarding the detection of circulating T. solium antigens in humans, since when the prevalence in residents of three villages in Burkina Faso was obtained, the results indicated that there can be large variation of human seropositivity to the presence of the larval stages of T. solium cysticercosis among rural areas of the same country and, specially, that the serological level of the antigen, not just whether it is positive or negative, must be considered when assessing prevalence of human cysticercosis antigens (Carabin *et al.* 2009).

Risk of porcine cysticercosis

Presence of a human tapeworm carrier in a household (Sarti *et al.* 1988; Lescano *et al.* 2007); lack of latrine (Sarti *et al.* 1992, 1994; Allan *et al.* 1996b; Vazquez-Flores *et al.* 2001); presence of free-range backyard or wandering pigs in communities that practice home-slaughter (Rodriguez-Canul *et al.* 1998; 1999); a seropositive pig within 50–500 metres of a house with a *Taenia* carrier (Lescano *et al.* 2007).

Whilst transmission of *T. solium* occurs mainly in rural areas of under-developed regions where pig ownership is high (Flisser *et al.* 2003), transmission or outbreaks of human cysticercosis have also been described in urban foci in endemic countries such as Ecuador and Peru (Goodman *et al.* 1999; Huisa *et al.* 2005). Furthermore, serological surveys revealed 12–15% cysticercosis seropositivity in soldiers living in Tegucigalpa (capital city of Honduras) and in Mexico City (Sanchez *et al.* 1998; Garcia-Garcia *et al.* 1999). Also, NCC cases have occurred in extremely low risk individuals in affluent households in New York City as a result of transmission of *T. solium* eggs from tapeworm positive house-maids (Schantz *et al.* 1992).

As previously discussed, recent molecular genotypic analysis of mitochondrial DNA extracted from *T. solium* isolates from different world regions, indicated two main genotypes, clades or strains, i.e. an Asian type and an African/Latin American type (Nakao *et al.* 2002). These have since been confirmed in several studies. However, it is not yet clear if the two genotypes exhibit differing epidemiology, transmission patterns or pathology (Craig and Ito 2007).

Taenia saginata

The human beef tapeworm, *T. saginata*, is the commonest taeniid of humans with an estimated 60–70 million carriers worldwide (Flisser and Craig 2005; Craig and Ito 2007). In highly endemic regions, for example Ethiopia, Bali and Tibet, 22–27% prevalences of human *T. saginata* taeniosis have been recorded (Li *et al.* 2006; Wandra *et al.* 2006a, b; Craig and Ito 2007). In Europe and Australia beef tapeworm infection remains endemic, albeit at low prevalence (usually <0.05%), probably maintained in part due to the practice of application of sewage sludge on to pastures (Rickard *et al.* 1977; Cabaret *et al.* 2002). Human cysticercosis cannot be caused by ingestion of *T. saginata* eggs and therefore the public health impact for this parasite is limited to gut infection of humans (taeniosis). Consequently the epidemiology of this tapeworm species chiefly concerns transmission from human carriers to cattle, yak or other bovines. Bovine cysticercosis is however of economic importance because it may be responsible for condemnation or downgrading of meat, and even prevent development of potential beef export markets in resource-poor economies (Kebede 2008).

The risk factor for human *T. saginata* taeniosis is eating raw or under-cooked beef. Therefore *T. saginata* is more prevalent in communities or populations where dietary practices or cuisines include under-cooked and/or raw beef. For example in Sichuan and Yunnan provinces of SW China, and in Bali, Indonesia, raw beef is a delicacy. Consequently in their rural populations *T. saginata* taeniosis prevalence may be >20% (Li *et al.* 2006; Wandra *et al.* 2006b). In Bali, Indonesia 56/60 cases of suspected *T. saginata* were detected by questionnaire in a community study (n = 398) and confirmed as *T. saginata* by PCR. Males had a significantly higher prevalence and the risk age group was 30–44 years (Wandra *et al.* 2006a). A similar cross-sectional epidemiological study (n = 661) in a Tibetan area of western Sichuan Province (China) found that 31% of persons reported a history of proglottid expulsion, and 18 of 21 proglottid positives tested by PCR were confirmed as *T. saginata* and three as *T. asiatica*. Of the 21 faecal samples from *Taenia* carriers 18 were also coproantigen ELISA positive (Li *et al.* 2007). In these 2 studies risk factors for taeniosis were consumption of raw beef, a history of passing proglottids in the previous 1–2 years, owning cattle/yak, poor hygiene/hand-washing and low level of education. Mean age of first infection (anamnesis) in 26 *T. saginata* cases treated in Addis Ababa was 12.2 years (Tesfa-Yohannes 1990).

Taenia asiatica

Taenia asiatica has been found in Taiwan, Korea, China, Vietnam, Philippines, Indonesia and Thailand. It is expected to also occur in Lao PD, Cambodia and Myanmar (Ito *et al.* 2007, 2008). *T. asiatica* was only described formally as a new tapeworm of humans in 1993 (Eom and Rim 1993). Prior to that its occurrence in rural communities of south east Asia was attributed to *T. saginata*, to which it closely resembles morphologically, but was often described in patients that consumed raw pig liver but not beef (Isobe 1922; Huang *et al.* 1966; Chao *et al.* 1979; Fan 1988; Fan *et al.* 1990; Eom and Rim 1993; Ito *et al.* 2003). It appears that spontaneous release of motile segments occurs in *T. asiatica* infections in the same way as for *T. saginata* and similarly therefore *T. asiatica* carriers are usually aware of their infection (Craig and Ito 2007; Wandra *et al.* 2007).

There have been relatively few epidemiological studies in known *T. asiatica* endemic communities, because previous studies were unable to differentiate *T. asiatica* and *T. saginata*, and so the majority of infections were classed as *T. saginata* (Eom and Rim 2001; Ito *et al.* 2003). One recent specific epidemiologic study on *T. asiatica* was undertaken in a rural Batak ethnic community in Ambarita village on Samosir Island, Lake Toba, Sumatra (Wandra *et al.* 2006b). A total of 240 persons were voluntarily registered and answered a questionnaire, which indicated eight persons with a history of passing proglottids, and six (2.5% total prevalence) of these passed *T. asiatica* tapeworms (confirmed by PCR). Interestingly all six cases were coproparasitologically negative for *Taenia* eggs, but four that were tested by coproantigen ELISA were positive. Risk factors for *T. asiatica* taeniosis in the Lake Toba community were: consumption of pork (only 2.5% of population ate beef), home slaughter of pigs, predilection for raw pig liver and lack of sanitary facilities (Wandra *et al.* 2006b, 2007). Since experimental infections in pigs performed with eggs from *T. asiatica* (Lake Toba isolate) developed cysticerci in the liver and not in the muscles or other locations (Fan *et al.* 1990, 2006), it is likely that in parts of Southeast Asia the distribution of *T. asiatica* and *T. solium* will be sympatric. This appears to be the case, at least, in Tibetan and Bai ethnic groups in SW China (Li *et al.* 2006) and in Karen ethnic communities on the Thai-Myanmar border (Anantaphruti *et al.* 2007). In the latter study in Kanchanaburi Province Thailand, all three human *Taenia* species occurred in those communities where under-cooked pork and beef were consumed, and at least one dual infection with *T. solium* and *T. asiatica* adult tapeworms was confirmed after DNA analysis (Fig. 51.3).

Transmission dynamics

There have been relatively few quantitative studies in relation to the transmission dynamics of the human *Taenia* spp. In contrast, a significant number of experimental and field studies were used to construct transmission models for the common taeniid species of livestock. Animal studies with *Taenia* species can be used to understand transmission dynamics of *T. solium* (Lawson and Gemmell 1989).

At any one time a *Taenia* parasite population will be in one of three states: the egg, the metacestode (cysticercus), or the adult; all three states can happen simultaneously in one community and even in the same human host in the case of *T. solium*. The effects of environmental factors such as temperature, humidity, dispersal (rain, arthropods) on eggs in the environment were important in consideration of transmission of dog-sheep taeniid species (Lawson and Gemmell 1983). For *T. solium* however the rapid direct ingestion of human faeces by pigs is common so that eggs may not be exposed for long periods in an endemic environment (Martinez-Maya *et al.* 2000). A recent study based on experimental pig infections further indicates that pig-pig transmission may occur through coprophagy i.e. pig-human coprophagy followed by pig-pig coprophagy (Gonzalez *et al.* 2006). The distribution of cestode larvae in the pig intermediate host is usually over-dispersed, with acquired immunity stimulated by egg/oncosphere challenge and age-specific resistance also occurring probably within 15 days (Gemmell *et al.* 1987) the duration of immunity is not clear but probably lasts three months in the absence of egg challenge (Kyvsgaard *et al.* 2007). Pigs may be protected against *T. solium* egg infection from probably as little as 10 eggs, and immunity can be passively transferred from pregnant sow to new born piglets to provide up to 2–4 months protection (Gemmell *et al.* 1987; Gonzalez *et al.* 2002). In humans the biotic potential of a gravid adult *T. solium* tapeworm is relatively high with possibly 200,000 eggs passed per day, though the size (approximately 2–3 m) and life-span (probably months to a few years) of this species appears to be significantly below that for *T. saginata* (Allan *et al.* 1996a; Flisser 2006; Craig and Ito 2007). The basic reproductive number (Ro) for *T. solium* has been assumed to be close to one (Gonzalez *et al.* 2002), nevertheless a relatively low prevalence (~1%) of human taeniosis can still sustain transmission of *T. solium* (WHO/FAO/OIE, 2005). In addition to these parasite factors, transmission dynamics of *T. solium* will be affected by human/pig interrelations, pig behaviour, human sanitary habits and local socio-economic factors (Lawson and Gemmell 1989; Sarti *et al.* 1997; Gonzalez *et al.* 2002; Kyvsgaard *et al.* 2007). Knowledge of the transmission dynamics will assist in development of rational intervention simulations and control programs.

Prevention and control

In theory it should be relatively easy to prevent the occurrence of human taeniosis/cysticercosis and to break the parasitic life-cycle of the three human *Taenia* species. This is because humans are the only natural definitive hosts, and domestic pigs and cattle, the only important intermediate hosts. Consequently *T. solium* was added to the list of eradicable diseases (ITFDE 1993; Schantz *et al.* 1993). However, in practice it will be very difficult to implement control measures in poor rural areas of developing countries in which *T. solium* is highly endemic and where sanitation is poor or absent, where there exists cultural preference for under-cooked pork, where home-slaughter is the norm, and where pigs are bred unpenned and allowed to roam free. Furthermore, pork is the most popular meat consumed worldwide with at least 300 million pigs in endemic regions (Flisser *et al.* 2003, 2006). The demand for household pig rearing and pork protein is growing rapidly in resource-poor regions which will increase the transmission potential of *T. solium* and the probability of exposure to human taeniosis/cysticercosis (Lekule and Kyvsgaard 2003; WHO/DFID-AHP, 2006).

Prevention and control of cysticercosis/taeniosis can be considered as a long-term horizontal approach eg, improved sanitation, husbandry, slaughter regulations, meat inspection, and general education. Education is making a difference in Mexico. Recently, information to support the viewpoint that neurocysticercosis may

no longer be a public health problem in Mexico was published (Flisser and Correa 2010), based on the dramatic decrease in the frequency of cysticercosis and taeniosis available from the national surveillance system of the Mexican Ministry of Health. A possible explanation to the previous phenomenon is that publications of the Mexican scientific and medical community working on cysticercosis on imaging and immunological diagnosis, clinical studies, cestocidal treatments, epidemiological surveys and control interventions led to the publication and implementation of the Official Mexican Guidelines for the Control and Prevention of Taeniosis/Cysticercosis that establish criteria, strategies and operative techniques and are obligatory for the whole Mexican territory; importantly, they include treatment of tapeworm carriers. Another factor of major importance is the general improvement of living conditions in Mexico, which are illustrated in the PLoS paper. Control measures can be more focused or vertically directed interventions that aim to break the transmission cycle over shorter periods. There are 4 main options for such directed shorter-term intervention approaches:

1) Directed health/husbandry education,

2) Mass treatment against human taeniosis,

3) Mass chemotherapy against porcine cysticercosis,

4) Anti-cysticercosis livestock vaccines.

Of course combinations of some of the above interventions are likely to further improve control efficacy, especially against *T. solium*. In addition appropriate surveillance methods and systems, including modern computer simulations to model cost-effective intervention approaches, are required at local and regional scales to measure control effect and monitor progress.

Animal husbandry, meat inspection, sanitation and socio-economic development

Pork 'measles' was known in ancient Greece and described by Aristotle. Furthermore pork vendors in ancient Rome had to guarantee that pig meat was free of measles. In the Middle Ages the Ausburg Charter of 1276 stated, '*If a butcher kills a measly hog, he shall sell it to no one without a statement of this fact*' (Discussed in Viljoen 1937). An understanding of the life-cycle of *T. solium* after its elucidation and publication by Kuchenmeister in Germany in 1855, quickly resulted in formal recommendations about the dangers of eating under-cooked pork, and also clarified why the infection was rare in Jewish and Muslim communities (Grove 1990). Over the next 100 years the prevalence of human and porcine cysticercosis slowly declined across Western Europe, primarily through gradual improvements in sanitation, the adoption of formal meat inspection measures, less consumption of raw pork (in part because of historic outbreak of trichinellosis in continental Europe), and the move to more intensive rearing of pigs (Grove 1990; WHO/FAO/OIE 2005). Endemic foci of *T. solium* however remain today in parts of rural Portugal and Spain where free-range pig husbandry is still not uncommon (Overbosch 2002; WHO/FAO/OIE 2005).

The connection between bovine cysticercosis ('beef measles') and an outbreak of human taeniosis in soldiers in South Africa was noted by Knox in 1819 and, following these observations, the role of cattle in the life-cycle of *T. saginata* was elucidated in 1861 by Leuckart (Viljoen 1937). Several authors by the late nineteenth and early twentieth centuries already advocated the inspection of slaughtered cattle, treatment of measly beef by freezing (−10°C for

2–6 days), and cooking or heating infected beef (Grove 1990). For *T. solium*, cysticerci are killed at −20°C for 1–3 days (Sotelo *et al.* 1986; Garcia *et al.* 2007) and proper salting of pork (12–24 hours) is also effective (Rodriguez-Canul *et al.* 2002). In most of Europe the prevalence of *T. saginata* taeniosis has declined to levels below 0.1% (range 0.01–2%), while prevalence of bovine cysticercosis at meat inspection ranges between 0.02 and 7% (Cabaret *et al.* 2002). Improved sanitation in Europe has no doubt reduced the likelihood of direct contamination of grazing pastures. However indiscriminate defecation by campers, walkers, travellers etc., and the use of treated urban sewage sludge to irrigate pastures, has probably maintained transmission of *T. saginata* in several parts of the developed world (Rickard *et al.* 1977; Cabaret *et al.* 2002). In Switzerland during 2005 and 2006, 119 farms with infected cattle were identified at slaughter as compared to 66 randomly selected farms with cattle slaughtered in the same period but with no evidence or history of infection. The presence of a railway line or a car park close to areas grazed by cattle, leisure activities around these areas, use of purchased roughage and organized public activities on farms attracting visitors, were the risk factors, pointing to outdoor defecation by tapeworm carriers (Flutsch *et al.* 2008).

Routine meat inspection usually involves up to five knife cuts in specific sites on the carcass (e.g. masseters, upper foreleg, hind-leg, heart, tongue). However >30% of infected cattle or pig carcasses (especially with light infections) may not be detected by these methods (WHO/FAO/OIE 2005; Phiri *et al.* 2006; Geysen *et al.* 2007). Restraint or corralling of pigs in resource-poor settings is effective in preventing ingestion of human faeces (Vazquez-Flores *et al.* 2001). In practice this is not easy to implement because of economic constraints. Furthermore in parts on India, Indonesia and China pigs are restrained or penned deliberately under or close to latrines so that they are able to remove human faecal waste from the household environment (PS Craig, unpublished observation). Backyard-free-roaming pigs or semi-confined household pigs in southern Mexico had significantly higher *T. solium* seropositive rates compared to more intensively farmed animals (Sarti *et al.* 1994, 1997, 2000; Rodriguez-Canul *et al.* 1998). Reports of restraint of pigs that were normally free-roaming have indicated decrease in swine cysticercosis rates in Peru, Mexico and China (Bern *et al.* 1999; Vazquez-Flores *et al.* 2001; Pawlowski *et al.* 2005).

Health education

Humans can acquire cysticercosis after accidentally ingesting *T. solium* eggs. Furthermore, the prevalence of taeniosis among patients with neurocysticercosis is higher than previously reported. In addition, a clear association between the presence of taeniosis and the severity of neurocysticercosis was seen, since most massive cerebral infections (with more than 100 cysticerci) were present in patients who harboured the adult tapeworm in the intestine. Therefore, the perception that tapeworms are silent guests, causing no harm to humans, is erroneous and tapeworm carriers should be regarded as potential risks to themselves and to those living in their close environment (Gilman *et al.* 2000). Consequently, an important risk factor is the presence of a tapeworm carrier in the household or neighbourhood (Sarti *et al.* 1988; Flisser 2002b; Flisser and Gyorkos 2007). A study performed in a Mexican municipality with around 750,000 inhabitants showed that self-identification of tapeworm carriers is a feasible tool for control of *T. solium* (Flisser *et al.* 2005b). Also, identified tapeworm carriers can be treated with a high degree of efficacy (Jeri *et al.* 2004).

Health education in relation to taeniosis/cysticercosis could, in theory, lead to the acquisition of appropriate knowledge required to understand the life-cycle of the parasite. That knowledge could result in a change in risk-behaviours and/or husbandry practices that help propagate transmission, with a resultant reduction in human and livestock infection/exposure indices. There are only a few modern examples of specific education programmes in relation to *T. solium*, and very few, if any, reported for *T. saginata* or *T. asiatica*. In the late 1980s and early 1990s community based epidemiologic studies on *T. solium* in Mexico began to identify some of the sociological/behavioural risk factors for human and porcine infection (Sarti *et al.* 1988, 1992; Schantz *et al.* 1994). As a consequence, two educational intervention programs were developed and applied to rural communities in Mexico. In Guerrero State, 131 families were given health education about the parasite and associated risk factors, and after two years 76% of children but only 2% of adults acquired specific knowledge. Disappointingly the pre-intervention prevalence of tongue palpable cysticerci in one year old pigs increased from 6% to 11% (Keilbach *et al.* 1989). In Morelos State, a rural population (n = 1,931) was subjected to intense health education which used knowledge acquisition questionnaires, tongue palpation with immunoblot serology in pigs, and microscopy and coproantigen rates in humans, as pre-intervention and post-intervention indicators of transmission. Although there was no significant difference in human taeniosis rates before and after the educational programme, health education increased villagers' knowledge about the parasite and transmission, despite an apparent lack of observed major behavioural changes. Nevertheless in this case there was significantly reduced porcine infection and exposure rates after six months (Sarti *et al.* 1997), which remained up to 42 months (Flisser and Correa 2010).

A health education intervention trial was also recently applied in north eastern Tanzania-but differed from the Mexican one in that the study was a randomized control programme (n = 827 households, including 418 as household controls), targeted towards pig husbandry including building proper pig pens, as well as pit latrines, and safe disposal of human faeces; sentinel pigs were employed as transmission indicators over a one year period. Similar to the Morelos study, despite significant gain in knowledge acquisition, there was no improvement in observed risk practices amongst targeted or control households. However the porcine incidence rate based on tongue palpation and circulating antigen testing in sentinel pigs (given to each family) was significantly lower in the health education intervention household group, as was reported pork consumption (Ngowi *et al.* 2008). Interestingly, factors associated with the prevalence of circulating antigens to porcine cysticercosis in three villages of Burkina Faso were studied. The results of the logistic regression analyses suggest that people acquire knowledge of porcine cysticercosis, but this happens, following the infection of their animals (Ganaba *et al.* 2011). The authors conclude that education of pig farmers is urgently needed to reduce the prevalence of this infection. Long-term follow-up was not reported and it remains to be seen whether public health education alone could provide sustained decrease in transmission of *T. solium* in resource-poor communities in Latin America, Sub Saharan Africa or elsewhere. Interestingly rigorous health education programmes for cystic echinococcosis in resource-rich countries/regions were not always effective for long-term sustained reduction of transmission of *Echinococcus granulosus* (Craig and Larrieu 2006).

Taeniosis mass drug treatment

The life-cycles of *T. solium, T. saginata* and *Taenia asiatica* involve humans as the only obligatory definitive host. Therefore, effective anthelmintic mass treatment of human populations in endemic areas could result in control of transmission or even elimination of the parasite (Pawlowski 1990). Furthermore, the provision of annual or sub-annual mass treatment for school age children using albendazole for gastrointestinal nematode and other infections has been very successful in reducing the burden of chronic helminth infections in under-developed regions (Molyneux *et al.* 2005; Flisser *et al.* 2008). Consequently, the approach of mass treatment against human taeniosis has gained support. Furthermore, effective tapeworm treatment could remove any (or more than one) of the three *Taenia* species (as well as *Hymenolepis nana*) where they are sympatric (Allan *et al.* 2002; WHO/FAO/OIE 2005; Anantaphruti *et al.* 2007; Craig and Ito 2007).

There are several factors to consider in relation to mass treatment for human taeniosis however, that are different from directly transmitted gastrointestinal nematodes.

1) The age-specific prevalence of *T. solium* taeniosis is distributed mainly above the school-age group (ie. >15 years old) (Allan *et al.* 1996b; Sarti *et al.* 1997, 2000; Garcia *et al.* 2003b), and thus targeted treatment to schools would not be so effective.

2) The prevalence of human *T. solium* taeniosis is usually below 3.5% in endemic communities and therefore very high population coverage is required.

3) Pigs if untreated, act as a reservoir of infection back to the human population.

4) The most effective anthelmintic drug against human taeniosis is praziquantel (not albendazole the preferred drug in mass-treatment of gastrointestinal nematodes), but this drug is also used to treat neurocysticercosis and therefore has the potential to cause cerebral inflammation in asymptomatic neurocysticercosis cases. Despite that risk for mass administration of praziquantel such clinical effects have to date only rarely been reported (Cruz *et al.* 1989; Flisser *et al.*1993). In relation to praziquantel safety, that drug has been extensively used in China and Africa at higher dosage for mass treatment campaigns against schistosomosis without apparent adverse effects on asymptomatic neurocysticercosis (Pawlowski 2006).

At the present time (2011) only six studies have been reported internationally since 1989 in which mass drug administration was used to control *T. solium* transmission, and all of these were carried out in Latin America (summarized in Table 51.2). Five of these studies used praziquantel and one niclosamide as the taenicidal agent. Niclosamide is slightly less efficacious (85–90%) than praziquantel (>95%) and is five times more expensive and has a more limited shelf-life (Pawlowski *et al.* 2005). Niclosamide however has the advantage that the drug is poorly absorbed from the gut and therefore would not cause potential inadvertent effects on asymptomatic neurocysticercosis. Also *Taenia* tapeworms are usually passed intact after niclosamide treatment which facilitates identification (Allan *et al.* 1996b, 2002).

The endemic *T. solium* rural populations targeted ranged in size from <400 in Sinaloa Mexico to 10,000 in the Loja/El Oro region of south Ecuador. Follow-up occurred at various periods from four to 40 months but the average was one year. Pre and post intervention surveillance was mainly based on human taeniosis prevalence (stool examination and/or coproantigen test), and porcine cysticercosis prevalence/incidence in pig cohorts born after the intervention (necropsy, tongue palpation and/or serology). In one study in Peru the pig population was also subjected to mass treatment with the drug oxfendazole (Garcia *et al.* 2006). Other factors, such as health education and changes in behaviour as well as improved sanitation and pig husbandry may have occurred in parallel as a result of the programme design, or indirectly occurred in the community, and thus could have influenced the effect of taeniosis mass-treatment (Allan *et al.* 2002). Five of the six mass treatment programmes (see Table 51.2), where human taeniosis was monitored, showed a statistically significant decrease in the prevalence of taeniosis within one year of mass treatment, with no taeniosis

Table 51.2 Summary of 6 control programmes for *T. solium* in rural communities in Latin America where mass treatment of human taeniosis was applied

Country (site/start year of programme)	Human Pop.	Drug mg/kg, no. doses (% coverage)	Follow-up period	Taeniosis pre-tx (%)	Taeniosis post-tx (%)	Pig cysticercosis pre- (%)	Pig cysticercosis post- (%)	Ref.
Ecuador (Loja/1986)	10,000	PZQ 5mg/kg, x1 (76%)	1 year	1.6 °	0 (n = 539)	11.4*	2.6 (n = 113)	Cruz *et al.* (1989)
Mexico (Guerrero/1986)	530	PZQ 5mg/kg, x1 (60%)	4 months–1 year	3.2 °	0	6** (n = 440)	11	Keilbach *et al.* (1989)
Mexico (Sinaloa/1989)	339	PZQ 10mg/kg, x1 (71%)	1 year	1.3°	0 (n = 238)	ND	ND	Diaz-Camacho *et al.* (1991)
Mexico (Morelos/1991)	1865	PZQ 5mg/kg, x1 (87%)	3.5 years	1.1++	0.5 (n = 605)	1.2** 4.8+	0.6 3.4	Sarti *et al.* (2000)
Guatemala (Santa Gertrudis/1994)	1582	Niclosamide 1gm, x1 (75%)	10 months	3.5++	1.0	55+	7 (n = 330)	Allan *et al.* (1997)
Peru (Quilcas/1996)	2100	PZQ 5mg/kg, x1 (75%)	18 months	ND	ND	0.57+^ plus OXF	0.40	Garcia *et al.* (2006)

° Stool exam/worm recovery; ++ coproantigen/worm recovery; * pig necropsy.
** pig tongue palpation; + pig serology; ^ total mean sero-incidence; plus OXF additional treatment of two rounds oxfendazole in pigs (n = 3177) at 30mg/kg; PZQ praziquantel.

cases being detected post-intervention in three of those studies (Cruz *et al.* 1989; Keilbach *et al.* 1989; Diaz-Camacho *et al.* 1991). In all but one intervention study, porcine cysticercosis rates were also significantly reduced after 1–3.5 years follow-up, but pig infection was not eliminated (Sarti *et al.* 2000). Even when two rounds of oxfendazole dosing of pigs was included with a taeniosis mass treatment program for the human population, the parasite persisted in the pig population despite significant decrease in porcine seroprevalence and seroconversion rates (Garcia *et al.* 2006).

Taenicidal drug coverage of the human population was never above 70–90% in these six mass treatment programmes and therefore persistence of a handful of tapeworm carriers in a treated community could still maintain transmission because of the high biotic potential of the parasite. Nevertheless these studies demonstrate that at least short-term reduction (within one year) in transmission of *T. solium* may occur after taeniosis mass-treatment. Long term assessments have not been carried out except in Morelos (Mexico) where 42 months after mass administration with a single dose of praziquantel, human taeniosis prevalence remained 56% below the pre-intervention rate, pig tongue palpation rates were 52% lower and the seroprevalence of human cysticercus antibodies was 75% reduced (Sarti *et al.* 2000; Flisser and Correa 2010). In this study 5mg/kg instead of 10 mg/pg praziquantel were used (as recommended by WHO, Pawlowski 1990), and therefore drug efficacy was 50% instead of 95%. Mass treatment alone will therefore probably not be enough to interrupt transmission of *T. solium,* which appears to return to pre-intervention levels within 2–3 years (Garcia *et al.* 2007). Therefore options should consider more frequent drug administration and ensure that >95% of the population is treated (Gonzalez *et al.* 2002). Alternatively specific identification and treatment of tapeworm carriers should be also considered (Flisser *et al.* 2005b).

Mass treatment for *T. saginata* taeniosis is unlikely to be cost-effective because this parasite does not cause sufficient economic or public health impacts. However in some regions where *T. saginata* is common, self-medication on a large scale may occur; for example in Addis Ababa (Ethiopia) where >80% of the adult population regularly take taenicidal drugs (Tesfa-Yohannes 1990; Pawlowski 2006). Prophylactic use of taenicidal drugs by workers in cattle feed-lots may also reduce the risk of local outbreaks of bovine cysticercosis in both developed and resource-poor settings (Dorny *et al.* 2002).

Anthelmintic mass drug treatment of livestock

The possibility to use anti-metacestode drugs to control the transmission of *T. solium* from pigs to humans has also been investigated. Both praziquantel and albendazole can affect the viability of *T. solium* cysticerci in pigs, and the latter was 100% effective in killing muscle cysticerci (non viable cysts were present) though viable cysts remained in the brain (Flisser *et al.* 1990; Peniche-Cardenas *et al.* 2002). Praziquantel was highly effective even at one day treatment (Torres *et al.* 1992). The overall efficacy of both drugs, however, was not as great as oxfendazole for treatment of porcine cysticercosis (Gonzalez *et al.* 1996), although this latter drug was used at a higher dose than the one commercially available. A single dose (30mg/kg) of oxfendazole caused cyst death and disappearance within 3 months of treating infected pigs, and pigs also appeared refractory to further infection for another 3 months (Gonzalez *et al.* 1996; 2001). In rural Latin America and in other resource-poor regions, pigs are usually about 9 months old at slaughter, so a single dose of oxfendazole or praziquantel (or better two doses at 3 months and 6 months) could in theory keep pigs free of cysticerci for that period with the added advantage of full economic return on the carcass (Torres *et al.* 1992; Gonzalez *et al.* 2003). Despite these results, an intervention trial that used mass administration of oxfendazole to pigs in parallel with mass praziquantel administration to the human population in Peru, reduced transmission but did not eliminate human taeniosis or porcine cysticercosis after 18 months (Garcia *et al.* 2006).

Cysticercosis vaccines for livestock

The marked protective immune response of sheep and cattle to experimental egg challenge or vaccination with oncosphere antigen extracts of various *Taenia* species, lead the development of protective subunit vaccines against cysticercosis and echinococcosis (Lightowlers and Gauci 2001; Lightowlers 2003; 2006; reviewed by Flisser and Lightowlers 2001). In 1989 the first recombinant subunit anti-parasite vaccine (To45W) was developed, and this was for *Taenia ovis*, the cause of ovine cysticercosis, a non-zoonotic metacestode disease of economic importance (Johnson *et al.* 1989). Following that success, which was based on the use of a recombinant oncosphere peptide antigen, the homologous genes were identified in *T. saginata* and the expressed peptides (TSA-9/TSA-18) given intramuscularly with adjuvant to cattle resulted in 99% protection against oral challenge with *T. saginata* eggs (Lightowlers *et al.* 1996). Efforts were subsequently directed towards the scaling-up of both vaccines (for ovine and bovine cysticercosis) for production such that adequate quantities and quality-controlled vaccines are available for practical use (Lightowlers 2006).

A parallel approach using the homologous genes was subsequently adopted for development of a *T. solium* recombinant subunit oncosphere vaccine (TSOL18) against porcine cysticercosis which gave 99.5–100% protection against experimental egg challenge infection of pigs (Flisser *et al.* 2004b; Gonzalez *et al.* 2005). A field trial of TSOL18 in 240 community owned pigs 2–3 months old, carried out in an endemic area of Cameroon, resulted in 100% protection (cysticerci free) at 12 months slaughter compared to a 19.6% infection rate in control animals (Assava *et al.* 2010). There are other putative anti-infection vaccines for *T. solium* cysticercosis (Flisser and Lightowlers 2001; Hernandez *et al.* 2007), but it is likely that TSOL18 will provide the most effective protective vaccine in pigs for further assessment and eventual incorporation into *T. solium* control programmes (Gonzalez *et al.* 2003; Pawlowski *et al.* 2005). The more difficult proposition for the therapeutic vaccination of intermediate hosts against already established taeniid larval cysts has been considered but remains largely experimental (Bøgh *et al.* 1988; Craig and Zumbuehl 1988; Evans 2002).

Surveillance methods

Prevention and control of any infectious/parasitic disease cannot be reliably undertaken without appropriate surveillance tools. Several approaches and tools have been developed for taeniosis/cysticercosis, especially in relation to epidemiological and intervention studies for *T. solium*. Surveillance is important in the human population for taeniosis and cysticercosis, and in the pig population for cysticercosis. In addition, health education acquisition by the target population can be measured by questionnaires and observational studies. A number of diagnostic or detection methods have been developed for *T. solium* (Schantz and Sarti 1989; Garcia *et al.* 2003a).

Johnson, K.S. *et al.* (1989). Vaccination against ovine cysticercosis using a defined recombinant antigen. *Nature*, **338**: 585–87.

Jongwutiwes, S. *et al.* (2004). Jejunal perforation caused by morphologically abnormal *Taenia saginata* infection. *J. Infect.*, **49**: 324–28.

Jung, R.C. *et al.* (1981). Racemose cysticercus in human brain. A case report. *Am. J. Trop. Med. Hyg.*, **30**: 620–24.

Jung, H. *et al.* (2008). Medical treatment for neurocysticercosis: drugs, indications and perspectives. *Curr. Topics Med. Chem.*, **8**: 424–33.

Karanikas, I.D. *et al.* (2007). Taenia saginata: a rare cause of bowel obstruction. *Trans. R. Soc. Trop. Med. Hyg.*, **101**: 527–28.

Kebede, N. (2008). Cysticercosis of slaughtered cattle in northwestern Ethiopia. *Res. Vet. Sci.*, **85**: 522–26.

Keilbach, N.M. *et al.* (1989). A program to control taeniasis-cysticercosis (*T.solium*): experiences in a Mexican village. *Acta Leid.*, **57**: 181–89.

Kosin, E. *et al.* (1972). Taeniasis di Pulau Samosir. *Maj. Kedok. Universitat.*, **3**: 5–11.

Kyvsgaard, N.C. *et al.* (2007). Simulating transmission and control of *Taenia solium* infections using a Reed-Frost stochastic model. *Int. J. Parasitol.*, **37**: 547–58.

Laclette, J.P. *et al.* (1982). *Ultrastructure of the surrounding envelopes of Taenia solium eggs*. In: A. Flisser *et al.* (eds.) *Cysticercosis. Present state of knowledge and perspectives*, pp. 375–87. NY: Academic Press.

Lawson, J.R. and Gemmell, M.A. (1983). Hydatidosis and cysticercosis: the dynamics of transmission. *Adv. Parasitol.*, **22**: 261–308.

Lawson, J.R. and Gemmell, M.A. (1989). The ovine cysticercosis as models for research into the epidemiology and control of the human and porcine cysticercosis *Taenia solium*: II. The application of control. *Acta Leiden.*, **57**: 173–80.

Lekule, F.P. and Kyvsgaard, N.C. (2003). Improving pig husbandry in tropical resource-poor communities and its potential to reduce risk of porcine cysticercosis. *Acta Trop.*, **87**: 111–17.

Lescano, A.G. *et al.* (2007). Swine cysticercosis hotspots surrounding *Taenia solium* tapeworm carriers. *Am. J. Trop. Med. Hyg.*, **76**: 376–83.

Li, T. *et al.* (2006). Taeniasis/cysticercosis in a Tibetan population in Sichuan Province, China. *Acta Trop.*, **100**: 223–31.

Li, T. *et al.* (2007). Taeniasis/cysticercosis in China. *Southeast Asian J. Trop. Med. Pub. Health*, **38** (Suppl 1): 1–9.

Lightowlers, M.W. (2003). Vaccines for prevention of cysticercosis. *Acta Trop.*, **87**: 129–35.

Lightowlers, M.W. (2006). Vaccines against cysticercosis and hydatidosis: foundations in taeniid cestode immunology. *Parasitol. Int.*, **55**: S30–43.

Lightowlers, M.W. and Gauci, C.G. (2001). Vaccines against cysticercosis and hydatidosis. *Veterinary Parasit.*, **101**: 337–52.

Lightowlers, M.W. *et al.* (1996). *Taenia saginata*: vaccination against cysticercosis in cattle with recombinant oncosphere antigens. *Exp. Parasitol.*, **84**: 330–38.

Liu, Y.M. *et al.* (2005). Acute pancreatitis caused by tapeworm in the biliary tract. *Am. J. Trop. Med. Hyg.*, **73**: 377–80.

Maravilla, P. *et al.* (1998). Comparative development of *Taenia solium* in experimental models. *J. Parasitol.*, **84**: 882–86.

Maravilla, P. *et al.* (2003). Detection of genetic variation in *Taenia solium*. *J. Parasitol.*, **89**: 1250–54.

Maravilla, P. *et al.* (2008). Genetic polymorphism in *Taenia solium* cysticerci recovered from experimental infections in pigs. *Infect. Genet. Evol.*, **8**: 213–16.

Margono, S.S. *et al.* (2006). Taeniasis/cysticercosis in Papua (Irian Jaya), Indonesia. *Parasitol. Int.*, **55**: S143–48.

Martinez-Maya, J.J. *et al.* (2000). Failure to incriminate domestic flies (Diptera: Muscidae) as mechanical vectors of *Taenia* eggs (Cyclophillidea: Taeniidae) in rural Mexico. *J. Med. Entom.*, **37**: 489–91.

McManus, D.P. (2006). Molecular discrimination of taeniid cestodes. *Parasitol. Int.*, **55**: S31–37.

McManus, D.P. and Bowles J. (1994). Asian (Taiwan) *Taenia*: species or strain. *Parasitol. Today*, **10**: 273–75.

McManus, D.P. and Ito, A. (2005). Application of molecular techniques for identification of human *Taenia* spp. In: K.D. Murrell (ed.) *WHO/FAO/OIE Guidelines for the surveillance, prevention and control of taeniosis/cysticercosis*, pp. 52–55. Paris: OIE.

Medina-Escutia, E. *et al.* (2001). Cellular immune response and Th1/Th2 cytokines in human neurocysticercosis: Lack of immune suppression. *Parasitology*, **87**: 587–90.

Merchant, M.T. *et al.* (1997). Autoradiographic analysis of the germinative tissue in evaginated *Taenia solium* metacestodes. *J. Parasitol.*, **83**: 363–7.

Merchant, M.T. *et al.* (1998). *Taenia solium* description of the intestinal implantation sites in experimental hamster infections. *J. Parasitol.*, **84**: 681–85.

Meza-Lucas, A. *et al.* (2003). Limited and short-lasting humoral response in *Taenia solium*: seropositive households compared with patients with neurocysticercosis. *Am. J. Trop. Med. Hyg.*, **69**: 223–27.

Molyneux, D.H. *et al.* (2005). Rapid-impact interventions: how a policy of integrated control for Africa's neglected tropical diseases could benefit the poor. *PloS Med.*, **2**: 101–7.

Myadagsuren, N. *et al.* (2007). Taeniasis in Mongolia, 2002–2006. *Am. J. Trop. Med. Hyg.*, **77**: 342–46.

Nakao, M. *et al.* (2002). A phylogenetic hypothesis for the distribution of 2 genotypes of the pig tapeworm *Taenia solium* worldwide. *Parasitology*, **124**: 657–62.

Nelson, G.S. *et al.* (1965). The significance of wild animals in the transmission of cestodes of medical importance in Kenya. *Trans. R. Soc. Trop. Med. Hyg.*, **59**: 507–24.

Ngowi, H.A. *et al.* (2008). A health-education intervention trial to reduce porcine cysticercosis in Mbulu District, Tanzania. *Prev. Vet. Med.*, **85**: 52–67.

Ngowi, H.A. *et al.* (2010). Spatial clustering of porcine cysticercosis in Mbulu district, northern Tanzania. *PLoS Negl Trop Dis.*, **4**(4): e652.

Okamoto, M. *et al.* (2007). Asian *Taenia*: species or subspecies? *Southeast Asian J. Trop. Med. Pub. Health*, **38**S1: 125–30.

Overbosch, D. *et al.* (2002). Neurocysticercosis in Europe. In: P. Craig and Z. Pawlowski (eds.) *Cestode zoonoses: echinococcosis and cysticercosis. An emergent and global problem*, Vol. 5, pp. 33–40, NATO Science Series. Amsterdam: IOS Press.

Pawlowski, Z. (1990). Perspectives on the control of *Taenia solium*. *Parasitol. Today*, **6**: 371–73.

Pawlowski, Z. (2006). Role of chemotherapy of taeniasis in prevention of neurocysticercosis. *Parasitol. Int.*, **55**: S105–09.

Pawlowski, Z. *et al.* (2005). Control of taeniasis/cysticercosis: from research towards implementation. *Int. J. Parasitol.*, **35**: 1221–32.

Pawlowski, Z. and Schultz, M.G. (1972). Taeniasis and cysticercosis (*Taenia saginata*). *Adv. Parasitol.*, **10**: 269–343.

Peniche-Cardenas, A. *et al.* (2002). Chemotherapy of porcine cysticercosis with albendazole sulphoxide. *Vet. Parasitol.*, **108**: 63–73.

Phiri, I.K. *et al.* (2006). Assesssment of routine inspection methods for porcine cysticercosis in Zambian village pigs. *J. Helminthol.*, **80**: 69–72.

Praet, N. *et al.* (2009). The disease burden of Taenia solium cysticercosis in Cameroon.. *PLoS Negl Trop Dis.*, **3**(3):e406.

Praet, N. *et al.* (2010). Infection with versus exposure to *Taenia solium*: What do serological test results tell us? *Am. J. Trop. Med. Hyg.*, **83**: 413–15.

Psarros, T.G. *et al.* (2003). Endoscopic management of supratentorial ventricular neurocysticercosis: case series and review of the literature. *Mini. Invas. Neurosurg.*, **46**: 331–334.

Rabiela, M.T. *et al.* (1989). Morphological types of *Taenia solium* cysticerci. *Parasitol. Today*, **5**: 357–59.

Rabiela, M.T. *et al.* (2000). Evagination of *Taenia solium* cysticerci: a histologic and electron microscopy study. *Arch. Med. Res.*, **31**: 605–7.

Rajkotia, Y. *et al.* (2007). Economic burden of neurocysticercosis: results from Peru. *Trans. R. Soc. Trop. Med. Hyg.*, **101**: 840–46.

Rickard, M.D. *et al.* (1977). The prevalence of cysticerci of *Taenia saginata* in cattle reared on sewage-irrigated pasture. *Med. J. Aus.*, **1**: 525–27.

Rodriguez-Canul, R. *et al.* (1998). Application of an immunoassay to determine risk factors associated with porcine cysticercosis in rural areas of Yucatan, Mexico. *Vet. Parasitol.*, **79**: 165–80.

Rodriguez-Canul, R. *et al.* (1999). Epidemiological study of *Taenia solium* taeniasis/cysticercosis in a rural village in Yucatan State, Mexico. *Ann. Trop. Med. Parasitol.*, **93**: 57–67.

Rodriguez-Canul, R. *et al.* (2002). *Taenia solium* metacestode viability in infected pork after preparation with salt pickling or cooking methods common in Yucatan, Mexico. *J. Food Prod.*, **65**: 666–69.

Rodriguez-Hidalgo, R. *et al.* (2002). Comparison of conventional techniques to differentiate between *Taenia solium* and *Taenia saginata* and an improved polymerase chain reaction-restriction fragment length polymorphism assay using a mitochondrial 12S r DNA fragment. *J. Parasitol.*, **88**: 1007–11.

Roman, G. *et al.* (2000). A proposal to declare neurocysticercosis an international reportable disease. *Bull. WHO*, **78**: 399–406.

Saenz, B. *et al.* (2006). Neurocysticercosis: clinical, radiologic, and inflammatory differences between children and adults. *Pediat. Infect. Dis. J.*, **25**: 801–03.

Sako, Y. *et al.* (2000). Molecular characterization and diagnostic value of *Taenia solium* low-molecular-weight antigen genes. *J. Clin. Microbiol.*, **38**: 4439–44.

Sanchez, A.L. *et al.* (1998). Prevalence of taeniasis and cysticercosis in a population of urban residence in Honduras. *Acta Trop.*, **69**: 141–49.

Sarti, E. *et al.* (1988). *Taenia solium* taeniasis and cysticercosis in a Mexican village. *Trop. Med. Parasitol.* , **39**: 194–98.

Sarti, E. *et al.* (1992). Prevalence and risk factors for *Taenia solium* taeniasis and cysticercosis in humans and pigs in a village in Morelos, Mexico. *Am. J. Trop. Med. Hyg.*, **46**: 677–85.

Sarti, E. *et al.* (1994). Epidemiologic investigation of *Taenia solium* taeniasis and cysticercosis in a rural village of Michoacan State, Mexico. *Trans. R. Soc. Trop. Med. Hyg.*, **88**: 49–52.

Sarti, E. *et al.* (1997). Development and evaluation of a health education intervention against *Taenia solium* in a rural community in Mexico. *Am. J. Trop. Med. Hyg.*, **56**: 127–32.

Sarti, E. *et al.* (2000). Mass treatment against human taeniasis for the control of cysticercosis: a population-based intervention study. *Trans. R. Soc. Trop. Med. Hyg.*, **94**: 85–89.

Sato, M.O. *et al.* (2003). Evaluation of tongue inspection and serology for diagnosis of *Taenia solium* cysticercosis in swine: usefulness of ELISA using purified glycoproteins and recombinant antigen. *Vet. Parasitol.*, **111**: 309–22.

Sato, M.O. *et al.* (2006). Evaluation of purified *Taenia solium* glycoproteins and recombinant antigens in the serologic detection of human and swine cysticercosis. *J. Infect. Dis.*, **194**: 1783–90.

Schantz, P.M. and Sarti, E. (1989). Diagnostic methods and epidemiologic surveillance of *Taenia solium* infection. *Acta Leiden.*, **57**: 153–63.

Schantz, P.M. *et al.* (1992). Neurocysticercosis in an orthodox Jewish community in New York City. *N. Eng. J. Med.*, **327**: 692–95.

Schantz, P.M. *et al.* (1993). Potential eradicability of taeniasis and cysticercosis. *Bull. PAHO*, **27**: 397–403.

Schantz, P.M. *et al.* (1994). Community–based epidemiological investigations of cysticercosis due to *Taenia solium*: comparison of serological screening tests and clinical findings in two populations in Mexico. *Clin. Infect. Dis.*, **18**: 879–85.

Sikasunge, C.S. *et al.* (2008). Prevalence of *Taenia solium* porcine cysticercosis in the Eastern, Southern and Western provinces of Zambia. *Vet. J.*, **176**: 240–4.

Simanjuntak, G.M. *et al.* (1997). Taeniasis/cysticercosis in Indonesia as an emerging disease. *Parasitol. Today*, **13**: 321–23.

Singh, G. *et al.* (2002). *Taenia solium* taeniasis and cysticercosis in Asia. In: G. Singh and S. Prabhakar (eds.) *Taenia solium cysticercosis*, pp. 111–27. Oxon, UK: CAB International.

Sorvillo, F. *et al.* (2011). Public health implications of cysticercosis acquired in the United States. *Emerg Infect Dis.*, **17**: 1–6.

Sotelo, J. and Del Brutto, O.H. (2000). Brain cysticercosis. *Arch. Med. Res.*, **31**: 3–14.

Sotelo, J. and Del Brutto, O.H. (2002). Review of neurocysticercosis. *Neurosurg. Focus*, **12**: e1.

Sotelo, J. *et al.* (1986). Freezing of infested pork muscle kills cysticerci. *J. Am. Med. Ass.*, **256**: 893–94.

Sudewi, A.A. *et al.* (2008). *Taenia solium* cysticercosis in Bali, Indonesia: serology and mtDNA analysis. *Trans. R. Soc. Trop. Med. Hyg.*, **102**: 96–98.

Suri, A. *et al.* (2008). Transventricular, transaqueductal scope-in-scope endoscopic excision of fourth ventricular neurocysticercosis: a series of 13 cases and a review. *J. Neurosurg. Ped.*, **1**: 35–39.

Tesfa-Yohannes, T. (1990). Effectiveness of praziquantel against *Taenia saginata* infections in Ethiopia. *Ann. Trop. Med. Parasitol.*, **84**: 581–85.

Torres, A. *et al.* (1992). Praziquantel treatment of porcine brain and muscle *Taenia solium* cysticercosis. 3. *Effect of 1-day treatment. Parasit. Res.*, **78**: 161–64.

Tsang, V.C.W. *et al.* (1989). An enzyme-linked immunoelectrotransfer blot assay by glycoprotein antigens for diagnosing human cysticercosis (*Taenia solium*). *J. Infect. Dis.*, **159**: 50–59.

Vázquez-Flores, S. *et al.* (2001). Hygiene and restraint of pigs associated with absence of *Taenia solium* cysticercosis in a rural community of Mexico. *Salud Pública de México*, **43**: 574–76.

Verster, A. (1965). *Taenia solium* Linnaeus (1758) in the chacma babbon. *Papio ursinus*, (Kerr 1792). *J. South Afri. Vet. Med. Ass.*, **36**: 580.

Verster, A. (1974). The golden hamster as a definitive host of *Taenia solium* and *Taenia saginata*. *Onderstepoort J. Vet. Res.*, **41**: 23–28.

Viljoen, N.F. (1937). Cysticercosis in swine and bovines, with special reference to South African conditions. *Onderstepoort J. Vet. Sci. Anim. Indust.*, **9**: 337–570.

Wandra, T. *et al.* (2006a). Taeniasis and cysticercosis in Bali and North Sumatra, Indonesia. *Parasitol. Int.*, **55**: S155–60.

Wandra, T. *et al.* (2006b). High prevalence of *Taenia saginata* taeniasis and status of *Taenia solium* cysticercosis in Bali, Indonesia, 2002–2004. *Trans. R. Soc. Trop. Med. Hyg.*, **100**: 346–53.

Wandra, T. *et al.* (2007). Current situation of taeniasis and cysticercosis in Indonesia. *Trop. Med. Health*, **35**: 323–28.

WHO (1983). *Guidelines for surveillance, prevention and control of taeniasis/ cysticercosis*, (eds. M. Gemmell, Z. Matyas, Z. Pawlowski, and E.J.L. Soulsby), VPH/83.49, pp. 207. Geneva: World Health Organization.

WHO/DFID-AHP (2006). *The control of neglected zoonotic diseases*. WHO/ SDE/FOS/2006. pp. 1, 54. Geneva: World Health Organization.

WHO/FAO/OIE (2005). *Guidelines for the surveillance, prevention and control of taeniosis/cysticercosis*. (ed. K.D. Murrell), pp. 139. Paris: OIE.

Wilson, M. *et al.* (1991). Clinical evaluation of the cysticercosis enzyme linked immunoelectrotransfer blot in patients with neurocysticercosis. *J. Infect. Dis.*, **164**: 1007–8.

Wilkins, P.P. *et al.* (1999). Development of a serologic assay to detect *Taenia solium* taeniasis. *Am. J. Trop. Med. Hyg.*, **60**: 199–204.

Willingham, A.L. and Engels, D. (2006). Control of *Taenia solium* cysticercosis/taeniosis. *Adv. Parasitol.*, **61**: 509–66.

Yamasaki, H. *et al.* (2004). DNA differential diagnosis of taeniasis and cysticercosis by multiplex PCR. *J. Clin. Microbiol.*, **42**: 548–53.

Yoshino, K. (1933a). Studies on the post-embryonal development of *Taenia solium*. Part I. On the hatching of the egg of *Taenia solium*. *J. Med. Ass. Form.*, **32**: 139–41.

Yoshino, K. (1933b). Studies on the post-embryonal development of *Taenia solium*. Part II. On the migration course of the oncosphere of Taenia solium within the intermediate host. *J. Med. Ass. Form.*, **32**: 155–58.

Yoshino, K. (1933c). Studies on the post-embryonal development of *Taenia solium*. Part III. On the development of cysticercus cellulosae within the definite intermediate host. *J. Med. Ass. Form.*, **32**: 166–69.

Zinsstag, J. *et al.* (2005). Potential of cooperation between human and animal health to strengthen health systems. *Lancet*, **366**: 2142–45.

CHAPTER 52

Other adult and larval cestodes

Sheelagh Lloyd

Summary

Adult *Diphyllobothrium latum* is acquired by consumption of raw fish by persons living around lakes/reservoirs/rivers. *Hymenolepis nana* can have a direct life cycle so eggs produced by adults in man are important in transfer between humans. The contribution of rodents and the indirect life cycle through arthropods need re-evaluation. Other minor adult cestode infections are described.

Man can be an intermediate host for tissue metacestodes. *Taenia multiceps* and related species are that acquired from canids and produce a coenurus. *Spirometra* spp. pleurocercoids are acquired from copepod or reptile/amphibian/mammalian intermediate hosts. Other metacestode infections are very rare.

Adult cestode infections

Diphyllobothrium latum (Linnaeus 1758) Lühe 1910 and related species

History

The Swiss physician, Dunus, was the first to draw attention to *Diphyllobothrium latum* but it was not until 1881/82 that Braun fed fish plerocercoids to dogs and man and 1917 when Rosen completed the life cycle in *Cyclops* and fish (Grove 1990). *Diplogonoporus balaenopterae* Loennberg, 1892 (syn *D. grandis*) was described in man earlier than in its whale host.

The agents

Diphyllobothrium latum and *D. nihonkaiense*, previously 'D. latum of Japan' are the most common in man. *Diphyllobothrium dendriticum*, *D. klebanovskii* and *D. pacificum* and some 10 other species are recorded rarely in man from marine- and fresh-water fishes but morphological identification is difficult as there is considerable structural plasticity in plerocercoids and adults (Devos *et al.* 1990). Keys and descriptions for some plerocercoids and adults have been given by Yamane *et al.* (1981), Muratov and Posokhov (1988), and Andersen and Gibson (1989). Molecular analyses of *cytochrome c oxidase 1 (cox1), NADH dehydrogenase subunit 3 (ND3), 18S rRNA, Internal Spacer 1 (ITS1)* and/or *ITS2* genes have differentiated human infections (Yera *et al.* 2006; Skerikova *et al.* 2006; Nakao *et al.* 2007; Arizono *et al.* 2007; Wicht *et al.* 2007; 2008a; b).

Adult *D. latum* ivory in colour are up to 10 m long. The spoon-shaped scolex, 1 x 2.5 mm, has two long, weak grooves, the bothria. Proglottids are broader than long with numerous lateral testes and vitellaria. From the posterior ovary a central brown rosette is the uterus containing eggs that are released from a central genital pore and passed in faeces. Proglottids disintegrate, but occasionally strings of proglottids, with their dark, central uterus markings, are passed in faeces. Eggs, 70 x 45 μm, with rounded ends, are light brown and operculate. Eggs in water develop and hatch as 6-hooked, ciliated oncospheres, the coracidia. Procercoids in copepods retain the six hooks. Plerocercoids in fish commonly are 1–4 cm long with a glistening, opaque, furrowed body; others species translucent bluish-white.

Diplogonoporus balaenopterae can reach 20 m in whales. It and its eggs are very similar to *D. latum* but both are keyhole-shaped and reproductive organs are paired with two dark uteri in each proglottid.

Hosts

Diphyllobothrium latum: the broad fish tapeworm

Procercoid: >40 species of copepods (*Eudiaptomus, Diaptomus, Cyclops*, etc.),

Plerocercoid: freshwater fishes, including burbot, pike, perch, ruff, charr, redlip mullet, brown trout, and in Canada *Oncorhynchus* spp. salmon, though the role for salmonids needs re-evaluation (Scholtz *et al.* 2009),

Adult tapeworm: piscivorous mammals, e.g. man, dog, cat, fox, bear, lynx, wolf, etc.

Diphyllobothrium dendriticum

Plerocercoid: freshwater fishes, primarily salmonids and coregonids, burbot, etc.,

Adult tapeworm: piscivorous birds, particularly seagulls and terns; mammals, e.g. dog, man.

Diphyllobothrium nihonkaiense

Plerocercoid: a variety of anadromous *Oncorhynchus* spp. northern Pacific salmon,

Adult tapeworm: brown bear; man.

Diphyllobothrium klebanovskii

Plerocercoid: *Oncorhynchus* salmon,

Adult tapeworm: brown bear, dog, cat, man.

Diphyllobothrium pacificum and *Diphyllobothrium* spp.

Plerocercoid: a variety of marine fishes,

Adult tapeworm: sea lion, seal, other marine mammals; piscivorous birds; man.

Diplogonoporus balaenopterae

Plerocercoid: anchovy, presumably other marine fish,

Definitive host: whales; man.

Life cycle

Dipyllobothrium latum can mature in 4–6 weeks, may live 7–10 years, and produce up to 1,000,000 eggs/day. Eggs hatch in 5–12 days at 25–16°C. *Diphyllobothrium latum* and *D. dendriticum* survive in fresh water; *D. klebanovskii* was differentiated as its eggs survive only in sea water; other species are marine. Coracidia ingested by copepods develop in 2–3 weeks to procercoids. Fish eat the planktonic crustacea and plerocercoids are long-lived and can transfer from prey fish to accumulate in older, bigger, predator fish. *Diphyllobothrium latum* is more prevalent in man as their plerocercoids' predilection site is muscle versus *D. dendriticum* in viscera, though in rockeye salmon the latter may be in muscles.

Geographic distribution and epidemiology

Diphyllobothrium latum, with an estimated 9–20 million cases, is circumpolar in northern temperate and subarctic countries with many lakes. Foci of infection stretch east from France, northern Italy, the Baltic States, through northern Russia into China, Japan, and North America, but also South America, i.e. Patagonia, Argentina, and Chile and Peru. Sporadic infections are described in other countries, i.e. Brazil, Cuba, Korea, Australia, and 1% prevalence recently was described in six to 10 year old children in Karnataka, India. Genetic analyses are required to confirm *D. latum* at all its reported locations.

Reports from Russia found effluent from a town sewage plant contained eggs that also were found in canals and ditches, all draining into a reservoir. However, infection did not establish in water near very large human settlements as industrial pollution greatly decreased zooplankton levels. Reduced *D. latum* prevalence now is recorded in many areas with improved sewage treatments and reduced human sewage outflow to lakes although egg content may be reduced only 95–99% . Flooding events could increase contamination. Direct contamination of lakes occurs through faecal contamination by fishermen and while boating. Dogs and foxes are infected but only 0–0.5% were infected in surveys in Finland, Germany, and Switzerland, and they may be poor hosts.

Prevalence in Europe has declined markedly. Infection persists with >10 cases a year in Scandinavia (10–50 cases a year in Sweden, 400 cases in Finland). Infection is re-emerging with >10 cases a year around many Swiss, Italo-Swiss and Franco-Swiss sub-alpine lakes. Two to 10 cases are recorded in France, Italy, Poland, and Romania, with sporadic cases in some other European countries (Dupouy-Camet and Peduzzi 2004). Re-emergence is related to greater interest in 'ancestral' and 'new' culinary habits and the 'nutritive value' of fish eaten rare, raw, salted, marinated as gravalax and strogonini in Scandinavia, carpaccio in Italy and France, plus cerviche, tartare, sushi, and sashimi. Further, fish from infected lakes is supplied fresh to an often increasing number of local restaurants and homes. A recent outbreak affecting eight of

26 wedding guests involved raw, marinated perch fillets caught that day in Lake Geneva. Increased diagnosis may contribute to re-emergence.

Since the 1980s infection continues in 4–33% of perch and pike in sub-alpine lakes (Dupouy-Camet and Peduzzi 2004) and in 90–95% of pike and 14% perch in foci in rivers and lakes in Russia. In Chile, on the River Valdiva, 0–1.2% of humans and 5–10% of dogs were infected as were 2.8% and 4.5%, respectively, in Choshuenko, Lake Panguipulli. *Diphyllobothrium latum* was present in 28% of rainbow trout in Lake Moreno, Argentina, One to 10 and occasionally more pleurocercoids are recorded/fish.

Diphyllobothrium nihonkaiense is described in humans in Asia, particularly Japan (with declining rural but increasing urban cases) and far east Russia, acquired from salmon in northern Pacific waters, and infection has been described in man in Canada, Europe and New Zealand.

Diphyllobothrium klebanovskii occurs in far east Russia (Seas of Japan, Okhotsk, Bering and major inland river regions) and was found in 3% of humans and dogs and 10.5% of cats in the southern areas. In inland Amur Region, 0.4–4.2% of people living along rivers were infected; infection acquired in June to October when salmon, having acquired infection (30–46%) in the marine littoral environment, migrate inland to spawn. Brown bear were important definitive hosts, 47% infected.

Diphyllobothrium pacificum infects man in Peru and Chile but also occurs in salmon in northern Pacific waters. El Niño is said to affect fish and sea lion behaviour to increase human infection in northern Chile.

Diphyllobothrium dendriticum is common in fish in many of the same areas as *D. latum*. In the 1980s, it was recorded in 30–100% of various fish in Lake Baikal, Russia and Great Central Lake, Canada, and recently 58% of rainbow trout in Lake Moreno. Although present in wild and not farmed salmon in the Puget Sound, it is recorded in farmed salmon and trout in lakes/reservoirs with an abundant zooplankton in Scotland and trout in northwestern Ireland. It is not common in man as many plerocercoids are in the viscera.

The other *Diphyllobothrium* species are recorded primarily in Japan and SE Asia but are recorded in seamen, so possibly acquired elsewhere.

About 200 cases of *D. balaenopterae* are reported primarily in Japan, with highest prevalence in Kochi Prefecture where raw immature anchovies are eaten as a tonic by elderly males (Arizono et al. 2007). Two other *Diplogonoporus* spp. are described in humans in Japan.

Increased demand for fresh fish may further increase global diphyllobothriosis. Recent cases of *D. nihonkaiense* in France and Switzerland were associated with salmon imported fresh chilled from the American Pacific coast and *Diphyllobothrium* cases in Western USA from Alaskan salmon and in Brazil from Chilean fish (Yera et al. 2006; Wicht et al. 2007; 2008b). Other cases of *D. latum,* *D. nihonkaiense* and *D. dendriticum* could have been acquired during travel. Whether or not *D. latum* pre-existed in North America or arrived with European immigrants, immigration was responsible for establishment of *D. latum* in copepods and imported fish in lakes and rivers in Argentina and Chile; the parasite recently has moved north in Chile (Cabello 2007). Ten years after the Krasnoyarsk reservoir was built, *Diphyllobothrium* infection had established in 90 and 14% of pike and perch, in 27% of dogs, and 8–12% of humans. There is potential for similar establishment of imported parasites elsewhere. Known hosts, i.e. trout for *D. dendriticum*, may be present in lakes while colonization of other hosts of the same genus must be considered (Torres *et al.* 2004; Yera *et al.* 2006; Wicht *et al.* 2008a).

Clinical signs

Many human infections are asymptomatic, but abdominal pain, dizziness, fatigue, transient diarrhoea, dyspepsia, and vomiting may occur. There is preferential intrinsic factor and vitamin B_{12} uptake by *D. latum*. Regarded as a classic sign, pernicious anaemia was considered due to a more anterior intestinal attachment of the worm or a genetic or familial basis in the Baltics, but, with improved diets, while 40% of patients may have low vitamin B_{12}, anaemia occurs only in 2%.

Diagnosis

Faeces is examined for eggs. Sometimes a patient notices chains of proglottids with their central, brown rosette. A coproantigen test would be useful as there can be quite long periods without eggs in faeces. Molecular tests have improved differentiation of *Diphyllobothrium* species.

Treatment

Praziquantel as a single oral dose of 10–25 mg/kg is highly effective, 50 mg for *D. nihonkaiense*. Vitamin B_{12} is supportive. Niclosamide as a single or divided dose is useful. Other drugs, often followed by a saline purgative, should be replaced.

Control

Culinary habits and the importance of fish in human diets in coastal areas of seas/lakes/rivers makes education on the correct processing of fish and reduced consumption of raw fish important. It is difficult though to alter cultural behaviour that is changing in favour of consumption of raw fish anyway. Thorough cooking, 55°C for ≥5 mins or freezing to −10 to −20°C in the centre for at least 6–24 hours kills plerocercoids. In some countries all fish to be eaten raw must be frozen but increased desire for fresh and locally caught fish makes monitoring difficult. Salt content of >7% is lethal; times required for dry or wet salting at different temperatures are given by Dovgalev (1988).

Improved sanitation and treatment of effluents to remove eggs are being achieved at many rivers and lakes. However, this does not prevent indiscriminate human defaecation and contamination by animal definitive hosts, e.g. brown bear, dog, cat, etc., whose role must be assessed. Species with piscivorous birds, marine mammals, etc., as main definitive hosts cannot be controlled. An obstacle to understanding epidemiology has been the difficulty in differentiating *D. latum* from non- or rarely-zoonotic species in definitive and intermediate hosts, e.g. *D. detrimum* of birds and the myriad of marine species. Continued development of molecular tests will be useful. Consideration must be given to hosts when inland bodies of water are developed because a wide variety of freshwater copepods and fish act as hosts and foci of infection can develop rapidly.

Related diphyllobothriids

There have been a few records in man of *Ligula intestinalis* and *Schistocephalus solidus* of piscivorous birds and dogs in Central Europe or northern America from freshwater fish; *Pyramicocephalus* anthrocephalus of dogs and mammals from marine fish in North America; and probable adult *Spirometra erinaceieuropaei* in Japan.

Hymenolepis nana (von Siebold 1852) and *Hymenolepis diminuta* Rudolphi 1819

History

Hymenolepis diminuta was described from rodents by Rudolphi (1819), and then a child in the USA (Grove 1990). Bilharz observed *Hymenolepis nana* in a child in Egypt in 1851.

The agents

Hymenolepis (syn *Rodentolepis*) *nana*, the dwarf tapeworm, is 2.5–4 cm long. The scolex has four suckers and one row of 20–30 rostellar hooks. Proglottids, wider than long, have a single set of genital organs and unilateral genital pores. Gravid proglottids have a sac-like uterus. Oval eggs, 45 by 30 μm, contain an oncosphere with three pairs of hooks surrounded by two smooth membranes, the outer thin and clear, the inner with two polar thickenings each bearing 4–8 filaments. *Hymenolepis* (*Rodentolepis*) *microstoma*, with very similar eggs, recently was identified in man by molecular means (Macnish *et al.* 2003), however, its presence elsewhere in man requires investigation. *Hymenolepis diminuta* can reach 60 cm, the rostellum lacks hooks, the eggs are 60–70 μm long, the polar thickenings without filaments, and the thicker, darker outer membrane may have striations.

The hosts

Hymenolepis nana

Adult: man, rodents—small intestine,

Metacestode: man, rodents, stored food beetles (meal worms) *Tenebrio*, *Tribolium* spp., flea larvae, moths, etc.

Hymenolepis diminuta

Adult: rats, man—small intestine,

Metacestode: many arthropods.

Hymenolepis microstoma

Adult: rodents, man—biliary system,

Metacestode: *Tribolium* spp.

Life cycle and epidemiology

Hymenolepis nana is a unique tapeworm with its direct life cycle—eggs eaten by humans or rodents develop to cysticercoids within the villi, emerge in 4–6 days and develop to adults in the lumen by 16–28 days. *Hymenolepis microstoma* possibly has a direct life cycle (Andreassen *et al.* 2004).

Hymenolepis nana is common in man (possibly >50 million infections) and cosmopolitan in distribution, but most common in South America, Africa, Asia, and southeastern Europe. Direct faeco-oral, human-human transfer is important, so highest prevalence occurs in children in poor areas and in institutions. Rodent hosts also are likely to be prevalent in these areas and fly transfer of eggs to food is possible. Prevalences of 0.1–28% in children and 0–4% in adults were described in the 1980s and 1–9% of food handlers in institutions were infected. Food-borne clustering of cases in households is likely. Internal autoinfection is described but needs confirmation. Infection can continue in these ways in any country, infection persisted at least two years in south east Asian refugees in the USA.

The level of transfer of infection between rodents and humans requires confirmation as analysis of *cox1* indicated divergence between northwestern Australian mouse and human isolates with human-human transfer and an absence of close contact between mice and humans (Macnish *et al.* 2002a). A human specific life cycle was suggested as 51 isolates of human Australian *H. nana* failed to infect laboratory animals; but then only one of 24 of these infected *Tribolium* (Macnish *et al.* 2002b). Elsewhere there can be close contact between rodents and man and Fan (2005) in China and Ferretti *et al.* (1981) in Italy successfully transferred human parasites to mice.

An indirect life cycle is optional for *H. nana* but required for *H. diminuta.* Rodent faecal contamination of cereal foods infested with beetles is likely to be prevalent and insect larvae might eat human faeces in areas with poor sanitation. Humans then may eat cysticercoids in insects in uncooked food or accidentally. Although *H. diminuta* is common in rats in tropical and sub-tropical regions, there are only some 500 documented human infections mainly in Africa, Asia, and the USA. High prevalence of *H. nana* versus *H. diminuta* may not point to low importance of the indirect life cycle as humans could be non-permissive hosts for *H. diminuta* as are mice.

Clinical signs

Many *Hymenolepis* infections are asymptomatic but heavy *H. nana* infections can develop through poor hygiene (faeco-oral autoinfection). In Chile, infected children had abdominal pain (75%), bloating, diarrhoea, poor weight gain, and eosinophilia (33–53%). Nausea, vomiting and urticaria manifested occasionally. In Moscow, 26% of infected adults showed signs.

Hymenolepis diminuta is being examined for amelioration of Th1-mediated Crohn's disease and ulcerative colitis. Expulsion of *H. diminuta* reduced intestinal disease, particularly secretory effects, in the mouse model induced with dextran sodium sulphate; however, an oxazalone-induced Th2 colitis was exacerbated (Hunter *et al.* 2007).

Diagnosis

Ethyl acetate extraction or Kato-Katz are common techniques; >10,000 eggs/gm considered a heavy infection (Chero *et al.* 2006). Egg production can be sporadic. Low frequency of disease and infection in the West has not promoted development of immunodiagnosis.

Treatment

All family members should be examined for infection or treated. Praziquantel (10–15 mg/kg) has high efficacy (91–98%) against adult tapeworms and cysticercoids. Niclosamide has low efficacy against cysticercoids so is given daily for 5–7 days (2 g for adults; 1.5 g for children > 35 kg; 1.0 g for children of 11–35 kg) for about 70–90% efficacy. Benzimidazoles have lower efficacy but give the advantage of broad-spectrum activity against possible concurrent *Enterobius vermicularis*. Nitazoxanide has 75–95% efficacy (Chero *et al.* 2006) and also is effective against intestinal nematodes. Natural, indigenous products, powdered *Nigella sativa* seeds, garlic, etc., are used but need testing.

Control

In an Azerbaijan suburb, niclosamide treatment, improved sanitation, and public health education reduced prevalence from 5–9%

to zero at six months, but such measures must be sustained. Rodent colonies should be destroyed. Cereals that are eaten uncooked must be protected from rodents and insects.

Other adult cestodes

Other genera, found occasionally in man usually are asymptomatic. Praziquantel must be the treatment of choice with good efficacy against these or related species in animals.

Mesocestoides lineatus (Goeze 1782) Railliet 1893 and *Mesocestoides variabilis* Mueller 1928

Adults, variable in length, occur in birds and mammals, particularly wild carnivores, but also dogs and cats, in Asia, Europe, Africa, and North America. Speciation is uncertain. The scolex is unarmed; proglottids have a central genital pore; eggs enter a central, fibrous-walled paruterine organ. The life cycle first involves cysticercoids in unidentified coprophagous arthropods, possibly mites or ants (Padgett and Boyce 2005). Second intermediate hosts, amphibia, reptiles, birds, and mammals, contain tetrathyridia with four suckers that multiply asexually in body cavities. Tetrathyridia eaten by definitive hosts develop to adults, but may first multiply in the peritoneal cavity.

Human infection

About 30 cases of adult *Mesocestoides* are documented mainly in Japan, recently China, and Korea, but also the USA, Ruanda-Urundi and Greenland (Fuentes *et al.* 2003). Infection is acquired by ingesting raw, usually wild animal, viscera containing tetrathyridia, or consuming snake meat and blood. Infection is recognized by white segments in the faeces.

Bertiella studeri (Blanchard 1891) and *Bertiella mucronata* (Meyner 1895)

Adults, recognized by morphological differences (Bhagwant 2004) may be a species complex (Galán-Puchades *et al.* 2000), and are common in Old and New World primates, respectively, in sub-tropical and tropical regions. Unarmed adults reach 45 cm. Proglottids, excreted in chains of 3–24, are fleshy, much wider than long (6–10 x 0.5 mm), and the uterus is a transverse tube. Eggs are spherical, about 45–50 μm, with a well-developed pyriform apparatus (the innermost membrane pear-shaped due to a pair of hooked projections on one side). Free-living oribatid mites are intermediate hosts.

Human infection

Cases of *B. studeri* continue to be reported in countries in Asia, particularly the Indian subcontinent, China, Far East, and South East Asia, Africa, Mauritius, and Yemen. *Bertiella mucronata* is reported occasionally in Latin America and Cuba. Most cases occur in children accidentally ingesting mites on food or by geophagia pica. Patients come from villages where monkeys are bred, or that are visited by monkeys, or families have foraged for fruits in the forest.

Other adult anoplocephalids include: *Inermicapsifer* spp., tapeworms of rodents and hyraxes, reported in man in Africa, Cuba and South America, infection probably acquired from a mite intermediate host; *Mathevotaenia symmetrica* of rodents and mealworm insects in Thailand; *Moniezia expansa* of ruminants and oribatid mites described once in Russia.

Dipylidium caninum (Linnaeus 1758) Leuckart 1863

Common in Canidae and Felidae, adults reach 10–50 cm long, have four suckers, and up to 150 rose-thorn-shaped rostellar hooks. Two sets of genital organs open in two mid-lateral genital pores. Gravid proglottids are 'cucumber seed' shaped and filled with egg packets each containing up to 30 thin-walled eggs. Proglottids passed in faeces can migrate off the faeces or migrate from the anus and in the perianal area to drop to the floor particularly in the sleeping area of the dog/cat. *Ctenocephalides felis* of cats and dogs are the most efficient intermediate host; the role of lice needs re-evaluation. Flea larvae, common where the dog or cat sleeps, eat proglottids. In tropical areas at ≥32°C the cysticercoids can be infective in mature fleas emerging from the pupae. In cooler climates cysticercoids complete development in the flea only at >32°C on the host. Adult fleas are eaten accidentally when the dog/cat grooms its coat.

Human infection

Although prevalent worldwide in pets, human infection is uncommon (<200 reports) but underestimated as 43 cases were reported in the USA in 5 years when drug use could be recorded. Infection occurs usually in children under 6–12 months of age. Infected fleas may be ingested accidentally in the environment in hot climates or through close contact with an infested pet; dog(s) licking children could transfer fleas in saliva but this coincidence seems low.

Infection usually is noted by white, motile segments drying to rice grains on underclothes, bedclothes and on/in faeces. Anal pruritis, sleeplessness, and irritability may necessitate differentiation from pinworms. Pets in the household must be treated for tapeworms and flea control instituted, both on the animal and in the environment.

Other adults

Raillietina spp. of rodents have been recorded occasionally in humans in China, the Far East, Asian Pacific region, Cuba, and the Americas; intermediate hosts may be ants, beetles, cockroaches. Odd cases of *Multiceps longihamatus* are recorded in Japan. A possible or spurious case of *T. taeniaeformis* was described in child who vomited worms.

Metacestodes in tissues

A variety of metacestodes while not common need differentiation from *Taenia solium*, tumours, and other tissue helminths.

Coenurosis: *Taenia multiceps* Leske 1980, *Taenia serialis* (Gervais 1847) Baillet 1863, and *Taenia brauni* (Setti 1897) Fain et al. 1956

History

The many protoscolices in the coenurus led to the name *multiceps* (many-headed). Coenurosis in ruminants was mentioned by Hippocrates and a full description of disease given by Wepfer in 1658. 'Operations' to remove cysts and the life cycle were described in the nineteenth century. The first human case was reported in 1913 in France.

The agents

Adult Taenia tapeworms in Canidae are difficult to differentiate (Loos-Frank 2000). The coenurus of *T. multiceps* in sheep, goats, cattle, and other ruminants, can reach 5 or more cm in diameter with up to 400 protoscolices clustered in groups on the wall. The coenurus of *T. serialis* in lagomorphs, rarely rodents and the cat, is smaller with protoscolices in radiating rows. *Taenia brauni* in rodents and primates is very similar.

Life cycle and epidemiology

Dogs pass eggs and segments. Eggs remain viable on pasture for probably several months and fly-borne transmission of eggs should occur. *Taenia multiceps* oncospheres migrate in all tissues, but commonly only those in the CNS develop; the neurological signs undoubtedly increase scavenging by dogs. *Taenia serialis* and *T. brauni* in musculature restricting movement also would increase predation.

Taenia multiceps is common in sheep rearing areas but has disappeared from some, e.g. the USA and New Zealand; *Taenia serialis* is recorded worldwide; *T. brauni* in Africa. In endemic areas, e.g. mid-Wales and North Africa, prevalence varies greatly, reaching up to 27% in canids and 6% in sheep.

Human infection

The species in man commonly is not identified. Recent analysis of *ND1* aided identification of *T. serialis* in France (Collomb *et al.* 2007). In the USA only *T. serialis* is encountered producing mainly subcutaneous/intramuscular cysts but it must account for the central nervous system (CNS) lesions in man there. In Europe CNS infections usually are ascribed to *T. multiceps* with recent cases in Italy and Sardinia; subcutaneous cysts to *T. serialis*; intraocular cases could be either. Infections in Africa are primarily subcutaneous or intraocular and ascribed to *T. brauni*; CNS involvement is less common. A possible case of *Multiceps glomeratus* in muscle is described in Nigeria.

There are only a few hundred human cases in the literature, although many tissue nodules undoubtedly remain undiagnosed and unreported; ocular and neurological cases more frequently documented. Infectivity of *T. multiceps* for man seems low as there is very low incidence compared with higher human prevalence of *E. granulosus,* that has similar hosts in the same areas.

Clinical signs

CNS cysts are space-occupying and, in man, they have some predilection for the subarachnoid space, basal cisterns, and ventricular cavities causing disturbances in cerebrospinal fluid (CSF) pathways. Cranial hypertension and hydrocephalus present as violent headache, nausea, and movement disorders. Blockage of the fourth ventricular foramina can be rapidly fatal. Cysts in the brain parenchyma produce signs varying with site, e.g. seizures, limb weakness, paralysis, etc. Spinal cysts are recorded. Subcutaneous/intramuscular nodules may be painless or slightly tender. Cysts in the eye usually are unilateral in the vitreous and affect visual acuity, with perhaps pain, and occasionally severe endophthalmitis.

Diagnosis and treatment

Subcutaneous/intramuscular cysts are palpable, recognized by radiology or ultrasound and likely to be removed for differentiation from cysts and tumours.

Intravitreal cysts are visible on echography or fundoscopy. Inflammation can obscure cysts so tests comparable to those used for ocular larva migrans may be useful. As severe endophthalmitis has been observed on death of the cyst, cysts should be removed immediately on diagnosis without anthelmintic treatment.

CT and MRI are valuable in patients presenting with neurocoen-urosis evaluating cyst(s') size and location (Pau *et al.* 1987). Coenuri in the ventricular system may present the same problems with diagnosis as ventricular neurocysticercosis. Immunodiagnosis is not available. Surgical intervention is important as a ventricular cyst may move and cause acute onset blockage of CSF pathways; removal of parenchymal cysts immediately relieves the pressure atrophy.

Control

Measures that curb freedom of and numbers of dogs, regulate disposal of sheep carcasses, and give regular praziquantel treatments to dogs, as in *Echinococcus* control programmes, curb transmission of *T. multiceps.*

Spirometra mansoni Joyeux and Houdemer 1927, *Spirometra erinaceieuropaei* Rudolphi 1819, *Spirometra mansonoides* Mueller 1935

Spirometra mansoni occurs in Asia and South America; *S. erina-ceieuropaei* in Europe, Asia and Australia; *S. mansonoides* in the Americas; *S. theileri* in Africa south of the Sahara; although speciation is debated. Adult tapeworms in wild carnivores, dogs and cats resemble *Diphyllobothrium*. Procercoid larvae develop in *Cyclops* in ponds; plerocercoids in amphibia, reptiles, small mammals, birds, and in large game animals in Africa. The plerocercoids (spargana) are ribbon-like, white, wrinkled and is mm to 30–40 cm long. They can transfer from one to another intermediate host.

Human infection

Man can be a second intermediate host for all the species. New cases are reported each year most commonly in south east Asia, Japan, Korea, elsewhere in Asia, including China, and occasionally Europe, Africa and the Americas (Pampiglione *et al.* 2003).

Humans acquire infection by ingesting procercoids in *Cyclops* in unpurified water, plerocercoids in raw flesh of snakes, frogs, rodent meat, etc., or wild pig paratenic hosts. While in China and south east Asia, muscles of amphibia still are applied as a poultice in traditional self-treatment of ulcers, infected eyes, etc. which allows spargana to then wander across to the human tissues. Ingested parasites penetrate the intestine and wander to be found intraperitoneally, in other body cavities including the scrotum, in the viscera or bone, or they commonly migrate to subcutaneous, muscular and periocular sites. They elicit a recurrent inflammatory response or encyst in a fibrous nodule that may be painful and a sparganum can persist in the tissues for 20–30 years. CNS signs include headaches and intermittent seizures, ocular sparganosis can cause intense pain, oedema, and ulceration and these represent 50 and 15%, respectively, of infections in Thai literature reflecting documentation of unusual cases (Wiwanitkit 2005). Occasional proliferating spargana, seen mainly in Asia, break into segments each capable of further development, and can be serious and fatal.

Diagnosis and treatment

Treatment usually is surgery; diagnosis confirmed after surgical removal or biopsy of the organism. The sparganum is identified as cestode by the lack of body cavity, laminated, basophilic calcareous corpuscles, and acellular, syncytial tegument. Bead-shaped enhancement was the most MRI common finding. Characteristic on post contrast images was a tunnel-sign (hollow tube) up to several cms representing the migratory track (Song *et al.* 2007).

CT may reveal small calcifications. Changes in location suggest sparganum aetiology. ELISA is available in some areas and positive serum and CSF results are very useful in diagnosis of neurosparg0-nosis (Lee *et al.* 2003). Little information is available on anthelmintic therapy.

Other tissue metacestodes

A case of fatal, disseminated invasion by *H. nana* cysticercoids in an AIDS patient has been described (Olson *et al.* 2003). *Taenia crassiceps,* of foxes proliferates as cysticeri in rodents and has been reported in the human eye (Canada) but recently subcutaneous/intramuscular growths that have potential to spread rapidly have been described in AIDS patients and in an immunosuppressed patient in Europe (Klinker *et al.* 1992; Maillard *et al.* 1998; Heldwein *et al.* 2006). *Taenia taeniaeformis* has been described twice in human liver.

References

Andersen, K.I. and Gibson, D.I. (1989). A key to 3 species of larval *Diphyllobothrium* Cobbold, 1858 (Cestoda, Pseudophyllidea) occurring in European and North American fresh water fishes. *Syst. Parasitol.,* **13:** 3–9.

Andreassen, J., Ito, A., Ito, M., Nakao, M. and Nakaya, K. (2004). *Hymenolepis microstoma*: direct life cycle in immunodeficient mice. *J. Helminthol.,* **78:** 1–5.

Arizono, N., Fukumoto, S., Tademoto, S., *et al.* (2007). Diplogonoporiasis in Japan: Genetic analyses of five clinical isolates. *Parasitol. Int.,* **57:** 212–16.

Bhagwant, S. (2004). Human *Bertiella studeri* (family Anoplocephalidae) infection of probable Southeast Asian origin in Mauritian children and an adult. *Am. J. Trop. Med. Hyg.,* **70:** 225–28.

Cabello, F.C. (2007). Aquaculture and public health. The emergence of diphyllobothriasis in Chile and the world. *Rev. Med. Chil.,* **135:** 1064–71.

Chero, J.C., Saito, M., Bustos, J.A., *et al.* (2006). *Hymenolepis nana* infection: symptoms and response to nitazoxanide in field conditions. *Trans. R. Soc. Trop. Med. Hyg.,* **101:** 203–5.

Collomb, J., Machouart, M., Blava, M.F., *et al.* (2007). Contribution of NADH dehydrogenase subunit 1 and cytochrome C oxidase subunit 1 sequences toward identifying a case of human coenurosis in France. *J. Parasitol.,* **93:** 934–37.

Devos, T., Szalai, A.J. and Dick, T.A. (1990). Genetic and morphological variability in a population of *D.* dendriticum (Nitzsch, 1824). *Syst. Parasitol.,* **16:** 99–105.

Dovgalev, A.S. (1988). Decontamination of Pacific salmon from type F plerocercoids. *Meditsinsk. Parazitol. Parazit. Bolezni,* **5:** 88–91.

Dupouy-Camet, J. and Peduzzi, R. (2004). Current situation of human diphyllobothriasis in Europe. *Euro Surveill.,* **9:** 31–35.

Fan, P.C. (2005). Infectivity and development of the human strain of *Hymenolepis nana* in ICR mice. *Southeast Asian J. Trop. Med. Public Health,* **36:** 97–102.

Ferretti, G., Gabriele, F. and Palmas, C. (1981). Development of human and mouse strain of *Hymenolepis nana* in mice. *Int. J. Parasitol.,* **11:** 425–30.

Fuentes, M.V., Galán-Puchades, M.T. and Malone, J.B. (2003). Short report: a new case report of human *Mesocestoides* infection in the United States. *Am. J. Trop. Med. Hyg.,* **68:** 566–67.

Galán-Puchades, M.T., Fuentes, M.V. and Mas-Coma, S. (2000). Morphology of *Bertiella studeri* (Blanchard, 1891) sensu Stunkard (1940) (Cestoda: Anoplocephalidae) of human origin and a proposal of criteria for the specific diagnosis of bertiellosis. *Folia Parasitol.,* **47:** 23–28.

Grove, D.I. (1990). *A History of Human Helminthology.* Wallingford: CAB International.

Heldwein, K., Biedermann, H-G., Hamperl, W-D., *et al.* (2006). Subcutaneous *Taenia crassiceps* infection in a patient with non-Hodgkin's lymphoma. *Am. J. Trop. Med. Hyg.,* **75**: 108–11.

Hunter, M.M., Wang, A. and McKay, D.M. (2007). Helminth infection enhances disease in a murine TH2 model of colitis. *Gastroenterology,* **132**: 1320–30.

Klinker, H., Tintelnot, K., Joeres, R., *et al.* (1992). *Taenia crassiceps* in AIDS. *Dtsch Med. Wochenschr.,* **24**: 133–38.

Lee, S-H., Kim, M-N., Back, B-Y., Choi, J-Y., Kim. T-H. and Hwang, Y-S. (2003). Analysis of parasite-specific-antibody positive patients for *Clonorchis sinensis, Paragonimus westermanni, Cysticerosis* and *Sparganum* using ELISA. *Korean J. Lab. Med.,* **23**: 126–31.

Loos-Frank, B. (2000). An up-date of Verster's (1969) 'Taxonomic revision of the genus *Taenia*' (Cestoda) in table format. *Syst. Parasitol.,* **45**: 155–83.

Macnish, M.G., Morgan-Ryan, U.M., Monis, P.T., *et al.* (2002a). A molecular phylogeny of nuclear and mitochondrial sequences in *Hymenolepis nana* (Cestoda) supports the existence of a cryptic species. *Parasitology,* **125**: 567–75.

Macnish, M.G., Morgan, U.M., Behnke, J.M. and Thompson, R.C.A. (2002b). Failure to infect laboratory rodent hosts with human isolates of *Rodentolepis* (= *Hymenolepis*) *nana. J. Helminthol.,* **76**: 37–43.

Macnish, M.G., Ryan, U.M., Behnke, J.M. and Thompson, R.C.A. (2003). Detection of the rodent tapeworm *Rodentolepis* (=*Hymenolepis*) *microstoma* in humans. A new zoonosis? *Intern. J. Parasitol.,* **33**: 1079–85.

Maillard, H., Marionneau, J., Prophette, B., Boyer, E. and Célerier, O. (1998). *Taenia crassiceps* cysticercosis and AIDS. *AIDS,* **12**: 1551–52.

Muratov, I.V. and Posokhov, P.S. (1988). Aspects of the epidemiology of diphyllobothriasis in the lower Pri-Amur region. *Meditsinsk. Parazitol., Parazit. Bolezni,* **4**: 53–57.

Nakao, M., Abmed, D., Yamasaki, H. and Ito, A. (2007). Mitochondrial genomes of the human broad tapeworms *Diphyllobothrium latum* and *Diphyllobothrium nihonkaiense* (Cestoda: Diphyllobothriidae). *Parasitol. Res.,* **101**: 233–36.

Olson, P.D., Yoder, K., Fajardo, L.F., *et al.* (2003). Lethal invasive cestodiasis in immunosuppressed patients. *J. Infect. Dis.,* **187**: 1962–66.

Padgett, K.A. and Boyce, W.M. (2005). Ants as first intermediate hosts for *Mesocestoides* on San Miguel Island, USA. *J. Helminthol.,* **79**: 67–73.

Pampiglione, S., Fioravanti, M.L. and Rivasi, F. (2003). Human sparganosis in Italy. Case report and review of the European cases. *Acta Pathol., Microbiol. Immunol. Scand.,* **111**: 349–54.

Pau, A., Turtas, S., Brambilla, M., *et al.* (1987). Computed-tomography and magnetic resonance imaging of cerebral coenurosis. *Surg. Neurol.,* **27**: 548–52.

Scholtz, T., Garcia, H.H., Kuchta, R. and Wicht, B. (2009). Update on the human broad tapeworm (genus *Diphillobothrium*), including clinical relevance. *Clin. Microbiol. Rev.,* **22**: 146–60.

Skerikova, A., Brabec, J., Kuchta, R., Jimenez, J.A., Garcia, H.H. and Scholtz, T. (2006). Is the human-infecting *Diphyllobothrium pacificum* a valid species or just a South American population of the holarctic fish broad tapeworm, *D. latum? Am. J. Trop. Med. Hyg.,* **75**: 307–10.

Song, T., Wang, W-S., Zhou, B.R., *et al.* (2007). CT and MR characteristics of cerebral sparganosis. *Am. J. Neuroradiol.,* **28**: 1700–1705.

Torres, P., Cuevas, C., Moying, T., *et al.* (2004). Introduced and native fishes as infection foci of *Dipyllobothrium* spp. in humans and dogs from two localities at lake Panguipulli in southern Chile. *Comp. Parasitol.,* **71**: 111–17.

Wicht, B., de Marval, F. and Peduzzi, R. (2007). *Diphyllobothrium nihonkaiense* (Yamane *et al.* 1986) in Switzerland: first molecular evidence and case reports. *Parasitol. Int.,* **56**: 195–99.

Wicht, B., de Marval, F., Gottstein, B. and Peduzzi, R. (2008a). Imported diphyllobothriasis in Switzerland: molecular evidence of *Diphyllobothrium dendriticum* (Nitsch, 1824). *Parasitol. Res.,* **102**: 201–4.

Wicht, B., Scholz, T., Peduzzi, R. and Kuchta, R. (2008b). First record of human infection with the tapeworm *Diphyllobothrium nihonkaiense* in North America. *Am. J. Trop. Med. Hyg.,* **78**: 235–38.

Wiwanitkit, V. (2005). A review of human sparganosis in Thailand. *Int. J. Infect. Dis.,* **9**: 312–16.

Yamane, Y., Kamo, H., Yazaki, S., Fukumoto, S., and Maejima, J. (1981). On a new marine species of the genus *Diphyllobothrium* (Cestoda, Pseudophyllidea) found from a man in Japan. *Japanese J. Parasitol.,* **30**: 101–11.

Yera, H., Estran, C., Delaunay, P, Gari-Toussaint, M., *et al.* (2006). Putative *Diphyllobothrium nihonkaiense* acquired from a Pacific salmon (*Oncorhynchus keta*) eaten in France; genomic identification and case report. *Parasitol. Int.,* **55**: 45–49.

CHAPTER 53

Cystic echinococcosis

Paul R. Torgerson, C. N. L. Macpherson and D. A. Vuitton

Summary

Cystic echinococcosis (CE)\cystic hydatid disease is one of the most widespread and important global helminth zoonoses. The parasite *Echinococcus granulosus* is maintained in a wide spectrum of intermediate hosts, including sheep, goats, camels, cattle, pigs and equines. A number of wild intermediate hosts occur, including cervids in the northern part of the North American continent and Eurasia, marsupials in Australia and wild herbivores in East and southern Africa. The application of a range of molecular techniques to the characterization of the parasite has confirmed the existence of mostly host-adapted strains and genotypes of the parasite and several new species have been proposed. The ubiquitous domestic dog serves as the most important definitive host for the transmission of the parasite throughout its wide geographical range.

A wide range of diagnostic techniques, including necropsy, arecoline purgation, coproantigen ELISA and DNA based tests are available for detecting *E. granulosus* infection in the definitive host. In intermediate animal hosts, diagnosis at *post mortem* still remains the most reliable option. In humans, imaging techniques including ultrasound, nuclear magnetic resonance (NMR) or computer aided tomography (CAT-scan) provide not only a method of diagnosis but also reveal important clinical information on the location, condition, number and size of the hydatid cysts in man. Of these ultrasound is the most widely used diagnostic technique and is the only imaging technique for screening of populations in rural areas, where the disease is most common. A classification system has been developed which can be used to assess the likely development of a cyst and hence guide the clinician in treatment options for the patient. Treatment relies on surgery and/or percutaneous interventions, especially 'Puncture, Aspiration, Injection, Re-aspiration' (PAIR) and/or antiparasitic treatment with albendazole (and alternatively mebendazole).

CE is largely a preventable disease. Successful elimination programmes have focused on frequent periodic treatments of dogs with anthelmintics and the control of slaughter of domestic livestock. In many regions elimination or even control remains a problem as the parasite is endemic over vast areas of low income countries where there may be limited resources for control. In some areas, such as former communist administered countries, the parasite is resurgent. New tools are becoming available to control the parasite, including a highly effective vaccine in sheep which prevents the infection in sheep and breaks the transmission cycle. In addition cost effective methods are being developed which may be appropriate in low income countries where financial resources are not available for intensive control programmes that have been successful in high income countries.

Introduction and historical considerations

Perhaps one of the first references to hydatid disease may be that of Hippocrates (379 BC) with other early references including the works of Galen (AD 139–200), Aretaeus (AD 7–79), and Rhazes (AD 860–932). The cyst was often regarded as enlarged degenerating glands, pus, or end blood vessels (reviewed in Dew (1928); Schwabe (1986)).

Discovery and investigations of the life cycle from the seventeenth century

Redi (1624–94) first recognized that the cyst was of animal origin followed by Pallas who considered them to be a bladder forming parasite. Goeze divided this genus into visceral and intestinal taeniasis. The name *Echinococcus* was introduced into zoology by Rudolphi in 1801. In 1808, Rudolphi described three species within the genus *Echinococcus*: *E. hominis*, *E. simiae*, and *E. veterinorum*. In 1855, Kuchenmeister described two forms of *Echinococcus*: *E. scolicipariens* and *E. altricipariens* in which protoscolices and daughter cysts were formed, respectively. Von Siebold first experimentally infected dogs with *Echinococcus veterinorum* = *Taenia echinococcus* (Von Siebold 1853). This was followed by Naunyn in 1863 in Berlin and Krabbé in Iceland who independently infected dogs with adult worms derived from human protoscolex material. Haubner in 1855 first infected sheep. At that time, Virchow recognized that the condition known as colloid carcinoma was caused by a larval cestode. Subsequently, Leuckart described a form nominated as *Taenia multilocularis*, but did not regard it as a distinct species. Although Leuckart provided the first clear account of the life cycle before the end of the nineteenth century, speciation within the genus *Echinococcus* (Rudolphi 1801) was not solved until the mid-twentieth century.

Epidemiology and control up to the first half of the twentieth century

In Iceland in 1864 Krabbé wrote a 16-page pamphlet which explained the life cycle. Control was initiated in 1869. Dog numbers were limited by taxation and some were treated with areca nut, but the two most important factors in reducing prevalence were a change from wool to lamb production and the reading of Krabbé's pamphlet. Of 15,888 autopsies carried out between 1932 and 1982, 214 had CE. All but eight were born before 1900. The last non-latent case was found in 1960 in a 23 year old woman, but the last two latent cases were found in 1984 and 1988: born respectively in 1905 and 1920. The last two cases of ovine echinococcosis were observed in 1979 (Dungal 1957; Schwabe 1969; Beard 1973a, b).

The introduction of *E. granulosus* into Australia preceded knowledge of the life cycle, and it was considered prior to 1867 that 'hydatids' in humans was caused by eating undercooked sheep meats. From that time, information from Europe spread rapidly and it was recommended in 1898 in the sixth Annual Report of the New Zealand Department of Agriculture that all dogs should be treated with areca nut. Several attempts were made to introduce control there and elsewhere, but, except for Iceland, they were without success until the second half of the twentieth century (Gemmell 1990).

Systematics and biology in the twentieth century

For the first half of the twentieth century controversy existed if the alveolar form of *Echinococcus* was a separate species. It was not until the 1950s that the cestode observed in a rodent on St Lawrence Island by Rausch and Schiller (Rausch and Schiller 1951) was considered to be conspecific with the parasite causing alveolar hydatid disease in Eurasia (Rausch 1953). Initially nominated as *E. sibericensis* this was re-nominated as *E. multilocularis* Leuckart, 1863 (Vogel 1955). Two further species have been regarded as valid. *Taenia oligartha* Diesing, 1863 was transferred to the genus *Echinococcus* in 1910 by Lühe and the life cycle of *E. oligarthrus* was determined experimentally (Sousa and Thatcher 1969). A fourth species, *E. vogeli*, was subsequently described by Rausch and Bernstein (1972) in Ecuador.

Several species which were nominated during the twentieth century are now considered synonymous with *E. granulosus* (Schantz *et al.* 1975, 1976). In addition a further species has been described from the Tibetan plateau, *E. shiquicus* (Xiao *et al.* 2005).

There is also strain variation in the species now recognized as *E. granulosus* and there are proposals for taxonomic revision. This chapter will be primarily concerned with CE, caused by the larval stage of *E. granulosus,* and possibly some of the other newly elevated species of *Echinococcus* which were previously considered part of the taxon *E. granulosus.*

Current concepts in systematic of the genus *Echinococcus*

The suborder, Taeniata Skriabin (Schults 1937) and (subclass Eucestoda, order Cyclophyllidae) consists of a single family, Taeniidae (Ludwig 1886), to which belong the eucestodes of the greatest medical significance (Rausch 1993). Two monotypic subfamilies, Taeniinae (Stiles 1896) and Echinococcinae (Abuladze 1960) are recognized. The latter subfamily contains a single genus *Echinococcus* (Rudolphi 1801).

Recent proposals for speciation and intraspecific variation

Recently using molecular techniques, the phylogeny of *E. granulosus* has advanced considerably. Findings may vary depending on which gene is sequenced and if mitochondrial DNA or nuclear DNA is used for strain typing. The various strains/subspecies defined by molecular biology are often named after their main intermediate host (e.g. sheep strain, cattle strain etc.). However except for the horse strain, host specificity of each strain/subspecies or newly identified species does not occur. Until recently 10 strains of *E. granulosus* were proposed: G1–G10 (Thompson and McManus 2002; Thompson 2008) (Table 53.1). A taxonomic revision has now been recommended with some of these strains being elevated to species. *E. granulosus* strains G1 (the common sheep strain), G2 (Tasmanian sheep strain) and G3 (the buffalo strain) are very close genetically, with no more than 6 base pair variation in the cox1 gene and one variant between G2 and G3. This compares to at least 30 base pair differences between these and other genotypes. Likewise 12s Ribosomal DNA does not discriminate between G2 and G3 strains (Vural *et al.* 2008; Rinaldi *et al.* 2008). Consequently these may turn out to be minor variations of *E. granulosus sensu stricto*. Indeed from an epidemiogical and biological point of view each of these strains readily infects sheep, buffalo and man and a number of other species. In cattle they often produce non fertile cysts. Globally the G1 strain is the most widespread and is responsible for the vast majority of cases of human CE.

Molecular evidence now places the G4 strain in a separate species: *E. equinus*. The molecular variation between *E. equinus* and *E. granulosus sensu stricto* appears to be at least as great as that between *E. multilocularis* and *E. granulosus*. In addition *E. equinus* appears to infect only one group of intermediate hosts—equines and there are no reported cases of human infection with this parasite (Thompson 2008).

E. granulosus G5 strain (the cattle strain) has major genetic differences from *E. granulosus sensu stricto* and elevation to species status—*E. ortleppi* has been proposed. *E. ortleppi* produces highly fertile hydatid cysts in cattle and infects humans. The proposal to elevate this parasite to the status of *E. ortleppi* confirms the original taxonomic proposal in 1943 (Lopez-Neyra and Soler Planas 1943).

E. granulosus strains G6 (the camel strain), G7 (the pig strain), G8 (North American cervid strain) and G10 (the Scandanavian cervid strain) appear to be a genetic clade. *E. granulosus* G9 was reported from a series of patients in Poland (Scott *et al.* 1997). Further studies suggested no significant differences between the mitochondrial sequence data between this strain and the pig strain (G7) (Kedra *et al.* 1999). Presently these strains are still considered strains of *E. granulosus* although there may be sufficient genetic to justify elevating this group to species status. *E. canadensis* has been proposed for G6, G7 and G8 strains (Nakao *et al.* 2007). Alternatively the cervid strains G8 and G10 may represent one species (*E. canadensis*) with G6 and G7 a second species (*E. intermedius*) (Thompson 2008). Recent studies of the nuclear genome tend to confirm the findings of the mitochondrial genome analysis and support the proposal that the strains G6-G10 should be two species with G6, G7 and G9 being *E. intermedius* with G8 and G10 being *E. canadensis* (Saarma *et al.* 2009). The taxonomic status, however, is not settled and other proposals may be made with new molecular tools and a greater understanding of the parasites' biology. All these strains appear to be infective to man. Human CE caused by the pig strain has been reported from Europe and Turkey (Turcekova *et al.* 2003; Pawlowski and Stefaniak 2003; Schneider *et al.* 2007; Snabel *et al.* 2009,). The camel strain G6 has been isolated from an increasing number of human CE cases including from Africa

Table 53.1 Latest proposals for the taxonomic revision of *E. granulosus*

Proposed *Echinococcus* species	Previously recognised *Echinococcus granulosus* strains (genotypes)	Definitive hosts	Intermediate hosts	Infective to man	Geographic distribution
E. granulosus sensu stricto	Sheep strain (G1, G2, G3)	Dog, fox, dingo, jackal, hyena	Sheep, cattle, buffalo, pigs, camel, goats, macropods	Yes	Cosmopolitan: Eurasia, Africa, north and south America, Australia
E. equinus	Horse strain (G4)	Dog	Equines	No evidence	Europe, middle east, south Africa,
E. ortleppi	Cattle strain (G5)	Dog	Cattle, buffalo, sheep, goats	Yes	Europe, South Africa, India, Nepal, Sri Lanka, Russia, South America?
E. intermedius	Camel strain (G6) Pig strain (G7), (G9)	Dog	Pigs, goat, camel, cattle	Yes	Middle East, Iran, Africa, China, Nepal central Asia, Eastern Europe, Argentina
E. canadensis	Cervid strain (G8, G10)	Wolf, Dog	Cervids	Yes, but relatively benign	Northern Eurasia, North America
E. felidis	Lion strain	Lion	Warthogs, zebra, cape buffalo, wildebeest	Unknown	East and southern Africa

(Dinkel *et al.* 2004; Casulli *et al.* 2009), the Middle East (Sadijadi 2006) western China (Bart *et al.* 2006) and South America (Guarnera *et al.* 2004) The cervid strains, whilst infective to humans appear to be relatively benign (Castrodale *et al.* 2002).

A further development has confirmed that lions are definitive hosts for a genotype of *Echinococcus*, provisionally designated *E. felidis*. This parasite appears to be identical to the *E. felidis* isolated from lions previously by Ortlepp (1937). To date, hydatid cysts of the *E. felidis* genotype have only been reported in warthogs (*Phaeoceros* spp) (Huttner *et al.* 2009). It is unknown if *E. felidis* is infective to man.

These *Echinococcus* genotypes have a global distribution (Fig. 53.1)

Host range

Echinococcus spp. are small tapeworms 2–7 mm in length rarely possessing more than five proglottids. They require a definitive (final) host in which the adult develops in the small intestine, and an intermediate host in which the metacestode usually develops in the visceral organs. The principal definitive host of *E. granulosus* is the domestic dog with domestic animals, such as sheep, goats, cattle, camels, and pigs, as intermediate hosts. Several wild life

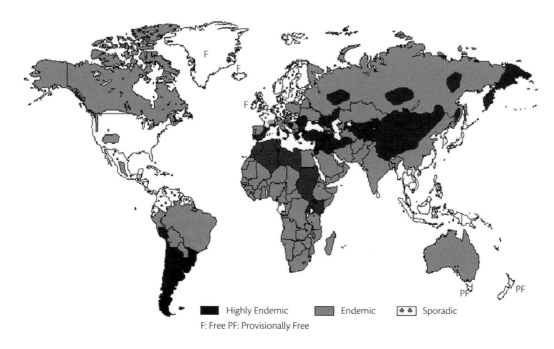

Fig. 53.1 Approximate geographical distribution of the zoonotic strains of *E. granulosus*.
Adapted from Eckert *et al.* (2000, 2001). © Institute für Parasitologie, Universität Zürich. Ireland is free of zoonotic *Echinococcus* spp, but is endemic for *E. equinus*.

cycles exist including for example the dingo (*Canis familiaris dingo*) and macropodid marsupials, particularly the swamp wallaby (*Wallabia bicolour*) in Australia (Jenkins 2006), the wolf and wild cervidae in the northern hemisphere (Thompson 2008) and the lion and warthog in Africa (Hüttner and Romig 2009) (Fig. 53.2). Humans are aberrant intermediate hosts and become infected by ingestion of *Echinococcus* spp. eggs.

Definitive host

Ingested protoscolices develop as tapeworms in the small intestine. Reproduction is sexual. Development involves proglottidization and formation of new reproductive units or proglottids and their maturation. Onset of egg production is between 34 to 58 days. It has been estimated that gravid proglottids are shed every 7–14 days.

The number of eggs per proglottid is variable ranging between 100 and 1,500 but possibly averages about 600 eggs. Limited studies on the longevity of the worms in dogs suggest it to be approximately 8 months to 1 year (Aminzhanov 1975). Indirectly the longevity has also been estimated through transmission models which also suggests approximately 1 year (Torgerson *et al.* 2003b).

The egg

Taeniid eggs are similar in size (30–40 μm), shape, and structure, and cannot be differentiated morphologically. Taeniid eggs are immediately infective after being passed by a definitive host and the larval stage or oncosphere of *Echinococcus* hatch in the small intestine and rapidly and actively penetrate it, aided by hook movement and possibly secretions. It has been suggested that transfer

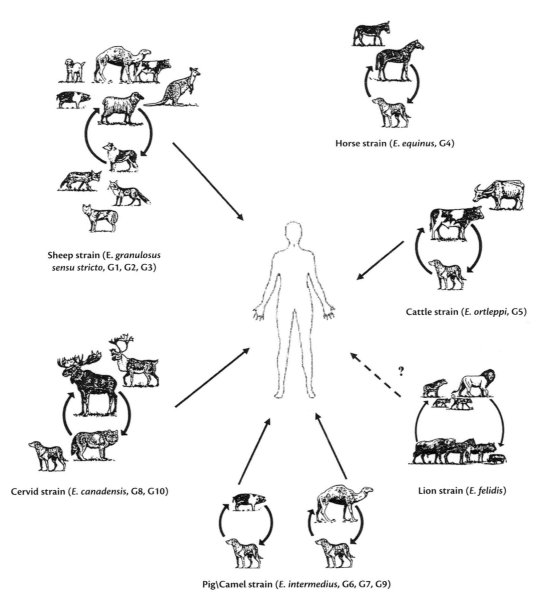

Horse strain (*E. equinus*, G4)

Sheep strain (E. *granulosus sensu stricto*, G1, G2, G3)

Cattle strain (*E. ortleppi*, G5)

?

Cervid strain (*E. canadensis*, G8, G10)

Lion strain (*E. felidis*)

Pig\Camel strain (*E. intermedius*, G6, G7, G9)

Fig. 53.2 Life cycle of *Echinococcus granulosus* illustrating host assemblages of genetically distinct strains and their proposed species designation. The straight arrows indicate those strains which have been found to occur in humans.

may occur via lymphatic or venous migration (Heath 1971). Once established, the oncosphere rapidly undergoes a series of changes to develop into a metacestode (Thompson 1995).

The metacestode

The metacestode of *E. granulosus* is typically unilocular, subspherical and fluid-filled. It consists of a thin germinal layer supported by a strong acellular laminated layer of variable thickness. Asexual proliferation of the germinal layer and brood capsule formation takes place endogenously. Pouching of the wall may give rise to secondary chambers and a multilocular appearance. In some cases daughter cysts may develop within the primary cyst (Rogan *et al.* 2006). Reproduction is asexual and thus has an almost unlimited generative capacity (Whitfield and Evans 1983). Brood capsules develop in the perinuclear layer and within them protoscolices are generated. Fertile cysts may occur in about 195 days in mice, 10–12 months in pigs, or 1 year in sheep.

Clinical aspects in animal hosts

There are no clinical signs of *E. granulosus* infection in dogs. In intermediate hosts there are often no obvious clinical signs, but evidence suggests that *E. granulosus* may cause significant reductions in productivity such as reduce fertility and wool, meat and milk production (Torgerson 2003a). Although many studies that suggest such losses were not well designed, such potential losses should be considered when examining the societal burden of echinococcosis (Carabin *et al.* 2005).

Diagnosis in definitive hosts

Necropsy

The sedimentation and counting technique (SCT) is considered the gold standard (Eckert *et al.* 2001a). The carnivore intestine is opened, incubated in physiological saline and the intestinal mucosa is scraped with a spatula. For mass screening, the intestinal scraping technique (IST), is a less laborious method with a sensitivity of 78% compared to the SCT (Eckert 2003). Deep mucosal scrapings (total 15 per intestine) are squashed into a thin layer and examined microscopically: semi quantitative estimation of the worm burden is possible. Safety precautions must be strictly followed using both these diagnostic strategies (Eckert *et al.* 2001c). An obvious major disadvantage of necropsy is it requires the killing of the dog and is therefore only useful for surveillance in strays and unwanted dogs.

Arecoline purgation

Oral administration of arecoline hydrobromide results in the purgation of intestinal contents after 30–60 minutes. This material can then be examined for the presence of *Echinococcus*. This technique was used during the eradication campaign in New Zealand for mass surveillance (Gemmell 1990). The technique has nearly 100% specificity and has been used for quantitative studies. Safety precautions during field work and parasite identification in the laboratory are essential and time consuming (Eckert *et al.* 2001c). Arecoline can also cause serious, adverse reactions in dogs requiring strict veterinary supervision. The sensitivity is poor with reports of 38% and 65% (Schantz 1997; Ziadinov *et al.* 2008). Nevertheless, it is a potentially useful technique, particularly when evaluating other diagnostic procedures as it can prove the presence of infection.

Coproantigen ELISA

The development of ELISA for the detection of antigens in the faeces of dogs was initially developed by several groups (Allan *et al.* 1992; Deplazes *et al.* 1992). Sensitivity of coproantigen assays is generally good with moderate to high worm burdens (>100 worms), but less in animals with low burdens. Coproantigens can also detect pre-patent infections (Jenkins *et al.* 2000; Allan and Craig 2006). Although sensitivity and specificity have often been defined in select groups of animals (e.g. experimentally infected animals), the actual field performance is less certain because of cross reactivity with antigens from other helminths. Test parameters will also vary with the population on which the test is used. Today coproantigen tests remain a useful procedure for population studies providing the potential pitfalls are fully understood when utilizing such tests.

DNA based tests

Highly specific polymerase chain reactions (PCR) have been developed for use on faeces or isolated eggs to confirm the presence of *Echinococcus* spp. (Stefanic *et al.* 2004; Mathis and Deplazes 2006; Trachsel *et al.* 2007). As PCR is costly and time-consuming, it cannot presently be considered suitable for routine diagnostic or large-scale purposes. Copro-PCR is best used for confirmatory purposes of coproantigen-positive samples. Alternatively, it can be used as the method of choice for identification of the morphologically indistinguishable taeniid eggs recovered from faecal or environmental samples.

A significant problem is that large volumes of faeces are required to obtain a high sensitivity. PCR procedures may also suffer from significant inhibition (Mathis and Deplazes 2006). One approach, to overcome these limitations is to undertake the PCR on isolated taeniid eggs (Mathis *et al.* 1996). A study in Kyrgyzstan suggests the sensitivity of egg isolation followed by PCR is 78% for *E. granulosus* infections. Attempts to improve the sensitivity beyond this could include repeated faecal sampling and/or using PCR techniques that do not rely on egg isolation thus detecting pre-patent infections (Al-Sabi *et al.* 2007). The dynamics of copro-DNA excretion is dependent on loss of parasite stages (protoscoleces during the first days after inoculation and immature stages at the end of pre-patency) whereas coproantigen concentrations are related in this infection period to parasite metabolic activity (Al-Sabi *et al.* 2007). Direct detection of DNA in faeces of *E. granulosus* infected dogs revealed 15 dogs positive by copro-PCR during the prepatent period of 58 dogs proven to be infected by *E. granulosus* indicating a sensitivity of 26% during this phase of the infection (Lahmar *et al.* 2007b). A further important limitation of copro-PCR is that formalin-fixed faecal material is not suitable due to DNA degradation. However, faecal material stored in 70% ethanol or at −20 °C or −80 ° can be used (Al-Sabi *et al.* 2007).

Serology in definitive hosts

Serology in dogs for intestinal *E. granulosus* infections (Gasser *et al.* 1990) has been investigated. Problems reported with sensitivity, specificity and previous infections have prevented serology being employed in surveillance studies (Gasser *et al.* 1993; Craig *et al.* 2003; Eckert *et al.* 2001b).

Diagnosis in intermediate hosts

Diagnosis is rarely indicated in the individual intermediate hosts but population surveys are important to obtain baseline epidemiological information, particularly in respect of control (Torgerson and Heath 2003). Generally, it is undertaken at post mortem (Torgerson et al. 1998). Sheep slaughtered for meat are often young which inevitably have a lower prevalence than older animals (Torgerson and Heath 2003). Furthermore, the better conditioned animals are sent to the abattoir with a smaller likelihood of infection. Thus, abattoir studies, especially if not age-stratified can produce substantial underestimates of the true prevalence. Ultrasound (US) examination can be used in sheep to detect hepatic cysts but the sensitivity is poor (Sage et al. 1998; Lahmar et al. 2007a).

Immunodiagnosis in sheep presents problems of sensitivity and specificity, limiting its applicability. Indirect haemaglutination, double diffusion and ELISA have all been attempted (Gatti et al. 2007). Poor specificity can often be attributed to cross reactivity with other taeniids (such as Taenia ovis and T. hydatigena). Recent studies using hydatid fluid antigen have reported a sensitivity and specificity of 89 and 90%, respectively. The specificity could be improved by using purified fractions of hydatid cyst fluid (S2B) but the sensitivity was decreased (Gatti et al. 2007). Previous studies using either hydatid cyst fluid, antigen B (AgB) purified from hydatid cyst fluid or protoscolex antigens have reported sensitivities ranging from 36% to 90% and specificities ranging from 65% to 96% (Yong et al. 1984; Ibrahem et al. 1996; Kittelberger et al. 2002).

Treatment by drugs

Definitive host

At the end of the nineteenth century, the only drug available to treat dogs for tapeworms was the areca nut, Areca catechu. In 1924, a synthetic salt, arecoline hydrobromide, was developed and used for treating dogs. Up to 11 treatments may be needed to free some dogs from worms. Praziquantel was evaluated in the 1970s and found to be highly effective (Gemmell and Johnstone 1981). The drug was equally effective when given with or without food and can be successfully incorporated into a medicated dog food of high acceptability (Pu-Sheng 1993). It can also be given by injection. The drug does not have a practical ovacidal effect. Praziquantel has now been used in millions of doses without toxicity or drug resistance (Gemmell and Johnstone 1981). Praziquantel remains the drug of choice and cheap supplies of the product are now available as the patent has expired. Although other effective products, such as epsiprantal (Arru et al. 1990) have become available, there appears to be no reason not to continue recommending praziquantel as the drug of choice to treat Echinococcus infections in dogs.

Intermediate hosts

Benzimadazoles such as mebendazole have been shown to be effective in sheep and pigs if treated daily 50 mg/kg for 3 months (Gemmell et al. 1981). It has been observed that in some areas CE in sheep has declined following the widespread introduction of albendazole for the control of nematodes (Santos et al. 2008) resulting in revived interest in using such products for the control of CE in livestock. There have been promising results with albendazole (Santos et al. 2008) and with oxfendazole combined with nitazoxanide (Gavidia et al. 2009).

Immunization

Definitive hosts

Population studies suggest that if dogs are exposed to E. granulosus they will develop a protective immunity (Torgerson 2006a) and exploiting this with a vaccine could be a valuable control tool. Early research with crude antigens to vaccinate dogs resulted in little demonstrable success (Gemmell et al. 1986b). More recently claims were made for significant protection using experimental vaccines (Zhang and McManus 2008). Detailed analysis of these claims (Torgerson 2008) demonstrated that to date there is little progress in developing a vaccine in dogs.

Intermediate hosts

There has been substantial progress in the development of an effective vaccine against E. granulosus in the intermediate host, particularly in sheep using the EG95 oncosphere antigen (Lightowlers et al. 2003). Presently the vaccine comprises a single recombinant oncosphere antigen that is expressed in E. coli and the adjuvant Quil A. It induces complement-fixing antibodies that kill the invading oncosphere early in an infection. In the majority of vaccinated animals, no hydatid cysts occur following a challenge infection but a small number of viable cysts may occur in some vaccinated animals. Animals are vaccinated subcutaneously on two occasions 1 month or more apart, and induce protection against infection which lasts for at least 12 months. A third injection given 6–12 months later induces a high and long-lasting protection against challenge infections. The vaccine has proved effective in vaccine trials carried out in ruminants in New Zealand, Australia, Argentina, Chile and China. GMP production scale-up of the vaccine has been undertaken in New Zealand and China and it is expected that the vaccine will be become available through these sources for implementation as part of hydatid control programs worldwide (Lightowlers and Heath 2004).

Human host

Incubation period and sites of predeliction

Human infection has been recorded in one year old children and in adults of more than 80 years of age (Drolshammer et al. 1973; Chaouachi et al. 1989; Utrilla et al. 1991). Abdominal CE infection is positively correlated with age, whilst surgical pulmonary cases are not (Macpherson et al. 2004). The peak age at the time of diagnosis is 30–50 years with females often over represented (Romig 1990; Schantz et al. 2003; Yang et al. 2006; Yolasigmaz et al. 2006; Yu et al. 2006). The incubation period and clinical picture is dependent on the organ involved (Grossi et al. 1991). The sites of predilection of 1,802 cysts recorded in the Australian Hydatid Register were liver (63%), lung (25%), muscles, (5%), bones (3%), kidney (2%); spleen, brain (1%), and heart, breast, prostate, parotid and pancreas (< 1%) (Grove et al. 1976). Similar figures are given from a series of 3,736 cases hospitalized in Western China: liver (65%), lung (27%), abdominal cavity (2%), brain (3%) and other locations (3%) (Wen and Yang 1997). Most patients have single cysts and the right lobe is more commonly affected than the left lobe of the liver (Romig 1990; Ammann and Eckert 1995). 'Collossal' cysts have been recorded particularly in patients with limited access to health care but the average size may be 1–10 cm (Todorov et al. 1992a).

Cysts have been reported to grow 1–50 mm per year (30%), 6–15 mm per year (43%)or > 30mm per year (11%) or to persist without change for years, or even collapse (4/75 cysts) (Romig *et al.* 1986; Mufit *et al.* 1998). Ultrasound (US) follow-up after mass surveys showed that half of the cysts failed to change in size despite having been diagnosed during the so-called evolutionary growth phase; in the other 50% increases were variable, ranging from a few millimetres to some centimetres (Wang *et al.* 2006). Cysts can spontaneously rupture collapse or disappear. A number of studies indicate that liver cysts grow at a slower rate than lung cysts (Larrieu and Frider 2001). The exact sequence of qualitative cyst changes during its natural history is still unclear (Rogan *et al.* 2006). Protoscolices may be found in daughter cysts of diameter 0.5 cm (Alvarez *et al.* 1991).

Symptoms, signs and complications

Symptomatology depends on:

1) The organ involved,

2) The size and location of the cyst within the invaded organ(s),

3) Pressure induced within organ(s),

4) Complications such as rupture and spread of larval tissue with formation of secondary cysts and possible sepsis.

Leakage following diagnostic puncture or spontaneous or post-traumatic rupture or fissure may induce mild or serious complications, such as urticaria, asthma, or anaphylaxis shock, due to allergic reaction to *Echinococcus* antigens (Vuitton 2004). Membrane nephropathy has also been described (Ammann and Eckert 1995). Secondary peritoneal echinococcosis may result from spontaneous, traumatic rupture, or rupture during surgery of a hepatic cyst, but is rare from a pulmonary cyst (Ammann and Eckert 1995). The consequences of secondary CE are recognized several years later. Cysts that become encapsulated and calcified, although potentially viable, may remain asymptomatic indefinitely accounting for a relatively high proportion of cases being asymptomatic during ultrasound surveys (Ammann and Eckert 1995). Spontaneous cure of CE does occur due to collapse and resolution, calcification, or cyst rupture into the bronchial tree or bile ducts (Ammann and Eckert 1995).

Diagnosis

Non-invasive methods

Ultrasound examination (US), a widely used technique, can confirm the diagnosis of abdominal echinococcosis and indicate if lesions are active. Further information can be found in many sources (WHO-IGWE 2003; Macpherson *et al.* 2003; Rogan *et al.* 2006; Kern *et al.* 2006; Bresson-Hadni *et al.* 2006). Pulmonary echinococcosis cannot normally be detected by US. US for mass screening is generally considered to have a sensitivity of 88–98% and a specificity of 93–100% for abdominal lesions (Macpherson and Milner 2003; Macpherson *et al.* 2003b). However, the sensitivity of this technique for detecting all forms of echinococcosis is somewhat lower. Using technical modifications, a proportion of lung cysts might be detected (El Fortia *et al.* 2006).

Nuclear magnetic resonance (NMR) or computer aided tomography (CAT-scan) can be used to confirm the diagnosis, especially for lung and brain cysts, and to perform a pre-therapeutic assessment of the lesions, for all locations (Turgut *et al.* 2007). Unfortunately, in many remote endemic areas such facilities are not available. In this case, serological back-up tests may be required to give additional information regarding the nature of the lesion detected by US.

WHO classification of cysts found on US

US has been used to study the evolution of cysts over time, the structural integrity of cysts following chemotherapy (WHO-IWGE 2003) and for use in screening and surveillance programmes (Macpherson *et al.* 2003a). A classification system has been developed which can be used to assess the likely development of a cyst and hence guide the clinician in treatment options for the patient (Fig. 53.3) (WHO-IWGE 2003).

The widespread use of the WHO classification provides a better understanding of the epidemiology, biology, public health importance, control and treatment of CE globally, through:

1) Standardization of the diagnostic values of US examination (sensitivity and specificity; positive and negative predictive values) by universal application of the classification to mass screening data collected in field studies.

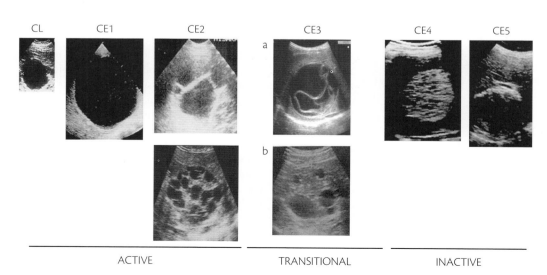

Fig. 53.3 WHO-IWGE classification of ultrasound images of the different CE cyst types (CE1–5). CL = cystic lesion of unknown aetiology which may include being early undifferentiated CE cysts (WHO-IWGE, 2003).

2) Evaluation and comparison of cyst types and locations as well as treatment outcomes of different CE types from different parts of the world (thus giving an insight into biological variations within the parasite species and/or transmission characteristics).

3) Evaluation and comparison of the changes and rates of change in cyst types from different studies in patients who receive chemotherapy or those who remain untreated.

4) Evaluation of standard treatment options which are currently recommended by the WHO-IWGE for each cyst type and group.

The WHO classification differs from Gharbi's original classification (Gharbi et al.1981) by introducing a cystic lesion (CL) stage and by reversing the order of CE Types 2 and 3 (Table 53.2; WHO-IWGE 2003; Brunetti et al. 2009). The number of cyst types remains unchanged from Gharbi's classification and the types are readily categorized into active, transitional and inactive stages. The inclusion of the CL stage reflects the detection of early, undifferentiated cysts found during mass screening. CL cysts are not included as a Type of CE as they have to be further evaluated before being classified as CE. The first CE Types are CE1 and 2 and such cysts are active, usually fertile cysts containing viable protoscoleces. CE3 are cysts entering a transitional stage where the integrity of the cyst has been compromised either by the host or by chemotherapy. CE4 and 5 are inactive cysts that have normally lost their fertility and are degenerative. Data on long-term follow-up of cysts treated with albendazole and percutaneous puncture (PAIR) provide ground for a further sub-classification of CE3 transitional cysts into CE3a (detached endocyst) and CE3b (predominantly solid with daughter cysts) (Junghanss et al. 2008). This has important implications for clinical decision making and prognosis.

Serology

A large number of serological assays have been developed for the diagnosis of human echinococcosis (reviewed in Carmena et al. 2006). Native crude antigens such as hydatid cyst fluid have generally proved to be sensitive. In a variable proportion of CE patients, no specific antibodies could be demonstrated with a variety of tests, especially those with lung cysts. The highest sensitivity, observed for liver cysts, may be due to complex parasite-host interactions modulating the immune system (Riganò et al. 2001) Specificity is a problem with cross reactions with other helminths (Eckert and Deplazes 2004). Specificity was considerably increased on genus or even species level by purification of components such as AgB in hydatid cyst fluid of E. granulosus metacestode material. Various groups have developed diagnostic tests based on recombinant AgB with better test performance than native AgB (reviewed by Mamuti et al. 2005; Carmena et al. 2006), and synthetic peptides mimicking defined epitopes have also been investigated. Sensitivity and specificity of tests based on AgB have largely been evaluated on known hydatid disease patients or known healthy individuals where sensitivity has varied between 0.45 and 0.92. Specificity is reported as between 0.71 and 1 with cross reactivity against AE, cysticercosis, Schistosoma and Toxocara (Carmena et al. 2006).

Serology also detects exposure to the parasite before disease development and exposure without parasite establishment. This, with the less than ideal level of test specificity explains why sometimes positive serological results are found during mass screening in endemic areas in patients without any cyst disclosed by US. The problems associated with detecting false positives prevent serology alone from being used for screening for CE.

Treatment

There are numerous important reviews on the therapeutic management of CE. However, it still is a controversial subject (Dziri et al. 2004). Few controlled studies on the treatment of CE with a proper follow-up of patients are available (Vuitton and Wen 2007). Consensus opinion was reached within the WHO-IWGE and the main conclusions published in 1996 (WHO-IWGE 1996) with updated recommendations published in 2009 (Vuitton 2009; Brunetti et al. 2009). Surgery was the only option until the late 1970s. Complementary or alternative options are now available, which include non-surgical interventions and chemotherapy with anti-parasitic drugs. Treatment indication should be based on a multidisciplinary discussion and depends on cyst type, number and location, and presence or absence of cyst complication. A proper and long-term follow-up of the patients should assess the efficacy of the treatment, detect treatment complications, and timely disclose recurrences.

Pre-operative treatment

To avoid protoscolex spillage during operation, viable components of the parasitic cyst must be inactivated with hypersaline solution or hydrogen peroxide prior to any cyst opening. Use of formalin must be totally forbidden; but none of the protoscolicides are totally safe (Ammann and Eckert 1995).

The main complication is sclerosing cholangitis, which is possible when there is communication between the cyst and the biliary tree (Ammann and Eckert 1995). There is still debate on the necessity, modalities and time schedule of anti-parasitic chemotherapy before and/or after interventional treatments, including surgery (Vuitton and Wen 2007).

Surgery

The principal methods include hepatic resection; pericystectomy and cystectomy for hepatic cysts; and opening, sterilization and partial removal of the cysts, also called partial cystectomy; pericystectomy and lobectomy for pulmonary cysts (Ming-Quian 1993). Laparoscopic surgery is a technical option in selected cases but possibly increases protoscolex spillage. Cysts should be removed as

Table 53.2 Prevalence of postoperative complications in 63/212 patients with cystic echinococcosis (CE)

Complication	Number of cases	%
Death	8	3.8
External bile fistula	8	3.8
Infection of residual cavity	3	1.4
Intraperitoneal abscess	5	2.8
Wound infection	10	4.7
Pneumonia	11	5.2
Recurrent CE	18	8.5

After Barros (1978)

much as possible; however, the more radical the intervention the higher the operative risk, but with the likelihood of fewer relapses, and vice versa (WHO-IGWE 1996). Following the cleavage plane between the inner layer of host's reaction facing towards the parasite and the outer layer, or 'adventitia', limits the damage to liver parenchyma when dissecting around the cyst and allows a safer removal of the cyst by total cystectomy (Wu et al. 2004). Postoperative complications may occur in between 10 and 25% of cases (Kammerer and Schantz 1993). Some of the untoward sequelae that may be expected are summarized in Table 53.2. Recurrence rates vary from 2 to 25% (Romig 1990; Todorov et al. 1992b) and are more frequent after partial operations. Absence of long-term follow-up and/or studies restricted to small series, in selected patients, and/or in highly specialized settings of developed countries, usually explains the most optimistic results. In an extensive review in China, 92, 7, 0.8 and 0.2% had 1, 2, 3, and 4 or more operations (Menghebat et al. 1993). In a study in Kenya, among 663 patients, there were 2 deaths, one intraoperative and one postoperative, after surgery, and 47 patients had repeated operations because of postoperative complications and/or recurrences (Cooney et al. 2004).

Besides recurrence, biliary leakage is the most frequent complication and the most difficult to manage. Lethality associated with the first operation is about 2% (Kammerer and Schantz 1993), but it increases substantially after subsequent surgery (Amir-Jahed et al. 1975).

Non-surgical management

Percutaneous puncture (PAIR) for inoperable cases is currently accepted as an alternative to surgery in selected cases. This includes puncture of the cyst, aspiration of the fluid content of the cyst, introduction of a protoscolicide, such as hypertonic saline or, preferably, alcohol and re-aspiration. It is carried out under ultrasonic guidance (Kammerer and Schantz 1993; Ammann and Eckert 1995; Filice et al. 2000). Detailed practical guidelines have been published by the WHO-Informal Working Group (WHO-IWGE 2001). In experienced hands, PAIR represents the first choice of treatment in middle-sized non-complicated cysts (Filice et al. 1990). Long term follow-up of patients is now available (Akhan et al. 1996). A meta-analysis has supported the efficiency, safety and usefulness of the procedure, in selected indications (Smego et al. 2003). A very limited number of anaphylactic shocks, usually reversible with appropriate resuscitation, have been reported. In most series, recurrence of the cysts is lower than after surgery. PAIR can be proposed for type CE1, and selected cases among CE2, and CE3 cysts. It is contraindicated if there is communication of the cyst with the biliary tree. Drainage may be associated with PAIR for large cysts (Filice et al. 1990). To treat cysts with numerous daughter cysts, modified techniques using larger tubes and vacuum aspiration through a small surgical incision have been described, but the rate of long-term recurrences seems to be high (Brunetti et al. 2009). Prior to, and for a period following percutaneous interventions, benzimidazoles should be administered. In the most accepted administration schedule, albendazole (ABZ) is given the day before and during 1 month after (Brunetti et al. 2009). ABZ should not be given when PAIR is performed during pregnancy.

Chemotherapy

Benzimidazole compounds are potential parasitocidal agents against E. granulosus. ABZ is currently the drug of choice to treat CE, either alone or as an adjunctive/prophylactic therapy together with surgery or percutaneous interventions. The drug is given orally at a dosage of 10–15 mg/kg/day (normally rounded to 400mg twice daily), accompanied by a fat-rich meal to increase bioavailability. It should be given continuously (Brunetti et al. 2009). Alternatively, mebendazole (MBZ) is another benzimidazole compound which may be used if ABZ is not available or not tolerated by the patient. MBZ daily dosage is of 50 mg/kg body weight, in three divided doses during fat-rich meals. Both drugs should be avoided during pregnancy, especially for the first trimester (WHO-IWGE 1996). Main side-effects are haematological and hepatic toxicity, and alopecia. Blood count and serum aminotransferases should be monitored every 2 weeks for the first 3 months, then monthly. Optimal dosage and optimal durations have never been formally assessed for either of the drugs (WHO-IWGE 1996; Ammann and Eckert 1996). Serum blood levels of ABZ sulfoxide or of MBZ should be monitored 1 month after commencement of treatment and then every 3 months (WHO-IWGE 1996).

Most studies have used echographic methods to assess benzimidazole efficiency (el-Mufti et al. 1993; Wen et al. 1993). Difficulties have been found in ascribing death of cysts to the treatment. Efficacy with standard 800 mg ABZ daily for 3–6 months produces an average of 30% cure and 45% response. It is more effective in younger patients and for small CE1 and CE3a cysts with a thin wall without infection or communication. It may be less effective for CE2 (Horton 1997). Three available randomized controlled trials showed that ABZ alone had a better effect on hydatid cysts than placebo or MBZ (Gil-Grande et al. 1993; Franchi et al. 1999; Keshmiri et al. 2001). Complete disappearance of all cysts was never reached and therefore chemotherapy is not the ideal treatment when used alone. In addition, its efficacy is lower for lung cysts or bone cysts than for liver cysts. This therapeutic option is indicated for inoperable patients, for patients with multiple cysts in liver or in two or more organs, and for patients with peritoneal cysts (Brunetti et al. 2009).

Praziquantel has been tested for protoscolicidal efficacy in vitro. In one in vivo study involving 101 patients, there was very little difference in the viability of protoscolices between the treated and untreated patients as determined at surgery (Jia-Zhong et al. 1993). One prospective controlled trial compared ABZ and praziquantel (25mg/kg/d) versus ABZ alone (Mohamed et al. 1998) and concluded that the combined treatment was more effective than ABZ alone. Combined treatment is usually administered in severe cases with multiple cysts and/or several locations, and in bone CE.

Epidemiology and transmission to man

E. granulosus has both sylvatic and domestic cycles. It is the latter transmission cycle that is the most common and poses the greatest threat to human health. The highest incidences in man are seen where there is a close association with man and domestic livestock, often using working dogs. A common source of infection for dogs is offal from infected sheep. The resultant high infection levels in these dogs then pose a risk to humans. The cohabitation with dogs and feeding of uncooked viscera is a known risk factor for human CE (Campos-Bueno et al. 2000).

The potential for domestic transmission of E. granulosus is highest in countries where the level of education may be poor, veterinary and medical services inadequate and where home slaughter is commonly practiced. In such circumstances, the rates of infection in dogs can reach between 20 and 50% with perhaps an excess of 50% of the sheep population being infected. Dog contact is a major risk factor as they are the definitive host (Tiaoying *et al.* 2005; Yu *et al.* 2006; Moro *et al.* 2008). Dogs themselves are more likely to become infected if they are young, allowed to roam, fed on raw offal, offal in the community is not disposed of properly, the dogs not receiving anthelmintic treatment or the dogs' owners being ignorant of the disease (Macpherson 2005; Budke *et al.* 2005a, b; Buishi *et al.* 2005, 2008; Ziadinov *et al.* 2008).

As a generalization, human CE is linked to the prevalence in domestic livestock, particularly sheep and livestock husbandry practices (Bai *et al.* 2002; Torgerson *et al.* 2002; Schantz *et al.* 2003; Moro *et al.* 2008; Ahmadi and Hamidi 2008). Occasionally other species, such as camels and pigs, may also be intermediate important hosts (Kedra *et al.* 1999). In Europe, autothochonous CE is generally rare in central and northern Europe, although there are some foci in eastern Europe which are believed to be mainly through transmission of the pig strain (Romig *et al.* 2006). The most intensely infected areas are Spain, where in some districts human incidence rates are 1.1–3.4/100,000/year (Carmena *et al.* 2008) and Italy, particularly Sardinia where annual human incidence rates are 3.5/100,000 (Castiglia *et al.* 2004). CE is also an emerging problem in Greece, Bulgaria and Romania where incidences of 3.3/100,000/year have been recorded (Todorov and Boeva 1999). There is also a small focus in Wales in the UK.

CE is a significant problem across much of the Middle East and North Africa. In Jordan the annual incidence is 2.9/100,000 (Kamhawi 1995), in Tunisia 15/100,000 (Majorowski *et al.* 2005), 10–30/100,000 in rural parts of and in Turkey 0.67–6.6/100,000 (Altintas 2003). In Central Asia surgical incidence rates are commonly between 10 and 20/100,000 (Torgerson *et al.* 2006).

Certain communities in Tibet have some of the highest incidences of CE. In some villages US prevalences range between 5–10% (Budke *et al.* 2004; Yu *et al.* 2008). Similar disease burdens have also been recorded in transhumant pastoral communities in East Africa, such as the Turkana and Masai in Kenya and Tanzania, Toposa in Sudan and the Dassanetch and Nyangatom in southern Ethiopia (Macpherson *et al.* 1989; Magambo *et al.* 2006).

In Latin America there are large endemic areas throughout the Andean regions of Peru, Argentina, Chile, Uruguay southern Brazil and sporadic cases being reported elsewhere such as Mexico (Moro and Schantz 2006).

In the US and Canada, CE tends to be sporadic and rare with cases occasionally being reported in certain groups of native Americans or particular ethnic groups (Moro and Schantz 2006).

In Australasia CE was introduced with European colonization (Jenkins 2005) and became a problem in large sheep rearing areas. Successful control programmes have resulted in the elimination of the parasite from New Zealand and Tasmania (Craig and Larrieu 2006). In continental Australia the parasite has established a wild life cycle between macropod marsupials and dingoes. Therefore prospects for elimination are now considered bleak. There are frequent descriptions of transmission within the domestic cycle and human CE is recorded not uncommonly (Jenkins 2005, 2006).

The risks associated with infection are illustrated by the deteriorating situation in Central Asia. Prior to the breakup of the Soviet Union, CE in man was at relatively low levels. Following independence of the Central Asian republics there was widespread structural and economic reform. This resulted in privatization of farms, abandonment of centralized meat processing facilities and a return to small subsistence-type agricultural practices. Veterinary services collapsed due to a lack of government funding. This resulted in an epidemic of human CE, with the annual incidence of surgical cases reported by hospitals in excess of 4–5 times the number reported prior to 1991 (Torgerson *et al.* 2006). A similar pattern is also emerging in other former communist countries like Bulgaria (Todorov and Boeva 1999). Unregulated slaughtering of domestic animals results in greater possibilities for dogs to become infected. Dogs are more numerous than previously as livestock units are smaller and greater numbers of dogs are required for shepherding. Small farms are also generally located closer to human population centers compared to the large state run farms previously. Thus there are more dogs with a higher prevalence of infection in greater contact with humans (Torgerson *et al.* 2006; Shaikenov *et al.* 2003). Another noticeable feature of these emerging epidemics in former socialist countries is the high numbers of children with the disease, with perhaps up to one third of surgeries in children under 14, indicating recent transmission (Torgerson *et al.* 2003a; 2006).

There is a growing body of evidence that CE may be a cause and consequence of poverty within endemic zones (Torgerson *et al.* 2001, 2003a, 2009b; Budke *et al.* 2004, 2005c). It is uncertain if this is cause and effect. Greater poverty may render individuals more susceptible to infection or as CE is a devastating disease, infection may lead to poverty such as through loss of employment.

Surprisingly dog contact is not always a risk factor for transmission of CE, especially in climates where eggs may survive in the environment for long periods of time (Carmona *et al.* 1998; Bai *et al.* 2002; Torgerson *et al.* 2003a). Lack of association with contact may be a consequence of infection occurring many years earlier and recall is difficult for subjects of epidemiological studies. Also of importance is the fact that in many highly endemic regions dog ownership and dog contact is almost universal, so this factor cannot discriminate between infected and non infected individuals (Torgerson *et al.* 2009) and hence it is the epidemiology of infection of the dog (see above) that becomes important. In some societies, such as in North Africa, the Middle East and Turkey dogs are considered unclean and hence there is a reluctance to have close contact with them (Dowling *et al.* 2000). Despite this CE infection amongst many of these people is evidence for indirect transmission of echinococcosis to man through contaminated food or water supplies (Carmona *et al.* 1998; Dowling *et al.* 2000; Larrieu *et al.* 2002; Torgerson *et al.* 2003a; Tiaoying *et al.* 2005). Epidemiological and experimental evidence has demonstrated that taeniid eggs can be transmitted considerable distances by mechanical carriers such as insects (Gemmell 1990). Thus, in highly endemic areas it is quite possible for individuals to contract CE even in the absence of dog contact.

Women are often reported to have a higher incidence of infection than men (Romig 1990; Schantz *et al.* 2003; Yang *et al.* 2006; Yolasigmaz *et al.* 2006; Yu *et al.* 2006) and this may be because they are more likely to tend to the household dogs and be involved with food preparation. In some populations men are found to have a higher incidence (Torgerson *et al.* 2003a) and this may reflect that in some societies men are more likely to be treated because they are more economically active, rather than an actual increased risk for men. Increasing age is also often reported as a risk factor (Romig 1990; Yu *et al.* 2006; Ahmadi and Hamidi 2008) with the peak age being 30–50 years. This is most likely due to continuous infection opportunities over time and the chronic and asymptomatic nature of abdominal CE (Macpherson *et al.* 2004).

Absence of CE in children may indicate that transmission has ceased following successful implementation of control measures (Zanini *et al.* 2009). Changes over time to more advanced cyst types seen in all age groups, following the introduction of control measures may also suggest cessation of transmission. Increasing numbers of paediatric cases and or small early cyst types in various age groups may indicate a breakdown of control measures (Torgerson *et al.* 2002, 2003a).

Economics and societal burden

CE presents a considerable societal and economic burden to a number of societies where *E. granulosus* is endemic. In terms of animal health the disease can lead to significant losses of production due to liver condemnations, lowered milk, meat and wool production or decreased fertility in animals (Torgerson 2003a). This particularly impacts on societies with low socio economic development which have the highest prevalences in livestock.

The societal burden in terms of human health is also of major consideration. In financial terms the costs of the disease include costs of surgical and medical treatment, the costs of convalescence such as loss of income and the costs of providing supportive care for individuals with chronic ill health. The direct treatment costs can vary depending on the country in which treatment is received. This can be as low as US$524 in a country such as Jordan (Torgerson *et al.* 2001) (2001 figures), to >$13,000 in the UK (Torgerson and Dowling 2001). This high variation reflects the different costs of medical care in different countries. In high income countries the costs of treatment are greater. However, the impact to individuals of such costs is likely to be much greater in countries where incomes are low as even the relatively low costs (by international comparison), may still be beyond the resources of patients from these areas. One of the consequences is that the incidence of CE in low income countries is much more likely to be underreported.

A number of studies have estimated the economic costs of CE in various countries and it is often considerable (Torgerson *et al.* 2000, 2001; Torgerson and Dowling 2001; Majorowski *et al.* 2005). There is also a financial estimate of the global costs of CE which suggests it could be as much as $3 billion annually (Budke *et al.* 2006) if estimates for underreporting of the disease are accounted for.

Although financial estimates of societal burden are important for zoonoses that have major impacts on both livestock productivity and animal health, other measures have also been calculated. The WHO preferred measure is the Disability Adjusted Life Year (DALY) (see Chapter 4, this volume). Estimates for DALYs have been made in a highly endemic region of the Chinese province of Sichuan and this indicates a loss of 0.81 DALYs per person in the population due to echinococcosis (Budke *et al.* 2004). Thus the health impact is considerable as the average numbers of DALYs lost to Chinese residents due to all causes is 0.18 DALYs. A preliminary estimate of the global burden on echinococcosis has also been made which indicates a loss of approximately 1 million DALYs (Budke *et al.* 2006). This is of a similar magnitude to the global burden of Trypanosomosis and considerably more than diseases such as Dengue or Leprosy.

Burden estimates present important methods in developing cost effective means of controlling this often neglected zoonoses.

Prevention and control

Some experience has now been gained on applying control based on studies of field trials, control programmes and, more recently, mathematical modelling (Craig and Larrieu 2006).

- **Control** describes the 'active implementation of a programme by a recognized authority on an instruction from the legislature to limit prevalence of a specific disease'.

- **Eradication** is the reduction of CE prevalence in the global human or animal host population to zero. This is not believed to be feasible at the present time.

- **Elimination** describes either the reduction of the prevalence of CE in a regional population to zero, or the reduction of the global prevalence to a negligible amount. In some islands this has been achieved such as Iceland, Tasmania and New Zealand.

Priority status for control include:

(1) Prevalence of disease,

(2) Morbidity or severity of disability,

(3) Risk of mortality,

(4) Feasibility of control or elimination, including relative efficiency and cost of intervention,

(5) Absence of adverse ecological factors,

(6) Adequate administration, operational and financial resources,

(7) Availability of effective tools,

(8) Favourable epidemiological features,

(9) Socio-economic importance,

(10) Specific reasons for preferring eradication over control.

It should always be remembered that these two goals are not the same.

Legislation, administration and funding

There are two models. The first creates, through specific legislation, a national or regional executive authority with responsibility for the control programme. The second utilizes an existing government organization (e.g. Ministry of Health or Agriculture). To an extent, the former is likely to be funded through a dog tax and latter through the legislature.

Depending on the programme to be adopted, areas in which legislation may be needed include:

(1) Meat inspection and effective disposal of offal at abattoirs and prevention of clandestine leakage of offal,

(2) Banning dogs from abattoirs and closure if necessary,

(3) Prevention of feeding raw offal to dogs, including inspection of offal disposal facilities on farms or other premises where sheep are killed,

(4) Control of dogs, including registration, submission of dogs for dosing, and elimination of unwanted dogs,

(5) Quarantine of premises with infected livestock.

Options and phases of control

Control of CE has always involved a combination of routine anthelmintic treatment of dogs, control and reduction of stray dog populations, supervision of the slaughter of livestock and subsequent disposal of offal, and education of the public. Gemmell and Roberts (1996) have previously described 5 options. The option of do nothing may be considered if there are more pressing public health issues that demand the use of resources. A slow track approach may focus on education and upgrading of facilities and development and possibly supplying drugs to treat dogs and such an approach may take many decades to complete. A third approach using arecoline testing as an educational approach is no longer appropriate due to the advent of better diagnostic technologies and the hazards and welfare issues surrounding the use of arecoline. The fourth option was combining this with dog euthanasia, which may also have substantial resistance in many societies. The fifth option was based on the intensive treatment of dogs with praziquantel. The pre-patent period of *E. granulosus* is approximately 6 weeks and hence this has usually been the recommended treatment interval.

With new technology (e.g. the sheep vaccine) additional options are becoming available. Mathematical models have been developed to simulate control options (Torgerson and Heath 2003). Six weekly anthelmintic treatment is highly effective but is expensive and therefore less suitable for use in poor countries. Simulation models suggest it may be possible to lengthen the interval between anthelmintic treatments to at least 3 months and still reduce prevalence rates in dogs and livestock to less than 1% within 10–15 years (Torgerson 2003b). This does depend on treating perhaps 75% or more of the dog population. If only 60% or less is treated then failure to eliminate the parasite is possible. This idea has been supported by field studies in Uruguay (Cabrera *et al.* 2002) and New Zealand (Gemmell 1990). The lengthening of the treatment intervals to beyond the pre-patent period can work because the mean time to reinfection is often considerably longer than six weeks. Six monthly anthelmintic treatment only reduces the levels of echinococcosis substantially if the treatment rate is well in excess of 90%, which is unlikely to occur in practice.

Providing at least 75% of sheep are vaccinated, echinococcosis will be reduced considerably, but not for several years after implementation and intensive vaccination of sheep may become an option when the EG95 vaccine is commercially available. Alternatively an option of twice yearly anthelmintic treatment of dogs and vaccination of sheep should be considered. Providing 60% of sheep are vaccinated and 60% of dogs treated there is high probability of success within a time frame of 15–20 years (Torgerson and Heath 2003).

Recent work has demonstrated that old sheep contain most of the infective larval biomass (Torgerson *et al.* 2009c). This presents opportunities for a faster track approach to control by culling old sheep and hence instantly reduce the infection pressure to dogs by 80–90% resulting in a rapid cessation of transmission (Fig. 53.4). Alternatively suitable chemotherapy in sheep (Gavidia *et al.* 2009) might achieve a similar effect. Economic analysis should be an important priority before control is initiated (Torgerson 2003a) to develop the most cost-effective means of control.

Four phases of control can be recognized: a 'preparatory' and/or 'planning' phase; 'attack'; 'consolidation' and, where appropriate, 'maintenance of elimination' phase (Gemmell 1987). During the

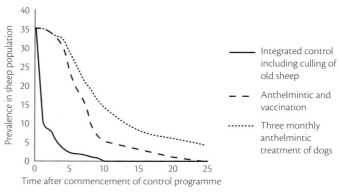

Fig. 53.4 The expected decline in prevalence in sheep during the attack phase In this scenario, pre-control prevalence is approximately 35% in sheep. If 75% or more of dogs are treated just 4 times a year (dotted line) effective control and possible elimination will only be achieved after a considerable period of time. If vaccination of sheep is included then elimination can be expected after 25 years (dashed line) even if a substantial proportion of dogs avoid treatment. If old sheep are removed this not only rapidly decreases the prevalence, but as most of the biomass of the parasite is removed, dogs will not be reinfected and hence there are rapid further declines in the prevalence in sheep. This should decrease the attack period to as little as 5 years or less (solid line).

costly 'attack' phase, the control measures are applied non-discriminately to the entire host population at risk. As soon as the parasite reaches certain low level it becomes more cost-effective to cease the overall attack and to target control in the 'consolidation' phase. If appropriate, once the parasite has been almost eliminated, the 'maintenance of elimination' phase may be entered. Here all specific activities are suspended or disbanded and 'vigilance' is permanently maintained through the normal meat inspection services.

Review of control programmes

The control programmes selected for review in this section, differ from one another in administration, resources used, methods applied, and rate of decline in transmission. The changes that occurred in the prevalence of *E. granulosus* in adult sheep are illustrated in Fig. 53.5.

Option 2 with evidence of success over 100 years

The successful programme initiated in the nineteenth century in Iceland has been described previously.

Option 2 with no evidence of success over 20 years
Island model

In New Zealand in 1908, it was made compulsory for owners to register their dogs. In 1935, a strong educational campaign was introduced. In 1937 by an amendment to the Dog Act (1908), all owners who registered their dogs received sufficient arecoline hydrobromide to treat them four times a year. In 1940, it was made illegal to feed raw offal to dogs. No change was detected in the prevalence of echinococcosis in animals or humans 20 years later (Gemmell 1990).

Continental model

Control in Uruguay was initiated in 1965 with the creation of a National Commission. Funding was initially provided by a dog tax

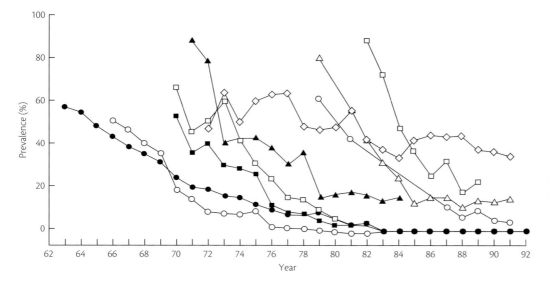

Fig. 53.5 Changes in the prevalence of E. granulosus in adult sheep during control in Uruguay (◊, Option 2); New Zealand (●) and Tasmania (◻) (Option 3); Cyprus (□); and the Falkland Island (■), Argentina (Nequén, ▲; Rio Negro ○), and Chile (Region 11, (□; Region 12△) Option 5)
From Gemmell and Roberts (1996).

and owners were also expected to purchase tablets and treat their dogs. No evidence could be found that any of the activities attempted between 1965 and 1991 modified the level of transmission of echinococcosis between dogs and sheep (Cabrera *et al.* 1995; Parada *et al.* 1995). Recent evidence from serological and ultrasound surveys also suggests that in some departments, up to 2% of the rural population may have asymptomatic CE (Bonifacino *et al.* 1991; Paolillo *et al.* 1991; Cohen *et al.* 1991). Since 1990, the programme has been transformed to Option 5).

Option 3 with evidence of success within 30 years
Island models

Two programmes using a 'slow-track' approach have been completed in New Zealand and Tasmania (Craig and Larrieu 2006).

In both programmes, transmission of CE (Tables 53.3 and 53.4) ceased to children within about 7–12 years of their introduction, although the 'maintenance of eradication' phase was not reached until about 35 years of their introduction. Both New Zealand and Tasmania are now believed to be free of *Echinococcus*.

Option 4 with evidence of success within 15 years
Island model

Cyprus initiated stray dog euthanasia in 1970 and a dog-testing programme with arecoline surveillance in 1972. In 1974, partition occurred, but control continued in the government-controlled area. There, transmission between animals rapidly ceased and in 1985 eradication was assumed (Economides *et al.* 1998). More recently, small foci have reappeared confirming the need to maintain 'vigilance' even when the parasite becomes difficult to find with current diagnostic tools (Christofi *et al.* 2002).

Option 5 with evidence of success within 15 years
Island model

The Falkland Islands introduced a 6 weekly dog-dosing programme in 1970 with praziquantel. Here the slope of the decline in the prevalence of *E. granulosus* in sheep and duration of the 'attack' phase was similar to that in Cyprus without a dog euthanasia programme.

In this programme, farm owners assumed responsibility for regular dog treatments. While transmission of CE to humans has ceased, it is not yet known whether or not elimination has been achieved (Craig and Larrieu 2006).

Continental model

In Chile, programmes with Option 5 were introduced in Region 12 in 1979 and Region 11 in 1982. The results obtained are illustrated in Fig. 53.5 and show clearly that this option is being successfully pursued (Anon. 1994) and should lead to the transformation from the costly 'attack' programme to a permanent 'consolidation' phase within 20 years.

Option 5 with limited evidence of success within 15 years
Continental models

In Argentina, control programmes using Option 5 have been funded by provincial ministries of health (Gemmell and Varela Diaz 1973). Few have been sustained, but three have demonstrated

Table 53.3 Age distribution of new hospital cases of CE in New Zealand 1958–1962 and 1963–1967

Age groups	Number of cases		Total cases	% reduction
	1958–1962	1963–1967		
0–4	19	3	22	84.2
5–14	98	35	133	64.3
15–24	82	46	128	43.9
25–44	112	64	176	42.9
45–64	98	48	146	51.0
>65	44	25	69	43.2
Total	453	221	674	51.2

From Gemmell and Roberts (1996)

Table 53.4 Age-specific annual surgical incidence (per 100 000) of CE in Tasmania 1966–1970 and 1971–1975 with the percentage reduction in the second 5-year period

	All ages	0–4	5–14	15–24	25–44	45–64	> 65
1960–1970	3.1	1.5	2.7	2.9	3.2	4.4	3.4
1971–1975	1.4	0.0	1.0	2.0	1.5	2.0	1.3
Percentage reduction	55	100	63	31	53	55	62

From Gemmell and Roberts (1996)

that control is feasible. For example, in a pilot trial in the Province of Neuquén in 1970, 28% of the dogs, 71.4% of sheep, and 90% of cattle harboured *E. granulosus*, but 17 years later when the trial was terminated, these prevalences were 2.1%, 6.9%, and 13.8% respectively, and transmission of CE to children had almost ceased (Kaczorkiewicz 1988). Similar programmes have been undertaken in the Provinces of Rio Negro (Craig and Larrieu 2006) with evidence of a reduction in prevalence in humans or animals or both.

Evaluation of control policies

Comparing the results obtained from programmes using Options 2 with 3, it seems that little progress is likely to be made in echinococcosis control simply by introducing legislation directing owners to treat their dogs and preventing them from gaining access to raw offal, even if a substantial educational programme is involved. From the results of the island programmes using Option 3, it is clear that control and even elimination is not only feasible, but also rapidly benefits the whole community. The important contributing factors include:

(1) Adequate funding,

(2) Education of the public through community participation,

(3) Supervision of the dog population, their treatment, and prevention of access to raw offal by technical personnel.

Comparing results obtained from programmes selecting Options 3, 4, and 5, it is clear that the costly 'attack' phase may be shorter with options 4 and 5 than with 3, provided that this phase can be transformed to the 'Consolidation' phase. It seems that this can only readily be achieved if effective survey and surveillance policies and animal health movement legislation can be applied. In their absence, there may be a trend to relax the dosing programme with unpredictable results. It seems that the most rapid progress can best be achieved by using animal health rather than human health administrations. Advantages also include:

(1) Experience with control of other animal diseases,

(2) Use of established laboratory and field services,

(3) Access to specialized services,

(4) Uniformity in staff training,

(5) Establishment of effective trace forward and trace back surveillance systems.

In conclusion, control is expensive and long-term and the 'planning' phase is now regarded as essential if the legislature is to be expected to support a programme financially. Modelling provides a criterion for deciding if a control programme can succeed in

eliminating the parasite and underpins a benefit–cost analysis of control options (Lawson 1994; Torgerson 2003a, b; Budke *et al.* 2005c). Several indicators of economic performance are available, including the net present value, the internal rate of return, but the most usual method is the benefit–cost ratio including the cost per DALY averted. This is calculated as the total discounted benefit over a fixed time period. If the benefit–cost ratio is greater than unity and/or the cost per DALY averted is low, then the benefits of a control action outweigh its costs and the programme can be recommended to the legislature as efficient from an economic point of view, with a relatively high priority as control has now been shown to be feasible.

References

Akhan, O., Ozmen, M. N., Dinçer, A., Sayek, I. and Goçmen, A. (1996). Liver hydatid disease: long term results of percutaneous treatment. *Radiology*, **198**: 259–64.

Al-Sabi, M. N., Kapel, C. M., Deplazes, P. and Mathis, A. (2007). Comparative copro-diagnosis of Echinococcus multilocularis in experimentally infected foxes. *Parasit. Res.*, **101**: 731–36.

Allan, J. C. and Craig, P. S. (2006). Coproantigens in taeniasis and echinococcosis. *Parasitol. Int.*, **55**: S75–80.

Allan, J. C., Craig, P. S., Garcia, N. J., Mencos, F., *et al.* (1992). Coproantigen detection for immunodiagnosis of echinococcosis and taeniasis in dogs and humans. *Parasitology*, **104**: 347–56.

Altintas, N. (2003). Past to present: echinococcosis in Turkey. *Acta Trop.*, **85**: 105–12.

Alvarez, C., Latourette, F., Geninazzi, H. and Perdomo, R. (1991). True and false relapses in hepatic hydatid disease. Usefulness of per-operatory control of parasitary sterilization. *Arch. Hidatidosis*, **30**: 599–607.

Aminzhanov, M. (1975). Duration of the life of Echinococcus granulosus in the organism of dogs. [Russian]. *Veterinariia*, 70–72.

Amir-Jahed, A. K., Fardin, R., Farzad, A. and Bakshandeh, K. (1975). Clinical echinococcosis. *Ann. Surg.*, **182**: 541–46.

Ammann, R. W. and Eckert, J. (1996). Cestodes. Echinococcus *Gastroenterol. Clin. N. Am.*, **25**: 655–89.

Anon. (1994). *Evaluacion proyecto de control de la hidatidosis en la XI1 Region de Chile*, periodo 83/87. Santiago, Chile.: Servicio d'Agricola y Ganadero, Ministerio de Agricultura.

Arru, E., Garippa, G. and Manger, B. R. (1990). Efficacy of epsiprantel against Echinococcus granulosus infections in dogs. *Res. Vet. Sci.*, **49**: 378–79.

Bai, Y., Cheng, N., Jiang, C., Wang, Q. and Cao, D. (2002). Survey on cystic echinococcosis in Tibetans, West China. *Acta Trop.*, **82**: 381–85.

Barros, J. L. (1978). Hydatid disease of the liver. *Am. J. Surg.*, **135**: 597–600.

Bart, J. M., Abdukader, M., Zhang, Y. L., *et al.* (2006). Genotyping of human cystic echinococcosis in Xinjiang, PR China. *Parasitology*, **133**: 571–79.

Beard, T. C. (1973a). Observations for Icelanders on hydatids and precautions against them. *Aust. Vet. J.*, **49**: 396–401.

Beard, T. C. (1973b). The elimination of echinococcosis from Iceland. *Bull. WHO*, **48:** 653–60.

Bonifacino, R., Malgor, R., Barbeito, R., *et al.* (1991). Seroprevalence of *Echinococcus granulosus* infection in a Uruguayan rural human population. *Trans. R. Soc. Trop. Med. Hyg.*, **85:** 769–72.

Brunetti, E., Kern, P., Vuitton, D. A.; Writing Panel for the WHO-IWGE. (2010). Expert consensus for the diagnosis and treatment of cystic and alveolar echinococcosis in humans. *Acta Trop.*, **114:** 1–16.

Budke, C. M., Deplazes, P. and Torgerson, P. R. (2006). Global socioeconomic impact of cystic echinococcosis. *Emerg. Infect. Dis.*, **12:** 296–303.

Budke, C. M., Campos-Ponce, M., Qian, W. and Torgerson, P. R. (2005a). A canine purgation study and risk factor analysis for echinococcosis in a high endemic region of the Tibetan plateau. *Vet. Parasitol.*, **127:** 43–49.

Budke, C. M., Jiamin, Q., Craig, P. S. and Torgerson, P. R. (2005b). Modeling the transmission of *Echinococcus granulosus* and *Echinococcus multilocularis* in dogs for a high endemic region of the Tibetan plateau. *Int. J. Parasitol*, **35:** 163–70.

Budke, C. M., Jiamin, Q., Qian, W. and Torgerson, P. R. (2005c). Economic effects of echinococcosis in a disease-endemic region of the Tibetan Plateau. *Am. J. Trop. Med. Hyg.*, **73:** 2–10.

Budke, C. M., Jiamin, Q., Zinsstag, J., Qian, W. and Torgerson, P. R. (2004). Use of disability adjusted life years in the estimation of the disease burden of echinococcosis for a high endemic region of the Tibetan plateau. *Am. J. Trop. Med. Hyg.*, **71:** 56–64.

Buishi, I., Njoroge, E., Zeyhle, E., Rogan, M. T. and Craig, P. S. (2008). Canine echinococcosis in Turkana (north-western Kenya): A coproantigen survey in the previous hydatid-control area and an analysis of risk factors. *Ann. Trop. Med. Parasitol.*, **100:** 601–10.

Buishi, I. E., Njoroge, E. M., Bouamra, O. and Craig, P. S. (2005). Canine echinococcosis in northwest Libya: Assessment of coproantigen ELISA, and a survey of infection with analysis of risk-factors. *Vet. Parasitol.*, **205**(3–4): 223–32.

Cabrera, P. A., Haran, G., Benavidez, U., Valledor, S., *et al.* (1995). Transmission dynamics of *Echinococcus granulosus*, *Taenia hydatigena* and *Taenia ovis* in sheep in Uruguay. *Int. J. Parasitol.*, **25:** 807–13.

Cabrera, P. A., Lloyd, S., Haran, G., Pineyro, L., *et al.* (2002). Control of *Echinococcus granulosus* in Uruguay: evaluation of different treatment intervals for dogs. *Vet. Parasitol.*, **103:** 333–40.

Campos-Bueno, A., Lopez-Abente, G. and Andres-Cercadillo, A. M. (2000). Risk factors for *Echinococcus granulosus* infection: a case-control study. *Am. J. Trop. Med. Hyg.*, **62:** 329–34.

Carabin, H., Budke, C. M., Cowan, L. D., *et al.* (2005). Methods for assessing the burden of parasitic zoonoses: echinococcosis and cysticercosis. *Trends Parasitol.*, **21:** 327–33.

Carmena, D., Benito, A. & Eraso, E. (2006). Antigens for the immunodiagnosis of *Echinococcus granulosus* infection: an update. *Acta Trop.*, **98:** 74–86.

Carmena, D., Sanchez-Serrano, L. P. & Barbero-Martinez, I. (2008). *Echinococcus granulosus* infection in Spain. *Zoon. Pub. Health*, **55:** 156–65.

Carmona, C., Perdomo, R., Carbo, A., Alvarez, C., *et al.* (1998). Risk factors associated with human cystic echinococcosis in Florida, Uruguay: results of a mass screening study using ultrasound and serology. *Am. J. Trop. Med. Hyg.*, **58:** 599–605.

Castiglia, P., Solinas, G., Sotgiu, G., Palmieri, A., Maida, A. and Dettori, M. (2004). Epidemiology of hydatidosis in the province of Sassari, Italy. *Parassitologia*, **46:** 371–73.

Castrodale, L. J., Beller, M., Wilson, J. F., Schantz, P. M., *et al.* (2002). Two atypical cases of cystic echinococcosis (*Echinococcus granulosus*) in Alaska, 1999. *Am. J. Trop. Med. Hyg.*, **66:** 325–27.

Casulli, A., Zeyhle, E., Brunetti, E., Pozio, E., *et al.* (2010). Molecular evidence of the camel strain (G6 genotype) of *Echinococcus granulosus* in humans from Turkana, Kenya. *Trans. R. Soc. Trop. Med. Hyg.*,**104:** 29–32.

Chaouachi, B., Ben Salah, S., Lakhoua, R., Hammou, A., *et al.* (1989). Hydatid cysts in children. Diagnostic and therapeutic aspects. A propos of 1195 cases. *Ann. Pediat.*, **36:** 441–44.

Christofi, G., Deplazes, P., Christofi, N., Tanner, I., *et al.* (2002). Screening of dogs for *Echinococcus granulosus* coproantigen in a low endemic situation in Cyprus. *Vet. Parasitol.*, **104:** 299–306.

Cohen, H. & Al., E. (1991). Hidatidosis en area rural: estudio simultaneo en tres hospederos. Capitulo seres humanos. *Arch. Hidatidosis*, **30:** 935–36.

Cooney, R. M., Flanagan, K. P. and Zehyle, E. (2004). Review of surgical management of cystic hydatid disease in a resource limited setting: Turkana, Kenya. *Eur. J. Gastroenterol. Hepatol.*, **16:** 1233–36.

Craig, P. S. and Larrieu, E. (2006). Control of cystic echinococcosis/hydatidosis: 1863–2002. *Adv. Parasitol.*, **61:** 443–508.

Craig, P. S., Rogan, M. T. and Campos-Ponce, M. (2003). Echinococcosis: disease, detection and transmission. *Parasitology*, **127:** S5–20.

Craig, P. S., Gasser, R. B., Parada, L., Cabrera, P., *et al.* (1995). Diagnosis of canine echinococcosis: comparison of coproantigen and serum antibody tests with arecoline purgation in Uruguay. *Vet. Parasitol.*, **56:** 293–301.

Deplazes, P., Gottstein, B., Eckert, J., Jenkins, D. J., *et al.* (1992). Detection of *Echinococcus coproantigens* by enzyme-linked immunosorbent assay in dogs, dingoes and foxes. *Parasit. Res.*, **78:** 303–8.

Dew, H. R. (1928). *Hydatid Disease*. Sydney: Australian Medical Publishing Company.

Dinkel, A., Von Nickisch-Rosenegk, M., Bilger, B., *et al.* (1998). Detection of Echinococcus multilocularis in the definitive host: coprodiagnosis by PCR as an alternative to necropsy. *J. Clin. Microbiol.*, **36:** 1871–76.

Dinkel, A., Njoroge, E. M., Zimmermann, A., Walz, M., *et al.* (2004). A PCR system for detection of species and genotypes of the Echinococcus granulosus-complex, with reference to the epidemiological situation in eastern Africa. *Int. J. Parasitol.*, **34:** 645–53.

Dowling, P. M., Abo-Shehada, M. N. and Torgerson, P. R. (2000). Risk factors associated with human cystic echinococcosis in Jordan: results of a case-control study. *Ann. Trop. Med. Parasitol.*, **94:** 69–75.

Drolshammer, I., Wiesmann, E. and Eckert, J. (1973). Echinokokkose beim Menschen in der Schweiz 1956–1969. *Schweizeris. Mediz. Wochensch.*, **103:** 1337–92.

Dungal, N. (1957). Eradication of hydatid disease in Iceland. *New Zealand Med. J.*, **56:** 213–22.

Dziri, C., Haouet, K. and Fingerhut, A. T. (2004). Treatment of hydatid cyst of the liver: where is the evidence? *World J. Surg.*, **28:** 731–36.

Eckert, J. (2003). Predictive values and quality control of techniques for the diagnosis of *Echinococcus multilocularis* in definitive hosts. *Acta Trop.*, **85:** 157–63.

Eckert, J. and Deplazes, P. (2004). Biological, epidemiological and clinical aspects of echinococcosis: a zoonosis of increasing concern. *Clin. Microbiol. Rev.*, **17:** 107–35.

Eckert, J., Deplazes, P. and Al., E. (2001a). Echinococcosis in animals: clinical aspects, diagnosis and treatment. In: J. Eckert *et al.* (eds.) *WHO/OIE manual on echinococcosis in humans and animals: a public health problem of global concern.* Paris: WHO/OIE.

Eckert, J., Deplazes, P., Craig, P. S., *et al.* (2001b). Echinococcus in animals: clinical aspects, diagnosis and treatment. In: J. Eckert *et al.* (eds.) *WHO/OIE Manual on echinococcosis in humans and animals.* Paris: WHO/OIE.

Eckert, J., Gottstein, B., Heath, D. and Liu, F. J. (2001c). Prevention of echinococcosis in humans and safety precautions. In: J. Eckert *et al.* (eds.) *WHO/OIE Manual on Echinococcosis in Humans and Animals: a Public Health Problem of Global Concern.* Paris: WHO/OIE.

Economides, P., Christofi, G. and Gemmell, M. A. (1998). Control of *Echinococcus granulosus* in Cyprus and comparison with other island models. *Vet. Parasitol.*, **79:** 151–63.

El-Mufti, M., Kamag, A., Ibrahim, H., Taktuk, S., *et al.* (1993). Albendazole therapy of hydatid disease: 2-year follow-up of 40 cases. *Ann. Trop. Med. Parasitol.*, **87:** 241–46.

El Fortia, M., El Gatit, A. and Bendaoud, M. (2006). Ultrasound wall-sign in pulmonary echinococcosis (new application). *Ultraschall Med.*, **27:** 553–57.

Filice, C., Brunetti, E., Bruno, R. and Crippa, F. G. (2000). Percutaneous drainage of echinococcal cysts (PAIR—puncture, aspiration, injection, reaspiration): results of a worldwide survey for assessment of its safety and efficacy. WHO-Informal Working Group on Echinococcosis-Pair Network [letter; comment]. *Gut,* **47:** 156–57.

Filice, C., Pirola, F., Brunetti, E., Dughetti, S., *et al.* (1990). A new therapeutic approach for hydatid liver cysts. *Gastroenterol.,* **98:** 1366–68.

Franchi, C., Di Vico, B. and Teggi, A. (1999). Long-term evaluation of patients with hydatidosis treated with benzimidazole. *Clin. Infect. Dis.,* **29:** 304–9.

Gasser, R. B., Lightowlers, M. W., Rickard, M. D., *et al.* (1990). Serological screening of farm dogs for Echinococcus granulosus infection in an endemic region. *Aus. Vet. J.,* **67:** 145–47.

Gasser, R. B., Jenkins, D. J., Paolillo, E., *et al.* (1993). Serum Antibodies in Canine Echinococcosis. *Int. J. Parasitol.,* **23:** 579–86.

Gatti, A., Alvarez, A. R., Araya, D., *et al.* (2007). Ovine echinococcosis I. *Immunological diagnosis by enzyme immunoassay. Vet. Parasitol.,* **143:** 112–21.

Gavidia, C. M., Gonzalez, A. E., Lopera, L., *et al.* (2009). Evaluation of nitazoxanide and oxfendazole efficacy against cystic echinococcosis in naturally infected sheep. *Am. J. Trop. Med. Hyg.,* **80:** 367–72.

Gemmell, M. A. (1987). A critical approach to the concepts of control and eradication of echinococcosis/hydatidosis and taeniasis/cysticercosis. *Int. J. Parasitol.,* **17:** 465–72.

Gemmell, M. A. (1990). Australasian contributions to an understanding of the epidemiology and control of hydatid disease caused by *Echinococcus granulosus*—past, present and future (published erratum appears in Intern. J. Parasit., (1990) 20(6):819). *Int. J. Parasitol.,* **20:** 431–56.

Gemmell, M. A. and Johnstone, P. D. (1981). Cestodes. *Antibiot. Chemother.,* **30:** 54–114.

Gemmell, M. A. and Roberts, M. G. (1996). Cystic echinococcosis (*Echinococcus granulosus*). In: S. R. Palmer *et al.* (eds.) *Zoonoses, Biology, Clinical Practice and Public Health Control,* pp. 665–87. Oxford: Oxford University Press.

Gemmell, M. A. and Varela Diaz, V. M. (1973). Review of Programs for the Control of Hydatidosis/Echinococcosis up to 1974. *Series of Scientific Technical Monographs, CPZ 8.* Buenos Aires, Argentina: Pan American Zoonoses Center.

Gemmell, M. A., Lawson, J. R. and Roberts, M. G. (1986a). Control of echinococcosis/hydatidosis: present status of worldwide progress. *Bull. WHO,* **64:** 333–39.

Gemmell, M. A., Lawson, J. R. and Roberts, M. G. (1986b). Population dynamics in echinococcosis and cysticercosis: biological parameters of *Echinococcus granulosus* in dogs and sheep. *Parasitology,* **92:** 599–620.

Gemmell, M. A., Parmeter, S. N., Sutton, R. J. and Khan, N. (1981). Effect of mebendazole against *Echinococcus granulosus* and *Taenia hydatigena* cysts in naturally infected sheep and relevance to larval tapeworm infections in man. *Zeitschr. Parasitenk.,* **64:** 135–47.

Gemmell, M. A., Lawson, J. R., Roberts, M. G., Kerin, B. R. and Mason, C. J. (1986c). Population dynamics in echinococcosis and cysticercosis: comparison of the response of *Echinococcus granulosus, Taenia hydatigena* and *T. ovis* to control. *Parasitology,* **93:** 357–69.

Gharbi, H. A., Hassine, W., Brauner, M. W. and Dupuch, K. (1981). Ultrasound examination of the hydatic liver. *Radiology,* **139:** 459–63.

Gil-Grande, L. A., Rodriguez-Caabeiro, F., *et al.* (1993). Randomised controlled trial of efficacy of albendazole in intra- abdominal hydatid disease. *Lancet,* **342:** 1269–72.

Grove, D. I., Warren, K. S. and Mahmoud, A. A. (1976). Algorithms in the diagnosis and management of exotic diseases. X. Echinococcosis. *J. Infect. Dis.,* **133:** 354–58.

Guarnera, E. A., Parra, A., Kamenetzky, L., Garcia, G. E. and Gutierrez, A. (2004). Cystic echinococcosis in Argentina: evolution of metacestode and clinical expression in various *Echinococcus granulosus* strains. *Acta Trop.,* **92:** 153–59.

Heath, D. D. (1971). The migration of oncospheres of *Taenia pisiformis, T. serialis* and *Echinococcus granulosus* within the intermediate host. *Int. J. Parasitol.,* **1:** 145–52.

Horton, R. J. (1997). Albendazole in the treatment of human cystic echinococcosis: 12 years of experience. *Acta Trop.,* **64:** 79–93.

Hüttner, M. and Romig, T. (2009). Echinococcus species in African wildlife. *Parasitology,* **136:** 1089–95.

Ibrahem, M. M., Craig, P. S., McVie, A., Ersfeld, K. and Rogan, M. T. (1996). *Echinococcus granulosus* antigen B and seroreactivity in natural ovine hydatidosis. *Res, Vet. Sci.,* **61:** 102–6.

Jenkins, D. J. (2005). Hydatid control in Australia: Where it began, what we have achieved and where to from here. *Int. J. Parasitol.,* **35:** 733–40.

Jenkins, D. J. (2006). *Echinococcus granulosus* in Australia, widespread and doing well! *Parasitol. Int.,* **55:** S203–6.

Jenkins, D. J., Fraser, A., Bradshaw, H. and Craig, P. S. (2000). Detection of *Echinococcus granulosus* coproantigens in Australian canids with natural or experimental infection. *J. Parasit.,* **86:** 140–45.

Jia-Zhong, T., Wei, P. and Chang, Q. (1993). Recent investigations on the pharmacotherapy of cystic echinococcosis in the Xingjiang Uygur Autonomous Region, P. R. C. In: F. L. Andersen (ed.) *Compendium on Cystic Echinococcosis.* Utah: Brigham Young University Print Services.

Junghanss, T., Da Silva, A. M., Horton, J., *et al.* (2008). Clinical management of cystic echinococcosis: state of the art, problems, and perspectives. *Am. J. Trop. Med. Hyg.,* **79:** 301–11.

Kaczorkiewicz, A. (1988). Lineamientos generales del Ministerio de Salud Publica del Neuquen en materia de control de la hidatidosis. *Bol. Intern. Ass. Hidatidosis,* **11:** 53–57.

Kamhawi, S. (1995). A retrospective study of human cystic echinococcosis in Jordan. *Ann. Trop. Med. Parasitol.,* **89:** 409–14.

Kammerer, W. S. and Schantz, P. M. (1993). Echinococcal disease. *Infect. Dis. Clin. N. Am.,* **7:** 605–18.

Kedra, A. H., Swiderski, Z., Tkach, V. V., Dubinsky, P., *et al.* (1999). Genetic analysis of Echinococcus granulosus from humans and pigs in Poland, Slovakia and Ukraine. A multicenter study. *Acta Parasitol.,* **44:** 248–54.

Kern, P., Wen, H., Sato, N., Vuitton, D. A., *et al.* (2006). WHO classification of alveolar echinococcosis: Principles and application. *Parasitol. Int.,* **55:** S283–87.

Keshmiri, M., Baharvahdat, F., Fattahi, S. H., *et al.* (2001). Albendazole versus placebo in the treatment of echinococcosis. *Trans. R. Soc. Trop. Med. Hyg.,* **95:** 190–91.

Kittelberger, R., Reichel, M. P., Jenner, J., Heath, D. D., *et al.* (2002). Evaluation of three enzyme-linked immunoabsorbent assays (ELISA) for the detection of serum antibodies in sheep infected with *Echinococcus granulosus. Vet. Parasitol.,* **110:** 57–76.

Lahmar, S., Ben Chéhida, F., Pétavy, A. F., *et al.* (2007a). Ultrasonic screening for cystic echinococcosis in sheep in Tunisia. *Vet. Parasitol.,* **143:** 42–49.

Lahmar, S., Lahmar, S., Boufana, B., *et al.* (2007b). Screening for *Echinococcus granulosus* in dogs: Comparison between arecoline purgation, coproELISA and coproPCR with necropsy in pre-patent infections. *Vet. Parasitol.,* **144:** 287–92.

Larrieu, E. J., Costa, M. T., Del Carpio, M., *et al.* (2002). A case-control study of the risk factors for cystic echinococcosis among the children of Rio Negro province, Argentina. *Ann. Trop. Med. Parasit.,* **96:** 43–52.

Lawson, J. R. (1994). Hydatid disease and sheep measles: the history of their control and the economics of a recent change of control policy. *New Zealand J. Zool.,* **21:** 83–89.

Lawson, J. R., Roberts, M. G., Gemmell, M. A. and Best, S. J. (1988). Population dynamics in echinococcosis and cysticercosis: economic assessment of control strategies for *Echinococcus granulosus, Taenia ovis* and *T. hydatigena. Parasitology,* **97:** 177–91.

Lightowlers, M. W. and Heath, D. D. (2004). Immunity and vaccine control of *Echinococcus granulosus* infection in animal intermediate hosts. *Parassitologia,* **46:** 27–31.

Lightowlers, M. W., Colebrook, A. L., Gauci, C. G., *et al.* (2003). Vaccination against cestode parasites: anti-helminth vaccines that work and why. *Vet. Parasitol.,* **115:** 83–123.

Lopez-Neyra, C. R. and Soler Planas, M. A. (1943). Revision del genero Echinococcosis Rud y descrption de una especie nueva Parasita intestinal del porro en Almeria. *Rev. Iberica Parasitol.,* **3:** 169–94.

Macpherson, C. N. L. (2005). Human behaviour and the epidemiology of parasitic zoonoses. *Int. J. Parasitol.,* **35:** 1319–31.

Macpherson, C. N. L. and Milner, R. (2003). Performance characteristics and quality control of community based ultrasound surveys for cystic and alveolar echinococcosis. *Acta Trop.,* **85:** 203–9.

Macpherson, C. N. L., Romig, T., Zeyhle, E, Rees, P. H. and Were, J. B. O. (1987). Portable ultrasound scanner verses serology in screening for hydatid cysts in a nomadic population. *Lancet,* **I:** 259–61.

Macpherson, C. N. L., Spoerry, A., Zeyhle, E., Romig, T. and Gorfe, M. (1989). Pastoralists and hydatid disease: an ultrasound scanning prevalence survey in East Africa. *Trans. R. Soc. Trop. Med. Hyg.,* **84:** 243–47.

Macpherson, C. N. L., Bartholomot, B. and Frider, B. (2003). Application of ultrasound in diagnosis, treatment, epidemiology, public health and control of *Echinococcus granulosus* and *E. multilocularis. Parasitology,* **127:** S21–35.

Macpherson, C. N., Kachani, M., Lyagoubi, M., *et al.* (2004). Cystic echinococcosis in the Berber of the Mid Atlas mountains, Morocco: new insights into the natural history of the disease in humans. *Ann. Trop. Med. Parasitol.,* **98:** 481–90.

Magambo, J., Njoroge, E. and Zeyhle, E. (2006). Epidemiology and control of echinococcosis in sub-Saharan Africa. *Parasitol. Int.,* **55:** S193–95.

Majorowski, M. M., Carabin, H., Kilani, M. and Bendsalah, A. (2005). Echinococcosis in Tunisia: a cost analysis. *Trans. R. Soc. Trop. Med. Hyg.,* **99:** 268–78.

Mamuti, W., Sako, Y., Nakao, M., Xiao, N., *et al.* (2005). Recent advances in charecterization of *Echinococcus* antigen B. *Parasitol. Int.,* **55:** s57–62.

Mathis, A. and Deplazes, P. (2006). Copro-DNA tests for diagnosis of animal taeniid cestodes. *Parasitol. Int.,* **55:** S87–90.

Menghebat, L., Jiang, L. and Chai, J-J. (1993). A retrospective survey for surgical cases of cystic echinococcosis in the Xingjiang Uygur Autonomous Region, P. R. C. (1951–90). In: F. L. Andersen(ed.) *Compendium on cystic echinococcosis.* Utah: Brigham Young University Print Services.

Ming-Quian, X. (1993). Diagnosis and complications of cystic echinococcosis, and surgical procedures for removal of hydatid cysts in the Xinxiang Uygur Autonomous Region, PRC. In: F. L. Andersen (ed.) *Compendium on cystic echinococcosis.* Utah: Brigham Young University Print Services.

Mohamed, A. E., Yasawy, M. I. and Al Karawi, M. A. (1998). Combined albendazole and praziquantel versus albendazole alone in the treatment of hydatid disease. *Hepatogastroenterology,* **45:** 1690–94.

Moro, P. L. and Schantz, P. M. (2006). Cystic echinococcosis in the Americas. *Parasitol. Int.,* **55:** S181–86.

Moro, P. L., Cavero, C. L., Tambini, M., *et al.* (2008). Identification of risk factors for cystic echinococcosis in a peri-urban population of Peru. *Trans. R. Soc. Trop. Med. Hyg.,* **102:** 75–78.

Mufit, K., Nejat, I., Mercan, S., Ibrahim, K., *et al.* (1998). Growth of multiple hydatid cysts evaluated by computed tomography. *J. Clin. Neurosci.,* **5**(2): 215–17.

Nakao, M., McManus, D. P., Schantz, P. M., Craig, P. S. and Ito, A. (2007). A molecular phylogeny of the genus *Echinococcus* inferred from complete mitochondrial genomes. *Parasitology,* **134:** 713–22.

Ortlepp, R. J. (1937). South African Helminths, Part 1. *Onderstepoort J. Vet. Sci. Anim. Ind.,* **9:** 311–36.

Paolillo, E. and Al., E. (1991). Hidatidosis un problema de attencion primaria de salud. *Rev. Med. Uruguay,* **7:** 32–37.

Parada, L., Cabrera, P., Burges, C., Acuna, A., *et al.* (1995). *Echinococcus granulosus* infections of dogs in the Durazno region of Uruguay. *Vet. Rec.,* **136:** 389–91.

Pawlowski, Z. & Stefaniak, J. (2003). The pig strain of *Echinococcus granulosus* in humans: a neglected issue? *Trends Parasitol.,* **19:** 439.

Pu-Sheng, C. (1993). Use of praziquantel-medicated tablets for control of cystic echinococcosis in the Xinjiang Uygur Autonomous Region, P. R. C. In: F. L. Andersen (ed.) *Compendium on Cystic Echinococcosis,* pp. 190–95. Utah: Brigham Young University Print Services.

Rausch, R. L. and Schiller, E. (1951). Hydatid disease (echinococcosis) in Alaska and the importance of rodent intermediate hosts. *Science,* **113:** 58.

Rausch, R. L. (1953). The taxonomic value and variability of certain structures in the cestode genus Echinococcus (Rud., 1801) and a review of recognized species. In: J. Dayal, J. and S. Singh (eds.) *Thapar Commemorative Volume, Lucknow University.* Lucknow: Prem Printing Press.

Rausch, R. L. and Bernstein, J. J. (1972). *Echinococcus vogeli* sp. n. (Cestoda: Taeniidae) from the bush dog, Speothos venaticus (Lund). *Zeitschr. Prakt. Anasth. Wiederbel. Intensivther.,* **23:** 25–34.

Rausch, R. L. (1993). The biology of *Echinococcus granulosus.* In: F. L. Andersen (ed.) *Compendium of cystic echinococcosis. With special reference to the Xinjiang Uygur Autonomous Region, the People's Republic of China,* pp. 27–56. Provo, Utah: Brigham Young University Print Services.

Riganò, R., Profumo, E., Bruschi, F., *et al.* (2001). Modulation of human immune response by *Echinococcus granulosus* antigen B and its possible role in evading host defenses. *Infect. Immun.,* **69:** 288–96.

Rinaldi, L., Maurelli, M. P., Capuano, F., *et al.* (2008). Molecular update on cystic echinococcosis in cattle and water buffaloes of southern Italy. *Zoon. Pub. Health,* **55:** 119–23.

Rogan, M. T., Hai, W. Y., Richardson, R., Zeyhle, E. and Craig, P. S. (2006). Hydatid cysts: does every picture tell a story? *Trends Parasitol.,* **22:** 431–38.

Romig, T. (1990). *Beobachtungen zur zystischen Echinokokkose des Menschen im Turkana-Gebiet, Kenia* : University of Hohenheim.

Romig, T., Dinkel, A. and Mackenstedt, U. (2006). The present situation of echinococcosis in Europe. *Parasitol. Int.,* **55:** S187–91.

Romig, T., Zeyhle, E., Macpherson, C. N. L., *et al.* (1986). Cyst growth and spontaneous cure in hydatid disease. *Lancet,* **i:** 861.

Saarma, U., Jõgisalu, I., Moks, E., Varcasia, A., *et al.* (2009). A novel phylogeny for the genus Echinococcus, based on nuclear data, challenges relationships based on mitochondrial evidence. *Parasitology,* **136:** 317–28.

Sadjjadi, S. M. (2006). Present situation of echinococcosis in the Middle East and Arabic North Africa. *Parasitol. Int.,* **55:** S197–202.

Sage, A. M., Wachira, T. M., Zeyhle, E. E., *et al.* (1998). Evaluation of diagnostic ultrasound as a mass screening technique for the detection of hydatid cysts in the liver and lung of sheep and goats. *Int. J. Parasitol.,* **28:** 349–53.

Santos, H. T., Santos, A. F. and De La Rue, M. L. (2008). The action of albendazole on hydatid cysts in sheep experimentally infected with eggs of *Echinococcus granulosus. J. Helminthol.,* **82:** 109–12.

Schantz, P. M. (1997). Sources and uses of surveillance data for cystic echinococcosis. In: F. L. Anderson *et al.* (eds.) *Compendium on cystic echinococcosis in Africa and in middle eastern countries with special reference to Morocco.* Provo, Utah, USA: Brigham Young University Print Services.

Schantz, P. M., Cruz-Reyes, A., Colli, C. and Lord, R. D. (1975). Sylvatic echinococcosis in Argentina. I. On the morphology and biology of strobilar *Echinococcus* granulosus (Batsch, 1786) from domestic and sylvatic animal hosts. *Tropenmed. Parasit.,* **26:** 334–44.

Schantz, P. M., Colli, C., Cruz-Reyes, A. and Prezioso, U. (1976). Sylvatic echinococcosis in Argentina. II. Susceptibility of wild carnivores to Echinococcus granulosus (Batsch, 1786) and host-induced morphological variation. *Tropenmed. Parasit.,* **27:** 70–78.

Schantz, P. M., Wang, H., Qiu, J., Liu, F. J., *et al.* (2003). Echinococcosis on the Tibetan Plateau: prevalence and risk factors for cystic and alveolar echinococcosis in Tibetan populations in Qinghai Province, China. *Parasitology,* **127:** S109–20.

Schneider, R., Gollackner, B., Edel, B., *et al.* (2007). Development of a new PCR protocol for the detection of species and genotypes (strains) of Echinococcus in formalin-fixed, paraffin-embedded tissues. *Intern. J. Parasitol.*, **38**: 1065–71.

Schwabe, C. W. (1969). *Veterinary Medicine and Human Health.* Baltimore: Williams and Wilkins.

Schwabe, C. W. (1986). Current status of hydatid disease: a zoonosis of increasing importance. In: R. C. A. Thompson (ed.) *The biology of echinococcus and hydatid disease.* London: George Allen.

Scott, J. C., Stefaniak, J., Pawlowski, Z. S. and Mcmanus, D. P. (1997). Molecular genetic analysis of human cystic hydatid cases from Poland: identification of a new genotypic group (G9) of *Echinococcus granulosus. Parasitology,* **114**: 37–43.

Shaikenov, B. S., Torgerson, P. R., *et al.* (2003). The changing epidemiology of echinococcosis in Kazakhstan due to transformation of farming practices. *Acta Trop.,* **85**: 287–93.

Smego, R. A. J., Bhatti, S., Khaliq, A. A. and Beg, M. A. (2003). Percutaneous aspiration-injection-reaspiration drainage plus albendazole or mebendazole for hepatic cystic echinococcosis: a meta-analysis. *Clin. Infect. Dis.,* **37**: 1073–83.

Snabel, V., Altintas, N., D'Amelio, S., Nakao, M., *et al.* (2009). Cystic echinococcosis in Turkey: genetic variability and first record of the pig strain (G7) in the country. *Parasitol. Res.,* **105**: 145–54.

Sousa, O. E. and Thatcher, V. E. (1969). Observations on the life-cycle of Echinococcus oligarthrus (Diesing, 1863) in the Republic of Panama. *Ann. Trop. Med. Parasitol.,* **63**: 165–75.

Stefanic, S., Shaikenov, B. S., Deplazes, P., *et al.* (2004). Polymerase chain reaction for detection of patent infections of *Echinococcus granulosus* ('sheep strain') in naturally infected dogs. *Parasitol. Res.,* **92**: 347–51.

Thompson, R. C. A. (1986). Biology and systematics of *Echinococcus.* In: R. C. A. Thompson (ed.) *The biology of Echinococcus and hydatid disease,* pp. 5–43. London: Allen & Unwin.

Thompson, R. C. A. (1995). Biology and Systematics of *Echinococcus multilocularis.* In: R. C. A. Thompson and A. J. Lymbery (eds.) *Echinococcus and Hydatid Disease.* Oxon, UK: CAB International.

Thompson, R. C. A. (2008). The taxonomy, phylogeny and transmission of Echinococcus. *Exp. Parasitol.,* **119**: 439–46.

Thompson, R. C. & McManus, D. P. (2002). Towards a taxonomic revision of the genus *Echinococcus. Trends Parasitol.,* **18**: 452–57.

Tiaoying, L., Jiamin, Q., Wen, Y., Craig, P. S., *et al.* (2005). Echinococcosis in Tibetan populations, western Sichuan Province, China. *Emerg. Infect. Dis.,* **11**: 1866–73.

Todorov, T., Vutova, K., Mechkov, G., Tonchev, Z., *et al.* (1992a). Experience in the chemotherapy of severe, inoperable echinococcosis in man. *Infection,* **20**: 19–24.

Todorov, T., Vutova, K., Mechkov, G., *et al.* (1992b). Experience in the chemotherapy of severe, inoperable echinococcosis in man. *Infection,* **20**: 19–24.

Todorov, T. and Boeva, V. (1999). Human echinococcosis in Bulgaria: a comparative epidemiogical analysis. *Bull. WHO,* **77**: 110–18.

Torgerson, P. R. (2003a). Economic effects of echinococcosis. *Acta Trop.,* **85**: 113–18.

Torgerson, P. R. (2003b). The use of mathematical models to simulate control options for echinococcosis. *Acta Trop.,* **85**: 211–21.

Torgerson, P. R. (2006). Canid immunity to Echinococcus spp.: impact on transmission. *Parasite Immunol.,* **28**: 295.

Torgerson, P. R. (2008). Dogs vaccines and Echinococcus. *Trends Parasitol.,* **25**: 57–58.

Torgerson, P. R. and Dowling, P. M. (2001). Estimating the economic effects of cystic echinococcosis. Part 2: an endemic region in the United Kingdom, a wealthy, industrialized economy. *Ann. Trop. Med. Parasitol.,* **95**: 177–85.

Torgerson, P. R. and Heath, D. D. (2003). Transmission dynamics and control options for *Echinococcus granulosus. Parasitology,* **127**: S143–58.

Torgerson, P. R., Williams, D. H. and Abo-Shehada, M. N. (1998). Modelling the prevalence of *Echinococcus* and *Taenia* species in small ruminants of different ages in northern Jordan. *Vet. Parasitol.,* **79**: 35–51.

Torgerson, P. R., Carmona, C. and Bonifacino, R. (2000). Estimating the economic effects of cystic echinococcosis: Uruguay, a developing country with upper-middle income. *Ann. Trop. Med. Parasitol.,* **94**: 703–13.

Torgerson, P. R., Dowling, P. M. and Abo-Shehada, M. N. (2001). Estimating the economic effects of cystic echinococcosis. Part 3: Jordan, a developing country with lower-middle income. *Ann. Trop. Med. Parasitol.,* **95**: 595–603.

Torgerson, P. R., Shaikenov, B. S., Baitursinov, K. K. and Abdybekova, A. M. (2002). The emerging epidemic of echinococcosis in Kazakhstan. *Trans. R. Soc. Trop. Med. Hyg.,* **96**: 124–28.

Torgerson, P. R., Karaeva, R. R., Corkeri, N., *et al.* (2003a). Human cystic echinococcosis in Kyrgystan: an epidemiological study. *Acta Trop.,* **85**: 51–61.

Torgerson, P. R., Shaikenov, B. S., *et al.* (2003b). Modelling the transmission dynamics of *Echinococcus granulosus* in dogs in rural Kazakhstan. *Parasitology,* **126**: 417–24.

Torgerson, P. R., Oguljahan, B., *et al.* (2006). Present situation of cystic echinococcosis in Central Asia. *Parasitol. Int.,* **55**: S207–12.

Torgerson, P. R., Rosenheim, K., Tanner, I., *et al.* (2009). Echinococcosis, toxocarosis and toxoplasmosis screening in a rural community in eastern Kazakhstan. *Trop. Med. Int. Health,* **14**: 341–48.

Torgerson, P. R., Ziadinov, I., Aknazarov, D., *et al.* (2009c). Modelling the age variation of larval protoscoleces of *Echinococcus granulosus. Int. J. Parasitol.,* **39**: 1031–35.

Trachsel, D., Deplazes, P. and Mathis, A. (2007). Identification of eggs of canine taeniids by multiplex PCR. *Parasitology,* **134**: 911–20.

Turcekova, L., Sanbel, V., D'Amelio, S., Busi, M. and Dubinsky, P. (2003). Morphological and genetic characterization of *Echinococcus* in the Slovak Republic. *Acta Trop.,* **85**: 223–29.

Turgut, A. T., Altin, L., Topcu, S., Kilicoglu, B., *et al.* (2007). Unusual imaging characteristics of complicated hydatid disease. *Eur. J. Radiol.,* **63**: 84–93.

Utrilla, J. G., Eyre, F. P., Muguerza, R., Alami, H. and Bueno, J. (1991). Hidatidosis en la infancia. *Arch. Hidatidosis,* **30**: 721–30.

Vogel, H. (1955). Über den Entwicklungszyklus und die Artzugehörigkeit des Europáischen Alveolarechinococcus *Deuts. Mediz. Wochensch.,* **80**: 931–32.

Vuitton, D. A. (2004). Echinococcosis and allergy. *Clin. Rev. Aller. Immun.,* **26**: 93–104.

Vuitton, D. A. (2009). Benzimidazoles for the treatment of cystic and alveolar echinococcosis: what is the consensus? *Expert Rev. Anti-Infect. Ther.,* **7**: 145–49.

Vuitton, D. A. and Wen, H. (2007). Treatment of cystic echinococcosis: a combination of general goals and rules, individual decisions and indications. *Netherlands J. Med.,* **65**: 86–88.

Vural, G., Baca, A. U., Gauci, C. G., *et al.* (2008). Variability in the *Echinococcus granulosus* Cytochrome C oxidase 1 mitochondrial gene sequence from livestock in Turkey and a re-appraisal of the G1-3 genotype cluster. *Vet. Parasitol.,* **154**: 347–50.

Wang, Y., He, T., Wen, X., Li, T., *et al.* (2006). Post-survey follow-up for human cystic echinococcosis in northwest China. *Acta Trop.,* **98**: 43–51.

Wen, H., New, R. R. and Craig, P. S. (1993). Diagnosis and treatment of human hydatidosis. *Br. J. Clin. Pharmacol.,* **35**: 565–74.

Whitfield, P. J. and Evans, N. A. (1983). Parthenogenesis and asexual multiplication among parasitic platyhelminths. *Parasitology,* **86**: 121–60.

WHO-IWGE (1996). Guidelines for treatment of cystic and alveolar echinococcosis in humans. WHO Informal Working Group on Echinococcosis. *Bull. WHO,* **74**: 231–42.

WHO-IWGE (2001). *PAIR: a new option for the treatment of cystic echinococcosis.* WHO Geneva, WHO/CDS/CSR/APH/2001.6. (http://whqlibdoc.who.int/hq/2001/WHO_CDS_CSR_APH_2001.6.pdf; accessed Dec. 16, 2009)

WHO-IWGE (2003). International classification of ultrasound images in cystic echinococcosis for application in clinical and field epidemiological settings. *Acta Trop.,* **85**: 253–61.

Wu, X. W., Peng, X. Y., Zhang, S. J., Niu, J. H., Sun, H. and Xi, Y. (2004). Formation mechanisms of the fibrous capsule around hepatic and splenic hydatid cyst, *Zhongguo Sheng Chong Chong Bing Za Zhi.,* **22**: 1–4. (in Chinese).

Xiao, N., Qiu, J., Nakao, M., Li, T., Yang, W., *et al.* (2005). *Echinococcus shiquicus* n. sp., a taeniid cestode from Tibetan fox and plateau pika in China. *Int. J. Parasitol.,* **35**: 693–701.

Yang, Y. R., Williams, G. M., Craig, P. S., Sun, T., *et al.* (2006). Hospital and community surveys reveal the severe public health problem and socio-economic impact of human echinococcosis in Ningxia Hui Autonomous Region, China. *Trop. Med. Int. Health,* **11**: 880–88.

Yolasigmaz, A., Reiterová, K., Turk, M., *et al.* (2006). Comparison of serological and clinical findings in turkish patients with cystic echinococcosis. *Helminthologia,* **43**: 220–25.

Yong, W. K., Heath, D. D. and Van Knapen, F. (1984). Comparison of cestode antigens in an enzyme-linked immunosorbent assay for the diagnosis of *Echinococcus granulosus, Taenia hydatigena* and *T. ovis* infections in sheep. *Res. Vet. Sci.,* **36**: 24–31.

Yu, R. Y., Sun, T., Li, Z., Zhang, J., Teng, J., *et al.* (2006). Community surveys and risk factor analysis of human alveolar and cystic echinococcosis in Ningxia Hui Autonomous Region, China. *Bull. WHO,* **84**: 714–21.

Yu, S. H., Wang, H., Wu, X. H., Ma, X., *et al.* (2008). Cystic and alveolar echinococcosis: an epidemiological survey in a Tibetan population in southeast Qinghai, China. *Japanese J. Infect. Dis.,* **61**: 242–46.

Zanini, F., Suárez, C., Pérez, H. and Elissondo, M. C. (2009). Epidemiological surveillance of cystic echinococcosis in rural population of Tierra del Fuego, Argentina, 1997–2006. *Parasitol. Int.,* **58**: 69–71.

Zhang, W. and McManus, D. P. (2008). Vaccination of dogs against *Echinococcus granulosus*: a means to control hydatid disease? *Trends Parasitol.,* **24**: 419–24.

Ziadinov, I., Mathis, A., Trachsel, D., *et al.* (2008). Canine echinococcosis in Kyrgyzstan: epidemiology and transmission analysis incorporting diagnostic uncertainty. *Int. J. Parasitol.,* **38**: 1179–90.

CHAPTER 54

Alveolar echinococcosis (*Echinococcus multilocularis*)

and neotropical forms of echinococcosis (*Echinococcus vogeli* and *Echinococcus oligarthrus*)

J. Eckert, P. Deplazes and P. Kern

Summary

In this chapter three forms of echinococcosis in humans are described that are caused by a larval stage (metacestode) of *Echinococcus multilocularis* Leuckart, 1863, *Echinococcus oligarthrus* (Diesing, 1863) or *Echinococcus vogeli* Rausch and Bernstein, 1972. *E. multilocularis* is the causative agent of alveolar echinococcosis (AE). In the human host the metacestode of *E. multilocularis* behaves like a malignant tumour, characterized by infiltrative proliferation and the potential to induce serious disease. The liver is nearly exclusively the primary site of metacestode development, but metastases may by formed in adjacent and distant organs. Typically AE exhibits a chronic progressive clinical course, which finally leads to death in up to 90% of untreated patients within 10 year after diagnosis. An undefined proportion of cases are abortive with inactivation of the parasite. Evidence has accumulated in recent years that anti-parasitic therapy with benzimidazoles (albendazole or mebendazole) over many years or lifelong, if necessary combined with interventional procedures, can inhibit disease progression and improve or stabilse the patient's clinical condition. Radical surgery in an early stage of the infection combined with anti-parasitic therapy for two years may lead to cure. The introduction of benzimidazole therapy of AE (1977), combined with improved diagnostic and surgical procedures, has resulted in significantly increased life-expectancies of adequately treated AE patients. In highly endemic areas ultrasound population screening (partially combined with antibody detecetion) has been successfully used for early detection of AE cases. Countrywide annual AE incidence rates are mostly low at approximately < 0.1 to 2.0 per 100,000 inhabitants, but they can be much higher locally. Furthermore, there are indications of emerging case numbers in some areas of Europe and Asia. In spite of relatively low case numbers, AE is a significant disease due to its severity and high costs of treatment (median costs of approximately €182,000 per case).

E. multilocularis occurs in at least 43 countries of the northern hemisphere (North America and Eurasia). Recent studies in Europe and Asia have shown that the endemic area of *E. multilocularis* is larger than previously known and has regionally expanded from rural to urban areas. *E. multilocularis* is predominately perpetuated in a wildlife cycle with canids (mainly foxes) as definitive hosts and small mammals (mainly rodents) as intermediate hosts. Humans acquire the infection by accidental ingestion of eggs released by infected definitive hosts to the environment. During the last two decades new immunological and molecular techniques have been developed allowing not only a quick and precise diagnosis of the intestinal *E. multilocularis* infection in living or dead definitive hosts but also the determination of the environmental contamination with infective parasite eggs. New studies suggest that in endemic areas increasing fox populations may be associated with a higher infection risk for humans. Recent controlled studies indicate that this riks can be reduced in confined regions, such as periurban areas, by baiting of foxes with praziquantel.

E. vogeli and *E. oligarthrus* are restricted to the neotropical region (Latinamerica), causing in humans a highly pathogenic polycystic (PE) and a less aggressive unicystic form of echinococcosis (UE), respectively. Total numbers of recorded human cases of PE and AE are currently low (< 200), but they may represent only the 'tip of the iceberg'. *Echinococcus shiquicus* n. sp., recently described from China, shares several features with *E. multilocualris* but currently it is not known whether this species can infect humans.

History

Echinococcus multilocularis

A first case of hepatic human alveolar echinococcosis (AE) was reported in 1852 by Buhl in Munich who diagnosed it initially as 'alveolar colloid' and identified it later as 'composed echinococcosis tumor' (Buhl 1856). In 1856 the German pathologist Virchow described another case from Würzburg as 'multilocular, ulcerating echinococcosis tumour of the liver' (Virchow 1856). At this time, it was unclear whether this form of echinococcosis was caused by *E. granulosus* or another *Echinococcus* species. In 1901 Posselt in Austria (Posselt 1928) infected a dog with alveolar parasite material containing protoscoleces from a human liver and found in the dog's intestine small tapeworms clearly differing from *E. granulosus* and showing characteristics of *Echinococcus multilocularis* described by Leuckart in 1863 (denominated by Posselt as *Taenia echinococcus alveolaris*). Posselt and some other authors provided further biological, clinical and epidemiological evidence for a 'dualistic' aetiology of cystic and alveolar echinococcosis opposing the 'monistic' view of Dévé and adherents that only a single species, *E. granulosus*, is the causative agent of both forms of echinococcosis (Posselt 1928; Rausch 1986). In 1928 Posselt recorded approximately 650 human cases of AE from Austria, southern Germany, Switzerland and adjoining areas, from Russia and some other regions (France, northern Italy, USA). He regarded southern Germany, Switzerland, the Austrian alpine regions and some parts of Russia as the 'classical distribution area' of AE. Some of his cases were observed in central and northern Germany (Posselt 1928). About 100 years after the detection of the first human cases of AE the 'dualistic' view was finally accepted based on results of the classical studies by Rausch and Schiller (1954) in Alaska and by Vogel (1957) in Germany who unequivocally demonstrated that *E. granulosus* and *E. multilocularis* are distinct species and that the latter is the causative agent of human AE (see Tappe *et al.* 2010a for review).

Echinococcus oligarthrus and *E. vogeli*

E. oligarthrus, isolated from the cougar (*Felis concolor L.*) in Brazil, and originally described as *Taenia oligarthra* by Diesing in 1863 was redescribed by Lühe in 1910 and transferred to the genus *Echinococcus*. The life cycle of *E. oligarthrus*, involving wild felids as definitive hosts and rodents as intermediate hosts, was experimentally determined by Sousa and Thatcher in 1969 (Sousa and Thatcher 1969; Rausch 1986; Tappe *et al.* 2008). A first human case of an *E. oligarthrus* infection ('unicystic echinococosis') was reported in 1989 from Venezuela (Lopera *et al.* 1989). *Echinococcus vogeli*, recovered from a bush dog, *Speothos venaticus*, which had been captured in Ecuador and kept in the Los Angeles zoo, was described as a new species by Rausch and Bernstein (1972). First observations on the natural cycle of this species involving bush dogs as definitive hosts and pacas as intermediate hosts were already reported in the 1960s by Cabrera *et al.* (cited in D'Alessandro and Rausch 2008).

Phylogeny and taxonomy

Current concepts in systematics of the genus *Echinococcus* and the *Echinococcus granulosus*-complex are described in chapter on cystic echinococcosis (see Chapter 53). Based on morphological, biological and genetic criteria *E. multilocularis* Leuckart, 1863, *Echinococcus oligarthrus* (Diesing 1863) and *Echinococcus vogeli* (Rausch and Bernstein 1972) are recognized as distinct species (Table 54.1) (Nakao *et al.* 2007; Thompson 2008; D'Alessandro and Rausch 2008; Saarma *et al.* 2009). Studies on phylogenetic relationships within the genus *Echinococcus*, based on mitochondrial DNA (mitochondrial phylogeny), have identified *E. oligarthrus* and *E. vogeli* as clades clearly separated from the *E. granulosus*-complex, but allocated *E. multilocularis* and *E. shiquicus* within this complex between *E. equinus* and *E. ortleppi* (Nakao *et al.* 2007; Saarma *et al.* 2009). Sequence data from 5 nuclear genes (nuclear phylogeny) have identified *E. multilocularis* as basal taxon with *E. shiquicus* next to it, followed by *E. oligarthrus* and *E. vogeli* (Saarma *et al.* 2009). In view of the characteristic morphological, biological and epidemiological features of these species the nuclear phylogeny appears to be more plausible then the mitochondrial phylogeny. *E. multilocularis* and *E. shiquicus* are genetically closely related, the adult stages are similar,

Table 54.1 Alveolar and neotropical forms of echinococcosis in humans

Echinococcus species	Name, (abbreviation) and synonym of disease	Geographical distribution
Echinococcus multilocularis	Alveolar echinococcosis (AE)	Northern hemisphere (Eurasia, North America)
Echinococcus oligarthrus	Unicystic echinococcosis (UE) *E. oligarthrus* echinococcosis	Central and South America
Echinococcus vogeli	Polycystic echinococcosis (PE) *E. vogeli* echinococcosis	Central and South America

both species occur sympatrically in Tibet and use foxes and pikas as hosts. However, the metacestode stage of *E. shiquicus* is described as 'unilocular' whereas *E. multilocularis* has a multilocular and proliferating metacestode stage. In view of limited information on *E. shiquicus* (Xiao *et al.* 2005) its recognition as a distinct species has been regarded as premature (Thompson 2008), but genetic data support the species status (McManus 2006; Saarma *et al.* 2009).

Alveolar echinococcosis

The causative agent, *Echinococcus multilocularis*

Alveolar echinococcosis of humans and other mammals is caused by the metacestode stage of *E. multilocularis* which has, like other *Echinococcus* species, a complex life cycle and epidemiology.

Life cycle of the parasite

E. multilocularis is predominantly perpetuated in a wildlife-cycle with carnivores as definitive and small mammals as intermediate hosts. The adult (strobilar) stage inhabits the small intestine of definitive hosts, primarily of foxes (genera *Vulpes* and *Alopex*), but also of domestic dogs, other canids and occasionally of felids (Fig. 54.1). Sexually mature worms produce eggs which are released to the environment, either enclosed in the terminal segment of the parasite or free in the intestinal content. The prepatent period can be as short as 26–28 days (Thompson and Eckert 1983; Kapel *et al.* 2006; Matsumoto and Yagi 2008). Upon release from the definitive host, the eggs normally contain a fully developed larval stage, the oncosphere, and are infective. If mature eggs are ingested by susceptible intermediate host animals, primarily arvicolid and cricetid rodents, oncospheres hatch in the stomach and small intestine, they are activated under the influence of host factors, penetrate the epithelial layer and migrate to the lamina propria within 30–120 min. after hatching (Thompson 1995). After invasion of venous or lymphatic vessels, the oncospheres are transported to the liver which is a primary site of further development to the metacestode stage. In susceptible intermediate hosts the metacestode produces by asexual proliferation and differentiation a variable number of protoscoleces within 40–60 days after infection or later (Sakamoto and Sugimura 1970; Vogel 1977). If an intermediate host, containing metacestodes with mature protoscoleces is eaten by a definitive host the cycle is closed.

Besides natural intermediate hosts, humans and several mammalian animal species, which do not play a role in parasite transmission, can accidentally acquire the infection ('accidental hosts') with subsequent establishment of metacestodes in the liver and other internal organs (Fig. 54.1).

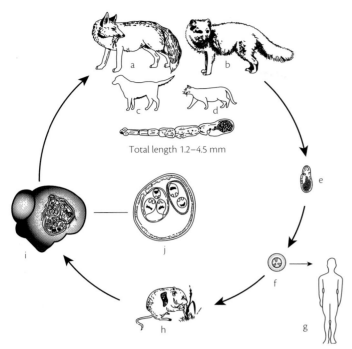

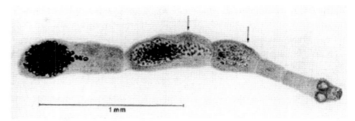

Fig. 54.2 Adult stage of *Echinococcus multilocularis* with sac-like uterus in the tertminal segment containing eggs. Arrows point to genital pores.
Photograph: © Institute of Parasitology, Zurich.

Fig. 54.1 Life cycle of Echonococcus *multilocularis* (a) Red fox (*Vulpes vulpes*) and (b) arctic fox (*Alopex lagopus*) as principle definitive hosts in wildlife cycles; (c) domestic dog as definitive host in synanthropic cycles; (d) domestic cat as occasional definitive host of low significance; (e) terminal segment of the parasite with eggs; (f) egg; (g) man as accidental host; (h) common vole (*Microtus arvalis*) as representative of many species of intermediate hosts; (i) liver of a rodent with metacestodes of the parasite; (j) magnification of (i), showing one cyst with two brood capsules and protoscoleces.
© Institute of Parasitology, Zurich.

The adult stage, its host range and biology
Morphology
E. multilocularis is a small tapeworm with a total body length between 1.2 and 4.5 mm and typically 5 (2–6) segments (Thompson 1995) (Fig. 54.2). The scolex is equipped with 4 suckers and a double row of large and small hooks with a mean length of 31.0 μm (range: 24.9–34.0 μm) and 27.0 μm (range: 20.4–31.0 μm), respectively. In comparison *to E. granulosus*, characteristic diagnostic features of *E. multilocularis* are the sac-like uterus without lateral sacculations in the gravid (terminal) segment and the position of the genital pore anterior to the middle of both the mature and the gravid segments (details see Vogel 1957; Thompson 1995). Morphologically *E. multilocularis* has similarities with *E. shiquicus*. Gravid segments of *E. multilocularis* contain between 200 and 300 eggs.

Host range and biology
Natural defintive hosts of *E. multilocularis* are predominantly carnivores of the family Canidae, including the red fox (*Vulpes vulpes*), arctic fox (*Alopex lagopus*), Tibet fox (*Vulpes ferrilata*) corsac fox (*Vulpes corsac*), wolf (*Canis lupus*), coyote (*Canis latrans*), domestic dog (*Canis lupus f. familiaris*) and the raccoon-dog (*Nyctereutes procyonoides*). Other hosts belonging to the family Felidae are Lynx (*Lynx lynx*), wildcat (*Felis silvestris*) and domestic cat (*Felis silvestris f. catus*) (Rausch 1995; Eckert et al. 2001a). The epidemiological

significance of various definitive host species is discussed below and examples are presented in Table 54.2.

Whereas members of the family Canidae (foxes, domestic dogs, raccoon-dogs) are highly susceptible to *E. multilocularis*, domestic cats have a much lower and more variable susceptibility (references in Eckert and Deplazes 2004; Thompson *et al.* 2003, 2006; Matsumoto and Yagi 2008). In a recent study, Kapel *et al.* (2006) inoculated groups, each of 5 animals, of naive red foxes, raccoon dogs, domestic dogs and domestic cats with 20,000 *E. multilocularis* protoscoleces (Swiss isolate) per animal. At day 35 post inoculation all animals, except one cat, were infected and harboured average intestinal worm burdens representing 84% of the infective dose in foxes, 40% in raccoon dogs, 12% in dogs and only 3% in cats. At day 90 post inoculation the parasite burdens in foxes and raccoon dogs had declined to low levels (1% of the 35 day burdens), but remained relatively high in domestic dogs (63%). At this time cats had also reduced worm burdens (9% of the 35 day burdens). In this study worms in cats produced low numbers of thick-shelled eggs, however, these eggs were not infective for mice (Kapel *et al.* 2006).

In definitive hosts *E. multilocularis* can attach to the mucosa of the small intestine at any region but the predominant sites of the parasites are the middle and distant sections (Thompson *et al.* 2006). Pre-patent periods of 26 days in dogs and of 29–33 days in foxes, raccoon dogs and cats were observed after experimental infections with *E. multilocularis* protoscoleces (Japanese and Swiss isolates) (Kapel *et al.* 2006; Matsumoto and Yagi 2008). The average duration of egg excretion (patent period during which 95% of the total egg mass was excreted) has been calculated comparatively in the study of Kapel *et al.* (2006) to 27 days for foxes, 30 days for raccoon dogs, 43 days for dogs, and 13 days for cats. An evaluation of faecal egg counts (carried out at 3 day intervals from day 25 post inoculation) revealed that after inoculation with 20,000 protoscoleces the mean egg production per animal during patency was high in foxes, raccoon dogs and dogs (approximately 280,000 to 345,000 eggs) but low in cats (573 eggs) (Kapel *et al.* 2006). In a Japanese study one heavily infected dog excreted about 10,000,000 eggs during a patent period of 132 days. The duration of the patent period was 2–5 months in dogs and approximately 2–3 months in foxes (Matsumoto and Yagi 2008).

The egg stage
E. multilocularis eggs are spherical in shape and range in size from 30–40 x 28–39 μm (Vogel 1957) (Fig. 54.1f). The egg is composed of a centrally located oncosphere, surrounded by an embryophore, consisting of a thin inner and a thick outer layer, the latter being

Table 54.2. *Echinococcus multilocularis*: Selected examples of definitive and intermediate host animals in various geographic regions and of parasite prevalences[1]. Names of hosts with special significance in bold letters

Region	Definitive hosts	Intermediate hosts
Western and central Europe (3, 5, 10, 11, 12, 13)[1]	**Red fox** (*Vulpes vulpes*) Raccoon dog (*Nyctereutes procyonoides*) Wolf (*Canis lupus*) Lynx (*Lynx* spp.) Domestic dog (*Canis familiaris*) Domestic cat (*Felis catus*) Prevalence rates: Foxes: < 1 – > 70%, dogs and cats: generally < 1%, in dogs focally up to 7%.	**Common vole** (*Microtus arvalis*) Snow vole (*Microtus nivalis*) Earth vole (*Pitymys subterraneus*) Red-backed vole (*Myodes* glareolus*) **Water vole** (*Arvicola terrestris*) Muskrat (*Ondatra zibethicus*) and others Prevalence rates: generally low: < 1% to 6%, rarely higher, notably in muskrats.
Northern Europe ◆ (Svalbard) (4)	**Arctic fox** (*Alopex lagopus*)	**Southern vole** (*Microtus rossiaemeridionalis*)
Eurasia ◆ Russia (2, 3, 10)	**Arctic fox** (*Alopex lagopus*) **Red fox** (*Vulpes vulpes*) Corsac fox (*Vulpes corsac*) Wolf (*Canis lupus*) Raccoon dog (*Nyctereutes procyonoides*) Wildcat (*Felis silvestris*) Domestic dog (*Canis familiaris*)	Northern vole (*Microtus oeconomus*) Common vole (*Microtus arvalis*) Voles (*Microtus* spp.) Brown lemming (*Lemmus sibiricus*) Red-backed voles (*Myodes** spp.) Jirds (*Meriones* spp.) Muskrat (*Ondatra zibethicus*) etc. Prevalence rates: around 1–11%, in some foci up to 50%
Asia ◆ Kazakhstan (7, 8)	**Red fox** (*Vulpes vulpes*) Prevalence rates: 5–33%	Grey marmot (*Marmota baibacina*) Steppe marmot (*Marmota bobac*) Northern red-backed vole (*Myodes** rutilus*) Red-tailed gerbil (*Meriones lybicus*) Root vole (*Microtus oeconomus*) Water vole (*Arvicola terrestris*) Muskrat (*Ondatra zibethicus*) etc. Prevalence rates: 0.05–6.5%
Asia ◆ China (1, 3, 10, 11)	**Red fox** (*Vulpes vulpes*) Wolf (*Canis lupus*) **Domestic dog** (*Canis familiaris*).	Brandt's vole (*Microtus brandti*) Pika (*Ochotona* sp.) Tibetan hare (*Lepus oiostolus*) Jird (*Meriones unguiculatus*) and others
Asia ◆ Japan (9, 11, 13, 14)	**Red fox** (*Vulpes vulpes*) Domestic dog (*Canis familiaris*) Domestic cat (*Felis catus*) Raccoon dog (*Nyctereutes procynoides*). *Prevalence rates:* (averages 1965–1991): Foxes: 14%, Dogs: 1%, cats: up to 5.5%.	Red-backed vole (*Myodes** glareolus*) **Gray Red-backed vole** (*Myodes** rufocanus*) Red- backed vole (*Myodes**rutilus*) etc. *Prevalence rates:* (averages 1965–1991): generally low with average around 1%.
North America: ◆ Northern tundra zone (1, 3, 6) ◆ Central North America (1, 3, 6)	**Arctic fox** (*Alopex lagopus*) **Domestic dog** (*Canis familiaris*) *Prevalence rates:* Artic foxes: 40 –100%, 12% **Red fox** (*Vulpes vulpes*) Coyote (*Canis latrans*) Grey fox (*Urocyon cineroargenteus*). *Prevalence rates:* Foxes: < 1 – > 65% Coyotes: 6– 35% Cats: focally 1– 5%	Northern vole (*Microtus oeconomus*) Brown lemming (*Lemmus sibiricus*) Red-backed vole (*Myodes**rutilus*) etc. *Prevalence rates:* generally high: 42–83%. Deer mouse (*Peromyscus maniculatus*) Meadow vole (*Microtus pennsylvanicus*) Muskrat (*Ondatra zibethicus*) Woodrat (*Neotoma cinerea*) House mouse (*Mus musculus*) *Prevalence rates:* generally low: about 0.5– 6%, rarely higher.

[1] Selected key references: (1) Schantz *et al.* (1995), (2) Bessonov (1998), (3) Eckert *et al.* (2001a), (4) Henttonen *et al.* (2001), (5) Malczewski (2002), (6) Rausch and Fay (2002), (7) Shaikenov and Torgerson (2002), (8) Shaikenov (2006), (9) Ito *et al.* (2003), (10) Vuitton *et al.* (2003), (11) Jenkins *et al.* (2005), (12) Moks *et al.* (2005), (13) Romig *et al.* (2006a), (14) Matsumoto and Yagi (2008),
* Previous name of the genus: *Clethrionomys*

covered with an outer vitelline layer ('egg shell') which is normally lost during egg release. In the light microscope the embryophore has a striped appearance due to its composition of blocks of a keratin-like protein which are held together by a cementing substance (Swiderski 1983; Thompson 1995). Morphologically eggs of *E. multilocularis* are indistinguishable from eggs of other *Echinococcus* and of *Taenia* species. However, they can be distinguished from each other by molecular techniques (see Chapter 53).

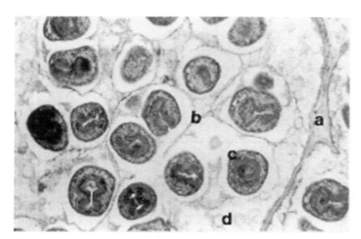

Fig. 54.3 Histological section of *Echinococcus multilocularis* metacestode from a rodent: (a) cyst wall; (b) wall of brood capsule; (c) protoscolex; (d) calcareous corpuscle. Scale ⊢————⊣ 100 micrometer.
Photograph: © Institute of Parasitology, Zurich.

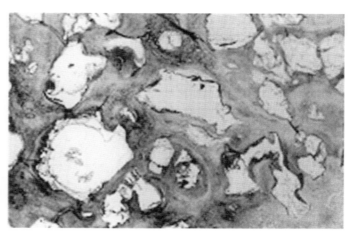

Fig. 54.4 Histological section of *Echinococcus multilocularis* metacestode in a human liver: cysts without brood capsule and protoscolex formation. Scale ⊢————⊣ 100 micrometer.
Photograph: © Institute of Parasitology, Zurich.

The oncosphere is a spherical, fully differentiated, infective larval stage, about 25 μm in diameter. As documented for *E. granulosus* (Swiderski 1983) the oncosphere is covered with a confluent nucleated tegument, it is armed with three pairs of hooks, and contains various groups of cells, including 10 germinal cells located in the posterior pole of the body. Germinal cells (= germinative cells, 'neoblasts') of cestodes are regarded as totipotent stem cells with mitotic activity and the capacity to directly differentiate to somatic cells (reviewed by Brehm and Spiliotis 2008; Brehm 2010). *Echinococcus* germinal cells (diameter 3–5 μm)–characterized by a pale nucleus with a conspicuous large nucleolus and a scant basophilic cyctoplasm–can be distinguished from differentiated cestode cells by light and electron microscopy (Sakamoto and Sugimura 1970; Vogel 1977; Mehlhorn *et al.* 1983). Germinal cells occur also in the neck region and in proglottids of adult cestodes. In the neck region they are involved in production of proglottids, and in proglottids they play a role in forming genital organs and oncospheres (Reuter and Kreshchenko 2004; Brehm and Spiliotis 2008; Brehm 2010). Some features of the eggs that are relevant to epidemiology are discussed below.

The metacestode, its biology and host range
Morphology and biology
The origin of the metacestode stage is the oncosphere that has travelled from the intestine in the blood stream to the primary target organ, mostly the liver. In rodents perorally infected with *E. multilocularis* eggs, oncospheres and perivascular aggregations of host cells can be microscopically detected in the liver as early as 4 hours and 8 hours, respectively, and tiny macroscopic foci are visible after 2–5 days (Ohbayashi 1960; Vogel 1977; Bosch 1982). These foci are found nearby the branches of the portal vein and liver sinusoids indicating the invasion of the liver by the portal circulation (Yamashita, 1960; Vogel 1977). After having attained an infection site in the liver, the oncosphere transforms to a unilocular vesicle (diameter between 15 and 70 μm) within 1–7 days by a ring-shaped arrangement of germinal cells in one layer and central cavity formation; the hooks disappear rapidly (Sakamoto and

Sugimura 1970; Vogel 1977; Bosch 1982). According to Sakamoto and Sugimura (1970) the vesicle wall is composed of germinal cells and immature 'cyst-wall-forming cells', but it is discussed whether germinal cells alone could be responsible for cyst wall formation (Brehm 2010). In the early stages of development oncospheres and initial vesicles are directly attached to surrounding intact or degenerating host cells (Sakamoto and Sugimura 1970; Vogel 1977). Multilocular vesiculation starts within 5–7 days post infection. At this stage the vesicles are made up of a thin cytoplasmic layer containing prominent germinal cells ('germinal layer'). Beginning 5 days after infection a thin outer acellular laminated ('cuticular') layer can be detected in histological sections in parts of the cysts (Sakamoto and Sugimura 1970; Vogel 1977). This layer is produced by the parasite as confirmed by *in vitro* studies (Deplazes and Gottstein 1991; Brehm and Spiliotis 2008). About 20–35 days

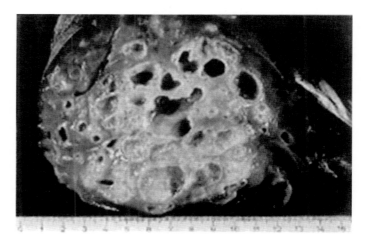

Fig. 54.5 Macroscopic appearance of human liver with *Echinococcus multilocularis*: multiple small and larger vesicles (maximum diameter 3 cm), partially interconnected.
Photograph: © Institute of Parasitology, Zurich.

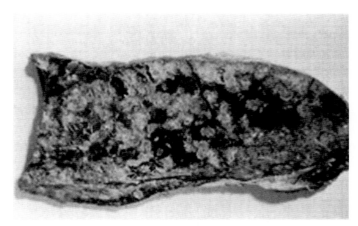

Fig. 54.6 Macroscopic appearance of human lung with multiple metastases of *Echinococcus multilocularis*.
Photograph: © University Hospital Zurich.

after infection the germinal layer begins to produce brood capsules and protoscoleces by asexual proliferation, and mature protoscoleces are found 40–60 days or later after infection (Sakamoto and Sugimura 1970; Vogel 1977; Bosch 1982, Matsumoto and Yagi 2008). Metacestode development and protoscolex production are highly variable depending on the host species (Figs. 54.1 i–j and 54.3). In humans, protoscolex formation is rare (Fig. 54.4).

The fully developed metacestode stage of *E. multilocularis* differs from that of *E. granulosus*. In macroscopic liver sections of infected intermediate or accidental hosts, the metacestode of *E. multilocularis* exhibits an alveolar structure consisting of numerous single or interconnected vesicles of irregular shapes and sizes between < 1 mm and 30 mm (Ammann and Eckert 1995; Eckert and Deplazes 2004) (Fig. 54.5). The individual cyst has a wall composed of a thin inner cellular 'germinal layer' and an outer acellular laminated (PAS-positive) layer and contains fluid or a jelly-like mass. The space between cysts is initially filled with various types of host cells and later with connective tissue or necrotic material. In the human liver, the metacestode can proliferate initially from minor lesions to diameters of 15 to 20 cm. Due to reduced supply with nutrients, the central parts of large metacestodes may become necrotic so that cavities are formed, containing necrotic masses, liquid material and small parasite vesicles (Posselt 1928; Ammann and Eckert 1996; Eckert and Deplazes 2004).

A characteristic feature of the *E. multilocularis* metacestode is its proliferative growth and metastasis formation (Fig. 54.6). Various forms of proliferation have been described, including exogenous budding of vesicles and the production of solid protrusions of the germinal layer, devoid of a laminated layer, which are extruded out of vesicles to the surrounding tissue (Fig. 54.7) (Vogel 1978; Ali-Khan et al. 1983; Mehlhorn et al. 1983). Protrusions, observed in experimentally infected jirds (*Meriones unguiculatus*), have been found by electron microscopy in intimate contact with surrounding host cells. The protrusions may later transform to cystic and tube-like structures both covered by a laminated layer (Vogel 1978; Eckert et al. 1983; Mehlhorn et al. 1983) (Fig. 54.7). Studies in jirds have shown that after subcutaneous transplantation of metacestode tissue into the neck region, metastatic lesions are first

detectable in regional lymph nodes and 10–12 weeks after infection in the lungs of 88% of the animals (Eckert et al. 1983). It is thought that germinal cells may detach from the metacestode tissue being then disseminated via lymph or blood vessels to other sites where metastases are formed (Vogel 1978; Ali-Khan et al. 1983; Eckert et al. 1983; Mehlhorn et al. 1983; Buttenschoen et al. 2009a). The fact that novel vesicles can be formed *in vitro* from isolated germinal cells supports the hypothesis of metastasis formation by disseminated germinal cells (Brehm and Spiliotis 2008). Dissemination of tiny vesicles (covered with a laminated layer) after infiltration of metacestodes into lymph or blood vessels has to be considered as another potential mechanism of metastasis formation.

Host range

Natural intermediate hosts of *E. multilocularis* are predominantly rodents, representing at least 7 families (Sciuridae, Cricetidae, Arviculidae, Muridae, Dipodidae, Ochotonidae, Myocastoridae) including numerous species. Furthermore, insectivores (Talpidae, Sorcidae) and lagomorphs (Leporidae) can also be involved in the cycle (Rausch 1995; WHO/OIE 2001; Vuitton et al. 2003). Parasite development and numbers of protoscoleces can vary considerably in the intermediate host species (Ohbayashi et al. 1971; Rausch 1986; Kroeze and Tanner 1987; Matsumoto and Yagi 2008; Burlet et al. 2011). Highly variable and overdispersed protoscolex burdens were found in Switzerland in a population of *Arvicola terrestris* with protoscolex numbers between 14 and 244,400 (Stieger et al. 2002). High individual protoscolex burdens have also been found in other intermediate hosts species, for example 3,700,000 protoscolces in a gray-sided vole (*Myodes*[= *Clethrionomys*] *rufocanus bedfordiae*) in Japan (Matsumoto and Yagi 2008), and 108,000 in a *Myodes* (= *Clethrionomys*) *glareolus* in Switzerland (Stieger et al. 2002). Great diversity exists between geographical regions and local endemic foci regarding the epidemiological role of intermediate hosts species. Examples are shown in Table 54.2.

Accidentally, metacestodes may establish in hosts that are not normally involved in the transmission cycle, including humans,

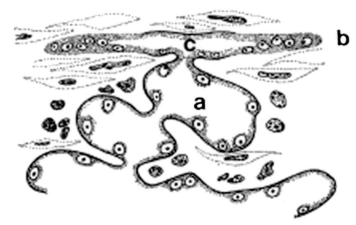

Fig. 54.7 Scheme of proliferation of *Echinococcus multilocularis* metacestode (a) cyst with inner nucleated germinal and outer laminated layer; (b) solid protrusion of the germinal layer (devoid of laminated layer) infiltrating surrounding host tissue; (c) formation of central lumen and outer laminated layer in a protrusion. After Vogel (1978), Eckert et al. (1983), Mehlhorn et al. (1983).
© Institute of Parasitology, Zurich.

domestic dogs, pigs and horses or the wild boar (*Sus scrofa*), nutria (*Myocastor coypus*), various genera of monkeys (in captivity, *Gorilla*, *Macaca*, *Lemur* etc.) (WHO/OIE 2001; Deplazes and Eckert 2001; Rehmann *et al.* 2003; Eckert and Deplazes 2004) and Chinchilla (*Chinchilla laniger*) (in captivity), (Staebler *et al.* 2007). Some reports on metacestodes of *E. multilocularis* in cattle and sheep are due to confusion with the well known atypical polycystic metacestodes of *E. granulosus* (Rausch 1995), as described by Sakamoto *et al.* (1987).

Biochemistry and molecular biology

Progress in biochemical and molecular research on *Echinococcus* has recently been reviewed by McManus (2009) and Brehm (2010). Only a few aspects can be discussed here.

Biochemistry

Studies on protoscoleces of *E. granulosus* and *E. mulilocularis* have demonstrated the presence of a glycolytic pathway and the complete set of tricarboxylic acid cycle enzymes with relatively high levels of activity (McManus 2009). Fermentative pathways yielding acetic, succinic and lactic acids as metabolic endproducts are active under anaerobic and even aerobic conditions. The tricarboxycic cycle is at least in part functional in *E. granulosus,* but its role is still unclear (McManus 2009). Matsumoto *et al.* (2008) found that protoscoleces of *E. multilocularis* possess a mitochondrial respiratory system involving the NADH-fumarate reductase system that is highly adapted to anaerobic conditions. This system occurs in many anaerobic organisms including parasitic helminths, but does not normally function in mammals (Matsumoto *et al.* 2008). The detection of the NADH-fumarate reductase system is consistent with observations that division and aggregation of *E. multilocularis* germinal cells *in vitro* depend on anaerobic and reducing conditions (Brehm and Spiliotis 2008).

Molecular biology

E. multilocularis and *E. granulosus* have chromosome sets of 2n = 18 with 2 larger rod-like and 16 smaller dot-like chromosomes (Frosch and Lucius 1994). The genome of *E. multilocularis* is estimated to be approximately 270 Mb. Several genes of *E. multilocularis* have been cloned and sequenced. Sequence data are available from the Echinococcus Genome Project (www.sanger.ac.uk/Projects/Echinococcus).

Molecular techniques allow phylogenetic studies based on the mitochondrial genome (Nakao *et al.* 2007) and on nuclear genes (Saarma *et al.* 2009). In contrast to *E. granulosus* only slight intraspecific genetic variation has previously been found in *E. multilocularis* (Thompson 2008). Analyses of mitochondrial genes revealed minor differences of each 2 nucleotides between two groups of *E. multilocularis* isolates (Europe versus North America and China) (Bowles and McManus 1993). Variability within NADH dehydrogenase sequences between *E. multilocularis* isolates from Poland and Japan has been described by Kędra *et al.* (2000). Recently, a tandemly repeated multilocus microsatellite called EmsB, exhibiting a higher level of intraspecific polymorphism, enabled new molecular epidemiological investigations on spatial and temporal scales (Knapp *et al.* 2009a)**.**

Molecular methods have opened new ways for the development of DNA-based diagnostic strategies and for addressing important basic questions, such as the host-parasite communication by cytokines and hormones or the oncogenic transformation of *E. multilocularis* germinal cells (reviewed by Brehm and Spiliotis 2008; Brehm 2010).

Parasite maintenance *in vivo* or *in vitro* and cryopreservation

Metacestode maintenance in the laboratory by serial passages in rodents and experimental infections of rodents with eggs or of definitive hosts with protoscoleces have been described in the previous edition of this book (Eckert 1998). Handling of infective *E. multilocularis* stages requires strict safety precautions (WHO/OIE 2001).

In vitro cultivation

Maintenance of the complete cycle of *E. multilocularis in vitro* is currently not possible. Immature unsegmented or segmented intestinal stages of *E. multilocularis* could be produced *in vitro* from protoscoleces (Thompson *et al.* 1990; Howell and Smyth 1995), and maturation of the parasites with development of thick-shelled eggs was achieved by cultivation of intestinal stages following partial development in the dog for 20–21 days (Thompson and Eckert 1982). *In vitro* maintenance of adult stages during a few weeks has been employed for collecting excretory/secretory antigens (Deplazes *et al.* 1999).

Great progress has been achieved in recent years by improving *in vitro* methods for the production of cysts from metacestode tissue blocks (Hemphill *et al.* 2010) and by axenic cultivation of metacestode vesicles. A break-through is the isolation of *E. multilocularis* germinal cells (from cysts obtained from cultures), their separation from host cells, their maintenance *in vitro* over several weeks and the induction of vesicle formation in these cultures under specific conditions (substances released by hepatoma cells through a membrane, anaerobic and reducing conditions) (Brehm and Spiliotis 2008; Spiliotis and Brehm 2008). These studies have shown that metacestode vesicles can be formed in a fluid medium from isolated germinal cells that divide, aggregate and develop by fusion to a small vesicle with a central cavity after 2 to 3 weeks. After having reached diameters of 50–100 μm a laminated layer is formed after 5 to 6 weeks of incubation (Brehm and Spiliotis 2008). These findings are consistent with previous observations that oncospheres developed *in vitro* to vesicles surrounded by a laminated layer containing the Em2G11 antigen (Deplazes and Gottstein 1991; Gottstein *et al.* 1992).

Cryopreservation

Metacestode tissue blocks of *E. multilocularis* can be cryopreserved and maintained in a viable state for at least 1 to 2 years by appropriate deep-freezing and storage in liquid nitrogen (Eckert 1988). Cryopreservation can reduce the number of serial passages in rodents needed for strain maintenance and preserve metacestode isolates in an original state for a prolonged period.

The infection in animals: definitive hosts

Pathological and clinical aspects

In the intestine of dogs *E. multilocularis* attaches between the villi, and worms extend the apical region of the rostellum deeply into crypts of Lieberkühn (Thompson and Eckert 1983) (Fig. 54.8). The hooks superficially penetrate the epithelium, and the suckers may grasp substantial plugs of host tissue. Although the epithelium of parasitized crypts is commonly flattened, no evidence of breakdown in the integrity of the crypts is normally seen (Thompson and Eckert 1983). Typically, relevant inflammatory reactions do not occur so that infections remain asymptomatic during the prepatent and patent period, even if dogs (or foxes) harbour burdens between 10,000 and 150,000 worms (Eckert *et al.* 2001b; Kapel *et al.* 2006) (Fig. 54.9).

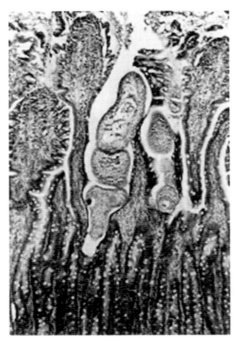

Fig. 54.8 Histological section of dog intestine with immature stages of *Echinococcus multilocularis* penetrating between intestinal villi. Scale ├───────┤ 1 mm.
Photograph: © Institute of Parasitology, Zurich.

Immunity

There are indications from experimental studies that foxes may develop some degree of immunity to intestinal *E. multilocularis* infections, but detailed knowledge is lacking (Al-Sabi *et al.* 2008; Matsumoto and Yagi 2008). Field observations revealed that young red foxes (< 1 year) had significantly higher worm burdens than older foxes (Hofer *et al.* 2000). However, it is unclear whether these differences are due to immunity in older animals or a higher exposure of young foxes (Deplazes and Eckert 2001).

Diagnosis

Procedures for diagnosing the *E. multilocularis* infection in definitive hosts are associated with an infection risk for personnel. Therefore, safety precautions have to be observed during handling of potentially infected animals and of diagnostic materials (WHO/OIE 2001).

Necropsy and parasitological examination

A reliable technique for the diagnosis of *E. multilocularis* infections in foxes and other definitive hosts is the parasitological examination of the small intestine at necropsy. In order to exclude an infection risk for personal, the carcasses or intestines of the definitive hosts should be deep-frozen at −70°C for one week prior to necropsy (Deplazes and Eckert 1996; WHO/OIE 2001). This procedure kills eggs of *E. multilocularis* if −70°C are retained in all parts of the material for at least 4 days (Veit al. 1995; Hildreth *et al.* 2004). Two techniques for parasite detection are preferably used, namely the intestinal scraping technique (IST) and the sedimentation and counting technique (SCT) that are described in detail elsewhere (Deplazes and Eckert 1996; Hofer *et al.* 2000; WHO/OIE 2001). The SCT is regarded as 'gold standard' having a sensitivity

and specificity close to 100%, compared to approximately 78% sensitivity and ~ 100% specificity of the IST (Hofer *et al.* 2000; Deplazes *et al.* 2003; Tackmann *et al.* 2006). Examinations of foxes in Austria revealed sensitivities of 73% for the IST and of 96% for a modified technique similar to SCT (Duscher *et al.* 2005).

The IST has been widely used for mass screening of fox populations for *E. multilocularis*. However, the SCT and IST techniques are time consuming, they can only be applied in dead animals, and material sampling is associated with high logistic expenditure. Furthermore, sampling can be influenced by various factors (for example by the numbers foxes killed by hunters or in accidents in a given area).

Arecoline hydrobromide purgation

This method for detecting the infection in living dogs has been an important diagnostic tool in control campaigns against *E. granulosus*. It was also applied in a few epidemiological studies on the prevalence of *E. multilocularis* in dogs (Stefanić *et al.* 2004; Budke *et al.* 2005), but sensitivity may be as low as 21% (Ziadinov *et al.* 2008). It can now be replaced in most situations by immunological and molecular techniques.

Detection of E. multilocularis eggs

Eggs of *E. multilocularis* can be detected in faecal samples of definitive hosts by routine flotation techniques and rarely on the perianal skin using clear adhesive tape. Effective isolation of taeniid eggs from faecal samples was achieved by a flotation method combined with sequential sieving (F/Si-method) (Mathis *et al.* 1996; Deplazes *et al.* 2003). Eggs of *E. multilocularis* and *Taenia* species are morphologically indistinguishable, but they can be differentiated by amplification of egg-DNA using polymerase chain reaction (PCR).

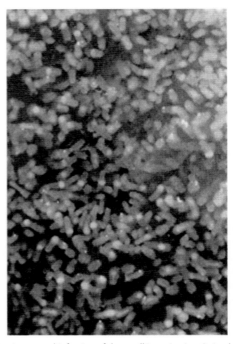

Fig. 54.9 Massive natural infection of the small intestine in a Swiss dog with *Echinococcus multilocularis* (about 45,000 specimens). Aggregation of eggs in sac-like uterus are visble as white spots. Scales ├───────┤ 2 mm.
Photograph: © Institute of Parasitology, Zurich.

In foxes with low egg excretion the sensitivities of the F/Si-method and a modified McMaster egg-counting technique were 89% and 5%, respectively (Al-Sabi *et al.* 2007).

Detection of coproantigens

Coproantigen-ELISAs (CA-ELISAs) using monoclonal or polyclonal antibodies directed against intestinal stages of *Echinococcus* spp. for the detection of antigens released by *E. multilocularis* to the intestinal contents (coproantigens) have been developed independently in Switzerland and Japan (Deplazes *et al.* 1992; Kohno *et al.* 1995; Sakai *et al.* 1998; Deplazes *et al.* 1999). Sensitivities (compared with SCT) are around 80–87% and specificities regarding other helminths genera approximately 70–95% (Deplazes *et al.* 2003). Coproantigens are already detectable in the prepatent period (beginning around 2 weeks post infection) and later during patency; antigen excretion declines to negative levels within 3–5 days after elimination of the parasites from definitive hosts by chemotherapy (Deplazes *et al.* 2003). CA-ELISAs can be employed for detecting *E. multilocularis* copro-antigens in faeces taken from the rectum at necropsy or deposited by foxes or other definitive hosts to the environment. Examination of fox faeces, collected in the field, by CA-ELISAs can identify risk areas contaminated with faeces of infected definitive hosts and discriminate areas of low and high endemicity (Deplazes *et al.* 1999; Raoul *et al.* 2001; Stieger *et al.* 2002; Raoul *et al.* 2003; Hegglin and Deplazes 2008). Therefore, this method can serve for large-scale surveillance in fox and dog populations, as an alternative to necropsy.

Detection of copro- or egg-DNA (C-DNA-test)

Two different *E. multilocularis* genes have so far been targeted in diagnostic PCR for the detection of intestinal *E. multilocularis* infection in faecal samples of foxes, the U1 snRNA gene (Bretagne *et al.* 1993) and the mt 12S rRNA gene (Dinkel *et al.* 1998). Initially, a problem of DNA detection was inhibition of PCR by substances in faecal samples. A successful approach to overcome this obstacle was to first concentrate taeniid eggs from the faecal samples by a flotation and sieving technique (see above) with subsequent egg identification by PCR (Deplazes *et al.* 2003). A recently developed multiplex PCR, based on targets in mitochondrial genes, allows the differentiation between *E. multilocularis*, *E. granulosus* (all genetic variants) and *Taenia* spp. infections; this method has been used in several epidemiological studies (Trachsel *et al.* 2007).

Selection of techniques for individual diagnosis and populations studies

The CA-ELISA, if carefully evaluated, is sensitive, highly specific, cheap and fast and can be used for detecting *E. multilocularis* in definitive hosts, both in individual cases and in populations. Furthermore, this method is suitable for epidemiological studies using faecal samples collected from the environment. DNA-detection is laborious and expensive and is mostly employed for re-evaluation of coproantigen-positive samples, but also as primary method in individual cases (Deplazes *et al.* 2003; Mathis and Deplazes 2006; Davidson *et al.* 2009). Epidemiological studies may include the CA-ELISA as a primary screeing test and a C-DNA-PCR as a confirmatory test. Parallel screening using two (or more) tests on populations is another option (Torgerson and Deplazes 2009).

Detection of serum antibodies

Echinococcus-specific circulating serum antibodies can be detected in a proportion of dogs and foxes with *E. granulosus* or *E. multilocularis* infections, respectively (reviewed by Lightowlers and Gottstein 1995; Deplazes and Eckert 1996). As there is no correlation between prevalence rates of serum antibodies and intestinal worm burdens, this method has no practical value.

Treatment

Dogs and cats with confirmed patent intestinal *E. multilocularis* burdens pose an infection risk to humans, notably to persons in close contact with these animals or their contaminated environment. If treatment of such animals is indicated, it must be carried out with a highly efficacious cestodicide under special safety precautions (WHO/OIE 2001). Well tolerated isoquinoline-derivatives are used in this indication, namely praziquantel (perorally 5 mg/kg body weight in dogs and cats) or epsiprantel (perorally 5.5 mg/kg in dogs, 2.75 mg/kg in cats) which are highly efficient against *E. multilocularis* and *E. granulosus* (WHO/OIE 2001; www.esccap.org). Although the likelihood of small residual worm burdens after a single-dose treatment with these drugs is low, it cannot be completely excluded, especially if the drug was not properly administered. Therefore, it is advisable to treat infected dogs or cats on two consecutive days. The result can be assessed by faecal examinations using adequate methods (egg detection, coproantigen ELISA, PCR) (WHO/OIE 2001). Shampooing and washing of the animal after treatment is recommended in order to remove parasite eggs adherent to the coat. Persons handling infected hosts should wear protective clothing, gloves and face mask (WHO/OIE 2001). Treatment of dogs or cats at risk and treatment of dog and fox populations can be part of strategies of prevention or control and are discussed below.

Infection in animals: intermediate and accidental hosts
Pathological, clinical and immunological aspects
Intermediate hosts

Various species of natural intermediate hosts differ in their susceptibility to *E. multilocularis* infection (Obayashi *et al.* 1971; Kroeze and Tanner 1987). This applies also to laboratory rodents. For example, jirds (*Meriones unguiculatus*), cotton rats (*Sigmodon hispidus*) and some strains of mice (AKR, Balb/c, C57BL/6J) are particularly susceptible, while some other mouse strains (C57BL/10, C3H/HeJ, CB-17) are relatively resistant (Playford *et al.* 1993; Gottstein and Felleisen 1995).

In recent years progress has been achieved in our understanding of the host-parasite interplay (reviewed by Gottstein *et al.* 2006; Siles-Lucas *et al.* 2008; Gottstein *et al.* 2010; Meijri *et al.* 2010). Cellular immunity plays an important role in controlling metacestode proliferation in mice and other hosts, as indicated by an intensive granulomatous infiltration around the parasite and by an extensive parasite proliferation in immunodeficient mice (athymic nude mice and SCID mice) and in AIDS patients. On the other hand, the metacestode can utilize various strategies of evasion and defence. For instance, in mice carbohydrate components (Em2/G11 and Em492) of the laminated layer and other parasite metabolites yield immunosuppressive and other immunomodulatory effects that support parasite survival in the host. A high nitric oxide (NO) production of peritoneal exsudate cells appears to contribute to immunosuppression. NO, produced by periparasitic macrophages and dendritic cells, could damage the parasite, but is has been proposed that the laminated layer protects the germinal layer from this toxic molecule and also from immune reactions of the host. Furthermore, macrophages from metacestode-infected

Table 54.3 Sites of *E. multilocularis* metacestodes with single and multiple organ involvement

Patients from Switzerland (n:70) (Mesarina-Wicki, cited in Ammann and Eckert 1995)		European Registry Cases (n: 554)[1] (Kern *et al.* 2003)	
Organ	No. of cases (%)	Organ	No. of cases (%)
Liver only	47 (67%)	Liver only	351 (63%)
Liver and adjacent organs:	14 (20%)	Liver and adjacent organs:	124 (22%)
◆ abdominal	1	◆ Diaphragm	59
◆ retroperitoneal	4	◆ Kidney and adrenal glands	26
◆ thoracic	6		
◆ thoracic and abdominal	1	◆ Lungs and pleura	15
◆ thoracic and retroperitoneal	2		
Liver and distant metastases:	9 (13%)	Liver and distant metastases:	66 (12%)
◆ brain	3	◆ lungs	39
◆ lungs	4	◆ brain	17
◆ bones	2	◆ spleen	10
Extrahepatic sites only:	0	Extrahepatic sites only: Spleen, peritoneum, lung, vertebra, brain, kidneys, heart	13 (2%)

[1] Total number of cases was 559, including 5 cases without data.

mice are impaired in antigen presentation and appear to trigger an unresponsiveness of T cells leading to suppression of their clonal expansion during the chronic phase of the infection (Gottstein *et al.* 2006, 2010; Meijri *et al.* 2009).

Accidental hosts

As mentioned above, a variety of mammalian animal species have been identified as accidental hosts of the metacestode stage of *E. multilocularis*. For example, severe clinical cases of AE occurred in dogs and monkeys with symptoms and pathological changes very similar to those of human AE (Deplazes and Eckert 2001; Scharf *et al.* 2004; Staebler *et al.* 2006; Heier *et al.* 2007; van Riel *et al.* 2007). Two dogs had an unusual dual infection with metacestodes of *E. multilocularis* in the liver and intestinal stages in the intestine (Deplazes and Eckert 2001). On the other hand, asymptomatic infections with abortive lesions have been observed in European wild boars and in domestic pigs in Japan and Europe (Deplazes and Eckert 2001; Deplazes *et al.* 2005).

Diagnosis
Intermediate hosts

Intermediate hosts of *E. multilocularis* are mainly arvicolid rodents and other small mammals (Table 54.2). Such animals have to be collected for epidemiological studies by specific methods of trapping under consideration of national regulations of animal protection. At necropsy metacestodes of *E. multilocularis* can often be visually detected in organs, notably in the liver, and diagnosed by microscopic examination of fresh material or histological sections. Molecular techniques allow a species-specific diagnosis, even in case of small and calcified lesions (Deplazes *et al.* 2003; Reperant *et al.* 2009).

Accidental hosts

The diagnosis of the *E. multilocularis* infection is possible by post mortem examination. In living larger animals, such as dogs and

monkeys, the diagnosis can be based on the examination of abdominal organs by ultrasound or computer tomography in combination with detection of *E. multilocularis*-specific serum antibodies (Deplazes and Eckert 2001; Scharf *et al.* 2004; Staebler *et al.* 2006).

Treatment

Dogs, monkeys or other accidental host animals are not normally treated because of an uncertain prognosis and difficulties of therapy. In some cases of hepatic AE in dogs surgical resection of liver lesions followed by postoperative chomotherapy with albendazole resulted in long-term clinical remission (Scharf *et al.* 2004).

The infection in humans

In humans the metacestodes of *E. multilocularis* may cause the alveolar form of echinococcosis, a chronic cancer-like disease with high lethality rates in untreated patients. Since the 1980's clinical aspects of the disease have received much attention, such as description of large patient cohorts, refinement of case definition, classification of disease, guidance for best treatment as well as for follow-up examinations (Ammann and Eckert 1995; Wilson *et al.* 1995; WHO 1996; Bresson-Hadni *et al.* 2000; Pawlowski *et al.* 2001; Eckert and Deplazes 2004; Kern *et al.* 2006; Brunetti *et al.* 2010; Li *et al.* 2010).

Biological and clinical aspects
Organ localization of metacestodes

After peroral infection with eggs of *E. multilocularis*, metacestodes almost exclusively develop primarily in the liver. Primary extrahepatic sites of metacestodes without detectable liver involvement are rare (Drolshammer *et al.* 1973; Kern *et al.* 2003;) (see Table 54.3). In the liver only one lobe, both lobes, only the hilus or the hilus and one or two lobes may be affected by the parasite (Ammann and Eckert 1995). From the primary site of development, the liver, metacestodes tend to spread to adjacent and distant organs by continuous proliferation or by metastasis formation (Buttenschoen *et al.* 2009a). Therefore, 34% of patients have metacestode lesions in the liver and simultaneously in one ore more extrahepatic organs at the time when the cases reach medical attention (Kern *et al.* 2003).

Course of infection and symptomatology

In the course of the infection two main clinical phases may be distinguished, an initial and a progressive phase.

The ***initial phase*** is always asymptomatic. Estimates of the incubation period vary between 5 and 15 years (Sato *et al.* 1993a; Ammann and Eckert 1995, 1996). The infection can persist for years within this phase, and might be detected by chance only. It may be cured spontaneously (see below: abortive lesions), persist as an undefined suspicious hepatic lesion, or may turn to a progressive phase.

Data from 1982–2000 revealed a median age of European patients at diagnosis of 56 years, (range 5 to 86, mean 52.5 years) and a gender ratio of 1:1.2 (male: female) (Kern *et al.* 2003).

The median age of AE patients in Western China was 43.4 years (age range 6–81 years), associated with a gender ratio of 1:1.4, respectively (reviewed by Vuitton *et al.* 2003).

In the ***progressive phase*** symptoms may occur, including abdominal pain, jaundice, sometimes fever and anaemia. The advanced stage is characterized by severe hepatic dysfunction, and is often associated with portal hypertension (Sato *et al.* 1993a). In 71.0% of cases from the European Registry, diagnosis was made after the patients reported symptoms; 11.8% were disclosed by chance in the course related to other diseases, and 3.2% of cases were found during screening programs for AE (no data available in 14%) (no data available in 14%) (Kern *et al.* 2003). Most of the Chinese investigations disclosed patients after mass ultrasound surveys, and 31.4% of patients suffered from a far advanced stage of the disease (Li *et al.* 2010).

The duration of the disease is variable between weeks and years. In an older Swiss study including 64 patients the mean duration was 3.7 years (2 weeks to 18 years) (Drolshammer *et al.* 1973). Lethality rates in untreated or inadequately treated patients are high and may reach 94% to 100% within 10 to 15 years after diagnosis (Ammann and Eckert 1996). Current treatment has substantially improved the prognosis of patients compared to the 1970s (see page 681).

Immunity and natural resistance

The following account is a brief summary of some relevant aspects. For further information the reader is referred to recent reviews (Siles-Lucas and Gottstein 2001; Zhang *et al.* 2008a,b; Mejri *et al.* 2010; Brehm 2010).

The majority of patients with alveolar echinococcosis respond to the infection with the production of antibodies of all isotypes which can be detected in serological tests. Most of the diagnostic tests are based on IgG detection (Siles-Lukas and Gottstein 2001). A direct role of antibodies in controlling metacestode proliferation has not been demonstrated but they may be involved in immunopathological processes (Gottstein and Felleisen 1995; Mejri *et al.* 2010). Accumulating evidence suggests that both the innate and the adaptive arms of the immune response play an important role regarding the outcome of the infection. *E.multilocularis* antigens modulate both regulatory and inflammatory Th1 and Th2 cytokines

and chemokines (Hübner *et al.* 2006; Kocherscheidt *et al.* 2008). It has been found that patients with the 'abortive' form of the infection or patients after radical resection of the lesions had high lymphoproliferative and low antibody responses, while in patients in advanced stages of the disease lymphoproliferative reactions were low and antibody responses high (Ammann *et al.* 2004). This may be an indication that in advanced stages of the disease lymphoproliverative responses are increasingly suppressed (Gottstein and Felleisen 1995). Immunosuppression is accompanied by spontaneous secretion of IL-10 by peripheral blood mononuclear cells which was suggested to be the immunological hallmark of patients with progressive forms as compared to abortive forms of AE (Godot *et al.* 1997; Kilwinski *et al.* 1999; Godot *et al.* 2000). In fact, the *E.multilocularis* metacestode seems to influence the pattern of immune responses that are beneficial not only to the parasite, but also to its intermediate host (Brehm 2010). These mechanisms facilitate the intrahepatic proliferation and maturation of the metacestode, and at the same time may limit the immunopathology in the human host. As indicated by the slow development of the metacestode, the immunological response, the very limited capacity of protoscolex formation and other features, humans have a relatively low susceptibility to *E. multilocularis*, and therefore a high natural resistance. Markers of the degree of resistance are possibly lymphoid cell-surface proteins encoded in the HLA region (Eiermann *et al.* 1998).

Pathology

Lesions of the liver

The lesions caused by the metacestode in the human liver vary from minor foci of a few millimetres in size up to extensive areas of infiltration occupying large parts of the liver. The World Health Organization – Informal Working Group on Echinococcosis (WHO-IWGE) PNM classification system denotes the extension of the parasitic mass in the liver (P), the involvement of neighbouring organs (N) and metastases (M) (Kern *et al.* 2006). Lesions often develop along large vessels and spread from there into the liver, in the draining lymph nodes or in neighbouring tissue structures (Buttenschoen *et al.* 2009a). In large screening programs of western China the diameter, the number and the character of the lesions were recorded as categories AE1 to AE3, depending on size, as well as using a prefix *s* for single lesion, *m* for multiple lesions or *f* for lesions encompassing a central necrotic liquid, respectively (Li *et al.* 2010).

In macroscopic sections of the human liver, the metacestodes of *E. multilocularis* exhibit an alveolar spongy structure composed of numerous irregular vesicles with diameters between < 1 mm and 30 mm (Fig. 54.5). Due to necrosis, cavities filled with liquid and necrotic material may be formed in central parts of the lesion reaching diameters of 15 to 20 cm or more (Ammann and Eckert 1996; Bresson-Hadni *et al.* 2000). Imaging reports may describe a cystic lesion which could then be misinterpreted as a manifestation of cystic echinococcosis. Thus, pseudocyst(s) can be a morphological feature of AE.

Microscopically single vesicles of *E. multilocularis* in the human host have a rather thin laminated layer in contrast to a mostly thick layer of E. *granulosus*. The germinal layer of vesicles in the human liver is a single, syncytial cell-layer with only a few nuclei, so called germinal cells or neoblasts (Brehm 2010). Brood capsules and protoscoleces are formed in much less than 10% of the cases

(Ammann and Eckert 1996) (Fig. 54.4). The metacestode proliferates actively into the liver parenchyma comparable to a sponge, the lesions are surrounded by an inner necrotic zone and outer layers of histiocytes and lymphocytes. In later phases, tissue reactions of chronic inflammation, often with giant-cell foreign body reaction, fibrous tissue, calcifications or necrotic areas are seen around cysts (Fujioka *et al.* 1993). In the human liver fibrous proliferation is often so intense that cysts are embedded in a very dense and hard fibrous stroma (Ammann and Eckert 1996). Most notably, the metacestode as a whole is not demarcated at its outer limits by a fibrous capsule like cysts of *E. granulosus*, except in cases of abortive lesions.

Lesions of other organs and metastases formation

The metacestode of *E. multilocularis* is characterized by a tumour-like proliferation and the potential of metastasis formation (Buttenschoen *et al.* 2009a). In the human host metastases may be formed in organs adjacent to the liver (gall bladder, pancreas, diaphragm etc.) or in distant localizations (lungs, bones, muscles, skin, brain, spine etc.) (Posselt 1928). In the European Registry of 554 patients 66 (12%) had distant metastases, wheras in Japan 11% of 156 patients (Kern *et al.* 2003; Sato *et al.* 1997a). The morphological structure of the *E. multilocularis* metacestode in other organs is essentially similar to those in the liver but may differ in certain localizations. In bones it might be especially difficult to differentiate *E. granulosus* and *E. multilocularis* infections as the former may exhibit an unusual small-vesicular structure if the parasite is restricted to the network of the spongiosa of the bones.

Abortive lesions

Although during the course of infection active metacestodes of *E. multilocularis* can partially degenerate centrally and calcify, it was previously believed that they would retain an unlimited proliferative capacity. However, several years ago spontaneous death of the *E. multilocularis* metacestode in the human liver was documented in 5 asymptomatic patients in Alaska (Rausch *et al.* 1987) with calcified dead parasite lesions (diameters 0.5–9.0 cm), having a mineralized wall and a cavity filled with amorphous necrotic material, containing in some cases also folded parasite membranes. Such cases have later on also been observed in France (Bresson-Hadni *et al.* 1994) and in Switzerland (Gottstein *et al.* 2001).

Clinical diagnosis

The clinical diagnosis of AE is based on:

(a) clinical findings and epidemiological data,

(b) lesion morphology identified by imaging techniques,

(c) serology,

(d) histopathology and/or DNA detection.

Details have recently been summarized by the WHO-IWGE as a result of a consensus meeting (Brunetti *et al.* 2010). Various techniques are used in the diagnostic procedure.

Imaging

Lesions of the liver are best visualized by ultrasonography (US), computer tomography (CT) and magnetic resonance imaging (MRI). Pulmonary and cerebral lesions can be detected by CT-scan. The morphological criteria, however, are not clear-cut, and experienced examiners should be consulted.

Ultrasound examination (US)

Typical findings by US (70% of cases) include (a) juxtaposition of hyper- and hypoechogenic areas in a pseudo-tumour with irregular limit and scattered calcification; (b) pseudo-cystic appearances due to a large area of central necrosis surrounded by an irregular hyperechogenic ring. Less typical features (30% of cases) include: haemangioma-like hyperechogenic nodules as the initial lesion; small calcified lesions due either to a dead or a small-sized developing parasite (Bresson-Hadni *et al.* 2000). US with colour Doppler provides information on biliary and vascular involvement (Kratzer *et al.* 2005; Ehrhardt *et al.* 2007).

Imaging techniques other than US

CT gives an anatomical and morphological characterization of lesions and best depicts the characteristic pattern of calcification (Reuter *et al.* 2001). In cases of diagnostic uncertainty, MRI uncovers the multivesicular morphology of the lesions, thereby supporting the diagnosis. It is the best technique to demonstrate the extension of AE lesions to adjacent tissue structures. Cholangio-MRI depicts the relationship between the AE lesion(s) and the biliary tree (Bresson-Hadni *et al.* 2006).

[18F]-Fluoro-Deoxyglucose-Positron-Emission-Tomography (FDG-PET)

FDG-PET scanning indirectly demarcates areas of parasitic activity. If combined with CT (PET/CT) or MRI (PET/MRI), it may show active lesions at a time when clinical symptoms are absent and recurring disease is not yet detectable by conventional imaging (Reuter *et al.* 2004; Stumpe *et al.* 2007). However, lack of detectable metabolic activity does not confirm parasite death, but indicates suppression of periparasitic inflammatory activity (Reuter *et al.* 2008; Crouzet *et al.* 2009).

Direct assessment of E. multilocularis and its viability

Diagnostic puncture of liver lesions should be avoided in any case as it may possibly lead to dissemination of parasite material and local metastases formation (Ammann and Eckert 1996). However, it may be necessary in seronegative cases with unclear imaging results. Histopathological examination shows the parasitic vesicles delineated by a Periodic-Acid-Schiff (PAS+) laminated layer. The periparasitic granuloma is composed of epithelioid cells lining the parasitic vesicles, macrophages, fibroblasts and myofibroblasts, giant multinucleated cells, and various cells of the nonspecific immune response, usually surrounded by lymphocytes. Also present are collagen and other extracellular matrix protein deposits. Polymerase chain reaction (PCR) can detect *Echinococcus*-specific nucleic acids in tissue specimens resected or biopsied from patients, and RT-PCR may assess viability (Ito and Craig 2003). However, a negative result on a thin needle aspiration sample does not rule out disease and a negative finding using RT-PCR does not indicate complete inactivity of a lesion (Kern *et al.* 1995).

The WHO-IWGE PNM-classification system

The WHO-IWGE PNM-classification system based on the above mentioned imaging findings, has been established as the international benchmark for standardized evaluation of diagnostic and therapeutic measures (Kern *et al.* 2006). It denotes the extension of the parasitic mass in the liver (P), the involvement of neighbouring organs (N), and metastases (M).

Laboratory diagnosis

Immunodiagnostic tests

Immunodiagnostic tests for primary diagnosis or confirmation of imaging results are more reliable in the diagnosis of AE than of CE (Carmena et al. 2007). The use of purified and/or recombinant, or in vitro-produced E. multilocularis antigens (Em2, Em2plus, Em18) have high diagnostic sensitivities (90–100%), with a specificity range between of 95 and 100% (Siles-Lukas and Gottstein 2001). Most of the purified antigens allow discrimination between AE and CE in 80 to 95% of cases. Immunoblotting tests are used for confirmation or as a first-line investigation if available (Ito and Craig 2003). Long term serologic analyses with affinity-purified and recombinant antigens have shown a promising correlation with disease activity in cohorts of patients (Ammann et al. 2004, Fujimoto et al. 2005), but the interpretation of the results in individual cases can be difficult. Recent data indicate that the Em18 assay shows the best performance for follow-up examinations (Tappe et al. 2009; 2010b).

Other laboratory tests

Routine laboratory tests do not yield specific etiological findings (Ammann and Eckert 1995) but they have to be performed for diagnosing the general clinical condition of the patient and to identify certain pathological changes, such as cholestasis or bilirubinaemia.

Definition of AE cases

According to Brunetti et al. (2010) patients can be diagnosed and classified as follows:

- Possible cases: patients with epidemiological history, and (a) species specific serology positive for AE, but without imaging findings, or (b) with imaging findings compatible with AE and negative serology.
- Probable cases: patients with epidemiological history, with imaging findings and serology positive for AE.
- Confirmed cases: imaging pattern for AE, histopathology compatible with AE and/or detection of E.multilocularis DNA in a tissue specimen.

Screening of populations

Systematic screening of different populations has been performed in Japan, western Europe, and recently in western China including the Tibetan plateau (Li et al. 2010). Earlier surveys have used ELISA's either alone or in combination with immunoblot analysis for serological screening (Gottstein et al. 1987; Craig et al. 1992; Sato et al. 1993b; Bresson-Hadni et al. 1994). Positive cases underwent subsequent ultrasound examination. In contrast, in most of the recent studies, ultrasound mass screening was first performed, and cases were then further characterized by several serological tests (Romig et al. 1999; Haenle et al. 2006; Hänle 2009; Yang et al. 2008; Li et al. 2010). However, accurate diagnosis of echinococcosis in population studies is challenging. In humans, a screening test of high sensitivity should ensure that most cases are detected, but confirmation with a highly specific test is then indicated. Surveillance on human populations with serology as the single diagnostic test must be undertaken with extreme caution, if at all (Torgerson and Deplazes 2009). Population-based studies should fully respect ethical requirements and be beneficial for individual participants (WHO/OIE 2001).

Treatment

General aspects

Treatment should be planned in a multidisciplinary discussion, taking all elements of pre-treatment imaging into account. In addition to antiparasitic therapy, early diagnosis, improved surgery, and medical care of the patients have contributed to the success of treatment and to the increase in patients' survival time during the past 3 decades (Torgerson et al. 2008). The success is based on defined rules in recognized national treatment centers, or by guidance of treatment through such centers. Guidelines for treatment of human AE, published previously (WHO 1996; WHO/OIE 2001), have recently been updated by the WHO-IWGE (Brunetti et al. 2010) and are summarized here.

The following rules should be followed:

(a) Treatment with benzimidazoles (preferably albendazole) is mandatory in all patients, temporarily after complete resection of the lesions, and for life in all other cases,

(b) interventional procedures should be preferred to palliative surgery whenever possible,

(c) radical surgery is the first choice in all cases suitable for total resection of the lesion.

Based on the WHO-PNM classification of AE cases (Kern et al. 2006) and international group of experts has recently suggested various approaches of therapeutic procedures depending on the stage of the disease and on the available resources (Brunetti et al. 2010).

Long-term therapy with benzimidazoles (BMZs) was introduced in 1976 based on animal studies (Eckert 1986), and can actually be seen as the backbone of the comprehensive treatment of human AE (Ammann et al. 1994; Reuter et al. 2000; Bresson-Hadni et al. 2000). Mebendazole, a benzimidazole derivative with high efficacy against metacestodes in rodents (see below), was the first drug successfully used for treatment of human AE (reviewed by Ammann and Eckert 1995; WHO/OIE 2001; Torgerson et al. 2008). Albendazole has an efficacy similar to mebendazole combined with some pharmacokinetic advantages. At present albendazole (ABZ) is recommended as the drug of choice (Horton 2003; Brunetti et al. 2010).

Although effective treatment schedules are in current use (see below), the optimal duration of treatment with BMZs and the criteria of cure have yet to be determined. The duration of treatment will depend on a number of factors, including early or late phase presentation, size of the lesions and status of immunity. Criteria of cure for a patient with initially inoperable lesion are still unsettled, but should include a negative PET/CT scan, calcified component of the AE lesion of more than 50% as well a significant decline or disappearance of specific antibodies (Crouzet et al. 2009; Tappe et al. 2009a).

Indications and contraindications for benzimidazole (BMZ) therapy

The current consensus strategy is the use of albendazole (ABZ) for treating (a) inoperable cases, (b) cases after incomplete surgical resection of parasitic lesions, (c) cases after presumed radical surgery (R-0 resection) and after liver transplantation (LT). Since residual parasite tissue may remain undetected at radical surgery, including liver transplantation (LT), ABZ should be given for at least 2 years. These patients should be monitored for a minimum of 10 years for possible recurrence (WHO 1996; Reuter et al. 2000).

Pre-surgical ABZ administration is not recommended except in the case of LT.

In view of the bad prognosis of untreated AE and the rather moderate toxicity of ABZ, there are only a few contraindications or limitations of treatment (WHO 1996). Examinations for adverse reactions are necessary initially every 2 weeks (first 3 months), then monthly (first year), then every 3 to 6 months. If a significant increase of aminotransferases (5 times the upper limit of normal = ULN) is observed, the following steps are recommended: check for other causes of the increase (other medication, viral hepatitis, AE-related biliary obstruction or liver abscess); monitor drug levels; if ABZ-sulphoxide plasma levels are higher than the recommended range of concentrations (0.5 to 1.70 mg/L, 4 hours after morning drug intake), decrease ABZ dosage; shift to the alternative BMZ (MBZ if ABZ and vice-versa); if an increase over 5 x ULN persists, consult a reference center. Leukocyte counts should be checked at 2 week intervals during the first 3 months. Decrease of leukocyte count under $1.0 \times 10^9/L$ indicates ABZ toxicity. In view of the teratogenic potential of BMZ's expert advice is needed for chemotherapy of women in child bearing age or in pregnancy.

Albendazole (Zentel®, Eskazole®) is given continuously at daily doses of 10–12 mg/kg b.w. in two divided doses together with a fat-enriched meal (WHO 1996; Brunetti et al. 2010). The long-term treatment has been established in many centers in Europe as well as in China (Reuter et al. 2004; Liu et al. 2009). Follow-up observations support the safety and tolerance of the drug for the majority of the patients. Toxic hepatitis, blood dyscrasia, and alopecia may occur in a sub-group of patients, necessitating regular medical supervision (Brunetti et al. 2010).

Mebendazole (Vermox forte®) is used as a second line drug, in particular in cases with drug intolerance to ABZ. The drug is given continuously at daily doses of 30–50 mg/kg b.w. in three divided doses together with a fat-enriched meal. Side effects and precautions are similar as to those of ABZ (WHO 1996).

Drug efficacy

The substances with anti-parasitic properties are MBZ and the main metabolite of ABZ, albendazole sulphoxid. Animal experiments have shown that long-term treatment with mebendazole, albendazole, fenbendazole and some other benzimidazole carbamates has the following effects against the metacestode of *E. multilocularis* (Eckert 1986; Ammann and Eckert 1995):

◆ Inhibition of metacestode proliferation resulting in reduction of parasite masses,

◆ Destruction of protoscoleces and partial destruction of the germinal layer and of the cystic structure of the metacestode,

◆ Prevention or suppression of metastasis formation; prolongation of animal host survival.

The parasites are normally not killed but only inhibited in proliferation during treatment. The effect of the drugs in animals is therefore not parasiticidal but parasitostatic.

Several studies with a total of > 150 patients with AE have shown that long-term treatment with MBZ or ABZ was beneficial in a high proportion of patients (Ammann and Eckert 1996; Bresson-Hadni et al. 2000; Reuter et al. 2000; Kadry et al. 2005) as indicated by clinical improvement, increased body weight, regression of cholestasis and decrease of the size of the liver lesion. Long-term

observations have revealed that treatment with BMZ alone or in combination with surgery has resulted in significant improved life-expectancy of AE patients. In a Swiss study based on 155 patient records, spanning the period 1967–2005, it was shown that life-expectancy of a 54 year old AE patient diagnosed in 1970 was estimated to be reduced by 18.2 and 21.3 years for men and women, respectively. By 2005 the loss of life time was reduced to 3.5 and 2.6 years, respectively (Torgerson et al. 2008).

Other drugs

Unfortunately, at present there are no alternative drugs available for the treatment of AE. However, drug discoveries have been reported or are envisaged using the metacestode vesicle as laboratory tool for sceening of drugs (Hemphill et al. 2010). Praziquantel, an isochinoline derivative, has no place in the treatment of human AE, based on experimental data (Eckert 1986; Marchiondo et al. 1994). Conventional and liposomal amphotericin B preparations have been used as a salvage treatment in a few patients who did not tolerate BMZ (Reuter et al. 2003). Some stabilization could be achieved. Nitazoxanide, a broad spectrum anti-infective drug, showed remarkable *in vitro* efficacy against metacestode vesicles (Stettler et al. 2004), but could not convince yet in case studies (Kern et al. 2008; Tappe et al. 2009b). Regrettably, *in vitro* screening of drugs has not yet resulted in the development of new compounds for clinical application (Hemphill et al. 2010).

Surgical treatment
Radical resection

Radical resection should always be the goal. The entire parasitic lesion is excised following the rules of tumour surgery including a 2 cm safety margin, and has to be classified according to the quality of resection by histopathology: R-0: no residue; R-1: microscopic residue; R-2: macroscopic residue. Non-radical liver surgery, previously regarded as beneficial for reducing the parasitic mass, does not appear to offer advantages over conservative treatment (Kadry et al. 2005; Buttenschoen et al. 2009b). Lesions not confined to the liver are not a contraindication to surgery per se, but curative procedures have to meet the criteria for R-0-resections as well. Lesions in other organs (e.g. brain) should be managed either by surgery or by alternative measures. Irrespective of the type of procedure, concomitant BMZ treatment is mandatory for at least two years. No staging system can judge 'resectability', but the WHO-IWGE PNM classification gives a rough estimation and enables comparison of results from different groups (Kern et al. 2006).

Whenever possible, complete resection of AE lesions should be performed. The potential for resection and whether there is disease dissemination must be assessed carefully by pre-operative imaging techniques. In principle, radical surgery should be avoided when R-0-resection is not achievable.

Palliative surgery

Palliative surgery ('debulking') should be avoided as it has little benefit, except in rare selected cases (Kadry et al. 2005). However, the diversity of AE manifestations sometimes results in individual solutions. R-1- or even R-2-resections might be necessary to effectively deal with a septic focus, if R-0-resection is impossible and/or if percutaneous drainage (see below) is not effective (Buttenschoen et al. 2009c). Palliative resection combined with BMZ has proven to be effective in treating skin lesions (Bresson-Hadni et al. 1996).

Table 54.4 Geographic distribution of *Echinococcus multilocularis* and human cases of alveolar echinococcosis (AE)[1]

Region	Occurrence *E. multilocularis* in animals (definitive and/or intermediate hosts)	Reports of human AE cases
North America	Alaska, Canada (CDN), northern and central US states (USA)	Alaska, USA
Western Europe	Belgium (B), Netherlands (NL), France (F)	B, NL, F
Central Europe	Germany (D), Duchy of Luxembourg (L) Switzerland (CH), Principality of Liechtenstein (FL), Austria (A), Italy (I), Czech Republic (CZ), Slovak Republic (SK), Slovenia (SLO), Poland (PL), Hungary (H), Estonia, (EST) Latvia (LV), Lithuania (LT)	D, CH, FL, A, CZ, PL, SLO[2], PL, LT
Northern Europe	Norway (Svalbard Archipelago) (N), Denmark (DK), Sweden (S)*	
South-eastern Europe and Turkey	Bulgaria (BU), Romania (RO), Turkey (TR)	RO, TR
Eastern Europe and Russian Federation	Belarus (BY), Ukraine (UA), Moldova (MD), Russian Federation (RUS)[3]	BY, UA, RUS
Caucasian Region and Middle East	Armenia (AR), Georgia (GE), Azerbaijan (AZ), Iraq (IRQ), Iran (IR)	AZ, IRQ[4], IR
Asia	Afghanistan (AFG) Kazakhstan (KZ), Turkmenistan (TM), Uzbekistan (UZB), Tajikistan (TJ), Kyrgyzstan (KS), Mongolia (MNG), PR China (VRC), Japan (J)	AFG[5], KS, KZ, MNG, VRC, J

[1] References see Torgerson *et al.* (2010) and text. [2] Cases identified by serology. [3] Endemic areas in both European and Asian parts. [4] Single case. [5] Case diagnosed in an Afghan immigrant in UK
* Two infected foxes detected 2010/11 in south-west Sweden (Osterman Lind *et al.*: Eurosurveillance 16 (14), April 2011).

Liver transplantation (LT)

LT has been performed in France and a few other countries in approximately 60 patients with inoperable lesions and/or chronic liver failure (Koch *et al.* 2003). Indications for LT are severe liver insufficiency (secondary biliary cirrhosis or Budd-Chiari syndrome) or life-threatening cholangitis for patients who, in addition, cannot undergo a radical liver resection, and have no extrahepatic manifestation. Cases with residual AE in lung or abdominal cavity should be regarded as exceptional indications, balancing all the pros and cons (Scheuring *et al.* 2003). In highly selected cases, LT save AE patients' lives: in 45 AE-patients 5 year survival was 71% and 5 year disease-free survival was 58% (Bresson-Hadni *et al.* 2003). Post-operative immunosuppression favours regrowth of larval remnants and formation or increase in size of metastases (reviewed by Vuitton *et al.* 2006). Thus, LT is contraindicated in the presence of extra-hepatic locations, and if immunosuppressive drugs and/or BMZ are contraindicated. Invisible or unrecognized parasitic remnants may re-grow and disseminate to other organs, even after years have passed.

Other interventions

Interventional procedures have to be considered for a number of complications of progressive AE (Bresson-Hadni *et al.* 2006): if surgery is felt to pose a high risk and total resection of the lesions cannot be safely performed. Further indications include liver abscess due to bacterial infection of large necrotic lesions, jaundice due to bile duct obstruction with or without acute cholangitis, hepatic or portal vein thrombosis or bleeding of oesophageal varices secondary to portal hypertension. The procedures may lead to a spread of parasitic material and should be avoided if post-interventional BMZ is not possible.

Percutaneous bile (Schantz *et al.* 1995; Eckert and Deplazes 2004) or abscess drainage has now advantageously replaced palliative surgery with jejuno-biliary anastomosis to treat life threatening cholangitis or liver abscess (Bresson-Hadni *et al.* 2000; Bresson-Hadni *et al.* 2006). However, bile drainage necessitates a permanent external drain, and regular changes to prevent

obstruction. Radical resection which was not possible initially may become feasible following the shrinkage of a necrotic cavity after percutaneous drainage. Endoscopic dilation of bile duct strictures followed by insertion of multiple plastic stents is an alternative to percutaneous intervention since it immediately allows internal bile drainage (Vogel *et al.* 1996; Bresson-Hadni *et al.* 2006). Additional treatment with ursodeoxycholic acid is given in some centres; its usefulness in preventing stent obstruction must be awaited for in prospective studies.

Epidemiology

Geographic distribution, parasite-host assemblages and AE in humans

E. multilocularis occurs in the northern hemisphere within a large belt stretching from the Arctic (80^0 N) southward to some regions around the 30th degree of northern latitude. The currently known endemic zone includes regions in Europe, Asia (extending eastward to Japan) and North America (Fig. 54.10). In previous years, a few human AE cases were recorded from northern India (1 case) and northern Tunisia (2 cases), but these countries are not regarded as endemic as supporting data are lacking (WHO/OIE 2001). By the end of 2010, autochthonous *E. multilocularis* infections in natural definitive and/or intermediate hosts were known to occur in at least 43 countries. Epidemiological aspects of *E. multilocularis* and AE, including detailed data on geographical distribution and prevalences, have been reported by WHO/OIE (2001). Further information can be obtained from several global reviews (Craig and Pawlowski 2002; Vuitton *et al.* 2003; Eckert and Deplazes 2004; Jenkins *et al.* 2005; Torgerson *et al.* 2010). Table 54.4 provides an overview of countries with endemic *E. multilocularis* in animals and on records of human AE cases. Examples of prevalences of *E. multilocularis* in definitive and intermediate hosts and selected incidence rates of AE in humans are presented in Table 54.2 and Table 54.5, respectively. The global burden of AE has been estimated by Torgerson *et al.* (2010).

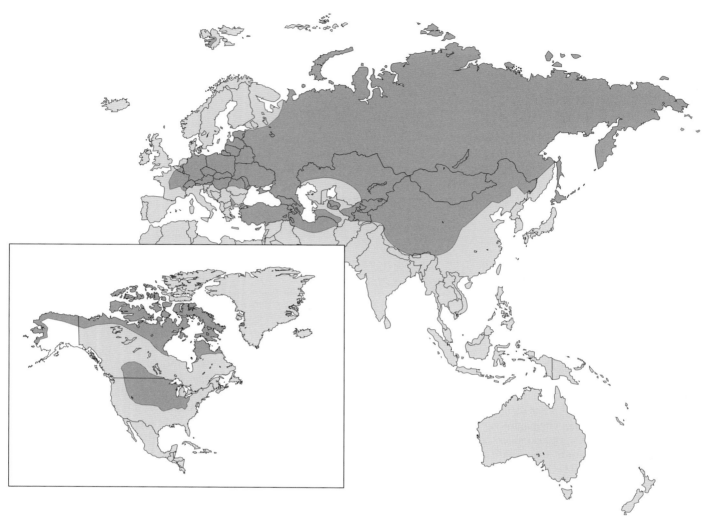

Fig. 54.10 Approximate geographic distribution of *Echinococcus multilocularis* (dark shaded areas). Modified after WHO/OIE 2001. © Institute of Parasitology, Zurich.

North America

In North America the geographical range of *E. multilocularis* extends from some islands in the Bering Sea along the Alaskan coast from the mouth of the Kuskokwim River north, east and southward to Canada (Fig. 54.10) (Schantz *et al.* 1995, 1996; WHO/OIE 2001). Prior to the 1960s *E. multilocularis* apparently spread from the northern tundra zone to southern Manitoba (Canada) and North Dakota (USA). By the mid 1990s the parasite was known to occur in the Canadian provinces of Manitoba, Saskatchewan and Alberta and in the following states of the USA (west to east): Montana, Wyoming, North Dakota, South Dakota, Nebraska, Minnesota, Iowa, Wisconsin, Illinois, Indiana, Ohio and Missouri (Rausch 1995; Schantz *et al.* 1995, 1996; WHO/OIE 2001).

In the northern tundra zone *E. multilocularis* is mainly transmitted between foxes, predominantly artic foxes (*Alopex lagopus*), and rodents. The northern vole (*Microtus oeconomus*) is the main intermediate host in western Alaska and on St Lawrence Island and the brown lemming (*Lemnus sibiricus*) in northern mainland Alaska and on some islands. In certain villages inhabited by indigenous people of the Artic, domestic dogs with access to rodents were frequently infected with *E. multilocularis* (12% on St Lawrence Island) thus representing an important infection source for humans (Schantz *et al.* 1995; WHO/OIE 2001). In central north America the red fox, the coyote (*Canis latrans*) and rarely the gray fox (*Urocyon cineroargenteus*) have been identified as definitive hosts and several species of rodents as intermediate hosts (Table 54.2).

Throughout 1947–1990, St Lawrence Island in the northern tundra zone had a high incidence of human AE in some villages with 53 cases, theoretically corresponding to annual incidence rates of 7–98 per 100,000 inhabitants. Only two human AE cases were diagnosed in central North America between 1937 and 1995 (Schantz *et al.* 1995) (see Table 54.4). Updated information is not available.

Western and central Europe

Until the 1980s it was anticipated that the geographical range of *E. multilocularis* was restricted to the 'classical distribution area' of human AE (Posselt 1928), including southern Germany, Switzerland, parts of Austria, eastern France, and a few adjoining areas.

Since the late 1980s numerous epidemiological studies have revealed that the range of *E. multilocularis* extends further north, east and south than previously known (reviewed by Eckert and Deplazes 1999; Eckert *et al*. 2000; Malczewski 2002; Vuitton *et al*. 2003; Eckert and Deplazes 2004; Jenkins *et al*. 2005; Romig *et al*. 2006a). By the end of 2010, the presence of the parasite in definitive and/or intermediate hosts was documented in 17 countries of western and central Europe (Table 54.4). The currently known endemic area in this part of Europe ranges from central France in the west to the Baltic States in the east and from northern Germany and Poland to southern regions, including Switzerland, Liechtenstein, northern Italy, Austria, Hungary (Sréter *et al*. 2004; Casulli *et al*. 2010) and possibly Slovenia. From the latter country rodents infected with *E. multilocularis* (Kolarova 1999) and suspected human AE cases have been reported (Logar *et al*. 2007).

Since the 1990s *E. multilocularis* has been found in final hosts of several areas and countries previously regarded as non-endemic (data see WHO/OIE 2001). Whether these findings are results of recent spatial parasite expansion or intensive investigations using adequate methods, is not known because of the lack of historical data (Jenkins *et al*. 2005). Based on the results of a recent study on microsatellite markers in populations of *E. multilocularis* from various European regions the authors speculated that the parasite has expanded 'at least many decades ago' from the core area–located in Switzerland and southern Germany–by migrating foxes that exported some genetic clusters to new areas (Knapp *et al*. 2009a).

In western and central Europe, *E. multilocularis* is typically perpetuated in a wildlife cycle, involving red foxes (*Vulpes vulpes*) as definitive hosts and rodents (*Microtus arvalis*, *Arvicola terrestris*, *Myodes* [= *Clethrionomys*] *glareolus* and other species) as intermediate hosts. Prevalences of *E. multilocularis* in red foxes range from about 1% to more than 60% in various regions (reviewed in WHO/OIE 2001; Romig 2002). Since worm numbers per fox are highly aggregated, a few foxes harbouring a large proportion of the total biomass can effectively contaminate the environment with parasite eggs (Deplazes *et al*. 2004). In some areas other carnivores have been identified as additional definitive hosts, such as the wolf (*Canis lupus*) in Latvia (Bagrade *et al*. 2009) and the raccoon dog (*Nyctereutes procyonoides*) in northern Germany (Thiess *et al*. 2001) and Poland (Machnicka *et al*. 2003).

In Switzerland 0.30% and 0.38%, respectively, of randomly selected dogs (n: 660) and cats (n: 263) were found to be infected with *E. multilocularis* (Deplazes *et al*. 1999), but in another more focal study 7% of 86 dogs were parasite carriers (Gottstein *et al*. 2001). Large population studies in Germany revealed that 0.24% of dogs (n: 17,894) and 0.25% of cats (n: 9,064) excreted *E. multilocularis* eggs as confirmed by egg-DNA identification (Dyachenko *et al*. 2008). Assessments of the potential epidemiological roles of various definitive hosts have to consider the much higher egg production of *E. multilocularis* in foxes, dogs and raccoon dogs as compared to cats.

A relatively new development, observed in central Europe since the middle of the 1980s, is the establishment of fox populations in urban habitats with densities similar or even higher than in rural areas. Spatial segregation between rural and urban fox populations has been demonstrated by food analyses of their stomachs and toxicological investigations (reviewed by Deplazes *et al*. 2004). Moreover, microsatellite analyses revealed a reduced gene flow between urban and rural populations (Wandeler *et al*. 2003). In small communities a different pattern has been observed, where foxes foraged during night in the peripheries of the settlements and slept during day in the rural surroundings (reviewed by Deplazes *et al*. 2004).

The existence of an urban cycle of *E. multilocularis* involving foxes and voles (*Arvicola terrestris* and other species) has been demonstrated in several cities (Deplazes *et al*. 2004). In Zurich and Geneva (Switzerland) prevalences of *E. multilocualris* in foxes significantly decreased from the periurban ares to the urban zones, along a gradient of increasing urbanization within a distance of few km (63 and 52% versus 16 and 30%, respectively (Hegglin *et al*. 2007; Reperant *et al*. 2007). In parallel, the predation of voles by foxes decreased towards the city centre of Zurich (Hegglin *et al*. 2007). In the borderland between a rural and urban habitat, high fox population densities intersect with suitable habitats for voles (Giraudoux *et al*. 2002). In these transition zones high fox densities combined with high *E. multilocularis* prevalences lead to an extraordinary environmental contamination with infective *E. multilocularis* eggs (Deplazes *et al*. 2004). For instance, in the outskirts of Zurich 10–60% of 647 fox droppings were positive for *E. multilocularis* as revealed by molecular methods (Stieger *et al*. 2002). Just in these areas up to 23% of *Arviocala terrestris* were infected with metacestodes of *E. multilocularis* (Stieger *et al*. 2002; Reperant *et al*. 2009). These data indicate that urban and peri-urban cycles of *E. multilocularis* have to be regarded as infection risks for humans and for domestic pets preying on rodents (Deplazes *et al*. 2004).

Cases of AE in humans are known from at least 12 countries in western and central Europe (Table 54.4). Core areas of AE with the highest incidence rates include central and eastern France, southern Germany, Switzerland parts of Austria and Lithuania (Kern *et al*. 2003; Eckert and Deplazes 2004; Bružinskaite *et al*. 2007). In these areas prevalences of *E. multilocularis* in foxes are consistently high at approximately 35–65% (Deplazes *et al*. 2004; Bružinskaite *et al*. 2007). Examples of AE incidences are presented in Table 54.5.

Active case finding studies covering the entire country have been performed in Switzerland for more than 50 years. As indicated in Table 54.5, between 1956 and 2000 the annual incidences of human AE varied in Switzerland between 0.10 and 0.18 per 100,000 inhabitants. During the period 2001–2005 a significant increase to 0.26 was observed (Schweiger *et al*. 2007). In 1998, a central surveillance for AE on a voluntary basis was initiated in Europe and denominated as 'European Echinococcis Registry' (EuEchinoReg) (Kern *et al*. 2003). Case numbers reported between 1981 and 2000 from Austria, Germany, France and Switzerland to EuEchinoReg are presented in Table 54.5. Further autochthonous cases from Belgium (3), Poland (14) and Greece (1) were registered (Kern *et al*. 2003). Incidences recorded in EuEchinoReg should be regarded as minimum values. For instance, EuEchinoReg recorded 75 cases from Switzerland for the period 1981–2000, but active case finding has revealed for a shorter period (1984–2000) 131 cases (Table 54.5). Hence, the EuEchinoReg has underestimated the case numbers approximately 1.7-fold. In 2001, reporting of AE became mandatory in Germany. Using a 'multiple source capture-recapture' method, it was estimated that this system is underreporting the AE incidence 3-fold (Jorgensen *et al*. 2008). Although a rare disease, AE has a considerable economic impact with median costs (in Switzerland) per case (if saved pension costs are not deduced) of approximately €182,600 (C.I. 144,800–231,400) (Torgerson *et al*. 2008).

Table 54.5 Selected incidence data on alveolar echinococcosis in humans

Region, country	Period	Number of new cases	Average per year	Annual incidence rate per 100,000 individuals	Reference
Eurasia	1956-1969	122	8.7	0.15	Schweiger et al. (2007)
Switzerland	1970-1983	145	10.4	0.16	
- (entire country)	1984-1992	71[1]	7.8	0.12	
	1993-2000	60	7.5	0.10	
	2001-2005	96	19.2	0.26	
Switzerland - (EurEchinoReg)	1981-2000	75	3.7	—	Kern et al. (2003)
Austria - (entire country)	1985-1999	38	2.5	0.03	Auer and Aspöck (2001)
Austria - (EurEchinoReg)	1981-2000	46	0.9	—	Kern et al. (2003)
Germany - (EurEchinoReg)	1981-2000	102	5.1	—	Kern et al. (2003)
France - (EurEchinoReg)	1981-2000	212	10.6	—	Kern et al. (2003)
Lithuania - (referenece hospital)	1997-2006[1]	80	8.4	—	Bružinskaite et al. (2007)
Turkey - entire country	1980-1998	202	10.6	—	Altintas (2003)
China	see text for prevalence rates				
Japan - Hokkaido	1997-2002 since 1995	9-27	≈ 10-20 15.5	≈ 1.0 - 2.0	Ito et al. 2003 Matsumoto and Yagi (2008)

[1] until July.

Northern Europe

In 1999 *E. multilocularis* was detected in rodents (*Microtus rossiaeme-ridionalis*) in the **Norwegian Svalbard Archipelago** located in the Arctic Ocean (74ºN). The rodents have probably been introduced from Russia with forage for cattle and horses. According to recent studies 8.5% of 353 artic foxes and 51% of the voles were found to be infected with *E. multilocularis* (Hennttonen *et al.* 2001; Stien *et al.* 2010). The parasite has never been recorded from the **Norwegian mainland** or **Finland** (Henttonen *et al.* 2001). After the first discovery of *E. multilocularis* in **Denmark** 1999, the parasite was found in 0.9% of 340 red foxes from an area near Copenhagen (Zealand) (Saeed *et al.* 2006), and recently in 1 of 169 cats (Dyachenko *et al.* 2008). Recently, infected foxes have been detected in Sweden (see Table 54.4).

South-eastern Europe and Turkey

Several species of rodents infected with metacestodes of *E. multilocularis* were recorded from **Bulgaria** (Genov *et al.* 1980; Kolarova 1999). Recent investigations in **Romania** revealed the occurrence of *E. multilocularis* in rodents and foxes in some central counties and in the north-western part of the country, including the border-counties to Hungary and the Ukraine (Kolarova 1999; Siko *et al.* 2010). **Turkey** is a well known endemic area of human AE with cases from all provinces, including the European Marmara province, but most of them originating from eastern and central Anatolia (WHO/OIE 2001). Between 1980 and 1998, a total of 202 new AE cases were recorded (Altintas 2003). Further cases were described in more recent publications, for instance by Ozturk *et al.* (2009).

Eastern Europe and Russian Federation

In these regions *E. multilocularis* is widely distributed, according to older data (reviewed by Bessonov 1998; Kolarova 1999; WHO/OIE 2001; Bessonov 2002). In eastern Europe the endemic zone includes **Belarus**, the **Ukraine** (Kharchenko *et al.* 2008) and **Moldova**. In the northern **Russian Federation**, the endemic zone extends from the area of the north western Barents Sea (Archangelsk) to the Chukotka region, Bering Strait, Kamchatka peninsula and northern Kuriles in the far east, and in the south from the region between the Black Sea and the Caspian Sea through Omsk, Novosibirsk, Irkutsk areas to the Amur region, Chabarovsk and the island of Sachalin. As updated information is lacking, it can only be assumed that the parasite is still endemic in wide areas of the Russian Federation (WHO/OIE 2001). This view is supported by records of human AE from at least 33 regions of Russia during the period 1983–1993; the total number of 2,863 human echinococcosis cases (CE and AE) included approximately 35% AE cases (Bessonov 2002).

Caucasian region and Middle East

Georgia, **Armenia** and **Azerbaijan** are regarded as endemic for *E. multilocularis* (Bessonov 1998), but details are not known. A report from northern **Iraq** on AE in a patient who had never left the region, may be an indication for an *E. multilocularis* focus (Al-Attar *et al.* 1983). In **Iran** *E. multilocularis* is known to occur in red foxes, jackals and in voles (*Microtus socialis*); 28 human cases of AE have been recorded between 1946 and 1993 (Mobedi *et al.* 1971; Rokni 2008).

Asia

According to previous reports, *E. multilocularis* was known to occur in **Kazakhstan, Turkmenistan, Uzbekistan, Tajikistan and Kyrgyzstan** (Bessonov 1998; WHO/OIE 2001). Recent data from **Kazakhstan** indicate a patchy distribution of *E. multilocularis* foci in various parts of the country, mainly depending on different habitat types (desert, steppe, shores of lakes etc.) with stable and high-density rodent populations (Shaikenov 2006). *E. multilocularis* has been found in the red fox (*Vulpes vulpes*), corsac fox (*Vulpes corsac*), spotty cat (*Felis lybica*), domestic dog (*Canis familiaris*) and in 18 rodent species, for instance the great gerbil (*Rhombomys opimus*). Parasite prevalences were high in foxes and dogs (up to ≈ 30%); a few dissected spotty cats harboured individual worm burdens up to 200,000 (Shaikenov and Torgerson 2002; Shaikenov 2006). Human AE has been recorded in most parts of the country with about 20 cases per year (Shaikenov and Torgerson 2002). In **Kyrgyzstan**, 11% of 466 dogs and 64% of 151 red foxes were found to be carriers of *E. multilocularis* (Ziadinov *et al.* 2008; Ziadinov *et al.* 2010). In **Uzbekistan** and **Turkmenistan** *E. multilocularis* occurs in red foxes, corsac foxes, jakals, and rodents (Shaikenov 2006). A case of AE, diagnosed in an Afghan immigrant in the UK (Graham *et al.* 2002) could be an indication for the occurrence of *E. multilocularis* in **Afghanistan**. A first case of human AE was reported from **Mongolia** in 1982 and a second in 2002. Three further cases, confirmed by DNA-tests, were found between 2006 and 2009 (Ito *et al.* 2010).

In the **People's Republic of China**, alveolar echinococcosis occurs mainly in western and central provinces and regions, including Xinjang Uygur AR, Tibet (Xizang), Qinghai, Gansu, Ningxia Hui AR, and Sichuan. Sporadic cases of AE in humans have previously been recorded from the northern provinces Inner Mongolia and Heilongjiang, but little information exists on these areas (reviewed in WHO/OIE 2001; Vuitton *et al.* 2003; Jenkins *et al.* 2005; Craig 2006). The red fox (*Vulpes vulpes*), corasc fox (*Vulpes corsac*), Tibet fox (*Vulpes ferrilata*), wolf (*Canis lupus*) and domestic dog (*Canis familiaris*) have been identified as definitive hosts, and voles (*Microtus brandti*), the pika (*Ochotona curzoniae*), the woolly hare (*Lepus oiostolus*) and some other small mammals as intermediate hosts (reviewed in WHO/OIE 2001; Vuitton *et al.* 2003; Jenkins *et al.* 2005). Endemic foci with human cases of AE are often associated with high prevalences of *E. multilocularis* in domestic dogs having access to voles or other intermediate hosts. For instance, 10% of 58 dogs were infected with *E. multilocularis* in Gansu (Craig *et al.* 1992) and 12% of 371 dogs in Shiqu County, Sichuan Province (Budke *et al.* 2005).

Surveys, using abdominal ultrasound examinations combined with serology (ELISA) for diagnosis, have revealed remarkably high prevalences of AE in human populations of endemic areas. For instance, in nine community surveys (1988–1998) performed in Ningxia, Gansu, Sichuan, Qinghai and Tibet (eight surveys each involving approximately 1,000–4,000 persons, one study with 394 persons), average AE prevalence between 0.29% and 5.9% were found (reviewed by Vuitton *et al.* 2003). A more recent study in the Shiqu County (western Sichuan) has shown that cystic and alveolar echinococcosis occurred in the same population of 3,199 persons; AE was diagnosed in 198 (6.2%) persons and CE in 216 (6.8%). Risk factors associated with both forms were the number of owned dogs, frequency of contact with dogs, and sources of drinking water (Tiaoying *et al.* 2005). Group prevalences around 5% are extremely high, theoretically corresponding to 5,000 cases/100,000 individuals. However, it has to be considered that studies from highly endemic foci may not be representative for larger regions (WHO/OIE 2001). Furthermore, the surveys include inactive and abortive AE cases; 39% of the AE cases belonged to this group in the study of Tiaoying *et al.* (2005). Sero-epidemiological studies in Europe have revealed much lower group prevalences with 2 confirmed AE cases among 17,166 individuals in Switzerland, and 13 cases among 7,884 persons in France, corresponding to group prevalences of 12 and 165 per 100,000 individuals, respectively (reviewed in WHO/OIE 2001). Recent countrywide data on incidence rates of human AE cases in China are apparently not available.

In **Japan,** the endemic area of alveolar echinococcosis is restricted to the northern island Hokkaido (Vuitton *et al.* 2003; Nonaka *et al.* 2009), but cases of human AE have been also reported on other islands, most of them with a history of previous residence in an endemic area (Ito *et al.* 2003). On the main island Honshu a stray dog was found to be positive for *E. multilocularis* by PCR, and the infection was documented in domestic pigs (Kamiya *et al.* 2007), but the significance of these findings is unclear. *E. multilocularis* is predominantly perpetuated in a wildlife cyle, involving red foxes (*Vulpes vulpes*) and gray-sided voles (*Clethrionomys rufocanus bedfordiae*) (Matsumoto and Yagi 2008). Since the 1980s the prevalence of the parasite in foxes has increased to around 40–55% (Kamiya *et al.* 2006; Kamiya *et al.* 2007). Dogs (0.4%) and rarely cats have been identified as parasite carriers which can excrete *E. multilocularis* eggs to the environment (Nonaka *et al.* 2008; Nonaka *et al.* 2009). The epidemiological situation is similar to that in Europe with increasing parasite prevalences in foxes and invasion of cities by foxes. Risk areas are now identified by the diagnosis of *E. mulilocularis* eggs in fox faeces using DNA-techniques (Lagapa *et al.* 2009). According to an official report of the Hokkaido Government approximately 500 cases of human AE were recorded during the period 1936–2005. Since 1995, 9–27 new cases have been reported each year with an annual average of 15.5 cases (Matsumoto and Yagi 2008).

Transmission dynamics

The dynamics of the *E. multilocularis* cycle and the transmission of parasite eggs to humans depend upon many factors, such as species composition and numeric density of definitive and intermediate hosts, interactions between these populations, prevalence and intensity of the infection with *E. multilocularis* in final hosts, egg dispersion, landscape characters, climate and weather conditions, human behaviour etc. Important knowledge on these factors has been published in recent years (Giraudoux *et al.* 2002; Romig 2002; Giraudoux 2003; Ito *et al.* 2003; Deplazes *et al.* 2004; Romig *et al.* 2006a; Hegglin *et al.* 2007), but our understanding of this complex matter is still incomplete. Only a few aspects can be discussed here.

Role of definitive and intermediate hosts

As described above, a great variety exists in the assemblages of definitive and intermediate host species of *E. multilocularis* in different endemic regions and within smaller areas (Rausch 1995). Examples are presented in Table 54.2. Two types of cycles are epidemiologically relevant: the wildlife and the synanthropic cycle. By definition, the wildlife cycle of *E. multilocularis* involves wild animal hosts, for example foxes and rodents. Typically, this cycle is restricted to rural or unpopulated regions, but it also occurs close to or within villages or even in urban areas (Deplazes *et al.* 2004; Ito *et al.* 2003).

In the synanthropic cycle domestic animals, predominantly dogs, are involved as definitive hosts. In recent years, some factors of potential epidemiological relevance have been identified.

In parts of continental Europe, since the mid 1980s a distinct increase of fox numbers, the establishment of urban fox populations and the existence of urban cycles of *E. multilocularis* have been recorded (Hofer *et al.* 2000; Deplazes *et al.* 2004; Hegglin *et al.* 2007). Furthermore, increasing prevalence rates of *E. multilocularis* in fox populations during the period 1991–2005, have been reported from some areas, for instance in the north German province Lower Saxony (Berke *et al.* 2008), whereas this tendency could not be observed in Austria (Duscher *et al.* 2006). The successful control of rabies by vaccination is regarded as the main cause for the increase of fox populations (Gloor *et al.* 2006), but reasons for increasing parasite prevalences are obscure. Our knowledge on the possible impact of changing risk factors on the incidence of human AE is still limited. In Switzerland the mean annual incidence rates of new human AE cases varied between 0.10 and 0.16 per 100,000 individuals during at least 45 years, suggesting a high degree of epidemiological stability (Schweiger *et al.* 2007). However, approximately 10–15 years (corresponding to the incubation time of AE) after a distinct numeric increase of fox populations, a higher incidence rate of 0.25 per 100,000 was recorded (Schweiger *et al.* 2007) (see Table 54.5).

Other risk factors include migration and expanding ranges of definitive hosts (i.e. migration of red foxes to urban areas or raccoon dogs to new regions), transportation of definitive host (i.e. dogs from endemic to non-endemic areas), expanding ranges of intermediate hosts (i.e. muskrats along rivers) (Mathy *et al.* 2009) or introduction of intermediate hosts to new territories.

Impact of landscape characters

Landscape characters and environmental conditions, such as humidity, may influence host populations and disease transmission in various ways. For instance, in China the distribution of grassland coincided with the occurrence of human AE in some areas, but not in others (Romig *et al.* 2006b). In central Europe, transmission of *E. multilocularis* is most intense in areas dominated by grassland or agricultural altered areas (Romig *et al.* 2006b). The persistence of transmission foci depend on landscape characters and climatic conditions, as described in Kazakhstan (Shaikenov and Torgerson 2002). For more details see Giraudoux *et al.* (2002, 2003) and Romig *et al.* (2006b).

Role of eggs

Eggs of *E. multilocularis*, deposited with droppings of foxes or other definitive hosts, can remain an infection reservoir for intermediate and accidental hosts during prolonged periods due to their considerable resistance to environmental conditions (reviewed in WHO/OIE 2001). In southern Germany maximum survival of *E. multilocularis* eggs under natural conditions was 8 months between August and May with air temperature extremes between $-15°C$ and $+27°C$. Eggs suspended in tap water at $+4°C$ survived for almost 16 months (478 days) (Veit *et al.* 1995). The eggs are highly resistant to lower temperatures. For instance, $-18°C$ for 240 days or $-27°C$ for 54 days are not lethal, but they are killed at $-70°C$ within 4 days (Veit *et al.* 1995; WHO/OIE 2001; Hildreth *et al.* 2004). Temperatures of $+60–80°C$ are lethal to eggs of *E. granulosus* within 5 min. Eggs of *E. multilocularis* are sensitive to desiccation (Veit *et al.* 1995; Matsumoto and Yagi 2009). In air of 27% relative humidity (r.h.) at $+25°C$ they lost infectivity within 48 hours, and at 15% r.h. at $+43°C$ within 2 hours (Veit *et al.* 1995).

Eggs of *E. multilocularis* are resistant to a variety of commercially available antiparasitic disinfectants containing phenol derivatives, aldehydes or ethanol (Veit *et al.* 1995). Sodium hypochlorite (NaOCl) kills eggs of *E. granulosus* within 10 min if applied at room temperature in concentrations of at least 3.75% NaOCl (Craig and MacPherson 1988). However, the effect of this disinfectant may vary (Craig and MacPherson 1988; Veit *et al.* 1995). Eggs of *E. multilocularis* were not killed in 10–40% ethanol within 24 hours (Veit *et al.* 1995), and eggs of *Taenia pisiformis* survived in 10% formalin for 3 weeks (ref. see WHO/OIE 2001).

Definitive hosts disperse *E. multilocularis* eggs with their droppings. In Europe, territories of red foxes vary in sizes between approximately 18 ha and 16 km^2 (Labhardt 1990; Deplazes *et al.* 2004). Within these areas, the spatial distribution of fox droppings containing *E. multilocularis* eggs underlies wide variations, including concentration to small foci such as vole ground systems (Stieger *et al.* 2000). From sites of deposition *Echinococcus* eggs can be dispersed by flies or other factors at least for several meters (Gemmell and Lawson 1986). The eggs can be distributed with contaminated plants as documented by an AE outbreak in a monkey colony in a zoo after feeding of grass harvested from meadows accessible to foxes infected with *E. multilocularis* (Deplazes and Eckert 2001). Eggs, adhering to shoes contaminated with fox faeces, may be carried to human dwellings. Migrations or transportation of definitive hosts can also contribute to egg dispersal, even over long distances. For instance, *E. multilocularis* was apparently introduced to Hokkaido/Japan by foxes imported from the Kurile Islands (Ito *et al.* 2003).

Disease transmission to humans

It is generally assumed that humans can become exposed to the eggs of *E. multilocularis* by handling of infected definitive hosts, or by food contaminated with eggs. Some reports suggested that egg transmission may occur by waterborne routes (Schantz *et al.* 1995; Tiaoying *et al.* 2005). Compared to the high prevalences of *E. multilocularis* in definitive hosts the incidence rates of AE in humans are relatively low in most of the endemic areas (Table 54.5). Possible reasons are low risks of exposure and high resistance to the infection.

In most epidemiological situations *E. multilocularis* is restricted to the wildlife cycle and thereby to some degree ecologically separated from humans. However, the degree of separation may vary from region to region from high in isolated and sparsely populated areas to moderate or low where infected foxes or other definitive hosts live in close proximity or even within villages and cities, for example in Europe or in Hokkaido (Japan) (Deplazes *et al.* 2004; Ito *et al.* 2003; Matsumoto and Yagi 2008). Recent studies have shown that recreational areas in the outskirts of cities can be heavily contaminated with *E. multilocularis* eggs by foxes (Deplazes *et al.* 2004; Matsumoto and Yagi 2008). Ecological separation does not exist if infected dogs live in close association with humans. In parts of Alaska and China, high prevalence or incidence rates of AE in humans were associated with high parasite prevalences in dogs (Schantz *et al.* 1995; Vuitton *et al.* 2003). In a recent study in China, the number of owned dogs, frequency of contact with dogs, and sources of drinking water were identified as risk factors for human AE (Tiaoying *et al.* 2005). Exposure to eggs can be influenced by occupational and behavioural factors. Hunters, trappers and persons who work with fur may frequently be exposed to eggs of *E. multilocularis* but there is little evidence that these groups are at increased risk (Schantz *et al.* 1995; Kern *et al.* 2004). Among 210 AE patients from the European Registry 21.9% were farmers and another 39.5% were engaged in farming, hunting or working in forestry in part time; 70.5% of all patients kept dogs and cats (Kern *et al.* 2003). Living in the countryside in close proximity to infected foxes and/or frequent contacts with egg-contaminated food or soil may be reasons for a higher infections risk, but exact information is not available.

Humans have a relatively high degree of resistance to infection with eggs of *E. multilocularis* as indicated by the slow development of the metacestode stage in the liver and other organs, the reduced capacity of protoscolex formation, the degree and type of histopathological reactions, and the occurrence of abortive cases of AE. In contrast, AIDS patients exhibit a reduced resistance to the infection (Mejri *et al.* 2010).

Prevention and control

In view of the fact that human AE is a potentially lethal disease, causing high costs of treatment and other losses, and the persisting infection risks in endemic areas, health authorities should establish coordinated systems of surveillance and risk assessment, in combination with measures to reduce morbidity and mortality of AE in the human population (Eckert and Deplazes 1999). Basic measures for endemic areas should include education, mandatory reporting of human AE cases, and designation and support of competence centres or networks for continued surveillance, and–if necessary– for treatment of human cases. Primary objectives of preventive and control measures include the reduction of infection risks for humans and the early diagnosis of human AE cases.

Measures in animal populations
The only possible targets of control measures are definitive hosts as carriers of intestinal *E. multilocularis* stages, whereas the parasite in intermediate hosts is currently not accessible to interventions.

Wild carnivores
Experience from rabies control programs has shown that a persistent and substantial numeric reduction of foxes by hunting cannot be achieved in most situations. Since the early 1990s large field trials have been conducted in Central Europe for mass treatment of red fox populations with 'baits' containing 50 mg praziquantel distributed to the environment at a density of 15–50 per km². In one recent trial 20 baits/km² were initially distributed at intervals of six to twelve weeks by aircraft in a 3000 km² area of southwestern Germany. The pre-baiting prevalence of *E. multilocularis* of 64% (95% C.I. 59–69), was reduced to a level of 15% (C.I. 10–21) after 18 months (Romig *et al.* 2007).

In an area of 5,000 km² in northern Germany 14 treatment campaigns were conducted (20 baits/km²) with delivery intervals of 6 (1st year) and 12 weeks (2nd and 3rd year). Prevalences of *E. multilocularis* in foxes during three pre-control years in two sub-areas of 12.5–36.6% and 3.4–8.2% were reduced to 2.4–6.2% and 0.6–0.9%, respectively, by the end of the intervention period (Tackmann *et al.* 2001). A mathematical evaluation of these data indicated that continued treatment of definitive hosts would be required to eliminate the parasite (Takumi and van der Giessen 2005). Similar studies resulting in reduced parasite prevalences in foxes during or after the control campaign have been carried out in other areas, for example in Bavaria (Germany) (König *et al.* 2008).

Urban peripheries where high fox numbers and suitable habitats for intermediate host intersect in densely populated areas are supposed to play a crucial role for the human infection risk (Deplazes *et al.* 2004). A small-scale study in the city of Zurich, Switzerland, demonstrated the feasibility for locally targeted interventions in periurban areas by manual bait distribution. Within six bait areas of 1 km² (monthly 50 baits per km² during 19 months) the proportion of coproantigen-positive faecal samples from foxes decreased from 24.6% to 5.5%, and the parasite prevalence in *Arvicola terrestris* from 6.7% to 2.1% (Hegglin *et al.* 2003). In six control areas (each 1 km²) the indicator parameters remained essentially unchanged (Hegglin *et al.* 2003). The infection pressure in the 1 km² areas recovered after the intervention within 2 years to the pre-control level. However, in one additional area of 2 km² with monthly baiting during a 3.5-year period, the infection pressure was still very low 3 years after the last delivery of baits (Hegglin and Deplazes 2008).

These studies have shown that intensive control programs can considerably reduce for certain periods both the prevalence of *E. multilocularis* in definitive or intermediate hosts and the environmental contamination with eggs. However, in view of a high reemergence and re-introduction potential after the end of control measures, it is unlikely that eradication of the parasite in large endemic areas could be achieved, except in island situations like on Hokkaido, Japan. On the other hand, in small and well defined, densely populated areas (i.e. urban or periurban areas) long-lasting control programs may reduce an existing high infection risk for humans and contribute to prevention of human AE (Deplazes *et al.* 2004).

Dogs and cats
In situations where dogs and cats are under close supervision by their owners the risk of acquiring *E. multilocularis* infections can be reduced by preventing the animals to prey on small mammals by training (dogs) or by indoor housing of cats. Another option is regular treatment with praziquantel or epsiprantel in intervals of 4 weeks (minimum pre-patent period: 26–28 days). In endemic areas, dogs at risk (those having access to rodents) should be treated continuously. This measure cannot exclude human exposure to eggs dispersed by foxes, other wild carnivores or untreated domestic carnivores. Treatment of individual dogs (or other susceptible carnivores) is recommended and compulsory in several countries if they are transferred from an endemic to a nonendemic area. According to a recent risk assessment, treatment of dogs against *E. multilocularis* on importation into the UK (Pet Travel Scheme, PETS) has a high probability of preventing the introduction of the parasite into the country (Torgerson and Craig 2009).

If domestic dogs play a significant epidemiological role, for example in China (see page 687), education of the population, the elimination of stray dogs and regular treatment of dogs can be considered. Mass treatment of isolated dog populations was evaluated in a 10 year field trial in St Lawrence Island, Alaska, where *E. multilocularis* occurs in a cycle involving domestic dogs and arctic foxes as definitive hosts and voles as intermediate hosts. Dogs were treated with praziquantel at 5 mg/kg body weight at monthly intervals. Infection rates of voles with *E. multilocularis* metacestodes declined from 29% to less than 5% but the infection rate rebounded rapidly toward pre-treatment levels after discontinuation of mass treatment (Schantz *et al.* 1995).

Measures in human populations
Individual prophylaxis
Individual prophylaxis (modified after WHO/OIE 2001):

♦ In endemic areas, vegetables, other edible plants and fruits from locations accessible to contamination with eggs of *E. multilocularis* should be thoroughly washed or better boiled before consumption. Deep-freezing at −20°C does not kill eggs of *E. multilocularis* (they loose their infectivity after deep-freezing at −70° for 4 days).

♦ After agricultural or gardening work including contact with potentially egg-contaminated soil, and after handling of dogs, hands should be thoroughly washed.

♦ Shoes or boots possibly contaminated with soil or faecal material should be cleaned and not be used in living areas.

♦ Living or dead foxes or other definitive hosts potentially infected with *E. multilocularis* should be handled with great care, always using disposable plastic gloves.

♦ If gardens or playgrounds are contaminated with fox droppings, faeces should be collected in a plastic bag and disposed in the garbage or by incineration. If contamination occurs regularly the elimination of foxes by authorized hunters should be considered.

♦ Special recommendations have been worked out for personnel concerned with examinations on *E. multilocularis* (WHO/OIE 2001).

Persons who had contact with infected definitive hosts or egg-contaminated materials (for example fox faeces) should be submitted to serological examinations for species specific anti-*E. multilocularis* antibodies: as soon as possible after the suspected contact and 6, 12 and 24 months thereafter. Highly sensitive and specific tests have to be employed for this purpose. Individuals with continuous infection risk (for example fox hunters, laboratory personnel etc.) should be serologically examined once a year. In unclear cases additional US examinations should be performed (WHO/OIE 2001). The aims of such examinations are exclusion or early diagnosis of an infection.

Measures for human populations
In Japan, China and some other endemic areas screening of large populations by abdominal ultrasound examination, combined with serology, has been successfully used for early detection of AE cases (Sato *et al.* 1997a, b; Vuitton *et al.* 2003; Tiaoying *et al.* 2005). If diagnosis is followed by adequate treatment and medical care, morbidity and mortality can be reduced considerably.

Neotropical forms of echinococcosis

The neotropical forms of echinococcosis, caused by *Echinococcus oligarthrus* or *Echinococcus vogeli*, are confined to Central and South America. By March 2007 in 12 Latin American countries 171 human cases of neotropical echinococcosis have been recorded (D'Alessando and Rausch 2008). Recently, reports on 7 further cases from Brazil (Siqueira *et al.* 2007; Siqueira *et al.* 2010) and 1 from French Guiana (Knapp *et al.* 2009b) were published. These numbers may represent only the 'tip of the iceberg' (D'Alessando and Rausch 2008). Previously, the forms of echinococcosis in humans, caused either by *E. oligarthrus* or *E. vogeli*, were denominated

as 'polycystic echinococcosis' (D'Alessandro 1997; WHO/OIE 2001). In a recent review D'Alessandro and Rausch (2008) have proposed 'unicystic echinococcosis' and 'polycystic echinococcosis' for the forms caused by *E. oligarthus* and *E. vogeli*, respectively. Although uncertainty remains on the species-specific diagnosis of most of the reported cases these terms are used in this chapter (Table 54.1).

Unicystic echinococcosis (UE)
The causative agent (*Echinococcus oligarthrus*) and life cycle
The adult stage of *E. oligarthrus* is only 2–3 mm long, typically composed of 3 segments, with a sac-like uterus in the gravid segment (Thompson 1995; D'Alessando and Rausch 2008). The natural life cycle involves wild Felidae as definitive hosts and several mammalian species as intermediate hosts (Fig. 54.11). Of 10 felid species indigenous to Central and South America 6 have been identified as definitive hosts of *E. oligarthrus*: pampas cat (*Felis colocolo*), Geoffroy's cat (*F. geoffroyi*), ocelot (*F. pardalis*), jaguarundi (*F. yagouaroundi*), jaguar (*Panthera onca*), and puma (*Puma concolor*). *E. oligarthrus* was also found in a bobcat (*Lynx rufus*) in northern Mexico (Rausch and D'Alessandro 2002). Furthermore, a domestic dog in Colombia had a dual intestinal infection with gravid *E. vogeli*

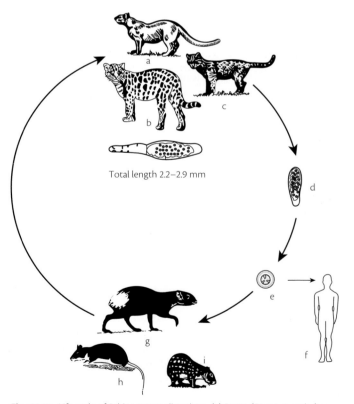

Total length 2.2–2.9 mm

Fig. 54.11 Life cycle of *Echinococcus oligarthrus*. (a) Puma (*Puma concolor*) as type definitive host; (b) jaguar (*Panthera onca*) and (c) ocelot (*Felis pardalis*) as representatives of other definitive hosts; (d) terminal segment of the parasite with eggs (e) egg; (f) man as accidental host; (g) agouti (*Dasyprocta* sp.); (h) spiny rat (*Proechimys* spp.) and (i) paca (*Cuniculus paca*) as intermediate hosts. Modified after Schantz *et al.* 1995. © Institute of Parasitology, Zurich.

and immature *E. oligarthrus* specimens. *E. oligarthrus* developed to maturity in experimentally infected house cats, egg excretion began 86 to 87 days post infection (D'Alessandro and Rausch 2008).

Natural infections with metacacestodes of *E. oligarthrus* were detected in rodents,including several species of agoutis (*Dasyprocta* spp.) and spiny rats (*Proechimys* spp.) and the paca (*Cuniculus paca*), marsupials opossum, (*Didelphis marsupialis*) and lagomorphs (*Sylvilagus floridanus*) (D'Alessandro *et al.* 1981; Rausch and D'Alessandro 2002; D'Alessandro and Rausch 2008).

In natural intermediate hosts metacestodes of *E. oligarthrus* are most commonly located in muscles (of the skin, extremities, psoas region, diaphragm, heart), in the abdominal cavity as well as in liver, lung, and spleen. Typically, the metacestode vesicles are 'unicystic' with a tendency to become multichambered, they have subspherical or irregular forms and diametres up to 3 cm. Growth of vesicles is expansive, external budding has not been recorded (Rausch and D'Alessandro 1999; D'Alessandro and Rausch 2008). The cysts, characterized by a thin laminated layer and a thick germinal layer, contain numerous brood capsules and protoscoleces when fertile. The protoscolex hooks can be distinguished from those of *E. vogeli* metacestodes by differences in size and shape (Rausch *et al.* 1978).

The infection in humans

To date only three confirmed human cases of UE are known from South American countries. However, it cannot be excluded that some further cases, clinically diagnosed as PE, were caused by *E. oligarthrus*. In two of the confirmed UE cases (Venezuela, Suriname) single cysts were located in the orbit of the eye, and in the third case (Brazil) two cysts (1.5 cm diameter) were attached to the myocardium in the heart ventricle (D'Alessandro 1997; D'Alessandro and Rausch 2008). In one of the ocular cases (6 year old boy in Surinam) a large cyst (2.7x 3.2 cm, filled with 10 ml fluid) surrounded by a thick fibrotic capsule was located at the apex of the orbit and had caused exophthalmus, other symptoms and blindness of the affected eye (Basset *et al.* 1998). Aspects of diagnosis and treatment are discussed under PE.

Epidemiology and geographic distribution

Little information exists on the prevalence of *E. oligarthrus* in wild felids. In older studies (predominantly published 1966–1979) *E. oligarthrus* has been found in 5 of 8 pumas (Costa Rica, Panama, Colombia, Brazil) 1 of 3 jaguars (Panama), 4 of 11 jaguarundis (Panama, Colombia) 1 of 11 Ocelots (Colombia), 7 of 46 Geoffroy's cats and in 1 pampas cat (Argentina). Worm burdens, as determined in a few animals, ranged from < 100 up to 100,000 (D'Alessandro *et al.* 1981).

Metacestode prevalences in natural intermediate hosts found in several countries varied between 7.8% (3 of 39) in agoutis (*Dasyprocta punctata*) (Panama), 0.17% (2 of 1,168) in spiny rats (Colombia) and 0.92% (3 of 325) in pacas (Colombia) (Rausch *et al.* 1981). In view of the low number of cases in humans it is assumed that humans may only rarely be exposed to infective eggs in the habitat of wild felids.

The geographic range of *E. oligarthrus* includes a wide area from Costa Rica in the north to La Pampas Province/Argentina in the south (Schantz *et al.* 1995). According to a single report the parasite was found in a bobcat in north-east Mexico, approximately 100 km south of the border of Texas (Salinas-Lopez *et al.* 1996).

Polycystic echinococcosis (PE)

The causative agent (*Echinococcus vogeli*) and life cycle

E. vogeli has typically three segments, but up to 6 proglottids can be present in fully developed specimens. The total length of the parasite varies between 3.9 and 5.5 mm, but may reach up to 12 mm (D'Alessandro and Rausch 2008). The gravid segment is very long in relation to the anterior part of the strobila and contains a long, tubular and sac-like uterus (Fig. 54.12). The prepatent period in the domestic dog is approximately 90 days (D'Alessandro and Rausch 2008).

E. vogeli is perpetuated in a life cycle with the bush dog (*Spoethos venaticus*) as natural definitive host and the paca (*Cuniculus papca*) as principle intermediate host (Fig. 54.12). Agoutis (*Dasyprocta aguti*) may also serve as intermediate hosts (D'Alessandro and Rausch 1981). Adult cestodes have also been found in a naturally infected domestic dog, and dogs could be experimentally infected. Intestinal stages of *E. vogeli* apparently do not develop in cats or in other felids (D'Alessandro and Rausch 2008).

In natural intermediate hosts the metacestode develops mostly in the liver in form of a few to numerous spherical or subspherical vesicles, isolated or contiguous. It appears that each vesicle arises from a single oncosphere and proliferation with production of new cysts does not play a role in natural intermediate hosts (D'Alessandro and Rausch 2008). In contrast, proliferation occurs in primates

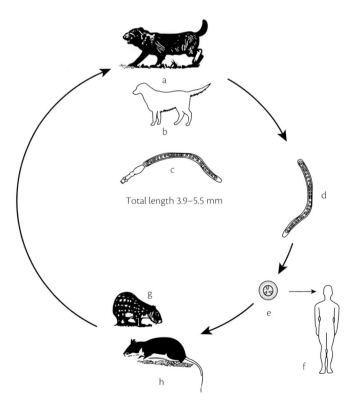

Total length 3.9–5.5 mm

Fig. 54.12 Life cycle of *Echinococcus vogeli* (a) Bush dog (*Speothos venaticus*) as principle definitive host; (b) domestic dog as occasional definitive host; (c) adult parasite (d) terminal segment of the parasite with eggs; (e) egg; (f) man as accidental host; (g) paca (*Cuniculus paca*) and (h) spiny rat (*Proechimys* sp.) as representatives of intermediate hosts.
Modified after Schantz *et al.* 1995. © Institute of Parasitology, Zurich.

(see below). In a survey in Columbia 73 (22%) of 325 pacas were found to be infected with the metacestode stage of *E. vogeli* (D'Alessandro *et al.* 1981).

The infection in humans

Pathological and clinical aspects

In hosts other than the natural intermediate hosts, a primary meta-cestode vesicle proliferates by successive production of new vesicles leading to polycystic parasite masses and infiltration of surrounding tissues (Rausch and D'Alessandro 1999; D'Alessandro and Rausch 2008). Among 42 confirmed human PE cases the liver was involved in 33 cases (79%), always with simultaneous parasite proliferation in the abdominal cavity and lung; in 9 (21%) cases metacestodes were only found in the mesenteries of the intestine and stomach (D'Alessandro and Rausch 2008). Six cases of PE without liver involvement have been recently reported from Brazil (Siqueira *et al.* 2010). After primary proliferation in the liver (the focus may remain undetected), the parasite can invade the peritoneal cavity eventually affecting various abdominal and chest organs (omentum, spleen, pancreas, uterus, ovaries, diaphragm, intercostal muscles, pericardium, lungs etc.) (D'Alessandro 1997; Rausch and D'Alessandro 1999). Vascular invasion is also possible (Siqueira *et al.* 2010). The exogenous proliferation of the *E. vogeli* metacestode accounts for its considerable pathogenicity in other hosts than natural intermediate hosts, including humans and nonhuman primates (Rausch and D'Alessandro 1999). Single cysts usually vary in diameter between 0,5 and 6 cm, but larger cysts (> 15 cm) may also occur (Oostbrurg *et al.* 2000). Cyst aggregates can attain much larger dimensions: in one case a total of 2 kg of cysts was surgically excised (D'Alessandro 1997). Caseous degeneration, partial necrosis and calcifications of cyst masses have been observed in several patients (D'Alessandro 1997; Siqueira *et al.* 2010).

Typically PE is a chronic disease lasting for long periods. In a group of 59 patients the duration of illness reported at the first consultation ranged between 1 month and 22 years; the median age of 51 patients was 44 years (range 6–78 years) without gender specificity (D'Alessandro 1997). The main clinical manifestations include abdominal pain, palpable abdominal masses, loss of weight, jaundice, hepatomegaly, anaemia, fever, haemoptysis (in cases of lung involvement), and in about 25% of the cases signs of portal hypertension and biliary obstruction. In some cases laboratory tests revealed high serum levels of bilirubin, γ-globulin and liver enzymes, eosinophilia and low levels of albumin (Meneghelli *et al.* 1992a, b; Ferreira *et al.* 1995; D'Alessandro 1997; Oostburg *et al.* 2000). In a series of 78 PE patients 23 (29%) died during the observation period due to the disease or complications associated with surgery. These data and fatal cases of PE in monkeys kept in zoos indicate that this form of neotropical echinococcosis is a serious and life-threatening disease (D'Alessandro and Rausch 2008).

Diagnosis and treatment

Diagnosis

Cystic structures can be detected by ultrasound imaging, X-ray examination or computer tomography. The imaging presentations of PE can be similar to infections with multiple cysts of *E. granulosus*. Discrimination between cystic echinococcosis (*E. granulosus*) and the neotropical forms on the one hand, and differential diagnosis between UE and PE depends on isolation of protoscoleces and morphological hook characteristics which allow a species-specific diagnosis (Rausch *et al.* 1978). Anti-*Echinococcus* antibodies can be detected by various serological tests but most of them are not specific enough for a differential diagnosis of UE and PE. However, an ELISA using an antigen fraction of *E. vogeli* (Ev2 antigen) allowed the discrimination between cases of cystic echinococcosis and neotropical polycystic echinococcosis (Gottstein *et al.* 1995). In the future, the use of molecular methods for the examination of metacestode material (isolated at biopsy, surgery or necropsy) may open new options for species-specific diagnoses.

Treatment

Surgery is the treatment of choice, although the rates of complications and recurrencies are high (mainly because of delayed diagnosis) (Siqueira *et al.* 2007). Experience with albendazole treatment of PE is limited. In a few cases improvement of clinical symptoms or cure have been reported (Meneghelli *et al.* 1992a; Siqueira *et al.* 2007; D'Alessandro and Rausch 2008), but the available data do not allow general conclusions on the efficacy of chemotherapy in cases of neotropical echinococcosis.

Epidemiology and geographic distribution

By March 2007 a total of 54 human confirmed cases of PE has been recorded from Latin American countries (group A). Further 114 cases were caused by polycystic metacestodes, but the *Echinococcus* species could not be determined as hooks required for identification were not available (group B) (D'Alessandro and Rausch 2008). Recently, a further case of group A has been diagnosed in French Guiana (Knapp *et al.* 2009b), and 7 cases of group B were reported from Brazil (Siqueira *et al.* 2007, 2010). These numbers accumulate to a total of 176 cases of human PE.

Human PE cases of groups A and B have been diagnosed in a large area, including Nicaragua, Costa Rica and Panama in Central America and in most of the South American states. The highest case numbers were recorded from Colombia (29), Brazil (105) and Argentina (11). As PE cases were also recorded from areas outside the geographic range of the bush dog (Nicaragua, Costa Rica, Uruguay, most of Argentina and Chile), it has been speculated that a proportion of cases from group B could have been caused by *E. oligarthrus* or that other canids may be involved in the transmission cycle, for instance the coyote in Central America (D'Alessandro and Rausch 2008). As the bush dog is a rarely observed wild animal, its role as source of human infections remains obscure. It is assumed that domestic dogs may play a role in transmission of parasite eggs to humans. Dogs are probably unable to capture pacas but they may become infected with metacestodes when fed viscera of pacas at the hunting site or at home (Basset *et al.* 1998; Rausch and D'Alessandro 2002; D'Alessandro and Rausch 2008).

Prevention of neotropical echinococcosis

There are no evaluated measures of prevention or control available, but education is essential. Viscera of potential intermediate hosts of *E. vogeli* should not be fed to domestic dogs.

References

Al-Attar, H.K., Al-Irhayim, B., and Al-Habbal, M.J. (1983). Alveolar hydatid disease of the liver: first case report from man in Iraq. *Ann. Trop. Med. Parasitol.*, **77**: 595–97.

Al-Sabi, M.N.S., Kapel, C.M.O., Deplazes, P., Mathis, A. (2007). Comparative copro-diagnosis of *Echinococcus multilocularis* in experimentally infected foxes. *Parasitol. Res.*, **101**: 731–36.

Al-Sabi, M.N., Kapel, C.M.O., Webster, P., and Deplazes, P. (2008). Reduced egg production of *Echinococcus multilocularis* in experimentally infected and re-infected red foxes (*Vulpes vulpes*). *Vet. Parasitol.*, 55: 59–66.

Ali-Khan, Z., Siboo, R., Gomersall, M., and Faucher, M. (1983). Cystolytic events and the possible role of germinal cells in metastasis in chronic alveolar hydatidosis. *Ann. Trop. Med. Parasitol.*, 77: 497–512.

Altintas, N. (2003). Past to present: echinococcosis in Turkey. *Acta Trop.*, 85: 105–12.

Ammann, R.W. and Eckert, J. (1995). Clinical diagnosis and treatment of echinococcosis in humans. In: R.C.A. Thompson and A.J. Lymbery (eds.) *Echinococcus and Hydatid Disease*, pp. 411–63. Wallingford, Oxon: CAB International.

Amman, R.W. and Eckert, J. (1996). Parasitic Diseases of the liver and intestine: Cestodes, *Echinococcus. Gastroenterol. Clin. N. Am.*, 25: 655–89.

Ammann, R.W., Ilitsch, N., Marincek, B., and Freiburghaus A.U. (1994). Effect of chemotherapy on the larval mass and the long-term course of alveolar echinococcosis. *Hepatology*, 19: 735–42.

Ammann, R.W., Renner, E.C., Gottstein, B., et al. (2004). Immunosurveillance of alveolar echinococcosis by specific humoral and cellular immune tests: long-term analysis of the Swiss chemotherapy trial (1976–2001). *J. Hepatol.*, 41: 551–69.

Auer, H. and Aspöck, H. (2001). Human alveolar echinococcosis and cystic echinococcosis in Austria: the recent epidemiological situation. *Helminthologia*, 38: 3–14.

Bagrade, G., Kirjusina, M., Vismanis, K., and Ozolins, J. (2009). Helminth parasites of the wolf *Canis lupus* from Latvia. *J. Helminthol.*, 83: 63–68.

Basset, D., Girou, C., Nozais, I.P., D'Hermies, F., et al. (1998). Neotropical echinococcosis in Suriname: *Echinococcus oligarthrus* in the orbit and *Echinococcus vogeli* in the abdomen. *Am. J. Trop. Med. Hyg.*, 59: 787–90.

Berke, O., Romig, T., and von Keyserlingk, M. (2008). Emergence of *Echinococcus multilocularis* among red foxes in northern Germany, 1991–2005. *Vet. Parasitol.*, 155: 319–22.

Bessonov, A.S. (1998). *Echinococcus multilocularis* infection in Russia and neighbouring countries. *Helminthologia*, 35: 73–78.

Bessonov, A.S. (2002). Echinococcosis of animals and humans in the Russian Federation. In: P. Craig and Z. Pawlowski (eds.) *Cestode Zoonoses: Echinococcosis and Cysticercosis*, pp. 91–98, Nato Science Series. Amsterdam: IOS Press.

Bosch, D. (1982). Tierexperimentelle Untersuchungen zur Entwicklung von *Echinococcus multilocularis*. In: R. Bähr (ed.) *Probleme der Echinokokkose unter Berücksichtigung parasitologischer und klinischer Aspekte*, pp. 36–40. Bern: H. Huber.

Bowles, J. and McManus, D.P. (1993). NADH dehydrogenase 1 gene sequences compared for species and strains of the genus *Echinococcus*. *Int. J. Parasitol.*, 23: 969–72.

Brehm, K. (2010). *Echinococcus multilocularis* as an experimental model in stem cell research and molecular host-parasite interaction. *Parasitology*, 137: 537–55.

Brehm, K. and Spiliotis, M. (2008). Recent advances in the *in vitro* cultivation of *Echinococcus multilocularis* metacestodes and germinal cells. *Exp. Parasitol.*, 119: 506–15.

Bretagne, S., Guillou, J.P., Morand, M., and Houin, R. (1993). Detection of *Echinococcus multilocularis* DNA in fox faeces using DNA amplification. *Parasitology*, 106: 193–99.

Bresson-Hadni, S., Laplante, J.J., Lenys, D., Rohmer, P., et al. (1994). Seroepidemiologic screening of *Echinococcus multilocularis* infection in an European area endemic for alveolar echinococcosis. *Am. J. Trop. Med. Hyg.*, 51: 837–46.

Bresson-Hadni, S., Humbert, P., Paintaud, G., et al. (1996). Skin localization of alveolar echinococcosis of the liver. *J. Am. Acad. Dermatol.*, 34: 873–77.

Bresson-Hadni, S., Vuitton, D.A., Bartholomot, B., et al. (2000). A twenty-year history of alveolar echinococcosis: analysis of a series of 117 patients from eastern France. *Eur. J. Gastroenterol. Hepatol.*, 12: 327–36.

Bresson-Hadni, S., Koch, S., Miguet, J.P., Gillet, M., et al. (2003). Indications and results of liver transplantation for *Echinococcus* alveolar infection: an overview. *Langenbeck's Arch. Surg.*, 388: 231–38.

Bresson-Hadni, S., Delabrousse, E., Blagosklonov, O., et al. (2006). Imaging aspects and non-surgical interventional treatment in human alveolar echinococcosis. *Parasitol. Int.*, 55: 267–72.

Brunetti, E., Kern, P., Vuitton, D.A., Writing Panel for the WHO-IWGE (2010). Expert consensus for the diagnosis and treatment of cystic and alveolar echinococcosis in humans. *Acta Trop.*, 114: 1–16.

Bruzinskaite, R., Marcinkute, A., Strupas, K., et al. (2007). Alveolar echinococcosis, Lithuania. *Emerg. Infect. Dis.*, 13: 1618–19.

Budke, C.M., Campos-Ponce, M., Qian, W., and Torgerson, P.R. (2005). A canine purgation study and risk factor analysis for echinococcosis in a high endemic region of the Tibetan plateau. *Vet. Parasitol.*, 127: 43–49.

Buhl, L. (1856). Über die zusammengesetzte Echinokokkengeschwulst der Leber. *Verhandl. Physic.-Med. Gesellsch. Würzburg*, 6: 428–29.

Burlet, P., Deplazes, P., and Hegglin, D. (2011). Age, season and spatio-temporal factors affecting the prevalence of *Echinococcus multilocularis* and *Taenia taeniaeformis* in *Arvicola terrestris*. *Parasit. Vectors*, 19(4): 6 (Epub ahead of print).

Buttenschoen, K., Kern, P., Reuter, S., and Barth, T. (2009a). Hepatic infestation of *Echinococcus multilocularis* with extension to regional lymph nodes. *Langenbeck's Arch. Surg.*, 394: 699–704.

Buttenschoen, K., Buttenschoen, D.C., Gruener, B., et al. (2009b). Long-term experience on surgical treatment of alveolar echinococcosis. *Langenbeck's Arch. Surg.*, 394: 689–98.

Buttenschoen, K., Gruener, B., Carli Buttenschoen, D., et al. (2009c). Palliative operation for the treatment of alveolar echinococcosis. *Langenbeck's Arch. Surg.*, 394: 199–204.

Carmena, D., Benito, A., and Eraso, E. (2007). The immunodiagnosis of *Echinococcus multilocularis* infection. *Clin. Microbiol. Infect.*, 13: 460–75.

Casulli, A., Széll, Z., Pozio, E., and Sréter, T. (2010). Spatial distribution and genetic diversity of *Echinococcus multilocularis* in Hungary. *Vet. Parasitol.*, 174: 241–6.

Craig, P.S. (2006). Epidemiology of human alveolar echinococcosis in China. *Parasitol. Int.*, 55: S 221–25.

Craig, P.S. and Macpherson, C.N.L. (1988). Sodium hypochlorite as an ovicide for *Echinococcus*. *Ann. Trop. Med. Parasitol.*, 82: 211–13.

Craig, P. and Pawlowski, Z. (eds.) (2002). *Cestode Zoonoses: Echinococcosis and Cysticercosis. An Emergent and Global Problem*, Nato Science Series. Amsterdam: IOS Press.

Craig, P.S., Deshan, L., MacPherson, C.N., et al. (1992). A large focus of alveolar echinococcosis in central China. *Lancet*, 340: 826–31.

Crouzet, J., Grenouillet, F., Delabrousse, E., et al. (2009). Personalized management of patients with inoperable alveolar echinococcosis undergoing treatment with albendazole : usefulness of positron-emission-tomography combined with serological and computed tomography follow-up. *Clin. Microbiol. Infect.*, 16: 788–91.

D'Alessandro, A. (1997). Polycystic echinococcosis in tropical America: *Echinococcus vogeli* and *E. oligarthrus*. *Acta Trop.*, 67: 43–65.

D'Alessandro, A. and Rausch, R.L. (2008). New aspects of neotropical polycystic (*Echinococcus vogeli*) and unicystic (*Echinococcus oligarthrus*) echinococcosis. *Clin. Microbiol. Rev.*, 21: 380–401.

D'Alessandro, A., Rausch, R.L., Morales, G.A., Collet, S., and Angel, D. (1981). *Echinococcus* infections in Colombian animals. *Am. J. Trop. Med. Hyg.*, 30: 1263–76.

Davidson, R.K., Oines, O., Madslien, K., and Mathis, A. (2009). *Echinococcus multilocularis*—adaptation of worm egg isolation procedure coupled with a multiplex PCR assay to carry out large-scale screening of red foxes (*Vulpes vulpes*) in Norway. *Parasitol. Res.*, 104: 509–14.

Deplazes, P. and Eckert, J. (1996). Diagnosis of the *Echinococcus multilocularis* infection in final hosts. *Appl. Parasitol.*, 37: 245–52.

Deplazes, P. and Eckert, J. (2001). Veterinary aspects of alveolar echinococcosis - a zoonosis of public health significance. *Vet. Parasitol.,* **98:** 65–87.

Deplazes, P. and Gottstein, B. (1991). A monoclonal antibody against *Echinococcus multilocularis* Em2 antigen. *Parasitology,* 103 Pt 1: 41–49.

Deplazes, P., Gottstein, B., Eckert, J., Ewald, D., *et al.* (1992). Detection of *Echinococcus* coproantigens by ELISA in dogs, dingoes and foxes. *Parasitol. Res.,* **78:** 303–8.

Deplazes, P., Alther, P., Tanner, I., Thompson, R.C., and Eckert, J. (1999). *Echinococcus multilocularis* coproantigen detection by enzyme-linked immunosorbent assay in fox, dog, and cat populations. *J. Parasitol.,* **85:** 115–21.

Deplazes, P., Dinkel, A., and Mathis, A. (2003). Molecular tools for studies on the transmission biology of *Echinococcus multilocularis*. *Parasitology,* **127:** S53–61.

Deplazes, P., Hegglin, D., Gloor, S., and Romig, T. (2004). Wilderness in the city: the urbanization of *Echinococcus multilocularis*. *Trends Parasitol.,* **20:** 77–84.

Deplazes, P., Grimm, F., Sydler, T., Tanner, I., Kapel, C.M.O. (2005). Experimental alveolar echinococcosis in pigs, lesion development and serological follow up. *Vet. Parasitol.,* **130:** 213–22.

Dinkel, A., von Nickisch-Rosenegk, M., Bilger, B., *et al.* (1998). Detection of *Echinococcus multilocularis* in the definitive host: coprodiagnosis by PCR as an alternative to necropsy. *J. Clin. Microbiol.,* **36:** 1871–76.

Drolshammer, I., Wiesmann, E., and Eckert, J. (1973). [Echinococcosis of humans in Switzerland 1956–1669] (Article in German). *Schweiz. Med. Wochenschr.,* **103:** 1337–41 and 1386–92.

Duscher, G., Prosl, H. and Joachim, A. (2005). Scarping or shaking–a comparison of methods for the quantitative determination of *Echinococcus multilocularis* in fox intestines. *Parasitol. Res.,* **95:** 40–42.

Dyachenko, V., Pantchev, N., Gawlowska, S., Vrhovec, M.G., and Bauer C. (2008). *Echinococcus multilocularis* infections in domestic dogs and cats from Germany and other European countries. *Vet. Parasitol.,* **157:** 244–53.

Eckert, J. (1986). Prospects for treatment of the metacestode stage of *Echinococcus.* In: R.C.A. Thompson (ed.) *The Biology of Echinococcus and Hydatid Disease,* pp. 250–84. London: Allen and Unwin.

Eckert, J. (1988). Cryopreservation of parasites. *Experientia,* **44:** 873–77.

Eckert, J. (1998). Alveolar echinococcosis (*Echinococcus multilocularis*) and other forms of echinococcosis (*Echinococcus oligarthrus* and *Echinococcus vogeli*). In: S.R. Palmer, E.J.L. Soulsby, and D.I.H Simpson (eds.) *Zoonoses,* pp. 689–716. Oxford: Oxford University Press.

Eckert, J. and Deplazes, P. (1999). Alveolar echinococcosis in humans: the current situation in central Europe and the need for countermeasures. *Parasitol. Today,* **15:** 315–19.

Eckert, J. and Deplazes, P. (2004). Biological, epidemiological, and clinical aspects of echinococcosis, a zoonosis of increasing concern. *Clin. Microbiol. Rev.,* **17:** 107–35.

Eckert, J., Thompson, R.C.A., and Mehlhorn, H. (1983). Proliferation and metastases formation of larval *Echinococcus multilocularis*. I. Animal model, macroscopiocal and histological findings. *Zeitschr. Parasitenk.,* **69:** 737–48.

Eckert, J., Conraths, F.J., and Tackmann, K. (2000). Echinococcosis: an emerging or re-emerging zoonosis? *Int. J. Parasitol.,* **30:** 1283–94.

Eckert, J., Deplazes, P., Craig, P.S., Gemmell, M.A., *et al.* (2001a). Echinococcosis in animals: clinical aspects, diagnosis and treatment. In: J. Eckert *et al.* (eds.) *WHO/OIE Manual on Echinococcosis in Humans and Animals: a Public Health Problem of Global Concern,* pp. 72–99. Paris: World Organization of Animal Health, ISBN 92-9044-522-X.

Eckert, J., Thompson, R.C.A., Bucklar, H., Bilger, B., and Deplazes, P. (2001b). Prüfung der Wirkung von Epsiprantel (Cestex®) gegen *Echinococcus multilocularis* bei Hunden und Katzen. *Berlin. München. Tierärztl. Wochenschr.,* **114:** 121–26.

Ehrhardt, A.R., Reuter, S., Buck, A.K., *et al.* (2007). Assessment of disease activity in alveolar echinococcosis: a comparison of contrast-enhanced ultrasound, three-phase helica CT and 18-F-fluorodeoxyglucose positron-emission tomography. *Abdom. Imag.,* **32:** 730–36.

Eiermann, T.H., Bettens, F., Tiberghien, P., *et al.* (1998). HLA and alveolar echinococcosis. *Tissue Antigens,* **52:** 124–29.

Ferreira, M.S., Nishioka Sde, A., Rocha, A., and D'Alessandro, A. (1995). *Echinococcus vogeli* polycystic hydatid disease: report of two Brazilian cases outside the Amazon region. *Trans. R. Soc. Trop. Med. Hyg.,* **89:** 286–87.

Frosch, M. and Lucius, R. (1994). Echinokokkose. In: M. Röllinghoff and M. Rommel (eds.) *Immunologische und molekulare Parasitologie,* pp. 187–206. Jena: Gutstav Fischer Verlag.

Fujimoto, Y., Ito, A., Ishikawa, Y., Inoue, M., *et al.* (2005). Usefulness of recombinant Em18-ELISA to evaluate efficacy of treatment in patients with alveolar echinococcosis. *J. Gastroenterol.,* **40:** 26–31.

Fujioka, Y., Shigeru, A., Sato, N., Uchino, J. (1993). Pathology. In: J. Uchino and N. Sato (eds.) *Alveolar Echinococcosis of the Liver,* pp. 51–62. Sapporo, Japan: Hokkaido University School of Medicine.

Gemmell, M.A. and Lawson, A.J.R. (1986). Epidemiology and control of hydatid disease. In: R.C.A. Thompson (ed.) *The Biology of Echinococcus and Hydatid Disease,* pp. 189–216. London: G. Allen & Unwin.

Genov, T.P., Svilenov, K., and Polyakova-Krusteva, O.T. (1980). The natural occurrence of *Alveococcus multilocularis* in the *Microtus nivalis* in Bulgaria. *Comp. Rendus Acad. Bulgare Sci.,* **33:** 981–84.

Giraudoux, P., Delattre, P., Takahasi, K., *et al.* (2002). Transmisson ecology of *Echinococcus multilocularis* in wildlife: what can be learned from comparative studies and multiscale approches? In: P. Craig and Z. Pawlowski *(eds.) Cestode Zoononoses: Echinococcosis and Cysticercosis an Emergent and Global Problem,* pp. 251–85, Nato Science Series. Amsterdam: IOS Press.

Giraudoux, P., Craig, P.S., Delattre, P., Bao, G., *et al.* (2003). Interactions between landscape changes and host communities can regulate *Echinococcus multilocularis* transmission. *Parasitology,* **127:** S121–31.

Gloor, S., Bontadina, F. and Hegglin, D. (2006). *Stadtfüchse.* Bern: Haupt Verlag.

Godot, V., Harraga, S., Deschaseaux, M., *et al.* (1997). Increased basal production of interleukin-10 by peripheral blood mononuclear cells in human alveolar echinococcosis. *Eur. Cytok. Network,* **8:** 401–8.

Godot, V., Harraga, S., Beurton, I., Deschaseaux, M., *et al.* (2000). Resistance/susceptibility to *Echinococcus multilocularis* infection and cytokine profile in humans. I. Comparison of patients with progressive and abortive lesions. *Clin. Exp. Immunol.,* **121:** 484–90.

Gottstein, B. and Felleisen, R. (1995). Protective immune mechanisms against *Echinococcus multilocularis*. *Parasitol. Today,* **11:** 320–26.

Gottstein, B., Deplazes, P., and Aubert, M. (1992). *Echinococcus multilocularis*: immunological study on the 'Em2-positive' laminated layer during in vitro and in vivo post-oncospheral and larval development. *Parasitol. Res.,* **78:** 291–97.

Gottstein, B., D'Alessandro, A., and Rausch, R. L. (1995). Immunodiagnosis of polycystic hydatid disease/polycystic echinococcosis due to *Echinococcus vogeli*. *Am. J. Trop. Med. Hyg.,* **53:** 558–63.

Gottstein, B., Lengeler, C., Bachmann, P., *et al.* (1987). Sero-epidemiological survey for alveolar echinococcosis (by Em2-ELISA) of blood doners in an endemic area of Switzerland. *Trans. R. Soc. Trop. Med. Hyg.,* **81:** 960–64.

Gottstein, B., Saucy, F., Deplazes, P., *et al.* (2001). Is high prevalence of *Echinococcus multilocularis* in wild and domestic animals associated with disease incidence in humans? *Emerg. Infect. Dis.,* **7:** 408–12.

Gottstein, B., Haag, K., Walker, M., Matsumoto, J., Mejri. N., and Hemphill, A. (2006). Molecular survival strategies of *Echinococcus multilocularis* in the murine host. *Parasitol. Int.,* **55:** S45–49.

Gottstein, B., Wittwer, M., Schild, M., Merli, M., *et al.* (2010). Hepatic gene expression profile in mice perorally infected with *Echinococcus multilocularis* eggs. *PLoS One.* **5:** e9779.

Graham, J.C., Gunn, M., Hudson, M., Orr, K.E., and Craig, P.S. (2002). A mass in the liver. *J. Infect.*, **45**: 121–22.

Haenle, M., Brockmann, S., Kron, M., *et al.* (2006). Overweight, physical activity, tabacco and alcohol consumption in a cross-sectional random sample of German adults. *BMC Pub. Health*, **6**: 233.

Hänle, M. M., Banzhaf, H-M., Forsbach-Birk, V., *et al.* (2009). Screening methods in alveolar echinococcosis: a follow-up study comparing Emc- and Emf-ELISA with Em2plus-ELISA and ultrasonography. *Epidemiol. Infect.*, **137**: 139–44.

Hegglin, D. and Deplazes, P. (2008). Control strategy for *Echinococcus multilocularis*. *Emerg. Infect. Dis.*, **14**: 1626–28.

Hegglin, D., Ward, P.I., and Deplazes, P. (2003). Anthelmintic baiting of foxes against urban contamination with *Echinococcus multilocularis*. *Emerg. Infect. Dis.*, **9**: 1266–72.

Hegglin, D., Bontadina, F., Contesse, P., Gloor, S., and Deplazes, P. (2007). Plasticity of predation behaviour as a putative driving force for parasite life-cycle dynamics: the case of urban foxes and *Echinococcus multilocularis* tapeworm. *Funct. Ecol.*, **21**: 552–60.

Heier, A., Geissbühler, U., Sennhauser, D., Scharf, G., and Kühn, N. (2007). [A case of alveolar hydatid disease in a dog: domestic animals as rare incidental intermediate hosts for *Echinococcus multilocularis*] [Article in German]. *Schweiz. Arch. Tierheilk.*, **149**: 123–27.

Hemphill, A., Stadelmann, B., Scholl, S., *et al.* (2010). *Echinococcus* metacestodes as laboratory models for the screening of drugs against cestodes and trematodes. *Parasitology*, **137**: 569–87.

Henttonen, H., Fuglei, E., Gower, C.N., *et al.* (2001). *Echinococcus multilocularis* on Svalbard: introduction of an intermediate host has enabled the local life-cycle. *Parasitology*, **123**: 547–52.

Hildreth, M.B., Blunt, D.S., and Oaks, J.A. (2004). Lethal effects of freezing *Echinococcus multilocularis* eggs at ultralow temperatures. *J. Parasitol.*, **90**: 841–44.

Hofer, S., Gloor, S., Müller, U., Mathis, A., Hegglin, D., and Deplazes, P. (2000). High prevalence of *Echinococcus multilocularis* in urban red foxes (*Vulpes vulpes*) and voles (*Arvicola terrestris*) in the city of Zürich, Switzerland. *Parasitology*, **120**: 135–42.

Horton, J. (2003). Albendazole for the treatment of echinococcosis. *Fund. Clin. Pharmacol.*, **17**: 205–12.

Howell, M.J. and Smyth, J.D. (1995). Maintenance and cultivation of *Echinococcus* species in vivo and in vitro. In: R.C.A. Thompson and A.J. Lymbery (eds.) *Echinococcus and Hydatid Disease*, pp. 201–32. Wallingford, UK: CAB International.

Hübner, M.P., Manfras, B.J, Margos, M.C., *et al.* (2006). *Echinococcus multilocularis* metacestodes modulate cellular cytokine and chemokine release by peripheral blood mononuclear cells in alveolar echinococcosis patients. *Clin. Exp. Immunol.*, **145**: 243–51.

Ito, A., Craig, P.S. (2003). Immunodiagnostic and molecular approaches for the detection of taeniid cestode infections. *Trends Parasitol.*, **19**: 377–81.

Ito, A., Romig, T., and Takahashi, K. (2003). Perspective on control options for *Echinococcus multilocularis* with particular reference to Japan. *Parasitology*, **127**: S159–72.

Ito, A., Agvaandaram, G., Bat-Ochir, O.E., *et al.* (2010). Histopathological, serological, and molecular confirmation of indigenous alveolar echinococcosis cases in Mongolia. *Am. J. Trop. Med. Hyg.*, **82**: 266–69.

Jenkins, D.J., Romig, T., and Thompson, R.C.A. (2005). Emergence/re-emergence of *Echinococcus* spp.- a global update. *Int. J. Parasitol.*, **35**: 1205–19.

Jorgensen, P., an der Heiden, M., Kern, P., *et al.* (2008). Underreporting of human alveolar echinococcosis, Germany. *Emerg. Infect. Dis.*, **14**: 935–37.

Kadry, Z., Renner, E.C. Bachmann, L.M., *et al.* (2005). Evaluation of treatment and long-term follow-up in patients with hepatic alveolar echinococcosis. *Br. J. Surg.*, **92**: 1110–16.

Kamiya, M., Lagapa, J.T., Nonaka, N., Ganzorig, S., Oku, Y., and Kamiya, H. (2006). Current control strategies targeting sources of echinococcosis in Japan. *OIE Rev. Sci. Techn.*, **25**: 1055–65.

Kamiya, M., Lagapa, J.T., Ganzorig, S., Kobayashi, F., Nanoka, N., and Oku, Y. (2007). Echinococcosis risks among domestic definitive hosts, Japan. *Emerg. Infect. Dis.*, **13**: 346–47.

Kapel, C.M.O., Torgerson, P.R., Thompson, R.C.A., and Deplazes, P. (2006). Reproductive potential of *Echinococcus multilocularis* in experimentally infected foxes, dogs, raccoon dogs and cats. *Int. J. Parasitol.*, **36**: 79–86.

Kharchenko, V.A., Kornyushin, V.V, Varodi, E.I., and Malega, O.M. (2008). Occurrence of *Echinococcus multilocularis* (Cestoda, Taeniidae) in red foxes (*Vulpes vulpes*) from Western Ukraine. *Acta Parasitol.*, **53**: 36–40.

Kędra, A.H., Świderski, Z., Tkach, V.V., Rocki, B., Pawlowski, J., and Pawlowski, Z. (2000). Variability within NADH dehydrogenase sequences of *Echinococcus multilocularis*. *Acta Parasitol.*, **45**: 353–55.

Kern, P., Frosch, P., Helbig, M., Wechsler, J.G., *et al.* (1995). Diagnosis of *Echinococcus multilocularis* infection by reverse transcription polymerase chain reaction. *Gastroenterology*, **109**: 596–600.

Kern, P., Bardonnet, K., Renner, E., Auer, H., *et al.* (2003). European echinococcosis registry: human alveolar echinococcosis, Europe, 1982–2000. *Emerg. Infect. Dis.*, **9**: 343–49.

Kern, P., Ammon, A., Kron, M., *et al.* (2004). Risk factors for alveolar echinococcosis in humans. *Emerg. Infect. Dis.*, **10**: 2088–93.

Kern, P., Wen, H., Sato, N., *et al.* (2006). WHO classification of alveolar echinococcosis: principles and application. *Parasitol. Int.*, **55** Suppl.: 283–87.

Kern, P., Abboud, P., Kern, W., Stich, A., *et al.* (2008). Critical appraisal of nitazoxanide for the treatment of alveolar echinococcosis. (Abstract). *Am. J. Trop. Med. Hyg.*, **79**: 119.

Kilwinski, J., Jenne, L., Jellen-Ritter, A., Radloff, P.D., Flick, W., and Kern, P. (1999). T-lymphocyte cytokine profile at the single cell level in alveolar echinococcosis. *Cytokine*, **11**: 373–81.

Koch, S., Bresson-Hadni, S., Miguet, J.P., Crumbach, J.P., Gillet, M., Mantion, G.A. (2003). Experience of liver transplantation for incurable alveolar echinococcosis: a 45 case European collaborative report. *Transplantation*, **75**: 856–63.

Kratzer, W., Reuter, S., Hirschbuehl, K., *et al.* (2005). Comparison of contrast-enhanced power Doppler ultrasound (Levovist) and computed tomography in alveolar echinococcosis. *Abdom. Imag.*, **30**: 286–90.

Knapp, J., Bart, J.-M., Giraudoux, P., *et al.* (2009a). Genetic diversity of the cestode *Echinococcus multilocularis* in red foxes at a continental scale in Europe. *PLoS Negl. Trop. Dis.*, **3**: e452, 1–10.

Knapp, J., Chirica, M., Simonnet, C., *et al.* (2009b). *Echinococcus vogeli* infection in a hunter, French Guiana. *Emerg. Infect. Dis.*, **15**: 2029–31.

Kocherscheidt, L., Flakowski, A.K., Grüner, B., *et al.* (2008). *Echinococcus multilocularis*: inflammatory and regulatory chemokine responses in patients with progressive, stable and cured alveolar echinococcosis. *Exp. Parasitol.*, **119**: 467–74.

König, A., Romig, T., Janko, C., *et al.* (2008). Integrated-baiting concept against *Echinococcus multilocularis* in foxes is successful in southern Bavaria, Germany. *Eur. J. Wildl. Res.*, **54**: 439–47.

Kohno, H., Sakai, H., Okamoto, M., *et al.* (1995). Development and characterization of murine monoclonal antibodies to *Echinococcus multilocularis* adult worms and its use for coproantigen detection. *Japanese J. Parasitol.*, **44**: 404–12.

Kolářová, L. (1999). *Echinococcus multilocularis*: new epidemiological insights in Central and Eastern Europe. *Helminthologia*, **36**: 193–200.

Kroeze, W.K. and Tanner, C.E. (1987). *Echinococcus multilocularis*: susceptibility and responses to infection in inbred mice. *Int. J. Parasitol.*, **17**: 873–83.

Labhardt, F. (1990). *Der Rotfuchs*. Hamburg: P. Parey.

Lagapa, J.T., Oku, Y., Kaneko, M., Ganzorig, S., *et al.* (2009). Monitoring of environmental contamination by *Echinococcus multilocularis* in an urban fringe forest park in Hokkaido, Japan. *Environm. Health Prev. Med.*, **14**: 299–303.

Li, T., Chen, X., Zhen, R., Qiu, J., Qiu, D., *et al.* (2010). Widespread co-endemicity of human cystic and alveolar echinococcosis on the eastern Tibetan Plateau, northwest Sichuan/southeast Qinghai, China. *Acta Trop.*, **113**: 248–56.

Lightowlers, M.W. and Gottstein, B. (1995). Echinococcosis/Hydatidosis: Antigens, immunological and molecular diagnosis. In: R.C.A. Thompson and A.J. Lymbery (eds.) *Echinococcus and Hydatid Disease*, pp. 355–410. Wallingford, UK: CAB International.

Liu, Y.H., Wang, X.G., Gao, J.S., Yao, Y.Q., Horton, J. (2009). Continuous albendazole therapy in alveolar echinococcosis: long-term follow-up observation of 20 cases. *Trans. R. Soc. Trop. Med. Hyg.*, **103**: 768–78.

Logar, J., Šoba, B., Lejko-Zupanc, T., and Kotar, T. (2007). Human alveolar echinococcosis in Slovenia. *Clin. Microbiol. Infect.*, **13**: 544–46.

Lopera, R.D., Melendez, R.D., Fernandez, I., Sirit, J., and Perera, M.P. (1989). Orbital hydatid cyst of *Echinococcus oligarthrus* in a human in Venezuela. *J. Parasitol.*, **75**: 467–70.

Machnicka, B., Dziemian, E., Rocki, B., and Kołodziej-Sobocińska, M. (2003). Detection of *Echinococcus multilocularis* antigens in faeces by ELISA. *Parasitol. Res.*, **91**: 491–96.

Malczewski, A. (2002). CE and AE in Eastern Europe. In: P. Craig and Z. Pawlowski (eds.) *Cestode Zoononoses: Echinococcosis and Cysticercosis. An Emergent and Global Problem*, pp. 81–89, Nato Science Series. Amsterdam: IOS Press.

Marchiondo, A.A., Ming, R., Andersen, F.L., Slusser, J.H., Conder, G.A. (1994). Enhanced larval cyst growth of *Echinococcus multilocularis* in praziquantel-treated jirds (*Meriones unguiculatus*). *Am. J. Trop. Med. Hyg.*, **50**: 120–27.

Mathis, A., and Deplazes, P. (2006). Copro-DNA tests for diagnosis of animal taeniid cestodes. *Parasitol. Int.*, **55**: S87–90.

Mathis, A., Deplazes, P., and Eckert, J. (1996). Improved test system for PCR-based species specific detection of *Echinococcus multilocularis* eggs. *J. Helminthol.*, **70**: 219–22.

Matsumoto, J. and Yagi, K. (2008). Experimental studies on *Echinococcus multilocularis* in Japan, focusing on biohazardous stages of the parasite. *Exp. Parasitol.*, **119**: 534–41.

Matsumoto, J., Sakamoto, K., Shinjyo, N., Kido, Y., *et al.* (2008). Anaerobic NADH-fumarate reductase system is predominant in the respiratory chain of *Echinococcus multilocularis*, providing a novel target for the chemotherapy of alveolar echinococcosis. *Antimicrob. Agents Chemother.*, **52**: 164–70.

Mathy, A., Hanosset, R., Adant, S., and Losson, B. (2009). The carriage of larval *Echinococcus multilocularis* and other cestodes by the musk rat (*Ondatra zibethicus*) along the Ourthe River and its tributaries (Belgium). *J. Wildl. Dis.*, **45**: 279–87.

McManus, D.P. (2006). Molecular discrimination of taeniid cestodes. *Parasitol. Int.*, **55**: S31–37.

McManus, D.P. (2009). Reflections on the biochemistry of *Echinococcus*: past, present and future. *Parasitology*, **136**: 1643–52.

Mehlhorn, H., Eckert, J., and Thompson, R.C.A. (1983). Proliferation and metastases formation of larval *Echinococcus multilocularis*: II. Ultrastructural investigations. *Zeitschr. Parasitenk.*, **69**: 749–63.

Mejri, N., Hemphill, A., and Gottstein, B. (2010). Triggering and modulation of the host-parasite interplay by *Echinococcus multilocularis*: a review. *Parasitology*, **137**: 557–68.

Meneghelli, U.G., Martinelli, A.L., Bellucci, A.D., Llorach Velludo, M.A., *et al.* (1992a). Polycystic hydatid disease (*Echinococcus vogeli*). Treatment with albendazole. *Ann. Trop. Med. Parasitol.*, **86**: 151–56.

Meneghelli, U.G., Martinelli, A.L., Llorach Velludo, M.A., *et al.* (1992b). Polycystic hydatid disease (*Echinococcus vogeli*). Clinical, laboratory and morphological findings in nine Brazilian patients. *J. Hepatol.*, **14**: 203–10.

Mobedi, I., Sadighian, A. (1971). *Echinococcus multilocularis* Leuckart, 1863, in red foxes, *Vulpes vulpes* Linn., in Moghan, Azerbaijan Province, northwest of Iran. *J. Parasitol.*, **57**: 493.

Moks, E., Saarma, U., and Valdmann, H. (2005). *Echinococcus multilocularis* in Estonia. *Emerg. Infect. Dis.*, **11**: 1973–74.

Nakao, M., McManus, D.P., Schantz, P.M., *et al.* (2007). A molecular phylogeny of the genus *Echinococcus* inferred from complete mitochondrial genomes. *Parasitology*, **134**: 713–22.

Nonaka, N., Hirokawa, H., Inoue, T., *et al.* (2008). The first instance of a cat excreting *Echinococcus multilocularis* eggs in Japan. *Parasitol. Int.*, **57**: 519–20.

Nonaka, N., Kamiya, M., Kobayashi, F., *et al.* (2009). *Echinococcus multilocularis* infection in pet dogs in Japan. *Vector Borne Zoon. Dis.*, **9**: 201–6.

Ohbayashi, M. (1960). Studies on echinococcosis. X. Histological observations on experimental cases of multilocular echinococcosis. *Japanese J. Vet. Res.*, **8**: 134–60.

Ohbayashi, M., Rausch, R.L., and Fay, F.H. (1971). On the ecology and distribution of *Echinococcus* spp. (Cestoda: Taeniidae), and characteristics of their development in the intermediate host. II. Comparative studies on the development of larval *E. multilocularis* Leuckart, 1863, in the intermediate host. *Japanese J. Vet. Res.*, **19**: 1–63.

Oostburg, B.F.J., Vrede, M.A., and. Bergen, A.E. (2000). The occurrence of polycystic echinococcosis in Suriname. *Ann. Trop. Med. Parasit.*, **94**: 247–52.

Ozturk, G., Polat, K.Y., Yildirgan, M.I., Aydinli, B., Atamanalp, S.S., and Aydin, U. (2009). Endoscopic retrograde cholangiopancreatography in hepatic alveolar echinococcosis. *J. Gastroenterol. Hepatol.*, **24**: 1365–69.

Pawlowski, Z., Eckert, J., Vuitton, D.A., *et al.* (2001). Echinococcosis in humans: clinical aspects, diagnosis and treatment. In: J. Eckert *et al.* (eds.) *Manual on Echinococcosis in Humans and Animals: a Public Health Problem of Global Concern*, pp. 20–66. Paris: World Organisation of Animal Health. ISBN 92-9044-522-X.

Playford, M.C., Ooi, H.K., Oku, Y., and Kamiya, M. (1993). Rodent intermediate host models for alveolar echinococcosis: biology and immunology. In: J. Uchino and N. Sato (eds.) *Alveolar Echinococcosis of the Liver*, pp. 33–49. Sapporo, Japan: Hokkaido University School of Medicine.

Posselt, A. (1928). Der Alveolarechinokokkus und seine Chirurgie. In: G. Hosenmann *et al.* (eds.) *Die Echinokokkenkrankheit*, pp. 305–418. Stuttgart: Verlag F. Enke.

Raoul, F., Deplazes, P., Nonaka, N., Piarroux, R., Vuitton, D.A., and Giraudoux, P. (2001). Assessment of the epidemiological status of *Echinococcus multilocularis* in foxes in France using ELISA coprotests on fox faeces collected in the field. *Int. J. Parasitol.*, **14**: 1579–88.

Raoul, F., Michelat, D., Ordinaire, M., *et al.* (2003). *Echinococcus multilocularis*: secondary poisoning of fox population during a vole outbreak reduces environmental contamination in a high endemicity area. *Int. J. Parasitol.*, **33**: 945–54.

Rausch, R.L. (1986). Life-cycle patterns and geographic distribution of *Echinococcus* species. In: R.C.A. Thompson (ed.) *The Biology of Echinococcus and Hydatid Disease*, pp. 44–80. London: George Allen & Unwin.

Rausch, R.L. (1995). Life cycle patterns and geographic distribution of *Echinococcus* species. In : R.C.A. Thompson and A.J. Lymbery (eds.) *Echinococcus and Hydatid Disease*, pp. 88–134. Wallingford, UK: CAB International.

Rausch, R.L. and Bernstein, J.J. (1972). *Echinococcus vogeli* sp. n. (Cestoda: Taeniidae) from the bush dog, *Speothos venaticus* (Lund). *Zeitschr. Tropenmed. Parasitol.*, **23**: 25–34.

Rausch, R.L., and D'Alessandro, A. (1999). Histogenesis in the metacestode of *Echinococcus vogeli* and mechanism of pathogenesis in polycystic hydatid disease. *J. Parasitol.*, **85**: 410–18.

Rausch, R.L., and D'Alessandro, A. (2002). The epidemiology of echinococcosis caused by *Echinococcus oligarthrus* and *E. vogeli* in the Neotropics. In: P. Craig and Z. Pawlowski (eds.) *Cestode Zoononoses: Echinococcosis and Cysticercosis an Emergent and Global Problem*, pp. 107–13, Nato Science Series. Amsterdam: IOS Press.

Rausch, R.L., and Fay, F.H. (2002). Epidemiology of alveolar echinococcosis, with reference to St. Lawrence Island, Bering Sea. In: P. Craig and Z. Pawlowski (eds.)*Cestode Zoonoses: Echinococcosis and Cysticercosis an Emergent and Global Problem*, pp. 309–25, Nato Science series. Amsterdam: IOS Press.

Rausch, R. and Schiller, E.L. (1954). Studies on the helminth fauna of Alaska: XXIV. *Echinococcus sibiricensis* Rausch and Schiller, 1954 on St. Lawrence Island. *Parasitology*, **40**: 659–62.

Rausch, R.L., Rausch, V.R. and D'Alessandro, A. (1978). Discrimination of the larval stages of *Echinococcus oligarthrus* (Diesing, 1863) and *E. vogeli* Rausch and Bernstein, 1972 (Cestoda: Taeniidae). *Am. J. Trop. Med. Hyg.*, **27**: 1195–202.

Rausch, R.L., D'Alessandro, A., and Rausch, V.R. (1981). Characteristics of the larval *Echinococcus vogeli* (Rausch & Bernstein 1972) in the natural intermediate host, the paca, *Cuniculus paca* L. (Rodentia: Dasyproctidae). *Am. J. Trop. Med. Hyg.*, **30**: 1043–52.

Rausch, R.L., Wilson, J.F., Schantz, P.M., and McMahon, B.J. (1987). Spontaneous death of *Echinococus multilocularis*: cases diagnosed serologically (by Em2 ELISA) and clinical significance. *Am. J. Trop. Med. Hyg.*, **36**: 576–85.

Rehmann, P., Gröne, A., Lawrenz, A., Pagan, O., Gottstein, B., and Bacciarini, L.N. (2003). *Echinococcus multilocularis* in two lowland gorillas (*Gorilla g. gorilla*). *J. Comp. Pathol.*, **129**: 85–88.

Reperant, L.A., Hegglin, D., Fischer, C., Kohler, L., Weber J-M., and Deplazes, P. (2007). Influence of urbanization on the epidemiology of intestinal helminths of the red fox (*Vulpes vulpes*) in Geneva, Switzerland. *Parasitol. Res.*, **101**: 605–11.

Reperant, L.A., Hegglin, D., Tanner, I., Fischer, C., Deplazes, P. (2009). Rodents as shared indicators for zoonotic parasites of carnivores in urban environments. *Parasitology*, **136**: 329–37.

Reuter, M. and Kreshchenko, N. (2004). Flatworm asexual multiplication implicates stem cells and regeneration. *Can. J. Zool.*, **82**: 334–56.

Reuter, S., Jensen, B., Buttenschoen, K., Kratzer, W., and Kern, P. (2000). Benzimidazoles in the treatment of alveolar echinococcosis: a comparative study and review of the literature. *J. Antimicrob. Chemother.*, **46**: 451–56.

Reuter, S., Nüssle, K., Kolokythas, O., Haug, U., *et al.* (2001). Alveolar liver echinococcosis: a comparative study of three imaging techniques. *Infection*, **29**: 119–25.

Reuter, S., Merkle, M., Brehm, K., Kern, P., and Manfras, B. (2003). The effect of amphotericin B on the larval growth of *Echinococcus multilocularis*. *Antimicrob. Agents Chemother.*, **47**: 620–25.

Reuter, S., Buck, A., Manfras, B., Kratzer, W., Schirrmeister, H., Reske, S.N., and Kern, P. (2004). Structured treatment interruption in patients with alveolar echinococcosis. *Hepatology*, **39**: 509–517.

Reuter, S., Grüner, B., Buck, A.K., Blumstein, N., Kern, P., and Reske, S.N. (2008). Long-term follow-up of metabolic activity in human alveolar echinococcosis using FDG-PET. *Nuklearmed.*, **47**: 147–52.

Rokni, M.B. (2008). The present status of human helminthic diseases in Iran. *Ann. Trop. Med. Parasitol.*, **102**: 283–95.

Romig, T., Kratzer, W., Kimmig, P., *et al.* (1999). An epidemiological survey of human alveolar echinococcosis in southwestern Germany. *Am. J. Trop. Med. Hyg.*, **61**: 566–73.

Romig, T. (2002). Spread of *Echinococcus multiloculalis* in Europe?. In: P. Craig and Z. Pawlowski (eds.) *Cestode Zoononoses: Echinococcosis and Cysticercosis. An Emergent and Global Problem*, pp. 65–80, Nato Science Series. Amsterdam: IOS Press.

Romig, T., Dinkel, A., and Mackenstedt, U. (2006a). The present situation of echinococcosis in Europe. *Parasitol. Int.*, **55**: S187–91.

Romig, T., Thoma, D., and Weible, A.K. (2006b). *Echinococcus multilocularis*-a zoonosis of anthropogenic environments? *J. Helminthol.*, **80**: 207–12.

Romig, T., Bilger, B., Dinkel, A., *et al.* (2007). Impact of praziquantel baiting on intestinal helminths of foxes in southwestern Germany. *Helminthologia*, **44**: 137–44.

Saarma, U., Jõgisalu, I., Moks, E., *et al.* (2009). A novel phylogeny for the genus *Echinococcus*, based on nuclear data, challenges relationships based on mitochondrial evidence. *Parasitology*, **136**: 317–28.

Saeed, I., Maddox-Hyttel, C., Monrad. J., and Kapel, CM. (2006). Helminths of red foxes (*Vulpes vulpes*) in Denmark. *Vet. Parasitol.*, **139**: 168–79.

Sakamoto, T. and Sugimura, M. (1970). Studies on echinococcosis: XXIII. Electron microscopical observations on histogenesis of larval *Echinococcus multilocularis*. *Japanese J. Vet. Res.*, **17**: 131–44.

Sakamoto, T., Tani, S., Hutchinson, G.W., *et al.* (1987). Studies on echinococcosis in Australia. I. Histopathological observations on echinococcosis of cattle in Australia. *J. Fac. Agr., Iwate University*, **18**: 323–37.

Sakai, H., Nonaka, N., Yagi, K., Oku, Y., and Kamiya, M. (1998). Coproantigen detection in a survey of *Echinococcus multilocularis* infection among red foxes, *Vulpes vulpes* schrencki, in Hokkaido. *Japanese J. Vet. Med. Sci.*, **60**: 639–41.

Salinas-Lopez, N., Jimenez-Guzman, F., and Cruz-Reyes, A. (1996). Presence of *Echinococcus oligarthrus* (Diesing, 1863) Lühe, 1910 in *Lynx rufus texensis* Allen, 1895 from San Fernando, Tamaulipas State, in north-east Mexico. *Int. J. Parasitol.*, **26**: 793–96.

Sato, N., Aoki, S., Matsushita, M., and Uchino, J. (1993a). Clinical features. In: J. Uchino and N. Sato (eds.) *Alveolar Echinococcosis of the Liver*, pp. 63–98. Sapporo, Japan: Hokkaido University School of Medicine.

Sato, N., Uchino, J., Suzuki, K., Kamiyama, T., *et al.* (1993b). Mass screening. In: J. Uchino and N. Sato (eds.) *Alveolar Echinococcosis of the Liver*, pp. 121–29. Sapporo, Japan: Hokkaido University School of Medicine.

Sato, N., Uchino, J., Takahashi, M., Aoki, S., *et al.* (1997a). Surgery and outcome of alveolar echinococcosis of the liver: historical comparison of mass screening systems in Japan. *Int. Surg.*, **82**: 201–04.

Sato, N., Namieno, T., Furuya, K., Takahasi, H., *et al.* (1997b). Contribution of mass screening to resectability of hepatic lesions involving *Echinococcus multilocularis*. *J. Gastroenterol. Hepatol.*, **32**: 351–254.

Schantz, P.M., Chai, J., Craig, P.S., Eckert, J., Jenkins, D.J., Macpherson, C.N.L., and Thakur, A. (1995). Epidemiology and control of hydatid disease. In: R.C.A. Thompson and A.J. Lymbery (eds.) *Echinococcus and Hydatid Disease*, pp. 233–331. Wallingford, Oxon: CAB International.

Schantz, P.M., Eckert, J., Craig, P.S. (1996). Geographic distribution, epidemiology, and control of *Echinococcus multilocularis* and alveolar echinococcosis. In: J. Uchino and N. Sato (eds.) *Alveolar Echinococcosis*, pp. 1–25. Sapporo, Japan: Fuji Shoin.

Scharf, G., Deplazes, P., Kaser-Hotz, B., Borer, L., Hasler, A., Haller, M., Flückiger, M. (2004). Radiographic, ultrasonographic, and computed tomographic appearance of alveolar echinococcosis in dogs. *Vet. Radiol. Ultrasound*, **45**: 411–18.

Scheuring, U.J., Seitz, H.M., Wellmann, A., *et al.* (2003). Long-term benzimidazole treatment of alveolar echinococcosis with hematogenic subcutaneous and bone dissemination. *Med. Microbiol. Immunol.*, **192**: 193–95.

Schweiger, A., Ammann, R.W., Candinas, D., *et al.* (2007). Human alveolar echinococcosis after fox population increase, Switzerland. *Emerg. Infect. Dis.*, **13**: 878–82.

Shaikenov, B.S. (2006). Distribution and ecology of *Echinococcus multilocularis* in Central Asia. *Parasitol. Int.*, **55**: S213–19.

Shaikenov, B.S. and Torgerson P.R. (2002). Distribution of *Echinococcus multilocularis* in Kazakhstan. In: P. Craig and Z. Pawlowski (eds.) *Cestode Zonnoses: Echinococcosis and Cysticercosis. An Emergent and Global Problem*, pp. 299–307. Nato Science Series, Amsterdam: IOS Press.

Siko, S.B., Deplazes, P., Ceica, C., Tivadar, C.S. *et al.* (2010) *Echinococcus multilocularis* in south-eastern Europe (Romania). *Parasitol. Res.* Nov. 18. Epub.ahead of print.

Siles-Lucas, M.M. and Gottstein, B.B. (2001). Molecular tools for the diagnosis of cystic and alveolar echinococcosis. *Trop. Med. Int. Health,* **6:** 463–75.

Siles-Lucas, M., Merli, M., Gottstein, B. (2008). 14-3-3 proteins in *Echinococcus*: their role and potential as protective antigens. *Exp. Parasitol.,* **119:** 516–23.

Siqueira, N.G., de Almeida, F.B., Chalub, S.R., *et al.* (2007). Successful outcome of hepatic polycystic echinococcosis managed with surgery and chemotherapy. *Trans. R. Soc. Trop. Med. Hyg.,* **101:** 624–26.

Siqueira, N.G., Almeida, F.B., Suzuki, Y.A., *et al.* (2010). Atypical polycystic echinococcosis without liver involvement in Brazilian patients. *Trans. R. Soc. Trop. Med. Hyg.,* **104:** 230–33.

Sousa, O.E., and Thatcher, V.E. (1969). Observations on the life-cycle of *Echinococcus oligarthrus* (Diesing, 1863) in the Republic of Panama. *Ann. Trop. Med. Parasitol.,* **63:** 165–75.

Spiliotis, M. and Brehm. K. (2009). Axenic *in vitro* cultivation of *Echinococcus multilocularis* metacestode vesicles and the generation of primary cell cultures. In: S. Rupp and K. Sohn (eds.) *Methods in Molecular Biology: Host-Pathogen Interaction*, pp. 245–62. Totowa, NJ: Humana Press.

Sréter, T., Szell, Z., Egyed, Z., Varga, I. (2003). *Echinococcus multilocularis*: an emerging pathogen in Hungary and Central Eastern Europe? *Emerg. Infect. Dis.,* **9:** 384–86.

Štefanić, S., Shaikenov, B.S., Deplazes, P., *et al.* (2004). Polymerase chain reaction for detection of patent infections of *Echinococcus granulosus* ('sheep strain') in naturally infected dogs. *Parasitol. Res.,* **92:** 347–51.

Staebler, S., Grimm. F., Glaus, T., Kapel, C.M., *et al.* (2006). Serological diagnosis of canine alveolar echinococcosis. *Vet. Parasitol.,* **141:** 243–50.

Stettler, M., Rossignol, J.F., Fink, R., Walker, M., Gottstein, B., Merli, M., Theurillat, R., Thormann, W., Dricot, E., Segers, R., and Hemphill A. (2004). Secondary and primary murine alveolar echinococcosis, combined albendazole/nitazoxanide chemotherapy exhibits profound anti-parasitic activity. *Int. J. Parasitol.,* **34:** 615–24.

Stieger, C., Hegglin, D., Schwarzenbach, G., Mathis, A., and Deplazes, P. (2002). Spatial and temporal aspects of urban transmission of *Echinococcus multilocularis*. *Parasitology,* **124:** 631–40.

Stien, A., Voutilainen, L., Haukisalmi, V., *et al.* (2010). Intestinal parasites of the Arctic fox in relation to the abundance and distribution of intermediate hosts. *Parasitology,* **137:** 149–57.

Stumpe, K.D., Renner-Schneiter, E.C., Kuenzle, A.K., *et al.* (2007). F-18-fluorodeoxyglucose (FDG) positron-emission tomography of *Echinococcus multilocularis* liver lesions: prospective evaluation of its value for diagnosis and follow-up during benzimidazole therapy. *Infection,* **35:** 11–18.

Swiderski, Z. (1983). *Echinococcus granulosus*: hook-muscle systems and cellular organisation of infective oncospheres. *Int. J. Parasitol.,* **13:** 289–99.

Tackmann, K., Löschner, U., Mix, H., *et al.* (2001). A field study to control *Echinococcus multilocularis*-infections of the red fox (*Vulpes vulpes*) in an endemic focus. *Epidem. Infect.,* **127:** 577–87.

Tackmann, K., Mattis, R., and Conraths, F.J. (2006). Detection of *Echinococcus multilocularis* in foxes: evaluation of a protocol of intestinal scarping technique. *Vet. Med. B,* **53:** 395–98.

Takumi, K. and van der Giessen, J. (2005). Transmission dynamics of *Echinococcus multilocularis*; its reproduction number, persistence in an area of low rodent prevalence, and effectiveness of control. *Parasitology,* **131:** 133–40.

Tappe, D., Stich, A., and Frosch, M. (2008). Emergence of polycystic neotropical echinococcosis. *Emerg. Infect. Dis.,* **14:** 292–96.

Tappe, D., Frosch, M., Sako, Y., Itoh, S., *et al.* (2009). Close relationship between clinical regression and specific serology in the follow-up of patients with alveolar echinococcosis in different clinical stages. *Am. J. Trop. Med. Hyg.,* **80:** 792–97.

Tappe, D., Müller, A., Frosch, M., and Stich, A. (2009). Limitations of amphotericin B and nitazoxanide in the treatment of alveolar echinococcosis. *Ann. Trop. Med. Parasitol.,* **103:** 177–81.

Tappe, D., Kern, P., Frosch, M., and Kern, P. (2010a). A hundred years of controversy about the taxonomic status of *Echinococcus* species. *Acta Trop.* **115:**167–74.

Tappe, D., Sako, Y., Itoh, S., Frosch, M., Grüner, B., Kern, P., and Ito, A. (2010b). Immunoglobulin G subclass responses to recombinant Em18 in the follow-up of patients with alveolar echinococcosis in different clinical stages. *Clin. Vacc. Immunol.,***17:** 944–48.

Thiess, A., Schuster, R., Nöckler, K., and Mix, H. (2001). [Helminth findings in indigenous raccoon dogs *Nyctereutes procyonoides* (Gray, 1843)] [Article in German]. *Berlin. Münch. Tierärztl. Wochenschr.,* **114:** 273–76.

Thompson, R.C.A. (1995). Biology and systematics of Echinococcus. In: R.C.A. Thompson and A. J. Lymbery (eds.) *Biology and Hydatid Disease*, pp. 1–50. Wallingford, Oxon: CAB International.

Thompson, R.C.A. (2008). The taxonomy, phylogeny and transmission of *Echinococcus. Exp. Parasitol.,* **119:** 439–46.

Thompson, R.C.A. and Eckert, J. (1982). The production of eggs by *Echinococcus multilocularis* in the laboratory following *in vivo* and *in vitro* development. *Zeitschr. Parasitenk.,* **68:** 227–34.

Thompson, R.C.A. and Eckert, J. (1983). Observations on *Echinococcus multilocularis* in the definitive host. *Zeitschr. Parasitenk.,* **69:** 335–45.

Thompson, R.C.A., Deplazes, P., and Eckert, J. (1990). Uniform strobilar development of *Echinococcus multilocularis in vitro* from protoscolex to immature stages. *J. Parasitol.,* **76:** 240–47.

Thompson, R.C.A., Deplazes, P., and Eckert, J. (2003). Observations on the development of *Echinococcus multilocularis* in cats. *J. Parasitol.,* **89:** 1086–88.

Thompson, R.C.A., Kapel, C.M.O., Hobbs, R.P., and Deplazes, P. (2006). Comparative development of *Echinococcus multilocularis* in its definitive hosts. *Parasitology,* **132:** 709–16.

Tiaoying, L., Jiamin, Q., Wen, Y., Craig, P.S., Xingwang, C., Ning, X., Ito, A., Giraudoux, P., Wulamu, M., Wen, Y., and Schantz, P.M. (2005). Echinococcosis in Tibetan populations, western Sichuan Province, China. *Emerg. Infect. Dis.,* **11:** 1866–73.

Torgerson, P.R., and Craig, P.S. (2009). Risk assessment of importation of dogs infected with *Echinococcus multilocularis* into the UK. *Vet. Rec.,* **165:** 366–98.

Torgerson, P.R., and Deplazes, P. (2009). Echinococcosis: diagnosis and diagnostic interpretation in population studies. *Trends Parasitol.,* **25:** 164–70.

Torgerson, P.R., Schweiger, A., Deplazes, P., *et al.* (2008). Alveolar echinococcosis: from a deadly disease to a well-controlled infection. Relative survival and economic analysis in Switzerland over the last 35 years. *J. Hepatol.,* **49:** 72–77.

Torgerson, P.R., Keller, K., Magnotta, M., and Ragland, N. (2010). The global burden of alveolar echinococcosis. *PLoS Negl. Trop. Dis.,* **4:** e722.

Trachsel, D., Deplazes, P., and Mathis, A. (2007). Identification of taeniid eggs in the faeces from carnivores based on multiplex PCR using targets in mitochondrial DNA. *Parasitology,* **134:** 911–20.

van Riel, A., Sjollema, B., Klarenbeek, S., and van der Giessen, J. (2007). A dog with alveolar echinococcosis: the larval stage of the fox tapeworm. *(Article in Dutch) Tijdsch. Diergeneesk.* **132:** 828–31.

Veit, P., Bilger, B., Schad, V., Schafer, J., Frank, W., and Lucius, R. (1995). Influence of environmental factors on the infectivity of *Echinococcus multilocularis* eggs. *Parasitology,* **110:** 79–86.

Virchow, R. (1856). Die multiloculäre, ulcerierende Echinokokkengeschwulst der Leber. *Verhandl. Physic.-Med. Gesellsch. Würzburg,* **6:** 84–95.

Vogel, H. (1957). Über den *Echinococcus multilocularis* Süddeutschlands. l. Das Bandwurmstadium von Stämmen menschlicher und tierischer Herkunft. *Zeitschr. Tropenmed. Parasitol.,* **8:** 404–54.

Vogel, H. (1977). Über den *Echinococcus multilocularis* Süddeutschlands. II. Entwicklung der Larvenstadien und histologische Reaktionen in der Feldmaus, *Microtus arvalis. Tropenmed. Parasitol.,* **28:** 409–27.

Vogel, H. (1978). Wie wächst der Alveolarechinokokkus? *Tropenmed. Parasitol.,* **29:** 1–11.

Vogel, J., Görich, J., Kramme, E., Merkle, E., *et al.* (1996). Alveolar echinococcosis of the liver: percutaneous stent therapy in budd-chiari syndrome. *Gut,* **39:** 762–64.

Vuitton, D.A., Zhou, H., Bresson-Hadni, S., *et al.* (2003). Epidemiology of alveolar echinococcosis with particular reference to China and Europe. *Parasitology,* **127:** S87–107.

Vuitton, D.A., Zhang, S.L., Yang, Y., *et al.* (2006). Survival strategy of *Echinococcus multilocularis* in the human host. *Parasitol. Int.,* **55:** 51–55.

Wandeler, P., Funk, S.M., Largiader, C.R., *et al.* (2003). The city-fox phenomenon: genetic consequences of a recent colonization of urban habitat. *Mol. Ecol.,* **12:** 647–56.

WHO (1996). Guidelines for treatment of cystic and alveolar echinococcosis in humans. *Bull. WHO,* **74:** 231–42.

WHO/OIE (2001). *Manual on Echinococcosis in Humans and Animals: a Public Health Problem of Global Concern* (eds.) J. Eckert, M.A. Gemmell, F-X. Meslin, Z.S. Pawlowski). Paris: World Organisation of Animal Health, ISBN 92-9044-522-X.

Wilson, J.F., Rausch, R.L., Wilson, F.R. (1995). Alveolar hydatid disease. Review of the surgical experience in 42 cases of active disease among Alaskan Eskimos. *Ann. Surg.,* **221:** 315–23.

Xiao, N., Qiu, J., Nakao, M., Li, T., Yang, W., Chen, X., Schantz, P.M., Craig, P.S., and Ito, A. (2005). *Echinococcus shiquicus* n. sp., a taeniid cestode from Tibetan fox and plateau pika in China. *Int. J. Parasitol.,* **35:** 693–701.

Yamashita, J. (1960). On the susceptibility and histogenesis of *Echinococcus multilocularis* in the experimental mouse, with the state of echinococcosis in Japan. *Parassitologia,* **2:** 399–406.

Yang, Y.R., Craig, P.S., Sun, T., Vuitton, D.A., Giraudoux, P., Jones, M.K., Williams, G.M., McManus, D.P. (2008). Echinococcosis in Ningxia Hui Autonomous Region, northwest China. *Trans. R. Soc. Trop. Med. Hyg.,* **102:** 319–28.

Ziadinov, I., Mathis, A., Trachsel, D., *et al.* (2008). Canine echinococcosis in Kyrgyzstan: using prevalence data adjusted for measurement error to develop transmission dynamics models. *Int. J. Parasitol.,* **38:** 1179–90.

Ziadinov, I., Deplazes, P., Mathis, A., *et al.* (2010). Frequency distribution of *Echinococcus multilocularis* and other helminths of foxes in Kryrgyzstan. *Vet. Parasitol.,* **171:** 286–92.

Zhang, S., Hüe, S., Sène, D., Penfornis, A., *et al.* (2008a). Expression of major histocompatibility complex class I chain-related molecule A, NKG2D, and transforming growth factor-β in the liver of humans with alveolar echinococcosis: New actors in the tolerance to parasites? *J. Infect. Dis.,* **197:** 1341–49.

Zhang, W., Ross, A.G., and McManus, D.P. (2008b). Mechanism of immunity in hydatid disease: implications for vaccine development. *J. Immunol.,* **181:** 6679–85.

CHAPTER 55

Zoonotic schistosomosis (schistosomiasis)

Hélène Carabin, Maria V. Johansen, Jennifer F. Friedman, Stephen T. McGarvey, Henry Madsen, Zhou Xiao-Nong and Steven Riley

Summary

History

Asiatic schistosomosis is a very old disease with *Schistosoma japonicum* eggs found in human remains >2000 years old from Hunan and Hubei provinces in China (Mao and Shao 1982). The original description of Asiatic schistosomosis was made by Fujii in 1847 (Sasa 1972). The life cycle was first described by Kawanashi (1904) who noted trematode-like eggs in cat faeces. The same year, Katsurada recovered adult worms from a cat from Katayama, Japan (Okabe 1964). Fujinami and Nakamura (1909) first reported skin infection with *S. japonicum* cercariae of different mammals, and Miyairi and Suzuki (1914) discovered that *Oncomelania hupensis* served as intermediate host where miracidia developed into sporocysts and further into cercariae (Jordan 2000). The snail hosts of *S. japonicum* were discovered in China by Faust and Meleney (1923), the Philippines by Tubangui (1932) and in Indonesia by Carvey *et al.* (1973). In addition to the skin as the principal route of infection, Suda (1924) described oral infection and several authors described the intrauterine route of infection (Okabe 1964; Sasa 1972).

Following the understanding of the lifecycle, control measures including wearing closely woven clothing, composting of faeces with urine for at least 14 days, replacing cattle with horses, killing of rodents especially rats, killing of snails by lime, copper sulphate or salt water, were proven to have some efficacy. In Japan, an effective integrated control programme started after the Second World War with the last human case being reported in 1978 (Jordan 2000). The National Schistosomosis Control Programme in China started in 1955 and at that time more than 10 million people were infected with *S. japonicum* (Wu 2002). Emetine and antimony potassium tartrate were among the first drugs with proven efficacy against schistosomosis in humans. Later antimony and finally praziquantel and artemether have been introduced as highly effective drugs with only minor adverse effects (Wu 2002).

The agent

Taxonomy and anatomy

The zoonotic schistosomes all belong to the genera *Schistosoma* of the family Schistosomatidae which are dioecious Digenea belonging to the class Trematoda. The main zoonotic schistosomes are found in the *S. japonicum* species group, which comprises *S. japonicum* from the People's Republic of China, Taiwan, Japan, Sulawesi and the Philippines, *S. mekongi* from Laos and Cambodia, *S. malayensis* from the Malaysian Peninsula, *S. sinensium* from Thailand and China (Chilton *et al.* 1999), and *S. ovuncatum* from Thailand (Attwood *et al.* 2002). The former two are zoonotic. Molecular techniques suggest that an ancestral schistosome dispersed from Asia to Africa by mammal migration 12–19 million years ago (Morgan *et al.* 2001). In Asia, the ancestral *Schistosoma* branched as the *S. japonicum* group (Lockyer *et al.* 2003).

Sexual dimorphism in schistosomes is unique among trematodes. Adult females of *S. japonicum* and *S. mekongi* measure 15–30 mm in length whereas males are smaller (Rollingson and Simpson 1987). Both male and female worms have oral and ventral suckers, an oesophagus, a bifurcated intestine joins to form a blind caecum, and an oral mouth opening in the anterior end which also serves as the anus. But the oral suckers are much better developed in males. The male has a gynaecophoric (ventral groove) in which the female permanently resides. The male of *S. japonicum* has 7 testes located posterior to the ventral sucker. Female worms have a single ovary and a uterus which leads to a genital opening near the ventral sucker (Rollingson and Simpson 1987). All *S. japonicum* males have tubercules and bosses on the posterior area close to the tail tip, suckers and gynaecophoris canal, but not on their surface and spines (Rollingson and Simpson 1987).

Zoonotic potential of schistosomosis

Among the schistosomes infecting humans, *S. japonicum* alone has significant zoonotic transmission. It is unique among helminth zoonoses as the infection is transmitted naturally between man and other mammals and maintained by all species (Nelson 1975). Using microsatellite DNA markers, Wang *et al.* (2006) were able to demonstrate that the same *S. japonicum* population was shared among seven different mammalian species living in the same villages. Besides humans, 40 different mammalian species, belonging to 28 genera and seven orders, are considered reservoir hosts for *S. japonicum* (Chen 1993). However, it is likely that only about ten species play a significant role in transmission (Carabin *et al.* 2005; Wang *et al.* 2005, 2006). The epidemiological importance of each host is based on the actual contribution from each host species, which can be determined by number of hosts, prevalence and intensity of infection, amount of faeces produced, egg hatchability and habitat contamination potential (Wang *et al.* 2005). Transmission in a given area has been shown to be highly dynamic and complex and significantly influenced by local biological and cultural factors (Wang *et al.* 2005).

S. mansoni has frequently been found in rodents and non-human primates, and *S. haematobium* has also been detected in non-human primates, but these hosts are believed not to contribute significantly to infection of humans (Taylor 1987). The true zoonotic potential of *S. mekongi* has yet to be elucidated, but from P.R. Laos a prevalence of 10% in pigs has been reported (Standgaard *et al.* 2001).

Strain variation of S. japonicum

Important geographical variations in *S. japonicum* species have been found among China, the Philippines, Japan, Taiwan and Indonesia regarding morphological, biological, and immunological aspects and responses to chemotherapy (Cheever *et al.* 1980; Hsû and Hsû 1962; Kresina *et al.* 1991; Moloney *et al.* 1985; Ruff *et al.* 1973; Sobhon *et al.* 1986).

S. japonicum differ within mainland China regarding genetics, morphology, pathogenicity, and drug responses (Chilton *et al.* 1999; Gasser *et al.* 1996; He *et al.* 1991, 1994; Wang and Mao 1989). He *et al.* (1994) reviewed five *S. japonicum* isolates from China and found significant variation in worm size, testes number, eggs' size and shape, pre-patent period, snail infectivity, host/parasite compatibility, pathogenesis, immune responses and host response to chemotherapy. They concluded that at least four distinct strains (Yunnan, Guangxi, Sishuan, Anhui-Hubei) exist. These results were confirmed through random amplified polymorphic DNA technique (Gasser *et al.* 1996) and allozyme electrophoresis (Chilton *et al.* 1999) using seven isolates from different locations in China, leading Chilton *et al.* (1999) to suggest that a species complex exist. Strains from PR China are thought to be significantly different from strains found in the Philippines (Rudge *et al.* 2009).

Life cycle of S. japonicum

Adult schistosomes live in pairs in the mesenteric veins of the definitive host, specifically large intestinal veins for large animal hosts and small intestinal veins for rodents (Johansen *et al.* 2000). *S. japonicum* females produce 1,000–3,000 eggs per day. Each egg contains an embryo, which matures to a miracidium in 9–12 days and may survive for up to 3 weeks (see Fig. 55.1 for life cycle of *S. japonicum*). The miracidium excretes histolytic enzymes which facilitates its passage from the venules to the gut lumen. Eggs excreted with faeces may hatch in freshwater if temperature (15–30°C) and light conditions are favourable. Free swimming miracidia must penetrate an *Oncomelania* spp. snail host within hours to survive. Upon penetration, the miracidium develops to a primary sporocyst which yields fork-tailed cercariae-producing secondary sporocysts. Stimulated by light and water temperatures above 15°C, cercariae are shed from the snail. The pre-patent period in the snail is influenced by water temperature ranging from 48 days at 30°C to 160 days at 17°C. In freshwater, cercaria can survive for up to 2–3 days. Upon water contact cercariae penetrate the skin of a definitive host using proteolytic enzymes. The cercariae, called schistosomula following transformation in the epidermis, lose their tails and migrate via the venous circulation to

the lungs and systemic circulation. In about 4 weeks, they reach the liver where males and females mate and finally lodge in the mesenteric vessels. The pre-patent period for *S. japonicum* is 42 days in humans. The adult worms may survive in the host for many years (Chen and Mott 1980).

Both oral and congenital infections (natural and experimental) of the definitive hosts are reported from several animal species. Congenital transmission was first described in dogs in 1911 but has since been described in humans, cattle, goats, sheep, mice, guinea pigs, pigs, and rabbits (Okabe 1964; Sasa 1972; Johansen and Ørnbjerg 2005). Experimental infections of sows during mid to late pregnancy results in nearly 100% patent infection in piglets. Infection in early pregnancy results in high percentage of stillbirths and neonatal deaths (Willingham *et al.* 1999). Congenital infections also change the pathogenesis, and the host response to post-natal infections and to treatment after birth (Johansen and Ørnbjerg 2005).

The intermediate host of S. japonicum

The schistosome species in Southeast Asia are transmitted by prosobranch snails belonging to two subfamilies, Pomatiopsinae and the Triculinae, of the family Pomatiopsidae (Caenogastropoda: Rissooidea). Certain subspecies of *Oncomelania hupensis* (Pomatiopsidae: Pomatiopsinae) are known to transmit *S. japonicum* (Rollinson and Southgate 1987). Some of these subspecies, however, should be recognized as a full species, i.e. *O. quadrasi* (Woodruff *et al.* 1988; Hope and McManus 1994) and *O. lindoensis* (Woodruff *et al.* 1999). *S. mekongi*, which primarily infects humans

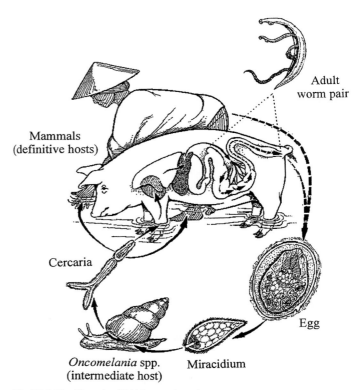

Fig. 55.1 The life cycle of *Schistosoma japonicum*

along the Mekong river of Laos and Cambodia, is transmitted by *Neotricula aperta* (Pomatiopsidae: Triculinae). Three strains of *N. aperta* have been identified (Davis *et al.* 1976). All three strains are able to act as host for *S. mekongi* but only the γ-strain is known to be epidemiologically significant (Attwood *et al.* 1997). In Malaysia, *S. malayensis* infects mainly rodents but can also infect humans and the intermediate hosts are species of *Robertsiella* (Pomatiopsidae: Triculinae) (Davis and Greer 1980; Attwood *et al.* 2005).

Oncomelania hupensis ssp. with some variation among subspecies are small, amphibious and dioecious snails. Females tend to be larger than males. Eggs are laid singly on solid objects. Hatching occurs after 10–25 days, depending on temperature, and newly-hatched snails pass through an aquatic stage of 1–2 weeks. Snails reach sexual maturity after 10–16 weeks and may live for 24–35 weeks. Their reproductive potential is low compared to the pulmonate snails and recolonization of sites treated with molluscicide may take 1–2 years. *Oncomelania hupensis* ssp. inhabit flood plains and especially man-made habitats, resulting from agricultural development, drainage channels, roadside ditches, rice fields, and small canals and drainage canals of irrigation works, are important. Snails are found primarily on the banks but some are also found in very shallow water (i.e. depth less than 20 cm). Habitats preferred by *O. hupensis* are shaded by vegetation, and the temperature is relatively constant and cool. Water current speeds above 0.14 m/s are generally unfavourable for *O. hupensis*.

Tricula aperta is found in parts of the Mekong and Mun rivers where it clings to rocks, twigs and other solid objects in running, well-aerated, clear water (Upatham *et al.* 1980). Population densities appear to be controlled by the annual variation in the water level of the river. During the rainy season the flow is torrential and the species seems to persist as eggs attached to the underside of stones. Female snails live less than a year and apparently lay large numbers of eggs prior to the onset of the rains. *Robertsiella kaporensis* may be found in small streams attached to rocks, leaves and twigs, but are most abundant in overgrown areas where they attach to roots (Greer *et al.* 1980).

Epidemiology of *S. japonicum*

Human distribution and risk factors

Schistosoma infections are reported from China, the Philippines and certain areas of Indonesia (King 2009).

Most risk factors for human *S. japonicum* infection are linked to water contact behaviour. Some studies report an association between the frequency and duration of water contact and infection (Maszle *et al.* 1998; Ross *et al.* 1998; Wu *et al.* 1993), although measurement of water contact is inconsistent (Payne *et al.* 2006). Occupations involving frequent water contact are thus associated with the highest prevalence of infection (Blas *et al.* 2004; Spear *et al.* 2004; Huang and Manderson 2005; Tarafder *et al.* 2006). The prevalence of infection tends to peak at adolescence (Domingo *et al.* 1980; Olveda *et al.* 1996) and is independent of water contact activities (Ross *et al.* 2001), due to the ubiquitous water contact in these resource-poor subsistence societies. Males generally show higher prevalences than females (Wu *et al.* 1993; Olveda *et al.* 1996; Ross *et al.* 1997; Acosta *et al.* 2002) and peaks of infection occur earlier in males than females (Olveda *et al.* 1983; Ross *et al.* 1997; Tarafder *et al.* 2006). Preventive factors include

high socio-economic status (household wealth and income, and education) (Huang and Manderson 2005; Spear *et al.* 2004) and a previous history of infection (Ellis *et al.* 2007; Olds *et al.* 1996; Olveda *et al.* 1996). Some large scale, community-based factors have also been found to be associated with the prevalence of infection. These include climate change and water management (Blas *et al.* 2004; Maszle *et al.* 1998; Yang *et al.* 2005; Zheng *et al.* 2002), and levels of infection in animals (Guo *et al.* 2006; Jiang *et al.* 1996; McGarvey *et al.* 2006; Wang *et al.* 2005).

Animal distribution and risk factors

It is believed that human contribution to schistosomosis transmission has been greatly reduced in China over the past decades, which has increased the relative contribution of primarily domestic animals. In China, cattle and water buffaloes play a major role in transmission due to the high number of animals, high prevalence, frequent contact with infested waters and large volume of faeces produced (Wang *et al.* 2005). In contrast, the prevalence of infection in water buffaloes was found to be very low in Samar Province of the Philippines (Fernandez *et al.* 2007), where there was a cross-sectional association between the village-level intensity of infection in cats and dogs and the intensity of infection in humans (McGarvey *et al.* 2006). In China, cattle are generally found with significantly higher prevalences compared to water buffaloes in areas where they are grazing together despite the fact that buffaloes have much more water contact than cattle (Dai *et al.* 2004). Age-related resistance is seen in mainly water buffaloes after repeated exposure in the second grazing season (Wang *et al.* 2005). However, it is possible that the role that these draught animals play in transmission will change as they are being replaced by tractors. Pigs are also important reservoirs in certain regions due to their numbers and size, relatively high prevalence and often free grazing in infested habitats (Shi *et al.* 1992). After approximately 3 months of an acute infection, pigs tend to undergo self-cure (Hurst *et al.* 2000). Goats are highly susceptible to *S. japonicum* and with an increase in goat farming, especially in China their importance for transmission of schistosomosis needs to be assessed (Zhang *et al.* 1998). In Samar province of the Philippines, Fernandez *et al.* (2007) found that the prevalence of infection in animals, when adjusted for misclassification error, was extremely variable from village to village. This suggests that there may be clustering of different strains in villages within the same province. In 29 of 50 villages studies, the prevalence was highest in rats, followed by dogs, and then by pigs and cats. The prevalence was highest in dogs in 18 villages. In China, Wang *et al.* (1998) found low prevalences of infection in cats and dogs. Although horses, mules and donkeys have been found naturally infected with *S. japonicum,* they are among the least susceptible livestock (Mao 1990).

More than 20 species of wild mammals have been found infected with *S. japonicum* of which the rat (*Rattus norvegicus*) has been found with the highest prevalence; 88% in China (Xu and Li 1992) and 29.5% in 50 villages of the Samar province of the Philippines (Fernandez *et al.* 2007).

Transmission dynamics

Mathematical transmission models have helped us to improve our understanding of schistosomosis epidemiology (Anderson and May 1992) and of the relative effectiveness of control programmes, by giving greater insight into available data.

The structure of models used and the degree of inference used with the models has varied widely for *S. japonicum*. Complex models of transmission have been produced using data from China (Spear *et al.* 2004), the Philippines (Ishikawa *et al.* 2006) and Cambodia for *S. mekongi* (Hisakane *et al.* 2008), producing useful region-specific results.

Three studies have assessed the role of non-human definitive hosts in transmission. Williams *et al.* (2002) used data from bovine and human infections in China to compare four control strategies. Initial human treatment combined with a 45% efficacious bovine vaccine and improvement in human sanitation or reduction in water contact was found to lead to the elimination of the parasite. In the Philippines, Riley *et al.* (2005) developed an initial transmission model using community data from 1981, before widespread praziquantel use, to provide an estimate of endemic equilibrium. This model suggested that differences in infection intensity between villages were caused by differences in both the infection and recovery processes in humans. In a more recent model, data from 50 villages in the Philippines on humans and other animals, and adjusted for specificities and sensitivities of the measurement techniques were used (Riley *et al.* 2008). The results suggested that human to human transmission was more important than transmission from other mammals to humans. Also, the process of infection from snails to mammals was found to drive differences in transmission between villages, rather than the process of infection from mammals to snails.

Pathology of *S. japonicum*

Pathogenesis and clinical manifestations in humans

The adult worms of *S. japonicum* live in the mesenteric veins. Pathology is mainly due to eggs that are swept up into the liver and eggs that damage the intestinal sub-mucosa as they migrate through the intestinal wall to be passed in stool.

Over half of the thousands of eggs released by mature female worms remain trapped in host tissues (Smith and Christie 1986). Eggs swept up into the liver cause the most significant pathology, inducing a granulomatous response that ultimately progresses to focal areas of fibrosis or scarring. Many host-specific factors including age, gender, and type of host immune response to egg antigens modify this risk (Coutinho *et al.* 2007; Booth *et al.* 2004). Though early stage liver fibrosis can be modified with treatment, late stage fibrosis is not reversible. Progressive liver fibrosis results in portal hypertension, which leads to splenomegaly, esophageal varices, and upper gastrointestinal bleeding, the latter being the most common cause of death. Even eggs that successfully leave the mesenteric veins en route to the gut lumen may cause organ pathology. Secretions of the miracidium contain proteolytic enzymes that lyse tissue, aiding migration to the sub-mucosa of the intestinal wall. Occasionally, eggs become trapped, leading to granulomatous inflammation and colonic and rectal polyposis, which can result in significant blood loss (Warren 1982).

This passage of eggs through the gut wall, even without development of significant polyps, is thought to contribute to schistosomosis-related anaemia from chronic, occult, gastrointestinal blood loss. However, extra-corporal blood loss, with attendant iron loss, likely contributes to anaemia among those with high egg burdens (Kanzaria *et al.* 2005; Ndamba *et al.* 1991). Recent studies have shown that increased inflammatory response to egg antigens increases the risk of anaemia, which suggest anaemia of

inflammation (Leenstra *et al.* 2006a; Leenstra *et al.* 2006b), rather than gastrointestinal blood loss or other potential mechanisms (Friedman *et al.* 2005). Regardless of the etiology, *S. japonicum*-associated anaemia is an important contributor to disability weights, as it is one of the main causes of schistosomosis-related disability (Finklestein *et al.* 2008; King *et al.* 2005).

The chronic inflammatory state driven by adult worms and eggs also contribute to under-nutrition. There are two primary ways in which cytokines may impact nutritional status. The first is through appetite suppression or anorexia induced by TNF-α and IL-6 (Arnalich *et al.* 1997; Mantovani *et al.* 1998). The second way in which these cytokines may impact nutritional status is through their potent catabolic effects, leading to weight loss and tissue wasting (Kotler 2000).

The three major schistosome species that infect humans have all been related to protein energy malnutrition in human populations (Stephenson 1993). A randomized clinical trial in Leyte, the Philippines, demonstrated a causal link between *S. japonicum* infection and decreased adiposity (McGarvey *et al.* 1996). Finally, longitudinal studies at the same site demonstrated improvement in body mass index Z-scores (BMIZ) following treatment after adjustment for confounders (Coutinho *et al.* 2006). High intensity reinfection at 18 months was associated with significantly less absolute growth from baseline compared to lower intensity and no reinfection.

A final important clinical manifestation of schistosomosis infection is decreased cognitive function. A randomized controlled trial of praziquantel among *S. japonicum* infected children in China found that younger children in the treatment group showed significant improvement in tests of cognitive function only three months after chemotherapeutic cure (Nokes *et al.* 1999). A separate, cross-sectional study conducted in the Philippines demonstrated that *S. japonicum* infection was associated with poor performance on tests of learning, after controlling for confounders (Ezeamama *et al.* 2005).

Clinical manifestations in animals

Schistosomosis japonica is a disease with a wide range of manifestations depending primarily on the host species, intensity of infection, time of first exposure, and acquired immunity. Cattle, sheep and goats are generally more susceptible than water buffaloes whereas horses and some rodent species are almost refractory (Mao 1990).

The main clinical symptoms are related to the early egg excretion phase and include fever, diarrhoea, anorexia, eosinophilia and anaemia. In heavy infections coughing, bloody diarrhoea, growth reduction, emaciation and death can be seen especially in young animals (Dumag *et al.* 1980; Hurst *et al.* 2000; Johansen *et al.* 2000). Gross pathological lesions, which are primarily associated with the tissue-deposited eggs, are seen in both the intestine and in the liver, correlate with intensity of infection, and peak around time of maximum egg excretion (Johansen *et al.* 2000). Lesions in the intestines include haemorrhages occasionally with ulcerations and thrombophlebitis in the mesenteric vessels (Hurst *et al.* 2000). In the liver, hepatomegaly, enlargement of lymph nodes, and disseminated small grey-white nodules are common findings as is portal and interlobular fibrosis. Ascites is another common chronic manifestation. Egg induced lesions may also be found in lungs, brain, spleen, kidney and lymph nodes (Cheever 1985).

Diagnosis of S. *japonicum* in animals and humans

There is no gold standard for the diagnosis of schistosomosis in humans or animals.

In humans, the most widely used method of diagnosis for large-scale epidemiological studies and surveillance is the Kato-Katz, which involves clearing a measured volume (weight) of faeces using a glycerine-impregnated cellophane coverslip (Feldmeier and Poggensee 1993). This technique detects current infection but presents obvious identification problems due to the uncharacteristic shape of the eggs resembling protozoan cysts, air bubbles, pollen and debris. Furthermore, the sensitivity of the test declines with decreasing intensity of infection (Yu *et al.* 1998; Lin *et al.* 2008; Tarafder *et al.* 2006). To overcome this problem, antibody detection in serum has been extensively used, especially indirect haemagglutination assay (IHA) and ELISA with soluble egg antigen (Wu 2002). The issue with this approach is that it detects both past and present infection and presents cross reactions with other helminth infections. A commonly used diagnostic strategy has therefore been to screen for antibodies and subsequently examine the stool of seropositive individuals using Kato-Katz or hatching test (Zhou *et al.* 2007). Polymerase Chain Reaction (PCR) test has the potential for high sensitivity and specificity. Lier *et al.* (2006) first published the development of a PCR for detection of S. *japonicum* and determined that the seroprevalence using an IHA was much higher (26.1%) than the prevalence in stool-based tests which were 5.3%, 3.2% and 3.0% for PCR, hatching test and Kato-Katz thick smear, respectively.

In animals, the hatching test for S. *japonicum* is exclusively used in China. The method has potentially high sensitivity as large samples are used but the method is difficult to standardize as hatching is influenced by a range of abiotic and biotic factors and immature eggs are not likely to hatch and eggs excreted from different host species have different hatching rates (Yu *et al.* 2007). The method

has primarily been used for cattle and water buffaloes but Wang *et al.* (2005) applied the method to a range of domestic animals and found that prevalence and intensity of the infection varied significantly between species and areas, highlighting the importance of more accurate data to determine cost-effective control strategies. Sedimentation tests are numerous, but are most often only qualitative, lack sensitivity and precision, are too time-consuming and not at all standardized. The tedious microscopy of the sediment makes this approach subject to tremendous potential reader-bias. Willingham *et al.* (1999) developed a combined filtration, sedimentation and centrifugation technique (DBL-method) for counting S. *japonicum* in pig faeces. The method is quantitative, uses no hazardous chemicals, is simple and as eggs remain alive, viability is easily assessed.

In all definitive hosts, it has been shown that the sensitivity of the stool examination increases with the number of stool samples provided over consecutive days while the specificity decreases (Table 55.1). This is because *Schistosoma* eggs are not shed regularly from day to day (Yu *et al.* 1998). The sensitivity of the test is particularly poor among subject providing one stool sample and with low intensity of infection (Zhang *et al.* 2009). The sensitivity and specificity of the Kato-Katz for S. *japonicum* with different numbers of stool samples has not been determined.

Treatment of S. *japonicum*

Human treatment

Praziquantel remains the mainstay of treatment for human schistosomosis globally. Praziquantel was released in 1979 and ultimately proved to be more efficacious and safer than its predecessors. Interestingly, praziquantel's mechanism of action against schistosomes remains poorly understood.

Two special populations warrant further consideration. First, praziquantel was never studied in pregnant or lactating women, thus necessitating its designation as a Pregnancy Class B drug,

Table 55.1 The sensitivity of the stool examination increases with the number of stool samples provided over consecutive days while the specificity decreases

| | | Species | | | | |
		Water buffaloes	Cats	Dogs	Pigs	Rats
Sensitivity	1 stool sample	78.0 (47.6–95.7)	65.0 (48.3–79.6)	75.0 (67.1–82.3)	77.1 (56.6–95.7)	76.8 (62.1–88.7)
	2 stool samples	95.2 (72.5–99.8)	87.7 (73.2–95.8)	93.8 (89.2–96.9)	94.8 (81.2–99.8)	94.6 (85.6–98.7)
	3 stool samples	98.9 (85.6–100)	95.7 (86.2–99.2)	98.4 (96.5–99.5)	98.8 (91.8–100)	98.7 (94.5–99.9)
	4 stool samples	99.8 (92.4–100)	99.5 (96.3–100)	99.6 (98.8–99.9)	99.9 (98.5–100)	99.7 (97.9–100)
	5 stool samples	100 (96.0–100)	99.5 (96.3–100)	100 (99.6–100)	99.9 (98.5–100)	100 (99.2–100)
Specificity	1 stool sample	98.7 (96.8–99.7)	97.2 (95.2–98.8)	97.0 (95.2–98.3)	99.1 (98.4–99.6)	92.6 (87.0–97.2)
	2 stool samples	97.4 (93.7–99.4)	94.4 (90.6–97.6)	94.1 (90.6–96.6)	98.2 (96.8–99.2)	85.7 (75.7–94.5)
	3 stool samples	96.2 (90.7–99.1)	91.8 (86.2–96.4)	91.3 (86.3–95.0)	97.3 (95.2–98.8)	79.4 (65.9–91.8)
	4 stool samples	94.9 (87.8–98.8)	89.3 (82.1–95.3)	88.5 (82.1–93.4)	96.4 (93.8–98.4)	73.5 (57.3–89.3)
	5 stool samples	93.7 (85.0–98.5)	86.8 (78.2–94.1)	85.9 (78.2–91.8)	95.6 (92.3–98.0)	68.0 (49.8–86.8)

Reproduced from Carabin *et al.* (2005), with permission from Elsevier.

which has led to withholding treatment in these women in most schistosomosis endemic countries. In 2002, WHO suggested that all schistosomosis infected pregnant and lactating women should be considered as a high-risk group and be offered treatment individually or during treatment campaigns (Allen *et al.* 2002). However, many nations have not adopted this strategy, and await results of ongoing studies in sub-Saharan Africa and the Philippines. Another group often excluded from treatment is young children. Most school based programs will miss children under the age of six, despite the growing realization that young children are infected and likely contribute to transmission (Stothard and Gabrielli 2007).

Animal treatment

Despite evidence that animals transmit and seriously suffer from zoonotic schistosomosis, only few examples of integration of animal treatment in schistosomosis control programmes exist (Chen 1971; Chen 2005; Jiang *et al.* 2002). Using a mathematical model, Williams *et al.* (2002) suggested a combination of human and bovine treatment as it would significantly reduce human prevalence and maintain the reduction for an extended period of time. Praziquantel has been shown to be highly effective against all zoonotic scistosomes in a range of animal species (King and Mahmoud 1989). The recommended dose of praziquantel varies depending on the animal host. Effective doses for water buffaloes are 25 mg/kg, cattle 30 mg/kg, pigs 40 mg/kg and goats require 60 mg/kg due to their very fast metabolism (King and Mahmoud 1989; Johansen 1996; Wang *et al.* 2006). Effectiveness of a single dose of praziquantel applied orally wrapped in tree leaves was assessed in lowland China. The drug efficacy was 97% but as reinfection after treatment was high and occurred throughout the year in both cattle and water buffaloes, the strategy did not effectively prevent transmission (Wang *et al.* 2006). New evidence-based strategies for integrated control of animal schistosomosis are needed to reduce transmission and improve the health and productivity of the animals. Promising DNA-based vaccines have recently been developed and tested showing reduction in both worm load and an anti-fecundity effect in cattle, water buffaloes and pigs (Shi *et al.* 2002; Wu *et al.* 2004).

Prevention and control of S. *japonicum*

Great control efforts have been made in all endemic countries to control and eliminate infection. Schistosomosis' elimination in Japan was achieved throught snail control strategy combined with social-economic development during the 1960s and 1970s (Tanaka and Tsuji 1997; WHO 2001). The snail control strategy involved environmental modification in isolated endemic areas, which was also applied to the Bohol island in the southern Philippines (Ebisawa 1998; Yasuraoka *et al.* 1989).

Schistosomosis control in China could be considered as exemplary (Wang *et al.* 2008a). The national control programme has achieved elimination of the disease from five out of 12 formerly endemic provinces by using several resources and approaches. Substantial progress has also been made in most of the remaining endemic areas (Wu *et al.* 2006) and the estimated total number of infected people has reduced by over 90% since 1950 (Wang *et al.*

2008b). A 2004 nationwide survey estimated that 720,000 people are infected (Zhou *et al.* 2007), while a 2008 study estimated that 412,000 people are infected (Hao *et al.* 2009). There is hope of future national elimination through treatment of water buffaloes in marshland and lake regions (Wang *et al.* 2009a; King 2009; Wang *et al.* 2009b).

Schistosomosis is believed to be endemic in 28 provinces in the Philippines, including most of the Mindanao region, the eastern part of the Visayas and a few provinces in Luzon. Before the 1980s, the government focused on health education, limiting human exposure to the infective form of the parasite, and efforts to break the parasite life cycle through control of the intermediate host snail using agro-engineering methods and environmental modification (Leonardo *et al.* 2002). Environmental modifications in combination with molluscicides were found to be too expensive. In 1978, community-based praziquantel treatment became the main approach to control schistosomosis. This period saw dramatic decreases in the national prevalence of *S. japonicum* infection (Olveda 2006). The most impressive impact was attributed to the implementation of the Philippines Health Development Plan in 1990–95. The National Schistosomosis Control Service was able to intensify case finding and treatment in all endemic areas and reduced the national prevalence from more than 10% before 1990 to less than 5% after 1995 (Hernandez 2003). However, the presence of animal reservoirs was believed to limit the effectiveness of chemotherapy alone at eliminating schistosomosis. Interruption of treatment for more than two years resulted in rebound morbidity and intensity of *S. japonicum* infection (Leonardo *et al.* 2002).

Only two isolated areas are endemic in Indonesia, namely Lindu valley and Napu valley, both located in the Province of Central Sulawesi (Hadidjaja 1985). Over the past six decades, schistosomosis control has been implemented and the average prevalence is now much lower. In 2006, the prevalences were 0.5% in seven villages in Lindu valley and 1.1% in 17 villages of Napu valley, respectively. The corresponding prevalence of infection in snails ranged from 0–13.4% and 0–9.1%, respectively (Garjito *et al.* 2008). The present data indicate that transmission of schistosomosis is ongoing despite regular surveillance and control activities covering the whole endemic area.

Strong political commitment is a key element in successful control, which requires persistent efforts and a systematic step-by-step approach with increasingly ambitious targets to reach elimination (Wang *et al.* 2009b). There are several limitations to the above-mentioned achievements. First, the successful snail control programmes in Japan were not duplicated elsewhere (Leonardo *et al.* 2008). Second, the case-detection and praziquantel treatment approach renewed hopes of achieving control with limited resources. Third, the poor sensitivity of the Kato-Katz analysis using a single stool sample underestimates the true prevalence of infection (Lin *et al.* 2008a; Zhou *et al.* 2008; Zhang *et al.* 2009). Fourth, a reduction in coverage of the treatment (Tallo *et al.* 2008) strongly suggests that chemotherapy-based programmes must be combined with other control measures until an alternative, more effective approach, has been developed (e.g. vaccination) (Utzinger *et al.* 2005). Fifth, schistosomosis japonica have re-emerged, in terms of the total number of infected cases, in areas where transmission control and interruption had been declared previously (Liang *et al.* 2006) following the termination of chemotherapy programmes (Utzinger *et al.* 2005). The ongoing transmission in other endemic areas, albeit at a lower level, is also of considerable concern as the situation is likely to deteriorate as soon as control efforts are scaled down (Utzinger *et al.* 2005; Wang *et al.* 2008b). It is crucial for continued success to maintain and sustain the current efforts to further reduce transmission, through integration with other diseases control programmes.

References

Acosta, L.P., Aligui, G.D., Tiu, W.U., McManus, D.P., Olveda, R.M. (2002). Immune correlate study on human *Schistosoma japonicum* in a well-defined population in Leyte, Philippines: I. Assessment of 'resistance' versus 'susceptibility' to *S. japonicum* infection. *Acta Trop.,* **84**: 127–36.

Allen, H.E., Crompton, D.W., De Silva, N., Loverde, P.T. & Olds, G.R. (2002). New policies for using anthelmintics in high risk groups. *Trends Parasitol.,* **18**: 381–82.

Anderson, R.M. & May, R.M. (1992). Infectious disease of humans: dynamics and control. Oxford: Oxford Science Publications.

Arnalich, F., Martinez, P., Hernanz, A. *et al.* (1997). Altered concentrations of appetite regulators may contribute to the development and maintenance of HIV-associated wasting. *Aids,* **11**: 1129–34.

Attwood, S.W., Fatih, F.A., Mondal, M.M. *et al.* (2007). A DNA sequence based study of the *Schistosoma indicum* (Trematoda: Digenea) group; population phylogeny, taxonomy and historical biogeography. *Parasitology,* **134**: 2009–20.

Attwood, S.W., Kitikoon, V., Southgate, V.R. (1997). Infectivity of a Cambodian isolate of *Schistosoma mekongi* to *Neotricula aperta* from Northeast Thailand. *J. helminthol.,* **71**: 183–87.

Attwood, S.W., Lokman, H.S., Ong, K.Y. (2005). *Robertsiella silvicola*, a new species of triculine snail (Caenogastropoda: Pomatiopsidae) from peninsular Malaysia, intermediate host of *Schistosoma malayensis* (Trematoda: Digenea). *J. Molluscan Stud.,* **71**: 379–91.

Attwood, S.W., Panasoponkul, C., Uptam, E.S. *et al.* (2002). *Schistosoma ovuncatum* n. sp. (Digenea: Schistosomatidae) from Northwest Thailand and the historical biogeography of Southeast Asian *Schistosoma* Weinland 1858. *System. Parasit.,* **51**: 1–19.

Blas, B.L., Rosales, M.I., Lipayon, I.L. *et al.* (2004). The schistosomosis problem in the Philippines: a review. *Parasitol. Int.,* **53**: 127–34.

Booth, M., Mwatha, J.K., Joseph, S. *et al.* (2004). Periportal fibrosis in human Schistosoma mansoni infection is associated with low IL-10, low IFN-gamma, high TNF-alpha, or low RANTES, depending on age and gender. *J. Immunol.,* **172**: 1295–303.

Carabin, H., Balolong, E., Joseph, L. *et al.* (2005). Estimating sensitivity and specificity of a faecal examination method for *Schistosoma japonicum* infection in cats, dogs, water buffaloes, pigs, and rats in Western Samar and Sorsogon Provinces, The Philippines. *Int. J. Parasitol.,* **35**: 1517–24.

Cheever, A.M. (1985). A review: *Schistosoma japonicum*: the pathology of experimental infection. *Exp. Parasitol.,* **59**: 1–11.

Cheever, A.W., Rodney, H., Duvall, H., Minker, R.G. (1980). Quantitative parasitologic findings in rabbits infected with Japanese and Philippine strains of *Schistosoma japonicum. Am. J. Trop. Med. Hyg.,* **29**: 1307–15.

Chen, M.G. (1993). *Schistosoma japonicum* and *S. japonicum*-like infections–epidemiology, clinical and pathological aspects. In: P. Jordan, G. Webbe, and R.F. Sturruck (ed.) *Human schistosomisis,* pp. 242–43. Oxford: CAB International.

Chen, M.G. (2005). Use of praziquantel for clinical treatment and morbidity control of schistosomosis japonica in China: a review of 30 years' experience. *Acta Trop.,* **96**: 168–76.

Chen, M.G. and Mott, K.E. (1988). Progress in assessment of morbidity due to *Schistosoma japonicum* infection. *Trop. Dis. Bull.,* **85**: 1–45.

Chen, T.H. (1971). Schistosomosis in mainland China, a review of research and control programmes since 1949. *Am. J. Trop. Med. Hyg.,* **20**: 26–53.

Chilton, N.B., Bao-Zhen, Q., Bøgh, H.O., Nansen, P. (1999). An electrophoretic comparison of *Schistosoma japonicum* (Trematoda) from different provinces in the Peoples Republic of China suggests the excistence of cryptic species. *Parasitology,* **119**: 375–83.

Coutinho, H.M., Acosta, L.P., McGarvey, S.T. *et al.* (2006). Nutritional status improves after treatment of schistosoma japonicum-infected children and adolescents. *J. Nutrition,* **136**: 183–81.

Coutinho, H.M., Acosta, L.P., Wu, H.W. *et al.* (2007). Th2 cytokines are associated with persistent hepatic fibrosis in human Schistosoma japonicum infection. *J. Infect. Dis.,* **195**: 288–95.

Dai, Z.J., Yan, J.B., Mao, G.Q., Xie, Z.M., Yang, A.G. (2004). Studies on the epidemiology and controlling methods of livestock schistosomosis in different mountainous epidemic districts. *Southwest China J. Agr. Sci.,* **17**: 393–98.

Davis, G.M. and Greer, G.J. (1980). A new genus and two new species of Triculinae (Gastropoda: Prosobranchia) and the transmission of a Malaysian Mammalian *Schistosoma* sp. *Proc. Acad. Natu. Sci. Philadelphia,* **132**: 245–76.

Davis, G.M., Kitikoon, V., Temcharoen. P. (1976). Monograph On *Lithoglyphopsis aperta* the snail host of Mekong River schistosomosis. *Malacologia,* **15**: 241–87.

Domingo, E.O., Tiu, E., Peters, P.A., Warren, K.S., Mahmoud, A.A., Houser, H.B. (1980). Morbidity in schistosomosis japonica in relation to intensity of infection: study of a community in Leyte, Philippines. *Am. J. Trop. Med. Hyg.,* **29**: 858–67.

Dumag, P.U., Gajudo, C.E., Sefia, C.Y., Cardenas, E.C., Fementira, E.B. (1980). Epidemiology of animal schistosomosis in the Philippines. *Philippine J. Anim. Ind.,* **35**: 1–23.

Ebisawa, I. (1998). Epidemiology and eradication of Schistosomosis japonica in Japan. *J.Travel Med.,* **5**: 33–35.

Ellis, M.K., Zhao, Z.Z., Chen, H.G., Montgomery, G.W., Li, Y.S., McManus, D.P. (2007). Analysis of the 5q31 33 locus shows an association between single nucleotide polymorphism variants in the IL-5 gene and symptomatic infection with the human blood fluke, *Schistosoma japonicum. J. Immunol.,* **179**: 8366–71.

Ezeamama, A.E., Friedman, J.F., Acosta, L.P. *et al.* (2005). Helminth infection and cognitive impairment among Filipino children. *Am. J. Trop. Med. Hyg.,* **72**: 540–81.

Feldmeier, H. and Poggensee, G. (1993). Diagnostic techniques in schistosomosis control. *Acta Trop.,* **55**: 205–20.

Fernandez, T.J., Tarafder, M.R., Balolong, E. *et al.* (2007). Prevalence of *Schistosoma japonicum* infection among animals in 50 villages of Samar Province, The Philippines. *Vector Borne and Zoon. Dis.,* **7**: 147–55.

Finkelstein, J.L., Schleinitz, M.D., Carabin, H., McGarvey, S.T. (2008). Decision-model estimation of the age-specific disability weight for endemic *Schistosoma japonicum* infection in humans. *PLoS Negl. Trop. Dis.,* **2**: e158.

Friedman, J.F., Kanzaria, H.K., McGarvey, S.T. (2005). Human schistosomosis and anemia: the relationship and potential mechanisms. *Trends Parasitol.,* **21**: 386–92.

Garjito, T.A., Sudomo, M., Abdullah, Dahlan, M., Nurwidayati, A. (2008). Schistosomosis in Indonesia: past and present. *Parasitol. Int.,* **57**: 277–80.

Gasser, R.B., Bao-Zhen, Q., Nansen, P., Johansen, M.V., Bøgh, H. (1996). Use of RAPD for the detection of genetic variation in the human blood fluke, *Schistosoma japonicum*, from mainland China. *Mol. Cell. Probes,* **10**: 353–58.

Gray, D.J., Williams, G.M., Li, Y., McManus, D.P. (2008). Transmission Dynamics of *Schistosoma japonicum* in the Lakes and Marshlands of China. *PLoS ONE,* **3**: e4058.

Greer, G.J., Lim, H.K., Ow-Yang, C.K. (1980). Report of a freshwater hydrobiid snail from Pahang, Malaysia: a possible host for schistososomes infecting man. *Southeast Asian J. Trop. Med. Pub. Health,* **11**: 146–47.

Guo, J., Li, Y., Gray, D. *et al.* (2006). A drug-based intervention study on the importance of buffaloes for human *Schistosoma japonicum* infection around Poyang Lake, People's Republic of China. *Am. J. Trop. Med. Hyg.,* **74**: 335–41.

Hadidjaja, P. (1985). *Schistosomosis in central Sulawesi, Indonesia.* Faculty of Medicine, University of Indonesia.

Hao, Y., Zhen, H., Zhu, R. *et al.* (2009). Schistosomosis status in People's Republic of China in 2008. *Chinese J. Schistomiasis Contr.,* **21**: 451–56.

He, Y.X., Hu, Y.Q., Yu, Q.F., *et al.* (1994). Strain complex of *Schistosoma japonicum* in the mainland of China. *Southeast Asian J. Trop. Med. Pub. Health,* **25**: 232–42.

He, Y.X., Li, X.W., Hu, Y.Q. and Yu, Q.F. (1991). Studies on strain differences of *Schistosoma japonicum* in the mainland of China. VI. Analysis with multilocus enzyme electrophoresis. *Chinese J. Parasit. Dis.,* **9**: 290–91.

Hernandez, L.M. (2003). International Symposium on Schistosomosis, September 11–12. Alabang, Muntinlupa City, The Philippines.

Hisakane, N., Kirinoki, M. Chigusa, Y. *et al.* (2008). The evaluation of control measures against Schistosoma mekongi in Cambodia by a mathematical model. *Parasitol. Int.,* **57**: 379–85.

Hope, M. and McManus, D.P. (1994). Genetic variation in geographically isolated populations and subspecies of *Oncomelania hupensis* determined by a PCR-based RFLP method. *Acta Trop.,* **57**: 75–82.

Hsû, H.F. and Hsû, S.Y.L. (1962). *Schistosoma japonicum* in Formosa: a critical review. *Exp. Parasitol.,* **12**: 459–62.

Huang, Y.X. and Manderson, L. (2005). The social and economic context and determinants of schistosomosis japonica. *Acta Trop.,* **96**: 223–31.

Hurst, M.H., Shi, Y.E. and Lindberg, R. (2000). Pathology and course of natural *Schistosoma japonicum* infection in pigs: results of a field study in Hubei province, China. *Ann. Trop. Med. Parasitol.,* **94**: 461–77.

Ishikawa, H., Ohmae, H., Pangilinan, R. *et al.* (2006). Modeling the dynamics and control of Schistosoma japonicum transmission on Bohol island, the Philippines. *Parasitol. Int.,* **55**: 23–29.

Jiang, Q., Zhang, S., Yuan, H., Liu, Z., Zhao, G., Brinkmann, U. (1996). The effect of a combined approach to schistosomosis control on the transmission of Schistosoma japonicum in Xingzi of Poyang Lake area, China. *Southeast Asian J. Trop. Med. Pub. Health,* **27**: 535–41.

Jiang, Q.W., Wang, L.Y., Guo, J.G., Chen, M.G., Zhou, X.N., Engels, D. (2002). Morbidity control of schistosomosis in China. *Acta Trop.,* **82**: 115–25.

Johansen, M.V. (1998). Effect of praziquantel treatment on experimental porcine *Schistosoma japonicum* infection. *Parasitology,* **116**: 519–24.

Johansen, M.V. and Ørnbjerg, N. (2005). Prenatal *Schistosoma japonicum* infection in piglets: effect of repeated exposure of the dams on treatment efficacy and susceptibility of challenge infections. *J. Parasitol.,* **90**: 392–96.

Johansen, M.V., Bøgh, H.O., Nansen, P., Christensen, N.Ø. (2000). *Schistosoma japonicum* infection in the pig as a model for human schistosomosis. *Acta Trop.,* **76**: 85–99.

Jordan, P. (2000). From Katayama to the Dekhla Oakhla Oasis: the beginning of epidemiology and control of bilharzia. *Acta Trop.,* **77**: 9–40.

Kanzaria, H., Acosta, L., Langdon, G. *et al.* (2005). Schistosoma *japonicum* and occult blood loss in endemic villages in Leyte, The Philippines. *Am. J. Trop. Med. Hyg.,* **72**: 115–18.

King, C.H. (2009). Toward the elimination of schistosomosis. *N. Eng. J. Med.,* **360**: 106–9.

King, C.H. and Mahmoud, A.F. (1989). Drugs five years later: praziquantel. *Ann. Intern. Med.,* **110**: 290–96.

King, C.H., Dickman, K., Tisch, D.J. (2005). Reassessment of the cost of chronic helmintic infection: a meta-analysis of disability-related outcomes in endemic schistosomosis. *Lancet,* **365**: 1561–69.

Kotler, D.P. (2000). Cachexia. *Annals of Internernal Medicine,* **133**: 622–34.

Kresina, T.F., Guan, X.H., Posner, M., Ramirez, B., Olds, G.R. (1991). Comparison of immune responses of Chinese and Philippine patients infected with *Schistosoma japonicum.* *Infect. Immun.,* **59**: 4698–700.

Leenstra, T., Acosta, L.P., Langdon, G.C. *et al.* (2006a). Schistosomosis japonica, anemia, and iron status in children, adolescents, and young adults in Leyte, Philippines 1. *Am. J. Clin. Nutr.,* **83**: 371–79.

Leenstra, T., Coutinho, H.M., Acosta, L.P. *et al.* (2006b) *Schistosoma japonicum* Reinfection after Praziquantel Treatment Causes Anemia Associated with Inflammation. *Infect. Immun.,* **74**: 6398–407.

Leonardo, L.R., Acosta, L.P., Olveda, R.M., Aligui, G.D. (2002). Difficulties and strategies in the control of schistosomosis in the Philippines. *Acta Trop.,* **82**: 295–99.

Leonardo, L.R., Rivera, P., Saniel, O. *et al.* (2008). Prevalence survey of schistosomosis in Mindanao and the Visayas, The Philippines. *Parasitol. Int.,* **57**: 246–51.

Liang, S., Yang, C., Zhong, B., and Qiu, D. (2006). Re-emerging schistosomosis in hilly and mountainous areas of Sichuan, China. *Bull. WHO,* **84**: 139–44.

Lier, T., Simonsen, G.S., Wang, T. *et al.* (2009). Real-Time Polymerase Chain Reaction for Detection of Low-Intensity *Schistosoma japonicum* Infections in China. *Am. J. Trop. Med. Hyg.,* **81**: 428–32.

Lier, T., Simonsen, G.S., Haaheim, H., Hjelmevoll, S.O., Vennervald, B.J., Johansen, M.V. (2006). Novel real-time PCR for detection of *Schistosoma japonicum* in stool. *Southeast Asian J. Trop. Med. Pub. Health,* **37**: 257–64.

Lin, D.D., Liu, J.X, Liu, Y.M. *et al.* (2008). Routine Kato-Katz technique underestimates the prevalence of *Schistosoma japonicum*: a case study in an endemic area of the People's Republic of China. *Parasitol. Int.,* **57**: 281–86.

Lockyer, A.E., Olson, P.D., Østergaard, P. *et al.* (2003). The phylogeny of the Schistosomatidae based on three genes with emphasis on the interrelationships of *Schistosoma* Weinland, 1858. *Parasitology,* **126**: 203–24.

Mantovani, G., Maccio, A., Lai, P., Massa, E., Ghiani, M., Santona, M.C. (1998). Cytokine involvement in cancer anorexia/cachexia: role of megestrol acetate and medroxyprogesterone acetate on cytokine downregulation and improvement of clinical symptoms. *Crit. Rev. Oncol.,* **9**: 99–106.

Maszle, D.R., Whitehead, P.G., Johnson, R.C., Spear, R.C. (1998). Hydrological studies of schistosomosis transport in Sichuan Province, China. *Sci. Total Environ.,* **216**: 193–203.

McGarvey, S.T., Aligui, G., Graham, K.K., Peters, P., Olds, G.R., Olveda, R. (1996). Schistosomosis japonica and childhood nutritional status in northeastern Leyte, the Philippines: a randomized trial of praziquantel versus placebo. *Am. J. Trop. Med. Hyg.,* **54**: 498–502.

McGarvey, S.T., Carabin, H., Balolong Jr., E. *et al.* (2006). Cross-sectional associations between intensity of animal and human infection with *Schistosoma japonicum* in Western Samar province, Philippines. *Bull. WHO,* **84**: 446–52.

Moloney, N.A., Garcia, E.G. and Webbe, G. (1985). The strain specificity of vaccination with ultraviolet attenuated cercariae of the Chinese strain of *Schistosoma japonicum.* *Trans. R. Soc. Trop. Med. Hyg.,* **79**: 245–47.

Morgan, J.A.T., De Jong, R.J., Snyder, S.D., Mkoji, G.M. and Loker, E.S. (2001). *Schistosoma mansoni* and *Biomphalaria*: past history and future trends. *Parasitology,* **123**: 211–28.

Ndamba, J., Makaza, N., Kaondera, K.C., Munjoma, M. (1991). Morbidity due to Schistosoma mansoni among sugar-cane cutters in Zimbabwe. *Int. J. Epidemiol.,* **20**: 787–95.

Nelson, G.S. (1975). Schistosomosis. In: W.T. Hubbert, W.F. McCulloch and P.R. Schnurrenberger (eds.) *Diseases transmitted from animals to man,* pp. 620–40. Springfield: Charles C. Thomas.

Nokes, C., McGarvey, S.T., Shiue, L. *et al.* (1999). Evidence for an improvement in cognitive function following treatment of Schistosoma japonicum infection in Chinese primary schoolchildren. *Am. J. Trop. Med. Hyg.,* **60**: 556–65.

Okabe, I. (1964). Biology and epidemiology of *Schistosoma japonicum* and schistosomosis. In: K. Morishita, Y. Komiya and H. Matsubayashi (eds.) *Progress of Medical Parasitology in Japan.* Tokyo: Meguro.

Olds, G.R., Olveda, R., Wu, G. *et al.* (1996). Immunity and morbidity in Schistosomosis japonicum infection. *Am. J. Trop. Med. Hyg.,* **55** (5 Suppl): 121–26.

Olveda, R. M. (2006). Schistosomosis in the Philippines: Accomplishments over the last 100 years. Presented at the International Symposium on Schistosomosis, September 11–12. Alabang, Muntinlupa City, the Philippines.

Olveda, R.M., Daniel, B.L., Ramirez, B.D. *et al.* (1996). Schistosomosis japonica in the Philippines: the long-term impact of population-based chemotherapy on infection, transmission, and morbidity. *J. Infect. Dis.,* **174:** 163–72.

Olveda, R.M., Tiu, E., Fevidal, P. *et al.* (1983). Relationship of prevalence and intensity of infection to morbidity in schistosomosis japonica: a study of three communities in Leyte, Philippines. *Am. J. Trop. Med. Hyg.,* **32:** 1312–21.

Payne, G., Carabin, H., Tallo, V. *et al.* (2006). Concurrent comparison of three water contact measurement tools in four endemic villages of the Philippines. *Trop. Med. Int. Health,* **11:** 834–42.

Riley, S., Carabin, H., Bélisle, P. *et al.* (2008). Multi-host transmission dynamics of Schistosoma japonicum in Samar province, the Philippines. *PLoS Medicine,* **5:** e18.

Riley, S., Carabin, H., Marshall, C. *et al.* (2005). Estimating and modeling the dynamics of the intensity of infection with schistosoma japonicum in villagers of leyte, Philippines. Part II: Intensity-specific transmission of S. japonicum. The schistosomosis transmission and ecology project. *Am. J. Trop. Med. Hyg.,* **72:** 754–61.

Rollingson, D. and Simpson, A.J.G. (1987). *The Biology of Schistosomes. From Genes to Latrines.* London: Academic Press.

Rollinson, D. and Southgate, V.R. (1987). The genus *Schistosoma*: a taxonomic appraisal. In: D. Rollinson and A.J. Simpson (eds.) *The Biology of Schistosomes: From Genes to Latrines*, pp. 149. London: Academic Press.

Ross, A.G., Sleigh, A.C., Li, Y. *et al.* (2001). Schistosomosis in the People's Republic of China: prospects and challenges for the 21st century. *Clin. Microbiol. Rev.,* **14:** 270–95.

Ross, A.G., Yuesheng, L., Sleigh, A.C. *et al.* (1998). Measuring exposure to S. japonicum in China. I. Activity diaries to assess water contact and comparison to other measures. *Acta Trop.,* **71:** 213–28.

Ross, A.G., Yuesheng, L., Sleigh, A.S. *et al.* (1997). Epidemiologic features of *Schistosoma japonicum* among fishermen and other occupational groups in the Dongting Lake region (Hunan Province) of China. *Am. J. Trop. Med. Hyg.,* **57:** 302–8.

Rudge, J.W., Carabin, H., Balolong, E. *et al.* (2008). Population Genetics of *Schistosoma japonicum* within the Philippines Suggest High Levels of Transmission between Humans and Dogs. *PLoS Negl. Trop. Dis.,* **2:** e340.

Ruff, M.D., Davis, G.M., Werner, G. (1973). *Schistosoma japonicum:* protein patterns of the Japanese, Philippine and Formosan strains. *Exp. Parasitol.,* **33:** 437–46.

Sasa, M. (1972). A historical review of the early Japanese contributions to the knowledge of schistosomosis japonica. In: M. Yokogawa (ed.) *Research in filariasis and schistosomosis*, pp. 235–61. Baltimore: University Park Press.

Shi, F., Zhang, Y., Lin, J. *et al.* (2002). Field testing of *Schistosoma japonicum* DNA vaccines in cattle in China. *Vaccine,* **20:** 3629–31.

Shi, Z.G., Hu, S.G., Zhou, Q.Y., Wang, Z.K. & Zhang, Z.G. (1992). The role of pigs in schistosomosis. transmission in Yujiang Village. *Chinese J. Schistosomosis Cont.,* **4:** 293–95.

Smith, J.H. and Christie, J.D. (1986). The pathobiology of Schistosoma haematobium infection in humans. *Human Pathol.,* **17:** 333–45.

Sobhon, P. Koonchornboon, T., Yuan, H.C. *et al.* (1986). Comparison of surphase morphology of adult *Schistosoma japonicum* (Chinese, Philippine and Indonesian strains) by scanning electron microscopy. *Int. J. Parasitol.,* **16:** 205–16.

Spear, R.C., Seto, E., Liang, S. *et al.* (2004). Factors influencing the transmission of *Schistosoma japonicum* in the mountains of Sichuan Province of China. *Am. J. Trop. Med. Hyg.,* **70:** 48–56.

Stephenson, L. (1993). The impact of schistosomosis on human nutrition. *Parasitology,* **107:** S107–23.

Stothard, J.R. and Gabrielli, A.F. (2007). Schistosomosis in African infants and preschool children: to treat or not to treat? *Trends in Parasit.,* **23:** 83–86.

Strandgaard, H., Johansen, M.V., Pholsena, K., Teixayavong, K., Christensen, N.Ø. (2001). The pig as a host for *Schistosoma mekongi* in Laos. *J. Parasitol.,* **87:** 708–9.

Tallo, V.T., Carabin, H., Alday, P., Olveda, R., McGarvey, S.T. (2008). Is mass treatment the appropriate schistosomosis elimination strategy?– Secondary analysis of data collected as part of the Schistosomosis Transmission and Ecology in the Philippines (STEP) project. *Bull. WHO,* **86:** 765–71.

Tanaka, H. and Tsuji, M. (1997). Discovery to eradication of schistosomosis in Japan 1847–1996. *Int. J. Parasitol.,* **27:** 1465–80.

Tarafder, M.R., Balolong Jr., E., Carabin, H. *et al.* (2006). A cross-sectional study of the prevalence of intensity of infection with *Schistosoma japonicum* in 50 irrigated and rain-fed villages in Samar Province, the Philippines. *BMC Pub. Health,* **6:** 61.

Taylor, M.T. (1987). Schistosomes in domestic animals: *Schistosoma bovis* and other animal forms. In: E.J.L. Soulsby (ed.) *Immunology, Immunoprophylaxis and Immunotherapy of Parasitic Infections*, pp. 50–90. Boca Raton: CRC Press.

Upatham, E.S., Sornmani, S., Thirachantra, S., Sitaputra, P. (1980). Field studies on the bionomics of alpha and gamma races of *Tricula aperta* in the Mekong River at Khemmarat, Ubol Ratchathani Province, Thailand. In: J.I. Bruce & S. Sornmani (eds.) The Mekong Schistosome, Malacological Review, 2, Supplement: 239–61.

Utzinger, J., Zhou, X.N., Chen, M.G., Bergquist, R. (2005). Conquering schistosomosis in China: the long march. *Acta Trop.,* **96:** 69–96.

Wang T.P., Shrivastava J., Johansen M.V., Zhang S.Q., Wang F.F., Webster J.P. (2006b). Do multiple hosts mean multiple parasites?: Population genetic structure of *Schistosoma japonicum* between definitive host species. *Int. J. Parasitol.,* **36:** 1317–25.

Wang, L.D., Chen, H.G., Guo, J.G. *et al.* (2009a). A strategy to control transmission of *Schistosoma japonicum* in China. *N. Eng. J. Med.,* **360:** 121–28.

Wang, L.D., Guo, J.G., Wu, X.H. *et al.* (2009b). China's new strategy to block Schistosoma japonicum transmission: experiences and impact beyond schistosomosis. *Trop. Med. Int. Health,* **14:** 1475–83.

Wang, L., Utzinger, J., Zhou, X-N. (2008). Schistosomosis control: experiences and lessons from China. *Lancet,* **372:** 1793–95.

Wang, T., Zhang, S., Wu, W. *et al.* (2006a). Treatment and re-infection of water buffalo and cattle infected with *Schistosoma japonicum* in the Yangtze River Valley, Anhui Province, P. R. China. *J. Parasitol.,* **92:** 1088–91.

Wang, T.P., Johansen, M.V., Zhang, S.Q. *et al.* (2005). Transmission of *Schistosoma japonicum* by man and domestic animals in the Yantze River Valley, Anhui Province, P.R. China. *Acta Trop.,* **96:** 198–204.

Wang, X.Q. and Mao, S.P. (1989). Comparison of the morphology, pathogenicity and drug response among three isolates of *Schistosoma japonicum* in the mainland of China. *Ann. Parasit. Hum. Comparée,* **64:** 110–19.

Warren, K.S. (1982). Schistosomosis: host-pathogen biology. *Rev. Infect. Dis.,* **4:** 771–75.

WHO (2001). Report of the WHO informal consultation on schistosomosis in low transmission areas: control strategies and criteria for elimination. WHO/CDS/CPE/SIP/2001.1.

Williams, G.M., Sleigh, A.C., Li, Y. *et al.* (2002). Mathematical modelling of schistosomosis japonica: comparison of control strategies in the People's Republic of China. *Acta Trop.,* **82:** 253–62.

Recent national prevalence of *C. sinensis* in Korea was 2.1% reaching 31% in peoples living near a tributary of the Nakdong river (Lim *et al.* 2006); 0.4–0.8% prevalence in China reaching 2.4% in 27 endemic provinces, particularly Guangdong Province with pockets of >28; in north west Vietnam 5% were infected (Dung *et al.* 2007). As many as 13–85% of fish can be infected.

In northern Thailand, infection with *O. viverrini* fell from 34–64% in 1981 to 16–19% in 2001 with national reported cases falling from 1.8 in 2001 to 0.7/100,000 in 2006 (Kaewpitoon *et al.* 2008) but 86% infection has been reported in Laos (Sayasone *et al.* 2009). *Opisthorchis felineus* is widespread but participation of man declines from high in central Russia to rare in Western Europe. Prevalence is high in western Siberia, 1.6% infection in the north reached 38% in the in the Ob river basin and increasing in Kemerovo Region where 11 and 33% of residents in Tomsk city and a nearby village, respectively, were seropositive. Up to 50% of cyprinid fish were infected. The six outbreaks in Italy since 2003 were associated with tench and white fish, 83% of the former infected with metacercariae (Armignacco *et al.* 2008).

Recently, nationwide in China, echinostomes were detected in 0.015%, but 5% in endemic Fujian and Guangdong Provinces (Zhou *et al.* 2008); 0.2% in Korea with pockets of 22% in some inland areas (Chai and Lee 2002; Shin *et al.* 2008); and, in a tribal community in Bandipore, India, 10% were passing echinostome eggs. Two to 41% of fish carry metacercariae.

Nationwide in Korea 1.2% were infected with *Metagonimus* in 1981 but this has fallen to 0.3–0.5% although 20–70% were positive along large and small streams in eastern and southern coastal areas where sweetfish are available, and 5% positive along upper reaches of large rivers where minnow and carp are caught (Chai and Lee 2002; Shin *et al.* 2008). Brackish water heterophyids were less common, i.e. *H. nocens* 0.1% reaching 11% on islands, and *G. seoi* 0.1% reaching 4% on southwestern islands. In the Nghia Hung district, Vietnam, and several districts in Laos, heterophyids particularly *Haplorchis* spp., but also *P. molenkampi*, infected some 65% of adults with poly-trematode infection common (Dung *et al.* 2007; Chai *et al.* 2007; Sayasone *et al.* 2009). Heterophyids were in 5% of fish in areas in Vietnam and 42–100% of mullet and goby in some coastal areas of Korea.

Fasciolopsis buski occurs in many Asian countries though, in many, prevalence has declined, i.e. infection has virtually disappeared from central Thailand. Infection persists in other areas, i.e. 7% in a village in north east Thailand and 4% in children near Dongting Lake, China, and may be re-emerging in Uttar Pradesh, northern India. Prevalence is highest among peoples living near water caltrop plantations.

Prevalence of *Paragonimus* in eight Provinces in China was 1–7% with 30% of children infected in rural Shangluo (Zhou *et al.* 2008). Prevalence can be high, up to 50–100%, in crabs and crayfish. In Sin Ho district, Vietnam, 7.4% were infected. In north east India, particularly Arunachai Pradesh, infection is emerging with 21% prevalence of *P. heterotremus* in children ≤15 years (Devi *et al.* 2007). In endemic areas of Nigeria, Cameroon, and Liberia up to 10–17% may be infected. Infection occurs in small foci from Mexico to Brazil and Peru. In the USA infection is sporadic. In Japan infection is re-emerging from eating wild boar but also immigration, travel, and importation of infected crab/crayfish from China.

Pathogenesis, pathology, symptoms and signs

Liver flukes

Liver flukes sucking blood produce ulceration, mechanical irritation, and desquamation in large and medium sized bile ducts, adenomatous hyperplasia of the epithelium, and goblet cell hyperplasia. Mucus rich bile, hyperplasic liver cells, and worms produce choleostasis and sludge in the gall bladder favouring secondary infection. Absorbed antigens and eggs lodged in walls induce granulomata, eosinophil and mononuclear cell infiltration with degranulation, cytokine production, and nitric oxide damage in the portal triad producing cholangitis, necrosis, and oedema. Periductal fibrosis becomes prominent around enlarged ducts. Eggs are a nidus for choleoliths. The extent of damage is related to intensity and chronicity of infection and multiple infections. Low numbers of flukes may be asymptomatic or induce abdominal discomfort and malaise. Higher levels (100–1,000 worms) have a more pronounced presentation.

Clonorchis sinensis and *O. felineus,* often asymptomatic, may present acutely 2–4 weeks after infection particularly in naive migrants, as fever, anorexia, right upper abdominal pain, weight loss, and sometimes allergic arthralgia, asthma, and urticaria. In the chronic phases hepatomegaly, portal hypertension, ascites, and jaundice may occur and sudden acute presentation may manifest due to obstruction from hyperplasia, periductal stenosis, worms, and choleoliths. Other severe complications include pyogenic cholangitis, pancreatitis, and cholangiocarcinoma (CHCA). *Clonorchis sinensis* is a Group 2A carcinogen (probably carcinogenic — International Agency for Research on Cancer). In Hong Kong and Korea, *C. sinensis* is considered responsible for 6% of liver cancers with risk also related to male sex, alcohol, and raw fish consumption.

Acute disease from *O. viverrini* is uncommon, infections mostly asymptomatic or benign. At any one time in a northeastern Thai village 5–10% of the population had some mild symptoms (malaise, flatulence, dyspepsia, pain) from gall bladder enlargement, dysfunction, and gallstones, with possibly hepatomegaly. Severe complications, although uncommon, are pyogenic cholangitis and importantly CHCA related to high intensity (>6,000 eggs/gm indicative of >120 worms) and duration of infection. *Opisthorchis viverrini* (Group 1 definite carcinogen) is associated with an increased incidence of bile duct CHCA (multicentric peripheral type), an important cause of death after 20–40 years of chronic, repeated infection (Kaewpitoon *et al.* 2008). Incidence of CHCA in endemic countries is high, i.e. 40–98/100,000 in Khon Kaen Province, Thailand, compared with 0.1–3 elsewhere in the world whereas hepatocellular carcinoma prevalences are comparable.

Experimental evidence reinforces the link between *O. viverrini* (and *C. sinensis*) and CHCA although mechanism(s) are not understood. Flukes may act as a promoter with hyperplastic epithelium susceptible to exogenous, endogenous or worm carcinogens. Excretions/secretions (ES) of *O. viverrini* induced cell proliferation *in vitro*. Tenascin, integral in epithelial cell interactions in tumourogenesis, is expressed in infected duct walls, surrounding tissues, and CHCA stroma. *Opisthorchis viverrini* cDNA has revealed potential mutagenic activity, i.e. progranulin, a cell-, including tumour cell-growth factor, and a kallikrein-like protease possibly associated with epithelial to mesenchymal cell progression (Laha *et al.* 2007).

There may be synergism between the flukes and dietary N-nitro compounds that occur in commonly eaten 'pla ra', fermented fish sauce, etc. High incidence of CHCA occurred in fluke infected hamsters treated with N-nitrosodimethyamine but not hamsters with either alone. An important role for host produced NO and rOI in DNA damage has been suggested. Increased NO synthase and the vigorous production of NO in the bile ducts could represent an endogenous genotoxic substance. Host genetics will contribute.

Intestinal flukes

Gastrodiscoides hominis seems well tolerated; in heavy infection inflammation of the large intestine causes diarrhoea. *Fasciolopsis buski* produces trauma of the anterior intestine, excess mucus production, ulceration, haemorrhage, and abscess formation, and possibly reduced vitamin B_{12} absorption. Heavy infections in children (100 to >1,000 worms) produce a protein-losing enteropathy, profuse diarrhoea, pain, nausea, and occasionally obstruction. Ascites and facial oedema may be due to hypoalbuminaemia but allergy or 'toxaemia' has been suggested.

The large echinostomes seem less pathogenic than small heterophyids, *N. seoulense* and other species. These latter enclose and penetrate between villi into crypts producing inflammation, villous atrophy, necrosis, oedema, ulceration, and petechial haemorrhages. There may be mild digestive disturbances, intermittent or continuous usually mucoid, but occasionally bloody, perhaps profuse diarrhoea, anaemia, and anorexia.

Some heterophyids, particularly *S. brevicaeca, H. heterophyes, M. yokogawai* and their eggs, may penetrate the mucosa and embolize to various organs. Granulomatous lesions, particularly noticeable in brain and heart, have been fatal. *Gymnophalloides seoi* may produce signs of pancreatitis making it very important (Chai *et al.* 2003).

Lung flukes

Paragonimus migrating in the pleural cavity induces pleural effusion, adhesions, pneumothorax, and focal haemorrhagic pneumonia with pain, cough, fever, fatigue, and marked eosinophilia. Greyish-white fibrous cysts, 1–3 cm in diameter, containing yellow-brown purulent fluid, open into a bronchus and produce chronic dry cough (97%), then rust-coloured sputum, haemoptysis, often with a 'fish-taste' (83–92%), chest and abdominal pain (42–70%), pleural effusion (26%), and eosinophilia (90%) (De *et al.* 2000; Devi *et al.* 2007).

Paragonimus skrjabini and *P. miyazakii* in particular migrate aberrantly to the chest, abdominal wall, liver, spleen, intestine, or extremities. The nodule or migrating mass often is painful inducing marked eosinophilia. Cerebral migration causes oedema, haemorrhage, and meningitis; severe headache, seizures, and hemiparesis manifest in 8% of patients.

Diagnosis

Clinical signs and imaging are not pathognomonic from other liver diseases, many diarrhoeas and tuberculosis, all prevalent in endemic areas. Eating habits can be useful.

Examinations for eggs

Faecal (sputum) samples examined by formalin-ether/ethyl acetate concentration, Stoll, or Kato thick smears can have sensitivity of 85–90% for *O. viverrini* and *C. sinensis* this reduced to 70% on a single examination of light infections (<20 worms). Duodenal aspiration may detect scarce eggs. Bile duct cannulation has been used. The eggs of many of the liver and minute intestinal flukes are very similar so skilful, time-consuming examinations are required. The operculum and egg length to width are useful but the considerable intraspecific variability usually divides eggs only into groups (Lee *et al.* 1984; Chai and Lee 2002). Recent advances include release of DNA from opisthorchid eggs and use of polymerase chain reaction (PCR) that detects the group (Müller *et al.* 2007), primers specific for different species also are now available. Eggs of echinostomes, *F. buski* and *G. hominis* are detected with detergent/sedimentation techniques and iodine or methylene green/blue stains. Worms can be expelled with praziquantel followed by a saline purgative (Chai *et al.* 2007). Pseudoparasitism, particularly by *D. dendriticum*, is ruled out by a controlled diet.

Imaging

Cholangeography may outline liver flukes and damaged, dilated bile ducts showing irregular filling defects. M-mode sonogram may detect fluke movement. On heavy infection ultrasonography and CT scan show dilation of particularly the distal ducts, highly echogenic thickened bile duct walls, and sludge in the gallbladder (Choi and Hong 2007; Lim *et al.* 2008). CHCA shows as a large irregular mass with low density stippled areas or powder-like high-density areas (Rim 2005). Radiography for *Paragonimus* may show patchy consolidation of haemorrhage from migration and linear shadows from the pleural surface, presumably migratory tunnels filled with pleural fluid/air as obvious when accompanied by pleural effusion or pneumothorax. Radiography may be negative in about 20% of patients early in infection. Calcified/fibrous cysts are evident. CT shows cloudy infiltration of the lungs and poorly marginated nodules, frequently subpleural or subfissural possibly with a low attenuation central area. Focal pleural thickening was common (84%) and linear opacities leading to the nodule (tracks) characteristic (48%) (Kim *et al.* 2005).

Immunodiagnosis

Serodiagnosis, particularly ELISA, is increasingly used for liver and lung flukes. ES, superior to crude extracts, of *Opisthorchis, Clonorchis* and *Paragonimus* gives >80% sensitivity although cross-reactions remain among the Opisthorchiidae and *Paragonimus* spp. (Choi *et al.* 2003). A *P. heterotremus* ES antigen band on immunoblot was 98% sensitive and 100% specific when detected with IgG_4 antibodies (Wongkham *et al.* 2005). A variety of recombinant antigens now are becoming available and have shown >80–96% specificity in ELISA and western blot (Nagano *et al.* 2004; Ruangsittichai *et al.* 2006; Zhao *et al.* 2004; Hu *et al.* 2007; Ma *et al.* 2007; Lee *et al.* 2007). Tests for circulating antigens generally have lower sensitivity but high specificity.

Treatment

Three 25 mg/kg doses of praziquantel given on 1 day, repeated on day 2 for heavy infections, has >90% efficacy against *Clonorchis* and *Opisthorchis* spp. Light infections may be treated with 40 mg/kg given once, producing fewer side-effects that are usually mild and transient (<24 hours), possibly severe if neurocysticercosis was present (Rim 2005).

A single dose of 10–15 up to 25 mg/kg praziquantel is highly effective against *F. buski* and other intestinal flukes. Triclabendazole has efficacy in pigs.

At least one course of praziquantel, 50–75 mg/kg as three divided doses for 3 days, had good efficacy (>87%) against pulmonary and ectopic *Paragonimus*, eggs disappearing in a few weeks, lesions clearing slowly. Triclabendazole, 10 mg/kg once or twice in a day or 5–10 mg/kg for 3 days, was >84% effective (Calvopinña *et al.* 2003).

In laboratory animals derivatives of artemisinin have shown promise against some liver and intestinal flukes and tribendimidine against liver flukes (Keiser and Utzinger 2007; Keiser *et al.* 2007).

Control

The cost of treatment and lost wages from opisthorchosis and CHCA was estimated at US$120 million a year in Thailand. Control should involve:

1) Education,

2) Targeted treatment,

3) Socio-economic development; to reduce faecal contamination of water and inadequate preparation of fish.

Education on life cycles and preparation of fish, shellfish, water plants is important though it may be difficult to change cultural habits. In a southern Chinese village, 27–57% had no knowledge of *C. sinensis*'s life cycle/disease, ate raw fish >1–2 times a month, and/or fed fish with human/animal faeces (Zhang *et al.* 2007). In northern Thailand, even after >10 years of the control programme, 40% continued to eat raw fish and defaecate promiscuously. However, in Taiwan, an aggressive education programme controlled *F. buski*. Some information on killing metacercariae is available. *Opisthorchis viverrini* metacercariae were killed at 80°C for 5 min, 70°C for 30 min, vinegar treatment for 1.5 hours, salting at 33.6% for 24 hours, or freezing at −10°C for >5 days though neither freezing for 3 days nor the common Russian 3-day wet salting or 1.7% dry salting killed *O. felineus*. Irradiation could be adopted commercially. Metacercariae of *F. buski* could remain viable on plants for perhaps 2–3 months in damp, cool weather but are killed by desiccation and boiling.

Treatments targeting infected individuals after faecal examination should markedly reduce egg output as 74% of *C. sinensis* were aggregated in 10% of the population. Reducing intensity and duration of infection should reduce severe disease and CHCA risk. Data is required concerning rates of reinfection and the relevance of eggs produced by lightly infected individuals and particularly reservoir hosts. Even where man was the most important definitive host, treatment once a year was insufficient to control *O. viverrini* due to reinfection. Treatment plus education has success however. The Public Health Development Plan in northern Thailand combined yearly targeted treatment, community preparation, and health education (Jongduksuntigul and Imsomboom 2003; Kaewpitoon *et al.* 2008). Infection and disease incidence declined significantly with increased knowledge of *Opisthorchis* and reported decrease in 'koi pla' fish consumption. Occasional treatments could be targeted to season as infection may peak after monsoon flooding when fish abound in ponds and paddy fields or, in countries with a cold season, in late summer/autumn.

Increased socio-economic status usually decreases infection with improvements in standard of living, sanitation, hygiene, and education. Migration of rural poor to urban areas will remove them from the source of infection. An increase in the price of fish (through export or supply) may decrease levels of infection. Increased wealth though may increase consumption of raw, ethnic dishes in restaurants and homes. The re-emergence of opisthorchosis in Italy has been associated with this.

Changes in the environment and agriculture can impact on transmission. Increased water pollution from factories and insecticides was linked to the decline of *C. sinensis* in Japan. A decline in *H. heterophyes* along the Nile was attributed to changed water nutrients due to the Aswan Dam. A north east Thailand water development programme increased water flow reducing snails and *O. viverrini*. Conversely, construction of dams and/or migration of infected people into areas increased prevalence of *O. felineus* and it is important to consider changes in water flow in the whole network of water bodies, not just the immediate vicinity. Migration of labourers, with often asymptomatic and long-lived infections, from endemic areas to new lakes and irrigation areas and to countries where control has been successful, could introduce infection.

Modern pig farming using commercial foods will break the cycle of flukes in pigs. Water plants should be dried, fish viscera cooked before feeding to pigs. Heat treatment (even composting) of faeces used as fertilizer in fish ponds is useful. Predator snails/ducks/fish, etc., can reduce numbers of cercariae and snails or bivalves, i.e. clams.

Aquaculture is the fastest growing method of protein production increasing from thousands to many millions of tons of fish, particularly cyprinids, but also crustaceans, particularly in China, but also other south east Asian trematode endemic areas (Keiser and Utzinger 2005). In the same areas small scale fish production and marketing to nearby areas also has increased exponentially. In China, *C. sinensis* prevalence increased three-fold in the face of a decline of soil-transmitted helminths and *S. japonicum*, the increase related to aquaculture expansion. In Korea, soil-transmitted helminths have fallen further than fish-borne trematodes.

The increased global trade in chilled, potentially infected fish could result in use in ethnic dishes among immigrant populations and residents eating novel dishes. Increasing numbers of *Paragonimus* cases in Japan occur in Chinese inhabitants, with travel and consumption of local, ethnic dishes in endemic areas and import of shellfish contributing.

References

Armignacco, O., Caterini, L., Marucci, G. *et al.* (2008). Human illnesses caused by *Opisthorchis felineus* flukes, Italy. *Emerg. Infect. Dis.*, **14:** 1902–5.

Blair, D. (2000). Genomes of *Paragonimus westermani* and related species: current state of knowledge. *Int. J. Parasitol.,,* **30:** 421–26.

Blair, D., Xu, Z-B. and Agatsuma, T. (1998). Paragonimiasis and the genus *Paragonimus. Adv. Parasitol.,* **48:** 113–222.

Calvopinña, M., Guderian, R.H., Paredes, W. and Cooper, P.J. (2003). Comparison of two single-day regimens of triclabendazole for the treatment of human pulmonary paragonimiasis. *Trans. R. Soc. Trop. Med. Hyg.,* **97:** 451–54.

Chai, J-Y. and Lee, S-H. (2002). Food-borne intestinal trematode infections in the Republic of Korea. *Parasitol. Int.,,* **51:** 129–54.

Chai, J-Y., Choi, M-H., Yu, J.R. and Lee, S-H. (2003). *Gymnophalloides seoi*: a new human intestinal trematode. *Trends Parasitol.,* **19:** 109–12.

Chai J-Y., Han, E-T., Guk, S-M. *et al.* (2007). High prevalence of liver and intestinal fluke infections among residents of Savannakhet Province in Laos. *Korean J. Parasitol.,* **45:** 213–18.

Choi, D. and Hong, S.T. (2007). Imaging diagnosis of clonorchiasis. *Korean J. Parasitol.*, **45**: 77–85.

Choi, M.H., Park, I.C., Li, S. and Hong, S.T. (2003). Excretory-secretory antigen is better than crude antigen for the serodiagnosis of clonorchiasis by ELISA. *Korean J. Parasitol.*, **41**: 35–39.

De, N.V., Cong, L.D., Kino, H., Son, D.T. and Vien, H.V. (2000). Epidemiology, symptoms and treatment of paragonimiasis in Sin Ho district, Lai Chau province, Vietnam. *Southeast Asian J. Trop. Med. Public Health*, **31** (Suppl 1): 26–30.

Devi, K.R., Narain, K., Bhattacharya, S. *et al.* (2007). Pleuropulmonary paragonimiasis due to *Paragonimus heterotremus*: molecular diagnosis, prevalence of infection and clinicoradiological features in an endemic area of northeastern India. *Trans. R. Soc. Trop. Med. Hyg.*, **101**: 786–92.

Dzikowski, R., Levy, M.G., Poore, M.F., Flowers, J.R. and Paperna, I. (2004). Use of rDNA polymorphism for identification of Heterophyidae infecting freshwater fishes. *Dis. Aquat. Organ.*, **21**: 35–41.

Dung, D.T., De, V.N., Waikagul, J. *et al.* (2007). Fishborne zoonotic intestinal trematodes, Vietnam. *Emerg. Infect. Dis.*, **13**: 1828–33.

Fried, B., Graeczyk, T.K. and Tamang, L. (2004). Food-borne intestinal trematodiases in humans. *Parasitol. Res.*, **93**: 159–70.

Grove, D.J. (1990). *A History of Human Helminthology*. Wallingford, Oxon: CAB International.

Hu, F., Yu, X., Ma, C. *et al.* (2007). *Clonorchis sinensis*: expression, characterization, immunolocalization and serological reactivity of one excretory/secretory antigen-LPAP homologue. *Exp. Parasitol.*, **117**: 157–64.

Intapan, P.M., Kosuwan, T., Wongkham, C. and Maleewong, W. (2004). Genomic characterization of lung flukes, *Paragonimus heterotremus*, *P. siamensis*, *P. harinasutai*, *P. westermani* and *P. bangkokensis* by RAPD markers. *Vet. Parasitol.*, **124**: 55–64.

Iwagami, M., Ho, L.Y., Su, K. *et al.* (2000). Molecular phylogeographic studies on *Paragonimus westermani* in Asia. *J. Helminthol.*, **74**: 315–22.

Jongsuksuntigul, P. and Imsomboon, T. (2003). Opisthorchiasis control in Thailand. *Acta Trop.*, **88**: 229–32.

Kaewpitoon, N., Kaewpitoon, S.J., Pensaa, P. and Sripa, B. (2008). *Opisthorchis viverrini*: the carcinogenic human liver fluke. *World J. Gastroenterol.*, **14**: 666–74.

Keiser, J. and Utzinger, J. (2005). Emerging foodborne trematodiasis. *Emerg. Infect. Dis.*, **11**: 1507–14.

Keiser, J. and Utzinger, J. (2007). Artemisinins and synthetic trioxolanes in the treatment of helminth infections. *Curr. Opin. Infect. Dis.*, **20**: 605–12.

Keiser, J., Shu-Hua, X., Chollet, J., Tanner, M. and Utzinger, J. (2007). Evaluation of the in vivo activity of tribendimidine against *Schistosoma mansoni*, *Fasciola hepatica*, *Clonorchis sinensis*, and *Opisthorchis viverrini*. *Antimicrob. Agents Chemother.*, **51**: 1096–98.

Kim, T.S., Han, J., Shim, S.S. *et al.* (2005). Pleuropulmonary paragonimiasis: CT findings in 31 patients. *Am. J. Roentgenol.*, **185**: 616–21.

Laha, T., Pinloar, P., Mulvenna, J. *et al.* (2007). Gene discovery for the carcinogenic liver fluke, *Opisthorchis viverrini*. *BMC Genomics*, 8: 189–203.

Lee, S.H., Hwang, S.W., Chai, J.Y. and Seo, B.S. (1984). Comparative morphology of eggs of heterophyids and *Clonorchis sinensis* causing human infections in Korea. *Korean J. Parasitol.*, **22**: 171–80.

Lee, J.S., Lee, J., Kim, S.H. and Yong, T.S. (2007). Molecular cloning and characterization of a major egg antigen in *Paragonimus westermani* and its use in ELISA for the immunodiagnosis of paragonimiasis. *Parasitol. Res.*, **100**: 677–81.

Lim, J.H., Mariang, E. and Ahn, G.H. (2008). Biliary parasitic diseases including clonorchiasis, opisthorchiasis and fascioliasis. *Abdom. Imaging*, **33**: 157–65.

Lim, M.K., Ju, Y.H., Franceschi, S. *et al.* (2006). *Clonorchis sinensis* infection and increasing risk of cholangiocarcinoma in the Republic of Korea. *Am. J. Trop. Med. Hyg.*, **75**: 93–96.

Ma, C., Hu, X., Hu, F. *et al.* (2007). Molecular characterization and serodiagnosis analysis of a novel lysophospholipase from *Clonorchis sinensis*. *Parasitol. Res.*, **101**: 419–25.

Mas-Coma, S., Batgues, M.D. and Valero, M.A. (2005). Fascioliasis and other plant-borne trematodes zoonoses. *Int. J. Parasitol.*, **35**: 1255–78.

Müller, B., Schmidt, J. and Mehlhorn, H. (2007). PCR diagnosis of infections with different species of Opisthorchiidae using a rapid clean-up procedure for stool samples and specific primers. *Parasitol. Res.*, **100**: 905–9.

Muller, R. and Wakelin, D. (2002). *Worms and Human Disease*. Wallingford, Oxon: CABI Publishing.

Nagano, I., Pei, F., Wu, Z. *et al.* (2004). Molecular expression of a cysteine proteinase of *Clonorchis sinensis* and its application to an enzyme-linked immunosorbent assay for immunodiagnosis of clonorchiasis. *Clin. Diagn. Lab. Immunol.*, **11**: 411–16.

Pearson, J.C. and Ow-Yang, C.K. (1982). New species of *Haplorchis* from Southeast Asia, together with keys to the *Haplorchis*-group of heterophyid trematodes of the region. *Southeast Asian J. Trop. Med. Public Health*, **13**: 35–60.

Ruangsittichai, J., Viyanant, V., Vichasri-Grams, S. *et al.* (2006). *Opisthorchis viverrini*: identification of a glycine-tyrosine rich eggshell protein and its potential as a diagnostic tool for human opisthorchiasis. *Int. J. Parasitol.*, **36**: 1329–39.

Rim, H.J. (2005). Clonorchiasis: an update. *J. Helminthol.*, **79**: 269–81.

Saijuntha, W., Sithithaworn, P., Wongkham, S. *et al.* (2007). Evidence of a species complex within the food-borne trematode *Opisthorchis viverrini* and possible co-evolution with their first intermediate hosts. *Int. J. Parasitol.*, **37**: 695–703.

Saito, S., Chai, J-Y., Kim, K.H., Lee, S.H. and Rim, H.J. (1997). *Metagonimus miyatai* sp. nov. (Digenea: Heterophyidae), a new intestinal trematode transmitted by freshwater fishes in Japan and Korea. *Korean J. Parasitol.*, **35**: 223–32.

Sayasone, S., Vonghajack, Y., Vanmany, M. *et al.* (2009). Diversity of human intestinal helminthiasis in Lao PDR. *Trans. R. Soc. Trop. Med. Hyg.*, **103**: 247–54.

Schuster, H., Agada, F.O., Anderson, A.R. *et al.* (2007). Otitis media and a neck lump—current diagnostic challenges for *Paragonimus*-like trematode infections. *J. Infect.*, **54**: 103–6.

Shin, E.H., Guk, S.M., Kim, H.J., Lee, S.H. and Chai, J.Y. (2008). Trends in parasitic diseases in the Republic of Korea. *Parasitology*, **24**: 143–50.

Soulsby, E.J.L. (1982). *Helminths, Arthropods and Protozoa of Domesticated Animals*. London: Baillière Tindall.

Sugiyama, H., Morishima, Y. *et al.* (2006). Application of multiplex PCR for species discrimination using individual metacercariae of *Paragonimus* occurring in Thailand. *Southeast Asian J. Trop. Med. Public Health*, **37** Suppl 3: 48–52.

Toledo, R., Esteban, J-G. and Fried, B. (2006). Immunology and pathology of intestinal nematodes in their definitive hosts. *Adv. Parasitol.*, **63**: 285–365.

Wongkham, C., Intapan, P.M., Maleewong, W. and Miwa, M. (2005). Evaluation of human IgG subclass antibodies in the serodiagnosis of *Paragonimus heterotremus*. *Asian Pac. J. Allergy. Immunol.*, **23**: 205–11.

Yang, H-J., Guk, S-M., Han, E-T. and Choi, J-Y. (2000). Molecular differentiation of three species of *Metagnimus* by simple sequence repeat anchored polymerase chain reaction (SSR-PCR) amplification. *J. Parasitol.*, **86**: 1170–72.

Zhao, Q.P., Moon, S.U., Lee, H.W. *et al.* (2004). Evaluation of *Clonorchis sinensis* recombinant 7-kilodalton antigen for serodiagnosis of clonorchiasis. *Clin. Diagn. Lab. Immunol.*, **11**: 814–17.

Zhang, R., Gao, S., Geng, Y. *et al.* (2007). Epidemiological study on *Clonorchis sinensis* infection in Shenzhen area of Zhujiang delta in China. *Parasitol. Res.*, **101**: 179–83.

Zhou, P., Chen, N., Zhang, R-L., Lin, R-Q. and Zhu, X-Q. (2008). Food-borne parasitic zoonoses in China: perspective for control. *Trends Parasitol.*, **24**: 190–96.

CHAPTER 57

Strongyloidosis

T. J. Nolan, T. B. Nutman and G. A. Schad

Summary

Strongyloidosis is an intestinal parasitism caused by the thread-worm, *Strongyloides stercoralis*. The parasite, occurring in dogs, primates and man, is found throughout the moist tropics, as well as in temperate areas where poor sanitation or other factors facilitate the occurrence of faecally transmitted organisms. In some parts of the world, notably Africa and New Guinea, human infections caused by *S. fülleborni* have been reported (Hira *et al.* 1980). In Africa, the latter is primarily a parasite of primates, but in New Guinea, no animal host is known. *S. stercoralis* is unique among zoonotic nematodes, in that larvae passing in the faeces can give rise to a free-living generation of worms which, in turn, give rise to infective larvae. This life history alternative (i.e. heterogonic development) acts as an amplification mechanism, increasing the population of infective larvae in the external environment. The infective larvae are active skin penetrators; infection *per os*, while possible, is probably of limited importance. Because the parasitic female's eggs hatch internally, a potential for autoinfection exists when precociously developing larvae attain infectivity while still in the host. This is another virtually unique feature of *S. stercoralis* infections in both its human and animal hosts. Autoinfection can occasionally escape control by the host, with massive re-penetration and larval migration. This can cause pulmonary or cerebro-spinal strongyloidosis as well as fulminant intestinal parasitism. Control of canine strongyloidosis has been achieved in kennels by strategic use of anthelmintics. Given the lack of epidemiological information community-based programs to control human strongyloidosis have not been attempted. The growing importance of human strongyloidosis depends upon the unique ability of *S. stercoralis* to replicate within its host and to behave as a potentially fatal opportunistic pathogen in immuno-compromised hosts, particularly in those receiving corticosteroids.

History

The history of strongyloidosis and of its etiological agent, *Strongyloides stercoralis*, is presented in detail by Grove (1989). The disease, originally called Cochin China Diarrhoea, was discovered by the French naval physician Louis Normand in 1876. Meanwhile the parasite, known only on the basis of the rhabditiform preinfective larvae passing in the faeces, was described by Bavay (1876), Normand's colleague and professor of pharmacy at the

naval hospital in Toulon. Bavay named the nematode *Anguillula stercoralis* and recognized that when the larvae were kept in faeces for a few days under favorable conditions, they developed into free-living adult male and female worms. Subsequently, in autopsies of soldiers returning from duty in Cochin China (presently Vietnam), Normand found larvae throughout the intestines, bile and pancreatic ducts and adult parasitic females in the intestines. Not surprisingly, given that the parasitic females (there are no parasitic males) differ markedly from the free-living adults in morphology, these parasitic females were considered a different species and named *Anguillula intestinalis* by Bavay (1877). Giving further credence to this deduction was the additional discovery of a second kind of larva, a filariform larva (subsequently recognized as the infective stage) which at that point in the history of strongyloidosis could logically be considered the larva of the putative second species, *A. intestinalis*. Thus, in the years immediately following the recognition of the disease and of the parasite, all the stages in the life of the parasite became known, but their relationship was confused because it appeared that there were two species with different life cycles, namely, *A. stercoralis* whose rhabditiform larva occurred in the stools and whose adults occurred in the external environment and *A. intestinalis* whose adults were intestinal parasites and whose progeny were filariform larvae.

Remarkably, Grassi and Parona (1878) almost immediately resolved some of the confusion and explained much of the unusual and complex life cycle of the parasite. They found that the parasitic female named *A. intestinalis* laid eggs which hatched rapidly, giving rise to the rhabditiform larvae that were known as *A. stercoralis*. Apparently, they had a homogonic strain of the parasite because all of the rhabditiform larvae developed to infective filariform larvae such as had been described for *A. intestinalis*. It remained for Perroncito in 1881 to complete the free-living part of the life cycle by showing that the rhabditiform larvae, as originally observed in faeces by Normand, do indeed develop into free-living males and females and, furthermore, that these in turn produce filariform larvae, the infective stage of the parasite. Perroncito, however, did not realize that the various life history stages he and others had observed were parts of a complex life cycle having facultatively alternating parasitic and free-living generations.

The French workers, Normand and Bavay, discovered the disease and described the parasite; the Italian workers, Perroncito and

Grassi and Parona, elucidated the free-living life cycle; and, subsequently, the German parasitologists, Looss (1905), and Fülleborn (1914), found, respectively, that infection occurred by skin penetration, and that larvae could migrate from the skin to intestines via the circulation, lungs and trachea. Finally, Gage (1911) reported the occurrence of autoinfection, i.e. that larvae hatching from eggs laid in the host can develop to infectivity precociously and reinfect the same host in which they were hatched. The host, parasite and environmental factors that determine the alternative developmental pathways of *S. stercoralis* in both man and animals remain poorly understood but are under active investigation (see Life History below).

The agent

Taxonomy

The family Strongyloididae (Class Secernentea, Order Rhabditida, Superfamily Rhabditoidea) is constituted of three genera, *Strongyloides* (Grassi 1879), *Parastrongyloides* (Morgan 1928), and *Leipernema* (Singh 1976). The members of the genus *Strongyloides*, also called threadworms, are heterogenetic, with both free-living and parasitic generations. The genus includes fifty-two named species. The majority of these are parasites of mammals, but some can be found in birds, reptiles and amphibians. The only species dealt with in detail in this chapter is *Strongyloides stercoralis* (Bavay 1876) (synonyms: *Anguillula stercoralis*, *S. intestinalis*, *S. canis*, *S. felis*) an intestinal parasite of dogs, primates and man. *Strongyloides fülleborni* (von Linstow 1905), is usually considered a parasite of primates that also infects humans, but, at least in some parts of its range, is transmitted in the absence of primates. Thus, its zoonotic status is presently uncertain and it is omitted here. Several species are important parasites of livestock (*S. ransomi*, *S. westeri*, *S. papillosus*) or are laboratory models of human strongyloidosis (*S. ratti*, *S. venezuelensis*). *Parastrongyloides trichosuri*, a parasite of Australian marsupials that is related to *Strongyloides*, is becoming an increasingly important laboratory model for some aspects of the *Strongyloides* life cycle, since it can be maintained in its free-living stages indefinitely as a microbiverous species on agar culture plates (Nolan *et al.* 2007).

Life history

The life history of *S. stercoralis* is complicated by a number of facultative alternatives. These alternatives include:

(1) direct (or homogonic) development with parasitic parthenogenetic females and only larval stages occurring in the free-living phase of the life cycle,

(2) indirect (or heterogonic) development with the inclusion of one generation free-living adult worms (i.e. with an alternation of parasitic and free-living generations),

(3) autoinfective development, with some of the larval progeny of the parasite population developing to infectivity precociously, while still in the intestines, and after parenteral migration returning to the intestines to mature.

The latter pathway, when constrained by still poorly understood host and/or parasite factors, is thought to lead to a slow turnover in the adult worm populations, thus maintaining highly persistent chronic infection. When these constraints fail, autoinfection is

explosive forming the basis for the fulminant hyper- and disseminated forms of the infection.

In its simplest homogonic form, the life cycle involves parthenogenetic females lying embedded in the crypts of the intestinal mucosa where they deposit their eggs. The egg hatches giving rise to a first-stage larva (L1), known as a rhabditiform larva in the parasitological literature. Just after hatching, the young L1 responds to environmental cues detected by 2 amphidial neurons to make the decision as to which pathway (homogonic vs heterogonic) by which it will develop (Ashton *et al.* 1998). If the homogonic route is selected, the actively feeding, microbiverous form leaves the crypts and moves down the intestines, and exits the body while still a pre-infective rhabditiform larva. During intestinal passage and in faecal deposits, this larva feeds, grows and moults so that two rhabditiform stages occur (L1, L2). Under favourable environmental conditions including a suitable faecal flora, warmth and moisture, the L2 grows and moults, giving rise to an infective filariform larva (L3), a long slender form, with a long slender oesophagus, hence the name filariform larva. It invades the host by active skin penetration.

In the heterogonic cycle, as in homogonic cycle, the larval progeny of the parthenogenetic parasitic females exit the host in the faeces. At this point (before the midpoint in the life span of the L1 (Nolan *et al.* 2004)) the larva again will use environmental cues sensed through its amphidial neurons to make a decision to follow the homogonic or heterogonic routes. For example at higher temperatures (above 34C) the worms tend to develop via the homogonic route (Nolan *et al.* 2004). If the heterogonic route is chosen the larvae will undergo 4 moults as they develop to the free-living adult male and female worms. These adults will mate and lay eggs, the larvae which hatch from the eggs will give rise to infective larva (L3) via the usual two rhabditiform stages. The infective forms leave the faeces or polluted soil in which they have developed and ascend surface particles to the extent permitted by soil or faecal moisture films (Sciacca *et al.* 2002). Here the larvae are positioned for contact with a host. The L3 will also respond to chemical (especially factors found in skin such as salt and urocanic acid (Forbes *et al.* 2003; Safer *et al.* 2007)) and heat gradients (Lopez *et al.* 2000) to move towards a host. After contact and percutaneous entry into a host, the larvae enter the circulation and migrate to the intestines. It is generally accepted that the migratory route involves the lung, trachea and oesophagus (pulmo-tracheal migration), but this route has been challenged by Wilson and by Schad and colleagues. After percutaneous infection of dogs, some larvae do follow the pulmonary route, but most do not. In fact, studies with radio labelled larvae have indicated that no predominant migratory route exists and that larvae reach the intestines via a number of different pathways (Mansfield *et al.* 1995).

Autoinfection is the third life history alternative. In this case, eggs hatch in the intestines as they normally do, but the larvae develop to infectivity precociously while still in the host. In this case the L1 not only choose the homogonic route of development, they also continue to develop as they move down the intestine, reaching the filariform L3 stage by the time they are in the colon. This autoinfective L3 (L3a) is morphologically distinct from the soil dwelling L3 (L3i) as it is smaller in size, slightly wider and has a less filariform oesophagus (Schad *et al.* 1993). The L3a penetrate the wall of the large intestine and from here migrate to many organs of the body, again, some use pulmonary migration, but others return to the intestine by other pathways. Upon return to the intestine, the L3a give rise to a fourth larval stage which in turn moults to give rise to the female adult worm.

Morphology

The parasitic female is one of the stages found in tissue sections of the small intestine; it is rarely seen in the stools of infected hosts. It measures 2.0–2.8 mm in length and 37 μ in width. It has a long cylindrical oesophagus, an intestine constituted of dorsal and ventral rows of 20 cells each. The tail is a short cone. The vulva is ventrally situated at 2/3 the body length from the anterior tip. Eggs are present in 2 single rows, one to either side of the vulva. The cuticle of the female worm is finely striated and, in tissue sections, is often wrinkled. In cross section, depending on the level, one may see a muscular oesophagus, intestine, ovaries and eggs. Reproduction is by parthenogenesis and, hence, there are no parasitic males.

The rhabditiform larva, the stage that hatches from the egg, is the form most commonly identified in faecal samples. It measures approximately 250 μ in length and 17 μ in diameter when passed in faeces, and is characterized by a bulbed oesophagus and a thinner, longer intestine (Schad 1989). In intestinal aspirates, the newly hatched larva is smaller, measuring 180–240 μ in length and 14–15 μ in width. In tissue sections they are often found in the intestinal submucosa and within small intestinal crypts, but only exceptionally in the lungs; they cannot be specifically identified based on their morphologic characteristics. The filariform (third stage) larva of autoinfective origin is the stage most frequently identified in parenteral tissues and body fluids (most often the sputum) in patients with disseminated infections. They are longer and more slender than rhabditiform larvae and have a cylindrical oesophagus that occupies one half the body length. In transverse sections the cuticle shows four characteristic lateral alae, which can be used for species identification. Filariform infective larvae arising as progeny of free-living adults are even longer and more slender, measuring up to 700 μ in length and 20 μ in width.

Disease mechanisms

Chronic infections are probably sustained by a relatively low number of adult worms, many of which may be barren (the so-called post-reproductive females), which reside in relative harmony within their host's intestine and the infection persists by means of periodic bouts of autoinfection (Schad et al. 1997). The occurrence and rate of autoinfection is generally believed to be regulated by the host's cell-mediated immunity. When this regulatory function becomes impaired during immunosuppression, increasing numbers of autoinfective larvae complete the cycle, and the population of parasitic adult worms increases (hyperinfection). Eventually, with extraordinary numbers of larvae migrating, large numbers deviate from the generally presumed route (intestine—> venous bed—> lungs—> trachea—> intestine) and disseminate to other organs, including meningeal spaces and brain, liver, kidneys, lymph nodes, cutaneous and subcutaneous tissues. In these organs the larvae cause haemorrhage by breaking capillaries, elicit inflammatory responses, and implant Gram-negative bacteria carried from faecal material. The resulting syndrome, known as disseminated strongyloidosis, is nearly always fatal.

The validity of the migratory pathways in the above widely accepted model has been questioned by Schad et al. Schad et al. (1989) used an experimental canine model of disseminated strongyloidosis to show that only a few larvae could be recovered from the lungs of dogs with massive hyperinfection. Later, in studies based on the organ specific distribution of radio-labelled larvae and compartmental analysis of the data, they presented strong evidence that, in young dogs, the pulmonary route was not used by the majority of the migrating larvae. Larvae that began their migration in the skin (primary infection) or in the distal ileum (autoinfection) were not more likely to pass through the lungs than through any other organ, suggesting that the migratory pathway involved random dissemination throughout the body. However, this conclusion has not been fully accepted because large numbers of larvae are frequently identified in bronchoalveolar lavage fluid from hyperinfected human patients. It may be that in hyperinfection, as distinct from a primary infection, pulmonary migration is more frequent (Kerlin et al. 1995).

The theory that host immunity controls the rate and mode of parasite development fails to consider the role that parasites themselves may play in this regulation. It is known that the free-living nematode *Caenorhabditis elegans* can sense the population density and uses this information to switch developmental pathways. In both the dog and gerbil model of strongyloidosis initially low numbers of worms will lead to the autoinfective development of some of the larvae, an event not seen in infections initiated by higher numbers of worms (Nolan et al. 1999; Schad et al. 1997). The adverse impact of increased parasite density on egg production and growth ('crowding effect') has been demonstrated for several intestinal nematodes. Although it may be difficult to distinguish between host resistance and direct parasite-to-parasite effects, it seems clear that in a normal host-parasite relationship, the parasite may reach a particular population size or a critical biomass, after which yet unknown regulatory mechanisms intervene to limit the population. However, results of investigations using the gerbil-based model of strongyloidosis have failed to provide support for this type of self regulation of worm burden by the parasite (Nolan et al. 2002).

Genta (1986) has proposed that, during the parallel evolution of humans and their parasites, *S. stercoralis* developed the ability to reach an optimal population size in the duodenum of a human. If the initial infective dose of larvae is low, a higher rate of intraluminal moulting occurs, enabling the parasite to attain the infective stage internally, reinfect and multiply. This occurs until the 'optimal' size of the adult population is reached. In this model, it is assumed that *S. stercoralis*, similar to other nematodes, transmit their moulting signal by moulting hormones (ecdysteroids). As the size of the parasite population reaches a certain level, adult females decrease their production of ecdysteroids, resulting in a lowered moulting rate, i.e. just sufficient to replace the dying adults. During the initial phase of infection, the host mounts humoral and cellular immune responses directed at all tissue stages of the parasite. These well characterized responses do not eradicate all the parasites, but limit the size of the parasite population. Impaired immune responses may allow the growth of larger numbers of parasites, as reported in agammaglobulinemic patients, but total dysregulation of the parasite population does not occur since worms, in part, regulate their own growth. Conversely, the presence of intact immune responses is not sufficient to prevent dissemination should the parasites' own regulatory mechanisms fail.

The level of ecdysteroid-like substances are generally negligible in healthy subjects. The administration of exogenous, or endogenous, corticosteroids may result in increased amounts of ecdysteroid-like substances in the host's tissues, including in the intestinal wall, where adult females reside. These substances may act as moulting signals for the eggs or rhabditiform larvae, which transform intraluminally into excessive numbers of filariform larvae (Genta 1992). Available data are not sufficient to prove a dose-dependent effect, but it is indeed remarkable that patients who develop fulminating hyperinfection after only a few days of steroid administration are usually those who have received intravenous methylprednisone. Once a population has become very large (for example 100,000 adult worms) it may continue to expand rapidly, even at low moulting rates, and the discontinuation of steroids may not be sufficient to arrest the relentless growth process which leads to the host's death. Some evidence from the gerbil model supports this as other immunosuppressive effectors are not as effective at inducing hyperinfection as is methyprednisolone and large worm burdens lead to hyperinfection in the absence of immunosuppression (Nolan et al. 2002).

Growth and survival requirements

Attempts to cultivate the parasitic stages of S. stercoralis in vitro have been unsuccessful. Infective larvae have been maintained for months under host-like conditions in tissue culture media (Chapman et al. 1994), but the larvae failed to grow or develop. Free-living stages are easily reared in standard parasitological cocultures. These stages can also be raised on agar plates seeded with bacteria or in liquid cultures consisting of bacteria in a nematode saline.

Hosts

These include dogs, various primates and humans. Cats, ferrets and gerbils (Nolan et al. 1993) have been infected experimentally. Transmissibility of S. stercoralis between host species varies geographically. The canine strain from North America is transmissible to humans (Georgi 1974), although molecular characterization using RFLP was able to distinguish a dog isolate from several human isolates (Ramachandran et al. 1997).

Animal hosts

Pre-patent period

In both primates and dogs the pre-patent period is short, rhabditiform larvae appearing in the faeces in 1–2 weeks.

Symptoms and signs

Symptoms and signs of infection vary markedly with respect to the individual. In primates there is also marked interspecific variation, monkeys being less susceptible than the anthropoid apes. Most cases in dogs are asymptomatic and become occult in 2–3 months. Although larvae disappear from the faeces, barren adult females may survive embedded in the intestinal mucosa for several months after the infection becomes inapparent (Schad et al. 1997). These infections can be reactivated by immunosuppression attributable to either chemotherapy or concurrent disease. Dogs that have expelled an infection are resistant to reinfection.

In young pups, hyperinfective strongyloidosis occurs spontaneously. Although these infections are usually mild and self-limiting, in some animals the worm burden may increase to clinically significant levels associated with watery or mucus diarrhoea and with signs of bronchopneumonia. Older dogs rarely become severely infected.

S. stercoralis occurs commonly in various monkeys. It is usually well tolerated, but in young Patas monkeys (Erythrocebus patas) it may produce severe hyperinfective strongyloidosis (Harper et al. 1982). These severely affected animals have diarrhoea, lose weight, and may die suddenly. Larvae may or may not be found in the faeces even in severely affected cases. Severe, often fatal strongyloidosis, occurs even more frequently in young anthropoid apes (Penner 1981). Gibbons are particularly susceptible to sudden death without a history of previous illness.

Diagnosis

Diagnosis of S. stercoralis infection is complicated by the fact that larvae may be absent from the faeces even in symptomatic cases. Additionally, larvae (not eggs) pass in the faeces, making concentration techniques using high density flotation solutions somewhat difficult to use. The Baermann apparatus is commonly used for finding larvae in faeces. The first-stage larvae are easily recognized, their genital primordium being exceptionally prominent. Many cases of this infection are probably first suspected when larvae are seen either in a direct smear or in a saturated salt flotation. The Baermann funnel is then used to obtain clean, intact larvae for a definitive diagnosis. However, faecal flotations done with zinc sulfate yield readily identifiable larvae provided that the preparation is examined promptly before the larvae shrink. In animals showing respiratory symptoms, a transtracheal wash may reveal migrating third-stage larvae. This stage is easily identifiable by its long filariform oesophagus and its notched tail. A small percentage of the larvae present in a faecal sample may be third-stage larvae, particularly in recently acquired infections. Infectious stools held at room temperature for 24 hours or more may contain a variety of stages, including free-living adults. Although rarely used with dogs, the agar plate method of Koga et al. (1990) can also be used (for details see 'Diagnosis' under 'Human hosts' below). However, care must be taken to distinguish the species of the larvae leaving the tracks on the agar as hookworms are common in dogs and will also be detected by this technique. In the USA this parasite is most commonly diagnosed in puppies recently acquired from a pet store or 'puppy mill'.

Pathology

Intestinal pathology varies with intensity of the infection which in turn varies with the strain of organism and the age and species of host. In asymptomatic infected dogs, the intestinal tissues may be grossly normal and worms and larvae exceedingly difficult to find by histological methods. In symptomatic cases, gross intestinal changes range from congestion of mucosal surface with an abnormal abundance of luminal mucus to confluent ulceration that may penetrate to the muscular layer. In cases of severe infection, parasites in great abundance will be present in the intestinal walls (Grove et al. 1983).

In primates a similar range of lesions has been observed; however, severe strongyloidosis with significant ulcerative enteritis is rare in monkeys but well known in gibbons and orangutans. Complicated strongyloidosis with severe hyperinfection occurs spontaneously in young Patas monkeys, gibbons and orangutans. Characteristic pathological lesions include the presence of the full spectrum of parasite life history stages in the gastrointestinal tract and the presence of filariform larvae in the lungs associated with pulmonary haemorrhage. The number of migrating larvae frequently does not correlate with the amount of pulmonary haemorrhage.

Treatment

Treatment of dogs with an active hyperinfection is difficult because available drugs do not kill the migrating autoinfective L3. However, unless a dog is very young or immunosuppressed, it is unlikely to have numerous migrating autoinfective larvae at any one time. The following anthelmintic treatments will remove adult *S. stercoralis* from dogs:

- Albendazole, twice daily for 3 consecutive days at 100 mg/kg.
- Thiabendazole, once a day for 3 consecutive days at 50 mg/kg,
- Fenbendazole, once a day for 3 days at 50 mg/kg;
- Ivermectin, one dose at 200 ug/kg.

In all cases, follow-up faecal examinations should be done weekly for 2 to 3 weeks to verify that no migrating larvae survived the treatment and matured. In cases where hyperinfection is suspected the following treatments can be used: fenbendazole, once daily for 7 to 14 days at 50 mg/kg or ivermectin once every 4 days for 3 or 4 doses at 200 ug/kg (Mansfield *et al.* 1992). Although these treatments will not kill migrating larvae, they will remove adults as they mature in the small intestine and therefore prevent new autoinfective larvae from being produced. The problem is that the life-span of migrating autoinfective larvae is unknown (although mathematical modelling suggests the migration should take no more than 5 days (Mansfield *et al.* 1995)), and, therefore, recommended treatments may continue for longer than necessary. Again, follow-up faecal examinations should be done to confirm that a parasitological cure has been achieved. Ivermectin and fenbendazole should also be effective against *S. stercoralis* infections in cats.

The possible occurrence of migrating autoinfective larvae must also be considered in treating primates for a *S. stercoralis* infection. In most animals, unless immunosuppressed, it is unlikely that numerous autoinfective larvae will be present, and, therefore, a single course of treatment should be curative. The following treatment regimes, each repeated after 2 weeks, have been used in primates:

- Thiabendazole, 50 to 100 mg/kg, PO, once a day for 2 days,
- Mebendazole, 50 mg/kg, PO, twice a day for 3 days,
- Fenbendazole, 25 mg/kg, PO, once a day for 3 days,
- Ivermectin, 0.2 mg/kg, PO, as a single dose.

However, in the anthropoid apes, i.e. gibbons, chimpanzees, gorillas, and the orangutan, fatal infections have occurred, especially in juveniles in the absence of immunosuppression. Fatal hyperinfections are also seen in otherwise normal Patas monkeys. Thus, in these animals a more extended course of treatment may be advisable. In all cases, follow-up faecal examinations should be done for an extended period to verify that treatment has completely eliminated the parasites.

Prognosis

The prognosis for dogs infected with *S. stercoralis* is good. Except in dogs infected with the Southeast Asian (Indochinese) strain of the parasite, the infection is usually self-limiting and infrequently attains a clinical level of intensity. The prognosis for infections in primates varies with the species of host. Most monkeys carry easily treated asymptomatic infections. Anthropoid apes, on the other hand, are more susceptible to severe strongyloidosis, and young gibbons and orangutans, in particular, may die suddenly without apparent previous illness. In anthropoid apes, partial clearing of the infection by most anthelmintics occurs, resulting in low-grade, sometimes occult, chronic infection which may be seriously exacerbated by subsequent immunosuppression.

Human hosts

Pre-patent period

The pre-patent period in humans has been reported to be between 23 and 28 days (Freedman 1991). This is about a week longer than the pre-patent period in animals.

Symptoms and signs

Acute infection

The clinical manifestations of acute strongyloidosis are generally associated with the path of larval migration to the small intestine. Infected individuals may experience irritation at the site of skin penetration by larvae, followed by tracheal irritation or dry cough and ultimately gastrointestinal symptoms such as diarrhoea, constipation, abdominal pain, or anorexia (Keiser 2004).

Chronic, uncomplicated infection

In uncomplicated strongyloidosis, many patients are asymptomatic or have mild cutaneous and/or abdominal symptoms.

Gastrointestinal manifestations

The gastrointestinal manifestations of chronic strongyloidosis are usually non-specific. Epigastric abdominal pain, post-prandial fullness or bloating, and heartburn are among the symptoms most commonly reported, episodes of diarrhoea alternating with constipation may also occur (Grove 1996; Milder *et al.* 1981). The diarrhoea usually consists of semi-formed non-bloody stools. Occult blood in the stool can occur in persons with chronic infections, and even massive colonic haemorrhage has been reported.

Physical examination of chronically infected patients is normal or reveals only mild abdominal tenderness on palpation. Less commonly, chronic strongyloidosis resembles inflammatory bowel disease, particularly ulcerative colitis, and the endoscopic appearance may be that of pseudopolyposis.

Cutaneous manifestations

Dermatologic manifestations such as recurrent urticaria can occur (Leighton 1990; Pelletier *et al.* 1988) as can *larva currens*, (pruritic linear streaks located along the lower trunk, thighs and buttocks) as a result of migrating larvae.

Other manifestations

Unusual manifestations of chronic strongyloidosis include arthritis (Richter *et al.* 2006), nephrotic syndrome (Hsieh *et al.* 2006), chronic malabsorption (Alam 1982; Atul *et al.* 2005; Garcia *et al.* 1977; Harish *et al.* 2005; Sturchler 1987), duodenal obstruction (Suvarna *et al.* 2005), focal hepatic lesions (Gulbas *et al.* 2004) and recurrent asthma (Tullis 1970).

Hyperinfection syndrome/disseminated Strongyloidosis

Hyperinfection describes the syndrome of accelerated autoinfection, generally the result of an alteration in immune status (Longworth *et al.* 1986). The distinction between autoinfection and hyperinfection is not strictly defined, but hyperinfection syndrome implies the presence of signs and symptoms attributable to increased larval migration. Development or exacerbation of gastrointestinal and pulmonary symptoms is seen, and the detection of increased numbers of larvae in stool and/or sputum is the hallmark of hyperinfection. Disseminated infection occurs when larvae migrate beyond the organs of the autoinfective cycle (lung and gastrointestinal tract), although this may occur at low levels in chronic strongyloidosis.

Hyperinfection syndrome has been described as late as 64 years after an individual has left a *Strongyloides*-endemic area.

Gastrointestinal

Gastrointestinal symptoms commonly occur and may include crampy abdominal pain or bloating, watery diarrhoea, constipation, anorexia, weight loss, difficulty swallowing, sore throat, nausea or vomiting. Diffuse abdominal tenderness and hypoactive bowel sounds may be due to ileus and small bowel obstruction. Protein losing enteropathy can give rise to hypoalbuminemia with peripheral oedema and ascites. Mesenteric lymphadenopathy has been reported to cause intestinal pseudo-obstruction in HIV infected patients with hyperinfection syndrome. Mucosal ulceration can occur in the small intestine as a result of direct invasion of larvae and may be associated with occult blood, haematochezia or life threatening gastrointestinal bleeding.

Infectious complications

Penetration of large numbers of larvae through the intestinal wall can be associated with gram negative sepsis as larvae carry organisms with them into the bloodstream. Organisms that have been reported to cause sepsis in such patients include Group D streptococci, *Streptococcus bovis* meningitis and bacteremia, *Escherichia coli*, *Klebsiella pneumoniae*, *Proteus mirabilis*, Pseudomonas, *Enterococcus faecalis*, coagulase negative staphylococci and *Streptococcus pneumonia* (Keiser 2004).

Either aseptic or gram negative meningitis can be associated with disseminated strongyloidosis. Larvae have been recovered from cerebrospinal fluid, meningeal vessels, dura, epidural, subdural and subarachnoid spaces.

Pulmonary manifestations, if present, include cough, wheezing, hoarseness, palpitations, atrial fibrillation, pleuritic chest pain, or dyspnea. Petechial haemorrhage, hyperemia of the bronchial mucosa or, rarely, massive haemoptysis have been reported. Chest radiographs most frequently demonstrate focal or bilateral interstitial infiltrates.

Cutaneous manifestations such as, Cutaneous periumbilical purpura has been described in patients with disseminated disease due to migration of larvae through vessel walls in the dermis (Salluh *et al.* 2005).

Neurologic/Central Nervous System manifestations

Apart from the meningitis (both bacterial and aseptic), a less common form of central nervous system manifestation is the formation of cerebral and cerebellar abscesses containing *S. stercoralis* larvae.

Infrequent manifestations such as cardiac arrhythmias and arrest are rare and have been attributed to a direct myocardial damage caused by the migrating larvae or to electrolyte imbalance precipitated by severe intestinal strongyloidosis. The passage of larvae in the sperm and the presence of genital lesions in association with strongyloidosis have also been described, however, Grove (1982) found no evidence that it could be transmitted through sexual contact.

Diagnosis

The stage of *S. stercoralis* most commonly identified in faeces is the rhabditiform larva, but filariform larvae, adult females and even eggs also may be identified. The sensitivity of a single stool examination for the detection of *S. stercoralis* ranges between 30% and 60%. The use of a Baermann apparatus allows a larger volume of faeces (up to several grams) to be examined and is more sensitive than direct microscopy. Culturing faeces mixed with bone charcoal or peat moss also increases the sensitivity of faecal examination. However, these procedures are not suited for routine diagnosis in the clinical laboratory. A detection method proposed by Koga *et al.* (1990) involves the use of nutrient agar plates and is very sensitive and easy to perform. This method depends on larval dispersal from a faecal sample applied to the surface of a 1.5% nutrient agar plate and the subsequent growth of bacteria along the tracks left by these larvae. This technique has been shown to be more sensitive than formalin-ether sedimentation, Harada-Mori filter paper cultures or the Baermann technique (Arakaki *et al.* 1990; Intapan *et al.* 2005; De Kaminsky 1993), and using a cheaper non-nutrient agar works almost as well (Sukhavat *et al.* 1994). Although the examination of duodenal aspirate is reportedly very sensitive, this invasive method is recommended only in the paediatric patient when it is necessary to achieve a rapid demonstration of parasites, as in an immunocompromised child with suspected overwhelming infection. The 'string test,' a gelatin capsule containing a string swallowed by the patient and retrieved after a few hours, enjoyed some popularity a few years ago, but currently is infrequently used. In disseminated infections larvae of all stages and adult parasites have been found in specimens of sputum and broncho-alveolar lavage, ascitic fluid, pancreatic aspirates, and cerebro-spinal fluid. In summary, stool examination is currently the primary technique for the detection of *S. stercoralis*. If special techniques are not available, several specimens collected on different days should be examined if the diagnosis is strongly suspected.

The only haematologic abnormality associated with chronic, uncomplicated strongyloidosis is eosinophilia. In most case series, *Strongyloides*-associated eosinophil levels ranged between 500 and 1,500 eosinophils/mm^3. Patients with disseminated strongyloidosis often have normal eosinophil counts likely related to either corticosteroid administration or endogenous factors (e.g. fever, endogenous steroids, stress, epinephrine).

Total serum IgE levels are elevated (> 200 IU/ml) in 50 to 70% of the patients with strongyloidosis. The diagnostic relevance of such elevation is similar to that of eosinophilia. Both eosinophilia and an elevated IgE level should be investigated, but the absence of elevation does not necessarily exclude strongyloidosis.

Enzyme linked immunosorbent assay (ELISA) has been increasingly used in conjunction with stool studies to increase diagnostic sensitivity. The high negative predictive value of the ELISA can be particularly useful in excluding strongyloidosis part of the differential diagnosis (Genta 1988). Despite its usefulness, serodiagnosis has several limitations including cross reactivity in patients with active filarial infections, lower sensitivity in patients with haematologic malignancies or HTLV-1 infection and inability to distinguish between current and past infection (Conway *et al.* 1993a, b). In addition, the current ELISA relies on the preparation of larval antigen from stool samples of heavily infected humans or experimentally infected animals.

Various techniques have been developed in an effort to improve on the drawbacks of the current immunoassays. Recombinant antigens, such as NIE, have been proposed as an alternative to the crude antigen currently in use (Ravi *et al.* 2002). An immediate hypersensitivity skin test has been used in a research setting quite effectively, although it may have limited utility in HTLV-1 infected patients (Neva *et al.* 2001). Most recently, a lucifease immunoprecipitation assays (LIPS) has been developed using two recombinant Strongyloides-specific recombinant construct that has provided a rapid, sensitive and specific method for diagnosis (Ramanathan *et al.* 2008).

Pathology

The pathologic lesions associated with chronic, uncomplicated *S. stercoralis* have received little attention, because only rarely have patients with such lesions come to autopsy. However, pathologic descriptions of the lesions in a few patients in whom strongyloidosis was an incidental finding and animal studies indicate that the worms can exist in the intestinal mucosa without causing significant inflammatory responses or tissue damage. The classic description of the pathology of strongyloidosis was made by De Paola in 1962, and later updated by Genta and Caymmi-Gomes. These authors proposed the subdivision of the intestinal lesions into three distinct forms.

In 'catarrhal enteritis' (presumably associated with light infections), the small intestine is congested, the mucosa is covered with abundant mucoid secretions, and scattered petechial haemorrhages are present. The most remarkable histologic feature is an increased mononuclear infiltrate in the submucosa, although parasites are rare. In the more severe 'oedematous enteritis', the intestinal wall is grossly thickened, the mucosal folds flattened, and the affected intestinal segments assume a rubbery consistency. Submucosal oedema, flattening of the villi, and parasites scattered throughout the lamina propria are observed microscopically. The most severe form 'ulcerative enteritis' is almost exclusively seen in association with hyperinfection. The intestinal walls may be rigid due to the oedema and fibrosis resulting from long-standing inflammation, the mucosa may be show atrophy, erosions and ulcerations. An abundant inflammatory infiltrate, most often consisting of neutrophils, as well as all stages of *S. stercoralis*, are present throughout the intestinal mucosa. Jejunal perforation has been reported in patients with the ulcerative enteritis form of strongyloidosis. Uncommonly, the mucosal damage occurs predominantly in the large intestine, simulating ulcerative colitis and pseudopolyposis. *S. stercoralis* larvae have been found in the appendix, and eosinophilic appendicitis apparently caused by this parasite has been reported. In patients with disseminated strongyloidosis, the intestinal lesions reflect the large number of worms dwelling within the small intestinal mucosa and penetrating the intestinal walls. In addition, the stomach and the peritoneal cavity may be invaded by migrating parasites. However, because most of these patients are receiving immunosuppressive doses of corticosteroids, inflammatory responses are often minimal in spite of extensive tissue damage. The gastrointestinal pathology is often overshadowed by the lesions found in other organs, particularly in patients who receive anthelminthic therapy before succumbing to disseminated strongyloidosis.

Migrating parasites may cause mechanical damage as well as inflammation. In human patients, the extra-intestinal organ most commonly affected by this migratory damage is the lung. In severe disseminated infection, when larger numbers of adult parasites dwell in the intestine and millions of larvae migrate throughout the body, alveolar microhaemorrhages may result in massive pulmonary bleeding. As larvae penetrate the large intestine, they create small breaks in the mucosa that facilitate the invasion of the bloodstream by enteric bacteria. The larvae themselves carry bacteria on their cuticle to distant sites. Regardless of the mechanism, the widespread dissemination of larvae is frequently associated with polymicrobial sepsis, diffuse or patchy bronchopneumonia, pulmonary and cerebral abscesses, and meningitis. Filariform larvae, and occasionally rhabditiform larvae and adult worms, also may disseminate to mesenteric lymph nodes, the biliary tract, as well as the liver, pancreas, spleen, heart, endocrine glands and ovaries. In these locations the parasite frequently induces a granulomatous response.

Treatment

To prevent the development of hyperinfection syndrome, chronically infected, asymptomatic individuals must be treated (Coulter *et al.* 1992). Because even one remaining adult female can multiply and cause disseminated disease, the goal of treatment is complete eradication of the parasite. The current treatment of choice for chronic strongyloidosis is single dose ivermectin (200ug/kg), although some studies have suggested that 2 doses of ivermectin 200 ug/kg given on consecutive days may have greater efficacy. Ivermectin has better efficacy when compared to thiabendazole in patients with chronic, uncomplicated strongyloidosis. In a randomized trial, up to 95% of patients on thiabendazole experienced side effects compared to 18% of ivermectin-treated patients. Side effects of thiabendazole include general fatigue, dizziness, headache, nausea, anorexia, abdominal pain, liver dysfunction and neuropsychiatric symptoms. Ivermectin has superior efficacy when compared to albendazole, a drug that has cure rates ranging from 45–77% (Archibald *et al.* 1993; Jorgensen *et al.* 1996).

For disseminated strongyloidosis, oral ivermectin should be given daily until stool examinations are negative for at least 2 weeks (the duration of the autoinfective cycle) or longer if patients remain immunosuppressed. Off label rectal administration of ivermectin or thiabendazole, while useful in some critically ill patients, can be problematic in patients with severe diarrhoea. Patients with paralytic ileus can have difficulty absorbing oral ivermectin due to tissue oedema, larger volume of distribution and increased clearance of unbound drug. Lower serum ivermectin levels than that achieved in normal subjects after oral administration have been demonstrated in patients with paralytic ileus. Parenteral formulations of ivermectin, however, are not currently approved for use in humans and have only been used under compassionate use INDs.

Prognosis

Except in cases of hyperinfection, the prognosis is good. Many infected persons are asymptomatic or have nonspecific minor complaints. In adults, these well-regulated infections may persist for decades without producing clinically significant strongyloidosis, and most will respond to anthelmintic treatment. However, because the risk of developing severe, hyperinfective strongyloidosis is always present, all infected persons must be considered at risk for fatal infection and treated with the goal of achieving a parasitological cure. Once hyperinfection occurs prognosis should be guarded.

Epidemiology

Although information regarding the worldwide prevalence of strongyloidosis is fragmentary, 3 million to 100 million are estimated to be infected worldwide. The unreliability of these estimates is reflected in the wide range of prevalence rates, varying between <1% and 85%, of populations living in adjacent regions of the same country. With these limitations in mind, one can assume that *S. stercoralis* is present in virtually all tropical and subtropical regions of the world. Pockets of low endemicity (<1% to 3%) exist in several industrialized countries of Western Europe (e.g. Italy, France, and Switzerland), Eastern Europe, the USA (the Appalachian region and the Southern states), Japan (Okinawa) and Australia (aboriginal populations). Significant prevalences of strongyloidosis have been found in institutionalized patients. Considering the long persistence of this parasite in its host and its relatively high prevalence among some populations, physicians practicing in industrialized countries should consider strongyloidosis in immigrant or refugee patients born in tropical or subtropical regions as well as in persons from local areas of endemicity (Genta 1989).

Immunocompromise and hyperinfection/dissemination

Corticosteroids

For reasons that are not entirely clear, corticosteroids have a particularly strong and specific association with the development of hyperinfection syndrome. Hyperinfection syndrome has been described regardless of dose, duration or route of administration. Even short courses of steroids in immunocompetent patients have led to hyperinfection syndrome and death. Other therapies or conditions may predispose to dissemination although the concomitant administration of steroids in most cases makes it difficult to assign a direct causal association (Ramanathan *et al.* 2008).

HTLV-1 Infection

A growing body of evidence points to the synergistic relationship between human T-cell lymphotropic virus type 1 (HTLV-1) and *Strongyloides*. Higher rates of Strongyloides infection have been found in HTLV-1/Strongyloides-co-infected patients (Arakaki *et al.* 1992). Relapsing *Strongyloides* infection despite treatment should prompt consideration of HTLV-1 infection. HTLV-1 enhances susceptibility to *Strongyloides* infection as a result of diminished IgE levels. *Strongyloides* may, in turn, facilitate HTLV-1 virus replication as suggested by a measurable decline in HTLV-1 mRNA levels in one patient after treatment with ivermectin. *Strongyloides* has been proposed to accelerate the progression of HTLV-1 to adult T-cell leukemia in that there is a more rapid development of leukemia in co-infected patients.

HIV

Hyperinfection syndrome has not been observed frequently with HIV infected patients despite vast numbers of co-infected individuals. A recent study postulates that lower CD4+ counts may favour indirect rather than direct development of *Strongyloides* larvae based on the proportion of free living adults and infective larvae in stools of co-infected patients. Whether immune reconstitution syndrome occurs after the initiation of antiretroviral therapy in *Strongyloides* infected patients remains unclear although this issue has been raised in case reports.

Other conditions

Several case reports have supported an association between *Strongyloides* infection and primary hypogammaglobulinemia. In these cases, prolonged recovery and refractoriness to therapy was noted. Haematologic malignancies such as lymphoma have been associated with hyperinfection syndrome in the absence of corticosteroid use. Relatively few cases of infection following bone marrow transplantation have been reported.

Prevention and control

Transmission of *S. stercoralis* among both humans and animals can be prevented by implementing measures aimed at ensuring proper disposal and treatment of excrement and by avoiding contact with contaminated substrata, i.e. soil, caging, etc. The free-living larval stages are susceptible to desiccation. Thus, maintaining a clean dry environment provides effective control. In human patients from endemic areas who may harbour asymptomatic chronic strongyloidosis, life-threatening disseminated hyperinfection may be prevented by seeking and eradicating the parasite before corticosteroid, immunosuppressive or anti-neoplastic therapy is started. Strongyloidosis in animal populations has been a problem in canine breeding kennels and in the primate colonies of zoos and research organizations. Both death losses and occurrences of clinical strongyloidosis can be reduced in breeding kennels by periodic mass treatment with thiabendazole or ivermectin, but this will not eradicate the parasitism in the dog population. Apparently, eradication has been achieved as a by-product of *Filaroides hirthi* control. This involved treating of brood bitches between pregnancies with albendazole given at the rate of 25 mg/kg orally twice daily for 5 days. Control of strongyloidosis in primate colonies has depended on creating a clean dry environment because the free-living larvae of strongyloides are highly susceptible to desiccation. It also depends on the detection of infected individuals by faecal examination and their treatment. Thiabendazole given orally by stomach tube or in food as a single dose of 100 mg/kg and repeated after 2 weeks is effective for control.

References

Alam, S.Z. and Purohit, D. (1982). A case report. Malabsorption secondary to S. *stercoralis* infestation. *Med. J. Zambia*, **16**: 85.

Arakaki, T., Iwanaga, M., Kinjo, F., Saito, A., Asato, R. and Ikeshiro, T. (1990). Efficacy of agar-plate culture in detection of *Strongyloides stercoralis* infection. *J. Parasitol.*, **76**: 425–28.

Arakaki, T., Asato, A.R., Ikeshiro, T., Sakiyama, K. and Iwanaga, M. (1992). Is the prevalence of HTLV-1 infection higher in *Strongyloides* carriers than in non-carriers? *Trop. Med. Parasit.*, **4**: 199–200.

Archibald, L.K., Beeching, N.J., Gill, G.V., Bailey, J.W. and Bell, D.R. (1993). Albendazole is an effective treatment for chronic strongyloidosis. *Queensland J. Med.*, **86**: 191–95.

Ashton, F.T., Bhopale, V.M., Holt, D., Smith, G. and Schad, G.A. (1998). Developmental switching in the parasitic nematode Strongyloides stercoralis is controlled by the ASF and ASI amphidial neurons. *J. Parasitol.*, **84**: 691–95.

Atul, S., Ajay, D., Ritambhara, N., Harsh, M. and Ashish, B. (2005). An unusual cause of malabsorption in an immunocompetent host. *J. Ayub Med. Coll., Abbottabad: JAMC*, **17**: 85–86.

Chapman, M.R., Hutchinson, G.W., Cenac, M.J. and Klei, T.R. (1994). In vitro culture of equine Strongylidae to the forth larval stage in a cell-free medium. *J. Parasitol.*, **80**: 225–31.

Conway, D.J., Atkins, N.S., Lillywhite, J.E., *et al.* (1993a). Immunodiagnosis of *Strongyloides stercoralis* infection: a method for increasing the specificity of the indirect ELISA. *Trans. R. Soc. Trop. Med. Hyg.*, **87**: 173–76.

Conway, D.J., Bailey, J.W., Lindo, J.F., *et al.* (1993b). Serum IgG reactivity with 41-, 31-, and 28-kDa larval proteins of *Strongyloides stercoralis* in individuals with strongyloidosis. *J. Infect. Dis.*, **168**: 784–87.

Coulter, C., Walker, D.G., Gunsberg, M., *et al.* (1992). Successful treatment of disseminated strongyloidosis. *Med. J. Aus.*, **157**: 331–32.

De Kaminsky, R.G. (1993). Evaluation of three methods for laboratory diagnosis of *Strongyloides stercoralis* infection. *J. Parasitol.*, **79**: 277–80.

Forbes, W.M., Ashton, F.T., Boston, R. and Schad, G.A. (2003). Chemotactic behaviour of *Strongyloides stercoralis* infective larvae on a sodium chloride gradient. *Parasitology*, **127**: 189–97.

Freedman, D.O. (1991). Experimental infection of human subject with *Strongyloides* species. *Rev. Infect. Dis.*, **13**: 1221–26.

Garcia, F.T., Sessions, J.T., Strum, W.B., *et al.* (1977). Intestinal function and morphology in strongyloidosis. *Am. J. Trop. Med. Hyg.*, **26**: 859–65.

Genta, R.M. (1986). *Strongyloides stercoralis*: immunobiological considerations on an unusual worm. *Parasit. Today*, **2**: 241–46.

Genta, R.M. (1988). Predictive value of an enzyme-linked immunosorbent assay (ELISA) for the serodiagnosis of strongyloidosis. *J. Clin. Path.*, **89**: 391–94.

Genta, R.M. (1989). Global prevalence of strongyloidosis: critical review with epidemiologic insights into the prevention of disseminated disease. *Rev. Infect. Dis.*, **11**: 755–67.

Genta, R.M. (1992). Dysregulation of strongyloidosis: a new hypothesis. *Clin. Microbiol. Rev.*, **5**: 345–55.

Georgi, J.R. and Sprinkle, C.L. (1974). A case of human strongyloidosis apparently contracted from asymptomatic colony dogs. *Am. J. Trop. Med. Hyg.*, **23**: 899–901.

Grove, D.I. (1982). Strongyloidosis: is it transmitted from husband to wife? *Br. J. Venereal Dis.*, **58**: 271–72.

Grove, D.I., Heenan, P.J. and Northern, C. (1983). Persistent and Disseminated Infections with *Strongyloides stercoralis* in immunosuppressed dogs. *Int. J. Parasitol.*, **13**: 483–90.

Grove, D.I. (1989). Historical introduction. *Strongyloidosis: a major roundworm infection of man*, pp. 1–9. London: Taylor & Francis.

Grove, D.I. (1996). Human strongyloidosis. *Adv. Parasit.*, **38**: 251–309.

Gulbas, Z., Kebapci, M., Pasaoglu, O. and Vardareli, E. (2004). Successful ivermectin treatment of hepatic strongyloidosis presenting with severe eosinophilia. *Southern Med. J.*, **97**: 907–10.

Harish, K., Sunilkumar, R., Varghese, T. and Feroze, M. (2005). Strongyloidosis presenting as duodenal obstruction. *Trop. Gastroenter.*, **26**: 201–2.

Harper, J.S., Rice, J.M., London, W.T., Sly, D.L., and Middleton, C. (1982). Disseminated Strongyloidosis in *Erythrocebus patas*. *Am. J. Primatol.*, **3**: 89–98.

Hira, P.R., and Patel, B.G. (1980). Human strongyloidosis due to the primate species *Strongyloides fuelleborni*. *Trop. Geograph. Med.*, **32**: 23–29.

Hsieh, Y.P., Wen, Y.K. and Chen, M.L. (2006). Minimal change nephrotic syndrome in association with strongyloidosis. *Clin. Nephr.*, **66**: 459–63.

Intapan, P.M., Maleewong, W., *et al.* (2005). Comparison of the quantitative formalin ethyl acetate concentration technique and agar plate culture for diagnosis of human strongyloidosis. *J. Clin. Microbiol.*, **43**: 1932–33.

Jorgensen, T., Montresor, A., and Savioli, L. (1996). Effectively controlling Strongyloidasis. *Parasitol. Today*, **12**: 164.

Kerlin, R.L., Nolan, T.J., and Schad, G.A. (1995). *Strongyloides stercoralis*: Histopathology of uncomplicated and hyperinfective strongyloidasis in the Mongolian gerbil, a rodent model for human strongyloidosis. *Int. J. Parasitol.*, **25**: 411–20.

Keiser, P.B. and Nutman, T.B. (2004). *Strongyloides stercoralis* in the immunocompromised population. *Clin. Microbiol. Rev.*, **17**: 208–17.

Koga, K., Kasuya, S., Khamboonruang, C., *et al.* (1990). An evaluation of the agar plate method for the detection of Strongyloides stercoralis in northern Thailand. *J. Trop. Med. Hyg.*, **93**: 183–88.

Leighton, P.M. and Macsween, H.M. (1990). *Strongyloides* stercoralis. The cause of an urticarial-like eruption of 65 years' duration. *Arch. Intern. Med.*, **150**: 1747–48.

Lopez, P.M., Boston, R., Ashton, F.T. and Schad, G.A. (2000). The neurons of class ALD mediate thermotaxis in the parasitic nematode, Strongyloides stercoralis. *Int. J. Parasitol.*, **30**: 1115–21.

Longworth, D.L., and Weller, P.F. (1986). Hyperinfection syndrome with strongylodiasis. In: J.S. Remington and M.N. Schwartz (eds.) *Current Clinical Topics in Infectious Diseases*, pp. 1–26. NY: McGraw Hill.

Mansfield, L.S., and Schad, G.A. (1992). Ivermectin treatment of naturally acquired and experimentally induced *Strongyloides stercoralis* infections in dogs. *J. Am. Vet. Med. Ass.*, **201**: 726–30.

Mansfield, L.S., Alavi, A., Wortman, J.A. and Schad, G.A. (1995). Gamma camera scintigraphy for direct visualization of larval migration in *Strongyloides stercoralis*-infected dogs. *Am. J. Trop. Med. Hyg.*, **52**: 236–40.

Milder, J.E., Walzer, P.D., Kilgore, G., Rutherford, I. and Klein, M. (1981). Clinical features of *Strongyloides stercoralis* infection in an endemic area of the United States. *Gastroenterology*, **80**: 1481–88.

Neva, F.A., Gam, A.A., Maxwell, C. and Pelletier, L.L. (2001). Skin test antigens for immediate hypersensitivity prepared from infective larvae of *Strongyloides stercoralis*. *Am. J. Trop. Med. Hyg.*, **65**: 567–72.

Nolan, T.J., Megyeri, Z., Bhopale, V.M., and Schad, A. (1993). *Strongyloides stercoralis*: The first rodent model for uncomplicated and hyperinfective strongyloidosis, the Mongolian gerbil (*Meriones unguiculatus*). *J. Infect. Dis.*, **168**: 1479–84.

Nolan, T.J., Rotman, H.L., Bhopale, V.M., Schad, G.A., and Abraham, D. (1995). Immunity to a challenge infection of *Strongyloides stercoralis* third-stage larvae in the jird. *Parasite Immunol.*, **17**: 599–604.

Nolan, T.J., Bhopale, V.M. and Schad, G.A. (1999). *Strongyloides stercoralis*: oral transfer of parasitic adult worms produces infection in mice and infection with subsequent autoinfection in gerbils. *Int. J. Parasitol.*, **29**: 1047–51.

Nolan, T.J., Bhopale, V.M., Rotman, H.L., *et al.* (2002). *Strongyloides stercoralis*: high worm population density leads to autoinfection in the jird (*Meriones ungui*culatus). *Exp. Parasitol.*, **100**: 173–78.

Nolan, T.J., Brenes, M., Ashton, F.T., *et al.* (2004). The amphidial neuron pair ALD controls the temperature-sensitive choice of alternative developmental pathways in the parasitic nematode, *Strongyloides stercoralis*. *Parasitology*, **129**: 753–59.

Nolan, T.J., Zhu, X., Ketschek, A., *et al.* (2007). The sugar glider (*Petaurus breviceps*): a laboratory host for the nematode *Parastrongyloides trichosuri*. *J. Parasitol.*, **93**: 1084–89.

Penner, L.R. (1981). Concerning Threadworm (Strongyloides stercoralis) in Great Apes-Lowland Gorillas (*Gorilla gorilla*) and Chimpanzees (*Pantroglodytes*). *J. Zoo Animal Med.*, **12**: 128–31.

Pelletier Jr., L.L., Baker, C.B., Gam, A.A., Nutman, T.B. and Neva, F.A. (1988). Diagnosis and evaluation of treatment of chronic strongyloidosis in ex-prisoners of war. *J. Infect.Dis.*, **157**: 573–76.

Ramachandran, S., Gam, A.A. and Neva, F.A. (1997). Molecular differences between several species of Strongyloides and comparison of selected isolates of S. stercoralis using a polymerase chain reaction-linked restriction fragment length polymorphism approach. *Am. J. Trop. Med. Hyg.*, **56**: 61–65.

Ramanathan, R., Burbelo, P.D., Groot, S., *et al.* (2008). Luciferase immunoprecipation systems assay enhances sensitivity and specificity of diagnosis in *Strongyloides stercoralis* infection. *J. Infect. Dis.*, **198**: 444–51.

Ravi, V., Ramachandran, S., Thompson, R.W., Andersen, J.F. and Neva, F.A. (2002). Characterization of a recombinant immunodiagnostic antigen (NIE) from *Strongyloides ste*rcoralis L3-stage larvae. *Mol. Biochem. Parasit.*, **125**: 73–81.

Richter, J., Muller-Stover, I., Strothmeyer, H., *et al.* (2006). Arthritis associated with *Strongyloides stercoralis* infection in HLA B-27-positive African. *Parasitol. Res.*, **99**: 706–7.

Safer, D., Brenes, M., Dunipace, S. and Schad, G. (2007). Urocanic acid is a major chemoattractant for the skin-penetrating parasitic nematode *Strongyloides stercoralis*. *Proc. Nat. Acad. Sci. USA*, **104**: 1627–30.

Salluh, J.I., Bozza, F.A., Pinto, T.S., Toscano, L., Weller, P.F. and Soares, M. (2005). Cutaneous periumbilical purpura in disseminated strongyloidosis in cancer patients: a pathognomonic feature of potentially lethal disease? *Brazilian J. Infect. Dis.*, **9**: 419–24.

Schad, G.A. (1989). Morphology and life history of *Strongyloides stercoralis*. *Strongyloidosis: a major roundworm infection of man,* pp. 85–104. London: Taylor & Francis.

Schad, G.A., Aikens, L.M. and Smith, G. (1989). *Strongyloides stercoralis*: is there a canonical migratory route through the host? *J. Parasitol.*, **75**(5): 740–49.

Schad, G.A., Smith, G., Megyeri, Z., Bhopale, V.M., Niamatali, S. and Maze, R. (1993). Strongyloides stercoralis: an initial autoinfective burst amplifies primary infection. *Am. J. Trop. Med. Hyg.*, **48**: 716–25.

Schad, G.A., Thompson, F., Talham, G., *et al.* (1997). Barren female *Strongyloides stercoralis* from occult chronic infections are rejuvenated by transfer to parasite-naive recipient hosts and give rise to an autoinfective burst. *J. Parasitol.*, **83**: 785–79.

Sciacca, J., Ketschek, A., Forbes, W.M., *et al.* (2002). Vertical migration by the infective larvae of three species of parasitic nematodes: is the behaviour really a response to gravity? *Parasitology,* **125**: 553–60.

Sukhavat, K., Morakote, N., Chaiwong, P., and Piangjai, S. (1994). Comparative efficacy of four methods for the detection of *Strongyloides stercoralis* in human stool specimens. *Ann. Trop. Med. Parasitol.*, **88**: 95–96.

Sturchler, D. (1987). Parasitic diseases of the small intestinal tract. *Bailliere's Clin. Gastroenter.*, **1**: 397–424.

Sukhavat, K., Morakote, N., Chaiwong, P. and Piangjai, S. (1994). Comparative efficacy of four methods for the detection of Strongyloides stercoralis in human stool specimens. *Ann. Trop. Med. Parasitol.*, **88**: 95–96.

Suvarna, D., Mehta, R., Sadasivan, S., Raj, V.V. and Balakrishnan, V. (2005). Infiltrating Strongyloides stercoralis presenting as duodenal obstruction. *Indian J. Gastroenter.*, **24**: 173–74.

Tullis, D.C. (1970). Bronchial asthma associated with intestinal parasites. *N. Eng. J. Med.*, **282**: 370–72.

CHAPTER 58

Capillariosis

Choosak Nithikathkul, Prasert Saichua,
Louis Royal and John H. Cross

Summary

Capillaria species are members of the superfamily Trichinelloidae. These worms have a filamentous thin anterior end and a slightly thicker oesophagus which is surrounded by glandular cells or stichocytes. This oesophageal pattern is called stichosomal oesophagus.

Capillaria species are parasites which are found in many vertebrate animals. More than two hundred species have been reported in several vertebrate species, including fish, amphibians, reptiles, birds, and mammals (Cross 1992; Chitwood *et al.* 1968), but only three species infect humans. These are *Capillaria hepatica, C. aerophila* and *C. philippinensis* (McCarthy and Moore 2000). Of these intestinal capillariosis, a fish-borne parasitic zoonoses caused by *C. philippinensis*, is the most important. Humans acquire the parasite, *C. philippinensis*, by eating uncooked or raw freshwater fish (Cross and Basaca-Sevilla 1991). The disease is endemic mainly in the Philippines and Thailand where there are many reported fatalities.

Although *C. hepatica* is found in rodents worldwide, only a few cases of hepatic capillariosis have been reported in humans from Europe, Asia, Africa, North and South America. The infection is acquired by the ingestion of embryonated eggs from the soil. Female worms deposit eggs in the liver tissue and granulomas develop around the egg. The eggs are released after the rodent is eaten and the liver digested. Eggs pass in the faeces and are deposited in the soil where they embryonate. Avoidance of contaminated soil would prevent human infection and destruction of rodents would control animal infections.

Only 12 cases of human infection caused by *Capillaria aerophila* have been reported, the majority from Russia. The parasite is found within tissue of the respiratory passages of canines and felines worldwide.

Anatrichosoma cutaneum (Nematoda, Trichosomoididae), also included in this chapter, is primarily a subcutaneous parasite of monkeys, but there are two reports of cutaneous infections in humans resulting in serpiginous lesions in the skin of the soles, palms, and nasal passages. In addition there is a further suspected case isolated from a breast nodule and a possible case of mucosal lesions in the mouth reported. Whole monkey colonies can be infected with this parasite and control is difficult.

Capillaria philippinensis

History

At the First International Congress of Parasitology in Rome in 1964, the case of a 29 year old male Philippine school teacher from Northern Luzon was presented. The patient had unremitting diarrhoea beginning 3 weeks prior to his admission to hospital. He died one week after admission, emaciated and with ascites, possibly related to his chronic alcoholism. Autopsy revealed intestinal worms, but with no definite identification of species. From 1965 to 1966, a large number of deaths related to symptoms of severe gastroenteritis were reported in Pudo West, a village some 150 km south of the school teacher's home. The cause was identified as infection with *Capillaria philippinensis* by the Philippine Department of Health. In subsequent reviews, it was found that more than 1,000 individuals were infected, with 77 deaths. Further infections were found in regions of the western and northern coasts of Luzon (Cross 1992).

In previous years, Cross reported the total numbers of intestinal capillariosis cases in Northern Luzon. From 1967 to 1990, there were 1,884 cases and 110 deaths (Cross 1992). In addition, sporadic cases have been reported from Japan (Nawa *et al.* 1988; Hong and Cross 2005), Korea (Lee *et al.* 1992; Hong *et al.* 1994), Taiwan (Hwang 1998; Lu *et al.* 2006; Bair *et al.* 2004), Indonesia (Chichino *et al.* 1992), Iran (Hoghooghi-Rad *et al.* 1987) and Egypt (Hong and Cross 2005). In humans, *C. philippinensis* causes intermittent or continuous diarrhoea leading to weight loss, abdominal pain, borborygmi, muscle wasting, weakness, and oedema. If the intestinal capillariosis patients are not treated, there will be more severe muscle wasting, cachexia, oedema and death. Most patients died from the fluid and electrolyte loss resulting in heart failure, or septicemia (Austin *et al.* 1999; El-Dib *et al.* 1999; el-Karaksky *et al.* 2004; Ahmed *et al.* 1999; Saichua *et al.* 2008).

Epidemiology

Intestinal capillariosis caused by *C. philippinensis* have been found in the Philippines, as well as in Thailand, Japan, Iran, Egypt and Taiwan. However, the major outbreaks have occurred in the Philippines and Thailand. Annual surveillance reports in Thailand from 1994 to 2005 showed 82 cases of intestinal capillariosis.

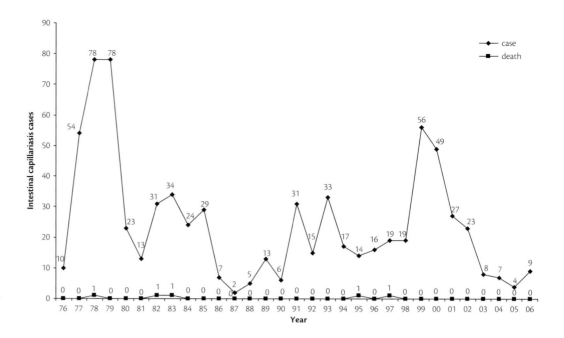

Fig. 58.1 Intestinal capillariosis cases in Thailand from 1976–2006
Data from Saichua *et al.*, 2008.

Nearly half of all these cases reported the consumption of raw or undercooked fish (Fig. 58.1) (Saichua *et al.* 2008).

In addition to the initial severe outbreak in the 1960s in Tagudin, Ilocos Sur in the Philippines, there was an epidemic in the early 1980s in Southern Leyte. Further outbreaks occurred in Monkayo in Compostela Valley Province, Philippines in the 1990s (Belizario *et al.* 2000).

Studies of these outbreaks have shown a preponderance of infected males, with about twice as many males as females infected. Early middle aged individuals were infected in the highest numbers. However, within family groups in which 2 or more were infected, subsequent new infections shifted to younger aged individuals and children (Detels *et al.* 1969).

Consumption of raw fish has been associated with the majority of infections (Cross 1992). Poor sanitation is another potential factor. Nevertheless, the distance between human epidemic locations also suggests the involvement of fish-eating birds in the infective cycle (Belizario *et al.* 2000).

In the first reports of capillariosis from Lao PDR, three patients were infected. These were unrelated, previously healthy young men: a 24 year old man from Vientiane, a 26 year old man from Vientiane, and a 27 year old man from southern Lao PDR. These infections occurred from September 2005 to December 2007 (Soukhathammavong *et al.* 2008).

Capillariosis was first reported in Japan in an adult male who was found in Hiroshima by Tsuji. In 1982 a second case was reported. This was in a 46 year old male laundry worker who initially complained of occasional abdominal pain in November 1986. In October, 1987, he was admitted because of intractable diarrhoea and hypoproteinemia (Nawa *et al.* 1988).

Thirty intestinal capillariosis cases were reported in Taiwan from January 1983 to December 2003. Two Taiwanese aboriginal tribes, the Ami and Paiwan, presented a high prevalence. The males and

elderly also had high rates of infection. About half of the 30 cases admitted having consumed raw or uncooked fish. All cases recovered full health after receiving medication, with no deaths or recurrence (Lu *et al.* 2006).

In 1991, there was the first reported case of intestinal capillariosis in the Republic of Korea, in a man infected by *Capillaria philippinensis*. He had chronic diarrhoea with severe loss of body weight. He enjoyed hunting and fishing and eating raw fish. An open full-thickness biopsy of the ileum showed a flat mucosal surface and sections of the round worm. Faecal examination revealed numerous elliptical helminth eggs. The worms and eggs were consistent with features of *C. philippinensis* (Lee *et al.* 1993). Further cases have been reported. These include a 41 year old man who was diagnosed by both eggs in the faeces and worms in the biopsy specimen of the ileum. This patient was supposedly infected in Indonesia. Another was in a 78 year old man, who had not been abroad. He suffered from intractable diarrhoea. He was diagnosed by eggs in the faeces, and several juvenile worms were collected after anti-helminthic treatment. In both cases, the treatment was successful using albendazole (Hong and Cross 2005).

The first reported case of intestinal capillariosis in Iran, Middle East, was diagnosed in a 30 year old fisherman from Malihan Village, Khoozestan Province, Iran. He reported a more than two month history of diarrhoea, borborygmus, muscular atrophy, and debility. Eggs, larvae, and adults of *Capillaria philippinensis* were found in his faeces (Hoghooghi-Rad *et al.* 1987).

Intestinal capillariosis in Indonesia was first reported in a 32 year old Italian man. After he made a trip to Indonesia that lasted approximately one month, he developed heartburn, abdominal pain, irregular bowel movements, headache, fatigue, weight loss, low-grade fever, and severe itching. The diagnosis was provided by the recovery of *Capillaria philippinensis* eggs in the stool (Chichino *et al.* 1992).

Causative agent: description and life cycle

The nematode (roundworm) *C. philippinensis* is one of over 250 species of *Capillaria*, found in fish, amphibians, reptiles, birds, and mammals. But only 3 species are known to infect humans: *C. hepatica*, *C. aerophila* and *C. philippinensis*.

C. philippinensis is of major importance for human populations because it has caused major epidemics and deaths in humans. Analysis of the life cycle of *C. philippinensis* shows that fish-eating birds have also been infected with larvae from infected fish. For this reason, such birds are considered the natural host in a fish-bird life cycle (Fig. 58.2). This would help to explain the wide dispersal in recorded human cases: humans can also be infected by eating the infected fish (Cross 1992).

The life cycle of *C. philippinensis* involves a small fresh water or brackish water fish harbouring the infective stages in the visceral organs. The *C. philippinensis* larvae from the digestive tract of a freshwater fish (*Hypselotris bipartita*) from an endemic area were given by stomach tube to Mongolian gerbils (*Meriones unguiculatus*). Ten to eleven days post infection larvae had developed to the adult stage and female worms generated larvae in 13–14 days. After that, these capillarid larvae developed to adults which could release unembryonated eggs within 22–24 days. Moreover, this experiment proposed that autoinfection could occur in gerbils.

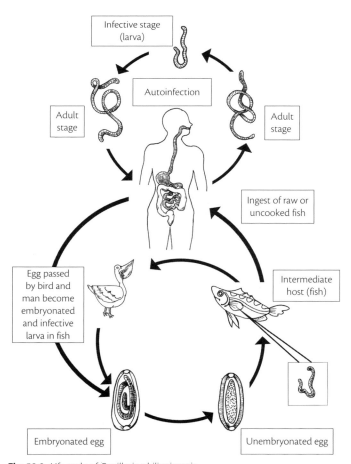

Fig. 58.2 Life cycle of *Capillaria philippinensis*.
Modified from http:/www.dpd.cdc.gov/dpdx

The gerbils were fed only two larvae from fish but 852 to 5,353 worms were recovered (Cross *et al.* 1978).

The biological aspect of fish as the intermediate host of *C. philippinensis* has been reported in several studies. In a study from Thailand, *Cyprinus carpio*, *Puntius gonionotus* and *Rasbora boraperensis* were fed *C. philippinensis* eggs by self feeding or forced feeding. After 10–30 days the results showed that the larvae of *C. philippinensis* were recovered from fish intestines and could develop to egg producing adults in gerbils by feeding the gerbils the same larvae (Bhaibulaya *et al.* 1979). Likewise, Cross *et al.* (1972) reported *Elotris melanosoma* (birut), *Ambassis commersoni* (bagsang) and *Apogon sp.* (bagsit), fresh water fish in the Philippines, as intermediate hosts in experimental infections. *C. philippinensis* larvae recovered from the digestive tracts of those fresh water fish led to intestinal capillariosis after being fed to monkeys. Moreover, two specimens of *Apogon sp.* were found naturally infected with *C. philippinensis* larvae but the mechanism of infection with *C. philippinensis* remains unknown. It was suggested that defecation from humans into water resources in the endemic area provided an excellent opportunity for *C. philippinensis* eggs to encounter and be ingested by naturally susceptible fish (Cross *et al.* 1972). Bhaibulaya *et al.* (1979) reported that fish-eating birds (*Amaurornis phoenicurus* and *Ardeola bacchus*) were susceptible to *C. philippinensis* infection; adults and larvae form were recovered from the birds' intestinal content. Therefore, fish-eating birds are a naturally occurring reservoir host that may contaminate water resources with *C. philippinensis* eggs in endemic areas. These mechanisms can maintain the parasite life cycle in nature (Saichua *et al.* 2008).

Morphology

The typical eggs of *C. philippinensis* are thick shelled without special capsules. They are bioperculate and contain one or more cells, with size ranges of 36–48μm x 18–μm. The adult female has a size of 2.7–3.7 cm in length and is divided into two parts of equal length. The anterior part contains an oesophagus and oesophageal gland, and the posterior part contains the intestinal and reproductive organs with a prominent vulva located behind the oesophagus. They are often found with embryonated eggs. The adult male size ranges from 2.3–32 mm in length. They are characterized by very long thin, cylindrical shaped bodies (Nawa *et al.* 1988).

Symptoms and pathology

Patients with advanced intestinal capillariosis usually present with watery diarrhoea, weight loss, abdominal pain, borborygmi, muscle wasting, weakness, and oedema. Laboratory examinations have shown low levels of potassium and albumin in blood (Pradatsundarasa *et al.* 1973; Manmanee *et al.* 1977; Tesana *et al.* 1983) and malabsorption of fats and sugar (Cross 1992; Chunlertrith *et al.* 1992). Those patterns may result from the secretion of a proteolytic substance by *C. philippinensis* or by direct penetration of the intestine causing cellular injury and dysfunction (Cross *et al.* 1978). Several studies have shown the intestinal pathological findings. In *C. philippinensis* infection crypts have atrophied, flattened villi, and leukocyte cell infiltration, which were considered signs of intestinal cell injury (Tesana *et al.* 1983; Sangchan *et al.* 2007; Wongsawasdi *et al.* 2002). Therefore, the destruction of intestinal wall cells may interrupt nutrient absorption, causing weight loss in intestinal capillariosis patients. Moreover, the intestinal cell destruction may lead to fluid, protein and electrolyte losses because the dysfunctional intestinal cells cannot control fluid and electrolyte balance in the body (Sun *et al.* 1974). This results in low levels of potassium and albumin in the blood of *C. philippinensis* infected patients. The oedema in patient is due to hypoalbuminemia (Tesana *et al.* 1983). Albumin is a plasma protein which controls fluid in blood vessels by maintaining the osmotic pressure. If the osmotic pressure decreases, the plasma fluid in the vessel will leak out of the capillaries to the interstitial space and lead to oedema in intestinal capillariosis patients (Porth 1998).

Clinical signs and symptoms

In contrast to most nematode infections which rarely cause death in the human host, infection with *C. philippinensis* causes severe illness and death if untreated. Although the initial infection may cause no obvious signs or symptoms, the infected person will become symptomatic as the parasite population increases. Symptoms often include long periods of abdominal pain, abdominal 'gurgling' (borborygmus), and recurring loose stools over several weeks. Less commonly, nausea and vomiting are reported. Throughout this duration of symptoms, the volume of stool becomes marked with an accompanying loss of body weight. Infection ultimately leads to fluid depletion and malabsorption, producing the physical findings of muscle wasting, weakness, hypotension, abdominal distension with tenderness to palpation, oedema and decreased reflexes (Whalen *et al.* 1969).

Diagnosis of intestinal capillariosis

The detection of *C. philippinensis* is based on the recovery of eggs, larvae and/or adult worms in the stool of the patients. Unembryonated *C. philippinensis* eggs are peanut-shaped with flattened bipolar plugs and a striated shell. Larvae are found in the faeces but identification may be difficult as in the case of *C. philippinensis* (Cross 1992). An inexperienced laboratory worker may confuse *C. philippinensis* with *Trichuris trichiura* eggs which have prominent mucoid bipolar plugs. The eggs of *C. philippinensis* are excreted sporadically in faeces and this may lead to a delay in the diagnoses of intestinal capillariosis. Therefore, multiple stool samples are important for early diagnosis (Cross 1992). In most of the cases of intestinal capillariosis reported in Thailand eggs, larvae or adult worms were found in faeces (El-Dib *et al.* 1999; El-Karaksy *et al.* 2004; Saichua *et al.* 2008; Belizario *et al.* 2000; Detels *et al.* 1969; Graczyk *et al.* 1999; Bhaibulaya *et al.* 1979; Whalen *et al.* 1969). But there were some patients who died from *C. philippinensis* infection in whom *Capillaria* eggs or larvae were not found in faeces (Tesana *et al.* 1983). Small intestinal aspiration or biopsy may be necessary to confirm *Capillaria* infection (Cross 1992). For example, gastroduodenoscopy in a 13 year old boy from central Thailand revealed *C. philippinensis* eggs in a jejunal biopsy (Wongsawasdi *et al.* 2002). Moreover, jejunal mucosal biopsy and microscopic jejunal content examinations were successfully used to identify intestinal capillariosis in a 27 year old Thai man who had repeated negative stool tests (Sangchan *et al.* 2007). Immunodiagnosis may be a supplementary diagnostic tool which helps to detect *C. philippinensis* infection. Recently, Intapan *et al.* (2006) investigated intestinal capillarias using *Trichinella spiralis* antigen. The study found that sera from intestinal capillariosis patients were positive with *T. spiralis* antigen. The antigenic patterns recognized by intestinal capillariosis sera varied with the molecular masses, ranging from less than 20.1 to more than 94 kDa.

The immune-blotting profiles of the trichinosis sera were similar to those of the intestinal capillariosis sera. The antigenic bands with 100% reactivity were located at 36.5, 40.5, and 54 kDa, respectively. This may be useful for screening of persons who have intestinal capillariosis like symptoms before discovering capillaria eggs or larvae in their stool. Parasitological stool examinations of the positive cases are necessary as second-tier laboratory tests for confirming the diagnosis (Intapan *et al.* 2006).

The first reported intestinal capillariosis identified by endoscopy was carried out to identify the cause of protein-losing enteropathy. Endogastroduodenoscopy (EGD) showed mild erythema of the gastric antrum and a thickening of small intestinal folds (Wongsawasdi *et al.* 2002). The biopsies indicated significant changes of intestinal villi: flattening, crypt proliferation, acute inflammation and eosinophilic granulomata. *Capillaria philippinensis* eggs were identified in the biopsy section (Fig. 58.3). The mucosal changes were related to mucosal invasion, lymphatic obstruction toxin and cytokine release and intestinal microflora changes by parasites.

Source of intestinal capillariosis

Capillaria philippinensis infections are found most often among individuals who reside in areas where raw fish are commonly eaten. For example, in the Philippines, residents of Ilocos Norte province like to eat raw bagsit (*Hypseleotris bipartita*). In fish containing *Capillaria* larvae, consumption of a single bite can lead to infection with *C. philippinensis* (Cross 1992). In an experimental study, fresh water fish in Thailand, such as *Cyprinus carpio*, *Puntius gonionotus*, *Aplocheilus panchax*, *Gambusia holbrookii*, *Rasbora boraperensis* and *Trichopsis vittatus*, could serve as intermediate hosts for *C. philippinensis* (Bhaibulaya *et al.* 1979). Moreover, some people usually chew the freshly caught fish because those fish are too small to eviscerate. So the raw fresh water fish eating behaviour is a major factor associated with intestinal capillariosis in Thailand.

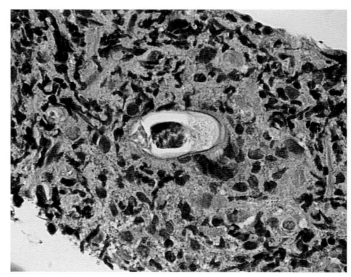

Fig. 58.3 Section of jejunal biopsy showing a *Capillaria philippinensis* egg and numerous histiocytes and eosiniphils.

Prevention: strategies for intestinal capillariosis control

Intestinal capillariosis is a potentially severe disease that may lead to death without early diagnosis and treatment. The symptoms of *C. philippinensis* infection include continuous or intermittent watery diarrhoea associated with severe weight loss, severe protein-loss and severe electrolyte depletion.

The epidemiology of this infection has shown that there is a reservoir host in birds and an intermediate host in fish, with the relationship of the naturally occurring cycle of bird-fish consumption. Ingestion by humans of infected fish will lead to *C. philippinensis* infection in humans, resulting in intestinal capillariosis and potentially, death. Based on this information, a primary strategy to fight the disease consists of avoidance of eating raw fish. Because humans may transmit the infection back to fish, additional efforts include improvement in overall sanitation and education about the risk of defecation in proximity to water sources, such as lakes, streams and rivers. Although the earliest cases were discovered in Southeast Asia, this infection has now been documented in several more distant countries. With increasing globalization and increasing travel in recent decades, it is essential to provide widespread education for the public at risk. Promotion of health education programs and early diagnosis are necessary to minimize and eradicate *C. philippinensis* infections.

The health education campaign aims to avoid the consumption of raw fish and to avoid defecation near or into water resources in order to control *C. philippinensis* infection. Early diagnosis is necessary in the treatment of intestinal capillariosis patients. In this regard improvement in the training of laboratory workers and the collection of multiple stool examinations are essential.

Treatment

In the early years, thiabendazole in a dose of 25mg/kg/day, or one gm/day for 30 days was reasonably effective and the therapeutic agent of choice. Due to high rates of relapse with thiabendazole, the preferred drug treatment changed to mebendazole in a dosage of 400 mg/day given in two divided doses for 20 days. Relapses were treated with mebendazole for 30 days. However, presently albendazole is the drug of choice, at 400mg/day in divided doses but for only 10 days. Insufficient duration of treatment results in a recurrence of infection, as determined by eggs and parasites in stool samples within 20–30 days.

In patients severely affected, dehydration may require IV hydration and electrolyte replacement. Agents to control diarrhoea and high protein diets are also helpful to re-establish adequate nutrition. Since some studies have shown the development of capillariosis in family members weeks to months after the identification of the initial case, it is very important to assess all family members initially, and again in one to two months to confirm that their eating habits no longer include raw fish.

Capillaria hepatica

History

Capillaria hepatica was first reported in 1850 in a rat liver. In the ensuing years capillarids were discovered in the livers of rats and other animals (Skrjabin *et al.* 1957). Bancroft (1893) described the parasite as *Trichocephalus hepatica* from worm fragments in the liver, and noted the encapsulated eggs in the liver parenchyma. The nematode was subsequently placed into the genera *Trichosoma*, *Hepaticola*, *Eucoleus*, *Thominx* and *Capillaria*. Moravec (1982) placed it into the genus *Calodium* and Anderson (1992) concurred and consider it *Calodium hepaticum*. The parasitological and medical literature continue to refer to the parasite as *Capillaria hepatica*, consequently it will remain in use in this chapter.

Human hepatic capillariosis was first reported by MacArthur (1924) in a English soldier who died after serving in India for 3 years. Eggs and adult worms were found in his liver at autopsy. McQuown (1950) discovered the parasitosis in a man who died in Louisiana, and Otto *et al.* (1954) found eggs and worms in a woman from Maryland. Human infection continued to be reported sporadically during the next 40 years and to date fewer than 30 cases of capillariosis hepatica have been documented worldwide. Spurious infections of eggs in human faeces are often reported, the eggs resulting from the ingestion of infected animal livers.

Hepatic capillarioasis is reported from rodents and other animals from all parts of the world; it is not uncommon, with prevalence rates varying from 0.7 to 85% of rodents examined. The parasite has also been found in livers of other rodent species and other wild animals, dogs, cats, pigs, ungulates, and monkeys. *C. hepatica* has also caused significant infections and deaths in the free-ranging population of endangered mountain gorillas (*Gorilla gorilla beringei*) in Rwanda (Graczyk *et al.* 1999).

Adult *C. hepatica* mature and reproduce in the liver of animals, and eggs are deposited into the surrounding tissue. The adults eventually die and the eggs become encapsulated. Mild infections are subclinical but in heavy infections there is hepatitis, splenomegaly, ascites, and eosinophilia. The eggs may elicit granuloma formation and fibrosis. The eggs remain in the tissue until the animal dies or is consumed by another animal.

Eggs reaching the soil after release from liver tissue, embryonate and become infectious. Humans accidentally acquire infection probably through geophagy or eating contaminated food. Control measures are difficult except for rodent control and education.

The agent

Capillaria hepatica has been placed in the superfamily Trichinelloidea, family Trichiuridae, subfamily Capillariinae. The adult worm is delicate when removed from the liver, is filariform and white. The cuticle is finely transversely striated. There are two wide bacillary bands, each occupying the circumference and dividing the muscle layer. The female is 5–8 cm long and 0.1 mm wide and the male about 2–4 cm long and 0.1 mm wide. The anterior of both sexes is narrow and is occupied by the oesophagus. The posterior end is wider and contains the intestines and reproductive organs. The oesophagus, like other members of the family, is surrounded by stichocytes. The vulva of the female opens near the end of the oesophagus. The male spicule is slightly chitinized and measures 0.4–0.5 mm in length; the sheath is membranous and without spines. Eggs are thick-shelled and minute pores give a striated appearance. There are two polar plugs and the eggs measure 50–68 by 30–35 μm (Fig 58.4).

The eggs remain undeveloped while in the liver tissue. Adults in the liver parenchyma eventually die and are destroyed by the inflammatory reaction. When the infected animals are eaten by another animal the eggs are digested out of the liver, pass out with the faeces and are dispersed in the soil. In a moist environment

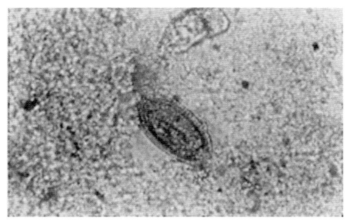

Fig. 58.4 Egg of *C. hepatica* (50–68 by 30–35 μm) recovered from human faeces from a spurious infection (×100).

with the right temperature the eggs mature and larvae develop in about 1 month. When the egg is ingested by a susceptible host it hatches in the intestines and the released larva (140–190 μm in length) penetrates the intestinal wall and is picked up by the hepatic portal system and carried to the liver. These larvae may reach the liver in 1 or 2 days and develop into adults within 18–20 days. Eggs are soon produced and the males die by 40 days but females live up to 59 days. The eggs and worms form yellow streaks or white patches on the liver surface. The liver becomes enlarged and soft in acute hepatic capillariosis and in chronic infection the liver becomes fibrotic. In the acute infection focal parenchymal destruction and granulomas may develop with mononuclear cells and eosinophils. In older infections some adults and eggs are scattered throughout the liver tissue, causing granulomatous inflammation (Fig. 58.5). Eggs continue to be produced and group together with bundles of fibrous connective tissue and cellular infiltration with lymphocytes and polymorphonuclear cells, espe-

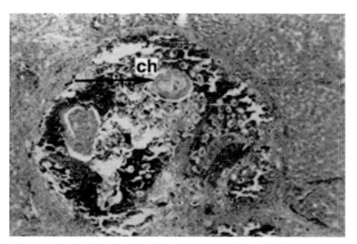

Fig. 58.5 Rodent liver showing *C. hepatica* worm sections (ch) and eggs surrounded by inflammatory reaction (×20).

cially eosinophils. Eggs continue to build up and the fibrosis increases. Giant cells will destroy adult worms and some eggs.

Survival of the parasite in nature depends upon the presence of a rodent or other animal species, and cannibalism among the animal groups. The eggs also contaminate the environment following death and decomposition of infected animals. Temperature and humidity are also important to survival. However, eggs can withstand cold weather and infections can be acquired in the winter time.

The host

Animal

The disease in the rodent host as well as other animals depends upon the degree of infection; the greater the number of eggs ingested, the more severe the disease. Hepatitis and hepatomegaly develop soon after *egg* deposition. There is an early onset of granuloma formation and cellular infiltration. Parenchymal alterations are characterized by degeneration, pycnosis and karyorrhexis of liver cells, and loss of typical structure of the liver. Increasing egg deposition causes an increase in weight and size of the liver. The weight of the spleen also increases. A chronic granulomatous response occurs when egg deposition ceases. Calcification occurs at a later stage, with dead parasites in the centre of the lesion. At about 100 days most lesions are non-reactive and surrounded by a thin layer of connective tissue. Although large numbers of inflammatory and giant cells are evident in early lesions, these clear later in the infection. The acute inflammatory reaction is replaced by a relative normalization of remaining hepatic sections with the retention of atrophic changes. Animals usually die in the acute stage in heavy infections.

There are also changes in enzyme activity in the first few weeks of infection, with the maximum increase in transaminase and dehydrogenases in the third week. Activity continues but plateaus at a lower level into the chronic stage.

The only means of diagnosing animal infection is by examination of liver tissue by open biopsy or by autopsy and histological examination of the tissue. Serological testing using immunofluorescence technique, haemagglutination tests, or ELISA should be possible. Several drugs (febantel, albendazole, mebendazole, oxfendazole) were reported to be effective in preventing deposition of *C. hepatica* eggs in mouse livers (Cheetham and Markus 1991). However the value of treatment after egg deposition is questionable.

Animals may survive light infections, with the development of acquired immunity. However, with heavy infection death may readily occur.

Human

People are accidental hosts of *C. hepatica* and usually the time of infection is not known. Many cases have been discovered at autopsy and ante-mortem by liver biopsy. Enlargement of the liver is first noticed by the patient. There may also be abdominal pain, fatigue, anorexia, high morning fever, nausea, and vomiting. Enlargement of the spleen, diarrhoea or constipation, abdominal distension, oedema of the extremities, and sometimes pneumonia are reported.

Laboratory findings show marked leucocytosis with eosinophilia, and moderate hyperchromic anaemia, and bone marrow examination may reveal a cellular marrow with normoblastic erythropoiesis and a marked proliferation of the eosinophilic series of leucocytes. Liver function tests and serum proteins may be abnormal.

The diagnosis is made by finding eggs, and at times adults, in liver tissues taken by needle biopsy or at autopsy (Fig. 58.6). The lesions taken early in the infection will show worms and eggs and some liver fibrosis. The eggs can be identified by the thick striated shell, and two polar plugs (Fig. 58.4). The adult worms can be identified by the presence of stichocytes and other characteristics listed above. Serological tests are being developed with promising results using immunofluorescence assays (Juncker-Voss *et al.* 2000; Assiss *et al.* 2004).

The pathology associated with human infections is similar to that found in animals, such as white to greying nodules on the surface of the liver. Microscopically, the principal lesions consist of necrotic foci and granuloma consisting of numerous eosinophils. As the disease progresses inflammatory changes continue, with eggs grouping together within bundles of fibrous connective tissue and eosinophils. Eventually there is extensive fibrosis and the eggs may become phagocytosed by multinucleated giant cells and destroyed.

Treatment of human capillariosis hepatica is not well documented. Anthelminthics would have little action on eggs but could affect adult worms in the liver. Choe *et al.* (1993) used thiabendazole and albendazole and found the drugs to be ineffective against the eggs but effective against the adults. Sodium antimony gluconate may have some effect.

The prognosis is not good for hepatic capillariosis, most infections are fatal. The prognosis is good if the diagnosis is made early and treatment initiated.

Epidemiology

Capillaria hepatica has a worldwide distribution, being found in the liver of rodents and a myriad of other mammals. It lacks host specificity, having been found in the dog, cat, beavers, rabbits, hyrax, peccary, prairie dog, shrew, skunk, and opossum. It was found in 12 different species of *Rattus* on several islands of Indonesia (Brown *et al.* 1975) and *C. hepatica*-like eggs were found in the liver of a short-nosed fruit bat (*Cynoptrus brachyotis*) and a sheath-tailed bat (*Emballonura alectro*) from Kalimantan Island (Borneo) Indonesia (Brown *et al.* 1974). Monkeys and the chimpanzee among the primates, have also been reported with hepatic capillariosis. The prevalence of infections is variable. Although animals other than rodents

have been found infected, the rates of infections have been low. However, in rodents, 90% of the animals examined have been found to be infected in some areas of the world.

Hepatic capillariosis is rare in humans and up to 2000 just 37 cases have been reported (reviewed by Li *et al.* 2010). Cases have been reported from India, the USA, Turkey, South Africa, Mexico, Brazil, Italy, Czechoslovakia, Nigeria, Switzerland, Japan, and Korea (Choe *et al.* 1993). Additional cases are reported from Germany (Pannenbecker *et al.* 1990), the former Yugoslavia (Kokai *et al.* 1990), China (Li *et al.* 2010) and Thailand (Tesana *et al.* 2007). Many spurious infections have also been reported with eggs being found in faeces (Fig. 58.4). *Capillaria hepatica*-like eggs were also found in the sputum of a woman on Taiwan (Liu *et al.* 1970). Spurious infections occur when the liver of infected animals is eaten raw or cooked. The eggs are digested out of the tissue and pass with the faeces.

Humans, as well as other animals, acquire hepatic infections by ingesting embryonated eggs in food or drink. The eggs are in the soil or on vegetation in areas where there is an abundance of rodents. Children more often than adults acquire infections because of their habit of geophagy. There is no known transmission of infections from humans to other animals.

Prevention and control

Hepatic capillariosis is so rare that extensive control measures would be difficult. However, rodent control and sanitary disposal of dead animals would be recommended. Education and improved hygiene would also be advisable and the training of children to avoid eating dirt.

Capillaria aerophila

History

Capillaria aerophila was described as *Trichosoma aerophila* by Creplin (1839) after finding the nematode in the trachea of a wolf in Germany. Dujardin (1845) placed it in the genus *Eucoleus* and Ramson (1911) referred to it as *Capillaria*. The name was changed many times over the years: *Capillaria*, *Thominx*, and *Eucoleus*, and Moravec (1982) and Anderson (1992) considered it *Eucoleus aerophilius*. However, most texts still refer to it as *Capillaria aerophila*.

It is a parasite of the respiratory tract of canines, felines, and mustellids. The parasite invades the respiratory mucosa causing irritation, increased mucosal secretion, and constriction of the lumen of the respiratory passages. There may be rhinitis, tracheitis, bronchitis, and bronchopneumonia. Secondary bacterial infection may cause death, especially in young animals.

The parasite has a widespread distribution in nature in North and South America, Europe, Russia, Asia, North Africa, and Australia. The prevalence of natural infection in wild and domestic animals is variable. Butterworth and Beverley-Burton (1981) reported prevalence rates of infection of 44% and 15% for the red fox and marten, respectively, and Skirnisson *et al.* (1993) found 6% of arctic foxes passing *C. aerophila* eggs. Control of these lungworm infections is nearly impossible in nature, but on farms for fur-bearing animals infections can be kept at a minimum by raising animals in cages suspended from the floor.

The agent

Capillaria aerophila is in the order Enoplida, superfamily Trichnelloidea, family Trichuridae, subfamily Capillarinae. The

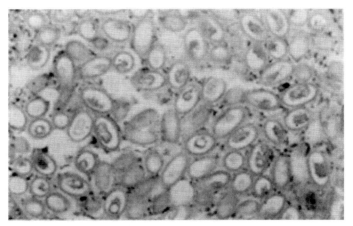

Fig. 58.6 Histological section of human liver taken at autopsy, showing cluster of *C. hepatica* eggs (×100).

males are 15–18 mm in length and 9 μm at the anterior end, 62 μm at the end of the oesophagus and 28 μm at the posterior end; the anus is subterminal; caudal alae absent; spicule moderately sclerotized, the spicular sheath long and densely covered with cuticular spines. The female is 18–20 mm in length with a maximum width of 96–105 μm; width at the anterior end, 12 μm; at the oesophagus, 86–99 μm; and at the posterior end, 27–49 μm. The anus is subterminal and the vulva is located behind the oesophagus and it is not elevated.

Eggs are deposited in the lungs, are coughed up, swallowed, and pass in the faeces. They are unsegmented but after 5–7 weeks in the soil become embryonated. The eggs may be ingested by earthworms where they hatch and the infection acquired by an animal after eating the earthworm. Infection may also be transmitted directly by the ingestion of embryonated eggs. Once in the host the larvae migrate to the respiratory passages and invade the mucosa. The migration route is not known but it is speculated that the larvae reach the respiratory passages via the blood and lymphatics. The parasite causes an increase in mucosal secretions by direct action on the tissue or provoked by products from the parasites metabolism. In addition the infection may also cause lobar, catarrhal purulent bronchopneumonia with mucosal haemorrhage of the respiratory tract. This occurs especially in young animals. The life span of *C. aerophila* in the fox is about 1 year.

The host

Animal

The prepatent period for capillariosis aerophila is variable, depending on the animal and may be 25–40 days, but the incubation period is not known. The most common symptoms are coughing, sneezing, rales, superficial respiration, weakness, loss of appetite, and progressive emaciation.

The parasite becomes established in tunnels in the respiratory mucosa, and there is leucocytosis and eosinophilia. At necropsy of infected animals the respiratory mucosa is swollen and covered with mucus and small haemorrhages. Some areas may be emphysematous with other areas in a state of atelectasis. The thoracic cavity may contain a brownish to red fluid containing fibrin. Abscesses sometimes occur in the lungs. Fatalities usually occur in animals less than 1 year of age. Adults do not suffer as much and can be reinfected. The diagnosis is made by finding characteristic eggs in the faeces. The eggs are barrel-shaped, measure 65 × 35 μm and are thick-shelled with polar plugs (Fig. 58.7). Biopsy of respiratory tissue may also reveal the parasite.

Intratracheal injection of aqueous iodine alone or with potassium iodide has been used in the past to treat pulmonary capillariosis. Tracheal brushes have also been used. The currently recommended anti-helminthics are thiabendazole or ivermectin (Kazacos and Cantwell 1985). Steroids can also be used to relieve symptoms. The prognosis is good if infections are light. Young animals may die with heavy infection while adults survive and become reinfected.

Humans

Human capillariosis caused by *C. aerophila* is very rare; only 12 cases have been reported — from Russia and Ukraine (8), Morocco (1), Iran (1), France (1) and Serbia (1) (Vilella *et al.* 1986; Lalosevic *et al.* 2008). The incubation period in humans is not known, but could be similar to the pre-patent period in animals, 25–40 days.

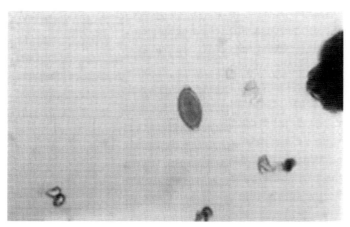

Fig. 58.7 Egg of *C. aerophila* (65 x 55 μm) recovered from the faeces of an arctic fox (x100).
Courtesy of Dr K. Skirnisson. U. of Iceland.

Most of the cases reported have been in adults and a few children. Infection in humans consists of bronchitis, coughing, mucoid or blood-tinged sputum, fevers, dyspnoea and eosinophilia. Some patients developed hepatomegaly, become cyanotic, and produced moist rales. Radiographs show infiltrates with reticulogranular patterns that progress to a honeycomb pattern. Lung biopsies have shown numerous granulomatous lesions with foreign body multinucleated giant cells containing the parasite surrounded by lymphocytes, plasma cells, eosinophils, and fibrin deposits. On one occasion the infection was misdiagnosed as bronchial carcinoma (Lalosevic *et al.* 2008).

The diagnosis of human pulmonary capillariosis is by finding characteristic eggs in sputum and or faeces. Eosinophils may also be present in the sputum. Biopsy of pulmonary tissue reveals the parasite.

Thiabendazole has been shown to be effective in treating human infections. Steroids may also be of value in relieving symptoms. Prognosis is good with treatment.

Epidemiology

Capillaria aerophila has been found in the respiratory passages of the dog, cat, wolf, marten, fox, ferret, opossum, badger, hedgehog, and humans in Europe, North and South America, Asia, Africa, and Australia. The prevalence rates are highly variable for species and geographic location. In the USA 0.8–9.6% of dogs and nearly 10% of the cats examined were found to be infected, while in Belgium 12% of the cats examined were positive for infection, but no dogs were infected. In England 20% of wild red foxes were positive, and on fur-breeding farms 30% of the red foxes and 50–100% of the silver foxes were infected. Epidemics of the parasitosis are serious problems on farms raising fur-bearing animals.

Infections are acquired by ingestion of embryonated eggs that are in the soil or by the ingestion of earthworms that have ingested embryonated eggs. The egg hatches in the earthworm and enters the body cavity. Transmission of the parasite to dogs, foxes, and cats has been accomplished by feeding infected earthworms. However, the major means of transmission is by ingestion of embryonated eggs since the susceptible animals do not usually include earthworms in their diets.

Human infections have been reported for the most part from the former USSR, Morocco, Iran, and France. The means of infection are unknown but most probably were through eating soil contaminated with embryonated eggs.

Prevention and control

Infections of *C. aerophila* are difficult to control in nature. Infection in foxes and other animals raised for fur can be prevented by keeping the animals elevated above the floor and by maintaining good sanitary practices. Anthelminthics routinely administered to the animals would also be beneficial. Intratracheal injection with aqueous solutions of iodine and potassium iodide have also been used in the past. The use of thiabendazole or ivermectin would make this treatment obsolete, however.

Human infections could be prevented by avoiding the ingestion of contaminated soil and preventing children from playing in areas that may have been contaminated with wild animal faeces.

Anatrichosoma cutaneum

History

Anatrichosoma species are found in the subcutaneous tissue of a number of animals. Swift *et al.* (1922) described *Trichosoma cutaneum* from skin lesion and nodules, and serpiginous tracts of the palms and soles of a *Macaca mulatta*, Smith and Chitwood (1954) and Chitwood and Smith (1958) described *A. cynamolae*. They transferred *T. cutaneum* to the genus *Anatrichosoma* and designated the species to *A. cutaneum*. Conrad and Wong (1973) described two other species, *A. rhina* and *A. nadpoli* from *M. mulatta* and reported *Anatrichosoma* spp. from other Asian monkeys. In the meantime Orihel (1970) reported finding *Anatrichosoma* spp. in the nasal epithelium of several monkeys and baboons. Breznock and Pulley (1975) found *Anatrichosoma* sp. in ears, eyes, noses, and eyelids of adult gibbons (*Hylobates lar*) originally from Thailand. *Anatrichosoma* spp. have also been reported from the opossum, cat, and dog. Two human cases of creeping eruption have been reported with *A. cutaneum*.

The agent

Anatrichosoma spp. are in the family Trichiuridae, subfamily Trichosomoidinae. The morphologic features are characteristic of the group: stichocytes surrounding the oesophagus, etc. The oesophagus extends from one-third to one-half of the body. Females measure 22–24 mm in length, width at the head 52 μm, at the oesophagus 100–110 μm, and at the posterior end 200 μm. The vulva is behind the oesophagus without a special appendage, the anus terminal. Very few worms have been extracted in their entirety. The males are about the same length as females but more slender. Males are without a spicule and spicular sheath, the posterior end has two sub-neutral papillae, and they have at least two pair of lateral papillae. During copulation the male inserts one-half of the posterior end of the spicule into the vagina of the female. Eggs produced by the females are ellipsoidal, thick walled, and have a smooth surface with polar plugs; they measure 56–70 by 37–42 μm and are embryonated when deposited (Fig. 58.8).

The worms are in serpiginous lesions in the subcutaneous tissue on the soles and palms and nasal mucosa of primates. The lesions may contain exudates and eggs are released in the exudate. The life cycle has not been determined but it is believed to be direct since

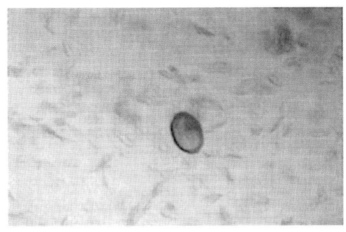

Fig. 58.8 Embryonated egg of *A. cutaneum* (56–70 by 42μ) recovered from the skin of the palm of a monkey (x100).

the eggs are embryonated and an intermediate host has not been found. Eggs probably hatch after ingestion and the larvae migrate to the subcutaneous tissue to mature.

The host
Animal

Little is known about the details of the life cycle, pre-patent period, or incubation period. Animals develop the infection and lesions begin to appear in the nasal tissue, feet, or palms. Swift *et al.* (1922) described the evolution of a nodule in the hands in which oedema first occurred with nodular thickening in the middle. The oedema disappeared and the nodule became more distinct. Tenderness of the nodules was not always present. Aside from oedema there was little evidence of acute inflammation. These small nodules eventually decreased in size. Larger swellings of irregular size were found over the muscle of the arm, involving both skin and subcutaneous tissues. These lesions were flat, 5–10 by 8–20 mm in size, would persist for 2–5 days, and quickly disappeared. They resembled urticarial wheals. Lesions also developed on the ankles and wrists. Blisters, 3–5 by 2–10 cm, developed on the palms and soles, they were serpiginous and filled with blood-tinged serous fluid. Microscopic examination of lesions would reveal cross-sections of the worm surrounded by epithelial cells and leucocytes, especially eosinophils. Oedema, a perivascular reaction, and diffuse infiltration with eosinophils were present in the surrounding tissue. Eggs in the tissue were surrounded by a thick pink shining hyaline structure two to three times the diameter of the egg.

In the nasal tissue the female worms become located in the squamous epithelial layer with eggs deposited in the epithelium and shed from the mucosal surface in plaques of exfoliating keratinized cells. Diffuse hyperplasia and parakeratosis are prominent changes in the mucosal epithelium (Allen 1960). Inflammatory reactions were also observed in the lamina propria with lymphocytes, plasma cells, and eosinophils. Some worms were within vessels of the lamina propria and the vessels exhibited focal necrosis and distension. Worms were also free in the connective tissue.

Human

The two human cases of Anatrichosomiosis caused by *A. cutaneum* reported were from Japan and Vietnam. Morishita and Tani (1960) reported cutaneous creeping eruption in a finger and ankle of a Japanese male. The patient noted redness that moved 5–10 mm/day causing severe pruritis. One female worm was removed from each lesion. The pruritis ceased after the surgery. In the second case three adult female worms were removed from superficial galleries in the skin of the hand, foot, and scrotum of a Vietnamese male (Le-Van-Hoa *et al.* 1963). A possible further case was found in a subcutaneous mammary nodule (Pampiglione *et al.* 2005). In addition lesions in the oral mucosa of a child in Brazil have also been suggested as being caused by this parasite (Nunez 2010).

In both monkeys and humans surgical removal of the worms is beneficial; however, anthelmintics such as thiabendazole, mebendazole, albendazole, and fen-bendazole given daily for 10–14 days may also relieve symptoms and provide cure. The prognosis appears to be good with treatment.

Epidemiology

It appears that *Anatrichosoma* spp. are not uncommon parasites of non human primates. Orihel (1970) reported 29% of 298 African monkeys belonging to five species infected with a species of *Anatrichosoma*. Conrad and Wong (1973) reported 5% of nasal swabs and 17% histological examinations of monkeys, positive for *Anatrichosoma*, while in other studies (Wong and Conrad 1978) 18% of 697 macaques were infected. Karr *et al.* (1979) examined 100 rhesus monkeys; 3% were positive from one geographic site and 68% from another site. Ulrich *et al.* (1981) found 54% of wild-caught macaques positive, and within 3 years they were negative for the parasite. Infants born to these monkeys after captivity never developed infection. Eggs were collected from the nasal epithelium by cotton swabs. Long *et al.* (1976) found 3.6% of 394 monkeys examined for *Anatrichosoma* sp. by nasal swab to be positive, and 13.9% positive by histological examination of tissue.

The means of transmission of *A. cutaneum* is not known but may be through the faecal-oral route, by fomites, or airborne. Captive primates should be maintained in clean cages and a clean environment. Infected animals should be isolated from uninfected ones and anthelminthics given. In the case of outbreaks, uninfected animals should be given prophylactic doses of an anthelminthic.

Prevention and control

It is not known how human infections are acquired but animal caretakers should be examined periodically when monkeys in their charge are infected. However, there have been no known human infections among those working in animal care facilities.

References

Ahmed *et al.* (1999). *Capillaria philippinensis*: an emerging parasite causing severe diarrhoea in Egypt. *J. Egypt Soc. Parasitol.*, **29**: 483–93.

Allen, A. M. (1960). Occurrence of the nematode, *Anatrichosoma cutaneum* in the nasal mucosae of *Macaca mulatta* monkeys. *Am. J. Vet. Res.*, **21**: 389–92.

Anderson, R. C. (1992). *Nematode parasites of vertebrates: Their development and transmission*, pp. 540–61. Wallingford, Oxon: CAB International.

Assiss, B. C. *et al.* (2004). A contribution to the diagnosis of *Capillaria hepatica* by indirect immunofluorescence test. *Mem. Inst. Oswaldo Cruz.*, **99**: 173–77.

Austin, D. N. *et al.* (1999). Intestinal capillariasis acquired in Egypt. *Eur. J. Gastroenter. Hepatol.*, **11**: 935–36.

Bair, M. J. *et al.* (2004). Clinical features of human intestinal capillariasis in Taiwan. *World J. Gastroenter*, **15**: 2391–93.

Belizario, V. Y. *et al.* (2000). Compostela Valley: A New Endemic Focus For *Capillariasis philippinensis*. *Southeast Asian J. Trop. Med. Pub. Health.*, **31**: 478–81.

Bhaibulaya, M., Indra-Ngarm, S. and Ananthapruti, M. (1979). Freshwater fishes of Thailand as experimental intermediate hosts for *Capillaria philippinensis*. *Int. J. Parasitol.*, **9**: 105–8.

Bhaibulaya, M. and Indra-Ngarm, S. (1979). *Amaurornis phoenicurus* and *Ardeola bacchus* as experimental definitive hosts for *Capillaria philippinensis* in Thailand. *Int. J. Parasitol.*, **9**: 321–22.

Butterworth, E. W. and Beverley-Burton, M. (1981). Observations on the prevalence and intensity of *Capillaria* spp. (Nematoda: Trichuroidea) in wild carnivora from Ontario, Canada. *Proc. Helminthol. Soc. Washington*, **48**: 24–37.

Breznock, A. and Pulley, L. T. (1975). *Anatrichosoma* infection in two white-handed gibbons. *J. Am. Vet. Med. Ass.*, **167**: 631–33.

Brown, R. J., Carney, W. P., Van Peenen, P. F. D., and Cross, J. H. (1975). Capillariasis in wild rats in Indonesia. *Southeast Asian J. Trop. Med. Pub. Health*, **6**: 219–22.

Cheetham, R. F. and Markus, M. B. (1991). Drug treatment of experimental Capillaria hepatica infection in mice. *Parasit. Res.*, **77**: 517–20.

Chichino, G. *et al.* (1992). Intestinal capillariasis (Capillaria philippinensis) acquired in Indonesia: a case report. *Am. J. Trop. Med. Hyg.*, **47**: 10–12.

Chitwood, M. G. and Smith, W. N. (1958). A redescription of *Anatrichosoma cynamolgi*, Smith and Chitwood, 1954. *Proc. Helminthol. Soc. Washington*, **25**: 112–17.

Chitwood, M. B., Valesquez, C., Salazar, N. G. (1968). *Capillaria philippinensis* sp. n. (Nematoda: Trichinellida), from the intestine of man in the Philippines. *J. Parasitol.*, **54**: 368–71.

Choe, C. Y. *et al.* (1993). Hepatic capillariasis: First case report in the Republic of Korea. *Am. J. Trop. Med. Hyg.*, **48**: 610–25.

Chunlertrith, K., Mairiang, P., and Sukeepaisarnjaroen, W. (1992). Intestinal capillariasis: a cause of chronic diarrhea and hypoalbuminemia. *Southeast Asian J. Trop. Med. Pub. Health.*, **23**: 433–36.

Creplin, F. C. H. (1839). Eingeweidewürmer, Binnenwüemer, Tierwürmer. *Allgem. Encyclop. Wissenschaften Kunste*, **32**: 277–392.

Cross, J. H. (1992). Intestinal capillariasis. *Clin. Microbiol. Rev.*, **5**: 120–29.

Cross, J. H. and Basaca-Sevilla, V. (1991). *Capillariasis philippinensis*: a fish-borne parasitic zoonosis. *Southeast Asian J. Trop. Med. Pub. Health*, **22**: S153–57.

Cross, J. H., Banzon, T. and Singson, C. (1978). Further studies on *Capillaria philippinensis*: development of the parasite in the Mongolian gerbil. *J. Parasitol.*, **64**: 208–13.

Cross, J. H. *et al.* (1972). Studies on the experimental transmission of *Capillaria philippinensis* in monkeys. *Trans. R. Soc. Trop. Med. Hyg.*, **66**: 819–27.

Conrad, H. D. and Wong, M. M. (1973). Studies on *Anatrichosoma* (Nematoda: Trichinellida) with descriptions of *Anatrichosoma rhina* sp. N and *Anatrichosoma nacepobi* sp.n. from the nasal mucosa of Macaca mulatta. *J. Helminthol.*, **47**: 289–302.

Dujardin, F. (1845). *Histoire naturelle des helminthes ou vers intestinaux.* Paris, 654 pp.

Detels, R. *et al.* (1969). An Epidemic of Intestinal Capillariasis in Man; A study in a Barrio in Northern Luzon. *Am. J. Trop. Med. Hyg.*, **18**: 676–82.

El-Dib, N. A. *et al.* (1999). Parasitological aspects of *Capillaria philippinensis* recovered from Egyptian patients. *J. Egypt Soc. Parasitol.*, **29**: 139–47.

El-Karaksy, H. *et al.* (2004). *Capillaria philippinensis*: a cause of fatal diarrhea in one of two infected Egyptian sisters. *J. Trop. Pediatr.*, **50**: 57–60.

Graczyk, T. K. *et al.* (1999). *Capillaria hepatica* (Nematoda) Infections in Human-Habituated Mountain Gorillas of the Parc National de Volans, Rwanda. *J. Parasitol.*, **85**: 1168–70.

Hong, S. and Cross, J. (2005). *Capillaria philippinensis* in Asia. In: N. Arizono *et al.* (eds.) *Asian Parasitology*, Food borne helminthiasis in Asia Chiba, Vol. 1, pp. 225–29. Japan: Federation of Asian Parasitologists.

Hong, S. T. *et al.* (1994). Two cases of intestinal capillariasis in Korea. *Korean J. Parasitol.*, **32**: 43–48.

Hoghooghi-Rad, N. (1987). *Capillaria philippinensis* infection in Khoozestan Province, Iran: case report. *Am. J. Trop. Med. Hyg.*, **37**: 135–37.

Hwang, K. P. (1998). Human intestinal capillariasis (*Capillaria philippinensis*) in Taiwan. *Acta. Paed. Sin.*, **39**: 82–85.

Intapan, P. M. *et al.* (2006). Potential use of *Trichinella spiralis* antigen for serodiagnosis of human *Capillariasis philippinensis* by immunoblot analysis. *Parasitol. Res.*, **98**: 227–31.

Junker-Voss, M. *et al.* (2000). Serological detection of *Capillaria hepatica* by indirect immunofluorescence assay. *J. Clin. Microbiol.*, 38: 431–33.

Karr, S. L., Henrickson, R. V., and Else, J. G. (1979). A survey for *Anatrichosoma* (Nematoda: Trichinellida) in wild caught *Macaca mulatta*. *Lab. Anim. Sci.*, **29**: 789–90.

Kazacos, K. R. and Gantwell, H. D. (1985). Ivermectin for treatment of nasal capillariasis in a dog. *J. Am. Vet. Med. Ass.*, **186**: 174–75.

Kokai, G. R., Misic, S., Perisic, V. N., and Grujovska, S. (1990). *Capillaria hepatica* infestation in a 2-year-old girl. *Histopathology*, **17**: 275–77.

Lalosevic, D. *et al.* (2008). Pulmonary capillariasis miming bronchial carcinoma. *Am. J. Trop. Med. Hyg.*, **78**: 14–16.

Lee, S. H. *et al.* (1993). A case of intestinal capillariasis in the Republic of Korea. *Am. J. Trop. Med. Hyg.*, **48**: 542–46.

Le-Van-Hoa, Dong-Hong-Mo, and Nguyen-Luu-Vien. (1963). Premier cas de capillariose cutanée humaine. *Bull. Soc. Pathol. Exotique*, **56**: 121–26.

Li, C. D., Yang, H. L., Wang, Y. (2010). *Capillaria hepatica* in China. *World J. Gastroenter.*, **16**: 698–702.

Liu, J. C, Whalen, G. E., and Cross, J. H. (1970). *Capillaria* ova in human sputum. *J. Form. Med. Ass.*, **69**: 80–82.

Long, G. G., Lichtenfels, J. R., and Stookey, J. L. (1976). *Anatrichosoma cynamolgi* (Nematoda: Trichinellida) in rhesus monkeys, *Macaca mulatta*. *J. Parasit.*, **62**: 111–15.

Lu, L. H. *et al.* (2006). Human intestinal capillariasis (*Capillaria philippinensis*) in Taiwan. *Am. J. Trop. Med. Hyg.*, **74**: 810–13.

MacArthur, W. P. (1924). A case of infestation of the human liver with *Hepaticola hepatica* (Bancroft, 1893), Hall, 1916. *Proc. R. Soc. Med.*, **17**: 83–84.

McCarthy, J. and Moore, T. A. (2000). Emerging helminth zoonoses. *Int. J. Parasitol.*, **30**: 1351–60.

McQuown, A. L. (1950). *Capillaria hepatica*. Report of genuine and spurious cases. *Am. J. Trop. Med.*, **30**: 761–67.

Mangmanee, L., Aswapokee, N. and Vanasin, B. (1977). Intestinal Capillariasis. Report of the fourth case in Thailand. *Siriraj Hosp Gaz.*, **29**: 439–49.

Moravec, F. (1982). Proposal of a new systematic arrangement of nematodes of the family Capillariidae. *Folia Parasit.*, **29**: 119–32.

Morishita, K. and Tani, T. (1960). A case of *Capillaria* infection causing cutaneous creeping eruption in man. *J. Parasit.*, **46**: 79–89.

Nawa, Y. *et al.* (1988). A case report of intestinal capillariasis- second case found in Japan. *Japanese J. Parasit.*, **37**: 113–18.

Nunez, F. A. (2010). *Trichuris*, *Capillaria* or *Anitrichosoma*? *Parasit. Intern.* (in press: *doi:10.1016/j.parint.2010.02.008*).

Otto, G. F., Berthrong, M., Appleby, R. D., Rawlings, J. C., and Wilber, D. (1954). Eosinophilia and hepatomegaly due to *Capillaria hepatica* (Bancroft, 1893) infection. *Bull. Johns Hopkins Hosp.*, **94**: 319–36.

Orihel, T. G. (1970). *Anatrichosoma* in African monkeys. *J. Parasitol.*, 56: 982–85.

Pampiglione, S. *et al.* (2005). An unusual parasitological finding in a subcutaneous mammary nodule. *Pathol. Res. Pract.*, **201**: 475–78.

Pannenbecker, J., Miller, T. C., Muller, J., and Jeschke, R. (1990). Schwerer leberbefall durch *Capillaria hepatica*. *Monatsschr. Kinderheil.*, **138**: 767–71.

Porth, C. (1998). *Pathophysiology: concepts of altered health states*. (5 edn.), pp. 590–91. New York: Lippincott.

Pradatsundarasar, A. *et al.* (1973). The first case of intestinal capillariasis in Thailand. *Southeast Asian J. Trop. Med. Pub. Health.*, **4**: 131–34.

Sangchan, A. *et al.* (2007). The endoscopic-pathologic findings in intestinal capillariais: a case report. *J. Med. Ass. Thai.*, **90**: 175–78.

Saichua, P., Nithikathkul, C. and Kaewpitoon, N. (2008). Human intestinal capillariasis in Thailand. *World J. Gastroenter.*, 28: 506–10.

Skirnisson, K., Eydal, M., Gunnarsson, E., and Hersteinsson, P. (1993). Parasites of the Artic fox (*Alopex lagopus*) in Iceland. *J. Wildl. Dis.*, **29**: 440–46.

Skrjabin, K. I., Shikhobalova, N. P., and Orlon, I. V. (1957). *Essentials of nematology. Trichocephalidae and Capillariidae of animals and man and the disease caused by them*, Vol. VI. (Israel Program for Scientific Translations, Jerusalem, 1970). Academy of Sciences of the USSR.

Smith, W. M. and Chitwood, M. B. (1954). *Anatrichosoma cynamolgi*, a new trichiurid nematode from monkeys. *J. Parasitol.*, **40** Sect. 2, (Suppl.): 12. (abstract).

Soukhathammavong, P. *et al.* (2008). Three cases of intestinal capillariasis in Lao People's Democratic Republic. *Am. J. Trop. Med. Hyg.*, **79**: 735–38.

Sun, S. C. *et al.* (1974). Ultrastructural studies of intestinal capillariasis *Capillaria philippinensis* in human and gerbil hosts. *Southeast Asian J. Trop. Med. Pub. Health.*, **5**: 524–33.

Swift, H. F., Boots, R. H., and Miller, C. P. (1922). A cutaneous nematode infection in monkeys. *J. Experim. Med.*, **35**: 599–620.

Tesana, S. *et al.* (1983). Intestinal capillariasis from Udon Thani province, northeastern part of Thailand: report of an autopsy case. *J. Med. Ass. Thai.*, **66**: 128–31.

Tesana, S., Puapairoj, A. and Saeseow, O. (2007). Granulomatous, hepatolithiasis and hepatomegaly caused by *Capillaria hepatica* infection: first report in Thailand. *Southeast Asian J. Trop. Med. Pub. Health*, **38**: 636–40.

Ulrich, C. P., Henrickson, R. V., and Karr, S. L. (1981). A epidemiological survey of wild caught and domestic born rhesus monkeys (*Macaca mulatto*) for *Anatrichosoma* (nematoda: Trichinellida). *Lab. Anim. Sci.*, **31**: 726–27.

Vilella, J. M., Desmaret, M. C., and Rouault, E. (1986). Gapillariose a *Capillaria aerophila* chez un adulte? *Méd. Mal. Infect.*, **1**: 35–36.

Whalen, G. E., *et al.* (1969). Intestinal capillariasis—a new disease in man. *Lancet*, **i**: 13–16.

Wongsawasdi, L. *et al.* (2002). The endoscopic diagnosis of intestinal capillariasis in a child: a case report. *Southeast Asian J. Trop. Med. Pub. Health.*, **33**: 730–32.

CHAPTER 59

Angiostrongylus cantonensis and Human angiostrongylosis

Qiao-Ping Wang and Zhao-Rong Lun

Summary

Introduction and historical aspects

Angiostrongylus cantonensis was first discovered in rats in Guangzhou (Canton), China in 1935 (Chen 1935). *A. cantonensis* is a zoonotic pathogen, which causes human angiostrongylosis with the main clinical manifestation of eosinophilic meningitis. The first case of human angiostrongylosis was reported in Taiwan in 1945. Subsequently several outbreaks of this disease occurred in Pacific Islands (Rosen *et al.* 1961; Kliks and Palumbo 1992). In the past decade, a number of outbreaks of human angiostrongylosis have emerged in some endemic regions, especially in China (Wang *et al.* 2008). Additionally, increasing numbers of travellers are diagnosed with eosinophilic meningitis caused by *A. cantonensis* after returning from endemic regions (Lo *et al.* 2001; Slom *et al.* 2002; Bartschi *et al.* 2004; Podwall *et al.* 2004; Kumar *et al.* 2005; Leone *et al.* 2007; Ali *et al.* 2008). The parasite continues to threaten human beings, especially people living in the Pacific Islands and Asia. So far, at least 2,825 cases have been recorded; of them, 1,337 were reported in Thailand, 769 in China (Hong Kong and Taiwan), 256 in Tahiti, 116 in the USA (Hawaii and Samoa) and 114 cases in Cuba (Wang *et al.* 2008).

Aetiology and pathology

The life cycle of *A. cantonensis* includes the rat definitive hosts and mollusk intermediate hosts (Fig. 59.1). Human *A. cantonensis* infections occur after eating mollusks or paratenic hosts such as prawns, frogs and monitor lizards, or vegetables, which contain or are contaminated by the infective larvae (the third stage) of the worm (Fig. 59.1). The larvae invade via intestine and enter bloodstream, and eventually reach the central nervous system (CNS) in about two weeks, causing eosinophilic meningitis. The external surface of brain and spinal cord are frequently normal without gross haemorrhage (Sonakul 1978; Chotmongkol and Sawanyawisuth 2002; Eamsobhana and Tungtrongchitr 2005). But physical lesions of tracks and microcavities caused by migrating parasites can be observed in the brain, and even the spinal cord. Infiltrations of lymphocytes, plasma cells and eosinophils are commonly revealed in the meninges and around intracerebral vessels (Sonakul 1978; Eamsobhana and Tungtrongchitr 2005).

Cellular infiltration around living worms is not prominent, but dead worms are usually surrounded by a granuloma, increased eosinophils and sometimes Charcot-Leyden crystals (Eamsobhana and Tungtrongchitr 2005). The larvae occasionally move to the eyes and cause ocular angiostrongylosis with visual disturbance such as diplopia or strabismus (Punyagupta *et al.* 1978; Sawanyawisuth *et al.* 2006).

Clinical features

The incubation of human angiostrongylosis is highly variable ranging from one day to several months (usually two weeks), depending on the number of parasites involved (Wang *et al.* 2008). Fig. 59.2 summarizes the clinical symptoms in 778 adult patients and 114 pediatric patients reported with eosinophilic meningitis caused by *A. cantonensis* (Wang *et al.* 2008). In adult patients, the common symptoms were headache (95%), stiff neck (46%), paresthesia (44%), vomiting (38%) and nausea (28%). Headache was frequently intermittent and can be relieved by repeated lumbar punctures (Punyagupta *et al.* 1975; Yii 1978). Neck stiffness usually was mild but nuchal rigidity has been observed in severe cases (Slom *et al.* 2002; Chau *et al.* 2003). Paresthesia occurred in a great variety of anatomical locations, usually in the extremities, and was expressed as pain, numbness, itching, or a sensation of worms crawling under the skin (Yii 1978). Vomiting and nausea probably were related to increased intracranial pressure and usually disappeared after the first lumbar puncture. Although a few adult patients suffering from visual disturbance or diplopia have been reported in China, this symptom was noted in 38% of patients in Thailand and 92% of patients in the USA (Punyagupta *et al.* 1978; Slom *et al.* 2002).

In children, stiff neck and paresthesia have been reported in 39% and 28% of cases. It was reported that 82% of pediatric patients had nausea and vomiting with 56% of the vomiting being projectile. The symptoms disappeared within one week in the most cases (Yii 1978). In addition, the incidence of fever (up to 80%), somnolence (82%), constipation (76%) and abdominal pain (34.2%) were relatively higher in children than among adults.

Patients may also develop additional clinical symptoms, including weakness of extremities, muscle weakness, muscle twitching, muscle pain, fatigue, diarrhoea, convulsions, and hyperesthesia. In heavy infections, coma and death may occur (Punyagupta *et al.* 1978; Chotmongkol and Sawanyawisuth 2002).

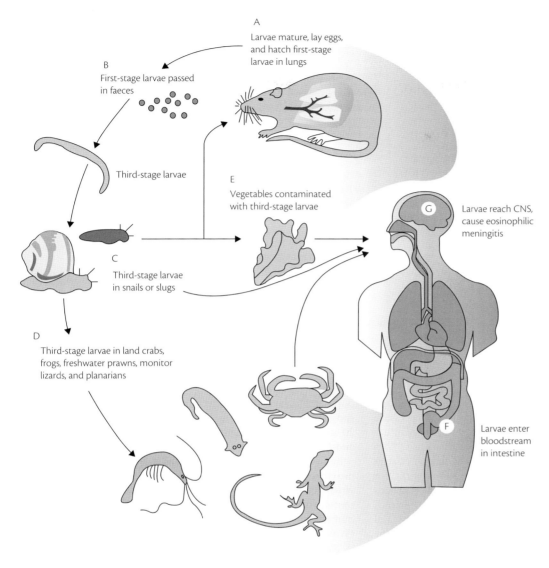

A
Larvae mature, lay eggs, and hatch first-stage larvae in lungs

B
First-stage larvae passed in faeces

Third-stage larvae

E
Vegetables contaminated with third-stage larvae

C
Third-stage larvae in snails or slugs

D
Third-stage larvae in land crabs, frogs, freshwater prawns, monitor lizards, and planarians

G
Larvae reach CNS, cause eosinophilic meningitis

F
Larvae enter bloodstream in intestine

Fig. 59.1 The life cycle of *Angiostrongylus cantonensis*. Rats, as definitive hosts, acquire *A. cantonensis* when the third-stage larvae are ingested. The larvae develop to sexual maturity and lay eggs in pulmonary arteries (A). Eggs hatch into first-stage larvae, which are excreted out with the faeces (B). The larvae in faeces are swallowed by intermediate host mollusks (snails or slugs) and develop into third-stage (infective) larvae (C). The third-stage larvae are then transmitted to the paratenic hosts such as shrimps, land crabs, predacious land planarians and monitor lizards (D). Humans occasionally acquire *A. cantonensis* when they eat snails, slugs and sometimes, land crabs, frogs, freshwater shrimps, monitor lizards, or vegetables, which contain the infective larvae (E). The larvae are digested from tissues and enter the bloodstream in intestine (F). The larvae finally reach the central nervous system (CNS) and cause eosinophilic meningitis (G) or move to the eye chamber and cause ocular angiostrongylosis.
Reproduced from Wang *et al.*, 2008, with permission from Elsevier.

Diagnosis and treatment

The recovery of *A. cantonensis* from patients confirms human angiostrongylosis. However, the frequency of the recovery is very low from clinical cases (2–11%) (Punyagupta *et al.* 1975; Yii 1978). For most cases, diagnoses of human angiostrongylosis are based on the clinical symptoms, medical history, laboratory findings in blood and cerebrospinal fluid (CSF), brain images and serological tests. The common clinical symptoms include headache, nausea and vomiting, neck stiffness, paresthesia and diplopia. However, a history of having eaten intermediate or paratenic hosts is very important for the diagnosis of this disease. In laboratory findings, eosinophils dominates in white cell counts in CSF (>10%) and peripheral blood (7–36%) (Yii 1978; Kuberski and Wallace 1979; Tsai *et al.* 2001; Slom *et al.* 2002). CNS images using MRI and CT can reveal lesions and are useful for differential diagnosis of angiostrongylosis from other parasitic diseases, such as cysticercosis, paragonimiasis, gnathostomiasis and schistosomiasis (Punyagupta *et al.* 1975, 1990; Ogawa *et al.* 1998;

Kanpittaya *et al.* 2000; Hasbun *et al.* 2001; Chau *et al.* 2003; Lo 2003; Jin *et al.* 2005).

Various enzyme-linked immunosorbant assay (ELISA) methods have been developed to detect antigens of, or antibodies against *A. cantonensis*, although none of them are commercially available (Cross and Chi 1982; Chen 1986; Eamsobhana *et al.* 1997, 2003). Antigens such as 29 kD, 31 kD and 32 kD have been found useful for development of ELISA detect (Nuamtanong 1996; Maleewong 2001; Li *et al.* 2005). The 29 kD antigen from female worms has showed potentiality to be a good marker for diagnosis with sensitivity and specificity 75% and 95%, respectively (Intapan *et al.* 2003). A dot-blot ELISA with 100% of sensitivity and specificity in laboratory tests has been developed to handle field samples for epidemiological surveys (Eamsobhana *et al.* 2003). *A. cantonensis* antigens can also be detected in serum by immuno-PCR (Chye *et al.* 2004).

Most patients with *A. cantonensis* infection are mild and self-limited, but death may occur in severe cases without prompt and appropriate treatment (Punyagupta *et al.* 1978; Chotmongkol and Sawanyawisuth 2002). Table 59.1 summarizes the treatment of

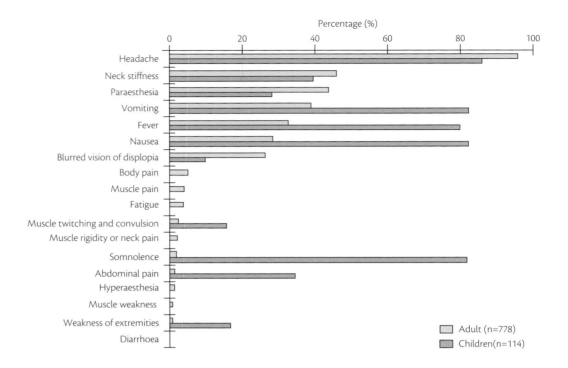

Fig. 59.2 Clinical features of human angiostrongylosis with eosinophilic meningitis

A. cantonesis infections in humans. Lumbar puncture was usually used to relieve headache caused by increasing intracranial pressure (Punyagupta *et al.* 1975; Yii 1978). Corticosteroids, anti-inflammatory agents are frequently effective in treating angiostrongylosis (Slom *et al.* 2002; Chotmongkol *et al.* 2006). However, anthelminthics, such as albendazole and mebendazole, usually are not recommended for treatment because of the theoretical possibility of exacerbating neurological symptoms (Hidelaratchi 2005). However these compounds have been used to treat this disease in Mainland China, Taiwan and Thailand where they appeared to relieve symptoms and reduce the duration of the disease (Chotmongkol *et al.* 2000, 2004). Sometimes, surgery is required to remove worms from eyes of patient with ocular angiostrongylosis (Kumar 2005; Sawanyawisuth *et al.* 2005).

Epidemiology

Human angiostrongylosis worldwide

Angiostrongylus cantonensis is mainly endemic in the Pacific Islands and Asia where it has been found as a main cause of eosinophilic meningitis. Many outbreaks of human *A. cantonensis* infections with cases from several to hundreds have been reported in these regions during the past decades. Over 2,800 cases of human angiostrongylosis have been reported in approximately 30 countries: Thailand, China (including Taiwan, Hong Kong), Tahiti, The USA (Hawaiian Islands, American Samoa), Cuba, Australia, Japan (Okinawa, Ryukyu Islands), New Caledonia, Vanuatu Republic (New Hebrides), India, Vietnam, Malaysia, Reunion Island, Egypt, Mayotte, Sri Lanka, Cambodia, Western Samoa, Costa Rica, Fiji, Indonesia, Ivory Coast, New Zealand, Papua New Guinea (New Britain), Germany, Italy, Belgium, Switzerland and the UK (Fig. 59.3 , in the colour plate section; Table 59.2).

So far, at least 1, 337 cases of human angiostrongylosis have been reported in Thailand. The main cause of this disease is the popular dietary habit of eating raw or undercooked snails (*Pila* spp.) with among young adult males: seventy percent were 20–40 years old (Punyagupta *et al.* 1978; Schmutzhard 1988; Cross and Chen 2007).

In Mainland China, *A. cantonensis* is endemic in at least seven provinces (Wang *et al.* 2007). The first case of human angiostrongylosis was documented in 1984. However, many outbreaks of *A. cantonensis* infections have emerged during the past decade. Nine outbreaks with a total of 319 cases have been reported since 1997 (Wang *et al.* 2008). Most of patients in these outbreaks were caused by eating raw or undercooked meat of an invasive freshwater snail *Pomacea canaliculata*. The snail, as a major infectious source in Taiwan, has also caused two outbreaks with a total of 17 human infections in 1998 and 2001 (Tsai *et al.* 2001; Tsai *et al.* 2004). Notably, an outbreak with 5 cases in Taiwan due to drinking vegetable juices was also reported (Tsai *et al.* 2004).

In pacific islands, most cases of human angiostrongylosis appeared in Tahiti, Samoa, New Caledonia, and Hawaii (Wang *et al.* 2008). The largest outbreak, with 202 cases, occurred in Tahiti in 1962 (Rosen *et al.* 1962). A further outbreak with 16 cases occurred in Samoa in 1982 (Kilks *et al.* 1982). Over 65 cases and 72 cases have been recorded in Hawaii and New Caledonia respectively (Hochberg *et al.* 2007; Wang *et al.* 2008).

Caribbean Islands and North American have become new endemic regions. The first case of human angiostrongylosis in the Caribbean Islands was reported in Cuba in 1973 (Pascual-Gispert *et al.* 1981), with a total of 114 cases recorded in this country since (Wang *et al.* 2008). Subsequently, many cases were reported in Costa Rica, and Jamaica (Vazquez *et al.* 1993; Lindo *et al.* 2004). Also, sporadic cases have been described in western travellers diagnosed with *A. cantonensis* after returning from Caribbean islands. The first case of human angiostrongylosis in North American was reported in New Orleans, Louisiana in 1985 (New *et al.* 1985).

Table 59.1 The treatments of human angiostrongylosis and their effectiveness

References	No. of Patients treated (ages*)	Treatment	Outcome
Chen *et al.* (2006)	22 (adults 15–43 years old)	Albendazole 400–1200 mg/day with dexamethasone 10–20 mg/day for 10–20 days	All recovered, serious side effects were not detected
	9 (adults 15–43 years old)	Praziquantel 400–1200 mg with dexamethasone 10–20 mg/day for 10–20 days	All recovered and serious side effects were not detected
Han *et al.* (2006)	28 (adults 25–63 years old)	Albendazole 15–20 mg/day with dexamethasone 10 mg/day for 9–27 days	All recovered, serious side effects were not detected, two recurred in a month
Tsai *et al.* (2004)	5 (adults 30–57 years old)	Dexamethasone 15 mg/day for 7 days, prednisolone 60 mg/day for another 7 days	All recovered in three weeks, but two cases had side effects
Tsai *et al.* (2001)	8 (adults 23–39 years old)	Mebendazole 200 mg/day with dexamethasone and prednisolone for 4–11 days	All recovered
Chotmongkol *et al.* (2006)	41 (adults 15 years old or over)	Mebendazole 10 mg/kg/day with prednisolone 60 mg/day for 14 days	Median duration of headache was 3 days; 7.8% had headache; no serious side effects
Jitpimolmard *et al.* (2006)	34 (adults 15 years old or over)	Albendazole 15 mg/kg/day	Mean duration of headache was 8.9 days; 20.5% of headaches persisted; no serious side effects
	32 (adults 15 years old or over)	Placebo	Mean duration of headache was 16.2 days
Chotmongkol *et al,* (2004)	26 (adults 15 years old or over)	Albendazole 15 mg/kg/day with prednisolone 60 mg/day for 14 days	Median duration of headache was 4 days; 11.5% had headache; no serious side effects
	32 (adults 15 years old or over)	Placebo	Mean duration of headache was 8.9 days; 40.6% had persistent headache; no serious side effects
Chotmongkol *et al.* (2000)	55 (adults 15 years old or over)	Albendazole 15 mg/kg/day for 14 days	Mean duration of headache was 5 days, 9% cases remained headache; no serious adverse effects
	55 (adults 15 years old or over)	No drug treatment	Mean duration of headache was 13 days; 45% cases had persistent headache
Punyagupta ea al. (1976)	284#	Analgesic for 14 days	35% patients had headache relief
	96#	Analgesic with prednisone 30–60 mg/day for 14 days	26% patients had headache relief
	56#	Penicillin 2.4–3.6 million U/day or tetracycline 2g/day for 14 days	34% of patients had headache relief
Slom *et al.* (2002)	9 (adults 21–28 years old)	Analgesic with or without nonsteroidal anti-inflammatory agents	All recovered, 67% had headache for at least four weeks
	3 (adults 21–28 years old)	Corticosteroid	Symptoms were markedly improved.

* No information regarding treatment in children was found in the published case series we reviewed.

The ages of these patients were not defined in the study. However, 82% of the patients were more than 20 years old.

Hosts for *A. cantonensis* and their prevalence as reservoirs of infection

The sources of human *A. cantonensis* infection are snails and slugs, crustaceans including freshwater shrimps and land crabs, and predacious land planarians such as flatworms in the genus *Platydemus*. Most species of mollusks are susceptible to and are capable of transmitting *A. cantonensis*. Terrestrial and some aquatic snails are the primary intermediate hosts (Cross and Chen 2007; Lv *et al.* 2008). However, in certain places, one or two species of snails are the main intermediate hosts and the intensity of infection in these hosts usually is very high. The giant African snail, *Achatina fulica*, is the major source of infection worldwide. The dispersal of *A. cantonensis* is associated with the spread of this snail from its native origin in Africa throughout the Pacific Islands and South Asia

(Kliks and Palumbo 1992). The golden apple snail, *P. canaliculata*, a very successfully invasive snail from South American, has a very wide distribution in Asia and has caused great damage to local agricultural systems (Hollingsworth and Cowie 2006). Unfortunately, this snail is also very susceptible to *A. cantonensis* and has replaced the African giant snail, *A. fulica*, as the major intermediate host of *A. cantonensis* and has become the main source of human infection in these regions (Wang *et al.* 2007). The infection rate in this snail is very high, 21% in Taiwan, 42–69.4% in Mainland China, and 10–39% in Okinawa.

There is little knowledge regarding the prevalence of *A. cantonensis* in reported paratenic hosts such as crustaceans (prawns and land crabs), predacious land planarians (flatworms in the genus *Platydemus*), fish, frogs or monitor lizards (Radomyos *et al.* 1994;

Table 59.2 Cases of human angiostrongylosis reported in countries or regions

Countries or Regions	Cases (%)
Thailand	1337 (47.3)
China including Taiwan and Hong Kong	769 (27.2)
Tahiti	256 (9.1)
The USA	116 (4.1)
Cuba	114 (4.0)
New Caledonia	72 (2.6)
Japan	63 (2.2)
Australia	24 (0.8)
Vanuatu Republic	19 (0.7)
India	10 (0.4)
Vietnam	8 (0.3)
Malaysia	6 (0.2)
Mayotte	6 (0.2)
Reunion island	4 (0.1)
Egypt	3 (0.1)
Sri Lanka	3 (0.1)
Cambodia	2 (0.1)
Western Samoa	2 (0.1)
Fiji	2 (0.1)
Belgium	1
Costa Rica	1
Germany	1
Indonesia	1
Jamaica	1
Italy	1
Ivory Coast	1
New Zealand	1
Papua New Guinea	1
Switzerland	1
The UK	1
Total	2825

Reproduced from Wang *et al.* (2008), with permission from Elsevier.

Panackel *et al.* 2004; Hidelaratchi *et al.* 2005). Small planarians may represent a very important but overlooked source for human infection, when they are consumed along with contaminated uncooked vegetables. Four outbreaks of human angiostrongylosis have been caused by eating contaminated vegetables or vegetable juice (Bowden 1981; Slom *et al.* 2002; Tsai *et al.* 2004). Frogs, monitor lizards and toads are also important reservoirs for *A. cantonensis*. In New Caledonia, 53.4% of frogs (*Hyla aurea*) were infected with the infective larvae (Ash *et al.* 1968). Eating raw frogs has been implicated in human infections in Taiwan, Mainland China and the USA. In Thailand, 95.5% of monitor lizards have been found infected with *A. cantonensis* and more than 18 cases of human angiostrongylosis in Thailand, Sri Lanka and India were attributed

to consumption of monitor lizard (Radomyos *et al.* 1994; Panackel *et al.* 2004; Hidelaratchi *et al.* 2005).

Rattus rattus and *R. norvegicus* have been considered the most common definitive hosts for *A. cantonensis*, but other species of rats found in rural and forested areas are also reported to be natural hosts (Cross and Chen 2007; Wu 2006). Rats are very necessary for the establishment of *A. cantonensis* foci in a local area. Table 59.3 summarizes the prevalence of *A. cantonensis* in definitive hosts *R. rattus*, *R. norvegicus* and *R. exulans* in some regions, where human infections or outbreaks have occurred.

Human beings and non-human primates can be accidental hosts for this parasite. It is unable to complete its development in either human or non-human primates and usually dies in the central nervous system of these hosts, causing eosinophilic meningitis or even death of the hosts. The worms have been reported as the cause of death of captive primates in the Bahamas, in Australia and in the USA (Gardiner *et al.* 1990; Prociv *et al.* 2000; Prociv *et al.* 2004).

Prevention and control

Because of the worldwide distribution of large numbers of rats and mollusks that are highly susceptible to this parasite, it would be very difficult to eliminate *A. cantonensis* from the environment. However, it is relatively easy to block the transmission pathway of this parasite to humans by educating susceptible populations not to eat raw or undercooked intermediate and paratenic hosts or potentially contaminated vegetables, particularly in endemic regions. Programs educating public health workers and physicians in endemic areas to be aware of this parasite, its hosts, and the dangers to the health of populations, and campaigns to warn against eating uncooked mollusks and paratenic hosts, are very useful, practical and achievable interventions for control of human *A. cantonensis* infection. The habit of eating raw snails and paratenic hosts should be strongly discouraged, although it is very difficult for people to abandon these customs that have existed for generations in some endemic regions, especially Thailand and China. Eating raw or undercooked snails with seasonings, such as pepper and pericarpium, is very popular, particularly in some Chinese restaurants. Several outbreaks of human *A. cantonensis* infections in China have been attributed to this method of preparing snails. So far, recommended measures for prevention in these endemic regions include:

1) Educating citizens to be aware of *A. cantonensis* and the disease caused by this parasite,

2) Only eating adequately cooked snails, slugs, small mollusks and paratenic hosts of *A. cantonensis* such as frogs, shrimps, land crabs, and monitor lizards,

3) Eradicating molluscan hosts near houses and vegetable gardens,

4) Not eating unwashed vegetables which may be contaminated with the infective stage larvae of *A. cantonensis*. Travellers heading to endemic regions must know the dangers of eating raw mollusks and vegetables from unknown sources and should avoid these foods.

Washing hands frequently, particularly after gardening, is also strongly recommended especially in endemic regions. For physicians in both non-endemic and endemic regions, it is very important to have good knowledge of the parasite in order to diagnose *A. cantonensis* infection in humans promptly.

Table 59.3 Primary definitive hosts of *A. cantonensis* and its prevalence in these reservoirs of infection in some severely endemic regions

Localities (Years)	Definitive hosts	Number examined	Prevalence (%)
Guangzhou, China (2005)	R. norvegicus	21375	1.7
Fujian, China (2001)	R. norvegicus	391	9.8
Zhejiang, China (2000)	R. norvegicus	351	20.4
Taiwan (1957–1962)	R. norvegicus	328	7.9
	R. rattus	792	3.3
Yoron Island, Japan (1979–1982)	R. rattus	108	28
Jamaica (2000)	R. rattus	74	27
	R. norvegicus	35	11
Queensland, Australia (1980)	R. rattus	174	21
	R. norvegicus	77	10
Fiji (1984)	R. rattus	54	29.6
	R. exulans	42	59.5
The Philippines (1965)	R. norvegicus	51	3.9
Cuba (1981)	R. norvegicus	20	60
New Orleans, USA (1986–1987)	R. norvegicus	94	21.4
The Dominican Republic	R. norvegicus	5	100
Indonesia (1978)	R. norvegicus	98	13.2
	R. exulans	14	28.6
Haiti (2003)	R. rattus.	4	75
	R. norvegicus	19	21
Papua New Guinea (1984)	R. norvegicus	7	14.2
Thailand (1997)	R. rattus	16	100
Thailand (1995)	R. rattus	22	77.3
Thailand (1995)	R. norvegicus	58	3.8

Reproduced from Wang *et al.* (2008), with permission from Elsevier.

Acknowledgements

Zhao-Rong Lun's laboratory was supported by grants from National Basic Research Program (973 project, #2010CB530000) and the National Nature and Science Foundation of China (30670275).

References

Ali, A.B., Van den Enden, E., Van Gompel, A. and Van Esbroeck, M. (2008). Eosinophilic meningitis due to *Angiostrongylus cantonensis* in a Belgian traveler. *Travel Med. Infect. Dis.*, **6**: 41–44.

Ash, L.R. (1968). The occurrence of *Angiostrongylus cantonensis* in frogs of New Caledonia with observations on paratenic hosts of metastrongyles. *J. Parasitol.*, **54**: 432–36.

Bartschi, E., Bordmann, G., Blum, J. and Rothen, M. (2004). Eosinophilic meningitis due to *Angiostrongylus cantonensis* in Switzerland. *Infection*, **32**: 116–18.

Bowden, D.K. (1981). Eosinophilic meningitis in the New Hebrides: two outbreaks and two deaths. *Am. J. Trop. Med. Hyg.*, **30**: 1141–43.

Chau, T.T., Thwaites, G.E., Chuong, L.V., Sinh, D.X. and Farrar, J.J. (2003). Headache and confusion: the dangers of a raw snail supper. *Lancet*, **361**: 1866.

Chen, H.T. (1935). Un nouveau nematode pulmonaire, *Pulmonema cantonensis* n.g., n. *sp. des rats de Canton. Ann. Parasit.*, **13**: 312–17.

Chen, S.N. (1986). Enzyme-linked immunosorbent assay (ELISA) for the detection of antibodies to *Angiostrongylus cantonensis. Trans. R. Soc. Trop. Med. Hyg.*, **80**: 398–405.

Chen, W.L., Zhong, J.M., Chen, H., Wu, S.Y. and Ding, L. (2006). Eosinophilic meningitis: 31 cases report. *Chinese J. Misdiagn.*, **6**: 4668–69.

Chotmongkol, V., Sawadpanitch, K., *et al.* (2006). Treatment of eosinophilic meningitis with a combination of prednisolone and mebendazole. *Am. J. Trop. Med. Hyg.*, **74**: 1122–24.

Chotmongkol, V., Sawanyawisuth, K. and Thavornpitak, Y. (2000). Corticosteroid treatment of eosinophilic meningitis. *Clin. Infect. Dis.*, **31**: 660–62.

Chotmongkol, V. and Sawanyawisuth, K. (2002). Clinical manifestations and outcome of patients with severe eosinophilic meningoencephalitis presumably caused by *Angiostrongylus cantonensis. Southeast Asian J. Trop. Med. Pub. Health*, **33**: 231–34.

Chotmongkol, V., Wongjitrat, C., Sawadpanit, K. and Sawanyawisuth, K. (2004). Treatment of eosinophilic meningitis with a combination of albendazole and corticosteroid. *Southeast Asian J. Trop. Med. Pub. Health*, **35**: 172–74.

Chye, S.M., Lin, S.R., Chen, Y.L., Chung, L.Y. and Yen, C.M. (2004). Immuno-PCR for detection of antigen to *Angiostrongylus cantonensis* circulating fifth-stage worms. *Clin. Chem.*, **50**: 51–57.

Cross, J.H. and Chen, E.R. (2007). Angiostrongyliasis, In: K.D. Murrell and B. Fried (eds.) *Food-Borne Parasitic Zoonoses*, pp. 263–90. USA: Springer.

Cross, J.H. and Chi, J.C. (1982). ELISA for the detection of *Angiostrongylus cantonensis* antibodies in patients with eosinophilic meningitis. *Southeast Asian J. Trop. Med. Pub. Health*, **13**: 73–76.

Cross, J.H. (1978). Clinical manifestations and laboratory diagnosis of eosinophilic meningitis syndrome associated with angiostrongyliasis. *Southeast Asian J. Trop. Med. Pub. Health*, **9**: 161–70.

Dorta-Contreras, A.J., Noris-Garcia, E., Escobar-Perez, X. and Padilla, D.B. (2005). IgG1,IgG2 and IgE intrathecal synthesis in *Angiostrongylus cantonensis* meningoencephalitis. *J. Neurol. Sci.*, **238**: 65–70.

Duffy, M.S., Miller, C.L., Kinsella, J.M. and de Lahunta, A. (2004). *Parastrongylus cantonensis* in a nonhuman primate, Florida. *Emerg. Infect. Dis.*, **10**: 2207–10.

Eamsobhana, P. and Tungtrongchitr, A. (2005). Angiostrongyliasis in Thailand. In: N. Arizono *et al.* (eds.) *Asian Parasitology*, Vol. 1, pp. 183–97. The Federation of Asian Parasitologists.

Eamsobhana, P., Yong, H.S., Mak, J.W. and Wattanakulpanich, D. (1997). Detection of circulating antigens of *Parastrongylus cantonensis* in human sera by dot-blot ELISA and sandwich ELISA using monoclonal antibody. *Southeast Asian J. Trop. Med. Pub. Health*, **28**: 624–28.

Eamsobhana, P., Yoolek, A. and Kreethapon, N. (2003). Blinded multi-laboratory evaluation of an in-house dot-blot ELISA kit for diagnosis of human parastrongyliasis. *Southeast Asian J. Trop. Med. Pub. Health*, **34**: 1–6.

Gardiner, C.H., Wells, S., Gutter, A.E., Fitzgerald, L., Anderson, D.C., Harris, R.K. and Nichols, D.K. (1990). Eosinophilic meningoencephalitis due to *Angiostrongylus cantonensis* as the cause of death in captive non-human primates. *Am. J. Trop. Med. Hyg.*, **42**: 70–74.

Han, J.H., Zhu, Y.H., Jie, W.Z., Li, Y., Yan, Y., Ying, M., Xiong, J. and Liu, Y.X. (2006). Eosinophilic meningitis: 28 cases report. *J. Pathol. Biol.*, **1**, Suppl.2–3.

Hasbun, R., Abrahams, J., Jekel, J. and Quagliarello, V.J. (2001). Computed tomography of the head before lumbar puncture in adults with suspected meningitis. *N. Eng. J. Med.*, **345**: 1727–33.

Hidelaratchi, M.D., Riffsy, M.T. and Wijesekera, J.C. (2005). A case of eosinophilic meningitis following monitor lizard meat consumption, exacerbated by anthelminthics. *Ceylon Med. J.*, **50**: 84–86.

Hochberg, N.S., Park, S.Y., Blackburn, B.G., et al. (2007). Distribution of eosinophilic meningitis cases attributable to *Angiostrongylus cantonensis*, Hawaii. *Emerg. Infect. Dis.*, **13**: 1675–80.

Hollingsworth, R.G. and Cowie, R.H. (2006). Apple snails as disease vectors. In: R.C. Joshi and L.C. Sebastian (eds.) *Global advances in ecology and management of golden apple snails*, pp. 121–32. Nueva Ecija, Philippines: Philippine Rice Institute.

Intapan, P.M., Maleewong, W., Sawanyawisuth, K. and Chotmongkol, V. (2003). Evaluation of human IgG subclass antibodies in the serodiagnosis of angiostrongyliasis. *Parasit. Res.*, **89**: 425–29.

Jin, E., Ma, D., Liang, Y., Ji, A. and Gan, S. (2005). MRI findings of eosinophilic myelomeningoencephalitis due to *Angiostrongylus cantonensis*. *Clin. Radiol.*, **60**: 242–50.

Jitpimolmard, S., Sawanyawisuth, K., et al. (2007). Albendazole therapy for eosinophilic meningitis caused by *Angiostrongylus cantonensis*. *Parasit. Res.*, **100**: 1293–96.

Kanpittaya, J., Jitpimolmard, S., Tiamkao, S. and Mairiang, E. (2000). MR findings of eosinophilic meningoencephalitis attributed to *Angiostrongylus cantonensis*. *Am. J. Neurorad.*, **21**: 1090–94.

Kliks, M.M., Kroenke, K. and Hardman, J.M. (1982). Eosinophilic radiculomyeloencephalitis: an angiostrongyliasis outbreak in American Samoa related to ingestion of *Achatina fulica* snails. *Am. J. Trop. Med. Hyg.*, **31**: 1114–22.

Kliks, M.M. and Palumbo, N.E. (1992). Eosinophilic meningitis beyond the Pacific Basin: the global dispersal of a peridomestic zoonosis caused by *Angiostrongylus cantonensis*, the nematode lungworm of rats. *Soc. Sci. & Med.*, **34**: 199–212.

Kuberski, T. and Wallace, G.D. (1979). Clinical manifestations of eosinophilic meningitis due to *Angiostrongylus cantonensis*. *Neurology*, **29**: 1566–70.

Kumar, V., Kyprianou, I. and Keenan, J.M. (2005). Ocular angiostrongyliasis: removal of a live nematode from the anterior chamber. *Eye*, **19**: 229–30.

Leone, S., De, M.M., Ghirga, P., Nicastri, E., Esposito, M. and Narciso, P. (2007). Eosinophilic meningitis in a returned traveler from Santo Domingo: case report and review. *J. Travel Med.*, **14**: 407–10.

Li, H., Chen, X.G., Shen, H.X., Peng, H.J. and Zhao, X.C. (2005). Antigen analysis of *Angiostrongylus cantonensis* in different developmental stages. *Chinese J. Parasitol. Parasitic Diss.*, **23**: 36–39.

Lindo, J.F., Escoffery, C.T., et al. (2004). Fatal autochthonous eosinophilic meningitis in a Jamaican child caused by *Angiostrongylus cantonensis*. *Am. J. Trop. Med. Hyg.*, **70**: 425–28.

Lo, R.V. and Gluckman, S.J. (2001). Eosinophilic meningitis due to *Angiostrongylus cantonensis* in a returned traveler: case report and review of the literature. *Clin. Infect. Dis.*, **33**: e112–15.

Lo, R.V. and Gluckman, S.J. (2003). Eosinophilic meningitis. *Am. J. Med.*, **114**: 217–23.

Lv, S., Zhang, Y., Steinmann, P., Zhou, X.N. (2008). Emerging angiostrongyliasis in Mainland China. *Emerg. Infect. Dis.*, **14**: 161–64.

Maleewong, W., Sombatsawat, P., et al. (2001). Immunoblot evaluation of the specificity of the 29-kDa antigen from young adult female worms *Angiostrongylus cantonensis* for immunodiagnosis of human angiostrongyliasis. *Asian Pacific J. Aller. Immun.*, **19**: 267–73.

Nakazawa, K., Kato, Y. and Sakai, H. (1992). A case of eosinophilic meningitis due to *Angiostrongylus cantonensis*. *Kansensh. Zasshi*, **66**: 998–1001. (In Japanese).

New, D., Little, M.D. and Cross, J. (1995). *Angiostrongylus cantonensis* infection from eating raw snails. *N. Eng. J. Med.*, **332**: 1105–6.

Noskin, G.A., McMenamin, M.B. and Grohmann, S.M. (1992). Eosinophilic meningitis due to *Angiostrongylus cantonensis*. *Neurology*, **42**: 1423–24.

Nuamtanong, S. (1996). The evaluation of the 29 and 31 kDa antigens in female *Angiostrongylus cantonensis* for serodiagnosis of human angiostrongyliasis. *Southeast Asian J. Trop. Med. Pub. Health*, **27**: 291–96.

Ogawa, K., Kishi, M., Ogawa, T., Wakata, N. and Kinoshita, M. (1998). A case of eosinophilic meningoencephalitis caused by *Angiostrongylus cantonensis* with unique brain MRI findings. *Rinsho Shink.*, **38**: 22–26.

Panackel, C., Cherian, G., Vijayakumar, K. and Sharma, R.N. (2006). Eosinophilic meningitis due to *Angiostrongylus cantonensis*. *Indian J. Med. Microbiol.*, **24**: 220–21.

Pascual Gispert, J.E., Aguilar Prieto, P.H. and Galvez Oviedo, M.D. (1981). Finding of *Angiostrongylus cantonensis* in the cerebrospinal fluid of a boy with eosinophilic meningoencephalitis. *Review Cubana Med. Trop.*, **33**: 92–95.

Podwall, D., Gupta, R., Furuya, E.Y., Sevigny, J. and Resor, S.R. (2004). *Angiostrongylus cantonensis* meningitis presenting with facial nerve palsy. *J. Neurol.*, **251**: 1280–81.

Prociv, P., Spratt, D.M. and Carlisle, M.S. (2000). Neuro-angiostrongyliasis: unresolved issues. *Intern. J. Parasit.*, **30**: 1295–1303.

Punyagupta, S., Bunnag, T., Juttijudata, P. and Rosen, L. (1970). Eosinophilic meningitis in Thailand. Epidemiologic studies of 484 typical cases and the etiologic role of *Angiostrongylus cantonensis*. *Am. J. Trop. Med. Hyg.*, **19**: 950–58.

Punyagupta, S., Bunnag, T. and Juttijudata, P. (1990). Eosinophilic meningitis in Thailand. Clinical and epidemiological characteristics of 162 patients with myeloencephalitis probably caused by *Gnathostoma spinigerum*. *J. Neurol. Sci.*, **96**: 241–56.

Punyagupta, S., Juttijudata, P. and Bunnag, T. (1975). Eosinophilic meningitis in Thailand. Clinical studies of 484 typical cases probably caused by *Angiostrongylus cantonensis*. *Am. J. Trop. Med. Hyg.*, **24**: 921–31.

Radomyos, P., Tungtrongchitr, A., et al. (1994). Occurrence of the infective stage of *Angiostrongylus cantonensis* in the yellow tree monitor (*Varanus bengalensis*) in five provinces of Thailand. *Southeast Asian J. Trop. Med. Pub. Health*, **25**: 498–500.

Rosen, L., Laigret, J. and Boils, P.L. (1961). Observation on an outbreak of eosinophilic meningitis on Tahiti, French Polynesia. *Am. J. Hyg.*, **74**: 26–42.

Sawanyawisuth, K., Kitthaweesin, K., et al. (2006). Intraocular angiostrongyliasis: clinical findings, treatments and outcomes. *Trans. R. Soc. Trop. Med. Hyg.*, **101**: 497–501.

Slom, T.J., Cortese, M.M., et al. (2002). An outbreak of eosinophilic meningitis caused by *Angiostrongylus cantonensis* in travelers returning from the Caribbean. *N. Eng. J. Med.*, **346**: 668–75.

Sonakul, D. (1978). Pathological findings in four cases of human angiostrongyliasis. *Southeast Asian J. Trop. Med. Pub. Health*, **9**: 220–27.

Tsai, H.C., Lee, S.S., Huang, C.K., Yen, C.M., Chen, E.R. and Liu, Y.C. (2004). Outbreak of eosinophilic meningitis associated with drinking raw vegetable juice in southern Taiwan. *Am. J. Trop. Med. Hyg.*, **71**: 222–26.

Tsai, H.C., Liu, Y.C., Kunin, C.M., et al. (2003). Eosinophilic meningitis caused by *Angiostrongylus cantonensis* associated with eating raw snails: correlation of brain magnetic resonance imaging scans with clinical findings. *Am. J. Trop. Med. Hyg.*, **68**: 281–85.

Tsai, H.C., Liu, Y.C., Kunin, C.M., Lee, S.S., et al. (2001). Eosinophilic meningitis caused by *Angiostrongylus cantonensis*: report of 17 cases. *Am. J. Med.*, **111**: 109–14.

Tsai, T.H., Liu, Y.C., Wann, S.R., et al. (2001). An outbreak of meningitis caused by *Angiostrongylus cantonensis* in Kaohsiung. *J. Microbiol., Immun. Infect.*, **34**: 50–56.

Vazquez, J.J., Boils, P.L., Sola, J.J., et al. (1993). Angiostrongyliasis in a European patient: a rare cause of gangrenous ischemic enterocolitis. *Gastroenterology*, **105**: 1544–49.

Wang, Q.P., Chen, X.G., Lun, Z.R. (2007). Invasive freshwater snail, China. *Emerg. Infect. Dis.*, **13**: 1119–20.

Wang, Q.P., Lai, D.H., Zhu, X.Q., Chen, X.G. and Lun, Z.R. (2008). Human angiostrongyliasis. *Lancet Infect. Dis.*, **8**: 621–30.

Wu, G.H. (2006). *Angiostrongylus cantonensis*. In: J.Q. Tang (ed.) *Nature-Borne Diseases.*, pp 1182–89. Beijing: Science Press.

Yii, C.Y. (1976). Clinical observations on eosinophilic meningitis and meningoencephalitis caused by *Angiostrongylus cantonensis* on Taiwan. *Am. J. Trop. Med. Hyg.*, **25**: 233–49.

CHAPTER 60

Zoonotic infections with filarial nematodes

Harman S. Paintal and Rajinder K. Chitkara

Summary

Filarial nematodes have been known to cause human disease for many centuries. Lymphatic filariasis is a common disease in the developing part of the world and much has been written about diagnosis and treatment of this scourge. *Wuchereria*, *Brugia* and *Onchocerca* (especially *O. volvulus*) have a wide pattern of distribution with severe morbidity. Given the years of scientific work in this field, many drugs that work against these parasites are available and being used to control these infections. In this chapter, we focus on filarial nematodes that do not use humans as their primary host. Instead, the filarial organisms that parasitize other animals and cause human infection due to a variety of factors are discussed. These factors include:

1. Proximity of humans to the primary host,

2. Proximity of humans to the vector,

3. Changing ecology with introduction of different animals (both host and vector) into new environments,

4. Increasing human mobility,

5. Special scenarios concerning humans, including altered immune function (immunosuppressed due to drugs, autoimmune illness, immunosuppressive diseases),

There has been an increased interest in this field as newer diagnostic techniques, including polymerase chain reaction (PCR) assays, DNA primers and electron microscopy have become widespread in use. This will eventually enhance our understanding of the pathophysiology of infections with these seemingly rare filarial organisms.

Much of the early work in this field was done in a few specialized centers. As information about these parasites (through the worldwide web) and diagnostic techniques are now widely available, it is our hope that more work regarding these nematodes will be carried out in the developing countries where these infections are common. In this chapter, we focus on *Dirofilaria*, *Meningonema*, *Loaina*, *Dipetalonema* and certain species of *Onchocerca* and *Brugia*.

Dirofilaria

History

Dirofilaria has been known to cause infections in humans for the last four centuries. João Rodrigues de Castelo Branco (better known as Amato Lucitano), a Portugese Jewish physician reported ocular filariasis in a three year old child most likely caused by *Dirofilaria repens* (Aldravando 1602), (Pampiglione 1995). In 1885, Addario reported the removal of a *Dirofilaria* worm from the eyelid of a woman (Addario 1885). Faust *et al*. (1952) were probably the first to report *Dirofilaria* infections in the USA.

Microbiology

The most common zoonotic species within the genus *Dirofilaria* that have been known to cause infections in humans are elucidated in Table 60.1.

Decades of advances in the field of imaging and parasitology have shed light on the structure and function of *Dirofilaria*. The anatomy of *D. tenuis* was first described in 1965 (Orihel and Beaver 1965; Orihel and Ash 1995). Recent work by Song *et al*. (2009) using both scanning and transmission electron microscopy elucidated the internal and external ultrastructure of *D. immitis* microfilaria.

Generally, the female worms are longer and larger than their male counterparts. The size of the worm is also dependent upon the host from which they are isolated. Identification of the particular worm species therefore depends primarily upon the size of the worm in conjunction with information regarding the host (see Table 60.1) from which it is isolated, the organ or body part from where the worm is recovered (*D. tenuis* is recovered from the subcutaneous tissues while *D. immitis* is usually found in the cardiovascular system), the geographic area in which the host is located and relevant travel history.

D. tenuis adult worms isolated from humans measure about 10 cm in length and 300 µ in outer diameter and have a beaded appearance given the presence of approximately 90 longitudinal ridges. The cross section and muscle morphology also helps differentiate various species, with *D. tenuis* possessing a 5–8 µ thick cuticle with a ridge that protrudes into the lateral chords and multiple longitudinal ridges that give the worm a rounded appearance. The number of tubes (two uterine tubes and one vaginal tube in the pseudocelom in females, one reproductive tube in the pseudocelom in males), presence of eggs (in females) or sperm (in males) helps differentiate the male from the female worm. The soft tissues including the coelomyarian muscles, lateral chords and tubular structures degenerate in the dead worm and the cuticle becomes oedematous making it difficult to accurately identify the worm.

Table 60.1 Most common species in the *Dirofilaria* genus that cause zoonotic disease

Dirofilaria species	Definitive animal host	Geographic region	Vector
D. immitis	Dogs	Widespread	Mosquito
D. repens	Dogs, cats	Africa, Asia, southern Europe	Mosquito
D. tenuis	Raccoons	North America	Mosquito
D. ursi	Bears	North America Asia	Blackfly (Simulium spp.)
D. subdermata	Porcupines	North America	Mosquito
D. striata	Felids	North America	Mosquito
D. magnilarvatum	Macaques	Malaysia	Mosquito
D. corynodes	Monkeys	Africa	Mosquito

The ridges tend to remain intact in the posthumous state (Orihel and Eberhard 1998; Eberhard 2006).

D. repens is a larger parasite with females reaching 17 cm in length and up to 650–660 μm in diameter, with males being much shorter (up to 7 cm) and thinner (up to 450 μm). These worms tend to have about 100 longitudinal ridges at the mid-body level, though this varies at the extremes (Pampiglione *et al.* 1995).

D. striata is one of the largest worms in this genus with females reaching 28 cm in length and up to 550 μm in diameter. The males can grow up to 8.5 cm in length and 380 μm in diameter. Important distinguishing features include the presence of lateral alae on the cuticular surface and the subtlety of the longitudinal ridges. *D. immitis* and *D. lutrae* can be differentiated morphologically from the rest due to the presence of a smooth cuticle. *D. ursi* worms have smaller cross sectional diameter than *D. tenuis* (up to 260 μm) and lesser number of longitudinal ridges (less than 90) (Gutierrez 1990).

It is also important to recognize that the worms vary in size depending upon their maturation when they are isolated. Some of these criteria are not met in the practice setting, and the worms are then categorized as *repens*-like, *ursi*-like and so on based on the closest match for the purpose of identification.

Life cycle of *dirofilaria*

As previously discussed, most species in this genus have a specific host and therefore a distinct life-cycle. We have attempted to describe this by mentioning the salient points of each while avoiding repetition of the commonalities.

D. immitis (also known as heartworm) is dependent upon the domestic dog (*Canis domesticus*) and the coyote (*Canis latrans*) as its primary host and reservoir. Canids known to become infected and subsequently transmit infection include the fox, maned wolf, timber wolf and the raccoon dog. Other animals that have been known to contract this infection include the domestic cat (*Felis domesticus*), raccoon, ferret, otter, black bear, orangutan, gibbon, red panda, California sea lion, seal, beaver and muskrat. Human infection is extremely rare. Mosquitoes serve as primary vectors for most species of *Dirofilaria* except *D. ursi* that is transmitted by the blackfly. Several species of mosquitoes belonging to the *Aedes*, *Anopheles* and *Culex* genera have been implicated. When a susceptible mosquito bites a microfilaremic host, it ingests these tiny

microfilariae (up to 360 μm long) into the midgut, where they stay for about 24 hours before migrating into the cells within the malphigian tubules. The microfilariae become short and thick like a sausage, hence that name for this stage. By day 5, differentiation within various parts of the gastrointestinal system is complete, leading to the subsequent migration of these filariae into the lumen of the Malphigian tubules over the next 2 days. Over the next 5 days, they molt twice to become third stage larvae (L3). These L3 larvae penetrate the malphigian tubules and reach the mouth parts after migrating through the body cavity of the mosquito. This cycle is temperature and moisture dependent, with high humidity and ambient temperature leading to shorter cycles (Abraham 1998; Cancrini and Kramer 2001).

These sexually differentiated L3 microfilariae are released (via rupture of the labellum) and transmitted onto the body of the primary host (domestic dog) by the mosquito while consuming its blood meal. These larvae initially occupy the subcutaneous tissue, and slowly make their way through the muscles and venous channels till they reach the right side of the heart within 70–120 days after the initial infection. This journey is accompanied by structural changes with initial molting within the first 3–12 days from L3 to L4 and subsequent molting to the final form between days 50–70. The worms entering the heart are usually small, and undergo rapid growth, especially in case of the female *Dirofilaria*. Sexual maturity is complete within 4 months of the initial infection. Dogs tend to have circulating microfilariae that may then be ingested by an uninfected susceptible mosquito thus completing the life cycle (Kotani and Powers 1982). The list of definitive hosts and the vectors involved in the life cycle of the various *Dirofilariae* is tabulated in Table 60.1.

Pathogenesis

Humans are not the definitive hosts for *Dirofilaria*. Almost universally, the infections are not patent (they cannot be transmitted back to the mosquito) and therefore the life cycle of the parasite generally ends in the human host. Rarely, sexually mature females (in the absence of males) or gravid females have been seen, as have isolated cases of microfilaremia in patients. The clinical manifestations of *Dirofilaria* infection are species specific, based on the geographic distribution of the parasite. The microfilariae of *D. immitis* extruded during the blood meal of the infected mosquito penetrate the subcutaneous tissue and elicit an inflammatory response. The mechanism of the immune response is not well understood. The prevailing hypotheses include a vigorous immune response killing the parasite to the immune system reacting to the release of various antigens by the dying parasite (Orihel and Eberhard 1998). Those that survive this vigorous immune response enter the venous channels and end their journey in the small-medium sized pulmonary vessels (Simon *et al.* 2005).

Most microfilariae are killed during this journey or upon lodging in the pulmonary arterial vasculature. The elicited response may cause vasculitis and often leads to a granuloma formation that can be seen on chest radiography (Theis 2005). Though uncommon, *D. immitis* has been isolated from other organ systems including the entero-hepatic system and the genito-urinary system. Therefore, the isolation of *Dirofilaria* species outside the cardiovascular system should not eliminate the possibility of finding *D. immitis*.

Most of the other *Dirofilariae* (including *D. tenuis*, *D. repens*, *D. ursi*, *D. striata* and *D. subdermata*) become lodged in the subcutaneous tissue in various parts of the body and their manifestations reflect this predisposition. *Dirofilaria* species (*D. immitis*, *D. repens* and *D. roemeri*) have also been isolated from subconjunctival, intraocular and orbital tissues.

Clinical presentation

Most patients infected with *Dirofilaria* are asymptomatic and therefore are never detected. Their presentations vary with parasite and the organs they get lodged in. It is fascinating to note that a majority of cases of human dirofilariasis in the USA and Japan involve the lungs, whereas in Europe, the majority of cases are subcutaneous or ocular in distribution (Simón *et al.* 2009). Given the widely accepted practice of taking chest radiographs and computer tomographic (CT) scans for a variety of reasons, coupled with the propensity of *Dirofilaria immitis* to go to the pulmonary arterial vasculature (to cause vasculitis and granuloma formation), it is easy to understand the current viewpoint that pulmonary nodules (coin lesions) are the most common presentation of human dirofilariasis. Most of the patients likely have radiographic imaging for unrelated reasons and have a solitary pulmonary nodule or multiple pulmonary nodules detected that then may lead to a workup for malignancy or infection. Serial CT scans on asymptomatic patients with *Dirofilaria* related nodules show radiographic stability and result in conservative follow-up rather than biopsies that may yield the diagnosis. Other associated pulmonary symptoms like cough, pleuritic chest discomfort and haemoptysis due to underlying pulmonary infarction are less common, but often lead to a more extensive diagnostic path. CT angiograms of the chest can detect obstruction of the pulmonary vasculature (but cannot differentiate a blood clot from a parasite causing the obstruction); echocardiograms can detect clots within the heart and elevated pressures that may suggest obstruction in the pulmonary arterial vasculature. Bronchoscopies for haemoptysis related to pulmonary embolism are often unrevealing. Since the parasite has also been isolated from vascular compartments of other organs, we are of the opinion that future imaging modalities will make it easier to detect the parasitic infestation in vascular compartments of other organs. Figures 60.1 and 60.2 illustrate the presence of microfilaria in the peripheral blood specimen.

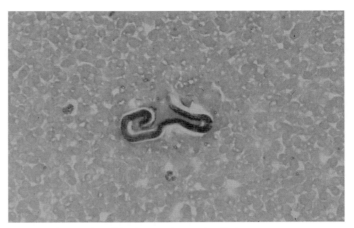

Fig. 60.1 This peripheral blood smear shows microfilaria.
Photo courtesy of Prof. Luis F. Fajardo, Stanford University School of Medicine.

Other species of *Dirofilaria* tend to occupy the subcutaneous tissue compartment and present with symptoms ranging from a nodule or a scar (merely cosmetic) to ulcerations (that are painful). These lesions may be pruritic and often contain eosinophils. *D. tenuis* is the most common parasite implicated; other members of the *Dirofilaria* family with a propensity for subcutaneous tissues include *D. repens*, *D. ursi* and *D. subdermata*. *D. repens* has been studied extensively and a review by Pampiglione and Trotti (1995) documented the presence of these parasites in the subcutaneous tissues of the body with the highest frequency noted in the orbital region (eyelids, conjunctiva and subconjunctival region). They were also detected in the male genitalia, peritoneal and omental cavities. Pampiglione *et al.* (2009) reported that most human infections in the Americas were related to *D. immitis* while those in the Old World were related to *D. repens*. The reasons for this are not entirely clear. A quick review of recent publications suggests that *Dirofilaria* related subcutaneous and ocular infections are

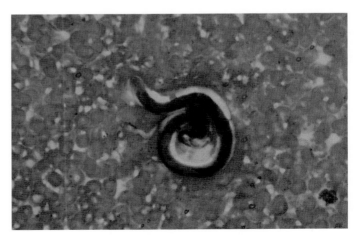

Fig. 60.2 Microfilaria in peripheral blood smear at higher magnification.
Photo courtesy of Prof. Luis F. Fajardo, Stanford University School of Medicine.

common and are being diagnosed with increasing frequency worldwide (Kramer *et al.* 2007; Szénási *et al.* 2008; Nath *et al.* 2010).

Cutaneous infestation with *Dirofilaria* causing meningeal involvement (including signs of meningeal irritation) and symptoms of meningoencephalitis has also been reported (Poppert *et al.* 2009).

Diagnosis

Patients tend to be asymptomatic and this underscores the difficulty in making a definitive diagnosis. Lab tests often reveal peripheral eosinophilia, an elevated erythrocyte sedimentation rate (ESR), a high C-reactive protein (CRP) with or without leukocytosis. These abnormalities are non-specific and should prompt reliance on history, physical and other pertinent tests. In the case of pulmonary involvement, most patients come under the radar with the incidental finding of stable pulmonary nodules on serial imaging. Recent studies that predict the requirement for continued radiographic follow up or invasive testing (for cancer and other significant diseases) may lead most physicians to ignore the presence of these stable nodules in asymptomatic patients. In order to make the diagnosis, pulmonary nodules must be excised surgically, a procedure that generally requires general anaesthesia and involves significant risks. Figs. 60.3 and 60.4 illustrate the anatomy of the adult dirofilarial parasite in the biopsy specimen of the human lung. Other diagnostic modalities like bronchoscopy and percutaneous CT guided biopsies are less helpful since diagnosis requires detection of the parasite generally appreciated better in the completely excised nodule.

Subcutaneous nodules can be excised and the parasite usually identified on sections. Serological tests to detect antibodies against these parasites have been used with limited success (Glickman *et al.* 1986; Morchón *et al.* 2006; Miyoshi *et al.* 2006).

Newer diagnostic molecular techniques including polymerase chain reaction, DNA probes and genetic primers have increased the sensitivity and specificity of diagnosing these infections and help increase understanding of how these parasites interact with humans (Scoles and Kambhapati 1995; Watts *et al.* 1999; Lee *et al.*

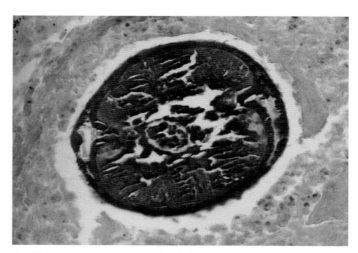

Fig. 60.4 Cross sectional image of Dirofilaria in lung.

2007). Serum measurements of thromboxane B2 may also prove to be helpful in diagnosing patients living in endemic areas (Morchón *et al.* 2006). Recent work on the presence of the bacterial endosymbiont *Wolbachia* in *D. repens* and its inflammatory reaction in the human body have led some to hypothesize that Immunoglobulin G (IgG) levels (against *Wolbachia*) can be used to both diagnose infections and gauge response to therapy against *D. repens* (Grandi *et al.* 2008).

Treatment

Most human infections with *Dirofilaria* do not require treatment since the parasite is destroyed as part of the immune response. In symptomatic patients, some experts recommend use of ivermectin and diethylcarbamazine or milbemycin though no large studies have validated this approach. Most of the drugs advocated by experts have been studied in filarial infections affecting humans as primary hosts. The addition of single dose albendazole to diethylcarbamazine was found to reduce the load of adult worms with no significant affect on microfilaremic load (Dreyer *et al.* 2006). Pharmacological trials against human filarial species have found that killing the bacterial endosymbiont *Wolbachia* can lead to death of the filarial parasite. An 8 week course of doxycycline (200 mg daily) was found to be effective against both the microfilaria and the adult worm (Taylor *et al.* 2005). In infected dogs, the arsenical compound melarsomine dihydrochloride is administered parenterally. The death of the worm leads to pulmonary thromboembolism that in canines requires treatment with heparin and steroids (McCall *et al.* 2008).

Ocular infections have been treated with removal of the worm. Painful nodules should be excised as the persistence of *Dirofilaria* may lead to a continuous inflammatory response.

Epidemiology

Climatic patterns and social habits of humans must be accounted for in order to understand the distribution of *Dirofilaria* infection in human settlements. Areas with ambient temperatures for vector proliferation and transmission and higher humidity lead to a much higher incidence of *Dirofilaria* infection (Genchi *et al.* 2009).

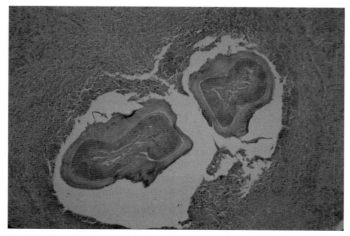

Fig. 60.3 Lung biopsy specimen showing cross-section of Dirofilaria (undetermined species).
Photo courtesy of Prof. Luis F. Fajardo, Stanford University School of Medicine.

It is intuitive that communities that encourage the domestication of dogs and those where *Dirofilaria* is endemic in dogs also have a higher incidence. The asymptomatic nature of the disease likely underestimates the true incidence of this public health problem (Simon and Lopez-Belmonte 2005). In the USA, the highest incidence is seen in the southeast part of the country. In a recent retrospective review of *D. immitis* infection in the USA from 1941 onwards Theis (2005) attempted to clear some falsely held notions regarding the parasite. The name heartworm makes most health care providers assume that this parasite literally lodges and lives in the heart, whereas it is primarily a vascular parasite usually found in the pulmonary arterial circulation though it has been isolated from the hepatic and testicular circulation. Theis also commented on the difficulty of trying to differentiate the spherical pulmonary nodules (granulomas formed after pulmonary artery/arteriole inflammation and resulting pneumonitis from the death of the worm) from other common causes of nodules. Vezzani *et al.* (2006) also recently published a historical review of *D. immitis* in South America. Miyoshi *et al.* (2006) published data regarding dirofilariasis in Japan. Such similar reports and case series have also been published in Europe from southern France, Spain and Italy (Muro *et al.* 1999).

Prevention and control

Universally accepted epidemiological control methods (including proper hygiene and sanitation) to control the spread of infections apply to preventing the spread of filarial nematode infections also. These include:

1. Avoidance of contact with the primary host (if feasible),

2. Prevention of contact with vector (including protection against bites with clothing, insect repellants and insecticide treated nets).

We recommend the following measures to owners of pets (especially dogs) for the prevention of dirofilariasis:

1. All pets should have regular visits to the veterinarian, receive routine vaccinations and be treated promptly if they exhibit symptoms and signs of any illness,

2. Dogs should be treated to prevent *Dirofilaria* infestation,

3. Pets should be fed well cooked or prepared food (no raw animal products). They should be prevented from scavenging garbage and from drinking non-potable water,

4. Pet owners should regularly wash their hands after contact with the animal.

Even though there is no evidence that dirofilariasis is a significant problem in immunocompromised hosts, pets can transmit other zoonotic illnesses in the immune-suppressed group (AIDS, post-splenectomy, post-transplant, pregnancy) (Trevejo *et al.* 2005; Kotton 2007).

Based on the U.S Public Health Service guidelines (Kaplan *et al.* 2002), we also recommend the following:

1. HIV infected patients should avoid pets aged less than 6 months (cats less than 1 year),

2. Avoid stray animals. Handle pets suffering from diarrhoea with extreme care and consider seeking a veterinarian,

3. Avoid contact with reptiles, birds or exotic birds,

4. Use gloves when cleaning animal excreta.

Meningonema

History

Meningonema peruzzi (Filarioidea Splendidofilariinae) is a zoonotic filarial parasite of African monkeys that is predominantly distributed around the central region of Africa. Given the geographic distribution of this nematode and lack of significant research, not much is known about the history and life cycle of this parasite (Orihel and Esslinger 1973).

Microbiology

Meningonema shares remarkable similarities with another filarial nematode, *Mansonella perstans* (also known as *Acanthocheilonema perstans*). The significant differences include the presence a outer tightly fitting sheath, four uterine branches (instead of two), an extremely thin body wall with weak musculature covering one third of the body circumference and lateral chords that occupy two-thirds of the body circumference.

Life cycle

Research suggests the cercopithecid monkey to be the likely definitive host. The vector for this worm is not known, though we think it important to mention that *Mansonella perstans*, which as stated above shares significant similarities with *Meningonema* is transmitted by tiny blood-sucking flies (biting midges of the genus *Culicoides*). Humans are probably infected by the bite of the flies or mosquitoes carrying this filarial parasite, and are not known to be involved in propagation (they are not patent hosts) (Orihel and Eberhard 1998).

Pathophysiology

Meningonema filariae are found both in the peripheral blood and in the central nervous system of the host monkey. The parasite derives its name from the propensity to cross the blood brain barrier and lodge in the subarachnoid space at the level of the medulla oblongata. The presence of this parasite in the spinal fluid of the human host causes an inflammatory reaction that may manifest with various neurological signs and symptoms.

Clinical presentation

Patients may present with signs of meningeal irritation that include headache, photophobia and meningismus. They may also have altered mentation depending upon the involvement of brain tissue. Seizures have been noted in patients with *Mansonella* and may occur with this parasite too.

Diagnosis

The presence of parasite in the cerebrospinal fluid is required to make the diagnosis. However, it is important that the clinician realize that this parasite may be present in the CSF asymptomatically (Boussinesq *et al.* 1995). Therefore, symptoms and signs of meningeal irritation are as important as the physical presence of *Meningonema* in CSF. We again stress the importance of differentiating this worm from *Mansonella*, a more commonly discovered parasite in patients from this part of the world (Duke and Gelfand 1968; Orihel 1973). It is likely that given the higher prevalence and greater experience in diagnosing *Mansonella* (along with the physical similarities), infection with *Meningonema* is an under-diagnosed problem. Staining with Mayer's Haemalum reveals a filarial nematode under 250 μm long with a small sheath (Denham 1975; Rosenblatt 2009). Patients may also have less specific laboratory abnormalities including peripheral eosinophilia, eosinophilia in the CSF (more specific for CNS parasite infection than peripheral eosinophilia), elevated ESR and CRP in the serum. Recent advances with serological markers, enhanced PCR techniques and DNA primers should help the physician make the diagnosis with increased accuracy.

Treatment

We could not identify any valid studies that have singularly reported or reviewed pharmacological treatment of *Meningonema* infections. However, given the similarities between *Mansonella* and *Meningonema*, it is believed that the same treatment regimen can potentially be tried (Coulibaly *et al.* 2009). This includes either a 3–4 week therapy using Mebendazole 100mg twice daily or Doxycycline 200 mg daily for 4–8 weeks (Simonsen *et al.* 2010).

Prevention and control

The relative lack of information regarding the life cycle of *Meningonema* prevents the institution of control measures. It is instructive to know that the blood-sucking flies of the genus *Culicoides* (vector for *Mansonella*) are too small to be caught in insecticide treated nets. Basic control measures against Meningonema thus include being well clad (to avoid insect bites) and using insect repellants.

Loaina

History

Even though this group of organisms has been known and studied since the late nineteenth century (1880s in the case of *Loaina scapiceps* and 1950s for *Loaina uniformis*), literature regarding human infections is scant. In fact it was only recently when Eberhard and Orihel (1984) proposed the name *Loaina* stating that certain species of *Dirofilaria* (*D. uniformis*, *Pelecitus scapiceps* and *D. roemeri*) were unique and unlike other *Dirofilaria* species both morphologically and biologically. They also share characteristics with *Loa* (Wisely and Howard 2008).

Microbiology

The *Loaina* group of parasites can be differentiated from dirofilarial parasites on account of a thin cuticle, large lateral chords and scant muscle cells. The reproductive system of both Loaina and Loa are similar. *L. scapiceps* has large lateral cuticular alae (Orihel and Eberhard 1998).

Life cycle

Certain species of rabbits are the primary hosts of *Loaina uniformis* and *Loaina scapiceps*, while kangaroos are primary hosts of *Dirofilaria roemeri* (*Loaina roemeri*). *Loaina* has been isolated in the eastern cottontail rabbit (*Sylvilagus floridanus*) and the snowshoe hare (*Lepus americanus*). The life cycle of *Loaina* is similar to that of *Dirofilaria* species barring some important distinctions. The parasite within the mosquito develops in the fat body and not in the malphigian tubules. The mosquitoes transmit the L3 microfilariae to the rabbit (or the kangaroo) during the blood meal. These then undergo a process of sequential molting, growth and

sexual maturity to reach the adult stage. The adult *L. scapiceps* worms (dead and alive) have been recovered from the tendons and the synovial sheaths around the ankle region of the hosts. Live worms and microfilaremia has been commonly observed in the eastern cottontail rabbit, while dead worms and an inflammatory response were noted in the tendons of the snowshoe hare. This allowed Bartlett to forward the hypothesis that the eastern cottontail rabbit was the primary host and the snowshoe hare was merely infected with the parasite (Bartlett 1983). Adult females produce microfilariae that may circulate in the vascular compartment of the host. The mosquito during its blood meal ingests these microfilariae, gets infected and thus completes the life cycle. Given the lack of literature regarding infections in humans, describing the process by which the microfilariae when introduced to the human body via the insect bite cause an infection would be mere conjecture. Humans are not known to be patent hosts.

Clinical presentation

The few reported cases of *Loaina* in humans have been intraocular infections. The worm(s) have been found in the anterior chamber of the eye and either removed surgically or isolated after enucleation (Van Duyse 1895; Gabrielides 1938). The cases reported have come from geographically and ecologically diverse regions (Australia, Greece and Colombia) (Botero *et al.* 1984; Beaver 1989). The signs and symptoms range from mild (ocular irritation, redness) to severe (decreased vision or blindness). Given the lack of published literature in this field, it is felt that many patients infected with *Loaina* are possibly asymptomatic and therefore never seek medical care.

Diagnosis

In humans, diagnosis is dependent upon a careful history regarding contact (or travel in areas) with animals that serve as primary hosts. Patient with ocular symptoms should have a comprehensive fundoscopic exam that may reveal the worm within the eye. Peripheral eosinophilia, elevated ESR and CRP should prompt physicians to seek more testing. Serological methods, PCR techniques and DNA primers should be utilized to identify this worm.

Treatment

Since very few cases of human infection with *Loaina* have been reported, it is difficult to proclaim any treatment provided in these cases to be the standard of care. Treatment of ocular infections depends upon the symptoms. Some patients complaining of pain may respond to mydriatics, while more significant symptoms necessitate removal of the worm. When patients present at later stages of ocular involvement with destruction of tissue, enucleation may be the only viable option.

Prevention and control

These measures are similar to those for Dirofilaria alluded to earlier in the chapter.

Dipetalonema

History

Worms of the genus *Dipetalonema* have been documented in medical literature from the late nineteenth century. *D. perstans* and *D. streptocerca* are commonly known to infect humans (that serve as primary hosts) (Wisely and Howard 2008). Other species of this genus affect a diverse range of mammals and there have been isolated reports of these zoonoses affecting humans. Some of these species are listed in Table 60.2.

Microbiology

These parasites can be distinguished from other filarial nematodes from the morphological differences in the cuticle, their reproductive system and nerve ring. The smooth cuticle lacks striae and ridges. Other differentiating features include a long tail with two or more papillae, a muscular oesophagus and on cross section the internal anatomy reveals cuticular ridges and tall coelomyarian muscle cells. Beaver *et al.* (1980) provided a detailed morphological description of *D. reconditum* isolated from the eye of a patient.

Life cycle

Dipetalonema is transmitted by fleas (of the genus *Pulex* and *Ctenocephalides*), ticks (*Rhipicephalus sanguineus*) and lice (*Linognathus*). *D. sprenti* and *D. arbuta* are transmitted via mosquitoes (Anderson 1992). The microfilariae can be detected in the serum of the primary host. At the end of the larval stage, the worm usually migrates into the subcutaneous tissues, and less commonly into the body cavities and kidneys. Given the very few reported cases of *Dipetalonema* infection in humans, it is difficult to describe with certainty its life cycle in the human host. It is probably safe to conjecture that humans are non-patent hosts and not involved in transmission of *Dipetalonema*. Microfilariae introduced into humans via the vector mature into adults and then likely die due to the inflammatory reaction generated by the immune system. It is hypothesized that most *Dipetalonema infections* in humans (just like in the primary mammalian hosts) are limited to the

Table 60.2 Potential zoonotic *Dipetalonema* species and their usual definitive hosts

Dipetalonema species	Definitive animal host
D. arbuta	Porcupine
D. sprenti	Beaver
D. dracunculoides	Dogs
D. evansi	Camels
D. gracile	Primates
D. marmasetae	Primates
D. obtuse	Primates
D. tamarinae	Primates
D. freitasi	White throated Capuchin monkey
D. yatesi	Peruvian spider monkey
D. vanhoofi	Chimpanzee
D. caudispina	Squirrel monkey
D. grassii	Dogs
D. loxodontis	African elephant
D. odendhali	California sea lion
D. reconditum	Dogs
D. spirocauda	Seals

subcutaneous tissues, even though literature supporting this is lacking. As we mention below, a few researchers have documented ocular infections with *Dipetalonema*.

Clinical presentation

Most case reports of *Dipetalonema* infections in humans involve the eye. Signs and symptoms ranged from a vague sensation of something moving within the eye, redness and pain to blurring of vision and decreased acuity (Huynh and Thean 2001). Beaver *et al.* (1980) reported a case in Oregon where a zoologist who had recently travelled to New Zealand and Fiji felt pain in his right eye along with an abnormal sensation. The fundoscopic exam revealed a worm that was removed via an irrigation aspiration procedure and identified as *Dipetalonema arbuta*, a species usually found in the body cavity of the American porcupine. They also reported on prior cases of ophthalmological involvement involving either *D. arbuta* or *D. sprenti* seen in the state of Oregon, USA. Serum tests may demonstrate eosinophilia with elevated ESR and CRP.

Diagnosis

Patients complaining of ocular symptoms should have a comprehensive eye exam including fundoscopy. Any suspicious subcutaneous nodules should be biopsied. Historically, diagnosis of *Dipetalonema* in humans has been made on the basis of morphological differences with other filarial nematodes. Recent advances, including the use of polymerase chain reaction assays and DNA primers have increased the diagnostic accuracy (Mar *et al.* 2002). This is however limited to a few laboratories worldwide, in hospitals that staff experienced parasitologists.

Treatment

The drugs diethylcarbamazine, praziquantel and ivermectin have been used experimentally in animals (primates) suffering from *Dipetalonema* infections with positive results (Zahner and Schares, 1993). However, no studies looking at effective treatment for *Dipetalonema* infections in humans have been conducted. Ocular involvement has traditionally been treated with removal of the worm with positive results (Huynh and Thean 2001).

Other zoonotic filarial parasites

While *Onchocerca volvulus* is a known parasite of humans, other zoonotic *Onchocerca* infections are being reported in literature with increasing frequency. This is related to close contact between humans and agricultural animals (cattle, horses and camels) that serve as natural hosts for many *Onchocerca* species (Table 60.3).

The adult blackfly (*Simulium nodosum*) has been found to carry *Onchocerca* larvae (Ishii *et al.* 2008). *Onchocerca* infections can be diagnosed on the basis of typical morphology of this genus. The female worm possesses a thick multilayered cuticle with annular ridges externally and transverse striae on the internal surface. The muscle cells are of coelomyarian type, with a loose, fibrillar and atrophied appearance. Males on the other hand have a thinner cuticle, internal striations that do not appear prominent and well developed muscle cells, hypodermis and lateral chords (Eberhard 2006).

Less than 20 cases of zoonotic *Onchocerca* have been reported and most are associated with subcutaneous tissue involvement (Hira *et al.* 2008). Patients have presented with nodular swelling in

Table 60.3 Potential zoonotic *Onchocerca* species and their usual animal host

Onchocerca species	Animal host
O. gutturosa	Cattle
O. gibsoni	Cattle
O. armillata	Cattle
O. lienalis	Cattle
O. fasciata	Camel
O. reticulata	Horses
O. cervicalis	Horses
O. dukei	Antelope
O. dewittei japonica	Wild boar
O. suzukii	Serows
O. skrjabini	Sika deer
O. eberhardi	Sika deer
O. jakutensis	Red deer
O. lupi	Dogs

various parts of their body, with the parasite being isolated from muscles, tendons and even ocular tissue (Burr *et al*. 1998; Sréter *et al*. 2002; Sallo *et al*. 2005). These nodules may be tender or completely asymptomatic. Patients with ocular involvement tend to present with vision loss, red eye or a sensation of something moving within the eye. Given the ubiquity of this genus and the abundance of the natural host around human dwellings, there is no geographic pattern to this zoonoses and infections have been reported from the USA, continental Europe, the Middle East and Japan. Species identification has been made on the basis of PCR techniques and use of genetic primers (Koehsler *et al*. 2007).

Sporadic cases of zoonotic *Brugia* infections transmitted by mosquitoes are found in medical literature (Orihel and Beaver 1989). Most cases involve lymph node enlargement in a subcutaneous distribution (Elenitoba-Johnson *et al*. 1996). While it has been challenging to determine the exact species of Brugia causing these zoonotic infections, in the USA, *Brugia leporis* (definitive host rabbits) and *Brugia beaveri* (definitive host raccoons and bobcats) are thought to be primarily responsible because of their wide geographic distribution (Eberhard *et al*. 1993).

Amongst filarial nematodes, lymph node involvement is limited to *Wuchereria* and *Brugia*. *Wuchereria* is a larger parasite is easy to differentiate morphologically (female *Brugia* are also larger than their male counterparts). *Brugia* parasites have a smooth cuticle without layers except over the lateral chords that occupy one-third of the circumference. The muscles (about 5 cells per quadrant) are divided into cytoplasmic and contractile zones. Besides these structural traits, diagnosis can be made with the help of special stains like the PASD, Grocott and Giemsa or with PCR techniques. A recent case report from Canada documented two cases of zoonotic *Brugia* infection causing subcutaneous nodules that on biopsy revealed granulomatous eosinophilic dermatitis (Kokta 2008). Ocular infection with zoonotic *Brugia ceylonensis* (parasite in dogs) has also been reported (Dissanaike *et al*. 2000).

A case report about ocular infections with *Setaria labiatopapillosa* has also been reported. This parasite infects the bovine species and is transmitted by mosquitoes (especially of the *Aedes* genus) (Panaitescu *et al*. 1999).

New treatment options

Scientists in India have reported on the antifilarial activity in the extract of stem portion of the plant *Lantana camara* against adult *Brugia malayi* and *Acanthocheilonema* (*Dipetalonema*) *viteae* and the activity of marine red alga *Botryocladia leptopoda* against *Litomosoides sigmodontis* and *Acanthocheilonema* (*Dipetalonema*) *viteae* (Misra *et al*. 2007; Lakshmi *et al*. 2004).

Conclusions

In this review, we have attempted to present to the reader, a detailed and distinctive review of various zoonotic infections with filarial nematodes. This review would be incomplete in the absence of a disclosure that all the above mentioned infections are diagnosed very infrequently and not much is known about the life cycle of these parasites in humans. The changing weather patterns (including global warming), ecological migration of both humans and animals, close contact between humans and various animal species, resistance of vectors to various control methods (including certain insecticides) have all led to an increase in such zoonotic infections. Newer diagnostic techniques like polymerase chain reactions and use of DNA primers have helped medical providers diagnose such infections with increasing frequency. However, given the lack of information about some of these parasites, more research especially in the field of diagnosis and pharmacological treatment is warranted. Till then, universally accepted and standard methods of control and prevention that limit contact between the humans and the primary host as well as the vector should be followed. Educating the public regarding the potential impact of such infections and the need for prevention is key.

It is important to recognize that experienced parasitologists are a prerequisite in making the diagnosis of these rare zoonoses. When physicians suspect these infections but lack the expertise or resources to make the diagnosis, we suggest that they contact either large university based hospitals (that specialize in infectious diseases) or national/international organizations that are responsible for data gathering and dissemination. In the Western hemisphere, we suggest the use of the following resources (not in the order of preference):

1. Tulane University School of Public Health and Tropical Medicine,
   Phone: (504) 988-3558; Fax: (504) 988-7313
   Email: tropmed@tulane.edu
   http://www.sph.tulane.edu/tropmed/ (accessed 24 February 2011)

2. London School of Hygiene and Tropical Medicine;
   Phone: +44 (0)20 7636 8636
   Fax: +44 (0)20 7436 5389
   http://www.lshtm.ac.uk/ (accessed 24 February 2011)

3. National Institute of Allergy and Infectious Diseases; http://www.niaid.nih.gov/topics/tropicaldiseases/Pages/Default.aspx (accessed 24 February 2011)

4. Centers for Disease Control and Prevention; National Center for Emerging and Zoonotic Infectious Diseases

Phone: +1(800) 232-4636
Email: cdcinfo@cdc.gov
http://www.cdc.gov/nczved/ (accessed 24 February 2011)
http://www.cdc.gov/ncezid/ (accessed 24 February 2011)

5. World Health Organization;
   Email: NTDnzdMail@who.int
   http://www.who.int/neglected_diseases/zoonoses/en/ (accessed 24 February 2011)

6. Neglected Tropical Disease Coalition
   Email: info@neglectedtropicaldiseases.org
   http://www.neglectedtropicaldiseases.org/ (accessed 24 February 2011)

References

Abraham, D. (1988). Biology of Dirofilaria immitis. In: P.F.L. Boreham and R.B. Atwell (eds.) *Dirofilariasis*, pp. 29–46. Boca Raton, Florida: CRC Press, Inc.

Addario, C. (1885). Su un nematode dell'occhio umano. *Ann. Ottalmolog.*, 13: 135–47.

Aldravando, U. 1602. De animalibus inssectis libri septem cum singulorum iconibus ad vivum expressis, in Boloniae apud Ioan Bapt. Bellagambaum., pp. 655–56.

Anderson, R.C. (1992). *Nematode parasites of vertebrates. Their development and transmission*. Wallingford, UK: CAB International.

Bartlett, C.M. (1983). Epizootiology, development and migration of *Dirofilaria scapiceps* (Nematoda: Filarioidea) of rabbits and hares. Paper read at the 58th Annual Meeting of the American Society of Parasitologists, 7 December 1983, San Antonio, Texas.

Bartlett, C.M. (1984). Pathology and epizootiology of *Dirofilaria scapiceps* (Leidy, 1886) (Nematoda: Filarioidea) in *Sylvilagus floridanus* (J.A. Allen) and *Lepus americanus erxleben*. *J Wildl. Dis.*, 20: 197–206.

Beaver, P.C. (1989). Intraocular filariasis: a brief review. *Am. J. Trop. Med. Hyg.*, 40: 40–45.

Beaver, P.C., Meyers, E.A., Jarroll, E.L., and Rosenquist, R.C. (1980). *Dipetalonema* from the eye of a man in Oregon. *Am. J. Trop. Med. Hyg.*, 29: 369–72.

Botero, D., Aguledo, L.M., Uribe, F.J., Esslinger, J.H., and Beaver, P.C. (1984). Intraocular filaria, a *Loaina* species, from man in Colombia. *Am. J. Trop. Med. Hyg.*, 33: 578–82.

Boussinesq, M., Bain O., Chabaud, A.G., et al. (1995). A new zoonosis of the cerebrospinal fluid of man probably caused by *Meningonema peruzzii*, filaria of the central nervous system of Cercopithecidae. *Parasite*, 2: 173–76.

Burr Jr., W.E., Brown, M.F., and Eberhard, M.L. (1998). Zoonotic *Onchocerca* (Nematoda:Filarioidea) in the cornea of a Colorado resident. *Ophthalmology*, 105: 1494–97.

Cancrini, G. and Kramer, L.H. (2001). Insect vectors of *Dirofilaria* spp. In: F. Simon and C. Genchi (eds.) *Heartworm Infection in Humans and Animals*, pp. 63–82. Salamanca, Spain: University of Salamanca.

Coulibaly, Y.I., Dembele, B., Diallo, A.A., et al. (2009). A randomized trial of doxycycline for Mansonella perstans infection. *N. Eng. J. Med.*, 361: 1448–48.

Denham, D.A. (1975). The diagnosis of filariasis. *Ann. Soc. Belge Med. Trop.*, 55: 517–24.

Dissanaike, A.S., Bandara, C.D., Padmini, H.H., and Ihalamulla, R.L., Naotunne, T.S. (2000). Recovery of a species of *Brugia*, probably *B. ceylonensis*, from the conjunctiva of a patient in Sri Lanka. *Ann. Trop. Med. Parasitol.*, 94: 83–86.

Dreyer, G., Addiss, D., Williamson, J., Norões, J. (2006). Efficacy of co-administered diethylcarbamazine and albendazole against adult *Wuchereria bancrofti*. *Trans. R. Soc. Trop. Med. Hyg.*, 100: 1118–25.

Dukes, D.C., Gelfand, M., Gadd, K.G., Clarke, V.D., and Goldsmid, J.M. (1968). Cerebral filariasis caused by *Acanthocheilonema perstans*. *Cent. Afr. J. Med.*, 14: 21–27.

Eberhard, M.L. (2006). Zoonotic filariasis. In: R.L. Guerrant, D.H. Walker, and P.F. Weller, (ed.) *Tropical Infectious Diseases, Principles, Pathogens, and Practice, (2nd edn.)*, pp. 1189–1203. Philadelphia: Elsevier.

Eberhard, M.L., DeMeester, L.J., Martin, B.W., and Lammie, P.J. (1993). *Zoonotic Brugia infection in western Michigan*. *Am. J. Surg. Pathol.*, 17: 1058–61.

Eberhard, M.L. and Orihel, T.C. (1984). *Loaina gen. n.* (Filarioidea: Onchocercidae) for the filariae parasitic in rabbits in *North America*. *Proc. Helminthol. Soc. Wash.*, 51: 49–53.

Elenitoba-Johnson, K.S., Eberhard, M.L., et al. (1996). Zoonotic Brugian lymphadenitis. An unusual case with florid monocytoid B-cell proliferation. *Am. J. Clin. Pathol.*, 105: 384–87.

Faust, E.C., Agosin, M., Garcia-Laverde, A., et al. (1952). Unusual findings of filarial infections in man. *Am. J. Trop. Med. Hyg.*, 1: 239–49.

Gabrielides (1938). Filaire dans le chambre anterieurede l'oeil. *Ann. Oculist (Paris)*, 175: 581.

Genchi, C., Rinaldi, L., Mortarino, M., Genchi, M., and Cringoli, G. (2009). Climate and Dirofilaria infection in Europe. *Vet. Parasitol.*, 163: 286–92.

Glickman, L.T., Grieve, R.B., Schantz, P.M. (1986). Serologic diagnosis of zoonotic pulmonary dirofilariasis. *Am. J. Med.*, 80: 161–64.

Grandi, G., Morchon, R., Kramer, L., Kartashev, V., and Simon, F. (2008). Wolbachia in Dirofilaria repens, an agent causing human subcutaneous dirofilariasis. *J. Parasitol.*, 94: 1421–23.

Gutierrez, Y. (1990). *Diagnostic pathology of parasitic infections with clinical correlations*, Philadelphia, Pa.: Lea & Febiger.

Hira, P.R., Al-Buloushi, A., Khalid, N., et al. (2008). Zoonotic filariasis in the Arabian Peninsula: autochthonous onchocerciasis and dirofilariasis. *Am. J. Trop. Med. Hyg.*, 79: 739–41.

Huynh, T., Thean, J., and Maini, R. (2001). *Dipetalonema reconditum* in the human eye. *Br. J. Ophthalmol.*, 85: 1391–92.

Ishii, Y., Choochote, W., Bain, O., et al. (2008). Seasonal and diurnal biting activities and zoonotic filarial infections of two *Simulium* species (Diptera: Simuliidae) in northern Thailand. *Parasite*, 15: 121–29.

Kaplan, J.E., Masur, H., and Holmes, K.K. (2002). Guidelines for preventing opportunistic infections among HIV-infected persons—2002. Recommendations of the U.S. Public Health Service and the Infectious Diseases Society of America. *MMWR Recom. Rep.*, 51: 152.

Koehsler, M., Soleiman, A., Aspöck, H., et al. (2007). Onchocerca jakutensis filariasis in humans. *Emerg. Infect. Dis.*, 13: 1749–52.

Kokta, V. (2008). Zoonotic deep cutaneous filariasis—three pediatric cases from Québec, Canada. *Pediatr. Dermatol.*, 25: 230–32.

Kotani, T., Powers, K.G. (1982). Developmental stages of *Dirofilaria immitis* in the dog. *Am. J. Vet. Res.*, 43: 2199–2206.

Kotton, C.N. (2007). Zoonoses in solid-organ and hematopoietic stem cell transplant recipients. *Clin. Infect. Dis.*, 44: 857–66.

Kramer, L.H., Kartashev, V.V., Grandi, G., et al. (2007). Human subcutaneous dirofilariasis, Russia. *Emerg. Infect. Dis.*, 13: 150–52.

Lakshmi, V., Kumar, R., and Gupta, P. (2004). The antifilarial activity of a marine red alga, *Botryocladia leptopoda*, against experimental infections with animal and human filariae. *Parasitol Res.*, 93: 468–74.

Lee, S.E., Kim, H.C., Chong, S.T., et al. (2007). Molecular survey of Dirofilaria immitis and Dirofilaria repens by direct PCR for wild caught mosquitoes in the Republic of Korea. *Vet. Parasitol.*, 148: 149–45.

Mar, P.H., Yang, I.C., Chang, G.N., and Fei, A.C. (2002). Specific polymerase chain reaction for differential diagnosis of Dirofilaria immitis and Dipetalonema reconditum using primers derived from internal transcribed spacer region 2 (ITS2). *Vet. Parasitol.*, 106: 243–52.

McCall, J.W., Genchi, C., Kramer, L.H., et al. (2008). Heartworm disease in animals and humans. *Adv. Parasitol.*, 66: 193–285.

Misra, N., Sharma, M., Raj, K., *et al.* (2007). Chemical constituents and antifilarial activity of *Lantana camara* against human lymphatic filariid *Brugia malayi* and rodent filariid *Acanthocheilonema viteae* maintained in rodent hosts. *Parasit. Res.*, **100**: 439–48.

Miyoshi, T., Tsubouchi, H., Iwasaki, A., *et al.* (2006). Human pulmonary dirofilariasis: A case report and review of the recent Japanese literature. *Respirology*, **11**: 343–47.

Morchón, R., López-Belmonte, J., *et al.* (2006). High levels of serum thromboxane B2 are generated during human pulmonary dirofilariosis. *Clin. Vacc. Immunol.*, **13**: 1175–76.

Muro, A., Genchi, C., Cordero, M., and Simón, F. (1999). Human dirofilariasis in the European Union. *Parasitol. Today*, **15**: 386–89.

Nath, R., Gogoi, R., Bordoloi, N., and Gogoi, T. (2010). Ocular dirofilariasis. *Indian J. Pathol. Microbiol.*, **53**: 157–59.

Orihel, T.C. (1973). Cerebral filariasis in Rhodesia - a zoonotic infection? *Am. J. Trop. Med. Hyg.*, **22**: 596–99.

Orihel, T.C., and Ash, L.R. (1995). Parasites in human tissues. American Society of Clinical Pathologists, Chicago, Ill.

Orihel, T.C. and Beaver, P.C. (1965). Morphology and relationship of *Dirofilaria tenuis* and *Dirofilaria conjunctivae*. *Am. J. Trop. Med. Hyg.*, **14**: 1030–43.

Orihel, T.C. and Beaver, P.C. (1989). Zoonotic *Brugia* infections in North and South America. *Am. J. Trop. Med. Hyg.*, **40**: 638–47.

Orihel, T.C. and Eberhard, M.L. (1998). Zoonotic filariasis. *Clin. Microbiol. Rev.*, **11**: 366–81.

Orihel, T.C. and Esslinger, J.H. (1973). *Meningonema peruzzii* gen. et sp. n. (Nematoda: Filarioidea) from the central nervous system of African monkeys. *J. Parasit.*, **59**: 437–41.

Pampiglione, S. (1995). Human sub-conjunctival dirofilariasis: a probable case seen in France by Amatus Lusitanus in the 16th century. *Parassitologia*, **37**: 75–78.

Pampiglione, S., Canestri Trotti, G., and Rivasi, F. (1995). Human dirofilariasis due to *Dirofilaria (Nochtiella) repens*: a review of world literature. *Parassitologia*, **37**: 149–93.

Pampiglione, S., Rivasi, F., and Gustinelli, A. (2009). Dirofilarial human cases in the Old World, attributed to Dirofilaria immitis: a critical analysis. *Histopathology*, **54**: 192–204.

Panaitescu, D., Preda, A., Bain, O., and Vasile-Bugarin, A.C. (1999). Four cases of human filariosis due to *Setaria labiatopapillosa* found in Bucharest, Romania. *Roum Arch. Microbiol. Immunol.*, **58**: 203–07.

Poppert, S., Hodapp, M., Krueger, A., *et al.* (2009). Dirofilaria repens infection and concomitant meningoencephalitis. *Emerg. Infect. Dis.*, **15**: 1844–46.

Rosenblatt, J.E. (2009). Laboratory diagnosis of infections due to blood and tissue parasites. *Clin. Infect. Dis.*, **49**: 1103–8.

Sallo, F., Eberhard, M.L., Fok, E., *et al.* (2005). Zoonotic intravitreal Onchocerca in Hungary. *Ophthalmology*, **112**: 502–4.

Simón, F., Lopez-Belmonte, J., *et al.* (2005). What is happening outside North America regarding human dirofilariasis? *Vet. Parasitol.*, **133**: 181–89.

Simón, F., Morchón, R., González-Miguel, J., *et al.* (2009). What is new about animal and human dirofilariosis? *Trends Parasitol.*, **25**: 404–9.

Simonsen, P.E., Onapa, A.W., and Asio, S.M. (2010). *Mansonella perstans filariasis in Africa. Acta Trop.* 2010 Feb 10 [Epub ahead of print].

Scoles, G.A., and Kambhampati, S. (1995). Polymerase chain reaction-based method for the detection of canine heartworm (Filarioidea: Onchocercidae) in mosquitoes (Diptera: Culicidae) and vertebrate hosts. *J. Med. Entomol.*, **32**: 864–69.

Song, K.H., Tanaka, S., and Hayasaki, M. (2009). Scanning Electron Microscopic Observation of Ultrastructure of Dirofilaria immitis Microfilaria. *J. Vet. Med. Sci.*, **71**: 779–83.

Sréter, T., Széll, Z., Egyed, Z., and Varga, I. (2002). Subconjunctival zoonotic onchocerciasis in man: aberrant infection with *Onchocerca lupi*? *Ann. Trop. Med. Parasitol.*, **96**: 497–502.

Szénási, Z., Kovács, A.H., and Pampiglione, S., *et al.* (2008). Human dirofilariosis in Hungary: an emerging zoonosis in central Europe. *Wien. Klin. Wochenschr.*, **120**: 96–102.

Taylor, M.J., Makunde, W.H., *et al.* (2005). Macrofilaricidal activity after doxycycline treatment of *Wuchereria bancrofti*: A double-blind, randomised placebo-controlled trial. *Lancet*, **365**: 2116–21.

Theis, J.H. (2005). Public health aspects of dirofilariasis in the United States. *Vet. Parasitol.*, **133**: 157–80.

Trevejo, R.T., Barr, M.C., Robinson, R.A. (2005). Important emerging bacterial zoonotic infections affecting the immunocompromised. *Vet. Res.*, **36**: 493–506.

Van Duyse (1895). Filaire dans la chambre anterieure. *Arch. Ophthalmol.*, **15**: 701–6.

Vezzani, D., Eiras, D.F., Wisnivesky, C. (2006). Dirofilariasis in Argentina: Historical review and first report of *Dirofilaria immitis* in a natural mosquito population. *Vet. Parasitol.*, **136**: 259–73.

Watts, K.J., Courteny, C.H., and Reddy, G.R. (1999). Development of a PCR- and probe-based test for the sensitive and specific detection of the dog heartworm, *Dirofilaria immitis*, in its mosquito intermediate host. *Mol. Cell. Probes.*, **13**: 425–30.

Wisely, S.M., Howard, J., and Williams, S.A., *et al.* (2008). An unidentified filarial species and its impact on fitness in wild populations of the black-footed ferret (*Mustela nigripes*). *J.Wildl. Dis.*, **44**: 53–64.

Zahner, H., and Schares, G. (1993). Experimental chemotherapy of filariasis: comparative evaluation of the efficacy of filaricidal compounds in *Mastomys coucha* infected with *Litomosoides carinii*, *Acanthocheilonema viteae*, *Brugia malayi* and *B. Pahangi*. *Acta Trop.*, **52**: 221–66.

CHAPTER 61

Trichinellosis

Edoardo Pozio

Summary

Trichinellosis is caused by nematodes of the genus *Trichinella*. These zoonotic parasites show a cosmopolitan distribution in all the continents, but Antarctica. They circulate in nature by synanthropic-domestic and sylvatic cycles. Today, eight species and four genotypes are recognized, all of which infect mammals, including humans, one species also infects birds, and two other species infect also reptiles.

Parasites of the genus *Trichinella* are unusual among the other nematodes in that the worm undergoes a complete developmental cycle, from larva to adult to larva, in the body of a single host, which has a profound influence on the epidemiology of trichinellosis. When the cycle is complete, the muscles of the infected animal contain a reservoir of larvae, capable of long-term survival. Humans and other hosts become infected by ingesting muscle tissues containing viable larvae.

The symptoms associated with trichinellosis vary with the severity of infection, i.e. the number of viable larvae ingested, and the time after infection. The capacity of the worm population to undergo massive multiplication in the body is a major determinant. Progression of disease follows the biological development of the parasite. Symptoms are associated first with the gastrointestinal tract, as the worms invade and establish in the small intestine, become more general as the body responds immunologically, and finally focus on the muscles as the larvae penetrate the muscle cells and develop there. Although *Trichinella* worms cause pathological changes directly by mechanical damage, most of the clinical features of trichinellosis are immunopathological in origin and can be related to the capacity of the parasite to induce allergic responses.

The main source of human infection is raw or under-cooked meat products from pig, wild boar, bear, walrus, and horses, but meat products from other animals have been implicated. In humans, the diagnosis of infection is made by immunological tests or by direct examination of muscle biopsies using microscopy or by recovery of larvae after artificial digestion. Treatment requires both the use of anthelmintic drugs to kill the parasite itself and symptomatic treatment to minimize inflammatory responses.

Both pre-slaughter prevention and post-slaughter control can be used to prevent *Trichinella* infections in animals. The first involves pig management control as well as continuous surveillance programmes. Meat inspection is a successful post-slaughter strategy. However, a continuous consumer education is of great importance in countries where meat inspection is not mandatory.

History

The unravelling of the nature of trichinellosis may reach back to antiquity as suggested by historical references to diseases that bear striking similarities to clinical aspects of *Trichinella* infection. The earliest such case involved a young Egyptian living along the Nile about 1200 B.C. (Gould 1970; Campbell 1983*a*). There is evidence of human infections even in prehistoric cultures (Owen *et al.* 2005). The modern history of trichinellosis, however, begins in 1835, with the discovery by microscopy of the larval stage of the parasite by James Paget and Richard Owen in London. It was Owen who coined its first name, *Trichina spiralis* (Owen 1835). The parasite was first found in animals by Leidy (1846), who identified larval cysts in muscles from a pig and realized that they were identical to those described in humans. Evidence that infection was acquired by ingestion of live larvae from infected muscles was obtained in the 1850s by feeding experiments using dogs and other animals (Virchow 1859). The first account of transmission to humans from infected pig meat, and association with a defined set of symptoms, was published by Zenker (1860) who made a detailed study of a patient who had been clinically diagnosed as having typhoid. Postmortem examination of muscle tissue, however, confirmed the presence of a heavy infection of *Trichinella*, and the symptoms recorded before death (fatigue, fever, oedema, muscle and joint pain) are now recognized as characteristic of trichinellosis and largely immunopathological in origin. The patient had eaten infected ham and sausages shortly before the onset of her symptoms, and similar symptoms also occurred in other members of the household who had eaten these items. Zenker's association of a defined pathogen with a defined disease was a milestone in medical microbiology, though it rarely receives the recognition it deserves, being overshadowed by later discoveries in bacteriology.

The agent

Taxonomy

For 150 years after its first scientific description, *Trichinella spiralis* was considered the sole member of the genus, having a phenomenally wide host range (Campbell 1983*b*). However, beginning in the 1950s and 1960s, scientists began reporting an increasing number of host-specific behaviours among different geographic isolates (Rausch *et al.* 1956; Nelson *et al.* 1966). These studies, conducted over the next 30 years, yielded a remarkable series of new findings on the genetic diversity within the genus resulting in a new *Trichinella* taxonomy encompassing eight species (Table 61.1), along with a more complete zoogeographical and epidemiological knowledge base (Pozio *et al.* 1992; Pozio and Zarlenga 2005; www.iss.it/site/Trichinella/index.asp).

The genus *Trichinella* comprises a monophyletic lineage in the family Trichinellidae, the putative sister to the Trichuridae (Capillariinae, Trichurinae and Trichosomoidinae). The superfamily Trichinelloidea to which *Trichinella* belongs is phylogenetically diagnosed by the stichosome, a region of the glandular oesophagus, and the bacillary bands, an assembly of structural characters unknown among the other nematodes. Today, two main clades are recognized in the genus *Trichinella*; one that encompasses species that encapsulate in host muscle tissue, and a second that does not encapsulate after muscle cell dedifferentiation (Pozio and Murrell 2006).

The encapsulated clade

Five species and four genotypes of undetermined taxonomic status infecting only mammals belong to this clade (Table 61.1).

Trichinella spiralis sensu stricto (Owen 1835) is the first species discovered and the most characterized because of its importance both as a cause of human disease and as a model for basic biological research investigations, due in large part to its relatively high frequency in both domestic and sylvatic animals and to its high infectivity for laboratory animals. Dissemination of the parasite

and its hosts was especially facilitated by the European colonization of North, Central and South America, New Zealand, Hawaii, and Egypt from the sixteenth to twentieth centuries. In many regions of the world this species has been transmitted to wildlife hosts through exposure to garbage dumps or foraging near human settlements, where pork scraps and offal from slaughtered animals were scattered in the environment (Pozio and Murrell 2006). At the world level, most of human infections are due to this species.

Trichinella nativa (Britov and Boev 1972) is usually named as the arctic or freeze resistant species and is widespread among wild carnivores of the arctic and subarctic areas of America, Europe and Asia. The main biological features of *T. nativa* are a very low infectivity to swine and a high resistance to freezing in muscles of carnivores (Pozio and Zarlenga 2005). Human populations living in frigid zones acquire *T. nativa* infection by eating raw meat from walruses, bears and other game animals. The genotype, *Trichinella* T6, phylogenetically related to *T. nativa*, is widespread in carnivores of Canada and Alaska, and along the Rocky Mountains and Appalachians in the USA. Sporadic infections in humans have been documented for the consumption of game meat.

Trichinella britovi (Pozio *et al.* 1992), is a Palearctic and African species. European and Asian isolates of this species were previously named *T. nelsoni* by Russian scientists (Pozio *et al.* 1992). Among sylvatic species, *T. britovi* has the widest geographical range, occurring in wild carnivores and wild boars of the temperate areas of Europe and Asia, and extending southward to northern and western Africa (Pozio *et al.* 2005a). This parasite can reach domestic pigs from extensive grazing systems or feed with scraps from sylvatic carnivores (Pozio and Zarlenga 2005). A percentage of human infections occurring in Europe, Asia, North and

Table 61.1 Main features of *Trichinella* species and genotypes recognized so far

Clade Species or genotype Encapsulated	Geographical distribution	Host range	Main source of infection for humans	Resistance of larvae in frozen muscles
T. spiralis	cosmopolitan	domestic and sylvatic mammals	domestic and sylvatic swine, horse	no
T. nativa	Arctic and subarctic areas of the Nearctic and Palearctic regions	sylvatic carnivores	bear, walrus	yes in carnivore muscles
Trichinella T6	Canada; Alaska, Rocky Mountains and Appalachian in the USA	sylvatic carnivores	carnivores	yes in carnivore muscles
T. britovi	Temperate areas of the Palearctic region, Northern and Western Africa	sylvatic mammals, seldom domestic pigs	wild boar, domestic pig	yes in carnivore muscles
Trichinella T8	South Africa and Namibia	sylvatic carnivores	non documented	no
T. murrelli	USA and Southern Canada	sylvatic carnivores	bear, horse	no
Trichinella T9	Japan	sylvatic carnivores	non documented	no
T. nelsoni	Eastern Southern Africa	sylvatic mammals	warthog, bush pig	no
Trichinella T12	Argentina	sylvatic carnivores	cougar	yes in carnivore muscles
Non-encapsulated				
T. pseudospiralis	cosmopolitan	sylvatic mammals and birds, domestic pigs	domestic and wild pigs	no
T. papuae	Papua New Guinea, Thailand	wild pig, saltwater crocodile	wild pig	no
T. zimbabwensis	Zimbabwe, Mozambique, Ethiopia, South Africa	Nile crocodile, monitor lizard lion	non documented	no

West Africa are caused by this species. The genotype *Trichinella* T8, very similar to *T. britovi*, has been identified in wild animals of South Africa and Namibia. No human case due to this genotype has been documented.

Trichinella murrelli (Pozio and La Rosa 2000), is spread among sylvatic carnivores across the USA and in some southern regions of Canada. This species does not develop in swine. It is the causative agent of infection in humans especially from consumption of meat from black bears. A great deal of clinical information on this species was gained from a 1985 outbreak in France due to the consumption of horse meat imported from USA (Ancelle 1998). *Trichinella* isolates from Japanese wildlife, originally identified as *T. britovi*, are now designated as a separate genotype, named *Trichinella* T9, which is phylogenetically related to *T. murrelli* (Pozio and Zarlenga 2005; Zarlenga *et al.* 2006).

Trichinella nelsoni (Britov and Boev 1972), *sensu stricto* (Pozio *et al.* 1992), has been detected in eastern Africa, from Kenya to South Africa. The host range includes sylvatic carnivores and, at least occasionally, bush pigs and warthogs, some of which have been the source of infection for humans. Less than 100 human infections have been documented for this species in Kenya and Tanzania (Pozio 2007).

Trichinella T12 is a new encapsulated species of *Trichinella*, recently detected in mountain lions (*Puma concolor*) from Patagonia, Río Negro, Argentina. The available information is the molecular structure of two non-coding and one coding sequences that are different from those of the eleven currently recognized species/genotypes of the genus *Trichinella* (Pozio *et al.* 2009).

The non-encapsulated clade

One species infecting mammals and birds, and two species infecting mammals and reptiles, compose this clade (Table 61.1). The main biological features of these parasites in comparison to those of the previous clade are the lack of a collagen capsule and their infectivity to other vertebrates in addition to mammals.

Trichinella pseudospiralis (Garkavi 1972) is a cosmopolitan species infecting both mammals and birds. Three populations, which can be distinguished on a molecular basis, have been detected in the Palaearctic, Nearctic, and Australian (Tasmania) regions (La Rosa *et al.* 2001). This parasite has been found in 14 mammalian species including domestic and sylvatic swine, and 13 avian species (Pozio 2005), where the number of reports in mammals is much higher than that in birds. Infections in humans, with some deaths, have been documented in Kamchatka, Thailand, and France (Pozio and Murrell 2006).

Trichinella papuae (Pozio *et al.* 1999), circulates in both mammals and reptiles (domestic sows, wild pigs, and farmed saltwater crocodiles) of Papua New Guinea and Thailand (Pozio *et al.* 2005b; Pozio 2007). Infections in humans have been documented (Owen *et al.* 2005; Kusolsuk *et al.* 2010).

Trichinella zimbabwensis (Pozio *et al.* 2002), very similar to *T. papuae*, has been detected in wild and farmed reptiles of Africa (Zimbabwe, Mozambique, South Africa, and Ethiopia), in experimentally infected mammals (Pozio and Murrell 2006) and in a lion. Human infections have yet to be reported.

Phylogeny

The phylogeny of species and genotypes of the genus *Trichinella* shows that the extant species of *Trichinella* diversified within the last 10 to 20 million years, which coincided with the divergence of Suidae from the Tayassuidae in the Lower Miocene in Eastern Asia. *Trichinella spiralis* appears to be the oldest of the encapsulated clade (Zarlenga *et al.* 2006; Pozio *et al.* 2009). The switch of non-encapsulated species to birds or reptiles occurred more recently. The introduction of *T. nelsoni*, *Trichinella* T8, and *T. britovi* into Africa is the result of three independent expansion events from Eurasia following the land connections that formed during upper Miocene and into the Pleistocene (Pozio *et al.* 2005a). According to Zarlenga *et al.* (2006), ursids, canids and felids are principally responsible for the radiation of Holarctic species throughout Europe and into North America through Beringia.

Biology

A peculiarity of the cycle of nematodes of the genus *Trichinella* is the development of two generations in the same host (Fig. 61.1). Larvae are released from the cysts by digestion in the stomach and pass into the small intestine, where they penetrate rapidly into the epithelial cells of the mucosa, occupying an intracellular niche. At this stage the larvae are about 1 mm long occupying some 40–50 enterocytes. Subsequent development is extremely rapid; the parasite undergoes four moults in about 30 hours to reach the immature adult stage and increases in length 2–3 times. As with all nematodes, the sexes are separate, and the female is the larger, reaching 3 mm in length.

Males and females mate in the small intestine, the eggs of the female are fertilized, develop rapidly in the uterus, and the female then begins lo release newborn larvae (NBL, the first larval stage) directly into the mucosa. Release continues for several days or possibly weeks, and is eventually terminated by the onset of immunity or by senility of the worm. The number of NBL produced during the lifetime of each female is dependent on many factors, and differs between the various species (100–1,500 per female). The severity of trichinellosis as a disease results largely from this capacity of the worm population to undergo massive multiplication in the body of the host.

After release from the female, NBL migrate into mucosal lymphatics, pass through the draining lymph nodes, enter blood vessels, and are carried around the body. Although they can complete their development only in striated skeletal muscles, larvae may attempt to penetrate other tissues, including the brain, heart, and kidneys. After penetration into striated muscle fibres the NBL lies free in the cytoplasm and induces a complex series of changes which result in the host cell becoming transformed into a quite different structure, the nurse cell that serves to ensure the growth, development, and survival of the parasite. With time the nurse cell becomes surrounded by a capsule of collagen and a network of capillaries to form the characteristic cyst. After 3–4 weeks the larva has grown considerably (from 100 μm to 1 mm), is resistant to digestion, and is capable of infecting another host to initiate a new infection cycle. Larvae can remain infective for very long periods (up to 20 years in bears and up to 40 years in humans); however, in some hosts with time, the cysts become calcified and the larvae die.

The 'free-living' stage

An important adaptation of the parasite, which facilitates its transmission, is the physiological mechanism utilized by muscle larvae

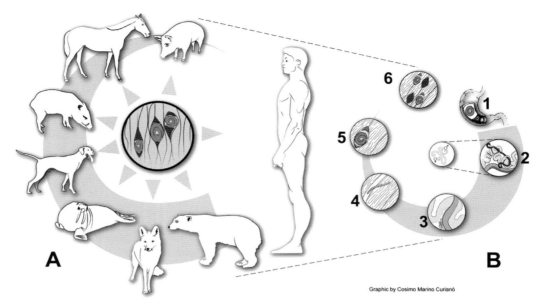

Fig. 61.1 *Trichinella* sp. life cycle. (A) Main sources of *Trichinella* spp. infections for humans; (B) *Trichinella* spp. cycle in the host body. Enteric phase: 1. muscle tissues are digested in the stomach and larvae are released; 2. larvae penetrate the intestinal mucosa of the small intestine, reach the adult stage within 48 h post infection, male and female mate; 3. female worm releases newborn larvae in the lymphatic vessels (from the fifth day post infection onwards; the length of newborn production, from one to several weeks, is under the influence of the host immunity). Parenteral phase: 4. the newborn larva reach the striated muscle and actively penetrate in the muscle cell; 5. the larva grows to the infective stage in the nurse cell (the former muscle cell); and 6. after a period of time (weeks, months or years) a calcification process occurs. Reproduced from www.iss.it/site/Trichinella/index.asp, with permission.

Graphic by Cosimo Marino Curianò

to promote their survival in decaying carcasses. The greater the persistence of larval viability, the higher the probability to induce infection when ingested by a scavenging host. In spite of the larva-induced angiogenic process that develops around the nurse cell after larval penetration of the muscle cell, larval metabolism is basically anaerobic (Despommier 1990), which favours its survival in decaying tissues. The persistence of larvae in putrefying flesh is, of course, also determined by the environment: high humidity and low temperatures favour survival of encapsulated larvae even when the muscle tissue is completely liquefied. This condition has been proposed as the environment of the 'free-living' stage, resembling the egg stage of most of other nematode species. The importance of this stage in the natural cycle of the parasite is underscored by the survival of muscle larvae in frozen muscles of carrion for one (*T. britovi*) or more years (*T. nativa* and *Trichinella* T6) (Pozio and Murrell 2006). It is important to stress that the survival of muscle larvae to freezing occurs mainly when these larvae parasitize striated muscles of carnivores, whereas the survival time to freezing is strongly reduced to a few days or weeks when muscle larvae of the same strain parasitize other mammalian hosts such as swine or rodents.

Epidemiology

Although *T. spiralis* was first discovered in domestic animals, the other species of this genus are primarily parasites of wildlife. When humans fail in the proper management of domestic animals and wildlife, *Trichinella* species are transmitted from the sylvatic environment to the domestic one, sometimes through synanthropic animals. In addition, they can transfer in a reversible path from domestic animals to wildlife.

The sylvatic cycle

The sylvatic cycle occurs in all continents with the exception of Antarctica, where there is neither a record of this nematode nor evidence of any searches for it in marine mammals and birds. *Trichinella* infections in wildlife have been documented in 66 (33.3%) countries of the world (Pozio 2007). These parasites have been reported in more than 100 species of mammals belonging to 11 orders, i.e. Marsupialia, Insectivora, Edentata, Primates, Lagomorpha, Rodentia, Cetacea, Carnivora, Perissodactyla, Artiodactyla, and Tylopoda (Pozio 2005). The transmission cycles of the different sylvatic species and genotypes are closely related to their host species ecologies. Among primates, only humans have been naturally infected with *Trichinella*. In spite of the potential broad host spectrum of *Trichinella* spp., the greatest biomass of these parasites occurs amongst the Carnivora and the artiodactylid family Suidae. The role of small mammals (mainly rodents and insectivores) in the sylvatic cycle is still uncertain due to the low number of infections in their populations and the lack of sufficient surveys on a large number of these mammals (Pozio and Zarlenga 2005). *Trichinella nativa* is commonly found in polar bears, and increasingly in walruses where it presents a significant zoonotic hazard. This has resulted in the implementation of food safety programmes in some arctic communities to test harvested walrus meat for *Trichinella* larvae prior to consumption (Proulx *et al.* 2002). *Trichinella* sp. has been reported very rarely in seals from the Arctic.

Seven species of birds are documented as hosts for *T. pseudospiralis*, and six other species suspected, but unconfirmed (Pozio 2005). Only three species of reptiles have been detected naturally infected in Africa (Nile crocodile and Nile monitor lizard) and in Papua New Guinea (saltwater crocodile). In addition, meat from a clouded monitor and a turtle has been implicated as the sources of infection of human trichinellosis outbreaks, which occurred in Thailand (Kambounruang 1991). A soft-shelled turtle has been implicated as a source of trichinellosis in Taiwan (Lo *et al.* 2009). There is a single report of an experimental infection of amphibians (frogs and axolotls) with *T. spiralis*, in which it was observed that the development of larvae in the muscles was incomplete. Attempts to infect fish with *T. spiralis*, *T. britovi*, *T. pseudospiralis*, *T. papuae* and *T. zimbabwensis* have also failed (Pozio and La Rosa 2005). The role of invertebrates as paratenic hosts of *Trichinella* species has been investigated in adult and larval stages of several insects and amphipods. The survival of *Trichinella* larvae in these paratenic hosts is under the influence of the environmental temperature, lower the temperature, longer the survival. The sylvatic cycle may be influenced by human actions such as the common habit of hunters of leaving animal carcasses in the field after skinning, or removing and discarding the entrails, which increases the probability of transmission to new hosts (Pozio *et al.* 2001).

The domestic cycle

This cycle has been documented in 43 (21.9%) countries of the world and it occurs where there are high risks farming practices such as the feeding of food waste containing pork scraps, or exposure to carcasses of dead swine, or wildlife (Gamble *et al.* 2000; Pozio and Murrell 2006; Pozio 2007). These risks are usually encountered in:

1. Pigs allowed to scavenge on garbage dumps,

2. Pigs feeding of wild game carcasses or scraps from hunting,

3. Horses fed with pork scraps or with carcasses of fur animals,

4. Sled dogs fed with carcasses of other dogs or of game in the arctic and fur animals fed with carcasses of slaughtered fur animals at the farm,

5. Farmed crocodiles fed with meat of slaughtered crocodiles.

The most common etiological agent of the domestic cycle is *T. spiralis*, which is well adapted to swine and synanthropic hosts, in which it exhibits a very high reproductive rate without inducing serious pathology. Occasionally, *T. britovi* and *T. pseudospiralis* have been transmitted in the domestic cycle, when humans feed pigs with game meat scraps or 'pasture' pigs in refuse dumps containing carcasses of sylvatic animals. Also *T. papuae* and *T. zimbabwensis* are transmitted among farmed crocodiles fed with scarps from slaughtered crocodiles (Pozio and Murrell 2006).

In the domestic habitat, the brown rat (*Rattus norvegicus*) is frequently found to be infected with *T. spiralis* and infrequently with *T. britovi* or *T. pseudospiralis* (Pozio and Zarlenga 2005). In the nineteenth century, Leuckart proposed a 'Rat Theory', which implicated rats as a major reservoir of *T. spiralis* for domestic pigs. In 1871, Zenker suggested that the infection in rats was merely an indicator of *Trichinella* exposure risk in the area and that the real source of infection for both pigs and rats was meat scraps and offal of infected pig carcasses. This is consistent with findings that the occurrence of *T. spiralis* in domestic pigs greatly decreased when feeding with uncooked garbage and offal was terminated (Pozio and Zarlenga 2005).

Trichinella sp. infections in horses

Between 1975 and 2005, human outbreaks of trichinellosis have occurred in France (2,296 infected people in eight outbreaks) and Italy (1,038 infected people in seven outbreaks), from the consumption of meat from horses imported from Canada, the Former Yugoslavia, Mexico, Poland, and the USA (Pozio and Zarlenga 2005). In addition infections in 21 horses, bred in the Former Yugoslavia, Mexico, Poland and Romania, have been detected at the slaughterhouses (Pozio and Zarlenga 2005). Worldwide, only 35 infections (horses that were the source of infection for human outbreaks and positive horses detected at the slaughterhouse) have been documented in horses since 1975, with a prevalence of infection of about one infected horse per 250 thousand slaughtered horses (Pozio 2001a; Murrell *et al.* 2004). Horse-meat outbreaks have important consequences for public health because of the high number of infected persons resulting from consumption of meat from a single horse. This has a high impact in terms of medical costs, horse-meat market economics, which collapses after each outbreak, and in legal and administrative terms related to the implementation of control measures at the national and international level (Ancelle 1998).

Trichinella infection in humans

Trichinellosis is the proper term for the human zoonotic disease also known as trichinosis or trichiniasis. Of 198 countries present in the world, 40 (20%) are small islands or city-states, where *Trichinella* sp. infections cannot develop for the lack of potential reservoirs. According to published data, clinical trichinellosis has been documented in people of 55 countries (27.8%) (Pozio 2007). On the basis of reports from these 55 countries, the yearly incidence of clinical trichinellosis has been estimated to 10,000 cases with 0.2% of deaths but the real figure of infections and contacts between these parasites and the human beings is rather unknown.

Trichinella infections in humans are more related to cultural food practices which include dishes based on raw or undercooked meat of different animal origins than to the presence of the parasite in the domestic and wild animals of the country. In France and in Italy, most of trichinellosis cases are due to the consumption of raw horse meat, because this food habit is strongly related to the French culture imported also in Italy (Boireau *et al.* 2000; Pozio 2001a).

In Finland, where there is a high prevalence of infection in animals, no infection leading to disease has been documented in humans, due to the practice of eating only well cooked meat (Pozio 2007). In Romania, the highest prevalence of trichinellosis in humans occurs in the Transylvanian region which was colonized by German people who have kept their food habits which are known to be risk factors for trichinellosis (Blaga *et al.* 2007). In Israel, Lebanon, and Syria, human outbreaks of trichinellosis have been documented following consumption of pork from wild boars only among the Christian populations or immigrants from Thailand (Pozio 2007). In Algeria and Senegal, where the majority of the human population is Muslim, trichinellosis has only been documented in expatriates from France and very seldom in the population (Gretillat and Vassiliades 1967; Nezri *et al.* 2006; Pozio 2007).

In most African countries south of the Sahara, human infection is seldomly documented in spite of the presence of *Trichinella*-infected wildlife, because about a third of all African populations are of the Bantu ethnic group, which rarely consumes meat and when they consume meat it is well cooked (Pozio 2007). In Indonesia, where most people are Muslims and do not eat pork, the island of Bali is one of the few areas of the country where the majority of people are Hindu and foreign tourists visiting this island acquired the infection (de Carneri and Di Matteo 1989). In South America, trichinellosis has been documented only in Argentina and Chile where a high percentage of the population consumes raw pork and pork products (Schenone *et al.* 2002; Ribicich *et al.* 2005).

Overall, the most important source of *Trichinella* infection for humans remains pork and its related products from domestic pigs. Important foci of human trichinellosis from pork occur in Central (Mexico) and South America (Argentina and Chile) (Ortega Pierres *et al.* 2000; Ribicich *et al.* 2005), in Asia (China, Laos, Myanmar, Thailand) (Takahashi *et al.* 2000; Pozio 2001*b*; Liu and Boireau 2002; Wang *et al.* 2006; 2007; Barennes *et al.* 2008) and Europe (Bosnia-Herzegovina, Bulgaria, Byelorussia, Croatia, Georgia, Latvia, Lithuania, Poland, Romania, Russia, Serbia, and Ukraine) (Pozio and Murrell 2006; Pozio 2007). The migration of persons from eastern to western countries of Europe, has resulted in several human outbreaks of trichinellosis in Denmark, Germany, Italy, Spain and the UK (Pozio and Marucci 2003; Gallardo *et al.* 2007; Stensvold *et al.* 2007). The increasing number of international travelers has resulted in many reports of tourists who acquired *Trichinella* infections for the consumption of pork from warthogs in Africa, of bear meat in Canada and Greenland, of pork from domestic pigs in China, Egypt, Indonesia (Bali Island), Laos and Malaysia, and wild boar meat in Turkey and Algeria (Pozio and Murrell 2006).

Pathology

The parasitic cycle can be divided into two phases: an intestinal (or enteric) phase and a muscular (or parenteral or systemic) phase, which can co-exist for a period lasting from a few days to weeks (Fig. 61.1). This cycle occurs in all mammals, including humans, in birds, and in reptiles. The larval penetration of the intestinal mucosa causes modifications in the brush border of villi, the lamina propria, and the smooth muscles of the jejunum. The migration of newborn larvae in the different organs provokes an immediate reaction, which causes immunological, pathological, and metabolic disturbances and the various clinical phenomena observed during the acute stage of the infection (Murrell and Bruschi 1994; Capo and Despommier 1996; Kociecka 2000). The immunological reaction consists of the production of inflammatory cells (i.e. mast cells, eosinophils, monocytes, and T and B lymphocytes), of cytokines, and antibodies.

The penetration and development of larvae in the muscle cells cause the acquisition by the cell of a new phenotype called 'nurse cell', accompanied by the disappearance of sarcomere myofibrils, the encapsulation of the larvae (in the case of encapsulated species), and the development of a capillary network surrounding the infected cell (Capo *et al.* 1998). In addition, the sarcoplasm becomes basophilic, the cell nucleus is displaced to the centre of the cell, and the nucleoli increase in both number and size. The cell becomes more permeable, resulting in an increased release of muscle enzymes. The parenteral or muscular phase is associated with inflammatory and allergic responses caused by invasion of the skeletal muscle cells by the migrating larvae.

This invasion can directly damage the muscle cells, or indirectly stimulate the infiltration of inflammatory cells. A correlation between the eosinophil levels and serum muscle enzymes such as lactate dehydrogenase (LDH) and creatine phosphokinase (CK) has been observed in people with trichinellosis, suggesting that muscle damage may be mediated indirectly by these activated granulocytes (Ferraccioli *et al.* 1988).

The presence of larvae in the central nervous system causes vasculitis and perivasculitis, with diffuse or focal lesions. The NBL tend to wander, causing tissue damage before re-entering the bloodstream, or remain trapped and destroyed by the following granulomatous reaction. Neural cells may also be damaged by eosinophil degranulation products such as eosinophil-derived neurotoxin and major basic proteins (Durack *et al.* 1979).

Moreover, heart and brain lesions are often associated and could result from the simultaneous intervention of local prothrombotic effects of eosinophil activation and vascular injury caused by the migrating larvae (Fourestié *et al.* 1993). Myocarditis is triggered initially by invasion of the migrating larvae, then from immunopathologic processes such as activated eosinophil infiltration and mast cell degranulation (Paolocci *et al.* 1998). The length of survival of the nurse-cell parasite complex in the host is known to vary greatly from one to two years to an undetermined number of years, although survival for up to 30 years has been reported in humans (Fröscher *et al.* 1988).

Symptomatology

In the early stage of the infection, the most common intestinal sign and symptom are diarrhoea and abdominal pain. This symptomatology usually precedes fever and myalgia by three to four days, and then disappears in less than one week. It has been observed that the shorter the duration between infection and the appearance of diarrhoea and fever, the longer the duration of both fever and facial oedema (Dupouy-Camet *et al.* 2002).

In most persons, the acute stage begins with the sudden appearance of general discomfort and severe headaches, an increase in fever, chills and excessive sweating. The major syndrome of the acute stage consists of persistent fever, periorbital or facial oedema, muscle pain, and severe asthenia, lasting for several weeks. Transient dizziness and nausea can also occur. Though less common, diarrhoea and conjunctival and sub-lingual haemorrhages are also observed. This is the stage during which the adults and the migrating larvae provoke the signs and symptoms of the disease. Fever is one of the earliest and most common sign of trichinellosis. Body temperature increases rapidly up to 39–40°C, and fever lasts from eight to ten days, although it can persist for up to three weeks when the disease is severe.

Oedemas are very typical signs of trichinellosis, although their intensity varies depending upon the intensity of the reaction to the infection. In the severe form of trichinellosis, oedema extends to the upper and lower extremities. The oedema is symmetrical. It usually vanishes rapidly following treatment with glucocorticosteroids. Muscle pain affects various muscle groups (cervix, trunk, masseters, and upper and lower extremities), and its intensity is related to the severity of the disease. The pain usually appears upon exertion, although most persons with severe trichinellosis or phlebitis associated with trichinellosis also experience myalgia at rest. Some persons with severe disease become disabled with a muscle weakness. The restriction of movement due to the pain associated with exertion leads to contractures of the upper and lower limbs, nuchal pseudorigidity, and trismus. Severe myalgia generally lasts 2–3 weeks.

Laboratory features

Eosinophilia has been observed in most case of trichinellosis, with few exceptions. It appears early, before the development of clinical signs and symptoms, and it increases between the 2–5 weeks after infection. Eosinophilia can be low (< 1,000/mm^3), moderate (1,000–3,000/mm^3), or high up to 19,000 cells per mm^3. It regresses slowly and can remain at lower levels for a period of several weeks to three months. The level of eosinophilia is correlated with the degree of myalgia and is higher in persons with neurological complications (Ferraccioli *et al.* 1988; Fourestié *et al.* 1993). The levels of muscle enzymes (CK, LDH, aldolase, and aspartate aminotransferase) in serum increase in 75–90% of infected persons between 2–5 weeks after the infection. In the course of trichinellosis, there is an increase in total IgE. Clinical observations suggest that *Trichinella*-specific IgE are responsible for allergic manifestations typical of the clinical picture of trichinellosis, such as cutaneous rash or oedemas (Watanabe *et al.* 2005).

Complications

Complications usually develop within the first two weeks in severe cases, but they have also been reported in moderate cases, in persons who were improperly treated (including those for whom treatment was begun too late) and, particularly, in the elderly. A positive correlation has been reported between age and the frequency and severity of complications (Dupouy-Camet *et al.* 2002). Encephalitis and myocarditis, which are both life-threatening, are often simultaneously present (Fourestié *et al.* 1993). Cardiovascular disturbances can occur in moderate or severe cases of trichinellosis, usually between the third and fourth week p.i.) (Bessoudo *et al.* 1981; Compton *et al.* 1993, Lazarevic *et al.* 1989; Puljz *et al.* 2005). Myocarditis develops in 5–20-% of all infected persons. The symptoms include pain in the heart region, tachycardia, and electrocardiogram abnormalities. Neurological complications include a variety of signs and symptoms (Fourestié *et al.* 1993). Neurological complications could be less frequent if the infected person is treated early. Ocular lesions appear during the acute stage of the disease and result from disturbances in microcirculation (Pozio *et al.* 2003). Dyspnea is relatively common and is caused primarily by parasite invasion and subsequent inflammation of respiratory muscles such as the diaphragm. Digestive complications occur during the acute stage of infection, and they consist of massive protein exudation leading to hypoalbuminemia and localized oedemas, acute intestinal necrosis, and prolonged diarrhoea (Pozio *et al.* 2003).

Severity of the disease

The severity of the disease depends on a number of variables which are often interrelated, including the number of larvae ingested, the frequency of consumption of infected meat; how the meat was cooked or treated (e.g. whether it was raw or rare or whether it had been smoked or salted); the amount of alcohol consumed at the time of meat consumption, given that alcohol could increase the resistance to the infection (Pawlowski 1983); the *Trichinella* species involved (the number of NBL shed by females differs by species); and individual susceptibility which depends on ethnic factors as well as sex, age, and the immune status of the host. The length of the incubation period depends upon the same variables as disease severity. Furthermore, it has been observed that for the more severe forms of trichinellosis, the incubation period is generally shorter, specifically: the incubation period lasts approximately one week for the severe form, two weeks for the moderately severe form, and at least three to four weeks for the benign and abortive forms.

Death

Death is rare. Of the more than 6,500 infections reported in the EU in the past 25 years, only five deaths have been observed, all of which were due to thromboembolic disease, in persons over 65 years of age; deaths has been reported in two outbreaks involving more than one thousand cases (Ancelle *et al.* 1988). Forty-two fatalities out of 70,987 cases were reported in a worldwide survey between 1986 and 2009. No death was reported in outbreaks caused by *T. britovi*.

Convalescent stage

The convalescent stage of trichinellosis begins when the adult females cease to release migrating larvae and the already established larvae have completed their development in the muscle cells. The transition to this stage is characterized by the progressive disappearance of the signs and symptoms of the disease and by the return of laboratory parameters to normal values. This stage usually begins between the sixth and the eight week p.i., and infected persons could still have a severe asthenia for several weeks and chronic muscular pain for up to six months. Most persons will then become asymptomatic, though live larvae will persist in their muscles for years.

Chronic trichinellosis

Whether or not a chronic form of trichinellosis actually exists is still under debate, and chronic trichinellosis could be difficult to distinguish from sequelae of the acute phase. However, its existence is supported by reports of persons who complain of chronic pain and a feeling of general discomfort and who show signs of paranoia and a syndrome of persecution, months or even years after the acute stage. The existence of a chronic form is supported by the presence of IgG antibodies in the serum, of bioelectric muscle disturbances, and of inflammatory cells in the muscles, all due to the chronic presence of live larvae. Moreover, this syndrome can also result from unnoticed brain localizations during the acute phase of the disease (Dupouy-Camet *et al.* 2002).

Immunopathology

Although it is certain that *Trichinella* cause pathological changes as a result of mechanical damage to the intestine and to muscle tissues, the majority of the clinical features of trichinellosis are immuno-pathological in origin and can be related to the capacity of *Trichinella* to induce allergic responses, a property shared by many helminth species. The molecular basis is still undefined, although clearly it must reflect particular characteristics of worm antigens and the manner in which they are presented to the host. Studies in mouse models show that *Trichinella* infections preferentially stimulate cells of the T helper 2 (Th2) subset of CD4+T lymphocytes (Grencis *et al.* 1991), which release the cytokines necessary for the development of many of the allergic components of the disease, and it can reasonably be assumed that a similar situation exists during human infections.

During the intestinal phase, there is a marked infiltration of inflammatory cells, including neutrophils, eosinophils, and mast cells into the gut mucosa. Significant changes take place in mucosal architecture (e.g. villous atrophy), fluid flux across the mucosa is disturbed, mucus production is increased, and intestinal transit time is decreased. All of these changes are the result of T-cell activity and all can be related to the symptoms appearing during the intestinal phase of infection, of which diarrhoea is the most characteristic. Eosinophilia is a consequence of T-cell responses to both the intestinal adult worms and the muscle larvae and is dependent upon release of the cytokine IL-5 (Herndon and Kayes 1992). It has been shown in rodents that infection stimulates both parasite-specific IgE and total IgE antibodies as well as IgG isotypes (IgGl) that are involved in hypersensitivity reactions (e.g. Gabriel and Justus 1979) and this is consistent with the dominance of the T-cell response by the Th2 subset. *Trichinella*-specific IgE responses have been detected in humans (Bruschi *et al.* 1990).

Diagnosis in humans

The diagnosis of trichinellosis should be based on the anamnesis (source of infection, amount of infected meat ingested, number of larvae present in the infected meat, and number of cases in the epidemic focus), clinical evaluation (recognition of the signs and symptoms of trichinellosis and definition of the form of the disease, which significantly affects the choice of treatment), and laboratory tests (immunodiagnosis and/or detection of larvae in a muscle biopsy). An algorithm which can be used for the diagnosis is shown in Table 61.2. The most highly recommended technique is ELISA with excretory/secretory antigens which have the highest ratio between sensitivity and specificity and is best used in combination with immunoblotting to confirm ELISA-positive samples. In regions with the circulation of other parasite infections, a high number of false positive reactions can be detected (Gomez Morales *et al.* 2008). Seroconversion occurs between 12 and 60 days post infection. For parasitological diagnosis, a muscle biopsy must be collected, preferably from the deltoid muscle, although any skeletal muscle could be used. The surgeon should carefully collect 0.2–0.5 g of muscle tissue (less than a pea size) without fat or skin. The sensitivity of the parasitological diagnosis depends on the amount of muscle sample tested and the number of larvae per gram. Larvae in the muscle biopsy can be detected by three methods.

1. Trichinelloscopy (small muscle samples are compressed between two microscopy slides, and examined under a light microscope at 20–40 X magnification). However, trichinelloscopy may fail when the larval density is low, when larvae are not yet encapsulated or with larvae from non-encapsulated species.

2. Digestion of muscle samples using pepsin and HCl digestion fluid is very useful for determining the number of larvae per gram of muscle tissue and for isolating larvae for molecular identification. However, if the muscle biopsy is taken too early after infection, the larvae can be destroyed by digestion. Only muscle larvae that are at least 15–18 days of age are not destroyed by artificial digestion.

3. The histological analysis of muscle tissue reveals fragments of larvae at various stages of development, the presence of the collagen capsule (for encapsulated species) or the remains of a destroyed capsule, the presence of muscle-cell basophilic transformation, and the type and composition of cellular infiltrates. The basophilic transformation of muscle cells represents a valuable diagnostic criterion of *Trichinella* invasion even when no larva has been detected. This method is more sensitive than trichinelloscopy in the early stage of muscle invasion, when larvae are very small and cannot be easily differentiated from the muscle fibres (Wranicz *et al.* 1998).

Treatment

In adults, mebendazole should be administered at a daily dose of 25 mg per kg body weight (administered in 2–3 doses) for 15 days.

Table 61.2 Algorithm for diagnosing the probability of being infected with acute *Trichinella* in humans

Group A	Group B	Group C	Group D
Fever	Diarrhoea	Eosinophilia (> 1,G/L) and/or increased total IgE level	Positive serology (with a highly specific test)
Eyelid and/or facial oedema	Neurological signs	Increased levels of muscular enzymes	Seroconversion
Myalgia	Cardiological signs Conjunctivitis Subungual haemorrhages		Positive muscular biopsy

The diagnosis is:
Very unlikely: one A or one B or one C
Suspected: one A or two B and one C
Probable: three A and one C
Highly probable: three A and two C
Confirmed: three A, two C, and one D; any of groups A or B and one C and one D

The efficacy of mebendazole against larvae in muscle tissues depends on the time between infection and treatment and could be dose-dependent. Albendazole should be used at a daily dose of 800 mg/day (15–20 mg/kg/day) administered in 2–3 doses, for 15 days; in children over two years of age, the drug is given at 10 mg per kg body weight. For severe infection, the treatment may be repeated after five days. Glucocorticosteroids are used by most physicians to treat the signs and symptoms. The most commonly-used glucocorticosteroid is prednisolone, which should be administered at 30–60 mg/day in multiple doses until the symptoms and signs disappear. They must always be used in combination with anthelmintics and never alone, since they could increase the larval burden by delaying the intestinal worm expulsion.

Trichinella infection in susceptible animals

The diagnosis of *Trichinella* infection in animals falls into two categories. Direct methods consist of identification and visualization of the first-stage muscle larvae encysted or free in striated muscle tissue. Indirect methods consist of detection of specific circulating antibodies.

Detection of *Trichinella* muscle larvae

The identification of *Trichinella* larvae in muscle samples is limited to post-mortem inspection of carcasses. In many countries, in order to prevent human trichinellosis, the examination of muscle samples from pigs and other susceptible animal species used for consumption (e.g. horses, wild boars, bears), should be a part of routine slaughter inspection (Gamble *et al.* 2000). Direct detection is also widely applied in wildlife epidemiology, where indicator animals (e.g. foxes, raccoon dogs, wild boars) are examined to assess the existence of infection among wildlife reservoirs. The sensitivity is greatly influenced by the muscle selected for sampling and the specific method used (Nöckler *et al.* 2000). Selection of muscles for sampling in meat inspection requires identification of predilection sites in a particular animal species. For routine meat inspection, it is necessary to ensure a sensitivity of approximately

1–3 larvae per g (lpg) as this is the level above which infection constitutes a food safety issue. Using the pooled sample digestion method, a minimum of a 1 g sample of tissue from a predilection site is examined. Using trichinoscopy, the examination of 28 oat kernel-size pieces of diaphragm muscle which corresponds to a 0.5 g sample, is recommended (Gamble *et al.* 2000). To ensure a high sensitivity in horse meat, 5 g samples should be examined by the pooled sample digestion method. For epidemiological studies in reservoir animals (wildlife), the sample size should also be adjusted upward to achieve a sensitivity of less than 1 lpg. Predilection muscles in carnivores may require a prolonged digestion time (up to 2 hours) (Kapel *et al.* 2005).

At least four artificial digestion methods are available:

1. The magnetic stirrer method,
2. The stomacher sedimentation method,
3. The stomacher filtration technique,
4. The 'Trichomatic 35' automated digestion method.

The magnetic stirrer method is considered the gold standard because it is a method specifically designed for pooled samples and it has been subjected to validation studies (Kapel *et al.* 2005). The International Commission on Trichinellosis (www.med.unipi.it/ict/welcome.htm) recommends that all slaughter testing methods for *Trichinella* detection in pigs, other livestock and game should be validated by standard procedures and any new method be subjected for evaluation by at least three reference laboratories (Gamble *et al.* 2000).

Detection of anti-*Trichinella* antibodies

Serological methods are used either for ante-mortem or post-mortem examination of serum samples for *Trichinella*-specific antibodies (World Organization for Animal Health (OIE) 2004). Serological methods are not recommended as a substitute for meat inspection of individual carcasses (Gamble *et al.* 2000). However, serological methods for detection of *Trichinella* infection are considered to be suitable for surveillance and epidemiological investigations in animal populations, where the prevalence of infection is high (Gamble *et al.* 2004). The ELISA method, the most commonly used method for the detection of *Trichinella* infection, provides an acceptable balance of sensitivity and specificity (OIE 2004). In many experimental and/or field studies, the successful use of an indirect ELISA for the detection of specific *Trichinella* antibodies in pig serum and meat juice samples has been demonstrated (Murrell *et al.* 1986; Nöckler *et al.* 2004).

The early stage of *Trichinella* infection is characterized by a 'diagnostic window' in which larvae have become encysted in muscle tissue as early as 17 d.p.i., but specific antibodies can not yet be detected in the host animal. In this case, false-negative results may occur when compared with direct tests (OIE 2004). Under normal conditions, serum antibodies decline slowly after an initial peak. In horses, specific antibody titres fell below cut-off levels of the ELISA as soon as 14 weeks p.i. (Soulé *et al.* 1989, 1993), and in naturally infected horses, specific circulating antibodies were not detected in spite of the presence of a high worm burden in muscles (Pozio *et al.* 1997, 1999). Considering the present state of knowledge, serological methods cannot be recommended to detect anti-*Trichinella* antibodies in this host (Gamble *et al.* 2004).

Prevention

In contrast to control measures, prevention of pig infection with *Trichinella* has received substantially less attention, and most gains in reducing infection in domestic pigs have been the by-product of other disease prevention initiatives. For example, the introduction of garbage cooking laws in the USA was intended to control vesicular exanthema and hog cholera (Zimmerman and Zinter 1971; Zimmerman *et al.* 1973). Likewise, improvements in swine husbandry, including the introduction of confinement housing systems, generally occurred without any intention to prevent exposure of pigs to *Trichinella*. Despite an overall reduction in the prevalence of *Trichinella* infection in domestic pigs in some countries, resulting from a transition to confined management systems and improved veterinary public health efforts, the increase in prevalence rates in other countries where organized farming systems have broken down, underscores the ongoing risk of infection with this parasite in domestic pigs. Although most pigs are produced in confinement, the production of free-ranging pigs has increased in many countries, and obviously such pigs have a higher risk of exposure.

Recently, in some eastern European countries, the breakdown of organized farming systems and a decline in the availability and quality of veterinary services have resulted in higher prevalence rates in pigs and outbreaks of trichinellosis in humans (Djordjevic *et al.* 2003; Cuperlovic *et al.* 2005; Blaga *et al.* 2007).

The risk of *Trichinella* infection for pigs raised in outdoor farming systems is clear in all parts of the world (Gamble *et al.* 1999; Liu and Boireau 2002; Nöckler *et al.* 2004; Ribicich *et al.* 2005). Nevertheless, the degree of risk to pigs raised outdoors depends in great part on the infection level in local wildlife, and this degree of risk is of substantial importance for 'organic' or 'green' pig producers, who provide products to consumers seeking meat from animals raised under natural conditions. The so-called 'backyard pigs' are often fed food scraps or other forms of meat-containing waste and have ready access to rodents and wildlife. To compound the problems, pigs raised in this manner are generally not sold through retail marketing channels, and therefore are not subjected to reliable methods of veterinary inspection. While this scenario might be more typical of developing countries, the situation exists to some extent in most countries of the world.

Certification of pig production systems

The knowledge of modes of transmission of *Trichinella* to domestic pigs, allows pig farmers/producers to design management systems which prevent or drastically reduce the risk of exposure. By following a series of good management practices, combined with documentation of these practices and regular official control to verify that these practices are effective, it is possible to certify the safety of pork without subsequent slaughter inspection or further processing. There are minimal requirements that need to be met for livestock to be considered *Trichinella*-free.

1. Architectural and environmental barriers, i.e. pig buildings are constructed to prevent rodents from entering buildings, areas within 100 meters of pig buildings are free from debris and rodent harbourage, and a 2 m perimeter consisting of gravel or vegetation mowed to a height of less than 10 cm is maintained around all pig buildings.

2. Feed is maintained in closed silos, which do not allow rodents to enter; it is purchased from an approved facility, which

produces feed by good production practices. Waste food, containing meat products is cooked in accordance with waste food laws intended to inactivate *Trichinella* larvae.

3. A documented rodent control programme is maintained by a recognized pest control provider and no evidence indicating the presence of rodents is observed by a recognized pest control provider.

4. Dead animals are disposed of within 24 hours and by sanitary means and no garbage dumps are present within a 2 km radius of the farm.

5. New animals which do not originate from *Trichinella*-free farms are held in quarantine and are tested serologically after three weeks to assure the absence of anti-*Trichinella* antibodies (Gamble *et al.* 2000; European Community 2005).

Programmes, which allow certification of pigs as free from *Trichinella* larvae should be administratively organized to allow proper documentation of certified herds. This is by developing a system of documentation of *Trichinella*-free production practices, which addresses issue certifications and maintain records of certified farms; periodically conducting spot audits of certified producers to assure the integrity of the system; and conducting periodic serology testing of pigs originating from certified farms to verify absence of infection (Forbes and Gajadhar 1999; Gajadhar and Forbes 2002; Forbes *et al.* 2005).

Recent legislation of the EU (European Commission 2005) describes requirements for certifying pigs from farms or categories of farms which raise pigs under certain conditions such as confinement housing, as free from risk of *Trichinella* infection. Pigs from these farms are exempt from requirements for *Trichinella* inspection at slaughter. In the USA, a system for certifying pig farms free from risk of exposure to *Trichinella* is in a pilot phase. This programme emphasizes auditing of good production practices which document the absence of risk factors that would exposure pigs to *Trichinella* in feed, rodents and wildlife (www.aphis.usda.gov/vs/trichinae). As part of the audit requirements, farms must maintain accurate records of animal movement, animal disposal, and rodent control logs. Further, it provides for education of veterinary practitioners who are responsible for conducting regular audits of farms seeking and maintaining *Trichinella*-free certification.

Trichinella-free regions

The International Commission on Trichinellosis does not endorse any programme for assuring pigs to be free from *Trichinella* based on geographic boundaries such as a region, state or country (OIE 2006). Indeed, *Trichinella* occurs in a wide range of wildlife reservoirs both in terrestrial and marine mammals and birds. The absence of *Trichinella* infection cannot be reliably documented in these various species.

References

Ancelle, T. (1998). History of trichinellosis outbreaks linked to horse meat consumption 1975–1998. *Euro. Surveill.*, **3**: 86–89.

Barennes, H., Saysone, S., Odermatt, P., *et al.* (2008). A major trichinellosis outbreak suggesting a high endemicity of *Trichinella* infection in northern Laos. *Am. J. Trop. Med. Hyg.*, **78**: 40–44.

Bessoudo, R., Marrie, T.J. and Smith, E.R. (1981). Cardiac involvement in trichinosis. *Chest*, **79**: 698–99.

Blaga, R., Durand, B., Antoniu, S., *et al.* (2007). Dramatic increase in the incidence of human trichinellosis in Romania over the past 25 years: impact of political changes and regional food habits. *Am. J. Trop. Med. Hyg.*, **76**: 983–86.

Boireau, P., Vallee, I., Roman, T., *et al.* (2000). *Trichinella* in horses: a low frequency infection with high human risk. *Vet. Parasit.*, **93**: 309–20.

Britov, V.A. and Boev, S.N. (1972). Taxonomic rank of various strains of *Trichinella* and their circulation in nature. *Vestnik. Akadem. Nauk. KSSR*, **28**: 27–32.

Bruschi, F., Tassi, C. and Pozio, E. (1990). Parasite-specific antibody response in *Trichinella* sp. 3 human infection: a one year follow-up. *Am. J. Trop. Med. Hyg.*, **43**: 186–93.

Campbell, W.C. (1983a). Historical introduction. In: W.C. Campbell (ed.) *Trichinella and Trichinosis*, pp. 1–30. New York and London: Plenum Press.

Campbell, W.C. (1983b). Modes of Transmission. In: W.C. Campbell (ed.) *Trichinella and Trichinosis*, pp. 425–44. New York and London: Plenum Press.

Capo, V. and Despommier, D. (1996). Clinical aspects of infection with *Trichinella* spp. *Clin. Microbiol. Rev.*, **9**: 47–54.

Capo, V., Despommier, D. and Polvere, R.I. (1998). *Trichinella spiralis*: vascular endothelial growth factor is up-regulated within the nurse cell during the early phase of its formation. *J. Parasitol.*, **84**: 209–14.

Compton, S.J., Celum, C.L., Lee, C., *et al.* (1993). Trichinosis with ventilatory failure and persistent myocarditis. *Clin. Infect. Dis.*, **16**: 500–504.

Cuperlovic, K., Djordjevic, M. and Pavlovic, S. (2005). Re-emergence of trichinellosis in southeastern Europe due to political and economic changes. *Vet. Parasit.*, **132**: 159–66.

De Carneri, I. and Di Matteo, L. (1989). Epidemiology of trichinellosis in Italy and in neighboring countries. *Ann. Istituto Super. Sanità*, **25**: 625–33. [in Italian].

Despommier, D.D. (1990). *Trichinella spiralis*: the worm that would be virus. *Parasit. Today*, **6**: 193–96.

Djordjevic, M., Bacic, M., Petricevic, M., *et al.* (2003). Social, political, and economic factors responsible for the reemergence of trichinellosis in Serbia: a case study. *J. Parasit.*, **89**: 226–31.

Dupouy-Camet, J., Kociecka, W., *et al.* (2002). Opinion on the diagnosis and treatment of human trichinellosis. *Exp. Opin. Pharmacother.*, **3**: 1117–30.

Durack, D.T., Sumi, S.M. and Klebanoff, S.J. (1979). Neurotoxicity of human eosinophils. *Proc. Nat. Acad. Sci. USA*, **76**: 1443–47.

European Commission (2005). Regulation (EC) No 2075/2005 of the European Parliament and of the Council of 5 December 2005 laying down specific rules on official controls for *Trichinella* in meat. *Offic. J. Euro. Comm.*, **L338**: 60–82.

Ferraccioli, G.F., Mercadanti, M., Salaffi, F., *et al.* (1988). Prospective rheumatological study of muscle and joint symptoms during *Trichinella nelsoni* infection. *Quart. J. Med.*, **69**: 973–84.

Fourestié, V., Douceron, H., *et al.* (1993). Neurotrichinosis. A cerebrovascular disease associated with myocardial injury and hypereosinophilia. *Brain*, **116**: 603–16.

Forbes, L.B. and Gajadhar, A.A. (1999). A validated *Trichinella* digestion assay and an associated sampling and quality assurance system for use in testing pork and horse meat. *J. Food Protect.*, **62**: 1308–13.

Forbes, L.B., Scandrett, W.B. and Gajadhar, A.A. (2005). A programme to accredit laboratories for reliable testing of pork and horsemeat for *Trichinella*. *Vet. Parasitol.*, **132**: 173–77.

Fröscher, W., Gullotta, F., Saathoff, M. and Tackmann, W. (1988). Chronic trichinosis. Clinical, bioptic, serological and electromyographic observations. *Eur. Neurol.*, **28**: 221–26.

Gabriel, B.W. and Justus, D.E. (1979). Quantitation of immediate and delayed hypersensitivity responses in *Trichinella*-infected mice. Correlation with worm expulsion. *Intern. Arch. Aller. Appl. Immun.*, **60**: 275–85.

Gajadhar, A.A. and Forbes, L.B. (2002). An internationally recognized quality assurance system for diagnostic parasitology in animal health and food safety, with example data on trichinellosis. *Vet. Parasitol.*, **103**: 133–40.

Gallardo, M.T., Mateos, L., Artieda, J., et al. (2007). Outbreak of trichinellosis in Spain and Sweden due to consumption of wild boar meat contaminated with *Trichinella britovi*. *Euro. Surveill.*, **12**: E070315.1.

Gamble, H.R., Brady, R.C., Bulaga, L.L., et al. (1999). Prevalence and risk factors for trichinellosis in domestic pigs in the north-eastern United States. *Vet. Parasitol.*, **82**: 59–69.

Gamble, H.R., Bessonov, A.S., Cuperlovic, K., et al. (2000). International Commission on Trichinellosis: recommendations on methods for the control of *Trichinella* in domestic and wild animals intended for human consumption. *Vet. Parasitol.*, **93**: 393–408.

Gamble, H.R., Pozio, E., Bruschi, F., et al. (2004). International Commission on Trichinellosis: recommendations on the use of serological tests for the detection of *Trichinella* infection in animals and man. *Parasite*, **11**: 3–13.

Garkavi, B.L. (1972). Species of *Trichinella* isolated from wild animals. *Veterinariya*, **10**: 90–91.

Gould, S.E. (1970). History. In: S.E. Gould (ed.) *Trichinosis in man and animals*, pp. 3–18. Springfield, Illinois: Charles C. Thomas Publisher.

Grencis, R.K., Hültner, L. and Else, K.J. (1991). Host protective immunity to *Trichinella spiralis* in mice: activation of Th cell subsets and lymphokine secretion in mice expressing different response phenotypes. *Immunology*, **74**: 329–32.

Gretillat, S. and Vassiliades, G. (1967). Presence of *Trichinella spiralis* (Owen, 1835) in wild carnivora and swine of the region of the Senegal river basin. *Comp. Rendus hebdom. seances de l'Acad. Sci.*, **264**: 1297–300.

Herndon, F.J. and Kayes, S.G. (1992). Depletion of eosinophils by anti-IL-5 monoclonal antibody treatment of mice infected with *Trichinella spiralis* does not alter parasite burden or immunologic resistance to reinfection. *J. Immunol.*, **149**: 3642–47.

Kapel, C.M.O. (2005). Changes in the EU legislation on *Trichinella* inspection – new challenges in the epidemiology. *Vet. Parasitol.*, **132**: 189–94.

Khamboonruang, C. (1991). The present status of trichinellosis in Thailand. *Southeast Asian J. Trop. Med. Pub. Health*, **22**: 312–15.

Kociecka, W. (2000). Trichinellosis: human disease, diagnosis and treatment. *Vet. Parasitol.*, **93**: 365–83.

Kusolsuk, T., Kamonrattanakun, S., Wesanonthawech, A., et al. (2010). The second outbreak of trichinellosis caused by *Trichinella papuae* in Thailand. *Trans. Roy. Soc. Trop. Med. Hyg.*, **104**: 433–37.

La Rosa, G., Marucci, G., Zarlenga, D.S. and Pozio, E. (2001). *Trichinella pseudospiralis* populations of the Palearctic region and their relationship with populations of the Nearctic and Australian regions. *Int. J. Parasitol.*, **31**: 297–305.

Lazarevic, A.M., Neskovic, A.N., Goronja, M., et al. (1999). Low incidence of cardiac abnormalities in treated trichinosis: a prospective study of 62 patients from a single-source outbreak. *Am. J. Med.*, **107**: 18–23.

Leidy, J. (1846). Remarks on trichina. *Proc. Acad. Anatomic Sci.*, **3**: 107–08.

Liu, M. and Boireau, P. (2002). Trichinellosis in China: epidemiology and control. *Trends Parasitol.*, **18**: 553–56.

Lo, Y.C., Hung, C.C., Lai, C.S., et al. (2009). Human trichinosis after consumption of soft-shelled turtles, Taiwan. *Emerg. Infect. Dis.*, **15**: 2056–58.

Murrell, K.D. and Bruschi, F. (1994). Clinical trichinellosis. In: T. Sun (ed.) *Prog. Clin. Parasit.*, pp. 117–50. FL, USA: CRC Press.

Murrell, K.D., Anderson, W.R., and Schad, G.A., et al. (1986). Field evaluation of the enzyme-linked immunosorbent assay for swine trichinellosis: efficacy of the excretory-secretory antigen. *Am. J. Vet. Res.*, **47**: 1046–49.

Murrell, K.D., Djordjevic, M., and Cuperlovic, K., et al. (2004). Epidemiology of *Trichinella* infection in the horse: the risk from animal product feeding practices. *Vet. Parasitol.*, **123**: 223–33.

Nelson, G.S., Blackie, E.J. and Mukundi, J. (1966). Comparative studies on geographical strains of *Trichinella spiralis*. *Trans. R. Soc. Trop. Med. Hyg.*, **60**: 471–80.

Nezri, M., Ruer, J., De Bruyne, A., et al. (2006). Premiere observation d'un cas de humain de trichinellose a *Trichinella britovi* en Algerie après consummation de viande de chacal (*Canis aureus*). *Bull. Soc. Pathol. Exotique*, **99**: 94–95.

Nöckler, K., Pozio, E., Voigt, W.P. and Heidrich, J. (2000). Detection of *Trichinella* infection in food animals. *Vet. Parasitol.*, **93**: 335–50.

Nöckler, K., Hamidi, A., Fries, R., et al. (2004). Influence of methods for *Trichinella* detection in pigs from endemic and non-endemic European region. *J. Vet. Med. B*, **51**: 297–301.

Ortega Pierres, M.G., Arriaga, C. and Yepez-Mulia, L. (2000). Epidemiology of trichinellosis in Mexico, Central and South America. *Vet. Parasitol.*, **93**: 201–25.

Owen, R. (1835). Description of a microscopic entozoon infesting the muscles of the human body. *Trans. Zool. Soc. Lond.*, **1**: 315–24.

Owen, I.L., Gomez Morales, M.A., et al. (2005). *Trichinella* infection in a hunting population of Papua New Guinea suggests an ancient relationship of *Trichinella* with human beings. *Trans. R. Soc. Trop. Med. Hyg.*, **99**: 618–24.

Paolocci, N., Sironi, M., Bettini, M., et al. (1998). Immunopathological mechanisms underlying the time course of *Trichinella spiralis* cardiomyopathy in rats. *Virch. Arch.*, **432**: 261–66.

Pawlowski, Z.S. (1983). Clinical aspects in man. In: W.C. Campbell (ed.) *Trichinella and trichinosis*, pp. 367–401. New York and London: Plenum Press.

Pozio, E. (2001a). New patterns of *Trichinella* infection. *Vet. Parasitol.*, **98**: 133–48.

Pozio, E. (2001b). Taxonomy of *Trichinella* and the epidemiology of the infection in the south-east Asia and Australian regions. *Southeast Asian J. Trop. Med. Pub. Health*, **32**(S2): 129–32.

Pozio, E. (2005). The broad spectrum of *Trichinella* hosts: From cold- to warm-blooded animals. *Vet. Parasitol.*, **132**: 3–11.

Pozio, E. (2007). World distribution of *Trichinella* spp. infections in animals and humans. *Vet. Parasitol.*, **149**: 3–21.

Pozio, E. and La Rosa, G. (2000). *Trichinella murrelli* n. sp: etiological agent of sylvatic trichinellosis in temperate areas of North America. *J. Parasitol.*, **86**: 134–39.

Pozio, E. and La Rosa, G. (2005). Evaluation of the infectivity of *Trichinella papuae* and *Trichinella zimbabwensis* for equatorial freshwater fishes. *Vet. Parasitol.*, **132**: 113–14.

Pozio, E. and Marucci, G. (2003). *Trichinella*-infected pork products: a dangerous gift. *Trends Parasitol.*, **19**: 338.

Pozio, E. and Murrell, K.D. (2006). Systematics and epidemiology of *Trichinella*. *Adv. Parasitol.*, **63**: 367–439.

Pozio, E. and Zarlenga, D.S. (2005). Recent advances on the taxonomy, systematics and epidemiology of *Trichinella*. *Int. J. Parasitol.*, **35**: 1191–204.

Pozio, E., La Rosa, G., Murrell, K.D. and Lichtenfels, J.R. (1992). Taxonomic revision of the genus *Trichinella*. *J. Parasitol.*, **78**: 654–59.

Pozio, E., Tamburrini, A., Sacchi L., et al. (1997). Detection of *Trichinella spiralis* in a horse during routine examination in Italy. *Int. J. Parasitol.*, **27**: 1613–21.

Pozio, E., Owen, I.L., La Rosa, G., Sacchi, L., Rossi, P. and Corona, S. (1999). *Trichinella papuae* n. sp. (Nematoda), a new non-encapsulated species from domestic and sylvatic swine of Papua New Guinea. *Int. J. Parasitol.*, **29**: 1825–39.

Pozio, E., Paterlini, F., Pedarra, C., et al. (1999). Predilection sites of *Trichinella spiralis* larvae in naturally infected horses. *J. Helminthol.*, **73**: 233–37.

Pozio, E., Casulli, A., Bologov, V.V., Marucci, G. and La Rosa, G. (2001). Hunting practices increase the prevalence of *Trichinella* infection in wolves from European Russia. *J. Parasitol.*, **87**: 1498–501.

Pozio, E., Foggin, C.M., Marucci, G., *et al.* (2002). *Trichinella zimbabwensis* n.sp. (Nematoda), a new non-encapsulated species from crocodiles (*Crocodylus niloticus*) in Zimbabwe also infecting mammals. *Int. J. Parasitol.*, **32:** 1787–99.

Pozio, E., Gomez Morales, M.A. and Dupouy-Camet, J. (2003). Clinical aspects, diagnosis and treatment of trichinellosis. *Exp. Rev. Anti-infect. Ther.*, **1:** 89–100.

Pozio, E., Pagani, P., Marucci, G., *et al.* (2005a). *Trichinella britovi* etiological agent of sylvatic trichinellosis in the Republic of Guinea (West Africa) and a re-evaluation of geographical distribution for encapsulated species in Africa. *Int. J. Parasitol.*, **35:** 955–60.

Pozio, E., Owen, I.L., Marucci, G. and La Rosa, G. (2005b). Inappropriate feeding practice favors the transmission of *Trichinella papuae* from wild pigs to saltwater crocodiles in Papua New Guinea. *Vet. Parasitol.*, **127:** 245–51.

Pozio, E., Hoberg, E., La Rosa, G. and Zarlenga, D.S. (2009). Molecular taxonomy, phylogeny and biogeography of nematodes belonging to the *Trichinella* genus. *Infect. Genet. Evol.*, **9:** 606–16.

Proulx, J.F., MacLean, J.D., Gyorkos, T.W., *et al.* (2002). Novel prevention program for trichinellosis in Inuit communities. *Clin. Infect. Dis.*, **34:** 1508–14.

Puljiz, I., Beus, A., Kuzman, I. and Seiwerth, S. (2005). Electrocardiographic changes and myocarditis in trichinellosis: a retrospective study of 154 patients. *Ann. Trop. Med. Parasitol.*, **99:** 403–11.

Ribicich, M., Gamble, H.R., Rosa, A., Bolpe, J. and Franco, A. (2005). Trichinellosis in Argentina: an historical review. *Vet. Parasitol.*, **132:** 137–42.

Rausch, R.L., Babero, B.B., Rausch, R.V. and Schiller, E.L. (1956). Studies on the helminth fauna of Alaska. XXVII. The occurrence of larvae of *Trichinella* spiralis in Alaskan mammals. *J. Parasitol.*, **42:** 259–71.

Schenone, H., Olea, A., Schenone, H., *et al.* (2002). Current epidemiological situation of trichinosis in Chile, 1991–2000. *Rev. Med. Chile*, **130:** 281–85. (in Spanish).

Soulé, C., Dupouy-Camet, J., Georges, P., *et al.* (1989). Experimental trichinellosis in horses: biological and parasitological evaluation. *Vet. Parasitol.*, **31:** 19–36.

Soulé, C., Dupouy-Camet, J., Georges, P., *et al.* (1993). Biological and parasitic variations in horses infested and reinfested by *Trichinella spiralis*. *Vet. Res.*, **24:** 21–31.

Stensvold, C.R., Nielsen, H.V. and Molbak, K. (2007). A case of trichinellosis in Denmark, imported from Poland, June 2007. *Eur. Surveill.*, **12:** E070809.3.

Takahashi, Y., Mingyuan, L. and Waikagul, J. (2000). Epidemiology of trichinellosis in Asia and Pacific Rim. *Vet. Parasitol.*, **93:** 227–39.

Virchow, R. (1859). Recherches sur le développement du *Trichina spiralis*. *Com. Rend. l'Acad. Sci.*, **49:** 660–62.

Wang, Z.Q., Cui, J. and Xu, B.L. (2006). The epidemiology of human trichinellosis in China during 2000–2003. *Acta Trop.*, **97:** 247–51.

Wang, Z.Q., Cui, J. and Shen, L.J. (2007). The epidemiology of animal trichinellosis in China. *Vet. J.*, **173:** 391–98.

Watanabe, N., Bruschi, F. and Korenaga, M. (2005). IgE: a question of protective immunity in *Trichinella spiralis* infection. *Trends Parasitol.*, **21:** 175–78.

World Organisation for Animal Health (2004). Trichinellosis. In: *Manual for Diagnostic Tests and Vaccines for Terrestrial Animals*, Chapter 2.2.9, (5th edn.). Paris, France: OIE.

World Organisation for Animal Health (2006). Trichinellosis. In: *Terrestrial Animal Health Code*, Chapter 2.2.9. Paris, France: OIE.

Wranicz, M.J., Gustowska, L., Gabryel, P., Kucharska, E. and Cabaj, W. (1998). *Trichinella spiralis*: induction of the basophilic transformation of muscle cells by synchronous newborn larvae. *Parasitol. Res.*, **84:** 403–7.

Zarlenga, D.S., Rosenthal, B., La Rosa, G., Pozio, E. and Hoberg, E.P. (2006). Post-Miocene expansion, colonization, and host switching drove speciation among extant nematodes of the archaic genus *Trichinella*. *Proc. Nat. Acad. Sci. USA*, **103:** 7354–59.

Zenker, F.A. (1860). Ueber die Trichinen-krankheit des Menschen. *Virch. Arch. Pathol. Anatomy*, **18:** 561–72.

Zenker, F.A. (1871). Zur Lehre von der Trichinenkrankheit. *Deutsche Arch. Klinische. Med.*, **8:** 387–421.

Zimmermann, W.J. and Zinter, D.E. (1971). The prevalence of trichiniasis in swine in the United States, 1966–1970. *Health Serv. Rep.*, **86:** 937–45.

Zimmermann, W.J., Steele, J.H. and Kagan, I.G. (1973). Trichiniasis in the US population, 1966–1970: prevalence and epidemiologic factors. *Health Serv. Rep.*, **88:** 606–23.

CHAPTER 62

Zoonotic hookworm infections

Dwight D. Bowman

Summary

Hookworms on occasion cause creeping lesions in the superficial layers of the human skin that have been designated as cutaneous larva migrans for the purpose of contrasting the condition with visceral larva migrans. Currently, the disease is presenting most commonly to physicians specializing in tropical or travel medicine in patients who have just visited a tropical beach and are presenting with serpiginous tracks in their skin. The serpiginous tracts can persist for week, and are often pruritic, may be associated with accompanying bulla, and can rarely lead to secondary sequelae. The larval are likely to penetrate ultimately to deeper tissues, where they may be persisting in the tissues of humans in the same fashion as they would within the tissues of any other vertebrate paratenic host.

Most hookworm larvae are capable of penetrating the skin and causing lesions that are similar to cutaneous larvae migrans. However, the geographic distribution of cases still seems to suggest that only one species, *A. braziliense*, is the offending species. The other species appear to spend less time in the skin of the human host, and if they do cause lesions, they appear to produce lesions that are more vesicular or that cause disease of a markedly shorter duration. It seems that the development of improved molecular methods will ultimately lead to the means of more carefully discrimination the geographical location of the offending species and may someday be able to identify specific larvae from lesions.

There are other manifestations of zoonotic hookworm infection. These include the infection of the human intestinal tract with the adults of the canine/feline hookworm *Ancylostoma ceylanicum*; the induction of cases of eosinophilic colitis in people with the canine hookworm, *Ancylostoma caninum*; suspected cases of ocular larva migrans due to hookworm larvae, and the rare case of cutaneous larva migrans due to hookworm species that are only rarely associated with human infections.

History of zoonotic hookworm disease and cutaneous larva migrans

The zoonotic hookworms typically associated with human disease are the common hookworm species of the dog and cat. Hookworm larvae are members of the superfamily Ancylostomatoidea. Therefore they are almost all capable of infecting the final host through skin penetration (Anderson 2000). Consequently it is likely that many of these larvae could cause skin penetration and infection in humans. However, most have been little studied in comparison to those of the dog and cat, and for the most part have not been of any reported significance in human zoonotic hookworm disease.

Zoonotic hookworm infections manifest in several different presentations. One species is responsible for hookworm infections of the small intestine in people and is similar to human hookworm species. In a second species, that infects dogs and cats, the larvae can cause significant human disease through the production of serpiginous pruritic tracts in the skin. A third form of infection is the development of canine hookworms to adulthood in people causing eosinophilic colitis. Hookworms that enter vertebrate paratenic hosts are capable of persisting in the tissues of these hosts for extended periods, and thus, after larvae penetrate the skin, they are capable of persisting in muscle and other tissues for very long times. There is some suggestion that the zoonotic hookworm infections are capable of causing ocular lesions, including retinochoroiditis. Finally, there have been skin lesions induced in people on rather rare occasions with the hookworms or ruminants or with other hookworm species of wildlife; these have typically presented as cutaneous lesions.

Looss was the first to show that hookworm larvae could penetrate the skin. First through the accidental spilling onto his own skin of a culture of third-stage larvae of the human hookworm, *Ancylostoma duodenale*, followed by careful work on the migratory behaviour of *Ancylostoma caninum* of the dog (Looss 1905). This led to the general elucidation of the hookworm life cycle. In hookworm endemic areas, the lesions induced in the skin of people by the penetrating human hookworm species, *Ancylostoma duodenale* and *Necator americanus*, was termed ground itch (Smith 1904). Working in Florida, USA, Kirby-Smith *et al.* (1926) recognized another condition wherein the larvae persisted in the skin for extended periods, and reported over 2,500 diagnosed cases that he distinguished from the ground itch of *N. americanus*. Not long afterward, it was shown in human volunteers that the larvae of the canine hookworm, *Ancylostoma braziliense*, caused lesions consistent with those of creeping eruption (cutaneous larva migrans) in human volunteers, while the larvae of the canine hookworm, *Ancylostoma caninum*, caused only transient papules, similar to that which occurred in ground itch (White and Dove 1928). Interestingly, there has only been one attempt to infect a person with the larvae of *Ancylostoma tubaeforme*, and this attempt proved unsuccessful (Kalkofen 1987).

Unfortunately, the two species, *Ancylostoma braziliense* and *Ancylostoma ceylanicum,* are very similar morphologically, and this caused significant confusion for a period. *A. braziliense* was described in 1910 by Gomes de Faria in Brazil from specimens recovered from cats and dogs. Looss (1911) described *A. ceylanicum* based on specimens recovered from a civet cat in Ceylon. Then, a few years later three human prisoners in India were found to have hookworms identified as *A. ceylanicum* (Grove 1990). The literature then became confused as to the existence and geographic distribution of the two species. Methods for distinguishing the two species were put forward by Biocca (1951), and single-sex cross-over experiments between the two species showed that fertile eggs were produced only when both sets of worms were either one species of the other. The distinction of the two species is also supported by the fact that human infections with *A. braziliense* have not been confirmed in areas where this is the only one of the two species present (Beaver 1956). *A. ceylanicum* is an important zoonotic agent in that it is capable of growing to adulthood in people, but it does not produce the same cutaneous larva migrans lesions as *A. braziliense.*

Cutaneous larva migrans in the south eastern USA has also been called 'plumber's itch', because the lesions appear on plumbers and other labourers who have crawled under the typical coastal-style house with a raised floor. They lie on their backs in the moist shaded sand to do their work, and many of them subsequently develop cutaneous serpiginous lesions. An outbreak, with lesions appearing on arms, legs, or back, involved eight pipe fitters and a painter working in a three-foot crawl space under a new hospital being built at Patrick Air Force Base in Florida (Fuller 1966). An outbreak of cutaneous larva migrans occurred in 22 campers and staff at a children's camp in the Miami area, attended by approximately 300 children (two to 15 years of age) and 80 staff members. Based on the higher proportion of infection among younger campers, the Miami-Dade County Health Department determined the outbreak was associated with a contaminated sandbox. Two feral cats had been observed at the camp and were removed from the premises (O'Connell *et al.* 2007).

The larvae of the zoonotic hookworms that succeed in penetrating the skin are likely to undergo a lung migration in the human host. Pneumonic radiographic lesions (Loeffler's syndrome) has been diagnosed in patients after creeping eruption, 26 of 76 such patients (Wright and Gold 1946). Muhleisen (1953) found hookworm larvae in the sputum of a person 12 to 36 days following exposure to soil heavily contaminated with dog faeces, and on the basis of the minimal lesions associated with the sites of penetration, believed that the infection was due to *A. caninum* rather than *A. braziliense*. Recently, a case of Loeffler's-like syndrome was reported in a person returning to France from Thailand with cutaneous larva migrans (Del Giudice *et al.* 2002).

The larvae in people who have suffered from cutaneous larva migrans and have not received treatment may possibly persist in muscle tissues as has been shown to occur in the paratenic hosts. In guinea pigs, larvae of *A. caninum* were recovered from skeletal muscle three years after infection, and larvae were recovered from swine belly fat 6 months after infection (Stone *et al.* 1979). In one human case where serial sections of a muscle biopsy was examined from a person three months after presenting with cutaneous larva migrans, a larva was found in the tissue (Little *et al.* 1983).

Human cases of cutaneous larva migrans are being reported most commonly at this time in travellers returning from areas where *A. braziliense* occurs. Thus, the cases are presented very typically to physicians specializing in tropical or traveller medicine. These cases are reported from around the world, but typically represent cases wherein people have returned home from an area where *A. braziliense* is known to be present (Biolcati and Alabiso 1997; Hochedez and Caumes 2007; Jensenius *et al.* 2008; Park *et al.* 2001; Prudhomme *et al.* 2002; Rivera-Roig *et al.* 2008; Senba *et al.* 2009; Veraldi and Arancio 2006). Fortunately, this is not a life threatening infection, but for a number of individuals, vacations are turned into tribulations. The problem is basically one of stray dogs and cats having access to beaches.

Treatment of cutaneous larva migrans can be quite successful. Cases are now treated with albendazole or ivermectin (Caumes *et al.* 1993; Hochedez and Caumes 2007; Senba *et al.* 2009), although thiabendazole is still used occasionally with very gratifying outcomes (Gourioto *et al.* 2001). In athletes, such as beach volleyball players, the concern is that the lesions can reduce performance and ability to enter competitions (Biolcati and Alabiso 1997).

The hookworm species in the dog and cat

It is the hookworms of the canine and feline companion animals that are most often associated with zoonotic hookworm disease. The hookworms commonly found in dogs are: *Ancylostoma caninum, A. braziliense, A. ceylanicum,* and *Uncinaria stenocephala.* The hookworms commonly found as adults in cats are: *Ancylostoma tubaeforme, A. braziliense, A. ceylanicum,* and *U. stenocephala.* However, *U. stenocephlala* rarely occurs in cats in the USA (Bowman *et al.* 2001). Except for *A. ceylanicum,* a species found in India and Southeast Asia, the parasites generally do not complete their life cycles in the human host (Beaver *et al.* 1984).

Hookworm life cycle and pathogenicity in the typical definitive host

The life of a hookworm begins with first-stage larvae hatching from eggs passed in the host's faeces. Eggs are not immediately infective but must first develop from the morula stage. There is then a period of development of the microbiverous larva in the soil to the infective, non-feeding third-stage larva. In the dog and cat hookworm larvae from the Ancylostomatidae branch enter the host mainly through skin penetration. However in the case of *Uncinaria stenocephala* and other members of the Bunostomidae the larvae are more likely to utilize oral infection of hosts (Anderson 2000).

After infective larvae enter the host, in adult dogs, a large proportion of *A. caninum* infective larvae undergo somatic migration and sequester in the tissues to be reactivated later, typically during lactation. Thus, puppies are often infected via the milk by the transmammary route. Transmammary infection does not routinely occur with other species such as *U. stenocephala, A. tubaeforme, A. ceylanicum,* and *A. braziliense.*

Hookworms of carnivores utilize paratenic hosts. The *Ancylostoma* spp. of dogs and cats are capable of being sequestered in the tissues of vertebrate paratenic hosts where they persist without any development, thus infection via hunting is a possibility with these species. It has also been shown that *A. caninum* is capable of persisting in the tissues of cockroaches and other insects, which probably aids in their reaching the tissues of paratenic hosts like rodents that are more likely to be eaten by the carnivorous final hosts.

Several species of the canine and feline hookworms cause significant blood loss into the intestine of the hosts, i.e. *A. caninum, A. tubaeforme, A. ceylanicum*. The blood loss due to the adult worms in the dog and cat (and people) can lead to hookworm associated disease related to anaemia. Peracute and acute disease from blood loss is particularly important and sometimes fatal in young puppies and kittens. Other hookworms such as *Uncinaria* and *A. braziliense* cause negligible blood loss (Miller 1971).

Zoonotic hookworm infection

Ancylostoma ceylanicum and intestinal infection in humans

A. ceylanicum is an infection that humans can share with dogs and cats. The infection is induced by larvae penetrating the skin. The lesions that develop at the penetration site resemble those of ground itch rather than those of *A. braziliense* induced cutaneous larva migrans (Bearup 1967; Haydon and Bearup 1963; Maplestone 1933; Wijers and Smit 1966). There is pain associated with the infection during the period when the adults first appear in the intestinal tract following an infection (Carrol and Grove 1986; Wijers and Smit 1966). In most people infected with *A. ceylanicum*, the infections are short lived and produce few if any eggs after the worms develop to adulthood (Chowdhury and Schad 1972; Carroll and Grove 1986). However, in New Guinea, people are infected with large numbers of these worms and develop anaemia from the infections (Anten and Zuidema 1964). Treatment of these infections is the same as for other intestinal dwelling hookworms of people.

A. caninum and eosinophilic enteritis

Several cases of eosinophilic enteritis have been attributed to infection with *A. caninum*, presumably following exposure to contaminated soil with infective larvae. Patients presented with mild to severe enteritis, abdominal pain, and peripheral eosinophilia as well as eosinophilic infiltration of the bowel wall. In some patients, immature adult *A. caninum* worms were found in the bowel lumen, indicating complete migration and attempted maturation within the gut (Croese *et al.* 1994a). Most reports of this infection have occurred in north-eastern Australia, where more than 200 cases were diagnosed clinically and serologically over a period of 4 years (Croese *et al.* 1994a, b). In these cases, solitary and immature adult hookworms were found in only 15 patients and identified as *A. caninum* in nine. Most of the cases had eosinophilic enteritis, but one was entirely asymptomatic.

In an attempt to reproduce the disease in a human volunteer, infections with *A. caninum* have been attempted (Langmann and Prociv 2003). In this study, a human volunteer was infected with small numbers of infective larvae that were administered orally and percutaneously to an informed healthy volunteer under medical supervision, over a period of a year. The volunteer was examined regularly for symptoms and weekly for blood eosinophil counts and the presence of eggs in the faeces by microscopy. The patient developed a marked blood eosinophilia followed a single oral exposure to 100 infective larvae, while faecal examination remained negative. Eosinophil counts then declined gradually, although a rapid, spontaneous rise several months later, at the beginning of the next spring did occur. Blood eosinophil numbers did not rise significantly after a secondary percutaneous infection with 200 larvae.

However, a subsequent, smaller, oral inoculum of 20 larvae provoked an eosinophil response similar to that of the first oral infection. It was concluded that following ingestion of larvae that some developed directly into adult worms in the human gut (as they do in dogs) and that the percutaneous route of exposure, while being the most common means of human exposure, leads mainly to subclinical infections, and that oral exposure might be the means of the induction of the symptoms of eosinophilic enteritis. Other studies in people have utilized percutaneous infections with *A. caninum*, and in the case of heavy exposure, perhaps with thousands of larvae, there was the induction of numerous papules and pustules, with some being accompanied with short, migratory tracts that can recur at variable intervals and widely separated sites, for up to 7 months (Hunter and Worth 1945; Miller *et al.* 1991). The application of *A. caninum* larvae to human skin have thus routinely failed to induce lesions similar to the continuous, intermittently migratory creeping eruptions of *A. braziliense*.

With the experimental infection of a human with oral *A. caninum* larvae (Langmann and Prociv 2003), the presentation of eosinophil enteritis remains variable and difficult to impossible to diagnose. The typical manifestations include recurrent abdominal pain. Severe cases have presented with an acute abdomen, sometimes with distal small bowel obstruction, with little choice but surgical intervention. In most cases, there is peripheral blood eosinophilia, but it may be absent in the early acute phase (Croese *et al.* 1990). Also, high serum IgE levels are a common non-specific feature. Radiographs may reveal, with and without contrast studies, small bowel thickening and obstruction.

In cases where laparotomies have been performed, they have revealed inflamed segments of distal ileum, varying in length from 2 to 100 cm, with intense serositis and, sometimes, turbid (eosinophilic) ascites. Occasionally, the colon, caecum and appendix are involved. Other patients will develop milder, intermittent, or chronic patterns of illness, which can persist for years. Occult or frank intestinal blood loss can occur, and presentation in these cases may be precipitated by rectal bleeding. Colonoscopy often reveals focal inflammation and or ulceration of the terminal ileum and colon. In subclinical, or chronic cases, small aphthous-like ulcers of the ileal and caecal mucosa suggest hookworm attachment site lesions (Croese *et al.* 1996). In most cases, symptoms are not severe enough to justify surgery or colonoscopy, but blood eosinophilia does suggest the diagnosis.

The histopathology of canine hookworm enteritis is described in detail elsewhere (Walker *et al.* 1995). The ileal segment may appear grossly inflamed and oedematous, and all layers of its wall may be heavily infiltrated with eosinophils. This undoubtedly represents a true allergic response, in people sensitized to secretory products of developing third- or fourth-stage larvae or adult worms. It seems unrelated to the intensity of exposure, although eosinophil enteritis has not yet been diagnosed in a patient known to have been exposed to large numbers of third-stage larvae. In not one case has there been evidence of preceding cutaneous larva migrans of Loeffler's syndrome.

Patent human infection with *A. caninum* has never been documented, making the diagnosis of eosinophilic enteritis very difficult, in the absence of a worm or a tissue specimen. Among patients with confirmed eosinophilic enteritis, or who have typical clinical features and blood eosinophilia, 70% have circulating IgG and IgE antibodies to adult *A. caninum* excretory-secretory antigens

(ES Ags) demonstrable by ELISA. In the city of Townsville, 30% of patients who complain of non-specific, recurrent abdominal pain but do not have blood eosinophilia are seropositive, compared with 8% of healthy controls (Croese *et al.* 1994a). A Western blot using ES antigens of *A. caninum* is more sensitive and specific than the ELISA; more than 80% of patients with eosinophilic enteritis demonstrate antibodies to a protein fraction of molecular weight 68 kDa (Ac68). Detection of specific IgG4 antibodies by immunoblot may be even more sensitive and specific (Loukas *et al.* 1996). However it is premature to incriminate Ac68 as the putative allergen, for the correlation between disease severity and specific antibody levels is poor.

One of the strongest IgE responses, both in Elisa and immunoblot, was from an asymptomatic man with a solitary adult *A. caninum*, whereas a woman with florid eosinophilic enteritis and a worm *in situ* was seronegative (Croese *et al.* 1994b). Monoclonal antibody studies indicate that Ac68 originates from the excretory glands of adult *A. caninum*, whereas sera from patients often bind more strongly to amphidial gland cytoplasm, suggesting that another molecule is allergenic (Sawangjaroen *et al.* 1995).

Hookworm eosinophilic enteritis can be diagnosed only if clinicians are aware of the disease. The histopathological diagnosis is confirmed by examining biopsy material, but rarely is a worm found to establish the etiology. Furthermore, even experienced pathologists can overlook the small, inconspicuous parasite embedded between oedematous mucosal folds (Walker *et al.* 1995). Present serology is neither adequately sensitive not specific for diagnosis acute cases, and the surgeon may not be able to await test results. Nether the ELISA nor Western blot distinguishes infections with *A. caninum* from those with anthropophilic hookworms (which can be diagnosed coprologically).

Treatment is simple: a single 300 mg dose of mebendazole usually brings about a dramatic resolution of symptoms within 24 hours. In fact, failure of response suggests a mistaken diagnosis. A smaller dose, or another anthelminthic, such as pyrantel, may also prove to be effective, but has not been clinically trialled. Having anti-inflammatory and anti-eosinophil activity, corticosteroids also rapidly suppress the symptoms, but are less specific in their action than anthelminthics. Many patients relapse, weeks or months later, apparently without re-exposure, to infection. This, and the seasonal incidence of eosinophilic enteritis (Croese 1995) suggest that sporadic activation of dormant larvae underlies the intermittent appearance of immature adult worms in the gut, but currently available anthelminthics are unlikely to eradicate hypobiotic third-stage larvae sequestered within muscle fibres.

There are a few other reports from outside Australia where hookworms suspected of being *A. caninum* were associated with eosinophilic enteritis (Khooshoo *et al.* 1994, 1995; Bahgat *et al.* 1999). Two reports occurred in New Orleans, LA, USA, but there have since been no additional reports from the USA. In the one other report, out of 95 patients within Egypt with eosinophilic enteritis and unexplained abdominal pain with peripheral eosinophilia, 11 patients were considered as being potentially infected with *A. caninum* on the basis of serotesting by IgG ELISA to detect antibodies to excretory/secretory (ES) antigens of adult *A. caninum* and by IgG and IgG4 Western blot (W.B.) to detect antibodies to Ac68 antigen. The 11 patients presented with acute abdomen (5), appendicitis (3), or recurrent mild to moderate abdominal pain (3). In other patients in this study with human hookworms, there was cross reaction in the antibody tests used and the only differential for the *A. caninum* suspected cases was the lack of hookworm eggs present in the stools.

Hookworm larvae and unilateral subacute neuroretinitis

Hookworm larvae are suspected, along with *Toxocara spp.*, *Baylisascaris spp.*, and possibly some other yet unidentified small nematode larvae, as a possible cause diffuse unilateral sub-acute neuroretinitis, a form of ocular larva migrans, which can lead to loss of vision, inflammation in the posterior eye, and retinal lesions. Two different size ranges of nematode larvae have been observed in the affected eyes of patients with diffuse unilateral subacute neuroretinitis; based on the size of observed larvae in some cases, *A. caninum* is considered a likely cause, along with *Toxocara* spp. and *Baylisascaris procyonis* (Goldberg *et al.* 1993; Sabrosa *et al.* 2001). As of yet, such infections have not been demonstrated by larval isolation as specifically being due to the larvae of zoonotic hookworms.

Atypical zoonotic infections with hookworms

There have been a number of reports of hookworms in people that have been due to hookworms that usually do not appear to cause disease in humans. These include *Necator suillus*, *Cyclodontostomum purvisi*, *Ancylostoma malayanum*, *Bunostomum phlebotomum*, and *Uncinaria stenocephala*.

Necator suillus Ackerrt and Payne, 1922, found in Trinidad and Central America, is a porcine hookworm very similar to *N. americanus*. While the latter does not develop in pigs, it probably evolved from *N. suillus* (Schad 1991) and its third-stage larvae can invade pig skin to cause ground itch (Ackert and Payne 1923). Buckley (1933) cultured eggs from adult *N. suillus* and infected himself percutaneously. Lesions developed at the entry site, and 54 days later, hookworm eggs appeared in his stools. Infection remained patent for four months, until treatment with oil of chenopodium expelled three adult *N. suillus*. He did not report abdominal symptoms, but speculated that this species may account for some presumed *N. americanus* infections in people living close to pigs.

Cylclodontostomum purvisi (Adams, 1933) is a parasite of the large intestine of rats in southeast Asia. Two adult specimens, a male and female, were found incidentally in the faeces of a 47 year old man in Thailand (Bhaibulaya and Indragarm 1975). No clinical significance could be attached to this case.

Ancylstoma malayanum (Alessandrini, 1905) infects bears in India and southeast Asia, and has a buccal capsule like that of *A. duodenale*. It is the largest member of the genus, with males growing to 15 mm and females to 19 mm. One case of human infection has been reported (Beaver *et al.* 1984).

Bunostomum phlebotomum occurs in cattle and related ungulates in most warm and temperate regions (Soulsby 1982; Anderson 2000), and can cause human cutaneous infection (Mayhew 1947).

Uncinaria stenocephala was reported as being able to cause percutaneous infection by Fülleborn in 1927 (Grove 1990).

Cases of cutaneous larva migrans have described in recent years from the UK, Germany, and Italy, but the agent(s) have not been clearly elucidated. One case in Great Britain was a 50 year old man who presented with a rash after paint-balling 3 weeks previously during the month of October (Diba *et al.* 2004). He had stored his fatigues in a shed where a dog was kept. Eight days after the event, there were approximately 40 lesions on the medial surface of his left forearm and his abdomen. He then noticed multiple itchy thread-like eruptions emanating from the marks, which also seemed to have shifted location. There was no recent history of travel abroad, but he had travelled to Sri Lanka 3 years previously. A biopsy did not reveal any hookworm larvae, but he did respond to treatment with oral albendazole at 400 mg twice a day for 5 days. It was assumed that the infection was due to *U. stenocephala* due to the lack of *A. caninum* in the area.

Two other cases of cutaneous larva migrans have been reported in the UK, both lesions appeared on the buttocks of individuals and have responded to therapy with either albendazole of ivermectin. There was also a report of cutaneous larva migrans acquired autochthonously in Germany (Klose *et al*. 1996) and cases from Italy (Albanese *et al*. 1995; Galanti *et al*. 2002) that included 6 persons that were infected with an association with potting soil used in flower arrangements. There have been 3 cases of autochthonous cutaneous larva migrans acquired in New Zealand, two in children in the northern town of Kaitaia and one in an 80 year old lady gardener in Christchurch (Bradley 1999; Manning *et al*. 2006). New Zealand is not known to have any *A. braziliense*, has only rare infections with *A. caninum* that was first observed in the country in 1976.

Epidemiology

Hookworms have been introduced with pet dogs and cats into areas that span the globe along with their hosts. Thus, the most common canine and feline hookworms, *A. caninum* and *A. tubaeforme*, respectively, occur to some extent in most areas where cats are found. Interestingly, both *A. braziliense* and *A. ceylanicum* which are capable of infecting both dogs and cats have a more limited geographical distribution than *A. caninum* and *A. tubaeforme*. *U. stenocephala* has a range that extends into colder climates than the *Ancylostoma* species, appears capable of infecting cats and dogs, has an egg that is morphologically distinguishable from that of the members of the genus *Ancylostoma*, but has a distribution that is more poorly described than that of the *Ancylostoma* species.

Ancylostoma braziliense

This is a parasite of dogs and cats that also occurs is various wild canids and felids. The geographic distribution of this parasite was recently re-examined relative to its presence around the world with the application of both morphologic and genetic methods (Traub *et al*. 2007). This species has been reported along the eastern Atlantic and Gulf coast of the USA, through the Caribbean islands, and on the east coast of Mexico into Surinam, Brazil, and Uruguay. In Asia, *A. braziliense* appears restricted to the south below latitude 10°N, being reported from Malaysia and Indonesia. The number of cases of cutaneous larva migrans in vacationers from Thailand would indicate that this worm is also highly prevalent in this country.

Ancylostoma ceylanicum

Again, a recent re-examination of the geographical distribution of this parasite of dogs and cats and wild relatives is reported from India, Taiwan, central Thailand, Malaysia, Borneo, Indonesia, and Surinam in South America with older reports of this worm in Papua New Guinea (Traub *et al*. 2007).

Ancylostoma caninum

This is a parasite of dogs and related canids and is present throughout most of the world where dogs are found. It is the most common of the canine parasites and also occurs frequently in wildlife species.

Ancylostoma tubaeforme

This is the common hookworm parasite of the cat and related felids around the world. This parasite has a worldwide distribution amongst felines around the world.

Uncinaria stenocephala

This parasite is common in dogs and foxes. It occurs in cats, but reports in naturally infected cats are fairly uncommon. It is considered to be a parasite that occurs in more temperature or cooler climates than the *Ancylostoma* species. It has been reported in the western hemisphere from Canada through Mexico into the northern countries in South America. It has been reported in northern Eurasia and around the Mediterranean (Bowman *et al*. 2001)

Control and prevention

Control and prevention of the transfer of infections with these pathogens from dogs and cats to people requires diligence on three fronts: minimization of the reservoir populations, control of the parasites in the companion animal population, and sanitation to protect public areas from faecal contamination.

There are massive efforts around the world to now reduce the number of unwanted and stray dogs and cats through a multitude of programs that rely strongly on spay and neuter programs. In some cases more draconian programs are used.

Parasite control in companion animals is having a marked effect on the parasites in well-cared for pets relative to the parasites present in shelter animals. Examination of shelter animals in the USA has shown that there are very high numbers of parasites prevalent in these hosts with 19.19% of shelter dogs and 11% of shelter cats having *Ancylostoma* spp. infections and the current prevalence in shelter dogs remaining similar in a second survey 10 years later (Blagburn *et al*. 1996; Blagburn personal communication) based on results from about 2/3 of the 10,000 target animal faecal samples from around the USA. Similar numbers for dogs seeing veterinarians was 4.5% for animals on their first visit (Mohamed *et al*. 2009). Thus, routine veterinary care seems to be capable of minimizing the risk of parasites being present in pets.

Veterinarians are taking a more and more active role in reducing pet infections for the purpose of protecting health and protecting the human animal bond through the minimization of zoonotic risk to client's from the pets under the veterinarian's care. In the USA this program has been helped by an interest in the Centers of Disease Control and Prevention in by informing the public as to the risk that these infections may bring and means of their control through proper veterinary attention. It seems that this is making a difference in the number of parasites in pets, and this is a major means of preventing environmental contamination.

The control of faecal waste material and limiting access to pets where faecal deposition can affect public health varies with community interest. However, it is a program that is gaining in the public's awareness. It is becoming more and more common for people to protect their own welfare and that of children through the proper management of dog and cat excrement. In the case of cutaneous larva migrans, a very large number of cases are associated with beaches, and this means that targeted control may be able to have a major positive outcome without the need to target the whole community.

Finally, there is the matter of wildlife. It seems highly unlikely that it will be possible to institute any significant control measures for wildlife reservoir hosts. However, it depends on the extent of the problem and the will of those involved. However, the process will probably involve the management of pets, then strays, and finally wildlife if the latter occurs at all.

People also need to have significant education as to how to protect themselves from these risks and to minimize the potential risks of others through the covering of sand filled play areas, laws limiting faecal deposition by pets, and the risk of contraction cutaneous larva migrans when on the beach. In discussions with Thai veterinarians, they feel that there are very few cases of cutaneous larva migrans in locals within Thailand while there are many in visitors to Thailand. This may be because local people are less likely to put themselves at risk lounging in areas where the larvae are liable to be prevalent.

Conclusions

Zoonotic hookworm infections appear to still be occurring throughout the world. Currently, the two major areas of increased incidence seems to be in cases amongst tourists from high income countries following visits to beach resorts that have *A. braziliense* present in the canine and feline population and in people who are somehow at risk of developing eosinophilic colitis due to *A. caninum*. It would seem that both these outcomes can be minimized through education, awareness, improved sanitation and targeted treatment of the animals that put people at risk.

The development of methods that will allow the determination of species present in a dog or cat through the characterization of faeces with molecular methods is going to provide a means of better delineating where the offending agents are in the world. Also, they may reach a point at sometime in the future where individual larvae if recovered in biopsies or biopsy sections will be able to be identified to actually verify the agents that are causing the observed lesions in people.

References

Ackert, J.E., and Payne, F.K. (1923). Investigations of the control of hookworm disease. XII. Studies of the occurrence, distribution, and morphology of *Necator suillus*, including descriptions of the other species of *Necator. Am. J. Hyg.*, **3**: 1–25.

Albanese, G., Di Cintio, R., Beneggi, M., *et al.* (1995). Larva migrans in Italy. *Int. J. Dermat.*, **34**: 464–65.

Anderson, R.C. (2000). *Nematode Parasites of Vertebrates: Their Development and Transmission*, (2nd edn.). Oxford: CABI.

Anten, J.F.G. and Zuidema, P.J. (1964). Hookworm infection in Dutch serviceman returning from West New Guinea. *Trop. Geograph. Med.*, **16**: 216–24.

Bahgat, M.A., El Gindy, A.E., Mahmoud, L.A., *et al.* (1999). Evaluation of the role of *Ancylostoma caninum* in humans as a cause of acute and recurrent abdominal pain. *J. Egypt. Soc. Parasit.,* **29**: 873–82.

Bearup, A.J. (1967). Correspondence: *A. braziliense. Trop. Geograph. Med.*, **19**: 161–62.

Beattie, P.E., and Fleming, C.J. (2002). Cutaneous larva migrans in the west coast of Scotland. *Clin. Experim. Dermat.*, **27**: 248–49.

Beaver, P.C. (1956). The record of *Ancylostoma braziliense* as an intestinal parasite of man in North America. *Am. J. Trop. Med. Hyg.*, **5**: 737–89.

Beaver, P.C., Jung, R.C., and Cupp, E.W. (1984). *Clinical Parasitology*. Philadelphia: Lea and Febiger.

Bhaibulaya, M. and Indragarm, S. (1975). Man, an accidental host of *Cyclodonostomum purvisi* (Adams, 1933), and the occurrence in rats in Thailand. *Southeast Asian J. Trop. Med. Pub. Health*, **6**: 391–94.

Biolcati, G., and Alabiso, A. (1997). Creeping eruption of larva migrans—a case report in a beach volley athlete. *Int. J. Sports Med.*, **18**: 612–13.

Biocca, E. (1951). On *Ancylostoma braziliense* and its morphological differentiation from *Ancylostoma ceylanicum. J. Helminthol.*, **25**: 1–10.

Blagburn, B.L., Lindsay, D.S., Vaughan, J.L., *et al.* (1996). Prevalence of canine parasites based on fecal flotation. *Comp. Cont. Educ. Pract. Vet.*, **18**: 483–509.

Bowman, D.D., Hendrix, C.M., Lindsay, D.S., and Barr, S.C. (2002). *Feline clinical parasitology*. Ames, Iowa: Iowa State University Press.

Bradley J. (1999). Home-grown cutaneous larva migrans. *N. Zealand Med. J.*, **112**: 241–42.

Carrol, S.M. and Grove, D.I. (1986). Experimental infedtion of humans with Ancylostoma ceylanicum: a model of human hookworm infection. *J. Infect. Dis.*, **150**: 284–94.

Caumes, E., Carrfiere, J., Datry, A., Gaxotte, P., *et al.* (1993). A randomized trial of ivermectin versus albendazole for the treatment of cutaneous larva migrans. *Am. J. Trop. Med. Hyg.*, **49**: 641–44.

Chowdhury, A.B. and Schad, G.A. (1972). *Ancylostoma ceylanicum*: a parasite of man in Calcutta and environs. *Am. J. Trop. Med. Hyg.*, **21**: 300–301.

Croese, J. (1995). Seasonal influence on human enteric infection with *Ancylostoma caninum. Am. J. Trop. Med. Hyg.*, **53**: 158–61.

Croese, J., Prociv, P., Maguire, E., and Crawford, A. (1990). Eosinohilic enteritis presenting as surgical emergencies: a report of six cases. *Med. J. Aust.*, **153**: 415–17.

Croese, J., Loukas, A., Opdebeeck, J., and Prociv, P. (1994a). Occult enteric infection by *Ancylostoma caninum*: a previously unrecognized zoonosis. *Gasteroenterology*, **106**: 3–13.

Croese, J., Loukas, S., Opdebeeck, J., Gariley, S., and Prociv, P. (1994b). Human eneteric infection with canine hookworms: an emerging problem in developed communities. *Ann. Internal Med.*, **120**: 369–74.

Croese, J., Fairley, S., Loukas, A., Hack, J., and Stonach, P. (1996). Ileal ulceration: and index of cryptic infection by *Ancylostoma caninum. Gasteroenter. Hepat.*, **11**: 524–31.

Del Giudice, P., Desalvador, F., Bernard, E., *et al.* (2002). Loeffler's syndrome and cutaneous larva migrans: a rare association. *Br. J. Dermat.*, **147**: 386–88.

Diba, V.C., Whitty, C.J., and Green, T. (2004). Cutaneous larva migrans acquired in Britain. *Clin. Experim. Dermat.*, **29**: 555–56.

Fuller, C.E. (1966). A common source outbreak of cutaneous larva migrans. *Pub. Health Rep.*, **81**: 186–90.

Galanti, B., Frusco, F.M., and Nardiello, S. (2002). Outbreak of cutaneous larva migrans in Naples, southern Italy. *Trans. R. Soc. Trop. Med. Hyg.*, **96**: 491–92.

Goldberg, M.A., Kazacos, K.R., Boyce, W.M., Ai, E., and Katz, B. (1993). Diffuse unilateral subacute neuroretinitis: morphometric, serologic, and epidemiologic support for *Baylisascaris* as a causative agent. *Ophthalmology,* **100**: 1695–1701.

Gourgiotou, K., Nicolaidou, E., *et al.* (2001). Treatment of widespread cutaneous larva migrans with thiabendazole. *Eur. Acad. Dermat. Venereol.*, **15**: 578–80.

Grove, D.I. (1990). *A history of helminthology.* Oxford: CAB International.

Hayden, G.A.M. and Bearup, A.J. (1963). *Ancylostoma braziliense* and *Ancylostoma ceylanicum. Trans. R. Soc. Trop. Med. Hyg.,* **57**: 76.

Hochedez, P. and Caumes, E. (2007). Hookworm-related cutaneous larva migrans. *J. Travel Med.,* **14**: 326–33.

Hunter, G.W. and Worth, C.B. (1945). Variations in response to filariform larvae of *Ancylostoma caninum* in the skin of man. *J. Parasitol.,* **31**: 366–72.

Jensenius, M., Maeland, A., and Brubakk, O. (2008). Extensive hookworm-related cutaneous larva migrans in Norwegian travellers to the tropics. *Travel Med. Infect. Dis.,* **6**: 45–47.

Kalkofen, U.P. (1987). Hookworms of dogs and cats. *Vet. Clin. N. Am.: Small Anim. Pract.,* **17**: 1341–54.

Khooshoo, V., Schantz, P., Craver, R., *et al.* (1994). Dog hookworm: a cause of eosinophilic enterocolitis in humans. *J. Pediat. Gasteroenter. Nut.,* **19**: 448–52.

Khooshoo, V., Craver, R., Schantz, P., Loukas, A., and Prociv, P. (1995). Abdominal pain, pan-gut eosinophilia, and dog hookworm infection. *J. Pediat. Gastoenter. Nut.,* **21**: 481.

Kirby-Smith, J.L., Dove, W.E., and White, G.E. (1926). Creeping eruption. *Arch. Dermat. Syphil.,* **13**: 137–75.

Klose, C., Mravak,. S., Geb, M., Bienzle, U., and Meyer, C.G. (1996). Autochthonous cutaneous larva migrans in Germany. *Trop. Med. Int. Health,* **1**: 503–4.

Langmann, J.K. and Prociv, P. (2003). Experimental human infection with the dog hookworm, *Ancylostoma caninum. Med. J. Aust.,* **178**: 69–71.

Little, M.D., Halsey, N.A., Cline, B.L., and Katz, S.P. (1983). *Ancylostoma* larva in muscle fiber of man following cutaneous larva migrans. *Am. J. Trop. Med. Hyg.,* **32**: 1285–88.

Looss, A. (1905). The anatomy and life history of *Achylostoma duodenale* Dub. *A monograph. Records of the Egyptian Government School of Medicine,* Vol III. National Printing Department, Cairo.

Looss, A. (1911). The anatomy and life history of *Agchylostoma duodenale* Dub. *A monograph. Records of the Egyptian Government School of Medicine,* Vol IV. National Printing Department, Cairo.

Loukas, A., Croese, J., Opdebeeck, J., and Prociv, P. (1992). Detection of antibodies to secretions of *Ancylostoma caninum* in human eosinophilic enteritis. *Trans. R. Soc. Trop. Med. Hyg.,* **86**: 650–53.

Manning, L., Chambers, S., Paltridge, G., and Maurice, P. (2006). Cutaneous larva migrans (hookworm) acquired in Christchurch, New Zealand. *N. Zealand Med. J.,* **119**(**1231**): 1–4.

Maplestone, P.A. (1933). Creeping eruption produced by hookworm larvae. *Indian Med. Gaz.,* **68**: 251–56.

Miller, T.A. (1971). Vaccination against the canine hookworm diseases. *Adv. Parasit.,* **9**: 153–83.

Mohamed, A.S., Moore, G. E. and Glickman, L.T. (2009). Prevalence of intestinal nematode parasitism among pet dogs in the United States (2003-2006). *J. Am. Vet. Med. Ass.,* **234**: 631–37.

Muhleisen, J.P. (1953). Demonstration of pulmonary migration of the causative agent of creeping eruption. *Ann. Internal Med.,* **38**: 595–600.

O'Connell, E., Suarez, J., Leguen, F., *et al.* (2007). Outbreak of cutaneous larva migrans at a children's camp–Miami, Florida, 2006. *Morb. Mort. Wkly. Rep.,* **56**: 1285–87.

Park, J.W., Kwon, S.J., and Ryu, J.S., *et al.* (2001). Two imported cases of cutaneous larva migrans. *Korean J. Parasitol.,* **39**: 77–81.

Prudhomme, H., Loche, F., Massip, P., and Marchou, B. (2002). Larva migrans cutanée: échect de l'ivermectine en dose unique. *Méd. Malad. Infectieuses,* **32**: 115–18.

Rivera-Roig, V., Sánchez, J.L., and Hillyer, G.V. (2008). Hookworm folliculitis. *Int. J. Dermat.,* **47**: 246–48.

Roest, M. and Ratnavel, R. (2001). Cutaneous larva migrans contracted in England: a reminder. *Clin. Experim. Dermat.,* **26**: 389–90.

Sabrosa, N.A. and Cunha de Souza, E. (2001). Nematode infections of the eye: toxocariasis and diffuse unilateral subacute neuroretinitis. *Curr. Opin. Ophthalm.,* **12**: 450–54.

Sawangjaroen, N., Opdebeeck, J.P., and Prociv, P. (1995). Imunohistochemical localization of excretory/secretory antigens in adult *Ancylostoma caninum* using monoclonal antibodies and infected human sera. *Exp. Parasit.,* **17**: 29–35.

Schad, G.A. (1991). The parasite. In: H.M. Gilles and P.A.J. Ball (eds.) *Hookworm infections, human parasitic disease,* Vol. 4, pp. 15–49. Amsterdam: Elsevier Science Publishers.

Senba, Y., Tsuda, K., Maruyama, H., *et al.* (2009). Case of creeping disease treated with ivermectin. *J. Dermatol.,* **36**: 86–89.

Smith, C.A. (1904). Uncinasriasis in the South, with special reference to mode of infection. *J. Am. Med. Ass.,* **91**: 608–9.

Soulsby, E.J.L. (1982). *Helminths, arthropods and protozoa of domesticated animals* (7th edn). London: Bailliere Tindall.

Stone, W.M., Stewart, T.B., and Smith, F. (1979). Infectivity of *Ancylostoma caninum* larvae from canine milk. *Am. J. Vet. Res.,* **31**: 1693–94.

Traub, R.J., Hobbs, R.P., Adams, P.J., *et al.* (2007). A case of mistaken identity–reappraisal of the species of canid and felid hookworms (*Ancylostoma*) present in Australia and India. *Parasit.,* **134**: 113–19.

Veraldi, S. and Arancio, L. (2006). Giant bullous cutaneous larva migrans. *Clin. Experim. Dermat.,* **31**: 613–14.

Walker, M.J., Croese, J., Loukas, A., Clouston, A., and Prociv, P. (1995). Eosinophilic enteritis in north-eastern Australia: pathology, association with *Ancylostoma caninum* and implications. *Am. J. Surg. Pathol.,* **19**: 328–37.

White, G.F. and Dove, W.E. (1928). The causation of creeping eruption. *J. Am. Med. Ass.,* **90**: 1701–4.

Wijers, D.O., and Smit, A.M. (1966). Early symptoms after experimental infection of man with *Ancylostoma braziliense* var. *ceylanicum. Trop. Geograph. Med.,* **18**: 48–52.

Wright, D.O. and Gold, E.M. (1946). Löffler's syndrome associated with creeping eruption (cutaneous helminthiasis): report of twenty-six cases. *Arch. Internal Med.,* **78**: 303–12.

CHAPTER 63

Anisakiosis (Anisakidosis)

Woon-Mok Sohn and Jong-Yil Chai

Summary

The term 'anisakiosis (anisakidosis)' or 'anisakiasis' collectively defines human infections caused by larval anisakids belonging to the nematode family Anisakidae or Raphidascarididae. *Anisakis simplex, Anisakis physeteris,* and *Pseudoteranova decipiens* are the three major species causing human anisakiosis. Various kinds of marine fish and cephalopods serve as the second intermediate hosts and the infection source. Ingestion of viable anisakid larvae in the fillet or viscera of these hosts is the primary cause of infection. The parasite does not develop further in humans as they are an accidental host. Clinical anisakiosis develops after the penetration of anisakid larvae into the mucosal wall of the alimentary tract, most frequently the stomach and the small intestine. The affected sites undergo erosion, ulceration, swelling, inflammation, and granuloma formation around the worm. The patients may suffer from acute abdominal pain, indigestion, nausea, vomiting, and in some instances, allergic hypersensitive reactions. Symptoms in gastric anisakiosis often resemble those seen in peptic ulcer or gastric cancer, and symptoms in intestinal anisakiosis resemble those of appendicitis or peritonitis. Treatments include removal of larval worms using a gastroendoscopic clipper or surgical resection of the mucosal tissue surrounding the worm. No confirmed effective anthelmintic drug has been introduced, though albendazole and ivermectin have been tried *in vivo* and *in vitro*. Prevention of human anisakiosis can be achieved by careful examination of fish fillet followed by removal of the worms in the restaurant or household kitchen. Immediate freezing of fish and cephalopods just after catching them on fishing boats was reported helpful for prevention of anisakiosis. It is noteworthy that anisakiosis is often associated with strong allergic and hypersensitivity reactions, with symptoms ranging from isolated angioedema to urticaria and life threatening anaphylactic shock.

Introduction

Anisakiosis is a food-borne parasitic zoonoses seen especially in localities where people have a custom of eating raw marine fish and squids, as dishes of *sushi, sashimi, ceviche,* or *lomi-lomi* (Sakanari and McKerrow 1989; Chai *et al.* 2005). Several ascaridoid (4 anisakid, 1 raphidascarid, and 1 toxocarid) species have been reported from human infections (Beaver *et al.* 1984; Garcia 2007; Fumarola *et al.* 2009); however, two anisakid genera, *Anisakis* and *Pseudoterranova,* are most frequently involved. Humans are accidental hosts, whereas marine mammals (dolphins, porpoises, whales, seals, sea lions, and walruses), fish, or birds are natural definitive hosts. Gastric, intestinal, or occasional extra-intestinal, anisakiosis occurs when people ingest third-stage larvae in the viscera or muscle of a wide range of marine fish or cephalopods (Chai *et al.* 2005). In acute cases, acute abdominal symptoms, including cramping pain, nausea, and vomiting, occur, and in chronic cases, symptoms, including intermittent epigastric tenderness, abdominal distention, and indigestion, occur.

Since the 1960s, when this disease was first discovered, increasing numbers of human cases have been recorded worldwide. The clinical importance of anisakiosis has also increased because allergy and hypersensitivity reactions are being attributed to anisakid larvae (Chai *et al.* 2005; Audicana and Kennedy 2008). In this review, the discovery and history of the disease; the causative agent, epidemiology, pathogenesis and clinical manifestations; and diagnosis, treatment, prevention and control of anisakiosis are briefly described.

Discovery and history of the disease

Prior to 1960, only two reports were available on the nematode family Anisakidae occurring in humans. Hitchcock (1950) first reported that 10% of 100 Eskimos examined in Alaska spontaneously expelled larval ascarid nematodes; one specimen among them was identified as *Porrocaecum* sp. (now considered to be *Pseudoterranova* sp.) and another was *Anisakis* sp. An immature *Porrocaecum* sp. worm (also now considered as *Pseudoterranova* sp.) was recovered from the mouth of a patient (Buckley 1951). In Japan, Otsuru *et al.* (1957) found that *Ascaris*-like nematode larvae provoked an intestinal disease different from those of the ordinary regional ileitis.

The concept of this zoonotic disease, now known as anisakiosis (= anisakidosis, anisakiasis, herring worm disease, or codworm disease), was first raised by van Thiel *et al.* (1960) reporting 11 patients in the Netherlands. A report of two such cases followed in England (Ashby *et al.* 1964). They found nematode larvae in eosinophilic lesions in the gastrointestinal tract of patients, who suffered from severe abdominal pain after eating salted herring. At that time, however, the causative agent was named erroneously as *Eustoma rotundatum* (van Thiel *et al.* 1960; Ashby *et al.* 1964). Asami *et al.* (1965) and Yokogawa and Yoshimura (1965) were the first who identified the causative nematode larvae as *Anisakis*-like larvae, and reported that their larvae were morphologically identical with those reported by van Thiel *et al.* (1960). The herring worm in the Netherlands was designated as the larva of *Anisakis marina* by van Thiel in 1966; however, it was later found to be synonym of *Anisakis simplex* (Davey 1971).

After these reports, anisakiosis has attracted considerable medical attention worldwide, including Japan, the Netherlands, the Republic of Korea, Spain, France, Italy, Germany, and the USA, and until now an estimated number of more than 50,000 human cases have been reported worldwide. Particularly in Japan, about 2,000 cases have been diagnosed annually by parasitological examinations (Chai *et al.* 2005; Fumarola *et al.* 2009). Now, anisakiosis is regarded as a serious zoonotic disease, and a dramatic increase in its prevalence is reported throughout the world during the last two or three decades (Chai *et al.* 2005).

An important event in relation to clinical aspects of anisakiosis was that since 1989–1990, it has been noted that *A. simplex* larvae are often associated with strong allergic responses, including anaphylactic shock (Kasuya *et al.* 1990; Audicana *et al.* 1995, 2002; Audicana and Kennedy 2008). These allergic responses were accompanied by elevated serum IgE levels against *A. simplex* antigen. Previous exposure to anisakid parasites and their antigens or allergens, either as living infection or by consumption of dead parasites in food fish, is considered as the main reason for the allergic reactions (Audicana and Kennedy 2008). The allergic symptoms were, however, provoked only in patients with current anisakid infection in the gastrointestinal tract (Alonso-Gomez *et al.* 2004).

Causative agent

Species causing human anisakiosis

The anisakid (including a few related raphidascarid and toxocarid species) nematodes of clinical importance so far known are *Anisakis simplex* (Rudolphi 1809) *sensu stricto*, *Anisakis pegreffii* Campana-Rouget and Biocca 1955, *Anisakis physeteris* Baylis 1923, *Pseudoterranova decipiens* (Krabbe 1878), *Contracaecum osculatum* (Rudolphi 1802), *Hysterothylacium aduncum* (Rudolphi 1802), and *Porrocaecum reticulatum* (Table 63.1) (Schaum and Müller 1967; Yagi *et al.* 1996; Garcia 2007; Umehara *et al.* 2007; Fumarola *et al.* 2009). The majority of human infections are caused by *A. simplex*, *A. physeteris*, and *P. decipiens*. In contrast, infections by *Contracaecum*, *Hysterothylacium*, and *Porrocaecum* are negligible because case reports attributed to these species are extremely rare.

The larvae of *A. simplex* (*Anisakis* type I larvae) are most frequently recovered from human cases worldwide (Audicana and Kennedy 2008). The larvae of *P. decipiens* (*Terranova* type A larvae) are less commonly found from humans (Seo *et al.* 1984; Sohn and Seol 1984; Oshima 1987; Ishikura and Namiki 1989). The larvae of *A. physeteris* (*Anisakis* type II larvae) are occasionally detected from human infections in Japan, Spain, and the Republic of Korea (Kagei *et al.* 1978; Claver *et al.* 1993; Im *et al.* 1995; Song *et al.* 1999; Yu *et al.* 2001).

Taxonomy

There have been debates in the taxonomy and nomenclature of ascaridoid nematodes (Smith and Wootten 1978; Gibson 1983; Mattiucci and Nascetti 2008; Iñiguez *et al.* 2009). It is now recognized that the superfamily Ascaridoidea contains more than 52 genera, among which several genera of medical and veterinary concern, and some of economic concern, are included (Mattiucci and Nascetti 2008). Recent molecular studies using mitochondrial DNA (mtDNA) and nuclear ribosomal DNA (rDNA) sequences provided provisional support for a monophyletic origin of the family Anisakidae, which includes the genera *Anisakis*, *Pseudoterranova*, and *Contracaecum* (plus *Phocascaris*) (Nadler and Hudspeth 2000; Nadler *et al.* 2005). *Hysterothylacium* is regarded as a member of the family Raphidascarididae, and *Porrocaecum* is included in the family Ascarididae (Fagerholm 1991; Fagerholm *et al.* 2004).

In the genus *Anisakis*, genetic studies using isozyme or PCR-RFLP analysis have revealed that at least 9 species are recognizable; (Mattiucci *et al.* 1997, 1998, 2005; Paggi *et al.* 1998; Pontes *et al.* 2005; D'Amelio *et al.* 2010).

A. simplex sensu stricto,

A. pegreffii,

A. simplex C Nascetti *et al.* 1986,

Table 63.1 Species of anisakid (= ascaridoid in strict sense) nematodes infecting humans* and natural definitive hosts†

Species	Type of larva (Koyama *et al.* 1969)	Major definitive host	Major infection source in human cases
Anisakis simple	*Anisakis* type I	blue-white dolphins, porpoises	sea eel, herring, mackerel, salmon
Anisakis physeteis	*Anisakis* type II	sperm whales	mackerel, moon fish, skipkach, bonito
Pseudoterranova decipiens	*Terranova* type A	seals, sealions, walruses	cod, halibut, greenling, rockfish, squid
Contracaecum osculatum	*Contracaecum* type B	fur seals	pollock, cod
Hysterothylacium aduncum	*Contracaecum* type A (?)	marine or freshwater fish	cod, salmon
Porrocaecum reticulatum	(?)	birds	(?)

* Garcia (2007).
† Oshima (1972, 1987), Yagi *et al.* (1996), Digiani and Sutton (2001).

A. typica (Diesing 1860),

A. ziphidarum (Paggi et al. 1998),

A. physeteris,

A. brevispiculata Dollfus 1968,

A. paggiae Mattiucci et al. 2005,
 Anisakis sp. A Pontes et al. 2005.

Two of them, A. simplex sensu lato (including A. pegreffi) and A. physeteris, are known to infect humans (Sakanari and Mckerrow 1989; Garcia 2007; Umehara et al. 2007; Fumarola et al. 2009).

Pseudoterranova decipiens (Krabbe 1878), known to infect humans, was originally described as Ascaris decipiens Krabbe 1878, which later became Porrocaecum decipiens Baylis and then Terranova decipiens Karokhin 1946 (Oshima 1987. Myers (1959) created a new genus Phocanema for this species, and proposed the name Phocanema decipiens. Before this, in 1951, the genus Pseudoterranova was erected by Mozgovoi for parasites from sperm whales (Mozgovoi 1953). Later, Gibson (1983) considered Phocanema as a synonym of Pseudoterranova, and began to use the name Pseudoterranova decipiens. Currently, at least 6 species are included in the genus Pseudoterranova; P. krabbei (Paggi et al. 2000), P. decipiens, P. bulbosa (Cobbold 1888) Mattiucci et al. 1998, P. azarasi (Yamaguti and Arima 1942) Mattiucci et al. 1998, P. cattani Geoge-Mascimento and Urrutia 2000, and P. decipiens E Bullini et al. 1997 (Mattiucci et al. 1998; Paggi et al. 2000; Mattiucci and Nascetti 2008). The validity of two other species, P. kogiae (Johnston and Mawson 1945) and P. ceticola (Deardoff and Overstreet 1981), is questioned (Mattiucci and Nascetti 2008).

The genus Contracaecum Railliet and Henry 1912 is big and presently contains more than 50 nominal species, most of which are adults in pinnipeds and fish-eating birds (Mattiucci and Nascetti 2008). Another genus Phocascaris Host, 1932, proposed for parasites of phocid seals rather than birds, is now considered monophyletic with Contracaecum (Nadler et al. 2000). In 1951, Contracaecum was divided into three subgenera; Contracaecum (Contracaecum), Contracaecum(Ornithocaecum),andContracaecum(Erschovicaecum) (Mozgovoi 1953). The former two were regarded as synonyms by Hartwich in 1975, and Contracaecum (Erschovicaecum) was transferred to Hysterothylacium Ward and Magath 1917 (Deardorff and Overstreet 1980). Contracaecum osculatum (Rudolphi 1802), the only know species infecting humans (Schaum and Müller 1967; Garcia 2007), includes a species complex consisting of 5 members; C. osculatum A Nascetti et al. 1993, C. osculatum B Nascetti et al. 1993, C. osculatum (Rudolphi 1802) sensu stricto, C. osculatum D (Orrechia et al. 1994), and C. osculatum E Orrechia et al. 1994 (Mattiucci and Nascetti 2008). Other species or subspecies of Contracaecum (plus Phocascaris) include C. osculatum baicalensis Mozgovoi and Ryzhykov 1950, C. orgmorhini Johnston and Mawson 1941, C. radiatum (v. Linstow 1907), C. mirounga Nikolskii 1974, P. phocae Host 1932, and P. cystophorae Berland 1964 (Mattiucci and Nascetti 2008).

Hysterothylacium aduncum (Rudolphi 1802), a fish intestinal parasite rarely infecting humans (Yagi et al. 1996), was described originally as Ascaris adunca, and then transferred to Contracaecum by Railliet and Henry in 1912 (Yagi et al. 1996). The genus

Thynnascaris was erected for Contracaecum-like ascaridoids of fishes by Dollfus in 1933 (Yagi et al. 1996). Because these nematodes mature into adults in fish, there were transferred to Thynnascaris Dollfus 1933 (Petter 1969). However, a review of Thynnascaris species revealed that they have the same generic features as an older genus Hysterothylacium Ward and Magath 1917, and a total of 47 species, including H. aduncum, were transferred to this genus (Deardorff and Overstreet 1980).

Life cycle

Adult anisakids, including Anisakis, Pseudoterranova, and Contracaecum, are parasitic in the stomach of marine mammals (definitive hosts), such as seals, sea lions, walruses, whales, and dolphins (Table 63.1). Adults of Hysterothylacium and Porrocaecum are parasites of marine fish and birds, respectively (Yagi et al. 1996; Digiani and Sutton 2001). Their eggs are discharged in the faeces from mature females, embryonate in the seawater, and hatch to liberate second-stage (L2) larvae. The sheathed L2 larvae swimming in sea water are ingested by eupausiid crustaceans, for example krills (= the first intermediate host), and then penetrate the gut wall and develop into the third-stage (L3) larvae in the abdominal cavity of the crustacean host. When infected crustaceans are eaten by fish or cephalopod hosts, including herring, mackerel, cod, sea eel, salmon, and squid (= the second intermediate host), the L3 larvae are liberated, penetrate into the body cavity, and encyst in the viscera of the hosts. The life cycle is completed when marine mammals ingest these infected fish or cephalopods. Human infections are principally the results of ingestion of fish or squids infected with the living L3 larvae (Miyazaki 1991).

Larval morphology

Morphological characteristics, especially oesophago-intestinal features, are useful for the identification of anisakid third-stage larvae. Oshima (1972) classified Anisakis larvae that may cause human infections into three types; Anisakis type I (Figs. 63.1 and 63.2), type II, and type III. The type I larvae, which are now recognized as larvae of A. simplex, are characterized by the presence of a prominent anteroventral boring tooth, a short tail with a caudal mucron (Table 63.2), and an oesophagus with a long ventriculus that ends obliquely at its junction with the intestine. Compared with P. decipiens larvae (Fig. 63.3), A. simplex larvae are smaller, slender, and somewhat more transparent (Chai et al. 1995). The type II larvae, which are now known as A. physeteris larvae, are characterized by a long tapered tail without a mucron, a short ventriculus, which has a horizontal junction with the intestine, and the presence of a prominent anteroventral boring tooth. The type III larvae are stout, each with a ventriculus similar to that of the type II larvae and a short tail with a tiny mucron. Their adult worm is yet unknown. The excretory pore of Anisakis larvae opens between subventral lips at the anterior end (Fig. 63.4) (Koyama et al. 1969). The characteristic features of L4 larvae are;

(1) Absence of the boring tooth at the anterior end and the mucron at the posterior end,

(2) The presence of the three well-defined lips,

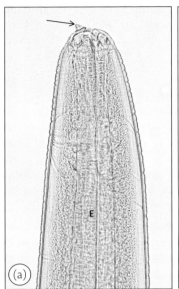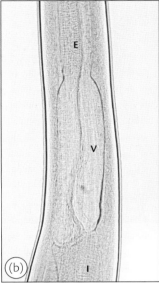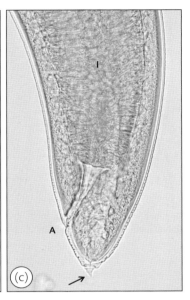

Fig. 63.1 A third stage larva of *Anisakis simplex* (*Anisakis* type I) recovered from a marine fish (yellow corvina, *Pseudosciaena manchurica*) (A) Anterior portion showing a prominent boring tooth (arrow) anteriorly x 200. (B) Ventriculus level showing simply connected esophagus, ventriculus, and intestine x 100. (C) Posterior portion showing a mucron (arrow) x 200. (E) oesophagus (muscular part). (I) intestine. (V) ventriculus.

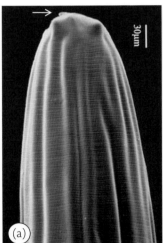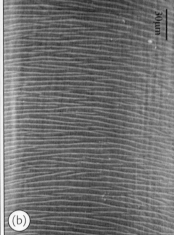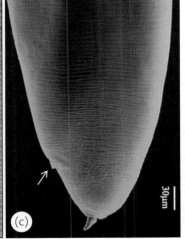

Fig. 63.2 Scanning electron microscopic (SEM) views of a third stage larva of *Anisakis simplex* collected from the viscera of a mackerel, *Scomber japonicus*. (A) Anterior portion with a boring tooth (arrow). (B) Cuticular surface with discontinuous wrinkles. (C) Posterior portion showing the anus (arrow) and a mucron.

Table 63.2 Diagnostic morphological characters* of anisakid larvae that can potentially infect humans (unit: mm)

Larval type	Length	Width (max.)	Preventriculus† (Oesophagus)	Ventriculus	Ventricular appendage	Intestinal caecum	Tail	Presence of mucron
Anisakis type I	13.4–36.0	0.23–0.58	1.25–2.78	0.57–1.50	–	–	0.07–0.16	+
Anisakis type II	21.6–31.9	0.53–0.71	1.80–2.51	0.47–0.71	–	–	0.21–0.38	–
Anisakis type III	23.8–38.4	0.65–0.97	1.46–2.33	0.47–0.73	–	–	0.10–0.20	+
Terranova type A	11.0–37.2	0.30–0.95	1.04–2.40	0.60–1.10	–	0.27–1.01	0.08–0.14	+
Terranova type B	6.6–6.7	0.14–0.16	0.82–0.92	0.66–0.67	–	0.76–0.86	0.12	–
Contracaecum type A	5.0–13.2	1.07–0.25	0.53–1.08	0.03–0.11	0.54–1.34	0.08–0.24	0.07–0.16	+
Contracaecum type B	10.3–27.2	0.29–0.74	0.93–1.66	0.05–0.17	0.61–1.60	0.46–1.10	0.12–0.24	–

* Descriptions are based on Koyama *et al.* (1969), Smith and Wooten (1978), and Chai *et al.* (1986).
† Muscular part of oesophagus.

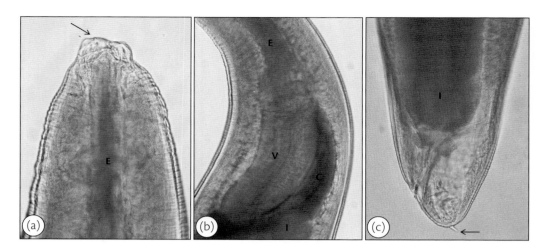

Fig. 63.3 A third stage larva of *Pseudoterranova decipiens* (*Terranova* type A) recovered from a marine fish (codfish, *Notothenia neglecta*) x 100. (A) Anterior portion showing a tiny boring tooth (arrow) x 200. (B) Ventriculus level x 100. (C) Posterior portion (arrow, mucron) x 200. (E) oesophagus (muscular part) (C) intestinal caecum. (I). intestine. (V). ventriculus.

(3) The appearance of transverse striations on the cuticular body surface,

(4) The appearance of a pair of small papillae at the cervical area,

(5) The appearance of altered ventriculus and intestine (Fig. 63.5) (Fujino *et al.* 1984; Weerasooriya *et al.* 1986; Sohn 1999).

Pseudoterranova decipiens larvae (= *Terranova* type A larvae) have an esophagus, ventriculus, and intestine with an anteriorly directed caecum (Table 63.2; Fig. 63.3). They commonly have the buccal cavity, three lips, and a boring tooth at the anterior end, and a tiny mucron at the posterior end. The excretory pore opens between subventral lips (Fig. 63.4). Their third-stage larvae are bigger, stouter, and darker in colour compared with those of *A. simplex* (Chai *et al.* 1995). *Terranova* type B larvae, of which adult is unknown, lack mucron (Koyama *et al.* 1969).

Contracaecum larvae have an oesophagus, ventriculus, ventricular appendage, and intestine with an anteriorly directed caecum (Table 63.2; Fig. 63.4). They have the buccal cavity, three lips, and a spine-like boring tooth at the anterior end, with or without a mucron at the posterior end. The excretory pore opens near the ventral interlabium. The larvae of *Hysterothylacium* are similar to those of *Contracaecum* but can be distinguished in that they have an excretory pore near the level of the nerve ring (Deardorff and Overstreet 1980).

Epidemiology

Distribution and prevalence

Human anisakiosis occurs throughout the world, with foci in eastern Asia and Western Europe, where there is widespread consumption of marine fish (Chai *et al.* 2005). Of more than 50,000 reported cases of anisakiosis, over 90% were from Japan, where approximately 2,000 cases are diagnosed annually. In the Republic of Korea more than 200 cases are estimated to occur annually. Most of the remainder are from the Netherlands, Germany, France, Spain, Italy, and the USA (Bouree *et al.* 1995; Mekerrow *et al.* 1988; Audicana *et al.* 2002; Pampiglione *et al.* 2002; Chai *et al.* 2005; Audicana and Kennedy 2008). As diagnostic methods improve, however, more cases are being reported from other areas of the world, including

Canada, Chile, New Zealand, and Egypt (Chai *et al.* 2005). The incidence of anisakiosis in Italy is probably higher than reported (Pampiglione *et al.* 2002). Up to 50 cases are reported per year in the USA and about 500 cases are recorded annually in Europe (Audicana *et al.* 2002).

Anisakiosis is generally more prevalent among coastal populations, particularly where people consume raw fish. However, the rapid progress of transportation and storage techniques allowed fish to be kept alive for a longer time and to be transported to remote inland areas, which resulted in an increase in the incidence of anisakiosis. However, in the Netherlands, human infections have decreased dramatically after the introduction of freezing regulations for green herring in 1968 (van Thiel 1976; Smith and Wooten 1978).

Source of infection

The prevalence of anisakiosis is clearly related to traditions of consuming raw, lightly cooked, or marinated fish, such as Japanese *sushi, sashimi* (sliced raw fish usually served with *wasabi* and vinegared red-pepper paste), *ikasashi* (sliced raw squid served with *shoga*, a kind of ginger), Dutch salted or smoked herring, Scandinavian gravlax, Hawaiian *lomi-lomi*, and Latin American *ceviche* (Sakanari and Mckerrow 1989). The risk of anisakiosis may be enhanced if the fish or squids are eaten whole, because worms are often found in the viscera rather than the flesh or if the fish have been kept whole for some time after capture, rather than gutted immediately. It has been reported that worms may migrate from the viscera to the flesh after death of the fish (Chai *et al.* 2005).

Various species of marine fish and cephalopods are the infection sources of human anisakiosis. In the Republic of Korea, the sea eel (*Astroconger myriaster*) was one of the most frequently consumed fish species by anisakiosis patients (Chai *et al.* 1992; Song *et al.* 1999). More than a half (57.5%) of the sea eels purchased from a market in Seoul was found to harbor anisakid larvae; the total number of larvae was 1,351, among which 564 were the larvae of *A. simplex* (as *Anisakis* type I larvae) and 615 were those of *Contracaecum* spp. (Chai *et al.* 1992). Similarly, the yellow corvina (*Pseudosciaena manchurica*) caught from the Yellow Sea, which is

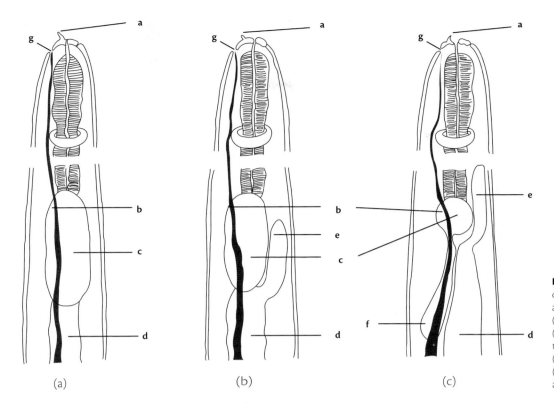

Fig. 63.4 Schematic drawing of oesophago-intestinal features of anisakid larvae. (A) *Anisakis* sp. Larva. (B) *Pseudoterranova* sp. Larva. (C) *Contracaecum* sp. larva. (a) boring tooth. (b) Renette (excretory) cell. (c) Ventriculus. (d) Intestine. (e) Intestinal caecum. (f) Ventricular appendage. (g) excretory pore.

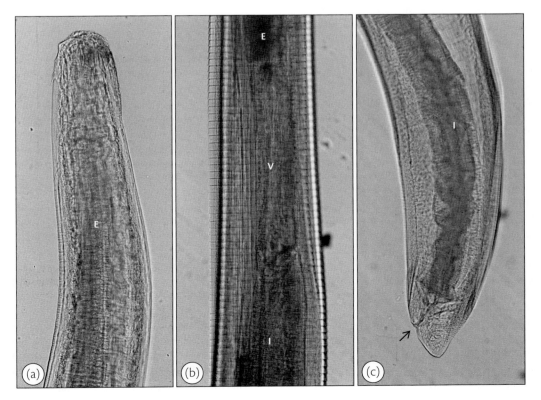

Fig. 63.5 A fourth stage larva of *Anisakis simplex* with cuticular striations recovered from a human case (this stage is occasionally found in humans) x 100. (A). Anterior portion. (B) Ventricular level. (C) Posterior portion showing the anus (arrow). (E) muscular esophagus. (V) ventriculus. (I) intestine.

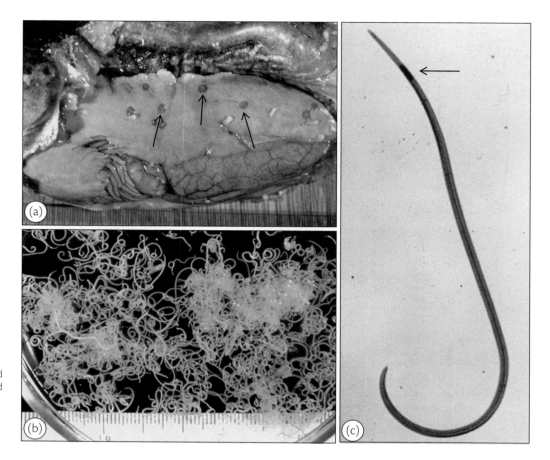

Fig. 63.6 Anisakid larvae (mostly *A. simplex*) in a marine fish, the walleye pollock (*Theragra chalcogramma*), caught from the Eastern Sea of the Republic of Korea. (A) Encysted larvae in the liver of a pollock, showing coiled larvae within cysts. (B) Larvae collected from the pollock. (C) Whole body of an *A. simplex* larva isolated from the viscera of a walleye pollock. Note the prominent ventriculus (arrow) x 10.

usually consumed after cooking, showed a 100% infection rate and a total of 1,068 anisakid larvae were detected (Chai *et al.* 1986). Among them, 80.4% were the larvae of *A. simplex* (as *Anisakis* type I larvae) (Fig. 63.6), and 15.5% were those of *Contracaecum* spp. (Chai *et al.* 1986).

In Japan, species of flounders, including the olive flounder (*Paralichthys olivaceus*), Japanese common squid (*Todarodes pacificus*), the Pacific cod (*Gadus macrocephalus*), and the bluefin tuna (*Thunnus thynnus*) have been reported to be the main sources in Hokkaido (Nagasawa and Moravec 1995; Ishikura *et al.* 1996). The spotted sardine (*Sardinops melanostictus*), the chub mackerel (*Scomber japonicum*), the horse mackerel (*Trachurus japonicas*), the oceanic bonito (*Katsuwonus pelamis*), and the chum salmon (*Oncorhynchus keta*) are important in Kyushu (Ishikura *et al.* 1996). In the Republic of Korea, the white-spotted conger (*Conger myriaster*), the olive flounder, Japanese common squid, Japanese amberjack (*Seriola quinqueradiata*), and some species of croakers (*Pseudosciaena* sp.) have been reported to be the important sources of anisakiosis (Im *et al.* 1995; Song *et al.* 1999). In the Netherlands, raw or pickled herring (*Clupea harengus*) is the primary source (van Thiel *et al.* 1960), and in Spain, raw or pickled hake (*Merluccius merluccius*), anchovy (*Engraulis encrasicholus*), and cod (*Gadus morhua*) are important sources (Audicana *et al.* 2002). Salmon, red snapper, herring, cod, halibut, mackerel, and squid are important sources of anisakiosis in North America and Hawaii (Oshima 1987; Sakanari and Mckerrow 1989).

Pathogenesis and clinical manifestations

Pathogenesis

When anisakid larvae are ingested they invade the stomach or intestinal wall. There is a tendency that *P. decipiens* is more often associated with gastric anisakiosis than intestinal asnisakiosis which is more commonly associated with *A. simplex* (Oshima 1987). Some larvae may remain in the gastrointestinal tract, without penetrating the mucosa, causing an asymptomatic infection which may only be discovered when the worms are expelled by coughing, vomiting, or defecating (Acha and Szyfres 1987). Most of the invaded larvae remain in the gastric or intestinal submucosa, which become a cause of granuloma formation in chronic stages. In rare instances, larvae may penetrate other sites, such as the throat (Kim *et al.* 1971; Beaver *et al.* 1984; Acha and Syfrez 1987; Amin *et al.* 2000). However, some larvae penetrate the gastrointestinal wall and escape, causing ectopic infections in the omentum, mesentery, and liver.

In acute gastric anisakiosis, invading worms give rise to oedema, hyperemia, and bleeding in the surrounding gastric mucosa, usually within 6 hours after the ingestion of raw marine fish or squid. In chronic infections in the gastrointestinal wall, eosinophilic granuloma may develop. Extra-gastrointestinal anisakiosis rarely occurs by the anisakid larvae that escape from the gastrointestinal tract to reach the peritoneum, liver, and lymph nodes in the abdominal cavity (Ishikura and Namiki 1989; Miyazaki 1991). Other ectopic foci of anisakid larvae include the abdominal cavity, omentum, mesentery, pancreas, ovary, and lung (Kobayashi *et al.* 1985; Matsuoka *et al.* 1994; Kagei *et al.* 1995; Kim *et al.* 1997; Lee *et al.* 1999; Cespedes *et al.* 2000; Yeum *et al.* 2002).

Pathology

Human anisakiosis takes a number of clinicopathological forms, depending on the location and histopathological lesions caused by the larvae. Histopathological examination of invasive anisakiosis usually reveals the worm embedded in a dense eosinophilic granuloma in the mucosa, often with localized or diffuse tumours in the stomach or intestinal wall (Beaver *et al.* 1984; Oshima 1987).

In acute infections, mild to severe gastric mucosal oedema occurs within 1–2 days after infection, and it is frequently accompanied by infiltrations of leukocytes and eosinophils. However, anisakid larvae may be invisible when they have already penetrated the gastric wall and have been transversely laid under the mucosa. Inflammation in the gastric wall invaded by larvae may proceed to a chronic stage and eosinophilic infiltration take place in the surrounding submucosa of worms. Granulation tissues are increased with the lapse of time, and then submucosal tumours are formed in the surroundings of worms. In most advanced chronic cases, only a granulomatous lesion with larval cuticular debris remains.

In chronic stages, the histopathologic lesions of gastric anisakiosis have been classified into four types according to the lapse of infection time (Kojima *et al.* 1966). Oshima (1972) added a fifth type, designated as the foreign body response type.

(1) Phlegmon-formation type: There may be edematous thickening of the submucosa with massive eosinophilic infiltration around invaded larvae.

(2) Abscess-formation type: There may be abscesses composed of eosinophils, neutrophils and lymphocytes around somewhat degenerated larvae.

(3) Abscess granuloma-formation type: About 6 months later in gastric anisakiosis, abscesses may be less extensive, and lymphocytes and granulation tissues may predominate.

(4) Granuloma-formation type: Abscess or granulomatous inflammation may be replaced by granulation tissue with some eosinophilic infiltration. Only remnant of the degenerated larvae is present in the center of the lesion.

(5) Foreign body response type: The histopathological features include infiltration and proliferation of neutrophils associated with a few eosinophils and giant cells. There is little or no oedema, but fibrin exudation, haemorrhage, and vascular damage usually occur. This type of response is associated with benign clinical symptoms and does not require surgery.

In intestinal anisakiosis, its pathological mechanisms are similar with those of gastric anisakiosis. However, it has some differences in the pathology from gastric anisakiosis. The inflammatory lesions formed around the invading larvae are more widely spread into the peritoneum, because the intestinal wall is not as thick as the stomach wall. Therefore, intestinal anisakiosis is frequently accompanied by signs of peritoneal irritation, and manifested by the abrupt onset of abdominal pain, nausea, vomiting, and diarrhoea 1–5 days after the ingestion of raw fish. Sometimes, the anisakid larvae are found in the intestinal tissues surgically removed from the patients under the diagnosis of acute abdomen, segmental inflammation,

and thickening of the intestinal wall (Kim *et al.* 1991; Takabe *et al.* 1998; Couture *et al.* 2003; Schuster *et al.* 2003).

Symptoms and signs

The clinical course of gastric anisakiosis is characterized by an abrupt onset of symptoms, such as intermittent epigastric pain, nausea, and vomiting, usually within 6 hours after the ingestion of raw marine fish or squid. Epigastric pain is often very severe and may not be relieved by analgesic medications (Sato 1992). Intestinal anisakiosis usually manifests symptoms 5 to 7 days after fish consumption (Acha and Szyfres 1987; Oshima 1987).

Acute gastric anisakiosis is roughly classified into two types, fulminant and mild types, according to the clinical features. In case of fulminant type, systemic allergic reactions such as anaphylaxis (IgE-mediated hypersensitivity), in addition to digestive symptoms, may be manifested in patients previously sensitized by anisakid antigens (see next section). In patients with fulminant type, emergency treatment may be required. The mild type is developed in patients infected for the first time with anisakid larvae (not sensitized by the anisakid antigen). This mild type, which was termed transient anisakidosis, mainly take place in non-endemic areas where people do not usually eat raw flesh of marine fish, and it is likely that many cases are under-diagnosed (Muraoka *et al.* 1996). In chronic infections, in which eosinophilic granuloma is frequently formed, symptoms, including intermittent epigastric tenderness, abdominal distention, and indigestion, may occur.

Allergic reactions

One of the most important findings about anisakiosis in recent years has been the discovery of allergic and hypersensitivity reactions to anisakid allergens (Audicana *et al.* 2002; Chai *et al.* 2005; Audicana and Kennedy 2008). Anaphylactoid reactions in gastric anisakiosis patients and mackerel-induced urticaria, possibly related with *Anisakis* worms, were first reported in Japan in 1989–1990 (Kasuya *et al.* 1990). After then, *A. simplex* was identified as an etiologic agent of allergic reactions in northern Spain (Audicana *et al.* 1995; del Pozo *et al.* 1996). The allergic responses were accompanied by elevated IgE responses to *A. simplex*, and clinical symptoms ranging from isolated angioedema to urticaria and life threatening anaphylactic shock (Alonso *et al.* 1997; Audicana *et al.* 2002; Audicana and Kennedy 2008). Now, patients of *Anisakis* allergy are reported from other regions of Spain (Añibarro *et al.* 2007), Italy (Purello-D'Ambrosio *et al.* 2000), South Africa (Nieuwenhuizen *et al.* 2006), and in the Republic of Korea (Kim *et al.* 2006; Choi *et al.* 2009).

Previous exposure to anisakid parasites and their antigens or allergens, either as living infection or by consumption of dead parasites in food fish, is considered as the main reason for the allergic reactions (Audicana and Kennedy 2008). The *A. simplex* allergens which invoke hypersensitivity reactions appear to be highly resistant to heat and freezing (Audicana *et al.* 2002). Hence, it was assumed that fish products which have been prepared in a way which would normally kill nematode larvae might not diminish the potency of their allergens to sensitize patients. Therefore, episodes of anaphylaxis associated with the consumption of *A. simplex* can occur without previously recognized infections. However, allergic symptoms were provoked only in patients with concurrent anisakid infection in the gastrointestinal tract (Alonso-Gomez *et al.* 2004).

The fact that serum IgE levels increase rapidly during the first few days of infection and remain high for months or years indicates the potential for type I hypersensitivity responses in acute anisakiosis (Audicana and Kennedy 2008). A total 8 types of *A. simplex* allergens have been found at the molecular level (Ani s 1 to Ani s 8); six were excretory-secretory products and two were somatic in origin (Audicana and Kennedy 2008). Allergens of other anisakid species have not been well characterized.

Diagnosis

The past history of ingesting raw flesh of marine fish within 6 hours prior to the onset of symptoms is helpful to make the diagnosis of acute gastric anisakiosis. However, definitive diagnosis is done by detection of anisakid larvae. Gastroendoscopy is highly useful for definitive diagnosis of gastric anisakiosis. Its application in patients at the onset of gastric symptoms often shows live larvae penetrating the mucosa (Fig. 63.7). The majority of cases are infected with 1–2 larvae, and rarely more than 10 larvae (Kagei and Isogaki 1992; Noh *et al.* 2003). In spite of the small number of worms infected, endoscopic findings are prominent and characteristic. Mucosal oedema is usually observed in most of the gastric anisakiosis patients, and hyperemia, erosion, and bleeding are found around the penetration site by the larvae. Larvae are found more frequently in the greater curvature than in the lesser curvature and preferentially in the body of the stomach (Kakizoe *et al.* 1995).

By gastroendoscopy, the worm itself may be seen and can be removed using biopsy forceps. Recovered worms should be fixed in 10% formalin, cleared in alcohol-glycerin or lactophenol, and

their species is identified based on morphological characteristics under a light microscope. The larvae of *A. simplex* (*Anisakis* type I larvae) are most frequently recovered from human cases (Kagei and Isogaki 1992; Seol *et al.* 1994; Song *et al.* 1999; Audicana and Kennedy 2008). The larvae of *P. decipiens* (*Terranova* type A larvae) are not infrequently found by gastroendoscopy (Oshima 1987; Ishikura and Namiki 1989; Koh *et al.* 1999; Song *et al.* 1999; Yu *et al.* 2001). The larvae of *A. physeteris* (*Anisakis* type II larvae) may also be detected by endoscopy or surgery (Oshima 1987; Claver *et al.* 1993).

Anisakiosis has been frequently misdiagnosed as gastric cancer, gastric ulcer, duodenal ulcer, appendicitis, or ileus. Recently, however, differential diagnosis can be done using radiologic techniques, including sonography (Matsumoto *et al.* 1992; Ido *et al.* 1998). Gastric submucosal tumours due to infections with anisakid larvae can be easily differentiated by endoscopic ultrasonography viewing from the thickness of the gastric wall (especially, a thickened third layer) and different echogenicity of the central area where a dead or degenerating worm body is located (Sakai *et al.* 1992; Kim *et al.* 2006). In some cases, gastric submucosal tumours caused by anisakid larvae may disappear after certain periods. In an analysis of vanishing gastric tumour masses, 41% of 71 cases were caused by anisakiosis (Takeuchi *et al.* 2000; Fujisawa *et al.* 2001).

In surgical specimens, the cross-sectional morphologies of worms, i.e. Y-shaped lateral cords, Renette cell, and high numbers of muscle cells in a quadrant, are useful clues for the diagnosis of chronic anisakidosis (Fig. 63.8). In addition, the histopathologic types of lesions defined by Kojima *et al.* (1966) are also helpful to make a diagnosis of chronic anisakiosis.

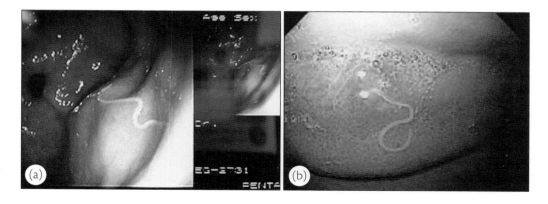

Fig. 63.7 Gastroendoscopic views of anisakiosis patients. (A) A whitish sigmoid-shaped larva penetrating the edematous mucosa of the greater curvature in the stomach of a patient. (B) A larva penetrated the edematous and hemorrhagic mucosa of the greater curvature in the lower body of the stomach of a patient.

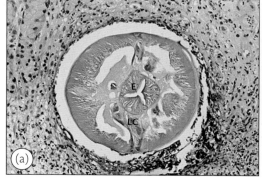
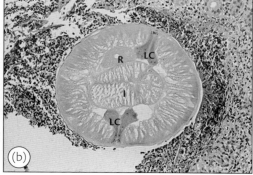

Fig. 63.8 Histopathological findings of anisakiosis due to *A. simplex* larvae. (A) Cross-sectional morphology of the oesophageal level of a larva. (B) Cross-sectional morphology of the intestinal level of a larva. (E) oesophagus; (LC), lateral cord. (I) intestine. (R) renette (excretory) cell.

Various monoclonal antibodies that recognize specific epitopes of *A. simplex* larvae have been produced for diagnosis of anisakiosis. Excretory-secretory products have been used for antigens in micro-ELISA. An immunoblot technique using the whole larval antigen to detect serum IgE is useful giving positive reactions after a few days (Garcia *et al.* 1997). An antigenic β–galactosidase helminth-derived recombinant fusion protein used in ELISA is completely specific in contrast to soluble antigens (Sugane *et al.* 1992). Detection of specific IgE directed toward a purified allergen, such as Ani s 1 (an excretory gland protein) from crude extracts is useful for the diagnosis of hypersensitivity as well as digestive tract anisakiosis (Caballero and Moneo 2002).

Treatment

The most effective treatment of acute gastric anisakiosis is removal of the worms under gastroendoscopy as early as possible (Oshima 1972). However, it is not always possible because worms are frequently not seen at endoscopy and have penetrated the gastric mucosa. In acute abdominal conditions, if diagnosis is not apparent, treatment is usually by surgery with resection of the affected part (Smith and Wootten 1978). In chronic gastric anisakiosis, the affected area should also be removed surgically in order to avoid possible future allergic exacerbation of the lesion (Oshima 1972). In intestinal aniaskiosis, if the diagnosis is definite, a conservative treatment is recommended with administration of antibiotics and isotonic glucose solution (Oshima 1972).

Anthelmintic treatment of anisakiosis patients with albendazole has been tried by several workers with considerable efficacy (Ioli *et al.* 1998; Moore *et al.* 2002; Pacios *et al.* 2005; Kim *et al.* 2006; Amato Neto *et al.* 2007). Albendazole was found also effective *in vitro* against *A. simplex* larvae and *in vivo* of experimental guinea pigs infected with *A. simplex* larvae (Dziekoñska-Rinko *et al.* 2002). Ivermectin was found to be highly effective *in vitro* against *P. decipiens* larvae collected from cod fish (Manley and Embil 1989).

Prevention and control

Control strategies for human anisakiosis include identification and removal of anisakid larvae from fish fillet. Candling is one of the most commonly employed technique for determining the presence or absence of anisakid larvae in fish fillet (Valdimarsson *et al.* 1985). This method involves shining a bright light through a piece of fish muscle and viewing it. Candling is not effective in the case of dark-fleshed fish.

Freezing is also effective for inactivation of anisakid larvae. It will take at least 24–52 hours to kill the parasites by freezing at −20°C (Bier 1976; Smith and Wootten 1987). Anisakid larvae in the gut and viscera of fish seem to migrate into the fillet when the fish are removed from the nets and dumped on the deck and the temperature is 30°C or higher (Cheng 1976). Rapid freezing immediately after capture of fish on the deck may prevent migration of larvae into the muscles of fish. Rapid gutting of captured fish before freezing can also reduce the incidence of human anisakiosis (Cheng 1976).

High temperatures, 50–60°C, will also kill anisakid larvae in fish fillet, although heating is not always a desirable method (Bier 1976), because fillets that had been heated have shorter shelf-lives. The effectiveness of smoking, pickling, or marination in destroying anisakid larvae in fish fillet has been studied, but these methods were found insufficient, with the possible exception of dry salting, provided the salt reaches all parts of the muscles in concentrated form (Bier 1976).

Radiation has been used to control of infectivity of various pathogens, including parasites (Farkas 1998). However, larvae of *A. simplex* were shown to be radio-resistant, possibly due to generation of a high superoxide dismutase activity (Seo *et al.* 2006).

References

Acha, P. and Szyfres, B. (1987). Zoonoses and Communicable Diseases Common to Man and Animals, (2nd edn.). Washington D. C.: Pan American Health Organization.

Alonso, A., Daschner, A. and Moreno-Ancillo, A. (1997). Anaphylaxis with *Anisakis simplex* in the gastric mucosa. *N. Eng. J. Med.*, **337**: 350–51.

Alonso-Gomez, A., Moreno-Ancillo, A., Lopez-Serrano, *et al.* (2004). *Anisakis simplex* only provokes allergic symptoms when the worm parasites the gastrointestinal tract. *Parasitol. Res.*, **93**: 378–84.

Amato Neto, V., Amato, J. G. P. and Amato, V. S. (2007). Probable recognition of human anisakiasis in Brazil. *Rev. Instit. Med. Trop. São Paulo*, **49**: 261–62.

Amin, O. M., Eidelman, W. S., Domke, W., Bailey, J. and Pfeifer, G. (2000). An unusual case of anisakiasis in California, USA. *Comp. Parasitol.*, **67**: 71–75.

Añibarro, B., Seoane, F.J. and Mugica, M.V. (2007). Involvement of hidden allergens in food allergic reactions. *J. Invest. Aller. Clin. Immun.*, **17**: 168–72.

Asami, K., Watanuki, T., Sakai, H., Imano, H. and Okamoto, R. (1965). Two cases of stomach granuloma caused by *Anisakis*-like larvae nematodes in Japan. *Am. J. Trop. Med. Hyg.*, **14**: 119–23.

Ashby, B. S., Appleton, P. J. and Dawson, I. (1964). Eosinophilic granuloma of gastro-intestinal tract caused by herring parasite *Eustoma rotundatum. BMJ*, **1**: 1141–45.

Audicana, M. T. and Kennedy, M. W. (2008). Anisakis simplex: from obscure infectious worm to inducer of immune hypersensitivity. *Clin. Microbiol. Rev.*, **21**: 360–79.

Audicana, M. T., Ansotegui, I. J., de Corres, L. F. and Kennedy, M. W. (2002). *Anisakis simplex*: dangerous-dead and alive? *Parasitol. Today*, **18**: 20–25.

Audicana, M. T., de Corres, L. F., Muñoz, D., *et al.* (1995). Recurrent anaphylaxis caused by *Anisakis simplex* parasitizing fish. *J. Aller. Clin. Immunol.*, **96**: 558–60.

Beaver, P. C., Jung, R. C. and Cupp, E. W. (1984). Clinical Parasitology, (9th edn). Philadelphia: Lea and Febiger.

Bier, J. W. (1976). Experimental anisakiasis: Cultivation and temperature tolerance determinations. *J. Milk Food Tech.*, **39**: 132–40.

Buckley, J. J. C. (1951). *Porrocaecum decipiens* in the month of a patient. *Trans. R. Soc. Trop. Med. Hyg.*, **44**: 362.

Bouree, P., Paugam, A. and Petithory, J. C. (1995). Anisakidosis: report of 25 cases and review of the literature. *Comp. Immun. Microbiol. Infect. Dis.*, **18**: 75–84.

Caballero, M. L. and Moneo, I. (2002). Specific IgE determination to Ani s 1, a major allergen from *Anisakis simplex*, is a useful tool for diagnosis. *Ann. Aller. Asth. Immun.*, **89**: 74–77.

Cespedes, M., Saez, A., Rodriguez, I., Pinto, J. M. and Rodriguez, R. (2000). Chronic anisakiasis presenting as a mesenteric mass. *Abdom. Imag.*, **25**: 548–50.

Chai, J. Y., Chu, Y. M., Sohn, W. M. and Lee, S. H. (1986). Larval anisakids collected from the yellow corvine in Korea. *Korean J. Parasitol.*, **24**: 1–11.

Chai, J. Y., Cho, S. R., Kook, J. and Lee, S. H. (1992). Infection status of the sea eel (*Astroconger myriaster*) purchased from the Noryangjin fish market with anisakid larvae. *Korean J. Parasitol.*, **30**: 157–62.

Chai, J. Y., Guk, S. M., Sung, J. J., *et al.* (1995). Recovery of *Pseudoterranova decipiens* (Anisakidae) larvae from codfish of the Antarctic Ocean. *Korean J. Parasitol.*, **33**: 231–34.

Chai, J. Y., Murrell, K. D. and Lymbery, A. J. (2005). Fish-borne parasitic zoonoses: Status and issues. *Int. J. Parasitol.*, **35**(11–12): 1233–54.

Cheng, T. C. (1976). The natural history of anisakiasis in animals. *J. Milk Food Tech.*, **39**: 32–46.

Choi, S. J., Lee, J. C., Kim, M. J., *et al.* (2009). The clinical characteristics of *Anisakis* allergy in Korea. *Korean J. Internal Med.*, **24**: 160–63.

Claver, A., Delgado, B., Sanchez-Acedo, C., *et al.* (1993). A live *Anisakis physeteris* larva found in the abdominal cavity of a woman in Zaragoza, Spain. *Jap. J. Parasitol.*, **42**: 445–48.

Couture, C., Measures, L., Gagnon, J. and Desbiens, C. (2003). Human intestinal anisakiosis due to consumption of raw salmon. *Am. J. Surg. Path.*, **27**: 1167–72.

Davey, J. T. (1971). A revision of the genus *Anisakis* Dujardin, 1845 (Nematoda: Ascaridata). *J. Helminthol.*, **45**: 51–72.

Dearforff, T. L. and Overstreet, R. M. (1980). Review of *Hysterothylacium* and *Iheringascaris* (both previously = *Thynnascaris*) (Nematoda: Anisakidae) from the northern gulf of Mexico. *Proc. Biolog. Soc. Washington*, **93**: 1035–79.

D'Amelio, S., Busi, M., Ingrosso, S., Paggi, L. and Giuffra, E. (2010). *Anisakis*. In: D. Lin (ed.) Molecular Detection of Foodborne Pathogens, pp. 757–68. Boca Raton, Florida: CRC Press.

del Pozo, M. D., Moneo, I., de Corres, L. F., *et al.* (1996). Laboratory determinations in *Anisakis simplex* allergy. *J. Aller. Clin. Immunol.*, **97**: 977–84.

Digiani, M. C. and Sutton, C. A. (2001). New reports and a redescription of *Porrocaecum heteropterum* (Diesing, 1851) (Ascarididae), a rare nematode parasitic in South American threskiornithid birds. *Sys. Parasitol.*, **49**: 1–6.

Dziekoñska-Rynko, J., Rokichi, J., and Jablonowski, Z. (2002). Effects of ivermectin and albendazole against *Anisakis simplex* in vitro and in guinea pigs. *J. Parasitol.*, **88**: 395–98.

Fagerholm, H. P. (1991). Systematic implications of male caudal morphology in ascaridoid nematode parasites. *Sys. Parasitol.*, **19**: 215–29.

Fagerholm, H. P., Brunanska, M., Roepstorff, A. and Eriksen, L. (2004). Phasmid ultrastructure of an ascaridoid nematode *Hysterothylacium auctum*. *J. Parasitol.*, **90**: 499–506.

Farkas, J. (1998). Irradiation as a method for decontaminating food–A review. *Intern. J. Food Microbiol.*, **44**: 189–200.

Fujino, T., Ooiwa, T. and Ishii, Y. (1984). Clinical, epidemiological and morphological studies on 150 cases of acute gastric anisakiasis in Fukuoka Prefecture. *Jap. J. Parasitol.*, **33**: 73–92 (in Japanese).

Fujisawa, K., Matsumoto, T., Yoshimura, R., Ayabe, S. and Tominage, M. (2001). Endoscopic finding of a large vanishing tumor. *Endoscopy*, **33**: 820.

Fumarola, L., Monno, R., Ieradi, E., *et al.* (2009). *Anisakis pegreffi* etiological agent of gastric infections in two Italian women. *Foodborne Path. Dis.*, **6**: 1–3.

Garcia, L. S. (2007). *Chapter 11. Tissue nematodes. Section: Anisakis simplex, A. physeteris, Pseudoterranova decipiens, Contracaecum osculatum, and Porrocaecum reticulatum (Larval Nematodes Acquired from Saltwater Fish)*. In: L. S. Garcia (ed.) Diagnostic Medical Parasitology, (5th edn.), pp. 312–14. Herndon, Virginia: ASM Press.

Garcia, M., Moneo, I., Audicana, M. T., *et al.* (1997). The use of IgE immunoblotting as a diagnostic tool in *Anisakis simplex* allergy. *J. Aller. Clin. Immunol.*, **99**: 497–501.

Gibson, D. I. (1983). *The systematics of ascaridoid nematodes-A current assessment* In: A. R. Stone, H. M. Platt, and L. F. Khalil (eds.) Concepts in Nematode Systematics, pp. 321–38. London: Academic Press.

Hitchcock, D. J. (1950). Parasitological study of the Eskimos in the Bethel area of Alaska. *J. Parasitol.*, **36**: 232–34.

Ido, K., Yuasa, H., Ide, M., Kimura, K., Tochimitsu, K. and Suzuki, T. (1998). Sonographic diagnosis of small intestinal anisakiasis. *J. Clin. Ultrasound*, **26**: 125–30.

Im, K. I., Shin, H. J., Kim, B. H. and Moon, S. I. (1995). Gastric anisakiasis cases in Cheju-do, Korea. *Korean J. Parasitol.*, **33**: 179–86 (in Korean).

Iñiguez, A. M., Santos, C. P. and Vicente, A. C. P. (2009). Genetic characterization of *Anisakis typica* and *Anisakis physeteris* from marine mammals and fish from the Atlantic Ocean off Brazil. *Vet. Parasitol.*, doi:10.1016/j.vet.par.2009.07.012.

Ioli, A., Leonaldi, R., Gangemi, C., *et al.* (1998). Apropos of 1 case of anisakiasis contracted in Sicily. *Bull. Soc. Path. Exotique*, **91**: 232–34 (in French).

Ishikura, H. and Namiki, M. (1989). *Gastric anisakiasis in Japan*. Epidemiology, diagnosis, treatment, pp. 1–141. Tokyo: Springer-Verlag.

Ishikura, H., Takahashi, S. and Ishikura, H. (1996). Anisakidae and anisakidosis in Japan. *Proceedings of the 2nd Japan-Korea Parasitologists' Seminar (Forum Cheju-2)*, 50–63.

Kagei, N. and Isogaki, H. (1992). A case of abdominal syndrome caused by the presence of a large number of *Anisakis* larvae. *Int. J. Parasitol.*, **22**: 251–53.

Kagei, N., Sano, M., Takahashi, Y., Tamura, Y. and Sakamoto, M. (1978). A case of acute abdominal syndrome caused by *Anisakis* type-II larva. *Jap. J. Parasitol.*, **27**: 427–31.

Kagei, N., Orikasa, H., Hori, E., Sannomiya, A. and Yasumura, Y. (1995). A case of hepatic anisakiasis with a literal survey for extra-gastrointestinal anisakiasis. *Jap. J. Parasitol.*, **44**: 346–51.

Kakizoe, S., Kakizoe, H., Kakizoe, K., *et al.* (1995). Endoscopic findings and clinical manifestation of gastric anisakiasis. *Am. J. Gastroenter.*, **90**: 761–63.

Kasuya, S., Hamano, H. and Izumi, S. (1990). Mackerel-induced urticercaria and *Anisakis*. *Lancet*, **335**: 665.

Kim, C. H., Chung, B. S., Moon, Y. I., Chun, S. H. (1971). A case report on human infection with *Anisakis* sp. in Korea. *Korean J. Parasitol.*, **9**: 39–43.

Kim, L. S., Lee, Y. H, Kim, S., Park, H. R. and Cho, S. Y. (1991). A case of anisakiasis causing intestinal obstruction. *Korean J. Parasitol.*, **29**: 93–96.

Kim, S. G., Jo, Y. J., Park, Y. S., *et al.* (2006). Four cases of gastric submucosal mass suspected as anisakiasis. *Korean J. Parasitol.*, **44**: 81–86.

Kim, S. H., Kim, H. U. and Lee, J. C. (2006). A case of gastroallergic anisakiasis. *Korean J. Med.*, **70**: 111–16.

Kobayashi, A., Tsuji, M. and Wilbur, D. l. (1985). Probable pulmonary anisakiasis accompanying pleural effusion. *Am. J. Trop. Med. Hyg.*, **34**: 310–13.

Koh, M. S., Huh, S. and Sohn, W. M. (1999). A case of gastric pseudoterranoviasis in a 43-year-old man in Korea. *Korean J. Parasitol.*, **37**: 47–49.

Kojima, K., Koyanagi, T. and Shiraki, K. (1966). Pathological studies of anisakiasis (parasitic abscess formation in gastrointestinal tracts). *Japanese J. Clin. Med.*, **24**: 134–43 (in Japanese).

Koyama, T., Kobayashi, A., Kumada, M., *et al.* (1969). Morphological and taxonomical studies of Anisakidae larvae found in marine fishes and squids. *Jap. J. Parasitol.*, **18**: 466–87 (in Japanese).

Lee, W. J., Lim, H. K., Lim, J. H., Kim, S. H., *et al.* (1999). Foci of eosinophil-related necrosis in the liver: Imaging findings and correlation with eosinophilia. *Am. J. Roentgen.*, **172**: 1255–61.

Manley, K. M., and Embil, J. A. (1989). *In vitro* effect of ivermectin on *Pseudoterranova decipiens* survival. *J. Helminthol.*, **63**: 72–74.

Matsumoto, T., Iida, M., Kimura, Y., Tanaka, K., *et al.* (1992). Anisakiasis of the colon: Radiologic and endoscopic features in six patients. *Radiology*, **183**: 97–99.

Matsuoka, H., Nakama, T., Kisanuki, H., *et al.* (1994). A case report of serologically diagnosed pulmonary anisakiasis with pleural effusion and multiple lesions. *Am. J. Trop. Med. Hyg.*, **51**: 819–22.

Mattiucci, M. and Nascetti, G. (2008). Advances and trends in the molecular systematics of anisakid nematodes, with implications for their evolutionary ecology and host-parasite co-evolutionary process. *Adv. Parasitol.*, **66**: 147–148.

Mattiucci, M., Nascetti, G., Cianchi, R., *et al.* (1997). Genetic and ecological data on the *Anisakis simplex* complex, with evidence for a new species (Nematoda, Ascaridoidea, Anisakidae). *J. Parasitol.*, **83**: 401–6.

Mattiucci, M., Paggi, L., Nascetti, G., *et al.* (1998). Allozyme and morphological identification of *Anisakis, Contracaecum* and *Pseudoterranova* from Japanese waters (Nematoda, Ascaridoidea). *Sys. Parasitol.*, **40**: 81–92.

Mattiucci, M., Nascetti, G., Daily, M., *et al.* (2005). Evidence for a new species of *Anisakis* Dujardin, 1845: morphological description and genetic relationships between congeners (Nematoda: Anisakidae). *Sys. Parasitol.*, **61**: 157–71.

Mckerrow, J. H., Sakanari, J. A. and Deardorff, T. L. (1988). Anisakiasis: Revenge of the sushi parasite. *N. Eng. J. Med.*, **319**: 1228–29.

Miyazaki, I. (1991). *Helminthic Zoonoses. Chaper 26.* Anisakiasis, pp. 314–27. Tokyo: International Medical Foundation of Japan.

Moore, D. A. J., Girdwood, R. W. A. and Chiodini, P. L. (2002). Treatment of anisakiasis with albendazole. *Lancet*, **360**: 54.

Mozgovoi, A. A. (1953). *Ascaridata of Animals and Man and the Diseases Caused by Them.* In: K. I. Skrjabin (ed.) Essentials of Nematodology, Vol. II. Moskvo: Izdatielstov AN SSSR.

Muraoka, A., Suehiro, I., Fujii, M., *et al.* (1996). Acute gastric anisakiasis: 28 cases during the last 10 years. *Digest. Dis. Sci.*, **41**: 2362–65.

Myers, B. J. (1959). *Phocanema*, a new genus for the anisakid nematode of seals. *Can. J. Zool.*, 37: 459–65.

Nadler, S. A. and Hudspeth, D. S. S. (2000). Phylogeny of the Ascaridoidea (Nematoda: Ascaridida) based on three genes and morphology: Hypotheses of structural and sequence evolution. *J. Parasitol.*, **86**: 380–93.

Nadler, S. A., D'Amelio, S., Fagerholm, H. P. *et al.* (2000). Phylogenetic relationships among species of *Contracaecum* Railliet & Henry, 1912 and Phocascaris Host, 1932 (Nematoda: Ascaridoidea) based on nuclear rDNA sequence data. *Parasitology*, **121**: 455–63.

Nadler, S. A., D'Amelio, S., Dailey, M. D., *et al.* (2005). Molecular phylogenetics and diagnosis of *Anisakis, Pseudoterranova,* and *Contracaecum* from northern Pacific marine mammals. *J. Parasitol.*, **91**: 1413–29.

Nagasawa, K. and Moravec, F. (1995). Larval anisakid nematodes of Japanese common squid (*Todarodes pacificus*) from the Sea of Japan. *J. Parasitol.*, **81**: 69–75.

Nieuwenhuizen, N., Lopata, A. L., Jeebhay, M. F., *et al.* (2006). Exposure to the fish parasite *Anisakis* causes allergic airway hyperreactivity and dermatitis. *J. Aller. Clin. Immunol.*, **117**: 1098–105.

Noh, J. H., Kim, B. J., Kim, S. M., Ock, M. S., *et al.* (2003). A case of acute gastric anisakiasis provoking severe clinical problems by multiple infection. *Korean J. Parasitol.*, **41**: 97–100.

Oshima, T. (1972). *Anisakis and anisakiasis in Japan and adjacent area,* In: K. Morishita, Y. Komiya and H. Matsubayashi (eds.) *Progress of Medical Parasitology in Japan,* Vol. 4, pp. 301–93. Tokyo, Japan: Meguro Parasitological Museum.

Oshima, T. (1987). Anisakiasis - Is the sushi bar guilty? *Parasitol. Today*, **3**: 44–48.

Otsuru, M., Ishizuke, F. and Hatsukano, T. (1957). Regional ileitis caused by the invasion of ascarid larva into the intestinal wall. *Nippon Ijishimpo*, No. 1775, 25–38 (in Japanese).

Pacios, E., Arias-Diaz, J., Zuloaga, J., *et al.* (2005). Albendazole for the treatment of anisakiasis ileus. *Clin. Infect. Dis.*, **41**: 1825–26.

Paggi, L., Nascetti, G., Webb, S. C., *et al.* (1998). A new species of Anisakis Dujardin, 1845 (Nematoda, Anisakidae) from beaked whales (Ziphiidae): alloenzyme and morphological evidence. *Sys. Parasitol.*, **40**: 161–74.

Paggi, L., Mattiucci, S., Gibson, D. I., *et al.* (2000). Pseudoterranova decipiens species A and B (Nematoda, Ascaridoidea): nomenclatural designation, morphological diagnostic characters and genetic markers. *Sys. Parasitol.*, **45**: 185–97.

Pampiglione, S., Rivasi, F., Criscuolo, M., *et al.* (2002). Human anisakiasis in Italy: a report of eleven new cases. *Patho. Res. Pract.*, **198**: 429–34.

Petter, A. J. (1969). Enquéte sur les Nématodes des pêchées dans la région nantaise. Rapport possible avec les granulomes éosinophies observés chez l'homme dans la région. *Ann. Parasitol. (Paris)*, **44**: 25–36.

Pontes, T., D'Amelio, S., Costa, G. and Paggi, L. (2005). Molecular characterization of larval anisakid nematodes from marine fishes of Madeira by a PCR-based approach, with evidence for a new species. *J. Parasitol.*, **91**: 1430–34.

Purello-D'Ambrosio, F., Pastorello, E., Gangemi, S., *et al.* (2000). Incidence of sensitivity to *Anisakis simplex* in a risk population of fisherman/ fishmongers. *Ann. Aller. Asth. Immunol.*, **84**: 439–44.

Sakai, K., Ohtani, A., Muta, H., *et al.* (1992). Endoscopic ultrasonography findings in acute gastric anisakiasis. *Am. J. Gastroenter.*, **87**: 1618–23.

Sakanari, J. A. and Mckerrow, J. H. (1989). Anisakiasis. *Clin. Microbiol. Rev.*, **2**: 278–84.

Sato, I. (1992). Clinical study of gastric anisakiasis. *Akita J. Med.*, **19**: 503–10.

Schaum, E. and Müller, W. (1967). Die Heterocheilidiasis. Eine Infektion des Menschen mit Larven von Fisch-Ascariden. *Deus. Mediz. Wochenschr.*, **92**: 2230–33.

Schuster, R., Petrini, J. L. and Choi, R. (2003). Anisakiasis of the colon presenting as bowel obstruction. *Am. Sur.*, **69**: 350–52.

Seo, M., Guk, S. M., Lee, S. H. and Chai, J. Y. (2006). Radioresistance of *Anisakis simplex* third-stage larvae and the possible role of superoxide dismutase. *J. Parasitol.*, **92**: 416–18.

Seo, B. S., Chai, J. Y., Lee, S. H., Hong, S. T., *et al.* (1984). A human case infected by the larva of *Terranova* type A in Korea. *Korean J. Parasitol.*, **22**: 248–52.

Seol, S. Y., Ok, S. C., Pyo, J. S., *et al.* (1994). Twenty cases of gastric anisakiasis caused by *Anisakis* type I larva. *Korean J. Gastroenter.*, **26**: 17–24.

Smith, J. W. and Wootten, R. (1978). *Anisakis* and anisakiasis. *Adv. Parasitol.*, **16**: 93–163.

Sohn, W. M. (1999). Ultrastructural changes on the cuticular surface, excretory and digestive organs of *Anisakis simplex* larvae chronologically recovered from experimental cats. *Korean J. Elect. Micros.*, **29**: 211–21. (in Korean).

Sohn, W. M. and Seol, S. Y. (1994). A human case of gastric anisakiasis by *Pseudoterranova decipens* larva. *Korean J. Parasitol.*, **32**: 53–56.

Song, T. J., Cho, S. W. and Joo, K. H. (1999). Endoscopic findings of acute gastric anisakiasis. Thirty-nine cases in Inchon City. *Korean J. Gastrointest. Endos.*, **19**: 878–84. (in Korean).

Sugane, K., Sin, S. and Matsuura, T. (1992). Molecular cloning of the cDNA encoding 2 42 kDa antigenic polypeptide of *Anisakis simplex* larvae. *J. Helminthol.*, **66**: 25–32.

Takabe, K., Ohki, S., Kunihiro, O., *et al.* (1998). Anisakidosis: a cause of intestinal obstruction from eating sushi. *American J. Gastroenter.*, **93**: 1172–73.

Takeuchi, K., Hanai, H., Iida, T., Suzuki, S. and Isobe, S. (2000). A bleeding gastric ulcer on a vanishing tumor caused by anisakiasis. *Gastrointest. Endos.*, **52**: 549–51.

Umehara, A., Kawakami, Y., Araki, J. and Uchida, A. (2007). Molecular identification of the etiological agent of the human anisakiasis in Japan. *Parasitol. Int.*, **56**: 211–15.

Valdimarsson, G., Einarsson, H., and King, F. J. (1985). Detection of parasites in fish muscle by candling technique. *J. Ass. Off. Analy. Chem.*, **68**: 549–55.

van Thiel, P.H. (1976). The present state of anisakiasis and its causative worms. *Trop. Geograph. Med.*, **21:** 75–85.

van Thiel, P. H., Kuiper, F. C., Roskam, R. T. (1960). A nematode parasitic to herring, causing acute abdominal syndromes in man. *Trop. Geograph. Med.*, **2:** 97–113.

Yagi, K., Nagasawa, K., Ishikura, H., *et al.* (1996). Female worm *Hysterothylacium aduncum* excreted from human: a case report. *Jap. J. Parasitol.*, **45:** 12–23.

Yeum, C. H., Ma, S. K., Kim, S. W., Kim, N. H., *et al.* (2002). Incidental detection of an Anisakis larva in continuous ambulatory peritoneal dialysis effluent. *Nephr. Dialy. Transplant.*, **17:** 1522–23.

Yokogawa, M. and Yoshimura, H. (1965). *Anisakis*-like larvae causing eosinophilic granuloma in the stomach of man. *Am. J. Trop. Med. Hyg.*, **14:** 770–73.

Yu, J. R., Seo, M., Kim, Y. W., Oh, M. H. and Sohn, W. M. (2001). A human case of gastric infection by *Pseudoterranova decipens larva*. *Korean J. Parasitol.*, **39:** 193–96.

Weerasooriya, M. V., Fujino, T., Ishii, Y. and Kagei, N. (1986). The value of external morphology in the identification of larval anisakid nematodes: A scanning electron microscope study. *Zeitschr. Parasit.*, **72:** 765–78.

CHAPTER 64

Toxocarosis

Sheelagh Lloyd and Eric R. Morgan

Summary

Toxocara canis and the syndromes of visceral and ocular larva migrans (VLM, OLM), covert toxocarosis, and neurological toxocarosis are described. Other potential agents, particularly *Toxocara cati* and *Baylisascaris procyonis*, are described. The transmission dynamics of toxocarosis to humans have never been fully elucidated, but the potential roles of pet and stray dogs, foxes, cats, and the influence of their population densities, and age demographies, are discussed in relation to contamination of the environment with eggs. Routes of infection with eggs by geophagia, poor hygiene outdoors and with dogs, and fly-borne contamination of food, and meat-borne ingestion of larvae are described. The development of prolonged *in vitro* culture and analyses of *T. canis* larval excretions/secretions (TES) and surface antigens helped explain the importance of the rapid production and shedding of TES in the prolonged course of infection and pathogenesis of disease. TES also have greatly improved serodiagnosis. However, we still have insufficient understanding of differences in the aetiology of the larvae or differences in immune responses among individuals to account for development of VLM, covert toxocarosis, or OLM in different individuals. Our understanding of the immunopathological response of the host to TES has emphasized the need for anti-inflammatory therapy in treatment; unfortunately, less information is available on the true efficacy of the anthelmintics available. The complexity of the *T. canis* life cycle in dogs is described and therapeutic regimens to prevent excretion of eggs by pet dogs are given. This, plus adequate control or exclusion of stray or wild canids from a property could prevent most cases of VLM. Control of infection from free-ranging stray dogs, cats and foxes, will be difficult and more data are needed to clarify the importance of these and of fly-borne and meat-borne transfer of infection to humans for control.

History

Toxocara canis was first described as *Ascaris canis* in 1782 and clinical VLM was initially ascribed in 1947 to *Ascaris lumbricoides*. Then Beaver in 1952 serially sectioned a larva from a patient, identified it as *Toxocara canis,* and later reproduced infection in two children.

Wilder reported 24 cases of ocular disease 1950, but only in 1956 were the larvae identified as *Toxocara* by Nichols. A milestone was de Savigny's prolonged *in vitro* culture of *T. canis* larvae to produce TES, improving diagnosis and allowing the considerable advances in our understanding of the cuticle of nematodes by Maizels and colleagues. The fact that *T. canis* can produce blindness, usually unilateral, in children creates considerable publicity, probably out of proportion compared with the importance of many other childhood or tropical parasitic diseases.

The agents and geographic distribution

Toxocara canis (Werner 1782) Stiles 1905

- Definitive host: dog, fox, other Canidae — small intestine,
- Paratenic host: essentially every species of mammal; bird; man — second stage larvae (L2) in parenteral tissues.

Toxocara canis is considered the most important species in toxocarosis. Adults are cream-white, thick-bodied, and reach 10–20 cm. The body bends ventrad anteriorly, has lanceolate, lateral, cervical alae, and there is a notch just before the end of the tail of the male. Eggs, 85 x 75 μm, with a thick, brown shell and pitted surface, are single celled when passed. L2 (second stage larvae) are 350–450 x 14–21μm with single lateral alae and an oesophageal ventriculus (Bowman 1987). *Toxocara canis* is virtually cosmopolitan in distribution; it is absent from the frigid Arctic region although it is found above 60°N; and low prevalences have been recorded in arid and semi-arid desert regions.

Toxocara cati (Schrank 1788) Brumpt 1927
syn *T. mystax*

- Definitive host: cats, other Felidae—small intestine,
- Paratenic host: rodents; birds; other mammals; man.

Adults are smaller than *T. canis* and their cervical alae arrowhead-shaped but their eggs are very similar. L2 are slightly smaller in diameter, e.g. 12–16 μm. It has a similar distribution. *Toxocara malaysiensis* is described in cats in Malaysia and China.

Baylisascaris procyonis (Stefanski and Zamowski 1951) Sprent 1958

- Definitive host: raccoons, dogs increasingly reported infected—small intestine

- paratenic host: rodents; other mammals; birds; man,

Adults reach 10–22 cms with vestigial cervical alae. Eggs are slightly smaller, with a granular shell, and are darker brown than *Toxocara* (Gavin *et al.* 2005). L2 grow in the host, reaching 1500 x 70–80 μm. It occurs in North America and was imported into Europe and Japan with raccoons and persists in raccoons. Other *Baylisascaris* spp. occur.

Ascaris suum of pigs and *Toxocara vitulorum* of cattle and buffalo can infect man but the larvae migrate for only about 3 weeks, at least in mice, although occasionally *A. suum* adults develop in man. Many other ascarids are proposed as potential zoonotic agents, e.g. *Toxocara pteropodis* (bats), *Toxascaris* (dogs, cats), *Lagochilascaris* (opossums), *Porrocaecum* (birds of prey), *Ophidascaris, Polydelphis, Travassoascaris* (snakes), etc., but any role is probably limited through short migratory times or lack of human contact with eggs.

Life cycle

The complex life cycle of *T. canis* with many options related to age, reproductive status, and dietary habits of the dog/fox, is summarized in Fig. 64.1. A similar life cycle undoubtedly occurs in all Canidae with infection transmitted between canids. The greatest number of eggs comes from the pivotal part of the life cycle involving the pregnant bitch/vixen and her pups/cubs. Adult dogs/foxes also produce eggs. The infective stage is an L2 whether in embryonated eggs or in tissues of paratenic hosts.

Somatic migration in adult dogs

In dogs 3–6 months of age, most L2 from ingested eggs migrate in the circulation through liver and lungs to somatic tissues where all organs are invaded. L2 continue to migrate for some time but later become dormant in the somatic tissues and remain alive probably for the life of the dog. Under certain circumstances L2 reactivate.

Transplacental migration from bitch to pups

L2 in a bitch begin to activate in the last 20 days of pregnancy and migrate across the placenta to foetal livers. From birth larvae migrate to the lungs, break out into the alveoli and undergo tracheal migration to be swallowed to start laying eggs about 2.5 weeks after birth; > 95% of L2 that a bitch transfers are transferred transplacentally.

Transmammary migration from bitch to pups

Some L2 activating in the bitch's tissues migrate to the mammary gland, as do L2 from eggs ingested in the peri-parturient period. The pup ingests these for up to 3–5 weeks to accrue more adults.

Tracheal migration in pups

L2 from eggs eaten by pups <3–6 months of age undergo tracheal migration to develop to adults with a pre-patent period of ≥ one month.

Puppy to bitch transfer of larvae

Some larvae entering the intestine of sucking puppies are swept out in their faeces. The bitch ingests her pups' fresh faeces while cleaning them and some larvae establish as adults in her intestine.

The mechanism(s) that allow re-activation of L2 and transplacental and transmammary transmission and the establishment of adults in the bitch have not been defined. Hormonal changes and/or depressed immunoreactivity may be involved. Adult *T. canis* in

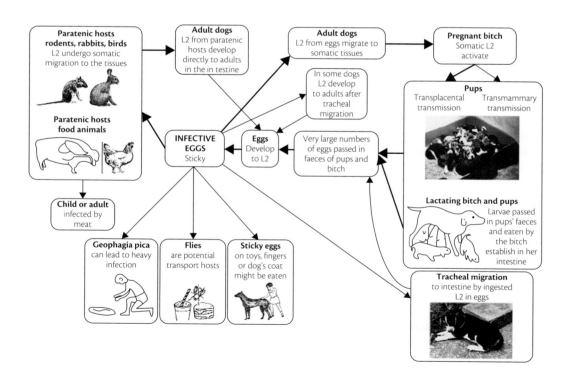

Fig. 64.1 The complex life cycle of *Toxocara canis.*

a pup will live two weeks to six months. Most adults in the bitch are expelled near to the end of lactation.

Tracheal migration in adults

In some adult dogs some L2 from eggs undergo tracheal migration to become adults. This is possibly related to breed/genetic susceptibility, hormonal changes, immunosuppression, and dose of eggs, and seems to be more common than previously realized. Low level egg administration has induced repeated infection in a number of juvenile and adult dogs/foxes with a pre-patent period of 1–2 months.

Transmission of L2 in paratenic hosts to dogs

L2 of *T. canis* hatch and migrate to the somatic tissues of all mammals, i.e. rodents, lagomorphs, birds, etc., but also domestic livestock. When eaten by dogs, the L2 from these paratenic hosts develop, without migration, to adults with a pre-patent period of ≥ one month.

Transmission of L2 between paratenic hosts

If one paratenic host is eaten by another, L2 can migrate from the tissues of the prey to the tissues of the new paratenic host.

When cats ingest eggs of *T. cati* there is tracheal migration of larvae with a pre-patent period of about 2 months. L2 in contrast to *T. canis*, do not seem not to persist in somatic tissues. There is vertical, lactogenic transmission to kittens but mainly only if the cat is infected in late pregnancy. Ingestion of paratenic hosts plays an important part in infection in adult cats.

Baylisascaris procyonis adults develop from ingested eggs in young raccoons and from eggs and paratenic hosts in adult raccoons. L2 of *T. vitulorum* accumulate in the tissues of adult bovines and transmammary transmission to calves occurs. L2 of *A. suum* undergo tracheal migration to the intestine in pigs.

Molecular biology, immune response, and immune evasion

Maizels and colleagues (reviewed by Maizels *et al.* 2006) confirmed the importance of *Toxocara* L2 TES and supplied considerable insight into the nematode glycocalyx and molecular structure, elaboration, and function of TES. The studies were facilitated by the remarkable ability of *Toxocara* L2 to survive in defined medium with a high rate of production of TES, an estimated 9 pg to 8 ng protein/larva/day. TES is highly glycosylated with 400 µg CHO per mg protein with a high proportion of O-linked galactose and N-acetylgalactosamine, like mucins. The major molecules are TES-26, -32, -45, -55, -70, -120, and -400 named for their apparent molecular weight on SDS-PAGE. Most of these are produced in the oesophageal and secretory glands and excreted through the buccal capsule and excretory pore. TES-32 seems to be transported through the cuticle. TES, with the exception of the 400 kDa molecule, then form the surface glycocalyx/coat about 10–20 nm wide and about 10 nm from the lipophilic epicuticle of *T. canis*. The glycocalyx is shed remarkably quickly, 25% of surface radiolabelled molecules are released into medium within one hour, with 80% released over 48 hours (Maizels *et al.* 1984).

The predominant surface product, TES-120, contains MUC-1, -2, and -3, part of a family of at least 5 mucins of which 1–3 are secreted. These glycans have novel trisaccharides with mono-or di-O-methylated groups on a terminal fucose (Khoo *et al.* 1991). TES 32 (CTL1) and TES-70 (CTL4) are C-type lectins. Other CTLs have been identified in expressed sequence tags (EST) of *T. canis*. TES-45 and -55 also might be lectins. rTES-32 binds to mannose and galactose in a Ca-dependent manner. TES-26 is a phosphatidylethanolamine-binding protein possibly associated with membrane restructuring.

Toxocara canis L2 have evolved to migrate and survive in the tissues of a wide variety of hosts in spite of the marked generalized antibody and inflammatory response they invoke. In man, leukocytosis, particularly marked eosinophila, and hyperglobulinaemia, including high titres of anti-*Toxocara* antibodies in all isotypes occur. Anti-heterophile antibodies are due to similar structure of the mucins to blood group antigens. IgM can persist rather than declining; this perhaps indicates a failure in isotype switching or an unusual configuration of the *T. canis* antigens, possibly the glycans, producing persistent IgM. IgE levels often are high. Eosinophilic, later becoming fibrotic granulomata develop in many tissues. This host response is not protective, however, as L2 can remain alive for years after infection.

TES are being related to the prolonged migration and survival of L2. EST identified 4 relatively large genes (abundant novel transcripts) that represented 18% of all the cDNA recovered (Tetteh *et al.* 1999) suppressed in the L2 *in vitro* and so possibly important for survival *in vivo* (Maizels *et al.* 2006). The glycocalyx is virtually absent from newly hatched larvae but appears within 24 hours in conditions mimicking the host. TES enzymes (elastase, acetylcholinesterase, metalloproteinase, cysteine proteases) could aid migration and survival. Superoxide dismutase might protect against reactive oxygen molecules.

TES molecules are shed spontaneously and, on attack by antibody and/or cells, surface antigen is aggregated and shed within three hours. The larva thereby could slough off and escape host effector mechanisms and re-migrate. Further, deposition of the immunodominant CHO of TES in granulomata or in immune complexes might divert the immune response from the larvae themselves. Sinuous tracts of antigen in tissues, the presence of extracellular antigen within granulomata, and the presence of granulomata that contain TES but no larva, all support this premise. With time though, in heavily infected mice proportionate to higher doses, an increasing proportion of larvae is found in eosinophilic granulomata in the liver. They do remain viable and can leave the increasingly fibrotic encapsulations (Kayes 2006). Encapsulation might reduce further damaging migration, or might increase predation through liver disease.

Despite the marked immune and eosinophilic granulomatous response, there is no evidence for eosinophil-mediated killing. The lack of an effective protective immune response may be due to TES up-regulating a possibly non-protective Th2 response and down-regulating Th1 as described with *Fasciola hepatica* (Chapter 72). *Toxocara* infection and injection of TES do induce a highly polarized Th2 response in mice. Cells from clinical toxocarosis patients have a higher than normal proportion of Th2 cells producing IL4 and IL5 and a lower than normal proportion of Th1 cells and clones of human T cells induced with TES had Th2 phenotype. Candidate molecules for down-regulation of protective immunity, in particular for modulating dendritic cells, are the glycans (Schabussova *et al.* 2007). TES could be like NES of *Nippostrongylus brasiliensis* adult worms that stimulated dendritic cells to induce a Th2 polarized response in naïve mice (Balic *et al.* 2004; Holland *et al.* 2005). The epicuticle binds lipids so it might bind host lipid to mask the L2.

Symptoms, pathogenesis, and pathology

Human disease

Seroprevalence of *Toxocara* is high at 2–10% of the population in industrialized countries and up to 80% or more in tropical developing countries, particularly in children. Records of disease though are not common. In part this may result from under-diagnosis due to mild and non-specific presentation and the non life threatening, self-limiting nature of some presenting with disease, but also a large majority of infected persons must be asymptomatic. Toxocarosis is not notifiable so numbers of cases/year must be estimated from laboratory records. In Austria 2–3.7% of the population were seropositive with 44, 17, 25, and 27% seropositivity in farmers, hunters, slaughterhouse staff, and veterinary surgeons; yet only several dozen cases are recorded each year (Deutz *et al.* 2005). Over a 10-year period in the USA, of 2,000–4,000 suspect samples submitted/year, 25–33% were positive of which an estimated 70% were OLM and 20% VLM. Ninety five per cent of the OLM cases had faulty vision, and 20% were blind in one or both eyes. In one 6-month period in England, of 1,182 sera, 150 were positive, one third being VLM patients.

A number of characteristic disease syndromes exist. Initially considered a disease primarily of children, increasingly disease is being recognized in adults due to increased diagnosis of covert toxocarosis and food-borne infection.

Asymptomatic

Positive toxocaral antibody and/or eosinophilia can occur in the absence of other clinical symptoms either currently or in the history, i.e. the 26% seropositive hydatid control officers in New Zealand that tested seropositive and 17–44% of rural workers seropositive in Austria. This is likely to be due to past and light infections or cross-reacting infections. The non-specific features of toxocarosis are likely to lead to under-diagnosis, while vision loss might go unnoticed in young children with later spontaneous resolution. Conversely, as positive serology is relatively common, it could mask an alternate diagnosis; for example, a case of retinoblastoma was masked by positive *Toxocara* titres.

Visceral larva migrans

This is an uncommon diagnosis in western industrialized countries although milder infections may be overlooked. VLM occurs when a large number of *T. canis* larvae continue to migrate for weeks and months through the liver and lungs and other tissues with symptoms related particularly to hepato-pulmonary migration. The L2 leave haemorrhagic tracts and a marked host inflammatory response. Commonly, but not exclusively, the patient is 2–7 years of age with a history of geophagia and contact with puppies. The classical signs are hepatosplenomegaly, abdominal pain, decreased appetite, fever, respiratory signs (cough, wheeze), restlessness, lymphadenopathy, pallor, and occasionally there may be urticarial skin lesions, neurological manifestations, heart problems, and ocular lesions. Leukocytosis including high eosinophilia (usually 30% or 2 x 10^9/L) is present and many patients have IgG/IgE hypergammaglobulinaemia. Gradually larvae become encapsulated in the musculature and liver and symptoms subside. High levels of IgM

antibodies have been associated with nephrosis. It is reasonable to assume that the disease is related to the migration of larvae and immune response to them.

Baylisascaris procyonis L2 migrate aggressively, increasing in size, and encapsulation is slow, but more commonly it presents neurologically. *Toxocara vitulorum* L2 are likely only to have a short-lived migration, but infection could induce cross-reacting antibody and eosinophilia and, in repeated infections, disease. While a large bolus of *A. suum* eggs given maliciously to students was pathogenic (severe pneumonia, eosinophilia), L2 have a short-lived migration and so are unlikely to cause disease in moderate or low numbers. Repeated exposure, e.g. in areas where intensive pig production and slurry disposal is common or where free-ranging pigs are reared, would induce an eosinophilia of unknown origin and possibly disease.

Covert or common toxocarosis

There is an increasing recognition of this milder form of toxocarosis first recognized in adult patients in the Midi-Pyrenees and in children in Ireland. Predominant symptoms vary somewhat between studies: this might relate to age or other factors. Commonly there is weakness/lethargy (in as many as 70%), abdominal pain (30–60%), lymphadenopathy (2–60%), skin lesions, pruritis (5–40%), respiratory features, cough/wheeze (12–70%), highest in a study group containing asthmatics), headache (23–48%), cervical adenitis, fever, anaemia, myalgia (particularly limb pains), nausea, anaemia, and other signs, including occasionally pica. There can be eosinophilia, high antibody titre and increased total IgE but one or more may be absent. It is postulated that covert patients are less able to encapsulate larvae permitting unlimited migration so that even a small number of larvae induce disease. Alternately, repeated light infection could account for the disease.

Ocular larva migrans

Loss in visual acuity is the most publicized and emotive manifestation, particularly as many patients come from non dog owning families. Patients are commonly, but not exclusively older children (8–15 years or more). The loss of visual acuity, usually related to the host response to a single larva, varies from blurring through to blindness, usually unilateral, rarely (1–3%) bilateral. Inflammation may be extensive with vitreal haze, chorioretinitis, endophthalmitis, uveitis, and also optic neuritis, but often no ocular pain. The impaired vision is related to the site of the eosinophilic and later fibrotic granuloma or to diffuse uveitis and leukoria. A granuloma on the posterior pole on or near the macula can cause severe visual loss. Granulomata on the peripheral retina are equally common and fibrotic repair of peripheral lesions can produce traction bands from the lesion to the posterior pole and lead to retinal traction, detachment and loss of vision. The impaired vision is related to the site of the eosinophilic and later fibrotic granuloma or to diffuse uveitis and leukoria. Vision loss may occur over days or weeks but many infections are subclinical. Patients seem to be lightly infected and only occasionally do OLM and VLM do occur concurrently; one suggestion is that the marked inflammatory response in VLM prevents migration to the eye. Little information is available on the incidence of OLM. Recently 1% of uveitis patients in San Francisco were diagnosed as OLM presenting with strabismus, failing vision, white eye (leukoria), etc., with vision loss due to vitritis, macular oedema and retinal detachment, although 7% were found at routine examination. One study found no OLM in 2,000 Irish schoolchildren with 31% seropositivity although Good *et al.* (2004), by questionnaire, described a prevalence per 100,000 of 6 Irish schoolchildren with a definite and 4 with a strongly suspected consultant diagnosis.

Baylisascaris procyonis has been implicated in diffuse unilateral neuroretinitis.

Neurological toxocarosis

Toxocara canis larvae accumulate in the brain of mice, and are found in the brain of man. Neurotoxocarosis though is rare (Moreira-Silva *et al.* 2004); about 30 cases of eosinophilic encephalitis/meningoencephalitis presenting as seizures, headaches, and other neurological manifestations. An association of *Toxocara* with subtle neuropsychological defects is postulated but not clear cut. Some, but not all studies suggest seropositive children have greater hyperactivity or lower cognitive function (Holland and Hamilton 2006). Similarly, a relationship between seropositivity and epilepsy is not confirmed but, in a small number of children, there was a strong association between history of a seizure and clinical diagnosis of OLM (Good *et al.* 2004).

Toxocara cati is less prone to migrate to the brain, at least in mice. *Baylisascaris procyonis*, while rare, elicits a progressive encephalopathy and a marked eosinophilic response, pathology is severe and the disease frequently fatal.

Allergic related disease

An association between *T. canis* seropositivity and asthma is suggested in studies in Holland and south-east Asia, but not in Connecticut, USA. Acute respiratory failure and bronchospasm have been recorded as a presenting symptoms of toxocarosis. Some laboratory studies provide credence for such an association, including the hyper-reactivity of mouse bronchial tissue to *Toxocara* antigen. Studies that standardize methodology, age, manifestation of asthma (acute or chronic) and the genetic influence of atopy are needed.

Allergic skin rash and pruritis are not uncommon in VLM and covert patients. A controlled study with improvement of chronic urticaria after treatment supported a *Toxocara* aetiology (Wolfrom *et al.* 1996) but other studies show no statistical association between antibody, disease, and efficacy of treatment.

Canine infections

Very large numbers of larvae migrating in newborn pups can produce haemorrhagic pneumonia. Adult *T. canis* in the intestine of pups induce hypertrophy of the tunica muscularis, villous atrophy, and malabsorption. A few worms will go unnoticed but, in larger numbers there will be poor growth or emaciation with a pot belly and variously diarrhoea and constipation. In very large numbers obstruction of the gut and death occasionally occur. Clinical signs of *T. canis* in adult dogs are very rare. Eye lesions might occur but are unnoticed or undiagnosed. One study in New Zealand described multifocal retinal disease of unknown aetiology in 39% of sheepdogs versus 6% of urban dogs and 4 of 70 necropsied dogs had ocular larvae.

Diagnosis

Human infection

Parasitological diagnosis (liver biopsy) is rarely undertaken as it is invasive, may not detect larvae, and morphological identification is unreliable. Bowman (1987) has provided keys for whole larvae or larvae in cross-section to aid differentiation of species in tissues.

The recent amplification of *ITS1* and/or *ITS2* rDNA and detection by PCR allows identification of several different ascarids (Jacobs *et al.* 1997, Zhu *et al.* 2001, Li *et al.* 2007) and could aid resolution of the importance of *T. cati* and other ascarids in soil and biopsy/post mortem samples (Borecka *et al.* 2008). Elevated eosinophils, globulins, anti-A and–B isohaemagglutins, and liver enzymes are useful but non-specific and may be absent in a proportion of covert cases.

Diagnosis was transformed by TES ELISA developed by de Savigny, now widely used, and commercially available. Differences in quality of product, age of larvae at TES harvest, cut off points, serum dilutions, and populations examined make it difficult to compare results (reviewed by Smith and Noordin 2006). Serum ELISA for VLM and usually covert toxocarosis has high sensitivity (88–100%), specificity (83–90%), and high predictive values in northern Europe and northern USA. The test though is only *Toxocara* genus specific and will not differentiate *T. cati* or *T. vitulorum*. Cross-reactions to *Ascaris, Anasakis,* and blood group antigens usually are ruled out by dilution of antigen and serum. In tropical populations polyparasitism with gastrointestinal helminths is prevalent and specificity falls to ≤50% but a competitive inhibition ELISA (using a cocktail of soluble heterologous parasite antigens) increased specificity. Recent developments have increased specificity in a tropical population: IgG4, although insensitive (46%), increased specificity to 79% (Noordin *et al.* 2005); IgG2 had sensitivity of 98% and specificity of 71% (Watthanakulpanich *et al.* 2008); IgE ELISA and possibly IgM ELISA are useful post-treatment to show a decline in titre. A recombinant TES-30 molecule produced sensitivity and specificity of 92 and 90%, respectively (Norhaida *et al.* 2008) with very good specificity if pre-absorbed with *Anasakis* (Yamasaki *et al.* 1998; 2000). Antibody to a 57 kDa *T. canis* antigen has shown potential, the band absent from *T. vitulorum* and not reacting with *T. cati* antibodies (Iddawela *et al.* 2007). rTc-MUC-1 also is available. All deserve additional testing.

Western blot using TES is reported as equally or more sensitive than ELISA and is used to confirm ELISA (Magnaval *et al.* 1991). Four low molecular weight bands (24, 28, 30, 35 kDa) were recorded as specific for toxocarosis; three high molecular weight bands (132, 147, 200 kDa) indicated cross-reactivity.

The signs of VLM and covert toxocarosis are non-specific and can be confused with other helminths, allergies, asthma, and malignancies. Equally, *Toxocara* infection and positive serology in healthy persons is not uncommon even in developed countries and antibody can persist at least 3–5 years (Magnaval and Glickman 2006). Positive serology therefore must be interpreted in light of clinical presentation and a careful history as symptoms often are acknowledged in history, rather than as presenting complaints (Taylor *et al.* 1987). In tropical areas particularly, stool examinations to rule out other often more pathogenic helminths is needed. Also, antibody titres in covert patients can be low and must be interpreted only in combination with the group of symptoms and signs that give a recognizable syndrome. Total IgE may be useful in covert toxocarosis, as may eosinophil cationic protein released from sequestered, degranulating, tissue eosinophils (Magnaval *et al.* 2001).

On MRI hepatic lesions are multiple, ill-defined oval or trapzoid nodules about 1–1.5 cm in diameter best observed on enhanced images in portal phase (Lim 2008). Lesions may be confluent in heavy infection. Lung lesions may have a ground glass opacity. Lesions may resolve spontaneously or number and positions may change. The lesions can resemble microabscesses, sarcoidosis, or those of *Capillaria hepatica*, *A. suum*, and *Fasciola* spp. that also produce eosinophilia. Liver ultrasound may reveal hypoechoic, small, oval areas with fuzzy margins.

As neurotoxocarosis is rare, CSF antibody tests are not standardized. Diagnosis should include high serum and CSF antibody and eosinophils in CSF. MRI reveals cortical or subcortical granulomata as diffuse lesions or circumscribed hyper-intense areas on T2-weighted images with resolution on treatment (Rüttinger and Hadidi 1991; Finsterer and Auer 2007). An experimental ELISA for *B. procyonis* using ES antigens is available in the USA.

OLM poses difficulties for diagnosis, particularly with the need for urgent differentiation from malignant retinoblastoma. Serum antibody titres may be low or absent in many OLM patients. Although invasive, *de novo* antibody production in vitreous and/or aqueous humour is confirmatory. Cytology reveals lymphocytes and eosinophils (often degranulated) in toxocarosis while elevated levels of lactic dehydrogenase and phosphoglucose isomerase occur in retinoblastoma. Echography can reveal a solid highly refractive granulomatous mass or traction bands or retinal detachment (Cella *et al.* 2004). Occasionally migratory tracts may be seen on the retina, or a larva may be visible.

Canine infection

Adult *Toxocara* infections are diagnosed by faecal flotation techniques; high specific gravity solutions, i.e. sodium nitrate, zinc sulphate, sucrose, combined NaCl/sucrose, are best used. High numbers of eggs will be found in puppies but the test is insensitive in adult dogs (perhaps only 50% compared with necropsy) as low levels of eggs are produced often intermittently.

Treatment

The source of infection must be identified and removed. As much of the pathology is due to the host inflammatory response to TES, therapy for VLM includes anti-inflammatory drugs. In severe cases cytotoxic immunosuppressants such as azathioprine have been used. Anthelmintic therapy (diethylcarbamazine [DEC], mebendazole [MBZ], albendazole [ABZ]) is included for acute VLM patients although evidence for efficacy is only moderate due to:

(i)   The relatively small number of cases,

(ii) The different treatment regimens begun after variable lengths of infection/disease,

(iii) Varying immunopathological responses between patients,

(iv) Spontaneous occurrence of remission.

Magnaval and Glickman (2006) compared the various trials and considered DEC more efficacious but only under experienced supervision due to side effects. DEC is given at 3–4 mg/kg for 21 days starting at 25 mg a day and progressively increasing; corticosteroids may partially inhibit DEC's activity and so are given sequentially. ABZ at 10–15 mg/kg or 400 mg bid both for 5 days is the treatment of choice for other physicians and has reported effect in neurotoxocarosis. ABZ does cross the blood-brain barrier. Patients should be monitored for liver side effects. Prognosis for *B. procyonis* with or without anthelmintic is poor and healing of the extensive migratory and inflammatory damage after treatment may worsen the disease.

Patients with covert toxocarosis should be monitored after reinfection is prevented. Many will improve and treatment need be initiated only in those that remain symptomatic (Magnaval and Glickman 2006).

No trials are available for treatment of OLM but options are discussed by Taylor (2006). Vigorous systemic and local anti-inflammatory therapy is required. Whether anthelmintics enter the eye is not known but possibly they could be included as potentially a larva may remain in a granuloma. Alternately, a living larva can be removed surgically. Vitrectomy for vitreal opacities and epiretinal dissection to relieve traction causing macular distortion and retinal detachment often improve vision. Laser photocoagulation has been used to destroy an intra-ocular parasite, to treat traction bands, and to eliminate choroidal neovascularization. Despite treatment, central lesions are likely to result in considerable, permanent visual deficit. However, in one study of 41 patients, final visual acuity was 20/20 in 50% and <20/200 in only 14% of patients.

Epidemiology

Egg contamination by animals

Prevalence in dogs varies widely irrespective of method of examination (faecal examination versus necropsy) and populations examined. Prevalence of infection is essentially 100% in most litters of puppies. Overall, prevalence and fecundity of worms decline in adult dogs and prevalence has declined in pets in industrialized countries in the last decade.

Prevalence in pets in recent studies was: in the UK, 30% in untreated ones and 1–4% in those treated every three months; in Germany, 0.7–22% were infected; in Kosice, Slovakia 7%; in Warsaw, Poland, 0.4% of pets in flats; and in Poznan, Poland, while 32% were positive, the majority of those infected were puppies (58%) versus adults (2.5%). In Australia there was only 0.4% prevalence in pets; in the USA 3%; and in Canada 3 and 14%, the latter study concentrating on at risk animals. In Ibadan and Ile-Ife, Nigeria, 9 and 34% of owned dogs were infected. In general, working dogs and strays show higher levels of infection than pets, i.e. 13% of working, hunting and military dogs in Greece and Turkey; 14–83% of farm and stray dogs in the USA, Estonia, a Province in China, townships in South Africa, and in urban Kosice and Dublin, Ireland. In studies in Poland, Slovakia, and Australia, prevalence in strays was 5 times higher than in pets.

Foxes are another source of infection with *T. canis* even for urban gardens. Fourteen to 73% of urban and rural foxes have been found infected in the UK, Germany, Denmark, Switzerland, Ireland, etc. Prevalence usually is higher in cubs (i.e. 87%) versus adults (52%) and, as the cubs examined are grouped as <6 mo, prevalence may be 100% as young cubs might lose worms at a few weeks to months of age as do puppies.

Prevalence of *T. cati* in stray cats ranged from 0.8% in Dohar, Qatar, through 4.9% in Australia, 20% in Spain, to 40–43% in Shiraz, Iran, and Dublin, Ireland. Twelve and 63% of farm cats in Spain and south west England, respectively, were infected. Prevalence in pet cats was lower, 1.7% in Australia and 11% in Spain but 21% of apartment cats and 49% of household cats in Mexico City.

High prevalence in foxes and stray dogs but also in free-roaming pet dogs and cats probably is due to diet in that these animals are free to hunt or scavenge paratenic small mammals or dead carcasses.

Adult *T. canis* can be extremely fecund. A female worm potentially can produce more than 100,000 eggs/day. Nonetheless, few data are available to quantify actual daily contribution of eggs by different hosts (dog, cat, fox, etc.) and age groups; most data presented as prevalence and not counts.

Normal, infected, adult, kennelled dogs in three studies in Belgium and the UK produced 1 and 2,145 eggs/gm faeces (epg). In a multi-country European study infected pets were passing geometric mean 423 epg (range 1 to 85,150 epg). Pet dogs in Nigeria showed around 400 (range 16–858) epg and stray dogs in Turkey 100–900 epg but up to 4,550 epg. There are few data for foxes. Young and adult silver and arctic foxes experimentally infected with eggs had epg ranging from 10s to nearly 4,000 and up to 11 adult worms. In the UK, wild foxes' epg ranged from 0.2 to 2,145. In Belgium, foxes were infected with an average of 3 but up to 16 worms.

Faecal egg counts in pups can reach 100,000/gm of faeces and total daily output from an experimentally heavily infected bitch and her pups was recorded as 1.5×10^7 eggs/day. Pets, however, are not as likely to be so heavily infected. In a study in Germany, nine bitches (3–9 months old) were exposed to infection by being walked for 3 h/day, 5 days/week, for 3 months, in an urban area with 150 dogs/km^2; the bitches acquired some tissue larvae as some pups in five litters were born infected; the levels of infection acquired were very low but then exposure of the dogs was limited. Kennelled Beagle bitches and their pups had geometric mean 72 and 52 epg (range 0 to 1,000) when examined 45 and 34 days after parturition with geometric mean worms in the pups of 3 (range 0 to 15). Kennelled greyhound pups were passing a mean of 1,200 to 34,000 epg when 3–7 weeks of age. No data are available concerning numbers of eggs being produced by a litter of cubs and their vixen.

The relative importance of different canid populations in contaminating the environment will depend not only on prevalence and intensity of infection, but also on the density of that population (strays, pets, foxes, etc.) in a given area. Up to 60% of households in the UK and USA may have a dog or a cat. Recent estimates are 63 and 61 million owned dogs and cats, respectively, in the USA and 10 and 6 million, respectively, in the UK. In Sweden numbers were lower, 15% of households estimated to own 800,000 dogs. Other surveys suggest 100–150 pet dogs/km^2 in various cities in the USA, UK, and Germany. Stray dogs were recorded at 330/km^2 in a high-density housing area in the UK and at 127–1304/km^2 in different areas in Valencia, Spain. The density of owned dogs in Zimbabwe was calculated as 3.4 dogs/km^2 rising to 68/km^2 in urban areas. In Lagos, Nigeria, figures for owned dogs were urban 131/km^2; rural 15/km^2. Dog densities were given as 3,000/km^2 in Sri Lanka and 1,922 km^2 in Dumagueti city, the Philippines. Fox densities in various cities and rural areas in the UK are described as 0.2–5.0 family groups (each group being two adults and 4.0–4.5 cubs)/km^2, 0.6–4 family groups/km^2 in Belgium and about 10 adult foxes/km^2 in Zurich.

Age distribution of populations will influence contamination; pups/cubs produce the highest numbers of eggs. Cubs make up a high proportion of the fox population in the spring and summer months, before they disperse in autumn/winter. In Zimbabwe, puppies <3-months-old were numerous; approximately 20% of the dog population. The percentage of dogs <1 year is much lower in the UK and USA. The territories used by animals also will influence contamination. Unconfined foxes and dogs will hunt over a territory of several kilometres. Pups/cubs usually remain confined to one area until 2–3 months of age. However, a lactating pet bitch, with her own worms, plus the eggs she acquired from cleaning her pups, will be walked for exercised in the garden or local area. Therefore, the number of breeding females in a canid population, and by implication rates of neutering, will be an important determinant of environmental contamination.

More than 70% of raccoons are infected with *B. procyonis* in the north east, mid-west and western USA. Expansion to Georgia (22%), Florida and Texas has occurred. Female worms can produce thousands of eggs each day.

Egg development and survival

Eggs develop to L2 in about 2–7 weeks at 25–15°C so development is seasonal in summer in temperate climates but year round in tropical areas. Unembryonated and embryonated eggs are very resistant and survive well over most winters. Only direct heat and desiccation kill them. From the data available in temperate climates eggs survive well for 6–12 months; some survive composting for at least a year; and a proportion survive in moist, cool conditions for 2–4 or possibly more years; conversely egg numbers declined to zero over 5 months in sandy soil in Australia. However, the actual proportion of deposited eggs that survive is unknown but probably is less than the ≤5% of *A. suum* eggs that survived 17 months in Central Europe.

Eggs in soil

Faeces are physically disrupted by rainfall, beetles, earthworms, slugs, etc. Eggs have been found on and in flies with potential for transfer to soil/lawns/food from faeces in neighbouring areas. Local dispersal in different soil and vegetation types is unknown bar that, in sandy soil in Poland one year after deposition most eggs were found in the top one cm (94% with 60–90% viability) and none were found 3 cm from the surface (Mizgajska-Wiktor and Uga 2006). Few eggs were recovered but lateral distribution was not reported. Studies on soil contamination usually give only the proportion of samples tested that proved positive and not the density of eggs. Also, methods of sampling and recovery differ markedly and usually only the genus *Toxocara* is reported. Mizgajska-Wiktor and Uga (2006) discuss the variable techniques and possible solutions. They also gave some differences between *T. canis* and *T. cati* eggs recovered from the uteri of females. *Toxocara canis* eggs were larger, 75% were 78–88 x 69–74 μm with maximum and minimum lengths 98 and 78 μm; *T. cati* were 59–74 x 54–69 μm (91%) with maximum and minimum 74 and 59 μm. *Toxocara canis* walls were thicker, less transparent, and had visible semi-circular cavities on the surface. Uga *et al.* (2000) however, considered that there was too much overlap in size between the species. They considered the topography of the egg surface, with *T. cati* having smaller and rounder pits compared with the polygonal pits of *T. canis*, useful in distinguishing the species with a 70–80% probability. Additional studies on field eggs are needed. PCR developed by Jacobs *et al.* (1997) efficiently differentiated eggs. *Toxocara vitulorum* has the finest pitting. *Baylisascaris procyonis* eggs also are finely granular.

Although techniques and areas studied vary, contamination of soil is prevalent. Recent studies have concentrated on squares, playgrounds, parks, sandpits, and backyards/gardens and have shown 1–60% samples positive. No clear geographic differences are necessarily present, i.e. 6 and 55% of samples contained eggs in recreational areas in Suba, Bogatá, Columbia, and Cuidad, Venezuela, respectively; in Maringá, southern Brazil, 52% of soil samples and 40–60% of grass samples in public squares were infected as were 21%, in São Paulo; in Kaduna, Nigeria, 50% of playground samples were contaminated. In Europe prevalence also varies: in Murcia, eastern Spain, and Salamanca, western Spain, one and 4–9% of samples from various recreational areas were positive; in Dublin County, Ireland, 6–15%; in the UK generally 5–10% although as many as 66% have been positive in the past; and several studies in Poland have revealed 10–50% prevalence. When urban versus rural village environments have been compared rural infection was more prevalent in Salamanca, Spain, and in Warsaw, Poland; conversely, in Poznan and Krakow, Poland, urban samples were more contaminated. Density and viability of eggs often are not recorded and density commonly is low <1 although up to 100 eggs/100 gm soil is recorded with a maximum of 700/100 gm. Infectivity can be low 1–2% of eggs, but up to 50–80% of eggs have been infective.

Few studies have identified species of eggs. In Poznan, one study described 90% of eggs from backyards as *T. cati* but there was an unusual marked divide with *T. canis* predominant February through May but *T. cati* very dominant June through January (Mizgajska-Wiktor and Uga 2006). A second study reported 97 per cent of eggs as *T. cati* in urban environments and 84% as *T. canis* in rural areas (Mizgajska-Wiktor and Jarosz 2007). Cats are considered responsible for the sometimes high *Toxocara* contamination in sandpits in recreational areas and gardens.

Eggs on animals

Contamination of dogs' hair recently has been reported as common. A careful study by Roddie *et al.* (2008) reported that 67% of dogs had eggs in their hair at up to 28 eggs/gm hair, this latter though in only one puppy. Only two of 71 adult dogs carried an embryonated egg/gm, the other 117 embryonated eggs being aggregated on puppies. It should be noted also that the dogs and puppies were mainly strays waiting to be euthanized at a rescue centre. The nature of the dogs, including the number of puppies, means the environment was likely to be heavily infected. Confined dogs having direct contact with faeces plus the difficulty in removing eggs from surfaces means infection pressure could have been high. Total (unembryonated and embryonated) eggs were comparable on the dorsum and the peri-anal area suggesting acquisition of sticky eggs from the environment rather than actual maintenance and embryonation on perianal hair. Studies on pets in The Netherlands and Ireland showed that while eggs were present on hair they were not embryonated and so not infective. Certainly, pet puppies would present risk but much of the faecal material will be removed by the bitch and deposited in her faeces to contaminate soil. In Turkey, where prevalence of infection is relatively high, only two of 51 pet dogs had embryonated eggs on their hair, one a puppy and one a 10 year old terrier (Aydnezizöz-Ozkayhan *et al.* 2008); it was not described whether the dogs were kennelled or not. Nonetheless, adult pet dogs could acquire eggs rolling in fox, cat or dog faeces.

Food-borne infection

Little information is available on food-borne *T. canis*. Free-ranging farm animals and birds have access to *Toxocara* eggs in farm, small-holding and backyard situations. Pigs and birds have been infected with L2 when fed raw viscera. *Toxocara canis* larvae persisted in pigs for more than one month but they have been described as dying relatively early in pigs. L2 persisted for 4.5 months in pigeons, 3.5 years in chickens and 7 months in lambs (Taira *et al.* 2004).

Larvae were found in all tissues, with highest numbers in the liver; viable larvae declined after slaughter but infective larvae still remained after 4 days at 4°C. On Welsh sheep farms where dogs were common, 7–13% of 6-month-old lambs and 47% of cull ewes were seropositive to TES though their infectivity was unknown (Lloyd 2006).

Acquisition of infection by humans

Humans potentially acquire *T. canis* by a number of routes. Risk factors include:

1 Geophagia pica,

2 Poor hygiene accompanied by access of dogs/foxes to gardens and play areas,

3 Poor hygiene and direct contact with dogs,

4 Consumption of L2 in raw/under-cooked meat or egg-contaminated food.

Socio-economic status will influence all these and the risks and levels of infection acquired vary between the human syndromes of disease. The most important risk factor for seroprevalence in a recent large scale study in the USA was the level of education of the head of household, with poverty, ethnicity, and dog ownership also having significant non-confounded effects (Won *et al.* 2008).

An important risk factor for VLM is geophagia pica that is common in about 10–25% of young children and may increase with nutritional deficiency. VLM requires heavy infection so a risk is ownership/contact with a puppy(ies) or fox cubs born in urban/village gardens in the last 6–12 months, these producing large numbers of eggs. These are most likely to be satisfied where children are outdoors unsupervised, thus, tropical climate, poverty, and low social status all contribute to VLM.

Smaller numbers of eggs in the soil may induce infection by geophagia and, with poor hygiene, the very sticky *Toxocara* eggs in soil may adhere to fingers, toys, food-stuffs, etc., that are placed in the mouth. These eggs might come from even well cared for pet dogs but also from contamination by dogs and foxes in gardens, parks, and other recreational areas. These risks have long been used to explain OLM that commonly is associated with low levels of infection and can occur in children that have no family pet or direct access to dogs. Regulations requiring leashing/kerbing/cleaning up after dogs, and provision of 'dog toilets', all point to the emphasis given to this route of infection by publicity and local government.

The importance of soil has been questioned with the alternate infection route eggs on dog hair perhaps deserving of more attention, though relative risk of pet dogs must be ascertained. For example, in the UK, more than 50% of patients with clinical toxocarosis had never owned a dog or had close contact with one. Conversely, high seroprevalence among agricultural workers and veterinary surgeons in Austria and hydatid control officers in New Zealand might support the importance of direct dog contact, but although these groups usually own dogs they generally work in rural areas so potentially could be infected through contact with land. Seropositivity in rural workers often is 3 times higher than in urban residents.

The relative importance of food-borne infection has never been ascertained. Where canids have access to unfenced vegetable gardens, transfer of eggs from faeces to salad greens could occur by rain splash. Food possibly could be contaminated with fly-borne eggs. VLM associated with consumption of raw liver was first described by Beaver in the 1950s. Now meat-borne disease is described particularly in Japan (Yoshikawa *et al.* 2008) but also elsewhere. Raw poultry, pig, lamb and beef liver and lightly cooked rabbit all have been incriminated. Eggs attached to snails collected in a meadow frequented by dogs were considered the cause of disease in an adult and consumption of an earthworm in a child.

The role of *T. cati* in VLM and OLM has never been reliably confirmed or refuted. Epidemiological data suggest that *T. cati* is not as important, e.g. people at risk included hydatid control officers and dog breeders but not cat breeders and, in Iceland where dog ownership was controlled, *Toxocara* antibody responses were negligible. A few histological studies also suggest *T. cati* is less important. However, higher antibody responses to *T. cati* than *T. canis* have been reported occasionally (Fisher 2003) and a recent case of adult VLM was related to ownership of a stray kitten. Nonetheless, *T. cati* larvae are less liable to either undergo somatic migration and/or persist in the tissues. Very occasionally adult *T. cati* have been described in children though it is not certain whether this represents true infection or pseudoparasitism from eating worms voided by cats.

Risk for *B. procyonis* is contact with raccoons that may be rescued or kept as pets or contact with 'racoon latrines' in wooded areas that create areas of very heavy contamination. Raccoons also will use rooftops, decking, sheds, etc. Chewing on fallen tree bark has induced disease.

Toxocara vitulorum eggs are likely to be ubiquitous in soil and water in tropical village environments; L2 potentially could also be consumed in milk.

Serological examinations in Holland have shown that children were seropositive to *Ascaris* as commonly as to *Toxocara*. As *A. lumbricoides* is uncommon in industrialized countries, these probably are *A. suum* infections from pig slurry/sludge that is commonly used as a fertilizer on farms and gardens. In developing countries exposure to both species is likely from soil in villages with free-roaming pigs and poor sanitation.

Control

Control of *T. canis* would be preferable to treatment of infection in humans because, even though the number of human cases is low, the time from infection to diagnosis may be prolonged, and effective therapy is not achieved in all cases. Costs of diagnosis and treatment of covert toxocarosis in adult patients were given as £620/patient by Magnaval and Baixench (1993). Costs for OLM are likely to be higher. Furthermore, these costs do not take into account the emotive aspects of disease or loss of vision in a child. Monetary and non-monetary methods by which the burden of toxocarosis and so the benefits of control could be calculated are given by Torgerson and Budke (2006).

The thick egg shell confers considerable resistance. On concrete, i.e. dry pavements exposed to sunlight, eggs will desiccate, but those in cracks will be protected. In kennels, while iodine and xylol have some effects, they are impractical. Hypochlorite (bleach) poured on flat surfaces can help by decoating the sticky surface of eggs so they can be washed away, but they will not be killed without prolonged contact. Only dry heat, e.g. a flame gun, is lethal. In damp, shaded soil eggs potentially will survive for years; detailed

studies on length of survival have never been performed. Only drastic measures will clean soil in gardens. Surface soil contaminated heavily with *B. procyonis* or *T. canis* theoretically could be broken up, turned and flamed several times or 10–20 cm of top soil removed and replaced (Kazacos 1991). Sand in sand-boxes can be steam sterilized or replaced and sand-boxes covered when not in use to prevent cat contamination but continued compliance was poor in a study in Japan.

Infection with *T. canis,* at least in pet dogs, is preventable by treatment, although unenforceable. Control of *Toxocara* in wild canids and roaming cats would be difficult. Regimens recommended for treatment of the bitch and puppies are:

1. The bitch and pups are treated every 2 weeks from 2 weeks after parturition until 8–12 weeks to kill worms developing in the intestine with one of many products with high efficacy against intestinal stages of *T. canis* though ease of administration to and licensing for the very young puppy are important considerations.

2. Bitches can be treated with 50 mg/kg/day fenbendazole from 22 days before to 2–20 days after parturition. This kills many of the L2 in the bitch as they migrate to the placenta/mammary gland and markedly reduces levels of infection in the puppies. The treatment must be repeated each pregnancy. Experimentally, selamectin and doramectin given twice in pregnancy also had good effect. The less frequent administration of these latter might increase owner compliance. Unfortunately, as the bitch and her pups, unless heavily infected, will appear perfectly healthy, many owners do not consider anthelmintic treatments.

While the rate of re-infection in dogs and so the treatment interval required has not been determined, susceptible animals theoretically could be re-infected immediately after treatment. Therefore, treatments at one or two month intervals for dogs and cats, respectively, must be appropriate, the interval increasing to 3–6 months only in dogs assessed as low risk. This should be a routine prophylactic public health programme as adult dogs infected with adult egg-laying *T. canis* are perfectly healthy and current parasitological diagnostic techniques have poor sensitivity and are time consuming. Resistance to the anthelmintics may not be a major problem as not all dogs and certainly foxes will be treated, treatment of individuals will not take place simultaneously, and a mosaic of drugs will be used. However, reports of pyrantel resistance in dog hookworms caution against complacency.

Education of pet owners is important but also additional education for veterinary surgeons is required. For example, in 1979 and 1989 in the USA and 2003 in western Canada fewer than 16% of vets recommended first worming of pups at <3 weeks although the majority (93–95%) had recommended worming at least once by 16 weeks. Recommendation to de-worm nursing bitches/queens improved in the three surveys from 16 to 64% though still remaining at only 72% in 2003 (Stull *et al.* 2007). A relatively high proportion of purchased pups will harbour infection so it is unfortunate that not every vet recommended worming when the pup presented for vaccination. Further, even in 2003 only 65% of vets recommended prophylactic deworming of dogs and cats and often only with a long interval of 4–6 months.

Legal cases pointing to egg contamination of parks as the source of infection have been recorded. Legislation has been invoked by many local councils for the restraint of dogs: exclusion of dogs from parks and beaches; requiring owners to collect their dog's faeces; provision of dog 'toilet areas'; and 'leash' laws for dogs. However, this is difficult to administer and often not enforced. Often the persons obeying the restrictions are the most responsible of pet owners whose dogs are the least likely to be infected; other owned dogs, stray dogs, and foxes remain uncontrolled. Further, methods for disposal of the faeces require evaluation. *Toxocara* eggs do survive composting and some would survive sewage processing, although the risk this poses is undetermined, while canine faeces place an additional burden on sewage disposal systems.

Treatment of stray dogs and foxes is not practical although measures put in place for rabies control and tested for *Echinococcus multilocularis* control in foxes (Chapter 54) could be put in place. These canid populations need to be controlled in number; control of stray dogs is necessary not only to prevent toxocarosis but also to reduce dog bites. Stray populations should be excluded from gardens, play areas, and playgrounds by fencing.

Good hand washing is necessary. Children at play should be supervised to encourage this and to prevent geophagia. Vegetables to be eaten raw should be well washed, but as the eggs are very sticky, vegetable gardens should preferably be fenced to exclude all canids although this will not exclude cats. The importance of fly-borne egg contamination of food requires evaluation, but fly control is required for other reasons also. While the importance of larvae in meat also is undetermined, meat, particularly liver, should be thoroughly cooked.

References

Aydnezizöz-Ozkayhan, M., Yagci, B.B. and Erat, S. (2008). The investigation of *Toxocara canis* eggs in coats of different dog breeds as a potential transmission route in human toxocariasis. *Vet. Parasitol.*, **152**: 94–100.

Balic, A., Harcus, Y., Holland, M.J. and Maizels, R.M. (2004). Selective maturation of dendritic cells by *Nippostrongylus brasiliensis*-secreted proteins drives Th2 immune responses. *Eur. J. Immun.*, **34**: 3047–59.

Bowman, D.D. (1987). Diagnostic morphology of four larval ascaridoid nematodes that may cause visceral larva migrans: *Toxascaris leonina, Baylisascaris procyonis, Lagochilascaris sprenti,* and *Hexametra leidyi. J. Parasitol.*, **73**: 1198–1215.

Borecka, A., Gawor, J., Niedworok, M. and Sordyl, B. (2008). Detection of *Toxocara canis* larvae by PCR in the liver of experimentally infected Mongolian gerbils (*Meriones unguiculatus*). *Helminthology*, **45**: 147–49.

Cella, W., Ferreira, E., Torigoe, A.M., *et al.* (2004). Ultrasound biomicroscopy findings in peripheral vitreoretinal toxocariasis. *Eur. J. Ophthalmol.*, **14**: 132–36.

Deutz, A., Fuchs, K., Auer, H., *et al.* (2005). *Toxocara*-infestations in Austria: a study on the risk of infection of farmers, slaughterhouse staff, hunters and veterinarians. *Parasitol. Res.*, **97**: 390–94.

Fisher, M. (2003). *Toxocara cati*: an underestimated zoonotic agent. *Trends Parasitol.*, **19**: 167–70.

Finsterer, J. and Auer, H. (2007). Neurotoxocarosis. *Rev. Instit. Med. Trop. Sao Paulo*, **49**: 279–87.

Gavin, P.J., Kazacos, K.R. and Shulman, S.T. (2005). Baylisascariasis. *Clin. Microbiol. Rev.*, **18**: 703–18.

Good, B., Holland, C.V., Taylor, M.R., *et al.* (2004). Ocular toxocariasis in schoolchildren. *Clin. Infect. Dis.*, **39**: 173–78.

Holland, C.V. and Hamilton, C. (2006). The significance of cerebral toxocariasis. In: C.V. Holland and H.V. Smith (eds.) *Toxocara: the Enigmatic Parasite*, pp. 58–73. Wallingford: CABI Publishing.

Holland, M.J., Harcus, Y.M., Balic, A. and Maizels, R.M. (2005). Th2 induction by *Nippostrongylus* secreted antigens in mice deficient in B cells, eosinophils or MHC Class I-related receptor. *Immun. Lett.*, **96**: 93–101.

Iddawela, R.D., Rajapakse, R.P., Perera, N.A. and Agatsuma, T. (2007). Characterization of a *Toxocara canis* species-specific excretory-secretory antigen (TcES-57) and development of a double sandwich ELISA for diagnosis of visceral larva migrans. *Korean J. Parasitol.*, **45**: 19–26.

Jacobs, D.E., Zhu, X., Gasser, R.B. and Chilton, N.B. (1997). PCR-based methods for identification of potentially zoonotic ascaridoid parasites of the dog, fox and cat. *Acta Trop.*, **68**: 191–200.

Kayes, S.G. (2006). Inflammatory and immunological responses to *Toxocara canis*. In: C.V. Holland and H.V. Smith (eds.) *Toxocara: the Enigmatic Parasite*, pp. 158–73. Wallingford: CABI Publishing.

Kazacos, K.R. (1991). Visceral and ocular larva migrans. *Semin. Vet. Med. Surg. (Small Animal)*, **6**: 227–35.

Khoo, K.-H., Maizels, R.M., Page, A.P., *et al.* (1991). Characterization of nematode glycoproteins: the major *O*-glycans of *Toxocara* excretory secretory antigens are methylated trisaccharides. *Glycobiology*, **1**: 163–71.

Li, M.W., Lin, R.Q., Chen, H.H., *et al.* (2007). PCR tools for the verification of the specific identity of ascaridoid nematodes form dogs and cats. *Mol. Cell. Probes*, **21**: 349–54.

Lim, J.H. (2008). Toxocariasis of the liver: visceral larva migrans. *Abdom. Imaging*, **33**: 151–56.

Lloyd, S. (2006). Seroprevalence of *Toxocara canis* in sheep in Wales. *Vet. Parasitol.*, **137**: 269–72.

Magnaval, J-F. and Baixench, M.T. (1993). Toxocariasis in the Mid-Pyrénées region. In: J.W. Lewis and R.W. Maizels (eds.) *Toxocara and Tococariasis. Clinical, Epidemiological and Medical Perspectives*, pp. 63–69. London: Institute of Biology.

Magnaval, J-F. and Glickman, L.T. (2006). Management and treatment options for human toxocariasis. In: C.V. Holland and H.V. Smith (eds.) *Toxocara: the Enigmatic Parasite*, pp. 113–26. Wallingford: CABI Publishing.

Magnaval, J.F., Fabre, R., Maurières, P., *et al.* (1991). Application of the western blotting procedure for the immunodiagnosis of human toxocariasis. *Parasitol. Res.*, **77**: 697–702.

Magnaval, J-F., Glickman, L.T., Dorchies, P. and Morassin, B. (2001). Highlights of human toxocariasis. *Korean J. Parasitol.*, **39**: 1–11.

Maizels, R.M., de Savigny, D. and Ogilvie, B.M. (1984). Characterization of surface and excretory-secretory antigens of *Toxocara canis* infective larvae. *Parasite Immunol.*, **6**: 23–37.

Maizels, R.M., Schabussova, I., Callister, D.M. and Nicoli, G. (2006). Molecular Biology and Immunology of *Toxocara canis*. In: C.V. Holland and H.V. Smith (eds.) *Toxocara: the Enigmatic Parasite*, pp. 3–17. Wallingford: CABI Publishing.

Mizgajska-Wiktor, H. and Uga, S. (2006). Exposure and environmental contamination. In: C.V. Holland and H.V. Smith (eds.) *Toxocara: the Enigmatic Parasite*, pp. 211–27. Wallingford: CABI Publishing.

Mizgajska-Wiktor, H. and Jarosz, W. (2007). A comparison of soil contamination with *Toxocara canis* and *Toxocara cati* eggs in rural and urban areas of Wielkopolska district in 2000–2005. *Wiad. Parazytol.*, **53**: 219–25.

Moreira-Silva, S.F., Rodrigues, M.G., Pimenta, J.L. *et al.* (2004). Toxocariasis of the central nervous system: with report of two cases. *Rev. Soc. Bras. Med. Trop.*, **37**: 169–74.

Noordin, R., Smith, H.V., Mohamad, S., Maizels, R.M. and Fong, M.Y. (2005). Comparison of IgG-ELISA and IgG4-ELISA for *Toxocara* serodiagnosis. *Acta Trop.*, **93**: 57–62.

Norhaida, A., Suharni, M., Sharmini, L.A.T. and Rahmah, N. (2008). rTES-30USM: cloning via assembly PCR, expression, and evaluation of usefulness in the detection of toxocariasis. *Ann. Trop. Med. Parasitol.*, **102**: 151–60.

Roddie, G., Stafford, P., Holland, C., and Wolfe, A. (2008). Contamination of dog hair with eggs of *Toxocara canis*. *Vet. Parasitol.*, **152:** 85–93.

Rüttinger, P. and Hadidi, H. (1991). MRI in cerebral toxocaral disease. *J. Neurol., Neurosurg. Psychiatry*, **54:** 361–62.

Schabussova, I., Amer, H., van Die, I., Kosma, P. and Maizels, R.M. (2007). *O*-methylated glycans from *Toxocara* are specific targets for antibody binding in human and animal infections. *Int. J. Parasitol.*, **37:** 97–107.

Smith, H. and Noordin, R. (2006). Diagnostic limitations and future trends in the diagnosis of human Toxocariasis. In: C.V. Holland and H.V. Smith (eds.) *Toxocara: the Enigmatic Parasite*, pp. 89–112. Wallingford: CABI Publishing.

Stull, J.W., Carr, A.P., Chomel, B.B., Berghaus, R.D. and Hird, D.W. (2007). Small animal deworming protocols, client education, and veterinarian perception of zoonotic parasites in western Canada. *Can. Vet. J.*, **48:** 269–76.

Taira, K., Saeed, I., Permin, A. and Kapel, C.M.O. (2004). Zoonotic risk of *Toxocara canis* infection through consumption of pig or poultry viscera. *Vet. Parasitol.*, **121:** 115–24.

Taylor, M.R.H. (2006). Ocular toxocariasis. In: C.V. Holland and H.V. Smith (eds.) *Toxocara: the Enigmatic Parasite*, pp. 127–44. Wallingford: CABI Publishing.

Taylor, M.R.H., Keane, C.T., O'Connor, P., *et al.* (1987). Clinical features of covert toxocariasis. *Scand. J. Infect. Dis.*, **19:** 693–96.

Tetteh, K.K.A., Loukas, A., Tripp, G. and Maizels, R.M. (1999). Identification of abundantly-expressed novel and conserved genes from infective stage larvae of *Toxocara canis* by and expressed sequence tag strategy. *Infect. Immun.*, **67:** 4771–79.

Torgerson, P.R. and Budke, C.M. (2006). Economic impact of *Toxocara* spp. In: C.V. Holland and H.V. Smith (eds.) *Toxocara: the Enigmatic Parasite*, pp. 281–93. Wallingford: CABI Publishing.

Uga, S., Matsuo, J., Kimura, D., Rai, S.K., *et al.* (2000). Differentiation of *Toxocara canis* and *T. cati* eggs by light and scanning electron microscopy. *Vet. Parasitol.*, **92:** 287–94.

Watthanakulpanich, D., Smith, H.V., Hobbs, G., Whalley, A.J. and Billington, D. (2008). Application of *Toxocara canis* excretory-secretory antigens and IgG subclass antibodies (IgG1-4) in serodiagnostic assays of human Toxocariasis. *Acta Trop.*, **106:** 90–95.

Won, K.Y., Kruszon-Moran, D., Schantz, P.M. and Jones, J.L. (2008). National seroprevalence and risk factors for zoonotic *Toxocara* spp. infection. *Am. J. Trop. Med. Hyg.*, **79:** 552–57.

Wolfe, A. and Wright, I.P. (2003). Human toxocariasis and direct contact with dogs. *Vet. Rec.*, **152:** 419–22.

Wolfrom, E., Chene, G., Lejoly-Boisseau, H., *et al.* (1996). Chronic urticaria and *Toxocara canis* infection. A case-control study. *Ann. Dermatol. Venereol.*, **123:** 240–46.

Yamasaki, H., Taib, R., Watanabe, Y.I., *et al.* (1998). Molecular characterization of a cDNA encoding a secretory-excretory antigen from *Toxocara canis* second stage larvae and its application to the immunodiagnosis of human Toxocariasis. *Parasitol. Int.*, **47:** 171–81.

Yamasaki, H., Araki, K., Lim, P.K.C., *et al.* (2000). Development of highly specific recombinant *Toxocara canis* second stage larva excretory-secretory antigens for immunodiagnosis of human toxocariasis. *J. Clin. Microb.*, **38:** 1409–13.

Yoshikawa, M., Nishiofuku, M., Moriya, K., *et al.* (2008). A famial case of visceral toxocariasis due to consumption of raw bovine liver. *Parasitol. Int.,*, **57:** 525–29.

Zhu, X.Q., Gasser, R.B., Chilton, N.B. and Jacobs, D.E. (2001). Molecular approaches for studying ascaridoid nematodes with zoonotic potential, with an emphasis on *Toxocara* species. *J. Helminthol.*, **75:** 101–8.

CHAPTER 65

Trichostrongylidosis

T. J. Nolan

Summary

Trichostrongylidosis is an infection involving nematodes of the superfamily Trichostrongyloidea, mainly those of the genus *Trichostrongylus*. Infections are usually asymptomatic, but when heavy, a variety of gastrointestinal symptoms, including abdominal pain and diarrhoea, can be present. Infections are initiated by the ingestion of third stage larvae. There is no parenteral migration and the adults are usually found in the mucosa of the duodenum. Eggs pass out with the faeces, hatch in about one day and the larvae develop to the infective stage in 4 to 6 days. Human infections with *Trichostrongylus* spp. have been reported worldwide, and are particularly common in southern Asia. Infections respond well to anthelmintics and periodic dosing of livestock is the chief method of control.

History

The type species for the Genus *Trichostrongylus* (*T. retortaeformis*) was described from rabbits in 1800 and *T. orientalis* was described from man in 1914 (Nagaty 1932). By 1927 human infections with animal-infecting species of *Trichostrongylus* were known well enough for Sandground (1929) to consider them in his differential diagnosis of a nematode infection found in a missionary from Africa. Evidence of human infections has been found in mummies dating to 1,000 BC (Goncalves *et al.* 2003).

In 1947 Stoll estimated that there were 5.5 million cases of human trichostrongylidiosis in the world, the vast majority of them being in Asia. In 1953 Watson revised Stoll's estimate using new reports of prevalence from India, Indonesia, China, the Middle East, and Africa as well as more up to date population estimates. He estimated that 58 million human cases occurred worldwide, with 30 million being found in Indonesia (based on a 41.2% incidence, more recent estimates of the prevalence (Oemijati 1971) put it in the range of 11% in this region). While Stoll's estimate was probably too conservative and Watson's may be skewed by the one prevalence estimate from Indonesia, the true number of cases today most likely is nearer to Watson's estimate than to Stoll's. With the increase in the human population in the areas with the highest prevalence rates that has occurred since 1953, coupled with the lack of any major change in the risk behavior of these

populations, Watson's estimate of 58 million cases appears reasonable. However, in some areas the general increase in sanitation or the use of anthelmintics for control of other diseases may have driven the prevalence of *T. orientalis* down, as seen in the Republic of Korea where the prevalence went from 7.7% in 1971 to zero in 1997 (Rim 2003).

Our knowledge of the life cycle parameters of *Trichostrongylus* spp. infections in humans comes from studies by Joe (1947) done in the 1940's. Using human volunteers and *T. colubriformis* and *T. axei* he was able to estimate the pre-patent period, some of the clinical signs, and the differences in infectivity of the different species for humans.

The agent

Taxonomy

Members of the genus *Trichostrongylus* are nematodes of the class Secernentea, order Strongylida, and superfamily Trichostrongyloidea. Adult *Trichostrongylus* spp. are slender, generally under 10 mm in length, and the male has a copulatory bursa at its posterior end. The adult worms lodge in the mucosa of the stomach or small intestine, the exact location varies depending on the species. The female worms lay thin walled 'strongyle-type' eggs which pass out with the faeces. Eggs hatch in 1 or 2 days in faeces or damp soil and the larvae eventually develop to the infective third stage, which is enclosed in the cuticle of the second stage. Infection takes place when these third stage larvae are swallowed by the host. These larvae invade the mucosa of the digestive tract and eventually develop to adults. There is no parenteral migration.

Ten species have been reported to infect humans: *Trichostrongylus axei*, *T. affinis*, *T. brevis*, *T. calcaratus*, *T. capricola*, *T. colubriformis*, *T. orientalis*, *T. probolurus*, *T. skrjabini*, and *T. vitrinus*. With the exceptions of *T. brevis* and *T. orientalis*, all are parasites of domestic and wild ruminants (Acha and Szyfres 1987). Humans are the natural host for *T. orientalis*, although it has also been found in sheep and camels. *T. brevis* is seen mainly in humans although it has been reported from goats in Turkey (Akkaya 1998). Other trichostrongylids of ruminants that have been found in man are *Haemonchus contortus*, *Ostertagia ostertagia*, *O. circumcincta*, and *Marshallagia marshalli* (Ghadirian and Arfaa 1973). These four nematodes have been reported on only a very few occasions despite their wide spread occurrence in domestic livestock.

Disease mechanisms

The adults of *Trichostrongylus* spp. feed on the mucosal tissue of the gastrointestinal tract. The resulting tissue destruction leads to the symptoms of the disease.

Growth and survival requirements

The eggs and larvae of *Trichostrongylus* spp. are resistant to cold and desiccation. Third stage larvae over-winter on pasture in Great Britain and in the southern hemisphere, after drought, the desiccated third stage larvae will rehydrate when the rains arrive and are still infective (Soulsby 1982). These parasites may also over-winter in the host as hypobiotic third stage larvae.

The hosts

Animal

Incubation period

In ruminants the time from ingestion of the third stage larvae to the passage of eggs in the faeces ranges from two to three weeks, depending on the species.

Clinical signs

Ruminants with heavy infections usually have diarrhoea and show a rapid weight loss. Signs in lighter infections range from none to soft faeces and a decline in the rate of weight gain. In most cases, ruminants infected with *Trichostrongylus* spp. are also infected with other nematodes and thus the clinical signs will reflect the mix of parasites and may therefore be different from those just described (Soulsby 1982).

Diagnosis

Trichostrongylus sp. infections in ruminants are usually diagnosed by finding the eggs in a faecal flotation using either a saturated sugar or salt solution. Because many ruminant nematode parasites produce 'strongyle-type' eggs a definitive diagnosis may require identification of larvae recovered from a faecal culture. But, because of the availability of broad spectrum anthelmintics, this larval identification procedure is rarely done.

Pathology

The third stage larvae penetrate the wall of the abomasum or intestine (the site depends on the species) and will tunnel within the mucosa. When the worms moult to the adult stage they break out of these tunnels, resulting in oedema and haemorrhage. Large numbers of adults can lead to erosion of the mucosal surface, with the subsequent development of diarrhoea. The heavily infected animal generally loses weight.

Treatment

Infected animals can be treated with ivermectin, levamisole or one of the benzimidazoles. However, drug resistance is now common in the *Trichostrongylus* spp. that infect ruminants, so the choice of drug will depend on the pattern of drug resistance seen in the local geographical area. Because the pasture is now contaminated with eggs and larvae, treated animals should be moved to new pasture after they are treated or treated prophylacticly for the rest of the grazing season.

Human

Incubation period

The time between ingesting the third stage larva and the development of the mature adult in humans has been reported to be 21 days (for *T. colubriformis*), although it might be expected that this time period will vary depending on the species of *Trichostrongylus* (Joe 1947). The adult worms can live for several years.

Symptoms

The symptoms and their severity depend on the number of worms present. Most infections are asymptomatic, but in heavy infections (over 100 adult worms) diarrhoea (sometimes tinged with blood), abdominal pain, nausea, mild anaemia, and weight loss have been reported (Boreham *et al.* 1995; Ralph *et al.* 2006). A transient or persistent eosinophilia may also be present. An accurate description of the symptoms present in a heavy infection is difficult as most people harbouring many adult *Trichostrongylus* sp. are also infected with other gastrointestinal nematodes.

Diagnosis

Diagnosis is usually made by examining the stools for eggs. The 'strongyle-type' eggs laid by *Trichostrongylus* spp. must be differentiated from hookworm eggs (Webb 1937). *Trichostrongylus* spp. eggs measure 73–95 m long and 40–50 m wide. They generally have dissimilar poles, one end is rounded while the other is somewhat pointed. Thus the eggs are larger than those of the hookworms and have a different shape. Hookworm and *Trichostrongylus* spp. infections can also be distinguished by examining the first stage larvae obtained by faecal culture. The most obvious difference between these first stage larvae is that those of *Trichostrongylus* spp. will have a beadlike swelling on the caudal tip of the tail while hookworm larvae have a tail that ends in a point. Specific diagnosis can be made by recovering adult male worms from the faeces after treatment. The spicules, gubernaculum, and bursal rays are used in making a species identification. At the research level, PCR primers have been developed with will distinguish *Trichostrongylus* from the human hookworms (Yong *et al.* 2007).

Pathology

Very little is known about the pathology of these worms in humans although it is thought to be similar to that seen in the animal host. Desquamation with haemorrhage has been reported at the intestinal sites infected by adult worms.

Treatment

Ivermectin, albendazole, thiabendazole, mebendazole, pyrantel embonate and bephenium hydroxynaphthoate have successfully cleared *Trichostrongylus* infections from humans (Ralph 2006; Bundy *et al.* 1985; Panasoponkul *et al.* 1985; Boreham *et al.* 1995; Markell 1968). A follow-up faecal examination should be done 2 to 4 weeks after treatment to verify that the infection has been cleared. It should be noted that *Trichostrongylus* spp. have developed resistance to various commonly used anthelmintics and before treating a patient, veterinary authorities should be consulted to see which class of drugs is still active in the local animals (Ralph 2006).

Prognosis

Patients cured of a *Trichostrongylus* infection make a rapid and complete recovery.

Epidemiology and epizoology

Occurrence

Members of the genus *Trichostrongylus* are common in ruminants worldwide and human infections have been reported from every continent except, of course, Antarctica. Human infections are common across southern Asia, as well as in Korea and some areas of Japan. Endemic areas are also found in Africa (Egypt, Ethiopia, Zaire, and Zimbabwe).

Sources, transmission and communicability

Many of the infections in Asia are due to *T. orientalis* and are the result of the use of human faeces as fertilizer. The infection is acquired while eating uncooked plant material on which the larvae are present. Of the remaining infections in these endemic areas the most common source of infection was domestic animals sharing living quarters with humans (Ghadirian and Arfaa 1975). Also, the use of animal faeces as fuel has been implicated in the infection of the people who gather and prepare the faeces for this purpose (Ghadirian and Arfaa 1975). The source of infections in non-endemic areas is most likely the accidental ingestion of larvae acquired from livestock pasture or the ingestion of unwashed vegetables grown with animal manure used as fertilizer (Boreham *et al.* 1995).

The human to human transmission of species of *Trichostrongylus*, other than *T. orientalis* and *T. brevis*, is probably low to nonexistent. Even the two species parasitizing humans are transmitted indirectly, and thus are not transmissible to people associated with infected humans, but who do not eat uncooked material from plants fertilized with human faeces.

Prevention and control

Prevention

In areas where *T. orientalis* is prevalent, uncooked plant material should not be eaten, especially vegetables and other crops that might have been fertilized with nightsoil. In endemic areas where other species of *Trichostrongylus* are found, hands should be washed before preparing or eating meals and vegetables should be thoroughly washed or cooked before eating. Animal manure should be composted at a high enough temperature to kill *Trichostrongylus* eggs before being used as a fertilizer. The practice of sharing living quarters with domestic livestock should be discouraged.

Control strategies

T. orientalis can be controlled by proper sanitation (i.e. removal of human faeces from areas where humans may come in contact with it) and the sterilization of faeces before its use as a fertilizer. Infections with *Trichostrongylus* spp. of animal origin can be controlled by periodic treatment of domestic livestock with anthelmintics. The time between treatments will depend on the local conditions. Since well nourished livestock are better able to reduce their parasite burdens, animals should be kept well fed and their diet supplemented with minerals. Particular care should be taken with animals under a year of age as they are still developing an immune response to the worms and therefore have higher worm burdens than older animals.

Since in warm weather larvae will survive on pasture for about one month, pasture rotation, with a period of greater than one month, will help to reduce worm burdens in livestock.

References

Acha, P.N. and Szyfres, B. (1987). Zoonoses and Communicable Diseases Common to Man and Animals, (2nd edn.). Washington DC: Pan American Health Organization.

Akkaya, H. (1998). Investigations on the trichostrongylid nematodes of hair goats slaughtered in Istanbul. *Acta Parasit. Turcica*, **22**: 77–87.

Boreham, R.E., McCowan, M.J., Ryan, A.E., *et al.* (1995). Human trichostrongyliasis in Queensland. *Pathology*, **27**: 182–85.

Bundy, D.A.P., Terry, S.I., Murphy, C.P. and Harris, E.A. (1985). First record of *Trichostrongylus* axei infection of man in the Caribbean region. *Trans. Roy. Soc. Trop. Med. Hyg.*, **79**: 562–63.

Ghadirian, E. and Arfaa, F. (1973). First report of human infection with *Haemonchus contortus*, *Ostertagia ostertagi*, and Marshallagia marshalli in Iran. *J. Parasitol.*, **59**: 1144–45.

Ghadirian, E. and Arfaa, F. (1975). Present status of trichostrongyliasis in Iran. *Am. J. Trop. Med. Hyg.*, **24**: 935–41.

Goncalves, M.L., Araujo, A., Ferreira, L.F. (2003). Human intestinal parasites in the past: new findings and a review. *Memor. Instit. Oswaldo Cruz.*, **98** Suppl 1: 103–18.

Joe, L.K. (1947). *Trichostrongylus* infections in man and domestic animals in Java. *J. Parasitol.*, **33**: 359–62.

Markell, E.K. (1968). Pseudohookworm infection- trichostrongyliasis. Treatment with thiabendazole. *N. Eng. J. Med.*, **278**: 831–32.

Nagaty, H.F. (1932). The Genus Trichostrongylus Looss, 1905. *Ann. Trop. Med. Parasitol.*, **26**: 457–518.

Oemijati, S. (1971). Gastrointestinal infections in Indonesia (a review). In: J. Cross (ed.) Proceedings of the seventh southeast Asian regional seminar on tropical medicine and public health: Infectious diseases of the gastrointestinal system in Southeast Asia and the Far East, pp. 153–61.

Panasoponkul, C., Radomyos, P. and Singhasivanon, V. (1985). *Trichostrongylus* infection in a Thai boy. *S.E. Asia. J. Trop. Med. Pub. Health*, **16**: 513–14.

Ralph, A., O'Sullivan, M.V., Sangster, N.C., Walker, J.C. (2006). Abdominal pain and eosinophilia in suburban goat keepers - trichostrongylosis. *Med. J. Aus.*, **184**: 467–69.

Rim, H.J. (2003). Experience and progress in controlling disease due to helminth infections in the Republic of Korea. IN: Controlling disease due to helminth infections. Crompton, D.W.T., *et al.* (eds). WHO, Geneva, Switzerland.

Sandground, J.H. (1929). *Ternidens deminutus* (Railliet and Henry) as a parasite of man in southern Rhodesia; together with observations and experimental infection studies on an unidentified nematode parasite of man from this region. *Ann. Trop. Med. Parasitol.*, **23**: 23–32.

Soulsby, E.J.L. (1982). Helminths, Arthropods and Protozoa of Domesticated Animals, (7th edn.). Philadelphia: Lea and Febiger.

Stoll, N.R. (1947). This wormy world. *J. Parasitol.*, **33**: 1–18.

Watson, J.M. (1953). Human trichostrongylosis and its relationship to ancylostomiasis in southern Iraq, with comments on world incidence. *Parasitology*, **43**: 102–9.

Webb, J.L. (1937). The helminths of the intestinal canal of man in Mauritius; and a first record of *Trichostrongylus axei* locally. *Parasitology*, **29**: 469–76.

Yong, T.S., Lee, J.H., Sim, S., *et al.* (2007). Differential diagnosis of *Trichostrongylus* and hookworm eggs via PCR using ITS-1 sequence. *Korean J. Parasitol.*, **45**: 69–74.

CHAPTER 66

Scabies and other mite infections

K. E. Mounsey and S. F. Walton

Summary

Acariasis in humans and animals is caused by a diversity of parasitic mites taxonomically grouped into the class Arachnida, subclass Acari. The zoonotic species that can transfer from birds and animals to man (e.g. *Cheyletiella* spp.; *Dermanyssus* spp. and *Ornithonyssus* spp.) are important in that they often cause major skin irritation or a hypersensitivity reactions or alternatively act as vectors of diseases such as scrub typhus. Like ticks the life cycle of mites involves four life stages of development. The female mite lays eggs on the host or in the environment; the eggs hatch into larvae and pass through two nymphal stages. All stages have eight legs except the six-legged larva. Transmission is predominantly via direct contact between hosts; however fomites have been recognized as a potential source of infestation although the importance of this is variable and dependent on the ability of the mite to survive in the environment. The geographic range of most zoonotic species is worldwide although some varieties may be rare or non-existent in some countries. No developmental change or propagation of the organism occurs during the transmission.

Introduction

While mites rarely transmit disease to humans, they definitely impact health in ways that range from simply being a nuisance, to inflicting severe skin irritation that can cause intense itching. The most commonly encountered mites, including those that can adversely affect human health, are listed below.

Sarcoptic mange

History

Scabies is one of the oldest diseases known to man, and was recognized from as early as 1,000 BC, with references to disease symptoms in the Old Testament of the Bible, and by Aristotle (384–322 BC). Several writers describe the condition of human scabies, including Tabarii (970AD), Saint Hillegard (1098–1179) and Avenzoar (1091–1162). However, until the early seventeenth century scabies was described as a 'corruption of flesh and blood', thought to originate from an internal illness rather than the presence of mites in the skin. In 1687, Bonomo and Cestoni first described the ectoparasitic association of scabies, making it one of the first diseases of man with a known causative agent. However, their revelation was largely ignored for nearly 200 years. In 1778, de Geer gave the first accurate description of the scabies mite, and to his credit the parasite was commonly referred to as *Sarcoptes scabiei* de Geer (Buxton 1941). In 1868, Hebra published a well received treatise on scabies, and acceptance of the origin of this disease was finally established. Alternative names for the mite through history include *Acarus siro* var. *scabiei*, *Acarus scabiei*, *Sarcoptes hominis*, *Sarcoptes communis*, and its present designation as *Sarcoptes scabiei*.

Biology

Sarcoptes scabiei belongs to the phylum Arthropoda, class Acari, order Astigmata and family Sarcoptidae. The family Sarcoptidae includes *Sarcoptes scabiei*, *Notoedres cati* and *Trixacarus caviae*. The mite infests up to 40 different mammalian hosts across 17 families (Elgart 1990). Common hosts include humans, dogs, pigs and foxes. It has been widely debated whether these variants represent separate species, or if one highly variable species exist. Although *S. scabiei* mites isolated from different hosts are morphologically similar, cross infectivity studies have demonstrated they are physiologically different and largely host specific. This is supported by genetic studies showing substantial genetic variation between human-derived and canine-derived *S. scabiei*, even in mites collected from the same household (Walton *et al.* 2004a). Limited gene flow and apparent lack of interbreeding between these populations supports designation of separate species, but current convention still involves sub-typing mites according to their host species, for example, *S. scabiei* var. *hominis* (human), *canis* (dog), *suis* (pig) etc.

S. scabiei is a tiny mite, its ovoid body measuring 0.2–0.5mm long and 0.16–0.42mm wide. Adult female mites are 0.3–0.5mm, just visible to the naked eye and easily observed with microscopy. The mite is an opaque, creamy white colour with brown legs and mouthparts. The convex dorsal surface of the body is covered with numerous spines, setae and striations, and the ventral surface is flattened. Adult and nymph *S. scabiei* have four pairs of legs, while larvae have three pairs. Male mites are smaller (0.2–0.3mm) and appear darker and than females. They also differ from females on leg IV (males have short stalked pulvilli whereas females have long setae).

Historically, it has been difficult to study the passage of the mite through various life stages in detail, due the difficulty in locating mites on the host. As a result, much of the information on the scabies life cycle has been largely anecdotal and sometimes contradictory. Much of this uncertainty was resolved by Arlian and colleagues in 1988, using a model of New Zealand white rabbits experimentally infested with *Sarcoptes scabiei* var. *canis* (Arlian and Vyszenski-Moher 1988). The fertilized adult female penetrates the horny layer of the skin to form a burrow. It is thought they achieve this by secreting a proteolytic saliva like substance which dissolves the host keratinocytes. The female begins to lay her eggs just hours after starting the burrow, and continues to lay 2–3 eggs per day for the rest of her life (around 4–6 weeks). It appears that very few of these eggs actually develop into adult mites. The eggs hatch after about 50 hours of incubation. The larvae find their way to the skin surface to seek food and shelter in the hair follicles, where they remain for 3–4 days. They then moult into protonymphs, then tritonymphs, from which an adult male or female emerges. Following fertilization of the female the cycle begins again. The development from egg to adult requires 10–13 days.

Mites are extremely sensitive to desiccation; therefore survival off the host is highly dependent on relative humidity and temperature. In general, mite survival is favoured by low temperature and high relative humidity. The ability of mites to survive off the host has important implications for disease transmission. Arlian found that mites held for 24–36 hours at room temperature were still capable of host penetration, although these experiments involved artificial transmission (Arlian *et al*. 1984). The experiments of Kenneth Mellanby in the 1940s provided fascinating insights into many aspects of the disease, using conscientious objectors to World War II as human subjects. Exchanging clothes and sleeping in beds previously occupied by infested patients failed to transmit scabies, despite intensive efforts. He found that the disease was most commonly transmitted by skin to skin contact, and that individuals with higher mite numbers were more likely to transmit the disease (Mellanby 1944). From this it appears that fomites are an insignificant source of transmission, except in cases of crusted scabies, where shed skin may contain enormous numbers of live mites.

Previous attempts to transfer canine mites to mice, rats, guinea pigs, pigs, cattle, goats or sheep were unsuccessful; likewise human or pig mites could not be transferred to New Zealand white rabbits. Human infestations of scabies derived from other animal hosts are commonly reported; however are almost always self limiting. Host immunity appears to play a role in this process, since sensitization to animal transmitted scabies is very different to a human infestation.

Scabies in animals

Scabies infestation in animals is referred to as sarcoptic mange. It affects many companion animals and livestock such as dogs, horses, pigs and camels. It is a particularly serious disease and cause of mortality in wild red foxes, wombats, rabbits, agile wallabies and alpacas. Sarcoptic mange causes significant losses to primary industries; especially in pig herds (Davies 1995), and in the UK, mange is increasingly reported as a cause of production losses in imported Camelid species.

Incubation period

This initial penetration of host skin takes less than 30 minutes (Arlian *et al*. 1984). In a primary mange infestation symptoms generally take 2–6 weeks to develop, consistent with a delayed hypersensitivity immune response. In subsequent infestations sensitization is rapid, generally less than 48 hours (Mellanby 1944).

Symptoms and signs

Clinical manifestations may vary according to species, but generally involve raised, red papules and vesicles. If infestation progresses to chronic mange, skin proliferation occurs, and mite-infested hyperkeratotic plaques form. The skin becomes thickened and wrinkled, and extensive alopecia results from a reduced supply of blood to the hair follicles. As with humans, intense pruritus is experienced and secondary bacterial infections may occur concomitantly with infestation. Mites appear to have a predilection for areas of thin skin, and sparse hair. Hence, in pigs, sheep and horses, sites first infected are generally the face and ears. In dogs, areas affected may include the muzzle, ears and face, legs, thighs, trunk and tail. Transmission of mites among a group of animals is most likely through direct contact or via contaminated bedding.

Diagnosis

While the presence of thickened skin crusts is distinctive of advanced or chronic mange, diagnosis is more difficult in earlier stages as symptoms may mimic other skin conditions such as eczema, insect bites, dermatitis, or other non-sarcoptic mange conditions. The obvious 'gold standard' for diagnosis is the identification of mites, their eggs, or faeces (Burgess 1996). Skin scrapings are performed by firmly scraping with a scalpel at right angles to the skin, to remove superficial layers. Paraffin or mineral oil may be used to assist collection. Scrapings can then be examined under low power microscopy. Treating the scraping with 10% potassium hydroxide is useful for dissolving skin and improving resolution of mites, however will also dissolve faecal pellets. This technique has poor sensitivity due to low numbers of mites present in many infections. Sensitivity of skin scrapings is also influenced by the scraping technique, number of sites sampled, size of the scraping and the type of lesion sampled. Mites may also be observed in histological sections of skin biopsies.

The ideal diagnostic test for scabies would involve serological tests where the identification of mites was not required. ELISAs using whole mite extract to detect sarcoptic mange in animal herds are commercially available, however a significant degree of variation exists in sensitivity between kits (Lowenstein *et al.* 2004). These tests are also only suitable for diagnosis of infected herds rather than individual animals. The use of whole mite extracts may be problematic due to the heterogeneous combination of both host and parasite antigens and potential for cross reactivity (Walton and Currie 2007).

Pathology

The disease progression of mange in pigs is well documented. Clinical symptoms are evident after about 2 weeks, by which time mites have begun to make numerous burrows in the skin. By four weeks keratinized crusts begin to appear. Crusts thicken as mites proliferate, which peak infestation at around 8–10 weeks. After this peak, crusts will become detached and regress three to four weeks later (Cargill and Dobson 1979). This natural regression suggests host immune responses act to inhibit growth of the mite population. Chronic mange appears to occur due to a failure to mount this protective immune response.

The humoral immune response in swine mange is well documented. Morsy and Gaafar (1989) reported high numbers of

IgG, IgM, and IgA secreting cells in the dermis of infected pigs, peaking at 3 weeks post infection. In another study, circulating antibody titres peaked at about 8 weeks (Wooten *et al.* 1986).

Histological sections of crusted mange lesions in swine showed tracts of necrotic material surrounded by eosinophils, neutrophils, lymphocytes and mast cells. Papular, erythmatous lesions also contained numerous eosinophils and lymphocytes. The eosinophilla observed in infected pigs appeared to be related to the degree of pruritus (Cargill and Dobson 1979).

Although these early studies have given great insights into swine immune responses to mange, there is still little understood regarding the temporality of cellular immune responses to infestation, nor the specific immune deficits predisposing animals to severe or chronic mange. Such information would assist the development of new immunodiagnostics and vaccines, of value for both animal and human populations.

Treatment

Traditional treatments for sarcoptic mange involved the application of topical agents such as sulphur, lindane, organophosphates and synthetic pyrethroids. Although many of these are effective, difficulties in application and potential side effects preclude their use in many settings.

Nowadays, treatment for mange largely relies on the macrocyclic lactone (ML) family of drugs. They offer flexibility of use as they can be administered both systemically and topically. Additionally, they offer broad spectrum coverage against a range of endo and ectoparasites. Commonly used MLs for sarcoptic mange include ivermectin, doramectin, selamectin, moxidectin and milbemycin. The pharmacokinetics of MLs vary substantially in animals according to species, sex, age, and physiological status (reviewed in Cerkvenik-Flajs and Grabnar 2002). Therefore the choice of drug is influenced by the animal. Caution is advised with use of ivermectin in certain breeds of dog, due to mutations in the *mdr1* gene. This mutation is present in dogs of the collie lineage, and results in a deficient P-glycoprotein pump, allowing the drug to cross the blood brain barrier. Signs of ivermectin toxicity in dogs include ataxia, increased salivation, depression, coma, or even death. Alternatives such as selamectin are reported to have a wider margin of safety. The recommended dosage of most MLs for sarcoptic mange is 200–400 μg/kg weekly for 4–6 weeks, depending on the severity of the condition. Moxidectin and doramectin are reported to be highly effective against mange in dogs, pigs and cattle.

Amitraz has been used successfully in camelid species which appear to be poorly responsive to MLs (Lau *et al.* 2007). For sarcoptic mange, the recommended dose is 0.25–0.5%, fortnightly for 4–6 weeks. Maximum effectiveness was obtained when acaricide therapy was combined with keratolytic bathing or clipping of hair to increase absorption. However, amitraz is contraindicated in pregnant and nursing bitches, as well as puppies. Reported side effects include depression, sedation, bradycardia (Curtis 2004).

Topical alternatives to amitraz include spot on formulations of fipronil, which may be useful for earlier stages of the disease, or where other treatments are contraindicated. A recently developed spot-on combination of imidicloprid and moxidectin, applied monthly for two months, was highly effective against canine mange (Fourie *et al.* 2006).

Prognosis

Prognosis depends on the severity of mange, the degree of secondary infection, and the host species. If treated promptly, and if re-infestation does not occur, the outcome is excellent in most animals. However in certain species, such as wombats, angora rabbits, and camelids, distress is significant and death may occur. Angorra rabbits may be particularly difficult to treat, and euthanasia is recommended in severe cases. Fortunately however, the new generation macrocyclic lactones have dramatically improved outcomes.

Scabies in man

The scabies mite infecting humans is referred to as *Sarcoptes scabiei* var. *hominis*. Animals infested with scabies can transmit infections to humans, but due to the host specificity of the mites, infestations are transient. People who work closely with farm animals may be affected, especially from cattle infected with *Sarcoptes scabiei* var. *bovis* ('dairyman's itch') or pigs with *S. scabiei* var. *suis* ('pig handlers itch'). In humans, animal transmitted scabies can be distinguished from other forms of scabies by rapid onset of sensitization (within 48 hours) and the absence of burrows. Furthermore, areas affected reflect where direct exposure to the animal occurred. The disease is self-limiting, and removal of the animal often leads to clearing of symptoms. The following section will focus solely on infection caused by the human mite variant.

Incubation

In a primary infestation of scabies, symptoms usually take 4–6 weeks to develop. This is thought to be due to delayed immune recognition, as sensitization is very rapid in subsequent infestations, generally less than 48 hours (Mellanby 1944). This delayed onset of symptoms contributes heavily to the spread of scabies, as people do not seek treatment until infestation and transmission is well established.

Symptoms and signs

Often referred to as 'classical' or 'uncomplicated' scabies, ordinary scabies is the most prevalent form of the disease. It is caused by infestation with surprisingly few parasites, with the average number of female mites per patient less than 15, reducing with repeat infestations. Infestation commonly involves the hands, particularly the wrists and interdigital spaces. Elbows, knees, feet and genitalia may also be affected. Symptoms may vary substantially in severity, but almost always include intense pruritus, often worsening at night. Visible symptoms may include papular or vesicular lesions related to the site of mite burrowing, in addition to a more generalized itchy rash assumed to be part of the allergic response to the mite products. Mite burrows, often regarded as the classical indicator of scabies, can be observed as a thin, greyish, line of 5–15mm (Buxton 1941). However, burrows can be very difficult see with the unaided eye, particularly on dark skin, and are not always present.

Scabies is easily transmitted to young infants and children, probably because of increased body contact during these years. Lesions reflect those of adults, but with a more widespread distribution over the body, commonly involving the palms, soles, midriff, face, neck and scalp. This is attributed to the mites' predilection for soft, folded areas of skin (Gordon and Unsworth, 1945). Vesicular and papular lesions are very common. Mellanby *et al.* (1942) noted a higher average number of mites in children, which may reflect underdevelopment of the immune system.

In addition to the symptoms described above, atypical manifestations of scabies may be observed. Nodular scabies involves the formation of extremely pruritic, reddish-brown nodules, which may persist for months following treatment. Mites are not found in nodules, making diagnosis difficult. In the elderly, inflammation of lesions may not be observed, although itching is intense. The distribution of mites may also involve the back, scalp, or behind the ears. The itching is commonly misdiagnosed, incorrectly attributed to dry skin, anxiety or senility. Scabies outbreaks in nursing homes are very common.

Akin to chronic mange in animals, crusted scabies is the most severe clinical manifestation of scabies, characterized by a proliferation of mites and formation of hyperkeratotic skin crusts. The condition was first described in 1848 as a variant of leprosy in Norway; and in 1851 mites were correctly identified as the causative agent. Thus, the condition is still commonly described as 'Norwegian scabies' despite having no inherent connection with this country. Crusted scabies in caused by the same mite as ordinary scabies, although it was once thought to be caused by a different variant, *S. scabiei* var. *crustosa* (Green 1989). It is now understood that crusted scabies results from the inability of the host immune system to control the mite burden, resulting in thousands to millions of mites present on a single patient in extreme cases. Areas affected differ to ordinary scabies and may include the soles of the feet and palms, back and buttocks. Crusting may be widespread or localized, with severe cases involving greater than 30% total body surface area. Crusts can range in thickness from 1–2mm up to 2–3cm and vary in their appearance. They can be loose, soft and spongy, containing many vacant burrows, and may be easily shed. Conversely, crusts can be very hard and adherent, with punch biopsies needed to reveal mites residing in the deep crusts. In many cases pruritus can be completely absent, but in other patients it may be extreme.

Diagnosis

Scabies has been referred to as one of the most difficult diagnoses in dermatology. As described previously, symptoms may closely resemble those of other skin conditions. For practical purposes, diagnosis relies largely on clinical presentation and the history of the patient and their contacts. Despite 100% specificity, skin scrapings have very poor sensitivity due to the low numbers of mites present in ordinary human scabies and the difficulty in identifying burrows in some cases. Even when performed by an expert, a negative skin scraping does not exclude scabies.

Epiluminesence microscopy and videodermatoscopy have been proposed as accurate and non-invasive techniques, however these require specialized equipment. Visibility of mite burrows may be improved by the use of India ink. The use of a PCR-ELISA method for detecting previously undiagnosed scabies has been reported, but due to the technical expertise required and hypothesized low levels of *S. scabiei* DNA present on the skin it is not currently a viable approach.

No immunodiagnostic tests are currently available for human scabies, with research in this area historically impeded due to the absence of an *in vitro* culture system and limited availability of purified recombinant mite antigens. However, through the establishment of *S. scabiei* expressed sequence tag libraries, several candidate *S. scabiei* antigens have been reported (Fischer *et al.* 2003).

The ability to produce a constant supply of purified recombinant antigen, facilitating detailed *in vitro* studies, suggests a highly specific diagnostic test for scabies may be a real possibility in the near future (Walton and Currie 2007).

Pathology

Crusted scabies usually results from an unknown underlying immunodeficiency. Predisposing conditions include substance abuse, HIV, HTLV-I, systemic lupus erythematosus, type 2 diabetes, previous leprosy and immunosuppression in transplant recipients. It also may be seen in patients with cognitive deficiency such as Down's syndrome, or in the elderly or institutionalized who may be unable to interpret the itch. Importantly, crusted scabies also occurs in people with no known immunological deficit. A recent clinical review of 78 crusted scabies patients in northern Australia found that 42% had no known risk factor (Roberts *et al.* 2005). These patients appear to have a specific, as yet unknown immune deficit predisposing them to crusted scabies.

Scabies patients generally have elevated levels of circulating antibodies, particularly IgG and IgE. The elevation of IgE in crusted scabies is striking and may be over 1,000 times higher than normal (Roberts *et al.* 2005). This dramatic, non-protective humoral response is probably due to the extreme antigenic load presented by the high mite burden. Specific antigens responsible for immune reactions include components of mite saliva and secretions, egg cases or faecal products.

Histopathological features of ordinary scabies include inflammatory infiltrates of eosinophils, lymphocytes and histiocytes. Whereas CD4+ T-lymphocytes were predominant in lesions of ordinary scabies patients, those from crusted scabies lesions were primarily CD8+ (Walton *et al.* 2008). Blood CD4+ and CD8+ levels and ratios were within normal limits in crusted scabies (Roberts *et al.* 2005), suggesting selective recruitment of these cells into the skin. Interestingly, no B-cells are observed in lesions of either crusted scabies or chronic mange, which may partially explain the lack of protective immune responses. Crusted scabies patients also have increased levels of inflammatory cytokines such as IL-4 (Walton *et al.* 2008). It is hypothesized that crusted scabies results from a preferential, non-protective Th-2 immune response, and interestingly IL-4 has been shown to stimulate keratinocyte proliferation (Yang *et al.* 1996). Similar Th-2 skewed responses have also been observed in atopic dermatitis and psoriasis.

Treatment

Sulphur compounds have been used as acaricides for centuries, and are still a relevant option in certain cases today. It is generally used as a 2–10% precipitate in a petrolatum base. It is considered safe for pregnant and lactating women, and for infants younger than two months. Although effective and inexpensive, sulphur compounds are messy, smelly and sometimes irritating. Furthermore, multiple applications are often required for successful treatment. Therefore, sulphur has largely been abandoned for more 'user friendly' alternatives.

Ten per cent crotamiton ointment has been used as an acaricide since 1946. It has antibacterial, antiparasitic and antipruritic activity, which coupled with low-toxicity, makes it a popular option for children. However, its clinical efficacy is questionable, with low cure rates reported. For successful treatment, multiple applications are required.

In areas where scrub typhus is a risk, insecticide treatment of vegetation will help to reduce mite populations. On a larger scale, burning or clearing of vegetation will confine mites to specific areas away from potential human contact.

Epidemiology of scrub typhus

Scrub typhus is commonly seen in the Asian-Pacific region, spreading from India and Pakistan in the East, Korea and Siberia in the North, and the Pacific Islands and northern Australia to the South. This region is sometimes referred to the 'tsutsugamushi triangle'. This endemic region is host to around 1 billion people, and an estimated 1 million cases of scrub typhus occur annually. Mortality rates range from <1% to 50%, depending on the rickettsial strain involved and treatment (Chattopadhyay and Richards 2007). Transmission of scrub typhus is dependent on the presence of the *Leptotrobium* vector, which can be found anywhere suitable for rodent populations and where ground moisture is sufficient for mite survival. Most common sites are the vegetation areas between woods and clearings, as these become re-colonized by scrub, trombiculid mites and their rodent hosts. The main risk factors for contracting scrub typhus are therefore occupational— outdoor related agricultural activities including fruit picking, chestnut gathering, or taking rest breaks amongst mite-infested vegetation (Kim *et al.* 2007).

Other mites affecting man

Dermanyssus and *Ornithonyssus* (=*Liponyssus*, =*Macronyssus*), poultry mites

Dermanyssus and *Ornithonyssus* are members of the order mesostigmata and family Dermanyssoidea. *D. gallinae* is a haematogphagous mite commonly known as the chicken or poultry red mite. *D. gallinae* mites were first described in 1834 by Duges. The mites are up to 0.7mm with a grey to dark red appearance (depending on time since blood meal). Mites feed at night for 0.5–1.5 hours, but generally live away from their host, residing in wall cracks, crevices and nesting boxes. They can survive around 8 months without feeding and are resistant to desiccation but do not survive well in humid conditions. With a very short life cycle of seven days, mite populations can grow exponentially and result in heavy infestations.

Poultry red mites result in substantial morbidity and loss of productivity to the industry, causing anaemia, restlessness, decreased egg production and egg quality. Heavy infestations may even cause death. It is also known that *D. gallinae* are reservoirs of several bacterial pathogens, which may have more serious implications for zoonotic disease transmission. Studies on *D. gallinae* have identified pathogens such as St-Louis encephalitis, *Pasturella multocida, Erysopelothrix rhusiopathiae, Coxiella burnetii* and *Listeria monocytogenes*. However presence is not indicative of vectorial capacity, and few studies have been able to demonstrate transmission in the field. Recent evidence however has shown that *D. gallinae* was implicated in the transmission of salmonellosis on poultry farms (Valiente Moro *et al.* 2009). As this is one of the most commonly encountered zoonotic diseases in man, control of the poultry mite is of increasing importance.

Ornithonyssus sp. are similar to *Dermanyssus* in appearance, differing in the shape of anal plates (*Dermnyssus* is triangular, while *Ornithonyssus* is pear-shaped). The two predominant species are *O. sylviarum* (northern fowl mite) and *O. bursa* (tropical fowl mite). *O. sylviarum* was first identified by Canestrini and Fanzago in 1877. The taxonomic position of *Ornithonyssus* has been variable through the years, having being placed in the genera *Macronyssus, Liponyssus* and *Bdellonyssusis. Ornithonyssus* infestations of poultry are more common in the USA, with *Dermanyssus* playing a minor role in this region. As opposed to *Dermanyssus, Ornithonyssus* mites lay eggs on the host, and feed during both day and night, and thus are a constant source of irritation.

Poultry mites can induce irritation in humans, and heavily infested flocks are a source of itching dermatitis to poultry workers. Like most other mite zoonoses, infestation is transient. Inhalation of *O. sylviarum* allergens may be a source of occupational asthma in personnel working in poultry premises (Lutsky and Bar-Sela 1982).

Control of poultry mites is problematic due to prolonged survival time off the host and niche habitats. Traditional control methods involved spraying of pens with agents such as carbamates, organophosphates and pyrethroids. The choice of acaricide is limited due to environmental and food-safety issues. Additionally, resistance has been reported for pyrethroids and organophosphates. Systemic acaricides such as ivermectin have been tested, but are only effective at extremely high doses (2–5 mg/kg), precluding its use due to toxicity and cost-effectiveness concerns. There is now an increasing research focus on the use of alternative control methods, such as natural product extracts and immunological approaches to combat this problematic group of mites.

Ornithnyssus (=*Macronyssus, Liponyssus*) Bacoti, tropical rat mite

Closely related to poultry mites are the haematophagous *Ornithnyssus bacoti*. The mite infests rodents, most commonly rats, mice, gerbils and hamsters. *O. bacoti* are morphologically similar to other macronyssid mites, but can be distinguished by the location and shape of genital shields, and are hairier when viewed by microscopy. Contrary to their common name, *O. bacoti* mites are prevalent in all continents where rodents are present. Like *D. gallinae*, the tropical rat mite lays eggs and spends time predominantly away from the host. They have low host-specificity and subsequently, in the absence of a rodent host they will readily seek out humans as opportunistic blood meals. Dermatitis associated with tropical rat mites was first described by Hirst in 1913, and has been frequently reported worldwide. Symptoms of rat mite dermatitis in humans resemble that of flea bites, with flat to raised erythmatous lesions. Mild pain may be felt upon biting, followed by intense pruritus. Lesions normally appear in linear configurations or in groups. Symptoms have been described in workers from animal laboratory facilities, and also in people occupying rodent-infested premises. Mites are rarely found on hosts but may be readily located in the host environment. Eradication of the mites through conventional acaricides will resolve symptoms. *O. bacoti* has also been shown to harbor organisms such as *Pastuerella tularensis,* but there have been no reports on transmission of diseases to humans, with the exception of a 1931 report implicating mites in the spread of human typhus.

Trixacarus caviae, the guinea pig mite

Trixacarus caviae is a burrowing Sacroptid mite closely related to *Sarcoptes scabiei*. It appears to be host specific for guinea pigs, causing intense pruritus, dermatitis, alopecia and crusting. Infestations may be associated with secondary bacterial infection, complications of which may lead to seizures and death of the animal. *Trixacarus* mites can be distinguished from the other Sarcoptid mites (*S. scabiei and Notoedres cati*) in their smaller size (females <200 µM) and differing appearance of dorsal setae and spines (Fuentealba and Hanna 1996). Guinea pigs with genetic resistance to infection with the nematode *Trichostrongylus colubriformis* are more susceptible to *T. caviae,* with higher mite numbers and increased hyperkeratosis (Rothwell *et al.* 1989). Pruritis and popular dermatitis has been reported in humans in contact with infested guinea pigs, but these are again transient and self limiting (Kummel *et al.* 1980).

Dermatophagoides, house dust mites

House dust mites are free living, astigmatid mites belonging to the family Pyroglyphidae. These mites include *Dermatophagoides farinae, D. pteronyssinus,* and *Euroglyphus maynei.* Mites feed on shed human and animal skin and organic debris, and are a common household occupant, thriving wherever dead skin may accumulate, such as carpets and pillows. Mites flourish in areas of high relative humidity, however even in drier climates proximity to humans provides the mite with adequate moisture levels. Mite faecal pellets are allergenic and can induce a range of hypersensitivity reactions, including asthma. Signs of house dust mite allergy include sneezing, itchiness, watery eyes, runny nose, and eczema. House dust mite allergy is diagnosed by determining IgE reactivity to various *Dermatophagoides* antigens.

Grain and storage mites

Grain and storage mites comprise over 10 genera, including *Acarus, Glycyphagus, Tyrophagus, Chortoglycphus* and *Blomia.* They are associated in grain and meal, stored products, and processed foods such as flour and cheese. They present an occupational hazard to humans exposed from straw, grain silos, bakeries, warehouses and other storage centres. Exposure can cause occupational asthma or various forms of allergic dermatitis, commonly known as 'grain itch', 'straw itch', 'bakers itch' etc.

References

Arlian, L. G., Runyan, R. A., Achar, S. and Estes, S. A. (1984). Survival and infestivity of *Sarcoptes scabiei* var. *canis* and var. *hominis. J. Am. Acad. Derm.,* **11:** 210–15.

Arlian, L. G. and Vyszenski-Moher, D. L. (1988). Life cycle of *Sarcoptes scabiei* var. *canis. J. Parasitol.,* **74:** 427–30.

Baima, B. and Sticherling, M. (2002). Demodicidosis revisited. *Acta Dermato-Venereol.,* **82:** 3–6.

Burgess, I. F. (1996). Diagnosing and treating scabies. *The Practitioner,* **240:** 739–43.

Buxton, P. A. (1941). The parasitology of scabies. *BMJ,* **1:** 397–400.

Carapetis, J. R., Connors, C., Yarmirr, D., *et al.* (1997). Success of a scabies control program in an Australian aboriginal community. *Pediat. Infect. Dis. J.,* **16:** 494–49.

Cargill, C. and Dobson, K. (1979). Experimental *Sacroptes scabiei* infection in pigs: (1) pathogenesis. *Vet. Rec.,* **104:** 11–14.

Cerkvenik-Flajs, V. and Grabnar, I. (2002). Ivermectin pharmacokinetics. *Slov. Vet. Res.,* **39:** 167–78.

Chattopadhyay, S. and Richards, A. (2007). Scrub typhus vaccines: Past history and recent developments. *Hum. Vacc.,* **3:** 47–54.

Currie, B. J., Harumal, P., Mckinnon, M. and Walton, S. F. (2004). First documentation of *in vivo* and *in vitro* ivermectin resistance in *Sarcoptes scabiei. Clin. Infect. Dis.,* **39:** e8–12.

Curtis, C. (2004). Current trends in the treatment of *Sarcoptes, Cheyletiella* and *Otodectes* mite infestations in dogs and cats. *Vet. Dermat.,* **15:** 108–14.

Davies, P. R. (1995). Sarcoptic mange and production performance of swine: A review of the literature and studies of associations between mite infestation, growth rate and measures of mange severity in growing pigs. *Vet. Parasitol.,* **60:** 249–64.

Elgart, M. L. (1990). Scabies. *Dermat. Clin.,* **8:** 253–63.

Fischer, K., Holt, D. C., Harumal, P., *et al.* (2003). Generation and characterization of cDNA clones from *Sarcoptes scabiei* var. *hominis* for an expressed sequence tag library: Identification of homologues of house dust mite allergens. *Am. J. Trop. Med. Hyg.,* **68:** 61–64.

Fondati, A., De Lucia, M., Furiani, N., *et al.* (2010). Prevalence of *Demodex canis*-positive healthy dogs at trichoscopic examination. *Vet. Dermat.,* **21:**146–51.

Forton, F. and Seys, B. (1993). Density of *Demodex folliculorum* in rosacea: A case-control study using standardized skin-surface biopsy. *Br. J. Dermatol.,* **128:** 650–59.

Fourie, J. J., Delport, P. C., Fourie, L. J., *et al.* (2009). Comparative efficacy and safety of two treatment regimens with a topically applied combination of imidacloprid and moxidectin (advocate) against generalised demodicosis in dogs. *Parasitol. Res.,* **105** (1): S115–24.

Fourie, L., Heine, J. and Horak, I. G. (2006). The efficacy of an imidacloprid/moxidectin combination against naturally acquired *Sarcoptes scabiei* infestations on dogs. *Aus. Vet. J.,* **84:** 17–21.

Fuentealba, C. and Hanna, P. (1996). Mange induced by *Trixacarus caviae* in a guinea pig. *Can. Vet. J.,* **37:** 749–50.

Gao, Y. Y., Di Pascuale, M. A., Li, W., *et al.* (2005). In vitro and in vivo killing of ocular *Demodex* by tea tree oil. *Br. J. Opthalm.,* **89:** 1468–73.

Georgala, S., Katoulis, A. C., Kylafis, G. D., *et al.* (2001). Increased density of *Demodex folliculorum* and evidence of delayed hypersensitivity reaction in subjects with papulopustular rosacea. *J. Eur. Acad. Dermat. Venereol.,* **15:** 441–44.

Ghubash, R. (2006). Parasitic miticidal therapy. *Clin. Techn. Small Anim. Pract.,* **21:** 135–44.

Gordon, R. M. and Unsworth, K. (1945). A review of scabies since 1939. *Br. Med. Bull.,* **3:** 209–15.

Green, M. S. (1989). Epidemiology of scabies. *Epidemiol. Rev.,* 11: 126–48.

Hillier, A. and Desch, C. E. (2002). Large-bodied *Demodex* mite infestation in four dogs. *J. Am. Vet. Med. Ass.,* **220:** 623–27.

Kim, D., Kim, K., Nam, H., *et al.* (2007). Risk factors for human infection with *Orientia tsutugamushi*: A case control study. *Clin. Microb. Infect.,* **14:** 174–77.

Kummel, B., Estes, S. and Arlian, L. (1980). *Trixacarus caviae* infestation of guinea pigs. *J. Am. Vet. Med. Ass.,* **177:** 903–8.

La Vincente, S., Kearns, T., Connors, C., *et al.* (2009). Community management of endemic scabies in remote aboriginal communities of northern Australia: Low treatment uptake and high ongoing aquisition. *PLoS Neg. Trop. Dis.,* **3:** e444.

Lau, P., Hill, P., Rybnicek, J. and Steel, L. (2007). Sarcoptic mange in three alpacas treated successfully with amitraz. *Vet. Dermatol.,* **18:** 272–77.

Lowenstein, M., Kahlbacher, H. and Peschke, R. (2004). On the substantial variation in serological responses in pigs to *Sarcoptes scabiei* var. *suis* using different commercially available indirect enzyme-linked immunosorbent assays. *Parasitol. Res.,* **94:** 24–30.

Lutsky, I. and Bar-Sela, S. (1982). Northern fowl mite (*Ornithonyssus sylviarum*) in occupational asthma of poultry workers. *Lancet,* 2: 874–75.

Mellanby, K. (1944). The development of symptoms, parasitic infection and immunity in human scabies. *Parasitology,* 35: 197–206.

Mellanby, K., Johnson, C. G., *et al.* (1942). Experiments on the survival and behaviour of the itch mite, *Sarcoptes scabiei* deGeer var. *hominis. Bull. Entomol. Res.,* **33:** 267–71.

Morsy, G. and Gaafar, S. (1989). Responses of immunoglobulin-secreting cells in the skin of pigs during *Sarcoptes scabiei* infestation. *Vet. Parasitol.,* **33:** 165–75.

Mounsey, K., Holt, D., Mccarthy, J., *et al.* (2009). Longitudanal evidence of increasing in vitro tolerance of scabies mites to ivermectin in scabies endemic communities. *Arch. Dermatol.,* **145:** 840.

Pasay, C., Arlian, L., Morgan, M., *et al.* (2009). The effect of insecticide synergists on the response of scabies mites to pyrethroid acaricides. *PLoS Neg. Trop. Dis.,* **3:** e354.

Paterson, W. D., Allen, B. R. and Beveridge, G. W. (1973). Norwegian scabies during immunosupressive therapy. *BMJ,* **4:** 211–12.

Roberts, L. J., Huffam, S. E., Walton, S. F. and Currie, B. J. (2005). Crusted scabies: Clinical and immunological findings in seventy-eight patients and a review of the literature. *J. Infect.,* **50:** 375–81.

Rothwell, T., Pope, S. and Collins, G. (1989). *Trixacarus caviae* infection of guinea pigs with genetically determined differences in susceptibility to *Tricostronglylus colubriformis* infection. *Int. J. Parasitol.,* **19:** 347–48.

Taplin, D., Porcelain, S. L., Meinking, T. L., *et al.* (1991). Community control of scabies: A model based on use of permethrin cream. *Lancet,* **337:** 1016–18.

Valiente Moro, C., De Luna, C., *et al.* (2009). The poultry red mite (*Dermanyssuss gallinae*): A potential vector of pathogenic agents. *Experim. Appl. Acarol.,* **48:** 93–104.

Walton, S., Dougall, A., Pizzutto, S., *et al.* (2004a). Genetic epidemiology of *Sarcoptes scabiei* (Acari: Sarcoptidae) in northern Australia. *Int. J. Parasitol.,* **34:** 839–49.

Walton, S. F., Beroukas, D., Roberts-Thomson, P. and Currie, B. (2008). New insights into disease pathogenesis in crusted (norwegian) scabies: The skin immune response in crusted scabies. *Br. J. Dermatol.,* **158:** 1247–55.

Walton, S. F. and Currie, B. J. (2007). Problems in diagnosing scabies, a global disease in human and animal populations. *Clin. Microb. Rev.,* **20:** 268–79.

Walton, S. F., McKinnon, M., Pizzutto, S., *et al.* (2004b). Acaricidal activity of *Melaleuca alternifolia* (tea tree) oil: *In vitro* sensitivity of *Sarcoptes scabiei* var. *hominis* to terpinen-4-ol. *Arch. Dermatol.,* **140:** 563–66.

Wooten, E., Blecha, F., Broce, A. and Pollmann, D. (1986). The effect of sarcoptic mange of growth performance, leukocytes and lymphocyte proliferative responses in pigs. *Vet. Parasitol.,* **22:** 315–24.

Yang, Y., Yoo, H. M., Choi, I., *et al.* (1996). Interleukin 4-induced proliferation in normal human keratinocytes is associated with c-myc gene expression and inhibited by genistein. *J. Investig. Derm.,* **107:** 367–72.

CHAPTER 67

Flea infestations

Heinz Mehlhorn

Summary

Fleas are wingless bloodsucking insects infesting a large variety of hosts. They can cause dermatological problems and act as zoonotic vectors transmitting very important agents of diseases in humans and in animals living close to humans. Among the agents of diseases occur: viruses, plaque bacteria or even worms etc. Thus flea control is an important target nowadays in order to protect human and animal health all over the world.

Introduction

Fleas (*German*: Flöhe, *Spanish*: pulgas, *French*: puces) exist at least since 50 million years, when they had been already enclosed in amber recently found in the Baltic Sea. Fleas are distributed worldwide infesting most species of mammal and birds. Infestation results in pruritis (Krämer and Mencke 2001; Mehlhorn 2008). In 1898 the French scientist Simond, discovered that fleas may transmit the plaque bacteria (*Yersinia pestis*). Subsequently fleas have been objects of constant scientific observation (Grüntzig and Mehlhorn 2010; Eckert *et al.* 2008). Today it is known that not only the tropical rat flea *Xenopsylla cheopis* is able to transmit *Yersinia pestis*, but also more than at least 30 other flea species (Rothschild and Clay 1957; Mehlhorn 2008; Krämer and Mencke 2001). Although most fleas remain for long periods on a host, feeding several times per day, they also may switch from one host to another if there is body contact or common use of a sleeping site. In addition there are two relatively non mobile species: *Tunga penetrans*, the so-called jigger flea (the female enters totally the skin and becomes considerably enlarged) and the so-called stick-tight flea, *Echidnophaga gallinacea*, where the mouthparts are fixed on the victim's skin. Control and prophylactic measures are needed with all flea species because of the often severe pruritis they cause and because they transmit other diseases that affect the health of animals and humans. Furthermore, flea infestation has a considerable economic impact on farm or pet animals (Mehlhorn and Mehlhorn 2009).

The parasites

There are about 3,000 species and subspecies of fleas described belonging to approximately 200 genera within 15 families.

Flea systematics have their origin in the Systema Naturae of Linnaeus (1758), who described *Pulex irritans* (the human flea) and *Tunga penetrans* (the sand flea, chigger). Further basic work was undertaken by Hopkins and Rothschild (see Lewis 1992; Peus 1938). However, modern investigations using molecular biological parameters will probably revise the systematic further.

The wingless adult fleas measure, depending on the species, from 1 to 6 mm in length. Their laterally compressed bodies (Figs. 67.1–67.3) are provided with six strong and rather long legs, which allow jumping over distances of more than 20 cm thus guaranteeing a high efficacy in host finding or switching from one host to another.

The body is covered by a thick chitineous ectoskeleton (with a light to dark brown colour) and shows the three body sections which are typical for insects (i.e. head = caput, breast = thorax and body = abdomen). The head is provided with a pair of simple lens eyes and a pair of antennae, which can be retracted into grooves. The mouthparts being composed of maxillary palps, laciniae, labial pulps and epipharynx form a double channel system. While saliva containing anticoagulants are injected via one channel, fluid blood is ingested via the second one. Species determination is often based

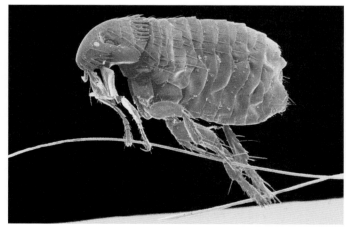

Fig. 67.1 Scanning electron micrograph of the cat flea *Ctenocephalides felis*. Note that the hind legs are larger than the others.

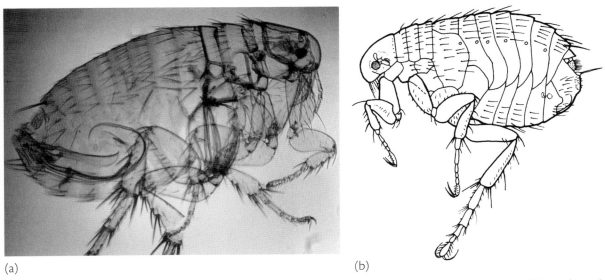

(a)   (b)

Fig. 67.2 Light micrograph (a) and diagrammatic representation (b) of *Pulex irritans*, the human flea, which nowadays is very rare in Central Europe due to the humidity inside human dwellings.

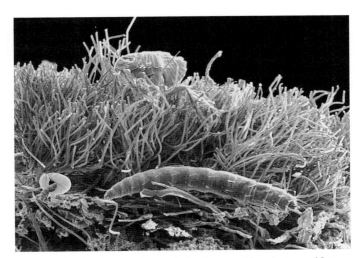

Fig. 67.3 Scanning electron micrograph showing some life cycle stages of fleas (egg, larva and an adult) in a carpet.

Table 67.1 Species with a differing presence of combs (ctenidia) at their head or pronotum (+ = present, − = absent).

Species	Size (mm)	Combs at head front	Combs at pronotum backside
Xenopsylla cheopis Tropical rat flea	2.5	−	−
Pulex irritans Human flea	4	−	−
Echidnophaga Sticktight chicken flea	1.5	−	−
Nosophyllus fasciatus Northern rat flea	2	−	+
Ceratophyllus gallinae Poultry flea	3.5	−	+
Diamanus montanus Ground squirrel flea	2.5	−	+
Archaeopsyllus erinacei Hedgehog flea	3.5	+ (only a few)	+ (many)
Spilopsylla cuniculis European rabbit flea	2.5	+ (many)	+ (many)
Leptospylla segnis European mouse flea	2	+ (many)	+ (many)
Ctenocephalides felis Cat flea	2.5–3.2	+ (many)	+ (many)
Ctenocephalides canis Dog flea	3–3.5	+ (many)	+ (many)
Tunga penetrans Sand flea = chigger	1	−	−

on the occurrence and shape of so-called ctenidia (spiny combs), which may occur at the front of the head and simultaneously at the back rim of the back shield of the first thoracic segment (= pronotum) or only at the pronotum (Table 67.1; Fig. 67.1) However, some species totally lack ctenidia.

Biology

The developmental cycle (Fig. 67.3) of most fleas is not very well understood. However, for those species of medical importance the details are clearer, since most of them can be cultured in the laboratory. Female fleas produce numerous 0.5 mm sized eggs per day (e.g. up to 46 in the case of *C. felis* or more than 200 in the case of *Tunga penetrans*). The first larva usually hatches from the egg after about 5 days. There are, in general, three larval stages

(*Tunga* has only two), which grow on organic debris and blood containing faeces that were excreted by adult fleas of both sexes. Once the larvae start feeding on adult faeces the colour of their gut turns into ruby-red or (later) black as can be seen from outside. The larvae move away from light (i.e. they are negatively phototactic), so that they are often not seen, although more than 80% of the larvae develop at the base of carpets in human habitations. Survival of flea larvae depends on temperature and humidity. Thus more than 90% of the larvae survive at temperatures between 21°C–32°C and at a relative humidity of 65–85%, while below 15°C no larval development occurred (Pospichil 1995). The total larval development needs from 5–12 days at optimum temperatures. After having reached a length of about 4–5 mm the third instar larva moves to a quiet place, voids its intestine and starts to spin a silk-like cocoon in which it pupates. The principal factors triggering pupation are declining levels of juvenile insect hormone. The silky pupal cocoon (produced by salivary glands) measures about 4 by 2 mm in size and becomes coated with dust and debris because of its stickiness thus giving rise to a perfect camouflage. Flea cocoons can be found in soil, on vegetation, in carpets, under furniture, on human or animal bedding, or depending on the species, in nests of birds. The duration of the pupal stage depends on the ambient temperature and usually takes one to two weeks. However, the adult fleas emerge from their pupal cuticle only after being stimulated by vibrations indicating the arrival of a potential host. In absence of such a stimulus the adult flea can wait within the cocoon long periods (often more than half a year). This behaviour explains why the first person or animal to enter a dwelling or a bird's nest, that had been uninhabited for a long period can suddenly be attacked by innumerable freshly hatched hungry fleas.

Adult fleas may also fast for a long time, if they do not find a host. About 60% of the adult fleas successfully emerge from cocoons held at only 13°C by day after eggs are collected from a culture (Silverman *et al.* 1981). In male pupae, it takes about 2–3 days longer.

After emerging from the cocoon the flea almost immediately begins to seek a host for a blood meal. Fleas are attracted by visual and thermal factors besides tactile stimuli, CO_2-concentrations and air currents. The adult fleas require periods between two and ten minutes to engorge and repeat this process several times per day. The amount of blood consumed by a female cat flea ranges between 10 and 16 µl per day representing an equivalent of about 15 times its body weight. Male fleas feed less than females. The maximum longevity of adult cat fleas has not been completely defined. Some studies describe a few weeks, other authors report periods of up to two years, if the flea was fed on dogs. The life span of fleas is characterized by active and inactive periods. Due to the optimum temperatures in human dwellings large flea populations may develop within weeks.

The life cycle of the sand flea, *Tunga penetrans,* also named jigger flea (Fig. 67.4) differs significantly from that of the human, cat or dog fleas. The tiny female flea enters into the host's epidermis with the help of its sword-like mouthparts and starts growing for about 3–4 weeks while drinking blood. The second and third abdominal segment become enormously enlarged so that the final stage reaches diameters of up to 1 cm (Fig. 67.4). Males copulate with females several times, and only after each copulation they suck blood. Six days after the first copulation the females start to eject

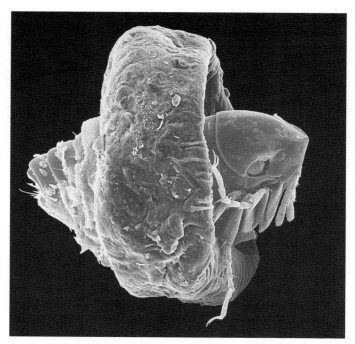

Fig. 67.4 Scanning electron micrograph of a female of *Tunga penetrans* extruded from human skin showing the typical central swelling of the body.

the 0.5 mm sized eggs, which fall to the ground, where the larval development in the eggs takes 3–4 days in sandy soils. The second larval stage is reached after 5–11 days, when pupation is initiated taking just 5–14 days. This flea species is found in dry regions of the tropics in South and Central America, Africa and in Australia. It is not very host specific and attacks many warm-blooded hosts such as humans, cats, rodents, bats, cattle, pigs and dog (Vobis *et al.* 2005a). Stray dogs are very important vectors inside human villages.

Medical importance

It is rare for flea bites alone, even in large number, to cause really severe clinical symptoms or death in animals or humans. However, the pruritis may be considerably and skin lesions may become secondarily infected bacteria (Figs. 67.5 and 67.6). Thus local reactions such as irritation of the skin, pruritus, an insignificant, transient invasion of lymphocytes and formation of 1 cm sized pustules are the most common dermal reactions representing a non-specific dermatitis. However, flea allergy dermatitis (FAD) (Fig. 67.7) is much more severe especially in hypersensitive dogs and cats and is associated with reactions that had been called 'summer eczema'. Similar phenomena may also occur in humans, where the identical symptoms were termed as papular urticaria. These may cause substantial problems in individuals which have a large exposure to fleas with additional signs such as hyperkeratosis, parakeratosis, severe pruritus, pyoderma and seborrhoea.

However, the medical importance of fleas is considerably increased in such cases where fleas act as vectors of agents of diseases (see Table 67.2) in humans and animals. A rather new finding is that fleas may transmit viruses via faeces or by blood sucking (Vobis *et al.* 2005b; Mencke *et al.* 2009).

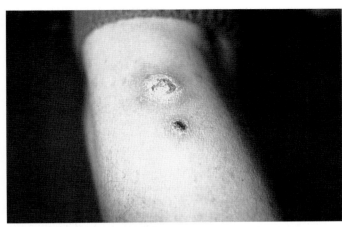

Fig. 67.5 Human arm with two flea bites, which are super infected by bacteria due to scratching.

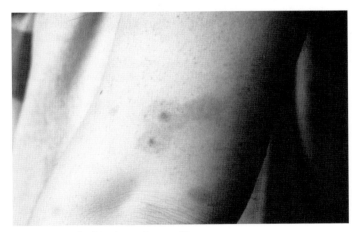

Fig. 67.6 Four flea bite sites on human skin.

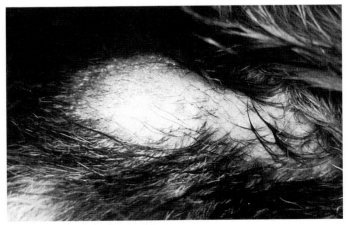

Fig. 67.7 Hairless skin spot of a dog due to FAD.

Table 67.2 Agents of diseases being transmitted by flea vectors (A= animals, B= bacteria, H= human, R= rickettsia, V= virus, W= worms)

Flea species	Agent of disease	Disease in humans (H) or animals (A)
Xenopsylla cheopis, Ctenocephalides species, Pulex irritans	Yersinia pestis (B)	Plaque (H, A)
Xenopsylla cheopis	Rickettsia typhi (mooseri) (R)	Murine spotted fever (H, A)
Ctenocephalides felis	Rickettsia conorii (R)	Boutonneuse fever (H)
Ctenocephalides felis	Feline lymphoma and feline calici virus (V)	FELV, FCV (A)
Ctenocephalides species	Tape worms: Dipylidium caninum, Hymenolepis species	Dipylidiasis, Hymenolepiasis (A, H)
Megabothris species Mouse flea	Franciscella Tularensis (B)	Tularaemia (H, A)
Mouse fleas	Erisipelothrix rhusopathiae (B)	Erysipeloid (H, A)
Rodent fleas	Omsk hemorrhagic fever virus (V)	Haemorrhagic fever (H)
Rodent fleas	Acanthocheilonema (W)	Filariasis (H, A)

Diagnosis

Diagnosis is not always straightforward as fleas may be difficult to see on infested animals or humans. However, the use of the indirect method of combing the hair and collecting the debris on a white paper is very helpful. The blood containing flea faeces will become apparent as dark dots which dissolve with a characteristic red stain if exposed to water. Intense combing will also show some adult fleas and/or their whitish eggs. Dogs and cats with FAD can be recognized by hairless spots (Fig. 67.7) at defined spots on the back (dog) or along the belly (cats). Furthermore the intense pruritus is also characteristic, although it may become masked by over-zealous grooming instead of scratching. The onset for flea allergy occurs mostly at an age of three to six years. Five stages of FAD are described.

Stage 1 A preclinical one — is bound to sensibilization,
Stages 2 until 4 are clinical ones and are characterized by retard hypersensibility.

(2) Immediate or retard hypersensibility,

(3) Immediate hypersensibility,

(4) While stage 5 (desensibilization) is rather rare.

Flea bite diagnosis in humans is fairly straightforward, since the typical bite reactions (Figs. 67.5 and 67.6) are easily recognizable due to the fact that the bites occurs in rows so that the papulae are lined up. This occurs because the fleas are easily disturbed during blood sucking and thus repeat the sucking act close to the first site.

Prophylaxis

There are a number of products to treat and control flea infestations. The most efficient method is the pour-on application of insecticides onto the neck of the animal. Products such as Advantage®, Advantix®, Advocate®, Capstar®, Exspot®, Frontline®, Practic®, Program®, Preventic®, Promeris Duo® or Stronghold® will protect dogs for at least four weeks. Cats do not tolerate products containing permethrin.

Insect repellents such as Viticks-Cool® or Autan® containing icaridin/saltidin or products containing Deet may be useful in humans who are in contact with a heavily infested environment.

To effectively control flea infestations it is also essential to treat the environment because of the developmental stages (eggs to pupae), which occur off the host. In general only 1% of the members of an active flea population are actually on the host. Indoor protection may be undertaken by spraying a non-toxic insect growth regulator such as methoprene, which block the moulting of larvae, on the beddings of animals or at the base of human beds etc., where flea larvae might hide. Methoprene is especially active against the third stage.

Adult fleas in rooms or beds are controlled by spraying insecticides into and around beds and animal sleeping sites. It is also recommended to wash the blankets and the covers of the animal and human bedding. This self-cure is only useful, if there are rather few fleas. In cases when dwellings are heavily infested with fleas, only the specialist can help by intensely fogging insecticides in closed rooms. Afterwards the room must be completely aerated and the surfaces must be cleaned of insectacides.

References

Eckert, J., Friedhoff, K.T., Zahner, H., Deplazes, P. (2008). Lehrbuch der Parasitologie für die Tiermedizin. 2. Stuttgart: Aufl. Enke.

Grüntzig, J., and Mehlhorn, H. (2010). Expedition into the empire of plagues. 2nd edition, Dusseldorf University Press.

Krämer, F., and Mencke, N. (2001). Flea Biology and Control. Heidelberg: Springer.

Lewis, R.E. (1992). Fleas (Siphonaptera). In: R.P. Lane and R.W. Crosskey (eds.) Medical insects and arachnids. London: Chapman Hall.

Linnaeus, E. (1758). Systema naturae. Stockholm: Stockholm University.

Martini, E. (1946). Lehrbuch der medizinischen Entomologie. Jena: G. Fischer.

Mehlhorn, B., and Mehlhorn, H. (2009). Gefahren für Hund und Halter. Dusseldorf: Dusseldorf University Press.

Mehlhorn, H. (2008). Encyclopedia of Parasitology. 3rd edition New York: Springer.

Mehlhorn, H., Eichenlaub, D., Löscher, T., and Peters, W. (1995). Diagnose und Therapie der Parasitosen des Menschen. Stuttgart: Fischer.

Mencke, N., Truyen, K., Vobis, M., and Mehlhorn, H. (2009). Transmission of Calici- and Feline leukaemia virus by fleas. Parasitol. Res., 105: 185–89.

Peus, F. (1938). Flöhe. Monographien zur hygienischen Zoologie. Bds. Leipzig: Schoeps.

Pospichil, R. (1995). Influence of temperature and relative humidity on the development of the cat flea. Proceedings Dt. Gesellsch. Parasit. Zbl. Bakt., 282: 193–94.

Rothschild, M., and Clay, T. (1957). Fleas, flukes and cuckoos. (3rd edn.). New Naturalist Series. London: Collins.

Silverman, J., Rust, M.K., and Reierson, D.A. (1981). Influence of temperature and humidity on survival and development of the cat flea. J. Med. Entomol., 18: 78–83.

Vobis, M., D'Haese, J., Mehlhorn, H., and Mencke, N. (2005a). Experimental quantification of the feline leukaemia virus in the cat flea (Ctenocephalides felis) and its feces. Parasit. Res., Supp: 102: 2–6.

Vobis, M., D'Haese, J., Mehlhorn, H., et al. (2005b). Molecular biological investigations of Brazilian Tunga sp. isolates from man, dogs, cats, pigs and rats. Parasitol. Res., 96: 107–12.

CHAPTER 68

The Myiases

Mahmoud N. Abo-Shehada

Summary

Human myiases can be caused by over 50 species of dipteran larvae. The numbers of human clinical myiasis reports, reflect their relative importance in the following order; cutaneous, ophthalmomyiases, nasal, oral, intestinal, ear, urogenital, and cerebral myiases. Myiasis producing flies are distributed worldwide, but most reported cases are from warm and developing countries. Molecular techniques have been applied to myiasis fly identification and classification, especially ostrids and calliphorines. Successful elimination programs have been carried out against *Hypoderma* spp. in the UK and *Cochliomyia hominivorax* in the USA, Mexico, Central America, Libya and the Caribbean Islands and another is ongoing against *Crysomya bezziana* in the Middle East. A beneficial myissis 'Biosurgery or maggot therapy' is the intentional use of *Lucilia sericata* larvae applied in specially designed dressings to chronic and MRSA infected wounds. The growing larvae execration/secretion facilitate wound debridement and successfully treated leg and pressure ulcers, wounds associated with diabetes, and many other types of infected wounds in a shorter time compared to conventional treatment. Now knowledge of myiases producing flies is accepted in many countries as a forensic tool.

Introduction

The biological term 'myiasis' was proposed by Hope (1840) to be used only in connection with dipterous larvae occasionally found in the human body. De la Torre-Bueno (1937) added clinical dimension to the term emphasizing the pathological effects of larvae to the definition 'disease or injury caused by the attack of dipterous larvae'. Zumpt (1965) argued 'the problem of myiasis must be considered from a biological aspect, and not only from a clinical one' and produced a more comprehensive definition for myiasis as 'the infestation of live human and vertebrate animals with the dipterous larvae, which, at least for a certain period, feed on the host's dead or living tissue, liquid body-substances, or ingested food'.

Dipterous larvae were separated biologically to obligate and facultative parasites. Obligatory parasites are those larvae which normally develop exclusively in or on living vertebrates. Obligatory myiases flies belong to Gastrophilidae, Cutterbridae, Ostridae and Hypodermatidae, such as *Gastrophilus* spp., *Dermatobia hominis*, *Oestrus ovis* and *Hypoderma bovis* respectively.

The facultative parasites are those larvae which are normally free-living and develop in decaying organic matter, including; carcasses, decomposing vegetables, faeces, manure and sewage. Occasionally and under certain circumstances, such larvae may gain access to the body of a living animal and infest it for a certain period of their life or complete its development. Examples for facultative parasites are blowflies which cause sheep strike (Fig. 68.1) or *Musca domestica* (House fly) and *Eristalis tenax* (Drone fly), which may be involved in rectal myiasis.

Also, myiasis producing flies can be classified into:

a) Primary flies which initiate strike by laying eggs on living animals,

b) Secondary flies which lay eggs on animal already struck,

c) Tertiary flies which lay their eggs when the carcass starts to dry.

Life cycles

The life cycles of most myiasis producing flies are provided by Zumpt (1965) and Beesley (1998). In general myiasis producing flies have similar life cycles which starts with attraction of the adult female fly to the host to deposit either her eggs or larvae on it. Usually attraction occurs due to the odour of decomposing matter, or wound. Bacterial activity appears to be important in preparing favourable conditions. In case of facultative flies (e.g. blowflies), the larvae can obtain the food from either dead carcasses or living animals. The female lays from a few hundred to a few thousands eggs. The larvae hatch after 8 hours to 3 days depending on temperature, humidity and fly species. They grow rapidly and pass two ecdyses. A few days later they will become mature third stage larvae (L3), when they will leave the host and pupate in the soil for three to seven days then hatch as adult flies (Fig. 68.1).

The life cycle of screw-worm blowfly (obligatory flies) is similar to other blowflies but differs in that the female attacks the wound of the live host only and not carcasses. The number of eggs laid by the female is 150–500 and the duration of the life cycle also varies.

The adult *Gastrophilus* spp. (Gastrophilidae) female fly lays 160–2400 eggs during persistent attacks causing annoyance to horses. They stick their eggs to the hairs of the host. The first stage larvae (L1) are stimulated to emerge by warmth and friction caused by the licking action of the host's tongue. In some species the hatched

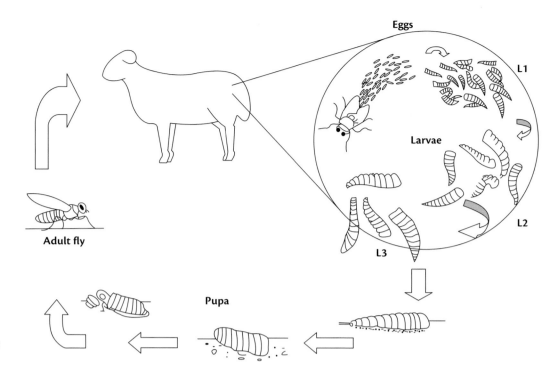

Fig. 68.1 The life cycle of **Blow-fly strike** caused by *Lucellia sericata* and *L. cuprina*.

L1 can penetrate unbroken skin. In *G. pecorum* the eggs are laid on the leaves of plants and are ingested by the host. *Gasterophilus* L1 may penetrate the tongue, lips or the inside of the cheek and begin migrating in tunnels until reaching the third stage larvae (L3) in the stomach, intestine, or rectum of the equine, depending upon the species.

The L1 of *G. pecorum* and *G. haemorrhoidalis* can penetrate human skin causing creeping myiasis as they move along under the skin resulting in a prominent indurated track in its course. L1 cannot develop further to the second stage (L2) in man.

The life cycle of *Dermatobia hominis* (Cutterbridae) is unusual. The female fly captures a day-flying mosquito, or another fly such as *Musca* spp. or *Stomoxys* spp., or even certain tick species, and glues its eggs to the other species's body. When this carrier host feeds on a suitable mammal host, the warmth stimulates the eggs to hatch and within 5–10 minutes the larvae penetrate the host's skin. Alternatively, the eggs are laid on vegetation or the ground and they hatch when a host brushes past them. A small nodule of host tissue subsequently develops around each larva, with a central breathing pore. As the larvae develop over the following 6–12 weeks they become quite large and a boil-like lesion forms at the site of infection. These lesions often attract screwworms with potentially fatal consequences. Once the larvae are mature they burrow out of the skin and drop to the ground where they pupate.

Females flies of the family Oesteridae, mainly *Oestrus ovis* are viviparous and deposit about 25 larvae on the nostrils of sheep. These larvae are about 1 mm long, and migrate through the nasal passages to reach the frontal sinuses, feeding on the mucus secretions which are stimulated by their movement. The first ecdysis occurs in the nasal passages and L2 crawl into the frontal sinuses where the final molt takes place. In the nasal sinuses the

larvae may remain several weeks before they migrate again to the nostrils and sneezed out to pupate on the ground and the adult fly is generated from the pupated larvae. The female survives only two weeks, but each can deposit up to 500 larvae in the nasal passages of the sheep.

The adult *Hypoderma* females attach eggs to the hairs of the underside of the body of cattle, the L1 then penetrate the skin via the hair follicles. After a migration of 5–6 months, through the connective tissues via the oesophagus (*H. lineatum*) or epidural fat (*H. bovis*) the larvae reach the skin of the back. They then feed for a further 4–6 weeks and moult into the second and third stages reaching the size of 25 mm in a boil. The L3 later falls to the ground to pupate. The larval migration described in cattle sometimes seen in man and horses. Humans usually suffer single larva infestations, and not 20–30 larvae as seen commonly in cattle. *H. lineatum* is the main species to infect humans and tends to occur in rural children. *Hypoderma* eggs are laid on the hairs of the body, probably the legs or arms, but L1 are usually seen in the gum or on the scalp, but may also appear in skin of the back, abdomen, chest, or genital region. The L3 can reach 20 mm in length in cattle but usually no more than 5–12 mm long in humans. Reported cases had a larva which broke the surface of the skin just above the right eyebrow, in the parietal and temporal regions of her head (Leclerq 1969). Twenty two cases of human myiasis with *Hypoderma* larvae causing painful swellings and abscesses were reported from Norway (Zumpt 1965). Intracranial haematomata due to migrating *Hypoderma* larvae have been recorded in humans and horses. *Hypoderma* spp. are also incriminated in many ophthalmomyiases cases.

Classification

Myiasis producing flies belong to seven families (Table 68.1).

Table 68.1 Classification, hosts (in addition to human), type of myiasis and geographical distribution of Dipteran human myiasis producing flies

Family	Fly name	Genera	Species	Host	Type of myiasis			Geographical distribution
Muscidae	Common house fly	*Musca*	*Musca domestica*	Animals	F	S	C,U,I,A,Or	Worldwide
			Musca sorbens	Animals	F	S	C	
	Latrine/lesser housefly	*Fannia*	*Fannia canicularis*	Animals	F	S	U,I	
			Fannia scalaris	Animals	F	S	U,I	
	Large house fly	*Muscina*	*M. stabulans*	Animals	F	S	U,I	
Calliphoridae	Congo floor maggot	*Auchmeromyia*	*A. luteola*	pig, hog, ant bears, hyenas	O	P	C, San	Africa south of the Sahara
	Tumbu/Mango fly	*Cordylobia*	*C. anthropophaga*	rats, dogs, cata, goats, mice, monkeys, chimpanzees, chicken	O	P	C,Oo,Or	Sub-Saharan Africa, Saudi Arabia
	Lund's fly		*C. rodhaini*	Antelopes, shrews, monkeys, gerbils, rats	O	P	C	Tropical Africa
	New-World screwworm	*Callitroga (Cochliomyia)*	*C. hominivorax*	Warm-blooded animals	O	S	C,Oo,U,A, Oo,N,Or C	From Belize and Guatemala to Uruguay and northern Chile, West Indies
	Secondary screwworm		*C. macellaria*		F	S	C	From south east Canada to Argentina
	Old-World screwworm	*Chrysomyia*	*C. bezziana*	Warm-blooded animals	O	S	C,Oo,U,A,Oo,Or	Africa, Middle East, Asia, from India and China to Papua New Guinea
			C. albiceps	Animals	F	T	C	Africa, Middle East, Asia
			C. megacephala		F	S	C	Africa, Middle East, Asia
			C. chloropyga		F	S		
			C. mallochi		F	S		
			C. putoria		F	S		
			C. inclinata		F	S		
	Sheep strike	*Lucilia*	*L. cuprina*	Sheep	F	P,S	C,I	Africa, Asia, Australia
	European sheep blow-flies, fleece-worms		*L. sericata*	Sheep	F	P,S	C,U,Or,I	Europe, USA
	Blowfly		*L. ampullacea*	Sheep	F	P,S	U	Europe, Japan
	Bluebottle flies	*Calliphora*	*C. erthyrocephala*	Sheep	F	P	C,I,U	Middle East
			C. vicina	Sheep	F	P	C,I,U	
			Microcaliphora varpis	Sheep	F	P	C,I,U	
			C. vomitoria	Sheep	F	S	C,Oo,U	
	Mack-blow flies	*Phormia*	*Ph. regina*	Sheep	F	P,S	C,I	North America
			Ph. terrae-novae	Sheep	F	P,S	C,I	North America, Europe
Sarcophagidae	Flesh flies	*Sarcophaga*	*S. haemoridalis,*	Warm-blooded animals	F	S	C,I,U	Worldwide
			S. tibials S. incisilobata		F	S	U	Central Europe, Ireland, Asia
		Wohlfahrtia	*W. magnifica*	Warm-blooded animals	O	P	C,Oo,Or,A,N	Mediterranean basin, Middle East, Asiatic Russia, China
					O	P		
			W. nuba		O	P	C	From west Africa to Pakistan
			W. vigil		O	P	C	Canada, Northern USA
Gastrophilidae	Horse bot fly	*Gastrophilus*	*G. pecorum,*	Equine	O	P	Cr	Global, especially the Mediterranean basin, Middle East, South Africa, Central America, Africa, USA
			G. haemorrhoidalis,				Cr	
			G. intermis				Cr	
			G. nigricornis,					

(Continued)

Table 68.1 (*Continued*)

Family	Fly name	Genera	Species	Host	Type of myiasis			Geographical distribution
Cuterebridae	Human bot	*Dermatobia*	*D. hominis*	Cattle, mammals	O	P	C,Oo,N,U,CC	Forested areas of the New-World tropics, West Indies
	Rodent botflies	*Cuterebra*	*C. emasculator*	Rodent	O	P	C,N	North America
Oestridae	Sheep nasal botflies	*Oestrus*	*O. ovis*	Sheep, goats	O	P	Eo,Or,A,N	Mediterranean basin, Middle East, India, Russia, South Africa, Central America, USA
	Horse nasal botflies	*Rhinoestrus*	*R. purpureus*	Equine			Eo	Russia, Italy, Africa
Hypodermatidae	Cattle grub	*Hypoderma*	*H. bovis*	Cattle	O	P	Io, CC	North temperate zone
	or warbles	*Hypoderma*	*H. lineatum*	Cattle, horse	O	P	C,Io,Cr, CC	South temporate zone
			H. diana	Red deer	O	P	C,Cr	Ireland, Scotland, Sweden, northern Europe
	Reindeer warble	*Oedemagena*	*O. tarandi*	Reindeer	O	P	Oo,Or	Scandinavia, Canada

F = Facultative myiases, O = Obligatory myiases, In = Incidental myiasis, P = Primary myiasis, S = Secondary myiasis, T = Tertiary myiasis, C = Cutaneous myiasis, Cr = Creeping myiasis, Eo = External ophthalmomyiasis, Io = Internal ophthalmomyiasis, Oo = Orbital ophthalmomyiasis, N = Nasal myiasis, Or = Oral myiasis, I = Intestinal myiasis, A = Ear myiasis, U = Urogenital myiasis, CC = Cerebral myiasis, San = Sanguinivorous.

Epidemiology

Geographical distribution

Myiasis causing flies are globally distributed, and some can fly considerable distances, e.g. *Cochliomyia hominvorax*, 300 km, and *Crysomya bezziana*, 100 km. Endemic areas of some of the more distinctive forms of myiasis are limited to parts of the tropics; however sporadic cases in returned travellers may be encountered in any part of the world (Hall and Wall 1995). Furthermore, with global warming many tropical flies, vectoring many infectious diseases are moving northwards.

Risk factors

Environmental factors

The presence of the myiasis producing fly in a locality supportive of fly abundance and activity are the main determining factors for the occurrence of myiases. The presence and the abundance of the animal hosts of the obligatory myiasis producing flies, the relative abundance of decaying biological materials for the facultative myiasis producing flies, and the suitable climate, mainly temperature and humidity are enhancing factors for the abundance of flies through shorter life cycles, and activities. *O. ovis* ophthalmomyiasis is prevalent in small ruminant raising areas and oral myiasis occurs mainly in the tropics (Chan *et al.* 2005).

Wound/cutaneous myiasis is known to be seasonal favouring warm seasons but not extreme temperatures of hot or cold. Cutaneous and wound myiases increase when animal diseases associated with skin lesions and natural opening inflammation and/or contamination with excreta, e.g. foot and mouth disease, diarrhoea, abortion, mange and wounds prevail. Inadequate or breakdown of medical services during wars and natural disasters is associated with human wound myiases.

Microclimate is equally important. For instance, areas detected as unsuitable for Old World Screwworm (OWS) by remote sensing were found to be heavily inhabited with the fly, e.g. Saudi intensive cattle farming, has brought thousands of cattle to the middle of the desert, provided concrete shades and humidifiers for cooling. These projects have changed the local climate, providing concrete resting places and suitable hosts for the fly.

Host factors

Cases of human infections with *Lucilia* spp. and other blowfly species are almost always associated with personal neglect and incapacity through old age, infancy, or disease. The flies are attracted by the smell of decay, they lay their eggs on the skin or soiled clothing.

People at high risk of myiases are the elderly, the bedridden, those suffering advanced dementia, the wounded, those with poor oral hygiene, those on tube feeding (Chan *et al.* 2005), those with diabetic foot ulcers, and the psychotic.

Oral Myiasis is associated with poor oral hygiene, alcoholism, senility, suppurating lesions, severe halitosis and other conditions (Droma *et al.* 2007). It has also been reported in males undertaking outdoor activities more than females (Droma *et al.* 2007). There are many underlying health disorders that predispose for myiases.

Socio-economic factors

While myiasis by saprophytic larvae is often indicative of poor environmental and personal hygiene, it can occur in unexpected places including well kept homes and hospitals. Nowadays, they are relatively uncommon in high income countries and most human cases are reported from low income countries.

Molecular epidemiology

In spite of the fact that genetic research has focused on diptera (Amendt *et al.* 2004) little attention was paid to the molecular epidemiology of myiasis producing flies. So far, the genes of subunite I and/or II of the mitochondrial encoded gene for cyto-chrome oxidase has been examined. The mitochondrial encoded 12S rRNA, COI and COII sequences of the two blowflies *L. cuprina* and *L. sericata* originating from different geographical regions throughout the world were studied by Stevens and Wall (1996). Morphologically proven *L. cuprina* specimens from Hawaii were assigned to *L. sericata* on the basis of mitochondrial sequence data. This result and the analysis of nuclear encoded 28S rDNA sequence reflect hybridization between the two species in Hawaii (Stevens *et al.* 2002). Specimens of *C. vomitoria* from the USA and the UK exhibited variability in the D1-D7 region of the nuclear encoded 28S rRNA sequences similar to that found between *C. vicina* and *C. vomitoria* in the UK (Stevens and Wall 2001). Recently, a small degree of genetic diversity was found between geographical populations of *C. bezziana* within the Arabian Gulf region suggesting that a single Gulf colony could be used to implement the sterile insect technique within an integrated control programme (Hall *et al.* 2009).

Human myiases

Only one fly species, the Congo floor maggot (*Aucheromyia leuteola*), is exclusively parasitic on man. Most species are zoonotic. With increased use of insecticides in agriculture the number of cases of human myiases has decreased and, at least in otherwise healthy individuals, they are usually restricted to agricultural workers or those living in close proximity to animals. The following clinical types of myiasis are reported with the numbers of the reported clinical cases of the different types of myiasis taken as a reflection of their importance (Table 68.2).

Cutaneous and wound myiases

D. hominis and *C. anthropophaga* are the main specific cutaneous myiasis flies. The majority of human cases are reported from endemic areas and travellers returning from those areas.

The common wound infesting fly species are; *Cochliomyia hominivorax, Chrysomya bezziana, Wahlfahrtia spp., Phormia regina, Phaenicia sericata, Sarcophaga sp., Calliphora sp.,* and *Musca*

Table 68.2 Number of myiasis reports of the different clinical types retrievable from Pub Med (accessed on 15 August 2009)

Type of myiasis	Number of myiases reports	
Key words	And myiasis	And human
Cutaneous	250	183
Ophthalmo	183	154
Ocular	64	47
Nose	129	66
Oral	122	69
Intestinal	122	68
Gastrointestinal	33	11
Ear	81	61
Auditory canal	15	13
External auricular	5	4
Urogenital	67	37
Cerebral	27	17
Pseudo	7	5
Hypodermic	2	2

domestica. The infestation is comparatively benign and sometimes beneficial, for the larvae feed on necrotic tissue and produce substances such as allantoin and deoxyribonuclease that facilitate healing. It is common in diabetic foot ulcers (Chan *et al.* 2005). The clinical signs are intense local reaction, wound widening, foul smell, itching, pricking sensation, induration of surrounding tissues, leakage of brownish serous to bloody exudates, redness and furuncular swelling. Also, first stage larvae may move along under the skin and cause prominent indurated track in its wake causing what is known as creeping myiasis.

Ophthalmomyiasis

Ophthalmomyiasis, or ocular myiasis, is the infestation of the human eye by the larval stage of certain flies of order diptera. This disease is classified into **internal**, **external**, and **orbital** forms, according to the location of the larvae (Kean *et al.* 1991).

Human external ophthalmomyiasis, ophthalmomyiasis externa

This form of ophthalmomyiasis involves mainly the conjunctiva, the eye lid and is most commonly caused by the larvae of *O. ovis* (Reingold *et al.* 1984; Harvey 1986; Heyde *et al.* 1986; Mazzeo *et al.* 1987; Amr *et al.* 1993). The larvae are barely able to penetrate the tissue and do not survive long. Most cases report one larva infestation, but 60 larvae were reported on one occasion (Victor and Bhargva 1998). Larvae were found in the conjunctiva, eye lids, lachrymal sac, and the cornea. The infestation occurs outdoors, in sheepherding areas (Heyde *et al.* 1986).

Other flies reported to cause ophthalmomyiasis externa are the human botfly, *D. hominis*, rodent botflies of genus Cuterebra (Wilhelmus 1986; Cogen *et al.* 1987) and horse botflies of various *Gastrophilus* species (Medownick *et al.* 1985). Gedoelstia, normaly a parasite of antelopes, causes a similar type of ocular myiasis in South Africa (Kean *et al.* 1991) and a case was caused by *Sarcophaga crassipalpis* (Uni *et al.* 1999). Clinical signs include; conjunctivitis of variable severity, sensation of suddenly moving foreign body with abrupt itching and lacrimation during warm months in endemic area, even without a history of fly strike. All reported cases, suffered from oedema, hyperaemia and unspecific irritation of the conjunctiva and some reported purulent conjunctivitis. Also, swollen eyelids with mild to severe oedema of the eye lids and cellulites were described. In addition, haemorrhage, ulceration, pain, larva protruding from an aperture in the eyelid, discharge, excoriation, erythema and laceration of the lacrimal drainage system. Ophthalmomyiasis was reported to associate with Herpes zoster ophthalmicus in a case caused by *C. bezziana* (Verma *et al.* 1990) and with short duration pre-septal cellulitis (Bali *et al.* 2007). Cornea involvement results in the reduction in vision.

Human internal ophthalmomyiasis, ophthalmomyiasis interna

Internal ophthalmomyiasis is most commonly caused by cattle botflies *H. bovis* and *H. lineatum* (Mason 1981; Vine and Schatz 1981; Syrdalen *et al.* 1982; Steahly and Peterson 1982; Edwards *et al.* 1984). The former is the common species in the cold temperate climatic zone while the latter is more prevalent in the warmer climatic zones, but the areas of distribution of these species overlap (Beaver *et al.* 1984). When *D. hominis* larvae enter the eye, signs of visual disturbance, redness of the eyes, haemorrhage of the fundus, retina and other parts of the eye occur and it may lead to unilateral or in severe cases bilateral-blindness. Other reported clinical signs are reversible severe decreased vision or vision loss, floaters (objects in the field of vision that originate in the vitreous), retinal haemorrhages in the funduscopic regions, pain, anterior uveitis and vitritis, mild panuveitis, diffuse stellate keratic precipitates, mild iris heterochromia and atrophy, fine neo-vascularization of the angle, and a mature cataract (Lagacé-Wiens *et al.* 2008). Also, an ophthalmomyiasis case was associated with Fuchs heterochromic iridocyclitis (Spirn *et al.* 2006).

Human orbital ophthalmomyiasis

This myiasis is caused by various species of the family calliphoridae. Obligatory species include *C. anthropophaga*, *C. bezziana*, *W. magnifica*, and *C. hominivorax*. Facultative species include *Calliphora vomitoria* and *C. macellaria* (Kean *et al.* 1991).

Symptoms are caused by the motion, feeding and excretory activity of the larvae and include foreign-body sensation and itching, trauma is the major cause of lachrymal apparatus lesions. Cases are refractive to antibiotics treatments only.

Diagnosis of ophthalmomyiasis is achieved by clinical examination and the use of slit-lamp bio-microscopy, ultrasonography and funduscopic examination.

Treatment is by removal of all larvae. Although some patients extract the fly larva by themselves, larvae may be removed by the cotton swab mounting technique. Suffocation of deeply seated larvae by the use of liberal amounts of topical antibiotic will facilitate their removal. No specific therapy is necessary in some cases. In contrast, surgical extraction may be needed in others. A successful treatment was achieved by oral ivermectin, in addition to antibiotic and topical steroids and cyclo-plegics. The treatment of choice is laser photocoagulation (Currier *et al.* 1995) or vitrectomy with larva removal and intraocular steroids. Larvae behind the retina could not be photocoagulated. Triamcinolone (0.4 mg) is administered for intraocular inflammation, and antibiotics are given as prophylaxis.

Nasal myiasis

The fly species reported to cause nasal myiasis are; *C. bezziana*, *C. hominivorax*, and *O. ovis* (Zhang *et al.* 2007). One case was reported to be caused by the fruit fly *Drosophila melanogaster* (Aydin *et al.* 2006) and another by *Calliphora erythrocephala* (Skibsted 1995). Infestation of ear, nose, and throat by the larvae of *C. bezziana* has been reported from the endemic areas. Among the predisposing factors, atrophic rhinitis is the most common (Kuruvill *et al.* 2006), followed by leprosy (Thami 1995) and upper respiratory tracts carcinoma (Gopalakrishnan *et al.* 2008). A case of Non Hodgkins lymphoma of ethmoidal sinus was associated with rhinoorbital myiasis (David *et al.* 1996).

Also, many nosocomial cases have been reported. The maggots burrow into delicate membranes and feed on underlying structures, causing considerable destruction of tissues, resulting in complications such as extensive erosion of the nose, face, and orbit, with rarely meningitis and death as a result of intracranial involvement (Sharma 1989). Reported complications include; pneumocephalus after atrophic rhinitis with nasal myiasis. Symptoms of rhinal myiasis are the same as in allergic rhinitis (Baldi 1990). Recurrent nasal myiasis was reported and treated successfully by permanent closure of the nostrils (Gupta 1978).

Oral myiasis

Oral myiasis cases have been reported worldwide from Asia, Europe and South America. Most of the cases were described in developing countries and in the tropics, and only rarely in developed countries.

Many fly species cause oral myiasis (Table 68.1). The larvae of *W. magnifica* were reported to be repeatedly recovered from the mouth and intubation tube of an unconscious patient (Yuca *et al.* 2005). Infestation may occur directly, by the fly deposition of eggs or larvae or indirectly, by ingestion of contaminated food such as meat. Breast-fed infants may suffer oral myiasis when suckling from mothers with breast myiasis caused by *C. anthropophaga* (Ogbalu *et al.* 2006).

A number of underlying medical disorders in patients are associated with oral myiasis. Most described cases had lesions located in the anterior part of the oral cavity, suggesting direct infestation. Other cases involved; the gingiva, lips and the floor of mouth (Droma *et al.* 2007).

Infestation by multiple larvae is common, though the number of cases is small (Chan *et al.* 2005). The number of infested larvae in the reported cases, ranged between 3 and > 50 larvae. The age of reported oral myiasis case ranged between 3 and 89 years with a median of 26 years.

Clinically, the patient suffers acute swelling in gingiva, lips, and/or other parts of the oral cavity (Faber and Hendrikx 2006). Although oral myiasis is uncommon, the dental surgeon should be aware of its existence, especially among patients returning from the tropical areas.

Intestinal myiases (Pseudomyiasis)

Reported species of intestinal myiasis where larvae were passed dead or alive on repeated occasions in carefully collected specimens include *Eristalis tenax*, *Musceina stabulans* and *Leptocera venalicia*. Intestinal myiasis may occur by one of the following: eggs or young larvae swallowed with contaminated food or water, faecal specimen may have been contaminated after it was passed and/or retroinfection from eggs or larvae deposited in the anus. The patient may suffer from diarrhoea, vomiting, abdominal pain, colic and fever. Symptoms of gastroenteritis subside after elimination of the larvae.

A whole range of species of diptera have been implicated although how many are cases of genuine parasitism is debatable. Many have undoubtedly arisen through maggots being present in food. During their passage through the gut they may set up some irritation and possibly even tissue damage but they are unable to establish themselves and cannot be considered to be parasitic. In other cases flies, such as *Eristalis tenax* which normally breed in faeces and rotting matter have laid their eggs around the anus and the larvae feed around the anal orifice and may even move into the rectum. They can cause irritation but they seldom cause physical damage and cannot be looked on as serious parasites. Cases of human myiasis such as these tend to occur among people who neglect personal hygiene through illness, extreme old age or infancy.

Aural myiasis

Aural myiasis is caused by *S. haemorrhoidalis, Wohlfahrtia magnifica*, screwworms and *Lucillia* spp. The majority of cases are reported from neonates and children. Cases reported in adults are associated with mental handicap, alcoholics, chronic otitis media, carcinoma and Alzheimer's disease patients. Symptoms include; purulent and haemorrhagic exudates in the external auditory canal, aural malodour, otalgia, aural itching, roaring sound, tinnitus, furuncle of the external ear, restlessness, and pain (Yuca *et al.* 2005). The treatment of aural myiasis requires removal of larvae, cleaning affected area with 70% alcohol, 10% chloroform, oil drops, topical ivermectin and normal saline (Yuca *et al.* 2005).

Uriogenital myiasis

Genuine cases of urinary tract myiasis are rare. Infection presumably occurs when flies oviposit around the urethral meatus. Species most frequently involved is *Fannia canicularis* (Table 68.1). The clinical signs include; frequent painful urination with pus, mucous and larvae in the urine, painful mixing, and bilateral costo-lumber pain.

Vaginal myiasis is infrequent and usually occurs when poor hygiene is combined with vaginal discharge. Vaginal myiasis has been associated with venereal diseases including trichomoniasis, candidiasis and gonorrhoea.

Cerebral myiasis

Cerebral myiasis is very rare. Three fly species have been described. Two cases involving children were caused by *Hypoderma bovis* and *H. lineatum* (Kalelioğlu *et al.* 1989; Semenov 1969). A fatal cerebral myiasis was also caused by *D. hominis* (Rossi and Zucoloto 1973).

Clinical signs

Clinical signs caused by the larvae vary depending on the causative fly species, and the site of infestation.

Diagnosis

The diagnosis of some myiases is often made by the patient or their carers. Clinical signs may be indicative of some myiasis. Unlike internal myiases, skin myiases are detected by palpation for warble fly in the expected sites. The larvae will appear as nodules of one cm in diameter in the skin which will cause a severe irritation and itching. *D. hominis* swellings can become itchy and painful, but unless they become infected with bacteria or the larvae enter the eye they are not serious.

Larval collection and preservation

Larvae must be collected from the lesion and include all morphological forms. Divide larvae to be sent to the laboratory to two equal groups. Place one group in water of 90° C for two minutes then transfer to a tube containing 70% alcohol or 10% formalin (Abo-Shehada 2005). Keep the remaining group in a perforated tube.

Label the tubes with the following:

- Place of collection,
- Species affected,
- Date of sample collection,
- Name of the veterinarian or physician in charge of the case.

Laboratory rearing of larvae

Larvae of several saprophytic species can be reared simply by putting them on blood agar plates kept at about 30° C. Larvae of most obligate parasitic species require special techniques of rearing.

Immunodiagnostic tools

Many tests (e.g. ELISAs) are easy and affordable tools for the detection of many myiasis-causing larvae on living animals, especially when larvae are undergoing migration and hence otherwise undetectable (rev. in Otranto 2001). However, information on the value of these methods for the diagnosis of nasal and gastrointestinal myiasis is unsatisfactory (Otranto 2001). Likewise, the value of immunodiagnosis of human myiases is questioned.

Other techniques used in myiasis diagnoses

Some techniques were reported to help in diagnosis of myiasis. The use of ultrasound in confirming the larval size and determine method of removal was described (Bowry and Cottingham 1997). The presence of *O. ovis* larvae in sheep sinuses can be detected by using rhinoscope (estroscope) and a third instar larvae were resolved after endoscopic examination of a nasal infestation (Badia and Lund 1994).

Fly identification

Morphological identification of the myiasis producing fly using early larval stages is very difficult. Identification keys for myiases producing flies are available (Zumpt 1965).

Molecular identification

To overcome the constraints of the classical morphological identification of some myiasis flies highly sensitive molecular assays were developed. Hypervariable DNA regions internal to some mitochondrial and nuclear ribosomal genes were used for the molecular identification of larvae belonging to the families oestridae (Otranto *et al.* 2003a,b; Otranto and Traversa 2004) and calliphoridae (Stevens and Wall 2001). Molecular identification using the mitochondrial encoded 12S rRNA, COI and COII sequences was achieved for *L. cuprina* and *L. sericata* (Stevens and Wall 1996). Similarly, the D1–D7 region of the nuclear encoded 28S rRNA sequences were used to identify *C. vicina* and *C. vomitoria* (Stevens and Wall 2001). Mitochondrial and nuclear genes of the four *Rhinoestrus* morphotypes affecting equids in Italy have been genetically characterized (Otranto *et al.* 2005a) and a seminested PCR assay employing mitochondrial genetic markers were used as molecular diagnostic tool in live animals.

A PCR-RFLP assay was used to differentiate between *H. bovis* and *H. lineatum* using the cytochrome oxidase I (COI) gene and restriction enzymes (Otranto *et al.* 2003) and similar assay was produced for *C. hominivorax* and *C. macellaria*. Also, PCR-RFLP assay provided a DNA-based method for identifying *C. hominivorax* individuals with a mutation in the esterase gene associated with organophosphate resistance (Carvalho *et al.* 2006).

As *R. purpureus* may cause ophthalmomyiasis in humans (Peyresblanques 1964), a seminested PCR assay employing a hyper-variable fragment (200 bp) internal to the *Rhinoestrus* cox1-gene encoding the region spanning from external loop 4 (E4) to the carboxy terminal (–COOH), was reported to differentiate between larvae of the two species. The fly DNA was extracted from nasal cotton swab samples.

Treatment

An effective treatment strategy consisted of mechanical removal of larva(e), dressing the affected tissues, and preventing re-infestation and secondary infections. Applying the treatment strategy will vary according to the infestation site. The complete removal of all larvae is essential. A foreign body response may occur against any part of the larvae remaining in the surgical site.

In superficial cases of myiasis, the larvae may be removed by irrigation and/or picked up with a cotton swap or forceps. Larvae in subcutaneous tissue can often be removed through a small incision after preliminary anesthesia of both host and parasite.

Deep infestations around the nose, eyes and ears require specialized surgical treatment. Wound occlusion and suffocation of deeply seated larvae can be achieved by the use of liberal amounts of topical antibiotics. The shape of *D. hominis* larvae and their curved body spines makes them difficult to extract. Covering the breathing hole of *D. hominis* with petroleum jelly, grease, fat, or Vaseline induce the larvae to force their own way out of the skin.

The treatment of oral myiasis is by surgical debridement under local anesthesia. Methods of wound occlusion and larvae suffocation were used in the treatment of cutaneous myiasis. Those methods aim at preventing air from the infesting larvae. Application of such methods may shift the aerobic larvae into a more superficial position where it is possible to remove them with ease and less tissue damage (Meinking *et al.* 2003). These methods are not easily applicable in the oral cavity. So far, lavage and surgical debridement are the only available treatment of choice for oral myiasis.

The patient's management include:

◆ Surgical exploration and search for larvae,

◆ Removal of all larvae and necrotic tissues,

◆ Topical application of gentian violet,

◆ Oral therapy with ivermectin (6 mg orally),

◆ Patient referred to plastic surgery to repair tissue damage.

Intestinal infestation usually responds to hexylresorcinol or tetrachlorethylene followed by purgation (Morris *et al.* 1996).

In cutaneous myiasis, the site of infestation may facilitate the entry of *Clostridium tetani* while removing the larvae using contaminated instruments and therefore vaccination is recommended. Research has shown that doramectin is capable of preventing infestation of wounds for at least 14 days after treatment.

Although many insecticides will kill *C. hominivorax* larvae, most of these require repeated applications before healing occurs. Under extensive grazing regimes, such as those practiced in parts of the Americas, treatment of individual animals is not practical.

Control and prevention

Provision of effective veterinary services and environmental hygiene are vital for the control and prevention of myiases in man. The veterinary services will provide the measures of controlling major animal diseases with cutaneous and natural orifices inflammation, e.g. FMD and diarrhoeal diseases and causes of wounds. Also, such services will provide treatment and prevention of specific myiasis producing fly infestation, e.g. *O. ovis*. In addition, the education of farmers to adopt the essential regular animal inspection for early detection of myiasis cases. Proper waste disposal will minimize the alternative breeding sites for the facultative myiasis producing flies, e.g. blowflies.

Quarantine measures, and international and regional cooperation

These measures aim to prevent the spread of fly species, such as screwworm flies, from endemic to non-endemic countries. This is especially important during period of mass importation of animals. For example during the annual Hajj season around seven million livestock are imported to Saudi Arabia over a 2 to 3 weeks period

from all over the world including screwworm endemic countries. Inspection of animals at ports of entry and insect control in ships and planes are important measures of control. Animal movements must be controlled during screwworm myiasis outbreaks.

Control of *D. hominis* has always been similar to that of other fly myiases and involves treatment of cattle with organophosphate or organochlorine insecticides. Trials of doramectin suggest that it may be a more effective and less toxic replacement. Treatment of human cases usually involves surgical removal of the larvae. Chemical control using effective insecticides is vital to reduce the number of flies and mass treat myiasis in infected farm animals. Regular animal inspection for myiasis cases must be done routinely in endemic countries, especially during outbreaks. The control of myiasis in wild animals is a difficult task.

The insect sterilization technique

Insect sterilization technique, also called sterile insect technique (SIT) is a proven effective biological method of control. As a biological method, SIT has attracted a great deal of interest for use in blowfly control because of increasing resistance to available insecticides as well as strict limits on the residual level of insecticides on wool imposed by the European Union. SIT has been proven to be effective in the field for the area-wide control of some insects (Knipling 1960; Krafsur 1998). SIT involves mass-rearing of insects that are then sterilized and released in sufficient numbers. This results in most of the wild females mating with the released sterile males and thus producing non viable eggs. This can result in suppression and subsequent elimination of the target insect population. For *C. capitata*, SIT has been shown to be most effective if only sterile males are released in the field (McInnis *et al.* 1994). The use of genetic engineering with the aim of developing a system for controlling female viability in a strain of *L. cuprina* that would allow a male-only sterile release program was attempted (Scott *et al.* 2004).

It may prove possible to eliminate or at least control some species by sterile male release and research was conducted towards this end in Australia. *C. bezziana* does not yet occur in Australia but it is present in Papua New Guinea and there is a real risk that it will be introduced in the near future.

The first major implementation of SIT was in the New World screwworm (NWS) Eradication Program, that successfully eliminated the NWS, from the Continental US, Mexico and much of Central America. Currently, ionizing radiation is used for sterilizing insects, but the safer, more cost-effective transgenic insect techniques could replace this method. Genetic transformation methods (GTM) have been demonstrated in NWS. GTMs help to identify genes and examine gene function in NWS (Allen *et al.* 2004).

C. hominivorax is restricted principally to North and South America, and the Caribbean Islands. An outbreak of NWS occurred in Libya during the late 1980s but this was eradicated using the sterile male release technique. Educating the public regarding myiasis may help preventing human myiasis (Abdo *et al.* 2006).

A significant number of human myiasis cases are acquired in nursing homes. Carers of the old and debilitated should be made aware of myiasis prevention measures, especially for those on tube feeding. The use of window screens and electrocuters in nursing homes should be adopted to prevent flies access and kill flies that do enter (Chan *et al.* 2005).

Medical personnel taking care of old or debilitated patients need to bear in mind the possibility of *C. bezziana* infestation to be able to make a prompt diagnosis and implement relevant intervention to prevent extensive tissue destruction (Chan *et al.* 2005).

Maggot therapy (Biosurgery)

Fly larvae can be used medically for the treatment of chronic (slow-healing) or badly-infected wounds. The intentional use of maggots to clean infected wounds has been practised for many years. Their use was first championed during the American Civil War and there was another burst of popularity during the 1920s and 1930s for the treatment of thousands of ex-soldiers from the First World War. The development of antibiotics in the 1940s saw a general demise in the use of maggot therapy (Chen *et al.* 2007). In the late 1990s, its value became increasingly recognized, at least in the UK, owing to problems of antibiotic resistance and methicillin resistant *Staphylococcus aureus* (MRSA). In the UK, maggot debridement therapy increased from two treatments a month in 1996 to more than 200 treatments per week in 2007. An estimated 30,000 people have been treated with sterile maggots since the mid 1990s and the demand is growing rapidly throughout the world.

The continual movement of the maggots was thought to stimulate the body to produce serous exudates that flush bacteria from the wound, and healing granulation tissue from viable cells. Likewise, the probing from the hooks was postulated to facilitate wound debridement. Recently, three proteolytic enzyme classes were identified in the maggot execrations/secretions (ES). The ES enzymes are capable of effective wound matrix digestion (Chen *et al.* 2007). The maggot ES also have inhibitory effect on bacteria including MRSA. In addition to the ammonia secreted by maggots is believed to increase the wound pH and hinder bacterial growth (Robinson 1940). Maggots also feed on and kill bacteria (Mumcuoglu *et al.* 2001). The ES have various substances which appear to enhance wound healing. For example, *in vitro* studies on cell cultures have identified substances capable of enhancing the proliferation and growth of human fibroblasts (Horobin *et al.* 2005).

In the UK, the main centre using maggot therapy is Bridgend General Hospital in South Wales. Currently, Bridgend-based biosurgical company *ZooBiotic*, is the only supplier of pharmaceutically produced maggots to the healthcare sector in UK and internationally.

Lucilia sericata is the species of fly used most frequently. The larvae are reared under stringently controlled conditions in three rooms. The adult flies are kept in a special room. The eggs are sterilized under aseptic conditions in another and the third room for breeding the larvae. The eggs are deposited on raw liver. Eggs are then transferred to flasks containing a sterile nutrient on which, after hatching, the larvae grow. When the larvae reach the required size (2 mm) they are tested for sterility by incubation in Tryptone Soya Broth and Thioglycollate Broth.

The larvae are applied to the wound in specially designed dressings which confine the larvae and protect the healthy skin from ES. After about 3 to 5 days the larvae reach about 13 mm and they are removed from the wound and destroyed. Some patients may require further treatment, and a fresh batch of larvae is applied.

Biosurgery has proved successful in the treatment of leg and pressure ulcers, wounds associated with diabetes, and many other types of infected wounds. While conventional treatments for these wounds can take months to achieve a successful outcome, maggot therapy usually takes one or two treatments, each lasting 5 days. Thus, it dramatically reduces treatment times and the associated costs (Bonn 2000). Evidence also suggests that it is successful in combating MRSA (Gupta 2008).

Forensic entomology

Another beneficial application of myiasis knowledge is in the field of forensic medicine. Insects including necrophagous dipteran species of the families; Calliphoridae, Fannidae, Muscidae and Sarcophagidae are attracted to the dead carcass within minutes. The presence of larvae on the dead body will provide a mean to estimate the postmortem interval (PMI). The minimum PMI is determined by the age of the insect stage. Now knowledge of myiases producing flies is accepted in many countries as a forensic tool (Amendt *et al.* 2004).

References

Abdo, E. N., Sette-Dias, A. C., *et al.* (2006). Oral myiasis: a case report. *Med. Oral, Patol. Oral Cirugía Bucal.*, **11**: E130–1.

Abo-Shehada, M. N. (2005). Incidence of *Chrysomya bezziana* screw-worm myiasis in Saudi Arabia, 1999/2000. *Vet. Rec.*, **156**: 354–56.

Allen, M. L., Handler, A. M., Berkebile, D. R. and Skoda, S. R. (2004). piggyBac transformation of the New World screwworm, *Cochliomyia hominivorax*, produces multiple distinct mutant strains. *Med. Vet. Entom.*, **18**: 1–9.

Amendt, J., Krettek, R. and Zehner, R. (2004). Forensic entomology. *Naturwissenschaften*, **91**: 51–65.

Amr, Z. S., Amr, B. A., and Abo-Shehada, M. N. (1993). Ophthalmomyiasis externa caused by *Oestrus ovis* L. in the Ajloun area of northern Jordan. *Ann. Trop. Med. Parasitol.*, **87**: 259–62.

Anaman, K. A., Atzeni, M. G., Mayer, D. G., and Walthall, J. C. (1994). Economic assessment of preparedness strategies to prevent the introduction or the permanent establishment of screwworm fly in Australia. *Prev. Vet. Med.*, **20**: 99–111.

Aydin, E., Uysal, S., Akkuzu, B. and Can, F. (2006). Nasal myiasis by fruit fly larvae: a case report. *Eur. Arch. Oto-Rhino-Laryng.*, **263**: 1142–43.

Badia, L., and Lund, V. J. (1994). Vile bodies: an endoscopic approach to nasal myiasis. *J. Laryng. Otol.*, **108**: 1083–85.

Baldi, E., Campadelli, G. and Mangiaracina, P. (1990). Rhinomyiasis. Considerations on a clinical case. *La Clin. Terapeut.*, **132**: 303–6.

Bali, J., Gupta, Y. K., Chowdhury, B., *et al.* (2007). Ophthalmomyiasis: a rare cause of short duration pre-septal cellulitis in a healthy non-compromised adult. *Singapore Med. J.*, **48**: 969–71.

Beesly, W. N. (1998). Myiases. In: S. R. Palmer, Lord Soulsby and D. I. H. Simpson (eds.) *Zoonoses*. Oxford: Oxford University Press.

Bonn, D. (2000). Maggot therapy: an alternative for wound infection. *Lancet*, **356**: 1174–78.

Bowry, R., and Cottingham, R. L. (1997). Use of ultrasound to aid management of late presentation of *Dermatobia hominis* larva infestation. *J. A&E Med.*, **14**: 177–78.

Chan, D. C., Fong, D. H., Leung, J. Y., *et al.* (2007). Maggot debridement therapy in chronic wound care. *Hong Kong Med. J.*, **13**: 382–86.

Chan, J. C., Lee, J. S., Dai, D. L., and Woo, J. (2005). Unusual cases of human myiasis due to Old World screwworm fly acquired indoors in Hong Kong. *Trans. R. Soc. Trop. Med. Hyg.*, **99**: 914–18.

Cogen, M. S., Hays, S. J., and Dixon, J. M. (1987). Cutaneous myiasis of the eyelid due to *Cuterebra* larva. *J. Am. Med. Ass.*, **258**: 1795–96.

Currier, R. W., Johnson, W. A., Rowley, W. A. and Laudenbach, C. W. (1995). Internal ophthalmomyiasis and treatment by laser photocoagulation: a case report. *Am. J. Trop. Med. Hyg.*, **52**: 311–13.

David, S., Rupa, V., Mathai, E. and Nair, S. (1996). Non Hodgkins lymphoma of ethmoidal sinus with rhinoorbital myiasis. *Indian J. Cancer*, **33**: 171–72.

de Carvalho, R. A., Torres, T. T., and de Azeredo-Espin, A. M. (2006). A survey of mutations in the *Cochliomyia hominivorax* (Diptera: Calliphoridae) esterase E3 gene associated with organophosphate resistance and the molecular identification of mutant alleles. *Vet. Parasitol.*, **140**: 344–51.

De La Torre-Bueno, J. R. (1937). *A glossary of entomology*. New York: Brooklyn Entomological Society.

Droma, E. B., Wilamowski, A., Schnur, H., *et al.* (2007). Oral myiasis: a case report and literature review. *Oral Surg. Med. Path. Radiol. Endod.*, **103**: 92–96.

Faber, T. E., Hendrikx, W. M. (2006). Oral myiasis in a child by the reindeer warble fly larva *Hypoderma tarandi*. *Med. Vet. Entomol.*, **20**: 345–46.

Gomez, R. S., Perdigão, P. F., Pimenta, F. J., *et al.* (2003). Oral myiasis by screwworm *Cochliomyia hominivorax*. *Br. J. Oral & Maxillof. Surg.*, **41**: 115–16.

Gopalakrishnan, S., Srinivasan, R., Saxena, S. K. and Shanmugapriya, J. (2008). Myiasis in different types of carcinoma cases in southern India. *Indian J. Med. Microb.*, **26**: 189–92.

Gupta, A. (2008). A review of the use of maggots in wound therapy. *Ann. Plas. Surg.*, **60**: 224–27.

Gupta, S. C. (1978). Permanent closure of the nostrils in recurrent nasal myiasis. *J. Laryng. Otol.*, **92**: 627–28.

Hall, M. and Wall, R. (1995). Myiasis of humans and domestic animals. *Adv. Parasitol.*, **35**: 257–334.

Hall, M. J., Wardhana, A. H., Shahhosseini, G., *et al.* (2009). Genetic diversity of populations of Old World screwworm fly, *Chrysomya bezziana*, causing traumatic myiasis of livestock in the Gulf region and implications for control by sterile insect technique. *Med. Vet. Entomol.*, **23**, Suppl 1: 51–58.

Harvey, J. T. (1986). Sheep botfly: ophthalmomyiasis externa. *Can. J. Ophthalm.*, **21**: 92–95.

Heath, A. C. G., and Bishop, D. M. (1995). Flystrike in New Zealand. *Surveillance*, **22**: 11–13.

Heyde, R. R., Seiff, S. R., and Mucia, J. (1986). Ophthalmomyiasis externa in California. *West J. Med.*, **144**: 80–81.

Hope, F. W. (1840). On insects and their larvae occasionally found in the human body. *Trans. R. Entom. Soc. London*, **2**: 256.

Horobin, A. J., Shakesheff, K. M. and Pritchard, D. I. (2005). Maggots and wound healing: an investigation of the effects of secretions from *Lucilia sericata* larvae upon the migration of human dermal fibroblasts over a fibronectin-coated surface. *Wound Rep. Regen*, **13**: 422–33.

James, M. T. (1948). *The flies that cause myiasis in man*. US Department of Agriculture Publication 6311947.

Kalelioglu, M., Akturk, G., Akturk, F., *et al.* (1989). Intracerebral myiasis from *Hypoderma bovis* larva in a child. *Case report. J. Neurosurg.*, **71**: 929–31.

Kean, B. H., Sun, T., Ellsworth, R. M. (1991). *Color Atlas/Text of Ophthalmic Parasitology*. New York: Igaku-Shoin.

Knipling, E. F. (1960). The eradication of the screw-worm fly. *Scient. Am.*, **203**: 54–61.

Krafsur, E. S. (1998). Sterile insect technique for suppressing and eradicating insect population: 55 years and counting. *J. Agri. Entom.*, **15**: 303–17.

Kuruvilla, G., Albert, R. R., Job, A., *et al.* (2006). Pneumocephalus: a rare complication of nasal myiasis. *Am. J. Otolaryng.*, **27**: 133–35.

Leclercq, M. (1969). *Entomological parasitology*. Oxford: Pergamon.

Lupi, O. (2006). Myiasis as a risk factor for prion diseases in humans. *J. Eur. Acad. Dermat.Venereol.*, **20**: 1037–45.

Mazzeo, V., Ercolani, D., Trombetti, D., *et al.* (1987). External ophthalmomyiasis. Report of four cases. *Intern. J. Ophthalm.*, **11**:73–76.

McInnis, D. O., Tam, S., Grace, C., and Miyashita, D. (1994). Population suppression and sterility induced by variable sex ratio, sterile insect releases of Ceratitis capitata (Diptera: Tephritidae) in Hawaii. *Ann. Entomol. Soc. Am.*, **87**: 231–40.

Medownick, M., Lazarus, M., Finkelstein, E., and Weiner, J. M. (1985). Human external ophthalmomyiasis caused by the horse bot fly larva (*Gasterophilus* spp.). *Aust N Z J. Ophthalm.*, **13**: 387–90.

Meinking, T. L., Burkhart, C. N., and Burkhart, C. G. (2003). Changing paradigms in parasitic infections: common dermatological helminthic infections and cutaneous myiasis. *Clin. Dermat.*, **21**: 407–16.

Minton, S. A. (1975). *Parasitism by miscellaneous invertebrates*. New York: Academic Press.

Morris, A. J. and Berry, M. A. (1996). Intestinal myiasis with Phaenicia cuprina. *Am. J. Gastroenter.*, **91**: 1290.

Mumcuoglu, I., Akarsu, G. A., Balaban, N., and Keles I. (2005). Eristalis tenax as a cause of urinary myiasis. *Scand. J. Infect. Dis.*, **37**: 942–43.

Mumcuoglu, K. Y., Miller, J., *et al.* (2001). Destruction of bacteria in the digestive tract of the maggot of *Lucilia sericata* (Diptera: Calliphoridae). *J. Med. Entom.*, **38**: 161–66.

Ng, S. O. and Yates, M. (1997). Cutaneous myiasis in a traveller returning from Africa. *Aus. J. Dermatol.*, **38**: 38–39.

Ogbalu, O. K., Achufusi, T. G. and Adibe, C. (2006). Incidence of multiple myiases in breasts of rural women and oral infection in infants from the human warble fly larvae in the humid Tropic-Niger Delta. *Int. J. Dermatol.*, **45**: 1069–70.

Otranto, D., Milillo, P., Traversa, D., and Colwell, D. D. (2005). Morphological variability and genetic identity in *Rhinoestrus* spp. causing horse nasal myiasis. *Med. Vet. Entomol.*, **19**: 96–100.

Otranto, D., Testini, G., Sottili, R., Capelli, G. and Puccini, V. (2001). Screening of commercial milk samples using ELISA for immuno-epidemiological evidence of infection by the cattle grub (Diptera: Oestridae). *Vet. Parasitol.*, **99**: 241–48.

Otranto, D., Traversa, D. and Giangaspero, A. (2004). [Myiasis caused by Oestridae: serological and molecular diagnosis]. *Parassitologia*, **46**: 169–72.

Otranto, D., Traversa, D., Guida, B., *et al.* (2003). Molecular characterization of the mitochondrial cytochrome oxidase I gene of Oestridae species causing obligate myiasis. *Med. Vet. Entomol.*, **17**: 307–15.

Otranto, D., Traversa, D., Milillo, P., *et al.* (2005). Utility of mitochondrial and ribosomal genes for differentiation and phylogenesis of species of gastrointestinal bot flies. *J. Econ. Entomol.*, **98**: 2235–45.

Otranto, D., Traversa, D., Tarsitano, E. and Stevens, J. (2003). Molecular differentiation of *Hypoderma bovis* and *Hypoderma lineatum* (Diptera, Oestridae) by polymerase chain reaction-restriction fragment length polymorphism (PCR-RFLP). *Vet. Parasitol.*, **112**: 197–201.

Peyresblanques, J. (1964). Ocular Myiasis. *Ann. d'oculist.*, **197**: 271–95.

Reingold, W. J., Robin, J. B., Leipa, D., *et al.* (1984). *Oestrus ovis* ophthalmomyiasis externa. *Am. J. Ophthalm.*, **97**: 7–10.

Robinson, W. (1940). Ammonium bicarbonate secreted by surgical maggots stimulates healing in purulent wounds. *Am. J. Surg.*, **47**: 111–15.

Rossi, M. A. and Zucoloto, S. (1973). Fatal cerebral myiasis caused by the tropical warble fly, *Dermatobia hominis*. *Am. J. Trop. Med. Hyg.*, **22**: 267–69.

Scott, M. J., Heinrich, J. C. and Li, X. (2004). Progress towards the development of a transgenic strain of the Australian sheep blowfly (*Lucilia cuprina*) suitable for a male-only sterile release program. *Insect Biochem. Mol. Biol.*, **34**: 185–92.

Semenov, P. V. (1969). A case of penetration of *Hypoderma lineatum* de Villers larva into the human brain. *Med. Parazit. i Parazitarnye Bolezni*, **38**: 612–13.

Sharma, H., Dayal, D. and Agrawal, S. P. (1989). Nasal myiasis: review of 10 years experience. *J. Laryng. Otol.*, **103**: 489–91.

Skibsted, R., Larsen, M. and Gomme, G. (1995). [Nasal myiasis]. *Ugeskr Laeger*, **157**: 2158–60.

Spirn, M. J., Hubbard, G. B., *et al.* (2006). Ophthalmomyiasis associated with Fuchs heterochromic iridocyclitis. *Retina*, **26:** 973–74.

Steahly, L. P. and Peterson, C. A. (1982). Ophthalmomyiasis. *Ann. Ophthalmol.*, **14:** 137–39.

Stevens, J. and Wall, R. (2001). Genetic relationships between blowflies (Calliphoridae) of forensic importance. *For. Sci. Int.*, **120:** 116–23.

Stevens, J. R., Wall, R. and Wells, J. D. (2002). Paraphyly in Hawaiian hybrid blowfly populations and the evolutionary history of anthropophilic species. *Insect Mol. Biol.*, **11:** 141–48.

Stevens, J. R., Wall, R. (1996). Species, sub-species and hybrid populations of the blowflies *Lucilia cuprina* and *Lucilia sericata* (Diptera: Caliphoridae). *Proc. R. Soc. London. Series B*, **263:** 1335–41.

Syrdalen, P., Nitter, T. and Mehl, R. (1982). Ophthalmomyiasis interna posterior: report of case caused by the reindeer warble fly larva and review of previous reported cases. *Br. J. Ophthalmol.*, **66:** 589–93.

Thami, G. P., Baruah, M. C., Sharmce, S. C. and Behera, N. K. (1995). Nasal myiasis in leprosy leading to unusual tissue destruction. *J. Dermatol.*, **22:** 348–50.

Tomita, M., Uchijima, Y., Okada, K. and Yamaguchi, N. (1984). [A report of self-amputation of the penis with subsequent complication of myiasis]. *Hinyokika Kiyo*, **30:** 1293–96.

Uni, S., Shinonaga, S., Nishio, Y., *et al.* (1999). Ophthalmomyiasis caused by *Sarcophaga crassipalpis* (Diptera: Sarcophagidae) in a hospital patient. *J. Med. Entomol.*, **36:** 906–8.

Verma, L., Pakrasi, S., Kumar, A., Sachdev, M. S. and Mandal, A. K. (1990). External ophthalmomyiasis associated with herpes zoster ophthalmicus. *Can. J. Ophthalmol.*, **25:** 42–43.

Victor, R. and Bhargva, K. (1998). Ophthalmomyiasis in Oman: a case report and comments. *Wilderness Environm. Med.*, **9:** 32–35.

Vine, A. K. and Schatz, H. (1981). Bilateral posterior internal ophthalmomyiasis. *Ann. Ophthalmol.*, **13:** 1041–43.

Wilhelmus, K. R. (1986). Myiasis palpebrarum. *Am. J. Ophthalmol.*, **101:** 496–98.

Yuca, K., Caksen, H., Sakin, Y. F., *et al.* (2005). Aural myiasis in children and literature review. *Tohoku J. Experim. Med.*, **206:** 125–30.

Zhang, X. C., Liu, X. D. and Lu, Z. M. (2007). [Myiasis of maxillary sinus and nasal cavity by the larvae of *Oestrus ovis*]. *Chinese J. Parasitol. & Parasit. Dis.*, **25:** pp. 1 preceding table of contents.

Zumpt, F. (1965). *Myiasis in Man and animals in the Old World.* London: Butterworth.

CHAPTER 69

Histoplasmosis

L. Joseph Wheat and Lynn Guptill

Summary

History

Histoplasma was initially described from a lesion in a horse by Rivolta in 1873, who named the organism *Cryptococcus farciminosum*. In 1905, Samuel Darling noted the presence of intracellular organisms in many tissues, including the lungs, of a patient suspected of succumbing to miliary tuberculosis (Darling 1906). Darling named the organism *Histoplasma capsulatum*, because it appeared to be an encapsulated protozoan-like organism. In 1912, mycologist Henrique da Rocha-Lima reviewed Darling's slides and noted the cytological similarities between Darling's *Histoplasma* organism and *Cryptococcus farciminosum*. *Cryptococcus farciminosum* was reclassified as *Histoplasma farciminosum* in 1934, and in 1985 it was again reclassified as a variant of *Histoplasma capsulatum* (var. *farciminosum*) (Weeks *et al.* 1985).

William De Monbreun cultured the organism from the blood of a child suffering from an unexplained febrile disease in 1934, and demonstrated it to be a dimorphic fungus (De Monbreun 1934). De Monbreun and others reported naturally occurring histoplasmosis in a dog in 1939, and subsequently demonstrated experimentally that clinically inapparent histoplasmosis occurred in dogs (De Monbreun 1939). De Monbreun and others speculated that animals might serve as the source of histoplasmosis in human beings. However, C.W. Emmons demonstrated in 1949 that *Histoplasma capsulatum* is a soil saprophyte, and that inhalation of aerosolized microconidia and mycelial fragments served as the source of infection (Emmons 1949).

The prevalence of histoplasmosis in endemic regions was estimated to be more than 50% based on positive skin tests for histoplasmin (Edwards *et al.* 1969). Active histoplasmosis has been identified in up to 50% of dogs in endemic regions based on culture at necropsy of healthy animals (Turner *et al.* 1972a). The case prevalence of disseminated histoplasmosis at a veterinary teaching hospital in an endemic region of the mid-western USA of 43 cases in cats and 12 cases in dogs per 100,000 hospital records per year has been estimated (Clinkenbeard *et al.* 1988; Kaplan 1973). Dogs and cats with outdoor exposure are reportedly at greater risk for histoplasmosis than those with minimal time outdoors. However, some completely indoor cats become ill with histoplasmosis (Davies and Troy 1996; Johnson *et al.* 2004). Young to middle-aged

dogs of hunting and sporting breeds have historically been reported at greatest risk for acquiring histoplasmosis (Selby *et al.* 1981). Risk factors for cats have not been systematically studied.

Infection by *Histoplasma capsulatum* var. *capsulatum* is not contagious except in unusual situations. Rare cases of horizontal transmission have been reported. Horizontal transmission is associated with conjugal contraction of individuals with cutaneous lesions of the genitalia (Sills *et al.* 1973) and by solid organ transplantation of infected organs (Limaye *et al.* 2000). No documented cases of transmission from animals to human beings or vice versa have been reported. In contrast to *Histoplasma capsulatum* var. *capsulatum*, equine infection by *Histoplasma capsulatum* var. *farciminosum* is contagious and is transmitted by bites of contaminated flies or ticks as well as through skin traumatized with contaminated tack (Kohn 2006).

Pathogenesis

Inhalation of microconidia and mycelial fragments is the route of natural *Histoplasma capsulatum* var. *capsulatum* infection. Once inhaled the conidia are engulfed by neutrophils, macrophages and dendritic cells, in which they proliferate until Th1 immunity develops. Over the 3–5 days the conidia transform into yeasts, which are the pathogenic form of the organism (Procknow *et al.* 1960). The yeasts multiply within macrophages, which spread the infection to extrapulmonary sites.

During the second week of infection cell-mediated immunity develops and halts progression in man and murine experimental models of histoplasmosis. Th1 lymhocytes and several cytokines are responsible for an effective immune response, which results in death of the organism. Interleukin-12, IL-18, tumour necrosis factor-α (TNF-α) and interferon-gamma play important roles in acquired immunity in histoplasmosis.

Progressive disseminated infection in humans is associated with conditions that reduce cell-mediated immunity (Assi *et al.* 2007; Wheat *et al.* 1982). Key among these are HIV infection, use of corticosteroids and other immunosuppressive medications, including tumour necrosis factor inhibitors, and rare immunodeficiency states (Steiner *et al.* 2009; Zerbe and Holland 2005). However, individuals of certain animal species, including dogs (Fattal *et al.* 1961; Rowley *et al.* 1954; Smith *et al.* 1976) cats (Rowley *et al.* 1954) and bats (Greer and McMurray 1981; Tesh and Schneidau 1967) fail to eradicate the infection in the absence of immunosuppression, suggesting inherent inability to develop immunity to *H. capsulatum*. Except for studies in murine and guinea pig models of histoplasmosis, immunity has not been studied extensively in animals.

Clinical findings in animals

Both natural and experimental histoplasmosis have been described in a variety of animals. While it has been possible to infect chickens, causing a localized infections of the feather (Tewari and Campbell 1965), histoplasmosis does not occur naturally in birds because of their higher body temperature. The natural disease caused by *Histoplasma capsulatum* var. *capsulatum* is most adequately described in dogs and cats. The prevalence of histoplasmosis is high in the endemic areas, as is indicated by the high percentage of dogs and cats with positive cultures from lungs or associated lymph nodes (Emmons *et al.* 1955; Emmons and Rowley 1955; Fattal *et al.* 1961; Turner *et al.* 1972a). The incubation period is approximately 7–14 days (Menges *et al.* 1954; Ward *et al.* 1979).

Most affected cats have disseminated histoplasmosis, a systemic disease, with clinical signs of weight loss, lethargy, fever, anorexia, and weakness (Clinkenbeard *et al.* 1987; Davies and Troy 1996). A review of medical records of 96 cats with histoplasmosis showed that, in contrast to previous reports, many cats with histoplasmosis are not presented for respiratory signs. In that study, the most common clinical signs of disease were lethargy, weakness, dehydration, pyrexia, and emaciation (67% of the cats). Thirty-nine percent of the cats had respiratory signs, 24% had ocular signs (chorioretinitis, anterior uveitis, retinal detachments), and 18% had evidence of skeletal involvement (Davies and Troy 1996). Skin lesions, oral ulcers, and diarrhoea are less common signs arising from focal tissue or organ dysfunction associated with disseminated histoplasmosis; mineralized pulmonary lesions are not commonly reported in cats (Clinkenbeard *et al.* 1987; Lamm *et al.* 2009; Pearce *et al.* 2007; Stark 1982; Vinayak *et al.* 2007). Bone marrow involvement is sometimes the only manifestation of histoplasmosis in cats. Thrombocytopenia, neutropenia, anemia, and mixed cytopenias are reported; evaluation of bone marrow aspirates or biopsies may be necessary for diagnosis (Clinkenbeard *et al.* 1987; Davies and Troy 1996; Gabbert *et al.* 1982; Hodges *et al.* 1994; Kerl 2003).

In dogs, pulmonary histoplasmosis can resolve with no sequelae, with mineralization of interstitial lung nodules and tracheobronchial lymph nodes, or with development of clinically apparent disseminated histoplasmosis (Burk *et al.* 1978; Schulman *et al.* 1999). Disseminated histoplasmosis is typically a subacute to chronic diarrhoeal disease of young to middle-aged dogs (Bromel and Sykes 2005; Clinkenbeard *et al.* 1989; Gingerich and Guptill 2008; Krohne 2000). Weight loss and anaemia are also common signs, fever, lymphadenopathy, hepatomegaly, splenomegaly, and respiratory signs are seen in up to 50% of dogs with systemic histoplasmosis. Focal signs or lesions other than diarrhoea are reported in fewer dogs with disseminated histoplasmosis, and these may include icterus, lameness, vomiting, oral ulcers, ocular lesions including retinal detachment and subretinal pyogranulomas which may lead to blindness, CNS signs, and rarely, skin lesions (Gingerich and Guptill 2008; Kabli *et al.* 1986; Kagawa *et al.* 1998; Krohne 2000; Nishifuji *et al.* 2005; Olson and Wowk 1981; Salfelder *et al.* 1965).

Clinical findings in humans

The clinical findings are generally similar, except that humans are more likely to have underlying conditions or be receiving medications that suppress their immunity, predisposing to progressive histoplasmosis. The clinical spectrum in humans may be somewhat broader than in animals, in part because of discovery of radiographic abnormalities as incidental findings during evaluation for other conditions. Also, manifestations causing mild symptoms, which are commonly noted in humans, may not be recognized in animals. The more common findings in humans include pulmonary or mediastinal manifestations and progressive disseminated disease.

Pulmonary histoplasmosis

In endemic areas, half to more than 80% of individuals have had histoplasmosis by age 20 (Edwards *et al.* 1969), and most are asymptomatic. About 5% of individuals develop a subacute pulmonary illness after low level exposure (Wheat 1989), and radiographs show enlarged hilar or mediastinal lymph nodes with patchy pulmonary infiltrates (Wheat *et al.* 1982). The illness usually is mild and evolves over several weeks to months before a diagnosis is established. Improvement occurs within a month (Brodsky *et al.* 1973), but fatigue may linger.

Pericarditis may occur as an immunological reaction to the adjacent and inflamed mediastinal nodes (Wheat *et al.* 1983). Outcome is excellent, with rare progression to constrictive pericarditis (Bilgi and Slesar 1976). Antifungal therapy is unnecessary (Picardi *et al.* 1976) unless the patient receives corticosteroids or has disseminated disease. Arthralga or arthritis, also occur as immunological reactions to the acute infection, and usually are associated with pulmonary complaints. The joint symptoms usually resolve in response to anti-inflammatory therapy (Medeiros *et al.* 1966).

An acute pulmonary illness follows heavy exposure. Patients usually present within two weeks of exposure with diffuse pulmonary involvement often causing respiratory difficulty (Loosli *et al.* 1952). Attack rates exceed 75% follow heavy exposure (Gustafson *et al.* 1981; Ward *et al.* 1979). Chest radiograms show diffuse reticulonodular or miliary pulmonary infiltrates, sometimes with mediastinal lymphadenopathy (Johnson *et al.* 1988). Some patients may manifest progressive extra pulmonary dissemination (Rubin *et al.* 1959). Although patients may recover without treatment (Rubin *et al.* 1959), the illness often is severe and recovery slow. Thus, treatment is advised. Adjunctive corticosteroid treatment may accelerate improvement in such cases, as the inflammatory response may contribute to the pathogenesis of the respiratory injury.

Chronic pulmonary histoplasmosis occurs in patients with underlying emphysema, and is characterized by cavitary upper lobe infiltrates similar to those typical of tuberculosis (Goodwin *et al.* 1976). The illness is chronic and progressive if left untreated.

Mediastinal granuloma

Enlarged mediastinal lymph nodes may impinge upon the airways, pulmonary vessels or vena cava, or the oesophagus, occurring in < 10% of patients with pulmonary histoplasmosis (Coss *et al.* 1987). These findings may first present years after the initial infection, as a result of smoldering inflammation and necrosis in the involved node. Symptoms include chest pain, cough, haemoptysis, dyspnea and dysphagia (Schowengerdt *et al.* 1969). Although enlarged nodes usually shrink and symptoms resolve without treatment (Sakulsky *et al.* 1967), obstructive syndromes may be severe (Greenwood and Holland 1972), and the masses may persist for years.

Fibrosing mediastinitis

Fibrosing mediastinitis is a fibrotic response to a prior episode of mediastinal histoplasmosis that is characterized by invasion and obstruction of mediastinal structures (Goodwin *et al.* 1972). The pathogenesis is thought to involve an excessive fibrotic response to *Histoplasma* antigens released from mediastinal lymph nodes. Obstruction may involve the superior vena cava, airways, pulmonary arteries or veins, or oesophagus. While the clinical impairments are chronic, they are not always progressive, and they do not respond to antifungal therapy. Surgery is associated with a high mortality, and is rarely indicated. Some patients may benefit from placement of stents in pulmonary or bronchial vessels, however.

Progressive disseminated histoplasmosis

Progressive disseminated histoplasmosis occurs mostly in immunodeficient patients and those at the extremes of age (Goodwin *et al.* 1980), and is characterized by a progressive infection involving extrapulmonary tissues. Fever and weight loss are the most common findings, accompanied by respiratory symptoms in most patients (Goodwin *et al.* 1980). Hepatomegaly, splenomegaly or lymphadenopathy occur in one to two-thirds of cases and, less frequently, adrenal, gastrointestinal, skin or mucosal lesions may be seen. The brain, spinal cord or meninges are involved in about 5% of cases (Wheat *et al.* 2005). Endocarditis is a rare complication of disseminated histoplasmosis (Bhatti *et al.* 2005). Any tissue may be involved. While the illness is progressive and ultimately fatal in 90% of cases (Sathapatayavongs *et al.* 1983), the untreated course may span a few months to several years, and some patients appear to recover spontaneously (Assi *et al.* 2007).

Diagnosis

Several tests are useful for diagnosis of histoplasmosis in humans, including serology, fungal stain of tissues, detection of antigen in body fluids, and fungal culture (Wheat 2009). In humans with acute pulmonary and progressive disseminated histoplasmosis the highest sensitivity is with antigen detection, which is most useful in patients with acute or severe disease. Serology is most useful in mild cases. Diagnosis in veterinary medicine is currently primarily based on detection of *Histoplasma* organisms upon cytologic or histopathologic evaluation of tissue aspirates, biopsies, or fluid obtained by tracheal wash or bronchoalveolar lavage (Figs. 69.1 and 69.2). Fungal culture of tissues or fluids is also useful. Polymerase chain reaction (PCR) testing may be applied to tissue samples, and fungal stains are also used when evaluating tissue samples (Bromel and Sykes 2005; Gingerich and Guptill 2008; Greene 2006; Nishifuji *et al.* 2005; Ueda *et al.* 2003). Serologic testing for antibody detection is not highly sensitive or specific for veterinary patients with focal or disseminated disease. Testing of serum or urine for the presence of fungal antigen has recently been introduced, but is not yet validated for veterinary patients.

Fungal stains

Histoplasma yeast measure 2–3 μm in diameter, and exhibit narrow-necked budding. In humans, fungal stain is less sensitive than

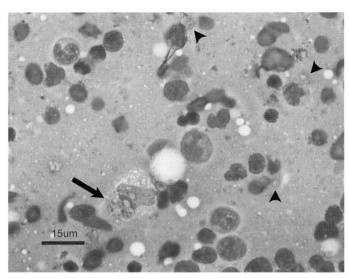

Fig. 69.1 Feline bone marrow aspirate demonstrating a single (arrow) macrophage containing several budding yeast. Several yeast are noted free in the background (arrow heads). Diff-Quik®, 100x objective.
Photomicrographs provided by Craig Thompson, DVM, DACVP.

antigen detection for diagnosis of disseminated and acute pulmonary histoplasmosis (Wheat 2009). One drawback of fungal stain is the requirement to perform invasive procedures to obtain specimens for evaluation. Also, the accuracy may vary depending upon the pathologist's experience with recognition of *Histoplasma* yeast, as other yeast or staining artefact may be mistaken as *Histoplasma* and small numbers of yeasts may be easily overlooked.

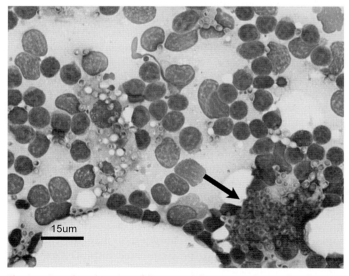

Fig. 69.2 Lymph node aspirate, feline. A single large macrophage is densely packed with yeast (arrow), and there are numerous yeast free in the background. Note the clear area surrounding the yeast, caused by shrinkage that occurs during fixation. Numerous small lymphocytes and a few bare nuclei are also present. Diff-Quik®, 100x objective.
Photomicrographs provided by Craig Thompson, DVM, DACVP.

Culture

Cultures are positive in many cases of disseminated histoplasmosis (Fattal *et al.* 1961; Turner *et al.* 1972b; Sathapatayavongs *et al.* 1983), but growth may be slow, requiring up to four weeks. The highest yield is from the lung, skin or mucosal lesions, or bone marrow, thus requiring invasive procedures to obtain specimens. In many cases in animals, cultures are not performed, however.

Antigen detection

A galactomannan antigen in the cell wall of proliferating *Histoplasma* yeast is released into the tissues and blood, and excreted in the urine. This antigen can be detected in an enzyme immunoassay. Antigen was detected in 95–99% of humans with disseminated histoplasmosis (Connolly *et al.* 2007), and in 83% of those with acute pneumonia (Swartzentruber *et al.* 2009). The greatest sensitivity for diagnosis required testing both urine and serum (Wheat 2009). Also, a negative result does not exclude the diagnosis. In cases with negative results, follow-up specimens may be positive in patients exhibiting progressive illness. Serology or culture may be positive in patients with negative antigen results. Antigen detection was sensitive when used to test stored samples from a bottlenose dolphin with disseminated histoplasmosis (Jensen *et al.* 1998). Prospective studies are needed to define sensitivity of antigen detection in animals.

Antigen may be detected in the respiratory secretions in humans with pulmonary histoplasmosis (Hage *et al.* 2010), occasionally permitting diagnosis in patients with negative results in urine and serum. Antigen also may be detected in the cerebrospinal fluid of humans with meningitis, offering a helpful method to diagnose this elusive manifestation (Wheat *et al.* 2005).

The galactomannan found in histoplasmosis cross reacts with that found in blastomycosis (Spector *et al.* 2008; Connolly *et al.* 2007). Furthermore, the clinical findings and endemic distribution overlap. Thus, differentiation of the two mycoses may be difficult via antigen detection alone.

Antigen levels decline during treatment and increase with relapse, providing a tool for monitoring therapy in humans. Again, the use of antigen detection for diagnosis or monitoring of histoplasmosis in animals requires further validation.

Serology

In humans, serologic tests are positive in over 90% of cases of subacute and chronic pulmonary histoplasmosis and often provide the basis for diagnosis (Wheat 2009). Serology is less useful in disseminated and acute pulmonary histoplasmosis, where tests may be falsely negative due to underlying immunosuppression in disseminated disease and because of the one to two month delay for antibodies to develop following acute infection.

The lack of sensitivity and specificity of available serologic tests for diagnosis of active histoplasmosis in animals is highlighted in reports of canine and feline histoplasmosis. Seventeen of 26 animals with culture, cytology, PCR, or necropsy-proven histoplasmosis had negative serologic test results (agar-gel immunodiffusion or complement fixation tests) (Clinkenbeard *et al.* 1987; Clinkenbeard *et al.* 1988; Hawkins and DeNicola 1990; Hodges *et al.* 1994; Johnson *et al.* 2004; Kowalewich *et al.* 1993; Mackie *et al.* 1997; Mitchell and Stark 1980; Nishifuji *et al.* 2005; Noxon *et al.* 1982; Olson and Wowk 1981). In those reports, some animals

with positive test results also had positive test results for other fungal pathogens; one animal with blastomycosis had a negative serologic test result for blastomycosis and a positive result for histoplasmosis, and two animals with negative tests for histoplasmosis had positive test results for other fungal pathogens. In a study evaluating naturally infected dogs, 51 dogs had positive *Histoplasma* cultures; 13 of those had positive serology for *Histoplasma* antigens, 10 were positive for *Blastomyces*, and 28 were positive for either *Blastomyces* or *Histoplasma* or both. Of 132 dogs with negative serologic tests, 23.5% had positive fungal cultures for *Histoplasma*, and of 125 dogs with positive complement fixation tests (using both *Blastomyces* and *Histoplasma* antigens), only 49% had positive fungal cultures for *Histoplasma* (Turner *et al.* 1972b).

Cross reactions by complement fixation may occur in patients with other endemic mycoses, and serum may be anti-complementary, preventing measurement of antibodies by complement fixation in some cases. H and M precipitin bands are specific for histoplasmosis and A precipitin bands for blastomycosis, assisting in differentiation of the two mycoses. However, the sensitivity of immunodiffusion is low (<20%) in dogs with blastomycosis (Spector *et al.* 2008) and <35% in dogs with histoplasmosis (Clinkenbeard *et al.* 1987, 1988; Hawkins and DeNicola 1990; Hodges *et al.* 1994; Johnson *et al.* 2004; Kowalewich *et al.* 1993; Mackie *et al.* 1997; Mitchell and Stark 1980; Nishifuji *et al.* 2005; Olson and Wowk 1981). Sensitivity may be improved using enzyme immunoassay, as described in blastomycosis, but the enzyme immunoassay may not be specific (Greene 2006; Spector *et al.* 2008).

Molecular methods

Molecular methods have not been tested extensively for diagnosis of histoplasmosis in humans or animals. Several PCR targets have been utilized, including the 18S ribosomal RNA gene, the rRNA internal transcribed spacer region, M and H antigens, and a 100 kDa protein, HC100, that is necessary for intracellular survival (Bialek *et al.* 2001, 2002; Bracca *et al.* 2003; Imhof *et al.* 2003; Sandhu *et al.* 1995; Tang *et al.* 2006). Specificity and sensitivity of these assays has not been extensively evaluated, however. PCR may be falsely-negative in specimens in which the organisms are seen by histopathology (Bialek 2002). More recently PCR assay was found to be less sensitive than antigen detection when applied to urine (Tang *et al.* 2006) or other body fluids (Wheat, unpublished observation, 2009). There are currently no commercially available PCR assays for diagnosis of histoplasmosis (Kauffman 2009). Molecular methods have not been widely used for diagnosis of histoplasmosis in dogs and cats (Nishifuji *et al.* 2005; Ueda *et al.* 2003).

Treatment

Amphotericin B

Amphotericin B is recommended for the first week or two in severe infections of small animals (Bromel and Sykes 2005; Gingerich and Guptill 2008; Grooters and Taboada 2003; Kerl 2003), as in humans (Wheat *et al.* 2007). Amphotericin B is recommended in humans who have more severe forms of histoplasmosis, requiring hospitalization. Liposomal amphotericin B (AmBisome) was more effective than the standard deoxycholate formulation, demonstrating a higher response rate (88% vs. 64%, respectively) and lower mortality (2% vs. 13%, respectively) in patients with progressive disseminated histoplasmosis (Wheat *et al.* 2007). Amphotericin B lipid complex may be preferred over liposomal amphotericin B because of lower cost. The deoxycholate formulation remains the standard formulation used in children. Amphotericin B is usually given for about a week, and then replaced with itraconazole in patients who have improved sufficiently to no longer require hospitalization. Nephrotoxicity remains a problem even with the lipid formulations of amphotericin B, and frequent monitoring of renal function, potassium and magnesium is required.

Amphotericin B lipid complex is currently recommended for small animal patients when amphotericin B treatment is required, rather than the deoxycholate form of the drug. The nephrotoxicity of the lipid complexed drug is significantly reduced compared with the deoxycholate form, giving it a markedly improved therapeutic index. However, monitoring of serum creatinine and urea nitrogen is still recommended (Grooters and Taboada 2003). Itraconazole is often administered concurrently with amphotericin B in small animals (Bromel and Sykes 2005; Gingerich and Guptill 2008; Greene 2006; Krohne 2000).

Itraconazole

Itraconazole is recommended for individuals with mild to moderate disease and after clinical improvement with amphotericin B in humans with severe disease (Wheat *et al.* 2007). Itraconazole capsules require an acid pH for maximum absorption, and should be taken with food. The suspension does not require an acidic environment, and should be taken on an empty stomach. Itraconazole is usually given for a year or more in patients with progressive disseminated or chronic pulmonary histoplasmosis and for six to 12 weeks in patients with other forms of pulmonary histoplasmosis.

Itraconazole is the treatment of choice for most mild to moderately severe infections in small animals. The bioavailability of the oral solution for cats is greater than that of the capsule form (Boothe *et al.* 1997), and it may be possible to reduce the dose when using the oral solution. The recommended duration of treatment varies with each small animal patient, but most patients are treated for at least three to six months, and it is advised that treatment continue until at least 60 days past the complete resolution of clinical signs and radiographic or ocular lesions. Treatment may be required for a year or longer, particularly for widely disseminated disease (Greene 2006; Krohne 2000).

Itraconazole is cleared by cytochrome P450:3A4 metabolism, and blood levels may be affected by medications that interact with that enzyme. Itraconazole blood level measurement is encouraged during the second week of treatment in humans, and if treatment failure or relapse is suspected. Target blood levels are 1.0–10 µg/mL. Target blood levels are not well-defined for treatment of histoplasmosis in animals. In cats, steady state was reached after 14–21 days of treatment, and in dogs steady state was reached after 14 days (Boothe *et al.* 1997; Legendre *et al.* 1996). Itraconazole may cause a variety of adverse effects, most commonly anorexia, vomiting, diarrhoea, lethargy, skin ulceration, or increased hepatic enzyme activities. Gastrointestinal side effects may be related to high blood levels in humans (Lestner *et al.* 2009). Bilirubin and hepatic enzymes should be monitored during therapy (Legendre *et al.* 1996; Wheat *et al.* 2007).

Other azoles

Several other azoles are active in histoplasmosis and provide alternatives in those unable to take or who have failed itraconazole.

Ketoconazole is infrequently used because it is less effective and causes more adverse effects than itraconazole, but its lower cost may be a reason to use it in some cases. Fluconazole is also less effective but may be used because of lower cost or reduced adverse effects compared with itraconazole. To prevent failure due to emergence of resistance to fluconazole (Wheat *et al.* 2001), doses of at least 10 mg/kg/day are recommended in human beings; similar data are not available for animals.

Posaconazole and voriconazole are more active than fluconazole and have been used successfully in humans with histoplasmosis (Wheat *et al.* 2007), but have not been evaluated extensively in animals and are expensive. These agents are reserved for patients unable to take or who have failed itraconazole and fluconazole. *H. capsulatum* also may become resistant to voriconazole (Wheat *et al.* 2006).

Prevention and control

Several aspects of histoplasmosis caused by *Histoplasma capsulatum* organisms make control strategies difficult. The exposure levels to *H. capsulatum* var. *capsulatum* vary by locale within endemic regions. An attempt to identify heavily contaminated sites should be made for sites with a high historical or scientific potential for heavy *Histoplasma* contamination, particularly where earth moving, demolition, or renovation will likely expose people and animals to dust or other debris from the site. Large bird roosts, or bat habitats are candidates for heavily contaminated sites.

Most bird roosts identified to be contaminated have been in use for at least three years (Chick *et al.* 1981; Weeks and Stickley Jr. 1984); but once contaminated, however, the organism may persist in the absence of continued roosting. Contaminated sites should be posted to warn of the risk for exposure to histoplasmosis. Preventing long-term use of roosting areas could decrease environmental contamination (D'Alessio *et al.* 1965), but the efficacy of dispersion techniques has been questioned (Weeks and Stickley Jr. 1984). Soil decontamination with formalin has been advocated, but is inconvenient, hazardous to those involved and the environment, of uncertain effectiveness, and expensive. Physical removal of the contaminated material may be appropriate if the area of contamination is small. Decontamination procedures should follow published guidelines (Lenhart *et al.* 1997), which include the use of respirators and other personal protection equipment, to reduce their risk of exposure during the removal or decontamination of sites containing *Histoplasma*.

Persons at high risk for histoplasmosis should be informed of the probability of high exposure in certain environments. Health-care workers should be educated of the increased risk for contraction of histoplasmosis for immunocompromised individuals. Unfortunately, in many instances the avoidance of insidious exposure by high-risk individuals may not be possible, but advising high-risk individuals to avoid areas of probable high *Histoplasma*-contamination is warranted (Wheat 1992).

Several strategies are available for control of equine epizootic lymphangitis. These include the control of biting flies and ticks, practice of general hygiene and disinfection, and quarantine or euthanasia of infected animals (Gabal *et al.* 1983). A killed vaccine to protect from *H. capsulatum* var. *farciminosum* is reportedly available for horses in endemic areas (Kohn 2006).

Acknowledgement

The authors thank Dr. Craig Thompson for the excellent photomicrographs.

References

Assi, M.A., Sandid, M.S., *et al.* (2007). Systemic histoplasmosis: A 15-year retrospective institutional review of 111 patients. *Medicine*, **86**: 162–69.

Bhatti, S., Vilenski, L., Tight, R., and Smego Jr., R.A. (2005). *Histoplasma* endocarditis: clinical and mycologic features and outcomes. *J. Infect.*, **51**: 2–9.

Bialek, R., Ernst, F., *et al.* (2002). Comparison of staining methods and a nested PCR assay to detect *Histoplasma capsulatum* in tissue sections. *Am. J. Clin. Path.*, **117**: 597–603.

Bialek, R., Fischer, J., Feucht, A., *et al.* (2001). Diagnosis and monitoring of murine histoplasmosis by a nested PCR assay. *J. Clin. Microb.*, **39**: 1506–9.

Bilgi, C. and Slesar, S. (1976). Constrictive pericarditis and pericardial calcification with positive histoplasmin skin test. *Can. Med. Ass. J.*, **114**: 877–82.

Boothe, D.M., Herring, I., Calvin, J., Way, N., and Dvorak, J. (1997). Itraconazole disposition after single oral and intravenous and multiple oral dosing in healthy cats. *Am. J. Vet. Res.*, **58**: 872–77.

Bracca, A., Tosello, M.E., *et al.* (2003). Molecular detection of *Histoplasma capsulatum* var. *capsulatum* in human clinical samples. *J. Clin. Microb.*, **41**: 1753–55.

Bradsher, R.W., Wickre, C.G., *et al.* (1980). *Histoplasma capsulatum* endocarditis cured by amphotericin B combined with surgery. *CHEST*, **78**: 791–95.

Brodsky, A.L., Gregg, M.B., Kaufman, L., and Mallison, G.F. (1973). Outbreak of histoplasmosis associated with the 1970 Earth Day activities. *Am. J. Med.*, **54**: 333–42.

Bromel, C., and Sykes., J.E. (2005). Histoplasmosis in dogs and cats. *Clin. Techn. Small Anim. Pract.*, **20**: 227–32.

Burk, R.L., Cornley, E.A., and Corwin, L.A. (1978). Radiographic appearance of pulmonary histoplasmosis in the dog and cat: a review of 37 case histories. *Vet. Rad. Soc. J.*, **19**: 2–6.

Chick, E.W., Compton, S.B., *et al.* (1981). Hitchcock's birds, or the increased rate of exposure to *Histoplasma* from blackbird roost sites. *Chest*, **80**: 434–38.

Clinkenbeard, K.D., Cowell, R.L., and Tyler, R.D. (1988). Disseminated histoplasmosis in dogs: 12 cases (1981–1986). *J. Am. Vet. Med. Ass.*, **193**: 1443–47.

Clinkenbeard, K.D., Cowell, R.L., and Tyler, R.D. (1987). Disseminated histoplasmosis in cats: 12 cases. *J. Am. Vet. Med. Ass.*, **190**: 1445–48.

Clinkenbeard, K.D., Wolf, A.M., Cowell, R.L., and Tyler, R.L. (1989). Canine disseminated histoplasmosis. *The Comp. Cont. Ed. Pract. Vet.*, **11**: 1347–60.

Connolly, P.A., Durkin, M.M., *et al.* (2007). Detection of *Histoplasma* antigen by a quantitative enzyme immunoassay. *Clin. Vacc. Immunol.*, **14**: 1587–911.

Coss, K.C., Wheat, L.J., *et al.* (1987). Esophageal fistula complicating mediastinal histoplasmosis: Response to amphotericin B. *Am. J. Med.*, **83**: 343–46.

D'Alessio, D.J., Heeren, R.H., Hendricks, S.L., *et al.* (1965). A starling roost as the source of urban epidemic histoplasmosis in an area of low incidence. *Am. Rev. Respir. Dis.*, **92**: 725–31.

Darling, S.T. (1906). A protozoan general infection producing pseudotubercules in the lungs and focal necroses in the liver, spleen, and lymph nodes. *J. Am. Med. Ass.*, 1283–85.

Davies, C. and Troy, G.C. (1996). Deep Mycotic Infections in Cats. *J. Am. Anim. Hosp. Ass.*, **32**: 380–31.

De Monbreun, W. (1939). The dog as a natural host for *Histoplasma capsulatum*. *Am. J. Trop. Med. Hyg.*, **14**: 565–87.

De Monbreun, W. (1934). The cultivation and cultural characteristics of Darling's *Histoplasma capsulatum*. *Am. J. Trop. Med. Hyg.*, **14**: 93–125.

Edwards, L.B., Acquaviva, F.A., *et al.* (1969). An atlas of sensitivity to tuberculin, PPD, and histoplasmin in the United States. *Am. Rev. Respir. Dis.*, **99**: 1–18.

Emmons, C.W. (1949). Isolation of *Histoplasma capsulatum* from soil. *Am. J. Pub. Health*, **64**: 892–96.

Emmons, C.W. and Rowley, D.A. (1955). Isolation of *Histoplasma capsulatum* from fresh and deep frozen peribronchial lymph nodes of dogs by mouse inoculation. *J. Lab. Clin. Med.*, **45**: 303–7.

Emmons, C.W., Rowley, D.A., *et al.* (1955). Histoplasmosis; proved occurrence of inapparent infection in dogs, cats and other animals. *Am. J. Hyg.*, **61**: 40–44.

Fattal, A.R., Schwarz, J., and Straub, M. (1961). Isolation of *Histoplasma capsulatum* from lymph nodes of spontaneously infected dogs. *Am. J. Clin. Path.*, **36**: 119–24.

Gabal, M.A., Hassan, F.K., Siad, A.A., and Karim, K.A. (1983). Study of equine histoplasmosis farciminosi and characterization of *Histoplasma farciminosum*. *Sabouraudia*, **21**: 121–27.

Gabbert, N.H., Campbell, T.W., and Beiermann, R.L. (1982). Pancytopenia associated with disseminated histoplasmosis in a cat. *J. Am. Anim. Hosp. Ass.*, **20**: 119–22.

Gingerich, K. and Guptill, L. (2008). Canine and feline histoplasmosis: A review of a widespread fungus. *Vet. Med.*, **103**: 248–64.

Goodwin, R.A., Nickell, J.A., and des Prez, R.M. (1972). Mediastinal fibrosis complicating healed primary histoplasmosis and tuberculosis. *Med. (Baltimore)*, **51**: 227–46.

Goodwin, R.A., Owens, F.T., Snell, J.D., and Buchanan, R.D. (1976). Chronic pulmonary histoplasmosis. *Medicine (Baltimore)*, **55**: 413–52.

Goodwin, R.A., Shapiro, J.L., Thurman, S.S., and des Prez, R.M. (1980). Disseminated histoplasmosis: Clinical and pathologic correlations. *Med. (Baltimore)*, **59**: 1–33.

Greene, C.E. (2006). Histoplasmosis. In: C.E. Greene (ed.) Infectious Diseases of the Dog and Cat, (3rd edn.), pp. 577–84. St Louis, USA: Elsevier Saunders.

Greenwood, M.F., and Holland, P. (1972). Tracheal obstruction secondary to *Histoplasma* mediastinal granuloma. *Chest*, 62: 642–45.

Greer, D.L., and McMurray, D.N. (1981). Pathogenesis of experimental histoplasmosis in the bat, *Artibeus lituratus*. *Am. J. Trop. Med. Hyg.*, **30**: 653–59.

Grooters, A.M., and Taboada, J. (2003). Update on antifungal therapy. *Vet. Clin. N. Am.: Small Anim. Pract.*, **33**: 749–58.

Gustafson, T.L., Kaufman, L., *et al.* (1981). Outbreak of pulmonary histoplasmosis and blastomycosis in members of a wagon train. *Am. J. Med.*, **71**: 759–65.

Hage, C.A., Davis, T.E., Fuller, D., *et al.* (2010). Diagnosis of histoplasmosis by antigen detection in BAL fluid. *Chest*, 137: 623–28.

Hawkins, E.C., and DeNicola, D.B. (1990). Cytologic analysis of tracheal wash specimens and bronchoalveolar lavage fluid in the diagnosis of mycotic infections in dogs. *J. Am. Vet. Med. Ass.*, **197**: 79–83.

Hodges, R.D., Legendre, A.M., *et al.* (1994). Itraconazole for the treatment of histoplasmosis in cats. *J. Vet. Intern. Med.*, **8**: 409–13.

Imhof, A., Schaer. C., *et al.* (2003). Rapid detection of pathogenic fungi from clinical specimens using LightCycler real-time fluorescence PCR. *Eur. J. Clin. Microb. Infect. Dis.*, **22**: 558–60.

Jensen, E.D., Lipscomb, T., *et al.* (1998). Disseminated histoplasmosis in an Atlantic bottlenose dolphin (*Tursiops truncatus*). *J. Zoo. Wildlife Med.*, **29**: 456–60.

Johnson, J., Kabler, J.D., *et al.* (1988). Cave-associated histoplasmosis: Costa Rica. *Morb. Mort. Wkly. Rep.*, **37**: 312–13.

Johnson, L.R., Fry, M.M., et al. (2004). Histoplasmosis infection in two cats from California. *J. Am. Anim. Hosp. Ass.*, **40**: 165–69.

Kabli, S., Koschmann, J.R., et al. (1986). Endemic canine and feline histoplasmosis in El Paso, Texas. *J. Med.Vet. Mycol.*, **24**: 41–50.

Kagawa, Y., Aoki, S., et al. (1998). Histoplasmosis in the skin and gingiva in a dog. *J. Vet. Med. Sci.*, **60**: 863–65.

Kaplan, W. (1973). Epidemiology of the principal systemic mycoses of man and lower animals and the ecology of their etiologic agents. *J. Am. Vet. Med. Ass.*, **163**: 1043–47.

Kauffman, C.A. (2009). Histoplasmosis. *Clin. Chest Med.*, **30**: 217–25.

Kerl, M.E. (2003). Update on canine and feline fungal diseases. *Vet. Clin. N. Am.: Small Anim. Pract.*, **33**: 721–47.

Kohn, C. (2006). Miscellaneous Fungal Diseases. In: D. Sellon and M. Long (eds.) Equine Infectious Diseases, pp. 431–45. St Louis, USA: Elsevier Saunders.

Kowalewich, N., Hawkins, E.C., Skowronek, A.J., and Clemo, F.A.S. (1993). Identification of *Histoplasma capsulatum* organisms in the pleural and peritoneal effusions of a dog. *J. Am. Vet. Med. Ass.*, **202**: 423–26.

Krohne, S.G. (2000). Canine systemic fungal infections. *Vet. Clin. N. Am.: Small Anim. Pract.*, **30**: 1063–90.

Lamm, C.G., Rizzi, T.E., Campbell, G.A., and Brunker, J.D. (2009). Pathology in practice. Histoplasma capsulatum infections. *J. Am. Vet. Med. Ass.*, **235**: 155–57.

Legendre, A.M., Rohrbach, B.W., et al. (1996). Treatment of blastomycosis with itraconazole in 112 dogs. *J. Vet. Intern. Med.*, **10**: 365–71.

Lenhart, S.W., Schafer, M.P., Singal, M., and Hajjeh, R.A. (1997). Histoplasmosis: Protecting workers at risk. U.S. Department of Health and Human Services Pamphlet.

Lestner, J.M., Roberts, S.A., et al. (2009). Toxicodynamics of itraconazole: implications for therapeutic drug monitoring. *Clin. Infect. Dis.*, **49**: 928–30.

Limaye, A.P., Connolly, P.A., et al. (2000). Transmission of *Histoplasma capsulatum* by organ transplantation. *N. Eng. J. Med.*, **343**: 1163–66.

Loosli, C.G., Grayston, J.T., et al. (1952). Some epidemiological and clinical aspects of pulmonary histoplasmosis in a farm family. *Trans. Ass. Am. Physic.*, **LXV**: 159–67.

Mackie, J.T., Kaufman, L., and Ellis, D. (1997). Confirmed histoplasmosis in an Australian dog. *Aus. Vet. J.*, **75**: 362–63.

Medeiros, A.A., Marty, S.D., Tosh, F.E., and Chin, T.D.Y. (1966). Erythema nodosum and erythema multiforme as clinical manifestations of histoplasmosis in a community outbreak. *N. Eng. J. Med.*, **274**: 415–20.

Menges, R.W., Furcolow, M.L., and Habermann, R.T. (1954). An outbreak of histoplasmosis involving animals and man. *Am. J. Vet. Res.*, **15**: 520–24.

Mitchell, M. and Stark, D.R. (1980). Disseminated canine histoplasmosis: A clinical survey of 24 cases in Texas. *Can. Vet. J.*, **21**: 95–100.

Nishifuji, K., Ueda, Y., et al. (2005). Interdigital involvement in a case of primary cutaneous canine histoplasmosis in Japan. *J. Vet. Med. Am*, **52**: 478–80.

Noxon, J.O., Digilio, K., and Schmidt, D.A. (1982). Disseminated histoplasmosis in a cat: Successful treatment with ketoconazole. *J. Am. Vet. Med. Ass.*, **181**: 817–20.

Olson, G.A., and Wowk, B.J. (1981). Oral lesions of histoplasmosis in a dog. *Vet. Med.*, 1449–51.

Pearce, J., Guiliano, E.A., et al. (2007). Management of bilateral uveitis in a *Toxoplasma gondii*-seropositive cat with histopathologic evidence of fungal panuveitis. *Vet. Ophthalm.*, **10**: 216–21.

Picardi, J.L., Kauffman, C.A., et al. (1976). Pericarditis caused by *Histoplasma capsulatum*. *Am. J. Cardio.*, **37**: 82–88.

Procknow, J.J., Page, M.I., and Loosli, C.G. (1960). Early pathogenesis of experimental histoplasmosis. *Arch. Path.*, **69**: 413–26.

Rowley, D.A., Haberman, R.T., and Emmons, C.W. (1954). Histoplasmosis: Pathologic studies of fifty cats and fifty dogs from Loudoun County, Virginia. *J. Infect. Dis.*, **95**: 98–108.

Rubin, H., Furcolow, M.L., Yates, M.L., and Brasher, C.A. (1959). The course and prognosis of histoplasmosis. *Am. J. Med.*, **27**: 278–88.

Sakulsky, S.B., Harrison, E.G., Dines, D.E., and Payne, W.S. (1967). Mediastinal granuloma. *J. Thorac. Cardiovasc. Surg.*, **54**: 280–90.

Salfelder, K., Schwarz, J., and Akbarian, M. (1965). Experimental ocular histoplasmosis in dogs. *Am. J. Opthalm.*, **59**: 290–99.

Sandhu, G.S., Kline, B.C., Stockman, L., and Roberts, G.D. (1995). Molecular probes for diagnosis of fungal infections. *J. Clin. Microb.*, **33**: 2913–19.

Sathapatayavongs, B., Batteiger, B.E., Wheat, J., Slama, T.G., and Wass, J.L. (1983). Clinical and laboratory features of disseminated histoplasmosis during two large urban outbreaks. *Med. (Baltimore)*, **62**: 263–70.

Schowengerdt, C.G., Suyemoto, R., and Beachley, F. (1969). Granulomatous and fibrous mediastinitis. *J. Thorac. Cardiovasc. Surg.*, **57**: 365–79.

Schulman, R.L., McKiernan, B.C., and Schaeffer, D.J. (1999). Use of corticosteroids for treating dogs with airway obstruction secondary to hilar lymphadenopathy caused by chronic histoplasmosis: 16 cases (1979–1997). *J. Am. Vet. Med. Ass.*, **214**: 1345–48.

Selby, L.A., Becker, S.V., and Hayes Jr., H.W. (1981). Epidemiologic risk factors associated with canine systemic mycoses. *Am. J. Epidem.*, **113**: 133–39.

Sills, M., Schwartz, A., and Weg, J.G. (1973). Conjugal histoplasmosis: A consequence of progressive disseminatino in the index case after steroid therapy. *Ann. Intern. Med.*, **79**: 221–24.

Smith, C.D., Furcolow, M.L., and Hulker, P. (1976). Effect of immunosuppressants on dogs exposed two and one-half years previously to *Blastomyces dermatitidis*. *Am. J. Epidem.*, **104**: 299–305.

Spector, D., Legendre, A.M., et al. (2008). Antigen and antibody testing for the diagnosis of blastomycosis in dogs. *J. Vet. Intern. Med.*, **22**: 839–43.

Stark, D.R. (1982). Primary gastrointestinal histoplasmosis in a cat. *J. Am. Anim. Hosp. Ass.*, 18: 154–56.

Steiner, S.J., Kleiman, M.B., Corkins, M.R., Christenson, J.C., and Wheat, L.J. (2009). Ileocecal histoplasmosis simulating Crohn disease in a patient with hyperimmunoglobulin E syndrome. *Pediatr. Infect. Dis. J.*, **28**: 744–46.

Swartzentruber, S., Rhodes, L., et al. (2009). Diagnosis of acute pulmonary histoplasmosis. *Clin. Infect. Dis.*, **49**: 1878–82.

Tang, Y.W., Li, H., et al. (2006). Urine polymerase chain reaction is not as sensitive as urine antigen for the diagnosis of disseminated histoplasmosis. *Diagn. Microb. Infect. Dis.*, **54**: 283–87.

Tesh, R.B. and Schneidau Jr., J.D. (1967). Naturally occurring histoplasmosis among bat colonies in the Southeastern United States. *Am. J. Epidem.*, **86**: 545–51.

Tewari, R.P. and Campbell, C.C. (1965). Isolation of *Histoplasma capsulatum* from the feathers of chickens inoculated intravenously and subcutaneously with the yeast phase of the organism. *Sabouraudia*, **4**: 17–22.

Turner, C., Smith, C.D., and Furcolow, M.L. (1972a). Frequency of isolation of *Histoplasma capsulatum* and *Blastomyces dermatitidis* from dogs in Kentucky. *Am. J. Vet. Res.*, **33**: 137–41.

Turner, C., Smith. C.D., and Furcolow, M.L. (1972b). The efficiency of serologic and cultural methods in the detection of infection with *Histoplasma* and *Blastomyces* in mongrel dogs. *Sabouraudia*, **10**: 1–5.

Ueda, Y., Sano, A., Tamura, M., Inomata, T., et al. (2003). Diagnosis of histoplasmosis by detection of the internal transcribed spacer region of fungal rRNA gene from a paraffin-embedded skin sample from a dog in Japan. *Vet. Microb.*, **94**: 219–24.

Vinayak, A., Kerwin, S.C., and Pool, R.R. (2007). Treatment of thoracolumbar spinal cord compression associated with *Histoplasma capsulatum* infection in a cat. *J. Am. Vet. Med. Ass.*, **230**: 1018–23.

Ward, J.I., Weeks, M., Allen, D., Hutcheson Jr., R.H., et al. (1979). Acute histoplasmosis: Clinical, epidemiologic and serologic findings of an outbreak associated with exposure to a fallen tree. *Am. J. Med.*, **66**: 587–95.

Weeks, R.J., Padhye, A.A., and Ajello, L. (1985). *Histoplasma capsulatum* var *farciminosum*: A new combination for *Histoplasma farciminosum*. *Mycologia*, **77**: 964–70.

Weeks, R.J. and Stickley Jr., A.R. (1984). Histoplasmosis and its relation to bird roosts: a review. *Bird Damage Research Report No. 330*, US Fish and Wildlife Service **897**: 31.

Wheat, L.J. (1992). Histoplasmosis in Indianapolis. *Clin. Infect. Dis.*, **14**: S91–99.

Wheat, L.J. (1989). Diagnosis and management of histoplasmosis. *Eur. J. Clin. Microb. Infect. Dis.*, **8**: 480–90.

Wheat, L.J. (2009). Approach to the diagnosis of the endemic mycoses. *Clin. Chest Med.*, **30**: 379–89.

Wheat, L.J., Connolly, P., Smedema, M., Brizendine, E., and Hafner, R. (2001). Emergence of resistance to fluconazole as a cause of failure during treatment of histoplasmosis in patients with acquired immunodeficiency disease syndrome. *Clin. Infect. Dis.*, **33**: 1910–13.

Wheat, L.J., Connolly, P., Smedema, M., Durkin, M., Brizendine, E., Mann, P., *et al.* (2006). Activity of newer triazoles against *Histoplasma capsulatum* from patients with AIDS who failed fluconazole. *J. Antimicrob. Chemother.*, **57**: 1235–39.

Wheat, L.J., Freifeld, A.G., Kleiman, M.B., *et al.* (2007). Clinical practice guidelines for the management of patients with histoplasmosis: 2007 update by the Infectious Diseases Society of America. *Clin. Infect. Dis.*, **45**: 807–25.

Wheat, L.J., Musial, C.E., and Jenny-Avital, E. (2005). Diagnosis and management of central nervous system histoplasmosis. *Clin. Infect. Dis.*, **40**: 844–52.

Wheat, L.J., Slama, T.G., Norton, J.A., *et al.* (1982). Risk factors for disseminated or fatal histoplasmosis. Analysis of a large urban outbreak. *Ann. Intern. Med.*, **96**: 159–63.

Wheat, L.J., Stein, L., Corya, B.C., *et al.* (1983). Pericarditis as a manifestation of histoplasmosis during two large urban outbreaks. *Med. (Baltimore)*, **62**: 110–19.

Zerbe, C.S. and Holland, S.M. (2005). Disseminated histoplasmosis in persons with interferon-gamma receptor 1 deficiency. *Clin. Infect. Dis.*, **41**: e38–41.

CHAPTER 70

Zoonotic infections with dermatophyte fungi

B. Mignon and M. Monod

Summary

Pathogenic dermatophytes are highly specialized fungi which are the most common agents of superficial mycoses. Most often, these fungi grow exclusively in the *stratum corneum*, nails or hair utilizing them as sole nitrogen and carbon sources. Dermatophyte species are recognized and classified as anthropophilic, zoophilic, or geophilic, depending on their major reservoir in nature (humans, animals, and soil, respectively). Zoophilic dermatophytes may result in zoonoses when humans are exposed to these organisms and dermatophytosis is considered to be one of the most common zoonotic diseases. The majority of zoonotic dermatophytoses are caused by four species:

Microsporum canis (usually derived from pet animals, particularly cats and dogs),

Trichophyton verrucosum (usually derived from cattle),

Arthroderma vanbreuseghemii (usually derived from cats and dogs),

Arthroderma benhamiae (usually derived from guinea pigs).

Infection results most often from direct contact with an infected animal, but may be also acquired indirectly through contact with a contaminated environment. While clinical disease is rarely serious, the lesions can result in disfigurement and pain. Diagnosis is based on history, clinical appearance and diagnostic procedures, e.g. direct microscopic examination of scales, hair or nail and fungal culture. Specific treatment is generally required to resolve lesions, and this may be prolonged depending on the fungal species and the host status. Identifying animals as the source of infection for people can help in the prevention of recurrence or new infections, especially in children, by adequately treating affected pets and their environments. Immunoprophylaxis is an attractive means of controlling infection in animals, and the development and widespread use of efficacious *T. verrucosum* vaccines in certain countries has already proved valuable in the management of cattle ringworm.

The agent

The dermatophytes are a highly specialized group of related, filamentous fungi that share (1) the unusual ability to digest and derive nutrition from keratin (Ajello 1974) and (2) morphological characteristics, i.e. the capacity to produce micro- and macroconidia. Three broad ecological groups of dermatophyte species are recognized, namely anthropophilic, zoophilic and geophilic (Weitzman and Summerbell 1995). Anthropophilic species typically colonize humans, while zoophilic species are found predominantly in animals. Geophilic species of dermatophytes are simply saprophytes existing in the soil without or sporadically causing disease (Table 70.1).

Taxonomy

Dermatophyte are ascomycete fungi, but only anamorphs (or asexual forms) are isolated from infected patients, animals or soil. Dermatophyte anamorphs are classified in three genera, *Trichophyton*, *Microsporum*, and *Epidermophyton*. *Microsporum* species make spindle-shaped thick-walled macroconidia (Fig. 70.1). *Trichophyton* species make macroconidia which are blunt at the ends, or do not make macroconidia. In *Epidermophyton* only one validated dermatophyte species (*E. floccosum*) has been described (Table 70.1).

Dermatophyte teleomorphs (or sexual forms) have been classified in the *Arthroderma* genus in the Ascomycotina subphylum. Teleomorphs of *Microsporum* species were previously classified in the *Nannizzia* genus but this has now been shown to be congeneric with *Arthroderma* (Weitzman *et al.* 1986). Most dermatophytes are heterothallic fungi. Therefore conjugation for sexual reproduction is possible only through the interaction of individual isolates of different mating type (designated as either '+' or '−'). In a number of zoophilic species like anthropophilic species sexual reproduction has not been observed. In some species clinical isolates tend to be of a single mating type as shown in other pathogenic fungi such as *Cryptococcus neoformans* (Idnurm *et al.* 2005). For example a bias of one particular mating type was observed in *M. canis*, *A. benhamiae* and *A. vanbreuseghemii*. The prevalence of '−' type for *M. canis* may, at least in some cases, be due to differences in the pathogenicity of the mating types (Rippon and Garber 1969).

Dermatophyte species identification

Dermatophyte identification is usually performed on the basis of macroscopic and microscopic characteristics of the organism grown in culture, but often remains difficult or uncertain because

Table 70.1 Ecological classification of dermatophytes into geophilic, zoophilic, and anthropophilic species (A: *Arthroderma*; M: *Microsporum*; T: *Trichophyton*; E: *Epidermophyton*)

Geophilic	Zoophilic	Anthropophilic
*M. gypseum** (*A. gypseum*, *A. fulvum*, *A. incurvatum*) (Stockdale 1961; 1963; Weitzman *et al.* 1986)	*M. canis* (*A. otae*) (Hasegawa and Usui 1975; Weitzman *et al.* 1986)	*M. audouinii*
*T. terrestre** (*A. quadrifidum*) (non pathogenic) (Dawson and Gentles 1961)	*M. equinum*	*M. ferrugineum*
T. ajelloi (*A. uncinatum*) (non pathogenic) (Dawson and Gentles 1959; 1961)	*M. persicolor* (*A. persicolor*) (Stockdale 1967; Weitzman *et al.* 1986)	*T. interdigitale*
	M. nanum (*A. obtusa*) (Dawson and Gentles 1961)	*T. tonsurans*
	A. benhamiae (formerly *T. mentagrophytes*) (Ajello and Cheng 1967)	*T. rubrum*
	T. erinacei	*T. violaceum*
	A. vanbreuseghemii (formerly *T. mentagrophytes*) (Takashio 1973)	*T. soudanense*
	T. equinum	*T. schoenleinii*
	T. simii (*A. simii*) (Stockdale *et al.* 1965)	*T. concentricum*
	T. verrucosum	*E. floccosum*
	T. gallinae	

* Species complex

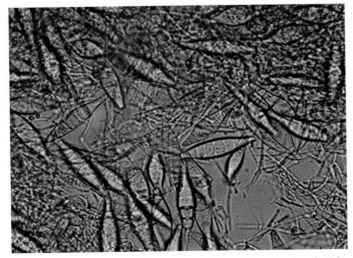

Fig. 70.1 Culture microscopy (*Microsporum canis*): typical spindle-shaped, thick-walled, spiny macroconidia composed of many cells.

there are variations from one isolate to another. Various techniques in molecular biology such as restriction fragment length polymorphism (RFLP), randomly amplified polymorphic DNA (RAPD) analysis, and DNA sequencing are useful tools for precise species delineation in this group of fungi (Mochizuki *et al.* 1997; Gräser *et al.* 1999; Kac *et al.* 1999; Ninet *et al.* 2003; Kamiya *et al.* 2004; Fréalle *et al.* 2007). The polymorphism of the ITS1 and ITS2 regions flanking the DNA sequence encoding the 5.8S rDNA is the most discriminating tool for distinguishing different species.

Current status of *Trichophyton mentagrophytes*

Several forms and varieties of dermatophytes, producing numerous pyriform or round microconidia but differing in macroscopic culture aspect and ecological preference, were named *Trichophyton mentagrophytes* (Vanbreuseghem *et al.* 1978; Kwong-Chung and Bennet 1992). However, mating strain experiments (Fig. 70.2) and recent work in molecular taxonomy showed that *T. mentagrophytes* contained different species which make teleomorphs (Table 70.2). *Arthroderma benhamiae* is the teleomorph obtained by mating strains isolated from rodents (Ajello and Cheng 1967) and *A. vanbreuseghemii* is the teleomorph obtained by mating strains isolated from humans, mice and chinchillas (Takashio 1973). In *A. vanbreuseghemii* were included zoophilic and anthropophilic strains (Nenoff *et al.* 2007). Zoophilic strains were named *T. mentagrophytes*, *T. mentagrophytes* var. *asteroides* or *Microides mentagrophytes* in many texts, and cause highly inflammatory tinea capitis, tinea corporis and tinea faciae. Anthropophilic strains were called *T. interdigitale*, *T. mentagrophytes* var. *interdigitale* or *Microides interdigitale*, and cause non inflammatory tinea pedis and tinea unguium. They do not mate with zoophilic strains (Symoens *et al.* 2011), and *T. interdigitale* should be considered as a separate species. Currently, *T. mentagrophytes* should be only used for the species designated by the reference strain CBS 318.56 designated as a neotype (Gräser *et al.* 1999). This *Trichophyton* resembles anthropophilic strains but has different ITS region and 28S sequences. It does not originate from Europe and is linked to a third teleomorphic species named *Arthroderma simii* (Gräser *et al.* 1999; Nenoff *et al.* 2007). For this reason, most *Trichophyton* spp. linked to the teleomorph *A. vanbreuseghemii* routinely isolated in veterinary medicine and human inflammatory mycosis should be called as such and not *T. mentagrophytes*.

Disease mechanisms

When compared to most other fungal diseases, host-fungus relationship in dermatophytic infections is remarkable. These fungi can affect immunocompetent individuals, but invade superficial keratinized structures. The non-invasive character of dermatophytes and the extraordinary variety of associated clinical signs are linked to pathophysiological mechanisms which remain broadly unknown (Vermout *et al.* 2008a). Nevertheless, these mechanisms depend on factors linked to the fungi themselves and on host reactions towards the dermatophytes and their metabolic products. Studies have been increasingly carried out to identify potential virulence factors (Vermout *et al.* 2008a; Monod 2008). Modern methods to study the various aspects of host reactions, including innate and specific immune responses have only been undertaken recently (Mignon *et al.* 2008).

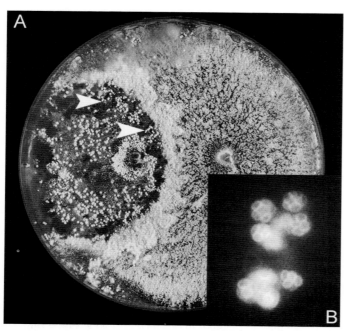

Fig. 70.2 (A) Mating of a + strain with a − strain of *Arthroderma benhamiae*. Cleistothecia are indicated by arrows. (B) Asci and ascospores from cleistothecia.

Dermatophyte virulence

The first stage in the development of dermatophytosis in a susceptible individual exposed to a sufficiently high level of inoculation is the adherence of arthrospores to corneocytes. These then germinate and hyphae penetrate the *stratum corneum*. Arthrospore

Table 70.2 Species in the *Trichophyton mentagrophytes* complex

Current species classification		Former species classification
Teleomorph*	Anamorph§	
Arthroderma benhamiae	*Trichophyton* sp. # (closely related to *Trichophyton erinacei*)	*Trichophyton mentagrophytes* (zoophilic strains)
Arthroderma vanbreuseghemii	*Trichophyton* sp. #	*Trichophyton mentagrophytes* var. *asteroides* (zoophilic strains)
	Trichophyton interdigitale	*Trichophyton mentagrophytes* var. *interdigitale* (anthropophilic strains)
Arthroderma simii	*Trichophyton mentagrophytes* (sensu stricto)	*Arthroderma simii*

* Sexual form of the fungus
§ Asexual or conidial form of the fungus
\# Anamorph names not given formally for *A. benhamiae* and *A. vanbreuseghemii*

germination, promoted by humidity, warmth, maceration and skin excoriation, must occur rapidly to avoid fungal elimination by a constantly desquamating epidermis. In haired areas, when a mycelial filament in the *stratum corneum* encounters a hair opening, it penetrates the keratinized external root sheath of the hair follicle up to the infundibulum, the internal root sheath (the external root sheath is no longer keratinized) and the hair. The fungus grows towards the hair bulb but is maintained in the newly formed keratin. Opposing growth of fungus and hair is balanced such that the dermatophyte does not reach the base of the hair follicle but stops at 'Adamson's fringe'. The aerial portion of the hair is progressively invaded by hyphae and arthroconidia. This makes the hair fragile, often causing it to break several millimeters above the skin surface with release of highly resistant spores into the environment. The dermatophyte can infect other adjacent hair follicles leading to centrifugal spread of lesions and the distinctive clinical appearance. Circular lesions are sometimes more inflammatory at the periphery and heal from the centre with hair re-growth. This description is valid only for anagen hair follicles. Some dermatophytes, such as *M. persicolor*, *E. floccosum* and *T. concentricum* are incapable of invading hair, even *in vitro*, and stay confined to interfollicular keratin. In glabrous skin, the infection process is basically similar, leading to centrifugal superficial lesions.

The kinetics of adherence of dermatophytes to the skin or nail surface was investigated in several *Trichophyton* and *Microsporum* species, using different experimental models and microscopy techniques (Baldo *et al.* 2007). These studies showed a time-dependent increase in the number of adhering spores, followed by germination and invasion of the *stratum corneum* by hyphae growing in multiple directions. Adherence of arthroconidia to keratinocytes generally begins by 2 hours and is still increasing by 6 hours (Baldo *et al.* 2008). The factors that mediate adherence of dermatophytes potentially include carbohydrate-specific adhesins, as shown in *T. rubrum* (Esquenazi *et al.* 2004). More recently, a keratinolytic protease from the family of the secreted subtilisins has been shown to be required for fungal adherence of *M. canis* to feline corneocytes (Baldo *et al.* 2010).

Since dermatophytes are almost exclusively localized in keratinized tissues and are able to secrete keratinolytic activity *in vitro*, research on mechanisms of the fungal invasion primarily focused on fungal secreted proteases, including subtilisins (serine endoproteases), fungalysins (metallo-endoproteases), dipeptidyl-peptidases and aminopeptidases (Monod 2008). Our knowledge about the range of potentially keratinolytic proteases produced by dermatophytes is constantly growing, several of them being characterized at the molecular level and having well known enzymatic properties (Monod 2008). Additionally, several of these proteases have been shown to be produced *in vivo* during infection (Mignon *et al.* 1998; Brouta *et al.* 2002; Descamps *et al.* 2002; Mathy *et al.* 2010; Staib *et al.* 2010). However, it is still not clear how dermatophytic fungi regulate the utilization of numerous proteases to obtain nutrients from the insoluble cornified substrate they invade (Kaufman *et al.* 2007), and which roles in virulence (Vermout *et al.* 2008b) and immunomodulation (Mignon *et al.* 2008) are played by these proteins.

Although the importance of dermatophytic keratinolytic proteases for pathogenicity is well established, efficient protein degradation of keratinous tissues by hydrolytic enzymes has to be accompanied by a simultaneous reduction of the cystine disulphide bridges, which are an important structural feature of keratin complexes. During infection, dermatophytes and filamentous fungi were shown to excrete sulphite as a reducing agent. Sulphite excretion is in the same time a detoxification pathway. In the presence of sulphite, disulphide bonds of the keratin substrate are directly cleaved to cysteine and S-sulphocysteine rendering structural protein complexes accessible for proteases (Monod 2008). In fungi, sulfite secretion is mediated by sulfite efflux pumps encoded by the gene *SSU1*, which belong to a small family of transporters. The relatively high expression of dermatophyte *SSU1* compared to that of *SSU1* in other fungi likely reflects a property of dermatophytes, which renders these fungi pathogenic in the *stratum corneum*, hair and nails.

Besides proteases, little information is available about other hydrolases, such as lipases and ceramidases, and other virulence factors. There is no doubt that they will be investigated in the near future, in light of new data on dermatophyte genomics.

Host defence mechanisms involved in pathogenesis

Non-immunological cutaneous defence mechanisms include exposure to ultraviolet rays, low humidity, competition with bacterial skin flora and *stratum corneum* turnover. Dermatophytes are thought unable to penetrate a normal intact epidermis (De Vroey 1985). However, once infection is established, the host develops an innate immune response which is essential for both the early defence against the fungus and the subsequent induction of a specific antibody and cellular immune response (Svejgaard 1985; Mignon *et al.* 2008).

Numerous studies have shown that the efficient and protective response against dermatophytes is a cell-mediated response of the Delayed Type Hypersensitivity (DTH) type, characterized namely by the action of macrophages and neutrophils as effectors, and thus by elevated activity of the key cytokines interleukine-12 (IL-12) and interferon-γ (IFN-γ) from the Th1 axis. However, the immune response that is raised, including the degree of inflammation, varies according to the dermatophyte species, to the host species, and to the physiopathological status of the host. The degree of inflammation is usually inversely related with the duration of infection. The more inflammatory are the lesions, the shorter time they persist with spontaneous resolution possible. Typically, a dermatophyte provokes a more intense inflammatory reaction on a host to which it is not adapted than it does on its natural host. This would explain certain chronic infections with little or no symptoms which are induced in humans and cats by *T. rubrum* and *M. canis* respectively. Similarly, this would explain the highly inflammatory lesions such as kerions caused by geophilic species in both humans and animals.

The factors responsible for the differential clinical expression of dermatophytosis caused by a given fungal strain in a given host species are not fully understood. However, the nature of the specific immune response that the host develops is critical. Most often, chronic persistent human infections are correlated with poor specific DTH, elevated specific IgE and IgG4, IgE-mediated immediate hypersensitivity (IH), and with the production of Th2 cytokines by mononuclear leukocytes (Woodfolk 2005; Mignon *et al.* 2008). The different ways in which dermatophytes may counter the immune system, or induce damage via immune defenses, include lymphocyte inhibition by cell wall mannans, macrophage function alteration, differential activation of keratinocytes and, putatively, differential secretion of proteases. For example, two dermatophytic secreted proteases, a subtilisin from *T. rubrum* (Tri r 2) and the dipeptidyl-peptidase V from *T. tonsurans* (Tri t 4), can induce dual immune responses. Acute dermatophytosis is associated with a DTH skin response against them, while persistent disease corresponds to IH responses.

The innate immune mechanisms involved in the different clinical presentations of dermatophytosis is now being investigated. These mechanisms are instrumental, notably because the receptors, the pathways and the cells which are involved have an instructive role on cells of the adaptive immune system, and thus on the induction or not of a Th1 cell mediated effector and protective response. Among crucial cells, keratinocytes are the first that dermatophytes encounter during the infection process and they have a pivotal role in the modulation of the host immune response. For example, upon exposure to dermatophytes they can produce a broad spectrum of cytokines (Shiraki *et al.* 2006), including IL-8, a potent chemo-attractant for neutrophils which can kill dermatophytes, and the proinflammatory tumour necrosis factor α (TNF-α) (Nakamura *et al.* 2002). However, dermatophyte species differ in their ability to induce cytokine production by keratinocytes. The zoophilic species stimulate the production of pro-inflammatory cytokines by human keratinocytes better than anthropophilic ones (Shiraki *et al.* 2006; Tani *et al.* 2007), and this correlates with the clinical aspects observed in both types of infection. Besides cytokines, human keratinocytes also secrete antimicrobial peptides (AMP), cathelicidins and defensins with potential antifungal activity. Their role in skin defence against dermatophytes was suggested by several authors who showed that human β-defensin (Jensen *et al.* 2007) and cathelicidin LL-37 (Lopez-Garcia *et al.* 2006) are either fungistatic or fungicidal *in vitro* against *T. rubrum* and that their expression is up-regulated *in vivo* in tinea corporis. An important future challenge would be to identify both the dermatophyte components interacting with keratinocytes and the pattern recognition receptors (PRR) stimulated in these sentinel cells.

Alongside keratinocytes, Langerhans cells (LC), a subtype of dendritic cells (DC), are another sentinel cells in contact with dermatophytes within the epidermis. They are antigen-presenting cells involved in both initiation and modulation of the adaptative anti-dermatophyte immune response. For example, dectin-2, a C-type lectin-like receptor constitutively expressed by mature DC, such as LC, was shown to be a PRR for fungi, including *M. andouinii* and *T. rubrum*, and to bind preferentially to hyphae rather than conidia, leading *in fine* to the up-regulated secretion of proinflammatory cytokines such as TNF-α (Sato *et al.* 2006). In contrast, upon phagocytosis by macrophages, *T. rubrum* conidia induce the secretion of the anti-inflammatory cytokine IL-10, while other factors related to enhancement of a relevant protective immune response are down-regulated, i.e. class II MHC, CD54 and CD80 co-stimulation molecules, nitric oxide and IL-12 (Campos *et al.* 2006). It appears that some immuno-modulation depends on which dermatophyte factors are produced in the course of infection, but also how they are detected by the host. The research on this topic is still ongoing. For example, a new PRR, DC-HIL, was found to be involved in the modulation of the immune response to dermatophytes. This PRR can both increase antigen presenting cell properties of DC, and negatively regulate T cell activation (Chung *et al.* 2009).

Besides keratinocytes and DC, neutrophils are important cells in innate anti-dermatophyte immunity. In mice, they were shown to accumulate as early as four to six hours after experimental infection with *T. mentagrophytes* (Hay *et al.* 1988). This is after adherence of conidia to the corneocytes, during the germination phase. Additionally, it is generally admitted that neutrophils are, in addition to macrophages, the effector cells allowing, via the Th1 dependent inflammatory response, the elimination of a dermatophytic infection.

Symptoms and signs

Clinical features in humans

Dermatophytoses vary depending on the causative agent and the body site affected. The disease is therefore described with the word 'tinea' followed by a term for the particular infected body site (Degreef 2008). Anthropophilic species (e.g. *T. rubrum*, *T. interdigitale*, and *T. tonsurans*), which typically colonize humans, tend to be associated with more chronic infections which are less inflammatory. In contrast, zoophilic and geophilic species of dermatophytes (e.g. *A. benhamiae*, *A. vanbreuseghemii*, *T. erinacei*, *T. verrucosum*, *M. canis* and *M. gypseum*) often cause highly inflamed lesions in humans (Fig. 70.3).

The classical ringworm lesions occur in tinea capitis, tinea corporis, and tinea barbae, which are the most common sites for zoophilic dermatophyte infections. The typical lesions are centrifugally growing, circumscribed, roughly circular areas of variable erythema, scaling, and desquamation, often having raised borders and either with or without a central healing area (Evans and Gentles 1985; Hay *et al.* 1992; Weedon 1992). Alopecia accompanies infection due to the increased fragility of infected hairs. The lesions vary in size and

may be solitary or multiple, and in the latter case affected areas may coalesce, giving irregular patches of infection. In areas such as the foot and in body folds lesions may be less circumscribed, and in tinea pedis and tinea manuum diffuse scaling is often the major sign, whereas tinea unguium usually leads to dystrophic nails.

The zoophilic dermatophytes that most commonly cause human dermatophytosis (*A. benhamiae*, *A. vanbreuseghemii*, *T. verrucosum*, and *M. canis*) tend to produce different degrees of inflammation. Infections with *M. canis* although variable, are generally moderately inflammatory and only rarely result in very severe inflammation (Marples 1956). In contrast, *T. verrucosum*, *A. benhamiae*, *A. vanbreuseghemii* frequently cause highly inflammatory lesions, which in tinea capitis and tinea barbae may be frequently accompanied by kerion formation—a suppurating, boggy, highly inflamed area of folliculitis (Hay *et al.* 1992; Weedon 1992).

Other distinct lesions, but most often associated with non zoonotic dermatophytes, are seen occasionally (Evans and Gentles 1985; Weedon 1992) including:

- Favus (chronic tinea capitis in which large crusts form over an erythematous base).

- Granulomatous dermatophytia (including Majocchi's and Wilson's granulomas, and circumscribed, nodular granulomatous perifolliculitis due to rupture of infected hair follicles).

- Dermatophytic pseudomycetoma.

Pseudomycetomas are rare lesions resembling true eumycotic mycetomas (discharging subcutaneous swellings containing granules or microcolonies of the aetiological agent in the pus), and may result from rupture of hair follicles followed by limited growth of the dermatophyte in the subcutaneous tissues, resulting in a severe host response with the formation of pseudogranules (Ajello *et al.* 1980).

Clinical features in animals

As in humans, the clinical appearance of dermatophytosis in animals is highly variable (Fig. 70.4). In most domestic animals the classical ringworm lesion is similar to tinea capitis in man, with a circular or irregular patch of alopecia, scaling and crusting, with central healing. Other common clinical signs include furunculosis, kerions, paronychia, generalized alopecia with scaling, and (particularly in some cats with *M. canis* infection) a chronic infection with minor lesions discernible only on close examination. In cats, dermatophytosis may occasionally present as 'miliary dermatitis' (Scott 1980), and mycetoma have also been described (Scott 1980). The zoophilic dermatophytes show variable host specificity, and a wide range of species have at times been isolated from most animal hosts (Table 70.3).

Diagnosis

A diagnosis of dermatophytosis cannot be made on the basis of clinical signs alone, and the three tests most widely used for the confirmation of a diagnosis are examination of hairs under ultraviolet light (Wood's lamp); direct microscopic examination of hairs, nails or scales; and fungal culture.

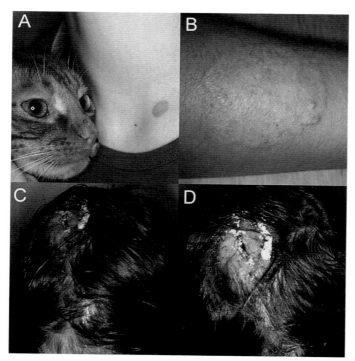

Fig. 70.3 Human dermatophytoses. (A) Tinea corporis with *Microsporum canis*, cat with periocular alopecia caused by the same agent. (B) Tinea corporis with *Arthroderma vanbreuseghemii*. (C and D) Tinea capitis (kerion) with *Arthroderma benhamiae*.

Examination using Wood's lamp

Under Wood's lamp illumination, hairs infected with *M. canis*, *M. audouinii*, *T. schoenleinii* or *M. ferrugineum* may produce a

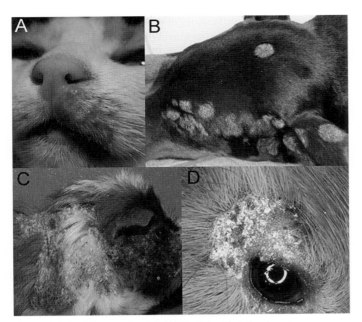

Fig. 70.4 Animal dermatophytoses. (A) Cheilitis with *Arthroderma vanbreuseghemii* in a cat. (B) Dog with multifocal patches of alopecia caused by *Arthroderma vanbreuseghemii*. (C and D) Extensive alopecia and scaling caused by *Arthroderma benhamiae* in guinea pigs.

characteristic yellow-green fluorescence (Rebell and Taplin 1970) and thus examination of lesions, or hairs plucked from lesions, can be valuable. The fluorescence induced by these dermatophytes is only present in the cortex and medulla of hairs infected *in vivo*, being absent from invading hyphae and arthrospores, infected scales and crusts, and from *in vitro* cultures including hairs infected *in vitro*. Not all infections caused by these dermatophytes result in fluorescence of hairs, and in both man and animals, a variable proportion of *M. canis* infections have been reported where fluorescence was not observed. Although fluorescence is only observed in a limited number of dermatophyte infections, examination under Wood's lamp is nevertheless very valuable as a rapid screening test in tinea capitis in man, and in canine and feline dermatophytosis

where *M. canis* is the major causal organism. Care should be taken during examination with a Wood's lamp to distinguish the true fluorescence associated with dermatophyte infections from the bluish fluorescence often produced by the topical use of various ointments or the presence of scales and crusts.

Direct mycological examination

Direct examination of skin, nail scrapings and hair samples for the presence of fungi is an essential step to confirm the clinical diagnosis of a cutaneous fungus infection and is one of the most widely practiced laboratory procedures in dermatology (Fig. 70.5). Simple clearing of the specimen with 10% potassium hydroxide or lactophenol, followed by microscopical examination is the traditional method still in use in many laboratories. However, when the light microscopy is used without contrasting, it can be difficult to detect fungal elements. Different techniques with Parker ink or histological staining dyes such chlorazol black E or Congo red give poor results (Monod *et al.* 1989). The use of fluorochromes such as Blankophor or Calcofluor White (Fluorescent Brightener 28, Sigma F3543) which specifically bind to vegetal and fungal cell wall polysaccharides allows a considerable improvement in the diagnostic of mycoses (Monheit *et al.* 1984; Holländer *et al.* 1984; Gip and Abelin 1987; Monod *et al.* 1989). The fluorescence techniques produce by far the best contrast in comparison to other techniques by allowing the immediate and sure detection of isolated spores and filaments (Monod *et al.* 1989). Whereas fluorescence microscopy is widely practiced in clinical laboratories, it is not generally used in private practice because of the high price of a microscope necessary to perform such analysis.

Fungal cultures

Fungal culture allows identification of the infecting dermatophyte by virtue of the macroscopic and microscopic morphology of the colony (Rebell and Taplin 1970). Dermatological sample is often seeded onto two media. The first one consists in Sabouraud's agar medium containing an antibacterial antibiotic, usually chloramphenicol (50 µg ml^{-1}), and the second one containing Sabouraud's agar medium with chloramphenicol plus cycloheximide (400 µg ml^{-1}). Cultures are normally maintained at 25–30°C and colonies will

Table 70.3 Major dermatophytes of the domestic animals and their reservoirs

Dermatophyte	Main animal reservoir(s)	Frequency on humans	Geographical distribution
M. canis	Cats, dogs	Common	Worldwide
T. verrucosum	Cattle	Common	Worldwide
A. benhamiae	Guinea pigs	Common	Worldwide
T. erinacei	Hedgehogs	Occasional	Europe, East Asia, New Zealand
A. vanbreuseghemii	Cats, dogs, mice	Common	Worldwide
T. equinum	Horses	Occasional	Worldwide
T. simii	Monkeys, chicken	Rare	India
M. equinum	Horses	Rare	Worldwide
T. gallinae	Chicken	Rare	Worldwide
M. persicolor	Voles	Rare	Europe, USA
M. nanum	Pigs	Rare	Worldwide

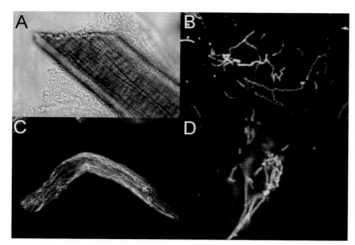

Fig. 70.5 Direct mycological examinations. (A) Light microscopy. Infected hair from a guinea pig, hyphae and arthrospores. (B-D) Fluorescence microscopy. (B) Tinea corporis, hyphae. (C) Tinea capitis, infected hair. (D) Hyphae and arthrospores from an infected cat.

often appear within 7 days, although cultures are typically maintained for 2–3 weeks before being discarded. The growth of most dermatophytes is inhibited at higher temperatures, but in the case of *T. verrucosum*, culture at 37°C is optimal for growth.

Dermatophyte test medium (DTM) was described by Taplin *et al.* (1969) and incorporates phenol red in the culture medium as a pH indicator. The medium works on the principle that fungal utilization of proteins results in the production of alkaline metabolites (turning the medium red in colour) whereas utilization of carbohydrates results in acidic metabolites (maintaining or turning the medium yellow in colour). Dermatophytes generally utilize proteins from the medium first, resulting in red colouration, before using carbohydrates and causing a return to yellow colouration later. In contrast, most other fungi utilize carbohydrates first, thus maintaining the yellow colour of the medium, and only later use proteins. Dermatophyte test medium was therefore designed to allow an evaluation of the colour change in the medium in relation to the appearance of fungal colonies for the diagnosis of dermatophytosis without the need for detailed knowledge of fungal morphology (Taplin *et al.* 1969). However, as DTM may alter the characteristic growth of dermatophytes, including suppression of conidia production, subculture on Sabouraud's dextrose agar may sometimes be required for confirmation of the nature of an isolate and identification of the species. Additionally, some dermatophytes, perhaps metabolically atypical strains, have been found not to cause an early colour change on DTM (Moriello and DeBoer 1991). Thus results of culture on DTM require careful interpretation, and this medium does not preclude the need for some mycological knowledge.

In some situations, such as tinea unguium, results of fungal culture are often negative, emphasizing the importance of other additional diagnostic techniques for direct identification of the fungus *in situ* in the collected sample. In the last few years, PCR assays have been developed for the detection of fungi directly from nail samples. These assays mainly focused on the identification of dermatophytes. However, recently developed PCR/sequencing/

RFLP assays allow identification, in addition to dermatophytes, of *Fusarium* spp. and other less frequently isolated non-dermatophyte fungi in onychomycoses (Monod *et al.* 2006).

Treatment

Treatment of infections in man

Treatment of dermatophytosis is adapted according to the clinical syndrome and the response to therapy. In general, recent focal lesions of the glabrous skin may be treated topically, whereas systemic treatment is recommended for chronic or widespread infections and in cases of tinea capitis and tinea unguium. Where systemic treatment is used, topical therapy may also be a useful adjunct and, for example in tinea capitis, may help reduce dissemination of infectious particles into the environment. To further reduce environmental contamination in tinea capitis, clipping of hair around the lesion has been advocated. Specific antifungal therapy should be combined with appropriate antibiotic therapy where secondary bacterial infection accompanies the dermatophytosis.

Griseofulvin deriving from *Penicillium griseofulvum* was the first systemic antifungal agent, being used in both man and animals from 1958. It exhibits fungistatic properties against the dermatophytes and, although the mechanism of action is incompletely understood, it inhibits fungal mitosis by disrupting the mitotic spindle through interaction with polymerized microtubules (Gull and Trinci 1973). Short-term responses to griseofulvin are generally good, but relapses after cessation of treatment may occur (Legendre and Steltz 1980; Hay 1990).

The azoles are generally considered to be fungistatic drugs and exert their effect by interfering with the cytochrome P450 enzymes, thereby inhibiting ergosterol synthesis, inhibiting cell proliferation, and affecting membrane permeability. Ketoconazole was the first systemic agent used as an alternative to griseofulvin for dermatophyte treatment, but despite showing equivalent or superior activity, the occurrence of hepatotoxicity and endocrine disturbances (due to interference with mammalian P450 activity) limits the value of this drug. The newer triazoles, and especially itraconazole, show a much greater specificity for fungal P450 and are safer, better tolerated, and free of the adverse endocrinological effects of ketoconazole.

The allylamines, like the azoles, interfere with ergosterol biosynthesis, but through blocking squalene epoxidation rather than cytochrome P450. There is a very narrow margin between the fungistatic and fungicidal concentration of terbinafine, and in clinical practice this drug is considered as a fungicidal agent.

Terbinafine and triazoles are commonly used for cutaneous dermatophytosis whatever is the dermatophyte species. However, in some clinical presentations such as tinea capitis, the therapeutic response may vary according to the incriminated dermatophyte species, which renders fungal identification necessary. The cure rate with terbinafine is excellent in cases of infection by the anthrophilic species *T. violaceum* and *T. soudanense*. However, griseofulvin remains the treatment of choice for tinea capitis caused by zoophilic species such as *M. canis*, *A. benhamiae* and *A. vanbreuseghemii* as well as the anthropophilic *M. langeroni* which show high resistance to treatment with terbinafine (Mock *et al.* 1998). Fluconazole may be useful in patients with a contraindication or intolerance to high-dose griseofulvin (Foster *et al.* 2005).

Treatment of infections in animals

Although infections can be self-limiting, treatment of dermatophytosis in animals is recommended (Chermette *et al.* 2008). It is aimed at stopping infection, speeding up resolution, preventing spread to other animals and man and avoiding fungal contamination of the environment. It consists of treating the deep follicular infection, destroying hyphae and spores in the hair shaft, decontaminating the environment and treating in-contact animals. The clinician often has little room for manoeuvre in his therapeutic approach because of the limited number of available effective drugs and the economic considerations, especially in farm animals. Additionally, he has to consider availability and local legislation applying to veterinary and human products which can be used.

The best therapeutic approach of a dermatophytic animal combines one or more of the following procedures: clipping, topical therapy, systemic therapy, therapeutic vaccination, environmental decontamination, hygiene measures for in-contact animals and monitoring of the treatment.

The aim of clipping is to limit spread of the fungus into the environment and to facilitate topical therapy especially in long- or medium-haired animals with extensive lesions. Total body clipping of hair has been advocated when lesions are extensive or generalized. However, the pros and cons of clipping need to be evaluated for each individual case. Indeed, this procedure may increase the severity of the dermatosis, presumably through microtrauma to the skin promoting spread of lesions. As dissemination of spores into the environment is a potential additional disadvantage, animals should be clipped in suitable premises easy to disinfect and hairs must be incinerated.

The main aim of topical therapy is to destroy fungal elements on distal hairs and reduce their dispersal. In farm animals and horses, topical therapy is frequently used as sole treatment, because systemic therapy is not economically viable. However, topical therapy alone should not be recommended, especially if generalized lesions are present. In practice, enilconazole, lime sulphur and an association of chlorhexidine-miconazole are the most suitable and effective drugs. They must be applied on the whole body if multifocal or generalized lesions are present, following the recommendations of the manufacturers. Creams, ointments, gels, lotions and other local antifungal preparations can be used only on a solitary lesion in a hairless region of skin.

The use of additional systemic therapy should always be considered. The most commonly used systemic antifungal agents are griseofulvin, ketoconazole and itraconazole, the two latter being used only in pets (Moriello 2004) for economic reasons. The fungistatic griseofulvin should be administered *per os* at an average daily dose of 50 mg/kg for several weeks, ideally with fatty meals. Absorption varies according to the degree of micronization of the product and also the individual, so that the dose has to be adapted for each case. Griseofulvin is teratogenic and should not be given to pregnant females. Side-effects (vomiting and diarrhoea) and idiosyncratic reactions (e.g. anaemia) may occur requiring clinical and haematological monitoring. Ketoconazole is a fungistatic diazole given *per os* at an average daily dose of 5–10 mg/kg with food for at least 4–6 weeks. It can be teratogenic and should be avoided in pregnant females. It frequently interacts with other drugs and great care should be taken if other medications are being used. It may have undesirable side-effects (mainly vomiting), especially at doses higher than the average recommended dose. Hepatotoxicity, well documented in man, is less common in dogs and cats. Itraconazole is a triazole used more and more in place of griseofulvin and ketoconazole. It is very effective and better tolerated than ketoconazole. It is given *per os* at an average daily dose of 5–10 mg/kg, with food, for several weeks. Its pharmacokinetic properties and very keratinophilic nature render it suitable for use in pulse therapy protocols, for example on alternate weeks, as it is recommended in cats. It can be teratogenic and should be avoided in pregnant females. Although the incidence of side-effects is less than with ketoconazole, itraconazole must be used with care in animals with liver disease. Terbinafine could be an alternative option for systemic therapy in pets, but additional scientific data are necessary.

There are no or too little scientific data supporting the benefits of vaccination against dermatophytosis as an effective curative option.

Whenever possible, contaminated premises should be vacuumed and cleaned, then disinfected to destroy as many spores as possible. Undiluted bleach and formalin are the most effective disinfectants. In practice, regular use of bleach, diluted 1:10, and enilconazole, as a spray or fogger, will decontaminate the environment.

In breeding units and multi-animal facilities, infected animals should be isolated from unaffected ones. Because asymptomatic infection or mechanical carriage is frequent in cats (Mignon and Losson 1997a), appropriate monitoring and treatment of apparently unaffected in-contact animals is necessary to eradicate feline dermatophytosis in catteries (Carlotti *et al.* 2010). Animals going into places where groups of animals are kept, e.g. cat shows, should be screened for dermatophytosis before reintegration into their environment.

An appropriate length of treatment is essential to achieve a complete cure. Monitoring is therefore absolutely needed. Generally, treatment must be pursued not only until a clinical cure has been obtained but also mycological cure. In practice, the duration of therapy is never less than one month, and should be continued until two negative fungal cultures, one month apart, have been obtained.

Prognosis

Dermatophytosis is a common disease in man, with infections generally being restricted to the *stratum corneum* where they may cause disfigurement, pruritus and pain. Infection is serious in rare cases. In many cases of dermatophytosis the disease is self-limiting, and humans infected with zoophilic dermatophyte species tend to undergo spontaneous resolution after a period of weeks to months. A good response to appropriate antimycotic therapy can generally be expected with these infections. In contrast, chronic dermatophyte infections, and particularly tinea unguium, do not always respond well to therapy, but these infections are usually produced by anthropophilic species. Spontaneous resolution of disease (due to the development of acquired immunity) is also typical of dermatophytosis in many animals, although as in man, chronic infections may occur in some cases.

Epidemiology

Occurrence

Dermatophytoses are widespread and are the most common cutaneous fungal infections in man. Although dermatophytes are closely related fungi each species has a predilection for certain body areas (Degreef 2008). *Trichophyton rubrum* is especially dominant in onychomycoses with 80% of the dermatophyte isolates. Zoophilic species are the main agents of inflammatory tinea capitis and tinea corporis. The prevalence of the different tineas recorded can change from one region to another. It depends on the repartition between urban and rural populations, on the mixing of populations from different origins and probably also on the importance given in different countries to the different tineas. Anthropophilic species are related to the geographical origin of the patients. *Trichophyton tonsurans* is highly prevalent in America and not frequently isolated in other part of the world. *Trichophyton violaceum* is isolated from patients of Mediterranean and African origin. *Trichophyton soudanense* and *M. langeroni* isolates are from black Africans. The transfer of a dermatophyte species from one population to another can be observed.

Although human dermatophytosis tends to be dominated by infection with anthropophilic species, zoophilic infections do form a substantial proportion of cases with *M. canis*, *A. vanbreuseghemii* and *A. benhamiae* most commonly implicated (Table 70.3). A marked rise in the incidence of zoophilic tinea capitis infections in recent years due to *M. canis* (Lunder and Lunder 1992; Seebacher *et al.* 2008) and, to a lesser extent, *A. vanbreuseghemii and A. benhamiae* (Fumeaux *et al.* 2004) may be explained by the increasing number of domestic animals as pets. In contrast, a decrease of frequency of *T. verrucosum* reflects the decrease of the rural population in some countries.

Worldwide, the vast majority of tinea capitis cases due to *M. canis* and other dermatophyte species occur in children, which may relate to lower levels of fungal-inhibitory fatty acids present in this age group (Kligman and Ginsberg 1950). Longer hair may help protect against infection by making penetration of infective spores to the scalp more difficult (McAleer 1980; De Vroey 1985). *Microsporum canis*, *A. vanbreuseghemii* and *A. benhamiae* rarely cause lesions other than tinea capitis and tinea corporis. In man, *T. verrucosum* infections are seen in both children and adults. *Trichophyton verrucosum* mainly is a cause of tinea corporis and tinea barbae in the rural population, and less commonly a cause of tinea capitis in children.

Sources and transmission

Human infection with zoophilic dermatophytes requires either direct contact with an infected animal, or indirect transmission through fomites and parasitized skin scales or hair shed into the environment. Although the former may be a more efficient means of transmission, the extensive contamination of the environment from clinical cases and the prolonged survival time of dermatophytes in infected material are of considerable epidemiological importance, and may contribute to indirect infection. Zoophilic dermatophytes apparently lose pathogenicity during serial passage in humans, and thus most infections are acquired directly from the animal or the environment rather than from human contact (Marples 1956).

The major hosts, the geographical occurrence and the frequency of the zoophilic dermatophytes are shown in Table 70.3. A different pattern of zoophilic infections is encountered in rural and urban populations which relates to the source of the infections. Infections with *T. verrucosum* occur almost exclusively in rural areas, being acquired directly or indirectly from infected cattle (Georg 1960; Chmel 1980). In urban populations, infection is more usually acquired from pet animals. *Microsporum canis* is most frequently implicated (Georg 1960; Chmel 1980), with cats considered the major reservoir for this species. In a recent study, the vast majority of cats from which *M. canis* was isolated were strictly indoor cats. In contrast, hunting cats, mainly European short hair cats, were found to be the reservoir of *A. vanbreuseghemii* which causes highly inflammatory tinea corporis and tinea capitis in humans. It can be suspected that the feline infections with *A. vanbreuseghemii* occurred from a soil and/or a rodent pray source during hunting (Drouot *et al.* 2008).

Pet rodents such as guinea pigs and rabbits are source of dermatophytosis with *A. benhamiae*. The occasional infections with the closely related *T. mentagrophytes* var. *erinacei* can usually be traced to contact with a hedgehog (Schauder *et al.* 2007).

Prevention and control

Almost all dermatophytes species infecting animals are zoonotic (Table 70.3). Because a sufficiently high level of inoculation is a prerequisite for establishment of skin invasion, close and repeated contacts with an infected animal represent the major risk of infection. Dermatophytes grow and produce lots of infective arthroconidia *in vivo* (Fig. 70.5A). However although they survive in the environment, they can neither reproduce nor produce macro- and microconidia off the host (De Vroey 1985). Consequently, zoonotic dermatophyte infections mainly occur after contact with infected wild or domestic animals and to a lesser extent through a contaminated environment. The best strategy to avoid human infections is therefore to prevent both direct and indirect infective contacts. This prophylactic strategy appears very simple but is not always feasible because infected animals do not systematically express obvious clinical signs. Asymptomatic carriers are frequent among small pets, especially guinea pigs, which become more and more popular as companion animals in Europe and America. These animals can harbour fungal elements in their coat for several months or years before expressing clinical disease. Cats infected with *M. canis*, especially long-haired ones, can express very subtle clinical signs (Mignon and Losson 1997a). In such animals, the diagnosis of dermatophytosis is frequently made after that a human infection has been diagnosed.

Screening for infection or carriage should be performed in newly acquired pets, especially rodents and cats obtained from pet shops or other potentially contaminated places. Feline ringworm represents an important problem in animal husbandry, chronically or asymptomatically infected individuals making it particularly difficult to eradicate, so that some breeders are not able to sell dermatophyte-free cats. Ideally, screening for carriage or infection should also be performed in cats after staying in boarding houses or participating to cat shows. Clinically and asymptomatic infected culture-positive animals should be appropriately treated and their environment cleaned and disinfected (see above).

To date, there is no commercial or standardized vaccine for preventing or eliminating any fungal infection in humans, including anthropohilic or zoophilic dermatophytosis (Mignon *et al.* 2008). In animals, effective live vaccines against dermatophytosis have been developed for cattle, but available inactivated vaccines for use in cats, dogs and horses have not proved to be a valuable mean to avoid fungal infection in these species and thus to prevent transmission to humans (see below).

Once a dermatophytic infection is diagnosed in a domestic animal, it is important to identify the causal agent by fungal culture.

As most often this agent is zoonotic, animal treatment and sanitary measures (see above) are critical to avoid human contamination. However, in a few cases, a geophilic species, e.g. *M. gypseum*, is isolated, which is not transmissible from animals to humans.

Although the risk of dermatophyte infection is greatest for young or old and debilitated animals, the infection is not strictly age- or health status-related. Consequently, the risk of infection and human transmission continues throughout life. People in contact with infected animals should be advised of the risks and made aware that there are specific risk groups in the society, notably immunocompromised individuals, elderly and young people, mentally disabled persons and people with specific occupational risks, e.g. veterinarians and cattle breeders (Seebacher *et al.* 2008).

In cases of highly inflammatory tinea corporis, tinea faciae and tinea capitis in humans, it is important to identify with certainty the precise etiologic agent and to examine pets as the possible source of infection. Identifying pets as the source of infection for people can help in the prevention of recurrence or new infections, especially in children, by adequately treating affected pets and their environments. Cooperation between the medical and veterinary professions is required in this situation. A planned and coordinated approach to the investigation is required though, so that pet animals are neither incorrectly blamed for human disease, nor overlooked as possible sources.

Prophylaxis against dermatophytosis in domestic animals

Control of the spread of dermatophytosis is difficult due to the movement of animals and the shedding of infectious particles from infected individuals. Maintaining animals in isolation is rarely practical and could not be justified simply as a measure to prevent dermatophytosis. However, the possibility of protection of individuals by immunoprophylaxis was suggested by the observation of acquired resistance to natural and experimental infections.

To be efficient, vaccination must prevent the development of clinical lesions, the transmission to other subjects and avoid contamination of the environment by infective fungal elements. In this respect, a remarkable success was obtained in cattle, using a live vaccine containing microconidia of an attenuated strain of *T. verrucosum*. Large-scale vaccination programmes carried out in Eastern Europe and Scandinavia in the past 35 years using this vaccine have dramatically reduced the incidence of both bovine ringworm and concurrent human infections. Protection was correlated with the induction of an immune response comparable with that induced by natural infections, which is considered as a cell-mediated Th1 immune response (Tornquist *et al.* 1985; Gudding and Naes 1986; Gudding *et al.* 1991; Mignon and Losson 1997b). This lyophilized live vaccine is not available in all the countries. It is administered by intramuscular injection after reconstitution with aqueous solvent. Two injections are necessary 10–14 days apart in order to elicit a good protection. Other similar products have been developed including a *T. mentagrophytes* vaccine for use in fox farms to prevent dermatophytosis by this agent, which is reported to be widespread in Russia and Eastern Europe (Rybnikar *et al.* 1991). Inactivated vaccines have also been developed and are currently marketed for use notably in cattle, horses and cats. One of their theoretical advantages over live vaccines is their potential use in already diseased animals, which is particularly relevant in veterinary medicine. However, data concerning their efficacy and the duration of the induced immune response are not firmly established. As a consequence, the use of these vaccines is currently not recommended either for prevention of ringworm in domestic animals or prevention of human transmission.

The need for safe and effective vaccines against dermatophytosis in companion animals, especially *M. canis* infection in cats, is obvious (Mignon *et al.* 2008). While dermatophytosis has been little studied compared to other fungal infections during the last 20 years, there has been a recent resurgence of interest in both dermatophytes and dermatophytic infection. The ongoing identification of major virulence factors, as well as the identification of host cells, cell receptors and cytokine pathways involved in both innate and specific immune responses against dermatophytes will undoubtedly contribute to a better understanding of the immunopathogenesis of dermatophytosis. In turn, sound strategies to induce protective specific immune responses through appropriate immunization should be developed and should contribute to a reduction of the zoonotic risk.

References

Ajello, L. (1974). Natural history of the dermatophytes and related fungi. *Mycopath. Mycol. Appl.*, **53:** 93–110.

Ajello, L. and Cheng, S-L. (1967). The perfect state of *Trichophyton mentagrophytes. Sabouraudia*, **5:** 230–34.

Ajello, L., Kaplan, W. and Chandler, F. W. (1980). Dermatophyte mycetomas: fact or fiction? In: *Proceedings of the fifth international conference of the mycoses - superficial, cutaneous and, sub-cutaneous infections*, pp. 135–40. Washington: Pan American Health Organization.

Baldo, A., Mathy, A., Tabart, J., Camponova, P., *et al.* (2010). Secreted subtilisins Sub3 from *Microsporum canis* is required for adherence to but not for invasion of the epidermis. *Br. J. Dermatol.*, **162:** 990–97.

Baldo, A., Mathy, A., Vermout, S., Tabart, J., *et al.* (2007). Les mécanismes d'adhérence des champignons responsables de mycoses superficielles. *Ann. Méd. Vétér.*, **151:** 192–99.

Baldo, A., Tabart, J., Vermout, S., *et al.* (2008). Secreted subtilisins of *Microsporum canis* are involved in adherence of arthroconidia to feline corneocytes. *J. Med. Microb.*, **57:** 1152–56.

Brouta, F., Descamps, F., Monod, M., *et al.* (2002). Secreted metalloprotease gene family of *Microsporum canis. Infect. Immun.*, **70:** 5676–83.

Campos, M. R. M., Russo, M., Gomes, E. and Almeida, S. R. (2006). Stimulation, inhibition and death of macrophages infected with *Trichophyton rubrum. Microb. Infect.*, **8:** 372–79.

Carlotti, D. N., Guinot, P., Meissonnier, E. and Germain, P. A. (2010). Eradication of feline dermatophytosis in a shelter: a field study. *Vet. Dermatol.*, **21:** 259–66.

Chermette, F., Ferreiro, L. and Guillot, J. (2008). Dermatophytoses in animals. *Mycopathologia*, **166:** 385–405.

Chmel, L. (1980). Zoophilic dermatophytes and infection in man. In: H. Preusser (ed.) *Medical Mycology*, pp. 61–66. Stuttgart: Gustav Fisher Verlag.

Chung, J. S., Yudate, T., Tomihari, M., *et al.* (2009). Binding of DC-HIL to dermatophytic fungi induces tyrosine phosphorylation and potentiates antigen presenting cell function. *J. Immunol.*, **183:** 5190–98.

Dawson, C. O. and Gentles, J. C. (1959). Perfect stage of *Keratinomyces ajelloi. Nature*, **183:** 1345–46.

Dawson, C. O. and Gentles, J. C. (1961). The perfect states of *Keratinocmyces ajelloi* Vanbreuseghem, *Trichophyton terrestre* Durie & Frey and *Microsporum nanum* Fuentes. *Sabouraudia*, **1:** 49–57.

Degreef, H. (2008). Clinical forms of dermatophytosis (ringworm infection). *Mycopathologia*, **166:** 257–65.

Descamps, F., Brouta, F., Monod, M., *et al.* (2002). Isolation of a *Microsporum canis* gene family encoding three subtilisin-like proteases expressed *in vivo*. *J. Investig. Dermatol.*, **119**: 830–35.

De Vroey, C. (1985). Epidemiology of ringworm (dermatophytosis). *Semin. Dermatol.*, **4**: 185–200.

Drouot, S., Mignon, B., Fratti, M., Roosje, P. and Monod, M. (2008). Pets as the main source of two zoonotic species of the *Trichophyton mentagrophytes* complex in Switzerland, *Arthroderma vanbreuseghemii* and *Arthroderma benhamiae*. *Vet. Dermatol.*, **20**: 13–18.

Esquenazi, D., Alviano, C. S., Souza, W. D. and Rozental, S. (2004). The influence of surface carbohydrates during in vitro infection of mammalian cells by the dermatophyte *Trichophyton rubrum*. *Res. Microb.*, **155**: 144–53.

Evans, E. G. and Gentles, J. C. (1985). *Essentials of medical mycology*. Edinburgh: Churchill Livingstone.

Foster, K. W., Friedlander, S. F., Panzer, H., Ghannoum, M. A. and Elewski, B. E. (2005). A randomized controlled trial assessing the efficacy of fluconazole in the treatment of pediatric tinea capitis. *J. Am. Acad. Dermat.*, **53**: 798–809.

Fréalle, E., Rodrigue, M., Gantois, N., *et al.* (2007). Phylogenetic analysis of *Trichophyton mentagrophytes* human and animal isolates based on MnSOD and ITS sequence comparison. *Microbiology*, **153**: 3466–77.

Fumeaux, J., Mock, M., Ninet, B., Jan, I., *et al.* (2004). First report of *Arthroderma benhamiae* in Switzerland. *Dermatology*, **208**: 244–50.

Georg, L. K. (1960). Epidemiology of the dermatophytoses sources of infection, modes of transmission and epidemicity. *Ann. N. Y. Acad. Sci.*, **89**: 69–77.

Gip, L. and Abelin, J. (1987). Differential staining of fungi in clinical specimens using fluorescent whitening agent (Blankophor). *Mykosen*, **30**: 21–24.

Gräser, Y., Kuijpers, A. F. A., Presber, W. and de Hoog, G. S. (1999). Molecular taxonomy of *Trichophyton mentagrophytes* and *T. tonsurans*. *Med. Mycol.*, **37**: 315–30.

Gudding, R. and Naess, B. (1986). Vaccination of cattle against ringworm caused by *Trichophyton verrucosum*. *Am. J. Vet. Res.*, **47**: 2415–17.

Gudding, R., Naess, B. and Aamodt, O. (1991). Immunisation against ringworm in cattle. *Vet. Rec.*, **128**: 84–85.

Gull, K. and Trinci, A. P. (1973). Griseofulvin inhibits fungal mitosis. *Nature*, **244**: 292–94.

Hasegawa, A. and Usui, K. (1975). *Nannizzia otae* sp. nov., the perfect state of *Microsporum canis* Bodin. *Japanese J. Med. Mycol.*, **16**: 148–53.

Hay, R. J. (1990). Antifungal drugs in dermatology. *Sem. Dermatol.*, **9**: 309–17.

Hay, R. J., Calderon, R. A. and Mackenzie, C. D. (1988). Experimental dermatophytosis in mice: correlation between light and electron microscopic changes in primary, secondary and chronic infections. *Br. J. Experim. Path.*, **69**: 703–16.

Hay, R. J., Roberts, S. O. B. and MacKenzie, D. W. R. (1992). Mycology. In: R. H. Champion, J. L. Burton and F. J. G. Ebling (eds.) *Textbook of Dermatology, Vol 2*, pp. 1127–216. Oxford: Blackwell Scientific Publications.

Holländer, H., Keilig, W., Bauer, J., Rothemund, E. (1984). A reliable fluorescent stain for fungi in tissue sections and clinical specimens. *Mycopathologia*, **88**: 131–34.

Idnurm, A., Bahn, Y. S., Nielsen, K., *et al.* (2005). Deciphering the model pathogenic fungus *Cryptococcus neoformans*. *Nature Rev. Microb.*, **3**: 753–64.

Jensen, J. M., Pfeiffer, S., Akaki, T., *et al.* (2007). Barrier function, epidermal differentiation, and human beta-defensin 2 expression in tinea corporis. *J. Investig. Dermatol.*, **127**: 1720–27.

Kac, G., Bougnoux, M. E., Chauvin, M. F. D., *et al.* (1999). Genetic diversity among *Trichophyton mentagrophytes* isolates using random amplified polymorphic DNA method. *Br. J. Dermatol.*, **140**: 839–44.

Kamiya, A., Kikuchi, A., Tomita, Y. and Kanbe, T. (2004). PCR and PCR-RFLP techniques targeting the DNA topoisomerase II gene for rapid clinical diagnosis of the etiologic agent of dermatophytosis. *J. Dermatol. Sci.*, **34**: 35–48.

Kaufman, G., Horwitz, B. A., Duek, L., Ullman, Y. and Berdicevsky, I. (2007). Infection stages of the dermatophyte pathogen *Trichophyton*: microscopic characterization and proteolytic enzymes. *Med. Mycol.*, **45**: 149–55.

Kligman, A. M. and Ginsberg, D. (1950). Immunity of the adult scalp to infection with *Microsporum audouinii*. *J. Investig. Dermatol.*, **14**: 345–58.

Kwong-Chung, K. J. and Bennet, J. E. (1992). *Medical Mycology*. Philadelphia & London: Lea and Febiger.

Legendre, R. and Steltz, M. (1980). A multi-center, double-blind comparison of ketoconazole and griseofulvin in the treatment of infections due to dermatophytes. *Rev. Infect. Dis.*, **2**: 586–91.

Lopez-Garcia, B., Lee, P. H. A. and Gallo, R. L. (2006). Expression and potential function of cathelicidin antimicrobial peptides in dermatophytosis and tinea versicolor. *J. Antimicrob. Chemother.*, **57**: 877–82.

Lunder, M. and Lunder, M. (1992). Is *Microsporum canis* infection about to become a serious dermatological problem? *Dermatology*, **184**: 87–89.

Marples, M. J. (1956). The ecology of *Microsporum canis* Bodin in New Zealand. *J. Hyg.*, **54**: 378–87.

Mathy, A., Baldo, A., Schoofs, L., Cambier, L., *et al.* (2010). Fungalysin and dipeptidyl-peptidase gene transcription in *Microsporum canis* strains isolated from symptomatic and asymptomatic cats. *Veterinary Microbiology*, **146**: 179–82.

McAleer, R. (1980). Fungal infections of the scalp in Western Australia. *Sabouraudia*, **18**: 185–90.

Mignon, B. R. and Losson, B. J. (1997a). Prevalence and characterization of *Microsporum canis* carriage in cats. *J. Med. Vet. Mycol.*, **35**: 249–56.

Mignon, B. and Losson, B. (1997b). Vaccination against ringworm in cattle. In: P. P. Pastoret, J. Blancou, P. Vannier, and C. Verschueren (eds.) *Veterinary Vaccinology*, pp. 490–91. Amsterdam: Elsevier Science.

Mignon, B., Swinnen, M., Bouchara, J. P., *et al.* (1998). Purification and characterization of a 31.5 kDa keratinolytic subtilisin-like serine protease from *Microsporum canis* and evidence of its secretion in naturally infected cats. *Med. Mycol.*, **36**: 395–404.

Mignon, B., Tabart, J., Baldo, A., *et al.* (2008). Immunization and dermatophytes. *Curr. Opin. Infect. Dis.*, **21**: 134–40.

Mochizuki, T., Sugie, N. and Uehara, M. (1997). Random amplification of polymorphic DNA is useful for the differentiation of several anthropophilic dermatophytes. *Mycoses*, **40**: 405–9.

Mock, M., Monod, M., Baudraz-Rosselet, F. and Panizzon, R. G. (1998). Tinea capitis dermatophytes: susceptibility to antifungal drugs tested *in vitro* and *in vivo*. *Dermatology*, **197**: 361–67.

Monheit, J. E., Cowan, D. F. and Moore, D. G. (1984). Rapid detection of fungi in tissues using calcofluor white and fluorescence microscopy. *Arch. Pathol. Lab. Med.*, **108**: 616–18.

Monod, M. (2008). Secreted proteases from dermatophytes. *Mycopathologia*, **166**: 285–94.

Monod, M., Baudraz-Rosselet, F., Ramelet, A. A. and Frenk, E. (1989). Direct mycological examination in dermatology: a comparison of different methods. *Dermatologica*, **179**: 183–86.

Monod, M., Bontems, O., Zaugg, C., *et al.* (2006). Fast and reliable PCR/sequencing/RFLP assay for identification of fungi in onychomycoses. *J. Med. Microb.*, **55**: 1211–16.

Moriello, K. A. (2004). Treatment of dermatophytosis in dogs and cats: review of published studies. *Vet. Dermatol.*, **15**: 99–107.

Moriello, K. A. and Deboer, D. J. (1991). Fungal flora of the haircoat of cats with and without dermatophytosis. *J. Med. Vet. Mycol.*, **29**: 285–92.

Nakamura, Y., Kano, R., Hasegawa, A. and Watanabe, S. (2002). Interleukin-8 and tumor necrosis factor alpha production in human epidermal keratinocytes induced by *Trichophyton mentagrophytes*. *Clin. Diagn. Lab. Immun.,* **9:** 935–37.

Nenoff, P., Herrmann, J. and Gräser, Y. (2007). *Trichophyton mentagrophytes sive interdigitale?* A dermatophyte in the course of time. *J. Deuts. Dermatol. Gesellsch.,* **5:** 198–202.

Ninet, B., Jan, I., Bontems, O., Lechenne, B., *et al.* (2003). Identification of dermatophyte species by 28S ribosomal DNA sequencing with a commercial kit. *J. Clin. Microb.,* **41:** 826–30.

Rebell, G. and Taplin, D. (1970). *Dermatophytes: Their recognition and identification.* Florida: University of Miami Press.

Rippon, J. W. and Garber, E. D. (1969). Dermatophyte pathogenicity as a function of mating type and associated enzymes. *J. Investig. Dermatol.,* **53:** 445–48.

Rybnikar, A., Chumela, J., Vrzal, V., Krys, F. and Janouskovcova, H. (1991). Prophylactic and therapeutic use of a vaccine against trichophytosis in a large herd of silver foxes and Arctic foxes. *Acta Vet. Brno.,* **60:** 285–88.

Sato, K., Yang, X. L., Yudate, T., *et al.* (2006). Dectin-2 is a pattern recognition receptor for fungi that couples with the Fc receptor gamma chain to induce innate immune responses. *J. Biol. Chem.,* **281:** 38854–66.

Schauder, S., Kirsch-Nietzki, M., Wegener, S., Switzer, E. and Qadripur, S. A. (2007). From hedgehogs to men. Zoophilic dermatophytosis caused by *Trichophyton erinacei* in eight patients. *Hautarzt,* **58:** 62–67.

Scott, D. W. (1980). Feline dermatology 1900–1978: a monograph. *J. Am. Anim. Hosp. Ass.,* **16:** 331–459.

Seebacher, C., Bouchara, J. P. and Mignon, B. (2008). Updates on the epidemiology of dermatophyte infections. *Mycopathologia,* **166:** 335–52.

Shiraki, Y., Ishibashi, Y., Hiruma, M., Nishikawa, A. and Ikeda, S. (2006). Cytokine secretion profiles of human keratinocytes during *Trichophyton tonsurans* and *Arthroderma benhamiae* infections. *J. Med. Microb.,* **55:** 1175–85.

Staib, P., Zaugg, C., Mignon, B., *et al.* (2010). Differential gene expression in the pathogenic dermatophyte *Arthroderma benhamiae in vitro* versus infection. *Microbiology,* **156:** 884–95.

Stockdale, P. M. (1961). *Nannizzia incurvata* gen. nov., sp. nov., a perfect state of *Microsporum gypseum* (Bodin) Guiart et Grigorakis. *Sabouraudia,* **1:** 41–48.

Stockdale, P. M. (1963). The *Microsporum gypseum* complex (*Nannizzia incurvata* Stockd., *N. gypseum* (Nann.) comb.nov., *N. fulva* sp.nov.). *Sabouraudia,* **3:** 114–26.

Stockdale, P. M. (1967). *Nannizzia persicolor* sp. nov., the perfect state of *Trichophyton persicolor* Sabouraud. *Sabouraudia,* **5:** 355–59.

Stockdale, P. M., Mackenzie, D. W. R. and Austwick, P. K. C. (1965). *Arthroderma simii* sp. nov., the perfect state of *Trichophyton simii* (Pinoy) comb. nov. *Sabouraudia,* **4:** 112–23.

Svejgaard, E. (1985). Immunologic investigations of dermatophytes and dermatophytosis. *Sem. Dermatol.,* **4:** 201–21.

Symoens, F., Jousson, O., Planard, C., *et al.* (2011). Molecular analysis and mating behaviour of the *Trichophyton mentagrophytes* species complex. *Int. J. Med. Microbiol.,* **301:** 260–66.

Takashio, M. (1973). Une nouvelle forme sexuée du complexe *Trichophyton mentagrophytes, Arthroderma vanbreuseghemii* sp. nov. *Ann. Parasit. Hum. Comp.,* **48:** 713–32.

Tani, K., Adachi, M., Nakamura, Y., *et al.* (2007). The effect of dermatophytes on cytokine production by human keratinocytes. *Arch. Dermatol. Res.,* **299:** 381–87.

Taplin, D., Zaias, N., Rebell, G. and Blank, H. (1969). Isolation and recognition of dermatophytes on a new medium (DTM). *Arch. Dermatol.,* **99:** 203–9.

Tornquist, M., Bendixen, P. H. and Pehrson, B. (1985). Vaccination against ringworm of calves in specialized beef production. *Acta Vet. Scand.,* **26:** 21–29.

Vanbreuseghem, R., De Vroey, C. and Takashio, M. (1978). *Guide pratique de mycologie médicale et vétérinaire,* pp. 1–264. Paris, New York, Barcelone, Milan: Masson.

Vermout, S., Tabart, J., Baldo, A., Mathy, A., Losson, B., Mignon, B. (2008a). Pathogenesis of dermatophytosis. *Mycopathologia,* **166:** 267–75.

Vermout, S., Baldo, A., Tabart, J., Losson, B. and Mignon, B. (2008b). Secreted dipeptidyl peptidases as potential virulence factors for *Microsporum canis*. *FEMS Immun. Med. Microb.,* **54:** 299–308.

Weedon, D. (1992). Mycoses and algal infections. In: D. Weedon (ed.) *The skin; systematic pathology, Vol 9,* pp. 639–76. Edinburgh: Churchill Livingstone.

Weitzman, I., McGinnis, M. R., Padhye, A. A. and Ajello, L. (1986). The genus *Arthroderma* and its later synonym *Nannizzia*. *Mycotaxon,* **25:** 505–18.

Weitzman, I. and Summerbell, R. C. (1995). The dermatophytes. *Clin. Microb. Rev.,* **8:** 240–59.

Woodfolk, J. A. (2005). Allergy and dermatophytes. *Clin. Microb. Rev.,* **18:** 30–43.

CHAPTER 71

Occasional, miscellaneous, and opportunistic parasites and fungi

Sheelagh Lloyd

Summary

A variety of organisms are mentioned and these are either not closely related to groups in earlier chapters or are free-living and can opportunistically infect man. The parasites presented are usually under their most important clinical presentation and the fungi are presented separately as a group. As they are usually rare, these infections do not often generate suspicion among health providers. Often they are difficult to differentiate from more common infections, and some can be fatal if misdiagnosed.

Neurological disease

Free-living amoebae causing amoebic encephalitis

Hosts and geographic distribution

Naegleria fowleri, at least 6 *Acanthamoeba* spp., i.e. *A. cuthbertsoni*, *A. castellani*, and *Balamuthia mandrillaris* are free-living and occur worldwide. *Naegleria fowleri*, an amoeboflagellate recently classified under Super Group Excavata: Vahlkampfiidae (Adl *et al.* 2005), causes acute, rapidly fatal meningoencephalitis usually in healthy children and young adults. *Acanthamoeba* spp. and *B. mandrillaris* amoebae, both in Super Group Amoebozoa: Acanthamoebidae, cause insidious, fatal encephalitis; *Acanthamoeba* mainly in immunosuppressed (HIV/AIDS, transplant patients, steroid recipients) or debilitated (drug, alcohol abusers) individuals; *Balamuthia* in these but also in immunocompetent individuals, though particularly the young, elderly and malnourished. All three amoebae contain bacteria including a number of pathogens, i.e. *Escherichia coli* 0157, *Legionella,* etc., but their role as reservoirs is undetermined.

Primary amoebic meningoencephalitis (PAM)

Naegleria fowleri, thermophilic (>30°C) in freshwater, is acquired in warm recreational water (lakes, ponds) particularly in the summer months, and in thermally heated rivers, as well as spas, pools, etc., inadequately treated with chlorine. It has been found in the nasal passages and throat of healthy individuals.

Contact with warm waters, particularly immersing the head, allows amoebae into the nostrils. Incubation may be 5–7 (1–14) days. Parasites enter the brain parenchyma through phagocytosis by olfactory neuroepithelial cells, the cribiform plate and sub-arachnoid space. The amoebae are highly destructive, producing haemorrhagic and necrotic meningoencephalitis involving particularly the olfactory and fronto-temporal regions. They feed on cells with amoebastome feeding cups, perforins and phospholipases disrupt membranes, and the amoebae may trigger apoptosis (Visvesvara *et al.* 2007). The cerebral hemispheres are swollen, oedematous, and congested. Fibrinopurulent exudates contain predominantly PMNs with large numbers of trophozoites but no cysts. Signs include sudden onset headache, fever, nuchal rigidity, nausea, vomiting, with later nerve palsies, seizures, and coma. Infection is rapidly fatal in 2–10 days from increased cranial pressure, brain herniation, and resultant cardiopulmonary problems.

The binucleate *Sappinia* probably *S. pedata* has been isolated from a patient with a haemorrhagic, necrotizing, inflamed lesion.

Granulomatous amoebic encephalitis (GAE)

Human infection occurs worldwide with no seasonal pattern. *Acanthamoeba* is ubiquitous in the environment and tolerates a wide range of osmolality and pH. Cysts survive desiccation for many years. *Acanthamoeba* are present in soil, dust, fresh and brackish water, including thermally heated water (cooling towers, ventilating systems, pools, tubs, spas, etc.), sewage, contact lens fluids, even sea water, etc., and cysts can be airborne (Khan 2006). *Acanthamoeba* can be cultured from the nasopharynx of 1–24% of healthy people. *Balamuthia mandrillaris* in contrast has been only occasionally isolated from soil. Human cases are recorded primarily in South and North America, (a preponderance of cases are in Hispanics for reasons unknown—contact with soil, genetic), but also in Asia, Australia, and Europe. Cases of either amoeba can present anywhere acquired elsewhere.

Infection possibly through olfactory nerves but entrance most probably is through broken skin and the respiratory tract (possibly intestinal tract) and, with or without cutaneous, nasopharangeal or repiratory tract lesions, subsequent haematogenous spread to the brain. *Acanthamoeba* binds to epithelial and endothelial cells with a 136 kDa mannose-binding protein, *Balamuthia* to laminin probably by a galactose-binding protein. There is apoptosis, amoebastomes aid engulfment of the cells, and proteinases, i.e. serine and metalloproteases, that cleave collagen, elastin, fibronectin, plasminogen, etc., and target tight junctions, facilitate invasion. IL6-mediated early inflammation increases permeability probably facilitating entry through cells (Khan 2007; Siddiqui and Khan 2008). Infection may have occurred weeks to months before the onset of central nervous system (CNS) disease. A few *Acanthamoeba* cases and >50% of *Balamuthia* cases may be preceded by cutaneous (occasionally respiratory) lesions that can persist for months before invasion of the CNS. The latter becomes rapidly fatal within days to weeks.

The lesion(s) is a single or multiple space–occupying mass(es) of necrosis, haemorrhage, oedema, and infarcts mainly in the cerebral hemispheres. Histology reveals multinucleated giant cells, necrosis, and neovascularization, suggestive of a tumour, but trophozoites and cysts are scattered through the tissues. There is thrombosis and cuffing with PMNs and amoebae. The giant cells may form granulomata particularly in fairly immunocompetent patients. Signs include headache, stiffness, mental changes, nausea, vomiting, ataxia, facial palsy, photophobia, seizures, coma, and death.

Diagnosis

Amoebic encephalitis is relatively rare and so does not generate suspicion being similar clinically to more common infections but rapid diagnosis and aggressive treatment is essential as mortality is exceedingly high.

The cerebrospinal fluid (CSF) of PAM patients may be grayish, with elevated PMNs, the number of rbc increases with disease progression, and an immediate CSF wet mount may show actively moving *N. fowleri* trophozoites. CSF of GAE patients very rarely reveals *Acanthamoeba* or *Balamuthia* but there is pleocytosis (increased lymphocytes and PMNs) and elevated protein.

Computerized tomography (CT) of GAE cases shows usually low density mass(es); magnetic resonance imaging (MRI) with enhancement, ring enhancing lesion(s); but these mimic abscesses, etc. Arterial occlusions and infarctions have been described. Images of PAM patients may show cerebral oedema and obliteration of cisternae and the subarachnoid space over the cerebral hemispheres (Singh *et al.* 2006). Particularly early in the disease the scan can be normal in as many as 40% of patients (Schumacher *et al.* 1995).

Circulating antibody tests (immunofluorescence, ELISA) must be interpreted with care. High titres against these organisms can be useful for diagnosis but then many patients have impaired immune systems and there rarely is time for antibody production to *Naegleria* although IgM might be useful. Antibody to any of the amoebae may be present in 3% to a high proportion of unaffected individuals.

Brain (or skin) biopsy will reveal trophozoites and cysts of *Acanthamoeba* or *Belamuthia* but no cysts in the case of *N. fowleri*, the organisms differentiated by immunostaining. *Acanthamoeba* and *Naegleria* are readily cultured on non-nutrient agar coated with enterobacteriaceae as food but may take days to develop. The latter grows at 45°C. *Balamuthia* usually requires mammalian cell culture (i.e. monkey kidney, human lung fibroblasts, human brain endothelial cells). All three are cytopathic to cell cultures. All three can be cultured axenically. *Naegleria* is 12 (10–25) μm with a single nucleus, large, central nucleolus, and moves with broad lobopodia. Under certain conditions (i.e. low osmolality) it becomes a temporary, pear-shaped, biflagellate possibly related to dispersal. *Acanthamoeba* and *Balamuthia* trophozoites are 12–60 μm, uninucleate, with a large central nucleolus (occasionally 2/3 in *Balamuthia*). *Acanthamoeba* has fine, tapering, thorn-like acanthopodia, *Belamuthia* pseudopodia are thicker and exhibit filamentous structures. The cysts are uninucleate and 10–30 μm with two (light microscopy) and three (EM) layers to the cyst wall.

Polymerase chain reaction (PCR) analysis of nuclear and mitochondrial SSU 18S, 16S rRNA, ITS1, ITS2, or nested PCR can be used to confirm diagnosis and for analysis of strain in patients and the environment (Réveiller *et al.* 2002; Schuster *et al.* 2003; Zhou *et al.* 2003; Booton *et al.* 2005). 18S rRNA has defined 3 morphological groups and 12 genotypes of *Acanthamoeba* of which T4 is the most frequently isolated from the environment (53%), keratitis cases (94%). and other body tissues (79%). A few brain isolates have been of rare genotypes (T1, 10, 12). Potentially T4 predominates in disease due to either virulence or abundance in the environment. PCR of 16S rRNA commonly is used to confirm *B. mandrillis* and nested PCR for *N. fowleri* infections. Recently, rapid real time multiplex PCR to simultaneously detect any of the three amoebae has been developed (Qvarnstrom *et al.* 2006).

Treatment and prevention

There are very few recoveries from amoebic encephalitis due to late diagnosis and relatively ineffective drugs. *Naegleria fowleri* has been treated with aggressive intravenous and intrathecal amphotericin B and miconazole. Azithromycin, rifampin and fluconazole have been used. *Acanthamoeba* and *Balamuthia* have been treated with combinations of flucytosine, pentamidine, sulphadiazine and fluconazole, or itraconazole and clarithromycin, and miltefosine, but the side effects of the drugs, particularly pentamidine, means discontinuance is likely (Khan 2006). Also, there is potential for re-activation of cysts in the brain at a later date. Surgical removal of any cutaneous lesion might reduce the parasite load but possibly is too late. Steroids could facilitate spread but then decrease cerebral oedema.

Naegleria fowleri can be killed by adequate chlorination (1 mg/L free chlorine) in well-run pools, spas, etc. (Visvervara and Schuster 2008). In some countries where problems could arise in recreational waters monitoring of water has been carried our (i.e. lakes in Australia, cooling tower heated river waters in France). Only advice, i.e. not putting your head underwater, can be given for rivers, ponds, lakes. *Acanthamoeba* are ubiquitous, resistant to chlorination, and can even multiply in water treatment sand and activated carbon filters so that adequate back-washing is essential (Thomas *et al.* 2008).

Meningoencephalitis—*Halicephalobus gingivalis*

Halicephalobus gingivalis, formally *Micronema (H) deletrix*, belongs to a group of usually free-living nematodes. Morphological descriptions and genetic identification of it come from soil isolates and infections with females, larvae and eggs in a few human cases in the USA, Europe, Japan, Egypt, and Columbia, and from CNS, viscera, jaw and nasal bones of horses (Nadler *et al.* 2003).

Halicephalobus gingivalis in man presents as a non-suppurative meningoencephalitis with rapid, fatal progression. There are multimodal necrotizing granulomata containing macrophages, multinucleate giant cells, lymphocytes, eosinophils, and parasites. Infection is thought to be through oral and nasal wounds, though other mucosa and the skin could be involved. Haematogenous spread is suggested as parasites frequently are found in and near blood vessels in the brain.

Nematodes are identified in sections or teased from tissues. Small (15–20 μm wide by 311–411 μm long) pathogenetic females have a rhabditiform oesophagus. The ovary is posterior with 9–12 oocytes and the terminal end curved ventrally. The anterior oviduct and uterus contain one egg and the terminal end is bent dorsally and posteriorly. Eggs, 50 x 18 μm, have flattened sides. First stage larvae (L1) and third stage larvae (L3) average 168 and 203 μm, respectively. The presence of females and eggs rather than just larvae differentiates *H. deletrix* from the closely related *Strongyloides*. Treatment has not been successful upon CNS involvement though high dose ivermectin given every 2 weeks had reported effect in a horse with a confined bone abscess.

The eye

Acanthamoeba spp. keratitis

Opportunistic *Acanthamoeba* spp. can cause vision-threatening keratitis and corneal ulceration. In developing countries amoebae gain access mainly through corneal abrasion/trauma. In the USA, UK, etc., infection occurs particularly in contact lens users with affected individuals more likely to use home-made solutions (amoebae present in home water tanks), disinfect lenses less frequently, and more likely to swim wearing lenses. The amoebae can bind to biofilms on the lens. Further, some strains are resistant to some commercially available solutions, particularly some more convenient, multipurpose solutions that were developed with reduced disinfection to decrease carcinogen risk (Polat *et al.* 2007; Patel and Hammersmith 2008). Tolerance of *Acanthamoeba* to high temperature and high osmolality correlated to pathogenicity in keratitis. Intense pain, photophobia, tearing, usually in one eye, occurs often within days of infection. Although several thousand cases are reported (about 0.15–2/100,000 with more in wearers of extended use lens) (Schuster and Visvesvara 2004; Khan 2006) infection may be misdiagnosed as herpes virus keratitis delaying the appropriate therapy.

Progression of the lesions is described by Patel and McGhee (2009). In the early stages the cornea is destroyed by the cytopathic amoebae with development of a characteristic, complete stromal ring of PMNs in as many as 50–80%. In the later stages there is ulceration, descemetocoele formation, and perforation. A non-healing ulcer, refractory to antibiotics, and the pain due to radial neuritis around the corneal nerve are indicative. Amoebae and cysts can be identified by confocal microscopy or corneal scraping (the highest likelihood of diagnosis is a combination of the two) and culture or PCR using 18S rRNA gene (Khan *et al.* 2001).

Presentation and duration at diagnosis are important. Rapid diagnosis and treatment gives good prognosis, the progressively deeper the disease the greater the treatment challenge and threat to vision. Awwad *et al.* (2007) reported five enucleations in a series of 118 patients where four had severe, ischaemic, posterior segment inflammation. Treatment must be aggressive and prolonged with polyhexamethylene biguanide, chlorhexadene gluconate, Brolene (propamidine/dibromopropamidine), or combinations of these and other drugs, i.e. micafungin, as they have good cysticidal activity reducing chances of recrudescence (Khan 2006; Visvesvara and Schuster 2008). Drug resistance does occur. Steroids can increase amoeba multiplication but decrease cyst formation, these resistant to drugs. Penetrating keratoplasty has been used to restore vision once amoebae have cleared. Corneal transplantation may be needed (Awwad *et al.* 2005). Cases do not progress to granulomatous amoebic encephalitis

although a case of uveitis was associated with the latter (Visvesvara *et al.* 2007). The involvement of opportunistic *Hartmannella* in keratitis is disputed.

Contact lens wearers and those with corneal damage must be warned that amoebae can be present even in potable water. Anywhere the water can heat up, i.e. in pipes outdoors, water tanks, etc., can aid growth. Disinfection of lenses must be thorough, lens cases cleaned and replaced regularly. Solutions containing hydrogen peroxide, i.e. 3%, were the most effective at killing trophozoites and cysts in 24 hours (Johnson *et al.* 2009). Contact lens wearers should continue to seek monitoring and expert advice to prevent complacency, change to possibly cheaper solutions, and reduction in hygiene; in one study the risk was poor hand-hygiene.

Conjunctival sac—adult *Thelazia* spp.

Thelazia callipaeda is common in the conjunctiva of dogs, cats, foxes and rabbits in Asia, and may remain undiagnosed in people in poor communities in China and is described in many areas of Asia. It can occur in 60% of dogs in southern Italy and is emerging in northern Italy, southeastern France, southern Germany, and southern Switzerland and is emerging in man (Otranto and Dutto 2008). *Thelazia californiensis* is described in western USA.

The fly host, drosophilid *Phortica* males (Otranto *et al.* 2006), acquires *T. callipaeda* L1 lapping and later the developed L3 migrates out of the mouthparts of a fly lapping secretions from the eyes of dogs and wild carnivores. *Fannia* spp. have been infected with *T. californiensis*. Human infection occurs at any age but is most common in young children. Worms on the conjunctiva cause floating filaments, pain, conjunctivitis, excess lachrymation, possibly keratitis and ulceration. Male only infections may be asymptomatic. Rare infections in the vitreous and subconjunctival space are described.

Adults, 0.5–1.7 cm, have a serrated cuticle and hexagonal buccal capsule. They can be removed physically with fine forceps. Topical moxidectin shows effect against some animal species.

Oestrus ovis is an occasional parasitic zoonoses of the conjunctival sac. This is covered in more detail in Chapter 68.

A *Cheilospirura* worm, normally in the gizzard of birds, possibly ingested in an insect intermediate host, was described in a conjunctival sac in man in the Philippines.

Cutaneous infections

Cutaneous amoebosis

Acanthamoeba dermatitis presentation is firm, often non-tender, erythematous nodules, possibly multiple chronic ulcers, and abscesses, seen mainly in HIV/AIDS patients particularly on the chest and limbs, and only rarely do CNS signs not develop concurrently or subsequently (Torno *et al.* 2000). *Balamuthia* dermatitis occurs as single, possibly multiple, plaques a few mm thick and up to several cms across that may ulcerate, particularly on the nose, face, and ear, but also on trunk and extremities. Skin lesions may be present in 50% of CNS disease patients, and are almost invariable in some South American patients, but North American patients present primarily with CNS signs. The lesions contain trophozoites and cysts. In addition to aggressive treatment with the antibiotics used for CNS disease, cutaneous application of chlorhexidine, ketoconazole and related creams have occasional reports of efficacy.

Skin blisters and ulcers—*Dracunculus* spp.

Dracunculus medinensis, 'the guinea worm', is one of the oldest known worms, probably depicted as the serpent and staff of Aesculapius, the Roman god of medicine. Formerly a scourge in arid and semiarid areas of Asia, the Middle East, and northern Africa, this parasite has been the subject of an intensive global eradication campaign. However, outbreaks still occur when clean water systems have failed in six countries from Mali to Ethiopia and Sudan. The dog and other mammals occasionally are infected but seem incidental to epidemiology. In North America rare human *Dracunculus* is due to *Dracunculus insignis* from raccoons, mink, and other carnivores.

Females protrude from skin ulcers to lay Ll in water. *Cyclops* are intermediate hosts, and tadpoles and frogs suitable paratenic hosts. Acquired mainly through drinking *Cyclops* in dirty water, parasites migrate through the peritoneal cavity and subcutaneous musculature for many months before moving to the extremities. The female emerging induces an allergic rash, red papule, then blister on an extremity. The long female is coiled near this. Secondary infection or worms that fail to emerge and degenerate cause severe abscessation.

L1 (500–760 µm with a very striated cuticle and long pointed tail) may be obtained after placing cold water on a ruptured blister. The worm is surgically excised or manually extracted. Histology reveals the female worm amid inflammation. For worms that are difficult to remove, corticosteroid therapy, perhaps with accompanying albendazole or ivermectin, might be helpful, though conclusive efficacy has not been demonstrated.

Migrating cutaneous swellings—*Gnathostoma* spp.

Hosts and geographic distribution

Gnathostoma spinigerum occurs in gastric nodules in wild and domestic Canidae, Felidae, and other carnivores, and is the most widespread species infecting man in south east Asia, China, Japan, the Indian subcontinent, and recently in Central Africa. Cases of human *G. hispidum* and *G. doloresi* of pigs and boars in Europe, Asia, Australia, and *G. nipponicum* of weasels, etc., in Japan are described. *Gnathostoma binucleatum* of opossums, etc., seems to be the species increasingly reported in man in northern Latin America and occasionally the USA.

Infection in humans

L1 hatch in water and develop in freshwater copepods. Mature L3 occur in viscera and muscles of fish intermediate hosts, i.e. swamp eels, eels, catfish, snook, cichlids, bream, trout. L3 also occur in amphibians, reptiles, rodents, pigs, and birds infected either from copepods or fish. In definitive hosts larvae migrate in the connective tissue and muscles to return to the stomach. Humans acquire infection primarily from raw fish in ethnic dishes such as 'hu-sae' in China and 'ceviche' in Mexico, but potentially from raw frogs, snakes, wild boar, poultry, etc., and possibly copepods in water. As many as 35% of villagers by a lake in Mexico were seropositive. Rare L3 skin penetration in food handlers and prenatal infection are described. Cases in immigrants and travellers from south east Asia and Latin America are increasing in frequency, and travellers are identifying infected areas, i.e. Zambia, Myanmar, infection previously unrealized as residents do not eat raw fish. Imported, chilled fish poses a threat. Infection in urban Japan was attributed to fish from Taiwan, Korea, or China, and in The Netherlands to imported trout.

In man, transient gastrointestinal symptoms (fever, anorexia, vomiting, pain) may occur within 24–48 hours for 2–3 weeks from the larva in the intestinal wall or liver (Herman and Chiodini 2009). Cutaneous gnathostomosis develops from a week to >5–12 months later and manifests primarily as episodes of migrating swelling, possibly with subcutaneous haemorrhages, cutaneous eruption or nodules mainly on the trunk but also involving the upper limbs, head, throat. etc., and lasting perhaps 1–2 weeks or more. Although intermittent, these signs can persist for years. Eosinophilia may be present. Occasionally an abscess develops. Systemic infection varies with organ, i.e. liver, lung, gut, etc. Neurological migration produces intracranial necrotic tracks and subarachnoid haemorrhage, severe radicular pain and/or headache and paralysis, and has long term side effects and 8–25% mortality. Ocular migration may occur sometimes years later.

Diagnosis

Migrating swellings, usually with eosinophilia, history of residence/travel, and dietary preferences are suggestive. Subcutaneous swellings differentiate gnathostomosis from other larva migrans (Herman and Chiodini 2009). The worm can be very difficult to recover from CNS or cutaneous lesions (it migrates as much as one cm/day) so blind excision may not be helpful although histopathology is described as useful (Magaña *et al.* 2004). An ocular larva is visible. Larvae are 2–15 mm long, reddish-white, with a characteristic head bulb bearing usually 3–4 rows of hooklets and rows of small cuticular spines. Larger parasites and their damage and migrating lesions might be visible on imaging. Serological diagnosis can be obtained in south east Asia. The fewest cross-reactions on ELISA were with IgG_2 antibodies (Herman and Chiodini 2009). On western blot, 24 and 21 kDa antigens of crude extracts, particularly using IgG_4 antibody, were considered specific for confirmation of IgG immunoblots (Anataphruti *et al.* 2005; Laummaunwai *et al.* 2007). A multi-immunodot test has been developed to differentiate some eosinophilic meningitides (Eamsobhana *et al.* 2006).

Treatment

The parasite can be removed surgically from the eye. Spontaneous recovery from cutaneous gnathostomiosis is possible but cutaneous migration, facial in particular, could lead to CNS or ocular complications. Albendazole (400 mg twice daily for 21 days) has been effective (Nontasut *et al.* 2005) and could be useful in cerebral gnathostomiosis. Ivermectin (200 µg/kg for two days) seems effective. Repeated treatment is advised as relapse can be 20–50%.

Neck abscesses—*Lagochilascaris minor*

Although only 50–100 cases of *Lagochilascaris minor* have been described, in rural, neotropical forest areas from Mexico to Brazil, Trinidad and Tobago, infection may be more common and infected dogs and cats are described further north and south than this. The normal hosts seem to be sylvatic Canidae, Felidae, opossums, with adults in the rhino-oro-pharynx and a wild rodent intermediate host.

Human infection probably is acquired by eating larvae in agouti or other rodents. Parasites mature and eggs and larvae develop in persistent, purulent, discharging abscess(es) in the soft tissues of the neck, ear, mastoid process, or throat. Fatal (6%) brain or lung infections are described.

Surgical debridement and excision will reveal rough-shelled eggs (55–80 µm long with a reticulate pattern) and larvae (Sakamoto and Cabrera 2002). Adult females up to 2 cm have three obvious lips and small lateral alae over most of the body. As many parasite stages are present and multiplying, anthelmintics should be given. Prolonged or repeated courses of ivermectin, levamisole, or albendazole are described as effective in individual cases.

Rhabditis dermatitis

Rhabditis (Pelodera) strongyloides is free living in organic matter but also is carried as a larva in the intestine of wood mice with related species in the skin of rodents, presumably using rodents for nourishment and dispersal. The larvae occasionally have been associated with dermatitis in varied domestic animals and several human cases now are recorded in Europe, the USA, and Japan. Skin scrapings show the large larvae (600–750 by 30–40 μm) distinguished by their rhabditiform oesophagus, distinct buccal capsule, and lateral alae (Saari and Nikander 2006).

Respiratory disease

Larynx and trachea—adult *Mammomonogamus* spp.

Over 100 human infections with mainly *Mammomonogamus laryngeus* and *M. nasicola* are recorded in the Caribbean and Brazil, but also Mexico, China, Thailand, and Korea. Infected ruminant definitive hosts are common in much of Central and South America, south east Asia, the Indian subcontinent, and tropical Africa. *Mammomonogamus gangguiensis* is described in China. Infection also is seen in primates.

Eggs in bovine faeces embryonate to L3. Probably eggs, or hatched L3, are eaten accidentally on vegetables. A paratenic host, e.g. earthworm, snail, might be involved and infection in China and Thailand was related to eating turtle meat or blood. Worms attach to the laryngeal/tracheal/bronchial mucosa and suck blood.

Patients have a 'crawling sensation' or 'lump in the throat' with chronic, non-productive cough, possibly paroxysmal with haemoptysis or vomiting. Some have severe 'asthma' symptoms because of obstruction of air passages. An unusual duodenal infection presented with pain and haemoptysis.

Patients in Western countries usually have a recent history of travel in the Caribbean. Eggs in sputum or faeces are ellipsoid and average 75–95 x 40–50 μm, larger than hookworm eggs, with a thicker shell and initially two cells. Males and females, up to 2 cm, are red/brown with a cup-shaped buccal cavity bearing basal teeth, and live in permanent copulo in a Y configuration. They can be visualized and removed by bronchoscopy from the larynx, trachea, and sometimes bronchi, but with their red colour may be difficult to discern against an inflamed mucosa. Benzimidazoles have been used.

Respiratory trichomonads

Originally considered site specific, human vaginal, intestinal, and particularly oral *Trichomonas* spp. have been identified in the respiratory tract of man, as have avian intestinal *Tetratrichomonas gallinarum* and bovine reproductive tract *Tritrichomonas foetus*. *Trichomonas foetus* also occurs in the intestine of diarrhoeic and normal cats, i.e. 31% at cat shows. *Pentatrichomonas hominis* has been found in cats', dogs' and pigs' intestines, human adapted strains are possible though (Duboucher *et al.* 2008).

Trichomonads have been found in 60–100% of *Pneumocystis* pneumonia (PCP) patients and in 30% of acute respiratory distress syndrome patients (and correlated with higher mortality), in cases of emphyaemia and in varied other respiratory diseases. Probably secondary contaminants the trichomonads seem able to establish and multiply in the more anaerobic respiratory tract, some trichomonads can damage cells and are pathogenic in their own site/host in their own right, so their potential contribution to the respiratory disease must be considered.

Identification is difficult and Duboucher *et al.* (2008) describe the amoeboid, non-flagellated forms that develop without revealing their flagellae or undulating membrane. Immunostaining or PCR (ITS1-5.8S rRNA-ITS2) are required (Duboucher *et al.* 2007). Trimethoprim-sulphamethoxazole for PCP is considered active against trichomonads. Metronidazole could be useful.

Alimentary tract infections

Nodules in oral mucosa—adult *Gongylonema pulchrum*

Gongylonema pulchrum adults lie in a zipper fashion in the oesophageal wall of ruminants, pigs, other ungulates, bear, and monkeys, in many countries. More than 50 human cases have been described worldwide, including Europe, Russia, Asia, Australia, and North Africa.

Beetle and cockroach intermediate hosts ingest eggs in ruminant faeces and humans presumably acquire infection eating these. Also, L3 are said to emerge from cockroaches in water. In man, *G. pulchrum* is found coiled in a filamentous nodule or blister in the oral epithelium and the lump often moves, patients describing a creeping sensation.

Some cases initially have been considered delusionary (Molavi *et al.* 2006). The worm is extracted surgically or by curette and patients themselves scratch them out. They are recognized by asymmetrical alae and cuticular bosses that lie in eight longitudinal series anteriorly.

Acanthocephala—'thorney headed worms'

Moniliformis moniliformis (normal hosts, rodents, particularly *Rattus* spp., dogs, cats, foxes) and *Macracanthorhynchus hirudinaceus* (domestic and wild pigs) have some 20 records in man (intestine) worldwide. Other records are: *Macracanthorhynchus ingens* (raccoon and skunk) in the southern USA, *Bolbosoma* spp. (Cetaceans, particularly seals) in Japan, *Acanthocephalus rauschi* (probably of marine fish) found in the peritoneum of an Eskimo in Alaska, *Corynosoma strumosum* (Cetaceans, Alaska) *and Pseudoacanthocephalus bufonis* (toads, south east Asia) may have been spurious infections.

A cystacanth develops in arthropod intermediate hosts (beetles, cockroaches, millipedes, for acanthocephalans parasitic in land animals; crustaceans for those in aquatic vertebrates). *Moniliformis moniliformis* in cockroaches may be accidentally eaten by children; other infections may be from beetles eaten as food in pig rearing areas in China and south east Asia; those of sea mammals in crustaceans. Cystacanths can re-encyst if eaten by non-definitive host vertebrates, so snake, frog or fish paratenic hosts could be responsible. Adults may cause weakness, abdominal pain, and diarrhoea from eosinophilic enteritis and occasional intestinal perforation by the proboscis with the worm entering the peritoneal cavity, but many infections do little harm.

Faecal eggs are ellipsoid or spindle-shaped, dark brown, and measure 110–120 by 56–60 μm *(M. moniliformis)* and 80–100 by

45–65 µm (*M. hirudinaceus*). They have four membranes of which, in terrestrial species, one is very thick and may be pitted. Eggs contain an 'acanthor' larva provided with an anterior circlet of hooks. Adults are cylindrical and 1–1,000 cm long with a 'thorny head', this a cylindrical or oval, invaginable proboscis armed with hooks.

In pigs, doramectin (300 µg/kg), or ivermectin (100–200 µg/kg in feed for 7 days) had good efficacy. Benzimidazoles have been used.

Oesophagostominae: *Oesophagostomum bifurcum* and *Ternidens deminutus* nematodes

Hosts and geographic distribution

Adults occur in the large intestine of non-human primates and *O. bifurcum* occurred at high prevalence in man in north west Ghana and north east Togo and sporadically elsewhere and *T. deminutus* is sporadic in man, particularly described in Zimbabwe, but also in East and Central Africa, Surinam, and Thailand. Recent molecular analyses of *O. bifurcum* cDNA in Ghana revealed 3 or 4 variants, in Patas or Mona monkeys, humans, or Olive baboons. This may indicate human-to-human transmission and certainly primate infections can be common in areas where there is no human infection (Gasser *et al.* 2006). However, additional cross infection studies are required as *O. bifurcum* from humans did infect primates, albeit relatively poorly, and non-human primates presumably remain a reservoir for sporadic infections in Africa and Asia. *Oesophagostomum aculeatum* in Indonesia and *O. stephanostomum* in Brazil and tropical Africa have been recorded rarely.

Infection in humans

Humans presumably eat L3 on vegetation or in soil. L3 have a remarkable ability to shrink on desiccation and revive months later. *Oesophagostomum* L3 enter the mucosa of the proximal colon but also terminal ileum and L4 develop in nodules and remain in the nodules or emerge to develop to adults in the lumen. *Ternidens* larvae develop in the lumen. Two types of pathology are produced by *O. bifurcum*. Uninodular disease comprises a single large (3–11 cm) nodule, frequently protruding into the lumen or adhering to the periumbilical abdominal wall ('Dapaong tumour'), containing thick pus around one or several larvae. Pain and fever are from intestinal obstruction or abscessation. Multinodular disease comprises hundreds of ≤ 1 cm mucosal/serosal nodules containing pus and a worm presenting as abdominal pain, diarrhoea, and weight loss in about 2%, most infections being asymptomatic. These latter on ultrasound usually having ≤10–15 visible nodules with possibly additional smaller, less pathogenic nodules. Rarely nodules occur elsewhere. Adult infections do little harm. Nodules become prevalent in the early dry and increase in size through the dry when disease is most likely to present, decreasing in number through the late dry to mid rainy season.

Diagnosis

Immature *O. bifurcum* (up to one cm) may be identified after surgical removal of a nodule. Faecal examination is a problem as eggs resemble hookworm eggs, *Ternidens* eggs slightly larger, 70–94 by 40–60 µm; *Oesophagostomum* differentiated on cultured L3 (700–950 µm)—larger than *Necator*, with prominent intestinal cells and a long 'hair-like' tail to the transversely striated sheath. Adults are about 1 cm long: *O. bifurcum* has a cylindrical buccal capsule, double leaf crown, cephalic vesicle, and distinct ventral groove; *T. deminutus* a globose buccal capsule, mouth collar, and leaf crown. Multiplex PCR has been used to simultaneously differentiate *O. bifurcum*, *Ancylostoma dudodenale* and *N. americanus* (Verweij *et al.* 2007).

Treatment

Surgery may be necessary for large abscesses. Albendazole, 400 mg for adults, is very effective. Experimentally, treatment twice in a year decreased prevalence from 53 to 5% and pathology from 38 to 6% changing to uninodular rather then multinodular (Ziem *et al.* 2006a, b). Four rounds of treatment decreased prevalence to 0.8%.

Ciliated *Balantidium coli* protozoa

Balantidium coli is cosmopolitan in pigs. In Europe infection can occur on >75% of farms and reach 60% in piglets and 100% in adults. Prevalence in free-roaming pigs and wild boar is from >19% to 100%. It infects captive and free-living non-human primates (13–100%) and occasionally other animal species.

Sporadic human infection is worldwide, and occasionally relatively common in farm workers and rural dwellers where free-ranging pigs occur, i.e. south east Asia, China, Western Pacific Islands, Latin America. Travellers to these areas may become infected. Infection is by ingestion of cysts from pig (occasionally primate) faeces, in soil or via contaminated food/water, occasionally inhalation. Infection may be from captive monkeys and human-to-human transmission in institutions has been reported. Recent prevalence has ranged from 0.02–1% and up to 30% in man, and 0.8–2.4% in diarrhoeic children. Infection usually is asymptomatic but acute, explosive diarrhoea and dysentery may present when trophozoites invade the large intestinal mucosa in an ulcer, mainly in the malnourished and immunocompromised. Intestinal perforation and occasional infection of the peritoneal cavity and genito-urinary tract are reported. Recent infections in the West have been respiratory, i.e. a thick-walled infected cavity in a farmer in contact with aerosolized pig manure, and pneumonia in immunosuppressed patients.

Cysts, 40–60 µm, or trophozoites, 60–70 µm long, are shed irregularly in the faeces. They have a large, kidney-shaped macronucleus, cilia, contractile vacuoles and large funnel-shaped peristome. Barium and biopsy define the ulcer and reveal trophozoites.

Metronidazole at 750 mg to 1.25 g (for adults) in three divided doses daily for 10 days is described as effective.

Entamoeba polecki—diarrhoea

Entamoeba polecki a parasite of pigs and monkeys, has foci of infection in man in south east Asia and Papua New Guinea. Infection is recorded sporadically in immigrants and in other countries, e.g. Venezuela, India, France, Tasmania. Infection is acquired as *B. coli*. Infection normally is asymptomatic, although rare reports of abdominal cramps, diarrhoea, and nausea were coincident with excretion of large numbers of cysts. Cysts are uninucleate, 14–16 µm in diameter, with a large, 3–4 µm nucleus and diffuse but central karyosome. Diloxanide furoate and metronidazole are used.

Non-invasive intestinal amoebae

Other amoebae live harmlessly in humans but must be differentiated from *Entamoeba histolytica*. Some also infect animals, particularly pigs and monkeys. Most are common worldwide. *Entamoeba dispar* is a commensal species identical to *E. histolytica* differentiated molecularly. *Entamoeba coli* has large (usually 20–30 μm) cysts with eight nuclei, an eccentric karyosome, coarse chromatin, and chromatoid bodies have a splintered, not rounded shape. *Entamoeba hartmanni* has small cysts (5–10 μm) with four nuclei and chromatoid bars of the *E. histolytica* type. *Endolimax nana* has a small oval cyst with small curved chromatoid bars, four nuclei, and a large, often eccentric, usually irregular, and sometimes fragmented karyosome. *Iodamoeba butschlii* is uninucleate with a large vacuole containing glycogen that stains brown with iodine. *Dientamoeba fragilis,* binucleate and occasionally associated with abdominal pain, is now considered a trichomonad flagellate. *Entamoeba gingivalis* in the mouth is a non-encysting amoeba, 10–20 μm, with a central karyosome.

Occasional parasites in the intestine

Several normally free-living *Rhabditis* spp. described occasionally in the intestine of man in Asia possibly are pseudoparasites after accidental ingestion. A *Reticularia* female worm of rodents or bats, presumably eaten in an insect intermediate host, was identified in the mucosa of the appendix at autopsy in New York.

Parenteral tissues

Viscera and nasopharynx—Pentastomida (arthropods)

Hosts and geographic distribution

Pentastomids now are considered modified crustaceans related to the branchurians. Human infection with *Linguatula serrata* is sporadic, but cosmopolitan. Incidence has been high where definitive host dogs fed viscera of ruminants carry adults in their nasal cavities, e.g. the Middle East, Turkey, parts of North Africa, the Indian subcontinent, and infection occurs occasionally in Latin America, but is rare in USA and southern Europe, although cases present in immigrants. *Armillifer armillatus* in West and Central Africa and *Armillifer moniliformis* and *Porocephalus* spp. in China and south east Asia, primarily Malaysia, can be common locally in humans. *Armillifer grandis* has been described occasionally in the Congo. Adults of these species normally occur in the trachea and lungs of large snakes, *Python, Bitis* spp. Individual cases of *Armillifer agkistrodontis* and *Pentastoma najae* of snakes in Asia and *Sebekia mississipiensis* (dermatitis) of alligators (Costa Rica) have been described. There is an unconfirmed report of *Leiperia cincinnalis* of crocodiles (Africa) and a subcutaneous creeping eruption from *Raillietella hemidactyli* of lizards (south east Asia).

Eggs are immediately infective in the secretions and faeces of canids and intestine and faeces of snakes. The clawed, oval, four to six-legged larva develops to a nymph in the MLN, liver, and occasionally peritoneum, omentum, and lungs of intermediate host lagomorphs or ruminants (*Linguatula*) or rodents and monkeys (*Armillifer*) or fish (*Sebekia* spp.).

Infection in humans

Man is usually an intermediate host. Water, food, and soil contaminated with faeces are sources of infection as is close contact with dog secretions. Heavy infections with *Armillifer* have been related to trapping snakes for skins and eating snake meat containing many eggs or an adult female worm. There is potential for infection when cleaning aquaria of pet snakes of unknown origin.

The nymphs develop under the peritoneum of the abdominal viscera and wall, in the liver, abdominal lymph nodes, mesenteries,

lungs, and on the pleural surface. Nymphs usually die and calcify within two years of infection. Most human infections (porocephalosis) are asymptomatic. Some present as abdominal pain or prolonged cough in heavy infection. Rare, acute, fatal cases have involved massive infection, including the brain. Rare ocular presentation has occurred.

Man also is a temporary definitive host for *L. serrata.* The nymph, acquired eating raw liver or lymph nodes of domestic ruminants and lagomorphs, attaches on to the nasopharyngeal mucosa and causes severe irritation and a Type I hypersensitivity reaction with coughing (perhaps paroxysmal) and sneezing within 1–24 hours. Symptoms (called 'halzoun' or 'marrara' in the Middle East and Sudan) are self-limiting after 1–7 (14 days) as the worm is discharged. As many as 20% may describe the symptoms. Very rarely, parasites develop to adulthood. In a few patients, possibly sensitized by previous adult or larval infection, acute congestion and oedema of the nasopharyngeal and laryngeal mucosae have more severe consequences.

Diagnosis and treatment

Nymphs have a ventral mouth and two pairs of cranial hooks, hence pentastomes. *Linguatula serrata* nymph(s) in the nasopharynx are tongue-shaped, slightly flattened anteroventrally, annulated with rows of spines, and up to 6–10 mm, and are physically removed by endoscopy. Most abdominal or lung nymph infections are diagnosed accidentally on surgery or radiography. Radiography can reveal crescent-shaped calcifications, 0.5–2 cm across. Occasionally nymphs are viable in cysts with little host reaction, commonly they are dead in a necrotic granuloma, or a scar contains remnants of cuticle/hooks, or crescent-shaped calcifications, 0.5–2 cm across, remain. The nymph, if still present, is or horseshoe-shaped. *Linguatulua* nymphs are like those in the nasopharynx. *Armillifer* nymphs are 12–20 mm and cylindrical with spiral rings resembling a screw (Tappe and Büttner 2009). Histology reveals ring-like sclerotized openings in the cuticle. Ivermectin might be useful in acute infection with large numbers of nymphal stages. Advice must be given on dietary habits, contact with dogs and snakes, and their treatment, perhaps with macrocyclic lactones, attempted.

Myositis—*Haycocknema perplexum*

This minute nematode (<500 μm long) in the Muspiceoidea occurs within myofibres. It multiplies here and larvae break out (Spratt *et al.* 1999; Basuroy *et al.* 2008). Myostitis and eosinophilia occur. Although related parasites occur in marsupials and mice, the source of infection for the few human cases in Australia is unknown. Diagnosis by biopsy and treatment with 400 mg albendazole/daily for 4–8 weeks has been successful. Steroids are not recommended.

Kidney—adult *Dioctophyma renale* (red scourge)

Only a few human cases are described, most in North America, but also Russia, China, Iran, south east Asia. Australia, and Spain. The parasite also occurs in South America. Normal hosts are piscivorous mustelids and canids, mainly mink in North America. A related *Eustrongylides* spp. of piscivorous birds has been described in eastern USA.

Eggs passed in urine develop in water and hatch when swallowed by an aquatic oligochaete annelid intermediate host. Oligochaetes in drinking water are infective, as are raw fish and frog paratenic hosts. Infective larvae penetrate the gut soon after infection and develop in the peritoneal cavity, then kidney. The adult worm in a thick-walled cyst containing haemorrhagic debris, usually found in or on the right kidney, has been confused with a tumour. Some are asymptomatic, others induce loin pain, haematuria, and worms have been expelled from the urethra. One lesion abscessed through the skin over the kidney. Worms might be found in the peritoneal cavity or liver. In two cases, a dioctophymid L3, possibly *Dioctophyma* or *Eustrongylides,* occurred in a subcutaneous nodule on the chest. *Eustrongylides,* acquired from minnows, usually migrate out of the oesophagus, stomach, and intestine causing peritonitis and abscesses.

At least one *D. renale* infection was detected by eggs (70–80 by 40–50 μm, barrel-shaped, brownish yellow with a thick, pitted shell and clear areas at the poles) in the urine. Ultrasound reveals echo-dense masses (the same echo-density as renal parenchyma). The blood-red worm reaches 1 m by 1 cm but seems to disintegrate after 1–3 years or more. Eggs remain in the granulomatous tissue of the cyst wall but the 'double-walled rings' of eggs can easily be confused with radially striated Liesegang-like rings.

The cyst and kidney (if atrophied) are removed surgically.

Opportunistic fungal infections

A very large number of fungi, growing mostly in soil enriched with decaying matter, induce opportunistic infections in man. Incidence has increased considerably in the last three decades as a result of a growing number of immunosuppressed patients (Cornely 2008). The fungi may remain localized, or disseminate though the infected organ, or disseminate to almost any organ, the most serious complication being CNS involvement. Risk increases with Human Immunodeficiency Virus (HIV) infection, newer aggressive therapies for stem cell and solid organ transplantation, haematological malignancies, neutropaenia, chemotherapy, corticosteroid use, new immunotherapies including TNF- and other cytokine-antagonists, and increased survival of critically ill patients. Concomitant diseases such as diabetes mellitus, COPD, liver cirrhosis, etc. also are risks. Infection in otherwise healthy persons, usually is asymptomatic, but can disseminate even in these. Mainly inhaled, a few infections enter through penetrating skin injury. Some produce surface lesions.

Some of these fungi occur worldwide, others are mainly tropical or subtropical, others occur in restricted geographic areas. The fungi might be common, but even in endemic areas, as opportunistic and uncommon, signs do not generate suspicion of a fungus, signs being similar to viral, and bacterial infections, and malignancies. Furthermore, increased travel and migration means disease presents in any country, particularly as some fungal infections may remain latent in healthy persons to activate and produce disease many years later. The diseases often have high mortality if untreated. Even if treated, the lack of suspicion and difficulties in diagnosis often mean diagnosis in delayed and, accompanied by drug efficacy often being limited with some species insusceptible to the drugs, and with the nature of the patients, mortality remains high (Cornely 2008).

Anti-fungals, particularly amphotericin B, the newer triazoles, i.e. itraconazole, voriconazole and the azole, fluconazole, and the echinocandins, i.e. caspafungin, micafungin, are the main therapeutic agents (reviewed by Cornely 2008). Maintenance therapy may be required for months, even years. Institution of prophylaxis in at risk patients increasingly has been shown useful in reducing incidence of infection but remains controversial. There is potential for increasing the rate of development of resistance to the limited number of groups of drugs, but this must be weighed against the poor prognosis associated with the infections. Combination therapy also remains controversial. In acquired immune deficiency syndrome (AIDS) patients, highly active anti-retroviral treatment (HAART), in others immunotherapy can be instituted. However, in some patients immune reconstitution inflammatory syndrome (IRIS) may ensue, the immunopathology, usually granulomatous inflammation, not understood, but associated with the developing immune response to usually the opportunistic infection that previously may have been clinical or subclinical (French 2009). Screening for opportunistic infections is important. Management of IRIS is described by Marais *et al.* (2009).

Pneumocystis pneumonia (PCP)

Taxonomy and development

Pneumocystis species now are considered to be host specific organisms but PCP still is included here to update the recent speciation and epidemiological studies versus the earlier supposition that *P. carinii* was an important zoonoses.

First described as a protozoan, DNA data has shown *Pneumocystis* to be an atypical fungus (Aliouat-Denis *et al.* 2008). Species status has been assigned on phenotypic and genetic differences and cross infection studies in severe combined immunodeficiency syndrome (SCID) mice (Frenkel 1999; Springer *et al.* 2002; Durand-Joly *et al.* 2002). *Pneumocystis jirovecii* is separated as host specific to humans, *P. carinii* specific to rats, and host specific species are being identified in other animals. Different strains also have been identified in man (Springer *et al.* 2002; Aliouat-Denis *et al.* 2008).

Cysts release uninucleate trophic forms that align, in the appropriate host, with Type I pneumocytes and produce filopodia to anchor to, deeply interdigitate with, but not penetrate the alveolar cell cytoplasm. Organisms of inappropriate species are eliminated within three days. Trophic forms evolve through sporocyte stages progressing from uninucleate to eight nucleate, to a thick or thin walled cyst containing eight spores. Consistent with possible inclusion in the ascomycetes perhaps the cyst should be renamed an ascus as most fungal asci contain eight ascospores. Binary fission of trophic forms and conjugation remain undetermined, most forms are haploid, but a few diploids and a meiotic pathway have been seen (Aliouat-Denis *et al.* 2008; Burgess 2008).

Infection in humans

Transmission is assumed to be airborne and *Pneumocystis* DNA has been identified in air outdoors and in patient rooms. The current hypothesis is a 'transient infection scenario', possibly with reinfection, with human to human transmission. Identification by PCR on deep nasal and oropharyngeal swabs now has identified *P. jirovecii* asymptomatic carriage in a variety of groups. While none of 28 and 30 healthy adults were infected in Chile and France, respectively, *P. jirovecii* DNA was found in 20% of 50 healthy adults in Spain and 20% of these were infected six months later.

Prevalence increases in different groups: 10–40% of people with chronic pulmonary disease revealed *P. jirovecii* DNA as did 15.5% of third trimester pregnant women, and prevalence increases in the elderly; these two groups potentially increasing infection in young children. Manifestation of severe disease occurs in the immunocompromised and transmission between them and to healthy care workers has important implications for health care centres. The immunocompromised also can be asymptomatic carriers.

First described as interstitial pneumonia in premature infants and occasionally patients with malignancies and transplants, PCP became a common presenting sign in AIDS and remains a major problem in those not receiving HAART or unaware of their HIV-status with CD4 cells <200/µl. The host response and mechanisms whereby *Pneumocystis* survives in the host are described by Thomas and Limper (2007). There is fever, progressive shortness of breath, non-productive cough, malaise, chest pain and sometime low fever. Alveoli are filled with foamy exudate containing organisms, immune cells (CD8 lymphocytes and macrophages), and necrotic tissue, and there is interstitial inflammation. Exudate and trophic forms on the alveoli prevent gas exchange resulting in hypoxaemia. In persons, immunosuppressed for solid organ transplants, cancer therapy, or receiving corticosteroids, the disease tends to be more fulminant and rapid in progression. Occasionally there can be a granulomatous response. Mortality can be up to 10–60%, highest in immunocompromised cancer patients.

Diagnosis

Giemsa, methamine silver or immunofluorescent antibody stains may reveal pleomorphic trophic forms (1–5 µm) and rounded cysts (5–10 µm) containing eight spores. Broncho-alveolar lavage (BAL) in HIV positive individuals shows abundant cysts and exudate, primarily lymphocytes and macrophages. BAL in HIV-negatives shows abundant inflammatory cells, particularly neutrophils, and cysts are present but less abundant. Molecular diagnosis by agarose gel separation and PCR amplification of diagnostic 346 and 550 bp bands is sensitive and specific. Radiography in HIV-positives reveals bilateral interstitial and alveolar infiltrates as ground glass opacities of particularly perihilar distribution. In HIV-negatives the exudates are diffuse. CT shows extensive ground glass opacities in the central, not peripheral lung, and there can be consolidated nodules, etc.

Treatment and prophylaxis

Trimethoprim-sulphamethoxazole remains the first choice for treatment and for prophylaxis in at risk patients (<200 CD4 cells/µl) although there is a relatively high rate of intolerance and treatment failure, i.e. sulpha-allergic persons and resistance due to mutation in dihydropteroate synthase. A generally preferred second line treatment is primaquine/clindamycin. Other treatments include pentamidine though with high toxicity, parfuramidine has proved less toxic in trials, dapsone-tirmethopim, atovaquone that also is used for prophylaxis, and dapsone-perimethamine used for prophylaxis (Thomas and Limper 2007). In persons receiving immunotherapy IRIS is a problem, 4–60% can develop this.

Human-to-human transfer has important implications in medical centres dealing with immunocompromised individuals and could promote spread of drug resistant strains. Strict isolation of *P. jirovecii* positive/suspected patients now seems important.

Dimorphic fungi associated with respiratory, disseminated, and CNS disease

While *Histoplasma* (Chapter 69) is the most common other dimorphic fungi can cause severe disease.

Cryptococcus neoformans and *Cryptococcus gatti*

Hosts and geographic distribution

Cryptococcus spp. are saprophytic, basidiomycetous, dimorphic fungi that develop from saprophytic hyphae to basidiospores (1.8–3 µm) and then yeast cells on infection. Hyphae are rarely seen in lesions. It is probably basidiospores that are inhaled in dust but cutaneous implantation also can initiate disease. Close human transfer might be possible as poorly encapsulated yeasts can be in sputum in large numbers during respiratory disease. Disease in lower animals manifests primarily in the nasal cavities, head and neck, so affected pets might be a risk. Transfer from humans or animals have only rarely been demonstrated (Ma and May 2009). *Cryptococcus neoformans* (serotypes A, D, and hybrids, A predominant) occurs worldwide, and produces disease primarily in immunosuppressed individuals, affected immunocompetent persons often have an underlying disease. *Cryptococcus neoformans* is found particularly in pigeon droppings and soils and debris enriched with these, but other birds can be involved; 27% of pet canaries in two Italian towns, and 10% of wild birds, particularly parrots, in Mexico, were infected. *Cryptococcus gatti* (serotypes B, C, hybrids), the main species seen in immunocompetent persons, is tropical and subtropical and found mainly in debris associated with red gum trees but also other trees, i.e. almonds, firs, so it is a rural disease in Africa, Australia, south east Asia, southern California, occasionally Europe, but now is emerging in temperate areas in Canada and north west and south east USA, for example. Occasionally, *C. gattii* x *neoformans* hybrids and other species are isolated from man.

Virulence is associated with ability to grow at 37°C, the capsule, melanin, mannnitol, and enzyme production, many of these secreted in vesicles, plus phenotypic switching from a smooth to more virulent mucoid form (Ma and May 2009). The thick polysaccharide capsule, composed of 90–95% galactoxylomannan (the structure of which defines the serotype) and connected to the yeast with glucans, has negative charge that inhibits phagocytosis and digestion, induces complement consumption, antibody unresponsiveness, and macrophage, dendritic cell, and cytokine dysregulation. Melanin, produced using for example dopamine in the brain, protects *Cryptococcus* as an anti-oxidant. Mannitol also protects against oxidative killing by PMNs and cell-free oxidants. Hydrolytic enzymes, particularly production of phospholipase that correlates with virulence, may promote destruction of membranes and lung surfactants.

Infection in humans

Incidence in immunocompetent persons is <1.5/100,000 in the USA. Disease occurs mainly in AIDS patients with an incidence of 2–7/1,000, and prevalence in Africa can reach 13–45% and in developed countries 5–10%. As many as 3% of solid organ transplant patients develop cryptococcosis. Mortality can be high particularly when CNS lesions develop.

The yeast enters small air passages and compresses tissue but induces little host response. Most infections remain latent and asymptomatic for many years in healthy persons and seroprevalence can be high. In mainly the immunocompromised, the yeast disseminates after reactivation or new infection. Disease due to *C. gattii* may occur 2–11 months after infection, *C. neoformans* may be longer. Although entry is respiratory, most patients present with CNS signs of severe headache, fever, nausea, vomiting, altered mental status, coma, etc. Reasons for CNS predilection are not known. There is chronic meningitis or focal parenchymal lesions, the latter being more common with *C. gatti*. Increased CSF pressure may in part be related to yeasts or capsules blocking CSF uptake by arachnoid villi but mannitol and the capsule increase osmolality and so promote brain oedema. About 20–50% of patients also show pulmonary disease, this more common in *C. gattii*. There may be asymptomatic pulmonary nodules or acute disease of cough, dyspnoea, fever, and there can be involvement of other tissues, joints, heart, skin, genitourinary tract, and eye. The skin, nodules, ulcers, molluscan-type lesions or cellulites, is involved in about 10% of patients.

Diagnosis

Diagnosis has been reviewed by Saha (2009). Because of the severity of CNS disease lumbar puncture is needed irrespective of presentation. In immunosuppressed patients direct examination of blood, urine, skin nodules, using indian ink or nigrosin stains, may reveal roundish, budding yeasts, 5–15 μm with a birefringent, polysaccharide capsule that stains red with mucicarmine. The yeast grows at 37°C, pseudohyphae are absent, it produces urease, and phenyloxidase, and a brown melanin like pigmentation on medium containing diphenolic compounds. Methenamine silver and PAS-stained histological sections are useful. These methods have 50–58 and 100% sensitivity and specificity, respectively. The sensitivity of latex agglutination and EIA antigen (galactomannan) detection tests in CSF, serum, urine, can be 93–99% in patients with culture-confirmed cryptococcal meningitis. Patients with *Aspergillus* or *Penicillium* may also react. PCR using primers for 18S rDNA can have high sensitivity and specificity. CT or MRI scans show ventricular enlargement and cerebral atrophy although, occasionally, the ventricles are small and there is cerebral oedema or a *Cryptococcus* mass.

Treatment

CNS disease is fatal if untreated and still has a high mortality with treatment (10–40% at 10 weeks). Liposomal amphotericin B accompanied by 5-flucytosine is a first line therapy. Resistance has developed in sub-Saharan Africa. Alternates are fluconazole, better for maintenance, or itraconazole. Lumbar puncture can relieve increased intracranial pressure. Subsequent maintenance therapy is important as a high percentage, will relapse. Immunotherapy may be considered.

Coccidioides immitis and *Coccidioides posadasii*

Coccidioides immitis affects persons particularly in California, and *C. psosdasii* elsewhere in south west USA, northern Mexico, and parts of Central and South America, particularly Argentina and Paraguay. The fungi are found in sandy soils and incidence in Arizona has increased to 60/100,000 with migration to the area and increased construction in desert areas. Ten to 50% of people in endemic areas may have been exposed and later activation is possible such that, should immunosuppressive, i.e. transplant therapy be considered in an inhabitant, they should be screened. A rainy summer for growth and dry and windy winter for dispersal is favourable for inhalation of arthroconidia.

Infection in humans

Infection was recognized first in agricultural workers as a progressive skin disease and then as an acute respiratory syndrome ('Valley fever'). In the terminal bronchioles the arthrospores transform to multinucleated spherules that grow to contain thousands of endospores. Rupture releases the endospores that transform to spherules and so on.

In immunocompetent persons coccidioidomycosis is asymptomatic in two thirds or produces mild or moderate flu-like respiratory disease (Parish and Blair 2008). There can be acute lobar or segmental pneumonia with headache, pleuritic chest pain, fever, cough, dyspnoea, etc. Cutaneous abnormalities, i.e. erythema nodosum, are more likely than in other pneumonias and indicate a favourable outcome reflecting an immune response. Diffuse pneumonia in heavy infection or in the immunocompromised produces severe illness. Most cases of acute pneumonia resolve spontaneously but a small proportion develop a chronic progressive pneumonia with consolidation and possibly cavitation, haemoptysis and weight loss. The residual effect of acute pneumonia is 1–2 cm nodules or walled cavities usually asymptomatic.

Disseminated disease occurs in <5% of immunocompetent persons but is likely in about 30% in HIV, transplant immunosuppression and haematological malignancies, with other risks including Filipino and African ancestry, age <1 year or the elderly, and late pregnancy. Disseminated disease may occur long after pulmonary infection and affects any organ but particularly skin, lymph nodes, bone, but infrequent CNS disease occurs with substantial morbidity despite treatment. There may be hydrocephalus, vasculitis, infarctions, and abscesses and headache, mental changes, and cranial nerve defects (Adam *et al.* 2009).

Diagnosis

Spherules may be seen on cytology or histology and culture is diagnostic. Immunodiffusion and latex agglutination to detect particularly IgM and IgG antibodies are useful; complement fixation titres reflect severity and response to treatment; but antibodies may be absent in as many as 50% of patients. The CSF usually is culture negative and must be diagnosed by CSF antibodies, elevated WBC and protein, and low glucose.

Treatment

Lipid formulations of amphotericin B are useful in severe disease, a triazole in moderate infections, and fluconazole in CNS disease (Parish and Blair 2008) with indefinite triazole therapy in immunocompromised patients as relapse on discontinuance of fluconazole is not uncommon. Nodular or cavitational lesions can remain untreated unless near pleural surfaces where rupture is a complication.

Paracoccidioides brasiliensis

This fungus occurs in soil in Latin America where it is the most prevalent systemic mycosis. There could be 10 million infected with disease in 2%, and again infection can remain dormant for many years to appear in immigrants in any country (Manns *et al.* 1996).

Children and young adults comprise <5% of cases but their disease can be severe with hypertrophy of the lymphoreticular system, bone marrow dysfunction, funginaemia, and infecting other organs, skin, bone, etc. This acute or subacute disease has high mortality if untreated and after treatment organisms may remain in lesions. Most cases are chronic and in males >30-years-old progressing slowly over months to years. Non-specific pulmonary signs occur in most, not uncommonly accompanied by other signs, most frequently oral and nasal mucosal ulcerations, skin lesions, lymph node and adrenals involvement, but occasionally these latter will be evident in the presence of a localized, asymptomatic lung lesion.

Diagnosis involves direct examination, histopathology, culture, and antibody and/or antigen detection using monoclonal antibodies to gp43 and/or gp70. Detection of antigen in CSF or BAL is more sensitive than in serum for CNS and lung disease. Radiography shows nodules, cavities and diffuse fibrotic pattern.

Treatment uses itraxonazole or amphotericin B. Trimethoprim-sulphamethoxazole, though used, seems less effective. A common sequel is fibrotic scarring particularly of the lung.

Blastomyces dermatitidis

Most common in foci in mid west, south east and south central USA, New York and Canada along the Great Lakes and St Lawrence, Missouri, Mississippi, and Ohio River regions, and northern Mexico, occasional cases occur in the Pacific regions, South America, Africa, India, and the Middle East. The fungus develops in moist soil containing decaying vegetation along rivers and streams and in forests. In Canada, exposure and inhalation occurred mainly in the summer. About 50% remained asymptomatic, but a peak occurred of either localized or acute pneumonic disease in autumn or diffuse chronic pneumonia with alveolar or interstitial infiltrates and mass lesions in spring. Dissemination occurs in up to 40% of those with chronic disease with manifestation primarily in the skin as verrucose and ulcerative lesions (entry through skin breaks is possible with chancre at the inoculation site), bone, genitourinary system, but also viscera. CNS involvement is rare except in AIDS patients where meningitis and mass lesions may occur in 40% (Mason et al. 2008).

The fungus is relatively easily recovered from BAL in lung disease, histopathology is used for other tissues. The bud attachment bases are fairly characteristic. An antigen detection test is described but there is cross-reaction, particularly with H. capsulatum (Durkin et al. 2004). Antibody tests are not recommended.

Guidelines for treatment (Chapman et al. 2008) are lipid amphotericin B for moderate to severe disease lung and disseminated disease, and itraconazole for mild to moderate disease, both followed by itraconazole for 6–12 months, possibly lifelong for immunosuppressed patients.

Penicillium marneffei

It is not certain whether P. marneffei is saprophytic or primarily a zoonoses from mainly bamboo rats in Asia (northern India, China, Taiwan, Thailand, and Vietnam) (Vanittanakom et al. 2006). It is the third most common opportunistic infection in Thailand and presents in immigrants in non-endemic areas. Fever, skin lesions (papules with central necrosis on the head and neck and elsewhere), anaemia, weight loss, lymphadenopathy, hepatosplenomegaly, and respiratory disease may occur. The yeast can be identified in scrapings or biopsies. It cross-reacts with antibodies to Aspergillus but they can be differentiated morphologically. Serological testing has been variable and PCR has been used in endemic areas. Even when treated with amphotericin B mortality can be high.

Other dimorphic and yeast-like fungi include *Sporothrix schenckii*, this a complex of species, on plants and soils that enters through pricks by roses and particularly through handling sphagnum moss. Lesions develop mainly in the skin and subcutaneous tissues 3 (1–12) weeks later, though spread to the bone is possible. A painless nodule is followed by others that resemble boils and ulcerate and are slow to heal. Inhalation and disseminated infections may occur. Terbinafine, itraconazole, and potassium iodide are useful. *Trichosporon* spp. are very invasive with funginaemia, pulmonary, skin, visceral, and eye infections. Break though infections have been seen in those with haemotological malignancies and neutropaenia on amphotericin B, fluconazole or echinocandins. Newer triazoles show *in vitro* efficacy. *Geotrichum* spp. (=*Blastoschizomyces capitatus*) is rare but seen mainly in Europe though reported elsewhere. Amphotericin B and voriconazole seem drugs of choice. *Rhodotorula* spp. induce funginaemia, endophthalmitis, peritonitis or meningitis and are susceptible to amphotericin B and flucytosine or ravuconazole versus other triazoles and echinocandins *in vitro*.

Some respiratory and disseminated opportunistic filamentous fungi

Aspergillus species

Aspergillus fumigatus is a very common cause of opportunistic fungal pneumonia. Bearing conidospores with large terminal, flask-shaped vesicles with sterimata on which conidia are formed and ubiquitous in decaying material means inhalation of the conidia is very common (Segal 2009). Other species are emerging, i.e. *A. flavus* and *A. nidulans* in sinus and granulomatous disease and *A. terreus* is resistant to amphotericin B.

Infection in man

Invasive aspergillosis presents acutely in the immunocompromised and can account for 90% of fungal infections in patients with haematological malignancies, 10–20% of stem cell transplants, and is seen in neutropaenia, bone marrow failure, and other transplant immunosuppression, AIDS, etc., and occasionally post-surgery. It is suggested that fluconazole prophylaxis increases colonization and that gene changes occur making *Aspergillus* more virulent. Hyphal invasion of vessels produces necrosis and tissue infarction particularly in the sinuses, also eroding local bone, and pulmonary infection produces fever, cough, dyspnoea, chest pain. Progression involves the mediastinum and chest wall with possible haematogenous spread to any organ. CNS involvement may be an abscess(es), meningitis or subarachnoid haemorrhage with seizures or focal neurologic changes.

In those less severely immunosuppressed and those with pre-existing lung disease there can be a slowly progressive pneumonia, over months or years, with variable levels of necrosis or cavitation or a fungal mass (aspergilloma) occupying a pre-existing lung cavity.

In immunocompetent persons, a sinusitis or chronic asthma from a Th2 allergic bronchopulmonary responses can manifest in 1–2% of patients with asthma and 1–5% of cystic fibrosis patients. There are pulmonary infiltrates and possibly bronchiectasis.

Diagnosis

Diagnosis still remains difficult (Maertens et al. 2009). Histologic demonstration of hyphae is useful. The septate, branched hyphae help differentiate *Aspergillus* from some, i.e. Zygomycetes, but not other fungi. Conidia, needing oxygen, are seen only in the lungs. Culture confirms diagnosis. Sandwich ELISA that detects fungal wall galactofuranose on galactomannan in serum or broncho-alveolar lavage (BAL) is more sensitive and specific than is EIA for glucans, though false positives with *Histoplasma* occur and the latter excludes *Pneumocystis*, *Cryptococcus* and the Zygomycetes. Complement fixation and immunodiffusion tests detect antibody. PCR analyses of ITS and 18S rRNA are used. Radiographs may show nodular lesions about 80% of which have a ground glass 'halo' sign of haemorrhagic inflammation, or cavitation, but these are not pathognomonic.

Treatment and prophylaxis

Voriconazole for CNS disease or posaconazole are first line treatments (Maertens *et al.* 2009). Fluconazole is not effective against moulds. Treatment failure can be high and multi-resistant *Aspergillus* have been described. Other treatments include liposomal amphotericin B and caspofungin. Surgical debridement or removal of localized lesions and fungal masses is important. Prophylaxis is controversial, also anti-fungals can decrease detection of galactomannan. Nonetheless, prophylactic amphotericin B decreased aspergillosis in neutropaenic patients from 14 to 4%. Oral azoles are more convenient with less nephrotoxicity; posaconazole was more efficient than fluconazole in stem cell transplant patients with GVHD and in neutropaenic patients though it did produce more adverse affects (Cornely *et al.* 2007).

Other filamentous fungi with septate hyphae also can be severe and fatal and are emerging causing 27% of fungal invasions in solid organ transplant patients in the USA and occurring elsewhere. *Fusarium* spp. are angioinvasive and tend to produce superficial or localized sinopulmonary disease in immunocompetent persons but have greater funginaemia and cutaneous manifestations than aspergillosis and also dissemination to the CNS in severely immunosuppressed and neutropaenic patients. Colonization of a hospital water system has been implicated in transmission. Relatively resistant to anti-fungals, six species were susceptible *in vitro* to terbinafine and one to amphotericin B. *Fusarium* can be fatal despite treatment related to the degree of immunosuppression and extent of invasion. Several genera of the the Zygomycetes in soil and decaying matter are pathogenic causing, depending on the group, an acute, rapid angioinvasive disease or a chronic, progressive disease. Infection occurs primarily in neutropaenic and immunosuppressed patients affecting sinuses, lungs, skin, also CNS, gastrointestinal tract, and a renal presentation. Diabetic patients are at risk. These infections have occurred as breakthrough infections in patients taking voriconazole and other anti-fungals including echinocandins. Lipid amphotericin B remains the therapy and posaconazole has been described as an effective salvage therapy though infection can be fatal despite aggressive treatment. Invasive *Acremonium*, *Paecilomyces* and *Trichoderma* species are resistant to amphotericin B.

Dematiaceous fungi

More than 100 species and 60 genera of septated filamentous dematiaceous fungi, with melanin pigmented, thick walls, found in soil and decaying material, cause infections worldwide but are more common in tropical and subtropical countries (Revankar 2006). Entrance is through penetrating injury.

Chromoblastomycosis in the skin and subcutaneous tissues occurs as verrucose, scaly plaques. The tuberculoid granulomata contain round sclerotic, 'muriform' bodies, 5–12 μm, in giant cells or microabscesses that can be revealed in scrapings and histologically. The organisms stain with Fontana-Masson for melanin and the hyphae in tissues are more fragmented than *Aspergillus*. Mycetoma ('Madura foot', fungal abscesses) is a deep infection usually of the lower extremities containing the mycotic granules. Phacohyphomycoses occurs as skin and subcutaneous cysts or abscesses containing hyphae. Pneumonia and CNS disease are uncommon but induced by some genera primarily in immunosuppressed patients. Several genera cause keratitis after trauma. Allergic sinusitis and pulmonary disease are caused by two genera. Different species and genera are resistant to amphotericin B and other anti-fungals. Surgery and newer triazoles seem effective.

Though not considered by all to be within this group as possibly not as melanized, *Scedosporium apiospermum* in soil and stagnant water enters a penetrating injury and causes subcutaneous mycetoma in immunocompetent patients and invades producing osteomyelitis and arthritis. It often colonizes cystic fibrosis patients. The immunosuppressed may show disseminated lung disease, multiple skin lesions, and CNS disease. This may occur early after transplant in those receiving amphotericin B or fluconazole, etc., prophylaxis. It is relatively insusceptible to most anti-fungals. New triazoles may be effective. *Scedosporium prolificans*, asymptomatic to invasive, also is relatively unaffected by anti-fungals. Surgery, immunotherapy and voriconazole or itraconazole plus terbinafine have been effective.

References

Adam, R.D., Elliott, S.P. and Taljanovic, M.S. (2009). The spectrum and presentation of disseminated coccidioidomycosis. *Am. J. Med.*, **122**: 770–77.

Adl, S.M., Simpson, A.G.B., Farmer, M.A. *et al.* (2005). The new higher level classification of eukaryotes with emphasis on the taxonomy of protists. *J. Eukaryot. Microbiol.*, **52**: 399–451.

Aliouat-Denis, C-M., Chabé, M., Demanche, C. *et al.* (2008). *Pneumocystis* species, co-evolution and pathogenic power. *Infect., Genet. Evol.*, **8**: 708–26.

Anataphruti, M.T., Numatanong, S. and Dekumyoy, P. (2005). Diagnostic values of IgG4 in human gnathostomaisis. *Trop. Med. Int. Health*, **10**: 1013–21.

Awwad, S.T., Parmar, D.N., Heilman, M. *et al.* (2005). Results of penetrating keratoplasty for visual rehabilitation after *Acanthamoeba* keratitis. *Am. J. Ophthalmol.*, **140**: 1080–84.

Awwad, S.T., Heilman, M., Hogan, R.N. *et al.* (2007). Severe reactive ischaemic posterior segment inflammation in acanthamoeba keratitis: a new potentially blinding syndrome. *Ophthalmology*, **114**: 313–20.

Basuroy, R., Pennisi, R., Robertson, T. *et al.* (2008). Parasitic myositis in tropical Australia. *Med. J. Aust.*, **188**: 254–56.

Booton, G.C., Visvesvara, G.S. *et al.* (2005). Identification and distribution of *Acanthamoeba* species genotypes associated with nonkeratitis infections. *J. Clin. Microbiol.*, **43**: 1689–93.

Burgess, J.W., Kottom, T.J. and Limper, A.H. (2008). *Pneumocystis* exhibits a conserved meiotic control pathway. *Infect. Immun.*, **76**: 417–25.

Chapman, S.W., Dismukes, W.E., Proia, L.A. *et al.* (2008). Clinical practice guidelines for the management of blastomycosis: 2008 update by the Infectious Diseases Society of America. *Clin. Infect. Dis.*, **46**: 1801–12.

Cornely, O.A. (2008). *Aspergillus* to Zygomycetes: causes, risk factors, prevention, and treatment of invasive fungal infections. *Infection.*, **36**: 296–313.

Cornely, O.A., Maertens, J., Winston, D.J. *et al.* (2007). Posaconazole vs. fluconazole or itraconazole prophylaxis in patients with neutropaenia. *N. Engl. J. Med.,* **356:** 348–59.

Duboucher, C., Barbier, C., Beltramini, A. *et al.* (2007). Pulmonary superinfection by trichomonads in the course of acute respiratory distress syndrome. *Lung,* **185:** 295–301.

Duboucher, C., Pierce, R.J., Capron, M., Dei-Cas, E. and Viscogliosi, E. (2008). Recent advances in pulmonary trichomonosis. *Trends Parasitol.,* **24:** 201–2.

Durand-Joly, I., el Aliouat, M., Recourt, C. *et al.* (2002). *Pneumocystis carinii* f. sp. *hominis* is not infectious for SCID mice. *J. Clin. Microbiol.,* **40:** 1862–65.

Durkin, M., Witt, J., Lemonte, A., Wheat, B. and Connolly, P. (2004). Antigen assay with the potential to aid in diagnosis of blastomycosis. *J. Clin. Microbiol.,* **42:** 4873–75.

Eamsobhana, P., Ongrotchanakun, J., Yoolek, A. *et al.* (2006). Multi-immunodot for rapid differential diagnosis of eosinophilic meningitis due to parasitic infections. *J. Helminthol.,* **80:** 2249–54.

French, M.A. (2009). HIV/AIDS: immune reconstitution inflammatory syndrome: a reappraisal. *Clin. Infect. Dis.,* **48:** 101–7.

Frenkel, J.K. (1999). *Pneumocystis* pneumonia, an immunodeficiency dependent disease (IDD): a critical historical overview. *J. Eukaryot. Microbiol.,* **46:** 895–925.

Gasser, R.B., de Gurijter, J.M. and Polderman, A.M. (2006). Insights into the epidemiology and genetic make-up of *Oesophagostomum bifurcum* from human and non-human primates using molecular tools. *Parasitology,* **132:** 453–60.

Goldani, L.Z., Aquino, V.R., Lunardi, L.W., Cunha, V.S, and Santos, R.P. (2009). Two specific strains of *Histoplasma capsulatum* causing mucocutaneous manifestations of histoplasmosis: preliminary analysis of a frequent manifestation of histoplasmosis in southern Brazil. *Mycopathologia,* **167:** 181–86.

Hainer, B.L. (2003). Dermatophyte infections. *Am. Fam. Physician,* **67:** 101–8.

Herman, J.S. and Chiodini, P.L. (2009). Gnathostomiasis, another emerging imported disease. *Clin. Microbiol. Rev.,* **22:** 484–92.

Johnston, S.P., Sriram, A., Qvarnstrom, Y. *et al.* (2009). Resistance of *Acanthamoeba* cysts to disinfection in multiple contact lens solutions. *J. Clin. Microbiol.,* **47:** 2040–45.

Khan, N.A. (2006). *Acanthamoeba*: biology and increasing importance in human health. *FEMS Microbiol. Rev.,* **30:** 564–95.

Khan, N.A. (2007). *Acanthamoeba* invasion of the central nervous system. *Int. J. Parasitol.,* **37:** 131–38.

Khan, N.A., Jarroll, E.L. and Paget, T.A. (2001). *Acanthamoeba* can be differentiated by polymerase chain reaction and simple plating assays. *Curr. Microbiol.,* **43:** 204–8.

Laummuanwai, P., Sawanyawisuth, K., Intapan, P.M. *et al.* (2007). Evaluation of human IgG class and subclass antibodies to a 24 kDa antigenic component of *Gnathostoma spinigerum* for the serodiagnosis of gnathostomiasis. *Parasitol. Res.,* **101:** 703–8.

Ma, H. and May, R.C. (2009). Virulence in *Cryptococcus* species. *Adv. Appl. Microbiol.,* **67:** 131–90.

Magaña, M., Messina, M., Bustamante, F. and Cazarín, J. (2004). Gnathostomiasis: clinicopathologic study. *Am. J. Dermatopathol.,* **26:** 91–95.

Maertens, J., Meersseman, W. and van Bleyenbergh, P. (2009). New therapies for fungal pneumonia. *Curr. Opin. Infect. Dis.,* **22:** 183–90.

Manns, B.J., Baylis, B.W., Urbanski, S.J., Gibb, A.P. and Rabin, H.R. (1996). Paracoccidioideomycosis: case report and review. *Clin. Infect. Dis.,* **23:** 1026–32.

Marais, S., Wilkinson, R.J., Pepper, D.J. and Meintjes, G. (2009). Management of patients with the immune reconstitution inflammatory syndrome. *Curr. HIV/AIDS Rep.,* **6:** 162–71.

Mason, A.R., Cortes, G.Y., Cook, J., Maixe, J.C. and Thiers, B.H. (2008). Cutaneous blastomycosis: a diagnostic challenge. *Int. J. Dermatol.,* **47:** 824–30.

McCully, J.P., Alizadeh, H. and Niederkorn, J.Y. (1995). *Acanthamoeba* keratitis. *CLAO J.,* **21:** 73–76.

Molavi, G.H., Massoud, J. and Gutierrez, Y. (2006). Human *Gongylonema* infection in Iran. *J. Helminthol.,* **80:** 425–28.

Nadler, S.A., Carreno, R.A. *et al.* (2003). Molecular phylogenetics and diagnosis of soil and clinical isolates of *Halicephalobus gingivalis* (Nematoda: Cephalobina: Panagrolaimoidea), an opportunistic pathogen of horses. *Int. J. Parasitol.,* **33:** 1115–25.

Nontasut, P., Claesson, B.A., Dekumyoy, P., Pakdee, W. and Chullawichit, S. (2005). Double-dose ivermectin vs albendazole for the treatment of gnathostomiasis. *Southeast Asian J. Trop. Med. Public Health,* **36:** 650–52.

Otranto, D. and Dutto, M. (2008). Human thelaziasis, Europe. *Emerg. Infect. Dis.,* **14:** 647–49.

Otranto, D., Cantacessi, C., Testine, G. and Lia, R.P. (2006). *Phortica variegata* as an intermediate host of *Thelazia callipaeda* under natural conditions: evidence for pathogen transmission by a male arthropod vector. *Int. J. Parasitol.,* **36:** 1167–75.

Parish, J.M. and Blair, J.E. (2008). Coccidioidomycosis. *Mayo Clin. Proc.,* **83:** 343–49.

Patel, A. and Hammersmith, K. (2008). Contact lens-related microbial keratitis. *Curr. Opin. Ophthalmol.,* **19:** 302–6.

Patel, D.V. and McGhee, C.N.J. (2009). *Acanthamoeba* keratitis: a comprehensive photographic reference of common and uncommon signs. *Clin. Experiment. Ophthalmol.,* **37:** 232–38.

Polat, Z.A., Vural, A. and Cetin, A. (2007). Efficacy of contact lens storage solutions against trophozoite and cyst of *Acanthamoeba castellanii* strain 1BU and their cytotoxic potential on corneal cells. *Parasitol. Res.,* **101:** 997–1001.

Qvarnstrom, Y., Visversvera, G.S., Sriram, R. and da Silva, A.J. (2006). Multiplex real-time PCR assay for simultaneous detection of *Acanthamoeba* spp., *Balamuthia mandrillaris,* and *Naegleia fowleri. J. Clin. Helminthol.,* **44:** 3589–95.

Revankar, S.G. (2006). Dematiaceous fungi. *Mycoses,* **50:** 91–101.

Réviller, F.L., Cabanes, P-A. and Marciano-Cabral, F. (2002). Development of a nested PCR assay to detect the pathogenic free-living amoeba *Naegleri fowleri. Parasitol. Res.,* **88:** 443–50.

Saari, S.A.M. and Nikander, S.E. (2006). *Pelodora* (syn. *Rhabditis*) *strongyloides* as a cause of dermatitis–a report of 11 dogs from Finland. *Acta Vet. Scand.,* **48:** 18–24.

Saha, D.C., Xess, I., Biswas, A., Bhowmik, D.M. and Padma, M.V. (2009). Detection of *Cryptococcus* by conventional, serological and molecular methods. *J. Med. Microbiol.,* **58:** 1098–105.

Sakamoto, T. and Cabrera, P.A. (2002). Subcutaneous infection of *Lagochilascaris minor* in domestic cats from Uruguay. *Vet. Parasitol.,* **108:** 145–52.

Schumacher, D.J., Tien, R.D. and Lane, K. (1995). Neuroimaging findings in rare amebic infections of the central nervous system. *Am. J. Neuroradiol.,* **16:** 930–35.

Schuster, F.L. and Visvesvara, G.S. (2004). Free-living amoebae as opportunistic and non-opportunistic pathogens of man and animals. *Int. J. Parasitol.,* **43:** 1001–27.

Schuster, F.L., Dunnebacke, T.H., Booton, G.C. *et al.* (2003). Environmental isolation of *Balamuthia mandrillaris* associated with a case of amebic encephalitis. *J. Clin. Microbiol.,* **41:** 3175–80.

Segal, B.H. (2009). Aspergillosis. *N. Engl. J. Med.,* **360:** 1870–84.

Siddiqui, R. and Khan, N.A. (2008). *Balamuthia* amoebic encephalitis: an emerging disease with fatal consequences. *Microb. Pathog.,* **44:** 89–97.

Singh, P., Kochhar, R., Vashishta, R.K. *et al.* (2006). Amebic meningoencephalitis: spectrum of imaging findings. *Am. J. Neuroradiol.,* **27:** 1217–21.

Spratt, D.M., Beveridge, I., Andrews, J.R.H. and Dennett, X. (1999). *Heycocknema perplexum* n.g., n.sp. (Nematoda: Robertdollfuscidae): and intramyofibre parasite in man. *Syst. Parasitol.,* **43:** 132–31.

Springer, J.R., Beard, C.B., Miller, R.F. and Wakefield, A.E. (2002). A new name (*Pneumocystis jiroveci*) for *Pneumocystis* from humans. *Emerg. Infect. Dis.,* **8:** 891–96.

Tappe, D. and Büttner, D.W. (2009). Diagnosis of human visceral pentastomiasis. *PLOS Neg. Trop. Dis.,* **5(2):** e320, online.

Thomas, C.F. and Limper, A.H. (2007). Current insights into the biology and pathogenesis of *Pneumocystis* pneumonia. *Nat. Rec. Microbiol.,* **5:** 298–308.

Thomas, V., Loret, J.F., Jousset, M. and Greub, G. (2008). Biodiversity of amoebae and amoebae-resisting bacteria in a drinking water treatment plant. *Environ. Microbiol.,* **10:** 2728–45.

Torno, M.S., Babapour, R., Gurevitch, A. and Witt, M.D. (2000). Cutaneous acanthamoebiasis in AIDS. *J. Am. Acad. Dermatol.,* **42:** 351–54.

Vanittanakom, N., Cooper, C.R., Fisher, M.C. and Sirisanthana, T. (2006). *Penicillium marneffei* infection and recent advances in the epidemiology and molecular biology aspects. *Clin. Microbiol. Rev.,* **19:** 95–110.

Verweij, J.J., Brienen, E.A., Ziem, J. *et al.* (2007). Simultaneous detection and quantification of *Ancylostoma duodenale, Necator americanus* and *Oesophagostomum bifurcum* in faecal samples using multiplex real-time PCR. *Am. J. Trop. Med. Hyg.,* **77:** 685–90.

Visvesvara, G.S. and Schuster, F.L. (2008). Opportunistic free-living amebae, Part I, Part II. *Clin. Microb. Newsl.,* **30:** 151–58, 59–66.

Visvesvara, G.S., Moura, H. and Schuster, F.L. (2007). Pathogenic and opportunistic freeliving amoebae: *Acanthamoeba* spp., *Balamuthia mandrillaris, Naegleria fowleri,* and *Sappinia diploidea. FEMS Immunol. Med. Microbiol.,* **50:** 1–26.

Wheat, L.J. (2003). Current diagnosis of histoplasmosis. *Trends Microbiol.,* **11:** 488–94.

Zhou, L., Sriram, R., Visvesvara, G.S. and Xiao, L. (2003). Genetic variations in the internal transcribed spacer and mitochondrial small subunit rRNA gene of *Naegleria* spp. *J. Eukaryot. Microbiol.,* **50:** S522–26.

Ziem, J.B., Magnussen, P., Olsen, A. *et al.* (2006a). Impact of repeated mass treatment on human *Oesophagostomum* and hookworm infections in northern Ghana. *Trop. Med. Int. Health,* **11:** 1764–72.

Ziem, J.B., Magnussen, P., Olsen, A. *et al.* (2006b). Mass treatment with albendazole reduces the prevalence and severity of *Oesophagostomum*-induced and hookworm infections in northern Ghana. *Trop. Med. Int. Health,* **11:** 1759–63.

CHAPTER 72

Fasciolosis

Michael Parkinson, John P. Dalton
and Sandra M. O'Neill

Summary

History of the disease

Liver fluke disease, or fasciolosis, of livestock and humans is caused by endoparasitic trematodes of the genus *Fasciola*. *Fasciola hepatica* is responsible for the disease in temperate climates whereas *F. gigantica* is found in tropical zones. Recently, hybrids between *F. hepatica* and *F. gigantica* have been described (Le *et al.* 2008; Periago *et al.* 2008). Fasciolosis is a true zoonoses as it is predominantly a disease of animals that can be transmitted to humans at a specific stage of the parasite's complex life cycle. There are a number of definitive hosts which includes sheep, cattle, and humans but this parasite has evolved to infect many other mammalian hosts including pigs, dogs, alpacas, llamas, rats, and goats (Apt *et al.* 1993; Chen and Mott 1990; Esteban *et al.* 1998). While prevalence of infection in humans may be relatively low in relation to animals, in specific geographic locations, for example in Bolivia, the prevalence of fasciolosis is so high in the human populations (hyperendemic) that it contributes to the spread of disease in animals (Esteban *et al.* 1999; Mas-Coma *et al.* 1999).

Archeological studies showing *Fasciola* eggs in ancient mummies in Egypt demonstrate that fasciolosis is an ancient human disease (David 1997). Sporadic cases of fasciolosis were reported in Egypt in 1958 (Kuntz *et al.* 1958). The first to carry out an extensive review on human fasciolosis were Chen and Mott (1990). They reported 2,595 cases in over 40 countries in Europe, the Americas, Asia, Africa and the western Pacific from 1970–1990. This review raised awareness of fasciolosis in humans and triggered a growth in epidemiological studies and a consequential dramatic increase in reporting of cases in the literature. Now human fasciolosis is recognized by the World Health Organization (WHO) as an important disease in humans with an estimated 2.4 million people infected annually and 180 million at risk to infection in over 61 countries (Haseeb *et al.* 2002). There have been several cases of large scale epidemics in France (Dauchy *et al.* 2007), Egypt (Curtale *et al.* 2007) and Iran (Rokni *et al.* 2002).

However, the only extensive epidemiological studies to determine the rate of infection have been carried out in Egypt and Bolivia (Curtale *et al.* 2003, 2007; Esteban *et al.* 2002; Parkinson *et al.* 2007). These studies have shown that co-infection with other diseases is a common occurrence and this may lead to under-reporting of the incidence of fasciolosis (Esteban *et al.* 2003; Maiga *et al.* 1991). In many countries, the overall rates of infection are extrapolated from sporadic reports of the disease and, consequently, worldwide disease prevalence is uncertain. In this chapter we will review the cause and effect of human fasciolosis, and particularly highlight important considerations in designing control strategies to reduce infection in at-risk communities.

Life cycle and human infection

Fasciola hepatica has an indirect life cycle, requiring both an invertebrate intermediate host, the snail *Galba truncatula* (formerly *Lymnaea truncatula*), and a definitive mammalian host (Andrews 1998) (Fig. 72.1). The sexually mature monoecious adult lives in the biliary tracts of the liver where it feeds on the lining of the bilary ducts and lays eggs that are carried by bile into the intestine. Eggs are void in faecal matter and embryonate in the presence of suitable conditions of moisture and temperature. Eggs hatch to release motile miracidia that seek out the intermediate host by chemotaxis (Christensen *et al.* 1976). The miracidia attach to the snail by its apical gland and cast off the cilia following the initial attachment to form a young sporocyst that migrates via the lymph or blood vessels to the digestive gland. One sporocyst has the potential to develop into 5–8 first generation rediae which in turn can give rise to 40 daughter rediae each of which has the potential to further develop into 600 cercariae. These are shed via the birth pore as cercariae that within 2 minutes to 2 hours lose their tail and develop a hard cyst following attachment to aquatic plants below the water surface. This encysted cercaria (termed a metacercaria) is the stage of the life cycle that is infectious to mammals (Smyth and Halton 1983). The means of development whereby one miracidium can give rise to hundreds of cercariae is a costly developmental trait but is vital to ensuring the successful completion of the life cycle since only a relatively few metacercariae will be ingested by the definitive host (Happich and Boray 1969).

Transmission to the definitive, mammalian host is passive, i.e. by the ingestion of aquatic plants or by drinking contaminated water (Esteban *et al.* 2002). The metacercariae exit their cysts as newly excysted juveniles in the duodenum of the host, a process initiated by high concentrations of carbon dioxide, reducing conditions and high temperatures (Dawes and Hughes 1964; Sukhdeo and Mettrick 1986). The NEJ parasites migrate through the intestinal wall into

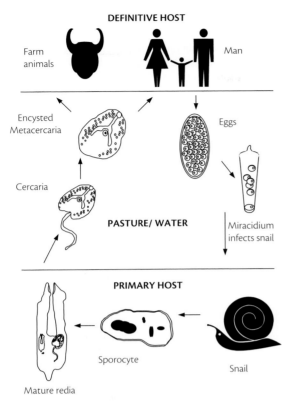

DEFINITIVE HOST

Farm animals

Man

Encysted Metacercaria

Eggs

Cercaria

PASTURE/ WATER

Miracidium infects snail

PRIMARY HOST

Sporocyte

Snail

Mature redia

Fig. 72.1 Life cycle of Fasciola hepatica.

(c) development of larval stages in the snail,

(d) release of cercariae from the snail (Schmidt and Roberts 1989)

(e) survival of the encysted metacercariae (Shaw 1932).

The availability of water is also important as the release of cercariae from the snail is stimulated by rainfall, and it is necessary for the miracidia to swim to the intermediate host. In the absence of sufficient water, eggs released from the host will desiccate rapidly. Precipitation of approximately 0.2mm in 24 hours (6mm per month) is a condition necessary for egg development. Other important factors which influence embryonation are oxygen tension and pH. Low oxygen tension inhibits embryonation (Rowcliffe and Ollerenshaw 1960) and pH 7.0 is optimum for egg development (Al-Habbib 1974). In the presence of sufficient water and at suitable temperatures infected snails will emerge and rapidly shed numerous cercariae. Once encysted on herbage 50% of metacercariae can survive a typical European winter (Ollerenshaw 1967). In dry spells snails can burrow into mud and survive for up to several months.

Climatic conditions are used as measurements to predict the incidence of fasciolosis in a region. Modelling using Geographical Information Systems and the importance of local precipitation has proved to be extremely useful for prediction of incidence of animal fasciolosis (Fuentes et al. 2005; Malone et al. 1998).

Snail distribution

The prevalence of animal and human fasciolosis corresponds to snail distribution (Mas-Coma et al. 1998). In Europe the snail is generally found at the side of the water sources. The miracidia must first seek out the snail and use a combination of phototropic properties to swim to the edge of the water source after which a chemotaxic gradient draws them to the snail (Christensen 1980). In Europe, larval development within the snail is halted in winter as low temperature influences the development of intra-molluscan stages of the lifecycle. Outbreaks recur in early spring as daytime temperature increase to greater than 9°C. In contrast, it was found that temperatures in Bolivia, where the all-year night-time and day-time temperatures range from 0–6°C and 18–22°C, respectively allowed transmission all year round (Oveido et al. 1995). Here, completion of the parasite life cycle occurs even during the dry season, a time when animals and humans collect around the shrinking water sources. Additionally, in Bolivia the snail resides almost wholly sub-aqua rather than in the mud and is observed on aquatic plants during the dry and rainy season.

Close association with livestock

The conditions that support endemic fasciolosis are predominantly associated with poorer rural communities (Curtale et al. 2003). In South America and Iran the prevalence of disease is mainly associated with subsistence farmers that rely on the land and their livestock to survive. Animals and humans feed on aquatic plants and algae that can be contaminated with metacercarial cysts. Free or mixed pasturing of livestock means that animals can roam freely amongst vegetation and release miracidia that infect snails. Failure to treat infected animals due to a lack of affordable flukicide treatment further contributes to disease transmission (Haseeb et al. 2002). It is not surprising therefore that infection of humans may occur at a distance from the source of infection as contaminated plants may be sold at local or distant markets.

the peritoneal cavity, subsequently penetrating the Gilson's capsule before migrating across the liver parenchyma to the biliary passages. This process takes almost 2 months in cattle, sheep and humans and once present in the bile duct the worms become sexually mature in 4–5 weeks and commence producing eggs (Dawes and Hughes 1964). After 2–4 months a fully mature egg laying adult fluke produces about 25,000 eggs per day (Happich and Boray 1969). Adults can successfully live in the bile ducts from several months to several years (Dan et al. 1981; Pantelouris 1965).

Factors that impact upon the life cycle

The successful completion of the life cycle is critical to the survival of any parasite and numerous factors can impact upon it. Understanding these factors will aid in the development of control strategies that interrupt the development and survival of the parasite at different stages of its life cycle. There are four main factors that influence the completion of the Fasciola life cycle: climatic factors, snail distribution, close association with livestock and dietary habits.

Climatic factors

Temperatures between 10°C and 26°C are necessary for completion of the life cycle in the intermediate snail host. Even within this temperature range small changes can influence the:

(a) embryonation of fluke eggs to form miracidia (Rowcliffe and Ollerenshaw 1960),

(b) liberation of the phototropic miracidia from the egg (Gold and Goldberg 1976; Roberts 1950; Rowan 1956),

Dietary habits

Transmission in humans is strongly associated with dietary habits, especially consumption of aquatic, leafy vegetables that are usually eaten raw (Marcos *et al.* 2006). The main types of aquatic plants in South America are 'berro berro' (watercress), 'algas' (algae), kjosco and totora (Bjorland *et al.* 1995). Eating seeds may also be a route of transmission (Curtale *et al.* 2003). In Europe, watercress is the main source of infection (Ashrafi *et al.* 2006; Mailles *et al.* 2006; Yilmaz and Godekmerdan 2004). Drinking alfalfa juice that contains contaminated leaves is also a source of infection in Peru (Marcos *et al.* 2006). Whilst drinking pumped water is not generally associated with infection, the consumption of surface water containing floating metacercariae can be (Caceres-Vega 1989). There are suggestions that the strain of *F. hepatica* in the Altiplano may have adapted to produce a greater proportion of free floating metacercariae (Esteban *et al.* 2002). Accordingly, vegetables washed in contaminated water may also become a source of infection. The incidence of infection is almost inevitably aggregated within familial groups that share contaminated food and drink from a common water source (Bjorland *et al.* 1995).

The causative agent

For the purpose of this chapter this section will be restricted to examining the biology of the causative agent within the definitive host. The adult fluke is leaf shaped, dorsoventrally flattened with fluted margins. At the tip of the parasite is an oral-cone and a highly muscular ventral sucker secures the fluke to the wall of the bile duct. A second muscular oral sucker forms the opening of a blind gut where food in the form of blood and cells enter. The gut is emptied approximately every three hours and a new blood-tissue meal ingested. The genital pore lies anterior to the ventral sucker and forms the opening of the male and female reproductive system.

The general body surface of the fluke is covered in numerous spines that function to secure the fluke to the bile duct. Distributed between these spines are chemoreceptors (with exposed cilia) and mechanoreceptors (with enclosed cilia). The surface or tegument forms the outer cuticle of the parasite and comprises of a surface syncytical layer of cytoplasm that is joined by cytoplasmic connections to nucleated tegumental bodies situated below. Below the cell bodies is a fibrous basal lamina and the main muscle layers consisting of an outer circular muscle and an inner longitudinal layer. The antagonistic action of these two muscles helps the fluke to migrate from the peritoneal cavity to the bile duct.

The tegument is metabolically active and its functions include the synthesis and secretion of substances, absorption of nutrients, osmoregulation, protection against host environment. The outside of the tegument is covered by a dense, carbohydrate-rich glycocalyx, while within the syncytium layer numerous secretory bodies (T0, T1, T2 and T3) that are synthesized in the cell bodies below move to the top and deliver their contents to the glycocalyx. The type of secretory body changes in the various stages of development within the mammalian host and since this alters the makeup of the glycocalyx at the host-parasite interface it may be an immune evasive strategy used by the parasite (Hanna 1980).

The fluke is made up of a number of organs that include muscular, nervous, digestive, cytoskeletal, excretory and reproductive system. Parenchymal cells separating each of these organ systems form tight junctions and have an important role in transportation.

The parenchyma also has a skeletal function as elastic fibers are found throughout the cells and may support the cytoskeleton to give the fluke its flexibility and shape. The parenchymal cells are also the main carbohydrate reserve for the fluke as they contain substantial quantities of α- and β-glycogen.

The cytoskeleton of the fluke is made up of three components, microtubules (based on tubulin), microfilaments (based on actin) and intermediate filaments. The most studied component is microtubules because they are considered targets of anthelmintics such as triclabendazole. The drugs may interrupt the important role that microtubules play in cell structure and movement, muscle contraction, cytoplasmic streaming, movement of secretory vesicles and cytokinesis. Microtubules and microfilaments seem to be involved in similar cell processes, but little is known about the intermediate filaments.

The fluke posses a central nervous system with two central ganglia situated on either side of the pharynx just behind the oral sucker. The main nerve cords form posteriorly along the main body. Three nerve cords run along each ganglion and the peripheral nervous system comprises of a plexus of cell bodies and nerve fibers, in the two suckers and is associated with various ducts. The structure of the nerve cell bodies is similar to other invertebrates and evidence suggests that the nerve cell bodies respond to a number of neurotransmitters. Indeed neurotransmitters such as acetylcholine, serotonin, dopamine and norepinephrine have been demonstrated in the fluke (Fairweather *et al.* 1987; Gianutsos and Bennett 1977; Holmes and Fairweather 1984).

The digestive system consists of a blind-ended gut divided into the foregut (with mouth or oral sucker), pharynx, oesophagus and a paired intestinal caeca made up of highly branched lateral diverticula. Digestion occurs in the lumen of the intestinal caeca which is lined by a single layer of cells that undergo fine structural changes at different stages of the absorptive and secretory phases. Digestion of protein macromolecules occurs as an extracellular process in the gut lumen and gives rise to small peptides that are transported into the surrounding cells for intracellular degradation to amino acids. The release of digestive enzymes reflects the diet of the fluke at different stages of development; the juvenile primarily feed on dead tissue while the adult is a blood feeder. Cysteine proteinases along with other proteinases are important in the digestion of haemoglobin (Dowd *et al.* 1994). The gut also secretes other molecules that are important to the fluke survival, for example proteases are released to break down the gut wall during migration, and antioxidants, such as GST and TPX, may neutralize the oxidative burst of immune cells (Cervi *et al.* 1999; Donnelly *et al.* 2005). The regulation of body fluid composition and waste excretion is controlled by the excretory system that consists of flame cells connected by fine tubules that lead into a primary ascending and descending duct which drains into a single bladder that opens via an excretory pore.

The fluke is hermaphrodite, and while it can self-fertilize, its preferred means of reproduction is by cross-fertilization. The male reproductive system is located centrally in the main body area and consists of highly branched testes in tandem. Two vas deferens exit from the testes to form a single duct—the seminal vesicle. This duct passes into an ejaculatory duct that leads into a protruding cirrus that opens into a common genital pore. The female reproductive system consists of a highly branched single ovary that is situated anterior to the testes with the vitelline glands. These glands are composed of numerous follicles that lie along the lateral margins of the body. A single oviduct leads from the ovaries to meet the ducts from the right and left vitelline glands and converge to form the vitelline reservoir. The vitelline reservoir joins the oviduct to give rise to the common ovovitelline duct leading to an egg producing chamber passing through a convoluted uterus leading to the common genital pore.

Pathogenesis

Fasciolosis rarely causes death in humans but causes extensive morbidity. The effect of morbidity due to fasciolosis has not been measured in terms of global disease burden and DALYs (disability adjusted life years). Humans are not a good host from the liver flukes' perspective since most flukes are trapped in the liver, rarely reaching the bile ducts. However, the trapping of flukes in the liver causes local haemorrhaging and inflammation that is associated with the major pathology of the disease (Aksoy et al. 2005; Chen and Mott 1990; Mas-Coma et al. 1998). The extent of this pathology is dependent upon the number of flukes that invade the liver. Inflammation results in an enlargement of the liver, with visible grey or white lesions distributed throughout the infected lobes. These lesions are formed by a collection of eosinophils that surround the dying flukes (Demirci et al. 2006). Haemorrhaging and inflammation is also caused by extensive tracts that are formed as the flukes migrate to the bile ducts. In addition to eosinophils, macrophages and lymphocytes are also found surrounding the trapped flukes and within the migratory tracts (Mulcahy et al. 1998).

Some pathology is also caused by the metacercariae penetrating the duodenum wall but this pathology is not always clinically evident. However, in the bile ducts there is significant pathology as flukes feed on the bile duct lining eventually causing hyperplasia and inflammation of the epithelium leading to thickening and dilation of the bile ducts and gallbladder. Blood loss into the bile is the major cause of anaemia found in this disease. Similar to that observed for the migratory tracts, the bile ducts are infiltrated with immune cells such as eosinophils, macrophages and lymphocytes. Several reports of egg granuloma have been reported but this is not extensive and does not contribute significantly to the overall pathogenesis (Acosta-Ferreira et al. 1979).

Clinical features

The clinical manifestation of liver fluke disease in man is similar to that exhibited by animals and for ease of reference can be divided into three stages; the invasive or acute stage, the pre-patent stage, and the chronic or obstructive stage. The invasive stage coincides with the migration of the juvenile flukes through the peritoneal cavity and across the liver parenchyma where they mature on reaching the bile duct. The precise mechanism for reaching the liver is not known but once the liver capsule is penetrated it burrows through the liver parenchyma causing extensive haemorrhaging and inflammation (Chen and Mott 1990; Garcia et al. 2007). The pre-patent or latent stage is the period when the mature fluke is laying eggs and the individual is asymptomatic. This stage commences 6–8 weeks after the initial infection. The chronic or obstructive stage occurs after several months to several years. The fluke feeds on the lining of the bile duct causing hyperplasia and inflammation of the epithelium. Thickening and dilation of the bile ducts and gallbladder ensue; the dilation of the common bile duct is reported to increase by 2–3 fold. The occurrence of cholangitis or cholecystitis coupled with the presence of flukes may result in mechanical obstruction resulting in an enlarged and oedematous gall bladder.

Abnormal laboratory findings are extremely useful in the diagnosis of all stages of human fasciolosis. As with most infectious agents changes in haematological parameters are associated with high leukocyte counts with eosonophilia, a characteristic cell marker during most helminth infections being typically within the range of 5–83% of total leucocytes. Leucocytosis and eosinophilia are usually greater in the acute phase but remain elevated in all stages. Anaemia is common but haemoglobin levels less than 7g dl^{-1} are rarely recorded. Abnormal liver function tests have been reported in both the acute and chronic stages of infection. Typically elevated liver enzymes such as glutamic pyruvic transaminase (GPT), glutamic oxalacetic transaminase (GOT) and Alkaline phosphatase (AKP) are associated with infection (Massoud et al. 2001). This can be observed in both the acute and obstructive phase of the diseases although in the acute phase GPT and GOT can be normal. Elevated serum bilirubin levels are observed during the obstructive phase when individuals are jaundiced and high bilirubin can also be detected in urine. Other hepatic markers measured during Fasciola infection include serum globulin with a high level of γ-globulins in particular.

In all stages of the disease raised immunoglobulins to parasite antigens are found. IgM is associated with early infection whereas elevated IgG is observed at all stages (Shehab et al. 2002). High IgE and IgG4 levels are typically associated with Fasciola infection in humans as with many helminth infections (O'Neill et al. 1998; Sampaio et al. 1985). IgE levels have been correlated with eosinophilia but not with faecal egg count and age of the individual infected (Sampaio et al. 1985). The particular isotype associated with protective immune responses in humans has not been determined, but in cattle IgG2 is considered protective, which is the counter isotype for human IgG1 (Mulcahy et al. 1998). IgG1 serum concentration is elevated in some but not all cases of human fasciolosis (unpublished data).

Symptoms and signs

The symptoms observed during Fasciola infection are due to the mechanical destruction of liver tissue and the initial symptoms include fever, sweating, abdominal pain and urticaria. The symptoms may be vague or absent in light infections. Respiratory symptoms have also been reported, the most common being bronchial wheeze, dysponea, dry cough, and chest pain. These symptoms are most often associated with the invasive or acute phase. Upon physical examination individuals present with hepatomegaly, splenomegaly and ascites. The liver is enlarged and tender. Ascites is yellow with high leucocyte count and eosinophilia. Anaemia is common in the acute stage and individuals may be pale, dizzy and weak but the duration of this stage is only approximately 6–8 weeks. Granuloma formation occurs around trapped flukes in the liver parcenchyma but this does not occur commonly (Arauco et al. 2007).

In the chronic or obstructive phase the clinical manifestations include right upper quadrant tenderness, epigastric pain, biliary colic, nausea, fatty food intolerance, jaundice and pruritus. Hepatic enlargement, splenomegaly and ascites are also common during this stage. The liver increases in size during the course of the disease and is more rigid on palpitation than in the acute stage. Splenomegaly occurs in a small number of individuals and ascites is more common in the acute stage. In the chronic stages individuals may appear jaundiced.

Development of cirrhosis and liver failure is observed in only a small proportion of cases. Ectopic fasciolosis is possible with flukes migrating to organs other than the liver, but is not common (Arjona *et al.* 1995; Zhou *et al.* 2007). The disease is mainly associated with morbidity but some mortality has been reported. There has been a link between liver fluke infection and the development of liver cancer (Sripa *et al.* 2007). Co-infections are not uncommon during infections and reports have shown an association with cryptosporidisis and schistosomiaisis (Esteban *et al.* 1997, 2003).

Diagnosis

Clinically, human fasciolosis is primarily diagnosed by coprological or serological analysis, particularly in large scale epidemiological studies. However, other methods of diagnosis that include invasive and non-invasive techniques are employed and will be briefly discussed at the end of this section. Early diagnosis is imperative because most of the disease pathogenesis is caused by the migrating flukes.

Parasitological examinations

Parasitological or coprological diagnosis is based upon the identification of *Fasciola* eggs in stool and is widely employed for the diagnosis of human and animal fasciolosis. *Fasciola* eggs have a distinctive operculated shape, are 130–150µm in length and 63–90µm in width making it possible to distinguish them from other helminth eggs. Coprological analysis is a rapid, reproducible and inexpensive means of diagnosis. While the presence of eggs in faeces is a definitive diagnosis, these are produced only when flukes are mature (after two months of infection) and therefore acute infection cannot be diagnosed by this method. Furthermore, since the release of eggs can be sporadic, several stool samples are required on different times on different days to ensure accuracy.

There are numerous techniques to diagnose the presence of eggs in stool and the sensitivity of coprological analysis is dependent upon the technique employed. Its specificity is heavily dependent also upon the experience of the technician performing the technique. The most rudimentary technique is the simple direct smear, an insensitive but rapid means of diagnosis. Egg concentration in the stool can be measured by various techniques including the sedimentation technique, the egg flotation technique and the Kato-Katz or cellophane faecal thick-smear technique (Katz *et al.* 1972). These latter methods are generally more accurate and sensitive.

A study performed by Munoz *et al.* (1987) compared three different coprological analysis techniques; Fast Sedimentation Method (FSM), the Teleman centrifugation technique (TM) and the gravity sedimentation technique (GS) (McNabb *et al.* 1985). Using TM only 33% of individuals were diagnosed correctly compared to 100% for the remaining two techniques. The most widely used methods are the Kato-Katz technique and the rapid sedimentation technique. The latter is highly sensitive but is expensive and laborious. The former is rapid, reproducible and economically viable making it suitable for large scale epidemiological surveys.

Immunological diagnosis

Immunological techniques are invaluable for disease diagnosis because they are inexpensive rapid, sensitive and allow for the diagnosis of a large number of individuals simultaneously. In human fasciolosis it has the added benefit of facilitating the diagnosis of acute infection since antibodies can be detected two weeks post infection. Immunological techniques exploit one of two immunological phenomena, a hypersensitivity reaction to antigen (skin test) or the formation of an antigen-antibody immune complex. The latter involves the detection of circulating liver fluke antigen, circulating immune complexes or the detection of specific antibodies to liver fluke antigen.

Skin tests were one of the first immunological tests employed to diagnose human fasciolosis and the antigen used was usually crude somatic liver fluke extract. Although this method is simple and cheap it is not highly sensitive and has limited diagnostic value. The detection of circulating antigen or circulating immune complexes (CIC) (Pelayo *et al.* 1998) has been tested in the diagnosis of fasciolosis in humans and animals. However, this can only be incorporated as a part of an experimental design in studies because low sensitivity means it has minimal clinical value and for a definitive diagnosis this test must be employed in conjunction with other techniques.

The earliest immunological methods used was the immunufluorescence assay (IFA) (Stork *et al.* 1973) where a cross section of liver fluke tissue was mounted on a slide and probed with serum. While sensitivity was good it was not very specific as cross reactivity was observed with other helminths such as schistosomes and ascaris or filarial worms. In addition, this method is cumbersome and impractical for use in large surveys. Other techniques for diagnosis of human fasciolosis include the indirect haematagglutination test (IHA) (Knobloch 1985), double diffusion, complement fixation (CF) (Biguet *et al.* 1965) and counter electrophoresis (CEP) (Hillyer *et al.* 1985). Enzyme linked immuno-electrotransfer blot (ETIB) (Hillyer *et al.* 1992) is highly sensitive and specific but the method is cumbersome, time consuming and only allows the diagnosis of a limited number of patients at any one time.

Enzyme linked immunosorbent assay (ELISA) is the current definitive immuno-diagnostic method for human fasciolosis since it can diagnose both the acute and chronic stages of disease. It is also highly specific and sensitive when compared to all other techniques. There are a number of assays based on different parasite antigen preparations and antibody combinations. The most successful assay to date is that based on a single recombinant protein Cathepsin L using IgG4 antibody as the detection antibody (O'Neill *et al.* 1998; Rokni *et al.* 2002). This assay was shown to be more specific and sensitive than crude somatic antigen and was comparable to assays employing excretory-secretory antigens. This assay has now been validated in several countries including Bolivia, Peru, Vietnam, Egypt, Iran and Iran (unpublished).

Non-invasive techniques

The majority of non-invasive diagnostic techniques are expensive and would not be employed in large epidemiological studies, particularly in countries where financial resources are limited. Radiological techniques employed in the diagnosis of fasciolosis include abdominal and chest X-ray, cholangiography and endoscopic retrograde cholangiopancreatography (ERCP) (Rana *et al.* 2007). Images obtained using these techniques show narrowing of the bile ducts, shadows and tracking in the liver tissue. Radioisotope scanning has also been employed as a useful tool in diagnosis since it illuminates the presence of 'cold areas' in the liver tissue where the liver fluke is present. Ultrasound (US) is also useful in diagnosis (Cosme *et al.* 2003; Zali *et al.* 2004), but has limited value as individual flukes are not visualized. Computed tomography scans have diagnosed the disease by identifying multiple hypodense areas in the liver tissue. It is a particularly useful in monitoring an individual's response to treatment (Marcos *et al.* 2008).

Invasive techniques

Invasive techniques for the diagnosis of fasciolosis include liver biopsy, laparoscopy and surgical intervention. Liver biopsy reveals eosinophilic abscess, granulation and charcot-leyden crystals. Eggs are sometimes present in the biopsy tissue (Kodama *et al.*1991). Laparoscopy is performed by placing a scope through the abdominal wall facilitating examination of the abdominal and liver tissue (Cosme *et al.* 1990). Lesions suggestive of liver fluke infection can be observed in the form of hepatic nodules of various shapes and sizes. Lesions may also be observed in Gilson's capsule and the peritoneal cavity. During exploratory laparatomy eggs may be found in the bilary ducts (Carrero *et al.* 1992). Finally, the symptoms of fasciolosis may be mistaken for cholecystitis, cholelthiasis or obstructive jaundice. During a cholecystectomy or choledochostomy, liver flukes or ova may be observed in the biliary ducts or the gall bladder. In a case reported by Chen and Mott (1990) over fifteen flukes were drained from the bile ducts during choledochostomy (Chen and Mott 1990).

Treatment and prognosis

Chemotherapeutic intervention is an important control strategy for human fasciolosis. For many years bithionol was the drug of choice but frequent and sometimes serious adverse effects meant that this drug could no longer be recommended. In addition, a number of studies demonstrated only moderate efficacy rates with this drug. Other chemotherapeutics like Emetine although highly effective were also highly toxic and serious adverse effects meant that it too can no longer be recommended. While Metronidazole has a high therapeutic index and is well tolerated with only mild side effects, this drug must be administered for a period of three weeks making compliance an issue. Other drugs examined for the treatment of fasciolosis include chloroquine, niclofan, albendazole and praziquantel (Chen and Mott 1990; Laird and Boray 1992; Price *et al.* 1993), but again these are not recommended because of toxic side effects or limited therapeutic value.

The current drug of choice for human fasciolosis is triclabendazole because its adverse effects are mild and treatment is successful following only one or two doses administered on consecutive days. Triclabendazole was first recorded as chemotherapy for human fasciolosis in 1988; prior to this the drug was more commonly used in veterinary medicine (Wessely *et al.* 1988). Triclabendazole is a halogenated benzimidazole derivative synthesized first in 1978 by Ciba-Geigy. It has two major metabolites, triclabendazole sulfoxide and triclabendazole sulfone that are attributed with its therapeutic action. The drug may act against the formation of microtubulin within the tegumental coat of the parasite by blocking the transport of microtubulin-dependent secretory bodies. The drug is also thought to inhibit mitotic division of spermatagenic cells and inhibit both RNA and protein synthesis.

There are several non-randomized studies in humans examining the efficacy rates of triclabendazole with cures typically in the region of 90–100%. The optimum therapeutic regime is 10mg/kg following one or two doses (Apt *et al.* 1995; Laird and Boray 1992). Concentrations less than 10mg/kg are only effective if more than once dose is given. Toxic side effects are mild with some gastrointestinal disturbances and tolerance of the drug is excellent with clinical symptoms associated with expulsion of the worm from the bile duct. Consumption of food with the drug is recommended as it increases it pharmokinetic parameters and administration with vitamins enhances its antioxidant capacity. Triclabendazole resistance is reported widely in livestock (Brennan *et al.* 2007) but only recently in Iran in humans where two cases were reported (Talaie *et al.* 2004). The success of the veterinary form of the drug in treating human fasciolosis led to the development of a tablet form for use in humans (Egaten, supplied by Novartis). Although this drug is no longer commercially available due to lack of commercial viability it is distributed by WHO to requesting government agencies (WHO).

Recent studies in Egypt have tested a drug called Myrazid as a new anti-flukacide. This drug is an oleo-resin extract of Myrrh from the *Commiphora molmol* tree and is used traditionally for many different conditions. A small study in children infected with *Fasciola* gave a complete cure (Soliman *et al.* 2004) and other small scale studies have reported similar findings with no adverse effects reported (Omar *et al.* 2005). However, large scale trials of Myrrh in Egypt for the treatment of schistosomiasis showed a lower response rate compared to a conventional treatment (Botros *et al.* 2005). Given that the target of the drug is likely to be the same in both parasites, further studies as part of a large scale randomized trial are required to confirm the therapeutic value of this drug and to establish fully its pharmacodynamic and pharmacokinetic parameters. Given the withdrawal of Egaten from the market, Myrazid could be important for the future treatment of the disease.

A variety of other drugs have shown promise for treatment of fascioliasis including: Artemether and OZ78 (highly effective in rats against triclabendazole resistant *F.hepatica*) (Keiser *et al.* 2007), Nitazoxanide (Rey and Debonne 2006) and Artesunate (in treating Triclabendazole resistant fasciolosis) (Hien *et al.* 2008).

Epidemiology

Every year an estimated 2.4 million people are infected worldwide and a further 180 million people are at risk of infection (Mas-Coma *et al.* 1998) with human infections reported in many countries including Iran, Peru, Cuba, Bolivia and Egypt (Bjorland *et al.* 1995; Chen and Mott 1990; Espino and Finlay 1994; Esteban *et al.* 2003; Haseeb *et al.* 2002; Hillyer *et al.* 1992; Massoud 1989; Rokni *et al.* 2002; Stork *et al.* 1973). Isolated incidents of fasciolosis due to imported cases or sporadic cases occur in many countries and will not be considered further. It is important to distinguish these from endemic fasciolosis where there is a constant level of fasciolosis or with a threat of periodic epidemics.

Iran, Peru, Cuba, Bolivia and Egypt are the countries with the highest incidence of disease reported worldwide (Table 72.1, only data from countries where detailed epidemiology is available was included). In Spain, Portugal and France the incidence is hypoendemic (since the rate of infection is monitored closely through health care systems for many years this is a true reflection of the incidence of the disease in these countries). Human fasciolosis is reported in many other countries in Asia (Vietnam, China and Thailand),

Table 72.1 The incidence of fasciolosis in endemic regions

Region	No. in study (year)	% infected/ cases	Reference
South America			
Bolivia	1951 (1939–1993)	1–95%	(Mas-Coma *et al.* 1995)
	2,723 (1993–1999)	14.4%	(Esteban *et al.* 1999)
	7,908 (meta-analysis)	18.53%	(Parkinson *et al.* 2007)
Peru	1011 (1973)	9%	(Stork *et al.* 1973)
	1226 (2005)	35%	(Espinoza *et al.* 2005)
	93 (2005)	33–51%	(Marcos *et al.* 2005)
	206 (2004)	21–30 cases	(Raymundo *et al.* 2004)
	338 (2002)	24%	(Esteban *et al.* 2002)
Ecuador	150	6%	(Trueba *et al.* 2000)
Cuba	40 (1983)	40 cases	(Espino *et al.* 1998)
	67 (1988)	67 cases	(Diaz *et al.* 1990)
Chile	5861 (1986–1990)	0.7%	(Apt *et al.* 1993)
Africa			
Egypt	1,350 (1995)	5.1%–17.1%	(Hassan *et al.* 1995)
	1,000 (2006)	0.2%–0.4%	(el-Shazly *et al.* 2006)
	1,035 (1998)	3%	(Curtale *et al.* 1998)
	21,477 (1998–2002)	0.043%	(Curtale *et al.* 2007)
	5,112 (2001)	7.47%	(el-Shazly *et al.* 2001)
	568 (2003)	12.8%	(Esteban *et al.* 2003)
	1,019 (2004)	1.7%	(Abo-Madyan *et al.* 2004)
	462 (2005)	2.83%	(Safar *et al.* 2005)
Europe			
Turkey	756 (2002)	6.1%	(Demirci *et al.* 2003)
	320 (2002)	0.9%	(Demirci *et al.* 2003)
	500 (2004)	1.8%	(Yilmaz and Godekmerdan 2004)
	415 (2006)	2.4%	(Kaya *et al.* 2006)
	171 (2006)	9.3%	(Kaya *et al.* 2006)
France	('50–82)	8,898 cases	Cited in: (Rondelaud *et al.* 2006)
	(99–06)	450 cases	
Iran	('99)	10,000 cases	(Rokni *et al.* 2002)
	('99–'02)	107 cases	(Moghaddam *et al.* 2004)
Portugal	('84–96)	1,115 cases	(Esteban *et al.* 1998)
Asia			
Thailand	(1984–1987)	63.3%	Cited in: (Kaewpitoon *et al.* 2007)
	(1988)	35.6%	
	(1901)	9.4%	
China	(1984)	44 cases	(Chen 1991)
	340 (1984)	0.005%	
	83 (1984)	0.02%	
Vietnam	(1978–2002)	500 cases	(Tranvinh *et al.* 2001)

South America (Chile, Cuba, Venezuela, Ecuador), Africa (Algeria, Tunisia and Mali) and Europe (Turkey) but since no epidemiological studies that focus upon fasciolosis detection in at-risk groups is available it is difficult to assess the true extent of the disease. In Australia and North America only a few reports of isolated cases of *F. hepatica* infection are made annually and many of these cases involve individuals that have recently travelled from endemic countries.

The highest prevalence of human fasciolosis is found in the Altiplano region of northern Bolivia, a high plain region situated between two Andean mountain ranges, approximately 3,700 metres above sea level. The Altiplano is the largest expanse of arable land in the Andes and is inhabited principally by the indigenous Aymaran population. A meta-analysis of 7,908 individual cases of human fascioliasis from 38 communities within these provinces surveyed over the last 11 years (Parkinson *et al.* 2007) gave a high overall recorded infection level (18.53%) over a long study period (infection has been recorded from 1984) showing that the disease is endemic. Human and bovine fasciolosis is associated with the communities lying in the plain from Lake Titicaca to La Paz, predominantly in the Los Andes province. In similar high plain regions throughout South America the incidence of this disease is also high (Raymundo *et al.* 2004). High prevalence of human fasciolosis was found at low level beside the Caspian Sea in Iran and in the Nile Delta of Egypt so the occurrence of Fasciola at high altitudes is currently only found in South America.

Factors associated with infection

There is a strong association of endemic fasciolosis with rural communities (Esteban *et al.* 1999; Parkinson *et al.* 2007; Raymundo *et al.* 2004). Fasciolosis is sporadically reported in urban communities where the incidence of infection is much lower and due to imported cases or consumption of contaminated raw vegetables. There is a correlation between infection rates in livestock and in humans in the same region (Parkinson *et al.* 2007). However, dietary habits and the availability of potable water strongly influence infection, and the intensity of infection in livestock does not always, therefore, directly correlate with the intensities in humans (Esteban *et al.* 1998). Studies in Egypt have shown that infection in sheep poses a greater risk than infection in cattle (Haseeb *et al.* 2002).

Age

Endemic fasciolosis is predominantly associated with children with peak infection associated with children of 8–11 years of age and progressively decreased thereafter (Curtale *et al.* 2003; Parkinson *et al.* 2007).

Gender

In Egypt, the incidence of infection was higher in girls than boys (Curtale *et al.* 2003; Curtale *et al.* 2007). This could be due to the fact that girls are removed from school to work on the farms and in these communities school attendance is greater for boys than girls.

Association with families

Given that individuals in families share similar dietary habits, the same drinking water source and are exposed to similar sanitation conditions it is no surprise to find clusters of infections in families. It is therefore important that programmes are directed at communities and that all family members are targeted (Marcos *et al.* 2005; Parkinson *et al.* 2007).

Strategies for prevention and control

It is apparent that human fasciolosis is endemic in a number of countries and in areas of high prevalence there is a need for a large regional control programmes (Table 72.2). Treatment of populations is expensive, and needs to be targeted. Large scale epidemiological studies have been performed in Egypt where the incidence

Table 72.2 Summary of control strategies

1. Preventing infection of the snail host

Molluscides to control snails is widely employed

Biological control of snail infection is also an option

2. Chemotherapeutic intervention

Treatment of farm animals to reduce pasture contamination

Treatment of human fasciolosis

3. Preventing metacercariae transmission

Pumped water

Good pasturing practices

Good food hygiene

Latrines

4. Education

Teaching parasitic life cycle

Information on mode of infection

Focused education of at-risk group

Education on public hygiene measures

of disease was found to range between 0.03% and 17.1%. From these epidemiological studies the Egyptian government introduced programmes and as a result of these interventions dramatically reduced the incidence of infection in high endemic regions (Curtale et al. 2005). The programme first focused upon identifying areas of high risk and determining the risk factors that are specific for this region. Similar programmes would have similar impact in countries such as Bolivia, Peru, Iran, and Vietnam.

Education programmes that focus upon eliminating risk factors should include changes in dietary habits, the introduction of proper water and sanitation facilities and better farming practices (or even separation of animals from water sources used by humans). Since fasciolosis is a true zoonoses, mass treatment of animals would have a significant impact on human infection. A control programme would, therefore, need to involve a combination of large-scale drug treatment of infected animals and humans.

Health education programmes need to be directed particularly at children since these have a higher risk of F. hepatica infection. The higher level of infection in children may be related to an increased exposure to the infective stages of the parasite as children commonly work in the fields minding livestock where the intensity of transmission would be expected to be higher. It is also believed that children are more likely to eat aquatic plants. Alternatively, the higher incidence of infection in children may indicate the existence of an age-related immunological resistance to infection by F. hepatica, a phenomenon that is well documented for the related digenetic trematode of the spp. Schistosoma (Hagan et al. 1991).

A safe and cost-effective means of controlling fasciolosis is the development of an effective vaccine that induces long-term protection. Vaccines need only focus on animals since breaking the cycle would prevent transmission to humans. Currently there are no commercially available liver fluke vaccines despite the fact that a number of candidate molecules have been identified including cathepsin L, glutathione S-tranferase, leucine aminopeptidase, fatty acid binding proteins and peroxiredoxin (Mulcahy et al. 1998; McManus and Dalton 2006).

References

Abo-Madyan, A.A., Morsy, T.A., Motawea, S.M. and Morsy, A.T. (2004). Clinical trial of Mirazid in treatment of human fascioliasis, Ezbet El-Bakly (Tamyia Center) Al-Fayoum Governorate. J. Egyptian Soc. Parasitol., 34: 807–18.

Acosta-Ferreira, W., Vercelli-Retta, J. and Falconi, L.M. (1979). Fasciola hepatica human infection. Histopathological study of sixteen cases, Virchows Archiv.A, Pathol. Anat. Histol., 383: 319–27.

Aksoy, D.Y., Kerimoglu, U., Oto, A., et al. (2005). Infection with Fasciola hepatica. Clin. Microb. Infect., 11: 859–61.

Al-Habbib, W.M.S. (1974). The effect of constant and changing temperatures on the development of the larval stages of Fasciola hepatica (L.). PhD Thesis, University of Dublin.

Andrews, S.J. (1998). The life cycle of Fasciola hepatica. In: J.P. Dalton (ed.) Fasciolosis, pp. 1–24. Wallingford, Oxon: CAB International.

Apt, W., Aguilera, X., Vega, F., Alcaino, H., et al. (1993). Prevalence of fascioliasis in humans, horses, pigs, and wild rabbits in 3 Chilean provinces, Boletin de la Oficina Sanitaria Panamericana. Pan American San. Bur., 115: 405–414.

Apt, W., Aguilera, X., Vega, F., et al. (1995). Treatment of human chronic fascioliasis with triclabendazole: drug efficacy and serologic response. American J. Trop. Med. Hyg., 52: 532–35.

Arauco, R., Zetola, N.M., Calderon, F. and Seas, C. (2007). Human fascioliasis: a case of hyperinfection and an update for clinicians. Foodborne Path. Dis., 4: 305–12.

Arjona, R., Riancho, J.A., Aguado, J.M., Salesa, R. & Gonzalez-Macias, J. (1995). Fasciliasis in developed countries: a review of classic and aberrant forms of the disease. Med. Anal. Rev. Gen. Med., Neurol., Psych., Dermat. Pediat., 74: 13–23.

Ashrafi, K., Valero, M.A., Massoud, J., et al. (2006). Plant-borne human contamination by fascioliasis. American J. Trop. Med. Hyg., 75: 295–302.

Biguet, J., Rose, G. and Capron, A. (1965). Diagnosis of distomatosis due to Fasciola hepatica by the hemagglutination reaction. Comparison with the results of immunoelectrophoresis and the hemolysis reaction. Bull. Soc. Path. Exotique et de Ses Fil., 58: 866–78.

Bjorland, J., Bryan, R.T., Strauss, W., Hillyer, G.V. and McAuley, J.B. (1995). An outbreak of acute fascioliasis among Aymara Indians in the Bolivian Altiplano. Clin. Infect. Dis., 21: 1228–33.

Botros, S., Sayed, H., El-Dusoki, H., et al. (2005). Efficacy of mirazid in comparison with praziquantel in Egyptian Schistosoma mansoni-infected school children and households. American J. Trop. Med. Hyg., 72: 119–23.

Brennan, G.P., Fairweather, I., Trudgett, A., et al. (2007). Understanding triclabendazole resistance. Experim. Mol. Pathol., 82: 104–109.

Caceres-Vega, E. (1989). Fasciola hepatica- 'Enfermedad y Pobreza campesina', pp. 202. Accion un Maestro Mas, La Paz, Bolivia: Imprenta Metodista.

Carrero, P.A., Gonzalez-Pastrana, M., et al. (1992). Parasitological discovery during exploratory surgery of the bile duct. Enferm. Infecciosas y Microbiol. Clin., 10: 497–98.

Cervi, L., Rossi, G. and Masih, D.T. (1999). Potential role for excretory-secretory forms of glutathione-S-transferase (GST) in Fasciola hepatica. Parasitology, 119: 627–33.

Chen, M.G. and Mott, K.E. (1990). Progress in morbidity due to Fasciola hepatica infection. Trop. Dis. Bull., 87: 1–37.

Chen, M.G. (1991). Fasciola hepatica infection in China. Southeast Asian J. Trop. Med. Pub. Health, 22 (S): 356–60.

Christensen, N.O. (1980). A review of the influence of host- and parasite-related factors and environmental conditions on the host-finding capacity of the trematode miracidium. Acta Trop., 37: 303–318.

Christensen, N.O., Nansen, P. and Frandsen, F. (1976). Molluscs interfering with the capacity of *Fasciola hepatica* miracidia to infect *Lymnaea truncatula*. *Parasitology*, **73**: 161–67.

Cosme, A., Alzate, L., Orive, V., Recasens, M., *et al.* (1990). Laparoscopic findings in liver fascioliasis. Study of 13 cases. *Rev. Espanola de Enferm. Digest.*, **78**: 359-62.

Cosme, A., Ojeda, E., Poch, M., *et al.* (2003). Sonographic findings of hepatic lesions in human fascioliasis. *J. Clin. Ultras.*, **31**: 358–63.

Curtale, F., Abd El-Wahab Hassanein, Y., *et al.* (2003). Distribution of human fascioliasis by age and gender among rural population in the Nile Delta, Egypt. *J. Trop. Pediat.*, **49**: 264–68.

Curtale, F., Hassanein, Y.A., Barduagni, P., *et al.* (2007). Human fascioliasis infection: gender differences within school-age children from endemic areas of the Nile Delta, Egypt. *Trans. R. Soc. Trop. Med. Hyg.*, **101**: 155–60.

Curtale, F., Hassanein, Y.A. and Savioli, L. (2005). Control of human fascioliasis by selective chemotherapy: design, cost and effect of the first public health, school-based intervention implemented in endemic areas of the Nile Delta, Egypt. *Trans. R. Soc. Trop. Med. Hyg.*, **99**: 599–609.

Curtale, F., Mas-Coma, S., Hassanein, Y.A., *et al.* (2003). Clinical signs and household characteristics associated with human fascioliasis among rural population in Egypt: a case-control study. *Parassitologia*, **45**: 5–11.

Curtale, F., Nabil, M., el Wakeel, A. and Shamy, M.Y. (1998). Anaemia and intestinal parasitic infections among school age children in Behera Governorate, Egypt. *Behera Survey Team. J. Trop. Pediat.*, **44**: 323–28.

Dan, M., Lichtenstein, D., Lavochkin, J., *et al.* (1981). Human fascioliasis in Israel. An imported case. *Israel J. Med. Sci.*, **17**: 430–32.

Dauchy, F.A., Laharie, D., Neau, D., *et al.* (2007). Fascioliasis: a 23-year retrospective study. *Presse Medicale*, **36**: 1545–49.

David, A.R. (1997). Disease in Egyptian mummies: the contribution of new technologies. *Lancet*, **349**: 1760–63.

Dawes, B. and Hughes, D.L. (1964). Fascioliasis: the Invasive Stages of *Fasciola hepatica* in Mammalian Hosts. *Adv. Parasitol.*, **2**: 97–168.

Demirci, M., Kaya, S., Cetin, E.S., *et al.* (2006). Eosinophil cationic protein in patients with fascioliasis: its probable effects on symptoms and signs. *Scan. J. Infect. Dis.*, **38**: 346–49.

Demirci, M., Korkmaz, M., Kaya, S. and Kuman, A. (2003). Fascioliasis in eosinophilic patients in the Isparta region of Turkey. *Infection*, **31**: 15–18.

Diaz, J., Pina, B., Lastre, M., Rivera, L. and Perez, O. (1990). Epidemic human fascioliasis. Cuba 1983. VI. Clinical study of 40 children in the Hospital Provincial of Sagua la Grande. *G.E.N,* **44**: 385–88.

Donnelly, S., O'Neill, S.M., Sekiya, M., Mulcahy, G. and Dalton, J.P. (2005). Thioredoxin peroxidase secreted by *Fasciola hepatica* induces the alternative activation of macrophages. *Infect. Immun.*, **73**: 166–73.

Dowd, A.J., Smith, A.M., McGonigle, S. and Dalton, J.P. (1994). Purification and characterisation of a second cathepsin L proteinase secreted by the parasitic trematode Fasciola hepatica. *Euro. J. Biochem./ FEBS*, **223**: 91–98.

el-Shazly, A.M., El-Nahas, H.A., Soliman, M., *et al.* (2006). The reflection of control programs of parasitic diseases upon gastrointestinal helminthiasis in Dakahlia Governature, Egypt. *J. Egypt Soc. Parasitol.*, **36**: 467–80.

el-Shazly, A.M., Soliman, M., Gabr, A., *et al.* (2001). Clinico-epidemiological study of human fascioliasis in an endemic focus in Dakahlia Governorate, Egypt, *J. Egypt. Soc. Parasit.*, **31**: 725–36.

Espino, A.M., Diaz, A., Perez, A. and Finlay, C.M. (1998). Dynamics of antigenemia and coproantigens during a human *Fasciola hepatica* outbreak. *J. Clin. Microb.*, **36**: 2723–26.

Espino, A.M. and Finlay, C.M. (1994). Sandwich enzyme-linked immunosorbent assay for detection of excretory secretory antigens in humans with fascioliasis, *J. Clin. Microb.*, **32**: 190–93.

Espinoza, J.R., Timoteo, O. and Herrera-Velit, P. (2005). Fas2-ELISA in the detection of human infection by Fasciola hepatica. *J. Helminthol.*, **79**: 235–40.

Esteban, J.G., Barques, M.D. and Mas-Coma, S. (1998). Geographical distribution, diagnosis and treatment of human fascioliasis: a review. *Res. Rev. Parasitol.*, **58**: 13–42.

Esteban, J.G., Flores, A., Aguirre, C., *et al.* (1997). Presence of very high prevalence and intensity of infection with Fasciola hepatica among Aymara children from the Northern Bolivian Altiplano. *Acta Trop.*, **66**: 1–14.

Esteban, J.G., Flores, A., Angles, R. and Mas-Coma, S. (1999). High endemicity of human fascioliasis between Lake Titicaca and La Paz valley, Bolivia. *Trans. R. Soc. Trop. Med. Hyg.*, **93**: 151–56.

Esteban, J.G., Gonzalez, C., Bargues, M.D., *et al.* (2002). High fascioliasis infection in children linked to a man-made irrigation zone in Peru. *Trop. Med. Int. Health*, **7**: 339–48.

Esteban, J.G., Gonzalez, C., Curtale, F., *et al.* (2003). Hyperendemic fasciolosis associated with schistosomiasis in villages in the Nile Delta of Egypt. *American J. Trop. Med. Hyg.*, **69**: 429–37.

Fairweather, I., Maule, A.G., Mitchell, S.H., *et al.* (1987). Immunocytochemical demonstration of 5-hydroxytryptamine (serotonin) in the nervous system of the liver fluke, Fasciola hepatica (Trematoda, Digenea). *Parasitol. Res.*, **73**: 255–58.

Fuentes, M.V., Sainz-Elipe, S., Nieto, P., *et al.* (2005). Geographical Information Systems risk assessment models for zoonotic fascioliasis in the South American Andes region. *Parassitologia*, **47**: 151–56.

Garcia, H.H., Moro, P.L. and Schantz, P.M. (2007). Zoonotic helminth infections of humans: echinococcosis, cysticercosis and fascioliasis. *Curr. Opin. Infect. Dis.*, **20**: 489–94.

Gianutsos, G. and Bennett, J.L. (1977). The regional distribution of dopamine and norepinephrine in *Schistosoma mansoni* and *Fasciola hepatica*. *Comp. Biochem. Physiol., C: Comp. Pharm.*, **58**: 157–59.

Gold, D. and Goldberg, M. (1976). Effect of light and temperature of hatching of *Fasciola hepatica* (Trematoda: Fasciolidae). *Israel J. Zool.*, **25**: 178–85.

Hagan, P., Blumenthal, U.J., Dunn, D., *et al.* (1991). Human IgE, IgG4 and resistance to reinfection with *Schistosoma haematobium*. *Nature*, **349**: 243–45.

Hanna, R.E. (1980). *Fasciola hepatica*: glycocalyx replacement in the juvenile as a possible mechanism for protection against host immunity. *Exp. Parasitol.*, **50**: 103–114.

Happich, F.A., Boray, J.C. (1969). Quantitative diagnosis of chronic fasciolosis. 2. The estimation of daily total egg production of *Fasciola hepatica* and the number of adult flukes in sheep by faecal egg counts. *Aust. Vet. J.*, **45**: 329–31.

Haseeb, A.N., el-Shazly, A.M., Arafa, M.A. and Morsy, A.T. (2002). A review on fascioliasis in Egypt. *J. Egypt. Soc. Parasitol.*, **32**: 317–54.

Hassan, M.M., Moustafa, N.E., *et al.* (1995). Prevalence of *Fasciola* infection among school children in Sharkia Governorate, Egypt, *J. Egypt. Soc. Parasitol.*, **25**: 543–49.

Hien, T.T., Truong, N.T., Minh, N.H., *et al.* (2008). A Randomized Controlled Pilot Study of Artesunate versus Triclabendazole for Human Fascioliasis in Central Vietnam. *American J. Trop. Med. Hyg.*, **78**: 388–92.

Hillyer, G.V., Sanchez, Z. and de Leon, D. (1985). Immunodiagnosis of bovine fascioliasis by enzyme-linked immunosorbent assay and immunoprecipitation methods. *J. Parasit.*, **71**: 449–54.

Hillyer, G.V., Soler de Galanes, M., *et al.* (1992). Use of the Falcon assay screening test—enzyme-linked immunosorbent assay (FAST-ELISA) and the enzyme-linked immunoelectrotransfer blot (EITB) to determine the prevalence of human fascioliasis in the Bolivian Altiplano. *American J. Trop. Med. Hyg.*, **46**: 603–9.

Holmes, S.D. and Fairweather, I. (1984). *Fasciola hepatica*: the effects of neuropharmacological agents upon in vitro motility. *Exp. Parasitol.*, **58**: 194–208.

Kaewpitoon, N., Kaewpitoon, S.J., Pengsaa, P. and Pilasri, C. (2007). Knowledge, attitude and practice related to liver fluke infection in northeast Thailand. *World J. Gastroenter.*, **13**: 1837–40.

Katz, N., Chaves, A. and Pellegrino, J. (1972). A simple device for quantitative stool thick-smear technique in *Schistosomiasis mansoni*. *Rev. Instituto de Med. Trop. de Sao Paulo*, **14**: 397–400.

Kaya, S., Demirci, M., Demirel, R., *et al.* (2006). Seroprevalence of fasciolosis and the difference of fasciolosis between rural area and city center in Isparta, Turkey. *Saudi Med. J.*, **27**: 1152–56.

Keiser, J., Utzinger, J., Vennerstrom, J.L., *et al.* (2007). Activity of artemether and OZ78 against triclabendazole-resistant Fasciola hepatica. *Trans. R. Soc. Trop. Med. Hyg.*, **101**: 1219–22.

Knobloch, J. (1985). Human fascioliasis in Cajamarca/Peru. II. Humoral antibody response and antigenaemia. *Trop. Med. Parasitol.*, **36**: 91–93.

Kodama, K., Ohnishi, H., Matsuo, T. and Matsumura, T. (1991). Three cases of human fascioliasis, *Kansenshogaku zasshi. J. Jap. Assoc. Infect. Dis.*, **65**: 1620–24.

Kuntz, R.E., Lawless, D.K., Langbehn, H.R. and Malakatis, G.M. (1958). Intestinal protozoa and helminths in the peoples of Egypt living in different type localities. *American J. Trop. Med. Hyg.*, **7**: 630–39.

Laird, P.P. and Boray, J.C. (1992). Human fascioliasis successfully treated with triclabendazole. *Aust. N. Zealand J. Med.*, **22**: 45–47.

Le, T.H., De, N.V., Agatsuma, T., *et al.* (2008). Human fascioliasis and the presence of hybrid/introgressed forms of *Fasciola hepatica* and *Fasciola gigantica* in Vietnam. *Intern. J. Parasitol.*, **38**: 725–30.

Maiga, Y.I., Maiga-Maiga, Z., Tembely, S., *et al.* (1991). Does human distomiasis due to *Fasiola gigantica* exist in the delta of the Niger river in Mali? (apropos of a serological survey). *Med. Trop.: Rev. Corps de Sante Colonial*, **51**: 275–81.

Mailles, A., Capek, I., Ajana, F., *et al.* (2006). Commercial watercress as an emerging source of fasciliasis in Northern France in 2002: results from an outbreak investigation. *Epidem. Infect.*, **134**: 942–45.

Malone, J.B., Gommes, R., Hansen, J., *et al.* (1998). A geographic information system on the potential distribution and abundance of *Fasciola hepatica* and *F. gigantica* in east Africa based on Food and Agriculture Organization databases. *Vet. Parasitol.*, **78**: 87–101.

Marcos, L., Maco, V., Samalvides, F., *et al.* (2006). Risk factors for *Fasciola hepatica* infection in children: a case-control study. *Trans. R. Soc. Trop. Med. Hyg.*, **100**: 158–66.

Marcos, L., Maco, V., Terashima, A., *et al.* (2005). Fascioliasis in relatives of patients with *Fasciola hepatica* infection in Peru. *Rev. Instituto Med. Trop. de Sao Paulo*, **47**: 219–22.

Marcos, L.A., Tagle, M., Terashima, A., *et al.* (2008). Natural history, clinicoradiologic correlates, and response to triclabendazole in acute massive fascioliasis. *American J. Trop. Med. Hyg.*, **78**: 222–27.

Mas-Coma, S., Angles, R., Strauss, W., *et al.* (1995). Human Fasciliasis in Bolivia: A general analysis and a critical review of existing data. *Res. Rev. Parasitol.*, **55**: 73–79.

Mas-Coma, S., Barques, M.D. and Esteban, J.G. (1998). Human Fasciolosis, In: J.P. Dalton (ed.) *Fasciolosis*, pp. 441–47. Wallingford, Oxon: CAB International.

Mas-Coma, S., Esteban, J.G. and Barques, M.D. (1999). Epidemiology of human fasciolosis: a review and proposed new classification. *Bull. World Health Organ.*, **77**(4): 340–46.

Mas-Coma, S., Rodrigues, A., Barques, M.D., *et al.* (1998). Secondary reservoir role of domestic animals other than sheep and cattle in fascioliasis transmission on the northern Bolivian Altiplano. *Res. Rev. Parasitol.*, **57**: 39–46.

Massoud, J. (1989). Fascioliasis outbreak in man and drug test (triclabendazole) in Caspian littoral, northern part of Iran. *Bull. Soc. Fran. Parasitol.*, **8**: 438.

Massoud, A., El Sisi, S., Salama, O. and Massoud, A. (2001). Preliminary study of therapeutic efficacy of a new fasciolicidal drug derived from Commiphora molmol (myrrh). *American J. Trop. Med. Hyg.*, **65**: 96–99.

McManus, D.P. and Dalton, J.P. (2006). Vaccines against the zoonotic trematodes *Schistosoma japonicum, Fasc. Hepat. Fasc. Gigan.*, *Parasit.*, **133**: S43–61.

McNabb, S.J., Hensel, D.M., Welch, D.F., *et al.* (1985). Comparison of sedimentation and flotation techniques for identification of Cryptosporidium sp. oocysts in a large outbreak of human diarrhea. *J. Clin. Microb.*, **22**: 587–89.

Moghaddam, A.S., Massoud, J., Mahmoodi, M., *et al.* (2004). Human and animal fasciolasis in Mazandaran province, northern Iran. *Parasit. Res.*, **94**: 61–69.

Mulcahy, G., Joyce, P. and Dalton, J.P. (1998). Immunology of *Fasciola hepatica* infection. In: J.P. Dalton (ed.) *Fasciolosis*, (1st edn.), pp. 341–410. Wallingford, Oxon: CAB Publishing.

Mulcahy, G., O'Connor, F., McGonigle, S., *et al.* (1998). Correlation of specific antibody titre and avidity with protection in cattle immunized against, *Fasc. Hepat. Vacc.*, **16**: 932–39.

Ollerenshaw, C.B. (1967). Some observations on the epidemiology and control of fasciliasis in Wales., *Proceedings of the Second international Liverfluke Colloquim*, pp. 103. Merck, Sharp and Dohme International, Wageningen.

Omar, A., Elmesallamy, G. and Eassa, S. (2005). Comparative study of the hepatotoxic, genotoxic and carcinogenic effects of praziquantel distocide & the natural myrrh extract Mirazid on adult male albino rats. *J. Egypt. Soc. Parasitol.*, **35**: 313–29.

O'Neill, S.M., Parkinson, M., Strauss, W., *et al.* (1998). Immunodiagnosis of *Fasciola hepatica* infection (fascioliasis) in a human population in the Bolivian Altiplano using purified cathepsin L cysteine proteinase. *American J. Trop. Med. Hyg.*, **58**: 417–23.

Oveido, J.A., Bargues, M.D. and Mas-Coma, S. (1995). Lymnaeid snails in the human Fasciolosis high endemic zone of Northern Bolivian Altiplano. *Res. Rev. Parasit.*, **55**: 35–43.

Pantelouris, E.M. (1965). *The Common Liver Fluke*. Oxford, London, New York, Paris and Frankfurt: Pergamon Press Ltd.

Parkinson, M., O'Neill, S.M. and Dalton, J.P. (2007). Controlling fasciolosis in the Bolivian Altiplano. *Trends Parasitol.*, **23**: 238–39.

Parkinson, M., O'Neill, S.M. and Dalton, J.P. (2007). Endemic human fasciolosis in the Bolivian Altiplano. *Epidem. Infect.*, **135**: 669–74.

Pelayo, L., Espino, A.M., Dumenigo Ripoll, B.E., *et al.* (1998). The detection of antibodies, antigens and circulating immune complexes in acute and chronic fasciolasis. Preliminary results. *Rev. Cubana de Med. Trop.*, **50**: 209–214.

Periago, M.V., Valero, M.A., El Sayed, M., *et al.* (2008). First phenotypic description of *Fasciola hepatica/Fasciola gigantica* intermediate forms from the human endemic area of the Nile Delta, Egypt. *Infect., Genet. Evol.*, **8**: 51–58.

Price, T.A., Tuazon, C.U. and Simon, G.L. (1993). Fascioliasis: case reports and review. *Clin. Infect. Dis.*, **17**: 426–30.

Rana, S.S., Bhasin, D.K., Nanda, M. and Singh, K. (2007). Parasitic infestations of the biliary tract. *Curr. Gastroenter. Rep.*, **9**: 156–64.

Raymundo, L.A., Flores, V.M., *et al.* (2004). Hyperendemicity of human fasciolosis in the Mantaro Valley, Peru: factors for infection with Fasciole hepatica. *Rev. Gastroenter. del Peru*, **24**: 158–64.

Rey, P. and Debonne, J.M. (2006). Therapeutic alternatives in case of failure of first-line treatment of intestinal helminthiasis in adults. *Med. Trop.: Rev. Corps de Sante Colon.*, **66**: 324–28.

Roberts, E.W. (1950). Studies on the lifecycle of *Fasciola hepatica* (Linnaeus) and its snail host *Lymnaea truncatula*, in the field and under controlled conditions in the laboratory. *Ann. Trop. Med. Parasitol.*, **44**: 187–206.

Rokni, M.B., Massoud, J., *et al.* (2002). Diagnosis of human fasciolosis in the Gilan province of Northern Iran: application of cathepsin L-ELISA. *Diagn. Microb. Infect. Dis.*, **44**: 175–79.

Rondelaud, D., Dreyfuss, G. and Vignoles, P. (2006). Clinical and biological abnormalities in patients after fasciolosis treatment. *Med. Malad. Infect.*, **36**: 466–68.

Rowan, W.B. (1956). The mode of hatching the egg of *Fasciola hepatica. Exp. Parasitol.*, **5**: 118–37.

Rowcliffe, S.A. and Ollerenshaw, C.B. (1960). Observations on the bionomics of the egg of *Fasciola hepatica. Ann. Trop. Med. Parasitol.*, **54**: 172–81.

Safar, E., Mikhail, E., Bassiouni, G., *et al.* (2005). Human fascioliasis in some areas in Cairo and Giza Governorates, Egypt. *J. Egypt. Soc. Parasitol.,* **35:** 181–92.

Sampaio Silva, M.L., Vindimian, M., *et al.* (1985). IgE antibodies in human *Fasciola hepatica* distomiasis. *Pathol. Biolog.,* **33:** 746–50.

Schmidt, G.D. and Roberts, L.S. (1989). *Foundations of Parasitology,* (4th edn,). St. Louis, Missouri: Time Mirror/Moseby College Publishing.

Shaw, J.N. (1932). Studies of the liver fluke (*Fasciola hepatica*). *J. American Vet. Med. Assoc.,* **34:** 76–82.

Shehab, A.Y., Allam, A.F. and el-Sayad, M.H. (2002). Serum IgM. Does it relate to the level of chronicity in fascioliasis? *J. Egypt. Soc. Parasitol.,* **32:** 373–80.

Smyth, J.P. and Halton, D.W. (1983). *The Physiology of Trematodes,* (2nd edn.). Cambridge: Cambridge University Press.

Soliman, O.E., El-Arman, M., *et al.* (2004). Evaluation of myrrh (Mirazid) therapy in fascioliasis and intestinal schistosomiasis in children: immunological and parasitological study. *J. Egypt. Soc. Parasitol.,* **34:** 941–66.

Sripa, B., Kaewkes, S., Sithithaworn, P., *et al.* (2007). Liver fluke induces cholangiocarcinoma. *PLoS Med.,* **4**(7): e201.

Stork, M.G., Venables, G.S., *et al.* (1973). An investigation of endemic fascioliasis in Peruvian village children. *J. Trop. Med. Hyg.,* **76:** 231–55.

Sukhdeo, M.V. and Mettrick, D.F. (1986). The behavior of juvenile *Fasciola hepatica. J. Parasitol.,* **72:** 492–97.

Talaie, H., Emami, H., *et al.* (2004). Randomized trial of a single, double and triple dose of 10 mg/kg of a human formulation of triclabendazole in patients with fascioliasis. *Clin. Experim. Pharm. Physiol.,* **31:** 777–82.

Tranvinh, H., Tran Thi, K.D., *et al.* (2001). Fascioliasis in Vietnam. *Southeast Asian J. Trop. Med. Public Health,* **32:** 48–50.

Trueba, G., Guerrero, T., Fornasini, M., *et al.* (2000). Detection of *Fasciola hepatica* infection in a community located in the Ecuadorian Andes. *American J. Trop. Med. Hyg.,* **62:** 518.

Wessely, K., Reischig, H.L., *et al.* (1988). Human fascioliasis treated with triclabendazole (Fasinex) for the first time. *Trans. R. Soc. Trop. Med. Hyg.,* **82:** 743–44.

WHO, *Fasciolosis.* Available: http://www.who.int/neglected_diseases/diseases/fascioliasis/en/index.html Accessed 2008, 04/30.

World Health Organisation (2006). *Report of the WHO Informal Meeting on use of triclabendazole in fasciliasis control. WHO headquarters, Geneva, Switzerland. 17–18 October 2006.* Available: www.who.int/neglected_diseases/preventive_chemotherapy/WHO_CDS_NTD_PCT_2007.1.pdf Accessed 2008, 04/01.

Yilmaz, H. and Godekmerdan, A. (2004). Human fasciolosis in Van province, Turkey. *Acta Trop.,* **92:** 161–62.

Zali, M.R., Ghaziani, T., Shahraz, S., *et al.* (2004). Liver, spleen, pancreas and kidney involvement by human fascioliasis: imaging findings. *BMC Gastroenter.,* **4:** 15.

Zhou, L., Luo, L., You, C., *et al.* (2008). Multiple brain hemorrhages and hematomas associated with ectopic fascioliasis in brain and eye. *Surg. Neurol.,* **69:** 516–21.

Index

Page numbers in *italic* indicate boxes, figures and tables.